Imaging of the Brain

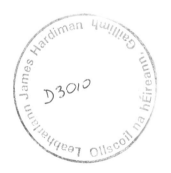

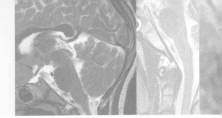

Imaging of the Brain

Editors

Thomas P. Naidich, MD
Professor of Radiology and Neurosurgery
Irving and Dorothy Regenstreif Research Professor of Neuroscience (Neuroimaging)
Director of Neuroradiology
Mount Sinai School of Medicine
New York, New York

Mauricio Castillo, MD
Professor of Radiology
Chief and Program Director, Neuroradiology
University of North Carolina School of Medicine
Chapel Hill, North Carolina

Soonmee Cha, MD
Professor of Radiology and Neurological Surgery
Program Director, Diagnostic Radiology Residency
Attending Neuroradiologist
University of California, San Francisco Medical Center
San Francisco, California

James G. Smirniotopoulos, MD
Chief Editor, MedPix®
Professor of Radiology, Neurology, and Biomedical Informatics
Uniformed Services University of the Health Sciences
Program Leader, Diagnostics and Imaging
Center for Neuroscience and Regenerative Medicine
Bethesda, Maryland

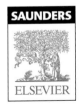

SAUNDERS

ELSEVIER

1600 John F. Kennedy Blvd.
Ste 1800
Philadelphia, PA 19103-2899

IMAGING OF THE BRAIN
ISBN: 978-1-4160-5009-4

Notices

Knowledge and best practice in this field are constantly changing. As new research and experience broaden our understanding, changes in research methods, professional practices, or medical treatment may become necessary.

Practitioners and researchers must always rely on their own experience and knowledge in evaluating and using any information, methods, compounds, or experiments described herein. In using such information or methods they should be mindful of their own safety and the safety of others, including parties for whom they have a professional responsibility.

With respect to any drug or pharmaceutical products identified, readers are advised to check the most current information provided (i) on procedures featured or (ii) by the manufacturer of each product to be administered, to verify the recommended dose or formula, the method and duration of administration, and contraindications. It is the responsibility of practitioners, relying on their own experience and knowledge of their patients, to make diagnoses, to determine dosages and the best treatment for each individual patient, and to take all appropriate safety precautions.

To the fullest extent of the law, neither the Publisher nor the authors, contributors, or editors, assume any liability for any injury and/or damage to persons or property as a matter of products liability, negligence or otherwise, or from any use or operation of any methods, products, instructions, or ideas contained in the material herein.

International Standard Book Number
978-1-4160-5009-4

Content Strategist: Helene Caprari
Senior Content Development Specialist: Jennifer Shreiner
Publishing Services Manager: Patricia Tannian
Senior Project Manager: Sarah Wunderly
Design Direction: Steven Stave

Printed in China

Last digit is the print number: 9 8 7 6 5 4 3 2

A book is an expression of the soul, revealing values and character.

To my loving and patient wife Michele and to our extended families.
You give meaning to my life.
Thomas P. Naidich

To Tom Naidich
Your knowledge, warmth, and caring personality
inspire us all to be the best we can be.
Your presence at any event elevates it to unprecedented heights.
Your friendship and mentoring are treasured gifts.
Mauricio Castillo

To Spencer, Shinae, and Peter, without whom I cease to exist.
Soonmee Cha

To my family and friends
and
to all the students, residents, and staff who have patiently listened
and then taught me through their curiosity and questions.
James G. Smirniotopoulos

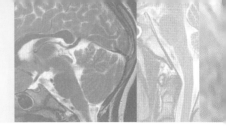

Contributors

Amit Aggarwal, MD
Fellow, Neuroradiology, Department of Radiology, Mount Sinai School of Medicine, New York, New York

Noriko Aida, MD, PhD
Director of Radiology, Kanagawa Children's Medical Center; Visiting Professor, Department of Radiology, Yokohama City University School of Medicine, Yokohama, Japan

Richard Ivan Aviv, MBChB, MRCP, FRCR(UK), FRCP(C)
Associate Professor, Division of Neuroradiology, Department of Medical Imaging, University of Toronto School of Medicine, Sunnybrook Health Sciences Centre, Toronto, Ontario, Canada

Marc Taiwo Awobuluyi, MD, PhD
Clinical Faculty, Department of Radiology, University of California, San Francisco School of Medicine, San Francisco, California

Richard Bitar, MD, PhD
Staff Radiologist, Department of Medical Imaging, Thunder Bay Regional Health Sciences Centre, Thunder Bay, Ontario, Canada

Avraham Y. Bluestone, MD, PhD
Neuroradiologist; Assistant Professor of Clinical Radiology, Stony Brook University Medical Center, Stony Brook, New York

Pascal Bou-Haidar, BMed, FRANZCR, MEngSc
Neuroradiologist, Department of Medical Imaging, St Vincent's Clinic, Darlinghurst, New South Wales, Australia

Richard A. Bronen, MD
Professor of Diagnostic Radiology and Neurosurgery; Vice Chair, Academic Affairs, Yale University School of Medicine, New Haven, Connecticut

Nicholas Butowski, MD
Associate Professor of Neurological Surgery; Director of Clinical Services, Neuro-Oncology Division, University of California, San Francisco Medical Center, San Francisco, California

Raymond Francis Carmody, MD, FACR
Professor of Radiology; Chief of Neuroradiology, University of Arizona Health Sciences Center, Tucson, Arizona

David M. Carpenter, PhD
Director of the Image Analysis Core, Translational and Molecular Imaging Institute, Mount Sinai Medical Center, New York, New York

Mauricio Castillo, MD
Professor of Radiology; Chief and Program Director, Neuroradiology, University of North Carolina School of Medicine, Chapel Hill, North Carolina

Soonmee Cha, MD
Professor of Radiology, University of California, San Francisco; Attending Neuroradiologist, University of California, San Francisco Medical Center, San Francisco, California

Bradley N. Delman, MD
Associate Professor of Radiology; Vice-Chairman for Quality, Performance Improvement & Clinical Research, Department of Radiology, Mount Sinai School of Medicine, New York, New York

Amish H. Doshi, MD
Assistant Professor; Associate Program Director, Neuroradiology; Associate Program Director, Radiology Residency, Department of Radiology, Mount Sinai School of Medicine, New York, New York

Patrick O. Emanuel, MB, ChB
Dermatopathologist, DML; Associate Professor of Pathology, School of Medical Sciences, University of Auckland, Auckland, New Zealand

Ramón E. Figueroa, MD, FACR
Professor of Radiology; Chief of Neuroradiology Service, Georgia Health Sciences University, Augusta, Georgia

Mary Elizabeth Fowkes, MD
Director of Clinical Neuropathology, Department of Pathology, Mount Sinai Medical Center, New York, New York

Allan J. Fox, MD, FRCP(C), FACR
Associate Professor, Division of Neuroradiology, Department of Medical Imaging, University of Toronto School of Medicine, Sunnybrook Health Sciences Centre, Toronto, Ontario, Canada

Merav W. Galper, MD
Resident in Radiology, Lahey Clinic, Burlington, Massachusetts

Sasikhan Geibprasert, MD
Lecturer, Department of Radiology, Mahidol University Faculty of Medicine, Ramathibodi Medical School Hospital, Bangkok, Thailand

Edward D. Greenberg, MD
Resident Physician, Department of Radiology, New York Presbyterian Hospital-Weill Cornell Medical Center, New York, New York

Christopher Paul Hess, MD, PhD
Associate Professor, Department of Radiology, University of California, San Francisco School of Medicine, San Francisco, California

Benjamin Y. Huang, MD, MPH
Assistant Professor, Department of Radiology, University of North Carolina, Chapel Hill, North Carolina

Pakorn Jiarakongmun, MD
Assistant Professor, Department of Radiology, Mahidol University Faculty of Medicine, Ramathibodi Medical School Hospital, Bangkok, Thailand

Blaise V. Jones, MD
Professor of Radiology, University of Cincinnati College of Medicine; Division Chief, Neuroradiology; Associate Director, Clinical Services, Department of Radiology, Cincinnati Children's Hospital Medical Center, Cincinnati, Ohio

Austin D. Jou, MD
Neuroradiologist; Co-Director, Neuroradiology, Kaiser Permanente Northwest, Portland, Oregon

Jane J. Kim, MD
Assistant Professor of Radiology, University of California, San Francisco School of Medicine; Radiologist, Kaiser Permanente, San Francisco, California

George M. Kleinman, MD
Pathologist, Stamford Pathology Group, PC, Stamford, Connecticut

Spyros Kollias, MD
Professor, Department of Radiology; Chief, Magnetic Resonance Imaging; Chief, MR Research Institute of Neuroradiology, University Hospital Zurich, Zurich, Switzerland

Niklaus Krayenbühl, MD
Department of Neurosurgery, University Hospital Zurich, Zurich, Switzerland

Timo Krings, MD, PhD, FRCP(C)
Professor of Radiology, University of Toronto; Program Director, Neuroradiology, Department of Medical Imaging, Toronto Western Hospital, Toronto, Canada

Pierre L. Lasjaunias, MD, PhD[†]
Professor of Neuroradiology, University Hospital Bicêtre, Paris, France

Benjamin C. Lee, MD
Clinical Instructor of Neuroradiology, Department of Radiology, University of California, San Francisco School of Medicine, San Francisco, California

Patrick A. Lento, MD
Professor of Clinical Medicine and Pathology, New York Medical College, Valhalla, New York.

Laurent Létourneau-Guillon, MD, FRCP(C)
Chief Fellow, Neuroradiology, Department of Medical Imaging, Division of Neuroradiology, University of Toronto, Toronto, Ontario, Canada

Jennifer Linn, MD
Associate Professor, Department of Neuroradiology, University Hospital Munich, Munich, Germany

Michael D. Luttrull, MD
Assistant Professor of Radiology, Wexner Medical Center at The Ohio State University, Columbus, Ohio

Luke A. Massey, MA, MRCP
Clinical Research Fellow, Sara Koe PSP Research Centre, Queen Square Brain Bank for Neurological Disorders, Reta Lila Westin Institute of Neurological Studies, University College London Institute of Neurology, London, United Kingdom

Xavier Montalban, MD, PhD
Professor of Neurology, Department of Medicine, Universitat Autònoma de Barcelona; Chair, Neurology/Neuroimmunology; Director, MS Center of Catalonia, Vall d'Hebron University Hospital, Barcelona, Spain

Pratik Mukherjee, MD, PhD
Associate Professor, Departments of Radiology and Bioengineering, University of California, San Francisco School of Medicine, San Francisco, California

Frances M. Murphy, MD, MPH
President, Sigma Health Consulting, LLC, Silver Spring, Maryland

Thomas P. Naidich, MD, FACR
Professor of Radiology and Neurosurgery
Irving and Dorothy Regenstreif Research Professor of Neuroscience (Neuroimaging)
Director of Neuroradiology
Mount Sinai School of Medicine
New York, New York

Johnny C. Ng, PhD
Researcher, Department of Radiology, Mount Sinai Medical Center, New York, New York

Esther A. Nimchinsky, MD, PhD
Department of Radiology, Mount Sinai School of Medicine, New York, New York

[†]Deceased.

Gen Nishimura, MD, PhD
Radiologist-in-Chief, Department of Radiology, Tokyo Metropolitan Kiyose Children's Hospital, Tokyo, Japan

Tetsu Niwa, MD, PhD
Staff Radiologist, Department of Radiology, Kanagawa Children's Medical Center, Yokohama, Japan

A. Orlando Ortiz, MD, MBA, FACR
Professor of Clinical Radiology, Stony Brook University School of Medicine, Stony Brook, New York; Chairman, Department of Radiology, Winthrop-University Hospital, Mineola, New York

Yoav Parag, MD
Assistant Clinical Professor, Department of Radiology, Mount Sinai School of Medicine, New York, New York

Ellen E. Parker, MD
Assistant Clinical Professor, Department of Radiology and Biomedical Imaging, University of California, San Francisco Medical School, San Francisco, California; Staff Radiologist, VHA National Teleradiology Program, San Bruno, California

Pedro Pasik, MD
Professor Emeritus of Neurology and Medical Education, Mount Sinai School of Medicine, New York, New York

Aman B. Patel, MD
Professor of Neurosurgery and Radiology; Vice-Chairman, Neurosurgery, Mount Sinai School of Medicine, New York, New York

Puneet S. Pawha, MD
Assistant Professor; Associate Program Director, Radiology, Department of Radiology, Mount Sinai School of Medicine, New York, New York

Vitor M. Pereira, MD, MSc
Head, Interventional Neuroradiology Unit, University Hospitals of Geneva, Geneva, Switzerland

Sirintara Pongpech, MD
Associate Professor of Radiology, Mahidol University Faculty of Medicine; Chief, Interventional Neuroradiology Unit, Ramathibodi Medical School Hospital, Bangkok, Thailand

Derk D. Purcell, MD
Assistant Clinical Professor, Department of Radiology, University of California, San Francisco School of Medicine; Staff Radiologist, California Pacific Medical Center, San Francisco, California

John H. Rees, MD
Assistant Professor of Radiology, Georgetown University, Washington, DC; Neuroradiologist, Sunshine Radiology, Sarasota, Florida

Basil H. Ridha, MD
Honorary Clinical Assistant, Dementia Research Centre, Institute of Neurology, University College London, London, United Kingdom

Jose C. Rios, MD, PhD
Attending Radiologist, Morristown Medical Center, Morristown, New Jersey

John L. Ritter, MD
Assistant Professor of Radiology and Radiological Sciences, Uniformed Services University of the Health Sciences; Staff Neuroradiologist, San Antonio Military Medical Center, Fort Sam Houston, Texas.

Nancy K. Rollins, MD
Professor of Radiology, University of Texas Southwestern Medical Center; Medical Director of Radiology, Children's Medical Center, Dallas, Texas

Lorne Rosenbloom, MDCM, FRCPC
Assistant Professor of Radiology, Sir Mortimer B. Davis-Jewish General Hospital, McGill University, Montreal, Quebec, Canada

Alex Rovira, MD
Associate Professor of Radiology, Universitat Autònoma de Barcelona; Co-Chair, Department of Radiology, Vall d'Hebron University Hospital, Barcelona, Spain

Mark E. Smethurst, MD
Neuropathology Fellow, Mount Sinai School of Medicine, New York, New York

James G. Smirniotopoulos, MD
Chief Editor, MedPix®; Professor of Radiology, Neurology, and Biomedical Informatics, Uniformed Services University of the Health Sciences; Program Leader, Diagnostics and Imaging, Center for Neuroscience and Regenerative Medicine, Bethesda, Maryland

Alice B. Smith, MD
Section Head, Neuroradiology, American Institute for Radiologic Pathology, Silver Spring, Maryland; Assistant Professor, Department of Radiology and Radiological Sciences, Uniformed Services University of the Health Sciences, Bethesda, Maryland

Evan G. Stein, MD, PhD
Attending Physician, Neuroradiology, Department of Radiology, Maimonides Medical Center, Brooklyn, New York

Jonathan D. Steinberger, MD
Department of Radiology, Mount Sinai Medical Center, New York, New York

Sean P. Symons, BASc, MPH, MD, FRCP(C)
Associate Professor of Medical Imaging and Otolaryngology-Head and Neck Surgery, University of Toronto; Division Head, Neuroradiology, Sunnybrook Health Sciences Centre, Toronto, Ontario, Canada

Cheuk Ying Tang, PhD
Director, Neurovascular Imaging Research; Director, In Vivo Molecular Imaging SRF; Associate Director, Imaging Science Laboratories; Associate Professor, Departments of Radiology and Psychiatry, Translational and Molecular Imaging Institute, Mount Sinai Medical Center, New York, New York

Majda M Thurnher, MD
Associate Professor of Radiology, Section of Neuroradiology and Musculoskeletal Radiology, Department of Radiology, Medical University of Vienna, University Hospital Vienna, Vienna, Austria

Cheng-Hong Toh, MD
Assistant Professor of Radiology, Department of Medical Imaging and Intervention, Chang Gung University College of Medicine, Chang Gung Memorial Hospital, Taipei, Taiwan

Vinodkumar Velayudhan, DO, DABR
Head, Neuroimaging, BAB Radiology, Long Island, New York

John D. Waselus, BS
Diagnostic Imaging Applications Specialist, Invivo Corporation, New York, New York

Robert Yeung, MD, FRCP(C)
Lecturer in Neuroradiology, Department of Medical Imaging, University of Toronto School of Medicine, Sunnybrook Health Sciences Centre, Toronto, Ontario, Canada

Tarek A. Yousry, Dr.Med.Habil, FRCR
Professor of Neuroradiology, Institute of Neurology; Head, Lysholm Department of Neuroradiology, The National Hospital for Neurology and Neurosurgery, London, United Kingdom

Robert D. Zimmerman, MD, FACR
Professor of Radiology; Vice Chair, Education and Faculty Development, Weill Medical College of Cornell University, New York Presbyterian Hospital, New York, New York

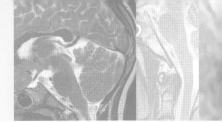

Preface

Fields of knowledge exist and advance because we find beauty and joy within them.

This volume attempts the dual task of providing a firm foundation for neuroimaging diagnosis and then illustrating the promise of things to come. It teaches the basics and then asks, "What's next?" and "Why not more?"

For the first task, we have carefully selected material and tailored discussions to teach the "core knowledge" that is the foundation for future growth. In this endeavor, we have tried to balance brevity with thoroughness, for efficient learning.

The initial sections of the text present concisely the techniques used for neuroimaging and systems for analyzing the densities and signal intensities of the images made. Following sections address in detail the anatomic bases for the images with extensive correlations to fresh and formalin-fixed human brain tissue. In sequence, serial sections then review the pathology and imaging of cerebrovascular disease, trauma, tumors and cysts, infection and inflammation, aging and degeneration, toxic and metabolic diseases, hydrocephalus, and epilepsy. In each section, data are presented in parallel format for completeness and ease of review. Where appropriate, illustrative cases and sample reports conclude each chapter.

The authors specifically include clinical and pathologic data for each entity, so readers may see how the imaging features explain the presentation and evolution of the clinical cases. With this understanding, they may discuss cases with clinical colleagues more usefully and provide more informed care to their patients. Since the book illustrates how neuroradiology aids patient care and contributes to scientific endeavor in all sister specialties, it is appropriate for all trainees and practitioners in the allied neurosciences—radiologists and neuroradiologists, neurologists and neurosurgeons, psychiatrists and neuroscientists.

For the second task, the authors have deliberately chosen to include novel material that entices, stimulates, or frankly confounds. All of us entered neuroradiology precisely because of what we did not know. We found joy in the challenge of puzzles to solve and satisfaction in the greater understanding that followed their solution. Decades later, we know vastly more, but still delight most in the puzzles ahead and the new questions posed by yesterday's solutions.

The authors and editors of this volume are all teachers, internationally recognized for their excellence in science and education. As teachers, we hope that this volume will help you to share in the beauty and joy we find in neuroradiology. We hope you may build upon the foundation we provide, accept the challenge of the unknown, and grow beyond us to advance the field into the future. We wish you—and your patients—every success.

THOMAS P. NAIDICH

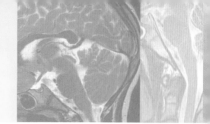

Acknowledgments

The editors would like to express their deep gratitude to the authors who prepared the chapters in this volume, to the residents, fellows, and nurses who worked with our patients, to the imaging supervisors, Mr. James D'Ambrosio and Mr. Thomas W. Eitel, and to the imaging technologists who actually made the images we display in this book.

We specifically acknowledge our debt to the neuropathologists, Drs. John H. Deck, Mary E. Fowkes, George M. Kleinman, Patrick A. Lento, Susan Morgello, Dushyant P. Purohit, and Mark Smethurst, and to the mortuary staff, Mr. Calvin Keys, Mr. Kevin Risby, and Ms. Claudia Delgado, for their help in preparing much of the anatomic and pathologic material that illustrates the chapters in this volume.

We thank, personally, Helene Caprari, Rebecca Gaertner, Pamela Hetherington, Jennifer Shreiner, Sarah Wunderly, and the other great staff at Elsevier for their advice, their expertise, and the hard work that enabled us to bring this volume to publication. We are grateful indeed for their contributions to this volume.

Finally, we would like to thank Ms. Elba Colman for her unfailing assistance in managing the myriad details that led to this publication.

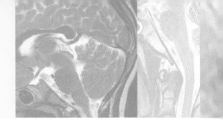

Contents

SECTION ONE

Techniques for Imaging

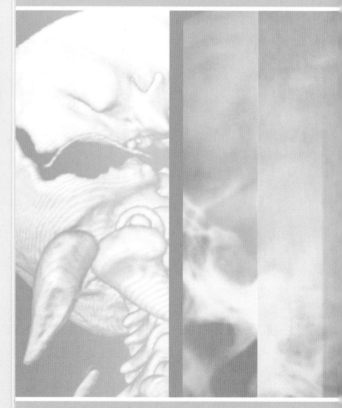

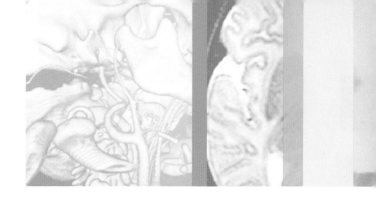

Static Anatomic Techniques

Jane J. Kim and Pratik Mukherjee

Computed tomography (CT) and magnetic resonance imaging (MRI) are the mainstays of anatomic neurologic imaging. CT was first introduced in the early 1970s and MRI in the early 1980s. Since then, CT and MRI have transformed medical diagnosis and proved essential in neuroimaging.

COMPUTED TOMOGRAPHY
Basic Concepts
CT relies on the differential attenuation of x-ray beams passing through tissues to produce an image. The patient lies on the CT table, with his or her long axis aligned along the longitudinal (z) axis of the scanner. The x-ray tube and detector, housed in a gantry, rotate 360 degrees around the patient so the x-ray beam strikes the patient in the transverse (x/y) axis. Conceptually, the slab of tissue imaged can be divided into many small volume elements (voxels), each with x, y, and z dimensions. The degree to which each of these voxels attenuates the x-ray beam is derived by analyzing the data from all the different angular projections, using a reconstruction method known as *convolution-backprojection.* The computed attenuation value of each voxel is then converted into a gray-scale value of Hounsfield units (HU) and displayed. The attenuation of distilled water at 0° Celsius and 1 bar of pressure is defined as 0 HU. The attenuation of air at the same standard pressure and temperature conditions is defined as −1000 HU.

The spatial resolution of the CT image depends in part on voxel size. Ideally, each voxel of data would be very small to provide high spatial resolution. Each voxel would also ideally be *isotropic* (having equal dimensions in all three planes) to provide for excellent image reconstructions in any arbitrary plane. It has been relatively easy to achieve high *in-plane resolution* (along the x/y axes), to the order of 0.5 to 0.7 mm.[1] It has proved difficult to achieve high resolution in the longitudinal or z-plane, because longitudinal resolution is determined by the slice thickness. Use of thin submillimeter slices reduces the length of tissue that can be scanned in a reasonable time or increases the scan time for equal lengths of tissue imaged. Evolution of CT technology over the years can be seen in part as the pursuit of this isotropic resolution.

Conventional CT
In early-generation CT scanners, each CT slice was acquired by one 360-degree rotation of the gantry around the patient. The scan table was then advanced one slice thickness and the process was repeated to obtain the adjacent slice. Because the electrical cables were attached directly to the gantry, the gantry had to stop after each scan to "unwind" the cabling before advancing to obtain the next slice. This type of scanning, known as step-by-step or conventional scanning, is relatively time consuming and prone to respiratory misregistration. It has largely been replaced by *spiral* or *helical* CT, which uses *slip ring technology* to eliminate the cable problem.

Spiral CT
Spiral CT was developed in the early 1990s to improve scan speed and flexibility. In spiral CT, the x-ray tube and detectors rotate continuously about the patient while the scan table advances the patient continuously through the gantry. As a result, the x-ray beam traces a helical path through the patient and provides a "spiral" of image data. Because the patient is intentionally moved through the gantry during scanning, there is significant motion artifact. However, computational methods known as *z-interpolation* were specifically developed to manage the spiral dataset and to eliminate the motion artifact caused by patient translation. For any image position along the z-axis of the patient, z-interpolation re-forms the spiral data to fit on a single plane. The conventional convolution-backprojection algorithm for data analysis can then be applied.

Spiral CT does not depend on direct, one-to-one correspondence between scan position and image slice, so image slices can be reconstructed *anywhere along the z-axis at different slice thicknesses and varying intervals.* This flexibility is an important advantage of spiral CT over conventional CT. Overlapping slices can be acquired with no increase in radiation dose to the patient, resulting in high-quality multiplanar reconstructions. Because scan time is fast, spiral CT examinations can be performed in a single breath-hold to reduce respiratory misregistration and motion artifact, and injected contrast agents can be imaged more quickly over greater lengths of tissue to perform CT angiography (CTA).

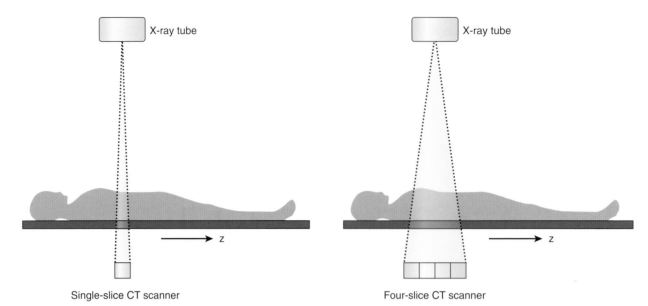

■ FIGURE 1-1   Single-slice versus multi-slice CT scanners. The four-slice scanner has multiple detector rows stacked along the z-axis of the patient.

One technical factor unique to spiral CT is pitch. Pitch is the ratio of table displacement per 360-degree gantry rotation to slice collimation or thickness (table speed × rotation time/slice collimation). A small pitch gives finer spatial resolution along the z-axis of the patient but covers less tissue in a given time and delivers a higher radiation dose to the patient. A large pitch reduces the radiation dose to the patient but also reduces spatial resolution in the z-axis.

Multislice Spiral CT

The next significant milestone in CT evolution was the introduction of scanners with multiple detector rows. In 1998, all major vendors introduced 4-slice CT scanners capable of acquiring up to four slices per gantry rotation. Instead of a single detector row, multiple detector rows were stacked in the gantry along the z-axis of the patient (Fig. 1-1). The time needed for the gantry to complete a 360-degree revolution (gantry rotation time) was also cut in half from 1 second to 0.5 second. For the same slice thickness, pitch, and scan time, a 4-slice CT scanner could image eight times the distance of a single-slice scanner. Alternatively, the 4-slice scanner could acquire four 1.25-mm slices in half the time that single-slice spiral CT acquired one 5-mm slice. Four-slice CT made higher z-axis resolution feasible for a reasonable anatomic length and scan time.

Subsequently, 16-, 40-, and 64-slice scanners were introduced widely for clinical use, the latter in 2004. As a result, slices as thin as 0.5 mm can now be acquired very quickly and over long distances to provide submillimeter resolution in the z-axis, truly isotropic voxels, and isotropic resolution. The advantages of multi-slice CT over single-slice imaging can be summarized as better spatial resolution in the z-axis, faster imaging time, and longer anatomic coverage.

Imaging
Scanning Parameters

A number of parameters must be specified for a spiral CT scan. Slice collimation, or nominal slice thickness, is typically 5 mm for a standard head CT and between 0.625 and 1.25 mm for both CTA and thin-section facial bone CT. Pitch is typically between 1 and 2. A pitch less than 1 implies overlapping images and high radiation dose, whereas a pitch greater than 2 causes gaps in object sampling along the z-axis. Gantry rotation times range

between 0.33 second and 1 second. Imaging of the brain is performed at approximately 120 kV and 200 to 400 mA for adults but uses reduced milliamperage for children.

Approximately 70 mL of nonionic contrast agent at a concentration of 300 to 350 mg of iodine per milliliter is administered for routine contrast-enhanced CT scans. If a contrast agent is to be administered intravenously for CTA, 70 to 100 mL of low/iso-osmolar nonionic contrast material with a concentration of 300 to 350 mg of iodine per milliliter is administered at an injection rate between 4 and 5 mL/s using a power injector.

Reconstruction Parameters

The data acquired during the scan are processed through convolution-backprojection algorithms to provide the CT images. Different algorithms or convolution kernels can be applied during convolution-backprojection to emphasize different tissues. Soft/smoothing or sharp/edge-enhancing algorithms will highlight different tissues such as soft tissue or bone, respectively.

Spiral CT slices can be reconstructed at different thicknesses. Images acquired at 1.25-mm collimation can be reconstructed at 2.5 mm, 3.75 mm, or 5.0 mm. However, slices cannot be reconstructed at thicknesses smaller than the original collimation. Slices can also be reconstructed with varying degrees of overlap, or *reconstruction intervals.* For a 1-mm thick slice, a reconstruction interval of 0.8 mm signifies 20% slice overlap, which is approximately the amount of overlap desired if slices are to be reformatted into other planes.

The CT data can be reprocessed in a number of useful ways. CT images obtained in the axial plane can be reformatted into coronal, sagittal, or oblique sections with *multiplanar reformation* (MPR), a two-dimensional (2D) technique that preserves all the data in the original source images. *Maximum intensity projection* (MIP) processing collects only the brightest voxels from a predefined volume and collapses this information onto a single slice. In this 2D technique, depth information is lost but attenuation data are retained. *Shaded surface display* (SSD) is a three-dimensional (3D) method for displaying the surfaces and shapes of objects, but with significant loss of attenuation information. *Volume rendering* (VR) is a superior 3D method to SSD and assigns color and opacity to each CT value.

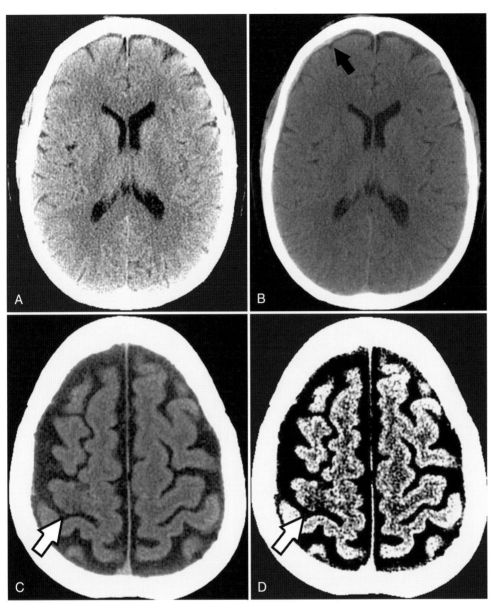

■ **FIGURE 1-2** Importance of window settings. **A,** Subdural hematomas can be easily missed with narrow window settings because hemorrhage may lie outside the window and appear as bright as adjacent bone. **B,** However, widening the window (width 150, level 80) shows a very small right frontal subdural hematoma (*arrow*). **C,** Normal brain window (width 80, level 40) shows very subtle loss of gray-white differentiation in the right motor cortex (*arrow*). **D,** The acute stroke is made more conspicuous (*arrow*) by narrowing the window (width 8, level 32) to emphasize the small attenuation difference between gray and white matter.

Display Parameters

The field of view (FOV) refers to the size of the area imaged. The viewing matrix, composed of individual picture elements or pixels, is typically 512 × 512. The pixel size can be determined by dividing the FOV by matrix size. For example, pixel size for a 512 × 512 matrix and a 25-cm FOV is 0.49 × 0.49 mm. At 0.5-mm collimated slices, voxel size is 0.49 × 0.49 × 0.5 mm, which is nearly isotropic.

Normal Appearance of Images

Attenuation is represented in Hounsfield units on a gray scale in which distilled water is set at 0 HU for standard temperature and pressure, and air is set at −1000 HU. Tissues such as bone, which attenuate the x-ray beam more than water, have positive HU values (approximately 1000 HU for bone) and appear very white. Tissues such as fat, which attenuate the x-ray beam less than water, have negative HU values and appear darker than water (−30 to −100 HU for fat).

The human eye can typically differentiate only 60 to 80 different levels of gray. In practice, therefore, the Hounsfield scale must be narrowed to illustrate specific structures of interest.

This is achieved by selecting a gray-scale *window* of displayed Hounsfield units and arbitrarily making all structures above the chosen window white and all structures below the window black. The *window width* describes the range of Hounsfield values displayed as shades of gray. The *window level* gives the center value of that gray-scale window. A head CT is typically viewed at window width of 80 HU and window level of 40 HU, which means that 0 HU and 80 HU are the lower and upper limits of the window, respectively, with 40 HU in the center. This relatively narrow window width successfully displays the small differences in attenuation values of the brain. Figure 1-2 emphasizes the importance of choosing appropriate windows to properly display structures of interest and to detect clinically important pathologic processes.

Artifacts

Common artifacts encountered in CT include patient motion, beam hardening, partial volume effects, and metallic object streak artifacts. *Patient motion* during scanning creates extensive blurring and misregistration of images. This can be partly mitigated by reducing scan times as much as possible. *Beam*

■ **FIGURE 1-3** Common CT artifacts. **A,** Beam hardening is seen between the petrous apices, limiting evaluation of the pons. **B,** Aneurysm clip causes extensive metallic streak artifact. **C,** Partial volume artifact is seen as streaks throughout the posterior fossa on this 5-mm thick slice. **D,** Reducing slice thickness to 2.5 mm significantly reduces partial volume artifact.

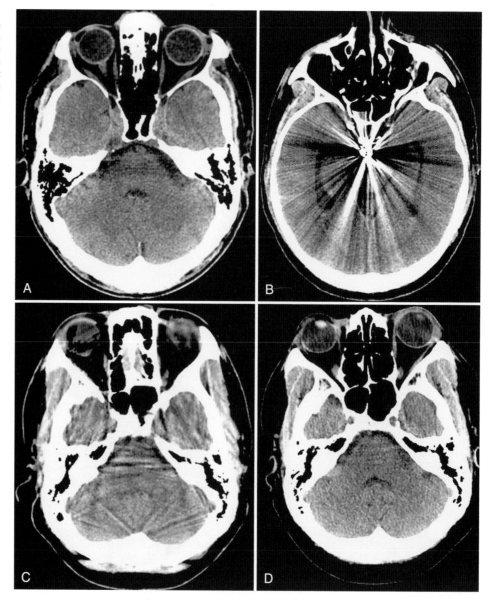

hardening occurs because the energy profile of the x-ray beam changes as it passes through dense objects such as bone. The softer (lower energy) x-rays are absorbed and filtered out by the bone, leaving a beam composed of only harder (higher energy) x-rays. On head CT, *beam hardening* typically occurs in the posterior fossa between the petrous apices, causing dark horizontal lines across the brain stem and limiting the utility of CT for assessing pathologic processes in this area. *Partial volume* artifacts ensue when an imaging voxel contains different types of tissue. The attenuation value of the voxel is a numerical average of the attenuation of all the tissues contained within that voxel. If a portion of the voxel has a very high (or low) Hounsfield unit value, that portion may influence the net attenuation of the voxel disproportionately and obscure the presence of other tissues. Like beam hardening, partial volume effects are most troublesome in the posterior fossa, where they cause streaks or bands of light and dark. Reducing scan thickness produces smaller voxels and helps to reduce partial volume effects. *Metallic objects* such as aneurysm clips or dental hardware generate intense streak artifacts because their exceptionally high density causes beam hardening and partial volume artifacts. The

streaks can completely obscure adjacent structures and prevent their evaluation. Figure 1-3 illustrates these typical artifacts.

Specific Uses

Brain CT is most useful in acute settings, especially emergency departments, because of its fast acquisition time, ready accessibility, and lower cost compared with MRI. As the first-line examination after trauma, CT is more sensitive than MRI for detecting skull fractures and radiopaque foreign bodies such as metal or glass.[2] CT readily identifies acute subdural/epidural and parenchymal hematomas and hemorrhagic contusions and is superior to MRI for detecting acute subarachnoid hemorrhage.[3] CT is particularly helpful for identifying calcification and assessing pathologic processes of bone, both of which may narrow a differential diagnosis. CT is indispensable for studying patients with cardiac pacemakers, defibrillators, intra-orbital metal, or other implants that contraindicate the use of MRI.

CT angiography (CTA) has become important in the initial evaluation of subarachnoid hemorrhage, achieving 90% to 93% sensitivity for detecting aneurysms according to meta-analyses of older studies.[4,5] The faster scan times available with 16- and

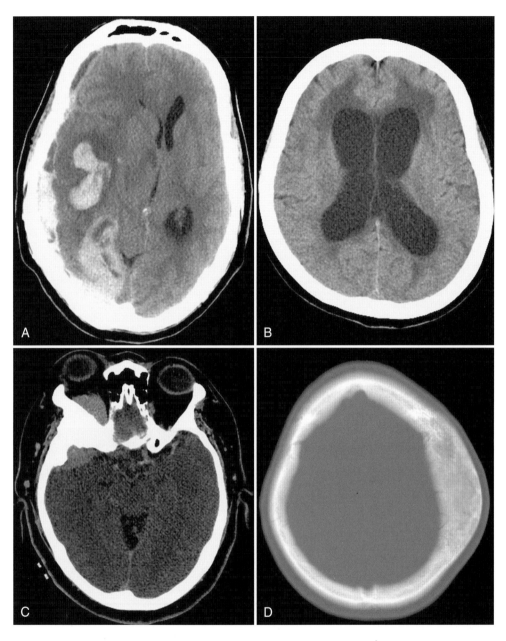

■ **FIGURE 1-4** Uses of CT. **A,** Extensive right parenchymal and subdural hematomas cause significant right-to-left midline shift, a neurosurgical emergency. **B,** Acute hydrocephalus with transependymal flow of CSF is seen as low attenuation of periventricular white matter. **C,** The sphenoid wing hyperostosis associated with this enhancing extra-axial mass is characteristic of meningioma. **D,** Fibrous dysplasia has a typical CT appearance as an expansile osseous lesion with ground-glass internal matrix.

64-slice scanners permit selective capture of the arterial phase of contrast opacification without venous contamination and provide images close to true angiograms. The fast, thinly collimated multi-slice acquisitions now permit CTA to be performed over long distances in short periods of time, so CTA can image the entire region from the base of the heart to the vertex of the skull to evaluate stroke patients for left atrial thrombi and potential occlusions in the cervical and intracranial circulations. Although digital subtraction angiography (DSA) remains the gold standard for angiography at present, the sensitivity and speed of CTA are constantly improving, so CTA will come to rival DSA in the near future.[6]

Analysis

In any acute setting, noncontrast head CT can be used to quickly assess for the three Hs—hemorrhage, herniation, and hydrocephalus—which may necessitate immediate neurosurgical intervention. Figure 1-4 illustrates the utility of CT in the acute setting, as well as its importance in the evaluation of bony lesions.

A sample report is shown in Box 1-1.

Pitfalls and Limitations

Several important problems do limit the utility of CT. In patients with renal impairment, the use of iodinated intravenous contrast is limited by concerns about contrast-induced nephropathy, generally identified as an increase in serum creatinine concentration after administration of a contrast agent, without an alternative explanation. Although there are no uniform diagnostic criteria (because creatinine levels are not necessarily precise), the two most important risk factors for developing nephropathy are preexisting renal impairment and diabetes.[7,8] Adequate hydration, acetylcysteine, and sodium bicarbonate may help prevent nephropathy in patients with borderline renal function.[9,10]

Radiologists are frequently asked what to do with patients who are "allergic" to shellfish or iodine. There is a mistaken

BOX 1-1   Sample Report: CT and CT Angiography of the Head (Fig. 1-5)

PATIENT HISTORY
A 53-year-old woman presented with subarachnoid hemorrhage.

COMPARISON STUDY
No study had been done.

TECHNIQUE
Contiguous axial 2.5-mm noncontrast images of the head were obtained from the vertex to the foramen magnum. After intravenous administration of 150 mL of Omnipaque-350, contiguous axial 0.625-mm images were obtained from the vertex to the upper neck. Maximum intensity projections were obtained in the coronal, axial, and sagittal planes. Finally, contiguous axial 2.5-mm postcontrast images of the head were obtained.

FINDINGS

Noncontrast CT of the Brain
A large 4.1 × 2.6 × 3.0-cm intraparenchymal hematoma is noted in the right insular region with surrounding vasogenic edema. There is mild associated right-to-left midline shift (0.3 cm) and trapping of the left lateral ventricle. Diffuse subarachnoid hemorrhage is seen throughout, including within the basilar cisterns and sylvian fissures bilaterally. Diffuse sulcal and cisternal effacement is compatible with extensive cerebral swelling.

CTA of the Intracranial Arteries
A 1 × 1 × 1.6-cm lobulated, saccular aneurysm is noted at the right middle cerebral artery (MCA) bifurcation, with surrounding hemorrhage indicating rupture. The aneurysm has a narrow neck measuring 0.3 cm and projects inferiorly. Two small 2-mm aneurysms are also seen arising from the anterior communicating artery (ACOM). The posterior circulation demonstrates codominant vertebral arteries. Normal bilateral posterior communicating arteries are present. Intracranial vessels are of normal caliber without narrowing to suggest vasospasm.

Postcontrast CT
The large right MCA bifurcation aneurysm is again demonstrated. There is no evidence of abnormal parenchymal or leptomeningeal enhancement. The dural venous sinuses are patent.

IMPRESSION
There is extensive right temporal intraparenchymal hematoma and diffuse subarachnoid hemorrhage associated with rupture of a large 1.6-cm saccular aneurysm at the right MCA bifurcation. This aneurysm has a narrow neck and projects inferiorly. Two additional small ACOM aneurysms are noted.

Also noted are associated mild right-to-left subfalcine herniation, trapping of the left lateral ventricle, and diffuse sulcal/cisternal effacement consistent with extensive cerebral swelling.

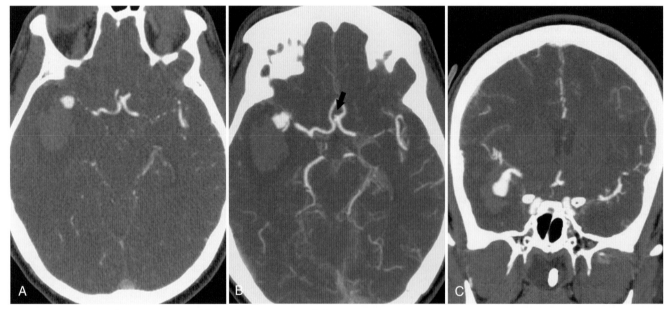

■ **FIGURE 1-5**   CTA of ruptured right middle cerebral artery (MCA) bifurcation aneurysm. **A,** The 0.625-mm collimated axial source images obtained on a 64-slice scanner demonstrate the saccular right MCA aneurysm with adjacent intraparenchymal hematoma. Axial (**B**) and coronal (**C**) maximum intensity projections (20-mm thickness with interval of 5 mm and 75% overlap) show more of the aneurysm and adjacent vessels with each slice than the thin source images. A small anterior communicating artery aneurysm is seen on the axial image (*arrow,* **B**).

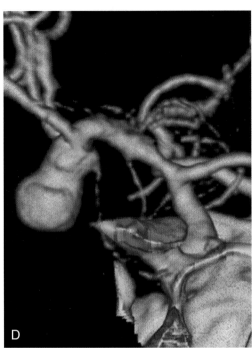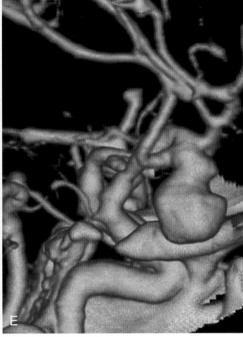

■ **FIGURE 1-5, cont'd** Coronal (**D**) and sagittal (**E**) volume-rendered images are useful to evaluate the relationship of the MCA branches to the aneurysm.

assumption that iodine in each of these compounds confers cross-reactivity to iodinated contrast agents. However, there is little to no evidence to indicate that the iodine itself triggers adverse reactions to contrast, seafood, or topical povidone-iodine.[11] In patients with a history of significant prior contrast reaction, premedication with histamine blockers and corticosteroids can be performed. Patients describing allergies to seafood should be questioned about the nature of the reaction but only insofar as a history of severe allergy to *any* food increases the risk of contrast reaction.

Pregnancy and lactation generate additional safety considerations for CT. The radiation dose to the fetus during the mother's head CT has been estimated at 0 to 1 mGy and is from scattered radiation only. It is generally believed that the risk to the fetus of teratogenesis or childhood cancer is negligible at radiation dosages less than 50 mGy.[12,13] Because the uterus lies outside the field of view and the radiation dose to the fetus is negligible, it is not clear that it is necessary to place lead shielding over the abdomen/pelvis. However, placing shielding may provide reassurance to the patient. Iodinated contrast material should be avoided if possible during pregnancy because of potential concern for fetal hypothyroidism. For lactating women, the traditional recommendation is to discontinue breast feeding for 12 to 24 hours after contrast agent administration and discard the milk.[14]

Current Research and Future Direction
CT scanners capable of up to 64-slice acquisitions are in common clinical use and afford submillimeter isotropic resolution, rapid scan times (<5 seconds for head CT), and good coverage (32 to 40 mm z-axis coverage with a single gantry rotation). Because the imaging parameters are now able to meet most clinical demands, it is not clear that increasing the number of slices acquired simultaneously is particularly useful or warranted. Instead, research has focused on meeting specific clinical needs, such as dynamic imaging for perfusion measurements and faster scan times for cardiac imaging.

Increasing the length of coverage along the z-axis may permit an entire organ to be imaged during a single gantry rotation, opening up the potential for dynamic perfusion imaging of individual organs. Ways of increasing the volume of coverage include using flat-panel detectors, manipulating the detector array, and increasing the number of detector rows. Indeed, 256- and 320-slice scanners have been developed and installed in limited capacity, providing 12 to 16 cm of z-axis coverage, although higher data load and cost burden are important considerations.

Dual-energy source CT is another promising area for future development. In this approach, two x-ray tubes and two detectors are housed in the same gantry and are used to deliver two x-ray beams at *different voltages* (e.g., 80 kV and 140 kV). Advantages of dual-source CT include much faster scan times and higher temporal resolution, which are invaluable for cardiac imaging. Dual-source scanning also has the potential to differentiate between specific tissues such as calcium and blood. This ability can be used to selectively depict a single tissue or selectively delete one tissue from the image. For example, one can accurately subtract bone from CTA images to clearly evaluate vessels at the skull base, an area that has traditionally been difficult to visualize.

MAGNETIC RESONANCE IMAGING
The U.S. Food and Drug Administration first cleared MRI for commercial use in 1984, and MRI has grown remarkably since that time. Most current MRI scanners have a magnetic field strength of 1.5 tesla (1.5 T), but units employing higher magnetic field strengths of 3 tesla (3 T) are coming into increasing use. Both the 1.5-T and newer magnets offer an unparalleled look at anatomic structures, with relative safety and freedom from the concerns about radiation dose that are inherent in CT.

MRI employs an astonishing array of sequences that are acquired by diverse means, are used for different purposes, and are designated by different acronyms by each manufacturer. Table 1-1 offers an overview of the major sequences commonly used in MRI (including their acronyms), which may be a useful reference during review of this chapter.

Basic Concepts
MR Signal Creation
Clinical MRI relies on the hydrogen nucleus. In their native state, the hydrogen nuclei exhibit random orientation and precess or

TABLE 1-1. Overview of Major MRI Sequences

	Sequence Types	Basics	Contrast
SE	Spin-echo (SE)	90-degree excitation pulse 180-degree refocusing pulse	T1 or T2
	Rapid acquisition with refocused echo (RARE): also known as fast spin-echo (FSE) or turbo spin-echo (TSE)	90-degree pulse Multiple 180-degree pulses	T1 or T2 (blurring increases with echo train length)
	Half-Fourier acquisition single-shot turbo spin-echo (HASTE), single-shot fast spin-echo (SSFSE)	90-degree pulse Multiple 180-degree pulses to fill half of k-space (other half inferred)	Usually T2 (severe T2 blurring due to very long echo train length)
	Inversion recovery: Fluid-attenuated inversion recovery (FLAIR) and short tau inversion recovery (STIR)	Preparatory 180-degree inversion pulse 90-degree pulse Single or multiple 180-degree pulses	Mix of T1 and T2
GRE	Gradient echo (GRE)	<90-degree pulse No 180-degree pulse	T1 or T2*
	Spoiled/incoherent: Spoiled gradient-recalled-echo (SPGR), T1-weighted fast field echo (T1-FFE), fast low-angle shot (FLASH)	Transverse magnetization is destroyed	T1
	Unspoiled/coherent: Gradient-recalled acquisition in steady state (GRASS), fast field-echo (FFE), fast imaging with steady-state free precession (FISP)	Steady-state free precession	Mix of T1, T2, T2*
	Balanced: Fast imaging employing steady-state acquisition (FIESTA), balanced FFE, trueFISP	Steady-state free precession	Mix of T1 and T2
	Echoplanar imaging (EPI)	Single excitation pulse to fill all of k-space	T2* (can also have T2 if spin-echo EPI)

rotate at varying rates. When an external magnetic field (B_0) is applied, the hydrogen nuclei begin to precess at a resonance frequency (designated the *Larmor frequency*) that is proportional to the magnetic field strength. Additionally, the external magnetic field prompts the hydrogen nuclei to align and precess along the axis of the magnetic field, creating a *net magnetization vector*. By convention, the direction of B_0 is designated the *longitudinal* or *z-axis*. The plane oriented perpendicular to the z-axis is designated the *transverse* or *x/y-axis*.

The precession of the hydrogen nuclei at the Larmor frequency creates a current, measured as the MR signal. This current cannot be detected in the z-axis; it can only be detected when its magnetization lies in the transverse plane. To measure the current, the net magnetization must be moved from the z-axis (where it cannot be measured) into the transverse x/y-axis (where it can be measured). To accomplish this, a radiofrequency (RF) pulse is applied to "flip" the net magnetization by a certain angle (the *flip angle*) into the transverse plane. Immediately after the RF pulse, nuclei in the transverse plane are *in phase*. They precess together at the same frequency and in the same direction, creating a signal known as the *free induction decay* (FID). However, the FID signal is rapidly lost as inhomogeneities in the magnetic field cause the nuclei to *dephase* and spin at different frequencies. The FID cannot be measured directly for imaging purposes. Instead, an echo of the FID—either a *spin echo* or *gradient echo*—must be produced by rephasing the nuclei. This is the basis for sequence design, as will be discussed later.

MR Signal Localization in 2D and 3D Imaging
To localize an echo within the body, one applies small magnetic fields called *gradients* that steadily increase in strength along a particular direction. Because of the gradients, a proton in one part of the body will feel a different magnetic field and will precess at a different Larmor frequency than a proton elsewhere. To localize protons within the body in all three orthogonal axes (x, y, and z), three different gradients are applied, designated the *frequency-encoding*, *phase-encoding*, and *slice-selection* gradients.

2D imaging acquires data from individual flat slices. In this technique, a specific RF pulse is used to excite a slice of tissue. The slice-selection gradient is turned on while the excitatory RF pulse is given, so that the only nuclei to respond will be those in the slice whose Larmor frequency matches that of the exciting RF pulse. The thickness of the slice that is excited depends largely on the strength of the slice-selection gradient: the stronger the slice-selection gradient, the thinner the excited slice. The frequency-encoding gradient is employed during detection or "readout" of the MR signal. The phase-encoding step, which is performed between slice selection and frequency-encoded readout, must be performed many times at different gradient strengths, making this one of the key determinants of the length of a scan. 2D imaging typically produces a series of slices that are not contiguous and greater than 1 mm in thickness.

In 3D imaging, the RF pulse and slice-selection gradient excite an entire *volume* of tissue along the z-axis, rather than a single thin slice. Phase encoding is performed in two directions, not just one as in 2D imaging, and is followed by the frequency-encoded readout. 3D imaging typically has a higher signal-to-noise ratio than 2D imaging because the MR signal is obtained from the entire volume of tissue rather than one slice. Therefore, the number of MR signals that forms each echo is much greater for 3D than for 2D imaging. 3D imaging also generates very thin slices (each <1 mm) that are contiguous with each other, permitting excellent multiplanar reconstructions. However, 3D imaging is slower than 2D imaging because it performs the relatively time-consuming process of phase encoding in two directions, not just one.

MR Image Creation
Generation of an actual image from an MR signal usually requires multiple excitations with an RF pulse to produce enough data for the image. The period between excitations is *TR* (time to repetition) while the period from excitation to echo readout is *TE* (time to echo).

The measured echoes from a particular slice are sampled and then encoded within *k-space*. *k-space* is a mathematical construct consisting of a blank grid or matrix onto which frequency

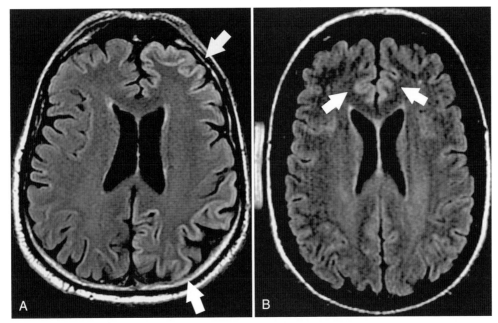

■ **FIGURE 1-6** Importance of proper coil selection. Patients with prion disorders such as Creutzfeldt-Jakob disease (CJD) may have high signal in the cerebral cortex, as was the case for the patient in **A,** who had bright cortical signal, particularly in the left cerebral hemisphere (*arrows*). The patient in **B** did not have CJD but was imaged in a surface coil, with high signal in the paramedian frontal cortex bilaterally (*arrows*). This is an artifact from closer proximity of superficial tissues to the surface coil. Because of the potential for confusion with artifactually inhomogeneous signal, diagnosis of CJD may be easier with a volume coil, which encircles the entire head and provides better signal uniformity.

and phase data can be mapped before their transformation into an MR image. In k-space, frequency information is typically mapped along the x-axis and phase information along the y-axis. In a conventional spin-echo sequence, one echo generates the data for a single line in k-space and corresponds to a single phase-encoding step. The center of k-space contains information about general form (low spatial resolution) at high image contrast. The periphery of k-space holds information about fine detail (high spatial resolution) at low image contrast. The data within k-space are rendered into an image by Fourier transformation, a computerized mathematical process of MR signal decoding that converts frequency information into the pixels of an image.

MR Hardware (Coils)

Radiofrequency antennas called *coils* are used to transmit the RF pulse and receive the MR signal. Separate coils can be used for transmission and reception, or the same coil can be used for both functions. MR coils may be constructed to have different regions of coverage: a *volume coil* is a circumferential structure that surrounds the body part completely, while a *surface coil* is typically flat or curved and placed on the skin surface overlying a specific region of interest. Volume coils both transmit and receive the MR signal. They encircle the body part completely, so they provide very uniform signal throughout the entire MR image. A typical volume coil used for neuroimaging is the bird-cage head coil. Surface coils are generally receive-only coils, so a separate volume head or body coil is needed to transmit the RF pulse. Surface coils have very high signal-to-noise ratio, especially for superficial structures close to the coil. However, they have a reduced FOV and are more prone to inhomogeneity of signal across an MR image, with signal loss for deeper tissues. *Phased-array* coils are composite coils composed of multiple small surface coils arranged to form an array. These have been developed to try to increase the FOV while maintaining the high signal-to-noise ratio of surface coils. Imaging for Creutzfeldt-

Jakob disease illustrates the importance of proper coil selection (Fig. 1-6).

Imaging
Tissue Weighting

T1, T2, and proton density are the fundamental parameters of MRI and determine the contrast between tissues. After the excitatory RF pulse and tilting of the net magnetization into the transverse or x/y-plane, the *transverse magnetization* is lost at a rate determined by a particular tissue's *T2 relaxation time*. Simultaneously, *longitudinal magnetization* along the z-axis is regained at a rate set by the tissue's *T1 relaxation time*.

Fat has a shorter T1 than cerebrospinal fluid (CSF) and recovers its longitudinal magnetization quickly after an RF pulse. If the TR is short, fat recovers more of its longitudinal magnetization than CSF and produces a stronger MR signal. More longitudinal magnetization leads to more transverse magnetization and stronger signal with the next RF pulse. Making *TR short* emphasizes the differences in the T1 relaxation times of tissues, so tissues with short T1 such as fat, melanin, and protein produce high signal. MR sequences that emphasize tissue differences in T1 relaxation are designated *T1-weighted* (T1W).

Fat has a shorter T2 relaxation time than CSF and loses its transverse magnetization (T2 signal) more rapidly. Making TE long provides greater time for the transverse magnetization to decay and emphasizes differences in the T2 relaxation times of tissues. When TE is long, tissues with short T2 relaxation times (fat) show greater loss of T2 signal and appear dark whereas tissues with long T2 relaxation times (CSF) retain a larger portion of their T2 signal and appear bright. MR sequences that use long TE to emphasize tissue differences in T2 relaxation times are designated *T2-weighted* (T2W).

If the TR is long and the TE is short, neither the T1 nor T2 difference between fat and CSF is emphasized. Any difference in contrast observed between the two tissues is then due to differences in the proton densities of the tissues. Tissues with higher proton density supply greater signal than tissues with lower proton density. MRI sequences that use long TR and short TE to capture differences in tissue proton density are designated *proton density–weighted* (PDW) sequences.

Image Quality

In MRI, image quality depends on spatial resolution and the signal-to-noise ratio. Like CT, spatial resolution reflects voxel size. Pixel size influences in-plane or x/y-axis spatial resolution, whereas slice thickness determines z-axis spatial resolution. Therefore, spatial resolution can be improved by reducing voxel size through decreasing the FOV, increasing the matrix size, or obtaining thinner slices. However, reducing voxel size to improve spatial resolution tends to increase the relative noise in an image. Spatial resolution and signal-to-noise ratio are competing considerations.

The *sampling bandwidth* refers to the rate at which an echo is sampled. A high bandwidth samples an echo quickly but requires a stronger frequency-encoding gradient and results in a greater range of frequencies. A low bandwidth takes longer to sample an echo but has a smaller range of frequencies and includes less sampling of noise. High bandwidths reduce acquisition time, so there is less opportunity for image degradation from signal decay. Low bandwidths prolong acquisition time but improve the signal-to-noise ratio.

Basic MRI Sequences

Spin echo and gradient echo are the only two basic sequences in MRI; all other sequences are variations of one of these two sequences. To create either a spin echo or gradient echo after the FID, a specific *pulse sequence* must be designed. A pulse sequence diagram illustrates the series and timing of requisite events, including application of the RF pulse and various gradients, to produce the sampled echo.

Spin Echo

The spin-echo (SE) sequence is created by following the 90-degree excitatory pulse with a 180-degree refocusing pulse at time TE/2. After the 90-degree RF pulse, transverse magnetization (FID) is quickly lost because of (1) *macroscopic* magnetic field inhomogeneities due to factors such as adjacent ferromagnetic objects, nonuniformities in the B_0 magnetic field, and tissue interfaces and (2) *microscopic* magnetic interactions among spinning nuclei. The loss of magnetization due to both microscopic and macroscopic factors is termed *T2* relaxation.* Signal loss due only to microscopic nuclear interactions is "true" T2 decay and occurs more slowly than T2* decay.

The 180-degree refocusing pulse is able to rephase nuclei that have begun precessing at different frequencies and can prevent the signal loss that is due to macroscopic factors. However, it cannot prevent the signal loss that is due to random, microscopic nuclear interactions, that is, T2 decay. The spin echo that results from the rephasing effects of the 180-degree pulse is still susceptible to T2 decay and therefore SE sequences with long TE are said to be T2 weighted (not T2* weighted).

Figure 1-7A illustrates the pulse sequence diagram for the SE technique.

Gradient Recalled Echo

If the 180-degree refocusing pulse is not given, an echo of the FID can still be produced by using gradients of opposite polarity (equal strength, opposite direction) to first dephase and then rephase the spins. Opposite-polarity lobes of the frequency-encoding gradient are used to bring spins together in phase and produce a gradient echo at time TE. Because they do not use a 180-degree refocusing pulse, gradient-recalled echo (GRE) images are prone to signal loss from both macroscopic and microscopic factors (T2* decay). Depending on various sequence

parameters, GRE sequences can be T1W or T2*W, but typically not T2W (see later for exceptions). Figure 1-7B illustrates the components of a GRE sequence.

Unlike SE, GRE sequences use small flip angles that are less than 90 degrees. These flip angles do not eliminate the longitudinal magnetization completely. Some longitudinal magnetization remains, so it recovers more completely before the next pulse. This permits use of a shorter TR and helps achieve faster scan time. In GRE sequences, the tissue weighting depends on TR, TE, and the value of the flip angle: larger flip angles accentuate differences in the T1 relaxation time, because more longitudinal magnetization must recover to produce the image. Larger flip angles therefore produce T1W images.

"Spoiling" or "refocusing" transverse magnetization provides another means of tissue weighting. To reduce scan times, GRE sequences frequently use very short TR (shorter than the T2 relaxation times of many tissues), so that the transverse magnetization does not have time to decay completely before the next excitatory pulse. In this situation, there is both residual transverse magnetization and recovered longitudinal magnetization just before the next RF pulse. If the residual transverse magnetization is "spoiled" or destroyed, only the longitudinal magnetization is left for the next RF pulse, resulting in *T1W images.* Spoiling of transverse magnetization is achieved by use of spoiler gradients or RF spoiling, a discussion of which is beyond the scope of this chapter. These T1W GRE sequences are known as *spoiled* or *incoherent GRE* sequences.

Alternatively, *unspoiled* or *coherent GRE* imaging preserves the transverse magnetization that accumulates between RF pulses in short TR sequences. The subsequent RF pulse rotates residual transverse magnetization into the longitudinal plane while flipping recovered longitudinal magnetization into the transverse plane. Over time and with successive RF pulses, there is an intricate mixing of transverse and longitudinal components known as *steady-state free precession.* Unlike spoiled GRE sequences, signal intensity in unspoiled sequences depends not only on the amount of longitudinal magnetization that has recovered but also on the amount of transverse magnetization that remains. Because recovery of longitudinal magnetization is determined by T1 and decay of transverse magnetization by T2, these sequences reflect a mixture of T1W and T2W imaging. Note that if TR is sufficiently long to allow complete decay of transverse magnetization and leave only longitudinal magnetization, the unspoiled/coherent sequence becomes T1 weighted much like a spoiled/incoherent GRE.

Another consequence of preserving residual transverse magnetization in unspoiled GRE imaging is the generation of a *spin echo* with the next excitatory RF pulse. The excitatory pulse behaves like a refocusing pulse on residual transverse magnetization and is conceptually similar to, although less effective than, the 180-degree refocusing pulse used in SE imaging. The residual transverse magnetization that was becoming dephased is suddenly refocused and generates an SE in addition to the usual FID that is created immediately after an RF pulse. Depending on sequence design, either the FID or SE can be favored to achieve more T2* or T2 weighting, respectively. *Balanced GRE* sequences are constructed so that all gradients are balanced and the FID and SE signals coincide, achieving a complex mix of T1 and T2 weighting.

Inversion Recovery Imaging

Inversion recovery (IR) imaging applies a preparatory pulse just before an SE or GRE sequence to emphasize T1 contrast or to eliminate signal from undesired tissues such as CSF or fat. A 180-degree inversion pulse is first given to flip the initial net magnetization vector from the +z axis to the −z axis. Nuclei recover longitudinal magnetization from −z to +z according to their T1 properties. If an excitatory 90-degree pulse is given during relax-

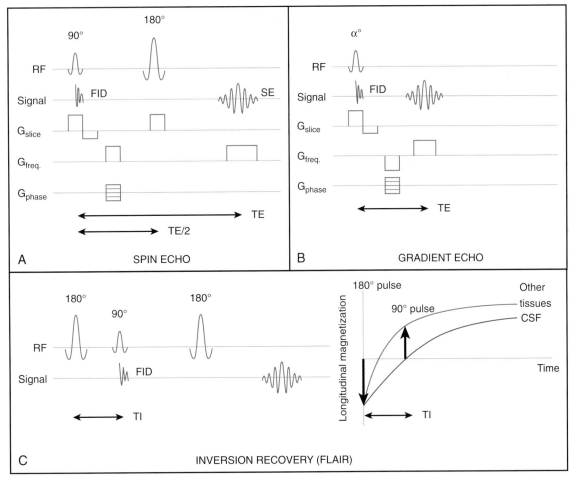

■ **FIGURE 1-7** Pulse sequence diagrams. **A,** Spin echo: Following the 90-degree excitation pulse, which occurs at the same time as the slice-selection gradient, the free induction decay (FID) quickly disappears. The 180-degree refocusing pulse given at time TE/2 rephases the spins to create the spin echo that is read out at time TE with application of the frequency-encoding gradient. The phase-encoding step must be performed many times at different gradient strengths so is pictured with multiple lines denoting different gradient amplitudes. **B,** Gradient echo: Following the RF pulse (with flip angle α < 90 degrees), the FID is rapidly lost. No 180-degree refocusing pulse is given; instead, opposing lobes of the frequency-encoding gradient are used to first dephase then rephase the spins, creating an echo at time TE. The negative (dephasing) lobe of the frequency-encoding gradient is shown below baseline, while the positive (rephasing) lobe is shown above baseline. **C,** Inversion recovery and FLAIR: A 180-degree pulse is given at the beginning of the sequence, which flips the net magnetization vector into the −z-axis. Tissues recover longitudinal magnetization according to their T1 properties and CSF, with long T1, regains magnetization more slowly than other tissues. The 90-degree excitatory pulse at time TI is given at the null point for CSF, when there is no longitudinal magnetization for CSF. However, other tissues have recovered longitudinal magnetization, which is flipped into the transverse plane with the excitatory pulse to generate the MR signal. FLAIR is performed on a spin-echo sequence.

ation (at *inversion time* TI), nuclei with shorter T1 will have recovered more longitudinal magnetization and thus produce greater transverse magnetization and MR signal. This creates T1 weighting.

As nuclei recover longitudinal magnetization from −z to +z after the 180-degree inversion pulse, they pass through a null point at which the net magnetization vector is zero. A 90-degree excitatory pulse given at this time for CSF (or fat) would have very little effect on and generate no MR signal from CSF (or fat). In this manner, specific tissues can be made dark on imaging. *STIR (short tau inversion recovery)* is the name of the sequence used for fat elimination. Because fat has a relatively short T1, STIR sequences typically employ inversion times of approximately 150 to 175 ms at 1.5T. *FLAIR (fluid-attenuated inversion recovery)* is the name of the sequence used for CSF suppression. Because water has a long T1, FLAIR sequences typically employ inversion times ranging from 1800 to 2400 ms at 1.5 T.[15] Figure 1-7C illustrates a typical IR sequence.

The concept of tissue contrast is more complex than simple T1 or T2 weighting for FLAIR. Although FLAIR sequences have long TE and are T2 weighted so that fluid other than CSF is bright, an element of T1 weighting is also present. The 180-degree inversion pulse introduces T1 weighting, because the degree to which tissues recover longitudinal magnetization before the excitation pulse is given depends on their T1 properties.

Fast Imaging Techniques

The main drawback of conventional SE imaging is its long imaging time. Long imaging time results because each excitatory RF pulse generates a single echo that fills only a single line of k-space, corresponding to a single phase-encoding step. The SE technique does not considerably lengthen the time required for obtaining T1W images, because T1W sequences use short TR and short TE. However, the SE technique significantly lengthens the time required for obtaining T2W images, because T2W sequences employ long TR and long TE. *Rapid acquisition with refocused echo* (RARE) sequences were developed to reduce imaging time. Commercially, these are known as fast spin-echo (FSE) or turbo spin-echo (TSE) sequences. In this approach, each

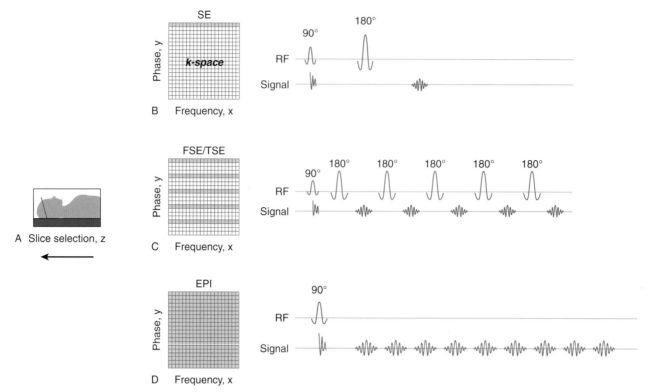

■ FIGURE 1-8   Comparison of single- and multiple-echo techniques, following a single excitatory pulse. **A,** An axial level in the brain is determined by the slice-selection gradient at the time of RF excitation. **B,** In conventional spin echo, a single 180° refocusing pulse after the excitatory pulse produces a spin echo that fills a single line of k-space (*shaded in green*). The sequence must be repeated, with phase encoding performed at a different amplitude, to generate another spin echo that fills a different line of k-space. **C,** In fast or turbo spin-echo, each excitatory pulse is followed by n number of 180 refocusing pulses (five in our case) that generate n echoes to fill n lines of k-space. The echo train length is 5 and scan time is 1/5 (1/ETL) of the conventional spin-echo sequence. Phase encoding is performed at a different amplitude for each echo, to fill a different line of k-space. **D,** In single-shot echoplanar imaging, the excitatory pulse is followed by rapid gradient switching that generates a long stream of gradient echoes, enough to fill all of k-space after a single pulse.

90-degree RF pulse is followed by multiple 180-degree refocusing pulses (not just one) to generate more spin echoes and fill multiple lines of k-space per excitation pulse. The number of echoes generated after each excitatory pulse is termed the *echo train length* (ETL) and corresponds to the number of phase encoding steps acquired in a single TR. Therefore, FSE or TSE reduces the scan time to 1/ETL of the time required for standard SE imaging.

k-space demonstrates a certain symmetry and redundancy of information that allows an image to be derived from a portion of the complete dataset. If enough echoes are collected to fill one-half of k-space after a single 90-degree excitatory pulse (designated a "shot"), the data in the other half of k-space can be inferred based on the known symmetry of k-space.[16] The technique used to produce images from a half-set of data is known as *single-shot RARE* (or commercially as half-Fourier acquisition single-shot turbo spin-echo [HASTE] or single-shot fast spin-echo [SSFSE]).

A similar rapid imaging technique using gradient echoes is designated *echoplanar imaging* (EPI). In EPI, the single excitatory pulse or shot is followed by a long stream of gradient echoes generated by rapidly switching gradients. The multiple gradient echoes fill all of k-space after a single shot.[17] EPI is one of the fastest MR sequences available, so it is used for diffusion-weighted imaging (DWI). Because DWI characterizes the microscopic movement or diffusion of water molecules through tissue, corruption by bulk macroscopic motion due to long scan time cannot be permitted.

Figure 1-8 summarizes the differences between single- and multiple-echo techniques. All multiple-echo techniques are

subject to image contrast blurring, because transverse magnetization decays over the course of the long echo train. This T1, T2, or T2* blurring increases with the ETL and reaches its extreme in the single-shot techniques (HASTE, SSFSE, and EPI).

Normal Appearance of Images

On T1W images of the normal adult brain, white matter is of slightly higher signal intensity than gray matter. However, the unmyelinated or partially myelinated white matter of infants younger than 2 years is hypointense to gray matter. Fat is bright and CSF is dark on T1W images, as previously discussed.

On T2W images of the normal adult brain, white matter is hypointense to gray matter. The unmyelinated or partially myelinated white matter of infants younger than 2 years is hyperintense to gray matter on T2W images. Fat is dark and CSF is bright on SE T2W images. However, fat may appear bright on FSE or TSE T2W images owing to a decrease in a phenomenon known as J-coupling. Any pathologic process increasing tissue water content will be readily seen on T2W sequences as bright signal.

Artifacts

Some of the common MRI artifacts are discussed here. Artifacts associated with specific MRI sequences are explained later in the chapter.

Wraparound/aliasing occurs when the body part imaged is larger than the FOV, causing "wraparound" of the data outside the FOV. This occurs along the phase-encoding direction(s) and can be eliminated by enlarging the FOV or by increasing the number of phase-encoding steps. *Truncation* or *Gibbs' ringing* artifact occurs because of undersampling or truncation of high-frequency data. It appears as alternating light and dark bands at high/low signal tissue interfaces, characteristically at the brain/skull interface and in the spine on sagittal images, where it can simulate a syrinx. Truncation artifact can be reduced by decreasing interface contrast (such as by using fat suppression) or by increasing matrix size. *Motion/ghost* artifacts typically occur in the phase-encoding direction, because time-consuming phase-encoding steps allow more time for motion to disrupt the MR signal and create artifact. Both patient and physiologic motion (such as CSF or blood pulsation) can cause artifact that may appear as blurred areas or as "ghosts" (discrete lines or objects). Motion artifact can be reduced by using fast imaging techniques or applying presaturation pulses to minimize signal from moving or pulsating structures. If the artifact obscures a structure of interest, swapping the phase- and frequency-encoding directions can redirect the artifact away from that specific structure.

Chemical-shift artifact occurs in the frequency-encoding direction. Frequency encoding spatially localizes the MR signal on the basis of frequency, and differences in frequency are automatically equated to differences in signal origin. The magnetic field experienced by a proton is influenced by the precise chemical environment in which it resides. Electron clouds of adjacent chemical groups may partially "shield" a proton from the applied gradient field, so that the proton experiences a slightly different magnetic field than its neighbor and responds by precessing at a slightly different frequency from its neighbor. The difference in precessional frequency caused by the different chemical environment is designated "chemical shift." Within the same voxel, the protons in fat and water precess at slightly different Larmor frequencies (chemical shift), because they experience different magnetic fields due to differential shielding by their electron clouds. Bright and dark signal at the fat/water interface results from mismapping of fat and water protons in the same voxel during frequency encoding and is known as chemical-shift artifact. Chemical-shift artifact can be reduced by suppressing signal from fat, by switching frequency- and phase-encoding directions to minimize disruption to a specific area, or by increasing the sampling bandwidth. Increasing the bandwidth increases the range of sampled frequencies and decreases the relative importance or conspicuity of the chemical shift difference. However, increasing the bandwidth will reduce the signal-to-noise ratio.

Susceptibility is a property of different materials that describes their interaction with a magnetic field. Certain materials, such as iron-containing hemorrhage or gadolinium-based contrast, weakly increase the local magnetic field and are known as *paramagnetic*. *Superparamagnetic* or *ferromagnetic* materials such as iron and various metal alloys more strongly increase and distort the local magnetic field, causing signal dropout and a warped appearance of the nearby tissues. GRE sequences are more prone to susceptibility artifact because they do not use a 180-degree refocusing pulse and signal dephases rapidly due to field inhomogeneities. Susceptibility artifact can be decreased by using SE rather than GRE technique (especially FSE or TSE with long ETLs), by using short TE (decreasing the time for dephasing to occur), and by increasing the sampling bandwidth (faster acquisition, decreasing the time for dephasing to occur). Alternatively, susceptibility artifact may be used to advantage to identify very small and otherwise easily overlooked foci of hemorrhage, such as those found with trauma, amyloid angiopathy, and cavernous malformations. These effects form the basis of susceptibility imaging and are especially prominent at higher field strengths.

Figure 1-9 illustrates several commonly encountered artifacts.

Specific Uses

MRI is the workhorse of neuroimaging for the adult brain and can be used to evaluate intracranial tumors, infection or inflammation, demyelinating processes, degenerative disease, ischemic injury, and developmental anomalies. Very small anatomic structures such as the sella turcica and cranial nerves can be depicted more precisely with MRI than CT. The following section highlights specific uses of MRI techniques for clinical neuroimaging.

Analysis
Spin Echo and Fast/Turbo Spin Echo
SE has traditionally been considered the mainstay of neuroimaging. T2-weighted SE or FSE/TSE highlights pathologic processes because of its sensitivity to fluid and changes in tissue cellularity. Appearance on T1W imaging can be helpful for identifying substances such as fat, melanin, and proteinaceous material, because they all appear bright. Hemorrhage has a variable appearance on T1W and T2W images depending on the age of the hematoma.

Gadolinium-based contrast material can be administered intravenously to highlight pathology. Gadolinium is a paramagnetic metal that, by itself, is toxic to the human body so must be tightly chelated to another substance such as diethylenetriaminepentaacetic acid (DTPA) before use. Gadolinium shortens T1 relaxation times, causing increased signal on T1W images wherever the blood-brain barrier has been breached and contrast material is able to enter (e.g., by a tumor).

Gradient Echo
The lack of a 180-degree refocusing pulse and the specific vulnerability to T2* decay can be exploited to detect intracranial hemorrhage. Paramagnetic blood products create local magnetic field inhomogeneities, cause adjacent spinning nuclei to dephase, and induce a striking, characteristic signal loss on GRE sequences (Fig. 1-10). In contrast, blood can be more difficult to detect on SE sequences, which are less sensitive to susceptibility effects due to the 180-degree refocusing pulse. FSE and TSE sequences are even less sensitive to hemorrhage than SE because they employ multiple refocusing pulses.

The faster imaging time of GRE is particularly useful in scanning uncooperative patients or in 3D imaging, which requires longer scan times than 2D. In particular, 3D spoiled GRE sequences provide T1W images and excellent anatomic detail. 3D GRE sequences are useful for evaluating subtle cortical abnormalities in seizure patients or for characterizing tumor extension in conjunction with gadolinium-based contrast.

Fluid-Attenuated Inversion Recovery
FLAIR is typically a T2-weighted FSE/TSE sequence that uses an inversion pulse to eliminate the signal from CSF. It is useful for highlighting lesions that lie close to ventricles or sulci and are not as conspicuous on T2W sequences, such as plaques of multiple sclerosis or small infarcts abutting the cortex.[18,19] Suppression of CSF signal allows for distinction between epidermoid cysts (bright) and arachnoid cysts (dark). Because FLAIR sequences normally suppress the signal of CSF within the sulci, failure of suppression of sulcal signal on FLAIR sequences suggests leptomeningeal disease with replacement of normal CSF by blood (subarachnoid hemorrhage), pus (meningitis), or tumor (leptomeningeal carcinomatosis). Because supplemental oxygen, especially at high concentrations, can artifactually create bright signal within the cisterns and sulci by reducing the T1 relaxation time of CSF, no diagnosis of cisternal abnormality on FLAIR images should be made before determining whether the patient was receiving oxygen during the MRI examination.

FLAIR imaging is also limited in evaluation of the posterior fossa because of CSF flow artifacts in the basilar cisterns and

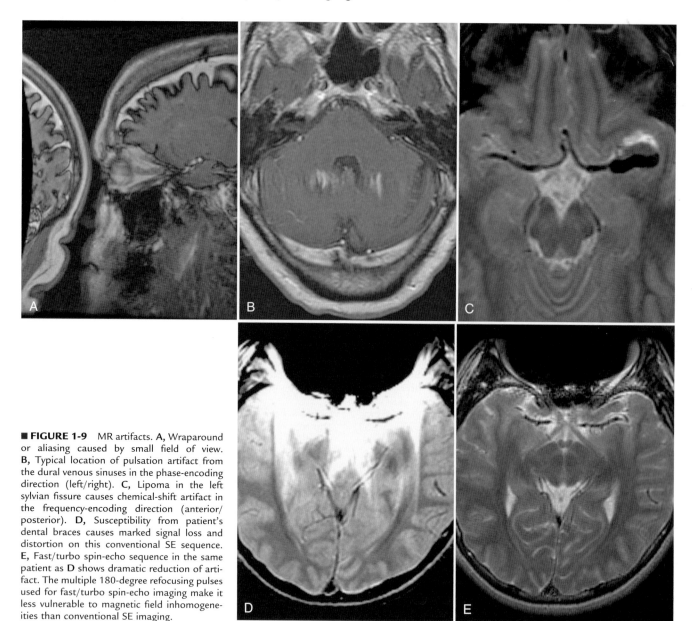

■ **FIGURE 1-9** MR artifacts. **A,** Wraparound or aliasing caused by small field of view. **B,** Typical location of pulsation artifact from the dural venous sinuses in the phase-encoding direction (left/right). **C,** Lipoma in the left sylvian fissure causes chemical-shift artifact in the frequency-encoding direction (anterior/posterior). **D,** Susceptibility from patient's dental braces causes marked signal loss and distortion on this conventional SE sequence. **E,** Fast/turbo spin-echo sequence in the same patient as **D** shows dramatic reduction of artifact. The multiple 180-degree refocusing pulses used for fast/turbo spin-echo imaging make it less vulnerable to magnetic field inhomogeneities than conventional SE imaging.

third/fourth ventricles. Unsuppressed CSF can flow into these narrow areas very rapidly, after the 180-degree inversion pulse but before signal sampling, creating bright FLAIR signal. 3D FLAIR is not as susceptible to CSF flow artifact as 2D FLAIR because the inversion pulse is applied to the entire volume imaged and not just a single slice. Figure 1-11 illustrates some important features of FLAIR.

Fat Saturation

Frequency-selective fat saturation (FS) is an alternative technique to STIR for eliminating signal from fat. FS exploits the chemical shift between protons in fat and those in water to reduce or remove the signal from the fat. In FS, a 90-degree saturation pulse specifically tuned to the Larmor frequency of fat is given to flip *only* the magnetization of fat into the transverse plane. This signal is then eliminated by a spoiler gradient. FS is clinically useful for diagnosing lipomas or dermoid cysts. Good FS requires that the main magnetic field be exactly uniform throughout. Field inconsistencies can make fat or water protons precess at slightly different frequencies from their Larmor frequency,

making the saturation pulse less effective (Fig. 1-12). Field inhomogeneities are especially pronounced along the periphery of the patient (farther from the isocenter of the magnet) and at air/tissue and bone/tissue interfaces, including the skull base and sinuses.

Diffusion-Weighted Imaging

DWI is a way to display the molecular motion or diffusion of water protons within tissue.[20] To achieve diffusion weighting, paired diffusion gradients of equal magnitude are added to an SE (T2W) echoplanar sequence. The first diffusion gradient is applied before the refocusing pulse, and the second gradient is applied after the refocusing pulse. If there is motion of water protons (diffusion is not restricted), the diffusion gradients cause *dynamic dephasing* of the moving nuclei that cannot be rephased, resulting in loss of MR signal that is proportional to the rate of water motion. This phenomenon is distinct from the static dephasing that can be rephased by the 180-degree refocusing pulse.

In the brain, diffusion of water varies in all directions (anisotropic) rather than occurring to the same degree in all directions

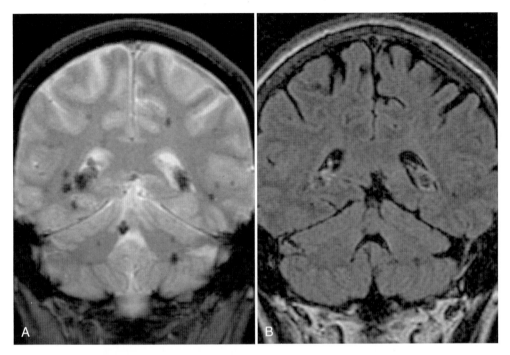

■ **FIGURE 1-10** Detecting hemorrhage with GRE sequences. **A,** Coronal refocused or coherent GRE (T2*W) shows numerous foci of susceptibility in this patient with familial multiple cavernous malformations. **B,** These lesions are much more difficult to appreciate on the coronal FLAIR, which is typically an FSE/TSE sequence and is less sensitive to hemorrhage because of multiple refocusing pulses.

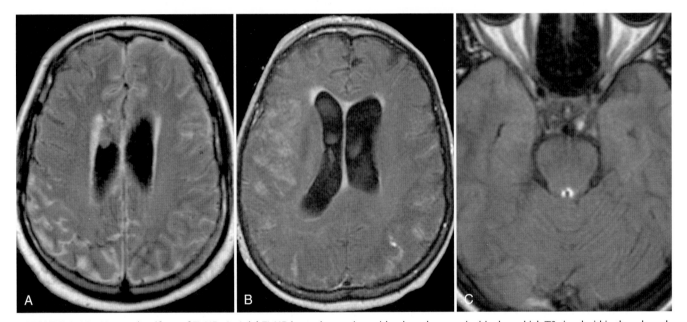

■ **FIGURE 1-11** Uses and artifacts of FLAIR. **A,** Axial FLAIR image in a patient with tuberculous meningitis shows high T2 signal within the subarachnoid space, particularly in the right parietal lobe, consistent with pus. **B,** Similar high T2 signal within the subarachnoid space is observed on axial FLAIR in this patient requiring general anesthesia for sedation, consistent with high flow oxygen artifact. This high FLAIR signal in the subarachnoid space will disappear within minutes after cessation of oxygen supplementation. **C,** High T2 signal around the cerebral aqueduct is typical of FLAIR artifact caused by incomplete CSF suppression.

(isotropic), because diffusion occurs more easily parallel to axon bundles rather than perpendicular to them. Because of anisotropy, diffusion is measured in multiple different orientations, for example, the x, y, and z gradient directions, and the results are combined into one "isotropic" image (Fig. 1-13).

MR signal intensity on DWI depends in part on the strength of the diffusion weighting, that is, the *b value*. When b = 0 s/mm^2, there is no diffusion weighting so the image displays only the effects of T2 weighting. As b is raised to 1000 s/mm^2, diffusion weighting increases and signal from CSF (which has unrestricted diffusion) decreases. However, T2 weighting does not

disappear entirely, even at high b values, so the T2 signal may still appear within the image *(T2 shine-through artifact)* and make it difficult to determine whether the bright signal seen on DWI represents restricted diffusion, T2 prolongation (T2 shine-through), or both in some proportion.

This difficulty is resolved by use of an *apparent diffusion coefficient* (ADC) map, which the computer derives mathematically by comparing the diffusion-weighted images obtained at two different b values (e.g., b = 0 s/mm^2 and b = 1000 s/mm^2). The ADC is a measure of the rate of diffusion, and the ADC map is a "pure diffusion map" free of T2 shine-through effects. On

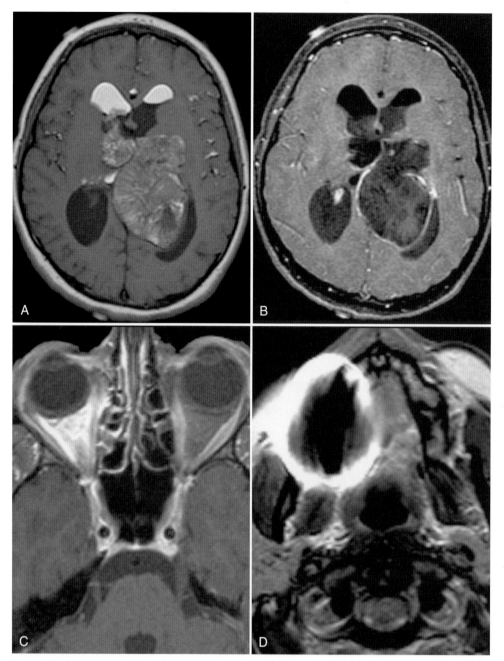

■ **FIGURE 1-12**   Uses and pitfalls of fat saturation. **A,** Axial unenhanced T1W image demonstrates a large lesion mostly in the region of the left lateral ventricle, with high signal layering nondependently in the frontal horns of both lateral ventricles as well as within the sulci bilaterally. The intrinsic T1 shortening is suspicious for fat-containing dermoid with rupture into the ventricular system and subarachnoid space. **B,** Loss of signal within the lesion, ventricles, and sulci after fat saturation confirms this diagnosis. **C,** Axial T1W post-gadolinium image with fat saturation demonstrates abnormal high signal within the right retrobulbar fat, which is of concern for enhancement. **D,** However, inspection of more caudal images shows there is extensive susceptibility from dental hardware. This creates magnetic field inhomogeneities, leading to failure of fat saturation in the right orbit that should not be mistaken for enhancement.

the ADC map, pixel intensity corresponds directly to the ADC value itself, so areas with high ADC (rapid diffusion) such as CSF will be bright, whereas areas with low ADC (slow diffusion) will be dark. Note that the signal intensities displayed on an ADC map are the inverse of what is seen on a diffusion-weighted image: areas of restricted diffusion will appear bright on DWI but dark on the ADC map.

Acute cerebral infarction (Fig. 1-14) is the most commonly encountered pathologic process to reduce diffusion (bright on DWI and dark on ADC), with MRI findings seen as early as 30

minutes after onset of ischemia.[21] Reduced diffusion can also be seen in pyogenic abscesses, epidermoid masses, herpes encephalitis, Creutzfeldt-Jakob disease, and tumors with high cellular density such as lymphoma. Limitations of DWI include susceptibility to field inhomogeneities, particularly at tissue/air interfaces, leading to signal dropout and image distortion near the skull base and posterior fossa.

An interesting application of DWI is *diffusion tensor imaging* (DTI), which assesses diffusion in at least six different directions. This yields a more complete set of diffusivity information that

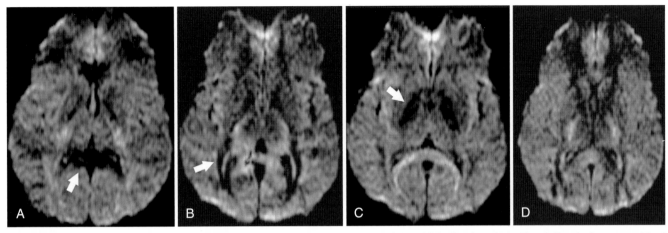

■ **FIGURE 1-13** The anisotropic nature of diffusion requires that diffusion be assessed in multiple directions (**A** to **C**) and then the images combined to yield an isotropic map (**D**). Signal loss is appreciated when diffusion occurs along the direction of the gradient. We can see that diffusion gradients were applied along the transverse (x, **A**), anterior/posterior (y, **B**) and craniocaudal (z, **C**) directions, as diffusion occurs along fibers of the splenium of the corpus callosum (*arrow*, **A**), frontoparietal white matter (*arrow*, **B**) and corticospinal tract (*arrow*, **C**).

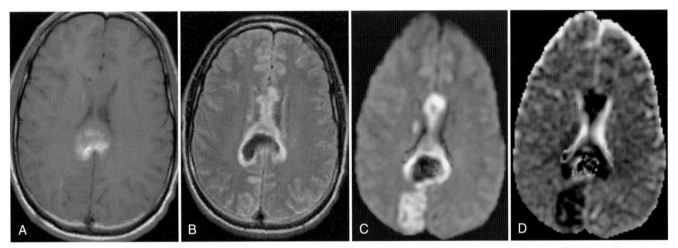

■ **FIGURE 1-14** **A,** Axial T1W SE image shows hyperintensity in the splenium of the corpus callosum, compatible with hemorrhage. **B,** Axial FLAIR image shows signal loss within the hemorrhage, as well as bright signal in the sulci posteriorly suggestive of subarachnoid hemorrhage. Increased signal is seen in the caudate body and along the body of the corpus callosum, with subtly increased signal in the right posteromedial parietal and occipital lobes. **C,** Axial DWI more dramatically demonstrates high signal in the right posterior parietal lobe, caudate body, and corpus callosum; this may reflect reduced diffusion due to acute infarction. DWI is prone to susceptibility effects, seen as signal loss within the hemorrhage. **D,** ADC map shows reduced diffusion in the right posterior cerebral artery territory and in the corpus callosum, consistent with acute infarction.

can be used to deduce axonal fiber orientation and thereby create 3D maps of white matter tracts in the brain.

Time of Flight MR Angiography

To visualize the intracranial vasculature, time of flight (TOF) imaging is most commonly used. TOF imaging provides an "MR angiogram" (MRA) of the circle of Willis by (1) minimizing signal from stationary background tissues and (2) maximizing signal from flowing blood.

GRE sequences with a rapid succession of RF pulses and very short TR are used. If the TR is shorter than the T1 of background tissue, the rapid RF pulses prevent the tissue spins from regaining their normal full longitudinal magnetization. Because the longitudinal magnetization is reduced to a minimum, the next RF pulse produces less transverse magnetization and the background tissue appears dark. In this state, the background tissue is described as *saturated*. Blood situated outside the imaging slice, however, is relatively unaffected by the successive RF pulses, retains its longitudinal magnetization, and remains *unsat-*

urated. When the unsaturated spins of the blood flow into the imaging plane with intact longitudinal magnetization, they generate a bright MR signal known as *flow-related enhancement*.

TOF MRA can be performed by both 2D and 3D techniques. 2D TOF MRA has higher sensitivity to slow blood flow than does 3D imaging, because 2D TOF imaging excites individual thin slices while 3D imaging excites entire slabs of tissue simultaneously. Because blood must travel a longer distance through a thicker slab with 3D imaging than with 2D imaging, the blood experiences some saturation effects from successive RF pulses and loses some signal. The signal loss is particularly pronounced for 3D imaging of slowly moving blood. For that reason, 3D TOF MRA may fail to display vessels with slow flow. However, 3D TOF MRA achieves thinner, contiguous imaging sections and much higher spatial resolution than does 2D TOF MRA. 3D TOF MRA is also less prone to signal loss from turbulent blood flow within an area of stenosis, so 3D TOF MRA is less likely to overestimate the severity of a stenosis. Cervical MRA for the carotid and vertebral arteries in the neck is typically performed with 2D

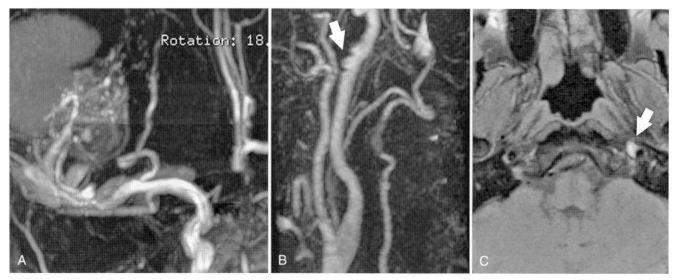

■ **FIGURE 1-15**   Intracranial and cervical MRA. **A,** 3-D TOF MRA of the circle of Willis shows a tangle of vessels with enlarged right middle cerebral and lenticulostriate artery branches, consistent with arteriovenous malformation and hemorrhage. **B,** Gadolinium-enhanced cervical MRA in a different patient shows focal lobular irregularity (*arrow*) of the left internal carotid artery (cervicopetrous junction), which is of concern for injury, such as dissection with pseudoaneurysm. **C,** Given the concern for dissection, axial unenhanced T1W fat-saturated sequence was obtained that shows crescentic high signal in the left internal carotid artery (*arrow*) consistent with methemoglobin in an intramural hematoma due to acute arterial dissection.

TOF because it is more sensitive for detecting slow flow within an area of stenosis. Intracranial MRA of the circle of Willis is typically performed with 3D TOF imaging because it provides better spatial resolution and depiction of small distal cerebral arteries (Fig. 1-15A).

Contrast-Enhanced MR Angiography

Contrast-enhanced MRA is often used for evaluation of cervical vessels (see Fig. 1-15B,C). A large coronal field of view can be employed to image the vessels from their origins at the aorta to their vascular territories within the brain in a fraction of the time required for conventional axial plane TOF MRA. Contrast-enhanced MRA also suffers less signal loss secondary to slow or turbulent flow.

Pitfalls and Limitations

Use of MRI is limited in several important situations. The magnetic field can induce voltages or currents in electrically conductive materials (wires, leads, implants), which may result in heating. Patients with medical implants or devices made of ferromagnetic materials, such as certain aneurysm clips, may be at risk of object displacement or heating. MRI should not be performed unless the specific type of implant or device can be documented to be MR compatible. Information regarding MR compatibility and safety testing of thousands of specific objects may be found online at www.MRIsafety.com. Cardiac pacemakers and defibrillators are considered a contraindication to MRI. Patients with such implants should be studied by MRI only after specific evaluation of risks and benefits and after consideration of alternative means of obtaining the data needed for care. Such studies should be performed only on a case-by-base basis and only if sufficient radiology and cardiology expertise is available.[22]

MRI can be performed at any stage of pregnancy, following thoughtful consideration of risks and benefits by appropriate attending radiologists, obstetricians, and perinatologists. Gadolinium-based contrast agents may be administered on a case-by-case basis but should *not* be given routinely in pregnancy, because their risks to the fetus are not known.[22,23] (Because gadolinium-based contrast agents can enter the amniotic fluid, there is theoretical potential for dissociation of the toxic gadolinium from its chelating compound and concern for fetal injury.) Again, any decision to administer a gadolinium-based contrast agent should be preceded by careful analysis of the risks and benefits by the team of attending physicians.

Much has been recently written about nephrogenic systemic fibrosis and its association with gadolinium-based contrast agents in patients with severe renal disease. Nephrogenic systemic fibrosis refers to tissue fibrosis with skin thickening and hardening, as well as fibrosis of other body parts, including the heart, lung, and skeletal muscles. It has been observed to occur after administration of a gadolinium-based contrast agent in 3% to 5% of patients with severe renal disease.[24,25] Although most published cases have been reported in patients who received gadodiamide (Omniscan, GE Healthcare), NSF has been associated with other gadolinium chelates such as gadopentetate dimeglumine (Magnevist, Bayer Schering) and gadoversetamide (OptiMARK, Mallinckrodt).[24] The most recent 2007 MR safety guidelines put forth by the American College of Radiology recommend that patients with chronic renal disease and glomerular filtration rates less than 60 mL/min/1.73 m^2 *not* receive a gadolinium-based contrast agent unless the benefits of contrast enhancement clearly exceed the risks. In those cases, the lowest possible dose necessary should be used and hemodialysis should be performed immediately after the scan (if the patient is already on dialysis). Patients with a glomerular filtration rate greater than 60 mL/min/1.73 m^2 need no special treatment, although gadodiamide should not be given to patients with any level of renal disease.[22,26]

Current Research and Future Direction

MRI at 1.5 T is the current clinical standard, although there has been an increasing shift to 3-T imaging for clinical use in the past few years. Systems at field strengths of 7 T and higher are now under investigation, although currently only used for research. The primary appeal of 3-T over 1.5-T imaging lies in its better signal-to-noise ratio. Field strength and MR signal are linearly related, with twice the MR signal at 3 T as 1.5 T for the same

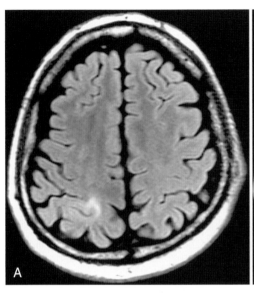
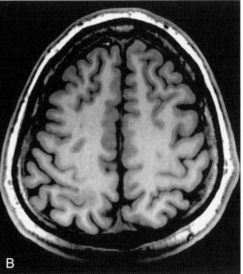

■ **FIGURE 1-16** Imaging at 3 T. A 29-year-old man with epilepsy was reported to have "abnormal FLAIR signal in the right parietal lobe" on prior outside MRI and presented for further workup. **A,** Imaging at 3 T demonstrates T2 prolongation in the right parietal lobe on axial FLAIR. **B,** Axial T1W spoiled GRE shows that the abnormal T2 signal corresponds to a focal area of cortical thickening and blurring. This is suggestive of a cortical dysplasia that, although subtle, can be better delineated at 3 T owing to its superior signal-to-noise ratio. The FLAIR and spoiled GRE sequences were 3D acquisitions to ensure thin, contiguous slices for detection of subtle abnormalities in this seizure patient.

scan time. Figure 1-16 illustrates the utility of imaging at higher field strength.

Higher field strengths prolong T1 recovery times but leave T2 relatively unaffected. This allows for higher-quality TOF MRA images at 3 T compared with 1.5 T, because the background is better suppressed at 3 T (less recovery of longitudinal magnetization) while inflowing, unsaturated blood has higher signal at 3 T (double the signal of 1.5 T). Longer T1 recovery times do result in poor tissue contrast between gray and white matter on T1-weighted SE or FSE/TSE sequences performed at 3 T if the same TR is used, but this can be avoided by using inversion-prepared sequences for T1 weighting. Higher field strengths also have greater chemical shift effects, allowing for more effective fat suppression but suffering from more chemical shift artifacts if a greater bandwidth is not used. Susceptibility effects increase with field strength, so sequence parameters must be optimized to decrease artifact. Figure 1-17 compares susceptibility effects at 3 T versus 7 T.

One of the chief concerns with high field imaging is the greater *specific absorption rate* (SAR), which is the energy absorbed by tissue after an RF pulse, potentially leading to tissue heating. SAR quadruples when field strength is doubled from 3 T to 1.5 T. SAR also increases with greater flip angles and more RF pulses during a given TR, so SAR is particularly high for FSE/TSE sequences where multiple 180-degree pulses are given. Modifications to limit SAR include decreasing the flip angle or refocusing pulse (although this also decreases MR signal). The synergistic and tandem development of *parallel imaging* techniques, which reduce scan time and limit energy exposure, has greatly facilitated imaging at 3 T.

In parallel imaging, k-space is undersampled by decreasing the number of phase-encoding steps. This reduces scan time. However, the resultant loss of spatial information is recovered by taking advantage of the redundant spatial information provided by the phased-array coils used for parallel imaging. Because signal strength varies according to distance from the receiver coil, spatial information afforded by differences in signal strength at the receiver coil can be used to complete the dataset for the MR image. Undersampling k-space reduces the FOV, which produces severe aliasing in the MR image. However, mathematical models have been developed to correct for aliasing and produce

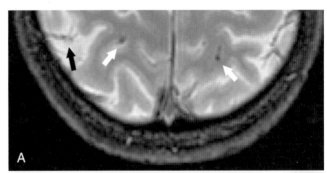
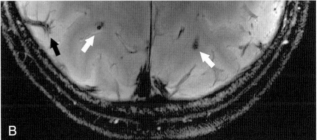

■ **FIGURE 1-17** Susceptibility effects at higher field strengths. **A,** A 3-T GRE sequence demonstrates two scattered foci of susceptibility near the gray-white junction (*white arrows*) compatible with hemorrhagic shear injury. **B,** A 7-T GRE sequence has markedly improved signal-to-noise ratio and more susceptibility artifact, better demonstrating shear injury (*white arrows*) as well as a deep venous anomaly that is difficult to appreciate at 3 T (*black arrow,* **A, B**).

a proper image; the two most commonly used techniques are sensitivity encoding (SENSE) and variants of the original simultaneous acquisition of spatial harmonics (SMASH) parallel imaging technique, such as generalized autocalibrating partially parallel acquisitions (GRAPPA).[27,28]

With these techniques, and newer developments to follow, MRI should remain the primary tool for neuroimaging for the foreseeable future. ●

SUGGESTED READINGS

Bitar R, Leung G, Perng R, et al. MR pulse sequences: what every radiologist wants to know but is afraid to ask. RadioGraphics 2006; 26:513-537.

Bushong S. Magnetic Resonance Imaging: Physical and Biological Principles, 3rd ed. St. Louis, Mosby, 2003.

DeLano MC, Fisher C. 3T MR imaging of the brain. Magn Reson Imaging Clin North Am 2006; 14:77-88.

Kalender WA. Computed Tomography: Fundamentals, System Technology, Image Quality, Applications, 2nd ed. Erlangen, Publicis Corporate Publishing, 2005.

Mitchell DG, Cohen MS. MRI Principles, 2nd ed. Philadelphia, WB Saunders, 2004.

REFERENCES

1. Kohl G. The evolution and state-of-the-art principles of multislice computed tomography. Proc Am Thorac Soc 2005; 2:470-476, 499-500.
2. Orrison WW, Gentry LR, Stimac GK, et al. Blinded comparison of cranial CT and MR in closed head injury evaluation. AJNR Am J Neuroradiol 1994; 15:351-356.
3. Gentry LR, Godersky JC, Thompson B, Dunn VD. Prospective comparative study of intermediate-field MR and CT in the evaluation of closed head trauma. AJR Am J Roentgenol 1988; 150:673-682.
4. Chappell ET, Moure FC, Good MC. Comparison of computed tomographic angiography with digital subtraction angiography in the diagnosis of cerebral aneurysms: a meta-analysis. Neurosurgery 2003; 52:624-631; discussion 630-631.
5. White PM, Wardlaw JM, Easton V. Can noninvasive imaging accurately depict intracranial aneurysms? A systematic review. Radiology 2000; 217:361-370.
6. Papke K, Kuhl CK, Fruth M, et al. Intracranial aneurysms: role of multidetector CT angiography in diagnosis and endovascular therapy planning. Radiology 2007; 244:532-540.
7. Barrett BJ, Parfrey PS, Vavasour HM, et al. Contrast nephropathy in patients with impaired renal function: high versus low osmolar media. Kidney Int 1992; 41:1274-1279.
8. Davidson CJ, Hlatky M, Morris KG, et al. Cardiovascular and renal toxicity of a nonionic radiographic contrast agent after cardiac catheterization: a prospective trial. Ann Intern Med 1989; 110:119-124.
9. Merten GJ, Burgess WP, Gray LV, et al. Prevention of contrast-induced nephropathy with sodium bicarbonate: a randomized controlled trial. JAMA 2004; 291:2328-2334.
10. Tepel M, van der Giet M, Schwarzfeld C, et al. Prevention of radiographic-contrast-agent-induced reductions in renal function by acetylcysteine. N Engl J Med 2000; 343:180-184.
11. Coakley FV, Panicek DM. Iodine allergy: an oyster without a pearl? AJR Am J Roentgenol 1997; 169:951-952.
12. McCollough CH, Schueler BA, Atwell TD, et al. Radiation exposure and pregnancy: when should we be concerned? RadioGraphics 2007; 27:909-917; discussion 917-918.
13. Ramchandren S, Cross BJ, Liebeskind DS. Emergent headaches during pregnancy: correlation between neurologic examination and neuroimaging. AJNR Am J Neuroradiol 2007; 28:1085-1087.
14. Bettmann MA. Frequently asked questions: iodinated contrast agents. RadioGraphics 2004;24(Suppl 1):S3-S10.
15. De Coene B, Hajnal JV, Gatehouse P, et al. MR of the brain using fluid-attenuated inversion recovery (FLAIR) pulse sequences. AJNR Am J Neuroradiol 1992; 13:1555-1564.
16. Feinberg DA, Hale JD, Watts JC, et al. Halving MR imaging time by conjugation: demonstration at 3.5 kG. Radiology 1986; 161:527-531.
17. Stehling MK, Turner R, Mansfield P. Echo-planar imaging: magnetic resonance imaging in a fraction of a second. Science 1991; 254:43-50.
18. Brant-Zawadzki M, Atkinson D, Detrick M, et al. Fluid-attenuated inversion recovery (FLAIR) for assessment of cerebral infarction: initial clinical experience in 50 patients. Stroke 1996; 27:1187-1191.
19. Hashemi RH, Bradley WG Jr, Chen DY, et al. Suspected multiple sclerosis: MR imaging with a thin-section fast FLAIR pulse sequence. Radiology 1995; 196:505-510.
20. Le Bihan D, Breton E, Lallemand D, et al. MR imaging of intravoxel incoherent motions: application to diffusion and perfusion in neurologic disorders. Radiology 1986; 161:401-407.
21. Warach S, Gaa J, Siewert B, et al. Acute human stroke studied by whole brain echo planar diffusion-weighted magnetic resonance imaging. Ann Neurol 1995; 37:231-241.
22. Kanal E, Barkovich AJ, Bell C, et al. ACR guidance document for safe MR practices: 2007. AJR Am J Roentgenol 2007; 188:1447-1474.
23. Webb JA, Thomsen HS, Morcos SK. The use of iodinated and gadolinium contrast media during pregnancy and lactation. Eur Radiol 2005; 15:1234-1240.
24. Kuo PH, Kanal E, Abu-Alfa AK, Cowper SE. Gadolinium-based MR contrast agents and nephrogenic systemic fibrosis. Radiology 2007; 242:647-649.
25. Sadowski EA, Bennett LK, Chan MR, et al. Nephrogenic systemic fibrosis: risk factors and incidence estimation. Radiology 2007; 243:148-157.
26. Thomsen HS. European Society of Urogenital Radiology guidelines on contrast media application. Curr Opin Urol 2007; 17:70-76.
27. Pruessmann KP, Weiger M, Scheidegger MB, Boesiger P. SENSE: sensitivity encoding for fast MRI. Magn Reson Med 1999; 42:952-962.
28. Sodickson DK, Manning WJ. Simultaneous acquisition of spatial harmonics (SMASH): fast imaging with radiofrequency coil arrays. Magn Reson Med 1997; 38:591-603.

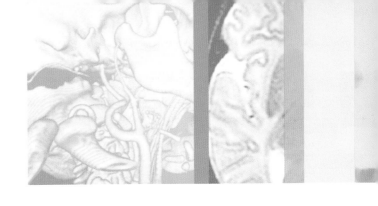

CHAPTER 2

Dynamic Functional and Physiological Techniques

Soonmee Cha

PHYSICAL PRINCIPLES

Diffusion-Weighted Imaging

Diffusion is defined as the process of random molecular thermal motion occurring at a microscopic scale. Diffusion of water in biologic systems, particularly within the brain, is affected not only by the complex interaction between the intracellular and extracellular compartments but also by the cytoarchitecture of the microstructures and permeability barriers. Diffusion of water molecules through the magnetic field gradient produces intravoxel dephasing and a loss of signal intensity. Because this microscopic diffusional motion is so small, a large gradient strength and/or duration is needed to produce observable signal loss from diffusion. By utilizing bipolar pulsed gradient methods, microscopic diffusional motion is detected by change in the magnitude of moving spins due to phase dispersion. To detect this highly sensitive motion, ultrafast imaging, such as the echoplanar imaging (EPI) technique, is needed to acquire a sufficient number of images in the range of milliseconds to produce meaningful information.[1]

The apparent diffusion coefficient (ADC) characterizes the rate of diffusional motion (given in millimeters squared per second). The ADC takes into consideration the heterogeneous environment of brain cytoarchitecture and factors other than diffusion, such as temperature, perfusion, and metabolic rates that can affect the measurement of microscopic thermal motion. High ADC implies relatively unrestricted water motion. Low ADC indicates restricted diffusional motion, as seen in acute cerebral ischemia. The diffusion sensitivity parameter, b value, is related to duration, strength, and time interval between the diffusion-sensitizing gradients. A typical b value used in clinical imaging is in the range of 900 to 1000 s/mm^2. The higher the b value, the more sensitive the diffusion imaging is for obtaining greater contrast and detecting areas of restricted water motion.[2]

Anisotropic diffusion is defined as having different diffusional motion in different directions, as is the case in normal myelinated white matter tracts in the brain. Diffusion of water mole-cules is far less restricted along the parallel plane of the axonal fibers than in perpendicular directions. White matter anisotropy can be demonstrated by comparing diffusion-weighted images with bipolar gradients placed in three orthogonal directions. By combining the information from the three orthogonal data sets, an orientation-independent image is created without the artifact from normal white matter anisotropy.[3]

EPI is currently the most widely used MRI technique for clinical application of diffusion-weighted imaging (DWI) for the diagnosis of acute stroke and other brain disorders such as abscess, epidermoid, traumatic shearing injury, or necrotic encephalitis. EPI is the fastest available MRI method. It allows the entire set of echoes needed to form an image to be collected within a single acquisition period of 25 to 100 ms.[4] The data are obtained by forming a train of gradient echoes by repeated reversal of a large gradient capable of very rapid polarity inversion to complete k-space filling after a single radiofrequency pulse. Each gradient echo is phase encoded separately by a very brief blipped gradient or a weak constant phase-encoding gradient. Although the long echo train renders the images sensitive to chemical shift and magnetic susceptibility artifacts, EPI virtually eliminates motion artifact. The chemical shift artifact is overcome by routine use of lipid suppression, whereas the magnetic susceptibility artifact is manifested prominently at air/bone/tissue interfaces such as those at the skull base, paranasal sinuses, orbits, and petrous temporal bone.[5-7]

Perfusion-Weighted MRI

Currently available perfusion-weighted imaging methods in clinical practice consist of arterial spin labeling (ASL), dynamic contrast-enhanced (DCE) MRI, and dynamic susceptibility-weighted contrast-enhanced (DSC) MRI. All three methods provide some type of a quantitative measurement of cerebral hemodynamic variables, such as cerebral blood flow (CBF), cerebral blood volume (CBV), and capillary permeability. Unlike DCE or DSC MRI, ASL is unique in that it does not require administration of exogenous contrast agent and uses tagged arterial blood spin as a source of endogenous contrast agent to measure CBF. A recent study has shown a promising role of ASL-derived CBF measurement as a complementary hemodynamic variable to more widely used DSC-derived CBV measurements in patients with glioblastoma multiforme.[8] DCE MRI proposes to quantify the steady-state exchange of MRI contrast agent, gadolinium (Gd-DTPA), between the intravascular and the interstitial tissue compartment and has emerged as a promising method for diagnosis and prognosis of glioblastoma multiforme.[9,10] K^{trans}, also known as a volume transfer constant, is the most widely used quantitative DCE MRI variable and reflects the rate of transfer of Gd-DTPA across the endothelial membrane. K^{trans} reflects the leakiness of tumor vasculature and has been used to grade gliomas.[11,12] Several recently published reports suggest that K^{trans} is capable of detecting the direct vascular effect of antiangiogenic therapy and thus is a promising candidate as a quantitative, clinically valid, endpoint for clinical trials.[13,14] Whereas DCE MRI measures Gd-DTPA in a steady-state, DSC MRI exploits the first-pass transit of Gd-DTPA within the intravascular compartment. Its most widely used hemodynamic variable, CBV, proposes to measure bulk vessel density.[15] DSC-derived CBV measurements have been extensively used to grade gliomas,[16,17] evaluate tumor vasculature,[18,19] differentiate recurrent tumor from treatment effect,[20] and assess prognosis of patients with glioma.[21] Other hemodynamic variables derived from DSC MRI such as the peak height and the percentage of signal recovery have shown their roles in further characterizing spatial heterogeneity of tumor vasculature[22] and in differentiating glioblastoma multiforme and single brain metastasis by virtue of fundamental difference in leakiness of tumor vessels between the two tumor types.[23]

Arterial Spin Labeling (ASL)

ASL is a noninvasive MRI method that provides quantitative measurements of CBF without the use of an exogenous contrast agent such as gadolinium. ASL images are based on differential sensitization of hydrogen spins to the effect of inflowing blood spins when the spins are in a different magnetic state to that of the static tissue. ASL images are acquired by magnetically labeling blood flowing into the slices of interest. Blood flowing into the imaging slice exchanges with tissue water, altering the tissue magnetization. A perfusion-weighted image can be generated by the subtraction of an image in which inflowing spins have been labeled from an image in which spin labeling has not been performed. Quantitative perfusion maps can be calculated if other parameters (such as tissue T1 and the efficiency of spin labeling) also are measured. The postprocessing of ASL image data typically involves several steps: subtraction of alternating tag and control image pairs, motion correction, segmentation of the anatomic T1-weighted (T1W) image, and voxel-wise computation of absolute CBF maps. The subtraction of magnetically "tagged" blood and control images (no tag) provides the perfusion-weighted signal intensity. Because the increase in signal intensity of label over control is on the order of only 1% to 2%, many repetitions of the control and label pairs are acquired during several minutes to provide the required signal to noise. The computation of absolute perfusion requires that the perfusion-weighted image be scaled by the mean signal intensity of the blood. This value is difficult to obtain, so the Mo (equilibrium) value of the white matter is used as a surrogate. A segmentation step is performed on the anatomic T1W images into gray and white matter, which is then applied to the Mo image from the perfusion data. The resulting absolute perfusion maps can be colorized with use of a standard scale.

Dynamic Contrast-Enhanced MRI (DCE MRI)

DCE MRI is a T1W, contrast-enhanced, gradient-echo imaging technique that can assess tumor perfusion, microvascular vessel wall permeability, and extravascular-extracellular volume fraction. It involves acquisition of serial images through the brain before, during, and after the injection of Gd-DTPA to evaluate the signal enhancement changes between intravascular and interstitial compartments. Either 2D or 3D gradient-echo sequences such as fast low angle shot (FLASH) or spoiled gradient-recalled at steady state (SPGR) techniques can be used for DCE MRI, but 3D volumetric methods provide better slice coverage with higher signal-to-noise ratio. DCE MRI exploits the equilibrium phase of Gd-DTPA in biologic tissues to maximize the evaluation of the Gd-DTPA extraction factors and compartmental equilibrium conditions. The signal intensity time curve of DCE MRI in the equilibrium method will rely on the local microvessel density, regional blood flow, microvessel permeability of Gd-DTPA, and size and physiochemical nature of the extracellular space accessible for Gd-DTPA.

Dynamic Susceptibility-Weighted MRI (DSC MRI)

DSC MRI is a fast, contrast-enhanced, EPI-based technique that exploits the first-pass effect of intravenous contrast agent within the intravascular compartment of the cerebrovascular system. When a paramagnetic agent such as Gd-DTPA passes through the cerebrovascular system, it produces T2* signal loss due to its local magnetic susceptibility. By exploiting the intravascular compartmentalization of Gd-DTPA and the resultant susceptibility effect, an indirect measure of bulk vessel density and hence CBV can be derived from the susceptibility signal intensity time curve. The passage of Gd-DTPA causes changes in both T2 and T2* so that both spin-echo and gradient-echo EPI sequences provide robust measurements of CBV. Gradient-echo sequences are, however, much more sensitive. When a paramagnetic contrast agent such as Gd-DTPA passes through the cerebrovascular system it induces differences in local magnetic susceptibility between vessels and the surrounding tissue. Although the vascular space is a small fraction of the total tissue blood volume (4%-5%), this compartmentalization of contrast agent causes targeted paramagnetism within the intravascular spins as well as the surrounding spins within a given voxel. Thus, both intravascular and extravascular spins experience a reduction of T2* that leads to a large transient signal loss of approximately 25% in normal white matter with a standard dose of contrast (0.1 mmol/kg). T2W spin-echo images are less sensitive and require double or even quadruple contrast agent doses to give substantial signal changes during the bolus passage. On the other hand, gradient-echo sequences are more prone to magnetic susceptibility artifacts. Asymmetric spin-echo EPI sequences provide a potentially useful compromise between gradient-echo and spin-echo EPI. In asymmetric spin-echo EPI sequences the echo center is displaced from the Hahn echo time, giving a mixture of T2 and T2* weighting. The degree of asymmetry can be adjusted to trade off sensitivity against susceptibility to artifacts.[20,21] Thus, when imaging lesions near brain/bone/air interfaces, such as the temporal or inferior frontal lobes where these artifacts are more pronounced, spin-echo sequences may be preferable. However, artifacts in gradient-echo images can be overcome to a large extent by reducing the slice thickness.[22] Although this reduces signal-to-noise ratio, we have found that this technique still provides diagnostic images. A second advantage of spin-echo sequences is that simulations and phantom experiments suggest spin-echo images will only be sensitive to contrast agent within the capillaries whereas gradient-echo sequences will be sensitive to contrast in both capillaries and larger vessels.[23] Although contamination by venous signals in gradient-echo images will potentially cause overestimates of CBV, it is relatively easy to identify the location of veins and make measurements of CBV in regions of interest that avoid them.

Proton MR Spectroscopy (MRS)

Magnetic resonance spectroscopy (MRS), the physical principle of which has been around since the 1940s, provides a measure of biochemical changes in the brain.[24] A small change in the Larmor resonance frequency of a nucleus (i.e., chemical shift) generated by circulating electrons surrounding the nuclei interacting with the main magnetic field can be measured and displayed as spectral format to detect alterations in chemical composition of brain.[25] The most common nuclei that are used are ^1H (proton), ^{23}Na (sodium), and ^{31}P (phosphorus). Proton spectroscopy (^1H MRS) is easier to perform and provides much higher signal-to-noise ratio than either sodium or phosphorus. For the scope of this textbook, only proton spectroscopy will be discussed.

^1H MRS can be performed within 10 to 15 minutes and can be added on to conventional MRI protocols. It can be used to serially monitor biochemical changes in tumors, stroke, epilepsy, metabolic disorders, infections, and neurodegenerative diseases. In the brain, several metabolites can be measured using ^1H MRS (Table 2-1). Each metabolite appears at a specific parts per million (ppm), and each reflects specific cellular and biochemical processes. In normal brain, different regions can have different chemical composition and hence variable amounts of each metabolite. Normal gray matter tends to have higher levels of choline than does white matter. N-acetyl-aspartate (NAA) is a neuronal marker and decreases with any process that compromises neuronal integrity. It can be markedly elevated in Canavan disease, a rare genetic leukodystrophy in which there is lack of an enzyme aspartoacylase, leading to abnormal accumulation of NAA. Choline is elevated in any disease that results in cellular membrane turnover, such as tumor or inflammatory process. Creatine reflects a measure of energetics in the brain. Lactate provides a measure of anaerobic metabolism and hypoxic condition. Lipid reflects an end product of tissue destruction and necrosis.[26] Myoinositol is considered to be an astrocyte marker and can be elevated in Alzheimer's disease.[27]

IMAGING

Parameters/Protocol

Table 2-2 lists the most widely accepted imaging parameters/protocol for DWI, three types of perfusion-weighted imaging, and proton MRS.

Several different types of DWI protocol can be used in clinical practice, but the most widely accepted and clinically used method is based on spin-echo EPI technique.

For the three different types of perfusion-weighted MR imaging, each requires specific imaging parameters, as listed in Table 2-2.

Proton MR spectroscopic (^1H MRS) imaging methods vary depending on the spatial coverage (single vs. multiple voxel), thickness (2D vs. 3D), and echo times (short, medium, and long) used.

Normal Appearance of Images by Technique

Diffusion-Weighted Imaging

In normal brain, there should not be any areas of reduced diffusion on DWI. The cerebrospinal fluid (CSF) within the ventricles has the lowest signal because the protons in CSF have the least restriction of motion, and normal white matter with highly organized axonal tracts such as the corpus callosum has the highest signal, as shown in Figure 2-1.

Perfusion-Weighted Imaging

Arterial Spin Labeling

In normal adult brain the cerebral blood flow to gray matter is approximately two to three times greater than that of white matter. In normal pediatric brain there is usually an increased signal-to-noise ratio as well as globally elevated absolute CBF when compared with adults. This globally increased signal intensity within normal pediatric brain has been attributed to higher baseline CBF, faster mean transit time, increased baseline magnetization values in gray and white matter, and increased T1 values in blood and tissue. ASL images of normal adult brain are shown in Figure 2-2.

Dynamic Contrast-Enhanced MRI

In normal brain with intact blood-brain barrier, the degree of leakage across the blood vessel is negligible. Therefore, DCE MRI of normal brain shows minimal enhancement, hence leakage of gadolinium contrast agent, whereas blood vessels are intensely enhancing. DCE images of normal adult brain are shown in Figure 2-3.

Dynamic Susceptibility-Weighted MRI

The normal appearance of DSC MRI through the brain resembles that of ASL images in that the gray matter, both superficial and deep, tends to have higher cerebral blood volume than does

TABLE 2-1. Proton MRS Metabolites

Parts Per Million	Metabolite	Biologic Correlate
0.9-1.4	Lipids	Tissue necrosis or destruction
1.3	Lactate	Anaerobic glycolysis
2.0	N-acetyl-aspartate (NAA)	Neuronal marker
2.2-2.4	Glutamine/GABA	Neurotransmitter
3.0	Creatine	Energy metabolism
3.2	Choline	Cell membrane turnover
3.5	Myoinositol	Glial/astrocyte marker

TABLE 2-2. MRI Parameters for 1.5-T Scanner

Name	Method	TR (ms)	TE (ms)	Slice Thickness/Skip (mm)	FOV (mm)	Matrix	NEX	Time (min)
DWI	SE EPI	8000	110 (b = 1000 s/mm²)	5/0	360	256	1	1.0
ASL	SE EPI	9.256	1.928	4/0	260	128	3	6.0
DCE	GE 3D vol	5.064	1.756 (flip θ = 10°)	3/0 (28 slices)	260	256 (12 phases)	1	6.0
DSC	GE EPI	1500	56	4/0	240	128	1	1.5
^1H MRS	Single voxel	1500	25, 144, 288	20	240	1	8	3
	2D multi-voxel	1100	25, 144, 288	20	240	18	1	6
	3D multi-voxel	1100	25, 144, 288	10	160	120 × 120 × 80 or 160 × 160 × 80	1	12-16

DWI, diffusion-weighted imaging; TR, repetition time; ASL, arterial spin labeling; TE, echo time; DCE, dynamic contrast-enhanced; b, diffusion sensitivity parameter; DSC, dynamic susceptibility-weighted contrast-enhanced; FOV, field of view; SE EPI, spin-echo/echoplanar imaging; NEX, number of acquisitions; GE 3D vol, gradient-echo 3D volumetric; GE EPI, gradient-echo/echoplanar imaging.

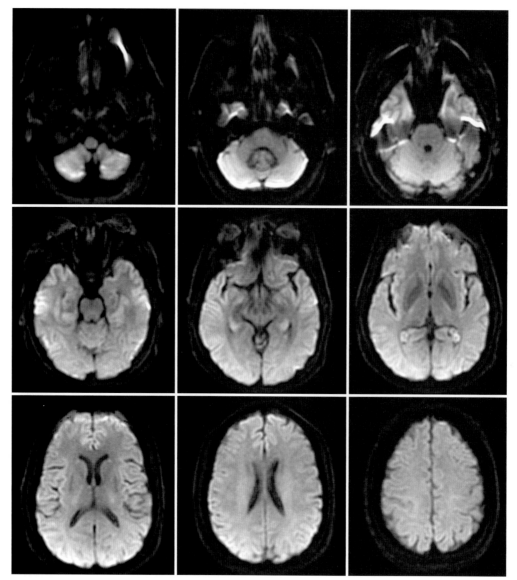

■ **FIGURE 2-1** Serial axial diffusion-weighted images through a normal brain show relative increase in water diffusion within the ventricle compared with the brain parenchyma.

white matter. DSC images of normal adult brain are shown in Figure 2-4.

Proton MR Spectroscopy
The spectroscopic appearance of normal brain can vary depending on the location where the spectroscopic information was obtained. For example, the deep gray matter and cerebellum tend to have higher levels of choline when compared with normal white matter. This may be, in part, related to higher metabolic demands in these regions, but the exact etiology remains unknown. Figure 2-5 shows single-voxel and 2D ^{1}H MRS images of normal brain. Figure 2-6 shows 3D multivoxel ^{1}H MRS images of normal brain.

Artifacts
The most common artifacts associated with DWI and perfusion-weighted MRI methods (ASL and DSC) are mostly related to the use of strong gradients and EPI technique.[28] On imaging, these artifacts are manifested as ghosting, distortion, and susceptibility artifact, especially in the presence of paramagnetic or ferromagnetic materials.[29] In the brain, blood products are the most common paramagnetic material that can cause mild to severe artifact on DWI and perfusion-weighted MRI. Ferromagnetic materials such as metals from surgery or trauma can often cause severe artifact and distortion. In addition, any ferromagnetic dental prosthesis can also cause impressive artifact and image distortion. Figures 2-7 and 2-8 illustrate examples of common artifacts associated with DWI and perfusion-weighted MR images, respectively.

The most common artifacts associated with ^{1}H MRS are related to technical factors such as shimming, degree of water suppression, partial volume averaging, and inclusion of unwanted peripheral fat (e.g., skull and scalp). Patient motion can also result in artifact.[30] Similar to DWI, the presence of susceptibility materials (e.g., blood products, metals) can lead to profound artifacts. Figure 2-9 illustrates lipid contamination artifact due to inclusion of bone marrow fat on 3D ^{1}H MRS.

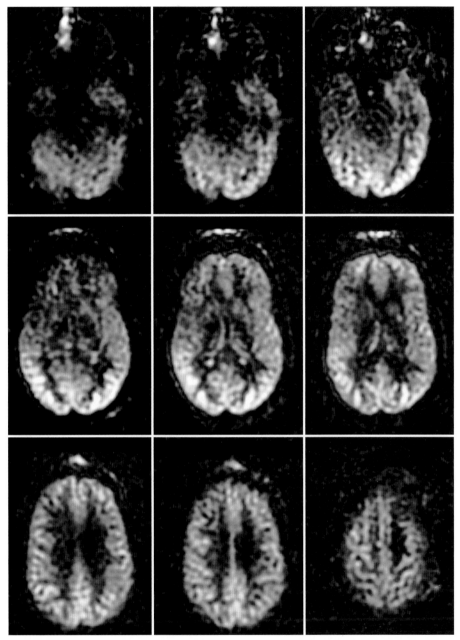

■ FIGURE 2-2 Serial axial arterial spin labeling images through a normal brain show greater cerebral blood flow to the gray matter compared with the white matter.

SPECIFIC USES
Diffusion-Weighted Imaging

DWI has made a great impact in the diagnosis and management of patients presenting with acute stroke. By its ability to detect acute ischemia within minutes of its onset, DWI can provide the location and extent of brain infarct and also suggest a possible source of the infarct. DWI is a fast imaging technique (usually acquired in less than 1 minute), which provides both qualitative and quantitative measure of relative water diffusion within the brain. The apparent diffusion coefficient (ADC) map, which provides the quantitative measure of water diffusion in biologic tissue, is calculated by acquiring two or more images with a different diffusion gradient duration and amplitude (b value, diffu-

sion sensitivity parameter). The contrast in the ADC map depends on the spatially distributed diffusion coefficient of the acquired tissues and does not contain T1 and T2* values. The increased sensitivity of DWI in detecting acute cerebral ischemia is thought to be the result of the water shift intracellularly restricting motion of water protons (cytotoxic edema), whereas the conventional T2-weighted (T2W) images show signal alteration mostly as a result of vasogenic edema. The reduced ADC value also could be the result of decreased temperature in the nonperfused tissues, loss of brain pulsations leading to a decrease in apparent proton motion, increased tissue osmolality associated with ischemia, or a combination of these factors. It is important

Text continued on page 33

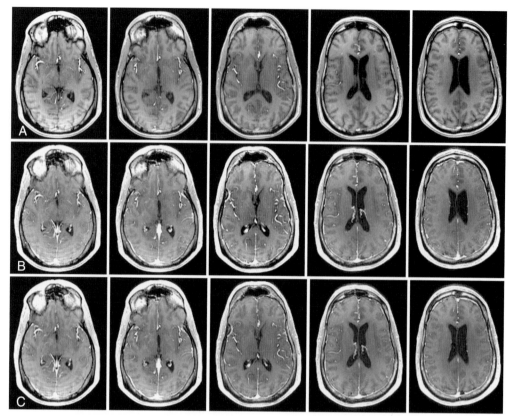

■ **FIGURE 2-3**   Serial axial images of dynamic contrast-enhanced MRI of a normal brain show prominent enhancement of the vessels. Because normal brain parenchyma has an intact blood-brain barrier there is no leakage of contrast agent, and hence, minimal contrast enhancement.

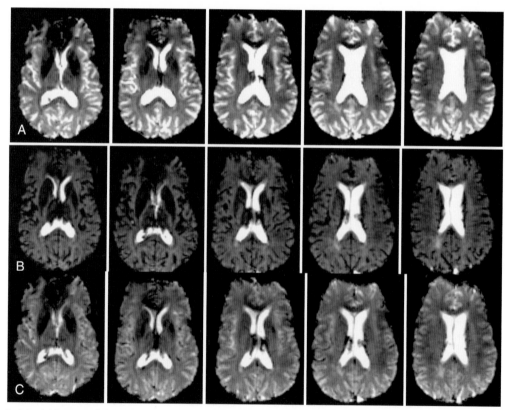

■ **FIGURE 2-4**   Serial axial images of dynamic susceptibility-weighted MRI through multiple levels before (**A**), during (**B**), and after (**C**) the bolus injection of intravenous contrast agent show T2* shortening within the vessels and choroid plexus and minimal changes within the normal brain parenchyma.

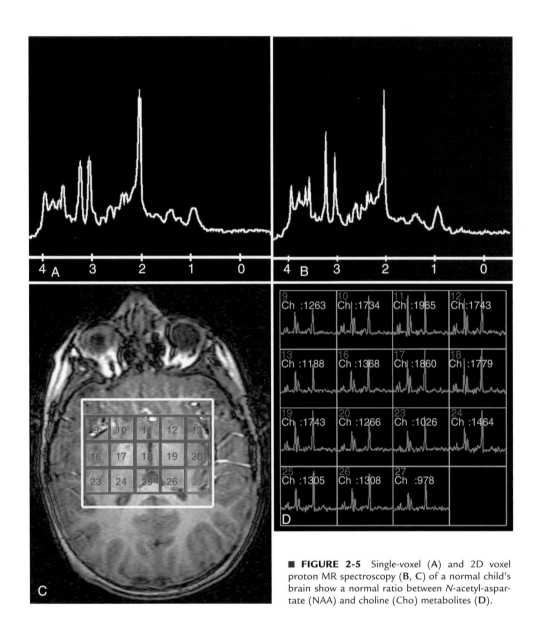

■ **FIGURE 2-5** Single-voxel (**A**) and 2D voxel proton MR spectroscopy (**B, C**) of a normal child's brain show a normal ratio between *N*-acetyl-aspartate (NAA) and choline (Cho) metabolites (**D**).

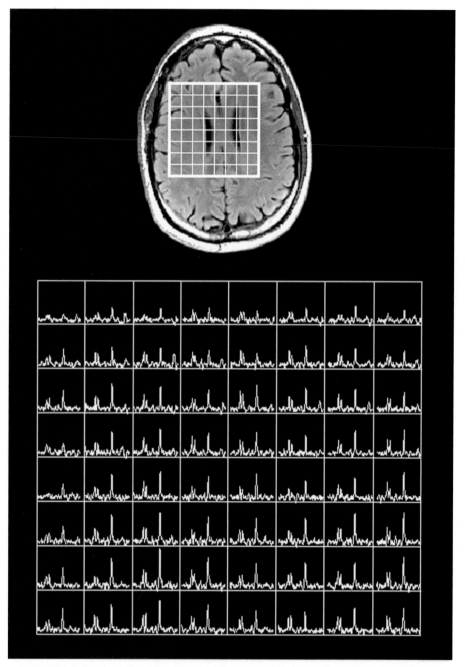

■ **FIGURE 2-6** Three-dimensional proton MR spectroscopic image shows normal metabolites.

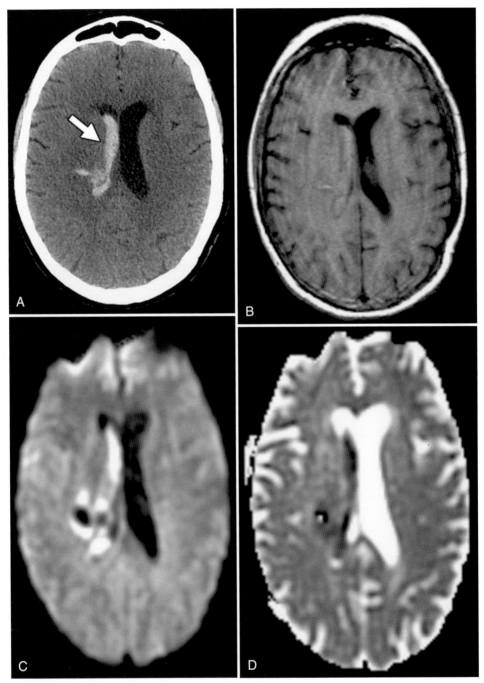

■ **FIGURE 2-7** Artifact on diffusion-weighted imaging. **A,** Noncontrast axial head CT shows blood within the right lateral ventricle (*arrow*). **B,** Axial T1W MR image confirms the presence of acute hemorrhage within the ventricle. Diffusion-weighted image (**C**) shows increased signal and ADC map (**D**) shows decreased signal corresponding to the intraventricular blood simulating a pathologically reduced diffusion.

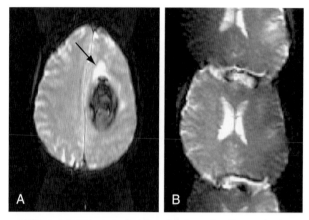

■ **FIGURE 2-8** Artifact on dynamic susceptibility-weighted images. **A,** A large left frontal melanoma brain metastasis (*arrow*) causes severe susceptibility artifact. **B,** A ghosting artifact is evident due to random phase variation.

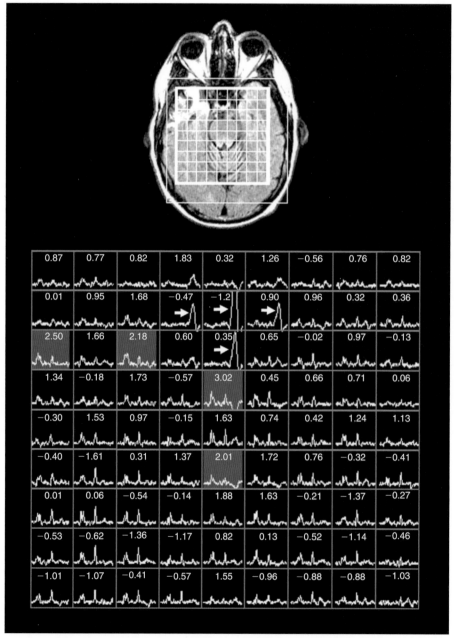

■ **FIGURE 2-9** Artifact on proton MR spectroscopy due to lipid contamination from the voxels (*arrows*) containing marrow fat of anterior clinoid bone.

TABLE 2-3. Brain Lesions with Abnormally Reduced Diffusion on DWI

Acute infarct
Toxic leukoencephalopathy
Axonal shearing injury
Herpes encephalitis
Epidermoid cyst
Pyogenic abscess
Postoperative injury
Increased tumor cellularity

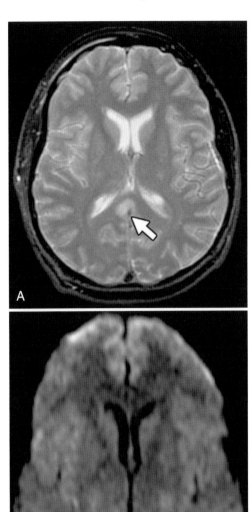

■ **FIGURE 2-11** Axonal shearing injury. **A,** Axial T2W image shows a subtle area of T2 prolongation within the right paramedian corpus callosum (*arrow*). **B,** Axial diffusion-weighted image more clearly demonstrates abnormal reduced diffusion within the callosal lesion (*arrow*).

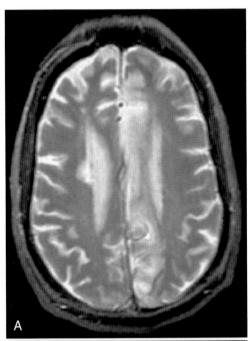

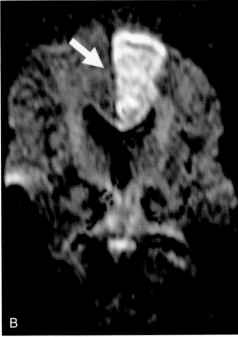

■ **FIGURE 2-10** Acute anterior cerebral artery infarct. **A,** Axial T2W image of the brain shows multiple areas of abnormal T2 prolongation. **B,** Coronal diffusion-weighted image shows clear evidence of acute infarct (*arrow*) in the anterior cerebral artery territory.

to emphasize that abnormally reduced diffusion is not unique to acute ischemia. As shown on Table 2-3, different types of brain disorders can result in abnormally reduced diffusion on DWI. Any process that involves alteration in water motion in the extracellular space of the brain can result in abnormally reduced diffusion. Examples of some of the disease entities listed in Table 2-3 are illustrated in Figures 2-10 to 2-16.

Perfusion-Weighted MRI

In clinical practice, perfusion-weighted imaging methods are used to assess, both qualitatively and quantitatively, the alterations in cerebral hemodynamics in diseased states, such as stroke, tumors, and inflammation. In acute stroke patients, DSC MRI has been used in conjunction with DWI to delineate areas

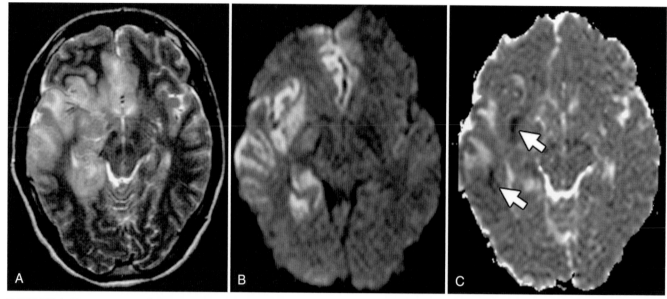

■ **FIGURE 2-12**   Herpes encephalitis. **A,** Axial T2W image shows diffuse T2 prolongation involving the right frontal and temporal lobes with cortical swelling and mass effect on the right midbrain. Axial diffusion-weighted image (**B**) and corresponding ADC map (**C**).

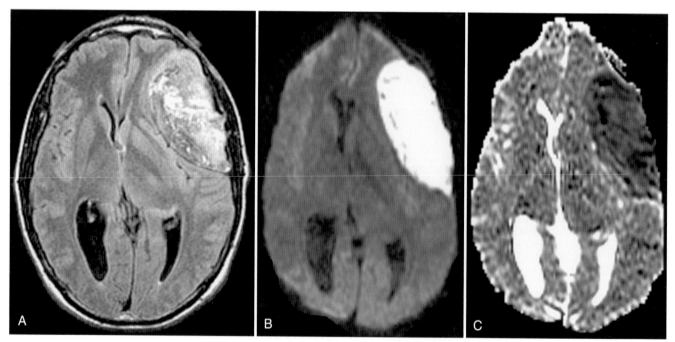

■ **FIGURE 2-13**   Epidermoid cyst. **A,** Axial FLAIR image shows a well-marginated extra-axial mass in the left frontal region. Axial diffusion-weighted image (**B**) and corresponding ADC map (**C**) show marked reduced diffusion associated with the mass.

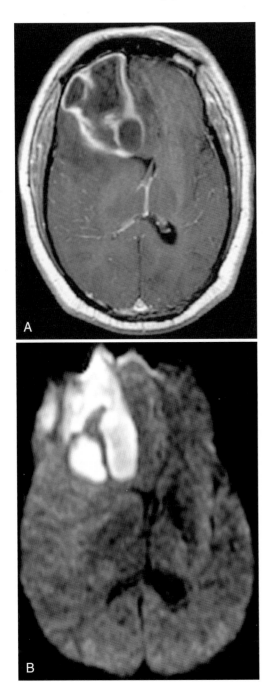

■ **FIGURE 2-14** Pyogenic abscess. **A,** Axial postcontrast T1W image shows a right frontal lobe mass with irregular rim and internal enhancement causing mass effect. **B,** Axial diffusion-weighted image shows marked reduced diffusion within the mass likely due to high viscosity of pus.

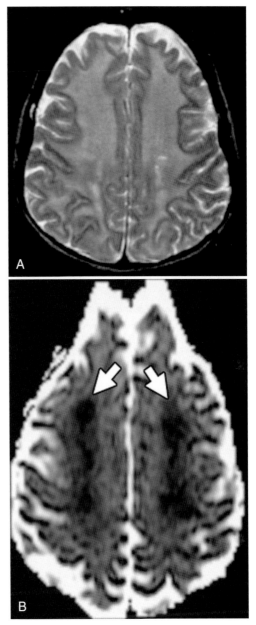

■ **FIGURE 2-15** Methotrexate necrotizing leukoencephalopathy. **A,** Axial T2W image shows bilateral confluent T2 prolongation within the cerebral white matter. **B,** ADC map through the same level shows marked reduced diffusion (*arrows*) within the areas of T2 prolongation.

of perfusion and diffusion mismatch, which in turn may predict ischemic penumbra. In brain tumors, the most commonly used perfusion MRI method is DSC MRI, owing to its short image acquisition time, ease of implementation, and vendor-supplied image postprocessing workstation for image interpretation. The relative cerebral blood volume (rCBV) map derived from DSC MRI has been used to grade astrocytoma and to differentiate low-grade oligodendroglioma and low-grade astrocytoma, recurrent glioma and treatment effect, brain tumor, and tumor-mimicking lesion.

DCE MRI is playing a bigger role in neuro-oncology because it is being used more commonly as the imaging test of choice to evaluate the efficacy of antiangiogenic drugs. Although the lack of standardization of imaging protocol and limited availability of postprocessing algorithms remain problematic, DCE MRI shows much promise in assessing tumor vasculature, especially in alterations in capillary permeability after antiangiogenic therapy.

ASL imaging offers the advantage over the other two perfusion MRI methods in that it does not require administration of gadolinium. However, ASL imaging requires more stringent hardware and software equipment, including a higher field magnet, which makes it more difficult to implement on standard clinical MR scanners. In addition, the image-processing algorithm for ASL is not widely available and requires physicists' expertise and support to derive any meaningful clinical information. ASL imaging has been used to depict blood flow abnormality

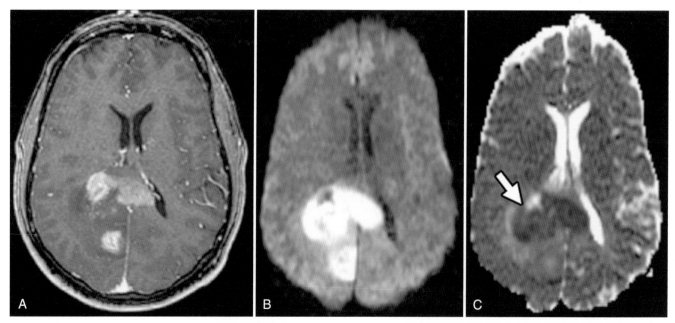

■ **FIGURE 2-16** Small cell glioblastoma multiforme. **A,** Axial postcontrast T1W image of the brain shows a heterogeneously enhancing corpus callosal and right medial parietal lobe mass. Axial diffusion-weighted image (**B**) and corresponding ADC map (**C**) show marked reduced diffusion within the mass (*arrow*) likely due to high cellular density within the mass.

TABLE 2-4. Brain Lesions with Abnormal Perfusion MRI

Disease	Perfusion MRI Findings
Acute infarct	Decreased rCBV and rCBF; increased MTT
Brain tumor	Increased rCBV and rCBF
Arteriovenous malformation	Increased rCBV, rCBF, MTT
Demyelinating lesion	Prominent venous enhancement within the lesion

rCBV, relative cerebral blood volume; rCBF, relative cerebral blood flow; MTT, mean transit time.

associated with brain tumors, vascular malformation, stroke, and other cerebrovascular diseases. As the availability and wider clinical application of 3-T MR scanners become more common, ASL imaging will be more widely used to evaluate intracranial diseases.

Examples of some of the disease entities listed in Table 2-4 are illustrated in Figures 2-17 to 2-19.

Proton MR Spectroscopy

Unique in its ability to detect metabolic changes within the brain, ^{1}H MRS is a powerful, noninvasive technique to assess a variety of intracranial disorders, including brain tumors, stroke, metabolic disease, and congenital disorders. Although the coverage of brain is limited in single-voxel ^{1}H MRS, this technique can provide unique and valuable information in certain clinical situations. For example, in pediatric patients with suspected ischemia, standard imaging, including DWI, may not show the abnormality, whereas single-voxel ^{1}H MRS may clearly demonstrate the presence of lactate within the brain parenchyma, which is indicative of hypoxic injury. In brain tumors, 2D or 3D ^{1}H MRS offers advantage over single-voxel ^{1}H MRS in terms of brain coverage. The 2D ^{1}H MRS can be done easily on any standard clinical magnet, but 3D ^{1}H MRS may require additional hardware. Similarly, the postprocessing of data is much simpler and can be done readily on an MR scanner for 2D but not 3D ^{1}H

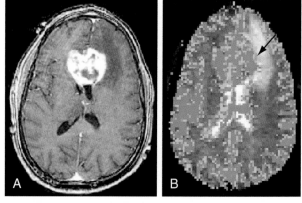

■ **FIGURE 2-17** Bifrontal glioblastoma multiforme. **A,** Axial postcontrast T1W image shows an avidly enhancing, centrally necrotic mass involving the corpus callosum and bifrontal lobes. **B,** Relative cerebral blood volume map shows markedly increased blood volume (*arrow*) associated with the mass.

MRS. For brain tumors, both 2D and 3D ^{1}H MRS can depict alterations in cellular metabolism and integrity of neuronal function. Elevation of choline indicates an abnormal increase in cell membrane turnover, and depression of NAA suggests either transient or permanent loss of neuronal integrity. Table 2-5 lists intracranial disease entities in which ^{1}H MRS can be useful in making the diagnosis. Figures 2-20 to 2-22 illustrate some examples of ^{1}H MRS abnormalities listed in Table 2-5.

PITFALLS AND LIMITATIONS
Diffusion-Weighted Imaging

The main pitfalls and limitations of DWI technique are related to the use of the strong gradient MR pulses that are necessary to encode the microscopic diffusional motion of water protons. First, the hardware used for the strong diffusion gradient can result in nonlinearity (which leads to distortion) and instability (which leads to ghost artifacts from random phase variations).

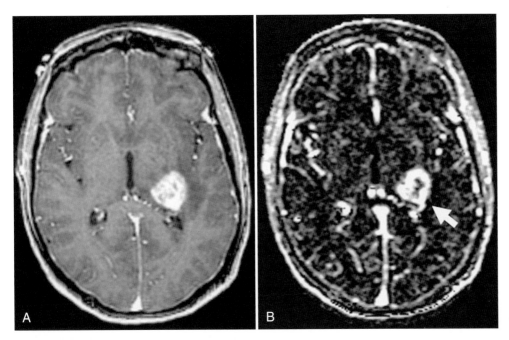

■ **FIGURE 2-18** Left thalamic glio-blastoma multiforme. **A,** Axial post-contrast T1W image shows an enhancing mass within the left posterior thalamus. **B,** Endothelial transfer constant (K^trans) map derived from DCE MRI shows highly leaky capillaries (*arrow*) associated with the mass.

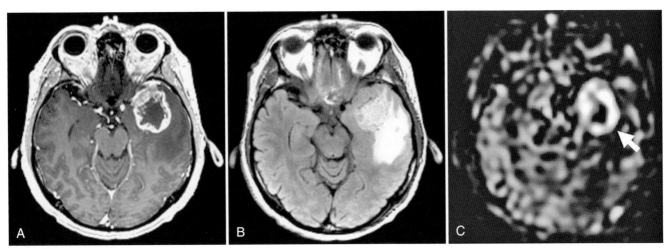

■ **FIGURE 2-19** Left temporal glioblastoma multiforme. **A,** Axial postcontrast T1W image shows an irregularly rim-enhancing, centrally necrotic mass within the left temporal lobe. **B,** Axial FLAIR image shows edema surrounding the enhancing mass. **C,** Axial cerebral blood flow map derived from arterial spin labeling shows marked increase in blood flow (*arrow*) within the peripheral aspect of the mass.

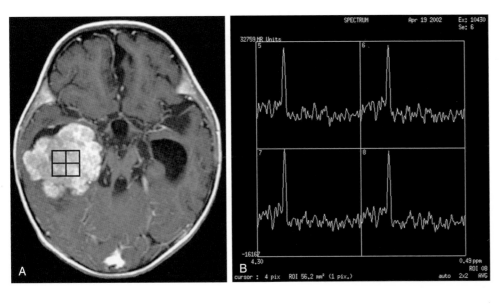

■ **FIGURE 2-20** Choroid plexus papilloma. **A,** Axial postcontrast T1W image shows an avidly enhancing intraventricular mass within the right temporal horn. **B,** 2D proton spectroscopy shows marked elevation of choline consistent with high membrane turnover.

TABLE 2-5. Brain Lesions with Abnormal ^{1}H MRS

Disease	^{1}H MRS Abnormality
Acute ischemia/infarct	Decreased NAA; presence of lipid and/or lactate
Brain tumor	Increased choline, decreased NAA
Malignant brain tumor	Lipid and/or lactate
Abscess	Increased acetate (1.92 ppm) and succinate (2.4 ppm)

NAA, *N*-acetyl-aspartate.

In addition, eddy currents, which can originate in any conductive part of the MRI scanner and scale upward with the strength of the gradient pulses, are induced when strong gradients are switched on and off rapidly. The artifacts related to eddy currents can appear as artifactual signal losses owing to an improper spin rephrasing or ghosting due to misalignment of the echoes in k-space. Although patient motion is a problem for all MRI, DWI is particularly sensitive to motion and can result in profound artifact manifested as ghosting and large signal variation across the image. Second, the EPI technique used in DWI can also result in eddy currents and the subsequent artifacts as well as artifacts related to chemical shift. EPI also requires a very homogeneous magnetic field, and magnetic interfaces result in local image distortion or signal dropout. The low bandwidth of EPI in the phase-encoding direction can cause severe shape distortion.[29]

Perfusion-Weighted MRI

The most common pitfalls associated with ASL and DSC perfusion-weighted MRI are related to the use of EPI techniques.[31] Similar to the pitfalls of DWI related to EPI, the perfusion images can be subject to ghosting artifacts, as shown in Figure 2-8B. In addition, any paramagnetic or ferromagnetic material will cause susceptibility artifact before the injection of gadolinium, thus limiting the application of these two perfusion MRI techniques in lesions with blood products, calcium, and melanin (see Fig. 2-8A) or near the skull or metallic material such as craniotomy screws or plates.

Proton MR Spectroscopy

The potential pitfalls and limitations of ^{1}H MRS revolve around both technical and practical issues relating to capturing metabolic information within the brain. Because of the bony skull that encases the brain, unwanted lipid contamination from calvarial fat can result in nondiagnostic spectral quality (see Fig. 2-9). Furthermore, because the spectroscopic interrogation volume is rectangular, the irregularly shaped brain lesions do not neatly fit into the spectroscopic volume of interest. Complete coverage of the lesion is often not possible and, in some instances, the critical areas of the abnormality may be completely missed. The absolute quantification of metabolite concentrations can be quite challenging and may not be feasible at all. For this reason, in most clinical practice, a ratio value of metabolites is often used to determine the degree of abnormality rather than the absolute measurement itself.

CURRENT RESEARCH AND FUTURE DIRECTION

Extensive research efforts are under way in numerous imaging laboratories around the world using the advanced MRI techniques that include DWI, perfusion-weighted imaging, and spectroscopic imaging techniques. Diffusion tensor imaging (DTI), which is a more extended version of DWI, is becoming one of the most highly researched imaging techniques to study the white matter integrity of neuronal connectivity of the brain. ASL techniques are becoming more widely used because there are more higher-field MR scanners available. DTI techniques are being used, both in the research arena as well as clinically, to evaluate neuronal connectivity and axonal integrity.

Perfusion-weighted MRI methods are being investigated as potential biomarkers of tumor vasculature and as endpoints for antiangiogenic therapy. In particular, the DCE MRI–derived parameter K^{trans} is being used as a marker of endothelial permeability and as a therapeutic endpoint for clinical trials involving anti–vascular endothelial growth factor agents. DSC MRI–derived parameters are being actively tested as potential surrogate markers of tumor vascularity and response to therapy.

MRS is being expanded beyond proton spectroscopy to include other nuclei, such as ^{13}C, ^{23}Na, and ^{31}P. Despite the challenges and technical limitations, the non-proton MRS methods are widely being investigated as research tools. It is anticipated that some of these non-proton MRS will be clinically applied to study the underlying chemical and metabolic derangements of brain disorders.

ANALYSIS

Diffusion-Weighted Imaging

The signal abnormalities on DWI must be interpreted along with the matching ADC map to determine whether a true reduced diffusion or a T2 shine-through effect is present. Because DWI is composed of both T2W spin-echo and diffusion-weighted sequences, any lesion that has high signal on T2W imaging can have apparent high signal on DWI, suggesting reduced diffusion. However, only when the ADC map shows a corresponding lesion to be of low signal is a true reduced diffusion present. In addition, true reduced diffusion is defined as ADC values less than or equal to 500×10^{-6} mm^2/s. In clinical practice, the most striking abnormalities on DWI are related to acute infarct. Reduced diffusion is not synonymous with acute infarct. Any process that leads to cytotoxic injury or reduced extracellular space or increase in viscosity can result in reduced diffusion. For example, herpes encephalitis is a viral encephalitis usually involving the temporal lobes and the limbic system heralded by aggressive tissue destruction that often leads to a fulminant hemorrhagic and necrotizing meningoencephalitis. On DWI, acute herpes encephalitis often shows marked reduced diffusion owing to frank tissue destruction and cellular swelling. A more benign entity can also have abnormally reduced diffusion. Epidermoid cyst of the brain is a benign, non-neoplastic lesion that typically shows marked reduced diffusion most likely due to an increase in viscosity of mucinous material. In highly cellular tumors such as lymphoma or medulloblastoma there is relative decrease in extracellular space due to increase in cell density.

Perfusion-Weighted MRI

Arterial Spin Labeling

Any intracranial process that involves alteration in CBF, such as acute stroke, vascular malformation, and brain tumor, demonstrates abnormality on ASL images. An example of increased CBF within a high-grade glioma is shown in Figure 2-17.

Dynamic Contrast-Enhanced MRI

Brain disorders that involve disruption or frank destruction of the blood-brain barrier will result in abnormal leakage of gadolinium on DCE MRI.[32,33] A highly vascular brain tumor whose tumor capillaries lack a blood-brain barrier shows avid contrast enhancement due to leakage of contrast agent, as shown in Figure 2-18.

Dynamic Susceptibility-Weighted MRI

In acute ischemia, there is often an increase in CBF and CBV, the so-called luxury perfusion, owing to recruitment of collateral

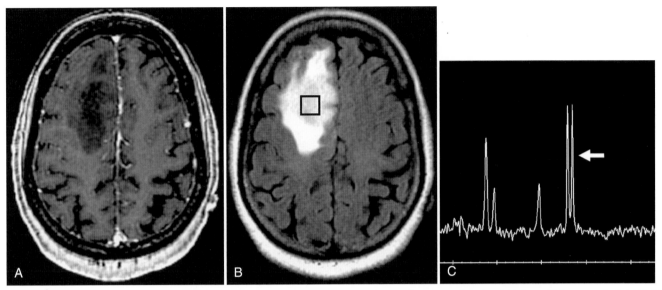

■ **FIGURE 2-21**   Right frontal anaplastic astrocytoma. **A,** Axial postcontrast T1W image shows nonenhancing right frontal lobe mass. **B,** Axial FLAIR image shows surrounding edema and a single-voxel spectroscopy laid over the mass. **C,** Single-voxel proton spectroscopy shows depression of NAA and marked elevation of lactate (*arrow*).

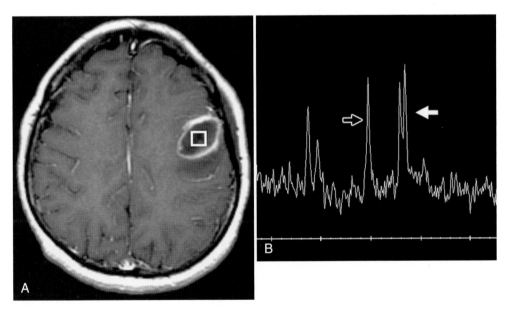

■ **FIGURE 2-22**   Left frontal pyogenic abscess. **A,** Axial postcontrast T1W image shows rim-enhancing left frontal lobe mass. **B,** Single-voxel proton spectroscopy shows elevation of lactate (*solid arrow*) and of acetate (*open arrow*).

vessels supplying the ischemic but viable tissues surrounding an infarcted core of brain. High-grade brain tumors with tumor angiogenesis tend to show prominent blood volume abnormality on DSC MRI,[34] as shown in Figure 2-21.

Proton MR Spectroscopy

^{1}H MRS can capture a variety of chemical and metabolic derangements associated with brain disorders. One of the most common uses of ^{1}H MRS is in brain tumor imaging to assess metabolic activity, degree of aggressiveness, and response to therapy. High-grade gliomas tend to have abnormal elevation of choline metabolite with depression of NAA as well as presence of lactate and/or lipid metabolites due to tumor hypoxia and necrosis. In pyogenic abscess of the brain, ^{1}H MRS can show acetate and lactate metabolites, as shown in Figure 2-22. In pediatric patients, ^{1}H MRS is often used to detect an abnormal presence of lactate in the setting of a metabolic or ischemic disorder.[35]

A sample report of a comprehensive MRI evaluation of the brain is presented in Box 2-1.

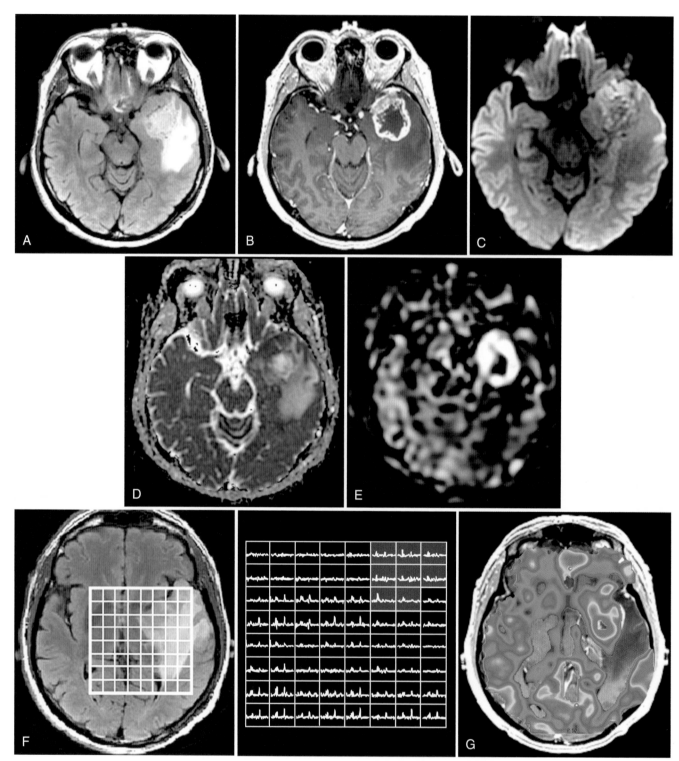

■ **FIGURE 2-23** Left temporal glioblastoma multiforme. **A,** Axial FLAIR image shows a large area of hyperintense signal abnormality within the left temporal lobe. **B,** Axial postcontrast T1W image reveals an irregularly rim-enhancing left temporal mass. Diffusion-weighted image (**C**) and the corresponding ADC map (**D**) demonstrate no evidence of reduced diffusion within the mass or the surrounding edema. **E,** Cerebral blood flow map derived from arterial spin labeling shows marked increase in blood flow within the peripheral aspect of the mass. **F,** 3D proton spectroscopic image shows elevation of choline and depression of *N*-acetyl-aspartate metabolites (*red shaded voxels*) within the FLAIR abnormality suggestive of tumor metabolism. **G,** Relative cerebral blood volume map derived from dynamic susceptibility-weighted imaging overlaid onto the corresponding axial post-contrast T1W image shows elevation of blood volume within the mass consistent with a hypervascular tumor.

BOX 2-1 Sample Report: MRI of Brain

PATIENT HISTORY

A 57-year-old man presented with progressive headache and witnessed seizure 1 week previously.

TECHNIQUE

MRI of the brain was obtained using the following MR sequences: 3-plane localizer, sagittal fast spoiled-gradient-recalled images, axial diffusion-weighted images, axial fluid-attenuated inversion recovery (FLAIR) images, axial fast spin-echo T2W images, axial ASL images, DCE images (before, during, and after the injection of Gd-DTPA [0.1 mmol/kg]), axial postcontrast spoiled-gradient-recalled images, DSC images (before, during, and after the injection of Gd-DTPA [0.1 mmol/kg]), and 3D proton MRS images.

FINDINGS

There is a large area of FLAIR abnormality within the left temporal lobe (Fig. 2-23A). Postcontrast T1W image (see Fig. 2-23B) shows an irregularly rim-enhancing intra-axial mass within the left temporal lobe measuring approximately $3 \times 3 \times 4$ cm (AP, TR, CC). The mass is surrounded by a large area of hyperintense signal abnormality on FLAIR images consistent with edema. DWI (see Fig. 2-23C) and the corresponding APC map (see Fig. 2-23D) do not demonstrate any evidence of abnormal reduced diffusion within the mass or the surrounding edema. The CBF map (see Fig. 2-23E) derived from ASL imaging shows marked increase in blood flow within the peripheral aspect of the mass. 3D proton MRS image (see Fig. 2-23F) demonstrates elevation of choline and depression of NAA metabolites within the FLAIR abnormality consistent with tumor metabolism. Relative CBV map derived from DSC image overlaid on postcontrast T1W image (see Fig. 2-23G) shows abnormal increase in CBV associated with the mass that is consistent with a hypervascular mass.

The remainder of the brain demonstrates no evidence of additional mass or signal abnormality. The ventricles and sulci are otherwise normal for the patient's stated age. Visualized portions of the orbits, paranasal sinuses, and skull base are normal. There is normal flow-void signal within the intracranial vasculature.

IMPRESSION

The overall MRI findings are most consistent with a primary high-grade glioma within the left temporal lobe associated with surrounding edema and mild mass effect.

SUGGESTED READINGS

Castillo M, Kwock L, Mukherji SK. Clinical applications of proton MR spectroscopy. AJNR Am J Neuroradiol 1996; 17:1-15.

Cha S, Knopp EA, Johnson G, et al. Intracranial mass lesions: dynamic contrast-enhanced susceptibility-weighted echo-planar perfusion MR imaging. Radiology 2002; 223:11-29.

Golay X, Petersen ET. Arterial spin labeling: benefits and pitfalls of high magnetic field. Neuroimaging Clin North Am 2006; 16:259-268.

Le Bihan D, Poupon C, Amadon A, Lethimonnier F. Artifacts and pitfalls in diffusion MRI. J Magn Reson Imaging 2006; 24:478-488.

O'Connor JP, Jackson A, Parker GJ, Jayson GC. DCE-MRI biomarkers in the clinical evaluation of antiangiogenic and vascular disrupting agents. Br J Cancer 2007; 96:189-195.

Schaefer PW, Grant PE, Gonzalez RG. Diffusion-weighted MR imaging of the brain. Radiology 2000; 217:331-345.

Taylor JS, Tofts PS, Port R, et al. MR imaging of tumor microcirculation: promise for the new millennium. J Magn Reson Imaging 1999; 10:903-907.

REFERENCES

1. Le Bihan D. Molecular diffusion nuclear magnetic resonance imaging. Magn Reson Q 1991; 7:1-30.
2. Sener RN. Diffusion MRI: apparent diffusion coefficient (ADC) values in the normal brain and a classification of brain disorders based on ADC values. Comput Med Imaging Graph 2001; 25:299-326.
3. Frank LR. Anisotropy in high angular resolution diffusion-weighted MRI. Magn Reson Med 2001; 45:935-939.
4. Edelman RR, Wielopolski P, Schmitt F. Echo-planar MR imaging. Radiology 1994; 192:600-612.
5. Castillo M, Mukherji SK. Diffusion-weighted imaging in the evaluation of intracranial lesions. Semin Ultrasound CT MR 2000; 21:405-416.
6. Schaefer PW, Grant PE, Gonzalez RG. Diffusion-weighted MR imaging of the brain. Radiology 2000; 217:331-345.
7. Holodny AI, Ollenschlager M. Diffusion imaging in brain tumors. Neuroimaging Clin North Am 2002; 12:107-124.
8. Warmuth C, Gunther M, Zimmer C. Quantification of blood flow in brain tumors: comparison of arterial spin labeling and dynamic susceptibility-weighted contrast-enhanced MR imaging. Radiology 2003; 228:523-532.
9. Roberts C, Issa B, Stone A, et al. Comparative study into the robustness of compartmental modeling and model-free analysis in DCE-MRI studies. J Magn Reson Imaging 2006; 23:554-563.
10. Strecker R, Scheffler K, Buchert M, et al. DCE-MRI in clinical trials: data acquisition techniques and analysis methods. Int J Clin Pharmacol Ther 2003; 41:603-605.
11. Cha S, Yang L, Johnson G, et al. Comparison of microvascular permeability measurements, K(trans), determined with conventional steady-state T1-weighted and first-pass T2*-weighted MR imaging methods in gliomas and meningiomas. AJNR Am J Neuroradiol 2006; 27:409-417.
12. Roberts HC, Roberts TP, Bollen AW, et al. Correlation of microvascular permeability derived from dynamic contrast-enhanced MR imaging with histologic grade and tumor labeling index: a study in human brain tumors. Acad Radiol 2001; 8:384-391.
13. Batchelor TT, Sorensen AG, di Tomaso E, et al. AZD2171, a pan-VEGF receptor tyrosine kinase inhibitor, normalizes tumor vasculature and alleviates edema in glioblastoma patients. Cancer Cell 2007; 11:83-95.
14. Gossmann A, Helbich TH, Kuriyama N, et al. Dynamic contrast-enhanced magnetic resonance imaging as a surrogate marker of tumor response to anti-angiogenic therapy in a xenograft model of glioblastoma multiforme. J Magn Reson Imaging 2002; 15:233-240.
15. Rosen BR, Belliveau JW, Vevea JM, Brady TJ. Perfusion imaging with NMR contrast agents. Magn Res Med 1990; 14:249-265.
16. Aronen HJ, Gazit IE, Louis DN, et al. Cerebral blood volume maps of gliomas: comparison with tumor grade and histologic findings. Radiology 1994; 191:41-51.
17. Knopp EA, Cha S, Johnson G, et al. Glial neoplasms: dynamic contrast-enhanced T2*-weighted MR imaging. Radiology 1999; 211:791-798.
18. Cha S, Johnson G, Wadghiri YZ, et al. Dynamic, contrast-enhanced perfusion MRI in mouse gliomas: Correlation with histopathology. Magn Reson Med 2003; 49:848-855.
19. Sugahara T, Korogi Y, Kochi M, et al. Correlation of MR imaging-determined cerebral blood volume maps with histologic and angiographic determination of vascularity of gliomas. AJR Am J Roentgenol 1998; 171:1479-1486.

20. Fuss M, Wenz F, Essig M, et al. Tumor angiogenesis of low-grade astrocytomas measured by dynamic susceptibility contrast-enhanced MRI (DSC-MRI) is predictive of local tumor control after radiation therapy. Int J Radiat Oncol Biol Phys 2001; 51:478-482.

21. Law M, Young R, Babb J, et al. Comparing perfusion metrics obtained from a single compartment versus pharmacokinetic modeling methods using dynamic susceptibility contrast-enhanced perfusion MR imaging with glioma grade. AJNR Am J Neuroradiol 2006; 27:1975-1982.

22. Lupo JM, Cha S, Chang SM, Nelson SJ. Dynamic susceptibility-weighted perfusion imaging of high-grade gliomas: characterization of spatial heterogeneity. AJNR Am J Neuroradiol 2005; 26:1446-1454.

23. Cha S, Lupo JM, Chen MH, et al. Differentiation of glioblastoma multiforme and single brain metastasis by peak height and percentage of signal intensity recovery derived from dynamic susceptibility-weighted contrast-enhanced perfusion MR imaging. AJNR Am J Neuroradiol 2007; 28:1078-1084.

24. Purcell EM, Torrey HC, Pound RV. Resonance absorption by nuclear magnetic moments in a solid. Phys Rev 1946; 69:37-38.

25. Proctor WG, Yu FC. The dependence of nuclear magnetic resonance frequency upon chemical shift. Physiol Rev 1950; 70:717.

26. Miller BL. A review of chemical issues in 1H NMR spectroscopy: N-acetyl-L-aspartate, creatine and choline. NMR Biomed 1991; 4:47-52.

27. Miller BL, Moats RA, Shonk T, et al. Alzheimer disease: depiction of increased cerebral myo-inositol with proton MR spectroscopy. Radiology 1993; 187:433-437.

28. Bitzer M, Klose U, Nagele T, et al. Echoplanar perfusion imaging with high spatial and temporal resolution: methodology and clinical aspects. Eur Radiol 1999; 9:221-229.

29. Le Bihan D, Poupon C, Amadon A, Lethimonnier F. Artifacts and pitfalls in diffusion MRI. J Magn Reson Imaging 2006; 24:478-488.

30. Young IR, Cox IJ, Coutts GA, Bydder GM. Some considerations concerning susceptibility, longitudinal relaxation time constants and motion artifacts in in vivo human spectroscopy. NMR Biomed 1989; 2:329-339.

31. Golay X, Petersen ET. Arterial spin labeling: benefits and pitfalls of high magnetic field. Neuroimaging Clin North Am 2006; 16:259-268.

32. Taylor JS, Tofts PS, Port R, et al. MR imaging of tumor microcirculation: promise for the new millennium. J Magn Reson Imaging 1999; 10:903-907.

33. O'Connor JP, Jackson A, Parker GJ, Jayson GC. DCE-MRI biomarkers in the clinical evaluation of antiangiogenic and vascular disrupting agents. Br J Cancer 2007; 96:189-195.

34. Cha S, Knopp EA, Johnson G, et al. Intracranial mass lesions: dynamic contrast-enhanced susceptibility-weighted echo-planar perfusion MR imaging. Radiology 2002; 223:11-29.

35. Castillo M, Kwock L, Mukherji SK. Clinical applications of proton MR spectroscopy. AJNR Am J Neuroradiol 1996; 17:1-15.

Image and Pattern Analysis

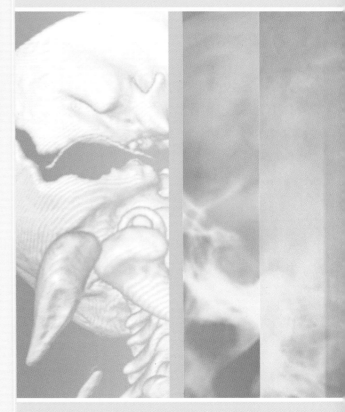

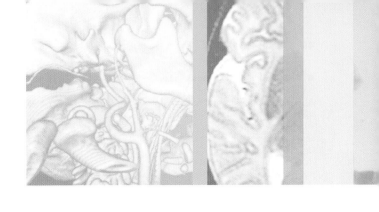

CHAPTER 3

Analysis of Density, Signal Intensity, and Echogenicity

Christopher Paul Hess and Derk D. Purcell

RADIOGRAPHIC/CT DENSITY
Standard Against Which to Measure Density

Conventional radiography and computed tomography are based on the differential attenuation of photons by tissues as they pass from an x-ray source on one side of the body to a detector on the opposite side. Mathematically, the measurement at the detector is determined by the sum of the values of the *linear attenuation coefficient*, μ, of each individual tissue along the course of the x-ray beam. At each point within an object, μ characterizes the rate at which x-rays are removed by scatter or absorption and thus reflects the biophysical interaction between photons emitted by the x-ray source and the tissue irradiated. For the relatively high photon energies used in diagnostic medical imaging and low atomic numbers of most organic matter, the primary determinant of μ is Compton scatter, which results in a magnitude of photon attenuation that is nearly linearly proportional to tissue density (mass per unit volume).[1] There are several additional contributors to x-ray attenuation that depend both on the x-ray source and the object being imaged, but in practice the primary basis of contrast in both radiography and CT can be considered to be tissue density.[2,3]

Planar projections of linear attenuation, the source of the imaging data depicted on plain films, reliably resolve only five different biologic densities: *air, fat, water, soft tissue,* and *bone.* Before the advent of tomographic imaging modalities such as CT and MRI, neuroradiologists went to great lengths to manipulate contrast in plain film radiography to make diagnoses, for example by purposefully introducing air or iodinated media into the subarachnoid space or blood vessels and thereby identify masses in the skull vault, spinal disc herniations, and intracranial aneurysms. Although important diagnoses can still be made from radiographic density abnormalities (Fig. 3-1), conventional radiographs have only limited application in modern neuroimaging and are commonly used at present for the gross evaluation of integrity of medical devices such as cerebrospinal fluid (CSF) shunts or spinal fusion hardware or in the detection of fractures or malalignment of the skull or spinal column.

Linear attenuation is a useful physical concept for understanding image formation in radiography and CT but is not directly applicable to the visual interpretation of images. Before display and storage, each pixel in a reconstructed CT image is normalized to an integer value termed the *Hounsfield unit* (HU) or *CT number.* This normalized attenuation scale arbitrarily assigns water an attenuation value of zero, such that a difference of 10 HU reflects approximately a 1% difference in linear attenuation. The maximum and minimum values of the Hounsfield scale depend on the numerical storage scheme of the manufacturer, but the range in attenuation that can be discriminated by most modern scanners is 4096 HU (from roughly −1000 HU to 3000 HU). Small numbers correspond to relatively radiolucent structures such as air and fat, and large numbers correspond to radiodense structures such as bone and calcium. There is considerable overlap between CT numbers for different tissues, but certain tissue densities can usually be distinguished based on their typical Hounsfield numbers (Table 3-1).

The dynamic range of the human visual system, which can reliably discriminate fewer than 100 shades of gray, is far less than the range in tissue density represented by the Hounsfield scale. To facilitate visual analysis of images on a digital workstation, different display windows are applied to the raw CT numbers to optimally visualize the different tissues of interest. The effect of windowing is to linearly map a subsegment of the Hounsfield scale to 256 shades of gray, a standard range of gray values between black and white depicted on a computer monitor. The central Hounsfield unit of the window is designated the *window level.* The *window width* determines the overall contrast of the displayed image, translating the values of the standard Hounsfield scale within the window to various shades of gray that are more easily interpreted by the human eye. Typical window parameters used to evaluate different tissues of interest are given in Table 3-2.

The recognition of abnormal density on CT images relies foremost on familiarity with the range of normal densities of the anatomic structures of the central nervous system (CNS) and its supporting structures. Brain regions where neuronal cell bodies are located comprise the gray matter of the cortex and deep gray nuclei, including the basal ganglia and thalami. These structures normally have CT numbers of 20 to 40 HU, which is slightly greater than those of white matter (20-35 HU), where the neuronal axons and their supporting glia are concentrated. As a consequence, optimal examination of the brain parenchyma requires a narrow display window that allows accurate discrimination between the densities of these two types of tissues. Any interruption of the normally homogenous density within a

45

■ **FIGURE 3-1** Diagnosis based on abnormal radiographic density. **A,** Facial trauma. Frontal radiograph of the face (Waters view) demonstrates low-density orbital emphysema (*arrowheads*) surrounding the right optic nerve (*arrow*) and high-density hemorrhage opacifying the right maxillary sinus. **B,** Calcified sellar mass. Lateral skull radiograph demonstrates enlargement of the sella turcica with ill-defined density (*asterisk*), suggesting the presence of a calcified pituitary tumor or craniopharyngioma. **C,** Hardware failure. Frontal radiograph of the lumbar spine demonstrates discontinuity (*arrow*) of a fusion rod that extends across a vertebral body compression fracture. **D,** Foreign bodies. Radiodense foreign bodies are readily seen on plain films, as in this psychiatric patient who complained of dysphagia after swallowing a safety pin (*arrowhead*).

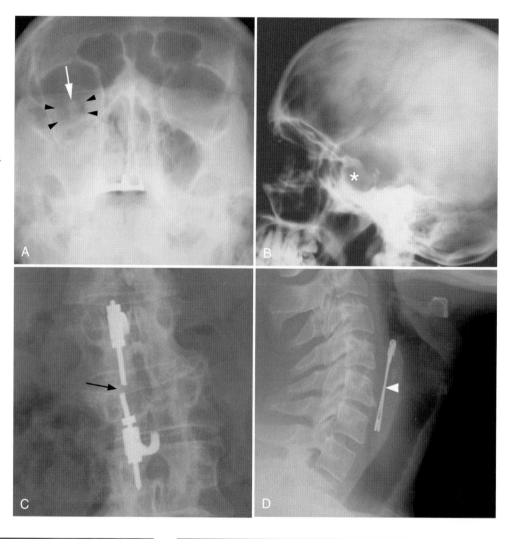

TABLE 3-1. Typical CT Numbers for Tissues of the CNS and Its Supporting Structures

Air	<−1000 HU
Adipose tissue	−20 to −100 HU
Water	−20-20 HU
White matter	20-35 HU
Gray matter	30-40 HU
Muscle	20-40 HU
Acute hemorrhage	50-100 HU
Calcification	>150 HU
Bone	800-1200 HU

HU, Hounsfield unit.

TABLE 3-2. Typical Window Parameters Used for Interpretation of CT Images

	Window Level	Window Width
Brain	40	80
Subdural	75	150
Bone	500	3500
CT angiography	120	700
Stroke	8	32
Soft tissue	0	225

Note that narrow CT windows, because they result in greater tissue contrast, are useful for displaying gray matter/white matter boundaries. Wider CT windows yield poor soft tissue contrast but allow more accurate delineation of bone/soft tissue interfaces and blood vessels. CT numbers that fall outside the window are displayed as black or white.

discrete white or gray matter structure implies a disruption in its normal physiology. The normal brain has sharp, well-defined boundaries between gray and white matter, and any regions where this distinction is lost should be viewed with suspicion.

CSF within the ventricular system and subarachnoid spaces of the brain and spinal cord normally has uniformly low attenuation that is nearly isodense to water. Inhomogeneity or altered attenuation in these regions is invariably abnormal. Similarly, the blood pool of the intracranial and extracranial vasculature is readily visualized within major arteries and veins and normally has homogeneous density that approximates the density of unclotted blood. Focal intravascular hyperdensity may be the only finding of acute stroke or dural venous thrombosis, and densely calcified vessels suggest atherosclerosis or an underlying

disorder in calcium metabolism that could predispose to arterial insufficiency.

Alternate Nomenclature

Because the CT number of a structure may vary[4] among different patients and scanners (and even in the same patient on the same scanner), it is important to interpret density abnormalities relative to an internal standard of reference. This is accomplished according to the type of tissue. The common nomenclature for describing radiodensity used in practice is as follows:

● Lesions within the brain or spinal cord parenchyma proper are described as *hypoattenuating (hypodense), isoattenuat-*

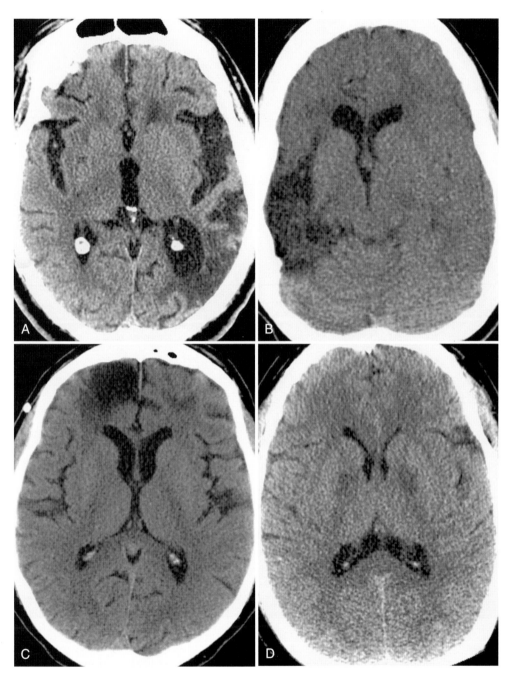

■ **FIGURE 3-2** CT appearance of encephalomalacia. Confluent areas of low density seen in association with focal loss of brain volume representing encephalomalacia and gliosis are nonspecific, but the location of the abnormality often points to an underlying cause. **A,** Remote stroke. Low density with volume loss, seen as ex-vacuo dilation of the left occipital horn, conforms to the territory of the posterior left middle cerebral artery. **B,** Encephalomalacia involving the cortical gray matter in multiple vascular territories can be caused by meningoencephalitis, as in this case of herpes encephalitis. Note ex-vacuo dilation of the frontal horn of the right lateral ventricle. **C,** Bifrontal encephalomalacia is most commonly caused by direct impact of the brain against the noncompliant calvaria years after the trauma. **D,** Chronic and symmetric low density within the deep gray nuclei is characteristic of toxic ingestion or metabolic abnormality, as seen within the globus pallidus of this patient who had previously attempted suicide by inhalation of carbon monoxide.

ing (*isodense*), or *hyperattenuating* (*hyperdense*) relative to normal adjacent structures.

● Soft tissue lesions outside the cranial vault or spinal column are best described in terms of their relative density with respect to muscle.

● Lesions within bone are described as *sclerotic* (*osteoblastic*) or *lucent* (*osteolytic*), depending on whether the density exceeds or is significantly less than that of normal cortical bone.

● Abnormalities that approximate the absolute density of water are characterized as *CSF density* or *water density*.

● Lesions with an attenuation consistent with fat are designated as *fat density*.

● A lesion is said to "enhance" when the difference in CT number between precontrast and postcontrast scans exceeds normal physiologic and technical variability between scans. For CT elsewhere in the body, this threshold has been taken as 10 HU.[5]

Causes of Decreased Density

Low density on CT is the manifestation of any of the acute or chronic pathologic endpoints of disorders that cause edema, necrosis, demyelination, or infarction. When it is chronic, low density usually implies an antecedent insult to the brain. After most serious injuries, there is a loss of tissue with time that results in involution of brain parenchyma, either by direct insult or autolysis of neurons. The process of encephalomalacia affects neurons in both gray and white matter and is characterized by a regional loss of brain volume that is primarily localized to the affected neuronal pathways. The ensuing reaction of the supporting white matter cells in this setting is gliosis, the formation of a dense fibrous network of scar tissue. On the cortical surface, encephalomalacia and gliosis are commonly the result of traumatic, infectious, or ischemic injuries and can be the source of recurrent seizures (Fig. 3-2). Within the structures of the deep gray matter, toxic and metabolic insults, intraparenchymal hemorrhage, infection, demyelinating disease, and lacunar ischemia

■ **FIGURE 3-3** Cortical low density. The CT finding of cortical low density results in a loss of the normally observed interfaces between gray matter and white matter. **A,** Acute stroke. In this patient with acute onset of left-sided hemiplegia, effacement of the normal subinsular gray matter/white matter interface (*arrows*) results in the "insular ribbon sign" of acute right middle cerebral artery infarction. **B,** Low density of the insular cortices and right cingulate gyrus (*arrow*) caused by herpes encephalitis, a neurologic emergency in this patient with altered mental status and fever. **C,** Bifrontal cortical low density extending into the lobar white matter without volume loss, typical of an acute traumatic injury. **D,** Anoxic encephalopathy. Diffuse cortical low density in this patient who was found unresponsive and hypotensive, giving the false impression of white matter hyperdensity.

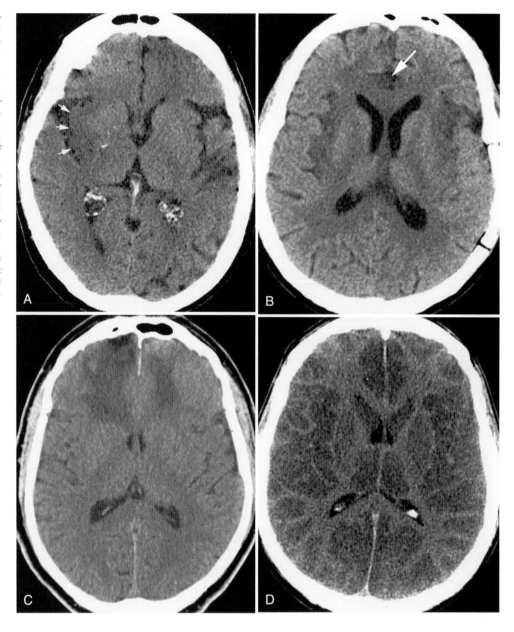

are common causes of encephalomalacia. Confluent areas of hypodensity seen on CT thus reflect the end stage of any type of brain injury and can usually be ascribed to a specific insult only in the context of appropriate clinical history or location within the brain.

Diseases that cause net changes in brain water content also give rise to confluent areas of hypodensity. In contrast to encephalomalacia, which is chronic and irreversible, most alterations in tissue water content reflect an acute disturbance in cerebral hemodynamics. Classically, cerebral edema has been categorized as cytotoxic or vasogenic.[6] Cytotoxic edema occurs in both gray and white matter and is the effect of the irreversible intracellular swelling of neurons and glia that occurs with cellular energy depletion. In contradistinction, vasogenic edema predominates in the white matter and reflects the potentially reversible shifts in water within the extracellular space that are due to alterations in the normal blood-brain barrier. Both cytotoxic and vasogenic edema are seen as hypodensity and are not readily distinguished on CT in the early stages of a disease. The identification of edema should prompt a search for its potential primary causes as well as its effects, because edema may secondarily lead to herniation. Edema that involves the entirety of the brain usually reflects hypoxic, traumatic, toxic, or metabolic injury, whereas localized edema suggests either a focal ischemic insult, infection, or a mass lesion inciting changes in the surrounding brain.

Hypodensity localizing to the gray matter of the brain surface (Fig. 3-3) warrants primary consideration of traumatic, infectious, or vascular causes. For example, brain contusion results when rapid acceleration or deceleration causes the cortical surface to come into direct contact with the rigid skull vault or dural reflections. Sources of cerebral infection, such as viral encephalitis and bacterial meningitis, also commonly involve cortical gray matter, usually as the result of direct spread of infection from the subarachnoid spaces. An important infectious cause of gray matter hypodensity that should be considered in the appropriate clinical context is herpes encephalitis. Subtle cortical low attenuation, particularly within the medial temporal lobes and cingulate cortex, can herald this disease and should prompt early treatment with intravenous antiviral chemother-

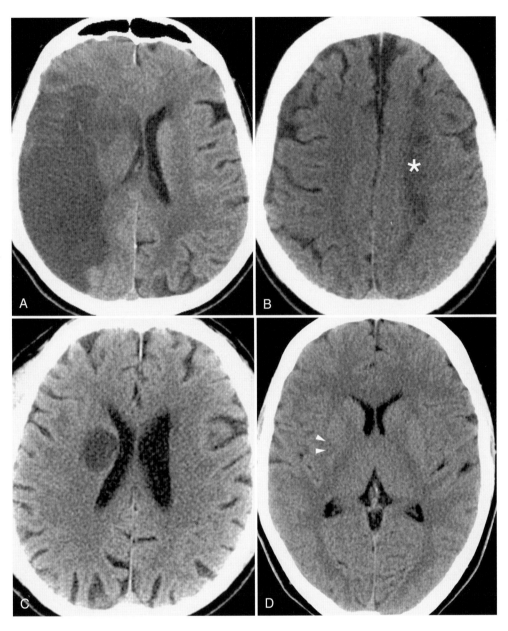

■ **FIGURE 3-4** The manifold appearances of ischemic injury on CT. **A,** Subacute stroke. Cortical and white matter low density in the distribution of the right middle cerebral artery, characteristic of subacute large vessel infarct. Note the accompanying mass effect, as evidenced by effacement of right hemispheric sulci, compression of the right lateral ventricle, and slight shift of the midline toward the left. **B,** Low density area (*asterisk*) conforming to the border zone between the left middle cerebral artery and anterior cerebral artery distributions, typical of watershed infarction. **C,** Low density and enlargement of the globus pallidus and putamen in this patient with altered mental status due to acute lenticulostriate infarct. It is important that this not be mistaken for a tumor, which could lead to unnecessary morbidity or mortality if surgical resection is attempted. **D,** Occlusion of the middle cerebral artery (*arrowheads*), because it also involves the lateral lenticulostriate arteries, may result in the loss of the normal comma-shaped morphology of the posterior putamen. This "comma sign" is a useful early sign of ischemia on noncontrast CT images.

apy. The regions of cortical gray matter hypodensity seen with both traumatic injury and infection are due to acute cellular and interstitial edema and are not infrequently accompanied by hemorrhage and interruption of the blood-brain barrier, the latter manifest by abnormal enhancement on administration of a contrast agent.

Acute interruption of the normal large- or small-vessel arterial supply to the brain and consequent ischemia may also yield hypodensity that involves both gray and white matter. The observation that hypodensity conforms to a vascular territory is central to this diagnosis (Fig. 3-4). In early ischemic injury, the attenuation of acutely ischemic brain parenchyma is inversely proportional to its water content. Specifically, a 1% total increase in tissue water content decreases its CT number by approximately 2.5 HU.[7] Interruption in blood flow causes the highly vascular gray matter to lose the ability to control neuronal permeability. As a result, neurons accumulate water and take on an intrinsic density that approximates that of white matter. This process results in the loss of the normal distinct boundaries between the involved gray matter and subjacent subcortical white matter, as well as local gyral swelling. A similar loss of density within isch-

emic deep gray matter nuclei also may be recognized only as a change in the normal shape of the nucleus. Infrequently, it is possible to detect acute small-vessel ischemia as a subtle focus of relative low density within white matter. To optimally discern the subtle changes in density that are due to acute ischemia, the level and width of the display window should be selected carefully.[8] With continued vessel occlusion, both gray and white matter hypodensity and swelling progressively increase and become more pronounced. With time, the infarcted brain tissue loses volume, ultimately resulting in encephalomalacia and glial scar within the involved vascular territory on follow-up imaging.

A number of acute and chronic disorders may produce large areas of hypodensity that are localized within the subcortical gray and white matter (Fig. 3-5). Hypodensity in these diseases selectively affects vulnerable brain tissues. For example, cardiopulmonary arrest, drug overdose, and other causes of acute global hypoxic injury preferentially injure tissues that have high metabolic demand. Early findings in this setting can be subtle on CT immediately after the insult, seen only as uniform low attenuation in white matter or effacement of normal gray-white

■ **FIGURE 3-5** White matter hypodensity. The relatively common CT finding of white matter hypodensity has a broad differential diagnosis but should be distinguished from hypodensity that involves both gray and white matter. **A,** Global hypoxic-ischemic injury. Uniform low density within the white matter of the supratentorial brain, with involvement of the deep gray nuclei, in a patient after an episode of hemorrhagic shock due to gastrointestinal bleeding. **B,** X-linked adrenoleukodystrophy. In this child there is a classic distribution of low density within the white matter of the occipital lobes and splenium of the corpus callosum. **C,** Transependymal edema. Low density "capping" the ventricular margins, combined with ventriculomegaly, is characteristic of the interstitial white matter edema that results when CSF outflow is obstructed. **D,** Microvascular leukariosis. Low density in the subcortical and periventricular white matter is a common finding in the aging brain and is thought to be due to the chronic ischemic effects of small vessels "pruned" by small vessel vasculopathies such as hypertension or diabetes.

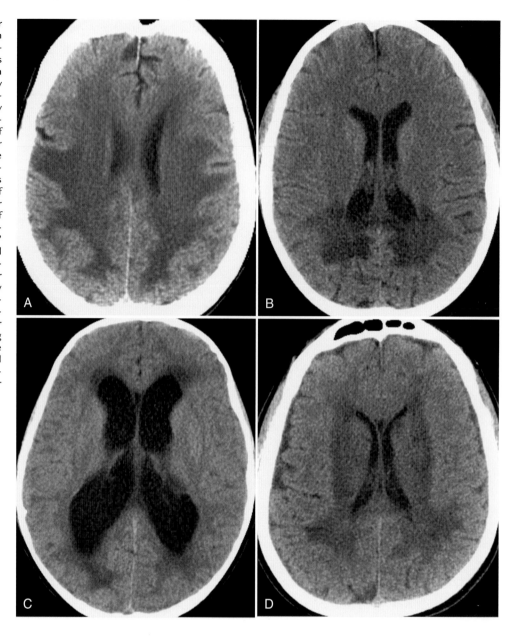

interfaces. Confluent periventricular low density is a common finding in the aging population, where small- and medium-sized vessels supplying the deep white matter of the brain are subject to chronic occlusive disease. In acute hydrocephalus, low density CSF may accumulate within the white matter surrounding the distended ventricles, a phenomenon referred to as *transependymal edema*. Metabolic leukodystrophies represent a broad class of dysmyelinating disorders that characteristically lead to varying distributions of low density within the subcortical white matter and often gray matter.

Benign and malignant tumors are a relatively common cause of altered density within both gray and white matter. Depending on the cell of origin, these may exhibit low or high density relative to normal brain anatomy. Most commonly, intra-axial tumors are seen as low attenuating lesions within white matter or as isoattenuating lesions within a larger region of surrounding vasogenic edema. As discussed later, low density within a tumor suggests necrosis, as may be seen with highly aggressive tumors such as glioblastoma multiforme or after treatment with chemotherapy or radiation. Sometimes mistaken for tumors, gray matter

heterotopias may be seen as discrete areas within white matter or along the ventricular margins that are isoattenuating to normal gray matter structures. The rare entity of gliomatosis cerebri should be considered when there are large areas of confluent hypodensity within white matter and clinical history points to an insidious course of cognitive deterioration or pyramidal tract signs. Finally, fat density within a CNS tumor is characteristic of few entities, including lipoma, dermoid, and lipomatous degeneration within certain tumors such as teratomas and rarely meningiomas.

Inflammatory demyelinating diseases such as multiple sclerosis and acute disseminated encephalomyelitis and intracranial infections represent another broad class of disease that should not be overlooked as a potentially reversible causes for low attenuation (Fig. 3-6). Small areas of circumscribed low density in white matter, especially around the margins of the lateral ventricles, may suggest the diagnosis of multiple sclerosis or other autoimmune demyelinating disease given the appropriate clinical history. A cerebral abscess is a cavity that contains pus, necrotic debris, and immune cells due to bacterial, fungal, or

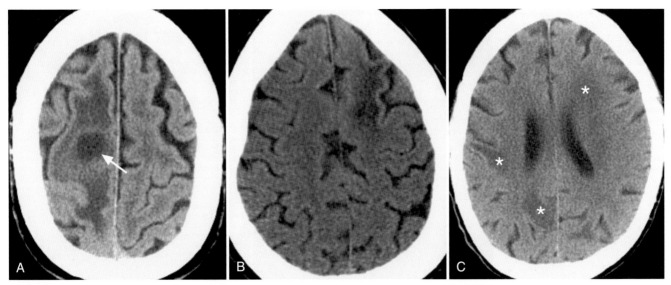

■ **FIGURE 3-6** Low density due to cerebral inflammatory disease. **A,** Typical appearance of a cerebral abscess: round, low-density cavity (*arrow*) surrounded by low-density vasogenic edema. Differentiation from other cavitary lesions such as radionecrotic cysts or cystic neoplasms often requires clinical/laboratory correlation, with help often provided by contrast-enhanced and diffusion weighted MRI. **B,** Progressive multifocal leukoencephalopathy. Whereas white matter low density is nonspecific, involvement of the subcortical U-shaped fibers in the AIDS patient can help differentiate this disorder from HIV encephalitis. **C,** Toxoplasmosis. Patchy white matter low density (*asterisks*) in an immunocompromised patient with altered mental status.

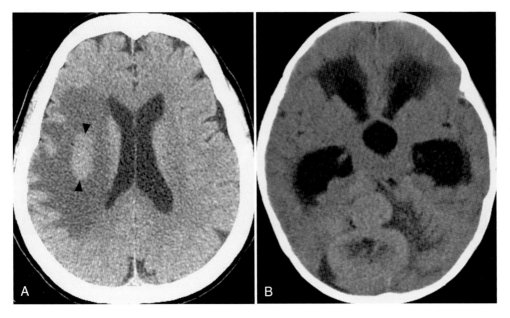

■ **FIGURE 3-7** Tumors of high cellularity. Tumors with densely packed cells and/or high nuclear-to-cytoplasmic ratios can demonstrate intrinsic hyperdensity at CT, even in the absence of calcification or hemorrhage. **A,** CNS lymphoma. Unenhanced CT demonstrating a circumscribed, hyperdense mass in the right hemispheric white matter (*arrowheads*) with surrounding low-density vasogenic edema. **B,** Medulloblastoma. Unenhanced CT demonstrating a lobulated, hyperdense mass in the posterior fossa.

parasitic infection that appears as a focal area of suppurative necrosis within the brain, usually with surrounding low density vasogenic edema. Progressive multifocal leukoencephalopathy, human immunodeficiency virus (HIV) encephalopathy, and infections such as those caused by *Toxoplasma*, cytomegalovirus, and *Cryptococcus* merit special consideration as causes for low density in the immunocompromised population.

Causes of Increased Density
High density on CT has a more limited differential diagnosis than low density. Specifically, high attenuation is characteristic of mineralization, blood products, iodinated contrast media, and certain neoplasms. Calcification is a feature of several primary brain tumors, including oligodendroglioma, ependymoma, and astrocytoma, as well as metastatic tumors such as renal cell

carcinoma, neuroblastoma, and mucinous tumors of the gastrointestinal tract. Extra-axial tumors such as meningioma may also calcify. Calcification may be the result of prior infection, such as neurocysticercosis or tuberculosis, or may be the residua of prior hemorrhage. Tumors of high cellularity referred to as "small round blue-cell neoplasms" including lymphoma, medulloblastoma, and primitive neuroectodermal tumors may have high density relative to normal brain parenchyma (Fig. 3-7).

Hemorrhage is a common cause of high density in the brain and extra-axial spaces in the acutely ill patient. Acute blood products have characteristic CT numbers ranging from 50 to 100 HU and often exert mass effect on adjacent structures. Within the brain parenchyma proper, high density due to acute hemorrhage may be the result of trauma, hypertension, hemorrhagic primary or metastatic brain tumor, vascular malformations

■ **FIGURE 3-8** CT appearance of intravascular hyperdensity. **A,** MCA thrombosis. The "dense MCA sign" is a specific but insensitive finding in acute stroke. **B,** Basilar artery thrombosis. Hyperdense basilar artery (*arrow*); compare with patent branches of the MCA. **C,** Venous thrombosis. Thrombus within the internal cerebral veins (*arrowheads*), resulting in bilateral thalamic ischemia (*asterisks*). **D,** Vascular malformations. Relative hyperdensity in this patent vein of Galen malformation.

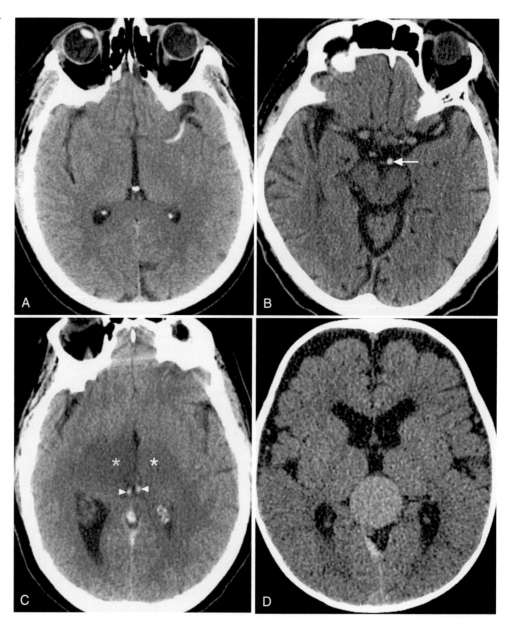

including arteriovenous and cavernous malformations, dural sinus thrombosis with venous ischemia, hemorrhagic infection such as from angioinvasive *Aspergillus*, coagulopathy, or amyloidosis. Intravenous administration of a contrast agent may allow discrimination between these causes by the observation of a primary enhancing tumor or vascular malformation or by detection of dural venous sinus occlusion.

High density confined to the lumen of an artery or vein has critical significance in that it suggests the presence of acute thrombosis. Clinical findings of acute hemiplegia, aphasia, visual field changes, or other symptoms of stroke should prompt a careful search for a hyperdense artery. Whereas this is a relatively infrequent finding seen in only approximately 22% of patients presenting with acute middle cerebral artery (MCA) stroke, it portends a poor long-term prognosis and may prompt early thrombolytic treatment.[9] The cause of high attenuation within acute thrombus has been posited to arise from accumulation of erythrocytes, fibrin, and cellular debris.[10] While originally described within the proximal or distal MCA, hyperdense thrombus can also be visualized within the anterior and posterior

cerebral and vertebrobasilar systems (Fig. 3-8). In the absence of a leading clinical history, arterial hyperdensity may alternatively suggest atherosclerotic calcification or hemoconcentration due to dehydration or polycythemia. Within the intracranial venous system, hyperdensity may be the only finding in patients with dural venous sinus or internal cerebral venous thrombosis. In patients with headache and venous hyperdensity, contrast-enhanced CT or MRI should be obtained urgently to guide prompt treatment with anticoagulation, because venous thrombosis remains a frequently missed diagnosis that often has disastrous consequences when missed.

The normal CSF spaces of the brain have an attenuation that is nearly that of water (Fig. 3-9). When high density is detected, it is usually caused by subarachnoid hemorrhage. However, meningitis, leptomeningeal tumor, and intrathecal contrast agents are alternative causes for hyperdensity that should be considered in the appropriate clinical setting. Intravenous administration of a contrast agent may help in differentiating among these causes, both for CT angiography in the search for a ruptured intracranial aneurysm and for the observation of enhancement. When hyper-

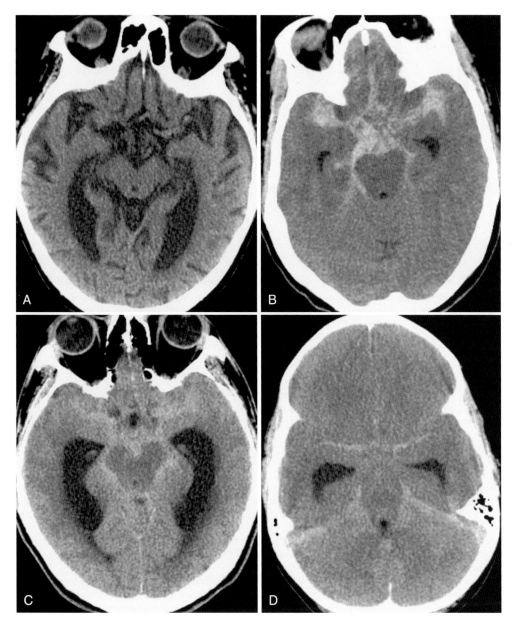

■ **FIGURE 3-9** Hyperdensity within the CSF spaces. The normal low density of normal CSF can be altered by any disease process that increases the protein/cell count. **A,** Normal basilar cisterns. Normal CSF has density that approximates that of water (0 HU). **B,** Subarachnoid hemorrhage. The location of hemorrhage may suggest the site of an aneurysm, although when diffuse the location may not be readily ascertained, as in this case of a ruptured posterior communicating artery aneurysm. **C,** Coccidiomycosis meningitis. High density CSF due to pus in the subarachnoid space is indistinguishable from acute subarachnoid hemorrhage, such that patient presentation and CSF analysis are required to differentiate these disorders. **D,** "Pseudo–subarachnoid hemorrhage." Diffuse cerebral edema displaces the normal hypodense CSF spaces and causes engorgement of pial vasculature that mimics the appearance of hemorrhage.

dense material in the subarachnoid space enhances, primary consideration should be given to bacterial, fungal, or mycobacterial meningitis or to leptomeningeal carcinomatosis. Intrathecal contrast media may be intentionally administered for myelography or for detection of CSF leak or may be present due to renal failure or compromise of the blood-brain barrier due to tumor or infection. The myelographic contrast agent Pantopaque may persist in the CSF many years after an examination.

Analysis of Mixed Patterns of Density

The pattern of mixed density within a lesion or in the structures adjacent to a lesion often provides additional clues as to the cause of a lesion. Low attenuation surrounding a solid lesion with a different dominant density suggests vasogenic edema and is most typical of primary glial tumors and metastases (Fig. 3-10). Variable density may also be due to necrosis, hemorrhage, edema, gliosis, and/or calcification within or incited by a lesion. Necrosis within a tumor is suggested by the presence of areas of low density within a solid lesion, resulting from tumor-induced hypoxia or apoptosis. It is a feature most characteristic of rapidly

growing malignancies such as glioblastoma multiforme or metastasis but can also be seen in many other tumors after irradiation or chemotherapy and in the setting of cerebral abscesses and tumefactive demyelinating lesions. Radiation necrosis may be especially difficult to differentiate from recurrent tumor after treatment, because both may demonstrate peripheral enhancement. Calcification may be seen in association with tumors, vascular malformations, and as a sequela of certain infections such as neurocysticercosis. Solid extra-axial tumors, the most common being meningioma, typically have intrinsic high density relative to the brain but also often exhibit some degree of calcification.

Hemorrhage within an intraparenchymal mass is commonly caused by tumors or vascular lesions. Bleeding is more common within metastases than primary brain tumors and may be marginal, diffuse, or heterogeneously scattered throughout different components of a tumor. Extensive tumor vascularity, vascular invasion, and rapid growth with resulting necrosis have all been cited as mechanisms for tumoral bleeding in both primary glioblastoma and metastases.[11] The presence of hemorrhage may

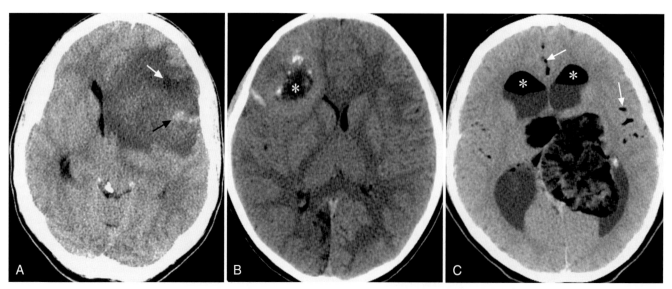

■ FIGURE 3-10 Variable density due to necrosis, hemorrhage, edema, gliosis, and/or calcification within or incited by a lesion. **A,** Glioblastoma multiforme. Large, heterogeneous mass with peritumoral vasogenic edema. High-density hemorrhage (*black arrow*) and low-density necrosis (*white arrow*) are signature features of this high-grade neoplasm. **B,** Anaplastic ependymoma. Coarse, hyperdense calcium along the periphery of region of central necrosis (*asterisk*). **C,** Ruptured dermoid cyst. Markedly heterogeneous tumor demonstrating densities ranging from fat to calcium. Note fat-fluid levels within the frontal horns (*asterisks*) and fat density within the sylvian and interhemispheric fissures (*arrows*).

suggest the primary origin of metastases, because melanoma, renal cell carcinoma, choriocarcinoma, and bronchogenic carcinoma have a greater propensity for hemorrhage than other metastases. Bleeding may also arise in vascular lesions such as arteriovenous malformations or cavernous angiomas, where adjacent calcifications (seen as focal high density), prominent vessels (seen as isodense to the normal blood pool), or gliosis from ischemic steal (seen as adjacent geographic hypodensity) can suggest the presence of an underlying vascular lesion (Fig. 3-11).

Several extra-axial lesions have characteristic mixed density appearances on CT. Heterogeneity in attenuation within a subdural hematoma may indicate acute or chronic hemorrhage or coagulopathy (Fig. 3-12). Hyperacute hemorrhage is suggested when areas of low density representing uncoagulated blood admix with high-density clotted blood, causing a "swirl sign." When present, fluid levels on CT indicate the presence of fluids of differing densities and can signal the presence of an underlying coagulopathy in patients with acute extra-axial hematomas. Sterile subdural collections should be distinguished from subdural empyema, a subdural collection of pus arising as a complication from meningitis, sinusitis, otitis media, or other infection. Heterogeneity within an extra-axial collection with other findings of infection should prompt primary consideration of subdural empyema.

MRI SIGNAL INTENSITY
Standard Against Which to Measure Signal Intensity

In contrast to the Hounsfield unit scale for CT there is no standard normalization of MR signal intensity that is in common use, and thus there is no absolute reference scale with which to quantify lesion intensity. Intensity is interpreted only through direct visual comparison with surrounding tissues. Such a comparison requires the application of a display window with suitable window width and level, set manually to visually facilitate interpretation rather than on absolute parameters as on CT. Similar to CT, however, the relative T1, T2, and T2* signal intensity of lesions is best described in reference to normal gray or

white matter in the brain, CSF in the extra-axial spaces or surrounding the spinal cord, or fat, muscle, or marrow outside the skull or spinal column.

Alternate Nomenclature
The following terms are used to describe MR signal intensity:

- Lesions that are brighter than the tissue of reference are referred to as *T1 hyperintense* or *T2 hyperintense*, depending on the dominant contrast weighting of the image. Because shorter T1 and longer T2 values yield higher signal intensities on T1- (T1W) and T2-weighted (T2W) images, hyperintensity can also be referred to as *T1 shortening* and *T2 prolongation*, respectively.
- Lesions that are less bright than the tissue of reference are designated *T1 hypointense* or *T2 hypointense*, or alternatively as causing relative *T1 prolongation* or *T2 shortening*, respectively.
- Lesions not discerned separately from surrounding structures are termed *T1 isointense* or *T2 isointense*, depending on the image weighting.
- Lesions that characteristically follow the signal intensity of gray matter, white matter, or CSF on all pulse sequences are described as being *isointense to* one of these tissues.

T1 versus T2 versus T2*
MR signal intensity is a complicated function of proton density (PD), T1 relaxation, T2 relaxation, magnetic susceptibility, and scan parameters, including flip angle, echo time (TE), and repetition time (TR). Proton density contributes to the signal intensity with all pulse sequences. Unless explicit water or fat saturating pulses are applied, the highest signal intensities in any MR image arise from proton-rich voxels containing water and/or fat. Air and cortical bone produce the low signal intensities in an image. Images obtained with long TR/short TE sequences are weighted predominantly by PD. However, because the concentration of protons is nearly homogeneous across different soft tissues, PD by itself does not usually provide appreciable tissue contrast. Two notable exceptions are in distinguishing between solid and cystic masses with high T2 signal intensity, where fluid tends to

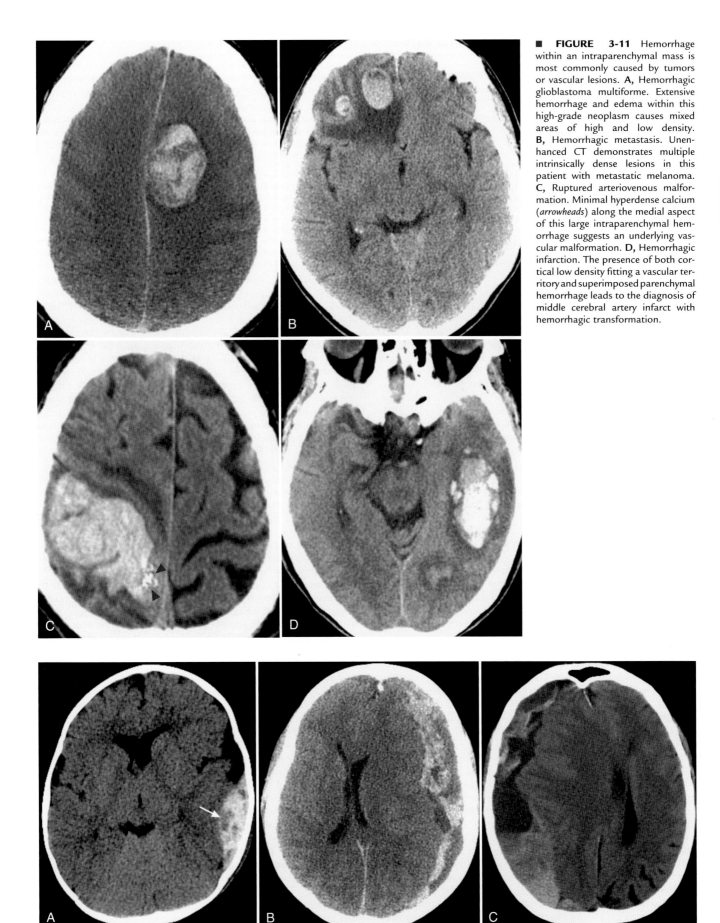

■ **FIGURE 3-11** Hemorrhage within an intraparenchymal mass is most commonly caused by tumors or vascular lesions. **A,** Hemorrhagic glioblastoma multiforme. Extensive hemorrhage and edema within this high-grade neoplasm causes mixed areas of high and low density. **B,** Hemorrhagic metastasis. Unenhanced CT demonstrates multiple intrinsically dense lesions in this patient with metastatic melanoma. **C,** Ruptured arteriovenous malformation. Minimal hyperdense calcium (*arrowheads*) along the medial aspect of this large intraparenchymal hemorrhage suggests an underlying vascular malformation. **D,** Hemorrhagic infarction. The presence of both cortical low density fitting a vascular territory and superimposed parenchymal hemorrhage leads to the diagnosis of middle cerebral artery infarct with hemorrhagic transformation.

■ **FIGURE 3-12** Mixed attenuation within extra-axial collections. **A,** Acute epidural hematoma. The finding of a "swirl sign" within a lentiform-shaped extra-axial collection should suggest active hemorrhage (*arrow*). **B,** Acute subdural hematoma in a patient with thrombocytopenia. Large hematomas with areas of hypodense unclotted blood may point to an underlying coagulopathy, as in this patient with thrombocytopenia. **C,** Acute on chronic subdural hematoma. Hyperdense blood indicates the presence of acute blood that when superimposed on mixed density suggests hemorrhage of varying ages, especially when there is layering over adhesions from previously clotted blood.

TABLE 3-3.　T1 and T2 Values* of Tissues at 1.5 T and 3.0 T

	1.5 T		3.0 T	
Tissue	**T1**	**T2**	**T1**	**T2**
Gray matter	1074-1174	87-103	1706-1934	92-106
White matter	834-934	68-76	1039-1129	66-72
Cerebrospinal fluid	2200-2400	500-1400	2360-2830	480-1200
Fat	240-250	60-80	360-400	64-72
Blood†	1321-1561	260-320	1847-2017	225-325
Muscle	988-1028	38-50	1399-1425	46-54

*Values given in milliseconds.
†Note that the T2 relaxation of whole blood varies according to relative oxygen concentration.

have low intensity on PD-weighted (PDW) images and solid lesions typically have high intensity, and the identification of chemical shift artifact, which signals the presence of fat. Differences in the values of T1 and T2 otherwise provide the dominant mechanism for soft tissue contrast, so that T1W and T2W images play a greater diagnostic role in MRI.

T1 (or spin-lattice) relaxation is the process by which protons return to their normal equilibrium magnetization in a static magnetic field after excitation by a radiofrequency pulse. In their return to the equilibrium state, protons exchange excess energy with the magnetic "lattice" of neighboring molecules. The value of T1 is a measure of the time that is required for spins to return to 63% of their baseline magnetization and is primarily determined by the size of the molecule to which spins are bound. Whereas macromolecules like proteins are subject to greater inertial forces in a magnetic field and thus have short T1 times, small molecules such as unbound water equilibrate rapidly and have long T1 times. On T1W images, tissues with large T1 have *low* signal intensity and tissues with short T1 have *high* signal intensity.

In contradistinction to T1, T2 (spin-spin) relaxation reflects the loss of magnetization that occurs as neighboring excited protons exchange energy not with the lattice but rather with one another. Protons excited by a radiofrequency pulse generate small magnetic fields that interfere with the normally homogeneous magnetic field on the molecular level. The microscopic inhomogeneities in magnetic field induced by differences in neighboring nuclei cause spins that were initially precessing in synchrony to lose coherence. The resulting loss of magnetization is quantified by the value of T2, which determines the length of time in which 37% of the magnetization is lost through this exchange of energy. On T2W images, tissues with large values of T2 have *high* signal intensities and tissues with short values of T2 have *low* signal intensity.

Nominal values for the T1 and T2 relaxation times of different tissues at 1.5 T and at 3.0 T are given in Table 3-3. Because the strength of the magnetic field of the lattice increases with the applied static magnetic field, T1 relaxation times increase gradually with magnetic field strength.[12,13] Normally, T2 values are much smaller than T1 values (and T2* values are much smaller than T2 values). Values of T2 are less dependent on field strength and range from 40 to 120 ms for most tissues, except in fluids with significant numbers of unbound protons such as CSF and blood where T2 values are normally up to 2700 ms.

Quantitative measurement of T1 and T2 can be done using specialized pulse sequences, but the longer imaging times required render these measurements of little value in practice. Instead, the different T1 and T2 characteristics of tissues are inferred by imposing deliberate T1- or T2-weighting on the acquired images. By choosing shorter values for the TR and TE of a spin-echo sequence or through the use of an inversion recovery technique, images with predominantly T1 weighting can be obtained. Long-TR/long-TE spin-echo sequences result in predominantly T2 weighting. Thus, through the judicious choice of scan parameters, the values in Table 3-3 impose characteristic signal intensities in images of the brain. CSF appears dark on T1W images but is very bright on T2W images. Because it has a longer T1 relaxation time in the adult brain, gray matter is normally hypointense relative to white matter on T1W images. In contrast, gray matter typically has greater signal intensity than white matter on T2W images in the adult brain. The signal intensities of gray and white matter depend on the stage of myelination in the developing brain, such that the normal gray matter/white matter relationship is reversed in the newborn. As with CT, inspection of both T1W and T2W images of the brain and spinal cord should show well-defined boundaries between gray and white matter. The identification of abnormalities requires the detection not only of focal variations in signal intensity but also of any effacement of the normal gray matter/white matter interfaces.

In general, T1 and T2 are heavily influenced by the viscosity of tissue. Tissues closer to fluid phase than solid phase have higher values of T1 and T2 and thus lower signal intensity on T1W images and higher signal intensity on T2W images. However, there are several circumstances when lesions on T2W images are solid, and it is not uncommon for lesions with low T2 signal intensity to represent fluid. When protons are bound to large molecules such as lipids or proteins they have short T2 times, and when protons in water molecules are unattached, as in the CSF spaces, they have long T2 times. As noted earlier, PDW images may suggest that a structure is solid or contains fluid, because the former has high signal intensity and the latter usually has lower signal intensity. The intravenous administration of a gadolinium chelate can more reliably make the distinction between solid and liquid phase. Solid tissues that are not composed primarily of bone or calcium usually enhance when the blood-brain barrier is disrupted. Liquids or devitalized tissue such as phlegmon should not enhance except at their margins, where they may be confined by viable vascularized tissue.

As excited protons return to their equilibrium magnetization, they are also subject to a loss of coherence that results from spin dephasing by local inhomogeneities in the main magnetic field. This effect, called magnetic susceptibility, is important when long values of TE are used and provides a third mechanism for image contrast. So-called T2* contrast is superimposed on the underlying T1 or T2 contrast mechanism of the sequence and can be used to detect disruptions in the normally homogeneous main magnetic field by metal, air, blood products, or mineralization. Alterations in magnetic susceptibility are visualized as either focal signal voids within normally homogeneous parenchymal architecture or as geometric distortion of the image. Gradient-echo sequences are especially sensitive to T2* effects, particularly when longer values of TE are used. T2* weighting should be included in any examination in which the detection of small areas of calcification or hemorrhage is necessary.

Causes of Decreased Signal Intensity on T1W, T2W, and T2*W Images

The initial step in the analysis of low MRI signal intensity is to determine the predominant mechanism for tissue contrast through examination of the pulse sequence parameters or relative tissue intensities. Low signal intensity implies that an object has longer T1, shorter T2, or shorter T2* relaxation times than surrounding tissues, depending on the predominant contrast mechanism used to weight the image.

Low T1 signal intensity is by itself nonspecific, because the large majority of pathologic lesions in the brain and spinal cord have long T1 relaxation times. The analysis of T1 hypointensity can be undertaken in a similar fashion to that of CT hypodensity

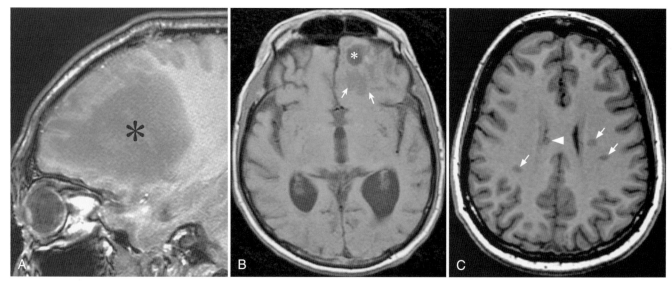

■ **FIGURE 3-13** T1 hypointensity, a nonspecific finding, is found in the large majority of pathologic lesions in the brain and spinal cord. **A,** Peritumoral vasogenic edema. Extensive, confluent white matter T1 hypointensity (*asterisk*) represents vasogenic edema in this patient with left frontal glioblastoma multiforme. **B,** Cerebral abscess. Round, hypointense parenchymal abscess (*asterisk*) with surrounding hypointense vasogenic edema (*arrows*). Contrast-enhanced and diffusion-weighted imaging will help confirm the diagnosis. **C,** Demyelination. Multifocal T1 hypointensity within the lobar white matter (*arrows*) and corpus callosum (*arrowhead*) are characteristic of demyelinating disease, as in this patient with long-standing symptoms of multiple sclerosis.

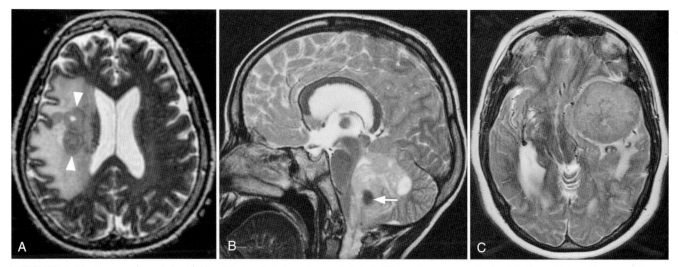

■ **FIGURE 3-14** Tumors characterized by low T2 signal. **A,** Lymphoma. Relatively T2 hypointense mass in the right frontal lobe white matter (*arrowheads*) with surrounding hyperintense vasogenic edema. **B,** Medulloblastoma. Central T2 hypointensity (*arrow*) within this posterior fossa mass enhanced avidly on postcontrast imaging, excluding the possibility of hemorrhage and/or calcium causing the low T2 signal. **C,** Meningioma. Large extra-axial mass, again demonstrating relative T2 hypointensity. In the case of meningioma, the T2 hypointensity is likely due to a combination of tumor calcification and high fibrous content.

(and, as discussed later, of T2 hyperintensity). Low T1 signal intensity may thus herald a variety of acute and chronic disorders and must be evaluated in conjunction with local mass effect and normal anatomy to determine whether it indicates the presence of edema, fluid collections, demyelination, and solid mass lesions (Fig. 3-13). In general, T1 prolongation is characteristic of fluids, cystic lesions, and solids. Fluid and cystic components of solid lesions commonly have very long T1 relaxation times and are thus seen to have signal intensity that approaches that of CSF on T1W images. Solid lesions including tumors and fibrosis also typically exhibit intermediate T1 signal between that of fluid and normal brain or soft tissue. The T1 signal intensity of protein-containing structures such as mucoceles is low at small protein

concentrations and gradually increases with higher concentrations and then falls again at even higher concentrations.[14] Low T1 signal can also be observed with flowing blood, hemosiderin, and calcification.

Low T2 signal intensity is characteristic of fat, tumors, fibrosis, certain blood products, mineralization, and gadolinium chelates in high concentrations. Lipid-containing lesions such as lipomas and dermoid cysts are suggested by relatively low T2 signal intensity in areas that have simultaneously high T1 signal intensity. Other intra-axial tumors are often seen as areas of relatively low T2 signal intensity surrounded by high-intensity vasogenic edema (Fig. 3-14). Tumors of high cellularity that have high density on CT images such as lymphoma, medulloblastoma, and

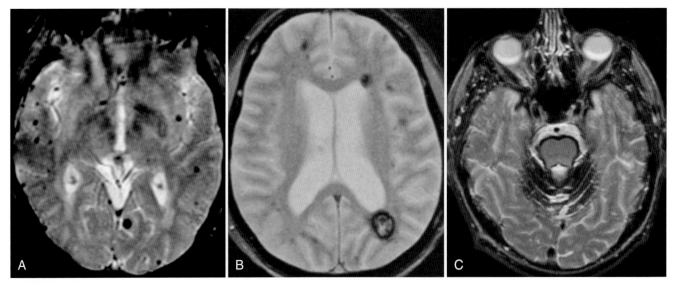

■ **FIGURE 3-15**   T2* hypointensity. The appearance of T2* hypointensity is due to magnetic susceptibility, increasing sensitivity to blood products at various stages of evolution. **A,** Amyloid angiopathy. Scattered T2* hypointense foci due to repeated microhemorrhages are characteristic but not diagnostic of this disease. **B,** Multiple cavernomas. Dominant mass centered posterior to the left ventricular trigone with peripheral T2 hypointensity, in conjunction with smaller hypointense lesions within the supratentorial white matter. **C,** Superficial siderosis. Diffuse T2* hypointensity "staining" the leptomeninges of the pons and vermis, owing to repeated hemorrhage in this patient with a spinal cord ependymoma.

other small round blue cell tumors are characterized by a relatively low signal intensity on T2W images. Meningiomas are often T2 hypointense, in part related to calcification and high fibrous content. Mature fibrosis with collagenous tissue, a common host response to prior surgery or trauma of tissue outside the CNS, has characteristic low T1 and T2 signal intensity. In contrast to other causes for T2 hypointensity, mature fibrosis is often seen to enhance in post-gadolinium T1W images. This can be useful, for example, in differentiating between recurrent disc herniation and scarring in the postoperative spine.

Hemorrhage has a complex temporal evolution in both T1 and T2 signal intensity. Both acute and chronic hemorrhage can be T2 hypointense. Shortly after hemorrhage occurs there is a shift in the oxygen dissociation curve of hemoglobin that causes oxyhemoglobin molecules to deoxygenate. Deoxyhemoglobin is highly paramagnetic and leads to a loss of MR signal intensity through its high magnetic susceptibility. Within the first week, however, the host inflammatory response causes deoxyhemoglobin within red blood cells within a hematoma to oxidize to methemoglobin, which has both high T1 and T2 signal intensity. This process typically starts at the margins of the hemorrhage, where phagocytic cells first encounter deoxygenated blood cells. Ultimately, metabolism of the blood cells by phagocytes results in resorption of fluid and protein. In this chronic stage of hematoma evolution, unbound iron released by the phagocytosis of methemoglobin is captured by hemosiderin molecules, which are insoluble in water and unable to cross the blood-brain barrier. The final residual of hemorrhage, the hemosiderin "stain" around the margins of the resorbed hematoma, has high iron content that appears dark on T2W images and gradient-echo images owing to magnetic susceptibility.

Decreased signal intensity on images sensitive to magnetic susceptibility indicates the presence of mineralization, blood products, or gadolinium chelate in high concentrations. These substances produce local disruptions in an otherwise homogeneous main magnetic field and give rise to signal voids on heavily T2*W images. T2*W imaging is especially sensitive for detection of hemosiderin and ferritin, the final products of hemoglobin metabolism that may be the only evidence for prior hemorrhage (Fig. 3-15). The presence of low T2* signal intensity on these images can be especially useful in suggesting the presence of small mineral deposits or blood products that would be other-

wise undetectable on standard T1W or T2W imaging. Parenchymal microhemorrhages are most commonly the result of chronic hypertension and amyloid angiopathy, the latter suggested by sparing of the deep gray nuclei and predominant distribution within the subcortical white matter of the frontal and parietal lobes. Cavernous malformations and post-traumatic shear injury can produce a similar pattern of punctate foci of low T2* signal. Less common causes for cerebral microhemorrhage on gradient-echo imaging include cerebral embolism, vasculitis, hemorrhagic micrometastasis, and radiation vasculopathy.[15,16]

Causes of Increased Signal Intensity on T1W, T2W, and T2*W Images

The identification of intrinsic high signal intensity within a lesion on T1W images raises a limited group of diagnostic considerations and usually implies the presence of lipid, methemoglobin, melanin, or proteinaceous fluid.[17] Lipid protons have short T1 relaxation times and may be uniquely identified when T1 hyperintensity is seen in association with chemical-shift artifact (Fig. 3-16). Lipid is characteristic of intracranial and spinal lipomas, dermoid cysts, surgical fat packing, and, rarely, lipomatous degeneration within tumors such as meningioma. Methemoglobin is a common cause of intrinsic T1 shortening that may be seen in the course of extra-axial, intraparenchymal and intraventricular hemorrhage, hemorrhagic infections and tumors, and vessel thrombosis. Gyriform high T1 signal is specific for cortical laminar necrosis, a finding that should suggest subacute infarct when it conforms to a vascular distribution. Interestingly, the mechanism of T1 shortening in laminar necrosis remains unclear. While initially believed to be the result of hemorrhagic infarction, histopathologic studies have failed to confirm the presence of methemoglobin and it is more likely the result of early reactive gliosis and deposition of fat-laden macrophages.[18]

Melanin is thought to reduce parenchymal or leptomeningeal T1 signal through a combination of paramagnetic free radicals in melanin and paramagnetic metal scavenging by melanoma cells. High T1 signal due to melanin is characteristic of melanoma and intracranial deposits of melanin in the phakomatosis neurocutaneous melanosis. Metastatic melanoma, while often hemorrhagic, often demonstrates high T1 signal even in the absence of hemorrhage unless the metastases are amelanotic[18] (Fig. 3-17). Both melanoma metastases and melanin deposits in

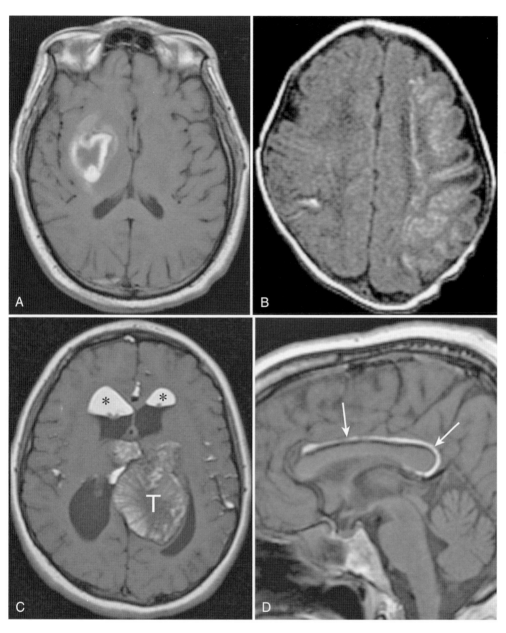

■ **FIGURE 3-16** Intrinsic T1 hyperintensity due to blood and fat. **A,** Intraparenchymal hematoma. Typical appearance of T1 hyperintensity from methemoglobin. **B,** Laminar necrosis. Gyriform T1 hyperintensity secondary to subacute left middle cerebral artery infarct. **C,** Ruptured dermoid cyst. T1 hyperintensity is demonstrated within the mass (T), layering within the ventricles (*asterisks*), and within the sylvian and interhemispheric fissures. **D,** Lipoma. Characteristic T1 hyperintensity along the superior margin of the corpus callosum (*arrows*).

neurocutaneous melanosis may be expected to enhance with administration of gadolinium. T1 shortening can also result from the interaction of water molecules with surrounding macromolecular proteins. Colloid cysts, Rathke's cleft cysts, craniopharyngiomas, and mucoceles may all contain proteinaceous fluids that demonstrate high intrinsic T1 signal. The posterior pituitary normally has intrinsic high T1 signal, most likely the result of proteins or phospholipids concentrated in this portion of the gland.

Flowing blood moves unsaturated spins from outside of a slice into the imaging plane and may result in high T1 signal within vessels. This phenomenon is the basis of flow-related enhancement in time-of-flight MR angiography techniques. Phase artifacts from circulating blood can also give rise to flow ghosts that, when superimposed on normal tissue, produce spurious T1 hyperintensity. Certain paramagnetic cations cause T1 hyperintensity in tissues. Specifically, intravenously administered gadolinium chelates at low concentrations and superparamagnetic iron oxide (SPIO) particle contrast agents deliberately exploit this property to enhance the signal intensity of the blood pool. Concentrations of particulate calcium up to 30% can reduce T1 relaxation times through a surface relaxation mechanism.[19]

Finally, manganese deposition from hepatic cirrhosis, parenteral nutrition, or industrial exposure is a rare cause for T1 shortening within the globi pallidi and midbrain.

The differential diagnosis for high T2 signal intensity is exceedingly broad, with a similar range of abnormalities encountered in the analysis of CT hypointensity and T1 hypointensity (Fig. 3-18). Confluent T2 hyperintensity in white matter may indicate edema or gliosis and may thus be a feature of both acute and chronic disease. High T2 signal should thus always be interpreted in conjunction with the presence or absence of local mass effect, because edema is often a secondary phenomenon associated with a mass or hemodynamic changes and gliosis is characterized by regional loss of parenchymal volume. Of note, although characteristic of liquids, T2 hyperintensity is also common to most brain tumors. To determine whether a lesion is truly cystic or necrotic it is necessary to administer gadolinium to document the absence of enhancement. Enhancement in a structure with high T2 signal intensity implies that it is vascular, and thus solid. Solid and cystic lesions with high T2 signal intensity can sometimes be differentiated by comparison with PDW images, where the former are usually bright and the latter are typically dark. Furthermore, "shading" or gravity-dependent

■ FIGURE 3-17 Intrinsic T1 hyperintensity due to melanin, proteinaceous fluids, and vasopressin. **A,** Orbital melanoma. Homogeneous T1 hyperintensity (*asterisk*) related to high melanin content within the globe in this patient with orbital melanoma. **B,** Neurocutaneous melanosis. T1 shortening within the mesial temporal lobes bilaterally (*arrows*) in a patient with a large dorsal cutaneous nevus on physical examination. **C,** Rathke cleft cyst. Large, cystic mass within the sella turcica. **D,** Ectopic pituitary. Punctate focus of T1 hyperintensity (*arrowhead*) related to storage of the hormone arginine vasopressin.

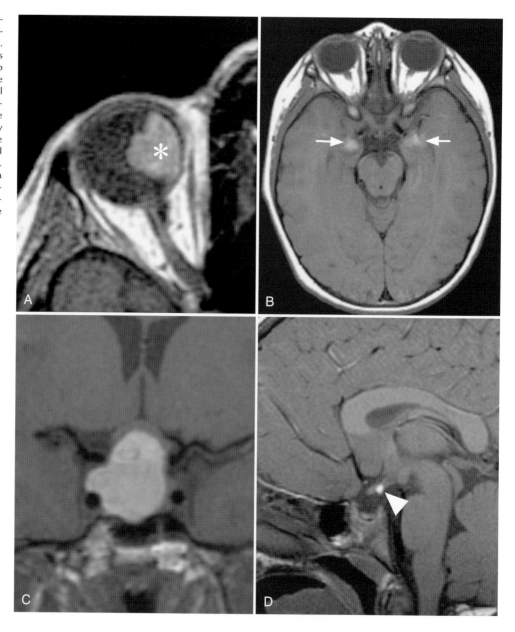

differentials in T2 signal intensity within a lesion suggest that the lesion is cystic, as may be seen with nodal metastasis of squamous cell carcinoma.[20]

ECHOGENICITY

Standard Against Which to Measure Echogenicity

Echogenicity refers to the ability to return a signal when tissue is in the path of a sound beam and is primarily a function of density and compressibility. Density, as with CT, depends on the mass of the molecules that constitute a tissue and their relative spacing. Compressibility reflects the degree to which molecules are displaced by ultrasonic energy and is the macroscopic correlate to the adherent forces between individual molecules. These intrinsic features of a tissue are characterized together as acoustic impedance, a physical constant that represents the balance of incident acoustic energy that is transmitted through a tissue and scattered back toward the transducer. Tissues with high acoustic impedance attenuate most of the energy of the sound beam, and tissues with low acoustic impedance allow most of the energy to pass through them unhindered. Among

biologic tissues, bone has the highest acoustic impedance, followed by muscle, fat, blood, water, and air. Thus, bone blocks the transmission of sound and serves as a poor acoustic window through which to evaluate deeper tissues. Echogenicity can only be adequately assessed for tissues of relatively low impedance such as muscle, blood vessels, and fluid collections. Furthermore, as impedance is proportional to the wavelength of the sound beam, high-frequency transducers are useful only for assessing structures close to the skin surface and it is necessary to use a lower-frequency transducer to interrogate deeper structures.

The relative fraction of energy transmitted and reflected at the interface between two different structures is determined by the transmission coefficient and reflection coefficients for the interface, as calculated from their acoustic impedance. A large difference in the magnitude of the impedance at an interface results in the majority of insonating energy being reflected, and smaller differences allow greater through-transmission of sound. The transmission coefficient is thus greater for air-muscle interfaces than muscle-bone interfaces. The latter produce acoustic shadows, points in the image beyond which there is no visualiza-

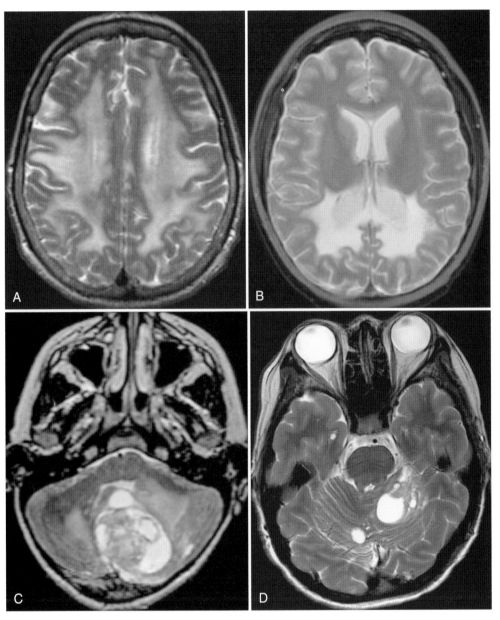

■ **FIGURE 3-18** T2 hyperintensity. Similar to hypodensity with CT, the relatively common MR finding of T2 hyperintensity has a broad differential diagnosis. **A,** Hashimoto's encephalopathy. Diffuse T2 hyperintensity within the supratentorial white matter due to acute inflammation. **B,** Typical distribution of T2 hyperintensity in this patient with X-linked adrenoleukodystrophy. **C,** Juvenile pilocytic astrocytoma. T2 hyperintense tumor cyst favors this diagnosis over that of other posterior fossa tumors in the pediatric population. **D,** Necrotic metastases. Central T2 hyperintensity suggests necrosis and cavitation within these breast cancer metastases.

tion of deeper tissues. Structures in the near field are thus more easily assessed than structures in the far field, which are interrogated by a sound beam of much lower energy that has been successively attenuated as it passes farther from the ultrasound transducer.

While there is some variation in the speed at which ultrasound travels through different tissues, a fixed speed of 1540 m/s is assumed by the scanner to spatially localize the source of reflected sound. As the acoustic beam encounters tissues of different impedance, velocities are altered such that returning echoes are received by the transducer at different times and have different intensities. This information, along with the values for sound wave velocities in different tissues, is synthesized to generate an ultrasound image. The intensities depicted in an ultrasound image should be interpreted as a map of the attenuation of the sound beam, modulated in the far field by the cumulative effects of sound attenuation in the near field.

Anatomic structures respond with characteristic features when insonated with an ultrasound beam. In comparison with neighboring tissues, the echo signature of bone, soft tissue, fluid, muscle, and fat can typically be uniquely distinguished. However, both the echogenicity and echotexture of a lesion are subjective rather than quantitative assessments that depend on the frequency of insonation, acoustic window, angle of insonation, and ultrasound scan parameters. In a similar approach to interpretation of cross-sectional modalities, the intensity (*echogenicity*) and pattern (*echotexture*) of echoes are usually described in reference to adjacent normal tissues.

Alternate Nomenclature

Several descriptive terms are commonly applied to the echogenicity of lesions:

- *Isoechoic* lesions are characterized by echogenicity that is identical to the tissue of reference, such that a lesion is not depicted separately when it is spatially contiguous with normal tissue. For example, subependymal heterotopias may be seen as solid masses along the ventricular margins that are isoechoic to gray matter.
- *Hypoechoic* structures such as infarcted brain appear less bright on ultrasound images than the tissue of reference, and *hyperechoic* (*echogenic*) lesions such as acute hemorrhage

■ **FIGURE 3-19** Vein of Galen malformation. Doppler imaging is used to confirm the vascular nature of hypo/anechoic masses. **A,** Gray-scale ultrasonography of the newborn brain demonstrating an anechoic, cystic-appearing mass (*asterisk*) located posterior to the thalamus. **B,** Color Doppler image demonstrating prominent flow within the "cystic" mass.

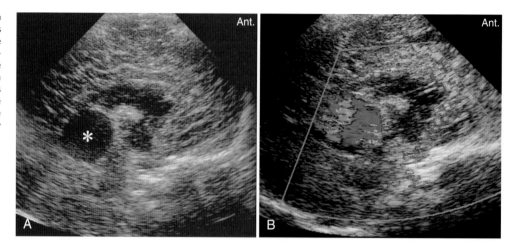

are brighter on ultrasound images than the tissue of reference.

- *Anechoic* or *sonolucent* structures such as CSF and cysts are characterized by an absence of internal echoes. The normal ventricular system is anechoic, as are uncomplicated cysts in the posterior fossa in the setting of Dandy-Walker malformations.

Echotexture may also aid in determining whether a lesion is solid or cystic when it is *homogeneous* (containing an internally uniform echo pattern) or *heterogeneous* (containing an internally irregular echo pattern). Homogeneous echotexture is typical of intracranial cysts and normal CSF, and heterogeneous echotexture is often found in intracranial neoplasms such as teratomas or blood products. Finally, the interaction of the sound wave with neighboring tissues is an additional diagnostic feature that may help in determining the nature of a lesion. In particular, the density of a lesion can be inferred from the degree to which it attenuates or enhances sound transmission. Dense structures such as bone and mineralization that dramatically attenuate sound cause *posterior acoustic shadowing*, and less dense structures such as cysts that readily transmit sound lead to *posterior acoustic enhancement (enhanced through-transmission)*.

Causes of Decreased Echogenicity

Ultrasound imaging has found limited clinical use in routine neuroradiology, in large part due to the poor penetration of sound through the skull and spinal column. However, because bone is less dense in neonates and open fontanelles provide an acoustic window through which to insonate the brain, neurosonography is widely used in the evaluation of the neonatal brain and spine. In this setting, ultrasound is highly sensitive for the detection of intracranial hemorrhage in infants born prematurely. The different echogenicity of normal white matter, basal ganglia, and the choroidal plexus make ultrasonography useful in screening for structural anomalies, periventricular leukomalacia, and hypoxic ischemic injury in the newborn brain, albeit with less sensitivity than MRI or CT. The incompletely ossified or unfused posterior elements of the spine also provide a clinically useful acoustic window, such that ultrasound plays a role in the assessment of the spinal cord in neonates suspected of having a tethered cord or myelomeningocele. Ultrasound imaging is also used in the evaluation of vessels in the neck and skull, the latter via transcranial Doppler ultrasonography. Finally, intraoperative ultrasonography is used in some institutions by surgeons during resection of brain and spinal cord tumors, both in adults and in children.

Decreased echogenicity in the newborn brain is characteristic of intracranial cysts or prior ischemic injury. Interhemispheric cysts and posterior fossa cysts appear as circumscribed regions that are isoechoic to normal CSF and may displace adjacent normal structures. While most often incidental, intracranial cysts are often the first finding in cases of an underlying congenital anomaly, such that their identification should prompt close investigation of the corpus callosum and cerebellum, respectively, to confidently make the diagnosis of callosal agenesis or the Dandy-Walker malformation. Subependymal cysts occur along the walls of the ventricles and reflect germinolysis due to congenital infection. In the late stage of intraparenchymal hemorrhage, hypoechoic areas or cystic cavities remain in areas of hemorrhage within the brain parenchyma, particularly around the margins of the ventricular system. Useful adjunct findings with intracranial cysts include posterior through-transmission and homogeneous echotexture.

Abnormalities primary to the intracranial vasculature are an important differential consideration in the evaluation of intracranial cysts (Fig. 3-19). The echogenicity of the blood pool is determined by the mechanical aggregation of red blood cells, which is directly related to blood flow velocity and inversely related to vessel diameter.[21] The internal echotexture and Doppler flow of hypoechoic or anechoic intracranial lesions should thus be carefully assessed to determine whether an apparently cystic lesion may actually represent a vascular malformation such as a dilated vein. Evaluation of the entirety of the abnormality may show hyperechoic areas that correspond to layering or flowing blood within the lesion.

Decreased echogenicity detected in the dorsum of the lumbar spine may be a subtle finding of myelomeningocele and spina bifida. Nonfusion of the posterior elements in this case allows a portion of the spinal canal to protrude through the defect, leading to the appearance of a rounded hypoechoic lesion within the soft tissues of the back superficial to the opening. A simple myelomeningocele is often associated with characteristic features of the type 2 Chiari malformation in the brain. Sacrococcygeal teratomas may also contain hypoechoic areas and may be included in the differential diagnosis of myelomeningocele.

Causes of Increased Echogenicity

Ultrasonography of the neonatal head has high sensitivity for the diagnosis of intracranial hemorrhage, which typically originates in the germinal matrix and extends into the ventricular system. At most institutions, infants born prematurely are routinely screened for this complication at 4 to 7 days after birth. Hemorrhage confined to the germinal matrix is readily identified as asymmetric increased echogenicity in the region of the

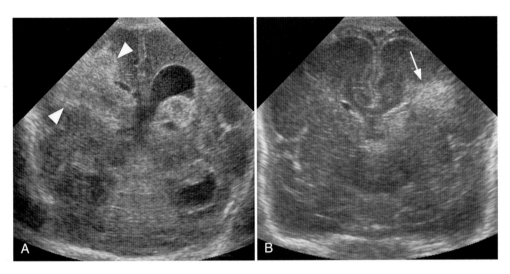

■FIGURE 3-20 Hyperechogenicity on neonatal neurosonography. **A,** Grade 4 germinal matrix hemorrhage. Hyperechoic bilateral germinal matrix hemorrhages (*arrowheads*) with parenchymal extension on the right in a newborn born at 28 weeks' gestation. **B,** Acute periventricular leukomalacia. Abnormal echogenic white matter surrounding the ventricles, more pronounced on the left (*arrow*) in a newborn with difficult delivery.

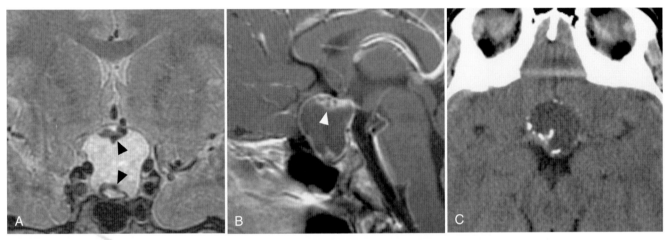

■ FIGURE 3-21 Multimodality characterization of a sellar mass (craniopharyngioma). **A,** Coronal T2-weighted imaging demonstrating a hyperintense mass with internal hypointense "debris" (*arrowheads*), suggesting the presence of blood and/or calcium. **B,** Sagittal gadolinium-enhanced imaging confirms the cystic nature of the lesion. Irregular enhancement of the cyst wall (*arrowhead*) suggests a neoplastic etiology. **C,** Axial, noncontrast CT confirms the presence of dense mural calcium, consistent with the diagnosis of craniopharyngioma.

caudothalamic notch, where the absence of choroid makes blood stand out from this normal tissue (Fig. 3-20). When blood extends into the ventricular system, ultrasonography is also useful for the detection of ventriculomegaly and accompanying intraventricular hemorrhage, which usually appears as focal areas of echogenicity in close proximity to the ventricular margins. Small subdural hemorrhages, which appear as thin lenticular extra-axial collections, are common after normal vaginal delivery and are usually considered normal incidental findings.

Acute periventricular leukomalacia can be diagnosed on ultrasound evaluation when increased echogenicity is seen within the superolateral periventricular brain parenchyma. When subtle, periventricular leukomalacia may be difficult to distinguish from the normal ring of hyperechoic white matter that surrounds the ventricles caused by the anisotropy effect of sound beam reflection from axons and vessels that emerge centripetally from the ventricles (see Fig. 3-20). When suggested by ultrasonography, this finding can be confirmed by neonatal MRI, which is diagnostic. Hypoxic-ischemic encephalopathy, in contrast, can be suggested by an overall increase in brain echogenicity or focal hyperechoic areas that conform to a vascular territory. The latter may also involve the thalami and lenticular nuclei, giving rise to more linear areas of echogenicity referred to as "thalamostriate vasculopathy." Similar to periventricular

leukomalacia, these findings can be exceedingly subtle and are best assessed using MRI.

RELATIVE SPECIFICITY OF DENSITY VERSUS SIGNAL INTENSITY VERSUS REFINING ANALYSIS BY USE OF MULTIPLE TECHNIQUES

There are certain circumstances when the complementary information about image intensity from more than one modality can be used to narrow the differential diagnosis among a longer list of considerations. For example, the MRI appearance of calcium is variable and nonspecific and the presence of calcium within a lesion may not be appreciated a priori on MRI.[22,23] Small particulate calcium seen on CT as fine or punctate may be subsumed by partial volume averaging in MR images and not visualized at all. When sufficiently large, calcium deposits may give rise to signal voids on T1W or T2W imaging, but their signal intensity is sufficiently variable that they may not be readily identified in all cases. CT can be used to increase diagnostic confidence in the differential diagnosis of tumors that commonly calcify, such as meningioma, oligodendroglioma, craniopharyngioma, and choroid plexus papilloma from other noncalcified tumors (Fig. 3-21). CT should also be considered in the workup

■ **FIGURE 3-22** Fibrous dysplasia. CT versus MRI characterization of bone lesions. **A,** Axial gadolinium-enhanced imaging demonstrating a enhancing lesion at the right orbital apex (*asterisk*). The list of differential considerations would include both neoplastic and inflammatory processes. **B,** Noncontrast CT demonstrates the bony origin of the lesion, with the characteristic "ground-glass" appearance (*asterisk*) of fibrous dysplasia.

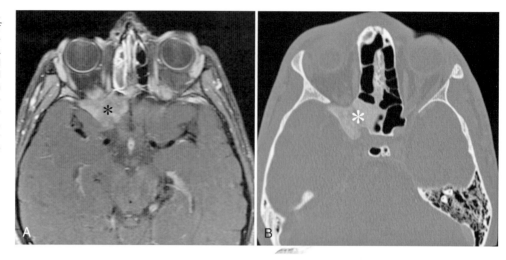

■ **FIGURE 3-23** Dark mucocele. Highly proteinaceous mucus within an obstructed sinus may be hypointense on both gadolinium-enhanced T1W (**A**) and fat-suppressed T2W (**B**) images, such that this mucosal disease of the paranasal sinuses may be overlooked on routine MRI. CT images at bone (**C**) and soft tissue (**D**) windows readily demonstrate relatively hyperdense material within an expanded, remodeled sphenoidal sinus, consistent with a mucocele.

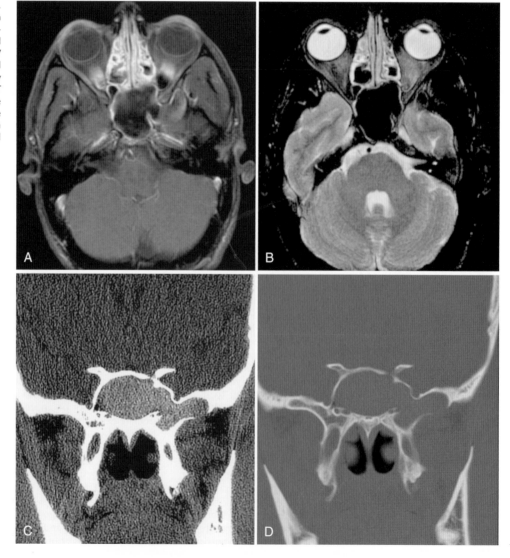

BOX 3-1   Sample Report: MRI of the Brain

PATIENT HISTORY

An 8-year-old boy presented with gradual onset of headaches and loss of vision over a 6-month period.

COMPARISON STUDY

Head CT was done a week earlier.

TECHNIQUE

Axial and sagittal T1W spin-echo, coronal T2W fast spin-echo, axial T2W FLAIR, coronal gradient-echo, and post-gadolinium axial and sagittal T1W spin-echo imaging of the brain performed at 1.5 T.

FINDINGS

There is a 2.4 × 1.2-cm circumscribed mass centered within both the sella and suprasellar cistern that is both solid and cystic. The lesion shows predominantly high T2 and low T1 signal intensity but contains several discrete areas of low T2 and high T1 signal that are consistent with blood products and/or proteinaceous debris. Thin peripheral linear areas of low intensity on T2W images correspond to susceptibility artifact on gradient-echo images, consistent with calcification as demonstrated on recent head CT.

Secondary enlargement of the sella is present, along with upward displacement of the overlying optic chiasm and flattening of an otherwise normal-appearing pituitary gland. The mass does not appear to involve the cavernous sinuses, and the normal flow voids of the internal carotid arteries are preserved. There is no reactive edema within the brain adjacent to the lesion, and although portions of the mass lie just below the foramen of Monroe there is no ventriculomegaly to indicate hydrocephalus.

On administration of gadolinium, the lesion shows several internal nodular areas of enhancement and demonstrates linear enhancement at its periphery. There is no suspicious enhancement of the brain parenchyma or leptomeninges.

IMPRESSION

This suprasellar solid and cystic mass is most consistent with craniopharyngioma, given the presence of internal T1 shortening, cyst wall enhancement, and calcification. Because the lesion is separate from the pituitary gland, this is unlikely to represent a hemorrhagic pituitary adenoma. The presence of calcification and internal solid enhancement also makes Rathke's cleft cyst and simple arachnoid cyst unlikely.

---

of non-neoplastic CNS disorders in which focal calcification is of diagnostic importance, including certain neoplasms and inflammatory/infectious processes such as granulomatous disease or neurocysticercosis, metabolic derangements such as Fabry's disease, and tuberous sclerosis or Sturge-Weber syndrome.

CT has far greater accuracy than MRI in the evaluation of most disease in or around the bones of the skull or spinal column. When MRI is the first study obtained in a patient with a benign or malignant lesion primary to bone, signal intensity on T1W and T2W images may not be sufficiently specific to arrive at a specific diagnosis. For example, the developmental disorder fibrous dysplasia leads to replacement of normal cancellous bone by immature osseous matrix and fibrous stroma. This has a nearly pathognomonic radiographic or CT appearance but has a variable appearance on MRI that may not be easily recognized (Fig. 3-22).[24] Concomitant T1 and T2 hypointensity, which is characteristic of fibrous tissue, is not usually seen in the entity. Instead, the majority of these lesions are isointense to muscle on T1W images and heterogeneously hyperintense on T2W images. Because identical imaging features can be found in malignant tumors of the brain or surrounding bones, plain film radiographs or CT should be considered when the MRI appearance is equivocal.

MRI may be particularly misleading in the evaluation of fluid collections. For example, the signal intensity of mucus contents within an obstructed paranasal sinus or mucocele depends on the relative protein content. On T1W images, fluid within a sinus is characteristically T1 hypointense. When the protein concentration exceeds roughly 25%, there is a T2-shortening effect that renders these inspissated secretions occult on T2W images. Furthermore, the diagnostic features of sinus expansion and osseous thinning are not easily recognized on MRI. To confidently diagnose the entity of a proteinaceous mucocele, CT should be obtained and correlated with the MRI findings, because the typical bony remodeling is readily visualized on CT (Fig. 3-23).

ANALYSIS

A sample formal imaging report is presented in Box 3-1 in which the description of how signal intensity and density are analyzed should lead the reader to the correct clinical diagnosis of craniopharyngioma. This report refers to the imaging example provided in Figure 3-21.

KEY POINTS

- Density, signal intensity, and echogenicity should be analyzed first in terms of location within gray matter, white matter, CSF spaces, bones, or elsewhere within the brain or spinal cord.
- CT number is an absolute measurement of density, but signal intensity on MRI and echogenicity in ultrasonography are relative and should be interpreted in reference to adjacent tissues.
- A suitable display window should be applied to both CT and MR images to detect subtle changes that may otherwise not be easily discerned.
- The intensity analysis of a lesion should initially focus on the lesion itself to determine its cause, but secondary changes in the intensity of adjacent tissues may provide additional clues.

SUGGESTED READINGS

Babcock DS. Sonography of the brain in infants: role in evaluating neurologic abnormalities. AJR Am J Roentgenol 1995; 165:417-423.

Barnes JE. AAPM Tutorial: characteristics and control of contrast in CT. RadioGraphics 1992; 12:825-837.

Mikulis DJ, Roberts TPL. Neuro MR: protocols. J Magn Reson Imaging 2007; 26:838-847.

Nitz WR, Reimer P. Contrast mechanisms in MR imaging. Eur Radiol 1999; 9:1032-1046.

Roberts TPL, Mikulis DJ. Neuro MR: principles. J Magn Reson Imaging 2007; 26:823-837.

REFERENCES

1. Phelps ME, Hoffman EJ, Ter-Pogossian MM. Attenuation coefficients of various body tissue, fluids, and lesions at photon energies of 18 to 136 keV. Radiology 1975; 117:573-583.

2. Mull RT. Mass estimates by computed tomography: physical density from CT numbers. AJR Am J Roentgenol 1984; 143: 1101-1104.

3. Brooks RA, Mitchell LG, O'Connor CM, Di Chiro G. On the relationship between computed tomography numbers and specific gravity. Phys Med Biol 1981; 26:141-147.

4. Levi C, Gray JE, McCullough EC, Hattery RR. The unreliability of CT numbers as absolute values. AJR Am J Roentgenol 1982; 139:443-447.

5. Bosniak MA. The small (<3.0 cm) renal parenchymal tumor: detection, diagnosis and controversies. Radiology 1991; 179:307-317.

6. Klatzo I. Presidential address: neuropathological aspects of brain edema. J Neuropathol Exp Neurol 1967; 26:1-14.

7. Marks MP, Holmgren EB, Fox AJ, et al. Evaluation of early computed tomographic findings in acute ischemic stroke. Stroke 1999; 30:389-392.

8. Lev MH, Farkas J, Gemmente JJ, et al. Acute stroke: improved nonenhanced CT detection- benefits of soft-copy interpretation by using variable level and center window settings. Radiology 1999; 213:150-155.

9. Somford DM, Nederkoorn PJ, Rutgers DR, et al. Proximal and distal hyperattenuating middle cerebral artery signs at CT: different prognostic implications. Radiology 2002; 223:667-671.

10. Rutgers DR, van der Grond J, Jansen GH, et al. Radiologic-pathologic correlation of the hyperdense middle cerebral artery sign. Acta Radiol 2001; 42:467-469.

11. Zimmerman RA, Bilaniuk LT. Computed tomography of acute intratumoral hemorrhage. Radiology 1980; 135:355-359.

12. Ethofer T, Mader I, Seeger U, et al. Comparison of longitudinal metabolite relaxation times in different regions of the human brain at 1.5 tesla and 3 tesla. Magn Reson Med 2003; 50:1296-1301.

13. Stanisz GJ, Odrobina EE, Pun J, et al. T1, T2 relaxation and magnetization transfer in tissue at 3T. Magn Reson Med 2005; 54: 507-512.

14. Som PM, Dillon WP, Fullerton GD, et al. Chronically obstructed sinonasal secretions: observations on T1 and T2 shortening. Radiology 1989; 172:515-520.

15. Tsushima Y, Aoki J, Endo K. Brain microhemorrhages detected on T2*-weighted gradient echo MR images. AJNR Am J Neuroradiol 2003; 24:88-96.

16. Blitstein MK, Tung GA. MRI of cerebral microhemorrhages. AJR Am J Roentgenol 2007; 189:720-725.

17. Cakirer S, Karaarslan E, Arslan A. Spontaneously T1-hyperintense lesions of the brain on MRI: a pictorial review. Curr Probl Diagn Radiol 2003; 32:194-217.

18. Boyko OB, Burger PC, Shelburne JD, Ingram P. Non-heme mechanisms for T1 shortening: pathologic, MR and CT elucidation. AJNR Am J Neuroradiol 1992; 13:1439-1445.

19. Henkelman RM, Watts JF, Kucharczyk W. High signal intensity in MR images of calcified brain tissue. Radiology 1991; 179:199-206.

20. Hetts SW, Urban JP, Quinones-Hinojosa A, et al. The shading sign in cerebral squamous cell metastases. AJR Am J Roentgenol 2004; 182:1087-1088.

21. Machi J, Sigel B, Beitler JC, et al. Relation of in vivo blood flow to ultrasound echogenicity. J Clin Ultrasound 1983; 11:3-10.

22. Holland BA, Kucharcyzk W, Brant-Zawadzki M. MR imaging of calcified intracranial lesions. Radiology 1985; 157:353-356.

23. Tsuchiya K, Makita K, Furui S, Nitta K. MRI appearance of calcified lesions within intracranial tumors. Neuroradiology 1993; 35:341-344.

24. Shah ZK, Peh WCG, Koh WL, Shek TWH. Magnetic resonance imaging appearance of fibrous dysplasia. Br J Radiol 2005; 78:1104-1115.

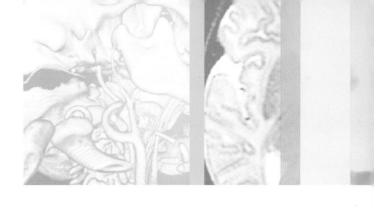

CHAPTER 4

Analysis of Mass Effect

Ellen E. Parker

Lesions or processes that cause *compression, distortion,* and/or *displacement* of intracranial contents may be said to have "mass effect." One important concept to understand is that mass effect is a manifestation on imaging of various intracranial processes (including tumor, hemorrhage, ischemia, and trauma) and not a diagnosis in itself. An analogy to clinical medicine is that vertigo is not a diagnosis in itself but rather a symptom with multiple possible underlying causes (such as posterior fossa infarct or vestibular abnormality). Detection and characterization of mass effect is a fundamental skill of neuroradiology. Accurate characterization of mass effect helps to precisely define the location of a lesion, which is crucial to forming an accurate differential diagnosis. In addition to diagnostic value, detection and prompt reporting of mass effect is also of great importance to the care of patients, especially those with life-threatening herniation. The goal of this chapter is to introduce key concepts and methods of analysis of mass effect to the beginning radiologist.

Prior to the advent of cross-sectional imaging, intracranial masses were localized and characterized by catheter angiography or other invasive techniques such as pneumoventriculography, pneumocisternography, and metrizamide ventriculography/cisternography.[1,2] CT and MRI are now the modalities of choice for evaluation of intracranial space-occupying lesions. Catheter angiography is now largely reserved for further characterization of and therapy for vascular intracranial lesions (e.g., preoperative evaluation and embolization of meningioma).

Although analysis of mass effect may be quantitative (e.g., measurement in centimeters of midline subfalcine herniation), mass effect is usually described in qualitative terms (e.g., severity of ventricular compression, hydrocephalus, sulcal effacement, obliteration of basal cisterns, or local tissue pressure effects).

Mass effect may be due to direct displacement of intracranial contents by discrete space-occupying lesions, such as benign and malignant neoplasms, non-neoplastic masses (e.g., arachnoid cyst), localized hemorrhage, or abscess. Mass effect may also be caused by brain swelling or *edema.* The pathophysiology of abnormal accumulation of fluid within the brain parenchyma is complex.[3] Edema may be described in terms of etiology (osmotic, hydrostatic, hyperemic), microscopic location (extracellular or intracellular), or macroscopic anatomic location (e.g., gray matter vs. white matter). In simple terms based on physical location with regard to cell membranes, brain edema may be classified as *vasogenic* (extracellular) or *cytotoxic* (intracellular).

Although these two descriptors of edema in reality often coexist and are not mutually exclusive, cerebral edema, on imaging, is often described as one or the other. In simple terms, cytotoxic edema demonstrates reduced diffusion (reduced apparent diffusion coefficient [ADC]) whereas vasogenic edema does not (normal or increased ADC). Cytotoxic edema is more prominently found in gray matter, whereas vasogenic edema is more prominent in white matter. The causes of cerebral edema are myriad. Examples include regional cytotoxic edema due to ischemic infarct, local or regional vasogenic edema associated with tumor or infection, post-traumatic edema, and generalized cerebral edema due to diffuse insult such as hypoxia/ischemia.[4]

According to the Monro-Kellie hypothesis, the intact calvaria creates a fixed intracranial space[5] that under normal conditions contains (1) *brain* (and its meningeal coverings), (2) *blood* (within vessels and dural venous sinuses), and (3) *cerebrospinal fluid* (within the subarachnoid space and ventricles).[6] Although the pathophysiology of intracranial pressure/volume relationships is indeed much more complex,[7] this basic understanding of the Monro-Kellie hypothesis is sufficient for the beginning radiologist. A corollary to this hypothesis for the radiologist is that under normal conditions the intracranial contents demonstrate a clearly defined midline with bilateral symmetry. Any disruption of this normal equilibrium (e.g., a space-occupying lesion and/or edema) may change the appearance of the contents of the intracranial space.

There are many factors contributing to mass effect. Some slow-growing large lesions may exhibit virtually no mass effect, whereas some small lesions may incite a surprisingly dramatic response.

ANATOMY

The discussion of analysis of mass effect may begin with a review of basic anatomic principles. Figure 4-1 presents a diagrammatic representation of the principles discussed here.

Brain Parenchyma: Gray and White Matter

The parenchyma of the brain may be divided into *gray matter,* consisting of unmyelinated neurons, and *white matter,* consisting of myelinated axons. The cortical mantles as well as deep nuclei of the cerebrum and cerebellum are composed of gray matter. White matter is characteristically located deep to the cortex and may be further described by location:

■ **FIGURE 4-1** Key anatomic concepts for discussion of mass effect.

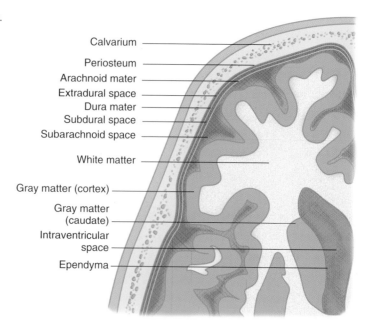

Calvarium
Periosteum
Arachnoid mater
Extradural space
Dura mater
Subdural space
Subarachnoid space
White matter
Gray matter (cortex)
Gray matter (caudate)
Intraventricular space
Ependyma

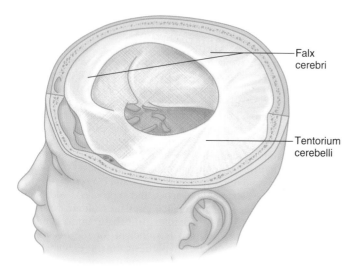

Falx cerebri

Tentorium cerebelli

■ **FIGURE 4-2** Gross specimen with dura retained in place to illustrate the falx cerebri and tentorium cerebelli. *(From Thibodeau GA, Patton KT. Anatomy and Physiology, 4th ed. St. Louis, Mosby, 1999, p 376.)*

subcortical, deep, and *periventricular.* The ventricles are lined by *ependyma.*

Meninges

The brain is held in place by the tough inelastic *dura mater* (also called *meninx fibrosa* or *pachymeninx* [plural, *pachymeninges*]), which under normal conditions is adherent to the periosteum of the inner surface of the calvaria. Reflections of the dura mater create fixed compartments within the intracranial space (Fig. 4-2). Named for its crescentic shape (L. *falx,* "sickle"), the *falx cerebri* separates the cerebral hemispheres along the interhemispheric fissure. The cerebrum and cerebellum are separated by the *tentorium cerebelli* (L. *tentorium,* "a shelter made of stretched skins"). The brain stem traverses an opening of the tentorium called the *tentorial incisura* (or *hiatus*).

The delicate *pia mater* and *arachnoid mater* comprise the *leptomeninges,* which cover the superficial cortical surfaces of the brain. The pia mater, adherent to the brain surface, follows the convolutions of the sulci and gyri. The arachnoid mater, external to the pia mater, covers the brain surface but follows the dural contours (i.e., it does not extend into the gyri and sulci). The reticulated inner surface of the arachnoid mater has fibers that intermingle with the surface of the pia. Free-flowing cerebrospinal fluid (CSF) is found in the *subarachnoid* space between the arachnoid mater and pia mater. Under normal conditions, the smooth outer surface of the arachnoid mater, overlying dura mater, and calvarial periosteum are in close approximation to each other with no discernible separation (i.e., the "subdural space" and "epidural space" are collapsed potential spaces).[8]

Localization as intra-axial or extra-axial is arguably the critical first step in evaluation of intracranial lesions.

Intra-axial versus Extra-axial

Lesions located within the brain parenchyma are termed *intraparenchymal* or *intra-axial.* It may be helpful for purposes of forming a differential diagnosis to further localize lesions with respect to gray and white matter. Lesions located external to the brain parenchyma are termed *extra-axial.*

Clues to the extra-axial location of a tumor (Fig. 4-3) may include displacement of pial vessels subjacent to the mass, buckling of the gray matter/white matter junction, widening of the adjacent subarachnoid space, a "cleft" of CSF between the brain parenchyma and the mass, a wide base along the dural or calvarial surface, and changes within the adjacent bone such as hyperostosis associated with meningioma (Fig. 4-4) or smooth scalloping associated with epidermoid (Fig. 4-5).[9,10]

Extra-axial lesions may be further characterized by their relationship to the meninges. Depending on the nature of the pathology, different descriptions for subdivisions of the extra-axial space may be used. Extra-axial intracranial *hemorrhage* may be described as subarachnoid, subdural, epidural, or intraventricular. Extra-axial intracranial *masses* are often described as intradural (rarely are they subdivided into subdural or subarachnoid categories), extradural, or intraventricular.

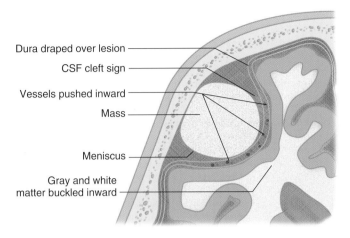

■ FIGURE 4-3 Clues to extra-axial location of a mass. *(From Grossman RI, Yousem DM [eds]. Neuroradiology Requisites. St. Louis, Mosby, 2004, p 275.)*

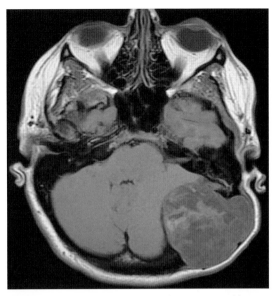

■ FIGURE 4-5 Posterior fossa epidermoid in a 40-year-old woman with palpable left occipital mass. Axial T1W noncontrast image demonstrates a heterogeneous extra-axial mass extending through the calvaria, with smooth scalloping of bone margins.

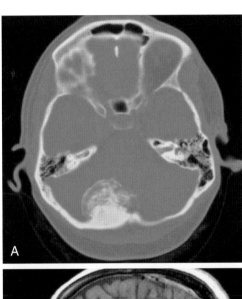

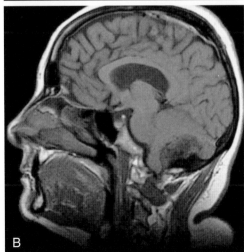

■ FIGURE 4-4 Posterior fossa meningioma in a 45-year-old woman with chronic headaches. **A,** Noncontrast CT (NCCT) demonstrates hyperostosis of the adjacent right occipital bone as well as calcification/ossification of the mass. **B,** Suggestion of hyperostosis and calcification (T1 lengthening) is evident on sagittal T1W precontrast MR image.

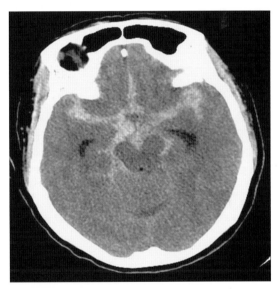

■ FIGURE 4-6 Acute subarachnoid hemorrhage in a 61-year-old woman with acute onset of headache and neck pain. NCCT demonstrates high density within the subarachnoid space, generalized cerebral edema with effacement of sulci, and early hydrocephalus with prominence of the temporal horns.

The *subarachnoid* space, between arachnoid and pia, normally contains CSF. The subarachnoid space (SAS) may be subdivided into the peripheral SAS and the basal cisterns. Subarachnoid hemorrhage may present as high density within these CSF spaces (Fig. 4-6). The *subdural* space, between dura and arachnoid, is normally a potential (collapsed) space. Subdural hematoma results from accumulation of blood products between the dura and arachnoid (Fig. 4-7). The dura is normally adherent to the periosteum of the inner table. Hematomas accumulating between the dura and periosteum are termed *epidural* or *extradural* (Fig. 4-8).

The *intraventricular space* (IVS) may also be considered a subdivision of the extra-axial compartment. The IVS contains CSF and choroid plexus and is lined by ependyma (in contrast to the peripheral SAS, which is lined by pia and arachnoid). Figure 4-9 demonstrates an intraventricular meningioma. CSF communicates between the IVS and SAS via the foramen of Luschka and choroid fissures.

TYPES OF HERNIATION

Under normal conditions, the brain rests within various compartments created by the rigid dural reflections just described. Brain swelling (cerebral edema) and/or discrete space-occupying lesions (e.g., tumor, hemorrhage) can cause parts of the brain at the margins of these dural reflections to be forced into another compartment. Damage to brain tissue may occur as a result of direct pressure of the herniating part against the dura, as a result of the herniating part causing pressure on another brain part (e.g., brain stem), or as a result of vascular damage as vessels are

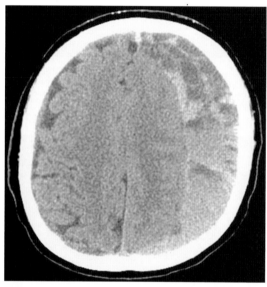

■ **FIGURE 4-7** Subdural hematoma in a 63-year-old man with altered mental status. NCCT demonstrates left holohemispheric crescentic mixed density fluid collection with compression and displacement of subjacent brain and effacement of sulci. On the right there is minimal dural thickening, but the dura is closely approximated to the calvarial periosteum.

compressed.[10-12] Prompt reporting of herniation may literally save a patient's life.

There are five classic descriptive patterns of herniation[10] (Fig. 4-10). Although these patterns are described as separate entities, different types of herniation may coexist in any given patient. In addition, please note that descriptions of these herniation syndromes slightly vary among authors.

1. *Subfalcine herniation* occurs when supratentorial mass effect is directed medially, causing the cingulate gyrus to shift below the falx cerebri. This is often reported as "midline shift" on CT examinations. The anterior cerebral arteries and internal cerebral veins may be compressed, causing infarcts. If the foramen of Monro is compressed, obstructive hydrocephalus involving one or both lateral ventricles may occur. This is often referred to as "entrapment" of the lateral ventricle(s). The lateral ventricle ipsilateral to the mass effect may be compressed (Fig. 4-11).

2. *Central caudal transtentorial herniation* occurs when supratentorial mass effect displaces the structures of the diencephalon (including the thalamus) and midbrain inferomedially. Obstructive hydrocephalus of the lateral and third ventricles may occur. *Duret's hemorrhage,* almost invariably an ominous sign, may occur within the midbrain and pontine tegmentum, presumably due to compression and shearing of perforating arterioles (Fig. 4-12).[13] Caudal transtentorial herniation usually occurs in the setting of bilateral uncal herniation.

3. *Temporal lobe (uncal) herniation* occurs when supratentorial mass effect displaces the temporal lobe medially and inferiorly over the medial free edge of the tentorium. (Note that some authors refer to this displacement of the uncus as "descending transtentorial herniation," not to be confused with central caudal transtentorial herniation of the thalamus and midbrain.) Uncal herniation may cause compression of the oculomotor nerve (cranial nerve III) with resultant ipsilateral pupillary dilatation, compression or occlusion of the posterior cerebral and anterior choroidal arteries leading to ischemic infarct in these territories, and midbrain compression. The suprasellar and perimesencephalic cisterns may be effaced (Fig. 4-13).

4. *Superior vermian transtentorial herniation* occurs when mass effect within the posterior fossa causes superior

■ **FIGURE 4-8** Acute epidural hematoma in a 6-month-old male infant with vomiting after a fall from a bed. **A** and **B,** NCCT of the brain reveals biconvex hyperdense hematoma with central low density overlying a subtle nondisplaced fracture of the squamous portion of the left temporal bone. Note normal appearance of the patent coronal and lambdoid sutures.

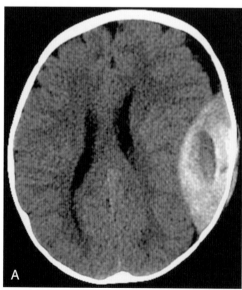

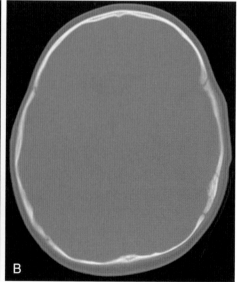

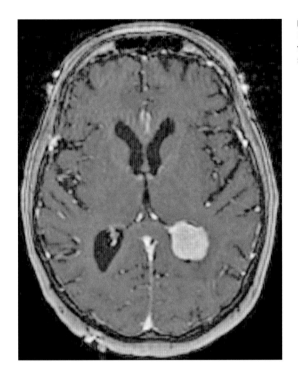

■ **FIGURE 4-9** Intraventricular meningioma in a 73-year-old woman with headache. Preoperative 3D FSPGR post-gadolinium MR image demonstrates an enhancing intraventricular mass, with subtle expansion of the trigone of the left lateral ventricle. Note subtle anterior displacement and enhancement of the choroid plexus.

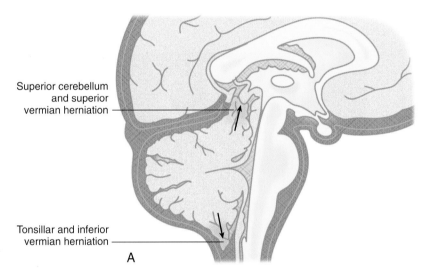

Superior cerebellum and superior vermian herniation

Tonsillar and inferior vermian herniation

A

■ **FIGURE 4-10** Herniations of the brain. **A,** Sagittal diagram of cerebellar herniation with the *upper arrow* demonstrating upward herniation of the superior cerebellum and superior vermis and the *lower arrow* demonstrating tonsillar and inferior vermian herniation. **B,** Coronal diagram, from the top downward, subfalcine herniation, central transtentorial herniation, downward transtentorial temporal lobe herniation and tonsillar herniation. Lines of force are demonstrated by the *arrows.* Note the pressure on the brain stem from these herniation patterns. *(From Grossman RI, Yousem DM. Neuroradiology Requisites. St. Louis, Mosby, 2004, p 261.)*

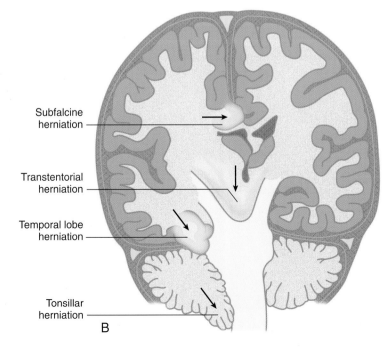

Subfalcine herniation

Transtentorial herniation

Temporal lobe herniation

Tonsillar herniation

B

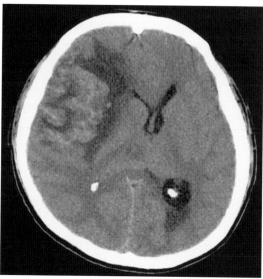

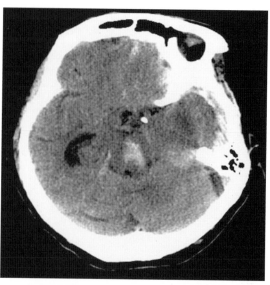

■ **FIGURE 4-11** Subfalcine herniation due to right middle cerebral artery infarct with hemorrhagic transformation in a 34-year-old man. Note compression of ipsilateral lateral ventricle and dilatation of the contralateral lateral ventricle due to entrapment.

■ **FIGURE 4-12** Duret's hemorrhage, due to compression or shearing of perforating arterioles with caudal transtentorial herniation, in an 80-year-old woman with altered mental status and blown right pupil. Also note traumatic left subdural hematoma and obstructive hydrocephalus.

■ **FIGURE 4-13** Isolated left uncal herniation due to glioblastoma multiforme in a 57-year-old man initially presenting with seizure. Effacement of the left perimesencephalic cistern and left aspect of the suprasellar cistern is apparent on NCCT (**A**) but is more conspicuous on MRI (**B** and **C**). Axial T2 MR image (**B**) more clearly shows the extent of mass-like T2 prolongation. Axial T1 FSPGR postcontrast image (**C**) shows the relatively small focus of enhancement in the setting of a much larger nonenhancing abnormality.

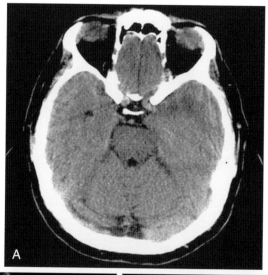

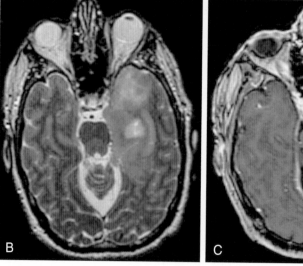

displacement of the vermis through the tentorial incisura, obliterating the superior vermian and quadrigeminal cisterns (Fig. 4-14). The midbrain and pons may be compressed. Obstructive hydrocephalus (typically involving the lateral and third ventricles) may occur if the cerebral aqueduct or fourth ventricle is compressed.[14,15]

5. Cerebellar (inferior tonsillar) herniation most commonly occurs when mass effect within the posterior fossa causes inferior displacement of the cerebellar tonsils through the foramen magnum (Fig. 4-15). This may cause compression of the cervicomedullary junction.[16] Mass effect within the posterior fossa may also cause compression of the fourth ventricle, with resultant obstructive hydrocephalus (typically involving the lateral and third ventricles). If the posterior inferior cerebellar arteries are compressed, cerebellar infarcts may occur.

Other types of herniation include *transalar* herniation and *transcalvarial* herniation.[12] Transalar (L. for "across the wing") refers to displacement of brain across the sphenoid wing or ridge. Transalar herniation may be "descending," involving posteroinferior displacement of the frontal lobe, with possible compromise of the middle cerebral artery, or "ascending," involving anterosuperior displacement of the temporal lobe, with possible compromise of the supraclinoid internal carotid artery. *Transcalvarial* (also known as *external calvarial, extracranial,* or *extracalvarial)* herniation occurs in the presence of an acquired, or much less commonly congenital, cranial defect, usually in the setting of a decompressive craniectomy (Fig. 4-16).

TECHNIQUES

Numerous techniques are available for detection and characterization of mass effect. The two primary imaging modalities, CT

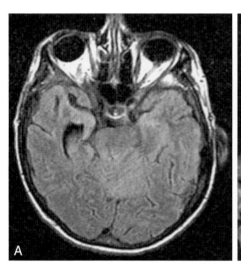
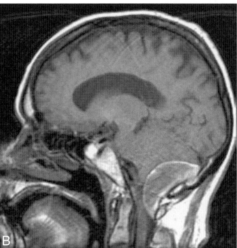

■ **FIGURE 4-14** Superior vermian transtentorial herniation due to posterior fossa epidural hematoma in a 57-year-old woman with new-onset somnolence and remote history of breast cancer. **A,** Axial FLAIR image demonstrates effacement of the superior vermian and quadrigeminal cisterns, with compression of the dorsal pons. **B,** Sagittal T1W MR image demonstrates the epidural hematoma as well as the cisternal effacement.

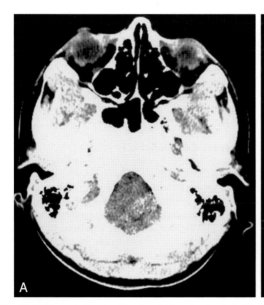
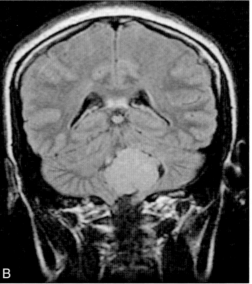

■ **FIGURE 4-15** Bilateral cerebellar tonsillar herniation due to choroid plexus papilloma in a 20-year-old woman presenting to the emergency department with headache. **A,** NCCT demonstrates crowding of the foramen magnum. **B,** Coronal FLAIR image shows downward displacement of the cerebellar tonsils due to a mass within the fourth ventricle.

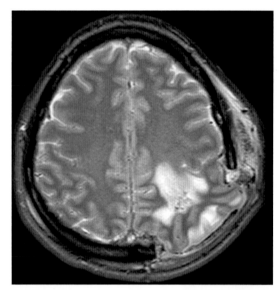

■ FIGURE 4-16 Transcalvarial herniation after decompressive craniectomy to relieve increased intracranial pressure due to left parietal venous infarct in a 19-year-old woman with postpartum dural venous sinus thrombosis. This type of herniation has sometimes been described as "fungal" owing to its mushroom-like appearance.

and MRI, are discussed here. Each modality has benefits as well as disadvantages. Selection of imaging studies for the care of any particular patient involves weighing risks and benefits in the context of that patient's needs.

CT

Noncontrast CT (NCCT) of the brain is an indispensable tool for neuroradiology. It is often the first examination performed for patients presenting with symptoms of increased intracranial pressure, such as nausea, vomiting, headache, and ataxia. NCCT is useful for detecting (or excluding) the "3 Hs": herniation, hemorrhage, and hydrocephalus. The ready availability and the rapidity of CT are very useful in critically ill patients, who may not tolerate either the wait for or duration of an MRI examination. In addition, CT is the study of choice for evaluation of features such as hyperostosis, bony erosion, and calcification.[17] NCCT is a useful tool for initial detection as well as for follow-up of certain pathologic processes.

Benefits of NCCT include relatively low cost, wide availability, rapid examination and interpretation, high sensitivity for acute intracranial hemorrhage, and excellent bone detail. Drawbacks to NCCT include the use of ionizing radiation, relatively poor soft tissue contrast compared with MRI, and artifacts within the posterior fossa.

In the setting of a negative NCCT of the brain, contrast-enhanced CT (CECT) is rarely indicated.[18,19] However, in patients with an abnormal brain NCCT, or a normal NCCT in certain clinical contexts, further investigation is usually required. Many indications for CECT of the brain have largely been replaced by MRI. However, CECT of the brain may be useful in the acute setting or for patients with contraindications to MRI. The utility of CECT must be weighed against the risks of ionizing radiation and iodinated contrast material.

MRI

With its excellent tissue contrast and characterization and multiplanar ability, MRI is superior to CT for precise intraparenchymal localization and is often superior to CT in defining extra-axial lesions as well. Lack of ionizing radiation is another benefit.

Gadolinium-diethylenetetraminepentaacetic acid (Gd-DTPA)–enhanced MRI has become the study of choice for evaluation of most space-occupying intracranial lesions. Gadolinium-enhanced MRI has been shown to be more sensitive for detection of metastases than enhanced CT, with multiple-dose gadolinium more sensitive than single-dose gadolinium.[20,21] However, recent recognition of a relationship of Gd-DTPA administration to an increased risk of development of nephrogenic systemic fibrosis presents a new challenge for imaging patients with impaired renal function.[22]

In addition to potential gadolinium complications, disadvantages of MRI (both contrast enhanced and noncontrast) include its relatively high cost, lesser availability, and longer acquisition time. The magnetic field presents a contraindication for patients with certain implants and pacemakers, as well as poses a safety hazard when ferromagnetic objects are introduced into the MRI suite.[23,24] A combination of these factors typically makes monitoring of critically ill patients more difficult during MRI than during CT.

ANALYSIS

One of the greatest challenges for the beginning radiologist is developing a comprehensive yet efficient search pattern for any particular study. A checklist of features that should be evaluated on every scan (CT and MRI) is provided. Although not inclusive of everything necessary to interpret studies, it provides a framework for developing a search pattern:

- Herniation
- Midline shift
- Effacement of ventricles, sulci, basilar cisterns, foramen magnum
- Hydrocephalus
- Hemorrhage
- Edema
- Bony changes

Noncontrast CT

Under normal conditions, axial NCCT images of the brain demonstrate a clearly defined midline with bilateral symmetry. The higher density of gray matter is easily differentiated from the lower density of white matter. CSF spaces (ventricles, sulci, basilar cisterns) demonstrate no effacement.

Manifestations of mass effect discernible on NCCT include displacement of brain parenchyma, low-density white matter edema, and effacement of sulci, ventricles, and basilar cisterns. Various herniation syndromes and their complications, such as ischemic infarct, may be diagnosed by NCCT. CT is the study of choice for evaluation of fine bony detail. Hyperostosis (e.g., meningioma) as well as scalloping and thinning (e.g., epidermoid) are usually better demonstrated on CT than MRI (see Fig. 4-4).

Contrast-Enhanced CT

Although indications for CECT have largely been supplanted by MRI, CECT is still commonly performed. Abnormal contrast enhancement of intracranial lesions increases their conspicuity. In addition, *normal* contrast enhancement of vascular structures may increase conspicuity of otherwise subtle or confusing intracranial lesions. For example, subdural hematoma may be more easily differentiated from brain parenchyma when the cortical veins are opacified (Fig. 4-17).

MRI

With its multiplanar capability and superior soft tissue contrast, MRI has largely replaced CT as the imaging modality of choice for evaluation of intracranial mass lesions.

The superior soft tissue contrast of MRI allows for more precise localization of both intra-axial and extra-axial lesions. In addition, the relationships of intracranial masses to vital structures (e.g., the relationship of parasagittal meningioma to the dural venous sinuses) are usually better evaluated on MRI. Herniation and hydrocephalus are readily identified

and evaluated. Extent of edema (manifest as FLAIR and T2 hyperintensity) is also well demonstrated. Although also sometimes discernible on CT, different degrees of mass effect (focal, local, and regional) are optimally evaluated by MRI (Figs. 4-18 to 4-20).

Sample reports are presented in Boxes 4-1 and 4-2.

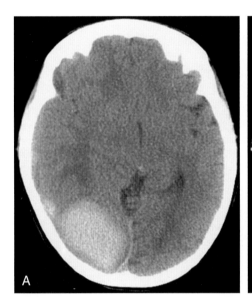 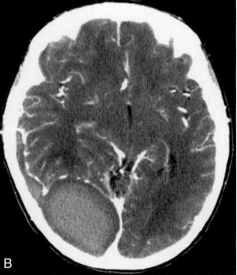

■ **FIGURE 4-17** Right parieto-occipital hematoma in a 20-year-old coagulopathic comatose woman with multisystem organ failure. **A,** NCCT reveals high density consistent with blood products. Localization of the hematoma as intra-axial or extra-axial is difficult on NCCT. **B,** CECT demonstrates displacement of cortical veins and buckling of cortex, clearly identifying the hematoma as extra-axial. Also note subfalcine herniation and generalized cerebral edema with sulcal effacement.

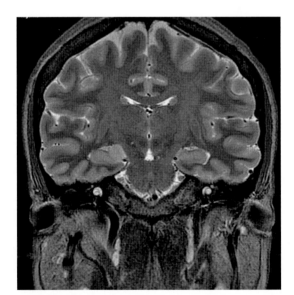

■ **FIGURE 4-18** Focal mass effect in a 30-year-old woman with seizures. Coronal T2W inversion recovery image reveals a focal mass, isointense to cortex, arising from the fimbria of the right hippocampus, with focal mass effect effacing the right choroid fissure. This mass was stable over 18 months of follow-up and is presumed to represent a low-grade glioma or hamartoma. Note lack of edema and lack of displacement of adjacent brain parenchyma.

BOX 4-1   Sample Report: Noncontrast CT of the Brain

PATIENT HISTORY

A 6-month-old presented after a fall.

COMPARISON STUDIES

None was available.

TECHNIQUE

CT with 5-mm contiguous transaxial images was performed from the skull base to the vertex without intravenous administration of a contrast agent (see Fig. 4-8).

FINDINGS

A left convexity extra-axial hemorrhagic collection, with lentiform shape, was found, suggestive of epidural hematoma. The hematoma demonstrates mixed densities, consistent with acute to subacute stage. There is an associated nondisplaced left temporal bone fracture involving the squamous portion. No other areas of hemorrhage are seen. The epidural hematoma exerts mass effect on the adjacent brain parenchyma. One centimeter of left-to-right midline shift is present. No areas of vascular infarct are evident. The gray matter/white matter differentiation is preserved.

IMPRESSION

A left convexity epidural hematoma measuring 3 cm transverse, with associated nondisplaced left temporal bone fracture involving the squamous portion, exerts mass effect on the adjacent frontotemporal lobe, with 1 cm of left-to-right subfalcine herniation.

■ **FIGURE 4-19** A 32-year-old woman presented with left-sided weakness. Axial FLAIR (**A**) and coronal T1W postcontrast (**B**) MR images demonstrate an expansile mass centered within the left insula, with minimal if any enhancement. At surgery, pathologic process was grade 2 astrocytoma. Note subtle local mass effect on the adjacent brain parenchyma but no edema and no subfalcine, uncal, or descending transtentorial herniation (compare with patient in Fig. 4-20). **C,** Axial T2W MR image from the same patient 19 years earlier; she underwent MRI at 13 years old for workup of dizziness. Note the subtle asymmetric T2 prolongation within the left insular cortex and subinsular white matter.

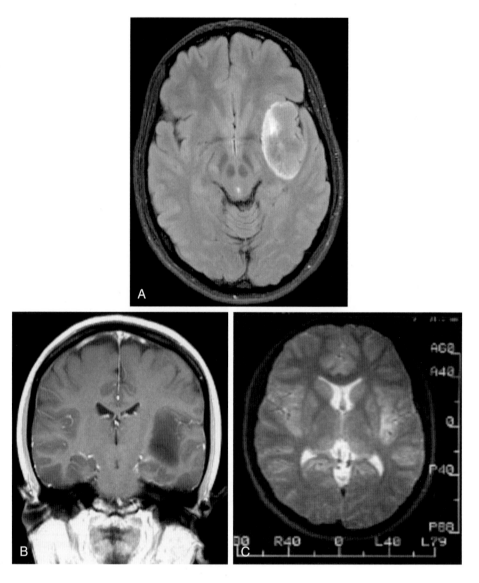

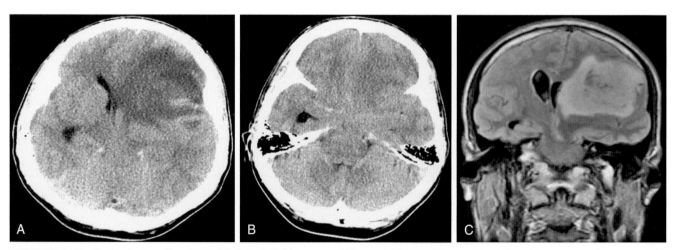

■ **FIGURE 4-20** Regional mass effect due to left frontal glioblastoma multiforme. A 31-year-old man presented to the emergency department with headache. NCCT images (**A** and **B**) and coronal FLAIR MR image (**C**) demonstrate a heterogeneous left frontal mass with subfalcine, uncal, and descending transtentorial herniation as well as entrapment of the left lateral ventricle.

BOX 4-2 Sample Report: MRI of the Brain

PATIENT HISTORY

A 53-year-old man presented with seizure and abnormal NCCT.

COMPARISON STUDY

NCCT of brain was done, but there was no previous MRI.

TECHNIQUE

The following sequences were used to image the brain on a 1.5-T magnet with fiducial markers in position: sagittal FSPGR, axial diffusion, axial FLAIR, axial 3D SPGR postcontrast and postcontrast axial 3D FSE T2 (see Fig. 4-13).

CONTRAST AGENT

Magnevist, 14 mL (0.1 mmol/kg; 0.2 mL/kg)

FINDINGS

An extensive amount of abnormal T2 prolongation and associated mass effect are identified within the mesial left temporal lobe with involvement of the left hippocampus and extension into the left parahippocampal gyrus. A more focal area of slightly less T2 prolongation is centered in the left hippocampus where irregular enhancement is noted after administration of the contrast agent. The remainder of the T2 abnormality is nonenhancing. This abnormal enhancement extends along the ependymal surface of the adjacent left temporal horn. There is associated uncal herniation and midbrain compression without evidence of transtentorial herniation. The ventricles are normal in size without hydrocephalus.

Several scattered foci of subcortical T2 prolongation are noted bilaterally, most likely representing small vessel ischemic disease. There are no areas of reduced diffusion to suggest acute ischemia. The major intracranial vessels are patent.

IMPRESSION

There is extensive abnormal T2 prolongation and associated mass effect within the left mesiotemporal lobe consistent with an infiltrative neoplasm. A more focal area of slightly less T2 prolongation centered in the left hippocampus is associated with irregular enhancement and is highly suggestive of an area of anaplastic transformation. Abnormal enhancement also extends along the ependyma of the adjacent right temporal horn.

KEY POINTS

■ Mass effect causes compression, displacement, or distortion of intracranial structures.

■ NCCT is a useful tool for screening or follow-up of mass effect.

■ CE MRI is the imaging study of choice for definitive characterization of intracranial masses.

SUGGESTED READINGS

Andrews PJ, Citerio G. Intracranial pressure: I. Historical overview and basic concepts. Intensive Care Med 2004; 30:1730-1733.

Citerio G, Andrews PJ. Intracranial pressure: II. Clinical applications and technology. Intensive Care Med 2004; 30:1882-1885.

Fisher CM. Brain herniation: a revision of classical concepts. Can J Neurol Sci 1995; 22:83-91.

Johnson PL, Eckard DA, et al. Imaging of acquired cerebral herniations. Neuroimaging Clin North Am 2002; 12:217-228.

Neff S, Subramaniam RP. Monro-Kellie doctrine. J Neurosurg 1996; 85:1195.

REFERENCES

1. Haddad FS, Hajjar J. [Pneumoventriculography in the localization of intracranial tumors]. Rev Med Moyen Orient 1956; 13:77-78.
2. Roberson GH, Taveras JM, Tadmor R, et al. Computed tomography in metrizamide cisternography—importance of coronal and axial views. J Comput Assist Tomogr 1977; 1:241-245.
3. Marmarou A, Signoretti S, Aygok G, et al. Traumatic brain edema in diffuse and focal injury: cellular or vasogenic? Acta Neurochir Suppl 2006; 96:24-29.
4. Marmarou A. A review of progress in understanding the pathophysiology and treatment of brain edema. Neurosurg Focus 2007; 22:E1.
5. Monro A. Observations on Structure and Functions of the Nervous System. Edinburgh, Creech and Johnson, 1783.
6. Mokri B. The Monro-Kellie hypothesis: applications in CSF volume depletion. Neurology 2001; 56:1746-1748.
7. Lakin WD, Stevens SA, Tranmer BI, Penar PL. A whole-body mathematical model for intracranial pressure dynamics. J Math Biol 2003; 46:347-383.
8. Greenberg RW, Lane EL, Cinnamon J, et al. The cranial meninges: anatomic considerations. Semin Ultrasound CT MR 1994; 15:454-465
9. Young RJ, Knopp EA. Brain MRI: tumor evaluation. J Magn Reson Imaging 2006; 24:709-724.
10. Grossman RI, Yousem DM. Neuroradiology: The Requisites, 2nd ed. Philadelphia, Mosby, 2003.
11. Castillo M. Neuroradiology: Core Curriculum. Philadelphia, Lippincott Williams & Wilkins, 2002.
12. Laine FJ, Shedden AI, Dunn MM, Ghatak NR. Acquired intracranial herniations: MR imaging findings. AJR Am J Roentgenol 1995; 165:967-973.
13. Parizel PM, Makkat S, Jorens PG, et al. Brainstem hemorrhage in descending transtentorial herniation (Duret hemorrhage). Intensive Care Med 2002; 28:85-88.
14. Hahn FJ, Witte RJ. CT signs of ascending transtentorial cerebellar herniation. J Comput Assist Tomogr 1989; 13:1091-1092.
15. Cuneo RA, Caronna JJ, Pitts L, et al. Upward transtentorial herniation: seven cases and a literature review. Arch Neurol 1979; 36:618-623.
16. Ishikawa M, Kikuchi H, Fujisawa I, Yonekawa Y. Tonsillar herniation on magnetic resonance imaging. Neurosurgery 1988; 22:77-81.

17. Loevner LA. Imaging features of posterior fossa neoplasms in children and adults. Semin Roentgenol 1999; 34:84-101.

18. Chishti FA, Al Saeed OM, Al-Khawari H, Shaikh M. Contrast-enhanced cranial computed tomography in magnetic resonance imaging era. Med Princ Pract 2003; 12:248-251.

19. Branson HM, Doria AS, Moineddin R, Shroff MM. The brain in children: is contrast enhancement really needed after obtaining normal unenhanced CT results? Radiology 2007; 244:838-844.

20. Kuhn MJ, Hammer GM, Swenson LC, et al. MRI evaluation of "solitary" brain metastases with triple-dose gadoteridol: comparison with contrast-enhanced CT and conventional-dose gadopentetate dimeglumine MRI studies in the same patients. Comput Med Imaging Graph 1994; 18:391-399.

21. Akeson P, Larsson EM, Kristoffersen DT, et al. Brain metastases—comparison of gadodiamide injection–enhanced MR imaging at standard and high dose, contrast-enhanced CT and non-contrast-enhanced MR imaging. Acta Radiol 1995; 36:300-306.

22. Broome DR, Girguis MS, Baron PW, et al. Gadodiamide-associated nephrogenic systemic fibrosis: why radiologists should be concerned. AJR Am J Roentgenol 2007; 188:586-592.

23. Price RR. The AAPM/RSNA physics tutorial for residents. MR imaging safety considerations. Radiological Society of North America. RadioGraphics 1999; 19:1641-1651.

24. Colletti PM. Size "H" oxygen cylinder: accidental MR projectile at 1.5 Tesla. J Magn Reson Imaging 2004; 19:141-143.

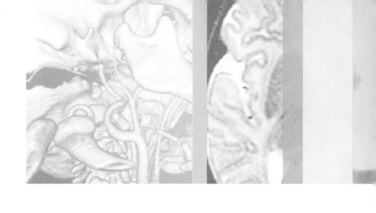

CHAPTER 5

Patterns of Contrast Enhancement

James G. Smirniotopoulos, Alice B. Smith, John H. Rees, and Frances M. Murphy

Contrast material has been essential to cross-sectional neuroimaging for almost 4 decades. The first intravascular contrast agents were U.S. Food and Drug Administration (FDA)–approved urographic and angiographic iodine-based compounds for parenteral injection. Modern iodine-based agents for CT are now usually low- and iso-osmolar compounds designed to lower the frequency of side effects and provide a higher safety margin. Multiple gadolinium-based contrast agents have been developed, and six have been approved by the FDA for intravascular injection for contrast-enhanced MRI: Vasovist Injection; Magnevist; MultiHance; Omniscan; OptiMARK; and ProHance.

In the central nervous system (CNS) contrast enhancement is produced by two related, yet independent, processes: interstitial (extravascular) enhancement and vascular (intravascular) enhancement.[1,2] The brain, spinal cord, and nerves are supplied by capillaries that have a selectively permeable membrane that creates a "blood-brain barrier." This selective barrier protects the nervous system from certain plasma proteins and limits inflammation by blocking inflammatory cells from entering the tissue. The primary structure of the blood-brain barrier is from endothelial cell specialization produced by cooperation between these cells and the astrocyte foot processes. The normal blood-brain barrier includes a continuous basement membrane, narrow intercellular gaps with junctional complexes, and only rare pinocytosis. The normal intact blood-brain barrier is far more permeable to lipophilic compounds (as measured by octanol/water partition fraction), and the blood-brain barrier retards lipophobic compounds. Some "desirable" compounds, such as glucose, are facilitated to cross the vessel wall or are actively transported out of the vessel and into the tissue compartment. Vascular enhancement is a combined product of blood volume, blood flow (delivery of contrast agent or "wash-in"), and "mean transit time" or time needed for "washout" of a contrast agent. In addition to neovascularity, which increases both blood volume and blood flow, vasodilatation of existing normal vessels (hyperemia) produces increased intravascular enhancement.

Parenteral contrast material is usually injected into a large peripheral vein, either slowly by a drip infusion or more rapidly by a short duration or bolus injection. A pressure injector may be used. When a contrast agent is injected as a bolus, the blood level rapidly rises to a peak concentration that pushes the contrast agent against the capillary endothelial membrane. If that capillary membrane is permeable to the contrast agent, it will rapidly leave the vessel and diffuse into the perivascular interstitial fluid space, driven by the concentration gradient. The higher the gradient, the greater the diffusion out of the vessel; thus, giving a double or triple dose of a contrast agent will increase enhancement. The spinal cord, brain, and spinal nerves have specialized capillary vessels with a blood-brain barrier, giving them special properties of selective permeability. Extravascular or interstitial enhancement will also depend on the permeability of these capillaries to the chosen agent. If you "choose wisely," enhancement will occur only in tissues without an intact blood-brain barrier. Interstitial enhancement is related to alterations in the permeability of the blood-brain barrier, whereas intravascular enhancement is proportional to increases in blood flow or blood volume. On CT, intravascular and interstitial enhancement may be seen simultaneously. When rapid dynamic CT images are obtained, as in CT angiography, most of the observed enhancement is intravascular. When CT is delayed for 10 to 15 minutes after a bolus infusion, most of the observed enhancement is interstitial. At intermediate times, or with a continuous drip infusion of contrast material, enhancement is a composite variable mixture of both intravascular and interstitial compartments.

MRI after administration of a contrast agent has several important differences, as compared with CT enhancement. Many MR pulse sequences create a "flow void phenomena"; thus, high-flow lesions such as aneurysms and vascular shunts (e.g., arteriovenous malformations) will have very low signal intensity.[3] The aneurysmal dilation of the vein of Galen, dural and pial fistulas, and the more common arteriovenous malformations will show as spherical, tubular, or serpentine signal voids.

The enhancement on MRI from blood-brain barrier breakdown and leakage of gadolinium out of the vessel requires a substrate of mobile water. Relative "dry" tissues, such as bone and normal dura, have very little interstitial free water. These tissues do not enhance well with gadolinium on routine T1-weighted (T1W) MR images—the gadolinium is in the tissues, but we cannot see a signal change without the water. This can be confusing, for example, when comparing an enhanced CT scan in which the falx and tentorium are brightly enhanced with an MR image in which there is only patchy and discontinuous enhancement.

Many different physiologic and pathologic conditions demonstrate contrast enhancement. Angiogenesis and neovascularity in neoplastic masses, breakdown of the blood-brain barrier in both infectious and noninfectious inflammation, physiologic changes from cerebral ischemia, and capillary pressure overload (eclampsia and hypertension) will all affect the blood-brain barrier and increase permeability. A paralysis of autoregulation—the primary cause of "malignant brain edema"—is actually a reactive hyperemia and will enhance on MRI, CT, and even at angiography. The newly created vessels from tumor angiogenesis will increase both blood volume and blood flow as compared with contralateral normal brain tissue. There will also be a short mean transit time.

All of these processes can produce enhancement on conventional angiograms, conventional T1W gadolinium-enhanced MR images, and iodine-enhanced CT scans. The old-fashioned "early draining vein" on the arteriogram is a direct correlate of the shortened mean transit time that can be calculated on perfusion MR and CT examinations.

EXTRA-AXIAL ENHANCEMENT

Extra-axial enhancement in the CNS may be classified as either pachymeningeal or leptomeningeal. The pachymeninges (from the Greek for "thick" meninges) are the dura mater, which comprises two fused membranes derived from the embryonic meninx primativa: the periosteum of the inner table of the skull and a meningeal layer. Pachymeningeal enhancement may be manifested up against the bone, or it may involve the dural reflections of the falx cerebri, tentorium cerebelli, falx cerebelli, and cavernous sinus. The leptomeninges (Greek for "skinny" meninges) are the pia and arachnoid. Leptomeningeal enhancement may occur on the surface of the brain or in the subarachnoid space. Because the normal, thin arachnoid membrane is attached to the inner surface of the dura mater, the pachymeningeal pattern of enhancement is also described as *dura-arachnoid enhancement* (Fig. 5-1). In comparison, enhancement on the surface of the brain is called pial or *pia-arachnoid enhancement*. The enhancement follows along the pial surface of the

brain and fills the subarachnoid spaces of the sulci and cisterns. This pattern is often referred to as leptomeningeal enhancement and is usually described as having a "gyriform" or "serpentine" appearance.

Pachymeningeal or Dura-Arachnoid Enhancement

Because the vessels supplying the dura do not have a blood-brain barrier, both endogenous and exogenous compounds (e.g., albumin, hemosiderin, contrast agents) readily leak into the interstitial space. Enhancement of the dura is normal on CT, typically uniform in the falx and tentorium. Enhancement of the dura against the skull is not readily noticed because of the adjacent dense white line of the cortical bone of the inner table of the skull. In contrast, on contrast-enhanced T1W MR images, the normal dura shows only thin, linear, and discontinuous enhancement.[4]

A variety of processes may accentuate dural enhancement, including vasocongestion and intradural edema, both of which may be nonspecific reactions to a wide variety of benign or malignant processes, including transient postoperative changes, intracranial hypotension (Fig. 5-2), neoplasms such as meningiomas, metastatic disease (from breast and prostate cancer), secondary CNS lymphoma, and granulomatous disease. Because of the Monro-Kellie doctrine,[5] when the cerebrospinal fluid pressure drops, there may be secondary fluid shifts that increase the volume of capacitance veins in the subarachnoid space. After neurosurgical intervention, even the placement of a shunt catheter or intracranial pressure bolt, meningeal enhancement is very frequent and occurs in a majority of patients. The postoperative enhancement may be pachymeningeal (dura-arachnoid) or leptomeningeal (pia-arachnoid)[6] and can be localized to the side of the procedure or diffuse (bilateral, supratentorial and infratentorial). Extra-axial enhancement may also occur after uncomplicated lumbar puncture in about 5% of patients.[7] Patients with spontaneous intracranial hypotension, with or

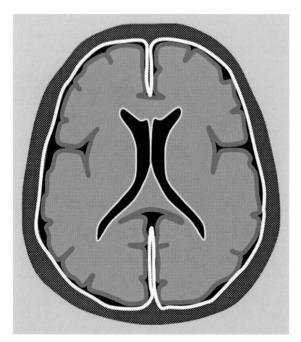

■ **FIGURE 5-1** Schematic diagram of dura-arachnoid enhancement on MRI. This is also called pachymeningeal enhancement. *(From Smirniotopoulos JG, Murphy FM, Rushing EJ, et al. Patterns of contrast enhancement in the brain and meninges. RadioGraphics 2007; 27:525-551.)*

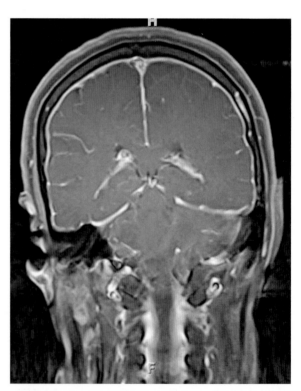

■ **FIGURE 5-2** Coronal T1W MR gadolinium-enhanced image of idiopathic intracranial hypotension. There is diffuse, smooth, and linear dura-arachnoid enhancement. Although veins may also enhance normally, there should be no other subarachnoid enhancement.

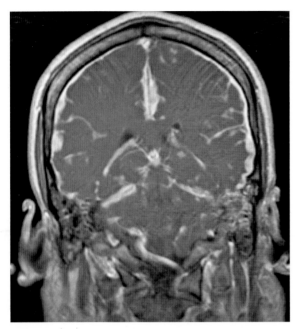

■ **FIGURE 5-3** Coronal T1W MR gadolinium-enhanced image of dural sarcoid. There is grossly abnormal diffuse thickening and enhancement of the dura including both the falx and the tentorium.

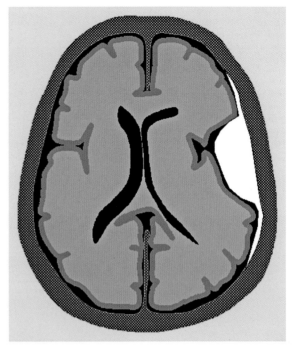

■ **FIGURE 5-4** Schematic diagram of dural-based enhancement limited to a mass growing against the inner table of the skull. This is a typical pattern for a meningioma, with linear tapering enhancement from the "dural tail." *(From Smirniotopoulos JG, Murphy FM, Rushing EJ, et al. Patterns of contrast enhancement in the brain and meninges. RadioGraphics 2007; 27:525-551.)*

without a cerebrospinal fluid leak, may show generalized diffuse pachymeningeal enhancement.[4,8,9] Prolonged intracranial hypotension may lead to vasocongestion and interstitial edema in the dura mater, findings similar to those seen in the dural tail of a meningioma. Rarely, a skull fracture may cause a cerebrospinal fluid leak and intracranial hypotension. More often intracranial hypotension may be related to a (seemingly) uncomplicated lumbar puncture. However, in most cases no definitive cause is ever found, and it is described as "idiopathic" intracranial hypotension.

MRI is relatively sensitive and specific in the detection of benign or spontaneous intracranial hypotension. A typical clinical feature of spontaneous intracranial hypotension is a headache that is orthostatic (postural) and worse when the patient is upright. Imaging findings include thickened dura with linear enhancement of the pachymeninges both above and below the tentorium, no enhancement of the sulci or brain surface, enlargement of the pituitary gland, and descent of the brain (low cerebellar tonsils and downward displacement of the iter of the third ventricle below the tentorial incisura line).[9] Some patients may have additional features of subdural effusions or even subdural hemorrhage. Other features of intracranial hypotension include dural thickening and an enlarged pituitary gland. Leptomeningeal enhancement (within the sulci) may be seen postoperatively but is not common with spontaneous intracranial hypotension and could suggest leptomeningitis, either inflammatory or neoplastic.

Extra-axial neoplasms may produce pachymeningeal enhancement. The most common primary dural neoplasm is meningioma, a benign tumor of meningothelial cells (Figs. 5-3 and 5-4). Meningiomas are slow-growing, well-localized, World Health Organization (WHO) grade 1 lesions that are usually resectable for cure.[10-12] They typically manifest in patients in the fourth to sixth decades of life, and they are roughly twice as common in women as in men. The typical meningioma is a localized lesion with a broad base of dural attachment (see Fig. 5-5B). This neoplasm actually arises from the arachnoid membrane that is attached to the inner layer of the dura mater. Even in the early days of CT, the accuracy of cross-sectional imaging in the

detection and characterization of meningioma was very good.[13] Contrast-enhanced MRI demonstrates a new finding (one not observed at CT): the dural tail or "dural flare." The dural tail is a curvilinear region of dural enhancement adjacent to the bulky hemispheric tumor (Figs. 5-5 to 5-7; see also Fig. 5-4).[14-16] The finding was originally thought to represent dural infiltration by tumor, and resection of all enhancing dura mater was thought to be appropriate.[17] Several studies have confirmed that in most cases of meningioma, linear dural enhancement is most likely a reactive process[18] rather than neoplastic, especially when it was more than a centimeter away from the bulky part of the tumor. The dural reaction may include a combination of increased extravascular spaces as well as small vessel vasocongestion. Both will thicken the dura, and the increased interstitial water allows visualization of contrast enhancement (see Fig. 5-5) because even normal dural capillaries do not form a blood-brain barrier. In addition to primary dural neoplasms, such as meningioma, hemangiopericytoma, and solitary fibrous tumor, metastases are possible. In women, breast carcinoma can cause a solitary dural metastasis; and in men, prostate cancer can do the same. Secondary CNS lymphoma is usually extra-axial and may be dural based or fill the subarachnoid space. Granulomatous inflammatory and infectious diseases including sarcoid, tuberculosis, Wegener's granulomatosus, luetic gummas, rheumatoid nodules, and fungal disease produce pachymeningeal enhancement usually involving the basilar meninges, including the suprasellar cistern and vessels of the circle of Willis. Sarcoid may produce focal or diffuse dural thickening (see Fig. 5-3).

Leptomeningeal or Pia-Arachnoid Enhancement

When the abnormal enhancement extends into the subarachnoid spaces of the sulci and cisterns it is called leptomeningeal or "pia-arachnoid" enhancement. Bacterial, viral, and even fungal meningitides may cause leptomeningeal enhancement (Fig. 5-8). The primary mechanism for this enhancement is a breakdown

■ **FIGURE 5-5** Axial (**A**) and coronal (**B**) T1W MR gadolinium-enhanced images of a meningioma. There is a brightly enhancing dural-based mass with a hemispheric shape. A long area of tapering linear enhancement—"dural tail"—extends away from the central bulky mass. Most of this linear enhancement is reactive rather than neoplastic. Axial T2W (**C**) and FLAIR (**D**) images show clearly that the lesion is extra-axial.

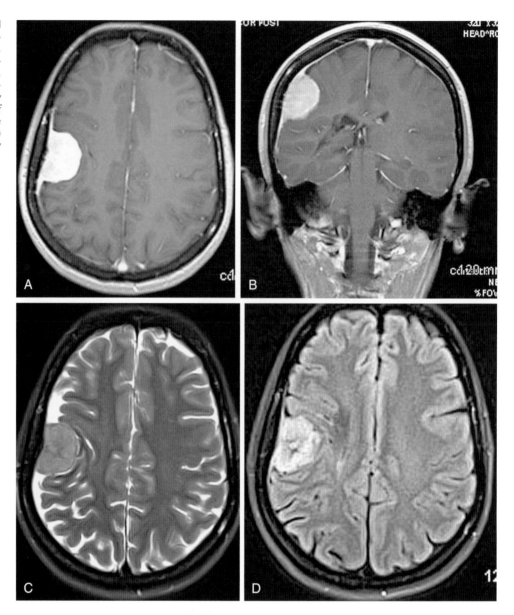

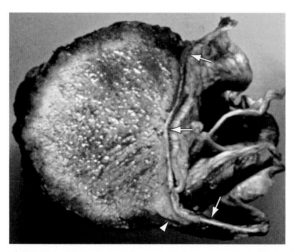

■ **FIGURE 5-6** Meningioma. The specimen has been cut in half, showing a hemispheric mass affixed to the underlying dura (*arrows*). There is a "claw" of tumor growing along the dura (*arrowhead*). However, the enhancement seen on MRI was far more extensive. *(From Smirniotopoulos JG, Murphy FM, Rushing EJ, et al. Patterns of contrast enhancement in the brain and meninges. RadioGraphics 2007; 27:525-551.)*

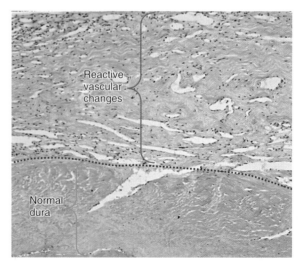

■ **FIGURE 5-7** Meningioma. Dural tail (H&E, original magnification, ×250). The lower half shows normal dura mater—mostly collagen. Vascular reactive changes and venous congestion, along with interstitial edema, contribute to contrast enhancement. *(From Smirniotopoulos JG, Murphy FM, Rushing EJ, et al. Patterns of contrast enhancement in the brain and meninges. RadioGraphics 2007; 27:525-551.)*

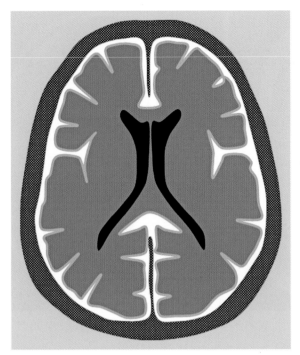

■ FIGURE 5-8 Schematic of pia-arachnoid (subarachnoid) enhancement. The contrast material fills the subarachnoid space and enters the sulci between the cerebral and cerebellar gyri. This pattern occurs in both bacterial meningitis and cerebrospinal fluid dissemination of neoplasms—"carcinomatous" meningitis. *(From Smirniotopoulos JG, Murphy FM, Rushing EJ, et al. Patterns of contrast enhancement in the brain and meninges. RadioGraphics 2007; 27:525-551.)*

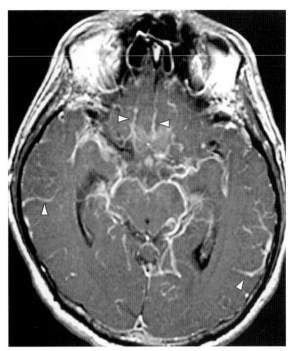

■ FIGURE 5-9 Axial T1W MR gadolinium-enhanced image of bacterial meningitis. There is diffuse linear superficial (pial) enhancement in the subarachnoid space, extending into sulci (*arrowheads*) and along the surface of the midbrain. *(From Smirniotopoulos JG, Murphy FM, Rushing EJ, et al. Patterns of contrast enhancement in the brain and meninges. RadioGraphics 2007; 27:525-551.)*

of the blood-brain barrier of the pial vessels themselves. In bacterial meningitis, glycoproteins released by bacteria cause breakdown of the blood-brain barrier and allow contrast material to leak from vessels into the cerebrospinal fluid. Bacterial and viral meningitis exhibit enhancement that is typically thin and linear (Figs. 5-9 and 5-10).[19] Some cases of fungal meningitis may produce nodular or "lumpy" enhancement.

Neoplasms that disseminate by spreading into the subarachnoid space—"carcinomatous meningitis"—also produce enhancement of the brain surface and subarachnoid space (Fig. 5-11). Primary brain tumors that reach the ventricular or pial surface may spread this way, including medulloblastoma, ependymoma, choroid plexus papilloma/carcinoma, glioblastoma, germinoma, and oligodendroglioma, as well as secondary tumors (e.g., lymphoma and breast cancer. We expect neoplastic disease in the subarachnoid space to produce thicker, lumpy, or nodular enhancement, similar to that of fungal disease. However, despite this logic, neoplastic meningitis can appear surprisingly thin and linear.

The clinical presentation should suggest an infectious cause with fever and meningismus. Spinal tap and cerebrospinal fluid sampling may reveal a reactive pleocytosis, and cerebrospinal fluid cultures may demonstrate the organism. Viral meningitis may be "culture negative," "aseptic," or "sterile." Normal cranial nerves never enhance within the subarachnoid space, and such enhancement is always abnormal. Viral encephalitis (as well as sarcoidosis) may also produce linear enhancement of the cranial nerves. Primary nerve sheath tumors (e.g., schwannoma) may show nerve enhancement in the subarachnoid space, but in the form of a lump or mass enlarging the nerve.

INTRA-AXIAL ENHANCEMENT

Intra-axial enhancement of the brain and spinal cord is never normal. There must be a vascular structure or a breakdown in

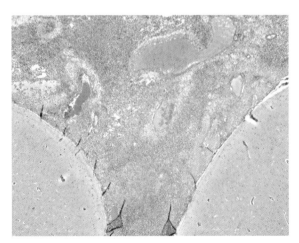

■ FIGURE 5-10 *Streptococcus pneumoniae* meningitis (H&E, original magnification, ×400). There is a dense inflammatory infiltrate along the surface of the brain that fills the subarachnoid space. *(From Smirniotopoulos JG, Murphy FM, Rushing EJ, et al. Patterns of contrast enhancement in the brain and meninges. RadioGraphics 2007; 27:525-551.)*

the blood-brain barrier. An abnormal increase in permeability may be reactive (gliosis), inflammatory (multiple sclerosis), infectious (encephalitis or abscess), and neoplastic. Intravascular enhancement may occur with developmental venous anomalies and cavernous malformations. Intravascular enhancement requires special MR pulse sequences, because of the "flow-void" effect of moving blood.

Gyral Enhancement

Gyral enhancement—along the surface of the brain—is almost always vascular or inflammatory and only rarely neoplastic

■ **FIGURE 5-11** Carcinomatous meningitis. This patient has diffuse subarachnoid spread of medulloblastoma. Axial contrast-enhanced CT scan (**A**) and axial T1W MR gadolinium-enhanced image (**B**) both show abnormal yet linear enhancement in the sulci of the cerebellum, forming a coating around the brain stem. *(From Smirniotopoulos JG, Murphy FM, Rushing EJ, et al. Patterns of contrast enhancement in the brain and meninges. RadioGraphics 2007; 27:525-551.)*

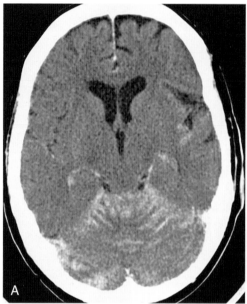
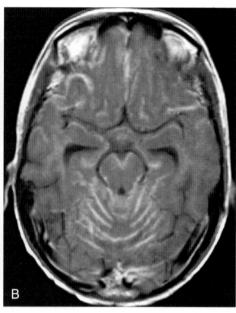

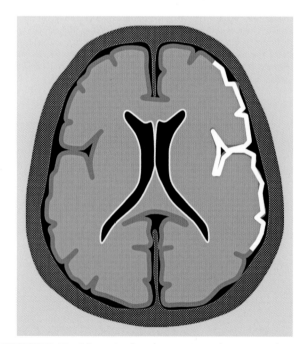

■ **FIGURE 5-12** Schematic of gyral gray matter enhancement. The cortical gray matter enhances while the underlying white matter does not. *(From Smirniotopoulos JG, Murphy FM, Rushing EJ, et al. Patterns of contrast enhancement in the brain and meninges. RadioGraphics 2007; 27:525-551.)*

(Fig. 5-12). Vascular causes of brain parenchymal gyral enhancement include causes of vasoactive hyperemia: migraine, loss of autoregulation, posterior-reversible encephalopathy syndrome, and reperfusion after thrombolysis or spontaneous clot lysis/migration. Gyral enhancement due to blood-brain barrier breakdown is also seen with reperfusion, during the subacute "healing" phase after cerebral infarction, and with vasculitis and encephalitis. Enhancement from hyperperfusion can be seen after seizures. The differential diagnosis between vascular and inflammatory causes of a superficial and serpentine pattern of enhancement requires clinical correlation and analysis of the enhancement topography. Embolic events and most thrombotic strokes have an abrupt onset of symptoms and involve regions that map to vascular territories. Migraine headache has a characteristic aura and throbbing pain. Fever, indolent history, and nonspecific headache or lethargy may suggest an encephalitis. Gyral lesions affecting the territory of a single artery are often vascular, whereas inflammatory lesions may affect multiple territories. The most common vascular processes affect the middle cerebral artery territory (up to 60% of cases). The lesions of posterior-reversible encephalopathy syndrome usually localize in the posterior cerebral artery territory, perhaps due to a deficiency in the sympathetic innervations (vaso nervorum).

Inflammatory Gyral Enhancement

The most common brain infection is caused by members of the herpesvirus family of viruses. Herpes encephalitis usually begins in the gray matter, causing swelling and altered signal intensity. Later, inflammatory breakdown of the blood-brain barrier will allow contrast enhancement in a cortical gyral pattern. The most common site of herpes encephalitis is the uncus of the medial temporal lobe and involvement of the cingulate gyrus of the medial frontal and parietal lobes (Fig. 5-13).[20,21] This distribution of lesions supports a route of infection from the nasal cavity, along the olfactory pathways to the brain. Because enhancement may be a lagging indicator of disease and because enhancement may be reduced by corticosteroids, the absence of enhancement cannot be used to rule out encephalitis.

Vascular Gyral Enhancement

Vascular gyral enhancement results from various mechanisms with variable time courses. The earliest enhancement can be caused by reversible blood-brain barrier changes when ischemia lasts for only several hours before reperfusion occurs.[22] Early reperfusion may also produce vasodilatation, with increased blood volume and shortened mean transit time. These features were first observed at conventional angiography; they were described as dynamic changes and were called "luxury perfusion" because of the increased blood flow.[23] The increased blood flow is caused by autoregulation mechanisms, which are "tricked" by the increased tissue Pco_2 that accumulates before reperfusion occurs. Ischemia or infarction may demonstrate gyral enhancement on both CT and MR images within minutes (with early reperfusion) (Fig. 5-14). In the healing phases of cerebral infarction, from several days (5 to 7 days) to several weeks after the event, there will be vascular proliferation or hypertrophy. Contrast enhancement usually fades away between 4 weeks and 4 months after the stroke, and enhancement is usually replaced by brain volume loss and encephalomalacia (Fig. 5-15).[24] The vascular changes facilitate the breakdown and removal of the dead brain tissue and lead to the encephalomalacia and atrophy characteristic of old "healed" infarction. The imaging appearance of postictal states may mimic the findings of cerebral infarction in several features, including gyral swelling, increased signal intensity on T2-weighted (T2W) images, and decreased signal intensity on T1W images, sulcal effacement, and gyral enhancement.[25] Reperfusion, whether

acute (e.g., after thrombolysis) or subacute to chronic ("healing" infarction), is required to deliver contrast material to produce enhancement.

Nodular Cortical and Subcortical Enhancement

Metastatic lesions are often small (<2 cm) circumscribed nodular lesions near the corticomedullary (gray matter/white matter) junction (Fig. 5-16). Metastatic disease usually reaches the brain hematogenously through the arteries and less commonly via the venous system. Metastatic deposits are distributed by blood flow. The majority of lesions are supratentorial in the cerebral hemispheres, often in the territory of the middle cerebral artery,[26] which has the widest distribution. Venous metastatic disease to the CNS is most often related to a primary pelvic malignancy (e.g., of the prostate or uterus) and travels through the prevertebral veins of the Batson venous plexus. This venous pathway connecting to the retroclival venous plexus partially accounts for the preferential distribution of some pelvic metastases to the posterior fossa (cerebellum and brain stem).

Metastatic lesions are typically juxtacortical, occurring in or near the gray matter/white matter (corticomedullary) junction. In contrast, most primary glial tumors arise deeper in the periventricular white matter. This peripheral dominant pattern of nodule distribution reflects where vessels branch and taper, acting as a sieve to filter intravascular tumor. Dissemination is only the beginning; the tumor emboli must establish themselves to grow into a macroscopic deposit. On gross pathologic inspection, as on imaging, metastatic nodules are circumscribed and have a "pushing margin," usually with significant surrounding perilesional vasogenic edema. Even small cortical or juxtacortical lesions may present as early symptoms, because of their ability to cause disruption of the sensory and motor cortex, and seizures are common. This early clinical presentation allows detection of small solid nodular lesions, often 0.5 to 2.5 cm in diameter (see Fig. 5-16). Primary glial tumors, both low-grade and high-grade astrocytomas, arise outside the cortex and deep in the white matter. They may infiltrate extensively without destruction or disruption and will usually present as much larger (2.5 to 5.0 cm in diameter) lesions by the time symptoms are reported.

We usually imagine that hematogenous metastasis is almost invariably multiple. However, in reality, roughly one half (40% to 60%) of patients will have only a single lesion on initial imaging. In these patients with a single lesion, double- and triple-dose gadolinium may reveal additional lesions. However, the

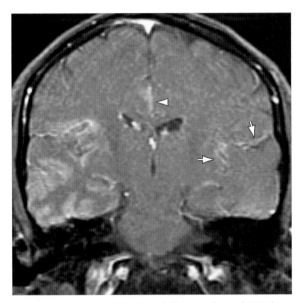

■ **FIGURE 5-13** Coronal T1W gadolinium-enhanced MR image of herpes type 2 encephalitis. Herpesvirus replicates within neurons, causing cortical destruction, inflammatory enhancement, and eventually destruction and atrophy. Ascending infection from the nasopharynx commonly affects the temporal lobes (*arrows*). However, involvement of the cingulate gyrus (*arrowhead*) is also frequent. *(From Smirniotopoulos JG, Murphy FM, Rushing EJ, et al. Patterns of contrast enhancement in the brain and meninges. RadioGraphics 2007; 27:525-551.)*

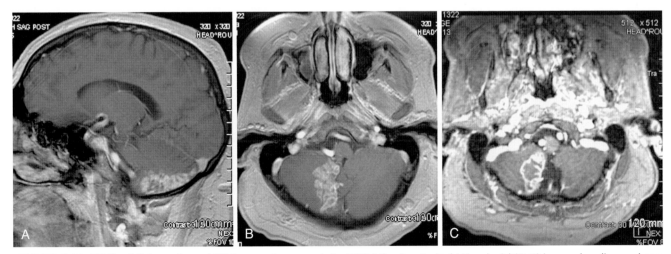

■ **FIGURE 5-14** T1W gadolinium-enhanced MR images of acute cerebellar PICA infarction. Sagittal (**A**) and axial (**B, C**) images show linear enhancement of the cerebellar folia in the right posterior inferior cerebellar artery territory. *Note:* In **C**, the lesion has ring enhancement.

same dosing scheme may also reveal single lesions in patients whose standard MR is negative. We should also remember that diffusely infiltrating astrocytomas may present as multifocal lesions in about 15% of cases. One point helpful in differential diagnosis: multifocal glioma lesions are usually not localized to the gray matter/white matter junction, whereas hematogenous metastases usually are. Thus, metastatic disease is often a solitary lesion and primary tumor can be multiple.

Deep and Periventricular Enhancement

Lesions that are localized deeper within the cerebral hemispheres are usually not caused by hematogenous dissemination. The most common exception is for lesions in the basal ganglia. Subcortical white matter and deeper lesions that involve the gray nuclei (e.g., basal ganglia and thalamus) are usually primary

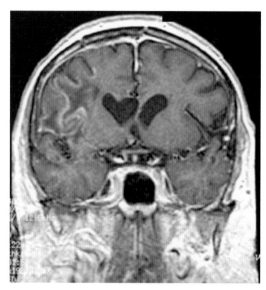

■ **FIGURE 5-15** This patient presented with an acute right middle cerebral artery infarction. Initial imaging noted a previously asymptomatic subependymoma. Postoperative imaging shows subacute middle cerebral artery cortical infarct enhancement, as well as postoperative dura-arachnoid enhancement.

processes within the CNS and may be non-neoplastic. Because of the cellular physiology of neurons, metabolic disease and both endogenous and exogenous toxins may preferentially affect the deep gray matter. The majority of diseases that affect myelin production or repair primarily damage the white matter and are called "leukoencephalopathies." Most leukoencephalopathies become destructive at some time during their natural evolution and will lead to a decreased volume ("atrophy") of the affected white matter. These changes may produce imaging changes from a loss of myelin lipids and an increased signal intensity from water on T2W and fluid-attenuated inversion recovery (FLAIR) MR images with correspondingly decreased attenuation on CT images. Many pathologic processes have inflammation that will produce enhancement localization similar to the location of the increased water signal. We look for these clear-cut distinctions between deep white matter lesions and deep gray matter lesions as a guide to differential diagnosis. However, many diseases affect both the deep gray matter and the white matter in the periventricular regions; and, some of these processes occur commonly in immunocompromised patients, such as toxoplasmosis and primary CNS lymphoma.

Deep Ring-Enhancing Lesions

Ring-enhancing lesions are uncommonly superficial. They are most commonly found either subcortical or deeper in the hemisphere (Fig. 5-17). In a review of 221 MR-enhancing ring lesions, Schwartz and colleagues[27] reported that 40% were gliomas, 30% were metastases, 8% were abscesses, and 6% were caused by demyelinating diseases. They also noted that almost one half (45%) of metastatic deposits were solitary whereas the majority (77%) of gliomas were single lesions. In contrast, both abscesses (75%) and multiple sclerosis lesions (85%) were multiple.[27] Because both necrotic metastases and hematogenous abscesses will be cortical or subcortical lesions with central cavitation, we must differentiate them by other means. Metastatic deposits are more often solid nodular lesions that may become ring enhancing because of necrosis (e.g., after chemotherapy or irradiation) (see Fig. 5-16). A history of known primary tumor would suggest metastasis. Additionally, fever, recent dental work, right-to-left shunt, bronchitis/bronchiectasis, intravenous drug use, subacute bacterial endocarditis, and indwelling catheters or other implanted devices such as cardiac valves would support ring-enhancing lesions with an infectious etiology (i.e., they

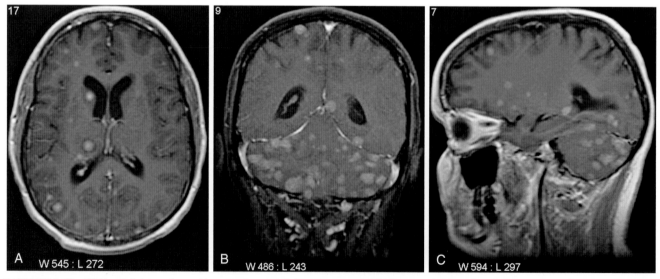

■ **FIGURE 5-16** T1W gadolinium-enhanced images of metastatic breast cancer. Axial (**A**), coronal (**B**), and sagittal (**C**) images all show multiple well-demarcated subcortical enhancing lesions.

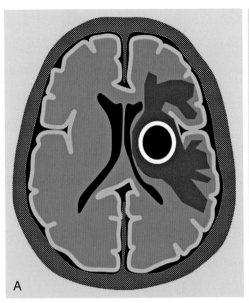
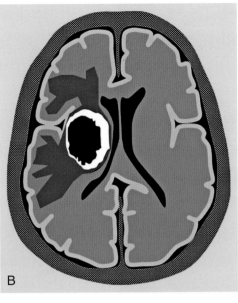

■ **FIGURE 5-17** Diagrams of ring lesions. **A,** Smooth ring suggesting abscess. **B,** Irregular ring with a "shaggy" inner margin suggestive of necrosis in a high-grade neoplasm (e.g., glioblastoma). Both of these lesions may have surrounding interstitial vasogenic edema that spreads away in a "finger-like" manner.

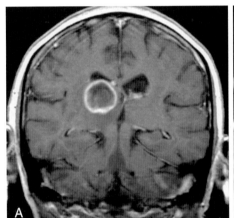
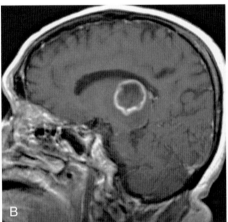
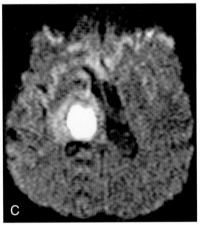

■ **FIGURE 5-18** Abscess. Coronal (**A**) and sagittal (**B**) T1W gadolinium-enhanced MR images and axial diffusion-weighted MR image (**C**). This ring-enhancing lesion has a thin, yet slightly irregular rim. The differential diagnosis would include a glioblastoma. However, the diffusion-weighted image shows hyperintensity from restricted diffusion, most characteristic for pus in an abscess. *(Case courtesy of J. Keith Smith.)*

represent brain abscesses). Deep white matter ring-enhancing lesions, especially those with mass effect and surrounding vasogenic edema, are most often either primary neoplasms (e.g., glioblastoma multiforme) or abscesses (Figs. 5-18 and 5-19; see also Fig. 5-17).

CNS Infections: Cerebritis and Abscess

Most pyogenic infections of the CNS develop from hematogenous septic emboli. Direct extension from adjacent sinus infections (sphenoidal, ethmoidal, frontal, and mastoid air cells) is also possible but requires transgression of the dura. Cerebritis is an acute inflammatory reaction with altered permeability of the native vessels but without angiogenesis or neovascularity. Brain inflammation or cerebritis begins with relatively poorly marginated hyperemia and breakdown of the blood-brain barrier. These reactive changes allow inflammatory white cells, such as neutrophils, and plasma proteins (antibodies and complement) to exit the intravascular space so they can reach the infected parenchyma. Before angiogenesis, the signal intensity and attenuation changes are directly caused by the inflammatory process. The perilesional vasogenic edema is variable and may be minimal.

Proliferation of the infecting organisms and necrosis of brain parenchyma create a zone of devitalized and avascular material. In the immunocompetent patient, cerebritis progresses to form an organized abscess with the formation of a capsule of granulation tissue (Figs. 5-20 and 5-21). The lesion now becomes more circumscribed by vascular changes (recruitment and neovascularity) along with a collagenous rim developing from vascular fibroblasts, thus creating a wall around the pus and dead brain, forming a classic abscess. Collagen in the wall reinforces it to localize and confine the infected brain and pus. Just outside the granulation tissue there is a layer of proliferating reactive astrocytes (astrogliosis) (see Figs. 5-20 and 5-21).[28,29]

The imaging appearance will change, just as the reaction and organization about the infection evolves. The enhancement in cerebritis is often diffuse and faint, whereas an organized abscess has a well-marginated rim of discrete enhancement (see Figs. 5-17 and 5-18). The peripheral rim enhancement in an abscess localizes the granulation tissue with its increased capillary permeability and increased perfusion/vascularity. An intermediate stage of transition from cerebritis to an organized abscess may be suspected when the lesion does not have a sharp margin or

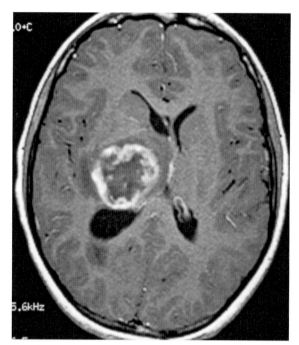

■ **FIGURE 5-19**   Necrotic ring pattern of high-grade neoplasm (glioblastoma multiforme— WHO grade 4). Axial gadolinium enhanced T1W MR image shows a large heterogeneous mass that displaces the frontal horn of the lateral ventricle. There is irregular and heterogeneous ring enhancement. The ring has a characteristically undulating or wavy margin, and its inner aspect is shaggy and irregular, all suggesting necrosis in a neoplasm.

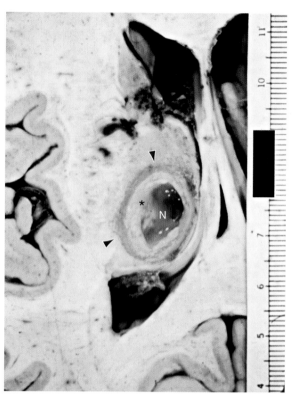

■ **FIGURE 5-20**   Cerebral abscess in a patient with AIDS who died of multiple brain abscesses from *Toxoplasma gondii*. Axially sectioned gross specimen shows an abscess in the thalamus with three macroscopic zones: a reddish region of neovascularity (*arrowheads*), a white region of extravascular white cells and pus (*asterisk*), and an inner zone of liquefaction necrosis (N). Liquefaction necrosis occurs in lipid-rich organs (e.g., the brain), when an exuberant leukocytic reaction brings lytic enzymes into the infected region. Scale is in centimeters. *(From Smirniotopoulos JG, Murphy FM, Rushing EJ, et al. Patterns of contrast enhancement in the brain and meninges. RadioGraphics 2007; 27:525-551.)*

has a wall that is less discrete. On initial CT and MR images, cerebritis will appear as a ring-enhancing lesion (see Fig. 5-18). In cerebritis without a collagen capsule, images obtained over 20 to 40 minutes may show "fill in" of the ring center.[30] This "filling in" does not occur in a well-organized abscess and suggests cerebritis.[30] Cerebritis is often treated nonsurgically with high doses of antibiotics.

It typically takes 2 to 4 weeks to create a well-formed abscess wall that separates the infection and necrosis from the relatively uninvolved surrounding brain. Pathologically, an organizing infection will develop concentric zones or layers: (1) necrotic brain in the innermost layer, (2) reactive white cells (macrophages, monocytes) and fibroblasts, (3) capillary vascular proliferation and collagen capsule formation, (4) neovascularity and active cerebritis, and (5) reactive astrogliosis and vasogenic edema in the outer margin (see Figs. 5-20 and 5-21).[28-30]

The classic abscess ring usually has both a smooth inner and outer margin and is typically less than 1 cm (usually about 5 mm) thick. During the transition from the diffuse inflammation of cerebritis to the organized wall of an abscess, the outer rim of enhancement may fade into the adjacent brain, like the corona of a solar eclipse (see Fig. 5-18B). On T2W MR images, the abscess wall is usually hypointense, contrasting to the bright necrotic center and the surrounding brain with vasogenic edema. Schwartz and colleagues reported that almost 90% of abscesses demonstrate a hypointense rim and 75% form a continuous hypointense rim.[27] Multiple theories have been proposed, including dense collagen, blood products (hemosiderin), and paramagnetic free radicals (e.g., atomic oxygen produced by leukocytes that are attacking the bacteria).[31] An abscess wall often appears thicker on the gray matter or "oxygen side" of the ring and thinner along the white matter or ventricular side. The tendency for an abscess to "point" toward the ventricular, deep, or medial aspect is a direct consequence of the thinner inner

margin. Rupture into the ventricle (pyocephalus) is usually devastating to the patient and often fatal.

We have seen that late stage cerebritis may produce ring enhancement. In addition, as organization progresses, the outer abscess rim may be thick or irregular. Extravascular enhancement (interstitial—from increased capillary permeability) localizes within millimeters of the abnormal vessels. Although extravascular, the contrast material cannot diffuse into the center of an organized abscess cavity, even on delayed images, owing to the viscosity of the pus and liquefaction necrosis. These same physical properties produce the high signal intensity on diffusion-weighted images (see Fig. 5-18C) and have a corresponding reduced apparent diffusion coefficient (ADC) and therefore are of low signal intensity on the maps of ADC values. Lastly, amino acids on proton MR spectroscopy (discussed in detail elsewhere) are seen in 80% of abscesses.[32]

Necrotic High-Grade Primary Neoplasms

Central necrosis within a neoplasm will also produce a ring-enhancing lesion. Remaining residual living tissue surrounds a central zone of necrotic tumor tissue. In general, rapidly growing tumors that become necrotic are usually, but not exclusively, malignant, either primary gliomas or metastases. Multilocular and complex ring patterns—lesions with a thick irregular rim (especially if > 10 mm) and those with an irregular or "shaggy" inner margin—usually represent necrotic high-grade neoplasms rather than abscess or cerebritis (Fig. 5-22; see also Fig. 5-19).

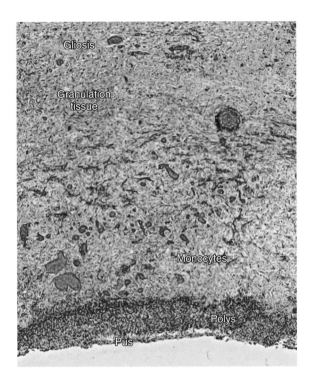

■ FIGURE 5-21 Brain abscess. Photomicrograph (H&E, original magnification, ×250) shows the microscopic layers from top to bottom: reactive gliosis and the brain margin, vascular proliferation with collagen formation (granulation tissue), migrating white blood cells (monocytes), and pus. polys, polymorphonuclear leukocytes. *(Courtesy of Joseph Parisi, MD, Mayo Clinic, Rochester, MN; from Smirniotopoulos JG, Murphy FM, Rushing EJ, et al. Patterns of contrast enhancement in the brain and meninges. RadioGraphics 2007; 27:525-551.)*

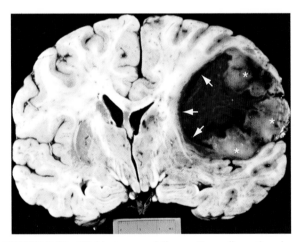

■ FIGURE 5-22 Glioblastoma multiforme. Coronally sectioned gross specimen shows the outer cortical region of the tumor with the more typical, thick irregular rim (*asterisk*) and shaggy inner margin, and the relatively smooth, thin, deep inner margin (*arrows*). Within the neoplasm is a region of hemorrhagic necrosis. Scale is in centimeters. *(From Smirniotopoulos JG, Murphy FM, Rushing EJ, et al. Patterns of contrast enhancement in the brain and meninges. RadioGraphics 2007; 27:525-551.)*

When these lesions are in the corpus callosum and thalamus, brain stem, or other deep parts of the brain, glioblastoma (diffuse astrocytoma, WHO grade 4) is more likely.

Histologically, grade 4 diffuse astrocytoma is characterized by aggressive features, including microscopic foci of necrosis with pseudopalisading. Larger lesions will have irregular geographic regions of necrotic cavitation.[33,34] These necrotic regions may

have increased diffusion rather than restricted diffusion, owing to the lysis of cell membranes and dissolution of boundaries. Glioblastomas vary from smaller unilocular rings to larger and more complex lobulated and multilocular rings, with thick rims of enhancement. They usually show angiographic and macroscopic neovascularity. This abnormal vascularity produces an increased regional cerebral blood volume and increased regional cerebral blood flow that combine to produce a short mean transit time. These findings are measurable on perfusion imaging, whether by MRI, CT, or even catheter angiography. The residual/remaining living tumor in the outer rim survives because it maintains a rich blood supply. This hypervascular rim can be several centimeters thick, may be irregular both outside and toward the central necrosis, and is often thicker toward the cortical gray matter or basal ganglia. The tumor is more likely to grow faster and thicker near the normally more vascular gray matter (see Fig. 5-22). Quite different from an abscess, delayed imaging in a necrotic neoplasm may show progression of enhancement toward the center, from islands of viable tumor that surround remaining patent vessels. Vascular endothelial growth factor has been implicated in the angiogenesis for most high-grade gliomas.[35] The high cellular density, rapid growth, and mitotic activity all require increased metabolism and corresponding increased perfusion. The newly recruited and co-opted vessels develop capillary endothelium with intercellular gaps, and they do not have a continuous basement membrane.

Fluid-Secreting Low-Grade Primary Neoplasms

Necrosis is a common feature of high-grade neoplasms, but all neoplastic "holes" are not formed by necrosis. Low-grade primary neoplasms may become heterogeneous not from necrosis but through accumulation of serous fluid. In addition, because fluid-secreting gliomas have well-defined "pushing margins," they may be resected completely, offering a cure. Because of features of slow growth, possible resection, and well-differentiated histology, most fluid-secreting brain neoplasms are WHO grade 1. The fluid must come from somewhere, so the periphery of the fluid spaces includes neoplastic tissue. Almost all "fluid-secreting" gliomas enhance on both MRI and CT. The two most familiar partially fluid brain tumors are the pilocytic astrocytoma and the hemangioblastoma. They are both most frequently located in the cerebellum (Fig. 5-23). Supratentorially, the differential diagnosis for "fluid-secreting" lesions includes pilocytic astrocytoma, pleomorphic xanthoastrocytoma, ganglioglioma, and extraventricular ependymoma. These lesions are not truly "cystic" because the fluid cavity is not lined by an epithelium. In the majority of cases, the neoplastic tissue is much smaller in volume compared with the fluid component, and either it forms a lump ("mural nodule") or comprises part of the rim. The remaining margin is normal, compressed, or gliotic brain tissue.

The fluid secreted in these low-grade neoplasms is not identical to tissue fluid or serum. It may have a high protein concentration and show increased signal compared with cerebrospinal fluid on T1W MRI and on CT but have lower signal intensity on T2W MR images. These low-grade lesions may have abnormal capillaries but usually do not show increased blood flow. There are limited (if any) changes in arteries and veins. With the exception of hemangioblastoma, these lesions are avascular on angiography. Although lacking increased perfusion, increased metabolism has been reported on metabolic studies.[36] Most authors believe that the abnormal capillaries in these lesions do not form a blood-brain barrier and that the increased permeability is related somehow to both fluid production and contrast material.[37] Histologically, the fluid is seen as microcysts within the "solid" tumor nodule. They may have high signal on FLAIR imaging and low attenuation on CT. The "cyst-with-nodule" appearance (Fig. 5-24; see also Fig. 5-23) is attributed to progressive fluid secretion that accumulates exophytically between the

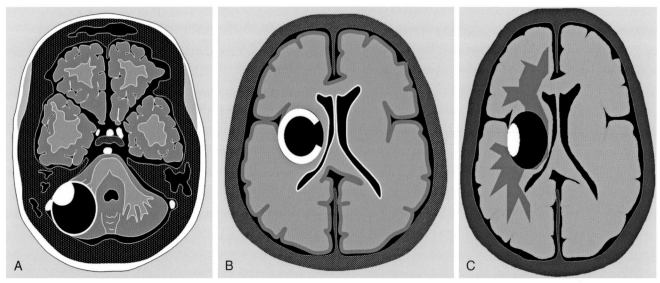

■ **FIGURE 5-23** Schematic fluid-secreting neoplasms and demyelination. **A,** Typical cerebellar "cyst with nodule" appearance for pilocytic astrocytoma and hemangioblastoma. **B,** Classic "open-ring" sign for tumefactive demyelinating lesions. **C,** Fluid secreting "cyst with nodule" neoplasms may produce interstitial vasogenic edema in the cerebral hemispheres. See also Figure 5-24.

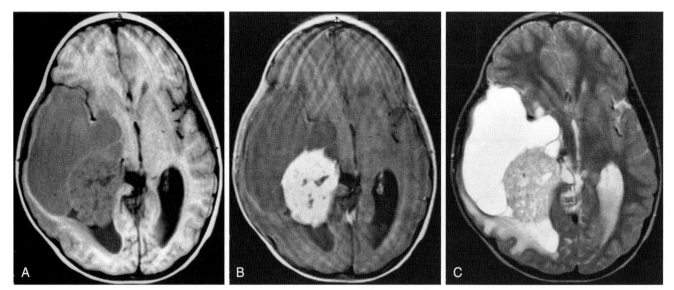

■ **FIGURE 5-24** Pilocytic astrocytoma—cerebral hemisphere. Axial MR images: T1W (**A**), T1W gadolinium-enhanced (**B**), and T2W (**C**). There is a large complex right hemispheric mass. Part of this is solid neoplasm (enhancing on **B**). Part of this is fluid secreted by the neoplasm. There is interstitial vasogenic edema surrounding the mass and extending into the posterior temporal and occipital lobes.

neoplastic nodule and the normal brain. Many fluid-secreting tumors have a more complex shape that cannot be simply described as a biphasic "cyst-with-nodule" shape. Roughly one third of hemangioblastomas show the classic unilocular fluid space with a single mural nodule.[38] The remaining two thirds vary in shape from almost completely solid to a large fluid space with only a tiny nodule. In pilocytic astrocytoma, with thinner slice thickness (<4 mm), MRI and CT frequently demonstrate that even the "solid" mural nodule is often heterogeneous with small fluid "lacunae" within the nodule itself, in addition to the larger fluid "cyst" (Fig. 5-25; see also Fig. 5-24). Reactive gliosis, which by conventional wisdom does not enhance, may nonetheless show contrast enhancement around the fluid in some pilocytic astrocytomas.[39] Enhancement of gliosis is variable and depends on the time delay between injection and imaging, the

contrast dose, and probably on the molecular weight of the contrast material. Lastly, the varying morphology of fluid-secreting neoplasms can produce the "open-ring sign," an incomplete rim of enhancement that is also a feature of some other benign lesions, such as demyelination.

White Matter Enhancement: Demyelination

The most common cause of neurologic disability in midlife is the leukoencephalopathy of multiple sclerosis. The demyelination is caused by a failure of the normal myelin physiology. Active destruction of myelin as well as faulty metabolism and repair by the oligodendrocytes will lead to denuded axons—the histologic hallmark of these diseases. There is gray matter involvement in many, if not most, patients, and axon destruction and neuronal loss occur in many cases. Multiple sclerosis is usually character-

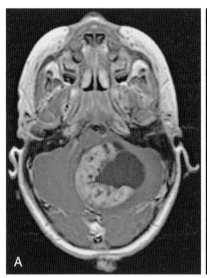 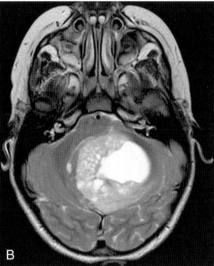 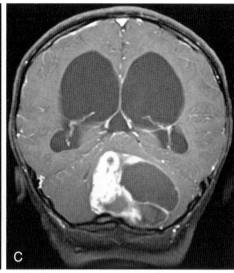

■ **FIGURE 5-25** Pilocytic astrocytoma. **A,** Axial T1W gadolinium-enhanced MR image. There is a heterogeneous C-shaped mass in the fourth ventricle. The right lateral wall enhances with a thick rim. However, the left margin does not. **B,** The axial T2W image shows the macroscopic fluid on the patient's left and heterogeneity from smaller fluid pockets within the mural mass. A fluid-secreting mass in the cerebellum is a classic indicator of a pilocytic astrocytoma in a child but would suggest a hemangioblastoma in an adult patient. **C,** Coronal gadolinium-enhanced T1W MR image shows intense thick enhancement of the right rim, but the left margin shows only very thin linear enhancement. The thin rim of enhancement was not neoplastic tissue; rather, it was reactive astrogliosis and that is why it showed only delayed enhancement on the coronal images.

ized by lesions separated in space and time, and the diagnosis (by the McDonald criteria) may now include imaging as well as clinical findings. Pathologically, the classic lesions of multiple sclerosis begin as a perivenular inflammatory reaction—"Dawson's fingers"—that produce a characteristic pattern of elongated lesions that are adjacent and perpendicular to the lateral ventricular margin. These are bright on T2W and FLAIR images because the normal myelin lipid has been destroyed and replaced by inflammation with macrophages and increased water. Contrast enhancement occurs in "active" demyelination and may be modulated by corticosteroids and other therapies. It may or may not be associated with correlating neurologic findings. Most active plaques will enhance for 2 to 6 weeks and only rarely longer.[40] Although we commonly think that the cause of the enhancement in demyelination is inflammation, it may be that the breakdown of the blood-brain barrier is a actually a necessary requirement and precursor for the self-destructive immune reaction that causes demyelination.

Classic demyelination does not cause angiogenesis nor necrosis. The blood-brain barrier changes are not associated with increased perfusion so that, unlike neoplasms and infection, the plaques usually do not show vasogenic edema beyond the rim of enhancement. The enhancing rim about an active zone may be discontinuous or "incomplete"[27,41] (Fig. 5-26), which may allow differentiation from necrotic neoplasm (which has a thick rim) or an abscess, both of which have surrounding vasogenic edema. Masdeu and associates[41] reported that an "open ring sign" is less common in abscess and neoplasm and may indicate demyelination. An "incomplete ring" or "open ring" may produce a "tumefactive demyelinating lesion" pattern[41] in multiple sclerosis, as well as other leukoencephalopathies, such as acute disseminated encephalomyelitis. The diagnosis of multiple sclerosis may be bolstered when MRI also demonstrates lesions in the spinal cord and/or optic nerve.[42]

Acute disseminated encephalomyelitis typically presents in children and younger patients (often < 13 years of age) within days of an immunologic event (infection or vaccination). The disease is monophasic with larger lesions that are more round and may be juxtacortical. There may be multiple ring-enhancing lesions with minimal mass effect and usually without spreading vasogenic edema. Once again, imaging the spinal cord may help narrow the differential diagnosis.

Periventricular Enhancement: Infection and Neoplasm
Periventricular enhancement may occur with inflammatory white matter disease, as described earlier. But, there may be true infection of the ventricle (ventriculitis) or its lining (ependymitis). Ependymitis may be caused by cytomegalovirus, a member of the herpesvirus family (herpesvirus type 5). Cytomegaloviral ependymitis often produces a thin (<2 mm, more often 1 mm) continuous linear enhancement of the ventricular lining on CT and MRI (Figs. 5-27 and 5-28). On coronal images, this will appear as thin linear enhancement along the ventricular (inferior) surface of the corpus callosum. Cytomegaloviral ependymitis is seen most often in immunocompromised patients, especially those with human immunodeficiency virus infection (see Fig. 5-28). Patients with infected ventricular diversion (shunt catheters) may also develop ventriculitis or meningitis. Some patients will also have a choroid plexitis, and a parenchymal abscess may "point" and drain into the ventricle, causing pyocephalus.

Primary glial neoplasms, usually astrocytoma grade 4 (glioblastoma), often infiltrate the corpus callosum, producing periventricular enhancement. However, they can also spread in the subependymal space or seed the ventricle directly from the surrounding white matter. Primary CNS lymphoma is also likely to both infiltrate the periventricular white matter and seed the ventricle. Almost all primary CNS lymphomas are malignant B-cell lymphomas. Previously a rare tumor, called "reticulum cell sarcoma" in the older literature, this lesion has become very common because of immune suppression for transplantation, treatment of immune-mediated diseases, and human immunodeficiency virus infection and acquired immunodeficiency syndrome. Periventricular CNS lymphomas may be multifocal or present as a lumpy periventricular mass, often with only mild to moderate surrounding cerebral edema. Because they are highly cellular "small round blue cell tumors," they usually have a characteristically "woolly" or "fluffy" high attenuation on

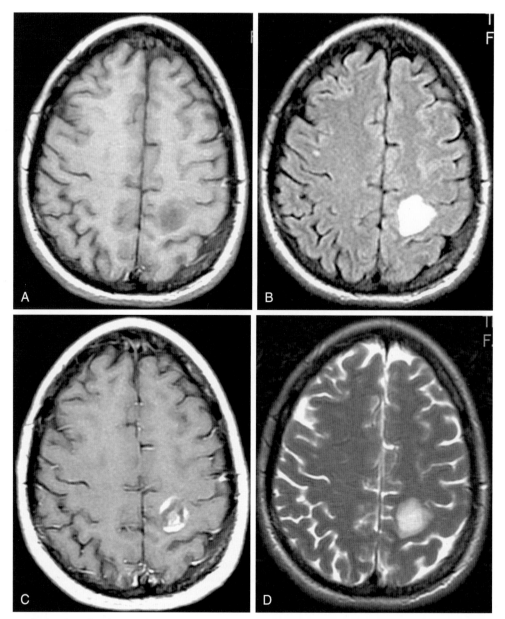

■ **FIGURE 5-26**   Tumefactive demyelination. Axial MR images: noncontrast T1W (**A**), T2W FLAIR (**B**), T1W gadolinium-enhanced (**C**), and T2W (**D**). The enhancement is both discontinuous ("open ring") as well internal. Most significantly, the enhancing rim is at the exact margin of the lesion's signal abnormality, that is, there is no perilesional white matter change. There is no vasogenic edema to suggest an abscess or a neoplasm.

noncontrast CT. There is correspondingly low signal on FLAIR and T2W images, which contrasts to the high signal of perilesional vasogenic edema (Fig. 5-29). Periventricular CNS lymphomas may have restricted diffusion with low signal on ADC map images. They almost invariably enhance, unless pretreated with corticosteroids or radiation. This periventricular pattern of enhancement is typical but not pathognomonic of the disease, with most cases of primary CNS lymphoma involving the corpus callosum, periventricular white matter, thalamus, or basal ganglia. Overall, the most common causes of tumefactive lesions of the corpus callosum are tumors with infiltrating cells: primary CNS lymphoma or astrocytomas.[33,43] Unlike primary CNS lymphoma, secondary CNS lymphoma is usually extra-axial, commonly affecting the dura and subarachnoid space.[43,44]

KEY POINTS

- Contrast enhancement may indicate increased blood volume and/or increased blood flow.
- Increased volume/flow can be physiologic (e.g., "luxury perfusion"), neoplastic (e.g., glioblastoma, metastasis), or reactive (abscess).
- Contrast enhancement may reflect altered permeability (i.e., blood-brain barrier breakdown).
- Altered permeability can be neoplastic (e.g., glioblastoma, metastasis) or inflammatory (e.g., infection, demyelination).
- Patterns of enhancement and surrounding edema may limit the differential diagnosis.

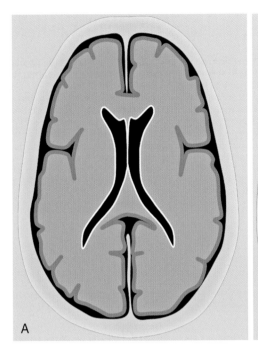
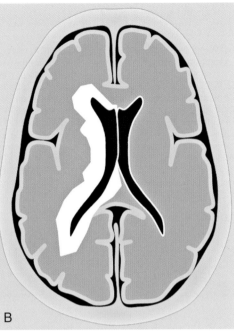

■ **FIGURE 5-27** Schematic periventricular enhancement. **A,** Ependymitis (e.g., from cytomegalovirus infection) usually produces only a very thin linear rim of enhancement. **B,** In contrast, periventricular lymphoma (usually primary B cell lymphoma) most often forms a mass or a thick irregular rind about the ventricle.

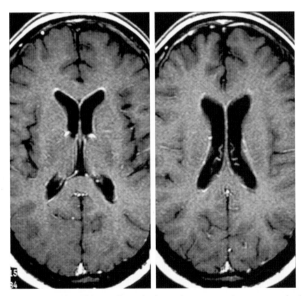

■ **FIGURE 5-28** Thin periventricular enhancement in cytomegaloviral ependymitis. Two axial gadolinium-enhanced T1W MR images show abnormal enhancement completely surrounding both lateral ventricles. The enhancement is thin and very uniform. Cytomegalovirus causes an inflammation of the ventricular lining and produces ependymitis. *(Courtesy of Vince Mathews, MD, University of Indiana, Indianapolis, IN; from Smirniotopoulos JG, Murphy FM, Rushing EJ, et al. Patterns of contrast enhancement in the brain and meninges. RadioGraphics 2007; 27:525-551.)*

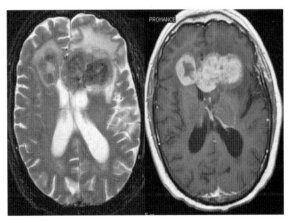

■ **FIGURE 5-29** Primary CNS lymphoma. Axial T2W (*left*) and T1W gadolinium-enhanced (*right*) MR images. The lesion is expansile and involves the corpus callosum. In this location, infiltrating gliomas (astrocytomas) and primary CNS lymphoma are the most common lesions. The low signal intensity on the T2W image (*left*) is highly consistent and also suggestive of lymphoma.

SUGGESTED READINGS

Chang KH, Han MH, Roh JK, et al. Gd-DTPA-enhanced MR imaging of the brain in patients with meningitis: comparison with CT. AJNR Am J Neuroradiol 1990; 11:69-76.

Elster AD, Jackels SC, Allen NS, Marrache RC. Dyke Award: Europium-DTPA: a gadolinium analogue traceable by fluorescence microscopy. AJNR Am J Neuroradiol 1989; 10:1137-1144.

Hesselink JR, Press GA. MR contrast enhancement of intracranial lesions with Gd-DTPA. Radiol Clin North Am 1988; 26:873-887.

Miller DH, Filippi M, Fazekas F, et al. Role of magnetic resonance imaging within diagnostic criteria for multiple sclerosis. Ann Neurol 2004; 56:273-278.

Muroff LR, Runge VM. The use of MR contrast in neoplastic disease of the brain. Top Magn Reson Imaging 1995; 7:137-157.

Polman CH, Reingold SC, Edan G, et al. Diagnostic criteria for multiple sclerosis: 2005 revisions to the "McDonald Criteria." Ann Neurol 2005; 58:840-846.

Rippe DJ, Boyko OB, Friedman HS, et al. Gd-DTPA-enhanced MR imaging of leptomeningeal spread of primary intracranial CNS tumor in children. AJNR Am J Neuroradiol 1990; 11:329-332.

Sage MR, Wilson AJ, Scroop R. Contrast media and the brain: the basis of CT and MR imaging enhancement. Neuroimaging Clin North Am 1998; 8:695-707.

Schmiedl UP, Kenney J, Maravilla KR. Dyke Award Paper: Kinetics of pathologic blood-brain-barrier permeability in an astrocytic glioma using contrast-enhanced MR. AJNR Am J Neuroradiol 1992; 13:5-14.

Spetzger U, Thron A, Gilsbach JM. Immediate postoperative CT contrast enhancement following surgery of cerebral tumoral lesions. J Comput Assist Tomogr 1998; 22:120-125.

REFERENCES

1. Provenzale JM, Mukundan S, Dewhirst M. The role of blood-brain barrier permeability in brain tumor imaging and therapeutics. AJR Am J Roentgenol 2005; 185:763-767.

2. Sage MR, Wilson AJ, Scroop R. Contrast media and the brain: the basis of CT and MR imaging enhancement. Neuroimaging Clin North Am 1998; 8:695-707.

3. Wilms G, Demaerel P, Bosmans H, Marchal G. MRI of non-ischemic vascular disease: aneurysms and vascular malformations. Eur Radiol 1999; 9:1055-1060.

4. Meltzer CC, Fukui MB, Kanal E, Smirniotopoulos JG. MR imaging of the meninges: I. Normal anatomic features and nonneoplastic disease. Radiology 1996; 201:297-308.

5. Mokri B. The Monro-Kellie hypothesis: applications in CSF volume depletion. Neurology 2001; 56:1746-1748.

6. Burke JW, Podrasky AE, Bradley WG Jr. Meninges: benign postoperative enhancement on MR images. Radiology 1990; 174:99-102.

7. Mittl RL Jr, Yousem DM. Frequency of unexplained meningeal enhancement in the brain after lumbar puncture. AJNR Am J Neuroradiol 1994; 15:633-638.

8. Phillips ME, Ryals TJ, Kambhu SA, Yuh WT. Neoplastic vs inflammatory meningeal enhancement with Gd-DTPA. J Comput Assist Tomogr 1990; 14:536-541.

9. Paldino M, Mogilner AY, Tenner MS. Intracranial hypotension syndrome: a comprehensive review. Neurosurg Focus 2003; 15:1-8.

10. Buetow MP, Buetow PC, Smirniotopoulos JG. Typical, atypical, and misleading features in meningioma. RadioGraphics 1991; 11:1087-1106.

11. Sheporaitis LA, Osborn AG, Smirniotopoulos JG, et al. Radiologic-pathologic correlation: intracranial meningioma. AJNR Am J Neuroradiol 1992; 13:29-37.

12. Elster AD, Challa VR, Gilbert TH, et al. Meningiomas: MR and histopathologic features. Radiology 1989; 170:857-862.

13. New PF, Aronow S, Hesselink JR. National Cancer Institute study: evaluation of computed tomography in the diagnosis of intracranial neoplasms: IV. Meningiomas. Radiology 1980; 136:665-675.

14. Aoki S, Sasaki Y, Machida T, Tanioka H. Contrast-enhanced MR images in patients with meningioma: importance of enhancement of the dura adjacent to the tumor. AJNR Am J Neuroradiol 1990; 11:935-938.

15. Gupta S, Gupta RK, Banerjee D, Gujral RB. Problems with the dural tail sign. Neuroradiology 1993; 35:541-542.

16. Tien RD, Yang PJ, Chu PK. Dural tail sign: a specific MR sign for meningioma? J Comput Assist Tomogr 1991; 15:64-66.

17. Nakau H, Miyazawa T, Tamai S, et al. Pathologic significance of meningeal enhancement ("flare sign") of meningiomas on MRI. Surg Neurol 1997; 48:584-590.

18. Nagele T, Petersen D, Klose U, et al. The dural tail adjacent to meningiomas studied by dynamic contrast-enhanced MRI: a comparison with histopathology. Neuroradiology 1994; 36:303-307.

19. Spellerberg B, Prasad S, Cabellos C, et al. Penetration of the blood-brain barrier: enhancement of drug delivery and imaging by bacterial glycopeptides. J Exp Med 1995; 182:1037-1043.

20. Burke JW, Mathews VP, Elster AD, et al. Contrast-enhanced magnetization transfer saturation imaging improves MR detection of herpes simplex encephalitis. AJNR Am J Neuroradiol 1996; 17:773-776.

21. Ametani M, Ogawa T, Tanabe Y, et al. Sequential MR imaging and SPECT studies in herpes simplex encephalitis with crossed cerebellar hyperperfusion. Ann Nucl Med 2005; 19:151-155.

22. Kinkel WR, Jacobs L, Kinkel PR. Gray matter enhancement: a computerized tomographic sign of cerebral hypoxia. Neurology 1980; 30:810-819.

23. Runge VM, Kirsch JE, Wells JW, et al. Visualization of blood-brain barrier disruption on MR images of cats with acute cerebral infarction: value of administering a high dose of contrast material. AJR Am J Roentgenol 1994; 162:431-435.

24. Norton GA, Kishore PR, Lin J. CT contrast enhancement in cerebral infarction. AJR Am J Roentgenol 1978; 131:881-885.

25. Silverstein AM, Alexander JA. Acute postictal cerebral imaging. AJNR Am J Neuroradiol 1998; 19:1485-1488.

26. Stark AM, Tscheslog H, Buhl R, et al. Surgical treatment for brain metastases: prognostic factors and survival in 177 patients. Neurosurg Rev 2005; 28:115-119.

27. Schwartz KM, Erickson BJ, Lucchinetti C. Pattern of T2 hypointensity associated with ring-enhancing brain lesions can help to differentiate pathology. Neuroradiology 2006; 48:143-149.

28. Brant-Zawadzki M, Enzmann DR, Placone RC Jr, et al. NMR imaging of experimental brain abscess: comparison with CT. AJNR Am J Neuroradiol 1983; 4:250-253.

29. Britt RH, Enzmann DR, Placone RC Jr, et al. Experimental anaerobic brain abscess. J Neurosurg 1984; 60:1148-1159.

30. Britt RH, Enzmann DR, Yeager AS. Neuropathological and computerized tomographic findings in experimental brain abscess. J Neurosurg 1981; 55:590-603.

31. Haimes AB, Zimmerman RD, Morgello S, et al. MR imaging of brain abscesses. AJR Am J Roentgenol 1989; 152:1073-1085.

32. Pal D, Bhattacharyya A, Husain M, et al. In vivo proton MR spectroscopy evaluation of pyogenic brain abscesses: a report of 194 cases. AJNR Am J Neuroradiol 2010; 31:360-366.

33. Rees JH, Smirniotopoulos JG, Jones RV, Wong K. Glioblastoma multiforme: radiologic-pathologic correlation. RadioGraphics 1996; 16:1413-1438.

34. Rong Y, Durden DL, Van Meir EG, Brat DJ. "Pseudopalisading" necrosis in glioblastoma: a familiar morphologic feature that links vascular pathology, hypoxia, and angiogenesis. J Neuropathol Exp Neurol 2006; 65:529-539.

35. Takano S, Kamiyama H, Tsuboi K, Matsumura A. Angiogenesis and antiangiogenic therapy for malignant gliomas. Brain Tumor Pathol 2004; 21:69-73.

36. Fulham MJ, Melisi JW, Nishimiya J, et al. Neuroimaging of juvenile pilocytic astrocytomas: an enigma. Radiology 1993; 189:221-225.

37. Takeuchi H, Kubota T, Sato K, Arishima H. Ultrastructure of capillary endothelium in pilocytic astrocytomas. Brain Tumor Pathol 2004; 21:23-26.

38. Ho VB, Smirniotopoulos JG, Murphy FM, Rushing EJ. Radiologic-pathologic correlation: hemangioblastoma. AJNR Am J Neuroradiol 1992; 13:1343-1352.

39. Beni-Adani L, Gomori M, Spektor S, Constantini S. Cyst wall enhancement in pilocytic astrocytoma: neoplastic or reactive phenomena. Pediatr Neurosurg 2000; 32:234-239.

40. Cotton F, Weiner HL, Jolesz FA, Guttmann CR. MRI contrast uptake in new lesions in relapsing-remitting MS followed at weekly intervals. Neurology 2003; 60:640-646.

41. Masdeu JC, Quinto C, Olivera C, et al. Open-ring imaging sign: highly specific for atypical brain demyelination. Neurology 2000; 54:1427-1433.

42. Bot JC, Barkhof F, Nijeholt G, et al. Differentiation of multiple sclerosis from other inflammatory disorders and cerebrovascular disease: value of spinal MR imaging. Radiology 2002;223:46-56.

43. Koeller KK, Smirniotopoulos JG, Jones RV. Primary central nervous system lymphoma: radiologic-pathologic correlation. RadioGraphics 1997; 17:1497-1526.

44. Tomlinson FH, Kurtin PJ, Suman VJ, et al. Primary intracerebral malignant lymphoma: a clinicopathological study of 89 patients. J Neurosurg 1995; 82:558-566.

Scalp, Skull, and Meninges

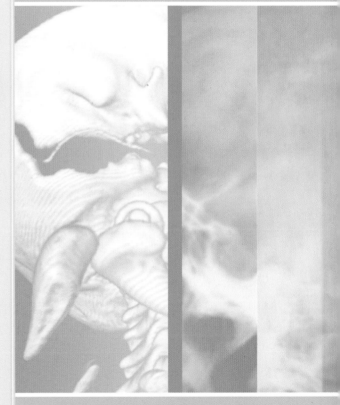

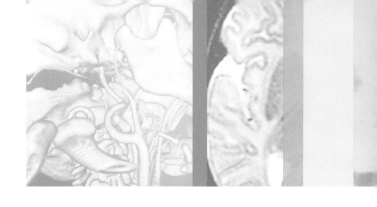

CHAPTER 6

Scalp

Yoav Parag, Thomas P. Naidich, and Patrick O. Emanuel

The scalp is the soft tissue covering of the calvarial vault. It extends from the eyebrows anteriorly to the external occipital protuberance and superior nuchal lines posteriorly to the zygomatic arches and external acoustic canals on both sides. It may also be designated the epicranium.

Grossly, the scalp has five layers.[1] From superficial to deep, these include:

- The skin proper, composed of the epidermis and dermis
- The superficial fascia, consisting of firm dense adipose tissue deep to and closely adherent to the skin
- The epicranial aponeurosis, a continuous fibromuscular sheet composed of the occipitofrontalis muscle, the temporoparietalis muscles, and their associated epicranial aponeurosis (synonym: galea aponeurotica)
- The loose subgaleal areolar tissue
- The pericranium (outer periosteum of the skull)

The scalp also contains the arteries, veins, lymphatics, and nerves that supply the soft tissue.

Thus far, imaging techniques clearly delineate only three of the five layers of the scalp, specifically, the skin, the dense adipose tissue of the superficial fascia, and the confluent galeal-subgaleal-pericranial complex.

On CT, the skin is usually isodense to soft tissue and measures 50 to 70 Hounsfield units. CT often displays the whorl pattern of the hair on broad-window images because air outlines the individual strands. On MRI, the skin is usually isointense to muscle on T1- and T2-weighted images. At present, imaging cannot demonstrate individual dermal adnexae such as hair follicles and sebaceous glands. However, in aggregate, normal hair follicles give the dermal-subcutaneous interface a serrated appearance, which can sometimes be appreciated as a rippled fat/soft tissue interface on high-field MRI. After administration of a contrast agent, the scalp shows intense enhancement owing to the presence of the rich network of blood vessels that have their origin from the underlying subcutaneous layer.

A full, illustrated discussion of the anatomy and imaging of the scalp is available online at www.expertconsult.com.

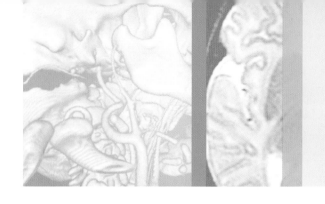

CHAPTER 7

Skull

A. Orlando Ortiz

The skull consists of multiple flat bones joined together by sutures. These flat bones have rounded margins that permit the formation of a vault that is located superior to the skull base. The skull surrounds the outer surface of the brain, whereas the skull base supports and covers the undersurface of the brain.

The skull vault comprises the neurocranium, which is bordered anteriorly by the facial bones or viscerocranium.[1] Multiple bones contribute to the formation of the skull vault. These include, in anterior to posterior direction, the frontal bone, the greater wing of the sphenoid bone, the frontal process of the zygoma, the squamous portion of the temporal bone, the parietal bone, and the occipital bone. These bones are connected by fibrous sutural membranes that initially allow for the expansion of the developing brain in early life. Growth of the brain and adjacent skull are also facilitated by the presence of anterior and posterior fontanelles. The anterior fontanelle is located between the frontal and parietal bones at the junction of the sagittal and coronal sutures. The posterior fontanelle is located between the parietal and occipital bones at the junction of the sagittal and lambdoid sutures.

Each of the skull bones is made up of an outer table of cortical bone, a middle table or diploë that contains bone marrow, and an inner table of cortical bone.[2] Periosteum covers the outer table of the skull. This periosteum is actually considered to be part of the deepest layer of the scalp. The periosteum is fairly adherent to the bony cortex and is tightly adherent at sutural

junctions between adjacent skull bones. The inner table is lined by the dura mater, the most superficial layer of the meninges. Periosteal dura is located immediately adjacent to the inner table cortex. A second layer of dura, the meningeal dura, is apposed to the periosteal dura except where these two dural leaves diverge to form the major dural venous sinuses, the sagittal and transverse sinuses, and the falx cerebri and cerebelli and tentorium cerebelli. Like the periosteum of the outer table, the periosteal dura is tightly adherent to the inner table at the cranial sutures. Despite this close apposition of these fibrous connective tissue structures, the periosteum and the periosteal dura, to their respective cortical layers, a potential space can be found beneath the periosteum, the subperiosteal space, and above or external to the periosteal dura, the epidural space. The subdural space is located deep to or beneath the meningeal layer of dura.

Scattered small vascular channels that transmit tiny vessels may be found anywhere about the skull vault but are most often seen in the vicinity of the major dural venous sinuses. These may involve one or both of the cortical tables of the skull. Arachnoid granulations may also be seen adjacent to the inner table often in the vicinity of the sagittal or transverse sinuses. These normal anatomic structures should not be mistaken for pathologic conditions.

For a full discussion of the imaging and analysis of the skull, please visit www.expertconsult.com.

CHAPTER 8

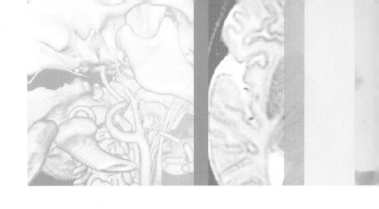

Cranial Meninges

Merav W. Galper, Thomas P. Naidich, George M. Kleinman, Evan G. Stein, and Patrick A. Lento

The term *cranial meninges* refers to the three tissue layers that ensheathe the brain deep to the skull. From superficial to deep, these are the dura mater, the arachnoid mater, and pia mater.

The dura mater is also termed the *pachymeninx* (thick meninx). The arachnoid and pia mater, together, are the *leptomeninges* (thin meninges).[1,2]

EMBRYOLOGY

The cranial dura is mesodermal in origin, derived from the sclerotomes. The leptomeninges are ectodermal in origin, derived from the neural crest.[1] The meninges form in three stages.[2,3]

Stage 1

From 22 to 40 days' gestation, migrating mesenchymal cells surround the neural tube to form a reticulum between the developing nervous system and the superficial ectoderm. A vascular tunic containing immature hematogenous elements forms within this mesenchymal layer, close to the developing neural tissue.[3] No distinct meninges are yet present.

Stage 2

The superficial portion of the reticulum condenses into a compact lamina that is three to four cells thick. Loosely organized mesenchyme remains deep to this lamina, between the lamina and the deeper vascular tunic. This mesenchyme is poorly cellular and has copious extracellular ground substance (glycosaminoglycans). From superficial to deep, the tissue layers are surface epithelium, compact cell lamina, poorly cellular loose mesenchyme, vascular tunic, and neuroepithelium.[3] With further development, the compact cellular layer will form the outer arachnoid membrane, the dura mater, and the skull. The poorly cellular loose layer will form the subarachnoid space. Primitive pia-arachnoid cells first begin to be seen at stage 2.[3]

Stage 3

There is growth of the meninges and increased tissue between blood vessels.[3] The compact cellular layer differentiates further into a deeper portion that will become the outer arachnoid layer and a more superficial portion that will become the dura mater. The outermost layer of the arachnoid (arachnoid barrier cell layer) is directly continuous with the innermost layer of the dura (dural border cell layer) throughout all further development. *No true subdural space can be identified between the dura mater and the arachnoid.*[3] There is no preexisting subdural space comparable to the pleural or peritoneal cavities.[4] In this stage, cerebrospinal fluid issues out from the ventricles into the poorly cellular loose mesenchyme, washes away the original extracellular ground substance, and replaces it with fluid, now designated cerebrospinal fluid (CSF). This process creates the "new" substantial, fluid-filled "layer" designated the subarachnoid space. That is, the subarachnoid space is really just a hugely expanded extracellular space. The primitive pia-arachnoid interface is organized in a simple laminar layer; in some areas, a single cell contributes different processes to both the pial surface and the inner portion of the arachnoid. Even in mature meninges, the distinction between these two layers remains difficult.[3] The pial cover of the cerebral surface is incomplete in many areas. At these sites, the basal lamina of the glia limitans comes into direct contact with the subarachnoid space.[3]

INTERNAL ORGANIZATION/LAYERS OF AREA

Dura Mater

The cranial dura forms the thick protective layer over the brain (Fig. 8-1). It is formed of an outer endosteal layer and an inner meningeal layer.[1] The outer endosteal layer is composed of elongated fibroblasts and osteoblasts. Large amounts of extracellular collagen give it strength.[1] This layer attaches directly to the inner table of the skull, forming the inner periosteum of the calvaria. With advancing age, this endosteal layer becomes progressively more adherent to the skull, may calcify, and may ossify into the inner table.[5]

The meningeal and endosteal layers of dura remain tightly fused over most of their surface but separate from each other at two major sites. Within the skull, the inner meningeal layer of each side delaminates from the endosteal dura, reflects inward, and merges with its mate to form the double-layered dural partitions, which include the falx cerebri (Fig. 8-2), the tentorium cerebelli, and the falx cerebelli. The dural venous sinuses form where the meningeal layers delaminate from the endosteal layer of dura (e.g., superior sagittal and transverse sinuses) and in spaces left between the two meningeal layers (e.g., inferior sagittal sinus, straight sinus). At the foramen magnum, the inner meningeal layer delaminates from the endosteal dura to form the thecal sac of the spinal canal while the outer endosteal layer remains with the bone to form the periosteum of the spinal column. The fat and vascular structures of the spinal epidural space lie between the inner meningeal layer (now thecal sac) and the outer endosteal layer of dura.

Falx Cerebri

The falx cerebri is a broad, "sickle-shaped" double fold of meningeal dura mater that reflects downward into the interhemispheric fissure (Fig. 8-3). The outer edge of the falx attaches to the inner table of the calvaria at or near the midline. Anteriorly, it adheres to the internal frontal crest and the crista galli. Posteriorly, it adheres to the internal occipital crest and the internal occipital protuberance.[6] The deep, inner edge of the falx presents a free inferior margin anteriorly but attaches strongly to the upper surface of the tentorium in the midline posteriorly. The anteriormost point at which the falx attaches to the tentorium lies at the apex of the incisura (see later) and is designated the confluence of the falx and tentorium. The superior sagittal

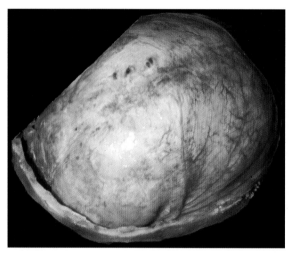

■ **FIGURE 8-1** Anterolateral aspect of the convexity dura seen in situ after removal of the calvaria. Fresh gross anatomic specimen.

sinus lies within the outer, attached margin of the falx superficially. The inferior sagittal sinus lies in the inner, free margin of the falx anteriorly. The straight sinus lies within the inferior margin of the falx along its attachment to the tentorium (see Fig. 8-3).[7]

The falx develops first as two anterior and posterior portions that become a single continuous structure later.[7] The anterior falx is typically shorter and thinner than the posterior portion (see Fig. 8-3) and may be perforated or even dehiscent when the posterior portion is robust (Figs. 8-4 and 8-5).[7] Rarely, the anterior falx may be completely absent.[7] The height of the falx varies from 28 to 48 mm anteriorly, from 41 to 62 mm in the middle, and from 40 to 62 mm posteriorly.[8] As a consequence, the opening beneath the falx (incisura of the falx) is far larger anteriorly and smaller posteriorly, permitting ready shift from side to side anteriorly but limited shift posteriorly.

The falx is partially calcified in 7% of normal adult skull radiographs and partially ossified in 11% of cases.[9-11] Complete ossification of the human falx is exceptionally rare.[10] The calcification and ossification typically appear at the periphery of the falx in relation to the superior sagittal sinus (Fig. 8-6) and/or as islands of bone on the lateral surface of the anterior falx.[9,10] These islands may contain bone marrow. Small fat deposits are found within the falx cerebri in 7.3% of cases.[12]

Falx Cerebelli

The falx cerebelli is a midline, sickle-shaped fold of the occipital dura mater that descends from the internal occipital protuberance into the posterior fossa. It attaches peripherally to the posterior inferior surface of the tentorium cerebelli and the internal occipital crest (Fig. 8-7). Its free margin projects into the posterior cerebellar notch between the left and right cerebellar hemispheres.[13,14] The falx cerebelli is typically 2.8 to 4.5 cm in length and 1 to 2 mm thick.[14] It is commonly "duplicated," even "triplicated," forming multiple dural folds in 15.4% to 76% of cadaver dissections.[14-16] The outer peripheral margin of the falx cerebelli encloses the occipital dural venous sinus.

Tentorium Cerebelli

The tentorium cerebelli ("tent") is a taut extension of the dura mater interposed between the cerebral hemispheres above and

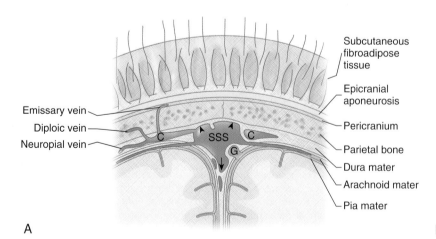

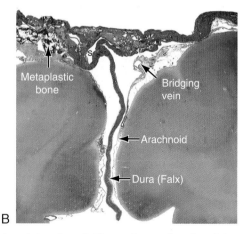

■ **FIGURE 8-2** **A,** Diagram of the separation of the endosteal dura (*arrowheads*) from the meningeal dura (*arrow*). The two layers of meningeal dura fold inward to establish the falx and enclose the superior sagittal sinus (SSS). The cerebral (neuropial) veins drain into the convexity dura lateral to the sinus and travel within intradural channels (C) to enter the lateral angles of the sinus. Specialized diverticula of the arachnoid designated arachnoid granulations (G) protrude into the SSS to help reabsorb cerebrospinal fluid into the general circulation. (See also Fig. 8-6.) **B,** Histologic specimen. Trichrome stain shows dura as bright blue, arachnoid and associated vessels as light blue and red, and the brain as deeper red (original magnification, ×100). The superior sagittal sinus (s) is partially collapsed. Metaplastic bone is seen formed along the inner aspect of the high convexity dura. The thin arachnoid and a bridging vein lie deep to the dura.

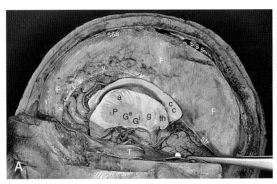
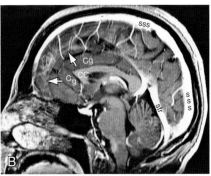

■ **FIGURE 8-3** Falx cerebri and falcine incisura. Anterior is to the reader's left. **A,** Formalin-fixed gross anatomic specimen in situ, viewed from the side after removal of much of the ipsilateral cerebral hemisphere. **B,** Contrast-enhanced T1W midsagittal MR image. The outer margin of the falx (F) attaches to the inner table of the skull along the superior sagittal sinus (sss) and to the tentorium along the straight sinus (str). The free margin of the falx (*open white arrowheads and white arrows*) descends into the interhemispheric fissure less deeply anteriorly and more deeply, posteriorly leaving a falcine incisura that is more widely open anteriorly and narrow posteriorly. The anterior cingulate gyrus (Cg), adjacent medial surface of the frontal lobe, and a large portion of the pericallosal artery lie just to each side of the falcine incisura. Further posteriorly, the free margin of the falx approximates the upper surface of the corpus callosum and the branches of the pericallosal artery pass superior to the free margin of the falx. As a consequence, midline shift is associated with greater displacement of the anterior than posterior cerebrum. In severe cases, compression ("pinching") of the pericallosal arteries against the free margin may lead to distal pericallosal infarctions. The veins of the medial surface of the brain drain upward into the superior sagittal sinus. In **A,** note the relationships among the corpus callosum (cc), the anterior limb (a) and genu (g) of the internal capsule, the putamen (P), external (e) and internal (i) nuclei of the globus pallidus (g), and the thalamus (th). T, remnant of the ipsilateral tentorial leaf. *(Specimen courtesy of Drs. B. Moriggl, Munich, and T. A. Yousry, London.)*

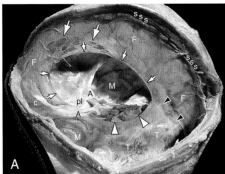
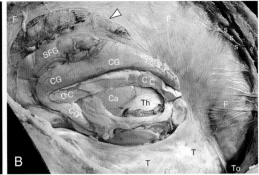

■ **FIGURE 8-4** Falx cerebri and falcine incisura. Fresh gross anatomic specimen in situ (same specimen as in Fig. 8-9). **A,** View from above and the side after removal of all the supratentorial brain tissue by section through the plane of the tentorial incisura. A midline "bucket handle" of bone remains to anchor the falx to the skull. Anteriorly, the sickle-shaped falx cerebri (F) attaches to the calvaria along the internal frontal crest and descends from there to insert onto the crista galli (c) and the floor of the anterior fossa in the midline. Posteriorly, the falx attaches to the superior midline segment of the tentorium (T), enclosing the straight sinus (*black arrowheads*). The superior sagittal sinus (sss) courses posteriorly along the periphery of the falx. The falx is thin, shallow, and widely fenestrated (*large white arrows*) anteriorly leaving a wide falcine incisura (*ring of small white arrows*). The anterolateral edge of the tentorium (T) attaches to the superior ridge of the petrous pyramid. The free medial border (*white arrowheads*) of the tentorium defines the tentorial incisura. The structures within the tentorial incisura are shown in Figure 8-9. A, anterior clinoid processes; M, middle cranial fossa on each side; pl, planum sphenoidale. **B,** Earlier stage in the same dissection and with external compression applied to the right hemisphere. Opening the cranium and resecting the ipsilateral cerebral hemisphere exposes the falx (F), the tentorium (T), and the superior sagittal sinus (sss) that drains posteriorly into the torcular Herophili (To). The medial surface of the contralateral hemisphere is seen through the incisura of the falx, including the corpus callosum (CC), cingulate gyrus (CG), and inferior portion of the superior frontal gyrus (SFG). Marked thinning and fenestration of the anterior falx (*white arrowhead*) exposes more of the medial surface than is usually observed (see Fig. 8-3). Because the vertical section through the brain entered the contralateral lateral ventricle, the head of the caudate nucleus (Ca), thalamus (Th), and choroid plexus of the opposite hemisphere are also visible. The strength of the falx and the variable relationship of its free inferior margin to the cingulate gyrus and corpus callosum determine how easily the brain may shift side to side and the point at which that shift will compress the pericallosal arteries to produce distal anterior cerebral artery infarction. *(Courtesy of John Deck, MD.)*

the cerebellar hemispheres below (Fig. 8-8). The tentorium is present only in mammals and birds. It is absent in fish, amphibians, and reptiles. Like the falx cerebri, the tentorium may be partially calcified or ossified.[17,18] In cats, and some other animals, the tentorium is completely ossified.[17]

Peripherally, the tentorium attaches to the rigid bony walls of the skull and encloses specific venous sinuses. The postero-lateral margins of the tentorium attach to the transverse occipital ridges and the internal occipital protuberance and enclose the paired transverse sinuses and the midline torcular Herophili (confluence of the sinuses).[18] The anterolateral margins of the tentorium attach to the superior surfaces of the petrous

pyramids along the petrous ridges and extend from there onto the *posterior* clinoid processes as the petroclinoid ligaments. The anterolateral margins of the tentorium enclose the superior petrosal sinuses. In the midline superiorly, the tentorium inserts into the inferior margin of the posterior falx cerebri and encloses the straight sinus. The vein of Galen typically joins the anterior end of the straight sinus at the confluence of the falx and tentorium. It then drains through the straight sinus and torcular Herophili into the transverse sinuses.[18]

Centrally, the free medial margins of the tentorium sweep forward and medially from the confluence of the falx and tentorium, pass just above and lateral to the petroclinoid ligaments

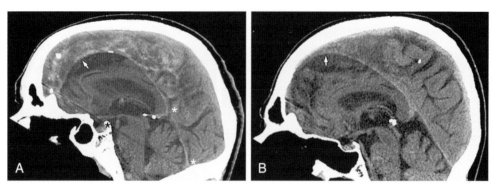

■ **FIGURE 8-5** Falx and falcine incisura. Midsagittal reformatted CT scans with faint residual contrast hours after unrelated thoracoabdominal studies in two patients. The size, position, and configuration of the falx and falcine incisura (*white arrows*) are displayed in relation to the structures of the medial surface of the cerebral hemispheres. **A,** The falx is typical in configuration. **B,** The anterior falx is markedly hypoplastic creating a very large falcine incisura. Coronal images (*not shown*) confirmed the near absence of the anterior falx. The tentorial index is measured as the length of the closed tentorium along the straight sinus (*between the two white asterisks*) divided by the length of the open tentorium from the dorsum sellae (*black asterisk*) to the confluence of the falx and tentorium (*upper white asterisk*).

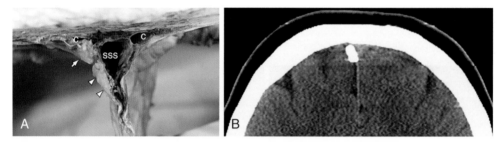

■ **FIGURE 8-6** Ossification of the lateral wall of the superior sagittal sinus (SSS). Coronal sections. **A,** Gross formalin-fixed specimen. The superior sagittal sinus is thrombosed in this specimen. **B,** Noncontrast reformatted CT scan of a different patient. The dural walls of the SSS commonly ossify at the angle between the convexity and the sinus (*arrow*) and along the side wall (*arrowheads*). The cerebral veins do not drain directly into the side or inferior angle of the sinus. Rather, they first drain into the dura lateral to the SSS and course within the dura to enter the sinus through channels (C) leading to the lateral angles of the sinus. (See also Fig. 8-2.) *(A, Courtesy of John Deck, MD.)*

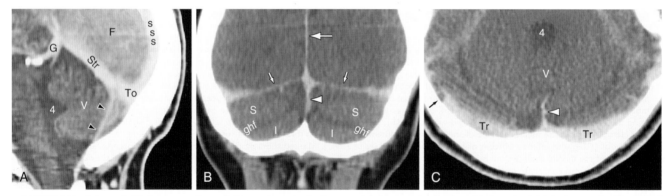

■ **FIGURE 8-7** Falx cerebelli. Contrast-enhanced CT scan in sagittal reformatted (**A**), coronal reformatted (**B**), and axial (**C**) planes. The falx cerebelli (*arrowheads*) attaches along the inferior margin of the torcular (To) and straight sinus (Str) above and along the internal occipital crest behind to project anteriorly into the posterior cerebellar notch. It lies inferior to the tentorium (*small arrows*), between the two cerebellar hemispheres, and posterior to the vermis (V). It aligns only imperfectly with the falx cerebri (F, *white arrow*) above. In C, the lateral aspect of the right transverse sinus (Tr) shows a filling defect (*small black arrow*) representing a pacchionian granulation. The superior semilunar lobule (S) is separated from the inferior semilunar lobule (I) by the great horizontal fissure (ghf). 4, fourth ventricle; G, vein of Galen; sss, superior sagittal sinus.

and posterior clinoid processes, and insert onto the anterior clinoid processes. This anatomic relationship is made possible because the interanterior clinoid distance is wider (22 to 32 mm) than the interposterior clinoid distance (17 to 25 mm) in each patient,[19] allowing the free margins of the tentorium to pass lateral to the posterior clinoid processes.

Tentorial Incisura

The tentorial incisura (tentorial hiatus, tentorial notch) is the gap between the two free margins of the tentorium. The incisura has the shape of a "gothic" arch, with its apex at the confluence of the falx and tentorium and its base on the anterior clinoid processes (Fig. 8-9; see also Fig. 8-8). Its anteroposterior length is

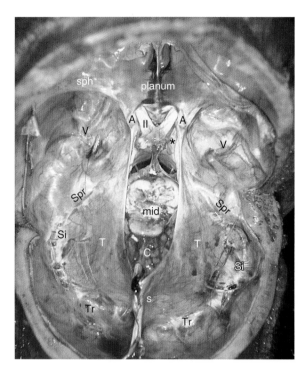

■ **FIGURE 8-8** Tentorium, incisura, and related dural venous sinuses. Fresh cadaver specimen seen from above after removing the cerebrum by section through the midbrain. The posterolateral borders of the two tentorial leaves (T) attach to the occipital bone along the transverse sinuses (Tr) and to the petrous ridges along the superior petrosal sinuses (Spr). The deoxygenated blood within the venous sinuses appears intensely blue. The free margins of the tentorium form a gothic arch that sweeps forward from its apex at the confluence of the falx and tentorium to insert into the anterior clinoid processes (A) bilaterally. The hiatus between the free margins is the tentorial incisura. It contains the culmen (C) of the vermis posteriorly, the midbrain (mid) and perimesencephalic cistern in the midportion, and the prepontine-suprasellar cistern anteriorly. The intracranial segments of the optic nerves (II) enter the suprasellar cistern medial to the anterior clinoid processes (A) and cross to form the optic chiasm (obscured here by residual hypothalamic tissue). Also seen are the cut anterior end of the straight sinus (s), the dura-covered veins (V) on the floor of the middle cranial fossae, the lesser wings of the sphenoid bone (sph), the planum sphenoidale (planum), and the sigmoid sinuses (Si).

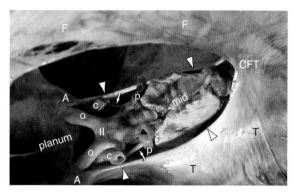

■ **FIGURE 8-9** Tentorial incisura. Fresh gross anatomic specimen in situ, viewed from above and the side. Anterior is to the reader's left (same specimen as Fig. 8-4). The free medial margins (*arrowheads*) of the tentorium (T) define the tentorial incisura. The incisura is shaped like a gothic arch with its apex at the confluence (CFT) of the falx (F) and tentorium (T) posteriorly and its base at the anterior clinoid processes (A) anteriorly. Because the width between the anterior clinoid processes is greater than the width between the posterior clinoid arteries, the free margins of the tentorium pass above and lateral to the posterior clinoid processes en route to the anterior clinoids. The anterior incisural space lies anterior to the midbrain (mid) and contains the prechiasmal intracranial optic nerves (o), the optic chiasm (II), the supraclinoid segments of the internal carotid arteries (c), the proximal posterior cerebral arteries (p), and the oculomotor nerves (*small white arrows*). The middle incisural space lies to each side of the midbrain. The posterior incisural space lies behind the midbrain. (*Courtesy of John Deck, MD.*)

46 to 75 mm (average, 52 mm) and its transverse width is 26 to 35 mm (average, 29.6 mm).[18] For comparative anatomy and human malformation, the length of the closed tentorium along the straight sinus may be compared with the length of the open tentorium along the incisura to indicate how completely the right and left leaves of the tentorium fused together in the midline. This proportion is given as a tentorial index, defined as the length of the straight sinus from the confluence of the falx and tentorium to the torcular divided by the length of the incisura from the dorsum sellae to the confluence of the falx and tentorium (see Fig. 8-5).[17] By this index the tentorium is best developed in the human and the vervet monkey.[17] Note, however, that the index specifically excludes the portion of the open tentorium anterior to the dorsum sellae.

The tentorial incisura provides the only path for CSF and brain structures to pass from the supratentorial to the infratentorial compartments in either direction (Fig. 8-10; see also Fig. 8-9). When viewed from above (after removal of the cerebrum), the incisura contains the sella turcica, the brain stem, the culmen of the vermis, and the related subarachnoid cisterns. When viewed from below (after removal of the cerebellum), the incisura contains the unci of the temporal lobes, the parahippocampal gyri, the brain stem, and the related subarachnoid cisterns.[18] The plane of the tentorium typically crosses the midbrain at the level

of the transverse intercollicular groove between the superior colliculi above and the inferior colliculi below.

The incisura is divided into anterior, middle and posterior incisural spaces in relation to the brain stem. The anterior incisural space lies anterior to the brain stem, the paired middle spaces lateral to the brain stem, and the posterior space behind the brain stem. The anterior incisural space lies anterior to the midbrain and pons. It includes the chiasmatic and interpeduncular cisterns, so it extends from the lamina terminalis above to the interpeduncular fossa below.[18] The posterior portions of the olfactory tracts (CN I), the optic nerves (CN II), and the oculomotor nerves (CN III) pass through this space. It also contains the circle of Willis, the proximal anterior choroidal arteries, the proximal superior cerebellar arteries, and the thalamoperforating arteries. The basal veins of Rosenthal course through the anterior space (and subsequently the middle and posterior spaces) to empty into the vein of Galen.[18]

The middle incisural space lies lateral to the brain stem and is intimately related to the hippocampal formations of the medial temporal lobes. The middle space includes the ambient and crural cisterns. The trochlear nerves (CN IV) and trigeminal nerves (CN V) pass through this space.[18,20-22]

The trochlear nerves arise from the dorsal surface of the brain stem just caudal to the inferior colliculi, inferior to the tentorium. They typically then course parallel to the free margins of the tentorium, immediately inferior to and 2 to 4 mm lateral to the free margins of the tentorium. This position places them at risk during surgery in the high cerebellopontine angle and incisura. The trigeminal nerves arise from the lateral surface of the pons, pass up and over the petrous apices (creating the trigeminal impressions), and then pass under the petroclinoid ligaments to enter Meckel's cave (see later). The major vessels traversing the middle incisural space are the anterior choroidal, posterior cerebral, and superior cerebellar arteries and the basal veins of Rosenthal.

The posterior incisural space is located behind the midbrain and corresponds to CSF cisterns, variably designated the quadrigeminal plate cistern, the peripineal cistern, or the cistern of the

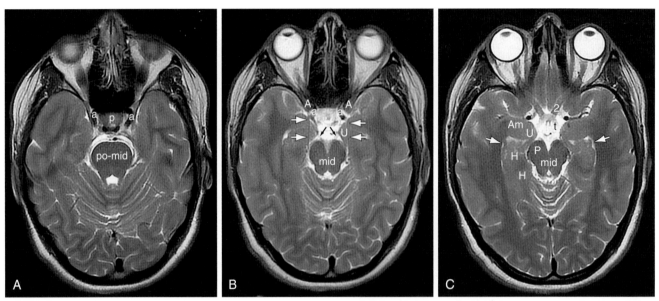

■ **FIGURE 8-10** Tentorial incisura and the incisural CSF spaces. Axial 3T T2W MR images displayed from caudal (**A**) to cranial (**C**). **A,** Just inferior to the plane of the incisura, the MR image displays the junction of the pons with the midbrain (po-mid), the sella turcica containing the pituitary gland (p), and the cavernous sinuses containing the cavernous segments of the internal carotid arteries (a). **B,** In the plane of the incisura, the free margins of the tentorium (*black lines indicated by white arrows*) insert onto the anterior clinoid processes (A). The posterior clinoid processes, seen faintly, clearly lie medial to the free margins. The oculomotor nerves (CN III) (*black arrows*) arise from the interpeduncular fossa of the midbrain (mid) and pass forward to run in the lateral walls of the cavernous sinus. The internal carotid arteries ascend immediately medial to the anterior clinoid processes to become the supraclinoid segments of the internal carotid arteries in the next-higher section. **C,** Just superior to the incisura, the optic nerves (2) decussate within the suprasellar cistern, giving rise to the optic tracts (t). The amygdala (Am) forms the anteriormost wall of the temporal horn (*white arrows*) of the lateral ventricle. The uncus (U) forms the lateral wall of the suprasellar cistern anterior to the temporal horn. The hippocampal formation (H) forms the inferior medial wall of the temporal horn and the medial surface of the temporal lobe. The perimesencephalic cistern surrounds the midbrain. It is often divided into a crural cistern situated between the uncus and the cerebral peduncle (P) and an ambient cistern situated between the hippocampal formation and the posterolateral surface of the midbrain.

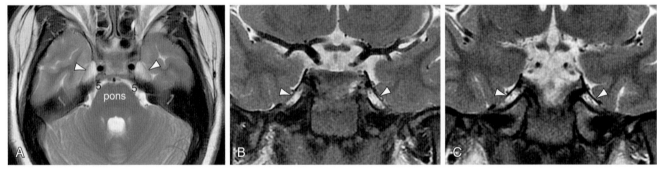

■ **FIGURE 8-11** Meckel's cave. Axial (**A**) and coronal (**B, C**) T2W MR images. The side walls of the sella turcica are the cavernous sinuses, containing the cavernous segments of the internal carotid arteries. Segments of cranial nerves III, IV, V₁, and V₂ run in the lateral wall of the cavernous sinus on each side. Meckel's caves (*white arrowheads*) lie lateral to the cavernous sinuses. The medial wall of Meckel's cave parallels the cavernous sinus. The lateral wall angles laterally, creating a triangular, CSF-filled pocket of dura situated lateral to and just slightly posterior and inferior to the cavernous sinus. The trigeminal ganglion lies along the anteroinferolateral wall of the cave. The trigeminal ganglion (CN V) gives rise to a spray of multiple thin fibers that course through the cave, join into a thick defined root (5) at the posterior aspect of the cave, and then cross the petrous apex to reach the side of the pons. The mandibular division of the trigeminal ganglion (V₃) is often seen to exit the skull through the foramen ovale just inferior to Meckel's cave.

vein of Galen. The trunks and branches of the posterior cerebral and superior cerebellar arteries traverse this space. In this space, the paired internal cerebral veins join the paired basal veins of Rosenthal, the pineal veins, and the superior (galenic) veins of the posterior fossa to enter the vein of Galen.[18]

Meckel's Cave

Meckel's cave is a dural pocket situated along the medial wall of the middle fossa. It contains the trigeminal ganglion (CN V), the central processes of the trigeminal ganglion that pass posteriorly to enter the pons, and a variably large pool of CSF designated the trigeminal cistern (Fig. 8-11).[22] The medial wall of Meckel's cave is dura propria. The lateral wall is the external periosteum. The opening into Meckel's cave lies just beneath the petroclinoid ligament where the anterolateral margin of the tentorium attaches to the posterior clinoid process. Therefore, the subarachnoid space extends into Meckel's cave from the lateral pontine cistern of the posterior fossa, even though the dural pocket itself lies within the middle fossa. The trigeminal ganglion is situated along the anteroinferolateral wall of Meckel's cave and there gives rise to the first (ophthalmic), second (maxillary), and third (mandibular) divisions of the trigeminal nerve.

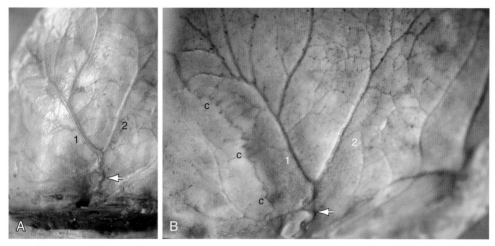

■ FIGURE 8-12 Epidural plane. Fresh gross postmortem specimen. **A,** Outer surface of the convexity dura. **B,** Inner surface of the apposing calvaria. The slight yellow cast is due to the patient's jaundice. The endosteal dura adheres to the bone, leaving no normal epidural space. The middle meningeal artery (*white arrow*) enters the skull base at the foramen spinosum, travels laterally across the middle fossa within the epidural plane, and ascends over the convexity on the outer surface of the dura just posterior to the coronal suture (c). This artery shows modest tortuosity over a short segment inferiorly and then divides into two straighter frontal (1) and parietal (2) branches. The middle meningeal veins parallel the artery. The middle meningeal grooves in the inner table of the calvaria mirror the vessel course.

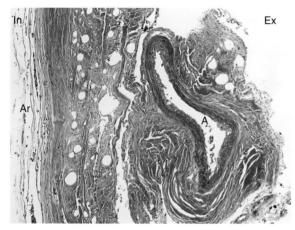

■ FIGURE 8-13 Histology of dura (trichrome stain, original magnification, ×100). From its external (Ex) to its internal (In) surfaces, the densely collagenous dura (intense blue stain) shows multiple parallel layers. The middle meningeal artery (A) lies at the external surface of the dura. Its adventitia is continuous with the outer layer of the dura. The loose arachnoid mater (Ar) is continuous with the internal aspect of the dura.

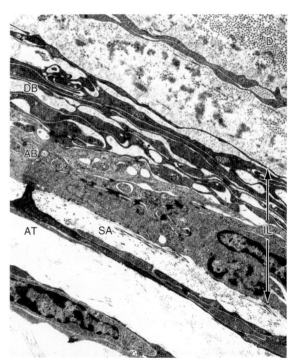

■ FIGURE 8-14 Undisturbed arachnoid-dural interface (fine structure, ×12,400). The interface layer (IL) lies between the subarachnoid space (SA) with its arachnoid trabeculae (AT) and the dura (D). This layer contains the arachnoid barrier (AB) cell layer and the dural border (DB) cell layer. The AB cell layer shows profuse junctional complexes with little extracellular space. The DB cell layer shows few junctional complexes. It lacks collagen and manifests multiple large empty extracellular cisterns. (*From Friede RL: Developmental Neuropathology, 2nd ed. Berlin, Springer-Verlag, 1989.*)

Epidural Space

Within the cranium, there is no preexisting epidural space. An intracranial epidural space is created only when the endosteal layer of the dura detaches from the bony skull. However, meningeal arteries and veins normally course between the dura and the calvaria, forming grooves in the inner table of the skull (Fig. 8-12).[1]

Subdural Space

There is no preexisting normal subdural space, potential or otherwise (Figs. 8-13 and 8-14).[4,23-28] Studies of human cranial meninges fixed in situ show that the outermost layer of the arachnoid (arachnoid barrier cell layer) is directly continuous with, and fused to, the innermost layer of the dura (dural border cell layer).[29] The dural border cell layer itself is characterized by an absence of collagen, by few intercellular connections, and by large extracellular spaces. The cells adhere very poorly to each other. Indeed, the cells of the dural border layer are more closely attached to the arachnoid barrier cell layer than to each other (see Fig. 8-14).[23] This anatomic arrangement provides little cellular cohesion.[29] When observed, the so-called subdural space actually results from tissue damage/trauma that shears along the dural border cell layer, creating a cleavage plane *within* the deepest layer of the dura.[26,28] Histologic study of "subdural" collections created in guinea pigs, with special care taken to remove the meninges intact, confirmed that there were no obvious fluid-filled spaces or gaps between the dura and the arachnoid.[27]

Arachnoid Mater

The cranial arachnoid mater is a very thin membrane situated between the dura mater and the pia mater. It ensheathes the brain and continues along the cranial nerves to their point of exit from the skull.[1] Grossly, the arachnoid appears lucent and glistening at the cerebral convexities. It is thicker and more opaque in the parasagittal region in relation to the arachnoid granulations and also thicker and more opaque along the skull base (Figs. 8-15 and 8-16). The arachnoid mater is avascular and receives nutrients by diffusion.

Histologically, the arachnoid consists of two or three tiers of flattened cells. The outer, arachnoid barrier cell layer is characterized by tightly spaced cells, cytoplasm that is more electrolucent than the cytoplasm of the overlying dural cells or the deeper arachnoid cells, many intercellular junctions, and a characteristic cytoplasmic "fuzz" on either side of these cell junctions. The inner arachnoid cell layer is composed of more loosely organized, less flattened cells connected by gap junctions and desmosomes. The junctions contain small lacunae of collagen fibrils with distinctly smaller diameter than the collagen fibrils of the dura (Fig. 8-17).[26]

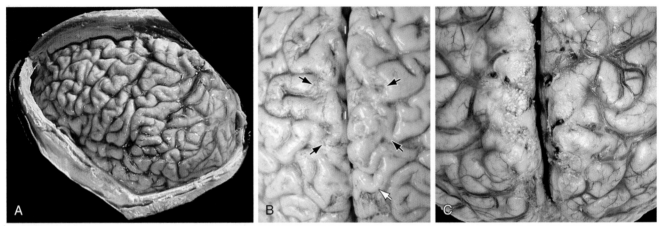

■ **FIGURE 8-15** Arachnoid and pia mater of the convexity. **A,** Fresh gross anatomic specimen in situ, viewed from above and the side after removal of the hemicalvarium and convexity dura. Anterior is to the reader's left (same specimen as in Fig. 8-4). The glistening arachnoid and pia mater ensheathe the brain. The arachnoid lies close to the crowns of the gyri and bridges over the sulci, creating cisterns. The pia mater is closely adherent to the brain surface and extends deeply into the depths of the sulci. The vessels tend to run within the sulci but do cross over the crowns of the gyri as they course over the brain. **B,** Young patient. Fresh gross anatomic specimen of the high convexity-parasagittal surfaces of the two hemispheres across the interhemispheric fissure (I). The parasagittal arachnoid (*black arrows*) is thicker and less translucent in the regions of the arachnoid villi than over the mid convexity. Opening (*white arrow*) of the arachnoid reveals the glistening pia deep to the subarachnoid space. **C,** Older patient. The parasagittal arachnoid displays thickening and prominent granulations resembling sesame seeds. (*A, Courtesy of John Deck, MD.*)

■ **FIGURE 8-16** Gross anatomic specimens of the outer surface of the dura (**A**) and corresponding inner surface of the calvaria (**B**). **A,** Formalin-fixed specimen. The parasagittal dura (*black arrows*) is thickened along the line of arachnoid granulations. **B,** Fresh specimen. The inner table of the skull shows multiple corresponding corticated impressions (*black arrows*) of variable depth to each side of the sagittal suture (s) and multiple ostia of emissary veins (*black arrowheads*). (See also Fig. 8-2.)

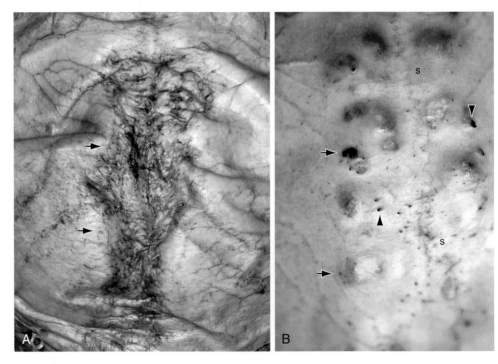

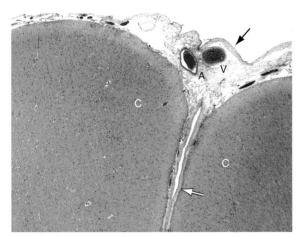

■ **FIGURE 8-17** Histology of the arachnoid and subarachnoid space (trichrome stain, original magnification, ×2). The outer condensed layer of arachnoid (*black arrow*) abuts the dura. Delicate strands of fibrous tissue cross the subjacent subarachnoid space to join the pia mater overlying the cerebral cortex (C). The cut cross sections of an artery (A) and vein (V) overlie the sulcus. A vein (*white arrow*) ascends within the sulcus toward the subarachnoid space.

CSF-Blood Barrier

The dural border cell layer lacks collagen, has large extracellular spaces with few intercellular connections, and has no tight junctions. Therefore, the dural border cell layer does not form a barrier to diffusion of materials.[26] Conversely, the arachnoid barrier cell layer is composed of larger cells with many different cell junctions (desmosomes, tight and gap junctions, hemidesmosomes, and intermediate junctions) and has very little extracellular space. The presence of numerous tight junctions is unique to the arachnoid barrier cell layer. It helps to create a barrier that is impermeable to the movement of fluids (including CSF), large molecular weight substances, and ions.[2,5,26]

Arachnoid Granulations

Arachnoid *villi* are microscopic structures that may be found within the superior sagittal sinus of fetuses and newborns. Arachnoid *granulations* (pacchionian granulations) are larger more complex protrusions of the arachnoid membrane and subarachnoid space into the dural venous sinus, usually at points where the veins enter the sinuses (Fig. 8-18).[30] They are most numerous along the lateral margins of the superior sagittal sinus, the transverse sinuses, and the sigmoid sinuses.[30-32]

Arachnoid granulations large enough to be visible to the naked eye are first seen at age 18 months at the midposterior portion of the superior sagittal sinus where the central and parieto-occipital veins drain into the sinus. The granulations increase in size and frequency with age, appear in the transverse sinuses by 3 years, and appear in other regions of the superior sagittal sinus by 4 years.[33] Ultimately, granulations are seen in 66% of cadaveric dissections and 90% or more of normal adults in vivo.[4,34-36]

The arachnoid granulations serve to resorb CSF into the vascular system and may help to dissipate the arterial pressure wave that enters the skull with each cardiac systole.[1] The size of each granulation varies as it functions, since the granulations distend and regress as they transport CSF from the subarachnoid space into the dural venous sinuses. On average, the mean diameter of the granulations is 1.5 mm at the superior sagittal sinus, 4.1 mm along the transverse sinuses, and 3.8 mm at the straight sinuses.[31] Their combined surface is 78.63 mm² over the whole brain.[30] Large arachnoid granulations commonly form depressions within the inner table and diploë of the skull (see Fig. 8-16). Very large

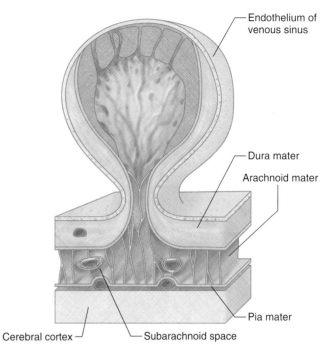

■ **FIGURE 8-18** Anatomy of the granulation. Diagram of the structure of an arachnoid granulation. A thin neck of arachnoid mater protrudes into the venous sinus through an ostium in the dura. This base expands into a series of channels within a core of collagenous trabeculae. A cap of arachnoid cells, approximately 150 μm thick, surrounds the core. The arachnoid cap is thin laterally and thickest at the apex of the granulation. Over most of the granulation, a fibrous dural cupola separates the core and arachnoid cap from the sinus endothelium. At the apex, however, the fibrous cupola thins out. The arachnoid cap thickens and attaches to the sinus endothelium over an area of approximately 300 μm. At this apex, small channels pass through the cap to reach the subendothelial layer of the granulation. *(From Standring S, et al. [eds]: Gray's Anatomy: The Anatomical Basis of Clinical Practice, 40th ed. Philadelphia, Elsevier, 2009.)*

granulations may even protrude through the skull to present beneath the pericranium.

Subarachnoid Space

The intracranial subarachnoid space is a true preexisting space situated between the arachnoid mater and the pia mater and entirely filled with CSF (see Figs. 8-17 and 8-18). Its size varies with location. The arachnoid lies relatively close to the pia over the convexities, so the convexity cisterns are relatively small.[1] The arachnoid is widely separated from the pia at the skull base, so the cisterns at the base are far larger. The arachnoid fuses with the pia at the level of the sella turcica (hypophyseal fossa).[1]

The subarachnoid space is in direct communication with the fourth ventricle by means of the median foramen of Magendie and the paired lateral foramina of Luschka. It is in direct communication with the spinal subarachnoid space via the foramen magnum. The size of the subarachnoid space varies widely among individuals. It definitely increases in size with advancing age beyond young adulthood. The specific subarachnoid cisterns, their relationships, and their contents are detailed in Chapter 13.

Pia Mater and the Perivascular (Virchow-Robin) Spaces

The pia mater consists of two layers: a superficial, epipial layer composed of collagenous fibers and an inner, intima pial layer composed of reticular and elastic fiber.[1] The superficial epipial layer is itself covered by a single layer of flattened mesothelial cells. The inner intima pial layer has a glial membrane that anchors the pia to the underlying cortex.[1] The intima pia, like

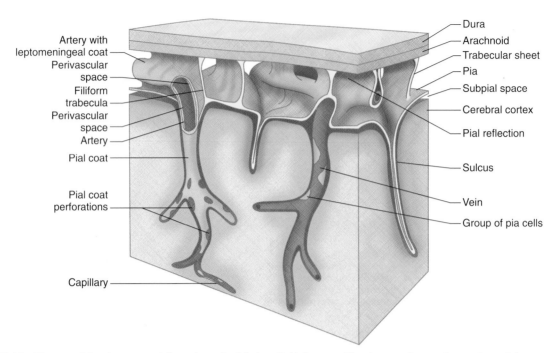

Artery with leptomeningeal coat
Perivascular space
Filiform trabecula
Perivascular space
Artery
Pial coat
Pial coat perforations
Capillary

Dura
Arachnoid
Trabecular sheet
Pia
Subpial space
Cerebral cortex
Pial reflection
Sulcus
Vein
Group of pia cells

■ **FIGURE 8-19** Diagram of the pia mater and the perivascular (Virchow-Robin) spaces. The pia mater invests the arteries and the cortex but is separated from both of these by a subpial space. As the arteries penetrate into the cortex, they carry with them their pial investment and its subpial space. Within the cortex, therefore, the periarterial space has two concentric portions: an outer epipial sleeve of fluid situated between the pia and the glial limiting membrane of the cortex and an inner subpial sleeve of fluid situated between the pia and the outer wall of the artery. As the arteries penetrate deeper into the cortex and morph into arterioles and capillaries, their pial sheath becomes progressively more perforated until it disappears. The smooth muscle and elastic lamina of the arterial wall gradually thin, dehisce focally, and then disappear at the capillary level. With increasing depth into the cortex, therefore, the periarterial-subpial spaces gradually become less well defined and then obliterated by fusion of the basement membrane of the vascular endothelium with the glia limitans of the cortex.[37] The pia mater invests the veins within the subarachnoid space but does not invest the veins within the cortex. Within the cortex, therefore, there is no subpial perivenous space. Instead, any perivenous space lies between the glia limitans of the cortex and the outer wall of the vein. *(From Standring S, et al. [eds]: Gray's Anatomy: The Anatomical Basis of Clinical Practice, 40th ed. Philadelphia, Elsevier, 2009.)*

the arachnoid, is avascular and derives its nutrients by diffusion from the CSF and the underlying nervous tissue.[26] The pial cells are flattened fibroblasts, similar to those of the arachnoid membrane but with thinner processes, on the surface of the brain. They have few or no cell junctions (gap junctions and desmosomes but no tight junctions). Water and low molecular weight solutes may pass freely through the pia, but erythrocytes from subarachnoid hemorrhage, particles, bacteria, and some metabolites are selectively blocked from entering the central nervous system through the pia mater.[5]

The pia mater invests the surface of the brain but is separated from the brain surface by a subpial layer (Fig. 8-19).[37] As the arteries and veins emerge from the brain, the pia encloses them in a perivascular pial sheath that isolates the vessels from the CSF. This leaves a subpial perivascular space between the pial sheath and the outer surface of these *traversing* vessels.[37] As the arteries and veins extend through the cortex, however, the pia forms two distinctly different relationships with the *intracortical* vessels.

Veins

The pial sheath does *not* extend into the brain along the veins. Within the brain, therefore, the veins lie within a space delimited by the glial basement membrane of the brain peripherally and the outer surface of the venous wall centrally.[37] At the surface, this space becomes confluent with the subpial layer of the brain surface. Within the brain, therefore, there is no perivenous pial sheath or subpial perivenous space.[37]

Arteries

The periarterial pial sheath and subpial periarterial space do extend into the brain with the penetrating artery. As a

consequence, the periarterial space consists of two concentric "hollow tubes": an outer tube situated between the glial basement membrane of the brain and the pial sheath and an inner tube situated between the pial sheath and the outer wall of the artery. This inner subpial periarterial space is directly continuous with the subpial periarterial space that surrounds the larger arteries traversing the subarachnoid space (see Fig. 8-19).[37] As the artery penetrates deeper into the brain and morphs into arterioles and capillaries, the arterial wall gradually loses its internal elastic lamina. The coat of smooth muscle thins and shows gaps, and then is lost at the capillary level. Concurrent with that change, the periarterial pial sheath gradually becomes perforated. The perforations become larger. The pial coat becomes incomplete and then disappears. The subpial periarterial space gradually becomes less well defined and is then obliterated by fusion of the basement membranes of the endothelium with the glia.[37] The role of the perivascular space is uncertain. One role may be to prevent peripherally produced catecholamines from entering the brain.[37]

Arterial Supply to the Dura

The dura receives arterial supply from multiple branches of both the anterior (carotid) and the posterior (vertebrobasilar) circulations.

Anterior Circulation

The anterior circulation supplies the cranial dura via five major routes:

1. The external carotid artery usually gives rise to the middle meningeal artery. This artery typically enters the skull through the foramen spinosum and courses extradurally along the

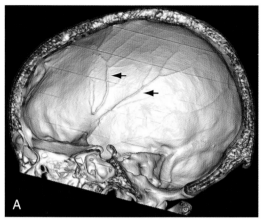

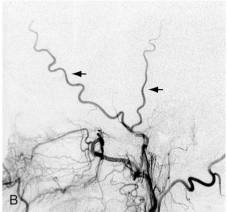

■ **FIGURE 8-20** Arterial supply to the dura: middle meningeal arteries. **A,** Three-dimensional CT reformatted image of the inner table of the skull (lateral view). The grooves (*black arrows*) for the middle meningeal artery pass upward and posteriorly, branching into progressively smaller channels. **B,** Selective external carotid arteriogram displays the proximal portion of the middle meningeal artery (*arrows*).

floor of the middle fossa to the external surface of the convexity dura (Fig. 8-20). There it typically divides into two branches: a larger frontal branch that supplies the outer surface of the dura from the frontoparietal convexity to the vertex and a smaller parietal branch that supplies the posterior dura and cranium only.[1] On occasion, the middle meningeal artery arises, instead, from the ophthalmic arterial branch of the internal carotid artery.

2. The external carotid artery may also give rise to an accessory meningeal artery that supplies the dura of the parasellar region and the trigeminal ganglion.[1]

3. The cavernous segment of the internal carotid artery gives rise to the meningohypophyseal trunk that divides into three major branches. The dorsal meningeal branch supplies the dura overlying the dorsum sellae and upper clivus and extends to the dura of the internal auditory canal. The tentorial branch extends along the medial free margin of the tentorium to supply that plus the adjacent dura. The inferior hypophyseal branch supplies the pituitary gland and adjacent portions of dura.[1]

4. The cavernous segment of the internal carotid artery supplies an anterior meningeal branch to the dura along the floor of the anterior fossa.[1]

5. The ophthalmic branch of the internal carotid artery gives rise to the lacrimal, posterior ethmoidal, and anterior ethmoidal arteries. The lacrimal artery gives off the recurrent meningeal artery to the dura of the anterior wall of the middle fossa. The posterior ethmoidal artery supplies the dura overlying the planum sphenoidale, the posterior half of the cribriform plate, and the ethmoidal air cells. The anterior ethmoidal artery gives off the anterior falcine branch to supply the anterior falx.[1]

Posterior Circulation

The posterior circulation supplies the cranial dura via two major routes (Fig. 8-21):

1. At approximately C2, the vertebral artery gives off an anterior meningeal branch to supply the dura of the anterior margin of the foramen magnum and the inferior clivus.

2. At approximately C1, the vertebral artery gives off a posterior meningeal branch to supply the dura along the posterior margin of the foramen magnum, the falx cerebelli, and the posterior medial portion of the wall of the posterior fossa. This artery may ascend external to the dural venous sinuses to supply the occipital dura superior to the tentorium.[1]

Venous Drainage

The dural venous sinuses lie between the inner meningeal layer of dura and the outer endosteal layer of dura mater (Figs. 8-22

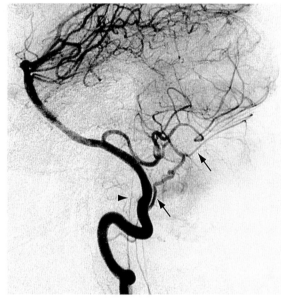

■ **FIGURE 8-21** Arterial supply to the dura: meningeal branches of the vertebral artery. Arterial phase lateral projection vertebral angiogram. The anterior meningeal branch (*arrowhead*) of the vertebral artery to the clivus arises at C2. The posterior meningeal branch (*black arrows*) of the vertebral artery to the occipital dura arises at C1.

and 8-23). They collect blood from the brain, meninges, and calvaria and deliver it to the internal jugular veins and the pterygoid venous plexus at the skull base. The sinuses contain thin (1 to 2 mm) uniform, non-nodular trabeculations (partial septations) first described by Willis and known as Willis cords.[38] These are seen most frequently in the superior sagittal sinus, then the transverse sinuses. They are postulated to tether the vessel walls to limit the expansion of the lumen or to serve as valves that prevent reflux of blood from the dural sinuses into the cortical veins.[38] The dural venous sinuses may be considered in two groups.

Superior Group

The superior group of venous sinuses drains the majority of the brain and skull. This group includes the superior and inferior sagittal sinuses, the straight sinus, the occipital sinus, the transverse sinuses, and the sigmoid sinuses.[39] These sinuses converge toward the torcular Herophili (confluence of the sinuses) just anterior to the internal occipital protuberance but do not necessarily merge together. Often these channels appear contiguous but are not confluent. That is, the flow through them is directed

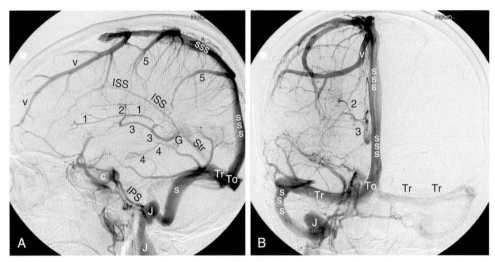

■ **FIGURE 8-22**   Dural venous sinuses. Lateral (**A**) and frontal (**B**) projections of right internal carotid arteriogram (venous phase). The superior sagittal sinus (sss) drains along the outer margin of the falx to reach the torcular (To). Blood then flows preferentially to the right transverse sinus (*white* Tr), sigmoid sinus (s) and jugular vein (J). At the torcular, some blood passes leftward into the smaller left transverse sinus (*black* Tr). A single sss may normally be absent anterior to the coronal suture. In such case, the frontal drainage passes via anterior longitudinal veins (v) to reach the sss behind the coronal suture. The inferior sagittal sinus (ISS) drains posteriorly along the free margin of the falx to reach the anterior end of the straight sinus (Str) at the confluence of the falx and tentorium. The cavernous sinus (c) drains into the jugular system via the inferior petrosal sinus (IPS). The deep venous system of the brain also drains to the straight sinus, including the septal vein (1), thalamostriate vein (2), internal cerebral vein (3), basal vein of Rosenthal (4) and the vein of Galen (G). The convexity veins (5) drain into the superior sagittal sinus (sss).

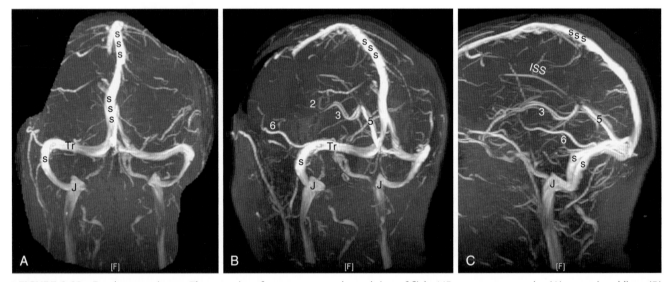

■ **FIGURE 8-23**   Dural venous sinuses. Three rotations from a contrast-enhanced time-of-flight MR venogram: posterior (**A**), posterior oblique (**B**), and lateral (**C**) views. The superior sagittal sinus (SSS) drains more nearly equally into the two transverse sinuses (Tr). The inferior sagittal sinus (ISS) and the thalamostriate (2) and internal cerebral (3) veins of the deep system drain through the straight sinus (5) to the "confluence" of the sinuses. The confluence more closely resembles a series of adjacent channels than a true merging of flows. The vein of Labbe (6) drains into the left transverse sinus. s, sigmoid sinus; J, jugular veins.

into isolated channels resembling the traffic through a cloverleaf interchange rather than into a parking lot.

The *superior sagittal sinus* courses along the midline where the periphery of the falx cerebri joins the inner table of the calvaria. It is triangular in cross section with a transverse diameter of 4 to 10 mm (see Figs. 8-3, 8-22, and 8-23). It receives the superior convexity veins, usually joins with the straight sinus at the torcular, and drains from there into the transverse sinuses (into the right three times more frequently than the left).[39] The precise pattern of drainage is variable. Often the superior sagittal sinus drains into the right transverse sinus near the torcular without actually forming a confluence with the other venous sinuses.[40]

The *inferior sagittal sinus* courses in the midline just inside the free margin of the falx (see Fig. 8-22). It begins above the anterior body of the corpus callosum. It receives tributaries from the superior surface of the corpus callosum, the medial cerebral hemispheres, and the falx cerebri. The inferior sagittal sinus then drains into the anterior end of the straight sinus to reach the torcular and the transverse sinuses. By petalia (see Imaging, later), the inferior sagittal sinus and the straight sinus often drain to the smaller transverse sinus on the left side while the superior sagittal sinus drains directly into the larger transverse sinus on the right side. The inferior sagittal sinus appears to be more pronounced in infants and young children.[39] It may communicate with the superior sagittal sinus via intrafalcine veins.[39]

The *straight sinus* lies along the union of the inferior margin of the falx cerebri with the upper surface of the tentorium cerebelli (see Figs. 8-3, 8-22, and 8-23). It receives drainage from the distal end of the inferior sagittal sinus and the vein of Galen. It may drain into the confluence of the sinuses or may be directed instead into one of the two transverse sinuses, usually the smaller left sinus.[39]

The *transverse sinuses* course along the outer margin of the tentorium cerebelli from the internal occipital protuberance to the lateral edge of the petrous temporal bone (see Figs. 8-22 and 8-23). The transverse sinuses receive blood flow from the superior and inferior sagittal sinuses, the straight sinus, veins along the inferior and lateral surfaces of the temporal and occipital lobes, including the vein of Labbe, and the veins of the cerebellar hemispheres. In turn, the transverse sinuses drain into the jugular veins at the jugular fossae.[39] By petalia (see Imaging, later), the left transverse sinus is typically lower than the right.[39] Overall, the transverse sinuses are estimated to be asymmetric in about half of cases. The right transverse sinus is larger than the left in 73% of asymmetric cases.[40] The left is atretic in up to 20% of cases.[40]

The *occipital sinus* is a common but inconstant venous sinus running along the inferior internal occipital crest from the torcular Herophili to the posterior edge of the foramen magnum. It may appear as a single midline sinus when the falx cerebelli is single or as paired paramedian sinuses when the falx cerebelli is duplicated. It is present in about 65% of cadavers.[41]

The *falcine sinus* is a midline channel between the posterior portion of the superior sagittal sinus and the inferior sagittal sinus or vein of Galen. It is normally present in embryonic life but becomes closed after birth.[42] On occasion, it persists into adult life as a normal variant, in addition to or replacing the straight sinus. It may also be seen in association with diverse congenital malformations.[42] Study of 610 patients undergoing CT angiograms of the head found falcine sinuses in 12 (2.1%) patients. Eleven of the 12 had no associated congenital anomaly or sinus occlusion.[42] One of the 12 had concurrent malposition of the proximal superior sagittal sinus.[42]

Inferior Group

The inferior group of venous sinuses drains the superficial sylvian veins, the basal and medial portions of the undersurface of the brain, and the orbits. This group includes the sphenoparietal sinuses, the cavernous sinuses, the superior and inferior petrosal sinuses, and the basal pterygoid venous plexus.[39]

The *sphenoparietal sinus* (sinus of Breschet) is the medial extension of the superficial middle cerebral vein along and beneath the lesser wing of the sphenoid. It may drain into the cavernous sinus, the pterygoid venous plexus, or the inferior petrosal sinus.[39]

The *cavernous sinuses* lie lateral to the body of the sphenoid bone and run from the superior orbital fissure to the petrous apex. They typically are compartmentalized sinuses, with different portions of the sinus receiving flow from different tributaries and directing the flow outward to different drainage fields. The anterior cavernous sinuses receive blood from the superior and inferior ophthalmic veins and the sphenoparietal sinus. The posterior cavernous sinuses receive flow from the superior petrosal sinus and drain through the inferior petrosal sinus into the jugular vein.[39]

The *superior petrosal sinuses* run along the petrous ridges where the tentorium cerebelli inserts onto the superior margin of the petrous temporal bone. These sinuses extend from the transverse sinus to the cavernous sinus on each side. The superior petrosal sinus receives the petrosal vein, the lateral mesencephalic vein, cerebellar veins, and veins draining the tympanic cavity.[39]

The *inferior petrosal sinuses* lie within the grooves between the clivus and the petrous apices on each side. They drain from the cavernous sinus into the anterosuperior portion of the jugular bulbs.

The *pterygoid venous plexus* lies around and partly within the lateral pterygoid muscle. Its tributaries correspond to the branches of the three parts of the maxillary artery. It communicates with the facial vein through the deep facial vein, with the cavernous sinus by means of one or more emissary veins passing through the foramen ovale, and with the inferior ophthalmic vein through the inferior orbital fissure. It drains through the maxillary vein. The plexus may be difficult to find in the cadaver where it is empty of blood but in the living subject is frequently a prominent feature.[43]

Intradural Venous Plexus

The dura mater itself contains a diffuse plexus of venous sinusoids that give it a sponge-like consistency. That is, the dura is not a fixed leathery sheet of collagen but an expansile structure. Engorgement of the intradural plexus of venous sinusoids may thicken the dura mater to greater than 1 cm over large expanses of the skull base, the dural partitions, and the convexity. The degree of sinus engorgement and the degree of dural thickening are directly related to the intracranial pressure and vary together, in both directions, with fluctuations in intracranial pressure. This phenomenon is particularly evident in patients with intracranial hypotension, in whom low CSF pressure is associated with marked thickening of the dura and in whom the dura decreases in thickness as the CSF pressure rises toward normal. It is thought that a small pressure gradient is needed to drive the CSF across the arachnoid granulation into the venous sinus. When the pressure in the CSF falls (intracranial hypotension), the body pools blood within the intradural venous plexus. This acts to reduce the intrasinus pressure below CSF pressure and maintain the gradient of pressure needed to resorb CSF.[44,45]

In the neonate, extensive dural venous plexi are found within the tentorium, posterior falx, and dura of the floor of the posterior cranial fossa.[34] These intrinsic dural plexi are thought to play a role in cases of nontraumatic infantile subdural hematoma.[4,34] Over time, these plexuses (of unknown function) disappear, leaving only the familiar major sinuses of the adult dura.[34]

Innervation of the Dura

The dura is innervated primarily by the three divisions of the trigeminal nerve (CN V), the dorsal sensory rami of the first three cervical spinal nerves, and the cranial sympathetic trunk. The recurrent branch of the ophthalmic nerve (V_1) supplies portions of the tentorium. The recurrent branch of the maxillary nerve (V_2) is distributed with the frontal branch of the middle meningeal artery to innervate the dura of the anterior portion of the middle fossa.[46] There are additional contributions from the facial (CN VII), glossopharyngeal (CN IX), vagus (CN X), and hypoglossal (CN XI) nerves.[1]

IMAGING

CT

Noncontrast CT has limited value for displaying the parietal dura of the convexity and skull base. It can display the inner dura of the falx and tentorium, especially when the subarachnoid cisterns are large, so the dura is surrounded by low-density CSF. Noncontrast CT does not display the normal pia or arachnoid mater. Dural calcification appears as linear to nodular foci of increased density along the planes of the dura (Fig. 8-24). Ossification appears as islands of increased density with corticated margins and lower-density centers (Fig. 8-25). Distinguishing dural calcification from ossification can be medically significant, because the marrow present within falcine ossifications may participate in extramedullary hematopoiesis, systemic

■ FIGURE 8-24 Calcification of the falx. **A,** Axial noncontrast CT shows increased density and slightly irregular thickening of the falx (*white arrowhead*). **B,** Corresponding T1W MR image shows paired parallel lines of increased signal flanking a midline low signal structure. Trace minerals in the calcific deposits outline the low signal fibrous falx.

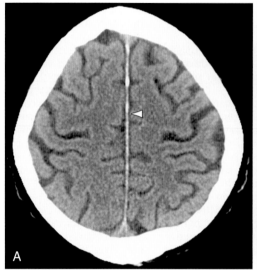
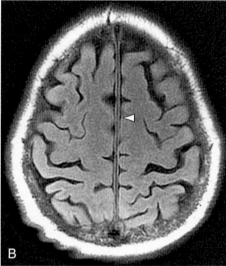

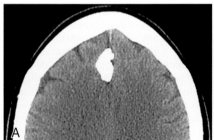
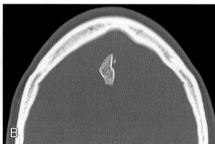
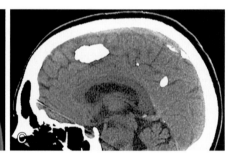

■ FIGURE 8-25 Ossification of the falx. Axial soft tissue (**A**) and bone (**B**) algorithm images display focal well-corticated, centrally less dense mineralization along the right lateral border and inferior margin of the anterior falx. **C,** Sagittal reformatted CT image displays the position of the mineralization with respect to the falcine incisura and medial surface of the hemisphere. Other smaller foci of ossification are also seen along the falx.

■ FIGURE 8-26 Fat deposits along the falx. Axial (**A**) and coronal reformatted (**B**) CT scans demonstrate a small, sharply marginated deposit of low density fat along the side of the falx. These are common, do not constitute "lipomas," and are not presently known to have pathologic significance.

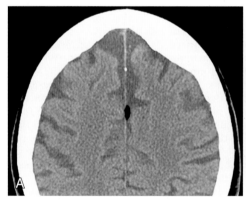
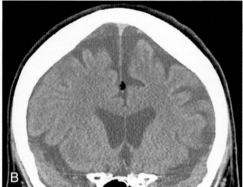

leukemias, and metastases to the marrow. Small deposits of fat appear as well-defined foci of low density along or within the dura (Fig. 8-26).

Contrast-enhanced CT displays all of the layers of the dura better than does noncontrast CT. The normal dura shows uniformly thick, homogeneous enhancement with a characteristic progression of anatomic features from superior to inferior in axial images (Figs. 8-27 and 8-28) and from anterior to posterior in coronal images (Fig. 8-29). Contrast-enhanced CT usually does not display the normal pia or arachnoid matter.

Petalia

The term *petalia* signifies the asymmetry of the dural partitions, venous drainage, and impressions on the inner table of the calvaria that arise because of cerebral dominance (Figs. 8-30 to 8-32).[47,48] Petalia is best understood through embryology, as follows:

1. Cerebral dominance is associated with asymmetric enlargement of the dominant parietal lobe. The larger dominant parietal lobe displaces the adjacent occipital lobe posteriorly

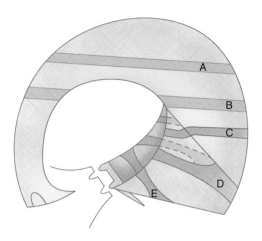

■ **FIGURE 8-27** Diagram of the relationships of serial axial CT sections to the falx and tentorium. View from above and lateral. From craniad to caudad, contrast-enhanced CT sections will display the following: *A,* An uninterrupted length of the falx in sections superior to the falcine incisura, *B,* Short anterior and long posterior *discontinuous* lengths of falx in sections through the falcine incisura but superior to the tentorium, *C,* Y to V "wine glass" shapes in sections through the upper tentorium superior to the torcular, *D,* An M shape in sections directly through the torcular, and, *E,* paired diverging lines of tentorium in sections wholly inferior to the torcular. The M shape is most obvious in patients with especially flat angles of the tentorium or in studies using thicker sections. It arises in sections through the torcular, because the upper portion of the section lies above the torcular, producing a deep V while the lower portion of the same section passes inferior to the torcular, producing diverging bands. Caught just right, these merge into an M.

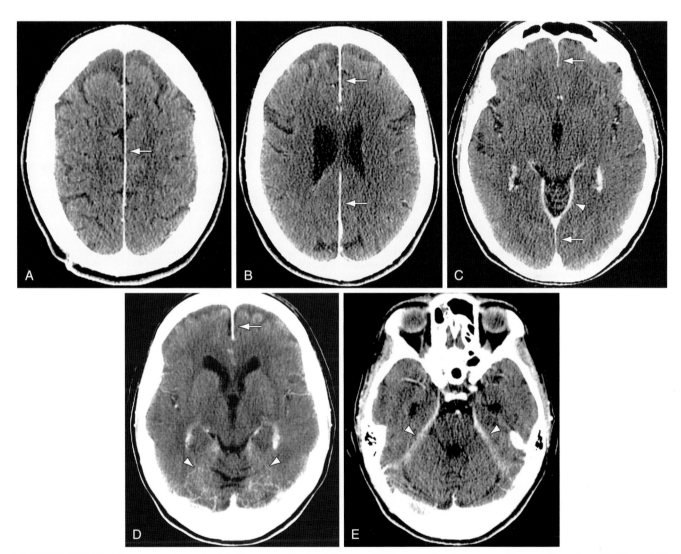

■ **FIGURE 8-28** Serial contrast-enhanced axial CT sections displayed from craniad to caudad and corresponding to sections **A** to **E** in Figure 8-27. *Arrows* indicate the falx cerebri. *Arrowheads* indicate the tentorium.

and, as seen on imaging, rotates it clockwise across the midline. The dominant hemisphere also bulges inferiorly, so the inferior surface of the temporo-occipital lobes lies lower on the dominant side. The frontal lobes are less affected and usually remain symmetric in size and position.

2. In right-handed individuals, and most left-handed individuals, the left parietal lobe is larger than the right.
3. The brain and meninges develop in a fixed embryologic order. The neural tissue (neuropil) begins to develop first. Then the vascular tunic begins to condense around the

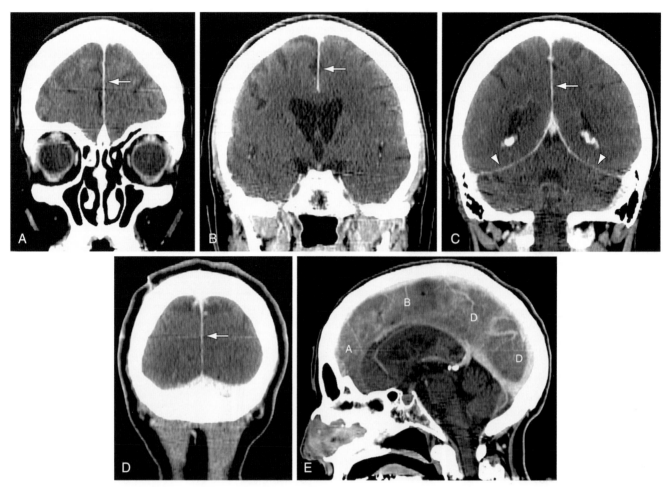

■ **FIGURE 8-29** Contrast-enhanced coronal CT sections through the falx and tentorium. From anterior to posterior, these display the uninterrupted falx anterior to the falcine incisura (**A**), the mid falx above the falcine incisura (**B**), the falx joining the tentorium in the midline (**C**), and the uninterrupted posterior falx behind the posterior fossa (**D**). **E**, Midsagittal reformatted contrast-enhanced CT. Letters indicate the positions of the four coronal sections. *Arrows* indicate the falx cerebri. *Arrowheads* indicate the tentorium.

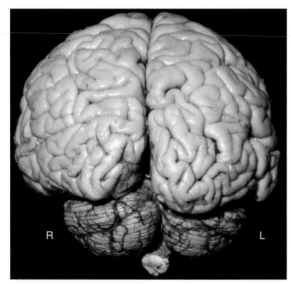

■ **FIGURE 8-30** Petalia. Formalin-fixed gross anatomic specimen. The left (L) and right (R) sides have been reversed, so that the sidedness conforms to the imaging convention. Posterior view of the occipital lobes and cerebellar hemispheres shows the asymmetric, posterior, and inferior position of the left occipital pole.

neuropil. Then the meninges begin to condense around both the neuropil and the vascular tunic, ultimately forming the pia, arachnoid, dura, and bone.

4. Because the neural tissue develops first and the dominant hemisphere shows asymmetric expansion, the meninges are forced to condense around an asymmetric brain.

Anatomically, the two frontal lobes are approximately symmetric up to the central sulci. Therefore, the mesenchyme that makes the anterior falx condenses in relation to the two symmetric frontal lobes and the *anterior* falx typically lies in the midline. The parietal and occipital lobes are asymmetric. The mesenchyme that makes the *posterior* falx condenses around the asymmetrically displaced occipital lobes, so the posterior falx typically deviates away from the midline toward the non-dominant side (Fig. 8-31). Similarly, the mesenchyme that makes the tentorium condenses under the asymmetric temporo-occipital lobes, so the tentorium forms in lower position on the left than the right sides (Fig. 8-32). The dural venous sinuses that course in the outer margins of the dura deviate with the dura. For the same reasons, therefore, the posterior portion of the superior sagittal sinus commonly deviates with the falx to the patient's nondominant right side and drains into a larger right jugular system. The transverse sinus is lower on the dominant left side. On occasion, the two frontal lobes are also affected by

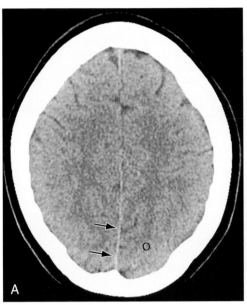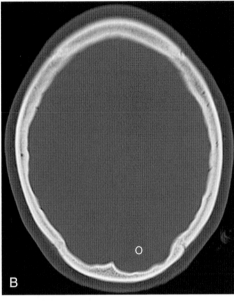

■ **FIGURE 8-31** Petalia. Axial non-contrast CT scan with brain (**A**) and bone (**B**) algorithm displays. The falx cerebri is midline anteriorly but breaks sharply to the right (*arrows*) posteriorly, in relation to the asymmetric position of the left occipital lobe (O). The inner table of the calvaria is scalloped focally in relation to the displaced occipital bone.

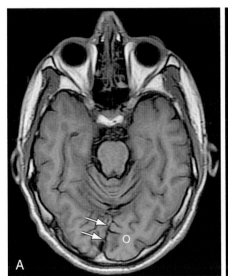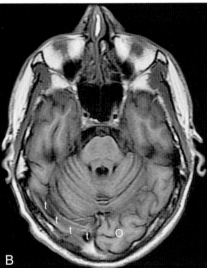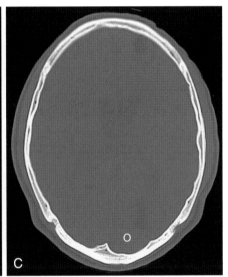

■ **FIGURE 8-32** Petalia. **A** and **B**, Axial T1W MR images. **C**, Bone algorithm CT. The posterior falx cerebri (*arrows*) deviates off midline to the right. The left occipital lobe (O) lies asymmetrically far posteriorly and inferiorly, scalloping the inner table of the left calvaria. In **B**, the left occipital lobe (O) is seen inferior to any portion of the right occipital lobe, in relation to the left cerebellar hemisphere and the large right transverse sinus (t).

this process. In those cases, they, too, exhibit clockwise rotation, displacing the right hemisphere across the midline to the left. In such cases, the nondominant frontal lobe and the anterior falx both deviate to the dominant left side, even though the dominant parieto-occipital lobes and posterior falx deviate to the opposite side. Similarly, the mesenchyme that condenses into the bone also condenses asymmetrically around the asymmetrically displaced hemisphere. As a result, the occipital bone is often thinner on the left side and the inner table of the occipital bone shows greater scalloping on the left than the right sides (see Figs. 8-31 and 8-32). Other significant effects of petalia such as asymmetries of the sylvian fissures are addressed in Chapter 9.

MRI
MRI is the best imaging modality to assess the intracranial meninges.[49-53] Noncontrast MRI shows the falx and tentorium by the

same criteria as for noncontrast CT (adjusted for the whiteness vs. blackness of the CSF on each pulse sequence). The contour and thickness of the dura may often be determined and followed serially. Contrast-enhanced MRI displays the parietal dura and the inner dural partitions very well. In patients with significant petalia, the sagittal MR images must be interpreted carefully. In that circumstance, the anterior and posterior ends of the same image may actually display two different hemispheres in the single sagittal image.

Arachnoid granulations are seen in 13% of patients by contrast-enhanced MRI and 24% by contrast-enhanced CT.[38,39] They appear hyperintense on T2-weighted (T2W) images and hypointense to isointense on T1-weighted (T1W) and fluid-attenuated inversion recovery T2W images. They are often observed in the posterior portion of the superior sagittal sinus near to the lambda and are often associated with small, smoothly corticated depressions (calvarial remodeling) in the adjacent bone. MRI frequently shows direct continuity of the granulation with the subarachnoid space and nearly always shows a small eccentric vein within the large arachnoid granulations (98% of cases).[38,39]

Thin linear bands or trabeculations termed *Willis cords* are commonly observed throughout the superior sagittal sinus. They arise in relation to the entry of cortical veins, so they are most frequent along the middle one third of the sagittal sinus, are less common in the transverse sinuses, and are not observed in the sigmoid sinuses.[38,39] The cords exhibit a broad (1-4 cm) base of attachment along the wall of the sinus, project a free inner margin into the sinus, and often extend from wall to wall as partial septations.[38,39] These cords appear to orient in multiple directions within the superior sagittal sinus but always align parallel to the long axis of the transverse sinuses.[35,38] Overall, Willis cords are found in up to 92% of sinuses on gadolinium-enhanced MR venography.[35,38]

The perivascular Virchow-Robin spaces contain interstitial fluid, not CSF, so their signal intensity differs slightly from CSF. Visually, the signal intensity of the interstitial fluid and CSF appear equal. Quantitatively the interstitial fluid is just slightly less intense than the CSF, no matter the pulse sequence utilized.[33] The mean T2W MR signal intensity of perivascular space has been approximated at 898, compared with 980 for subarachnoid space and 972 for intraventricular space.[54]

Perivascular spaces less than 2 mm appear in patients of all ages. They increase in frequency and size with advancing patient age (see Figs. 8-17, 8-19, and 8-33).[33] Perivascular spaces up to 5 mm are seen in approximately 1.6% of neurologically normal patients.[33,55] They appear as well-defined, bilateral, round, oval, or tubular structures that are isodense/isointense to CSF on all pulse sequences.[33] Prominent Virchow-Robin spaces are usually found in three classic locations. Type I Virchow-Robin spaces are frequently seen along the lenticulostriate arteries that enter the basal ganglia through the anterior perforated substance. Type II Virchow-Robin spaces are found along the perforating medullary arteries that pass through the cortical gray matter to penetrate into the underlying white matter. Type III Virchow-Robin spaces are seen in the midbrain, usually deep to the cerebral peduncles. Giant Virchow-Robin spaces are markedly enlarged, cause mass effect, and have unusual morphologies. When they border a ventricle or CSF conduits or are found in a noncharacteristic location, they may be considered pathologic.[33]

Special Procedures

The middle meningeal arteries and the dural venous sinuses are readily displayed by CT angiography, MR angiography, and conventional catheter angiography. The smaller meningeal arteries are best assessed by direct catheter angiography. The inferior petrosal sinus is often catheterized to sample the levels of pituitary hormones draining from the cavernous sinuses on the two sides. The difference between the two sides helps to lateralize an otherwise-occult pituitary adenoma for treatment by "blind" resection of one half of the pituitary gland.[39]

Altering of Normal Imaging Appearance by Pathologic Process

Pathology affecting the dura typically appears as abnormal thickening, nodularity, and increased enhancement of the dura. It may manifest focally, as in a dural-based meningioma or over broad reaches of the dura as in intradural (so-called subdural) hemorrhages and empyema. Pathology of the arachnoid and subarachnoid space usually manifests as meningeal inflammation that fibroses the space, perhaps causing hydrocephalus as well, or as meningeal filling processes that replace the CSF with blood (subarachnoid hemorrhage), pus (leptomeningitis), or tumor (leptomeningeal carcinomatosis).[50,51,56,57] Fluid-attenuated

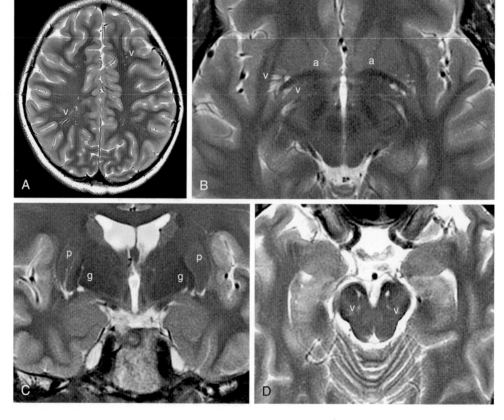

■ **FIGURE 8-33** Virchow-Robin (VR) perivascular spaces. In the cerebral hemispheres (**A**), prominent VR spaces appear as (curvi)linear high signal intensity strands aligned along the courses of the white matter veins. In the basal ganglia, axial (**B**) and coronal (**C**) T2W series show the VR spaces (v) ascending through the globus pallidus (g) and putamen (p) both medial and lateral to posterior curvature of the anterior commissure (a). In the midbrain (**D**), the VR spaces lie within the substantia nigra, course roughly perpendicular to the surface of the cerebral peduncle, and then curve gracefully into the parenchyma.

inversion recovery (FLAIR) T2W MRI may display subarachnoid processes as regions in which the subarachnoid space continues to exhibit high signal intensity instead of "nulling out" to low signal as would normal CSF. However, elevated partial pressures of oxygen within the CSF may also manifest as residual high CSF signal in FLAIR T2W series, presenting a diagnostic pitfall in patients receiving supplemental oxygen during MRI.

ANALYSIS

Modern CT scanners now provide "automatic" triplanar reconstructions, so CT and MR studies can be analyzed in much the same way. However, analysis of CT scans usually begins with axial images, whereas analysis of the MR images usually starts with the sagittal plane.

CT

1. First evaluate the overlying scalp for edema, mass, tracts, and so on.
2. Then analyze the calvaria and skull base for hyperostosis, erosion, permeation, fracture, vascularity, and other signs of disease. On noncontrast CT scans, asymmetric enlargement of a middle meningeal groove may be the sole sign of an otherwise occult meningioma or dural arteriovenous fistula.
3. Next, review the sulci and cisterns along the convexity, the interhemispheric fissure, and the interface between cerebrum and cerebellum for local or diffuse expansion, deflection, compression, effacement, or density change that may signify an adjacent dural or arachnoid pathologic process. Focal sulcal compression and displacement may be the sole clues to an adjacent isodense meningioma. Unexpectedly wide cisterns may reflect arachnoid, epidermoid, or other cysts.
4. On all cuts, specifically search along the inner table of the calvaria, the length of the interhemispheric fissure, the expected plane of the tentorium, and the incisura for evidence of meningeal disease. Identify deviations of the falx and tentorium that indicate petalia and confirm these by the correspondingly deep convolutional markings on the inner table of the occipital bone. Note the normal position and thickness of the dura and any calcifications, bone islands, fat deposits, and other variations present. Report any increased thickness, density, nodularity, or other abnormality that could represent dural pathology.
5. From knowledge of the changing appearance of the falx and tentorium on sequential axial, coronal, or sagittal images, note where deviations from that pattern suggest a pathologic process. In axial plane images, for example, the falx should appear as one continuous line superiorly but separate into discontinuous anterior and posterior portions further inferiorly where the section passes through the falcine incisura. Figures 8-3A and 8-4A document the wide variation in the depth of the falx and the site at which the falcine incisura may be expected, but persistence of a single "falx" below the level expected may be one sign of interhemispheric subdural or subarachnoid hemorrhage.[58]
6. Review the courses of the dural venous sinuses to understand the patterns of preferential drainage in that specific patient. Specifically search for any increased density that could signify sinus thrombosis.
7. On contrast-enhanced CTs, repeat the analysis above, specifically searching for regions of increased density and regions where expected increases in density fail to appear. Meningiomas, for example, may be isodense and undetectable on noncontrast CT but appreciable after contrast enhancement. Leptomeningeal inflammation and tumor may be identified most easily by a sulcal-cisternal pattern of contrast enhancement. Failure of a sinus to opacify may signify sinus thrombosis. Filling defects within an opacified venous

sinus are often pacchionian granulations but may be thrombi or tumor instead.
8. When triplanar images are available, deliberately review all of the coronal and sagittal images for anything that might have been missed on axial images. The sagittal images may be especially useful for the meningeal lesions such as small meningiomas along the skull base, especially the clivus.
9. Specifically review any older imaging studies for interval changes that help to understand the temporal evolution of any pathologic process discerned.

MRI

Analyze the MR images for the same features analyzed for CT, usually starting with the sagittal series. In addition, the analysis should continue and include those imaging features unique to MRI.

10. Review the diffusion-weighted series for restriction of diffusion by infarction, infection, and some tumors.
11. Review the T2*W images for abnormal magnetic susceptibility.
12. Consider use of high spatial resolution sequences such as General Electric's fast imaging employing steady-state acquisition (FIESTA) or Siemen's constructive interference in steady-state sequence (CISS) sequences to evaluate intracisternal pathology. Small arachnoid cysts and cisternal cysticercal cysts may become appreciable only on such series.

A sample report is presented in Box 8-1.

BOX 8-1 Sample Report: MRI for Postural Headache

PATIENT HISTORY

A 70-year-old woman presented with headache that was more severe when she was standing.

TECHNIQUE

Multisequence multidirectional MRI of the head was performed as noncontrast T1W sagittal; T1W, T2W, FLAIR T2W axial; and T1W, T2W and T2*W coronal plane series. Additional diffusion-weighted imaging with apparent diffusion coefficient maps was also performed. After determining that renal function was adequate, gadolinium-chelate contrast agent was administered in a dose of 0.1 mMol per kilogram of body weight. Thereafter, additional postcontrast T1W images were obtained in sagittal, axial, and coronal planes. The patient experienced no adverse reaction to the contrast agent.

FINDINGS

The axial T1W, T2W and FLAIR T2W images display uniform thickening and homogeneously increased signal of the pachymeninges along the convexity, falx, and tentorium (Fig. 8-34). There is no corresponding change in the leptomeninges. The contrast-enhanced images show markedly abnormal, uniformly thick contrast enhancement restricted to the dura. The ventricles and sulci are small for age. The brain parenchyma shows normal signal and normal contrast enhancement throughout. The visualized portions of the vascular tree are normal. A small well-defined perivascular space noted at the posterior right putamen is considered to be a normal variant.

IMPRESSION

There is diffuse uniform thickening, increased signal, and abnormal contrast enhancement restricted to the dura, sparing the leptomeninges. The size of the ventricles and sulci is subnormal for age. In a patient with postural headache, these findings most probably represent intracranial hypotension with compensatory dilatation of the intrinsic intradural venous plexus.

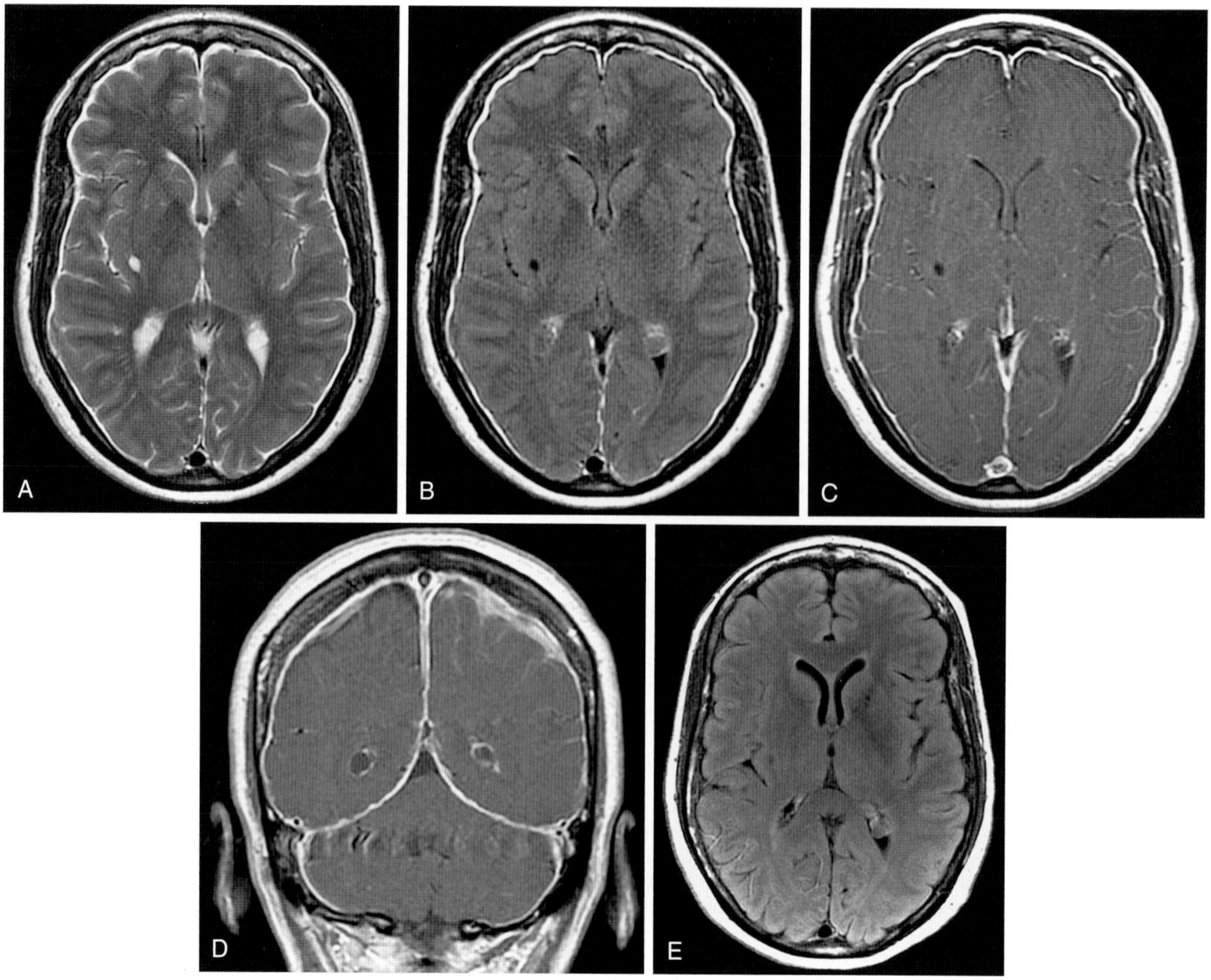

■ **FIGURE 8-34** A 70-year-old woman presented with a headache that is more severe in upright position. **A,** Noncontrast axial T2W MR image. **B,** Noncontrast axial FLAIR T2W MR image. **C** and **D,** Contrast-enhanced axial (**C**) and coronal (**D**) T1W MR images. **E,** Noncontrast FLAIR T2W MR image 6 days later. See sample report in Box 8-1. Blood patch repair of a post–lumbar puncture CSF leak corrected the leak, the headache, and the MR abnormalities simultaneously.

KEY POINTS

■ The falx is typically sickle shaped with a wide, anterior falcine incisura. Normal variations in the thickness, shape, and integrity of the falx alter the imaging appearance and influence the ease and extent of left-right subfalcine herniation and consequent distal anterior cerebral artery infarction.

■ The dural venous sinuses develop in the outer margins or the free edges of the falx and tentorium, establishing the positions of the superior and inferior sagittal sinuses, the straight sinus, the transverse and sigmoid sinuses, and the superior and inferior petrosal sinuses.

■ The torcular Herophili (confluence of the sinuses) may function as a true confluence of sinuses in which all flows merge. However, it often develops asymmetrically as partially separated, juxtaposed channels that direct flow preferentially toward specific routes. The superior sagittal sinus more commonly drains to the right transverse sinus, whereas the inferior sagittal/straight sinuses commonly drain to the left.

■ There is no true subdural space. Processes attributed to the subdural space appear to occur within the dural border cell layer instead.

■ The lateral edges of the tentorium insert into the occipital bone and the petrous ridges along the transverse and superior petrosal sinuses and then continue onto the posterior clinoid processes as the petroclinoid ligaments. The free medial margins of the tentorium extend from the confluence of the falx and tentorium posteriorly to insert onto the anterior clinoid processes anteriorly.

■ The tentorial incisura lies between the free medial margins of the tentorium and assumes the shape of a gothic arch, with its apex at the confluence of the falx and tentorium. It contains the brain stem and the culmen of the vermis.

■ The pia mater continues into the brain with the arteries but not the veins, so the intracerebral perivascular spaces surrounding the arteries differ from those about the veins. The intracerebral *periarterial* space is formed of two concentric sheaths: an outer epipial zone between the glia limitans of the brain and the pial sheath and an inner subpial zone between the pial sheath and the outer wall of the artery. The *perivenous* space consists of a single zone between the glia limitans and the outer wall of the vein.

■ The term *petalia* signifies a set of asymmetries in the brain, vasculature, meninges, and bone that result from asymmetric expansion of the dominant parietal lobe during embryogenesis. These commonly cause deviation of the posterior falx and superior sagittal sinus to the right, asymmetrically lower position of the tentorium, and transverse sinus on the left and preferential drainage of the inferior sagittal sinus through the straight sinus to the lower smaller left transverse sinus.

SUGGESTED READINGS

Carpenter MB, Sutin J. Human Neuroanatomy, 8th ed. Baltimore, Williams & Wilkins, 1983.

Nieuwenhuys R, Voogd J, van Huijzen C. The Human Central Nervous System, 4th ed. Berlin, Springer-Verlag, 2008.

Standring S, et al (eds). Ventricular system and subarachnoid space. In: Gray's Anatomy, 40th ed. Philadelphia, Elsevier, 2008, pp 237-245.

REFERENCES

1. Greenberg RW, Lane EL, Cinnamon J, et al. The cranial meninges: anatomic considerations. Semin Ultrasound CT MR 1994; 15:454-465.

2. Barshes N, Demopoulos A, Engelhard HH. Anatomy and physiology of the leptomeninges and CSF space. Cancer Treat Res 2005; 125:1-16.

3. McLone DG, Naidich TP. Developmental morphology of the subarachnoid space, brain vasculature, and contiguous structures, and the cause of the Chiari II malformation. AJNR Am J Neuroradiol 1992; 13:463-482.

4. Mack J, Squier W, Eastman JT. Anatomy and development of the meninges: implications for subdural collections and CSF circulation. Pediatr Radiol 2009; 39:200-210.

5. Weller RO. Microscopic morphology and histology of the human meninges. Morphologie 2005; 89:22-34.

6. Osborn AG, Anderson RE, Wing SD. The false falx sign. Radiology 1980; 134:421-425.

7. Hudson AJ. Bifrontopolar subdural hematoma and absence of the falx cerebri. Can Med Assoc J 1965; 93:761-764.

8. Galligioni F, Bernardi R, Mingrino S. Anatomic variation of the height of the falx cerebri: its relationship to displacement of the anterior cerebral artery in frontal space-occupying lesions. Am J Roentgenol Radium Ther Nucl Med 1969; 106:273-278.

9. Debnath J, Satija L, George RA, et al. Computed tomographic demonstration of unusual ossification of the falx cerebri: a case report. Surg Radiol Anat 2009; 31:211-213.

10. Tubbs RS, et al. Complete ossification of the human falx cerebri. Clin Anat 2006; 19:147-150.

11. Ohela K, Teir H. [Calcification of dura mater; medico-legal aspects of a case.] Dtsch Z Gesamte Gerichtl Med 1956; 45:488-491.

12. Chen S, Shao KN, Chiang JH, et al. Fat in the cerebral falx. Zhonghua Yi Xue Za Zhi (Taipei) 2000; 63:804-808.

13. Tubbs RS, Dockery SE, Salter G, et al. Absence of the falx cerebelli in a Chiari II malformation. Clin Anat 2002; 15:193-195.

14. D'Costa S, Krishnamurthy A, Nayak SR, et al. Duplication of falx cerebelli, occipital sinus, and internal occipital crest. Rom J Morphol Embryol 2009; 50:107-110.

15. Hasan M, Das AC. A note on the falx cerebelli. Acta Anat (Basel) 1969; 74:624-628.

16. Shoja MM, et al. A complex dural-venous variation in the posterior cranial fossa: a triplicate falx cerebelli and an aberrant venous sinus. Folia Morphol (Warsz) 2007; 66:148-151.

17. Klintworth GK. The comparative anatomy and phylogeny of the tentorium cerebelli. Anat Rec 1968; 160:635-642.

18. Rhoton AL Jr. Tentorial incisura. Neurosurgery 2000; 47(3 Suppl):S131-S153.

19. Bull JW. Tentorium cerebelli. Proc R Soc Med 1969; 62:1301-1310.

20. Yousry I, Moriggl B, Dieterich M, et al. MR anatomy of the proximal cisternal segment of the trochlear nerve: neurovascular relationships and landmarks. Radiology 2002; 223:31-38.

21. Yousry I, Moriggl B, Holtmannspoetter M, et al. Detailed anatomy of the motor and sensory roots of the trigeminal nerve and their neurovascular relationships: a magnetic resonance imaging study. J Neurosurg 2004; 101:427-434.

22. Yousry I, Moriggl B, Schmid UD, et al. Trigeminal ganglion and its divisions: detailed anatomic MR imaging with contrast-enhanced 3D constructive interference in the steady state sequences. AJNR Am J Neuroradiol 2005; 26:1128-1135.

23. Schachenmayr W, Friede RL. The origin of subdural neomembranes: I. Fine structure of the dura-arachnoid interface in man. Am J Pathol 1978; 92:53-68.

24. Haines DE. On the question of a subdural space. Anat Rec 1991; 230:3-21.

25. Haines DE, Harkey HL, al-Mefty O. The "subdural" space: a new look at an outdated concept. Neurosurgery 1993; 32:111-120.

26. Nabeshima S, Reese TS, Landis DM, Brightman MW. Junctions in the meninges and marginal glia. J Comp Neurol 1975; 164:127-169.

27. Frederickson RG. The subdural space interpreted as a cellular layer of meninges. Anat Rec 1991; 230:38-51.

28. Friede RL. Developmental Neurophatology, 2nd rev ed. Berlin, Springer-Verlag, 1989, p 577.

29. Schachenmayr W, Friede RL. Fine structure of arachnoid cysts. J Neuropathol Exp Neurol 1979; 38:434-446.

30. Grzybowski DM, Herderick EE, Kapoor KG, et al. Human arachnoid granulations: I. A technique for quantifying area and distribution on the superior surface of the cerebral cortex. Cerebrospinal Fluid Res 2007; 4:6.

31. Brodbelt A, Stoodley M. CSF pathways: a review. Br J Neurosurg 2007; 21:510-520.

32. Roche J, Warner D. Arachnoid granulations in the transverse and sigmoid sinuses: CT, MR, and MR angiographic appearance of a normal anatomic variation. AJNR Am J Neuroradiol 1996; 17:677-683.

33. Kwee RM, Kwee TC. Virchow-Robin spaces at MR imaging. RadioGraphics 2007; 27:1071-1086.

34. Squier W, Mack J. The neuropathology of infant subdural haemorrhage. Forensic Sci Int 2009; 187:6-13.

35. Liang L, Korogi Y, Sugahara T, et al. Normal structures in the intracranial dural sinuses: delineation with 3D contrast-enhanced magnetization prepared rapid acquisition gradient-echo imaging sequence. AJNR Am J Neuroradiol 2002; 23:1739-1746.

36. Leach JL, Jones BV, Tomsick TA, et al. Normal appearance of arachnoid granulations on contrast-enhanced CT and MR of the brain: differentiation from dural sinus disease. AJNR Am J Neuroradiol 1996; 17: 1523-1532.

37. Zhang ET, Inman CB, Weller RO. Interrelationships of the pia mater and the perivascular (Virchow-Robin) spaces in the human cerebrum. J Anat 1990; 170:111-123.

38. Farb RI. The dural venous sinuses: normal intraluminal architecture defined on contrast-enhanced MR venography. Neuroradiology 2007; 49:727-732.

39. Cure JK, Van Tassel P, Smith MT. Normal and variant anatomy of the dural venous sinuses. Semin Ultrasound CT MR 1994; 15:499-519.

40. Zouaoui A, Hidden G. Cerebral venous sinuses: anatomical variants or thrombosis? Acta Anat (Basel) 1988; 133:318-324.

41. Das AC, Hasan M. The occipital sinus. J Neurosurg 1970; 33:307-311.

42. Ryu CW. Persistent falcine sinus: is it really rare? AJNR Am J Neuroradiol 31:367-369.

43. Zamboni P, Consorti G, Galeotti R, et al. Venous collateral circulation of the extracranial cerebrospinal outflow routes. Curr Neurovasc Res 2009; 6:204-212.

44. Savoiardo M, Minati L, Farina L, et al. Spontaneous intracranial hypotension with deep brain swelling. Brain 2007; 130(pt 7):1884-1893.

45. Hochman MS, Naidich TP, Kobetz SA, Fernandez-Maitin A. Spontaneous intracranial hypotension with pachymeningeal enhancement on MRI. Neurology 1992; 42:1628-1630.

46. Larrier D, Lee A. Anatomy of headache and facial pain. Otolaryngol Clin North Am 2003; 36:1041-1053.

47. Lyttelton OC, Karama S, Ad-Dab'bagh Y, et al. Positional and surface area asymmetry of the human cerebral cortex. Neuroimage 2009; 46:895-903.

48. LeMay M. Asymmetries of the skull and handedness: phrenology revisited. J Neurol Sci 1977; 32:243-253.

49. Dietemann JL, Correia Bernardo R, Bogorin A, et al. [Normal and abnormal meningeal enhancement: MRI features.] J Radiol 2005; 86:1659-1683.

50. Sze G, Berry I, Brant-Zawadzki M, et al. Gadolinium-DTPA in the magnetic resonance evaluation of the postoperative patient: work in progress. Acta Radiol Suppl 1986; 369:568-571.

51. Kirmi O, Sheerin F, Patel N. Imaging of the meninges and the extra-axial spaces. Semin Ultrasound CT MR 2009; 30:565-593.

52. Quint DJ, Eldevik OP, Cohen JK. Magnetic resonance imaging of normal meningeal enhancement at 1.5 T. Acad Radiol 1996; 3:463-468.

53. Meltzer CC, Fukui MB, Kanal E, Smirniotopoulos JG. MR imaging of the meninges: I. Normal anatomic features and nonneoplastic disease. Radiology 1996; 201:297-308.

54. Ozturk MH, Aydingoz U. Comparison of MR signal intensities of cerebral perivascular (Virchow-Robin) and subarachnoid spaces. J Comput Assist Tomogr 2002; 26:902-904.

55. Groeschel S, Chong WK, Surtees R, Hanefeld F. Virchow-Robin spaces on magnetic resonance images: normative data, their dilatation, and a review of the literature. Neuroradiology 2006; 48:745-754.

56. Anzai Y, Ishikawa M, Shaw DW, et al. Paramagnetic effect of supplemental oxygen on CSF hyperintensity on fluid-attenuated inversion recovery MR images. AJNR Am J Neuroradiol 2004; 25:274-279.

57. Deliganis AV, Fisher DJ, Lam AM, Maravilla KR. Cerebrospinal fluid signal intensity increase on FLAIR MR images in patients under general anesthesia: the role of supplemental O_2. Radiology 2001; 218:152-156.

58. Dolinskas CA, Zimmerman RA, Bilaniuk LT. A sign of subarachnoid bleeding on cranial computed tomograms of pediatric head trauma patients. Radiology 1978; 126:409-411.

Normal Brain Anatomy

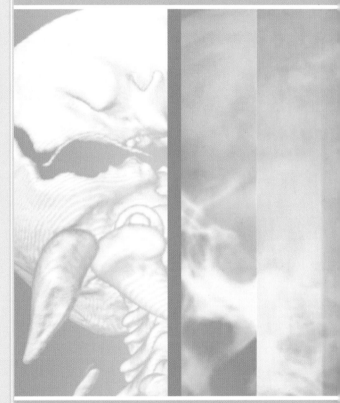

Supratentorial Brain

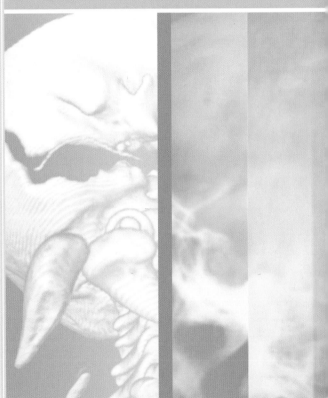

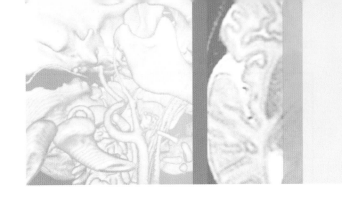

CHAPTER 9

Surface Anatomy of the Cerebrum

Thomas P. Naidich, Cheuk Ying Tang, Johnny C. Ng, and Bradley N. Delman

DESCRIPTIONS OF THE BRAIN SURFACE AND LABELING CODES USED IN THIS CHAPTER

Descriptions of the brain surface employ many synonyms and abbreviations. Some of those used in this chapter are cited here. Please note that the words "fissure" and "sulcus" are often used interchangeably, as in parieto-occipital sulcus = parieto-occipital fissure.

Anterior parolfactory sulcus = subcallosal sulcus
Central sulcus = fissure of Rolando, rolandic fissure
Inferior frontal gyrus = triangular gyrus
Insula = island of Reil
Intraparietal sulcus = interparietal sulcus
Lingual gyrus = medial occipitotemporal gyrus (MOTG)
Lateral occipitotemporal gyrus (LOTG) = overlaps with fusiform gyrus
Middle occipital sulcus = lateral occipital sulcus, prelunate sulcus
Preoccipital notch = temporo-occipital incisure, temporo-occipital arcus
Sylvian fissure = lateral fissure

A separate nomenclature is also used for the gyri of the surface.

Frontal lobe
F1: Superior frontal gyrus
F2: Middle frontal gyrus
F3: Inferior frontal gyrus

Parietal lobe
Pa: Ascending parietal gyrus (postcentral gyrus)
P1: Superior parietal lobule
P2: Inferior parietal lobule

Occipital lobe
O1: Superior occipital gyrus
O2: Middle occipital gyrus
O3: Inferior occipital gyrus
O4: Posterior intraoccipital portion of the LOTG
O5: Lingual gyrus (medial occipital-temporal gyrus)
O6: Cuneus

Temporal lobe
T1: Superior temporal gyrus
T2: Middle temporal gyrus
T3: Inferior temporal gyrus
T4: Anterior intratemporal portion of the LOTG
T5: Parahippocampal gyrus

Throughout this chapter, codes are used in images and text to identify the gyri and sulci. For reference, the codes are listed below. Please note that (1) an alternate designation may be used at times due to space constraints on the image or to use of illustrations reprinted by the kind permission of the authors and publishers; (2) the same structure may be given a second designation to fit the logic of the caption; and (3) other additional number/letter designations are used less commonly and are defined in context.

Gyri
1 = superior frontal gyrus, F1
2 = middle frontal gyrus, F2
3 = inferior frontal gyrus, F3
4 = precentral gyrus, PreCG, P
5 = postcentral gyrus, PostCG, p
6 = supramarginal gyrus, SMG
7 = angular gyrus, AG
8 = superior parietal lobule, SPL
9 = subcentral gyrus
10 = superior temporal gyrus, T1
11 = middle temporal gyrus, T2
12 = inferior temporal gyrus, T3
13 = anterior intratemporal portion of the lateral occipitotemporal gyrus, T4, LOTG
14 = parahippocamapal gyrus, T5
15 = superior occipital gyrus, O1
16 = middle occipital gyrus, O2
17 = inferior occipital gyrus, O3
18 = posterior intraoccipital portion of the lateral occipitotemporal gyrus, O4, LOTG

Continued

DESCRIPTIONS OF THE BRAIN SURFACE AND LABELING CODES USED IN THIS CHAPTER—cont'd

19 = lingual gyrus (medial occipitotemporal gyrus), O5, MOTG
20 = gyrus descendens (of Ecker)
21 = gyrus rectus
22 = subcallosal area
30 = cingulate gyrus
31 = isthmus of the cingulate gyrus
32 = paracentral lobule
33 = precuneus
34 = cuneus
35 = lingual gyrus (MOTG)
36 = lateral occipitotemporal gyrus, LOTG

Sulci
a = superior frontal sulcus, SFS
b = inferior frontal sulcus, IFS
c = precental sulcus, preCS
d = central sulcus, CS
e = postcentral sulcus, postCS
f = intraparietal sulcus, IPS
g = intra-occipital sulcus, IOS
h = lateral (middle) occipital sulcus
i = transverse occipital sulcus
ir = inferior rostral sulcus
j = intermediate sulci
k = parieto-occipital sulcus, POS
l = calcarine sulcus,

m = anterior calcarine sulcus
n = subparietal sulcus
o = cingulate sulcus
op = pars opercularis of F3
or = pars orbitalis of F3
p = superior temporal sulcus, STS
q = inferior temporal sulcus, ITS
r = paracentral sulcus
s = occipitotemporal sulcus
sr = superior rostral sulcus
t = rhinal sulcus
tr = pars triangularis of F3
u = collateral sulcus
v = pars marginalis of cingulate sulcus
w = superior occipital sulcus
x = supraorbital sulcus
y = intra-occipital sulcus, IOS
z = callosal sulcus

Other
B = Body of corpus callosum
G = Genu of corpus callosum
H = Hand motor area of the precentral gyrus *or* Heschle's transverse temporal gyrus, (in context)
R = Rostrum of corpus callosum
Sp = Splenium of corpus callosum

The surface of the brain comprises all of the features directly visible on the surface of the exposed brain after resection of the pia-arachnoid and the related vasculature.

The surface of the cerebrum is typically subdivided into lateral (convexity), medial, superior, and inferior surfaces, separated by angular edges designated margins.[1-3] The brain surface forms a continuous sheet of tissue that is folded and pleated to variable depths to form outwardly directed folds (the gyri), inwardly directed folds (the sulci), and large overhanging lips (the opercula) that cover the insula of each side. Individual gyri and sulci commonly continue from one surface across a margin onto an adjacent surface. The sulcal pattern shows wide variation among individuals, variation from side to side, and variation with patient handedness and language dominance (see section on petalia).[1] Overall, however, the pattern conforms to recognizable ranges of variation that permit ready identification of the sulci and gyri in most individuals.[1]

EMBRYOLOGY
The gyri and sulci mature in a reproducible pattern from fetal to infantile to adult age (Fig. 9-1).[4-9] Sulci first appear as linear depressions in the smooth brain surface (primary sulci). The primary sulci lengthen and deepen with time but retain relatively simple linear and curvilinear shapes. With maturation, the ends of the primary sulci typically bifurcate to form secondary sulci. These secondary sulci may later bifurcate to form tertiary sulci. The additional folds give the brain surface an increasingly complex appearance with age (see Fig. 9-1). Appreciation of this maturation pattern makes it simpler to understand the more complex folds, and variations, of the adult.[9-25]

ANATOMY
Lateral Surface
The lateral surface of the cerebrum includes the entire C-shaped convexity of the brain that extends around the sylvian fissure from the frontal pole anteriorly to the occipital pole posteriorly

to the temporal pole inferiorly (Figs. 9-2 and 9-3).[14,20,25] The lateral surface is subdivided into lobes by prominent intrinsic landmarks such as the central sulcus, sylvian fissure, and parieto-occipital sulcus; inconstant "landmarks" such as the preoccipital notch; and arbitrary lines including the lateral parietotemporal line and the temporo-occipital line (see Figs. 9-3 and 9-4).[1] The lateral parietotemporal line is drawn from the lateral end of the parieto-occipital sulcus superiorly to the preoccipital notch inferiorly. The temporo-occipital line is drawn from the posterior end of the sylvian fissure to the midpoint of the lateral parietotemporal line. The lateral surface of the cerebrum contains portions of the frontal, parietal, occipital, and temporal lobes, arrayed around the sylvian (lateral) fissure. With the just-noted landmarks, the lateral surface of the frontal lobe extends from the frontal pole to the central sulcus above the sylvian fissure. The lateral surface of the parietal lobe extends from the central sulcus to the parietotemporal line above the sylvian fissure and above the temporo-occipital line. The lateral surface of the temporal lobe extends from the temporal pole to the lateral parietotemporal line inferior to both the sylvian fissure and the temporo-occipital line. The lateral surface of the occipital lobe extends from the lateral parietotemporal line to the occipital pole. Because the occipital lobe curves sharply medially toward the occipital pole, true lateral views give a deceptively foreshortened impression of the size of the lateral occipital surface.

The lateral surface meets the medial surface of the brain at the superior margin. It meets the orbital surface of the brain at the orbital margin and meets the inferior surface at the inferior margin. The inferior margin shows a small, inconstant preoccipital notch that separates the inferior temporal margin anteriorly from the inferior occipital margin posteriorly.

Frontal Lobe
The convexity surface of the frontal lobe displays four major gyri (Figs. 9-2 to 9-6). Anteriorly, the longitudinally oriented superior

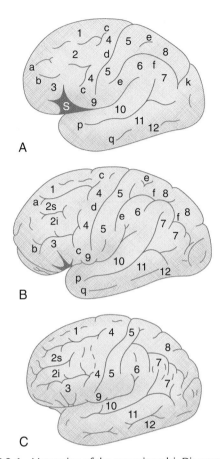

■ FIGURE 9-1 Maturation of the convexity sulci. Diagrammatic representations. *Gyri:* 1, Superior frontal gyrus; 2, middle frontal gyrus; 3, inferior frontal gyrus; 4, precentral gyrus; 5, postcentral gyrus; 6+7, inferior parietal lobule composed of the supramarginal gyrus (6) and the angular gyrus (7); 8, superior parietal lobule; 9, subcentral gyrus; 10, superior temporal gyrus; 11, middle temporal gyrus; 12, inferior temporal gyrus. **A,** At approximately 7 to 9 months' gestation. The opercula have not yet completed their folding, so the sylvian fissure (S) is widely open. The superior frontal sulcus (a) and inferior frontal sulcus (b) begin as a series of shallow longitudinal depressions on the convexity surface. The posterior ends of these sulci bifurcate forming separate upper and lower segments of the precentral sulcus (c). The central sulcus (d) is isolated from the sylvian fissure by the subcentral gyrus (9). The postcentral sulcus (e) also forms from two separate segments. The lower postcentral segment is simultaneously the upswing of the arcuate intraparietal sulcus (f). This sulcus presently describes a simple arc with little definition of the individual supramarginal (6) and angular (7) gyri. The parieto-occipital sulcus (k) is well developed. On the temporal convexity, the superior temporal sulcus (p) is best developed early. The inferior temporal sulcus (q) is immature. **B,** At approximately birth to 2 years of age. The opercula have closed together, narrowing the sylvian fissure. The individual segments of the superior (a) and inferior (b) frontal sulci have merged into unified lengths. The large middle frontal gyrus (2) is partially subdivided into superior and inferior segments (2s and 2i) by the middle frontal sulcus (*not labeled*). The posterior bifurcations of the superior and inferior frontal sulci form two separate segments of the precentral sulcus (c). These two segments do not merge together, leaving a gap through which the posterior portion of the middle frontal gyrus (2) unites with (was never separated from) the anterior face of the precentral gyrus (4). The intraparietal sulcus (f) is now better developed and lobulated, defining the supramarginal (6) and angular (7) gyri. The inferior temporal sulcus (q) has matured with greater length of its segments. **C,** After approximately age 2 years. With greater maturation, the sulci lengthen, deepen, and become deflected by the growth of the neighboring gyri. Their ends bifurcate to form secondary sulci, and the bifid ends bifurcate again to form tertiary sulci. Additional local folding creates unnamed folds over the surfaces of the named gyri. Further details are available in references 8 and 9. *(Based on data from Turner OA. Growth and development of the cerebral cortical pattern in man. Arch Neurol Psychiatry 1948; 59:1-12.)*

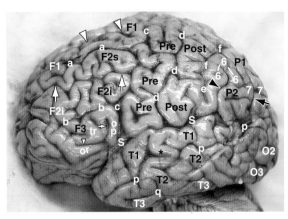

■ FIGURE 9-2 Surface features of the left hemisphere. Fresh gross specimen with pia-arachnoid and vessels intact. The convexity surface of the hemisphere displays four frontal gyri: the superior frontal gyrus (F1), middle frontal gyrus (F2), inferior frontal gyrus (F3), and the precentral gyrus (Pre); three temporal gyri: the superior temporal gyrus (T1), middle temporal gyrus (T2), and inferior temporal gyrus (T3); three subdivisions of the parietal lobe: the postcentral gyrus (Post), superior parietal lobule (P1), and inferior parietal lobule (P2); and three subdivisions of the occipital lobe: the superior occipital gyrus (*not seen from this view*), middle occipital gyrus (O2), and the inferior occipital gyrus (O3). Short inconstant medial frontal sulci (*large white arrowheads*) often groove F1. A longitudinal middle frontal sulcus (*large white arrows*) commonly divides F2 into superior (F2s) and inferior portions (F2i). These halves may unite with the adjacent F1 and/or F3 gyri in complex ways. The anterior horizontal ramus (*small white arrowhead*) and the anterior ascending ramus (*small white arrow*) of the sylvian fissure (S) extend into F3, dividing it into the pars orbitalis (or), pars triangularis (tr), and pars opercularis (op). They give F3 the shape of an upper case M. The superior frontal sulcus (a) separates F1 from F2 below. The inferior frontal sulcus (b) separates F2 from F3 below. The posterior end of the superior frontal sulcus (a) characteristically bifurcates to form the superior precentral sulcus (c) that separates F1 from the upper precentral gyrus (Pre). The posterior end of the inferior frontal sulcus (b) characteristically bifurcates to form the inferior precentral sulcus (c) that separates F3 from the lower precentral gyrus (Pre). F2 characteristically unites with the anterior face of the precentral gyrus (Pre) between the upper (c) and lower (c) portions of the precentral sulcus. The central sulcus (d) separates the precentral gyrus from the postcentral gyrus. The central sulcus is usually isolated from the sylvian fissure (S) by a subcentral gyrus, but not in this case. The upper and lower portions of the postcentral sulcus (e) separate the postcentral gyrus from the superior parietal (P1) and inferior parietal (P2) lobules. The lower portion of the postcentral sulcus is, simultaneously, the ascending portion of the arcuate intraparietal sulcus (f) that separates the superior parietal lobule (8) from the inferior parietal lobules (6+7). The ascending ramus (*black arrowhead*) of the sylvian fissure (S) angles upward into the inferior parietal lobule. The horseshoe-shaped gyrus draped over the posterior ascending ramus of the sylvian fissure is the supramarginal gyrus (6). The superior temporal sulcus (p) separates the superior temporal gyrus (T1) from the middle temporal gyrus (T2). The inferior temporal sulcus (q) separates the middle temporal gyrus (T2) from the inferior temporal gyrus (T3). Anteriorly, a short vertical gyrus (*black asterisk*) commonly extends between T1 and T2, interrupting the superior temporal sulcus (p) over a short segment. Posteriorly, the superior temporal sulcus angles upward in parallel with the posterior ascending ramus of the sylvian fissure over a segment designated the angular sulcus (*large black arrow*). The horseshoe-shaped gyrus draped over the angular sulcus is the angular gyrus (7). Together the supramarginal and angular gyri constitute most of the inferior parietal lobule.

frontal gyrus, middle frontal gyrus, and inferior frontal gyrus are separated from each other by the superior and inferior frontal sulci. The middle frontal gyrus is the largest of the three gyri and may be partially subdivided into upper and lower halves by an inconstant middle frontal sulcus. The convexity surface of the superior frontal gyrus may be grooved by short shallow sulci termed the *medial frontal sulci*. Posteriorly, the frontal lobe is formed by the precentral gyrus that courses vertically between

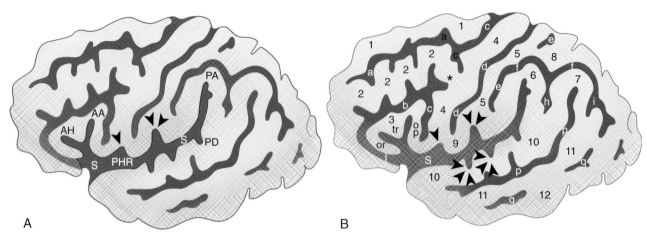

■ FIGURE 9-3   Convexity surface. Diagrammatic representation. **A,** The margins of the frontal, parietal and temporal opercula are defined by the sylvian fissure (S), by its five major rami (the anterior horizontal ramus [AH], anterior ascending ramus [AA], posterior horizontal ramus [PHR], posterior ascending ramus [PA] and posterior descending ramus [PD]) and by its minor arms (the anterior subcentral sulcus [*single arrowhead*], posterior subcentral sulcus [*double arrowheads*], and the transverse temporal sulci [*triple arrowheads* on **B**]). **B,** The configuration of the sylvian fissure then permits identification of the surface gyri and sulci. *Gyri:* 1, superior frontal; 2, middle frontal; 3, inferior frontal; 4, precentral; 5, postcentral; 6, supramarginal; 7, angular; 8, superior parietal lobule; 9, subcentral; 10, superior temporal, 11, middle temporal; 12, inferior temporal gyrus. *Asterisk* indicates junction of the middle frontal gyrus with the precentral gyrus. *Sulci:* a, superior frontal sulcus; b, inferior frontal sulcus; c, superior and inferior segments of the precentral sulcus; d, central sulcus; e, superior and inferior segments of the postcentral sulcus; f, intraparietal sulcus; p, superior temporal sulcus; q, inferior temporal sulcus; h, primary intermediate sulcus; i, secondary intermediate sulcus. *(Modified from Naidich TP, Valavanis AG, Kubik S, et al. Anatomic relationships along the low-middle convexity: II. Lesion localization. Int J Neuroradiol 1997; 3:393-409.)*

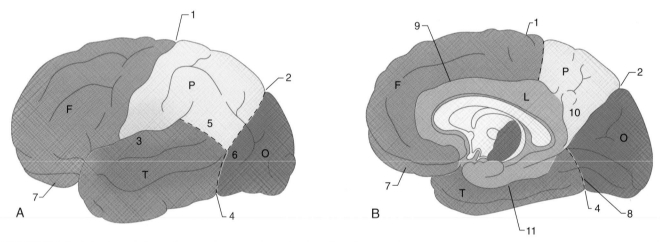

■ FIGURE 9-4   Lobar boundaries and nomenclature. **A,** Convexity (lateral) surface. On the convexity, the central sulcus (1) separates the frontal (F) from the parietal (P) lobes. The sylvian fissure (3) separates the frontal from the temporal (T) lobes. The demarcation of the temporal, parietal, and occipital lobes is arbitrary and inconstant from publication to publication. In one system, a *parietotemporal line* is drawn from the lateral edge of the parieto-occipital sulcus (2) to the preoccipital notch (temporo-occipital incisure) (4). This line sets the arbitrary anterior border of the occipital lobe (O), separating it from the parietal and temporal lobes anterior to it. A second arbitrary *temporo-occipital line* (5) is drawn from the posterior descending ramus of the sylvian fissure (3) to the middle of the parietotemporal line (6). This line sets the arbitrary parietotemporal boundary. **B,** Medial surface. On the medial surface, the central sulcus (1) usually curves onto the medial surface perpendicular to the marginal segment of the cingulate sulcus. A line drawn from the central sulcus to the cingulate sulcus establishes the frontoparietal border. The deep parieto-occipital sulcus (2) demarcates the parietal lobe from the occipital lobe. An arbitrary *basal parietotemporal line* (8) drawn from the inferior end of the parieto-occipital sulcus to the preoccipital notch establishes the temporal (T)/occipital (O) border. The limbic lobe (L) is delimited by the cingulate sulcus (9), the subparietal sulcus (10), and the collateral sulcus (11). Also labeled: 7, orbital surface.

the precentral sulcus anteriorly and the central sulcus posteriorly. The inferior end of the central sulcus usually does not intersect the sylvian fissure. Instead, a U-shaped subcentral gyrus is interposed between the inferior end of the central sulcus and the sylvian fissure.

Parietal Lobe

The convexity surface of the parietal lobe displays three major subdivisions (see Figs. 9-2 to 9-6). Anteriorly, the vertically

oriented postcentral gyrus lies between the central sulcus anteriorly and the postcentral sulcus posteriorly. Posteriorly, the deep, arcuate intraparietal sulcus subdivides the lateral surface of the parietal lobe into superior and inferior parietal lobules. The superior parietal lobule forms the superomedial portion of the parietal convexity between the superior margin of the hemisphere and the intraparietal sulcus. The inferior parietal lobule forms the inferolateral portion of the parietal convexity between the intraparietal sulcus and the temporo-occipital line. The

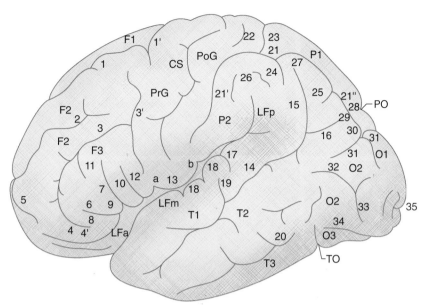

■ **FIGURE 9-5**   Surface features of the convexity. Diagrammatic representation.

Gyri: F1, F2, and F3, superior, middle, and inferior frontal gyri; P1 and P2, superior and inferior parietal lobules; T1, T2, and T3, superior, middle, and inferior temporal gyri; O1, O2, and O3, superior, middle, and inferior occipital gyri; PrG and PoG, precentral and postcentral gyri; PO, parieto-occipital fissure; TO, temporal-occipital incisure; LFa, LFm, and LFp, lateral fissure of Sylvius (anterior [a], middle [m] and posterior [p] segments).
Frontal lobe: 1, superior frontal sulcus; 1′, superior precentral sulcus; 2, inconstant middle frontal sulcus; 3, inferior frontal sulcus; 3′, inferior precentral sulcus; 4, lateral orbital sulcus; 4′, lateral orbital gyrus; 5, frontomarginal sulcus; 6, anterior horizontal ramus of the sylvian fissure; 7, anterior ascending ramus of the sylvian fissure; 8-10, partes orbitalis (8), triangularis (9), and opercularis (10) of the inferior frontal gyrus; 11, sulcus triangularis; 12, sulcus diagonalis within the pars opercularis; 13, subcentral gyrus delimited by the anterior (a) and posterior (b) subcentral sulci.
Temporal lobe: 14, superior temporal sulcus (parallel sulcus) anterior segment; 15, superior temporal sulcus, ascending posterior segment (synonym: angular sulcus); 16, superior temporal sulcus, horizontal posterior segment; 17, transverse temporal sulcus; 18, transverse temporal gyri; 19, sulcus acousticus; 20, inferior temporal sulcus.
Parietal lobe: 21, intraparietal sulcus, horizontal segment; 21′, intraparietal sulcus, ascending segment (coincident with inferior postcentral sulcus); 21″, intraparietal sulcus, descending segment; 22, superior postcentral sulcus; 23, transverse parietal sulcus; 24, primary intermediate sulcus (of Jensen); 25, secondary intermediate sulcus; 26, supramarginal gyrus; 27, angular gyrus; 28, first parieto-occipital arcus (first pli du passage of Gratiolet); 29, second parieto-occipital arcus (second pli du passage of Gratiolet).
Occipital lobe: 30, intraoccipital sulcus (superior occipital sulcus); 31, transverse occipital sulcus; 32, lateral (middle) occipital sulcus; 33, lunate sulcus; 34, inferior occipital sulcus; and 35, calcarine sulcus, here extending to the occipital pole. *(From Duvernoy HM. The Human Brain: Surface, Three-Dimensional Sectional Anatomy and MRI. New York, Springer, 1991.)*

inferior parietal lobule contains the supramarginal gyrus anteriorly and the angular gyrus posteriorly.

Occipital Lobe

The convexity surface of the occipital lobe displays three major gyri: the superior occipital gyrus, middle occipital gyrus, and inferior occipital gyrus, separated by the superior and inferior occipital sulci (see Figs. 9-3, 9-5, and 9-6). The superior occipital sulcus is usually seen as the posterior continuation of the intraparietal sulcus. The inferior occipital sulcus is usually seen as the posterior extension of the inferior temporal sulcus. The middle occipital gyrus is the largest of the three occipital gyri and may be partially subdivided into upper and lower halves by an inconstant middle (lateral) occipital sulcus. Far posteriorly, the convexity surface of the occipital lobe often displays a vertically oriented, arcuate lunate sulcus. The posterior end of the calcarine sulcus may extend around the occipital pole to lie on the convexity surface.

Temporal Lobe

The lateral surface of the temporal lobe displays three major gyri that course longitudinally inferior to the sylvian fissure and inferior to the temporo-occipital line (see Figs. 9-4, 9-5, and 9-6). The superior temporal, middle temporal, and inferior temporal gyri are separated by the superior and inferior temporal sulci. The transverse temporal gyrus of Heschl forms a focal protuberance

on the superior surface of the superior temporal gyrus (Figs. 9-7 and 9-8). This deflects the sylvian fissure upward focally. The inferior temporal gyrus forms the inferior margin of the hemisphere and curves onto the inferior surface of the hemisphere to form the lateralmost gyrus of the inferior temporal surface (Fig. 9-9). The preoccipital notch (temporo-occipital incisure) marks the transition from temporal lobe to occipital lobe along the inferior margin (see Figs. 9-5 and 9-6).

Opening the sylvian fissure discloses the superior surface of the temporal lobe, termed the *superior temporal plane.* This forms the inferior lip (temporal operculum) of the sylvian fissure. The transverse temporal gyrus of Heschl arises posteromedially immediately behind the insula and courses anterolaterally across the superior temporal plane to reach the lateral surface. Heschl's sulcus defines its posterior border (see Figs. 9-6 and 9-7). The portion of the superior temporal plane that lies between the temporal pole and the anterior surface of Heschl's gyrus is termed the *planum polare.* This is delimited medially by the circular sulcus of the insula (see later). The portion of the superior temporal plane that lies behind Heschl's gyrus and sulcus is termed the *planum temporale.* Because of the oblique course of Heschl's gyrus, the planum temporale appears triangular, with its base on the convexity surface and its apex directed posteromedially, immediately behind the origin of Heschl's gyrus. The planum temporale is usually larger on the side of language dominance.

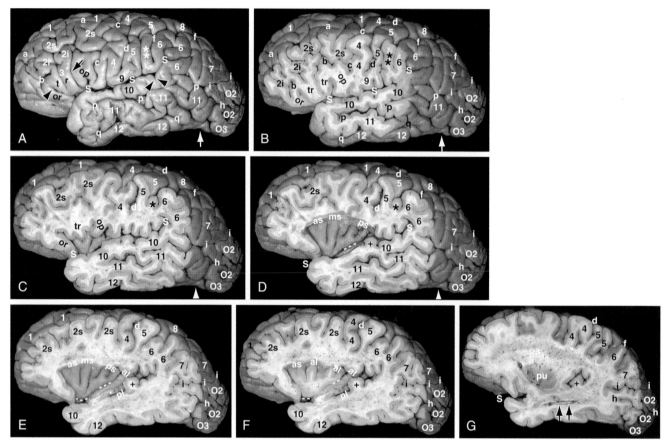

■ **FIGURE 9-6** Convexity surface of the brain with sequential sagittal sections. Formalin-fixed gross anatomic specimen after removal of the pia-arachnoid and vessels (same specimen as Fig. 9-10). **A** and **B,** The sylvian fissure (S) separates the frontal and parietal lobes superiorly from the temporal lobe inferiorly. At its anterior end, the anterior horizontal (*small black arrowhead*) and anterior ascending (*small black arrow*) rami subdivide the inferior frontal lobe into partes orbitalis (or), triangularis (tr), and opercularis (op). Posteriorly, the posterior ascending ramus (most posterior of the three S) deeply indents the supramarginal gyrus (6), giving it a horseshoe shape. The posterior descending ramus of the sylvian fissure (*two small black arrowheads*) is typically very small. The convexity surface of the frontal lobe is composed of the 1, superior frontal gyrus; 2s and 2i, superior and inferior segments of the middle frontal gyrus; 3, M-shaped inferior frontal gyrus; and 4, precentral gyrus. These are delimited by the superior frontal sulcus (a), the inferior frontal sulcus (b), and the precentral sulcus (c). A vertical triangular sulcus grooves the pars triangularis (*between the letters t and r*). The superior surface of pars triangularis commonly unites with the inferior segment of the middle frontal gyrus (2i) across the inferior frontal sulcus (b). The convexity surface of the parietal lobe is composed of the 5, postcentral gyrus; 6-7, the inferior parietal lobule formed by the supramarginal gyrus (6) and angular gyrus (7); and 8, the superior parietal lobule. These are delimited by the central sulcus (d), postcentral sulcus, intraparietal sulcus (f), middle (lateral) occipital sulcus (h), and the transverse occipital sulcus (i). The subcentral gyrus (9) links the inferior ends of the precentral (5) and postcentral (6) gyri inferior to the central sulcus (d). The inferior end of the postcentral gyrus (5) shows a deep partition. The posterior portion may be considered an accessory presupramarginal gyrus (*double asterisks*). The inferior portion of the postcentral sulcus constitutes the ascending segment of the arcuate intraparietal sulcus (f). The transverse occipital sulcus (i) separates the parietal lobe (7) from the middle occipital gyrus (O2). Just as the large middle frontal gyrus (2) is commonly divided into upper and lower portions by a middle frontal sulcus, the large middle occipital gyrus (O2) is often separated into upper and lower portions by a middle (lateral) occipital sulcus (h). **C,** This section just exposes the anterior lobule of the insula and the relationship of the partes orbitalis, triangularis, and opercularis to the insula. **D** to **F,** The insula is delimited by a circular (peri-insular) sulcus. The larger anterior lobule of the insula has three (or more) short insular gyri: anterior short (as), middle short (ms), and posterior short (ps). These converge inferiorly to form the apex of the anterior lobule. The posterior lobe has two long insular gyri: anterior long (al) and posterior long (pl). The central sulcus of the convexity (c) continues across the insula (*white dashes*) between the anterior and posterior insular lobules. It then swings immediately under the apex to pass medially toward the suprasellar cistern. Heschl's transverse temporal gyrus forms a distinct elevation (*black plus sign*) on the upper surface of the superior temporal gyrus. It characteristically arises immediately behind the posterior lobule of the insula and angles obliquely across the upper surface of the temporal lobe (see Fig. 9-7). **G,** This section cuts deep to the insula exposing the putamen (pu). Entry into the lateralmost portion of the temporal horn (*two black arrows*) exposes the lateral surface of the hippocampal formation that lies along the medial wall of the horn.

Insular Lobe

Opening the lips of the sylvian fissure discloses the insula (synonym: island of Reil) (see Figs. 9-6 and 9-7).[25] The insula is circumscribed by the circular (peri-insular) sulcus, which is subdivided into anterior, superior, and inferior peri-insular segments. The central sulcus of the convexity extends onto the insula, crosses the insular surface between the anterior insular lobule and the posterior insular lobule, and then curves medially into the deep sylvian fissure. The larger anterior insular lobule commonly displays three vertically oriented gyri referred to as

the anterior short, middle short, and posterior short insular gyri. Additional inconstant anterior insular gyri are common. Typically, the inferior ends of the anterior, middle, and posterior short insular gyri converge together to form the apex of the insula. The central sulcus courses immediately beneath the apex as it turns medially into the deep sylvian fissure. The anterior insular lobule connects directly with the posteromedial orbital lobule on the orbital surface of the frontal lobe (see Inferior Surface). The smaller posterior insular lobule typically displays two obliquely oriented gyri: the anterior long and posterior long

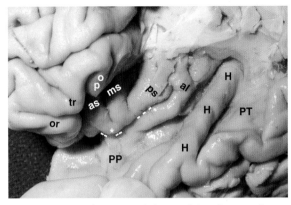

■ **FIGURE 9-7** Superior temporal plane and the primary auditory cortex (H). Formalin-fixed gross anatomic specimen. Resection of the frontal lobe posterior to the inferior frontal gyrus opens a view of the upper surface of the temporal lobe, designated the superior temporal plane, the transverse temporal gyrus of Heschl (H), Heschl's sulcus immediately behind the gyrus, and two broad flat planes of tissue anterior and posterior to Heschl's gyrus and sulcus. From the temporal pole anteriorly to the front of Heschl's gyrus, the flat surface is designated the planum polare (PP). From Heschl's sulcus to the posterior end of the temporal surface, the flat surface is designated the planum temporale (PT). The planum temporale is usually triangular, with its point medial and its base directed laterally. It is usually larger in the language-dominant temporal lobe. Note that Heschl's gyrus commonly bifurcates at its lateral end. The partes orbitalis (or), triangularis (tr), and opercularis (op) of the inferior frontal gyrus overhang the anterior lobule of the insula. The anterior lobule displays the anterior short (as), middle short (ms), and posterior short (ps) gyri. These converge to the apex (*asterisk*) of the insula inferiorly. The central sulcus of the insula (*dashed white lines*) separates the anterior lobe from the posterior lobe of the insula and then swings medially under the apex toward the suprasellar cistern.

insular gyri. In some ways, the transverse temporal gyrus of Heschl may be regarded as a third long insular gyrus that happened to be folded onto the superior surface of the temporal lobe by the development of the temporal operculum.

Central Lobe

The tissue surrounding the central sulcus has been proposed to form a separate lobe, referred to as the central lobe.[21] The tissue surrounding the central sulcus does form a continuous loop that can be followed, round and round, from the precentral gyrus anteriorly into the subcentral gyrus inferiorly, into the postcentral gyrus posteriorly into the paracentral lobule superiorly, and then back into the precentral gyrus, and so on. Because the pericentral gyri subserve sensorimotor function, the concept of a separate central lobe merits consideration, although it is not yet widely accepted.

Medial Surface

The medial surface of the cerebrum includes the flat medial surface of the cerebral hemisphere that abuts upon the midline. This surface is arrayed about the corpus callosum from the frontal pole anteriorly to the occipital pole posteriorly and extends for a short distance into the posterior temporal lobe inferiorly. The rest of the temporal lobe faces inferomedial, so it is considered with the inferior surface.

Like the lateral surface, the medial surface of the cerebrum is divided into lobes by prominent intrinsic landmarks such as the cingulate sulcus, central sulcus, parieto-occipital sulcus, and collateral sulcus; inconstant "landmarks" such as the preoccipital notch; and an arbitrary basal parietotemporal line drawn from the inferior end of the parieto-occipital sulcus superiorly to the preoccipital notch inferiorly.[1,2,17] Unlike the lateral surface, the

gyri and sulci of the medial surface are arranged in a radial coordinate system, in which all of the gyri form arcs of tissue that course co-curvilinear with the corpus callosum or perpendicular (radial) to the curvature of the corpus callosum. The central landmark of the medial surface is the corpus callosum, subdivided into the rostrum anteroinferiorly, the genu anteriorly, the body superiorly, and the splenium posteriorly (see Figs. 9-4 and 9-9). Grossly, the outer margin of the corpus callosum is delimited by the callosal sulcus Actually, however, the external surface of the corpus callosum is covered by a thin layer of gray matter: the indusium griseum superiorly and the paraterminal gyrus anteroinferiorly.

Limbic Lobe

The limbic lobe is the name given to that portion of the medial surface of the hemisphere that encircles the corpus callosum and extends along the superomedial surface of the temporal lobe to encircle the brain stem (Fig. 9-10). The portion of the limbic lobe on the medial surface consists of the paraterminal gyrus that lies on the rostrum of the corpus callosum posterior to the posterior parolfactory sulcus; the subcallosal area that lies anterior to the paraterminal gyrus between the anterior and posterior parolfactory sulci; the cingulate gyrus that circumscribes the corpus callosum between the callosal sulcus centrally and the cingulate sulcus peripherally; and the posterior portion of the cingulate gyrus that turns downward behind the splenium, narrows to the isthmus of the cingulate gyrus under the splenium, and swings forward to join the parahippocampal gyrus. These are delimited centrally by the callosal sulcus. They are delimited peripherally by the anterior parolfactory, cingulate, subparietal, anterior calcarine, and collateral sulci. The other portions of the limbic lobe that extend along the temporal surface are discussed later (see Inferior Surface).

Frontal Lobe

The medial surface of the frontal lobe is formed by the medial surface of the gyrus rectus and the medial surface of the superior frontal gyrus (synonym: medial frontal gyrus) (see Figs. 9-9 to 9-12). The gyri recti flank the midline at the anteroinferior extent of the hemisphere, between the inferior surface of the frontal lobe inferiorly, the rostral sulci superiorly, and the anterior parolfactory sulcus posteriorly. The gyri recti form the anterior portion of the inferomedial margin.

The superior frontal gyrus encircles the cingulate gyrus anterior to the anterior parolfactory sulcus, external to the cingulate sulcus, and posterior to the frontomarginal and transverse gyri of the frontal pole (see Poles). It swings back to reach the paracentral sulcus posteriorly. The cingulate sulcus delimits the peripheral surface of the cingulate gyrus. About two thirds of the way back along the corpus callosum, the cingulate sulcus sweeps upward to reach the superior margin of the hemisphere as the marginal segment of the cingulate sulcus. This marginal segment is termed the *pars marginalis* (singular) or *partes marginales* (plural). The paracentral lobule forms a broad ovoid on the medial surface of the brain just posterior to the superior frontal gyrus and external to the cingulate gyrus, between the paracentral sulcus anteriorly, the cingulate sulcus centrally, and the pars marginalis posteriorly. Together, the superior frontal gyrus and the paracentral lobule form the superior margin of the frontal lobe behind the frontal pole. The central sulcus extends superiorly across the convexity, cuts across the superior margin of the hemisphere, and then curves downward into the paracentral lobule just millimeters anterior to the pars marginalis. The upper end of the central sulcus characteristically aligns perpendicular to the oblique course of the pars marginalis. Because the central sulcus extends into the paracentral lobule, the most posterior portion of the paracentral lobule is technically part of the parietal lobe.

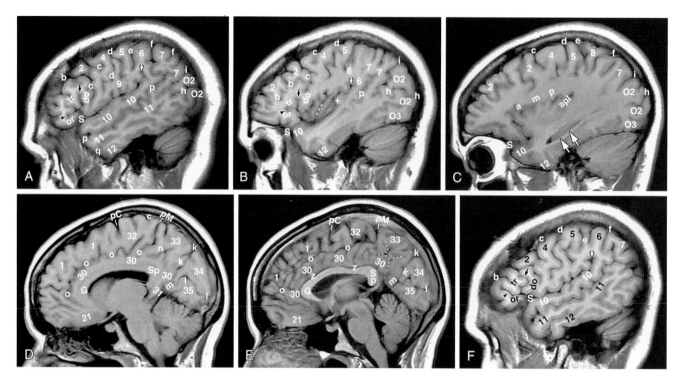

■ FIGURE 9-8 **A** to **C** and **F,** Lateral surface T1W MR images (labels as in Fig. 9-6). **D, E,** Medial surface T1W MR images (labels as in Fig. 9-10). MRI displays all of the surface features seen by gross inspection of the brain. The contralateral side of this same patient (see **F**) illustrates a common variation of the inferior frontal gyrus. Here, the anterior ascending ramus (*small black arrow*) of the sylvian fissure cuts completely through the gyrus, leaving pars opercularis as an anterior appendage of the lower precentral gyrus (4). Pars triangularis bridges across the inferior frontal sulcus to join the inferior portion of the middle frontal gyrus on the next section (*not shown*). In **C**, amp, short insular gyri; apl, long insular gyri.

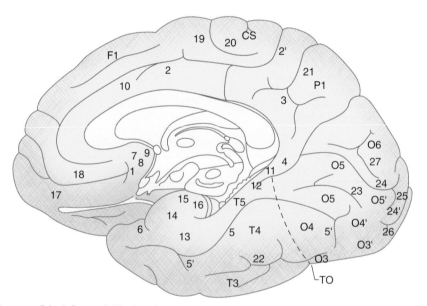

■ FIGURE 9-9 Surface features of the inferomedial brain. Diagrammatic representation.

Gyri: T3, T4, and T5, inferior temporal gyrus, temporal portion of the fusiform gyrus, parahippocampal gyrus; respectively; P1, medial aspect of the superior parietal lobule (precuneus); O3, O4, and O5, inferior occipital gyrus, occipital portion of the fusiform gyrus, lingual (medial occipitotemporal gyrus), respectively; O3 plus O4′ plus O5′, the caudal portions of O3, O4, and O5 merge into a common occipital cortex on the inferior aspect of the occipital pole. T4 plus O4 form the fusiform (lateral occipitotemporal) gyrus. TO, Temporo-occipital incisure. The limbic lobe is delimited, sequentially, by the 1, anterior parolfactory sulcus (subcallosal sulcus); 2, cingulate sulcus; 3, subparietal sulcus; 4, anterior calcarine sulcus; 5, collateral sulcus (medial occipitotemporal sulcus); and 6, rhinal sulcus. The limbic lobe is composed, sequentially, of the 7, subcallosal area; 8, posterior parolfactory sulcus; 9, paraterminal gyrus; 10, cingulate gyrus; 11, isthmus of the cingulate gyrus; 12, dentate gyrus; and 13, pyriform lobe (itself formed of the 14, gyrus ambiens; 15, semilunar gyrus; and 16, limbus [band] of Giacomini). Also labeled: 2′, marginal segment (pars marginalis) of the cingulate sulcus, and 5′, anterior and posterior transverse collateral sulci.

Medial frontal lobe: 17, gyrus rectus; 18, supraorbital sulcus; 19, paracentral sulcus; 20, paracentral lobule; CS, superior end of the central sulcus on the medial surface.

Medial parietal lobe: 21, transverse parietal sulcus.

Inferomedial temporal lobe: 22, lateral occipitotemporal sulcus.

Inferomedial occipital lobe: 23, inconstant lingual sulcus (when present it divides the lingual gyrus into upper and lower portions); 24, calcarine sulcus; 24′, retrocalcarine cortex; 25, gyrus descendens; 26, occipitopolar sulcus; 27, paracalcarine sulcus.

(From Duvernoy HM. The Human Brain: Surface, Three-Dimensional Sectional Anatomy and MRI. New York, Springer, 1991.)

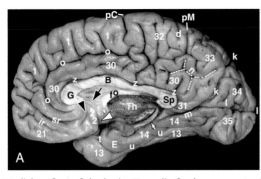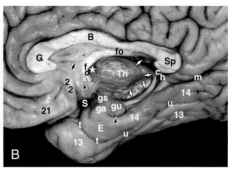

■ **FIGURE 9-10** Medial surface of the brain. Formalin-fixed gross anatomic specimen after removal of the pia-arachnoid, vessels, brain stem and obscuring portions of the thalami (Th). Same specimen as Figure 9-6. Compare with Figures 9-4B and 9-9. **A,** Full surface. From deep to superficial, the gyri and sulci of the medial surface are arrayed around the genu (G), body (B), and splenium (Sp) of the corpus callosum in successive co-curvilinear tiers of tissue and sulci, as follows: *Inner Tier 1* (mostly obscured in this view): paraterminal gyrus (*single black arrow*) closely applied to the rostrum of the corpus callosum, indusium griseum (closely applied to the outer surface of the corpus callosum and dentate gyrus [*not seen in this view*]). *Tier 2:* posterior parolfactory sulcus (*single white arrowhead*), pericallosal sulcus (z), and hippocampal fissure (*small white arrow*). *Tier 3:* subcallosal area (22), cingulate gyrus (30) and its isthmus (31), parahippocampal gyrus (14), and the uncus (labeled in **B**). *Tier 4:* anterior parolfactory sulcus (*single black arrowhead*), cingulate sulcus (o), subparietal sulcus (n and *dashed lines*), collateral sulcus (u), and rhinal sulcus (t). *Outer Tier 5:* gyrus rectus (21), superior frontal gyrus (1), paracentral lobule (32), precuneus (33), cuneus (34), lingual gyrus (35), and lateral occipitotemporal gyrus (13). The superiormost extent of the central sulcus (d) typically crosses the superior margin onto the medial surface a short distance anterior to the pars marginalis (pM). Anteriorly, the superior (sr) and inferior (ir) rostral sulci lie above the gyrus rectus (21). The anterior (*single black arrowhead*) and posterior (*single white arrowhead*) parolfactory sulci delimit the subcallosal area (22). The entorhinal cortex (E) lies inside the curvature of the rhinal sulcus along the medial face of the anterior parahippocampal gyrus. Posteriorly, the parieto-occipital sulcus (k) always joins the anterior end of the calcarine sulcus (horizontal sulcus below l) to form the anterior calcarine sulcus (m). This creates a lazy-Y configuration that is a powerful landmark for identifying the precuneus (33), cuneus (34), isthmus of the cingulate gyrus (31), and the lingual (synonym: medial occipitotemporal) gyrus (35). **B,** Magnified view of the limbic lobe. The anterior end of the parahippocampal gyrus (14) hooks superiorly, dorsally, and medially around the anterior end of the hippocampal fissure (*lower black arrowhead*) to form the uncus. Grossly, the hook of tissue contains the gyrus ambiens (ga), gyrus semilunaris (gs), and the gyrus uncinatus (gu). The fimbria of the fornix (*lower two white arrows*) arises from the hippocampal formation and arches upward (*middle white arrow*) as the crus of the fornix on each side. This passes anterior to the splenium (Sp) and inferior to the body (B) of the corpus callosum and unites with the opposite crus to form the body of the fornix (fo) under the body of the corpus callosum. The body then divides into paired anterior columns of the fornices that arch inferiorly along the anterior borders of the foramina of Monro (*asterisk*), immediately posterior to the anterior commissure (*upper black arrowhead*), en route to the mammillary bodies. Ch, choroid plexus partially obscuring the course of the fornix. S, sylvian fissure.

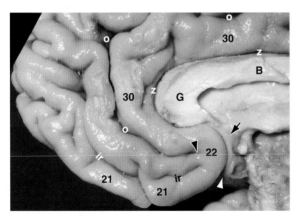

■ **FIGURE 9-11** Medial surface of the frontal lobe. Formalin-fixed gross anatomic specimen of the medial surface of the frontal lobe. The cingulate gyrus (30) arches around the body (B) and genu (G) of the corpus callosum between the callosal sulcus (z) on its deep aspect and the cingulate sulcus (o) superficially. The anterior cingulate gyrus turns downward to form the subcallosal area (22) between the anterior (*black arrowhead*) and posterior (*white arrowhead*) parolfactory sulci. The tenuous cap of gray matter on the superior surface of the corpus callosum (the indusium griseum), also turns downward immediately anterior to the genu and rostrum of the corpus callosum to form the paraterminal gyrus (*arrow*). The paraterminal gyrus lies behind the posterior parolfactory sulcus, closely applied to the rostrum of the corpus callosum. The inferior rostral sulcus (ir) delimits the upper border of the gyrus rectus (21).

Parietal Lobe

Posterior to the pars marginalis, the superior parietal lobule extends onto the medial surface of the hemisphere to form a surface termed the *precuneus* (see Figs. 9-10 and 9-12). Posterior to the splenium, the deep parieto-occipital sulcus separates the medial surface of the parietal lobe (precuneus) anteriorly from the medial surface of the occipital lobe (cuneus) posteriorly. The precuneus forms a roughly rectangular block of tissue between the pars marginalis anteriorly, the cingulate sulcus centrally, the parieto-occipital sulcus posteriorly, and the superior margin superficially. An H-shaped subparietal sulcus grooves the precuneus partially dividing the medial surface of the parietal lobe into three vertically oriented anterior, middle, and posterior bands. The horizontal portion of the H often aligns with the curvature of the cingulate sulcus and forms part of the sulcal arc that delimits the peripheral aspect of the limbic lobe.

Occipital Lobe

The parieto-occipital sulcus courses roughly parallel to the pars maginalis (see Figs. 9-10 and 9-12). It marks the anterior border of the upper occipital lobe. An arbitrary basal parietotemporal line drawn from the inferior end of the parieto-occipital sulcus to the preoccipital notch marks the anterior border of the lower occipital lobe. The deep upper end of the parieto-occipital sulcus extends laterally to notch the superior margin and convexity surface of the hemisphere. That notch serves as the superior landmark for the lateral temporoparietal line that marks the anterior border of the occipital lobe on the convexity surface of the hemisphere (see Figs. 9-4 and 9-9).

Behind the parieto-occipital sulcus, the calcarine sulcus forms a deep horizontal to zigzag sulcus that indents the occipital lobe (see Figs. 9-10 and 9-12). An inconstant paracalcarine sulcus

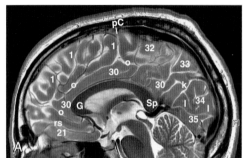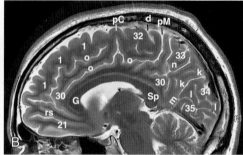

■ FIGURE 9-12   Medial surface. Sagittal T2W MRI in the midline (**A**) and just parasagittal (**B**) (labels as in Fig. 9-10). Sagittal T2W MR image displays the gross anatomic features of the medial surface arrayed around the corpus callosum, including the superior frontal gyrus (1), gyrus rectus (21), cingulate gyrus (30), paracentral lobule (32), precuneus (33), cuneus (34), and lingual gyrus (35). Sulci identified include: rostral sulcus (rs) anteriorly, cingulate sulcus (o), paracentral sulcus (pC), central sulcus (d), pars marginalis (pM), subparietal sulcus (n), parieto-occipital sulcus (k), calcarine sulcus (l), and anterior cingulate sulcus (m). In **B**, the cingulate sulcus (o) appears duplicated, a common normal variant.

(synonym: sagittal sulcus) may parallel the calcarine sulcus superiorly (see Fig. 9-9). An inconstant lingual sulcus may parallel the calcarine sulcus inferiorly. The posterior end of the calcarine sulcus is typically capped by the perpendicular retrocalcarine sulcus. The gyrus descendens of Ecker and the occipitopolar sulcus lie posterior to the retrocalcarine sulcus. The posterior end of the calcarine sulcus and these capping structures may remain on the medial surface of the hemisphere, extend onto the posterior convexity, or curve onto the postero-inferomedial surface of the hemisphere.

In all cases, the anterior end of the calcarine sulcus unites with the inferior end of the parieto-occipital sulcus to form an anterior calcarine sulcus, which courses anteroinferiorly onto the inferomedial surface of the brain. The portion of the medial occipital lobe behind the parieto-occipital sulcus but superior to the calcarine sulcus is termed the *cuneus*. The portion of the medial occipital lobe inferior to the calcarine sulcus and posterior to the anterior calcarine sulcus is the *lingual gyrus* (synonym: medial occipitotemporal gyrus).

Temporal Lobe

The parahippocampal gyrus forms the superomedial edge of most of the temporal lobe, from the rhinal sulcus anteriorly to the splenium posteriorly (see Figs. 9-9 and 9-10). Posteriorly, the cingulate gyrus swings around the splenium, narrows to the isthmus of the cingulate gyrus, and fuses with the posterior end of the parahippocampal gyrus. The lateral border of the parahippocampal gyrus is formed by the collateral sulcus (anteriorly) and the anterior calcarine sulcus (posteriorly). The lingual gyrus of the occipital lobe extends anteroinferiorly from the medial surface of the occipital lobe onto the inferomedial surface of the temporal lobe lateral to the anterior calcarine sulcus. The anatomy of this region is presented in greater detail in the sections on the inferior surface, including the section on the temporal lobe.

Superior Surface

The superior surface is the portion of the two convexities visible from above. It extends from the vertex down along both convexities to the widest portion of the brain, so it includes portions of both frontal lobes, both parietal lobes, and both occipital lobes. The temporal lobes typically lie inferior to the greatest dimension of the brain, so they are hidden from superior view. The specific structures seen vary slightly with the direction of view: anterosuperior versus direct superior versus posterosuperior. Only the superior margins of the hemispheres are displayed in superior view. Key landmarks along the frontal surface are depicted in Figures 9-13 and 9-14. These

landmarks help to identify the surface features in serial axial anatomic sections (Fig. 9-15) and MR images (Figs. 9-16 and 9-17).[10,12,15-20,23]

Frontal Lobes

The two frontal lobes form the anterior portion of the superior surface (see Figs. 9-15 to 9-17). The longitudinally oriented superior frontal gyri flank the midline anteriorly. They form the medial borders of the superior surface between the interhemispheric fissure medially, the superior frontal sulci laterally, and the paracentral sulci posteriorly. Behind the superior frontal gyri, the paracentral lobules form the medial surfaces of the frontal lobes between the paracentral sulci anteriorly and the central sulci posteriorly. Because the paracentral lobules end at the partes marginales, not the central sulci, the paracentral lobules also extend a short distance behind the central sulci into the parietal lobes. The middle frontal gyri lie lateral to the superior frontal sulci, forming the lateral borders of the superior surface. The superior frontal sulci typically extend posteriorly to end in the precentral sulci. The transversely oriented precentral gyri extend across the superior surface between the precentral sulci anteriorly and the central sulci posteriorly. The central sulci pass medially and cut across the superior margins of the hemispheres just millimeters anterior to the paired partes marginales. The hand motor areas of the precentral gyri form characteristic expansions of the posterior surfaces of the precentral gyri. These expansions deflect the central sulci posteriorly and indent the anterior surfaces of the postcentral gyri behind them.

Parietal Lobes

The two parietal lobes form the central portion of the superior surface behind the central sulci (see Figs. 9-15 to 9-17). The postcentral gyri extend across the whole superior surface of the brain between the central sulci anteriorly and the postcentral sulci posteriorly. The paired postcentral sulci approach the partes marginales to form "cups" or "parentheses" about the lateral borders of the partes marginales. The anterior surfaces of the postcentral gyri show characteristic concavities at the hand sensation area for vibration, joint position sense, and light touch.[11] Behind the postcentral sulci, the superior surface displays paired crescentic intraparietal sulci that divide the parietal lobes into medially placed superior parietal lobules and laterally placed inferior parietal lobules. Further posteriorly the prominent paired parieto-occipital sulci separate the parietal lobes anteriorly from the occipital lobes posteriorly. The medial surfaces of the two superior parietal lobules form the precunei between the partes marginales anteriorly and the parieto-occipital sulci posteriorly. When the subparietal sulci are deep,

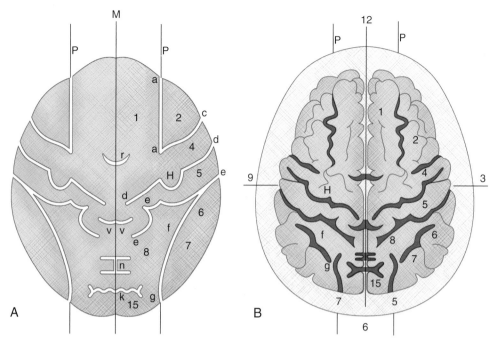

■ FIGURE 9-13 Key relationships along the superior surface of the brain. **A,** Template. In the midline (M) one finds the paracentral sulcus (r), pars marginalis (v), subparietal sulcus (n) and the parieto-occipital sulcus (k). Along the paramedian line (P), one finds the superior frontal sulcus (a), a sharp notch (inscription) in the central sulcus (d) just medial to the bump of the hand motor area (H), a corresponding usually shallower notch in the post-central sulcus, and the posterior end of the arcuate intraparietal (f)/intraoccipital (g) sulcus (IPS-IOS). Laterally, one finds the precentral sulcus (c), the central sulcus (d), and the postcentral sulcus (e). The lower portion of the postcentral sulcus is usually the initial ascending portion of the IPS-IOS. Archetypically, the paracentral sulcus (r) vaguely aligns with the precentral sulcus (c). The paired partes marginales (v v) from each side merge into a simple single curve designated the pars bracket or pars basket that always projects in relation to the anterior half of the IPS-IOS. The shape of the pars marginalis varies systematically from inferior to superior (see Fig. 9-26). The paired subparietal sulci (n) groove the medial surfaces of the two hemispheres to create a rough H shape. The paired parieto-occipital sulci (k) merge into a complex zigzag shape with bifid lateral ends ("fish tails"). The parieto-occipital sulci always align with the posterior half of the same IPS-IOS. The superior frontal sulcus (a) typically ends at the precentral sulcus (c). The central sulcus (d) forms the characteristic bump of the hand motor area (H) with its sharp medial notch roughly aligned along the superior frontal sulcus (a) and parasagittal line (P). Medially, the central sulcus (d) characteristically passes anterior to, and medial to, the lateral edge of the pars marginalis to "enter" the pars basket. The postcentral sulcus (e) parallels the course of the precentral sulcus (d) laterally but medially bifurcates to cup the pars marginalis (like two hands holding a heavy bowl with the fingers beneath the bowl and the thumbs on the rim). The anterior limbs of the postcentral bifurcation ("thumbs") do not enter the pars basket. The parieto-occipital sulci (k) separate the medial parietal lobe (8) anteriorly from the superior occipital gyrus (15) posteriorly. Laterally, the arcuate IPS-IOS separates the superior parietal lobule (8) superomedially from the inferior parietal lobule (6 and 7) inferolaterally. **B,** Actual tracings of the sulci on serial axial CT sections in one patient confirms the relationships diagrammed in the template. Considering the superior surface of the brain as a clock face, then the 12 to 6 o'clock line corresponds to the interhemispheric fissure. The 9 to 3 o'clock line is taken as the widest biparietal diameter of the head. That choice establishes a coordinate system that automatically corrects for the normal variations in individual head shape and the differing angles of the "axial" sections of CT and MRI. In that coordinate system, the IPS-IOS form arcuate curves along the 3 to 5 and 9 to 7 o'clock lines. The partes marginales fall at or posterior to the 9 to 3 line. *Gyri:* Superior frontal gyrus (1), middle frontal gyrus (2), precentral gyrus (4), postcentral gyrus (5), superior parietal lobule (8). *Sulci:* Superior frontal sulcus (a), precentral sulcus (c), central sulcus (d), postcentral sulcus (e), pars marginalis (v), subparietal sulcus (n), and parieto-occipital sulcus (k). *(Modified from Naidich TP, Brightbill TC. Vascular territories and watersheds: a zonal frequency analysis of the gyral and sulcal extent of cerebral infarcts: I. The anatomic template. Neuroradiology 2003; 45:536-540.)*

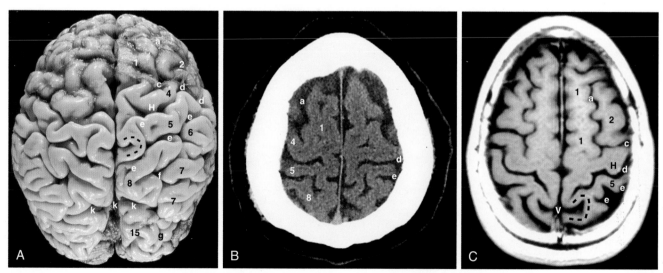

■ FIGURE 9-14 Key landmarks along the superior surface (labels as in Fig. 9-13). **A,** Formalin-fixed gross anatomic specimen after partial removal of the pia-arachnoid and vessels. **B,** Axial noncontrast CT section through the vertex. **C,** T1W axial MR image. The positions of the gyri and sulci appear to shift with the imaging modality and the angle of section. However, they remain constant with respect to the 9 to 3 o'clock line taken across the widest biparietal diameter of the brain. As a result, the pattern of the sulci and gyri at the vertex permits identification of most of the superior gyri in most patients.[15] The paired gyri (*dashed lines*) that enclose the pars bracket (v) resemble a small Halloween mask ("cat lady" sign). The hand motor area (H) forms the typical bump or "knob," and the inscription of the central sulcus just medial to it aligns with the superior frontal sulcus (a). The central sulcus (d) typically enters the pars bracket, whereas the postcentral sulcus (e) typically does not.

■ FIGURE 9-15 Superior surface of the brain with sequential axial sections. Formalin-fixed gross anatomic specimen after removal of the pia-arachnoid and vessels (labels as in Fig. 9-6). **A,** Uncut specimen, viewed from above and behind. The superior frontal gyrus (1) is often grooved by a series of unconnected shallow sulci, collectively designated the medial frontal sulcus (*white arrow*). The middle frontal gyrus (2) forms the perimeter of the frontal lobe in this view. Taking the interhemispheric fissure as the 12-6 o'clock line and the widest transverse dimension of the brain as the 9-3 o'clock line, then, at nearly all standard CT and MR angles, the intraparietal/intraoccipital sulci (f-g) form two arcs extending from 3 to 5 o'clock and from 9 to 7 o'clock. The pars marginalis (*paired black arrowheads*) falls at or behind the 9 to 3 o'clock line. **B to G,** Sequential axial sections with brain positioned slightly more horizontally. In this specimen, the postcentral sulci also enter the pars bracket at the very top of the brain (3% incidence only). H designates the hand motor area of the precentral gyrus (not Heschl's gyrus).

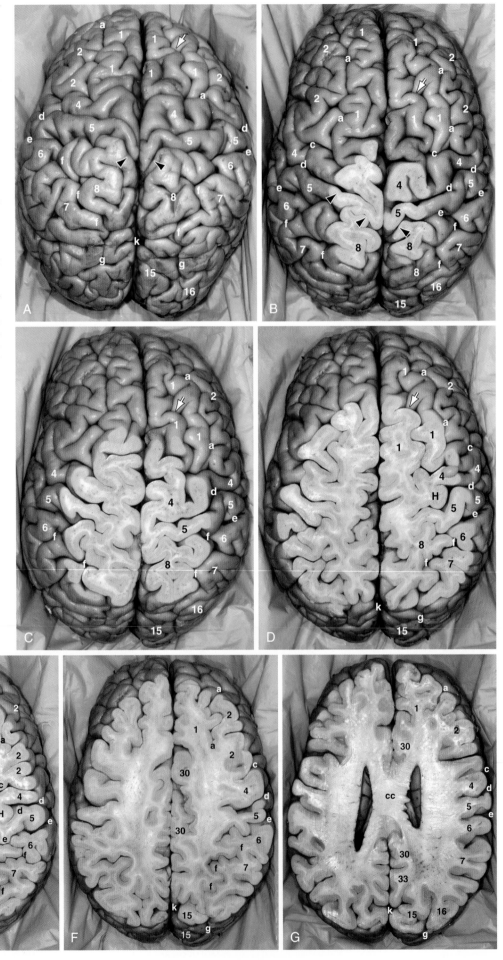

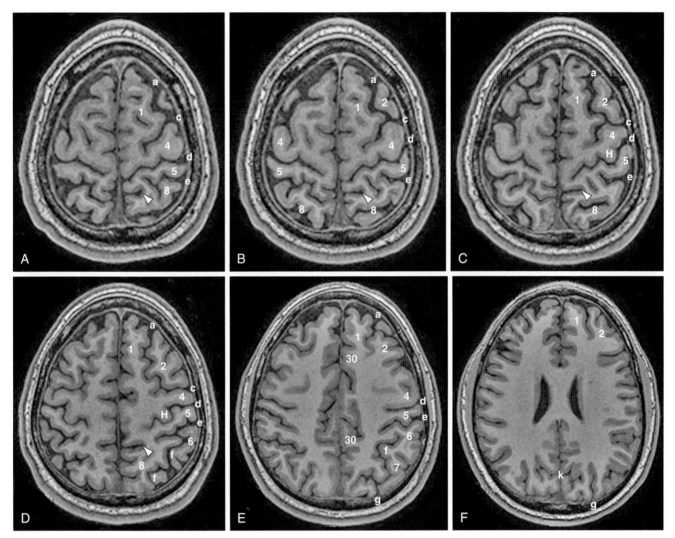

■ **FIGURE 9-16** A to F, Superior surface T1W MR images (labels as in Fig. 9-6). MRI displays all of the surface features seen by gross inspection of the brain. See analysis section for a systematic approach to identifying the gyri and sulci.

the grooves they form on the medial surfaces of the precunei become visible on the superior surface.

Occipital Lobes

The occipital lobes form the posterior portion of the superior surface behind the parieto-occipital sulci (see Figs. 9-15 to 9-17). The posterior ends of the arcuate intraparietal sulci pass into the occipital lobes, where they are renamed the intraoccipital sulci. The superior occipital gyri form the superior surface of the occipital lobe behind the parieto-occipital sulci and medial to the intraoccipital sulci. The medial face of each superior occipital gyrus is termed the *cuneus*. The middle occipital gyri form the lateral borders of the superior surface lateral to the intraoccipital sulci.

INFERIOR SURFACE

The inferior surface of the cerebrum is the portion of the brain visible from below after resection of the brain stem and cerebellum (Figs. 9-18 to 9-20). The inferior surface is divided into lobes by prominent intrinsic landmarks such as the sylvian fissure, rhinal-collateral sulci, and parieto-occipital sulci; inconstant "landmarks" such as the preoccipital notch; and arbitrary lines such as the basal parietotemporal line drawn from the inferior end of the parieto-occipital sulcus to the preoccipital notch.[1]

Frontal Lobes

The orbital surfaces of the two frontal lobes form the anterior portion of the inferior surface (see Figs. 9-18 and 9-19). Medially, the paired gyri recti form longitudinally oriented gyri that flank the interhemispheric fissure between the midline medially and the olfactory sulci laterally. Lateral to the olfactory sulci, four orbital gyri are arranged around roughly H-shaped orbital sulci as the medial orbital, lateral orbital, anterior orbital, and posterior orbital gyri on each side. The posterior ends of the orbital gyri form the frontal surface of the sylvian fissures. On each side, the posterior end of the medial orbital gyrus merges with the medial end of the posterior orbital gyrus to form a focal expansion referred to as the posteromedial orbital lobule. This connects directly with the anterior inferior medial aspect of the insula behind it.

Temporo-occipital Lobes

The inferior surface of the temporo-occipital lobe is a continuous sheet of tissue arbitrarily divided into temporal and occipital lobes by the basal parietotemporal line (see Figs. 9-4, 9-9, and 9-20). The lateral margin of this inferior surface is formed by the inferior temporal gyrus anterior to the preoccipital notch and by the inferior occipital gyrus behind the notch. The inferior temporal and occipital gyri are delimited medially by the

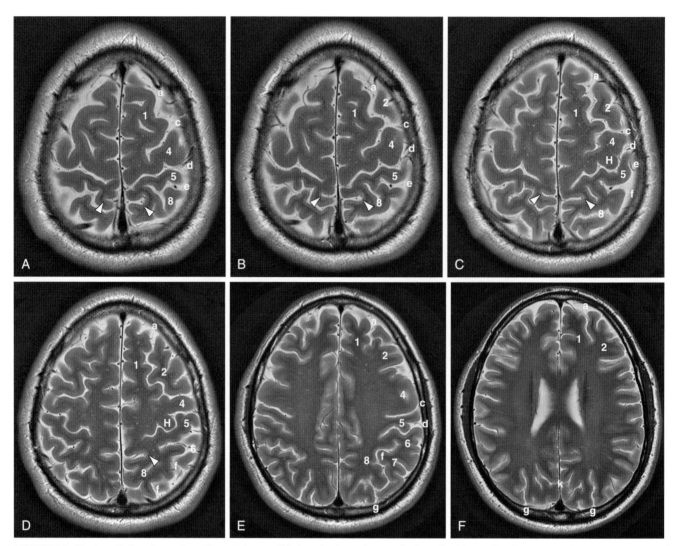

■ **FIGURE 9-17** **A** to **F,** Superior surface T2W MR images (labels as in Fig. 9-6). MRI displays all of the surface features seen by gross inspection of the brain. See analysis section for a systematic approach to identifying the gyri and sulci.

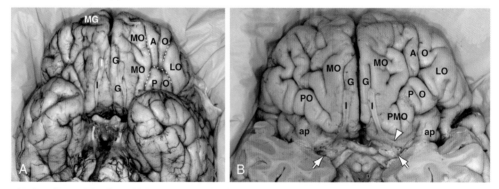

■ **FIGURE 9-18** Orbital surfaces of the frontal lobes. Formalin-fixed gross anatomic specimens. **A,** Intact meninges and vessels. The orbital surfaces of frontal lobe display five major gyri. The paired gyri recti (G) flank the midline and are delimited laterally by the olfactory sulci. The olfactory bulbs and tracts (CN I) (I) align along the olfactory sulci, partially obscuring them. The remaining orbital surface is composed of four major orbital gyri arrayed around a free-form H-shaped orbital sulcus (*dashed white lines*) as the medial orbital (MO), lateral orbital (LO), anterior orbital (AO), and posterior orbital (PO) gyri. Because the orbital roof is highly curved, the gyri recti and medial orbital gyri lie inferior to the others, largely between the orbits. At the anterior edge of the orbital surface, the transversely oriented frontomarginal gyri (MG) create the anterior orbitofrontal margin. The anterior temporal lobes and temporal poles overlie the olfactory bulbs and tracts. **B,** Different specimen (same as Fig. 9-20). Stripping the meninges and vessels and resecting the temporal poles exposes the posterior ends of the olfactory tracts (I) as they diverge into the medial and lateral (*white arrowhead*) olfactory striae. These define the anterior borders of the anterior perforated substance (*white arrows*). The posteromedial orbital lobule (PMO) merges laterally into the most anterior and inferior portion of the insula, near to the apex (ap) of the insula. Other labels as in **A,** above.

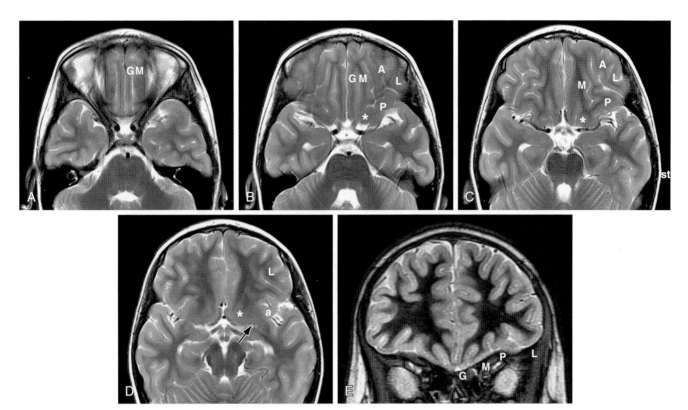

■ **FIGURE 9-19**   Orbital surface of frontal lobes. T2W MR images in the axial (**A to D**) and coronal (**E**) planes. Because the roof of the orbit is curved, with deep recesses between the orbits, serial axial sections display different portions of the orbital surface. **A,** Inferiorly, the paired parallel gyri recti (G) flank the midline with small portions of the medial orbital lobules (M) lateral to them. The gray cortices and central white cores are well differentiated. **B to C,** The next most superior sections show differing portions of all the gyri, but the lateral orbital gyrus (L) least well. The posterior end of the medial orbital gyrus (M) unites with the medial end of the posterior orbital gyrus (P) to form the posteromedial orbital lobule (PMOL) (*asterisk*). PMOL forms the anterolateral wall of the suprasellar cistern. At this level, the sylvian fissure and the middle cerebral vessels still separate the frontal from the temporal lobes. **D,** One section higher, immediately superior to the sylvian fissure, PMOL crosses over (*black arrow*) the top of the sylvian fissure to merge into the most anterior inferior portion of the insula near the apex (a). This is one route by which frontal and insular lesions may spread in either direction.

occipitotemporal sulcus. The long lateral occipitotemporal gyrus (LOTG) lies immediately medial to the inferior temporal and inferior occipital gyri, between the occipitotemporal sulcus laterally and the collateral sulcus medially. The collateral (i.e., collateral) sulcus defines the medial surface of the LOTG along its entire length. Short anterior and posterior transverse collateral sulci delimit a central portion of the LOTG, which may be designated separately as the fusiform gyrus. However, the definition and the location of the "fusiform gyrus" do not appear to be used uniformly. In the posterior portion of the inferior surface, the lingual gyrus (synonym: medial occipitotemporal gyrus [MOTG]) extends from the medial occipital surface onto the inferior surface just medial to the LOTG. It is delimited medially by the anterior calcarine sulcus. This gyrus and sulcus are not present anteriorly. The portion of the inferior surface situated medial to the collateral sulcus (anteriorly) and medial to the anterior calcarine sulcus (posteriorly) is the limbic lobe.

Limbic Lobe

The limbic lobe forms the medial margin of the inferior surface of the hemisphere (see Fig. 9-10). The portion of the limbic lobe on the inferior surface is delimited from the temporal pole by the rhinal sulcus, from the LOTG by the collateral sulcus, and from the lingual gyrus (MOTG) by the anterior calcarine sulcus. Typically, the rhinal sulcus runs parallel to or continuous with the collateral sulcus. Posteriorly, the limbic lobe turns up behind the splenium to become continuous with the cingulate gyrus.

The parahippocampal gyrus forms the medial edge of the inferior surface of the brain. At its anterior end, the parahippocampal gyrus hooks sharply medially, posteriorly, and superiorly around the hippocampal fissure to form the uncus (see Fig. 9-10). The uncus has anterior and posterior portions. The anterior portion of the uncus is part of the pyriform lobe and displays two small protrusions: the gyrus semilunaris and the gyrus ambiens, both of which overlie the amygdala. The posterior portion of the uncus contains three subdivisions: the gyrus uncinatus, the limbus Giacomini (tail of the dentate gyrus), and the gyrus intralimbicis. Lateral to the hippocampal formation, the medial surface of the parahippocampal gyrus contains the entorhinal cortex.

The term *hippocampal formation* is used to designate a structure composed of both gray matter and white matter that forms embryologically by in-rolling of the medial surface of the temporal lobe (Fig. 9-21). The gray matter components are the subiculum, dentate gyrus, and hippocampus proper. The white matter components are the alveus and fimbria, which together constitute the fornix. This anatomy is best shown in coronal sections, which display the subiculum below the hippocampal fissure, the dentate gyrus above the fissure, and the hippocampus proper (cornu ammonis) lateral to the hippocampal fissure, indenting the inferomedial surface of the temporal horn. Fibers arising from the entorhinal cortex and the hippocampal gyri form a thin sheet of white matter, the alveus, which lies between the ependyma of the temporal horn and the hippocampus proper. This sheet arches medially, above the hippocampus and

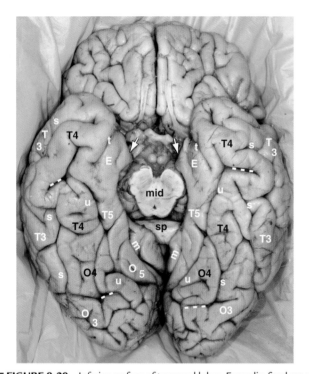

■ **FIGURE 9-20** Inferior surface of temporal lobes. Formalin-fixed gross anatomic specimen after removal of the meninges and vessels (same specimen as Fig. 9-18B). The inferior margin of each hemisphere is formed by the inferior temporal gyrus (T3) anteriorly and the inferior occipital gyrus (O3) posteriorly. The occipitotemporal sulcus (s) delimits the medial borders of these gyri. The midportion of each basal surface is formed by the composite *lateral* occipitotemporal gyrus (LOTG) (T4-O4). The LOTG extends the full length of the basal surface from the temporal pole to the occipital pole. It is delimited laterally by the occipitotemporal sulci (s) and medially by the rhinal (t) and collateral (u) sulci. The rhinal sulcus (t) separates the entorhinal cortex (E) medially from the neocortex of the LOTG (T4) laterally. The rhinal sulcus may align with, or merge with the collateral sulcus (u). The *collateral* sulcus should be thought of as the *collateral* sulcus, because it stays with the medial border of the LOTG throughout its length. Within the midportion of each LOTG, the anterior and posterior transverse collateral sulci (*four dashed white lines*) may be used to identify the fusiform gyri (also T4-O4). The entire medial edge of the temporal lobe is the parahippocampal gyrus (T5). Anteriorly, the parahippocampal gyrus hooks medially to form the uncus (*white arrows*). Posteriorly, the parahippocampal gyrus narrows to become the isthmus of the cingulate gyrus immediately behind the splenium (sp). The anterior and posterior halves of the temporal lobe show different arrangements of gyri. Anteriorly, the parahippocampal gyrus (T5) lies immediately adjacent to the LOTG (T4), separated by the rhinal-collateral sulci (t, u). Posteriorly, the lingual gyrus (medial occipitotemporal gyrus [MOTG]) (O5) intercalates itself between the parahippocampal gyrus and the LOTG (T4-O4). The anterior calcarine sulcus (m) marks its medial border. As a result, the order of the gyri and sulci in the posterior half, from lateral to medial, is inferior occipital gyrus (O3), occipitotemporal sulcus (s), LOTG (O4), collateral sulcus (u), lingual gyrus (MOTG) (O5), anterior calcarine sulcus (m), and the parahippocampal gyrus (T5) (which is merging into the isthmus of the cingulate gyrus under the splenium).

dentate gyrus, thickens by accrual of additional fibers, and separates from the dentate gyrus to form a free margin (the fimbria) that is visible on the medial surface (see Fig. 9-10).

Poles

The term *pole* designates the rounded end of a lobe and the adjoining tissue.

Frontal Pole

The frontal pole is formed by transversely oriented gyri interposed between the superior frontal gyrus and the orbital surface of frontal lobe. The frontomarginal gyrus forms the orbital margin of the frontal pole and is delimited superiorly by the frontomarginal sulcus. The superior and inferior transverse frontopolar gyri lie superior and posterior to the frontomarginal sulcus between the frontomarginal gyrus and the anterior end of the superior frontal gyrus.

Temporal Pole

The temporal pole is formed by the union of the superior, middle, and inferior temporal gyri. The temporal pole is separated from the parahippocampal gyrus behind it by the rhinal sulcus.

Occipital Pole

The occipital pole is formed by the merging of the superior, middle and inferior occipital gyri (Figs. 9-22 and 9-23). The posterior end of the calcarine sulcus and the retrocalcarine sulcus are sometimes seen at the occipital pole but may lie along the medial surface of the hemisphere or along the convexity laterally (see Fig. 9-9). The gyrus descendens of Ecker and the occipitopolar sulcus lie immediately behind the retrocalcarine sulcus.

IMAGING
Ultrasonography

All of the imaging modalities display the same anatomy. The differences among the images reflect the differing sensitivities of the studies to specific aspects of the anatomy and the differing planes of section used to make the images. Increasing utilization of CT scanners that automatically reformat images in three planes now enables the imager to use the same triplanar pattern analysis for CT and for MRI (Figs. 9-24 to 9-26).

The imaging appearance of the surface anatomy has already been illustrated immediately after the corresponding anatomic images, for easy comparison. A systematic approach to gyral-sulcal identification and lesion localization is presented in Analysis and illustrated in the case used for the sample report in Box 9-1.

ANALYSIS

Accurate localization requires seeing a structure in context and placing it in proper relationship to its neighbors. Correct localization of a single structure on the surface thus requires a broad overview of the brain surface to understand that structure in context. For that reason, the plane of imaging that is most useful for identifying structures varies with the structure to be identified. On average, sagittal images are most useful for identifying structures on the lateral and medial surfaces. Because of the landmarks used, convexity structures are best analyzed from lateral to medial, whereas midline and paramedian structures are best analyzed from medial to lateral. Axial plane images are most useful for localizing structures on the superior surface. These images are best analyzed from superior to inferior. Because the inferior frontal and temporo-occipital surfaces curve extensively, axial images section these surfaces only piecemeal. Therefore, the coronal and sagittal images are most useful for identifying structures on the inferior surface. In all planes, analysis proceeds systematically from anterior to posterior, because the range of normal variation is smaller frontally and larger at the confluence of the temporal, parietal and occipital lobes.

Correct analysis requires recognizing the patterns of anatomy described in this chapter and following the anatomy from landmark ("sign") to landmark to ensure that the patterns are appreciated properly. It must be understood at the outset that all of the signs to be described in this section are 85% to 98% reliable. Each sign fails in 2% to 15% of cases. Therefore, any localization made by using a single sign carries risk of error. Instead, it is appropriate to utilize all of the signs in concert, so that the imager can specify a location with confidence when multiple

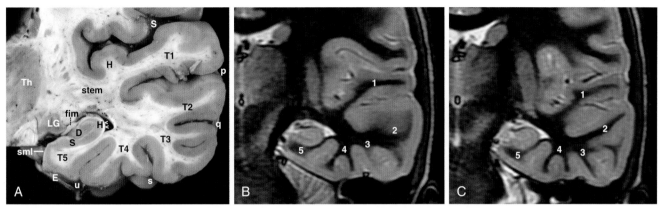

■ **FIGURE 9-21** Hippocampal formation. **A,** Formalin-fixed coronal anatomic section through the temporal lobe at the level of the lateral geniculate nucleus (LG). The temporal lobe expands outward from the temporal stem like a cauliflower on a stalk. The five major temporal gyri of the anterior temporal lobe are the superior temporal (T1), middle temporal (T2), inferior temporal (T3), lateral occipitotemporal (LOTG) (T4), and the parahippocampal (T5) gyri. The corresponding sulci are the superior temporal sulcus (p), inferior temporal sulcus (q), occipitotemporal sulcus (s), and collateral sulcus (u). Heschl's transverse temporal gyrus characteristically bulges upward above the superior temporal plane (*black* H). T3 makes the inferior margin of the temporal lobe. T4 characteristically displays a bifid (forked) white matter core and bifid surface. T5 makes the medial margin of the temporal lobe. The hippocampal formation is characteristically rolled into the temporal lobe to make the inferior medial wall of the temporal horn. The hippocampal formation is composed of the subiculum (*small black* S) situated below the hippocampal fissure (*unlabeled*), the dentate gyrus (D) above the fissure, and the hippocampus (*small black* H) lateral to the fissure and above the dentate gyrus. The superficial medullary lamina (sml) is a layer of white matter external to the gray matter seen with allocortex. It is thickest overlying the subiculum, extends into the hippocampal fissure with the subiculum, and is a landmark for the fissure. The alveus (*open white arrowheads*) is a thin well-defined layer of white matter situated between the ependymal lining of the temporal horn laterally and the hippocampus medially. It course posteriorly and medially to form a free medial margin, the fimbria (fim). Together, the alveus and the fimbria constitute the fornix. Also labeled: Th, thalamus. **B** and **C,** Sequential coronal inversion recovery MR images corresponding to **A** (with simplified labels).

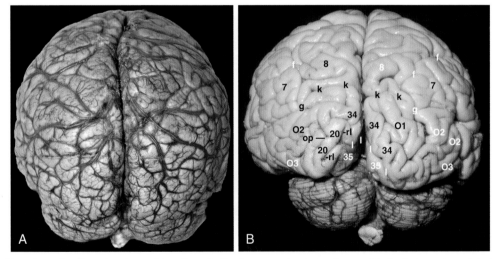

■ **FIGURE 9-22** Posterior poles. Posterior views of two formalin-fixed gross anatomic specimens with the leptomeninges intact (**A**) and after their removal (**B**). The specimen in **B** displays significant petalia. The deep parieto-occipital sulci (k) mark the anterior limits of the occipital lobes on the medial surface. Anterior to them lie the superior parietal lobule (8) and the angular gyrus (7) of the inferior parietal lobule. The occipital poles are often very asymmetric. The calcarine sulcus (l) courses horizontally between the cuneus (34) above and the lingual gyrus (medial occipitotemporal gyrus) (35) below. It is the first large horizontally oriented sulcus superior to the tentorium and cerebellum. The posterior end of the calcarine sulcus may remain on the medial surface, extend to the pole, or pass around the pole to the lateral or inferior surface of the hemisphere. The posterior end of the calcarine sulcus is capped by two concentric sulci and an intervening crescentic gyrus. The posterior end of the calcarine sulcus typically ends in a "fish tail" designated the retrocalcarine sulcus (rl). The gyrus descendens (20) encircles the retrocalcarine sulcus. The occipitopolar sulcus (op) encircles the outer border of the gyrus descendens. The superior occipital (O1), middle occipital (O2), and inferior occipital (O3) gyri converge to the occipital pole. The intraparietal sulci (f) demarcate the superior parietal lobule (8) from the inferior parietal lobule (7). The intraoccipital sulci (g) are the posterior portions of the intraparietal sulci, renamed intraoccipital when they pass posterior to the parieto-occipital sulcus (k) to enter the occipital lobes.

■ **FIGURE 9-23** Calcarine sulcus. Coronal T2W MR image. The calcarine sulcus (l) is the first large horizontal sulcus above the tentorium. Its lateral ends approximate and often indent the medial aspects of the occipital horns. Sections through the calcarine sulci may also display the cuneus (34) and lingual gyrus (35) that border the sulcus, the parieto-occipital sulcus (k), the superior parietal lobule (8), the intraparietal (f)/intraoccipital (g) sulci, and the angular gyri (7) of the inferior parietal lobules.

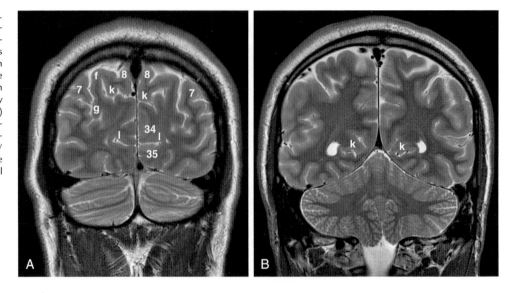

■ **FIGURE 9-24** Display of the gyri and sulci of the convexity by serial reformatted sagittal CT scans (labels as in Fig. 9-6). A single patient has been selected for Figures 9-24 to 9-26 to illustrate the same anatomy in three orthogonal planes and the utility of employing triplanar CT reformatted images. **B** shows the five rami of the sylvian fissure: anterior horizontal (*single black arrowhead*), anterior ascending (*dual black arrowheads*), posterior horizontal ramus (S), posterior ascending ramus (*dual white arrowheads*) and posterior descending (*single white arrowhead*). Compare the configuration of the sylvian fissure on sagittal CT with the anatomy shown in Figure 9-3. In **D**, the anterior (A) and posterior (P) lobes of the insula are delimited by the residual portion of the inferior frontal gyrus anteriorly, the serrated undersurface of the frontoparietal opercula superiorly, and the temporal lobe inferiorly. Other labels as defined in prior legends.

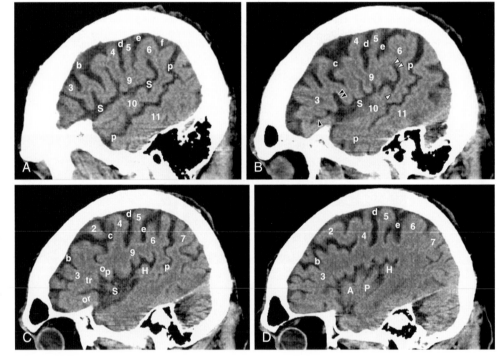

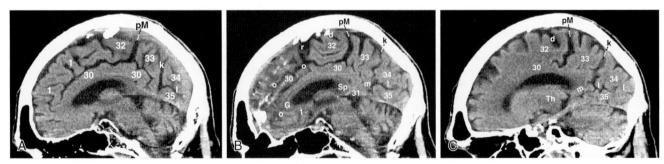

■ **FIGURE 9-25** Display of the gyri and sulci of the medial surface of the hemisphere by serial reformatted sagittal CT scans (labels as in Fig. 9-10). A and B, Reformatted images on both sides of the midline show side-to-side variations in fine detail but preservation of the basic pattern of anatomy. C, Off midline, the lazy-Y configuration of the parieto-occipital and calcarine sulci provides a useful landmark for anatomic localization. Th, thalamus. Other labels as defined in prior legends.

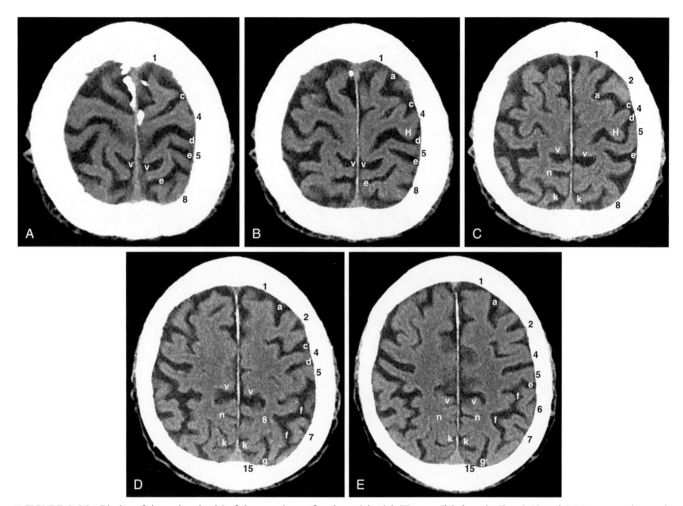

■ **FIGURE 9-26** Display of the gyri and sulci of the superior surface by serial axial CT scans (labels as in Figs. 9-13 and 9-14; same patient as in Figs. 9-24 and 9-25). H, Hand motor area of precentral gyrus.

signs give a concordant localization and, simultaneously, discard with confidence the one or two signs that are discordant. Furthermore, anatomic studies have shown that there is far less variation in gyral and sulcal anatomy in the frontal regions anteriorly than in the temporoparietal regions posteriorly. For that reason, it is prudent to begin identification of structures anteriorly and then count, gyrus by sulcus, from anterior to posterior to achieve a correct localization.

Lateral Surface

A simple algorithm provides accurate localization of the gyri and sulci of the lateral surface in nearly all cases (Fig. 9-27). This algorithm first identifies the arms of the sylvian fissure to establish the context and then localizes the specific gyri and sulci by their shape and their relation to the sylvian fissure and each other. For signs 13 to 16, see Fig. 9-6D-G.

1. *Start.* First, identify the five major rami of the sylvian fissure. The long oblique line typically called the sylvian fissure is actually designated the posterior horizontal ramus (arm) of the sylvian fissure. To simplify the language in this discussion, the term *sylvian fissure* will be used to designate this posterior horizontal ramus. Then, at the anterior end of the sylvian fissure, the anterior horizontal ramus and the anterior ascending ramus of the sylvian fissure take the shape of a capital letter V or Y that ascends into the frontal lobe. At the posterior end of the sylvian fissure, the posterior

ascending and posterior descending rami bifurcate to extend into the parietal and temporal lobes. On the upper surface of the sylvian fissure, two minor rami designated the *anterior subcentral ramus* and the *posterior subcentral ramus* delimit the anterior and posterior extent of the subcentral gyrus. On the lower surface of the sylvian fissure, several transverse temporal sulci delimit the posterior margin of the transverse temporal gyrus of Heschl. Identifying the arms of the sylvian fissure establishes the frame of reference and the proportions among the parts of the lateral surface (Fig. 9-27A and B).

2. *Triangular gyrus sign.* The inferior frontal gyrus has an overall triangular shape and may officially be designated the *triangular gyrus.* This shape is sufficiently different from the longitudinal and vertical shapes of the other frontal gyri that it helps to identify the inferior frontal gyrus (Fig. 9-27C).

3. *M sign.* The V or Y of the anterior horizontal and anterior ascending rami cut into the triangular inferior frontal gyrus, giving it the shape of the letter M. From anterior to posterior, the three parts of the M are the pars orbitalis that abuts onto the orbital gyri on the inferior surface of the frontal lobe, the pars triangularis in the middle, and the pars opercularis that contributes to the frontal operculum. A small triangular sulcus commonly grooves the pars triangularis. A small diagonal sulcus commonly grooves the pars opercularis (Fig. 9-27C).

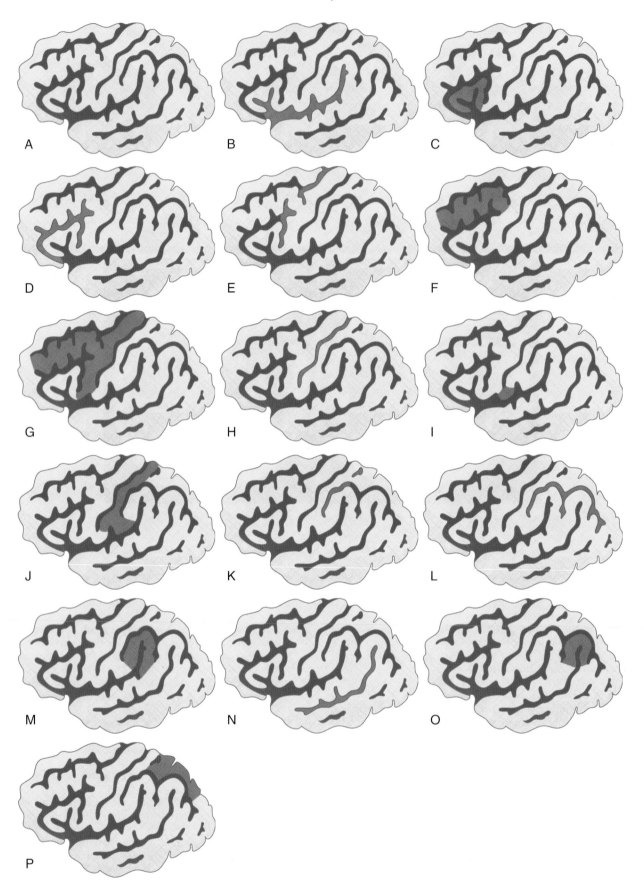

■ **FIGURE 9-27** A to P, Analysis of the gyri and sulci of the lateral surface. Diagram of the sequential steps for systematically reviewing the gyri and sulci of the lateral surface. The specific steps are detailed in the section on analysis. *(From Naidich TP, Valavanis AG, Kubik S, et al. Anatomic relationships along the low-middle convexity. Int J Neuroradiol 1997; 3:393-409.)*

4. *Inferior frontal sulcus sign.* The sulcus atop the triangular inferior frontal gyrus is the inferior frontal sulcus. This passes posteriorly and bifurcates into the vertical inferior precentral sulcus. Therefore, the gyrus superior to the inferior frontal sulcus is the middle frontal gyrus. The gyrus posterior to the inferior precentral sulcus is the inferior portion of the precentral gyrus. From there, one can simply count, sequentially, the precentral gyrus, central sulcus, postcentral gyrus, and postcentral sulcus to localize the gyri behind. A small bridge of tissue commonly connects the pars triangularis with the middle frontal gyrus across the inferior frontal sulcus. One must read past this small bridge to discern the overall shapes and relationships of the gyri and sulci (Fig. 9-27D-G).

5. *Zigzag middle frontal gyrus sign.* The middle frontal gyrus is very undulant and appears to wiggle or zigzag as it courses posteriorly above the inferior frontal sulcus. This undulance helps to identify the middle frontal gyrus (Fig. 9-27F).

6. *Union of middle frontal gyrus with the precentral gyrus.* Embryologically, the precentral sulcus is formed of two separate, upper and lower, portions. The posterior end of the superior frontal sulcus bifurcates to form a vertical ending that is called the superior precentral sulcus. The posterior end of the inferior frontal sulcus bifurcates to form a vertical ending that is called the inferior precentral sulcus. These verticals *do not meet* in the middle, so the middle frontal gyrus merges into the anterior surface of the precentral gyrus without interruption, identifying both gyri (Fig. 9-27G).

7. *Central sulcus gap sign.* Typically, the central sulcus is separated from the sylvian fissure by the U-shaped subcentral gyrus. The inferior surface of the subcentral gyrus is outlined by the anterior and posterior subcentral sulci of the sylvian fissure. Identification of the gap between the inferior end of a vertically oriented sulcus and the sylvian fissure helps to identify the central sulcus and the subcentral gyrus (Fig. 9-27H-I).

8. *Thin postcentral gyrus sign.* The sagittal dimension of the postcentral gyrus is thinner than the sagittal dimension of the precentral gyrus, so the thin vertical gyrus and sulcus posterior to the precentral gyrus and central sulcus are the postcentral gyrus and sulcus (Fig. 9-27J,K).

9. *Intraparietal sulcus sign.* The arcuate intraparietal sulcus begins anteriorly in the lower postcentral sulcus. From there it ascends, passes posteriorly across the parietal lobe, and then turns down into the occipital lobe. The inferior parietal lobule lies within the concavity of the sulcal arch. The superior parietal lobule lies along the convexity of the curve, superior to the arch. The long arcuate sulcus identifies the parietal lobe and the adjacent lobules (Fig. 9-27L-P).

10. *Posterior ascending ramus (of sylvian fissure) sign.* The posterior ascending ramus of the sylvian fissure extends into the anterior portion of the inferior parietal lobule. The "horseshoe" gyrus capping the posterior ascending ramus is the supramarginal gyrus (Fig. 9-27M).

11. *Angular gyrus sign.* The gyrus and sulcus just inferior to the sylvian fissure are the superior temporal gyrus and sulcus. The superior temporal sulcus courses co-curvilinear with both the sylvian fissure and its posterior ascending ramus, so the superior temporal sulcus may also be called the parallel sulcus. The posterior upswing of the superior temporal sulcus is termed the *angular sulcus*. The horseshoe gyrus capping the posterior end of the superior temporal sulcus (angular sulcus) is the *angular gyrus*. Because any single sulcus may bifurcate at its end, the "horseshoe" gyri just described as surrounding a simple sulcus may appear, instead, as "heart-shaped" gyri surrounding a bifid sulcus. This variance is especially common with the supramarginal

and angular gyri of the inferior parietal lobule (Fig. 9-27N-O).

12. *Longitudinal temporal gyri sign.* The temporal gyri course longitudinally parallel with the sylvian fissure and with each other. Therefore, one can simply count the gyri and sulci inferior to the sylvian fissure, one by one, to identify, in order, the sylvian fissure, superior temporal gyrus, superior temporal sulcus, middle temporal gyrus, inferior temporal sulcus, and the inferior temporal gyrus, which forms the margin and extends onto the inferior surface of the temporal lobe (Fig. 9-27O-P).

13. *Insular triangle sign.* The peri-insular sulcus takes the shape of a triangle with a nearly horizontal superior surface, a nearly vertical anterior surface, and an oblique inferior surface. The sulci forming the triangle are the superior, anterior, and inferior segments of the peri-insular (circular) sulcus (Fig. 9-6D-F).

14. *Hockey stick sign.* The central sulcus takes the form of a raised hockey stick as it crosses the insula. The superior segment is a short vertical. The inferior segment is a long oblique that descends anteroinferiorly. The large triangular lobule anterior to the hockey stick is the anterior lobule of the insula. The smaller lobule posteroinferior to the hockey stick is the posterior lobule of the insula (Fig. 9-6D-F).

15. *Three-finger (trident) sign.* The anterior short, middle short, and posterior short insular gyri form three verticals that converge to the apex of the insula just above the point at which the central sulcus curves medially toward the midline (Fig. 9-6D-F).

16. *Index thumb sign.* The anterior long and posterior long insular gyri usually take the shape of one's left index finger and thumb held together and extended in front of the face. The transverse temporal gyrus of Heschl fills in the gap inferior to the anterior long gyrus and posterior to the posterior long gyrus (Fig. 9-6D-G).

Medial Surface

A simple algorithm provides accurate localization of the gyri and sulci of the medial surface in nearly all cases (Fig. 9-28). This algorithm first identifies the four segments of the corpus callosum to establish the center of the medial surface and then considers the positions of the other gyri and sulci in relation to the corpus callosum. Overall, the medial surface is arrayed in a *radial* coordinate system with the major gyri and sulci arranged either co-curvilinear with or perpendicular (radial) to the corpus callosum.

1. *Start.* First, identify the rostrum, genu, body, and splenium of the corpus callosum. Then count the "parallel" curves from the corpus callosum outward toward the margin: callosal sulcus, cingulate gyrus, and cingulate sulcus (Fig. 9-28A-D).

2. *Pars marginalis sign.* Follow the cingulate sulcus posteriorly. About two thirds of the way back along the corpus callosum it swoops obliquely upward toward the superior margin of the hemisphere as the pars marginalis of the cingulate sulcus. The pars marginalis defines the posterior margin of the paracentral lobule and the anterior margin of the precuneus. The central sulcus crosses the superior margin of the hemisphere and then recurves posteriorly to run nearly perpendicular to the oblique pars marginalis, millimeters anterior to the pars marginalis. Therefore, the pars marginalis also localizes the expected position of the central sulcus. The precise location of the sulcus and its course perpendicular to the pars identifies that sulcus as the upper medial end of the central sulcus (Fig. 9-28D,E).

3. *Paracentral sulcus sign.* Feel the kinesthetics as you follow the curvature of the cingulate sulcus upward into the pars

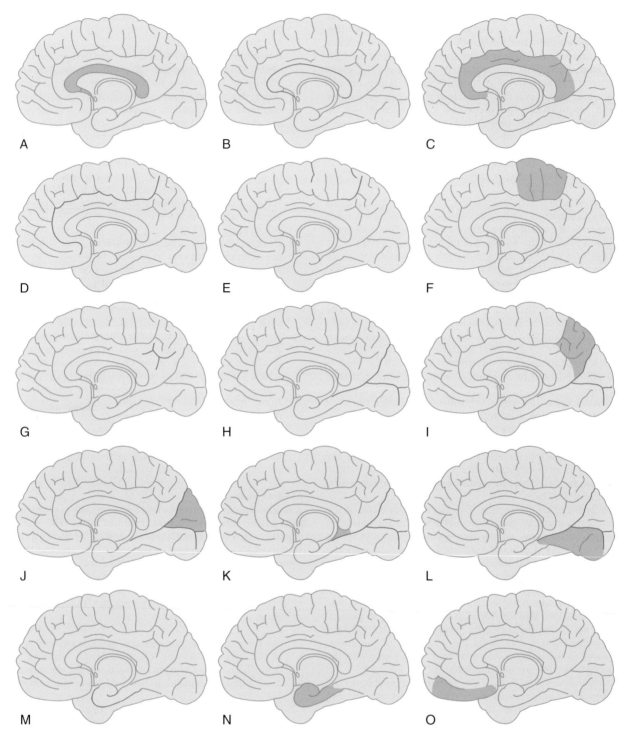

■ **FIGURE 9-28**   **A to S,** Analysis of the gyri and sulci of the medial surface. Diagram of the sequential steps for systematically reviewing the gyri and sulci of the medial surface. The specific steps are detailed in the section on analysis.

marginalis. Then, by kinesthetics reverse course, symmetrically, to swing down the pars marginalis, anterior along the cingulate sulcus, and back up to the margin at the variably prominent paracentral sulcus. The paracentral sulcus may ascend from the cingulate sulcus, descend from the superior margin, or do both together. The paracentral sulcus defines the posterior margin of the superior frontal gyrus and the anterior margin of the paracentral lobule (Fig. 9-28D-F).

4. *Subparietal sulcus sign.* Further posteriorly, above the posterior corpus callosum, a roughly H-shaped subparietal sulcus grooves the medial surface of the precuneus. The horizontal of the H usually aligns with the cingulate sulcus and appears to continue the curvature of the cingulate sulcus posterior to the pars marginalis. The H identifies the medial surface of the parietal lobe (precuneus) and the peripheral border of the cingulate gyrus (Fig. 9-28G).

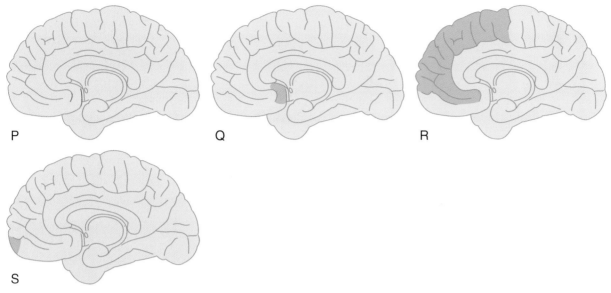

P   Q   R

S

■ **FIGURE 9-28, cont'd** For legend see opposite page.

5. *Lazy-Y sign.* Posterior to the splenium, the deep parieto-occipital sulcus runs obliquely, roughly parallel with the pars marginalis. In all normal individuals, the inferior end of the parieto-occipital sulcus merges with the anterior end of the calcarine sulcus to form an oblique anterior calcarine sulcus that continues onto the inferior surface of the hemisphere (Fig. 9-28H). The lazy-Y is a powerful landmark for identifying the gyri and lobules in this region. The precuneus of the parietal lobe lies anterior to the parieto-occipital sulcus above the splenium (Fig. 9-28I). The cuneus of the occipital lobe lies behind the parieto-occipital sulcus and above the calcarine sulcus (Fig. 9-28J). The cingulate gyrus thins and becomes the isthmus of the cingulate gyrus behind the splenium and anterior to the anterior calcarine sulcus (Fig. 9-28K). The lingual gyrus of the occipital lobe lies inferior to the calcarine sulcus and extends onto the inferior surface of the hemisphere posterolateral to the anterior calcarine sulcus (Fig. 9-28L). Because atrophy often widens the interhemispheric fissure, the lazy-Y sign may not be applicable in the true midline. However, the lazy-Y sign becomes very beneficial for identifying anatomy in the parasagittal sections just off midline (Fig. 9-28H-L).

6. *Collateral-rhinal sulcus sign.* The collateral sulcus of the temporal lobe sweeps forward and aligns (or unites) with the rhinal sulcus, outlining the parahippocampal gyrus and uncus (Fig. 9-28M-N).

7. *Gyrus rectus sign.* The gyrus rectus is readily identified as the longitudinally arrayed bar of tissue that forms the antero-inferior border of the medial surface between the inferior surface of the brain and the supraorbital sulcus (Fig. 9-28O).

8. *Subcallosal sign.* Inferior to the genu of corpus callosum and anterior to the rostrum, paired, vertical anterior and posterior parolfactory sulci define the anatomy of the infra-callosal region. The posterior end of the gyrus rectus appears to curve upward between these two sulci. The anterior parolfactory sulcus defines the posterior margin of the superior frontal gyrus. The subcallosal area lies between the anterior and posterior parolfactory sulci. The paraterminal gyrus lies posterior to the posterior parolfactory sulcus, applied to the rostrum (Fig. 9-28P-Q).

9. *Superior frontal gyrus sign.* The superior frontal gyrus forms the medial surface of the frontal lobe above the gyrus rectus, anterior to the subcallosal area and anterior to the paracentral lobule (Fig. 9-28R).

10. *Frontomarginal gyrus sign.* The frontomarginal gyrus forms the surface of the frontal lobe at the junction of the orbital surface with the convexity surface (Fig. 9-28S).

Superior Surface

A simple algorithm provides accurate localization of the gyri and sulci of the superior surface in nearly all cases (Fig. 9-29). Consider the ovoid axial section through the brain as a "clock face" with the midline interhemispheric fissure as the "12-6 line." Then take the *widest* biparietal dimension of the ovoid as the "9-3 line." Use of the *widest* dimension controls for differences in individual head shapes, scan angles, and modalities used for imaging.

1. *Start.* Start in the midline anteriorly and count from the midline laterally: interhemispheric fissure (IHF), superior frontal gyrus (SFG; 1), superior frontal sulcus (SFS; a), and middle frontal gyrus (MFG; 2) (Fig. 9-29A).

2. *Superior frontal sulcus sign.* Return to the SFS and trace the SFS posteriorly, saying: The SFS (a) ends in the precentral sulcus (c) (85% rule). By this rule, identify the precentral sulcus (preCS) at the posterior end of the SFS (Fig. 9-29B).

3. *Pericentral gyri and sulci.* Count from the posterior end of the SFS posteriorly: precentral sulcus (preCS; c), precentral gyrus (preCG; 4), central sulcus (CS; d), postcentral gyrus (postCG; 5), and postcentral sulcus (postCS; e) (Fig. 9-29C).

4. *Intraparietal sulcus sign.* Identify the intraparietal sulci (IPS; f) as paired crescents that form arcs along the clock face, convex medially, from 3 to 5 o'clock and from 9 to 7 o'clock. Because of the curved shape of the convexity, the superior parietal lobule (SPL; 8) lies superomedial to the IPS along the convexity of the IPS while the inferior parietal lobule (IPL; 6+7) lies inferolateral to the IPS within the concavity of the IPS. The SPL contains a large superior parietal lobule and a small additional arc of tissue posteriorly (the first parieto-occipital pli du passage of Gratiolet). The IPL contains two large gyri: the supramarginal gyrus (6) and the angular gyrus (7), plus a small additional arc of tissue posteriorly (the second parieto-occipital pli du passage of Gratiolet). These two parieto-occipital arches lie at the posterior

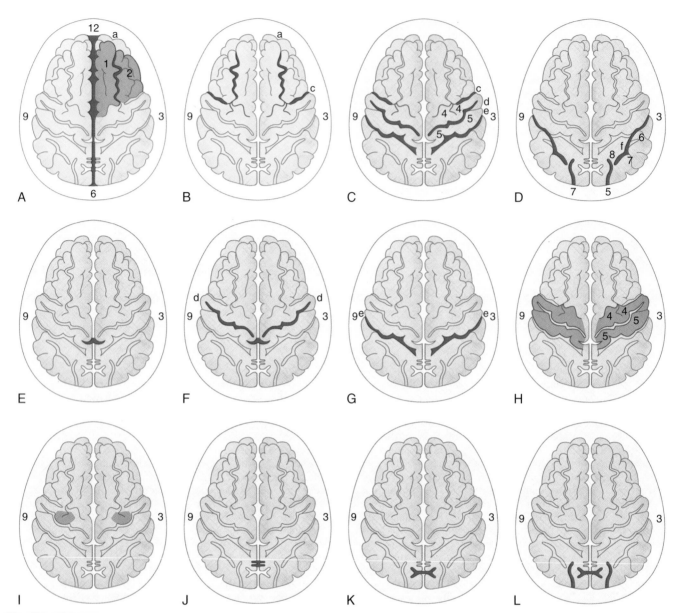

■ **FIGURE 9-29**   A to L, Analysis of the gyri and sulci of the superior surface. Diagram of the sequential steps for systematically reviewing the gyri and sulci of the superior surface. The specific steps are detailed in the section on analysis.

ends of the lobules, just anterior to the parieto-occipital sulcus (Fig. 9-29D).

5. *Pars marginalis.* Return to the 9-3 line. The small horizontal sulcus that resembles a "bracket" or mustache just behind the 9-3 line is formed by the pars marginalis of each side. In most cases the pars marginalis is readily identified by its relationship to the 9-3 line. As a further check, in axial images, the two partes together assume a characteristic shape that changes characteristically from lower to upper cuts. In four axial sections from inferior to superior, the partes resemble a "droopy" mustache, straight mustache, smiling mustache, and the mustache of Salvador Dali. Moreover, if one uses the mouse to scroll back and forth through the axial sections of the pars, the changing shapes of the partes resemble the beating of bird wings, up and down, until the pars flies away (Fig. 9-29E).

6. *Pars bracket sign.* The central sulcus (d) ascends along the convexity and nearly always reaches the superior margin of

the hemisphere just millimeters anterior to the pars marginalis. If one takes the full left-right extent of the two partes as the "pars bracket" or "pars basket," then the pars bracket sign for identifying the central sulcus is as follows: The central sulcus is the sulcus that, simultaneously, passes anterior to the pars marginalis on each side and passes medial to the lateral edge of the pars bracket. Put differently, the central sulcus "enters" the pars bracket (96% sign). The postcentral sulcus enters the bracket only rarely (3%) (Fig. 9-29F).

7. *Postcentral parenthesis.* The postcentral sulcus (e) characteristically courses "parallel" (i.e., co-curvilinear with) the central sulcus toward the pars marginalis. Near the pars, however, the postcentral sulcus typically bifurcates into a cup or "parenthesis" that encloses the pars bracket. The anterior aspect of this bifid segment passes anterior to the pars bracket, but *it does not pass medial to the lateral end of the pars marginalis* (i.e., it does not enter the bracket)

(97% rule). The posterior aspect of the sulcal bifurcation passes posterior to the pars marginalis and reaches toward or to the midline behind the pars marginalis. Together, the anterior and posterior aspects of the postcentral sulcus appear to enclose the pars marginalis (Fig. 9-29G).

8. *Intraparietal sulcus sign.* The anterior end of the intraparietal sulcus (f) is typically formed by the lower portion of the postcentral sulcus (e). Therefore, the anterior end of the intraparietal crescent should mark the postcentral sulcus and show concordant localization with the gyri and sulci identified by counting back from the posterior end of the superior frontal sulcus (Fig. 9-29, compare D with G).

9. *Thick-thin sign.* The precentral (4) and the postcentral (5) gyri form a parallel (co-curvilinear) pair of gyri, with the precentral gyrus anterior to the postcentral gyrus. The full sagittal dimension of the precentral gyrus is characteristically thicker than the full sagittal dimension of the postcentral gyrus. Furthermore, the thickness of the cortical gray matter along the posterior surface of the precentral gyrus is much greater than the thickness of the cortical gray matter along the anterior surface of the postcentral gyrus. Indeed, the greatest difference in cortical thickness between any two gyri abutting a single sulcus occurs at the central sulcus between the thick cortex of the precentral gyrus anteriorly and the thin cortex of the postcentral gyrus posteriorly[26] (Fig. 9-29H).

10. *Hand motor knob.* The posterior surface of the precentral gyrus (4) that abuts upon the central sulcus (d) shows a characteristic expansion that deflects the central sulcus posteriorly at the hand motor area (98% sign). This posteriorly directed "bump" may take the shape of a single bulge (omega shape) or a double bump (double-u shape). The bump of the hand motor area is identified as follows: View the length of the superior frontal sulcus (a) anteriorly and its alignment with the intraoccipital sulcus (in L) posteriorly. That line through the superior frontal sulcus and the intraoccipital sulcus is the parasagittal line.[23] The *medial* aspect of the hand motor bump characteristically lies at or very near the parasagittal line. The medial edge of the bump typically forms a sharp notch (inflection point) in line with the superior frontal sulcus. The portion of the central sulcus medial to the sharp notch then resembles a "lightning bolt" that strikes backward into the pars basket (Fig. 9-29I).

11. *Subparietal sulci.* Posterior to the partes marginales, the subparietal sulci form short horizontal lines (crossbars) across the interhemispheric fissure. These lines lie too far behind the 9-3 line to be mistaken for the partes marginales and bear the wrong relationship to the central sulcus. Typically, they are readily identified by their position between the partes marginales anteriorly and the parieto-occipital sulci posteriorly (see next sign) (Fig. 9-29J).

12. *Fish tail sign.* The parieto-occipital sulci appear in the posterior portion of the ovoid clock face at the same anteroposterior level as the posterior one thirds of the intraparietal sulci. The parieto-occipital sulci typically appear as high-frequency sulcal zigzags that extend laterally from the midline to terminate in broad fish tails on each side. Typically, the parieto-occipital sulci form more complex shapes than the simple brackets of the partes marginales. When there is concern about distinguishing the partes marginales from the parieto-occipital sulci, then a nearly 100% rule is that the partes are seen at the level of the anterior half of the intraparietal sulci, whereas the parieto-occipital sulci are seen at the levels of the posterior one third of the intraparietal sulci (Fig. 9-29K).

13. *Broken-M sign.* The intraparietal sulci form sulcal crescents along the 3-5 and 9-7 curves of the clock face (sign 4 above). Posteriorly, they extend across the border of the parietal

lobes to enter the occipital lobes. Properly, then, the posterior ends of these curves should be called the intraoccipital sulci and the full curves redesignated as the intraparietal-intraoccipital sulci (IPS-IOS). The posterior ends of the IPS-IOS curves come to lie parallel to the posterior end of the interhemispheric fissure. The two verticals of the IPS-IOS on each side of the midline and the fish tails of the parieto-occipital sulci between them resemble a broken letter M. The convexity face of the tissue within that broken M is termed the *superior occipital gyrus*. The medial surface of that tissue is designated the *cuneus* (Fig. 9-29L).

Inferior Surface
A simple algorithm provides accurate localization of the gyri and sulci of the superior surface in nearly all cases. Analysis of this region proceeds separately for the frontal lobe and for the temporo-occipital lobe.

Frontal Lobe
1. *Gyrus rectus sign.* The gyri recti are identified as paired longitudinal gyri that flank the interhemispheric fissure, falx, and crista galli between the midline medially and the olfactory sulci laterally. The olfactory sulci may run parallel with the midline, but their anterior ends often angle toward the midline. In coronal plane, the olfactory sulci are characteristically oriented obliquely, with the superior end situated farther lateral than the inferior end. The olfactory bulb and tract course inferior to and in line with the olfactory sulci. Because the cribriform plate lies inferior to the orbital roof, axial images display the gyri recti on sections obtained slightly below the orbital rim (Fig. 9-30).

2. *Orbital H sign.* Lateral to the olfactory sulcus, the roughly H-shaped orbital sulcus divides the orbital surface of the frontal lobe into medial orbital, lateral orbital, anterior orbital, and posterior orbital gyri. Because the roof of the orbit and the overlying orbital gyri are curved, the medial and lateral orbital gyri lie slightly inferior to the anterior and posterior orbital gyri. The posteromedial orbital lobule forms a prominence at the posteromedial edge of the orbital surface of the frontal lobe. In coronal sections, one may count outward from the midline, sequentially, to identify the midline, gyrus

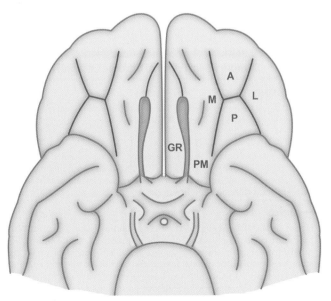

■ FIGURE 9-30 Analysis of the gyri and sulci of the inferior frontal surface. The specific steps are detailed in the section on analysis.

rectus, characteristically oblique olfactory sulcus with its olfactory bulb or tract, the medial orbital gyrus, the anterior (or posterior) orbital gyrus, and the lateral orbital gyrus. The structures in the orbit and the portion of the olfactory system (ovoid bulb vs. triangular tract) help to determine the antero-posterior position of the section and suggest whether the gyrus between the medial and lateral orbital gyri is the anterior or posterior orbital gyrus (see Figs. 9-19 and 9-30).

Temporo-occipital Lobes

1. *Five gyri sign.* Anteriorly, the temporal lobe displays five major gyri and four major sulci (see Fig. 9-21). One can identify these by counting each gyrus and sulcus in order from the sylvian fissure laterally into the parahippocampal gyrus medially. Specifically, these are the sylvian fissure, superior temporal gyrus, superior temporal sulcus, middle temporal gyrus, inferior temporal sulcus, inferior temporal gyrus curving onto the inferior surface of the temporal lobe, occipitotemporal sulcus, lateral occipitotemporal gyrus, collateral sulcus, and the parahippocampal gyri. The inferior temporal gyrus forms the inferolateral margin of the temporal lobe. The parahippocampal gyrus forms the medialmost surface of the temporal lobe. Good coronal images typically display the sulci well enough to identify each gyrus. When the sulci are ill defined, one must count the digitations of white matter that extend into each gyrus rather than the intervening sulci to achieve the same localization.
2. *Collateral sulcus sign.* Like the olfactory sulcus, the collateral sulcus is characteristically oblique with the superior end positioned lateral to the inferior end. The collateral sulcus also indents the inferior surface of the temporal horn and raises up the collateral eminence of the temporal horn. Thus, the oblique sulcus that aligns with and elevates the floor of the temporal horn is the collateral sulcus. This separate sign helps to confirm the localization made by counting the gyri.
3. *Six gyri sign.* In the posterior temporal lobe, the lingual gyrus intercalates itself between the lateral occipitotemporal gyrus laterally and the parahippocampal gyrus medially. The collateral sulcus still courses along the medial surface of the

lateral occipitotemporal gyrus. The anterior calcarine sulcus courses on the medial surface of the lingual gyrus between the lingual gyrus and the parahippocampal gyrus. Therefore, one must add the lingual gyrus and the anterior calcarine sulcus to those above to identify the gyri correctly by "counting" gyri along the posterior line.

Hippocampal Formation

Identification of the components of the hippocampal formation proceeds as a sequence rather than as a set of signs. It starts laterally at the collateral sulcus and proceeds medially and upward into the hippocampal formation (see Fig. 9-21).

Medial to the collateral sulcus, the entire medial surface of the temporal lobe is formed by the parahippocampal gyrus. Follow the curvature of the parahippocampal gyrus into the hippocampal fissure. This fissure appears as a shallow medial groove and a long closed line that extends deeply (laterally) into the tissue. The lower bank of the hippocampal fissure is the subiculum. The upper bank is the dentate gyrus. The hippocampus per se forms an arc of tissue around the deep lateral end of the hippocampal fissure. The external surface of the subiculum is covered by a layer of white matter designated the *superficial medullary lamina.* This layer identifies the subiculum and indicates that it is formed by allocortex, not neocortex. The dentate gyrus above the hippocampal fissure displays a sawtooth margin that gives it its name. The dentate gyrus contains the dentate granule cell layer in the shape of a basket. The hippocampus itself curves from lateral to medial, over and then into the dentate granule cell basket. The white matter of the parahippocampal gyrus and the hippocampal formation passes laterally to form a thin white lamina, the alveus, in the subependymal layer lateral to the hippocampus. The alveus then curves superomedially, above the dentate gyrus, detaches from the dentate gyrus, and forms a medially directed free margin (or elbow) of white matter referred to as the fimbria. Together the alveus and fimbria form the fornix. From the medial margin of the fimbria, the white matter then recurves laterally to help form the choroidal fissure and choroidal plexus (see Chapter 13).

A sample report is shown in Box 9-1.

BOX 9-1   Sample Report: MRI of Chronic Cerebral Infarctions

PATIENT HISTORY

A 72-year-old man presented with known prior cerebral infarctions and new left leg weakness of 24 hours' duration.

TECHNIQUE

Noncontrast multiplanar multi-sequence MRI was performed as sagittal T1W, axial T1W, T2W and FLAIR T2W, axial susceptibility-weighted (T2*), coronal T1W and T2W series, and diffusion-weighted imaging with apparent diffusion coefficient maps.

FINDINGS

Noncontrast MRI (Fig. 9-31) confirms the clinical history of prior cerebral infarctions. There is abnormally increased T2 signal in the left middle frontal gyrus, the posterior face of the left postcentral gyrus, the adjoining left superior parietal lobule, and patches of the right superior parietal lobule. There is additional involvement of the gray and the white matter of the left superior and inferior parietal lobules across the left intraparietal sulcus. These zones of infarction are well marginated and do not compress the adjacent sulci, indicating that they are chronic.

Further small foci of increased T2 signal are present within the white matter of both cerebral hemispheres. There is no evidence for old or new hemorrhage. Together, these findings indicate chronic vascular compromise with bilateral cerebral infarctions and bilateral microvascular ischemic white matter disease, with a predilection for the distal middle cerebral artery territories and the adjacent watersheds.

Diffusion-weighted imaging with apparent diffusion coefficient maps shows no evidence of acute infarction. There is no evidence of hemorrhage or mass. The major arterial trunks, deep cerebral veins, and venous sinuses show normal flow voids with no evidence for obstruction or occlusion.

The brain stem and cerebellum are normal. The visualized structures of the skull base, the paranasal sinuses and mastoids, and the soft tissue of the upper face and neck are normal.

IMPRESSION

This patient has chronic bilateral ischemic cerebral infarctions with bilateral ischemic white matter disease. There is no present evidence of acute infarction or hemorrhage.

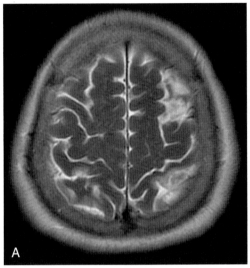
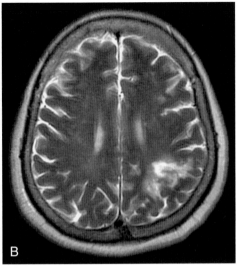

■ **FIGURE 9-31** Axial T2W MR images showing (**A**) the superior section and (**B**) the lower section. See the sample report in Box 9-1 for details.

SUGGESTED READINGS

Duvernoy H. The Human Brain: Surface, Three-Dimensional Sectional Anatomy and MRI. New York, Springer, 1991.

Ono M, Kubik S, Abernathey CD. Atlas of the Cerebral Sulci. Stuttgart, Georg Thieme, 1990.

Strandring S (ed). Gray's Anatomy: The Anatomical Basis of Clinical Practice, 39th ed. Philadelphia, Elsevier, 2005.

REFERENCES

1. Ono M, Kubik S, Abernathey CD. Atlas of the Cerebral Sulci. Stuttgart, Georg Thieme, 1990.
2. Duvernoy H. The Human Brain: Surface, Three-Dimensional Sectional Anatomy and MRI. New York, Springer, 1991.
3. Strandring S (ed). Gray's Anatomy: The Anatomical Basis of Clinical Practice, 39th ed. Philadelphia, Elsevier, 2005.
4. Bayer SA, Altman J. Atlas of the Human Central Nervous System, Vol 2, The Human Brain during the Third Trimester. Boca Raton, CRC Press, 2004.
5. Chi JG, Dooling EC, Gilles FH. Gyral development of the human brain. Ann Neurol 1977; 1:86.
6. Duvernoy HM. The Human Hippocampus. Functional Anatomy, Vascularization and Serial Sections with MRI, 3rd Edition. 2005 Berlin, Heidelberg, New York, Springer-Verlag, 2005.
7. Dooling EC, Chi JG, Gilles FH. Telencephalic development, changing gyral patterns. In Gilles FH (ed). The Developing Human Brain. Boston, Wright-PSG, 1983.
8. Turner OA. Growth and development of the cerebral cortical pattern in man. Arch Neurol Psychiatry 1948; 59:1-12.
9. Naidich TP, Grant JL, Altman N, et al. The developing cerebral surface. Neuroimaging Clin North Am 1994; 4:201-240.
10. Kido DK, LeMay M, Levinson AW, Benson WE. Computed tomographic localization of the precentral gyrus. Radiology 1980; 135:373-377.
11. Rumeau C, Tzourio N, Murayama N, et al. Location of hand function in the sensorimotor cortex: MR and functional correlation. AJNR Am J Roentgenol 1994; 15:567-572.
12. Yousry TA, Schmid UD, Jassoy AG, et al. Topography of the cortical motor hand area: Prospective study with functional MR imaging and direct motor mapping at surgery. Radiology 1995; 195:23-29.
13. Naidich TP, Brightbill TC. The intraparietal sulcus: a landmark for localization of pathology on axial CT scans. Int J Neuroradiol 1995; 1:3-16.
14. Naidich, TP, Valavanis AG, Kubik S. Anatomic relationships along the low-middle convexity: I. Normal specimens and MRI. Neurosurgery 1995; 36:517-532.
15. Naidich TP, Brightbill TC. The pars marginalis: I. A "bracket" sign for the central sulcus in axial plane CT and MRI. Int J Neuroradiol 1996; 2:3-19.
16. Naidich TP, Brightbill TC. The pars marginalis: II. A white matter pattern for identifying the pars marginalis in axial plane CT and MRI. Int J Neuroradiol 1996; 2:20-24.
17. Naidich TP, Brightbill TC. Systems for localizing fronto-parietal gyri and sulci on axial CT and MRI. Int J Neuroradiol 1996; 2:313-338.
18. Yousry TA, Schmid UD, Alkadhi H, et al. Localization of the hand motor area to a knob on the precentral gyrus: A new landmark. Brain 1997; 120:141-157.
19. Yousry TA, Fesl G, Büttner A, et al. Heschl's gyrus: anatomic description and methods of identification on magnetic resonance imaging. Int J Neuroradiol 1997; 3:2-12.
20. Naidich TP, Valavanis AG, Kubik S, et al. Anatomic relationships along the low-middle convexity: II. Lesion localization. Int J Neuroradiol 1997; 3:393-409.
21. Yousry TA. Historical perspective. The cerebral lobes and their boundaries. Int J Neuroradiol 1998; 4:342-348.
22. Valente M, Naidich TP Abrams KJ, Blum JT. Differentiating the pars marginalis from the parieto-occipital sulcus in axial computed tomography sections. Int J Neuroradiol 1998;4:105-111.
23. Naidich TP, Blum JT, Firestone MI. The parasagittal line: an anatomic landmark for axial imaging. AJNR Am J Neuroradiol 2001; 22:885-895.
24. Naidich TP, Brightbill TC. Vascular territories and watersheds: a zonal frequency analysis of the gyral and sulcal extent of cerebral infarcts: I. The anatomic template. Neuroradiology 2003; 45:536-540.
25. Naidich TP, Kang E, Fatterpekar GM, et al. The insula: anatomic-MR correlation at 1.5 tesla. AJNR Am J Neuroradiol 2004; 25:222-232.
26. Meyer J, Roychowdhury S, Russell EJ, et al. Location of the central sulcus via cortical thickness of the precentral and postcentral gyri on MR. AJNR Am J Neuroradiol 1996; 17:1699-1706.

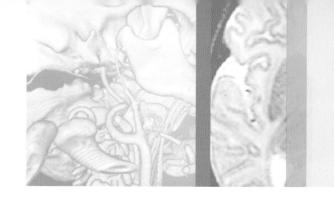

CHAPTER 10

Cerebral Cortex

Thomas P. Naidich, Esther A. Nimchinsky, and Pedro Pasik

The surface anatomy of the cerebral hemispheres is reviewed in Chapter 9. The anatomy of the thalami and basal ganglia is reviewed in Chapter 11. Here, the focus is on the architecture of the cerebral cortex, the thalamocortical interconnections, and cerebral function. The following is a list of definitions of the prominent structures to be discussed:

Telencephalon: the most rostral portion of the brain situated above a plane directed through the anterior commissure and the velum interpositum.[1] Practically, the term *telencephalon* equates to the cerebral hemispheres.

Cerebral cortex: the superficial layer of gray matter that extends along the surface of the two cerebral hemispheres.

Neocortex (isocortex): the pylogenetically newer portion of the cerebral cortex characterized by the presence of six predominant cell layers. The neocortex constitutes approximately 90% of the cerebral cortex (Fig 10-1).

Mesocortex: a transitional cortex interposed between the six-layered neocortex peripherally and the three-layered allocortex centrally (see later). Mesocortical tissue contains six cortical layers where it abuts the neocortex and three cortical layers where it abuts the allocortex.[2] Synonyms: juxta-allocortex; paralimbic cortex.

Allocortex: the portions of the cortex phylogenetically older than the neocortex. Allocortex is characterized by the presence of three predominant layers. It comprises approximately 10% of the cerebral cortex and has two divisions: the paleocortex and the archicortex (see Fig. 10-1).

Paleocortex: the portion of the allocortex that relates to the olfactory system. It includes the olfactory bulbs, olfactory tubercles, septal region, (pre)pyriform cortex, and part of the amygdala.

Archicortex: the portion of the allocortex that relates to the hippocampal formation. It includes the hippocampus, the subicular complex, and the entorhinal cortex.

Corticoid areas: the regions of gray matter with simple, poorly differentiated cortex and no clearly discernible cortical lamination.[2] The corticoid areas lie at the base of the forebrain and include the septal region deep to the paraterminal gyrus, the substantia innominata at the base of the frontal lobe, and parts of the amygdaloid complex. The corticoid regions utilize the same neurotransmitters as other cortical areas and exhibit similar interconnections.[2]

Limbic telencephalon: the combination of the allocortex and the corticoid areas.[2]

Perikaryon (plural: perikarya): the cytoplasm surrounding the nucleus of the cell (or cells).

Soma (plural: somata): the body of the cell(s), housing the nucleus and most of the protein-synthesizing apparatus.

Spine(s): dendritic protrusions that harbor excitatory synapses. Neurons that have large numbers of excitatory inputs bear large numbers of spines and are designated spiny neurons.

Cytoarchitectonics (cytoarchitecture): the systematic study of the arrangement of neuronal cell bodies within the cortex.

Myeloarchitectonics (myeloarchitecture): the systematic study of the arrangement of myelinated fibers within the cortex.[1]

Chemoarchitectonics (chemoarchitecture): the systematic study of the arrangement of the sources and receptors for the multiple different neurotransmitters.[3-6]

Radial: the direction perpendicular to both the superficial and the deep surfaces of the cerebral cortex at each point. Synonyms: vertical; perpendicular.

Tangential: the direction aligned with and coursing along the surface and laminae of the cortex at each point. Synonym: horizontal.

Unimodal: pertaining to one specific type of sensory input, such as auditory, visual, or somatosensory. Unimodal cortices receive one type of sensory input. Unimodal association areas process data received from one specific unimodal receptive cortex.

Multimodal (polymodal, heteromodal): pertaining to multiple different modalities simultaneously. Multimodal association cortices process data received from multiple different unimodal association cortices.

ANATOMY

In broad overview, the gray and white matter of the brain can be considered to be assembled into "sheets" of tissue, as in the cerebral cortex; into "blobs" of tissue as in the basal ganglia and thalami; or into mixed "sheet-like blobs" as in the olfactory bulbs, superior colliculi, and lateral geniculate nuclei. Although the mammalian brain is mostly sheet-like, other classes of vertebrates such as birds function with largely blob-like brains.

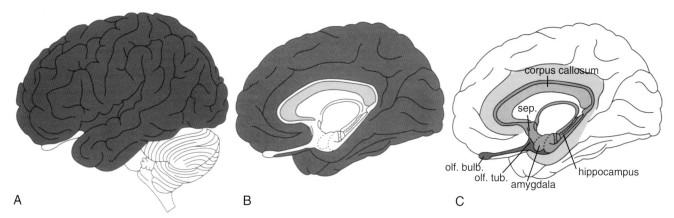

■ **FIGURE 10-1** Human cerebral cortex. **A** and **B,** The neocortex (*green*) of the lateral convexity (**A**) and mediobasal surface (**B**) comprises about 90% of the cerebral surface. **C,** The remaining 10% is composed of the paleocortex of the olfactory system and septum (*dark brown*), the inner limbic ring (*light brown*) and the outer limbic ring (*yellow orange*). In humans, the outer limbic ring lies along the cingulate and parahippocampal gyri. *(From Nieuwenhuys R. The human brain: an introductory survey. Med Mundi 1994; 39:64-79.)*

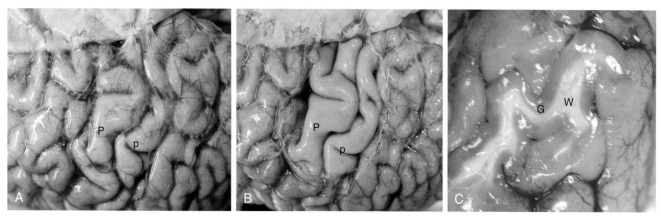

■ **FIGURE 10-2** Cerebral neocortex. **A** and **B,** High convexity. Fresh gross specimen of the precentral (P) and postcentral (p) gyri at the level of the hand motor and sensory cortices, seen through the intact pia-arachnoid (**A**) and then after removal of the leptomeninges and vessels (**B**). **C,** Shearing fracture of the lateral temporal cortex displays the gray matter (G), the white matter (W), and the distinct gray-white interface.

Gross Anatomy and Telencephalization

The *neocortex* is the phylogenetically newer portion of the cerebral cortex (Figs. 10-1 and 10-2). It comprises approximately 90% of the human cerebral cortex and is characterized by the presence of six predominant cell layers. The neocortex is especially large in humans versus other animals. On a standardized scale, the size of the neocortex is 1 in insectivores, 14.5 in prosimians, 45.5 in simians, and 156 in humans (Tables 10-1 and 10-2).[1] This disproportionate overgrowth of the neocortex of the cerebral hemispheres is designated *telencephalization.* The newly formed telencephalic cortex provides new neural tissue for associating and processing the information entering the brain via the sensory system and for formulating sophisticated responses before initiating motor action.[1]

Most of the cortex of other animals is devoted to projection areas that receive sensory data via the thalami or that help to steer motor activity.[1] In these animals, the primary sensory and motor areas are separated from each other only by narrow strips of other cortex. Telencephalization expands these narrow strips into large new association cortices in the temporoparietal lobes (for sensory integration) and in the frontal lobe (for motor integration).[1]

Light Microscopy
Cell Types

The neocortex contains three principal cell types: (1) pyramidal cells, (2) nonpyramidal spiny neurons, and (3) nonpyramidal nonspiny neurons.[11] Pyramidal cells are the most common cells of the neocortex. They are excitatory projection neurons that utilize glutamate as their neurotransmitter. Nonpyramidal spiny neurons are the next most common cell type. They are thought to be excitatory glutamatergic neurons. Nonpyramidal nonspiny neurons are the least common cell type. They are mostly inhibitory γ-aminobutyric acid (GABA)-ergic neurons.[11]

Pyramidal Cells

Pyramidal cells are characterized by a pyramid-shaped cell body that has its apex directed toward the surface and its base oriented tangentially, parallel to the underlying gray matter/white matter junction (Fig. 10-3).[11] The apex of the pyramidal cell gives rise to a single thick apical dendrite that extends radially into the most superficial layers of the cortex. There, the apical dendrite ramifies into terminal tufts called bouquets. The apical dendrites arising from adjacent cells organize into radially oriented bundles of dendrites.

The basal margin of the pyramidal cell gives rise to a fringe or "skirt" of tangentially oriented dendrites that extend outward and branch extensively into the adjacent tissue.

The basal surface of the pyramidal cell gives rise to a single slender axon[11] that extends into the underlying white matter. The axons of the pyramidal cells become myelinated shortly distal to the cell bodies and assemble into radially oriented bundles (radial fasciculi). The radial fasciculi increase in size as they descend toward the white matter and as additional axons

TABLE 10-1. The Human Cortex

Quantity	Value		Reference(s)
Volume of cortex (both hemispheres)	517 cm³ (males)		Pakkenberg and Gundersen[7]
	440 cm³ (females)		
Surface area of both hemispheres	1470-2275 cm²		Blinkov and Glezer[8]; Pakkenberg and Gundersen[7]
Total cortical surface	83,591 mm²	100.0%	Blinkov and Glezer[8]
Neocortex	80,202 mm²	95.9%	
Paleocortex	480 mm²	0.6%	
Archicortex	1,863 mm²	2.2%	
Intermediate cortex	1,040 mm²	1.3%	
Percent of total surface	*Child* %	*Adult* %	Blinkov and Glezer[8]
Frontal lobe	15.2	24.8	
Temporal lobe	16.2	23.4	
Inferior parietal lobe	6.7	9.3	
Superior parietal lobe	7.3	7.6	
Occipital lobe	13-14	12.5-13	
Precentral gyrus	10.6	9.2	
Insula	3.4	2.1	
Total number of neurons within both hemispheres	22.8×10^9		Pakkenberg and Gundersen[7]
Depth of neocortex	1.5-5.0 mm		von Economo and Koskinas[9]
Portion of the cortex situated within the sulci	Almost two thirds		Braak[10]

From Nieuwenhuys R, Voogd J, van Huijzen C. The Human Central Nervous System, 4th ed. Berlin, Springer-Verlag, 2008.

TABLE 10-2. Thickness of Cortex in Diverse Regions in Humans (mm)*

Cortical Layers	Frontal Region	Precentral Region	Postcentral Region	Inferior Parietal Region	Temporal Region	Occipital Region	Insula	Limbic Region
I	0.18	0.2	0.15	0.20	0.18	0.21	0.235	0.22
II	0.12	0.15	0.19	0.19	0.09	0.10	0.17	0.14
III	0.88	1.2	0.45	0.85	0.88	0.8	0.90	0.66
IV	0.12		0.20	0.30	0.12	0.36	0.18	0.10
V	0.54	0.55	0.25	0.54	0.49	0.33	0.61	0.45
VI-VII	0.71	1.15	0.35	0.75	0.85	0.56	0.9	0.75
Total	2.60	3.01	1.59	2.8	2.71	2.36	3.0	2.32

*Mean thickness of the areas constituting the region.
From Blinkov SM, Glezer II. The Human Brain in Figures and Tables: A Quantitative Handbook. New York, Basic Books, 1968.

■ **FIGURE 10-3** Pyramidal cells of the neocortex immunostained with an antibody (SMI-32) to the medium chain of the neurofilament. **A,** Large pyramidal cells of the motor cortex (BA 4). **B,** Large pyramidal cells of the parietal cortex. *(Courtesy of Dr. Patrick Hof, New York.)*

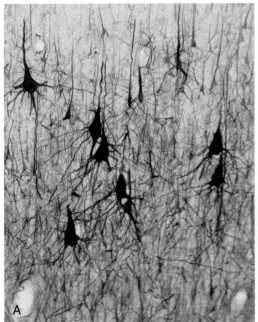
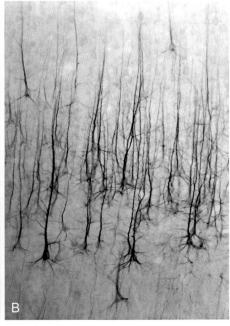

join the bundle.[1] The pyramidal cells form extensive collaterals within the cortex. Each pyramidal cell makes approximately 10,000 synapses with other cells.

Nonpyramidal Spiny Cells

Nonpyramidal spiny cells (synonyms: spiny granule cells; spiny stellate neurons) are small, multipolar cells that give rise to limited numbers of primary dendrites (Fig. 10-4). These den-

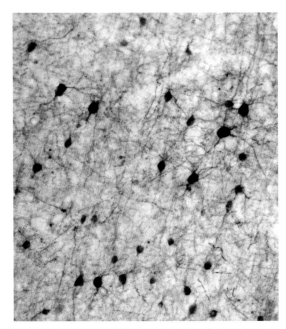

■ **FIGURE 10-4** Nonpyramidal (granule) cells of the prefrontal cortex, BA 46. *(Courtesy Dr. Patrick Hof, New York.)*

drites fan outward in multiple directions and are densely covered in spines. The axons arising from these cells branch outward, predominantly radially.[11]

Nonpyramidal Nonspiny Cells

The term *nonspiny (sparsely spiny) nonpyramidal cell* is used to designate any of a diverse set of interneurons whose axons extend radially or tangentially solely within the gray matter. Synonyms include *nonspiny granule cell* and *nonspiny stellate neuron.*[11]

Cortical Architecture

The architecture of the cortex shows distinct tangential and radial elements.

Lamination

The neocortex consists of six tangential zones or layers. Each layer is characterized by the number, type, and arrangement of the cell bodies (perikarya) within it and by the organization of the myelinated fibers that course through it (see Tables 10-2 and 10-3).[1] From superficial to deep, these layers are numbered I to VI and are designated by the cell type once thought to be predominant within each layer (Figs. 10-5 to 10-7).

Overview of the Cortical Layers

Layer I. The molecular layer may be thought of as the primordial input layer, because it receives axons from many early, highly conserved structures. These include the noradrenergic locus ceruleus, the serotonergic dorsal raphe nucleus, the dopaminergic ventral tegmental area, and cholinergic cells within the nucleus accumbens septi. None of these inputs is restricted to this layer. Layer I also receives corticocortical synapses from most other cell layers and projections from the anterior and intralaminar thalamic nuclei.

TABLE 10-3. Laminar Organization of the Neocortex

Cortical Layer		Cytoarchitectonics	Myeloarchitectonics
I	Molecular cell layer (cell sparse layer)	This layer contains very few cell bodies.*	The myelinated fibers form a narrow, densely populated plexus of tangentially oriented intrinsic and extrinsic fibers. These fibers contact the apical dendritic bouquets of the pyramidal cells situated within the deeper layers.
II	External granular cell layer	This layer is composed of a varying density of small, pyramidal and nonpyramidal cell bodies. Despite the name, most of the cells in this layer are small pyramidal neurons.†	The myelinated fibers orient predominantly radially as vertical fibers that pass perpendicularly through the layer.*
III	External pyramidal cell layer	This thick layer contains pyramidal cells of diverse size. Within the layer, the bodies of the pyramidal cells form a "gradient" with smaller pyramidal cell bodies at the superficial aspect of the layer and larger pyramidal cell bodies at the depth of the layer.*	The myelinated fibers course predominantly radially, perpendicular to the layer, as in layer II.*
IV	Internal granular cell layer	This layer contains small, round, densely packed, nonpyramidal cells and fewer small pyramidal cells. The internal granule cell layer is usually the thinnest cell layer of the neocortex.*	The myelinated fibers form a dense, tangentially oriented superficial band of horizontal fibers designated the external (outer) band of Baillarger.[11] In the visual cortex (Brodmann area 17) this band is so prominent that it is visible to the naked eye as the line of Gennari.†
V	Internal pyramidal cell layer	This layer contains loosely arranged medium-sized and large pyramidal cell bodies. The largest pyramidal cells of the neocortex usually lie within this layer.*	The myelinated fibers form a dense, tangentially oriented central band of horizontal fibers designated the internal (inner) band of Baillarger.*
VI	Multiform cell layer (fusiform or pleomorphic cell layer)	This layer typically contains small to medium-sized neurons of variable shape. The deep aspect of this layer merges imperceptibly into the underlying white matter, with no clear border.*	The myelinated fibers form tangential, progressively denser, bands of fibers that merge into the underlying white matter.*

*Data from Nieuwenhuys R, Voogd J, van Huijzen C. The Human Central Nervous System, 4th ed. Berlin, Springer-Verlag, 2008.
†Data from Standring S (ed). Cerebral hemisphere. In: Gray's Anatomy: The Anatomical Basis of Clinical Practice, 40th ed. Philadelphia, Churchill Livingstone Elsevier, 2008.

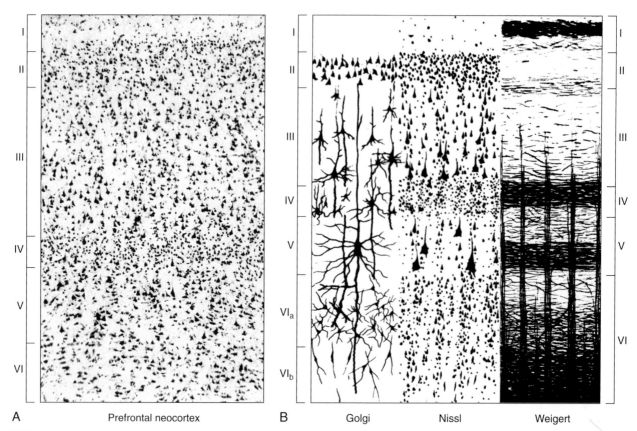

A   Prefrontal neocortex   B   Golgi   Nissl   Weigert

■ **FIGURE 10-5** Lamination of the neocortex: layers I to VI. **A,** Histologic section of the six-layered human neocortex. Nissl stain for neurons. **B,** Diagrammatic representation of the cytoarchitecture and myeloarchitecture of the six layers of the neocortex. Column 1. The Golgi stain impregnates the entire neuron, showing the location and full extent of the cells in each layer. Column 2. The Nissl stain demonstrates the cell bodies, showing the location and lamination of the somata of the cells. Column 3. The Weigert stain for myelinated nerve fibers demonstrates the radial (columnar) and horizontal (laminar) arrangement of nerve fibers in each layer. The myelinated plexi define sublayers within each of the six principal layers. *(**A,** Courtesy Dr. Patrick Hof, New York. **B,** From Carpenter MB, Sutin J. Human Neuroanatomy 8th Ed. 1983 Baltimore, Williams & Wilkins).*

Layer II. The external granular cell layer is the most superficial layer of corticocortical neurons. Because these cells lie closest to layer I, they have the shortest apical dendrites and look "granular." That appearance gave rise to the misnomer "external granular layer." Layer II contains many inhibitory interneurons, adding to its nonpyramidal appearance.

Layer III. The external pyramidal layer is composed of predominantly corticocortical pyramidal neurons and inhibitory interneurons.

Layer IV. The internal granular cell layer can be thought of as a major input layer of the cortex. It receives substantial thalamic inputs from phylogenetically more recent thalamic nuclei, such as the ventral posterolateral, ventral posteromedial, lateral geniculate, and medial geniculate nuclei. It also contains inhibitory interneurons. In cortical areas that primarily have "output" function, layer IV is very thin.

Layer V. The internal pyramidal layer is a major output layer of the cortex. It contains pyramidal neurons that project both cortically and subcortically.

Layer VI. The multiform layer contains neurons that project subcortically and corticocortically as well as interneurons.

Cortical Columns

The cortical neurons organize into radial columns that extend through all six cortical layers, superficial to deep (see Fig. 10-6).

These radially oriented cortical columns appear to be the fundamental units, or modules, for cortical function.

Within the *primary* sensory areas of the neocortex (i.e., the auditory, visual, and somatosensory cortices), the neurons are arranged as small radial columns that surround a radially oriented thalamic afferent fiber. In other areas of the neocortex, the neurons form radial columns organized around corticocortical afferents rather than thalamic inputs.[1] Within the visual cortex, for example, the radial organization establishes *orientation columns* approximately 300 to 500 μm in diameter, *ocular dominance columns* approximately 500 μm in width, and ellipsoidal *"blobs"* 150 to 200 μm in width. Within the motor cortex, radial cortical motor columns approximately 1 mm in diameter appear to control the contraction of specific muscles.[1] (See the later sections on myeloarchitecture, classification by thalamic connections, cortical afferents to the neocortex, and function.)

Parcellation of the Cortex

From area to area across the cerebral hemisphere, the cortex shows differences in the relative thickness of its gray matter; the thickness and cell density of each cortical layer; the nature and arrangement of the neuronal perikarya within the layers; the packing density and laminar arrangement of the myelinated fibers; and the density and laminar distribution of receptors for multiple neurotransmitters (see Figs. 10-5 to 10-7).[1] These differences are used to partition the cortex into cyto/myelo/chemo-architectonic areas that correspond to the different functions of each portion of cortex, at least in part.[9]

Korbinian Brodmann[12] parcellated the human cortex into 52 cytoarchitectonic areas now designated the Brodmann areas (BA). At present, this Brodmann map (Fig. 10-8) is the most widely used system for identifying functional areas, locations of pathologic processes on routine neuroimages, and sites of activation on functional MR images. Nieuwenhuys and colleagues estimate that there may actually be 150 juxtaposed structural (and potentially functional) areas present within the human cortex.[1] Other authors have described up to 200 separate cortical areas.[9,13]

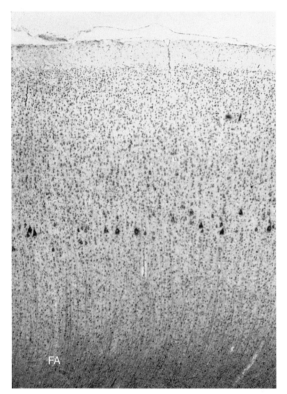

■ FIGURE 10-6 Cortical columns in the primary motor cortex (Klüver-Barrera stain) (non-human primate). The cerebral cortex displays distinct radial, columnar organization in addition to the laminar architecture. Note the large pyramidal (Betz) cells in the internal pyramidal cell layer V.

Gross Organization of the Cortex with Brodmann Designations

Frontal Lobe

Primary Motor Cortex (MI) (BA 4)

The primary motor cortex (MI) is a long "triangular" region situated along the length of the precentral gyrus (see Fig. 10-8). On the lateral surface, superiorly, MI occupies the full antero-posterior extent of the upper precentral gyrus. Inferiorly, MI tapers progressively, so its thin lower portion is confined to the posterior face of the precentral gyrus within the central sulcus. On the medial surface, MI occupies most of the paracentral lobule. Histologically, the primary motor cortex conforms to BA 4. In BA 4, the internal granule cell layer (IV) is nearly absent. The internal pyramidal cell layer V is thick and characteristically displays clusters of very large pyramidal cell bodies—the Betz cells—whose axons extend into the corticospinal and corticobulbar tracts.[11]

Premotor Cortex (PM) (BA 6)

The premotor cortex occupies a large portion of the frontal lobe immediately anterior to BA 4 (see Fig. 10-8).[11] On the convexity, BA 6 lateral extends over the frontal convexity and corresponds to the premotor (PM) area. This is subdivided into dorsal (d) and ventral (v) portions. The dorsal premotor area (PMd) receives input from the dorsolateral prefrontal region, whereas the ventral premotor area (PMv) receives input from the ventrolateral prefrontal region.[11] On the medial surface, BA 6 lies anterior to the paracentral lobule and extends from the superior margin of the hemisphere peripherally to the cingulate sulcus (BA 24) below.

Prefrontal Cortex (PF) (BA 9, BA 46, and BA 45)

The prefrontal cortex is also subdivided into dorsal and ventral portions (PFd and PFv) (see Fig. 10-8). PFd largely corresponds to BA 9 (and perhaps superior BA 46). PFv largely corresponds to inferior BA 46 and BA 45.[11] The medial prefrontal cortex includes BA 32 and 25. This region is similar to the anterior cingulate cortex (BA 24), so the two are often considered to be a single complex.[1]

Frontal Pole (FP) (BA 10)

BA 10 lies along the convexity and the medial surface of the superior frontal gyrus at the frontal pole (see Fig. 10-8). The human frontopolar cortex is specifically devoted to complex cognitive functions, such as integrating the outcomes of two or more separate cognitive operations directed toward a higher behavioral goal.[1]

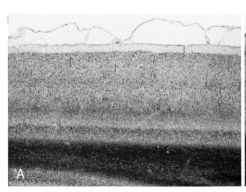
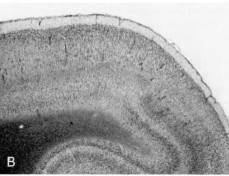

■ FIGURE 10-7 Differences in cortical lamination define distinct cytoarchitectonic zones within the cortex. (Klüver-Barrera stain) (non-human primate). **A,** Primary visual (striate) cortex (BA 17). **B,** Transition from primary visual cortex to visual association cortex (prestriate) (BA 18).

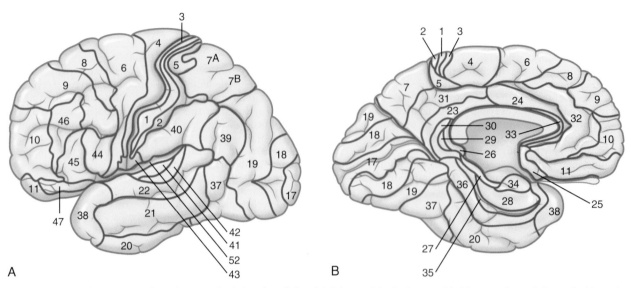

■ **FIGURE 10-8**   Brodmann areas along the convexity (**A**) and mediobasal (**B**) faces of the brain. *(Modified from Standring S [ed]. Cerebral hemisphere. In Gray's Anatomy: The Anatomical Basis of Clinical Practice, 40th ed. Philadelphia: Churchill Livingstone Elsevier, 2008.)*

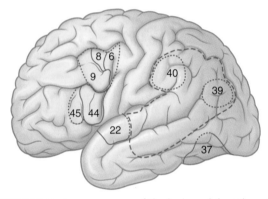

■ **FIGURE 10-9**   Language areas of the brain and frontal eye fields. Broca's motor speech area lies in the inferior frontal gyrus at the pars opercularis (BA 44) and the adjacent portion of the pars triangularis (BA 45). Wernicke's receptive area for speech has uncertain borders and may be highly individual. It appears to be included within the supramarginal (BA 40) and angular (BA 39) gyri of the inferior parietal lobule. BA 22 of the superior temporal gyrus is related to auditory processing of speech. BA 37 may have visuoauditory functions for speech recognition. The frontal eye field includes portions of BA 6, 8, and 9. *(Modified from Standring S [ed]. Cerebral hemisphere. In Gray's Anatomy: The Anatomical Basis of Clinical Practice, 40th ed. Philadelphia: Churchill Livingstone Elsevier, 2008.)*

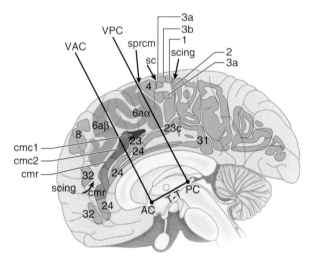

■ **FIGURE 10-10**   The supplementary motor area (SMA) and cingulate motor area. The supplementary motor area (BA 6aα) lies on the medial surface at the paracentral lobule between VAC and VPC (the verticals erected to the Talairach-Tournoux (T-T) baseline at the anterior commissure (VAC) and posterior commissure (VPC). The pre-SMA (negative SMA) (BA 6aβ) lies just anterior to the SMA. The cingulate motor cortex includes a rostral zone (cmr) that lies entirely rostral to VAC and a caudal zone (cmc) that flanks VAC but lies entirely rostral to VPC. Other labeled structures include the central sulcus (sc), cingulate sulcus (scing), medial precentral sulcus (sprcm), and the numbered Brodmann areas. *(From Zilles K, Schlag G, Geyer S, et al. Anatomy and transmitter receptors of the supplementary motor areas in the human and nonhuman primate brain. Adv Neurol 1996; 70:29-43.)*

Broca's Area (BA 44 and Part of BA 45)

In the dominant hemisphere, Broca's motor speech area is classically considered to lie within the inferior frontal gyrus at BA 44 and the adjacent portion of BA 45 (see Figs. 10-8 and 10-9). Some authorities now contest that localization and suggest that the true Broca motor speech area lies, instead, in the anterior lobule of the insula just deep to the inferior frontal gyrus.[11,14]

Supplementary Motor Area (MII) (SMA) (BA 6aα)

The SMA lies on the medial surface of the frontal lobe (Fig. 10-10). Zilles has localized the SMA to the portion of the medial cerebral cortex situated between two specific landmarks along the Talairach-Tournoux baseline. The Talairach-Tournoux baseline is the line drawn from the top of the anterior commissure (AC) to the bottom of the posterior commissure (PC). The anterior landmark, VAC (vertical at the anterior commissure), is the line raised perpendicular to the Talairach-Tournoux baseline at

the anterior commissure. The posterior landmark, VPC (vertical at the posterior commissure), is the line raised perpendicular to the Talairach-Tournoux baseline at the posterior commissure.[11,15] The supplementary motor area serves for learning and generating sequences of actions, for selecting the side to use for unilateral motor action, and for coordinating bimanual action and posture.[16]

Presupplementary Motor Area (pre-SMA) (BA 6aβ)

The pre-SMA lies on the medial surface of the frontal lobe anterior to the SMA (see Fig. 10-10). It is directly involved in motor inhibition. The pre-SMA is involved in selecting appropriate motor responses by suppressing automatic responses to environmental stimuli and stopping previously planned actions as new data indicate a need for change.[17]

Cingulate Gyrus

The cingulate cortex (see Fig. 10-10) contains multiple co-curvilinear regions that extend from beneath the genu of the corpus callosum (CC) (subgenual cingulate cortex), around and anterior to the CC (pregenual or perigenual cingulate cortex), then above the CC (supragenual cingulate cortex) to behind the splenium (retrosplenial cingulate cortex) (see Figs. 10-8, 10-10, and 10-11). These regions include BA 25 in the subgenual cingulate cortex; BA 33, 24 a/b/c, and 32 in the pregenual and supragenual cingulate cortex; caudal BA 32′ and caudal BA 24′ in the dorsal anterior cingulate cortex; BA 23 and 31 in the posterior cingulate cortex, and BA 29 and 30 in the retrosplenial cingulate cortex. As used in the neuropsychological and psychiatric literature (see Figs. 10-10 and 10-11), the term *rostral anterior cingulate cortex* conforms to the pregenual CC and includes BA 32 and inferior portions of BA 24. The subgenual anterior cingulate cortex lies inferior to the genu and includes BA 25 and caudal portions of BA 32 and 24. The dorsal anterior cingulate cortex includes caudal BA 24′ and 32′ and the cingulate motor area. The anterior cingulate region also contains affective and cognitive subdivisions.[18]

Frontal Eye Field (FEF, Portions of BA 6, BA 8, and BA 9)

Portions of BA 6, BA 8, and BA 9 form the frontal eye field along the posterior end of the middle frontal gyrus (see Fig. 10-9).[11]

Parietal Lobe
Somatosensory Cortex (S1) (BA 3a, BA 3b, BA 1, and BA 2)

S1 lies along the convexity surface and superior medial surface of the postcentral gyrus (see Fig. 10-8). At both sites, BA 3b, BA 1, and BA 2 form long vertical strips of tissue along the length of the postcentral gyrus. In order from anterior to posterior: BA 3b is buried within the central sulcus along the anterior face of the postcentral gyrus; BA 1 lies behind it along the posterior lip of the central sulcus; and BA 2 lies farther back along the crown of the postcentral gyrus. There may be serial, hierarchical processing of data from BA 3b through BA 1 to BA 2.[11] Parietal region BA 3a, which abuts directly on MI, is usually considered with the motor cortex.[1] Histologically, BA 1 through BA 3 are distinguished by the thinness of their cortices overall and by their especially thick, very compact layer IV.

Secondary Somatosensory Cortex (SII) (BA 5 and parts of BA 40 and BA 43)

SII lies along the upper margin of the sylvian fissure in the medial parietal operculum, just behind the central sulcus.[11] An additional parietal ventral area (PV), along the medial aspect of the parietal operculum, is also considered to be part of the somatosensory cortex.[1]

Vestibular Cortex

Vestibular cortex is found within three regions: (1) an elongated zone within the inferior portion of BA 3a; (2) a U-shaped zone 2v surrounding the anterior end of the intraparietal sulcus; and (3) the parietoinsular vestibular cortex (PIVC) situated within the posterosuperior insula and adjoining portions of the parietal lobe.[1]

Superior Parietal Lobule (BA 5, BA 7a, BA 7b)

BA 5 lies in the anterosuperior portion of the superior parietal lobule just across the postcentral sulcus from BA 2 (see Fig. 10-8).[11] It constitutes the unimodal somatosensory association cortex.[1] BA 7a and BA 7b lie along the superior parietal lobule posterior to BA 5, with BA 7a anterior to BA 7b.[11] BA 7 also extends onto the medial surface of the hemisphere at the precuneus. These regions are polymodal association cortices.[1] They are involved in spatial localization and appreciation of one's own body parts.

Inferior Parietal Lobule (BA 39, BA 40)

BA 40 and BA 39 form the inferior parietal polymodal association cortex (see Figs. 10-8 and 10-9).[1] BA 40 lies more anteriorly within the supramarginal gyrus.[11] It may participate in coordinated movements of the face and hand.[1] BA 39 lies more posteriorly within the angular gyrus. It may participate in the visual guidance of arm movements.[1]

Areas within the Intraparietal Sulcus (Intraparietal Areas)

Many polymodal association regions lie along the banks of the intraparietal sulcus (IPS). As a group, these regions serve as interfaces between the sensory input data and motor output response. That is, they receive combined sensory data from the surrounding visual, somatosensory, vestibular, and auditory cortices; send prominent feed-forward projections to specific regions of the premotor cortex; and receive feedback projections from the premotor cortex (Box 10-1).[1]

Temporal Lobe
Temporal Pole (BA 38)

BA 38 lies at the anterior extremity of the temporal lobe (see Fig. 10-8). This portion of the temporal cortex is considered to be paralimbic.[1]

Lateral Convexity (BA 22, BA 21, BA 20)

Behind the temporal pole, the lateral surface of the temporal lobe displays three parallel gyri: the superior temporal gyrus (BA 22), middle temporal gyrus (BA 21), and inferior temporal gyrus (BA 20) (see Fig. 10-8). BA 21 is a polysensory cortex. BA 20 is a visual association cortex. The middle temporal gyrus contains a motion-sensitive visual association area designated MT/V5 (middle temporal/V5).[11]

Medial Surface (BA 36, BA 37, and BA 38)

BA 36 lies on the medial surface of the temporal lobe between the rhinal-collateral sulci superiorly and the inferior temporal gyrus inferiorly (see Fig. 10-8). BA 37 lies along the lateral and the basomedial surfaces of the posterior temporal lobe.[1] BA 38 lies along the crown of the parahippocampal gyrus and covers the temporal pole.

BOX 10-1   Multimodal Areas Along the Intraparietal Sulcus (IPS) (extrapolated from macaque monkey)

- The anterior intraparietal area (AIP) on the lateral bank of the anterior IPS subserves tactile and visual object processing.
- The ventral intraparietal area (VIP) in the depth of the IPS subserves perception of self-movements and object movements in near extrapersonal space.
- The medial intraparietal area (MIP) in the intermediate portion of the medial bank of the IPS relates to planning, monitoring, and executing reaching movements.
- The lateral intraparietal area (LIP) in the medial lip of the IPS helps to mediate saccades.
- The caudal intraparietal area (CIP) in the medial bank of the posterior IPS functions in analyzing the axis, surface orientation, and three-dimensional features of objects.

Data from Nieuwenhuys R, Voogd J, van Huijzen C. The Human Central Nervous System, 4th ed. Berlin, Springer, 2008.

Primary Auditory Cortex (A1) (BA 41)

The superior surface of the temporal lobe displays one or more transverse temporal gyri (of Heschl). The most anterior Heschl gyrus and the adjoining superior temporal lobe contain BA 41 and correspond to the primary auditory area A1 (see Fig. 10-8).[1] Histologically, BA 41 is one of the thickest cortices. It displays a wide, poorly demarcated layer IV with myriad granule cells.

Auditory Association Cortex (BA 42 and BA 22)

The auditory association cortex lies directly posterior to A1 and partially surrounds it (see Figs. 10-8 and 10-9). It has two portions: a smaller belt and a larger parabelt. The belt (BA 42) borders directly on A1 and surrounds it anteriorly, laterally, and posteriorly. It lies predominantly on the medial opercular surface of the temporal lobe but also extends laterally onto the convexity surface of the superior temporal gyrus. The parabelt (BA 22) extends along the rest of the medial temporal operculum and along nearly all of the convexity surface of the superior temporal gyrus except for the temporal pole.[1]

Wernicke's Area

Wernicke's area in the dominant hemisphere is part of the auditory association cortex (see Figs. 10-8 and 10-9). It is centered in the planum temporale on the superior surface of the left temporal lobe just behind Heschl's gyrus and in the posterior portion of the superior temporal gyrus. From there, it extends over the inferior parietal lobule for a variable distance.[1,19,20]

Temporal Visual Association Cortex (BA 20, BA 21, and BA 37)

The temporal visual association cortex is an extension of the visual association cortex into the temporal lobe inferior to the superior temporal sulcus (see Figs. 10-8 and 10-9). Posteriorly, this area contains the middle temporal visual area (MTV5), the middle superior temporal area (MST), and the fusiform face area (FFA).[1]

Occipital Lobe
Primary Visual Cortex (V1) (BA 17)

BA 17 is the primary visual cortex (V1) (see Fig. 10-8). It surrounds the calcarine sulcus and extends forward for a variable distance along the anterior calcarine sulcus. Histologically, BA 17 is characterized by a complex layer IV, divided into sublayers A, B, Cα and Cβ. An especially dense, horizontally oriented layer of myelinated fibers in sublayer IVB is designated the stria

(stripe, line) of Gennari. For that reason, the primary visual cortex BA 17 is also designated the striate cortex. As with other primary sensory cortices, BA17 has a dense array of granule cells.

Extrastriate Cortex (V2, V3, and V4) (BA 18 and BA 19)

BA 18 and BA 19 surround BA 17, so they are designated the extrastriate cortices or parastriate belt (see Fig. 10-8). They form part of the visual association cortex, which also includes BA 20, BA 21, BA 37, and BA 39 in the parietal and temporal lobes.[1] BA 18 contains the visual areas V2, V3a, and V3b.[11] BA 19 contains the visual area V4 related to object recognition. Ultimately, perhaps one third of the human neocortex serves to process visual input.[1] (See also Temporal Lobe for information on the motion-sensitive visual association cortex MT/V5.)

Insula

The insula contains three cytoarchitectonic and functional areas arrayed from dorsolateral to ventromedial. Primary interoceptive representations are located in the dorsal posterior insula. They are then re-represented in a multimodal integrative zone in the mid insula and again in the anterior insular cortex.[21] The primary interoceptive, gustatory and vagal representations extend to the mid insula. The most ventral anterior portion of the insula lies adjacent to the frontal operculum.[21] The ventral anterior insula appears to be related to the limbic system and appears to be where the interoceptive sensations are given emotional valence.

Limbic Lobe

The limbic lobe includes the cingulate gyrus, parahippocampal gyrus, and hippocampal formation (see Figs. 10-1, 10-8, 10-10, and 10-11).[1]

Cingulate Gyrus (BA 23, BA 24, BA 25, BA 26, BA 29, BA 30, BA 31, BA 32, and BA 33)

The cingulate gyrus contains multiple Brodmann areas (see Figs. 10-8 and 10-10). From rostral to caudal these include the prelimbic cortex (BA 32), infralimbic cortex (BA 25), the anterior and posterior cingulate cortex (BA 24, BA 23) and part of the posterior cingulate-retrosplenial cortex (BA 31 and BA 29). BA 24 is a cingulate motor cortex.[1,11] Histologically, BA 24, BA 25, and BA 29 are considered more primitive cortices, with only three to five layers, and no clear layer IV. BA 23 displays a classic six-layered neocortex and is best thought of as a continuation of parietal cortex, with well-defined motor, oculomotor, and visual maps.

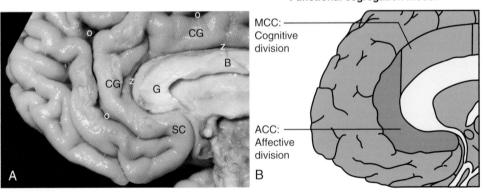

■ FIGURE 10-11   Cingulate gyrus. **A,** Medial brain surface. The cingulate gyrus (CG) extends around the body (B) and genu (G) of the corpus callosum between the callosal sulcus (z) centrally and the cingulate sulcus (o) superficially. The subgenual portion of the cingulate gyrus contains the subcallosal area (SC). **B,** On anatomic and physiologic grounds, the rostral cingulate cortex consists of functionally distinct regions: a rostroventral affective division (ACC or ventral ACC), and a dorsal cognitive division (MCC). (*B, Redrawn from Shackman AJ, Salomons TV, Slagter HA, et al. The integration of negative affect, pain, and cognitive control in the cingulate cortex. Nat Rev Neurosci 2011; 12:154-167; and based on data from Bush G, Luu P, Posner MI. Cognitive and emotional influences in anterior cingulate cortex. Trends Cogn Sci 2000; 4:215-222.*)

Parahippocampal Gyrus (BA 28, BA 35, and BA 36)

The entorhinal cortex (BA 28) occupies part of the surface of the parahippocampal gyrus (see Figs. 10-8 and 10-12). The perirhinal cortex (BA 35, BA 36) also lies within the parahippocampal gyrus.

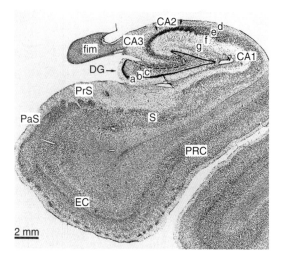

■ FIGURE 10-12 Coronal section of the human hippocampal formation (thionin stain) (see also Fig. 10-22). Dentate gyrus (DG): a, molecular layer; b, granule cell layer; c, plexiform layer. Hippocampal gyrus: CA, cornu ammonis fields 1, 2, and 3; d, stratum oriens; e, pyramidal cell layer; f, stratum radiatum; g, stratum lacunosum-moleculare. Subiculum (S): PrS, presubiculum; PaS, parasubiculum; EC, entorhinal cortex; PRC, perirhinal cortex. Measurement bar: 2 mm. *(From Standring S [ed]. Cerebral hemisphere. In Gray's Anatomy: The Anatomical Basis of Clinical Practice, 40th ed. Philadelphia: Churchill Livingstone Elsevier, 2008.)*

Hippocampal Formation

The hippocampal formation includes the dentate gyrus, the hippocampus proper (Ammon's horn), the subicular complex, and the entorhinal cortex (see Fig. 10-12).[11] The dentate gyrus shows a typical trilaminar architecture with a cellular layer interposed between two plexiform/fiber layers. From superficial to deep, the three layers of the dentate gyrus are designated the stratum moleculare, the stratum granulosum, and the polymorphic layer.[1] The hippocampus proper also displays an overall trilaminar architecture, but the horizontal laminations of the hippocampus are typically subdivided into named strata (see Fig. 10-12). The subicular complex is subdivided into the subiculum, presubiculum, and parasubiculum.[11] The subiculum is also a trilaminar cortex composed of a superficial molecular layer, a subjacent pyramidal cell layer and a deep polymorphic layer.[11] However, its cellular layer is especially wide with distinct superficial and deep zones.[1] The entorhinal cortex (BA 38) is defined by clusters of cells in layer II and a lamina dissecans unique to the entorhinal cortex.

Classification of Cortical Regions by Thalamic Afferents
By Nuclei of Origin

In many areas, there is close correlation between the cytoarchitecture of a cortical region and the specific thalamic relay nuclei that project to that portion of the cortex (Fig. 10-13). For that reason, cortical regions have also been classified by their relationship to the four major groups of thalamic relay nuclei: the sensory relay nuclei, the motor relay nuclei, the limbic nuclei, and the association nuclei of the thalamus.[1]

1. *Sensory relay nuclei.* The ventral posterior thalamic nucleus receives afferents from the somatosensory pathways and projects to BA 3, BA 1, and BA 2 of the primary somatosensory cortex (S1). The lateral geniculate nucleus receives

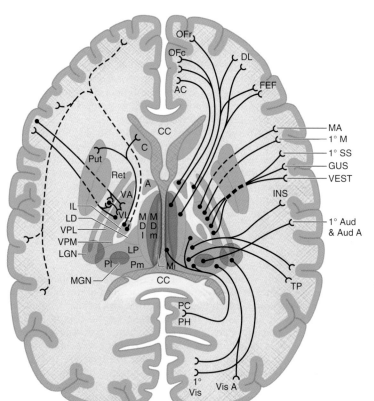

■ FIGURE 10-13 Diagram of thalamocortical connections. Reciprocal corticothalamic connections are not shown (see text for discussion). The internal medullary lamina (*light pink*) contains the intralaminar (IL) thalamic nuclei. These nuclei project to the striatum (including the ventral striatum) and diffusely to the frontal, parietal and temporal lobes. A, Anterior nuclear group; AC, anterior cingulate area; Aud, auditory cortex; Aud A, auditory association cortex; C, caudate nucleus; CC, corpus callosum; DL, dorsolateral prefrontal cortex; FEF, frontal eye fields; GUS, gustatory cortex; IL, intralaminar nuclei; INS, insula; LD, lateral dorsal nucleus; LGN, lateral geniculate nucleus; LP, lateral posterior nucleus; M, motor cortex; MA, motor association cortex; MDl, lateral part of the mediodorsal nucleus; MDm, medial part of the mediodorsal nucleus; MGN, medial geniculate nucleus; Mi, midline nuclei; OFc, orbitofrontal cortex; OFr, rostral orbitofrontal cortex; PC, posterior cingulate cortex; PH, parahippocampal cortex; Pl, lateral pulvinar; Pm, medial pulvinar; Put, putamen; Ret, reticular thalamic nuclei; SS, somatosensory cortex; TP, temporoparietal association cortex; VA, ventral anterior nucleus; VEST, vestibular cortex; Vis, visual cortex; Vis A, visual association cortex; VL, ventral lateral nucleus; VPL, ventral posterolateral nucleus; VPM, ventral posteromedial nucleus. *(Adapted from Nieuwenhuys R, Voogd J, van Huijzen C. The Human Central Nervous System, 4th ed. Berlin Heidelberg, Springer-Verlag, 2008.)*

TABLE 10-4. Nonthalamic Subcortical Afferents to the Neocortex

No.	Source of the Afferents	Afferents Pass to	Neurotransmitter Utilized
1	Claustrum		Glutamate
2	Basolateral amygdaloid nucleus		Glutamate
3, 4	Basal nucleus of Meynert (and other basal forebrain nuclei)		Acetylcholine
			γ-Aminobutyric acid
5	Hypothalamus		Orexin
			Histamine
			Melanin-concentrating hormone
6, 7	Midbrain (dorsal raphe nucleus and central superior nucleus)	Entire neocortex	Serotonin
8, 9	Ventral tegmental area and substantia nigra	Mainly to prefrontal cortex	Dopamine
10	Rostral pontine tegmentum (locus ceruleus)		Norepinephrine

From Nieuwenhuys R, Voogd J, van Huijzen C. The Human Central Nervous System, 4th ed. Berlin, Springer-Verlag, 2008.

afferents from the retina and projects to BA 17, the primary visual cortex (V1). The medial geniculate nucleus receives auditory data from the cochleae via the brain stem and projects to BA 41, the primary auditory cortex (A1).[1]

2. *Motor relay nuclei.* The motor relay nuclei of the thalamus include the ventral anterior nucleus (VA) and the anterior and posterior divisions of the ventral lateral nucleus (VLa and VLp). VA is the principal relay from the substantia nigra pars reticulata and projects to the frontal eye fields (BA 8) and adjacent portions of the prefrontal cortex. VLa is the relay for afferents from the internal segment of the globus pallidus and projects to the premotor cortex (BA 6). VLp receives a massive input from the cerebellar nuclei and projects to the primary motor cortex M1 (BA 4).[1]

3. *Limbic nuclei.* The limbic nuclei of the thalamus include the anterior nuclear complex and the lateral dorsal nucleus. These structures receive afferents from the subicular complex via the fornix, mammillary bodies, and mammillothalamic tracts. They project to the cingulate gyrus (BA 23, BA 24, BA 32), the retrosplenial area (BA 29, BA 30), and the presubiculum, parasubiculum, and the entorhinal cortex (BA 28).[1]

4. *Association nuclei.* The association nuclei of the thalamus include the multiple subnuclei within the mediodorsal (dorsomedial) nucleus and the pulvinar. The major afferents to these association nuclei arise from the cortex itself, so these nuclei appear to serve as relay stations in corticothalamocortical circuits. The mediodorsal (dorsomedial) nucleus projects to multiple areas including the prefrontal (anterior association) cortex. The pulvinar also projects to multiple areas, including the temporoparieto-occipital (posterior association) cortex.[1]

By the Neocortical Layers Innervated
Thalamic afferents to the cortex may also be classified into three different groups on the basis of the cortical layers to which the thalamic nuclei project:

Class 1 afferents arise from specific thalamic nuclei for somatic sensation, audition, and vision.[1] Their cortical projections end within layer IV, layer III or both.

Class 2 afferents arise from intralaminar thalamic nuclei. These cortical projections pass to deep cortical layers (V, VI, or both).[1]

Class 3 afferents arise from a number of paralaminar thalamic nuclei. These afferents show dense, widespread projections to layer I, with or without projections to other layers as well.[1]

Classification by Other Cortical Afferents
Corticocortical Afferents
Corticocortical afferents form a second major group of inputs to the neocortex, and, overall, tend to terminate in layers III and

IV.[1] Callosal fibers to the somatosensory cortex terminate in layers I to IV. Callosal fibers to the motor cortex terminate in a comparable pattern in layers I to III. Association fibers give off collaterals in the deep layers, especially VI, but are distributed mainly to layers I to IV, especially II and III.[1] These fibers pass radially through the cortex and issue relatively short branches at each layer.

Nonthalamic Subcortical Afferents to the Neocortex
Afferents to the neocortex also arise from at least 10 nonthalamic subcortical regions and utilize a wide variety of neurotransmitters (Table 10-4). Among these, the neocortical afferents from the basal forebrain, the hypothalamus, and the upper brain stem constitute the ventral branch of the ascending arousal system.[1]

The cholinergic, GABAergic, and monoaminergic inputs enhance or diminish the activity of limited neuronal ensembles during certain stages of information processing. By this, they modulate the responsiveness of cortical neurons that process sensory input, coordinate motor output, and integrate higher brain functions, such as mood, attention, motivation, cognition, learning, and memory.[1]

The *dopaminergic projections* to the neocortex are key modulators of motivational cognitive and motor functions.

The *serotoninergic projections* to the neocortex help regulate the sleep-wake cycle and modulate the sensory gating of behaviorally relevant cues in the environment.

The *cholinergic projections* to the neocortex are implicated in arousal, sleep-wake cycles, learning to process visual information, memory, and selective attention.

The *noradrenergic projections* from the locus ceruleus to the neocortex are thought to function in vigilance and in response to novel stimuli. Phasic activity of the locus ceruleus is related to the outcome of task-related decision processes and may help to optimize task performance (exploitation). The locus ceruleus appears to switch to tonic activity when disengaging from current task and searching for alternate behavior (exploration).[1]

Functional Divisions
Cortical Columns
The radially organized cells of a cortical column appear to function together to receive specific sensory data or to effect specific motor actions. Within the visual cortex, orientation columns are composed of cells that respond selectively to bars of light oriented along one specific axis and not other axes. The orientation of the light to which each cortical column responds preferentially changes by approximately 10 degrees every 300 to 1000 μm along the surface of the cortex. Ocular dominance columns receive input from either the ipsilateral or contralateral eye, not both.[1] These columns organize into alternating stripes 500 μm wide for receipt of visual input from one, then the other, eye.

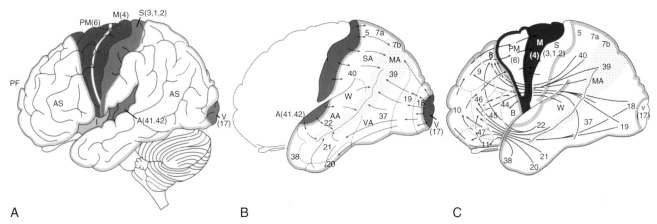

■ FIGURE 10-14 Association cortices. Dorsal and ventral data streams. **A,** In humans, the narrow primary sensory (*blue*) and motor (*red*) areas are widely separated by broad zones of association cortex (*outlined in yellow*). The insula (I) is colored *gray*. **B,** Core, belt, parabelt and multimodal association cortices. Sequential information processing. In one concept, primary data for single (unimodal) sensations reach the cortex at specific primary sensory cortical areas (e.g., S1, A1, and V1). These primary sensory areas are designated the "cores." From the cores, short association fibers convey the unimodal data to a surrounding unimodal association cortex (the "belt") for initial processing. The partially processed unimodal data are then conveyed farther to an adjoining association cortex designated the "parabelt." The more highly processed data from multiple different modalities then converge onto a multimodal association cortex (*dotted zone* MA) for integration of all relevant sensations. In humans, the multimodal association cortex on the lateral convexity extends along the superior temporal sulcus and parietal lobe from the lateral end of the parieto-occipital sulcus to the anterior temporal lobe. **C,** Information streams. From the unimodal and multimodal sensory association cortices, the data are passed anteriorly to the prefrontal cortex for motor decisions about how to respond to the sensory data received. On average, spatial data pass from the dorsal sensory areas to the dorsal prefrontal cortex in a dorsal "where" stream. Object data pass from the ventral sensory areas to the ventral prefrontal cortex in a ventral "what" stream. In turn, these data may then be passed to the medial frontal and orbitofrontal cortices where emotion/value judgments are made as to the significance of the data received. A, primary auditory area; AA, auditory association area; AS, association cortex; B, Broca's area; I, insula; M, primary motor cortex; MA, multimodal association area; PF, prefrontal cortex; PM, premotor cortex; S, primary somatosensory cortex; SA, somatosensory association area; V, primary visual cortex; VA, visual association area; WA, Wernicke's area. Numbers designate the Brodmann areas. *(From Nieuwenhuys R. The human brain: an introductory survey. Med Mundi 1994; 39:64-79.)*

"Blobs" are ellipsoidal columns in layers II and III, 150×200 microns in size, that respond selectively to specific colors, not orientations, of the light stimulus.[1] Together the orientation columns, ocular dominance columns, and blobs establish hypercolumns that serve to analyze discrete segments of the visual field.

Within the auditory cortex, analogous cortical columns respond selectively to one characteristic frequency, not others. Columns cluster into bands that do or do not receive strong contralateral auditory input. Bands with strong contralateral input serve as binaural summation units. Bands with weak contralateral input serve as binaural inhibition units.

Association Cortex

The association cortex can be divided into modality-specific (unimodal) regions and multimodality, higher-order (heteromodal) integration regions (Fig. 10-14). The unimodal areas are conceived of as roughly concentric zones designated the core, the belt, and the parabelt for each modality.

Unimodal Sensory Areas. Each separate primary sensation is considered a modality. The primary sensory cortex that receives the specific unimodal afferent data for that one sensation may be considered the "core" for that sensory modality (see Fig. 10-14A). Adjacent to each core, there is a modality-specific unimodal sensory association area (the "belt") that provides the initial "analysis" of the raw sensory input that was received by the core.[1] From the belts, the partially processed sensory data for each modality are conveyed onward to adjoining unimodal association cortices (the "parabelts") for additional processing.

The unimodal sensory association regions for somatic sensation, vision, and audition occupy most of the postcentral association cortex. The unimodal association cortex for somatic sensation lies within the superior parietal lobule, directly behind the primary sensory area S1. It corresponds to portions of BA 5

and BA 7 and, perhaps, parts of BA 40 in the anterior portion of the inferior parietal lobule.[1] The unimodal association cortex for vision surrounds the primary visual cortex (V1). It occupies a large part of the occipital lobe and extends forward into the inferior temporal lobe. It includes BA 18 to BA 21 and BA 37.[1] The unimodal association cortex for audition lies adjacent to the primary auditory cortex (A1) that lies in the transverse temporal gyrus of Heschl. The unimodal auditory association cortex covers much of the superior temporal gyrus and corresponds to BA 22.[1] The unimodal association cortex for olfaction may lie within the posterolateral orbital cortex and the anterior insula.

Heteromodal Association Areas. From the belts and parabelts, unimodal data from multiple different modalities converge onto a central heteromodal (multimodal) association cortex that integrates the partially processed data from many different unimodal association cortices. Geographically, the parietotemporal heteromodal association cortex lies between and adjoining the unimodal somatosensory, unimodal visual, and unimodal auditory association cortices.

On the convexity surface, the heteromodal sensory association area lies along an arc drawn from the lateral end of the parieto-occipital sulcus posteriorly downward and along the superior temporal sulcus to reach the anterior temporal lobe (see Fig. 10-14B). This heteromodal sensory association cortex includes the caudal portion of the superior parietal lobule (BA 7), most of the inferior parietal lobule (BA 39, BA 40), and the portions of the superior and middle temporal gyri facing the superior temporal sulcus at the junctions of BA 21 and BA 22. On the medial surface, the medial temporal heteromodal sensory association cortex lies along the anterior medial temporal lobe at BA 35 and BA 36, between the entorhinal area BA 28 and the visual association areas BA 19 to BA 37 and BA 20.[1]

Association areas in the frontal lobe appear to play a corresponding role for motor function. The premotor cortex (BA 6) anterior to the primary motor area (M1) may constitute a motor association cortex. This area includes the premotor cortex of BA 6 (with the supplementary motor area [M2]), posterior BA 8 and BA 44. The motor association cortex has reciprocal connections with the unimodal sensory association areas.[1]

The prefrontal heteromodal association cortex lies anterior to the motor association cortex and includes BA 9, BA 10, BA 45 to BA 47, as well as the anterior portions of BA 8, BA 11, and BA 12. This heteromodal association area receives afferents from the unimodal sensory association cortices and from the heteromodal parietotemporal and medial temporal zones. On average, data pertaining to spatial localization pass along a dorsal "where" stream to the dorsal prefrontal cortex.[22] Data pertaining to object identification pass along a ventral "what" stream to the ventral prefrontal cortex (see Fig. 10-14C).[22] The prefrontal heteromodal output is then transmitted via sequential, short-association fibers that pass to the anterior orbitofrontal cortex, the polar and lateral prefrontal areas BA 9, BA 10, and BA 46, the motor association cortex, and the primary motor cortex.[1]

Cortical Processing of Data

The processing of data across the cortex may proceed by hierarchical, feedback, and parallel processing circuits.[1]

Hierarchical Processing

Hierarchical processing is conceived of as a multisynaptic, feedforward system that passes data from primary unimodal sensory cortices, through successive heteromodal areas, to the premotor and motor cortices. These feed-forward systems originate mainly from pyramidal neurons in layer III and terminate in and around layer IV of the cortical area to which they pass.[1]

Feedback Fibers

Most (>75%) of the cortical feed-forward systems display reciprocal feedback fibers that project back to the cortex of origin. These feedback fibers nearly always arise from the infragranular layers V and VI and terminate largely in layers I and VI.[1]

Parallel Processing

At least some portions of the brain display parallel processing. The different components of the visual image, for example, remain segregated in the striate cortex and in their projections to the extrastriate visual association areas. The extrastriate visual association areas process data on spatial vision and movement via a different path than they do the data on object recognition.

Circuitry

Mental analysis and thought result from the functional integration of multiple regions of the brain, not from the activity of single isolated cortical regions. Increasingly, neural processes are conceptualized as occurring in circuits that subserve different functions.[1]

Thalamocortical Circuits

Nearly all the thalamic nuclei project to the cerebral cortex via thalamocortical fibers and receive back reciprocal afferent corticothalamic fibers from the cortical regions to which they project.[2] These reciprocal connections follow a topographic distribution with rostromedial and caudolateral portions of the thalamus connected with the corresponding portions of the cerebral cortex. Together, the connections establish corticothalamocortical circuits that subserve different functions.

Overall, in rostrocaudal order, the modality-specific areas of the frontal lobe (motor cortex), parietal lobe (somatosensory, taste, and vestibular cortices), temporal lobe (auditory cortex), and occipital lobe (visual cortex) interconnect with the ventral thalamic nuclei. The limbic and paralimbic cortices and

heteromodal portions of the prefrontal cortex interconnect with the midline, anterior, and medial nuclei of the thalamus. The heteromodal cortex of the parietal and temporal lobes and the unimodal association cortex for vision interconnect with the lateral nuclear group of the thalamus.[2]

Default and Task-Related Networks

Increasing evidence indicates that the brain contains both "default" and task-related (goal-directed, attentional) networks for data processing.[23] The two networks appear to function alternately, one, or the other, but not both simultaneously. External demands engage the task-related network and simultaneously deactivate the default network. Passive periods with no cognitive demand disengage the task-related network and activate the default network instead. The default network is conceived of as an intrinsically organized functional network that is associated with a variety of self-referential processes, including introspective processing, remembering the past and planning the future (Fig. 10-15).[18] Left alone, people tend to think about themselves in relation to significant past and future events. At those times, their minds wander and the default network engages in internal mentation.[24]

Anatomically, the task-positive network includes, among other areas, the dorsolateral prefrontal cortex (dLPFC), the dorsal anterior cingulate cortex (dACC), the cortical areas along the intraparietal sulcus (IPS), and the middle temporal area (MT). The default network (DN) consists of two subsystems that converge on a midline core with two hubs (Fig. 10-16)[24,25]:

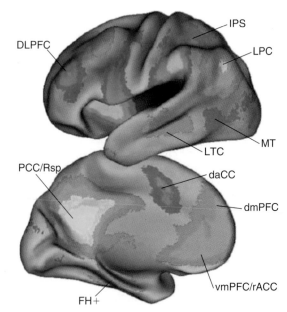

■ **FIGURE 10-15** Default mode network. The default network (*orange*) includes regions that *deactivate* during processing of external stimuli, including the ventral medial prefrontal cortex (vmPFC), rostral anterior cingulate cortex (rACC), posterior cingulate cortex (PCC), retrosplenial cortex (Rsp), lateral parietal cortex (LPC), lateral temporal cortex (LTC), dorsal medial prefrontal cortex (dmPFC), and hippocampal formation, including the entorhinal cortex and the surrounding cortex of the parahippocampal gyrus (FH+). The task positive network (*blue*) includes the dorsolateral prefrontal cortex (DLPFC), dorsal anterior cingulate cortex (daCC), intraparietal sulcus (IPS), and middle temporal area (MT). The task positive network becomes activated during tasks that require cognitive and attentional control. The *red* areas correlate positively with the default network. The *blue* task-related areas correlate negatively with the default network. (*Modified from Buckner RL, Andrews-Hanna JR, Schacter DL. The brain's default network: anatomy, function, and relevance to disease. Ann NY Acad Sci 2008; 1124:1-38.*)

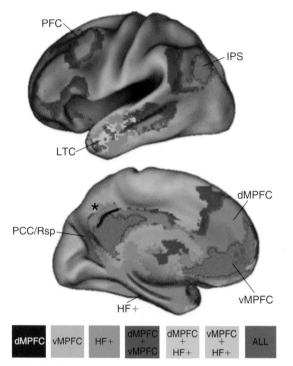

■ **FIGURE 10-16** Hubs and subsystems within the default network mapped by connectivity analysis. The posterior cingulate cortex (PCC)/ retrosplenial cortex (Rsp), inferior parietal lobule at the intraparietal sulcus (IPS), and ventral medial prefrontal cortex (vMPFC) are anatomic hubs in the default network to which all other regions are correlated. The dorsomedial prefrontal cortex (dMPFC) and the extended hippocampal region (HF+) both correlate strongly with the hubs but not with each other, indicating that they are part of distinct subsystems of the network. *(From Buckner RL, Andrews-Hanna JR, Schacter DL. The brain's default network: anatomy, function, and relevance to disease. Ann NY Acad Sci 2008; 1124:1-38.)*

Default subsystem 1. The dorsal medial prefrontal subsystem (dMPF) consists of the dorsal medial prefrontal cortex (dMPFC), the temporoparietal junction (TPJ), the lateral temporal cortex (LTC), and the temporal pole (TP).

Default subsystem 2. The medial temporal lobe (MTL) subsystem consists of the ventral medial prefrontal cortex (vMPFC), the posterior inferior parietal lobe (piPL), the retrosplenial cortex (RSpC), the parahippocampal cortex (PHC), and the hippocampal formation (HF⁺).

Default hubs. The two hubs are the anterior medial prefrontal cortex (aMPFC) and the posterior cingulate cortex (PCC).

Mentally, the default network activates when people are passive and left to think for themselves, undisturbed. The midline core of the default network responds most strongly to introspection about one's own mental state, to thoughts with personal significance, and to evoked emotion. The anterior hub (aMPFC), and often the posterior hub, also activates when people make judgments about themselves as compared with others. The dorsal medial prefrontal cortex (dMPFC) subsystem activates preferentially when people consider their present state and when they infer the mental states of others.[24] The medial temporal lobe (MTL) subsystem activates preferentially when people construct a mental scene based on memory and when they make self-relevant, affective decisions, especially about their future.

IMAGING

Routine CT displays the cortex as a cortical ribbon that is hyperdense to the underlying white matter. The cortex is thicker along the crowns of the gyri and thinner at the depths of the sulci. The gray matter/white matter interface is sharp (Fig. 10-17).

Routine clinical MRI displays the cortical ribbon in finer detail (Fig. 10-18). On T1-weighted (T1W) images, the cortex is hypointense to the myelinated white matter. On T2-weighted (T2W) images the cortical ribbon appears hyperintense to the myelinated white matter. Areas of greater cellularity such as the highly granular cortex of the transverse temporal gyrus (of Heschl)

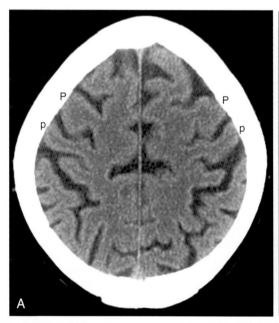
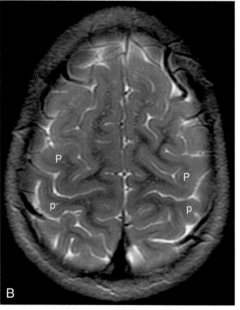

■ **FIGURE 10-17** Axial images through the cortex. **A,** Axial noncontrast CT of the neocortex. **B,** Axial T2W MR image. The gray matter of the cortical ribbon is distinctly different from the underlying digitations of white matter and shows a sharp gray-white interface. The cortex is thicker at the crowns of the gyri and thinner at the depths of the sulci. The agranular motor cortex along the posterior face of the precentral gyrus (P) is definitely thicker than the granular sensory cortex on the apposing anterior face of the postcentral gyrus (p). The greatest difference in cortical thickness between two adjacent gyri occurs between the posterior face of the precentral gyrus and the anterior face of the postcentral gyrus across the central sulcus.[26]

■ **FIGURE 10-18** Coronal MRI of the cortex. **A** and **B,** T1W MR images of the frontal (**A**) and temporal (**B**) lobes. **C** and **D,** T2W MR images of the frontal (**C**) and temporal (**D**) lobes. **A** and **C,** The cortex of the frontal and neocortical temporal lobes is hypointense to white matter on T1W images and hyperintense to white matter on T2W images. As on the CT, the cortex is thicker at the crowns of the gyri and thinnest at the depths of the sulci. The gray-white interface is sharp. **B** and **D,** Compared with the adjacent cortices, the highly granular cortex of Heschl's gyrus (*arrows*) appears brighter on T1W images and darker on T2W images.

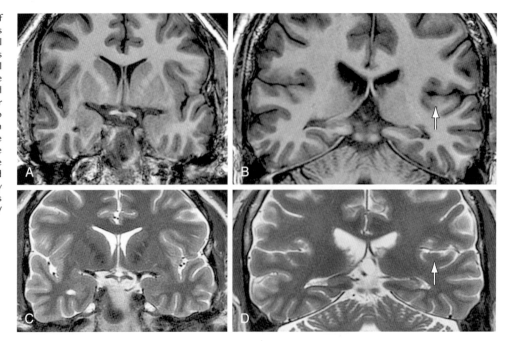

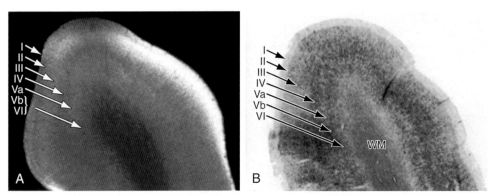

■ **FIGURE 10-19** Polar neocortex. **A,** A 9.4-T intermediate-weighted MR microscopic image of the frontal pole. **B,** Corresponding histologic section of the same specimen stained with Nissl stain for neurons. From superficial to deep, these images display the I, molecular layer; II, external granule cell layer; III, external pyramidal cell layer; IV, internal granule cell layer; V, internal pyramidal cell layer (subdivided into an outer sublayer Va and an inner sublayer Vb); and VI, multiforme layer. The signal intensity of each layer decreases with increasing cell density and increasing myelination. WM, white matter core of the gyrus (original magnification, ×8; in-plane resolution, 78 × 78 µm; slice thickness, 500 µm). *(From Fatterpekar GM, Naidich TP, Delman BN, et al. Cytoarchitecture of the human cerebral cortex: MR microscopy of excised specimens at 9.4 tesla. AJNR Am J Neuroradiol 2002; 23:1313-1321.)*

appear lower in signal than the adjacent cortex on T2W images. Meyer and colleagues showed that the greatest difference in cortical thickness across a single sulcus is at the central sulcus (see Fig. 10-17).[26] The marked difference between the thick agranular motor cortex of the precentral gyrus and the thin granular somatosensory cortex of the postcentral gyrus is one sign that helps to identify the central sulcus.

MR Microscopy

The internal architecture of the cortex can be displayed successfully using high-field (7.0 to 9.4 T) scanners, intermediate-weighted pulse sequences, and long scan times (Figs. 10-19 to 10-22).[27,28] These images demonstrate overall cortical thickness, display greater thickness of the cortex along the crown of the gyrus than at the depth of the sulcus, and begin to resolve the differing thicknesses and definition of the individual cortical layers. At present, MR microscopy may distinguish gross aspects of cortical architecture such as agranular versus granular cortices, demonstrate the transition from one to the other at the depth of the central sulcus, and demonstrate transitions from

allocortex to mesocortex at the medial temporal lobe and along the retrosplenial cingulate gyrus.

With intermediate-weighted pulse sequences, the signal intensity of the cortex is inversely proportional to both the degree of myelination and the cell density of the intracortical layers. Thus, low signal intensity is seen in two distinctly different settings: (1) the heavily myelinated layers such as the external band of Baillarger (stria of Gennari) (layer IVB) of the calcarine cortex and the subcortical U fibers (see Fig. 10-20) and (2) the highly cellular neuronal layers that are nearly devoid of myelin such as the granule cell layer of the dentate gyrus (see Fig. 10-22).[27,28] Regions with varying concentrations of myelin and varying cell density show intermediate signal intensity that varies in a complex fashion.

Voxel-Based Morphometry and Similar Computational Techniques

Voxel-based morphometry and similar in vivo techniques assess the volumes and thicknesses of tissue across a section or an organ. Application of these techniques to the human cortex

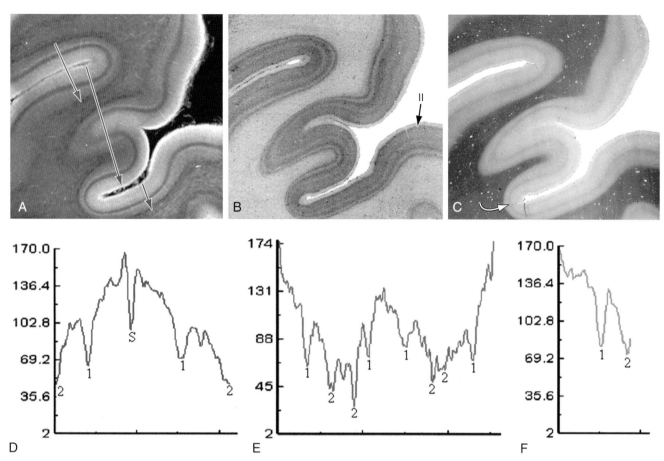

■ **FIGURE 10-20** Sensory isocortex. **A,** A 9.4-T intermediate-weighted MR microscopic image of the calcarine cortex. **B** and **C,** Corresponding histologic sections of the same specimen stained with Nissl stain for neurons (**B**) and Luxol fast blue for myelin with nuclear fast red counterstain (**C**). The thin prominent sharply defined intracortical band of low signal intensity in this region corresponds to the highly myelinated plexus of layer IVB (*curved arrow* in **C**) designated the external band of Baillarger. When seen in gross specimens, it is called the line (stria) of Gennari. The prominent granule cells of layer two (*long arrow* in **B**) appear as a gray band on the MR microscopic image (*long arrow* in **A**). Overall cortical thickness is substantially greater along the crowns of the gyri and thinner at the depths of the sulci. The variation in the thickness of the cortex between layer IVB and the underlying white matter (W) demonstrates that this variation in cortical thickness results mainly from thinning of the deep layers V and VI (original magnification, ×5). **D** to **F,** Color-coded density profiles across the calcarine cortex. In these profiles, the cortical layers crossed by each arrow are designated by their corresponding Arabic numbers. S, sulcus. *(From Fatterpekar GM, Naidich TP, Delman BN, et al. Cytoarchitecture of the human cerebral cortex: MR microscopy of excised specimens at 9.4 tesla. AJNR Am J Neuroradiol 2002; 23:1313-1321.)*

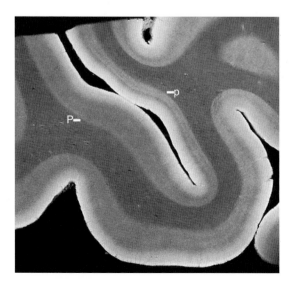

■ **FIGURE 10-21** Precentral and postcentral gyri across the central sulcus. Agranular (motor) and highly granular (sensory) neocortices. A 9.4-T intermediate-weighted MR microscopic image. The cortex of the precentral gyrus (P) is far thicker than the cortex of the postcentral gyrus (p). The greatest difference in the thickness of apposing cortices occurs across the central sulcus. The postcentral gyrus shows well defined external (II) and internal (IV) granule cell layers. The precentral gyrus shows loss of these well-defined layers with marked expansion and merging of the thick pyramidal cell layers (original magnification, ×8; in-plane resolution, 78 × 78 μm; slice thickness, 500 μm).

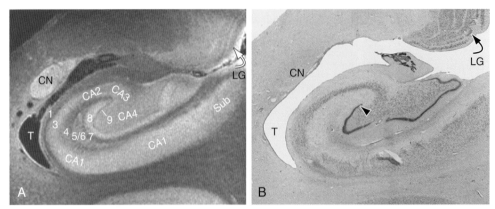

■ **FIGURE 10-22** Allocortex of the hippocampal formation (see also Fig. 10-12). **A** and **B**, A 9.4-T intermediate-weighted MR microscopy. **B**, Histologic section of the same specimen with Nissl stain for neurons. From lateral to medial, the MRM image displays the sequential histological layers of the hippocampal archicortex: 1, alveus; 2, stratum oriens (between 1 and 3); 3, stratum pyramidale; 4, stratum radiatum; 5, stratum lacunosum; 6, stratum moleculare of the denate gyrus; 7, hippocampal sulcus; 8, stratum moleculare of the hippocampal gyrus; 9, dentate granule cell layer (*arrowhead* in **B**). The fields of the hippocampal gyrus (cornu ammonis, CA) are labeled CA1 to CA4. Some authorities suggest grouping CA3 with CA4, but they are labeled separately in these images. Also seen are the tail of the caudate nucleus (CN), subiculum (Sub), and the lamellar retinotopic organization of the lateral geniculate body (LG, *curved arrow*). T, temporal horn (original magnification, ×6.25; in-plane resolution, 78 × 78 μm; slice thickness, 500 μm). *(From Fatterpekar GM, Naidich TP, Delman BN, et al. Cytoarchitecture of the human cerebral cortex: MR microscopy of excised specimens at 9.4 tesla. AJNR Am J Neuroradiol 2002; 23:1313-1321.)*

■ **FIGURE 10-23** Normal cortical asymmetry by gender and age. Voxel-based morphometry. **Upper row: Left,** Greater asymmetry in males. The color scale indicates the degrees of left-right cortical asymmetry in males versus females. Areas that are more asymmetric in males scale from dull red to white. Areas that are more asymmetric in females scale from blue to green. **Right,** Reduction in the normal male asymmetry with age. Areas that are more asymmetric in the aged scale from dull red to white. Areas that are less asymmetric in the aged scale from blue to green. The cortices show less asymmetry with age. **Lower row:** A smaller subset of the areas shown in the upper row are found to reach statistical significance ($P < 0.05$). *(From Kovalev VA, Kruggel F, von Cramon DY. Gender and age effects in structural brain asymmetry as measured by MRI textural analysis. NeuroImage 2003; 19:895-905.)*

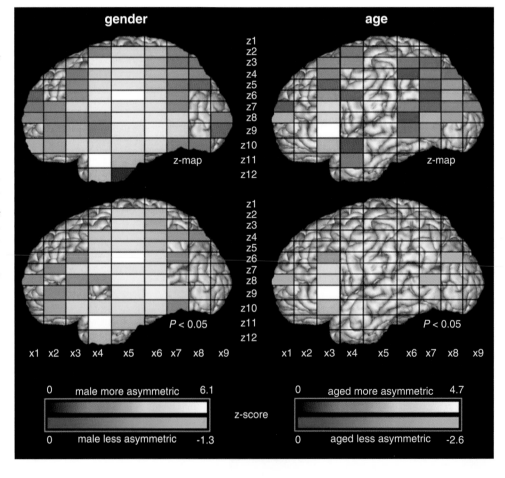

confirms the regional variations in cortical thickness shown histologically and displays the differences in the cortical thicknesses of the left versus the right hemispheres, the male versus female brain, and the younger versus aging brain (Fig. 10-23).[29,30] In 290 adults aged 18 to 32 years, Kovalev and colleagues documented that male brains are more asymmetric than female brains.[29] In 30 healthy young adults aged 20 to 30 years, Luders and associates showed that the cortex is thicker on the left side overall, with greater left-sided asymmetry in males than females. Regions showing significantly greater cortical thickness on the *left* include the precentral gyrus, middle frontal gyrus, anterior temporal lobe and superior parietal lobule along the convexity, and the medial surface of the hemisphere from the paracentral lobule forward (see Fig. 10-23). Regions showing significantly greater cortical thickness on the *right* include the posterior inferior temporal lobe and the inferior frontal lobe along the convexity and the medial surface posteriorly.[31]

The well-known age-related decrease in brain volume appears to be related more to the loss of gray matter than of white matter and affects some regions more than others (Table 10-5).[30] In 152 adults aged 18 to 70 years, Kovalev and colleagues demonstrated that the degree of cerebral asymmetry increases significantly with age in the anterior cingulate gyrus, the retrosplenial cortex, the parahippocampal gyrus, the anterior insula, and the inferior frontal gyrus. The degree of asymmetry decreases significantly with age in the precentral and angular gyri.[29]

f-MRI

The functional basis of MRI is still being debated. One concept of the physiology behind f-MRI is as follows: Throughout the

TABLE 10-5. Regional Analysis of Age-Related Involution of the Healthy Brain

Site	Percent Shrinkage per Decade
Gray Matter	
Lateral prefrontal cortex	5.36
Orbitofrontal cortex	3.35
Precentral gyrus	2.70
Anterior cingulate gyrus	0.43
Postcentral gyrus	3.07
Inferior temporal gyrus	2.29
Fusiform cortex	1.89
Hippocampus	3.09
Before age 50 years	0.71
After age 50 years	6.38
Inferior parietal lobule	+0.14
Visual cortex	1.70
White Matter	
Prefrontal white matter	2.97
Parietal white matter	+0.42

From Raz N, Gunning-Dixon F, Head D, et al. Aging, sexual dimorphism, and hemispheric asymmetry of the cerebral cortex: replicability of regional differences in volume. Neurobiol Aging 2004; 25:377-396.

brain, there is close coupling between the oxygen consumption in a region and the blood flow to that region. At rest, the delivery of oxygen and oxygen consumption are in balance. When brain activity increases *transiently,* above resting values, the flow of blood to the active region increases disproportionately. The oxygen delivered to the active region exceeds the oxygen consumed by that region, so the concentration of oxygen increases within the local blood vessels. Put differently, increased brain activity causes local increase in the oxygen concentration with consequent decrease in deoxyhemoglobin.

The blood oxygen level–dependent (BOLD) f-MRI technique measures the oxygen concentrations across the brain before, during, and after specific cognitive tasks and maps the work-related variations in oxygen concentration onto anatomic images of the brain. Those areas that display increased oxygen levels during the task are considered to have participated in the performance of the task and are said to have been activated by the task. Areas that show oxygen concentrations lower than baseline during the task are said to have been deactivated by the task. Multiple regions that act coherently to increase activity during a task are said to form networks that function together to perform or participate in the task.

In task-related f-MRI studies with block design, the activity of the brain in the "resting," "passive" state between tasks is characteristically taken as baseline for comparison with the "activations" induced by performance of the mental task. Broad experience with f-MRI, however, has disclosed a reproducible set of anatomic regions that show reduced activity during tasks. That is, one set of areas is clearly more active between tasks, during passive mentation, and that same set of areas "turns off" when the brain becomes engaged in performing an assigned task.[23] The set of areas more active during passive mentation and less active during task-related, goal-directed activity is now designated the default network (see Figs. 10-15 and 10-16).

CHEMOARCHITECTURE

Zilles, Amunts, and others are now working to establish the anatomic distribution of the neurotransmitters that act on the brain. The distribution of these multiple different receptors provides one map of the chemoarchitecture of the brain (Fig. 10-24).

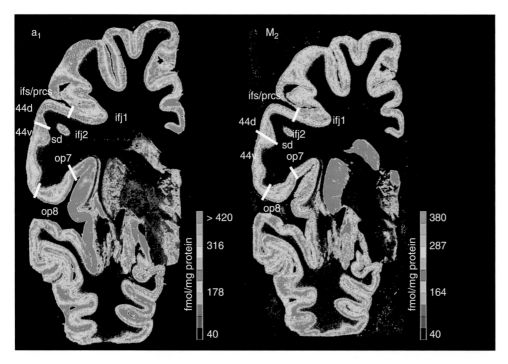

■ **FIGURE 10-24** Chemoarchitecture of the brain: Neuroreceptor distribution across the brain. The distribution of the noradrenergic receptor (left), and the cholinergic muscarinic M2 receptor (right) are shown in neighboring coronal sections of a complete human hemisphere. The receptor concentrations are indicated in femtomoles per milligram of protein and color-coded according to the color bar on the right of each section. The differences in receptor concentration are especially marked in the caudate nucleus, the putamen, the insular cortex, and the cingulate cortex. ifj1, inferior frontal junction area 1; ifj2, inferior frontal junction area 2; ifs, inferior frontal sulcus; op 7, opercular area 7; op 8, opercular area 8; prcs, precentral sulcus; sd, diagonal sulcus; 44d, dorsal area 44; 44v, ventral area 44. (*From Amunts K, Lenzen M, Friederici AD, et al. Broca's region: novel organizational principles and multiple receptor mapping. PLoS Biol 2010; 8:e1000489.*)

Differing subsets (or suites) of receptors help to differentiate among sensory, motor, and association cortices. In the future, ligands specific for each neurotransmitter may permit clinical mapping of the normal and deranged chemoarchitecture of the brain by positron emission tomography (PET).

ALTERING OF NORMAL IMAGING APPEARANCE BY PATHOLOGIC PROCESS

In the United States, 16.6% of individuals meet criteria for major depressive disorder at some time during their lives; 40% to 50% of such patients fail to respond to antidepressive medication.[18,32]

It is postulated that major depression is related to hyperactivity within the default network and inability to switch easily between the default and the task-related networks.[18] Increased resting regional blood flow in the rostral anterior cingulate cortex (rACC, BA 24a/b) predicts which patients will respond better to treatment for depression.

Imaging evidence indicates that one of the cortical regions affected early in Alzheimer's disease is the retrosplenial cortex, a region known to be part of the default network. Furthermore, major depression is known to be an independent risk factor for Alzheimer's disease. That relationship poses interesting questions.

SUGGESTED READINGS

Craig AD. How do you feel now? The anterior insula and human awareness. Nat Rev Neurosci 2009; 10:60.

Duvernoy HM, in collaboration with Cattin F, Fatterpekar G, Naidich T, et al. The Human Hippocampus: Anatomy, Vascularization and Serial Sections with MRI, 3rd ed. Berlin, Springer, 2005.

Fatterpekar GM, Naidich TP, Delman BN, et al. Cytoarchitecture of the human cerebral cortex: MR microscopy of excised specimens at 9.4 Tesla. AJNR Am J Neuroradiol 2002; 23:1313-1321.

Marsel Mesulam M. Principles of Behavior and Cognitive Neurology, 2nd ed. New York, Oxford University Press, 2000.

Mayberg HS, Brannan SK, Mahurin RK, et al. Cingulate function in depression: a potential predictor of treatment response. NeuroReport 1997; 8:1057-1061.

Naidich TP, Hof PR, Gannon PJ, et al. Anatomic substrates of language: emphasizing speech. Neuroimaging Clin North Am 2001; 11:305-341.

Naidich TP, Hof PR, Yousry TA, Yousry I. The motor cortex: anatomic substrates of function. Neuroimaging Clin North Am 2001; 11:171-193.

Nieuwenhuys R, Voogd J, van Huijzen C. The Human Central Nervous System, 4th ed. Berlin, Springer, 2008.

Price JL, Drevets WC. Neurocircuitry of mood disorders. Neuropsychopharmacol Rev 2010; 35:192-216.

Standring S (ed). The cerebral hemisphere. In Gray's Anatomy: The Anatomical Basis of Clinical Practice, 40th ed. Philadelphia, Elsevier, 2008.

REFERENCES

1. Nieuwenhuys R, Voogd J, van Huijzen C. The Human Central Nervous System, 4th ed. Berlin, Springer, 2008.
2. Gilman S, Newman SW. Manter and Gatz's Essentials of Clinical Neuroanatomy and Neurophysiology, 10th ed. Philadelphia, FA Davis, 2003.
3. Amunts K, Zilles K. Advances in cytoarchitectonic mapping of the human cerebral cortex. Neuroimaging Clin North Am 2001; 11:151-169.
4. Amunts K, Lenzen M, Friederici AD, et al. Broca's region: novel organizational principles and multiple receptor mapping. PLoS Biology 2010; 8:e1000489.
5. Nieuwenhuys R. The human brain: an introductory survey. Med Mundi 1994; 1994:64-79.
6. Zilles K, Amunts K. Centenary of Brodmann's map—conception and fate. Nature Rev Neurosci 2010; 11:139-145.
7. Pakkenberg B, Gundersen HJG. Neocortical neuron number in humans: effect of sex and age. J Comp Neurol 1997; 384:312-320.
8. Blinkov S, Glezer II. The Human Brain in Figures and Tables: A Quantitative Handbook. New York, Basic Books, 1968.
9. Von Economo C, Koskinas GN. Die Cytoarchitektonik der Hirnrinde des Erwachsenen Menshen. Berlin, Springer, 1925.
10. Braak H. Architectonics of the human telencephalic cortex. Berlin, Springer, 1980.
11. Standring S (ed). Cerebral hemisphere. In Gray's Anatomy: The Anatomical Basis of Clinical Practice, 40th ed. Philadelphia, Elsevier, 2008.
12. Brodmann K. Vergleichende Lokalisationlehre der Grosshirnrinde in Ihren Prinzipien Dargestellt auf Grund Des Zallenbaues [in German]. Leipzig, Barth, 1909.
13. Vogt BA, Vogt LJ, Nimchinsky EA, et al. Primate cingulate cortex cytoarchitecture and its disruption in Alzheimer's disease. In Bloom FE, Bjorkland A, Hökfelt T (eds). Handbook of Chemical Neuroanatomy, Vol 13: The Primate Nervous System. Part I. Amsterdam, Elsevier Science BV, 1997, pp 455-528.
14. Price CJ. The anatomy of language: contributions from functional neuroimaging. J Anat 2000; 197:335-359.
15. Zilles K, Schlag G, Geyer S, et al. Anatomy and transmitter receptors of the supplementary motor areas in the human and nonhuman primate brain. Adv Neurol 1996; 70:29-43.
16. Naidich TP, Hof P, Yousry TAT, Yousry I. The motor cortex: anatomic substrates of functional neuroimaging. Neuroimaging Clin North Am 2001, 11:171-193.
17. Hsu T-Y, Tseng L-Y, Yu J-X, et al. Modulating inhibitory control with direct current stimulation of the superior medial frontal cortex. Neuroimage 2011; 56:2249-2257.
18. Pizzagalli DA. Frontocingulate dysfunction in depression: toward biomarkers of treatment response. Neuropsychopharmacol Rev 2011; 36:183-206.
19. Ojemann GA. Brain organization for language from the perspective of brain stimulation mapping. Behav Brain Sci 1983; 6:189-230.
20. Ojemann GA, Ojemann J, Lettich E, et al. Cortical language localization in left, dominant hemisphere. J Neurosurg 1989; 71:316-326.
21. Craig AD. How do you feel now? The anterior insula and human awareness. Nat Rev Neurosci 2009; 10:60.
22. Mishkin M, Ungerleider LG, Macko KA. Object vision and spatial vision: two cortical pathways. Trends Neurosci 1983; 6:414-417.
23. Raichle ME, Snyder AZ. A default mode of brain function: a brief history of an evolving idea. NeuroImage 2007; 37:1083-1090.
24. Andrews-Hanna JR, Reidler JS, Sepulcre J, et al. Functional-anatomic fractionation of the brain's default network. Neuron 2010; 65:550-562.
25. Buckner RL, Andrews-Hanna JR, Schacter DL. The brain's default network anatomy, function, and relevance to disease. Ann NY Acad Sci 2008; 1124:1-38.
26. Meyer J, Roychowdhury S, Russell EJ, et al. Location of the central sulcus via cortical thickness of the precentral and postcentral gyri on MR. AJNR Am J Neurol 1996; 17:1699-1706.

27. Fatterpekar GM, Naidich TP, Delman BN, et al. Cytoarchitecture of the human cerebral cortex: MR microscopy of excised specimens at 9.4 Tesla. AJNR Am J Neuroradiol 2002; 23:1313-1321.

28. Fatterpekar GM, Delman BN, Boonn WW, et al. MR microscopy of the normal human brain. Neuroimaging Clin North Am 2003; 11:641-653.

29. Kovalev VA, Kruggel F, von Cramon DY. Gender and age effects in structural brain asymmetry as measured by MRI textural analysis. NeuroImage 2003; 19:895-905.

30. Raz N, Gunning-Dixon F, Head D, et al. Aging, sexual dimorphism, and hemispheric asymmetry of the cerebral cortex: replicability of regional differences in volume. Neurobiol Aging 2004; 25: 377-396.

31. Luders E, Narr KL, Thompson PM, et al. Hemispheric asymmetries in cortical thickness. Cerebral Cortex 2006; 16:1232-1238.

32. Mayberg HS, Brannan SK, Mahurin RK, et al. Cingulate function in depression: a potential predictor of treatment response. Neuro-Report 1997; 8:1057-1061.

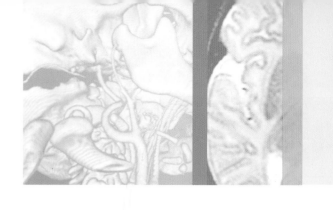

CHAPTER 11

Deep Gray Nuclei and Related Fiber Tracts

Thomas P. Naidich, Johnny C. Ng, John D. Waselus, Bradley N. Delman, and Cheuk Ying Tang

The deep gray nuclei are the central masses of gray matter arrayed around the lateral and third ventricles, including the basal ganglia and thalami (Figs. 11-1 and 11-2).[1-10] The specific nuclei within the deep gray matter have been grouped, reclassified, and designated by different names for different purposes.

EMBRYOLOGY

By the end of the fifth week of gestation, a longitudinal hypothalamic sulcus appears along the inner aspect of the developing diencephalon.[6,11,12] The hypothalamic sulcus delimits the future dorsal thalamus, metathalamus, and epithalamus that arise above the sulcus from the ventral thalamus and hypothalamus that arise below the sulcus. Ultimately, the dorsal thalamus will grow to form nearly all of the structure called thalamus in the adult. The ventral thalamus will remain small, forming the subthalamic nucleus, the reticular nuclei of the thalamus, and related fiber tracts.

By the end of the sixth week, an epithalamic swelling appears at the dorsal rim of the diencephalon separated from the thalamus by a dorsal (epithalamic) sulcus.[11] Initially, this epithalamus projects into the cavity of the ventricle and is larger than the dorsal thalamus.[6] A midline diverticulum of the epithalamic roof evaginates to form the pineal stalk. Proliferation of cells in the dorsal portion of that diverticulum forms the pineal gland. Paired paramedian habenular trigones with medial and lateral habenular nuclei develop in the lateral walls of the third ventricle, well inferior to their final position.

After the seventh week, the dorsal thalamus grows disproportionately to become the largest element of the diencephalon. This growth smooths out the dorsal (epithalamic) sulcus, displaces the epithalamus dorsally, and dwarfs the structures formed from the epithalamus.[11] The pineal stalk remains hollow, ultimately forming the pineal recess of the third ventricle. Fibers from the habenular nuclei decussate in the superior wall of the hollow pineal stalk to make the habenular commissure. Fibers from the accessory optic nuclei decussate in the inferior wall of the pineal stalk to make the posterior commissure.[6,9]

With continued growth of the thalamus the intervening third ventricle becomes narrow. The paired thalami meet in the midline and fuse together to form the massa intermedia (interthalamic adhesion).[6] Marked overgrowth of the telencephalic vesicles (future cerebral hemispheres) bulges them outward, so that they roll over and lateral to the thalami. The cleft between the telencephalic vesicles and the thalamus becomes narrowed and then obliterated, allowing the telencephalon to fuse with the dorsal surface of the diencephalon. The lamina affixa of the thalamus marks this line of fusion.

Inferior to the hypothalamic sulcus, the lateral walls of the diencephalon develop into the ventral thalamus and hypothalamus. The ventral thalamus remains small and is called the subthalamus. In the adult, this region is best conceptualized as a cephalic extension of the tegmentum of the midbrain.

The embryonic telencephalon is divided into pallial and subpallial regions. The pallium gives rise to the dorsal structures, including the cerebral cortex. The subpallium gives rise to the ventral structures such as the striatum and pallidum.[12] The future striatum appears during the sixth week as paired prominent swellings in the floors of the lateral ventricles. These ventricular eminences (synonym: ganglionic eminences) lie in the approximate position of the telencephalic-diencephalic fusion line.[6] The medial ventricular eminence appears first and is responsible for generating the cholinergic interneurons of the striatum, pallidum, and basal forebrain.[12] The lateral ventricular eminence develops later and is the principal source of GABAergic striatal neurons and mixed-transmitter striatal interneurons.[12] With later development of the cerebral cortex, fibers passing to and from the future cerebral cortex will extend along the line between the striatum and the thalamus to form the internal capsule.[6]

BASAL GANGLIA AND RELATED STRUCTURES

Gray Matter Structures: Descriptions and Definitions

Traditionally, the term *basal ganglia* has identified the caudate nucleus, putamen, globus pallidus, claustrum, and amygdaloid complex.[5,7] Some authors have also included the thalamus.[9] More recently, it has been restricted to the set of closely grouped, multiply interconnected, and functionally integrated cell masses composed of the caudate nucleus, putamen, external and internal nucleus of the globus pallidus (GPe and GPi), subthalamic nucleus, and substantia nigra.[9] The claustrum is now reclassified as a subinsular association area.[9] The amygdala is

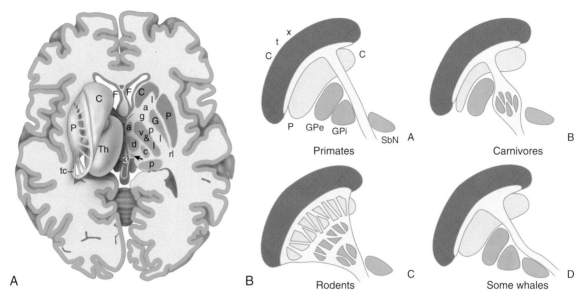

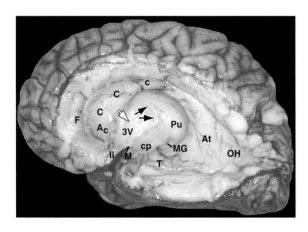

■ **FIGURE 11-1** Diagrammatic summaries of the relationships among principal components of the basal ganglia and thalami. **A,** The caudate nucleus (C) has a bulbous head that indents the frontal horn (F) of the lateral ventricle. It has a short body that lies above the thalamus (Th) and a long curving tail (tc) that passes laterally and inferiorly into the roof of the temporal horn (below the plane of this section). The putamen (P) lies lateral to the caudate nucleus but is connected to it by multiple bridges of gray matter. The gray bridges extend superior to and posterior to the central mass of the putamen. They are shorter, thicker, and more numerous anteriorly and longer, thinner, and sparser posteriorly. The individual white matter fascicles of the internal capsule arc through the gaps between the gray bridges medial to and behind the putamen. In axial cross section, these fibers describe an anterior limb (al), genu (g), and posterior limb (pl) of the internal capsule. The globus pallidus (G) lies medial to the putamen (P) within the arc of the internal capsule. Individual laminae of white matter separate the putamen from the globus pallidus and subdivide the globus pallidus (*not shown*). The thalamus contains multiple individual nuclei, separated by an internal medullary lamina. This lamina divides anteriorly to enclose the anterior nucleus (a) and splits centrally to enclose the intralaminar nuclei, one of which is the centromedian nucleus (c). The dorsomedial nucleus (d) lies medial to the internal medullary lamina. A larger number of individual ventral (v) and lateral (l) thalamic nuclei lie lateral to the lamina. The pulvinar (p) makes up the posterior pole of the thalamus. It arises as part of the lateral group but expands markedly, deflecting the internal medullary lamina anterior to it. At the posterior end of the midline third ventricle (3), paired medial and lateral habenular nuclei (*arrow*) form small masses of gray matter. The portion of the internal capsule behind the lenticular nucleus is the retrolenticular (rl) internal capsule. A sublenticular portion lies below the putamen. The structures of the basal ganglia are commonly grouped in two overlapping ways. Because the caudate nucleus and the putamen are connected, both anatomically and functionally, they may well be considered one structure, designated the striatum. Because the putamen and globus pallidus take a sector shape in cross section, they are often grouped together as the lenticular (lentiform) nucleus. Thus, the putamen falls into two commonly used groups. **B,** Coronal diagrams of the relationship of the internal capsule to the cerebral cortex (pallium) (Ctx), caudate nucleus (C), putamen (P), lateral (external) segment of the globus pallidus (GPe), medial (internal) segment of the globus pallidus (GPi), and the substantia nigra (SbN) pars reticulata. Comparative anatomy shows that the arrangement in primates (A) is just one of a number of known variations. The internal capsule may pass between GPi and SbN (primates), penetrate through one (carnivores) or both (rodents) of these nuclei or pass entirely medial to both the GPi and the SbN (some whales). Note that in rodents the internal capsule penetrates the combined caudate and putamen without forming a defined fiber bundle. (*A, Modified from Daniels DL, Haughton VM, Naidich TP. Cranial and Spinal Magnetic Resonance Imaging. An Atlas and Guide. New York, Raven Press,1987, based on an original drawing by the late Robert Albertin, 1984. B, Modified from Nauta HJW. A Simplified Perspective on the Basal Ganglia and Their Relationships to the Limbic System. New York, Raven Press, 1986.*)

■ **FIGURE 11-2** Relationship of the basal ganglia and thalamus to the lateral ventricle. Fresh gross anatomic specimen viewed from the midline toward the lateral walls of the third and lateral ventricles. The caudate nucleus resembles the convex outer surface of the head of a golf club (driver). The outer borders of the caudate and nucleus accumbens septi (Ac) form a single smooth curve that is convex anteriorly. Behind the optic chiasm (II), the mammillary body (M), cerebral peduncle (cp), medial geniculate nucleus (MG), and the pulvinar (Pu) create four distinct arcs along the undersurface of the hypothalamus-thalamus. Continuing around, the superior surface of the thalamus from the pulvinar back to the caudate head forms another smooth single curvature. Together, the basal ganglia and the thalami resemble a figure-of-eight (infinity sign) placed on its side enclosed within the arc of the frontal horn (F), atrium (At), occipital horn (OH), and temporal horn (T). The striae medullares thalamorum (*black arrows*) course posteriorly and inferiorly along the medial wall of the thalamus, defining the position of the roof of the third ventricle (3V). The optic chiasm (II) and mammillary body (M) define the floor of the third ventricle. The white arrow occupies the foramen of Monro.

better considered with the limbic system. The thalamus is described separately later in this chapter.

The *caudate nucleus* is an elongated C-shaped cell mass in the lateral wall of the lateral ventricle (Figs. 11-3 to 11-7; see also Figs. 11-1 and 11-2). Grossly, it has a bulbous head that indents the lateral wall of the frontal horn, a short body that lies along the lateral wall of the body of the lateral ventricle, and a long thin tail that curves along the lateral wall of the temporal horn to terminate in the posterior inferior putamen near the amygdala.[3,5] The C shape of the caudate nucleus recapitulates both the C shape of the cerebral cortex arrayed around the sylvian fissure and the C shape of the lateral ventricle. For much of its

claustrum

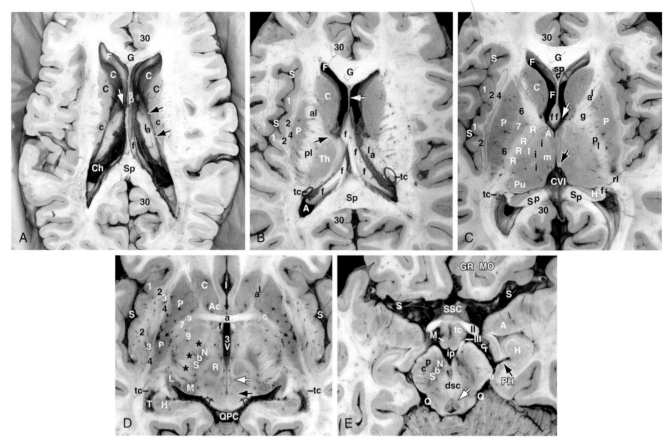

■ **FIGURE 11-3** Axial anatomic sections through the basal ganglia displayed from superior to inferior. Two specimens. **A,** Specimen 1. Section through the lateral ventricles and septum pellucidum (sp) discloses the genu (G) and splenium (Sp) of the corpus callosum, the ependyma-covered head of the caudate nucleus (*white* C) that indents the frontal horn (F) giving it its shape, the body of the caudate nucleus (*black* C, c) forming the caudate stripe along the upper lateral wall of the body of the lateral ventricle, the striothalamic (caudothalamic) groove (*black arrows*) at the junction of the caudate with the upper surface of the thalamus, the lamina affixa (la) that encloses the superior surface of the thalamus laterally (deep to the ependyma), the fornix (f) that rests atop the thalamus medially, and the choroid plexus (Ch) that passes through the choroidal fissure to emerge into the ventricle between the lateral edge of the fornix and the lamina affixa on each side. The fibers traversing the internal capsule are seen to ascend/descend through the brain just lateral to the caudate stripe. The superior lateral angles of the ventricles are enclosed only by ependyma and white matter, not gray matter. *White arrow,* foramen of Monro; 30, cingulate gyrus. **B** to **E,** Specimen 2. **B,** Asymmetric section through the frontal horns (F), atria (A), genu (G), and splenium (Sp) shows the relationship of the fornix (f) to the thalamus (Th) and choroid plexus at two levels. The tails (tc) of the caudate nuclei course along the lateral borders of the atria (A) before descending along the superior lateral margins of the temporal horns. The lamellae of the brain deep to the sylvian fissure include the insular cortex (1), extreme capsule (2), claustrum (*unlabeled*), external capsule (4), putamen (P), and the internal capsule with its anterior (al) and posterior (pl) limbs crossed by the caudatolenticular bridges of gray matter. *White arrow,* septum pellucidum; *black arrow,* striothalamic (caudothalamic) groove. **C,** Section through the thalami shows, in addition, the lateral medullary lamina of the lenticular nucleus (6), the lateral nucleus of the globus pallidus (GPe) (7), the reticular nuclei of the thalami (approximately along the row of Rs), the ventral/ lateral nuclear groups of the thalamus (*white* l), the internal medullary lamina (*black* i) of the thalamus, the anterior nucleus (A), medial nucleus (m) and pulvinar (Pu) of the thalamus, the striae medullares thalamorum (*black arrow*) along the medial wall of the thalami, the cistern of the velum interpositum (CVI), the anterior columns of the fornices (f, f) creating the anteromedial walls of the foramina of Monro (*white arrow*) at the caudal end of the septum pellucidum, and the retro-pulvinaric portions of the fornices (f) enclosing the retropulvinaric hippocampal formations (H). The thin tail (tc) of the caudate nucleus descends along the lateral wall of the atrium toward the temporal horn. spc, small cavum septi pellucidi within the anterior septum. **D,** Section through the anterior commissure shows the "π" configuration formed by the paired anterior columns of the fornices (f) descending behind the midline portion of the anterior commissure (a), the course of the anterior commissure through the lateral nucleus (7) of the globus pallidus, and the relation of the nucleus accumbens septi (Ac) and caudate nucleus to the anterior commissure (a) and anterior limb (al) of the internal capsule. The third ventricle (3V) transitions into the cerebral aqueduct. Posteriorly, the section shows the junction of the midbrain with the diencephalon and the transition (*row of asterisks*) from the internal capsule to the cerebral peduncle. The substantia nigra (SbN) and red nucleus (R) are ventral. The periaqueductal gray matter (*black arrow*) and oculomotor nucleus (CN III) (*white arrow*) lie more dorsally. The medial geniculate nucleus (M) lies at the side of the midbrain in the angle immediately posterior to the lateral edge of the cerebral peduncle. The lateral geniculate nucleus (L) lies further lateral and shows the characteristic notch in its inferior medial surface. The tails of the caudate nuclei (tc) descend along the lateral walls of the temporal horns. QPC, quadrigeminal plate cistern. **E,** Caudal section through the midbrain demonstrates the cerebral peduncle (cp) and substantia nigra (SbN) in relation to the decussation of the superior cerebellar peduncle (dsc), the aqueduct and periaqueductal gray matter, the oculomotor nucleus (*white arrow*), and the fibers of cranial nerve III (III) that emerge into the interpeduncular fossa (ip) along the medial border of the cerebral peduncle (cp). The optic chiasm (II), tuber cinereum (*white* tc), and mammillary bodies (M) lie within the suprasellar cistern (SSC). The perimesencephalic cistern comprises the interpeduncular fossa (ip) between the cerebral peduncles (cp), the crural cisterns (cr) between the midbrain and the uncus-hippocampal formation, the ambient cistern (a) between the midbrain and the parahippocampal gyrus (PH), and the quadrigeminal plate cistern (Q) between the midbrain and the medial cerebellum. GR, gyrus rectus; MO, medial orbital gyrus; S, sylvian fissure. The black arrow indicates the hippocampal fissure.

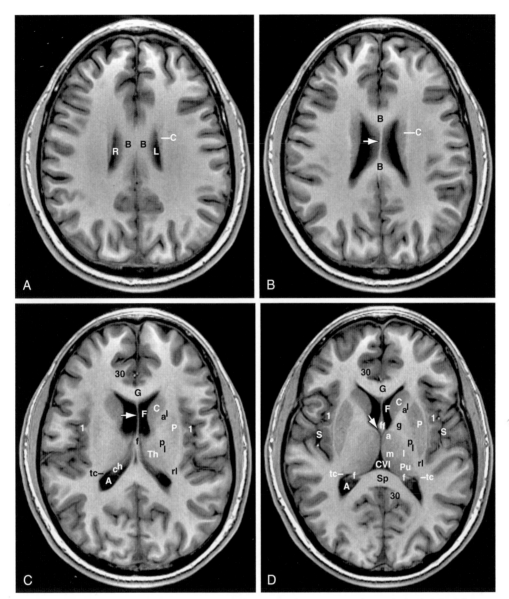

■ **FIGURE 11-4** Axial T1W MR images displayed from superior to inferior. **A** and **B,** Upper sections. The body (B) of the corpus callosum and the septum pellucidum (*single horizontal arrow*) form the medial walls of the left (L) and right (R) lateral ventricles. The body of the caudate nucleus (C) forms a thin stripe of gray matter along the upper lateral walls. **C** and **D,** The head of the caudate nucleus (C) and the thalamus (Th) lie medial to the anterior limb (al) and posterior limb (pl) of the internal capsule. The putamen (P) lies laterally, enclosed within the arc of the anterior limb, posterior limb, and retrolenticular (rl) portions of the internal capsule. The tail of the caudate nucleus (tc) runs along the lateral wall of the atrium (A) before descending into the temporal lobe. The paired fornices from each side converge to form a single body (*black* f) of the fornix inferior to the body of the corpus callosum. Nuclear groups within the thalamus (Th) include the anterior nuclei (a), the dorsomedial (mediodorsal) nucleus (m), and the combined ventral and lateral nuclei (l), which include the pulvinar (Pu). On each side, the foramen of Monro (*oblique arrow*) lies between the anterior column of the fornix and the anterior nuclei of the thalamus. The cortex of the insula (1) delimits the lateral wall of the cerebrum at the level of the third ventricle and basal ganglia. 30, cingulate gyrus; ch, choroid plexus; CVI, cistern of the velum interpositum; Sp, splenium; S, sylvian fissure.

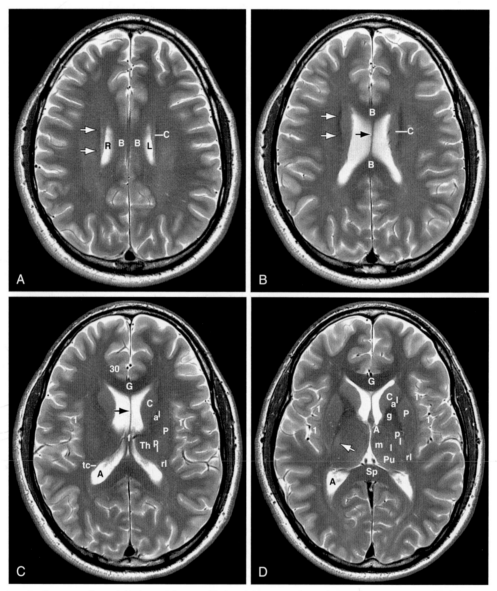

■ **FIGURE 11-5** A to D, Corresponding axial T2W MR images displayed from superior to inferior. In **B**, the superior occipitofrontal fasciculi (*white arrows*) appear as low signal stripes of compact myelinated fibers roughly parallel to the lateral walls of the ventricles. In addition to the structures labeled in Figure 11-4, T2W MR images show the capsular anatomy more clearly, including higher signal within the corticospinal tracts (*white arrow*) as they traverse the posterior limb of the internal capsule, and the flow voids of the two internal cerebral veins within the cistern of the velum interpositum just anterior to the splenium (Sp). The black arrow in **C** indicates the septum pellucidum.

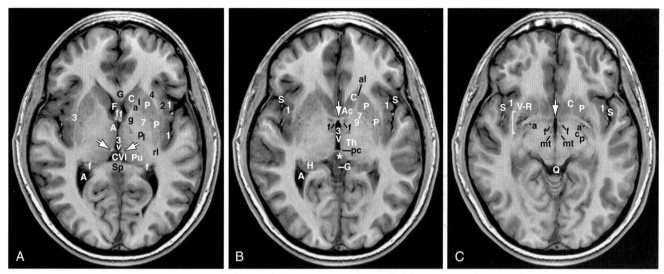

■ **FIGURE 11-6** **A** to **C,** Serial axial T1W MR images displayed from superior to inferior. **A,** The anterior columns of the fornix (f, f) appear as two adjacent well-defined white matter tracts that make up the medial walls of the foramina of Monro at the inferior ends of the septum pellucidum. The posterior portions of the fornices (f, f) lie behind the pulvinars (Pu). The habenular trigones (*paired white arrows*) lie along the side walls of the posterior third ventricle (3V) at the anterolateral margins of the cistern of the velum interpositum (CVI). **B,** The fornices (f, f) then diverge slightly and pass behind the anterior commissure (*vertical white arrow*) creating a characteristic shape resembling the Greek letter "π". The anterior limbs (al) of the internal capsule touch the lateral margins of the "π" at each side. The posterior commissure (pc) crosses the midline through the inferior wall of the stalk of the pineal gland (*asterisk*) at the posterior third ventricle. The axial plane through the top of the anterior commissure (AC) and the bottom of the posterior commissure (PC) is known as the AC-PC baseline of Talairach-Tournoux. G, vein of Galen; Ac, nucleus accumbens septi. **C,** From its midline segment (*white arrow*), the inferolateral portions (a, a) of the anterior commissure pass under the putamen in relation to the arteries and veins that pass through the anterior perforated substance to the basal ganglia. The perivascular (Virchow-Robin) spaces (*bracket:* V-R) surrounding these vessels characteristically encompass these specific segments (a, a) of the anterior commissure. The penetrating vessels and V-R spaces are characteristically more prominent anterolaterally than posteromedially. Behind the anterior commissure, the anterior columns of the fornices (f, f) continue inferiorly toward the mammillary bodies, and the mammillothalamic tracts (mt) ascend from the mammillary bodies toward the anterior nuclei of the thalami (*seen on more superior sections*). Q, quadrigeminal plate cistern. Other labels as indicated earlier.

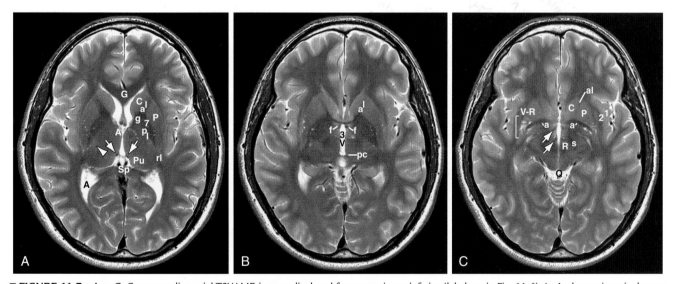

■ **FIGURE 11-7** **A** to **C,** Corresponding axial T2W MR images displayed from superior to inferior (labels as in Fig. 11-6). In **A,** the corticospinal tracts (*white arrowhead*) again display higher signal intensity, and the paired internal cerebral veins course through the cistern of the velum interpositum. In **C,** the two arrows indicate the anterior column of the fornix in front and the mammillothalamic tract behind. R, red nucleus; s, substantia nigra.

length, the caudate nucleus abuts onto the superior lateral thalamus. Their junction forms the striothalamic groove (synonyms: caudothalamic groove, sulcus terminalis) (see Fig. 11-2).[5] The stria and vena terminalis course along this groove deep to the ependyma.[5]

The *nucleus accumbens* is an inferomedial expansion of the caudate head. Grossly, it extends under the anterior portion of the lateral ventricle into the medial (septal) wall of the cerebral

hemisphere, forming a prominent bulge (Fig. 11-8; see also Figs. 11-3D and 11-6B).[9]

The *putamen* is the larger dark gray portion of the striatum that lies deep to the internal capsule and lateral to the globus pallidus (see later) (see Figs. 11-1 and 11-3 to 11-9).

The *olfactory tubercle* is the part of the anterior perforated substance that lies immediately posterior to the division of the olfactory tract into the medial and lateral olfactory striae on each

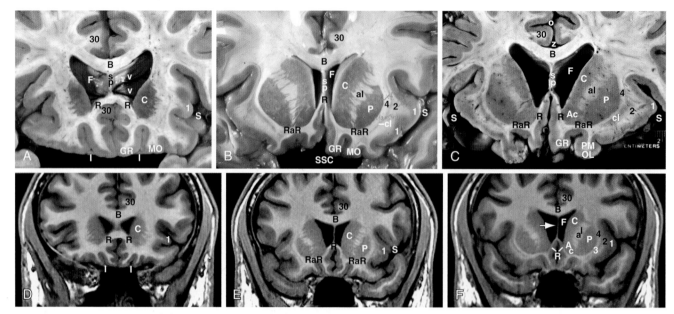

■ **FIGURE 11-8** **A** to **F,** Coronal plane images and gross anatomic sections displayed from anterior to posterior. **A,** Section through the frontal horns (F) displays the cingulate gyrus (30) encircling the body (B) and rostrum (R) of the corpus callosum. The smooth medial border of the head of the caudate nucleus (C) indents the frontal horn. The lateral border of the caudate head is characteristically serrated where it gives rise to the caudatolenticular bridges of gray matter (gray bridges) that pass to the putamen (*see next cuts*). Subependymal veins (v v) on the anterior wall of the frontal horn converge to the septum. Inferiorly, cranial nerve (CN) I lies along the inferior surface of the olfactory sulcus between the gyrus rectus (GR) and the medial orbital gyrus (MO). Laterally, the sylvian fissure (S) and insula (1) form the lateral surface of the deep brain. **B** and **C,** Coronal sections display the caudate head (C) united to the putamen (P) through the nucleus accumbens septi (Ac) anterior inferior and medial to the anterior limb (al) of the internal capsule. Fibers radiating (RaR) through the rostrum (R) pass inferior to the deep gray nuclei, defining the lower border of the ganglia. Superiorly, the body of the corpus callosum (B), pericallosal sulcus (z), cingulate gyrus (30) and cingulate sulcus (o) define the upper border of the deep brain. Further posteriorly, the anterior limb (al) of the internal capsule wedges between the caudate head (C) and the putamen (P) to just "kiss" the anterior commissure (a) on each side. Residual gray bridges interconnect the caudate with the putamen across the anterior limb. This far anteriorly, the lenticular nuclei display only the putamen (P). Postero-inferiorly, the posteromedial orbital lobule (PMOL) projects back into the suprasellar cistern (SSC). **D** to **F,** Corresponding T1W coronal plane MR images displayed from anterior to posterior.

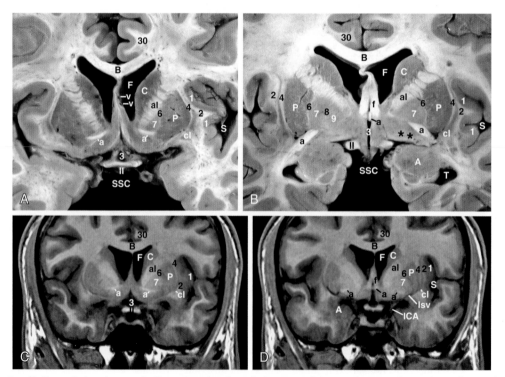

■ **FIGURE 11-9** **A** to **D,** Coronal plane images. **A,** Coronal section through the genus of the anterior commissure shows the anterior limbs (al) of the internal capsules touching the anterior commissure just medial to the genus. The anterior commissure passes through the bottom of the lateral nucleus (7) of the globus pallidus. Septal veins (v) are seen along the medial wall of the frontal horns (F). II, optic chiasm; 3, third ventricle; SSC, suprasellar cistern. **B,** Straight coronal section through the apex of the lenticular nucleus. From lateral to medial the layers of gray (*white numbers*) and white (*black numbers*) matter form a coherent series: sylvian fissure (S), cortex of insula (1), extreme capsule (2), claustrum (3), external capsule (4), putamen (P), lateral lamina of the lenticular nucleus (6), lateral nucleus of the globus pallidus (GPe) (7), medial lamina of the lenticular nucleus (8), medial nucleus of the globus pallidus (GPi) (9), and internal capsule. The claustrum (cl) becomes more prominent inferiorly and extends medially through the substantia innominata (*asterisks*) to the amygdala (A). **C** and **D,** Corresponding T1W coronal plane MR images. A, amygdala; ICA, internal carotid artery; lsv, lenticulostriate vessels (arteries and/or veins). The supraoptic recess of the third ventricle (3) lies immediately superior to the optic chiasm (II). Other labels as in **A** and **B.**

side.[9] The olfactory tubercle covers the superficial aspect of the nucleus accumbens and the head of the caudate nucleus. It receives direct sensory fibers from the olfactory bulb.

The term *corpus striatum* includes the caudate nucleus, the putamen, and the medial and lateral nuclei of the globus pallidus

(Figs. 11-9 to 11-11).[5] The name is said to derive from either the small-diameter, nonmyelinated to thinly myelinated striatal afferents and efferents that traverse these nuclei or the fiber bundles of the internal capsule that cross between the caudate nucleus and the putamen.

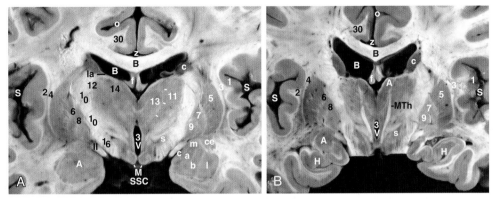

■ **FIGURE 11-10** Gross anatomic coronal plane images displayed from anterior to posterior. **A,** Section through the midthalami and midlenticular nuclei. The reticular nuclei of the thalami lie between the posterior limb (10) of the internal capsule laterally and the external medullary lamina of the thalamus medially (12). The internal medullary lamina of the thalamus (14 on right, *tick marks on left*) separates the ventral and lateral group of thalamic nuclei (11) from the medial group (13). The lamina affixa (la) delimits the upper surface of the thalamus laterally. In the midline, the bodies of the fornices overlie the medial thalami. The mammillary bodies (M) form part of the inferior wall of the third ventricle (3V). Their white matter capsule is just visible. The putamen is seen to be continuous with the amygdala (*upper A*) bilaterally. Multiple individual nuclei within the amygdala include the lateral nucleus (l), basal nucleus (b), accessory basal nucleus (a), cortical nucleus (c), medial nucleus (m), and central nucleus (ce). II, optic tract; 30, cingulate gyrus; o, cingulate sulcus; s, subthalamic nucleus; z, pericallosal sulcus. **B,** The mammillothalamic tracts (MTh) show their characteristic "antelope horn" configuration as they ascend from the mammillary bodies (*not present in this section*) to the anterior nuclei (*upper A*) of the thalamus. The anterior hippocampal formations (H) are now seen at the floor of the temporal horns. 30, cingulate gyrus; o, cingulate sulcus; s, subthalamic nucleus; z, pericallosal sulcus.

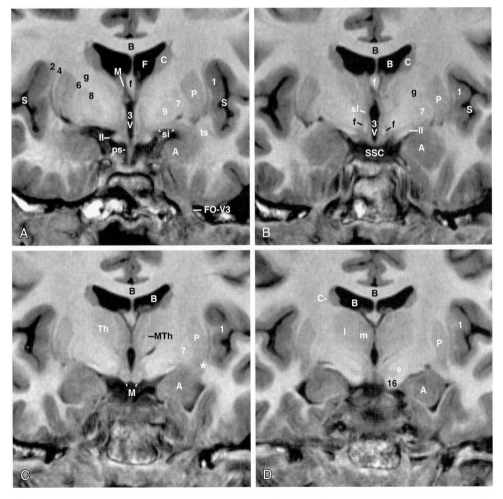

■ **FIGURE 11-11** Corresponding coronal T1W MR images displayed from anterior to posterior. **A,** The layered gray matter of the cortex and nuclei (*white odd numbers*) and white matter laminae (*black even numbers*) correspond to the anatomic images of Figure 11-9. The narrow temporal stem (ts) connects the temporal lobe with the deep frontal lobe. The mandibular division (V3) of the trigeminal nerve emerges from the skull through the foramen ovale (FO). **B,** The focal diamond-shaped widening of the third ventricle (3V) corresponds to the sulcus limitans (sl), a groove along the lateral wall of the diencephalon, which marks the division between the thalamus superiorly and the hypothalamus inferiorly. It corresponds directly to the sulcus limitans of the early neural tube, which separated the dorsal alar plate (sensory) from the ventral basal plate (motor). **C,** The mammillothalamic tracts (MTh) pass from the mammillary bodies (M) to the anterior nuclei of the thalami. (See also Figs. 11-10B and 11-24A.) A, amygdala; M, foramen of Monro; ps, pituitary stalk; si, substantia innominata. **D,** The internal medullary lamina divides the thalamus into medial (m) and combined ventral + lateral (l) nuclear groups. 16, cerebral peduncle.

The term *dorsal striatum* refers to the vast bulk of the caudate nucleus, putamen, and globus pallidus that is connected predominantly with motor and association areas of the cortex.[5,9]

The *ventral striatum* refers to the inferomedial portion of the striatum, including the nucleus accumbens and the greater portion of the olfactory tubercle. These connect predominantly with the limbic system, the orbitofrontal cortex, and the temporal cortex.[5]

The *globus pallidus* is a composite structure formed from the lateral (external) nucleus of the globus pallidus (GPe) and the medial (internal) nucleus of the globus pallidus (GPi) (see Figs. 11-1 and 11-9 to 11-11). Grossly, the globus pallidus is a conical structure situated within the hollow cone of the internal capsule, deep to the putamen. The widest portion of the cone is directed laterally, toward the insula, so the lateral nucleus of the globus pallidus is wider than the medial nucleus in all directions. The globus pallidus is traversed by numerous bundles of heavily myelinated fibers, which give it the lighter (pallid) color in fresh specimens.[9] The lateral and medial nuclei (GPe and GPi) have distinct afferents, efferents, and functions.[5] The anterior commissure traverses the inferior portion of the lateral pallidal nucleus (GPe).

The *dorsal pallidum* is the major portion of the globus pallidus situated superior to the anterior commissure.[5]

The *ventral pallidum* is the small portion of the pallidum situated inferior to the anterior commissure and extending inferiorly into the substantia innominata (see Fig. 11-9).[5]

The term *lenticular nucleus* (synonym: lentiform nucleus) refers to the combination of the putamen and the two portions of the globus pallidus (see Figs. 11-6 to 11-8). Because the putamen and globus pallidus lie within the cone of the internal capsule, axial and coronal sections through these nuclei give them a lenticular or sector shape, resembling a slice of pizza. Multiple medullary laminae separate and delimit the individual portions of the lenticular nucleus. These include the external (lateral) medullary lamina between the putamen and GPe, the internal (medial) medullary lamina between GPe and GPi, and the incomplete medullary lamina within the GPi.[9]

The *substantia innominata* is an ill-defined flattened cell mass situated immediately inferior to the putamen and globus pallidus (see Fig. 11-9). Grossly, it lies within the basal portion of the brain just above the basal cisterns and extends transversely between the lateral hypothalamus medially and amygdala laterally. It is partly separated from the putamen and globus pallidus by the anterior commissure.[9] It contains the basal nucleus of Meynert.

The *basal nucleus of Meynert* is a population of large cholinergic cells dispersed within the substantia innominata and projecting to the neocortex.[9] With other cholinergic nuclei, it provides excitatory input to the entire cerebral cortex, particularly the paralimbic areas.[13] The size of this cell population increases with the size of the telencephalon, so it is largest in primates and cetaceans.[9]

The *subthalamic nucleus* is a lenticular cell mass situated in the caudal (ventral) diencephalon.[1,4,6,9,10] Grossly, it lies just dorsal to the internal capsule where the internal capsule transitions into the cerebral peduncle (Figs. 11-12 to 11-17). The medial portion of the subthalamic nucleus overlaps the rostral portion of the substantia nigra.[9] It is encapsulated dorsally by axons, including fibers of the subthalamic fasciculus arising from the GPe.[5]

The *substantia nigra* is a large mesencephalic nucleus composed of a pars reticulata (SNr), a pars compacta (SNc), and a small pars lateralis (SNl) (Fig. 11-18). Grossly, the SNr and SNc form nearly separate cell layers oriented parallel with and immediately dorsal to the cerebral peduncle. The pars reticulata forms the layer immediately dorsal to the cerebral peduncle. The pars compacta forms the layer behind the pars reticulata, ventral to the tegmentum. The most rostral

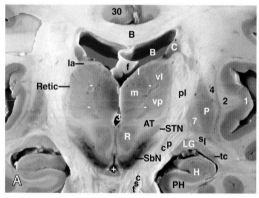
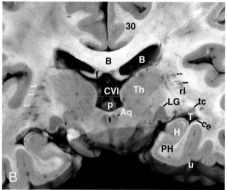

■ **FIGURE 11-12**   Gross anatomic coronal plane images displayed from anterior to posterior. **A,** Posterior lenticular section. The claustrum forms a thin sheet of gray matter between the extreme (2) and the external (4) capsules. This posterior section passes behind the medial nucleus of the globus pallidus, so the lenticular nucleus displays only the putamen (P) and lateral nucleus (7). The sublenticular portion (sl) of the internal capsule separates the lenticular nucleus from the lateral geniculate nucleus (LG) and the tail of the caudate nucleus (tc). The posterior limbs (pl) and cerebral peduncles (cp) continue into the corticospinal tracts (cst) on each side. These enclose the gray matter of the diencephalon and midbrain. Superiorly, the reticular nuclei (Retic) form a layer of gray matter just lateral to the external medullary lamina of the thalamus. The internal medullary laminae of the thalami (*white tick marks*) separate the thalamic nuclei into medial (m) and ventral groups. In this plane, the ventral group includes the ventrolateral (vl) and ventral posterior (vp) nuclei. The lateral dorsal nucleus (l) of the lateral group is situated superiorly. The lamina affixa (la) encloses the superolateral surface of the thalamus. Inferiorly, the lower third ventricle (3) and interpeduncular fossa (+) mark the midline. From lateral to medial, the cerebral peduncle (cp), substantia nigra (SbN), subthalamic nucleus (STN), area tegmentalis (AT), and red nucleus (R) present a characteristic appearance. The red nuclei resemble snake eyes. The subthalamic nucleus lies between the red nucleus and the substantia nigra, with the equator of the subthalamic nucleus approximately at the level of the upper pole of the red nucleus. The area tegmentalis (AT) flares upward and outward from the red nuclei to pass under the thalami. **B,** Retrolenticular section. The retrolenticular portion of the internal capsule is marked only by the caudatolenticular gray bridges (*white and black tick marks*) that pass through it. The cistern of the velum interpositum (CVI) and pineal gland (p) lie between the posterior thalami (Th) and above the aqueduct and periaqueductal gray matter (Aq) of the midbrain. The lateral geniculate nuclei (LG) show a characteristic "Napoleon's hat" configuration in coronal plane. The tail of the caudate nucleus (tc) lies at the roof of the temporal horn laterally. The hippocampal formation (H) indents the floor of the temporal horn inferomedially. The collateral sulcus (u) delimits the lateral border of the parahippocampal gyrus (PH). Deep invagination of the collateral sulcus elevates the floor of the temporal horn laterally, forming a bump designated the collateral eminence (ce).

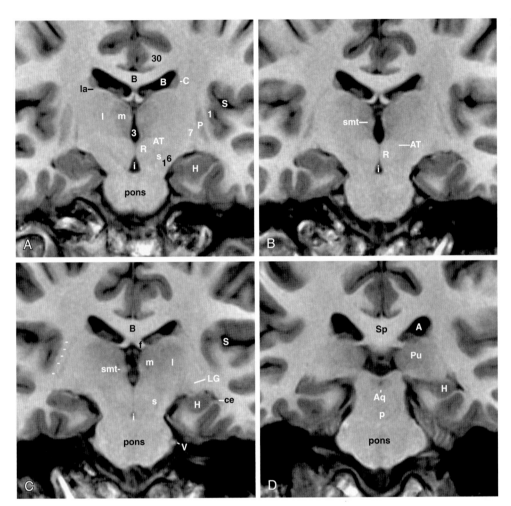

■ **FIGURE 11-13** A to D, Corresponding coronal T1W MR images displayed from anterior to posterior (labels as in Fig. 11-12).16, cerebral peduncle; i, interpeduncular fossa; s, substantia nigra; smt, stria medullaris thalami; V, fifth cranial nerve (trigeminal nerve) emerging from the side of the pons.

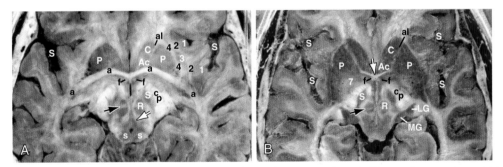

■ **FIGURE 11-14** A and B, Anterior commissure and brain stem. Axial cryomicrotome sections. **A,** The anterior commissure (a) is a highly compact fiber bundle that extends transversely across much of the brain in the shape of bicycle handlebars. From its midline position in the anterior wall of the third ventricle, the anterior commissure first passes anterolaterally to a genu (a). This first segment is related to the caudate nucleus (C) and the nucleus accumbens septi (Ac) anteriorly and to the anterior columns of the fornices (f, f) posteriorly. The anterior limb (al) of the internal capsule just touches the anterior superior surface of the anterior commissure immediately medial to the genu. The second segment of the anterior commissure (outer pair of "a") angles posteroinferolaterally through the temporal stem into the temporal lobe where it breaks up into individual fascicles too small to resolve. In the midbrain, the prominent habenulointerpeduncular tract (fasciculus retroflexus) (*black arrow*) grooves the red nucleus (R) on each side. The oculomotor nuclei (CN III) (*white arrow*) lie just anterolateral to the aqueduct of Sylvius and periaqueductal gray matter. Also labeled are the superior colliculi (small *white* s, s). **B,** The distinct discoids of the subthalamic nuclei (small *white* s in **B**) lie partially between the red nuclei (R) and the cerebral peduncle (cp). Also labeled are sylvian fissures (S), putamen (P), lateral nucleus of the globus pallidus (7), lateral geniculate nucleus (LG), and medial geniculate nucleus (MG). (*Modified from Naidich TP, Daniels DL, Haughton VM. Deep cerebral structures. In Daniels DL, Haughton VM, Naidich TP [eds]. Cranial and Spinal Magnetic Resonance Imaging: An Atlas and Guide. New York, Raven Press, 1987.*)

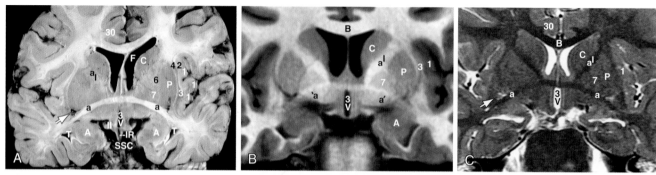

■ **FIGURE 11-15**   A to C, Oblique coronal plane images through the anterior commissure. **A,** Gross anatomic section through the anterior commissure (a) demonstrates its inferolateral path from the anterior wall of the third ventricle (3V) in the midline under the anterior limb of the internal capsule (al), through the inferior portion of the lateral nucleus of globus pallidus (GPe) (7), under the putamen (P), through the temporal stem, over the amygdala (A), and over the temporal horn (T) into the temporal lobe. Multiple vessels (*arrow*) penetrate the anterior perforated substance in relation to the segment of the anterior commissure just inferior to the putamen. Inferiorly, the infundibular recess (IR) of the third ventricle (3) passes downward just behind the optic chiasm (II). **B and C,** Corresponding T1W (**B**) and T2W (**C**) MR images in two different patients.

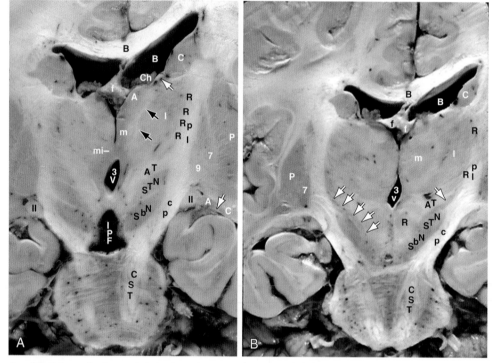

■ **FIGURE 11-16**   A and B, Substantia nigra, subthalamic nucleus, zona incerta, and thalamus. Gross coronal anatomic sections through the diencephalic-mesencephalic junction. **A,** Anterior section through the anterior thalamus, massa intermedia (mi), and interpeduncular fossa (IPF). Superiorly, the stria and vena terminalis (*white arrow*) lie at the floor of the body (B) of the lateral ventricle in the striothalamic (caudothalamic) groove. They both curve inferiorly along the ventricular wall into the roof of the temporal horn (*white arrow*). The mammillothalamic tract (*black arrows*) ascends from the mammillary body to the anterior nucleus of the thalamus on each side. The reticular nuclei of the thalamus (row of Rs) form a thin lamina deep to the posterior limb of the internal capsule (pl) and just lateral to the external medullary lamina of the thalamus. The corticospinal tract (CST) continues inferiorly from the posterior limb through the cerebral peduncle into the pons. The substantia nigra (SbN) and subthalamic nuclei (STN) form stacked tiers of gray matter, enclosed by the cerebral peduncle (cp) and area tegmentalis (AT). Here the term *area tegmentalis* is used as an umbrella term for the multiple tracts passing through this region to interconnect the roof nuclei of the cerebellum. the red nucleus, the thalamus, and the cerebral hemisphere. **B,** Posterior to the massa intermedia, in a section through the depths of the interpeduncular fossa, the substantia nigra and subthalamic nucleus have become smaller. The sinuous zona incerta (*white arrows*) curves through the area tegmentalis (AT) from the medial aspect of the subthalamic nucleus (STN) to the lateral aspect of the thalamus. The habenulointerpeduncular tract (fasciculus retroflexus) curves around the red nucleus (R), forming a prominent white matter tract along its margin. The fibers that arise from the globus pallidus to pass through the H, H1, and H2 fields of Forel are defined by their relation to the subthalamic nucleus and zona incerta (see Fig. 11-19). Superiorly, the internal medullary lamina of the thalamus is seen between the medial (m) and ventral/lateral (v & l) groups of thalamic nuclei.

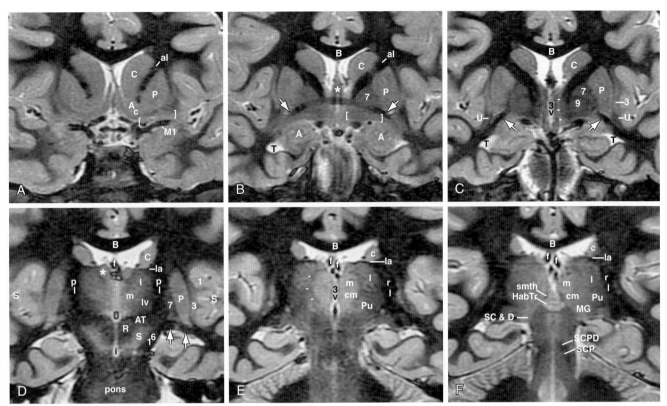

■ **FIGURE 11-17** A to F, Diencephalon. Coronal T2W inversion recovery MR images displayed from anterior to posterior. **A,** Anteriorly, the head of the caudate nucleus (C) is continuous with the putamen (P) through the nucleus accumbens septi (Ac) anterior and inferior to the anterior limb (al) of the internal capsule. The substantia innominata (*between white brackets*) lies within the inferior frontal lobe below the putamen and below the white matter that makes up the capsules of the basal ganglia and the radiations through the rostrum of the corpus callosum. The first segment of the middle cerebral artery (M1) runs in the sylvian fissure just below the substantia innominata. **B,** The anterior commissure (*white arrows*) forms a prominent landmark. From medial to lateral, the paired anterior columns of the fornices (*below asterisk*) pass behind the anterior commissure. The anterior limb (al) of the internal capsule just touches the top of the anterior commissure. The anterior commissure passes through the bottom of the lateral nucleus (7) of the globus pallidus, then under putamen (P), through the temporal stem, over the amygdala (A), and over the temporal horn (T) to disperse within the temporal lobe. The substantia innominata (*between the brackets*) largely lies inferior to the anterior commissure. **C,** Just behind the anterior commissure, the anterior columns of the fornices (*tick marks*) pass down to the mammillary bodies on both sides of the third ventricle (3V). The lateral portions of the anterior commissure (*white arrows*) pass through the temporal stem medial to the uncinate fasciculi (U). This plane passes through the full extent of the lenticular nucleus, including the putamen (P), lateral (7) and medial (9) nuclei of the globus pallidus, and the laminae between them. **D,** Section through the posterior lenticular nuclei, thalami, and upper brain stem shows the posterior limbs (pl) of the internal capsule and the cerebral peduncles (cp) as two arms of a parenthesis that encloses the paired thalami, red nuclei (R), and substantiae nigrae (S). Within the thalami, MR resolves the paired anterior nuclei (*white asterisk on right side*), medial (m), lateral (l), and lateral ventral (lv) nuclei. The heavily myelinated area tegmentalis (AT) (H field of Forel) forms a characteristic "upper butterfly wing" superolateral to the red nuclei. It contains a dense feltwork of fibers passing to, emerging from, or bypassing the red nucleus, including fibers from the dentate nucleus to the red nucleus, thalamus, and subthalamus, fibers from the red nucleus to the frontal lobes, and fibers passing from the lenticular nuclei to the thalami.[4] Lateral to the posterior limbs (pl) are the residual posterior portions of the insular cortex (1), claustrum (3), putamen (P), and lateral nucleus of the globus pallidus (GPe) (7). The interpeduncular fossa (i) identifies the midline of the midbrain anteriorly. **E,** Section behind lenticular nuclei shows the retrolenticular (rl) portion of the internal capsule, the lamina affixa (la) atop the thalamus laterally, and the internal medullary lamina (*white tick marks*) that divides the thalamus into nuclear compartments. At this level the thalamic nuclei include the medial (m), centromedian (cm), lateral (l), and pulvinar (Pu). **F,** Section through the posterior thalamus and superior colliculi shows the paired myelinated striae medullares thalamorum (smth) passing posteriorly to join the habenular trigones (HabTr). The superior colliculi (SC) and their decussation (D) lie just posteroinferior to the habenulae. Within the midbrain, the superior cerebellar peduncles (SCP) ascend and begin to bend medially toward their decussation (SCPD). The aqueduct and periaqueductal gray matter lie in the midline posterior and inferior to the habenulae and their commissure. MG, medial geniculate nucleus.

portion of the substantia nigra extends superiorly to approach the globus pallidus.[9]

The *pars reticulata* is composed of cells that strongly resemble the cells of the GPi. Histologically and functionally, the SNr is best regarded as a portion of the GPi that was isolated when the internal capsule developed and grew down into the cerebral peduncle.[9] The Gpi and the SNr provide the major motor output from the lenticular nucleus to the thalamus.

The *pars compacta* and the small pars lateralis are composed of large darkly pigmented cells that synthesize dopamine. Their dark color results from neuromelanin pigment that is synthesized as a by-product of catecholamine metabolism, so the pigment is

present even in albino patients.[9] The partes compacta and lateralis constitute the dopaminergic cell group A9. The A9 cells are continuous with each other through the ventral tegmental dopamine cell group A10 (synonym: paranigral nucleus).[5] SNc provides the dopaminergic supply to the ventral striatum, adjoining dorsal striatum, prefrontal cortex, and anterior cingulate cortex.[5]

The *zona incerta* is a thin sinuous, serpentine nucleus that lies within the ventral thalamus just dorsal to the subthalamic nucleus and inferior to the thalamus (Fig. 11-19; see also Fig. 11-16).[4,10] It represents a cephalic extension of the reticular nuclei of the brain stem and merges into the reticular nuclei of the ventral thalamus.

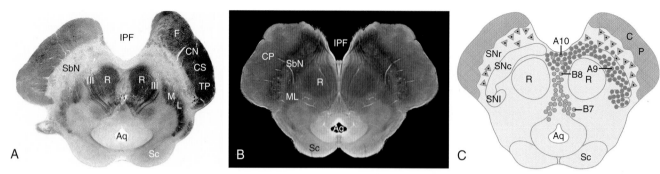

■ **FIGURE 11-18** **A** to **C,** Substantia nigra and neurotransmitters. Axial sections of the midbrain oriented with ventral anterior to correspond to standard MR display. **A,** Histologic section. Klüver-Barrera stain in which Luxol fast blue stains the myelin bright blue and cresyl violet stains Nissl bodies, nuclei, and nucleoli purplish. The *yellow dots* identify melanized neurons. **B,** Postmortem intermediate-weighted 9.4-T MR image of a formalin-fixed midbrain. **C,** Diagram of the distribution of the dopaminergic neurons (*blue dots*) of cell groups A9 and A10 and the serotoninergic cell groups of the raphe, B7 and B8 (*pink dots*). **A** to **C,** The substantia nigra (SbN) lies immediately dorsomedial to the cerebral peduncles (CP) and ventrolateral to the red nucleus (R) and the medial lemniscus (ML). Substantia nigra pars reticulata (SNr) lies ventrally, against the cerebral peduncle. Substantia nigra pars compacta (SNc) lies dorsomedial to SNr. A small dorsolateral component of substantia nigra is designated pars lateralis (SNl). The dopaminergic neurons of SNc and SNl form cell group A9 on each side. These are continuous with each other through the midline dopaminergic cell group A10. Serotonergic cell groups B7 and B8 (*pink dots*) occupy the raphe. Within the peduncle, the fibers are organized from medial to lateral as frontopontine fibers (F), corticonuclear fibers (CN), corticospinal fibers (CS), and temporoparietal pontine fibers (TP). The fibers of the oculomotor nerves (CN III) (III) describe beautiful reciprocal curves as they pass ventrally from the oculomotor nuclei at the ventral aspect of the periaqueductal gray matter through the red nuclei to emerge in the interpeduncular fossa (IPF) along the medial walls of the cerebral peduncles. Aq, cerebral aqueduct; Sc, superior colliculus. Yellow triangles, GABAergic neurons. (**A,** *courtesy of Dr. Tauba Pasik and Dr. Pedro Pasik, New York.*)

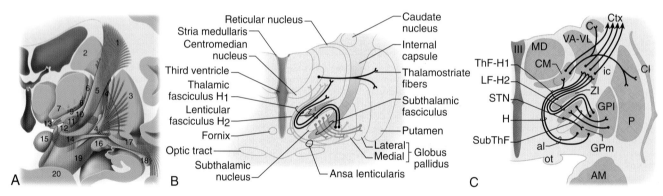

■ **FIGURE 11-19** **A** and **B,** Ansa lenticularis and Forel fields. **A,** Diagram of the anatomic relationships among the nuclei and some of the fiber tracts originating from, or passing near to, the basal ganglia. 1, Corona radiata; 2, body of the caudate nucleus; 3, putamen; 4, strionigral fibers; 5, posterior limb of the internal capsule; 6, reticular nuclei of the thalamus; 7, centromedian nucleus of the thalamus; 8, thalamic fasciculus (Forel field H1); 9, zona incerta; 10, lenticular fasciculus (Forel field H2); 11, subthalamic nucleus; 12, substantia nigra; 13, parafascicular nucleus; 14, ansa lenticularis; 15, red nucleus; 16, optic tract; 17, sublenticular portion of the internal capsule; 18, tail of the caudate nucleus; 19, cerebral peduncle; 20, pons. **B,** Classic diagram of the anatomic relationships of the fibers emerging from the globus pallidus and passing to target nuclei (pallidofugal system). The ansa lenticularis (*yellow*) arises from the outer portion of GPi, lateral to the incomplete medullary lamina of GPi and possibly GPe. These fibers pass ventrally, medially, and rostrally, around the internal capsule to enter the prerubral field (Forel field H; see label in **C**). Fibers of the lenticular fasciculus (*black*) (Forel field H2) arise from the dorsal side of the GPi, pass medially across the posterior limb of the internal capsule, and continue dorsal to the subthalamic nucleus to enter the prerubral field H. The ansa lenticularis and the lenticular fasciculus (H2) merge in the prerubral field H and project dorsolaterally as a component of the thalamic fasciculus (Forel field H1). The fibers in the thalamic fasciculus pass dorsomedial to the zona incerta (ZI) to reach the ventral anterior and ventral lateral nuclei of the thalamus. The subthalamic fasciculus (*blue*) consists of pallidosubthalamic fibers that cross through the internal capsule to GPi and GPe where they terminate in arrays parallel to the medullary lamina in both GPe and GPi. Thalamostriate fibers project from the thalamus to the putamen as part of a feedback system. **C,** Diagram of selected fiber bundles interconnecting the diencephalon with the telencephalon. AM, amygdaloid complex; al, ansa lenticularis; C, caudate nucleus; Cl, claustrum; CM, centromedian nucleus of the thalamus; Ctx, cerebral cortex; LF, lenticular fasciculus (H2); SubThF, subthalamic fasciculus; ThF, thalamic fasciculus (H1); GPl, lateral nucleus of globus pallidus; GPm, medial nucleus of globus pallidus; H, H1, and H2, tegmental fields of Forel; ic, internal capsule; ot, optic tract; P, putamen; STN, subthalamic nucleus; VA and VL, ventral anterior and ventral lateral nuclei of the thalamus; ZI, zona incerta; III, third ventricle. (**A** and **C,** *Modified from Nieuwenhuys R, Voogd J, van Huijzen C. The Human Central Nervous System, 4th ed. Berlin, Springer, 2008.* **B,** *From Carpenter MB, Sutin J. Human Neuroanatomy, 8th ed. Baltimore, Williams & Wilkins, 1983.*)

The *claustrum* is a thin sheet of gray matter that lies deep to the insular cortex. It has dorsal and ventral components. The compact dorsal (subinsular) portion is interposed between the extreme and external capsules (see Figs. 11-1, 11-8 to 11-10, 11-20 and 11-21). The more diffuse ventral (temporal) component extends inferolaterally into the temporal lobe to reach the amygdala. The ventral component is interrupted by the white fascicles of the anterior commissure and the uncinate fasciculus as they pass outward, lateral to the amygdaloid complex.[9]

White Matter Structures

The white matter structures of the cerebrum are discussed and illustrated in Chapter 12. The white matter structures specifically related anatomically and/or functionally to the deep gray nuclei are discussed here.

The term *internal capsule* designates the portions of the ascending and descending white matter fibers that are juxtaposed to the caudate nucleus and thalamus medially and to the lenticular nuclei laterally (see Figs. 11-1, 11-3, 11-8, 11-9, 11-12, 11-13, 11-20, and 11-21).[13] These fibers also pass superior and inferior to these nuclei but are given other names in those locations. Grossly, the internal capsule takes the shape of a hollow cone, with its open end directed laterally. The lenticular nucleus fills the hollow within the cone. The anterior limb of the internal capsule lies between the head of the caudate nucleus and the lenticular nucleus. The genu forms the most medial portion of the cone, enclosing the globus pallidus. The posterior limb lies between the thalamus and the lenticular nucleus. The retrolenticular and sublenticular portions lie posterior to and inferior to the putamen, respectively. Within the internal capsule, the corticobulbar fibers for the muscles of the head lie anterior to the corticospinal fibers for the body. The corticospinal tract traverses the posterior half of the posterior limb. The fibers for the upper extremity lie anterior to those for the lower extremity. The optic radiations cross through the retrolenticular internal capsule. The auditory radiations pass through the sublenticular internal capsule.

The term *comb system* designates the bundles of small striatal and coarse pallidal fibers passing through the internal capsule and cerebral peduncle, lending them a "tined" appearance.[9]

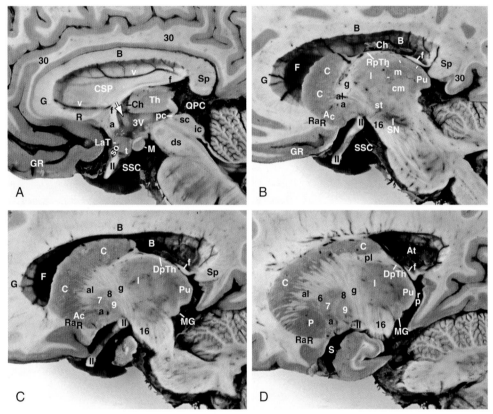

■ **FIGURE 11-20** A to H, Sagittal sections of a formalin-fixed gross anatomic specimen displayed from midline toward lateral. Refer to Figure 11-3. **A,** Midline sagittal section. There is a cavum septi pellucidi (CSP) with septal veins (v) coursing along its lateral wall. The foramen of Monro (*white arrow*) interconnects the lateral ventricle (*hidden by the cavum*) with the third ventricle (3V). The fornix (f) extends anteriorly from the undersurface of the corpus callosum, makes up the anteromedial wall of the foramen of Monro, and descends behind the anterior commissure (a) en route to the mammillary bodies (M). The supraoptic recess (so) of the third ventricle lies just superior to the optic chiasm (II). 30, cingulate gyrus; *black B*, body of the corpus callosum; Ch, choroid plexus at the foramen of Monro; Ds, decussation of the superior cerebellar peduncle; G, genu of the corpus callosum; GR, gyrus rectus; ic, inferior colliculus; QPC, quadrigeminal plate cistern; sc, superior colliculus; SSC, suprasellar cistern; t, tuber cinereum; Th, thalamus. **B,** The corpus callosum encircles the lateral ventricle. The radiations of the rostrum (RaR) define the bottom of the basal ganglia anteriorly. The anterior limb (al) and genu (g) form a narrow arc of white matter. The anterior limb just touches the anterior commissure (a). The rostral peduncle of the thalamus (RpTh) passes posterosuperiorly. The caudate nucleus (C) is continuous with the nucleus accumbens septi (Ac) anterior and inferior to the anterior limb. The internal medullary lamina of the thalamus (*arched group of 3 white ticks*) demarcates the lateral nuclei (l) from the medial (m) and centromedian (cm) nuclei. The pulvinar (pu) makes a prominent beak at the posterior pole of the thalamus. Inferiorly, the optic nerve and chiasm (II) cross the suprasellar cistern to reach the cerebral peduncle (16). The subthalamic nucleus (st) and substantia nigra (SN) lie at the ventral aspect of the midbrain. **C,** Farther laterally, the anterior limb (al) and genu (g) form a slightly wider arc enclosing the lateral (7) and medial (9) nuclei of the globus pallidus (Gpe and GPi). The caudate nucleus (C) and the nucleus accumbens septi (Ac) are coextensive anterior and inferior to the anterior limb. The medial geniculate nucleus (MG) now forms a distinctive curve along the posterior border of the brain stem inferior to the pulvinar (pu). **D,** The anterior limb (al) now reaches to the anterior margin of the gray matter separating the caudate (C) from the putamen (P). The anterior limb (al), genu (g), and posterior limb (pl) form a distinct shape resembling eyebrows and a nose (or a sea anchor upside down). The wider arc of the anterior limb and genu enclose, from anterior to posterior, the putamen (P), lateral lamina of the lenticular nucleus (6), lateral nucleus of the globus pallidus (GPe) (7), medial lamina of the lenticular nucleus (8), and medial nucleus of the globus pallidus (GPi) (9). The lateral and medial nucleus of globus pallidus "snug up" against the anterior wall of the genu. The anterior commissure (a) courses in the inferior aspect of the lateral nucleus of the globus pallidus, marking its location. The optic tract (II) circumscribes the lateral border of the cerebral peduncle (16). The ventral and lateral groups of thalamic nuclei (l) lie anterior to the pulvinar (Pu). The retropulvinaric cistern (rp) separates the pulvinar from the temporal lobe. At, atrium of the ventricle; DpTh, dorsal peduncle of the thalamus; F, frontal horn; *white B*, body of the lateral ventricle.

Continued

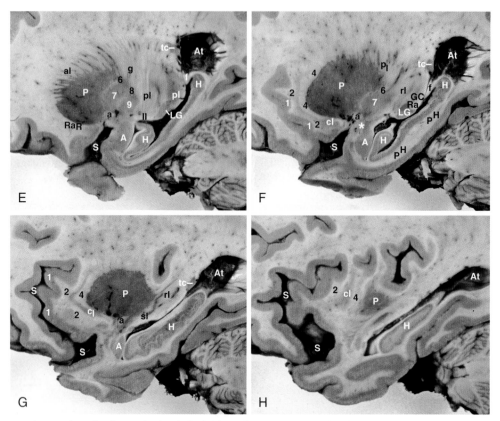

■ **FIGURE 11-20, cont'd** E, Far laterally, the caudatolenticular bridges of gray matter resemble the spines of a porcupine, localizing a wide arc of the internal capsule. Within the arc, from anterior to posterior, the lenticular nucleus displays distinct lamellae: anterior limb (al), putamen (P), lateral lamina (6), lateral nucleus (7), medial lamina (8), medial nucleus (9), and internal capsule (g: genu; pl: posterior limb). The thalamus is reduced to a small remnant of posterolateral nucleus (pl). The tail of the caudate nucleus (tc) lies along the anterior wall of the atrium (A). The optic tract (II) now leads into the lateral geniculate nucleus (LG). Inferiorly, the amygdala (A) and the hippocampal formation (H) cradle the ganglia and thalamus. **F,** The sylvian fissure (S) now opens into the peri-insular cistern. From anterior to posterior, the same laminae recur: cortex of insula (1), extreme capsule (2), claustrum that is widest inferiorly (cl), external capsule (4), putamen (P), lateral lamina (6), lateral nucleus of the globus pallidus (7), and internal capsule (here the retrolenticular portion [rl]). The tail of the caudate nucleus (tc) lies superiorly. The basal ganglia extend (*asterisk*) toward the amygdala (A) along the superior surface of the sylvian fissure. The lateral geniculate nucleus (LG) gives rise to the geniculocalcarine radiations (optic radiations) (GCRa) in relation to the retrolenticular portion of the internal capsule. The hippocampal formation (H) and the parahippocampal gyrus (PH) lie inferiorly. **G,** The peri-insular cistern opens more widely. The section passes lateral to the globus pallidus, so only the putamen (P) is displayed. The retrolenticular (rl) and sublenticular (sl) portions of the internal capsule form a distinct scimitar that delimits the posteroinferior margin of the putamen. Other labels are as in **F,** earlier. **H,** Far laterally, sagittal sections show the prominent peri-insular cistern (S) and insular cortex but only remnants of the extreme capsule (2), claustrum (cl), external capsule (4), and putamen (P).

The *medullary laminae of the lenticular nucleus* comprise thin laminae of white matter that partition the lenticular nucleus (see Figs. 11-8, 11-9, 11-20, and 11-21). The lateral (external) medullary lamina separates the putamen from the lateral nucleus of globus pallidus (GPe). The medial (internal) medullary lamina separates the lateral (GPe) from the medial (GPi) nucleus of the lenticular nucleus. The incomplete medullary lamina partially subdivides the medial nucleus.[4]

The term *anterior commissure* signifies a tightly packed ovoid bundle of fibers that cross the midline in the upper portion of the lamina terminalis to interconnect the olfactory bulbs and the temporal lobes (see Figs. 11-14, 11-15, 11-20, and 11-21).[14] The anterior limbs of the anterior commissure pass from the midline into the olfactory tracts in both directions to interconnect the two olfactory bulbs.[9] The posterior limbs of the anterior commissure pass from the midline through GPe, under the putamen, over the amygdala, and over the temporal horn to interconnect the temporal and occipital lobes of the two sides.[9] Because the anterior commissure crosses over nearly the full transverse dimension of the brain it is a useful landmark for imaging.

The term *ansa lenticularis* signifies the fibers of the globus pallidus that loop under (rostral and ventral to) the internal capsule and pass through Forel field H to join the lenticular fasciculus (see Fig. 11-19).[9]

The term *fields of Forel* is used to designate a dense mesh of fiber bundles that lie within the subthalamus rostral to the midbrain. These are named, H, H1, and H2 by their anatomic relationship to the zona incerta (see Figs. 11-16 and 11-19; see also later section on subthalamic structures).[9]

The *H field of Forel* is situated in the caudomedial portion of the subthalamic white matter, ventral to the zona incerta. Fibers of the ansa lenticularis traverse the H field. Fibers of the lenticular fasciculus arch medially from the H2 field through the H field into the H1 field en route to the thalamus. Ascending fibers from the contralateral cerebellar nuclei traverse the superior cerebellar peduncle and its decussation to pass into the H field.[4,6,7]

The *H2 field of Forel* signifies the portion of the subthalamic white matter situated ventrolateral to the zona incerta. The term *lenticular fasciculus* designates the fibers of the GPi that pass across the internal capsule, gather inferolateral to the zona

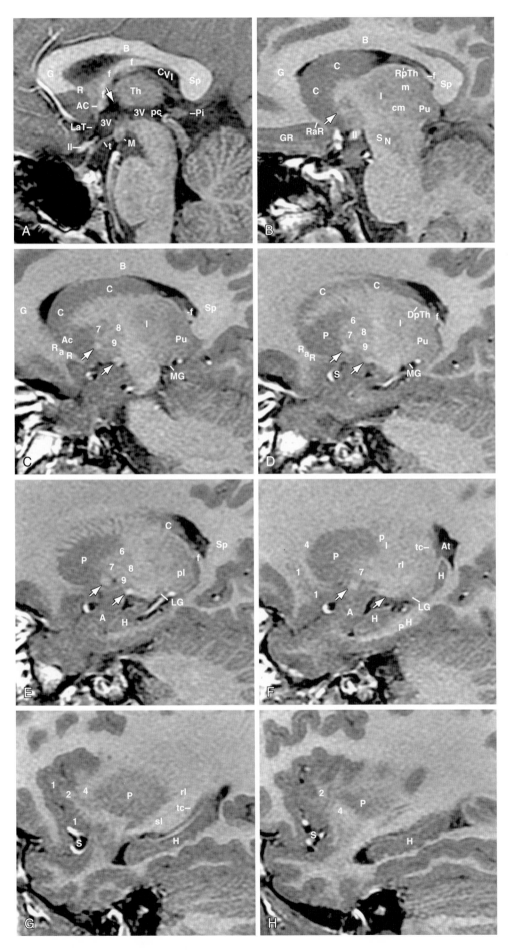

■ **FIGURE 11-21** A to H, Corresponding T1W sagittal MR images, selected and cropped to match Figure 11-20. In addition to the labels used in Fig. 11-20, other labels in **A** include AC, anterior commissure; CVI, cistern of the velum interpositum; Pi, pineal gland and in **C** to **F,** *upper white arrow,* anterior commissure; *lower white arrow,* optic tract.

incerta in field H2, make a hairpin turn around the medial border of the zona incerta, join the fibers of the ansa lenticularis, and, together, pass through field H1 dorsomedial to the zona incerta to reach the ventral anterior and ventral lateral nuclei of the thalamus.[4,6,7]

The *H1 field of Forel* signifies the portion of the tegmental white matter situated dorsomedial to the zona incerta. The term *thalamic fasciculus* designates the joint fiber bundles that pass through H1 between the zona incerta and the thalamus en route to the ventral anterior and ventral lateral nuclei of the thalamus.

The *stria terminalis* is a long, curved fiber tract that arises inferiorly from the amygdala and runs along the medial border of the caudate nucleus from the caudate tail in the temporal lobe to the caudate head at the level of the anterior commissure. There the stria terminalis divides into precommissural, commissural, and postcommissural portions (see Fig. 11-16A).[4] The stria terminalis conveys data to and from the amygdala.

Diencephalic Structures

Thalamus, Subthalamus, Epithalamus, Metathalamus, and Related Structures

Multiple subdivisions of the diencephalon are named for their relationship to the embryonic hypothalamic sulcus. These include the dorsal thalamus, subthalamus (ventral thalamus), epithalamus, metathalamus, and hypothalamus.

Thalamus (Dorsal Thalamus)

The term *thalamus* signifies an ovoid collection of multiple different nuclei situated in the lateral wall of the third ventricle, posterior and inferior to the foramen of Monro (Figs. 11-1, 11-2, and 11-22 to 11-24).[9] Embryologically, the structure commonly called the "thalamus" derives from the lateral wall of the diencephalon cephalic to the hypothalamic sulcus, making the proper name for it the "dorsal thalamus."

Gross Anatomy

The thalamic complex is subdivided into named compartments and nuclei by their relationship to the external and internal medullary laminae of the thalamus, by their reciprocal connections with specific cortical and subcortical structures, and by their histochemistry.[9] Overall, the external medullary lamina delimits the ventral/lateral surface of the thalamus. The internal medullary lamina compartmentalizes the internal structure of the thalamus into anterior, dorsomedial, ventral/lateral, and intercalated (intralaminar) groups of nuclei. For that reason, in this section we first discuss the thalamic laminae, return to the gray nuclei, and then address the interconnections of the thalamus with adjacent structures.

The *dorsal thalamus* is surrounded by a thin layer of myelinated fibers designated the external medullary lamina of the thalamus (see Figs. 11-22 to 11-24).[9] This lamina separates the dorsal thalamus medial to the lamina from the reticular nucleus lateral to it.[9]

The *internal medullary lamina* is a curved sheet of white matter that is convex laterally and divides the dorsal thalamus into the mediodorsal (dorsomedial) thalamic nucleus medially and the groups of ventral and lateral thalamic nuclei laterally (see Figs. 11-22 to 11-24).[9] Rostrally and dorsally, the internal medullary lamina splits around the anterior nuclear group of the thalamus. Centrally, the internal medullary lamina splits to enclose the intralaminar (intercalated) nuclei, including the centromedian and parafascicular nuclei. At the posterior pole of the thalamus, marked expansion of the lateral nuclear group forms the pulvinar and deviates the internal medullary lamina anteriorly. Important groups of thalamic gray matter nuclei are discussed in the next paragraphs.

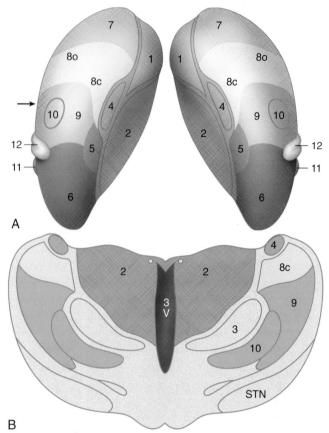

■ **FIGURE 11-22** A and B, Thalamus. Diagrams of the laminae and nuclei of the thalami. **A,** Top view. **B,** Coronal plane at the level shown by the *arrow* in A. The internal medullary lamina (*brown* division) splits anteriorly to enclose the anterior group of nuclei (1) and splits again in the middle to enclose the intralaminar (e.g., centromedian and parafascicular) nuclei (3). The far larger group of ventral and lateral nuclei includes the pulvinar (6), whose expansion deviates the internal medullary lamina medially. Twelve major thalamic nuclei may be considered in six groups: anterior, medial, intralaminar, lateral, ventral, and metathalamic. 1. Anterior nuclear group 2. Medial nuclear group: predominantly dorsomedial nucleus (synonym: mediodorsal nucleus) 3. Intralaminar nuclei (e.g., 3, centromedian nucleus [group also includes the parafascicular nucleus]) 4-6. Lateral nuclear group: 4, lateral dorsal nucleus; 5, lateral posterior nucleus; 6, pulvinar. 7-10.Ventral nuclear group: 7, ventral anterior nucleus; 8, ventral lateral nucleus; 9, ventral posterolateral nucleus; 10, ventral posteromedial nucleus. Within the ventral lateral nucleus, VLc is pars caudalis and VLo is pars oralis. 11-12. Metathalamic: 11, medial geniculate nucleus; 12, lateral geniculate nucleus. *(Modified from Carpenter MB, Sutin J. Human Neuroanatomy, 8th ed. Baltimore, Williams & Wilkins, 1983.)*

The *anterior nuclear group* consists of a number of anterior nuclei that lie within the split anterior end of the internal medullary lamina (see Figs. 11-22 to 11-24).[9] The lateral dorsal nucleus of the lateral group comes to lie in the same anterior compartment. The mammillothalamic tract terminates in the anterior nucleus (see Fig. 11-24A). This group is interconnected with the limbic cortex of the cingulate gyrus, retrosplenial area, and portions of the subicular complex.

The *posterior nuclear group* includes a diffuse posterior nucleus and two compact suprageniculate and limitans nuclei.[9] These nuclei receive input from the superior and inferior colliculi and from ascending fiber tracts, including the medial lemniscus, the spinothalamic tract, and the trigeminothalamic tract. The posterior nuclei project to the insular cortex and the

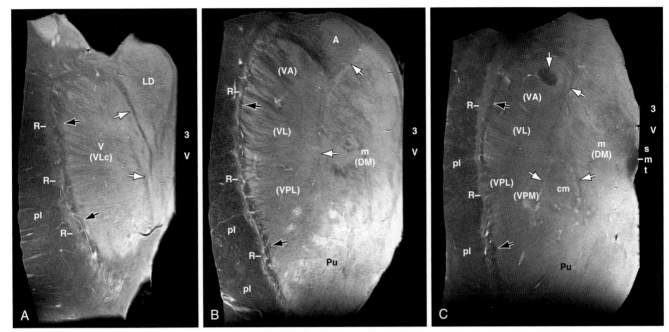

■ **FIGURE 11-23** A to C, Postmortem intermediate-weighted axial 9.4-T MR images of the formalin-fixed thalamus. The images are oriented to correspond to a right thalamus and displayed from superior to inferior. Compare with Figures 11-22 and 11-24. **A,** Near the superior margin, the lateral dorsal nucleus (LD) forms the anterior medial border of the thalamus, enclosed within the internal medullary lamina (*white arrows*). The ventral (V) nuclear group lies lateral to it. At this level, it is the ventral lateral nucleus pars caudalis. The reticular nuclei (R) form a thin layer of gray matter between the posterior limb (pl) of the internal capsule and the external medullary lamina (*black arrows*, A to C) of the thalamus. **B,** Inferior to the lateral dorsal nucleus, near to the lower margin of the anterior nucleus (A), the internal medullary lamina encloses the anterior nucleus and extends posteriorly to divide the dorsomedial nucleus (DM) of the medial (m) nuclear group from the ventral anterior (VA), ventral lateral (VL), and ventral posterolateral (VPL) nuclei of the ventral group and the pulvinar (Pu) of the lateral group. **C,** At the midthalamus, the mammillothalamic tract (*vertical down-pointing white arrow*) courses upward from the mammillary body to the ipsilateral anterior nucleus (*shown in* **B**). The internal medullary lamina (*white arrows*) splits posteriorly to enclose the centromedian nucleus (cm) of the intralaminar group. At this level the components of the ventral nuclear group include the ventral anterior (VA), ventral lateral (VL), ventral posterolateral (VPL), and ventral posteromedial (VPM) nuclei. The pulvinar (Pu) makes up the posterior pole of the thalamus. The white matter fibers of the stria medullaris thalami (smt) form a band of low signal on the medial wall of the thalamus.

adjacent retroinsular cortex surrounding the secondary somatosensory cortex (S2).

The *lateral nuclear group* comprises the lateral dorsal nucleus, the lateral posterior nucleus, and the massive pulvinar at the posterior pole of the thalamus (see Figs. 11-22 to 11-24).[9] The narrow lateral dorsal nucleus actually comes to lie within the internal medullary lamina. These nuclei are interconnected with the large association cortices of the temporal, parietal and occipital lobes.

The *ventral nuclear group* is subdivided into the ventral anterior, ventral lateral, and ventral posterior nuclei.[9] The *ventral anterior and ventral lateral thalamic nuclei* are situated rostrally and dorsally within the ventral nuclear group (see Figs. 11-22 to 11-24). They are motor relay nuclei that convey impulses from the cerebellum, substantia nigra, and basal ganglia to the motor and premotor cortices. The ventral lateral nucleus is the main termination of the superior cerebellar peduncle. *The ventral posterior group* lies in the posterior lateral portion of the thalamus (see Figs. 11-22 to 11-24). This group includes the somatosensory relay nuclei that receive deep sensation, nociceptive, thermoceptive, gustatory, and visceral sensations through the spinothalamic tract, trigeminothalamic tract, medial lemnisci, and the dorsal trigeminothalamic tract and relay them to the primary somatosensory cortex of the postcentral gyrus, the secondary somatosensory cortex in the parietal operculum, and the gustatory cortex situated in the insular operculum and the orbitofrontal cortex.[9] The ventral posterior nucleus is further subdivided into the ventral posterolateral (VPL) and the ventral

posteromedial (VPM) nuclei. The medial lemniscus and the spinothalamic tract that carry sensation from the contralateral body terminate in the VPL. The trigeminothalamic system that carries sensation from the face terminates in the VPM, ipsilaterally and contralaterally (in a complex fashion).

The *intralaminar (intercalated) nuclei* include the centromedian nucleus and the parafascicular nucleus that surrounds the fasciculus retroflexus (habenulointerpeduncular tract) (see Figs. 11-22 to 11-24).[9] These nuclei are regarded as different from other thalamic nuclei. They are believed to have a more diffuse connection to the brain than other thalamic nuclei. They receive convergent inputs from multiple sources rather than a single dominant source. They interconnect with wide areas of the reticular nucleus of the thalamus and project to more poorly defined regions of the cortex than other thalamic nuclei. In addition, they project to both the cortex and the striatum at sites that are then interconnected with each other via corticostriatal fibers.

The large *dorsomedial (mediodorsal) nucleus* lies medial to the internal medullary lamina (see Figs. 11-22 to 11-24). Its lateral portion interconnects with the frontal eye field and the prefrontal cortex. Its medial portion interconnects with olfactory regions of the prefrontal cortex and with the neocortical orbitofrontal cortex.

The *midline group of thalamic nuclei* includes a number of small named nuclei. Of these, the reunions nucleus is related to the massa intermedia.[9] These nuclei appear to distribute and function in a fashion similar to the intralaminar nuclei.

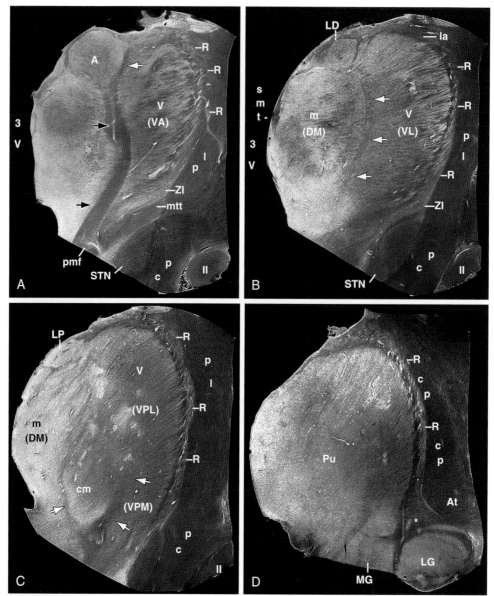

■ **FIGURE 11-24** A to D, Postmortem intermediate-weighted coronal 9.4-T MR images of the formalin-fixed thalamus. The images are oriented to correspond to a left thalamus and are displayed from anterior to posterior. Compare with Figures 11-22 and 11-23. **A,** Anterior section displays the anterior nucleus of the thalamus (A) enclosed within the internal medullary lamina (*white arrow*) at the anterior medial aspect of the superior surface and the ventral anterior nucleus (VA) of the ventral (V) group situated lateral to it. The external medullary lamina forms a well-defined layer of white matter that is perforated by the fibers passing into and out from the thalamus. The reticular nucleus (R) is a thin layer of gray matter situated between the external medullary lamina of the thalamus and the posterior limb (pl) of the internal capsule. The reticular nuclei (R) are believed to modulate the level of activity in the perforating fibers. Inferiorly, the mammillary body gives rise to the principal mammillary fasciculus (pmf) that ascends a short distance before it divides into the mammillothalamic tract (*black arrows*) to the anterior nucleus (A) and the mammillotegmental tract (mtt) that arches over the subthalamic nucleus (STN) to the brain stem. The zona incerta (ZI) appears as a thin sinuous nucleus that lies superior to the mammillotegmental tract and becomes continuous superolaterally with the reticular nucleus (R) of the thalamus. The H, H1, and H2 fields of Forel are related to the zona incerta (see Fig. 11-10B). II, optic tract. **B,** More posteriorly, the lateral dorsal nucleus (LD) forms the superior medial surface of the thalamus. The lamina affixa (LA) encloses the superior lateral surface of the thalamus. The internal medullary lamina (*white arrows*) encloses the lateral dorsal nucleus and divides the dorsomedial nucleus (DM) of the medial (m) group from the ventral lateral (VL) nucleus of the ventral (V) group. The sinuous zona incerta (ZI) curves over the subthalamic nucleus (STN) and ascends to merge with reticular nuclei (R). **C,** At the midthalamus, the lateral posterior nucleus (LP) forms the superior medial surface. The internal medullary lamina splits to enclose the centromedian nucleus (cm). The ventral group now includes the ventral posterolateral (VPL) and the ventral posteromedial (VPM) nuclei. Laterally, the posterior limb (pl) of the internal capsule continues inferiorly into the cerebral peduncle (cp). Myriad fibers traverse the thin lamina of the reticular nucleus (R) and the thin external medullary lamina to pass between the thalamus and the internal capsule. The optic tract (II) courses posteriorly around the cerebral peduncle toward the lateral geniculate nucleus. **D,** Posteriorly, coronal sections pass through the pulvinar (Pu), the medial geniculate nucleus (MG), the lateral geniculate nucleus (LG), and the geniculocalcarine radiations (*asterisk*). At, area tegmentalis.

A diffuse group of thalamic cells, designated *matrix cells*, is distributed widely throughout the thalamus, across nuclear borders. This group receives diffuse subcortical inputs.[9]

Reticular nuclei cells properly belong with the ventral thalamus rather than the dorsal thalamus and are discussed later.

Thalamic Peduncles

The term *thalamic peduncle* signifies a group of fibers that separate from the internal capsule and other major pathways and pass medially into the thalamus to convey impulses in both corticothalamic and thalamocortical directions.[9] The *anterior thalamic peduncle* separates from the anterior limb of the internal capsule to interconnect the thalamus with the prefrontal, orbitofrontal and cingulate cortices. The *superior and posterior thalamic peduncles* separate from the posterior limb of the internal capsule to interconnect the thalamus with the central parietal and occipitotemporal cortices. The *inferior thalamic peduncle* crosses medial to the posterior limb of the internal capsule to interconnect the ventromedial thalamus with the orbitofrontal, insular, and temporal cortices and the amygdaloid complex. It forms part of the ansa peduncularis.

Function

Functionally, the thalamic nuclei may also be classified as sensory relay nuclei, motor relay nuclei, association nuclei, and limbic nuclei.[9] The sensory relay nuclei include the ventral posterior nucleus (somatosensory), the medial geniculate nucleus (auditory), and the lateral geniculate nuclei (visual). These relay impulses onward to the primary somatosensory, visual, and auditory cortices. Motor relay nuclei include the ventral anterior and ventral lateral nuclei (VA-VL complex) that receive input from the basal ganglia and cerebellar nuclei and relay it to the motor and premotor cortices. The association nuclei are characterized by reciprocal interconnections with the cerebral association cortices. These include the dorsomedial (mediodorsal) nucleus that is connected with the prefrontal cortex and the lateral posterior and pulvinaric nuclei that are related to the association cortex of the temporal, parietal, and occipital lobes (TPO association cortex). The limbic nuclei include the anterior nucleus and the lateral dorsal nucleus situated within the internal medullary lamina. These relate to the cingulate and entorhinal cortices and portions of the subicular complex.

Subthalamus (Ventral Thalamus)

The ventral thalamus is the portion of the diencephalon that arises inferior to the hypothalamic sulcus. In the adult, it is best understood as a superior extension of the tegmentum of the midbrain and is usually designated the subthalamus.[6] The subthalamus marks the rostral limit of the red nucleus, the substantia nigra, the reticular nuclei, and feltwork of multiple ascending, descending and oblique fiber bundles.[6]

The term *subthalamus* signifies the region interposed between the dorsal thalamus and the hypothalamus (see Fig. 11-16).[9] It contains the zona incerta, the subthalamic nucleus, and the reticular nucleus of the thalamus and their associated fiber tracts.[10]

The *zona incerta* is an aggregate of small cells situated between the external medullary lamina of the thalamus and the cerebral peduncle (see Figs. 11-16 and 11-19).[5,6] It is the rostral continuation of the brain stem reticular formation and appears to link with the reticular nuclei of the ventral thalamus more rostrally.[9] The zona incerta is circumscribed on three sides by Forel fields H1, H, and H2.

The *subthalamic nucleus* is the largest mass of gray matter in the subthalamus (see earlier discussion).

The *reticular nucleus of the (ventral) thalamus* is a thin layer of cells that covers the rostral, ventral, and lateral faces of the dorsal thalamus (see Figs. 11-16, 11-22 to 11-24). It lies between the external medullary lamina of the thalamus medially and the internal capsule laterally. The cells of the reticular nucleus strongly modulate the activity of the corticothalamic and thalamocortical fibers that penetrate through the nucleus en route to the dorsal thalamic nuclei.[9]

The term *subthalamic fasciculus* signifies the fibers that cross through the internal capsule to interconnect the pallidum with the subthalamic nucleus (see Fig. 11-16).[9]

The *fields of Forel* were discussed in an earlier section on the white matter structures of the basal ganglia.

Epithalamus

The term *epithalamus* designates structures formed from the most dorsal division of the diencephalon. It includes the pineal body, medial and lateral habenular nuclei, habenular commissure, habenulointerpeduncular tract (fasciculus retroflexus), posterior commissure, striae medullares thalamorum, and the roof of the third ventricle (Fig. 11-25).[10,13,15]

The *pineal gland* (epiphysis) is the cone-shaped gland that diverticulates from the posterior wall of the third ventricle to overlie the tectal plate of the midbrain (see Fig. 11-25). It attaches to the third ventricle by the pineal stalk, which may contain a small dorsal extension of the third ventricle designated the pineal recess. The white matter fibers decussating in the upper wall of the pineal stalk constitute the habenular commissure. The white matter fibers decussating in the lower wall of the pineal stalk make up the posterior commissure. The pineal gland contains glial cells and pineocytes but no neurons. Instead, it has abundant terminals from postganglionic sympathetic neurons that lie within the superior cervical ganglion.[13]

The *habenular trigones* form a "duplicate horn" of paired medial and lateral habenular nuclei situated at each side of the posterior third ventricle (Figs. 11-25 and 11-26).[10] The medial and lateral habenular pathways appear to be strictly separate. The medial habenular pathway receives information from hippocampal, septal, and medial hypothalamic centers via the stria medullaris thalami and relays it via the habenulointerpeduncular tract to the interpeduncular nucleus of the midbrain.[9] The lateral habenular pathway receives information from the lateral hypothalamic region, substantia innominata, and GPi and relays it to diverse centers in the midbrain, including the substantia nigra pars compacta (SNc), the dorsal raphe, and the mesencephalic reticular centers.[9,16]

The *striae medullares thalamorum* are narrow tracts of white matter that course longitudinally along the medial walls of the thalami, just where the roof of the third ventricle inserts into the thalamus on each side (see Figs. 11-2 and 11-25). These striae interconnect the septal and rostral regions of the brain with the habenular nuclei and may cross to the contralateral habenular nuclei via the habenular commissure.[13]

The *habenulointerpeduncular tract* (fasciculus retroflexus) interconnects the habenular nuclei with the interpeduncular nucleus of the midbrain and with multiple raphe nuclei of the brain stem.[13] Seen together, the pair of tracts takes the shape of a lyre (see Fig. 11-26).

The *posterior commissure* conveys decussating fibers of the superior colliculi and the pretectum (visual reflex fibers) across the midline.[13]

Together, the striae medullares, the habenular nuclei, and the habenulointerpeduncular tract form a dorsal diencephalic conducting system for conveying limbic impulses from the telencephalon and the diencephalon to the rostral brain stem.[9]

Metathalamus

The term *metathalamus* designates the medial and lateral geniculate bodies (Fig. 11-27).[10] Embryologically, these arise in the lateral wall of the third ventricle superior to the hypothalamic sulcus and are rotated into their present horizontal alignment by

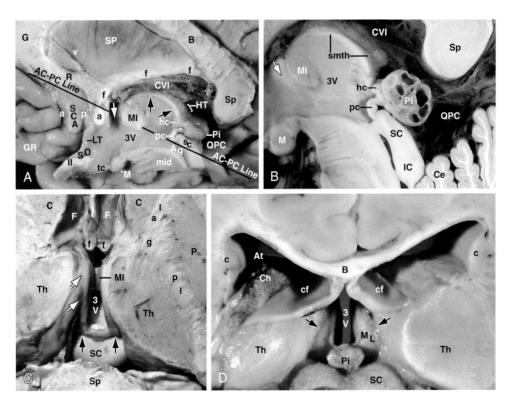

■ **FIGURE 11-25**   A to D, Epithalamus and third ventricle **A,** Midline section through the corpus callosum (Sp, B, G, R), septum pellucidum (SP), cistern of the velum interpositum (CVI), and third ventricle (3V). The septum pellucidum stretches between the undersurface of the corpus and the superior surface of the fornix (f). The CVI lies between the fornix (f) above and the roof of the third ventricle below. The stria medullaris thalami (*black arrows*) interconnects the septal region with the habenular trigone (*bracket,* HT). It runs along the medial wall of the thalamus, at the lateral edge of the third ventricular roof, and then characteristically turns sharply downward toward the habenular commissure (HC). The pineal gland (Pi) protrudes into the quadrigeminal plate cistern (QPC) to overlie the superior colliculi (sc). The pineal stalk shows an upper wall, a pineal recess (*asterisk*), and a lower wall. The fibers crossing in the upper wall of the pineal stalk are the habenular commissure (hc). The fibers crossing in the lower wall of the pineal stalk are the posterior commissure (pc). The PC forms the roof of the entry into the cerebral aqueduct (Aq). The line drawn from the top of the anterior commissure (a) to the bottom of the posterior commissure (pc) is the AC-PC baseline of Talairach and Tournoux (see Suggested Readings). Anteriorly, the gyrus rectus (GR) turns upward under the rostrum to form the subcallosal area (SCA) between the anterior (*white a*) and posterior (*white p*) paraolfactory sulci. The paraterminal gyrus (*not labeled*) lies behind the posterior paraolfactory sulcus, closely applied to the rostrum and lamina terminalis. The midline segment of the anterior commissure (a) runs in the anterior wall of the third ventricle and marks the transition between the rostrum (R) and the lamina terminalis (LT). The portion of the fornix immediately behind the anterior commissure forms the anterior medial wall of the foramen of Monro (*white arrow*). The massa intermedia (MI) is residual gray matter that interconnects the thalami across the third ventricle, not a white matter commissure. The mass intermedia is lacking in 25% to 30% of brains.[9] The prominent striothalamic groove between the caudate and the thalamus curves toward the foramen of Monro (*white arrow*). The stria medullaris thalami (*black arrows*) marks the line of attachment where the roof of the third ventricle (3V) inserts into the medial surface of the thalamus. **B,** Cystic pineal gland. Midsagittal section. The pineal gland is enlarged by multiple cysts of diverse size. Ce, central lobule of the vermis. **C,** Striae medullares thalamorum. Gross anatomic specimen. View into the third ventricle from above after resection of the body of the corpus callosum, the roof of the third ventricle, and associated vasculature/choroid plexus. The paired striae medullares thalamorum (*white arrows*) pass along the medial walls of the thalami (Th) from the septal region to the habenular trigones (*paired black arrows*). Their posterior ends turn sharply inferiorly to reach the habenulae. The habenular commissure (*between black arrows*) interconnects the two sides. The roughening of the surface of the commissure indicates the sites of the choroid plexus and the pineal gland (*lost in this specimen*). MI, massa intermedia. **D,** Habenular trigones. Gross anatomic specimen seen from above and behind. The habenular trigones (*black arrows*) lie just to each side of the posterior third ventricle (3V) where the thalami (Th) protrude posteriorly. They contain the medial (M) and lateral (L) habenular nuclei. The pineal gland (Pi) protrudes posteriorly to overlie the midline groove between the two superior colliculi (SC). The habenular commissure interconnects the two habenulae through the upper wall of the pineal stalk. The atrium (At) is delimited by the body (B) of the corpus callosum above, the caudate nucleus (c) superolaterally, and the crus of the fornix (cf) and thalami (Th) below. The choroidal fissure enters the ventricle between the fornix (cf) above and the thalami (Th) below, so the choroid plexus (Ch) enters the ventricle just lateral to the lateral edge of the fornix.

the growth and enlargement of the internal capsules and cerebral peduncles.

The *medial geniculate nuclei* form rounded elevations of gray matter at the cephalic end of the lateral mesencephalic sulci, just behind the lateral edges of the cerebral peduncles and just inferior to the overhanging pulvinars (see Fig. 11-27A, B). The medial geniculate nuclei receive auditory input from both ears via the lateral lemnisci that course superiorly at the lateral edges of the brain stem. The medial geniculate nuclei give rise to the auditory radiations that convey auditory data onward to the primary auditory cortex (A1) in the transverse temporal gyrus of Heschl.

The *lateral geniculate nuclei* form caret-shaped nuclei situated superolateral to the medial geniculate nuclei, just inferior to the overhanging pulvinars and just dorsal to the hippocampal formations of the underlying medial temporal lobes. In classical coronal anatomic sections, their shape is described as "Napoleon's hat" (see Figs. 11-12B and 11-27C, D). Each geniculate nucleus has six concentric layers, with two magnocellular layers near the hilus designated M1 and M2 and four parvocellular layers progressively closer to the dome designated P3-P6. The lateral geniculate nuclei receive visual data via the optic tracts that course around the ventral lateral margins of the cerebral peduncles to enter the hili of the lateral geniculate nuclei. Because the

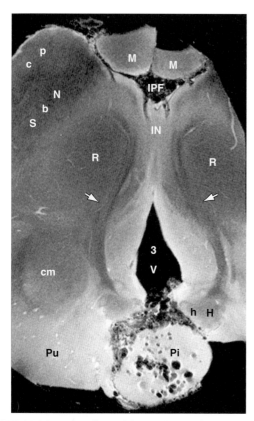

■ FIGURE 11-26 Habenulae. Axial 9.4-T intermediate-weighted postmortem MR image of the posterior third ventricle (3V) and pineal gland (Pi). The medial (h) and lateral (H) habenular nuclei lie to each side of the posterior third ventricle. The habenulointerpeduncular tract (*white arrows*) passes from the habenular nuclei medial to the centromedian nucleus (cm) of the thalamus and around the red nucleus (R) to reach the interpeduncular nucleus (IN) in the roof of the interpeduncular fossa (IPF): cp, cerebral peduncle; Pu, pulvinar; Sbn, substantia nigra. (*Modified from Naidich TP, Duvernoy HM, Delman BN, et al. High-field MRI: surface anatomy, internal structure, vascularization and 3D sectional anatomy. In: Duvernoy's Atlas of the Human Brain Stem and Cerebellum. New York, Springer, 2008.*)

optic fibers undergo *partial* decussation in the optic chiasm, each optic tract carries visual data from both eyes. The fibers from the ipsilateral eye pass to geniculate layers M2, P3, and P5 (remember 2 + 3 = 5), while the fibers from the contralateral eye pass to geniculate layers M1, P4, and P6. The lateral geniculate nuclei then relay the visual data onward through the optic radiations to the primary visual cortex (V1) in the medial occipital (striate) cortex. Other visual fibers diverge from the optic tract proximal to the lateral geniculate nuclei, form medial roots that bypass the lateral geniculate bodies, and enter the brachia of the superior colliculi to reach the tectal plate.[9]

Hypothalamus

The hypothalamus is the portion of the diencephalon situated ventral to the hypothalamic sulcus in the inferior wall of the third ventricle. This structure is discussed with the sellar/suprasellar structures in Chapter 14.

Functional Divisions

The basal ganglia and thalami are important to multiple brain functions, including motor preparation, action selection, action gating, and timing.[17] They also appear to be involved in reward-based learning, exploratory behavior, goal-oriented behavior, working memory, fatigue, and apathy.[17] Overall, the ganglia and

thalami may be regarded as having five functional divisions. Within each nucleus separately, and throughout the entire nuclear complex, these five divisions appear to be organized from dorsolateral to ventromedial as parallel tiers of sensorimotor, supplementary motor, premotor, association, and limbic territories. These divisions participate in functional cortical-basal ganglial-thalamocortical circuits (loops) (Fig. 11-28A).[18]

Evidence suggests that each of the major motor divisions of the basal ganglia and thalami is also organized somatotopically in a fashion that largely recapitulates the sensorimotor homunculus (see Fig. 11-28B).[19] The motor circuit appears to proceed from the cerebral cortex to the striatum, which projects in turn to the pallidum and the substantia nigra pars reticulata, from which efferents pass to the ventral anterior and ventral lateral nuclei of the thalamus (VA and VL) to influence the cortex.[5,6,17,19,20]

Figure 11-29 is a highly simplified schematic for the ganglio-thalamic control of motor function.* This may be conceptualized as follows.

1. The brain typically functions as a double negative system. It does not choose between "Go" and "No go." Instead it chooses between "No go" and "Not no go." This "no, not no" dichotomy may be likened to driving a car with both the gas and the brake depressed to the floor. Going forward is achieved by releasing the brake, not depressing the gas.

2. The natural state of a motor system is quietude, in order to conserve energy. Actions are (usually) a planned exception to quietude. For that reason, the motor system is tonically inhibited and actions result when inhibition is released.

3. The basal ganglia establish a motor plan that is expected to achieve the motor act. That is, they select and establish the strengths of agonists versus antagonists, establish the desired angles at each joint, and map out the physical factors that are *estimated* to achieve the anticipated motion.

4. The simple act of moving a limb automatically activates sensory receptors that report back the position of the limb in space. This returning information is called reafferent data.

5. For each action, the reafferent data are compared with the expected plan of action to adjust the motion made *both* for that one motion *and* for all similar motions made subsequently (motor learning).

6. The substantia nigra pars compacta (SNc) is the "comparator." It assesses any deviations between expectation (basal ganglial plan) and actuality (reafferent data) and releases dopamine *to minimize the difference* between expectation and action. The dopamine appears to confer plasticity on the multiple synapses that align along the dendrites of the spiny neurons of the striatum.

7. The major output of the basal ganglia is inhibitory (GABAergic).

8. The major output nuclei of the basal ganglia are the globus pallidus pars interna (GPi) and the substantia nigra pars reticulata (SNr). Phylogenetically, the GPi and SNr develop as a single nucleus that becomes accidentally subdivided by the downward growth of the internal capsule. GPi and SNr tonically inhibit the thalamus.

9. The subthalamic nucleus is the major excitatory (glutaminergic) nucleus of the basal ganglia. It activates the GPi/SNr, increasing their inhibition of the thalamus.

10. The striatum is overwhelmingly an inhibitory (GABAergic) nucleus. It acts on the GPi/SNr to inhibit their inhibition of the thalamus. It acts on the subthalamic nucleus to inhibit its activation of the Gi/SNr. By both actions, the striatum can reduce the inhibition of the thalamus, achieving a "not no" state.

---

*Courtesy of William Tatten, MD, personal communication.

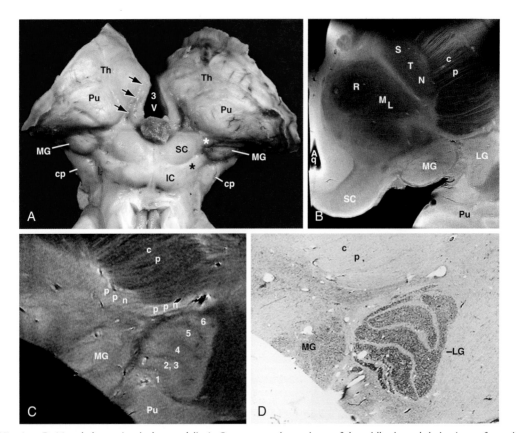

■ **FIGURE 11-27** **A** to **D**, Metathalamus (geniculate nuclei). **A**, Gross anatomic specimen of the midbrain and thalami seen from above and behind. The habenular trigones (*black arrows*) lie at the posterior end of the third ventricle (3V) medial to the thalami (Th). From the inferior colliculus (IC) fibers pass via the brachium (*black asterisk*) of the inferior colliculus, to the medial geniculate nucleus (MG). The medial geniculate nucleus lies at the side of the midbrain, just behind the posterolateral edge of the cerebral peduncle (cp) and beneath the overhanging pulvinar (Pu). From the superior colliculus (SC), the brachium (*white asterisk*) of the superior colliculus passes above and lateral to the medial geniculate nucleus to reach the lateral geniculate nucleus (*hidden beneath the pulvinar in this view*). **B**, Axial 9.4-T intermediate-weighted postmortem MR image of a half midbrain, oriented like the left half of a clinical MR scan. The medial geniculate nucleus (MG) lies just lateral to the superior colliculus (SC), posterior to the cerebral peduncle (cp), and inferior to the pulvinar (Pu) of the thalamus. The subthalamic nucleus (STN), superior pole of the red nucleus (R), and medial lemniscus (ML) lie ventral to the medial geniculate nucleus. Because the STN is centered superior to the red nucleus (R), the midportion of the STN is imaged here at the upper pole of the red nucleus (R). Aq, cerebral aqueduct. **C** and **D**, A 9.4-T intermediate-weighted postmortem MR image (**C**) and a Nissl-stained histologic section of the same specimen (**D**) display the lateral geniculate nucleus (LG) and part of the medial geniculate nucleus (MG) in relation to the cerebral peduncle (cp) and the pulvinar (Pu). MR resolves the six layers of the LG (two magnocellular layers at the base [1, 2] and the four parvocellular layers [3, 4, 5, 6] toward the apex). On each side, layers 2, 3 and 5 receive fibers from the ipsilateral retina whereas layers 2, 4, and 6 receive decussated fibers from the contralateral retina. The peripeduncular nucleus (ppn) partially circumscribes the posterior cerebral peduncle. (**A** to **D**, *Modified from Naidich TP, Duvernoy HM, Delman BN, et al. High-field MRI: surface anatomy, internal structure, vascularization and 3D sectional anatomy. In: Duvernoy's Atlas of the Human Brain Stem and Cerebellum. New York, Springer, 2008.*)

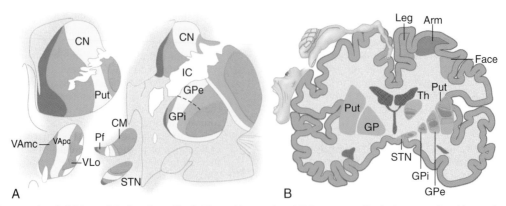

■ **FIGURE 11-28** Functional divisions of the basal ganglia. **A**, The caudate nucleus (CN), putamen (Put), the external and internal nuclei of the globus pallidus (GPe and GPi), the subthalamic nucleus (STN), and many motor nuclei of the thalamus are organized into parallel tiers for sensorimotor function (*orange*), supplementary motor function (*lilac*), premotor function (*yellow*), associative function (*pink*), and limbic function (*blue*). Within the thalamus the ventral anterior (VA) and the ventral lateral (VL) nuclei belong to the ventral group. The centromedian nucleus (CM) and the parafascicular nucleus (Pf) are intralaminar nuclei. **B**, The cortical orientation of leg, arm, and face is preserved within each nucleus of the basal ganglia and thalamus. (**A**, *From Nakano K, Kayahara T, Tsutsumi T, Ushiro H. Neural circuits and functional organization of the striatum. J Neurol 2000; 247[Suppl 5]:V/1-V/15.* **B**, *From Obeso JA, Rodríguez-Oroz MC, Benitez-Temino B, et al: Functional organization of the basal ganglia: therapeutic implications for Parkinson's disease. Mov Disord 2008;23[Suppl 3]:S548-S559.*)

11. Simplistically then, when a motor action is intended, the cortex (glutaminergic) activates the striatum. The striatum (GABAergic) plans out a motor program that inhibits the GPi/SNR and/or inhibits the activation of GPi/SNR by the subthalamic nucleus. Both actions reduce the activity of GPi/SNR so there is less inhibition of the thalamus,

12. Released from inhibition, the thalamus (glutaminergic) activates the cortex.

13. The cortex activates the spinal cord, achieving motion and automatically generating reafferent data.

14. The SNc compares the expected motor plan with the reafferent data and releases dopamine to adjust the synaptic connections in the striatum to achieve smooth motor action (one time) and improved motor performance over time (motor learning).[21]

The dopamine system that acts as a modulator of motor function may also modulate cognitive and emotional function, conferring flexibility of response. The nucleus accumbens receives a dopaminergic input from dopaminergic cell group A10 in the ventral tegmental area of the midbrain (see Fig. 11-18). This is believed to mediate the sense of "reward" associated with some recreational drugs and therefore to be a major factor in addiction.[5]

The lateral habenular nucleus functions in this complex and is one of the targets being tested for control of depression by deep brain stimulation. The function and interactions of the lateral habenular nuclei are summarized succinctly by Hikosaka and colleagues.[16]

The claustrum is presently regarded as a cortical satellite with multiple reciprocal overlapping somatotopic interconnections with the motor, premotor, and somatosensory visual and auditory association cortices.[9] Presumably, it functions in the integration of these overlapping inputs and outputs.

Overall, the basal ganglia and thalami work as an integrated system linked by direct axonal connections and coordinated by patterns of electrical oscillations and chemical signaling.[22] The reader is referred elsewhere for additional useful functional data beyond the scope of this chapter.[23,24]

IMAGING

All of the imaging modalities display the same anatomy. The differences among the images reflect only the differing sensitivities of the studies to specific aspects of the anatomy and the differing planes of section used to make the images. Increasing utilization of CT scanners that provide immediate reformatted images in three planes, for example, now enables the imager to analyze CTs with the same sagittal and coronal pattern analysis used for ultrasonography and MRI.

At times, the confluence of structures may create a pattern helpful in localizing structures, such as the "π" of the anterior commissure and anterior columns of the fornices in axial plane (see Figs. 11-6, 11-7, and 11-14) or the "Eiffel tower" sign (Fig. 11-30) for these same structures in coronal plane.

In addition to imaging of the gross anatomy, imaging of the basal ganglia is influenced by the progressive deposition of iron within specific nuclei over time (Fig. 11-31).[25-27] In broad terms, iron is normally deposited first within the globus pallidus, then the medial substantia nigra, then the red nucleus, and then the dentate nucleus of the cerebellum. With age, iron also accumulates progressively within the putamen and then the caudate nucleus (Figs. 11-32 and 11-33). Areas containing ferric iron show dephasing of the signal and low signal intensity on MR images.

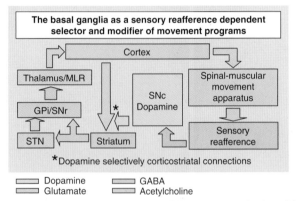

The basal ganglia as a sensory reafference dependent selector and modifier of movement programs

*Dopamine selectively corticostriatal connections

▢ Dopamine ▢ GABA
▢ Glutamate ▢ Acetylcholine

■ **FIGURE 11-29** Simplified schematic of the motor organization of the basal ganglia (see text for discussion). *(Courtesy of William Tatten, MD.)*

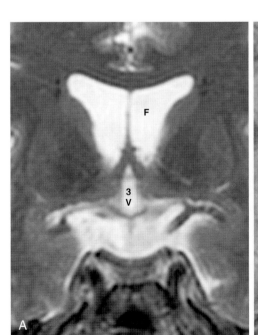

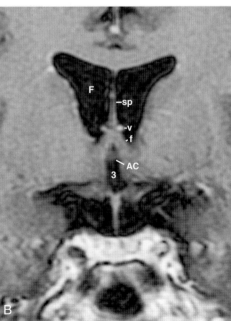

■ **FIGURE 11-30 A** and **B,** "Eiffel tower" sign. **A,** Noncontrast T2W MRI. **B,** Contrast-enhanced T1W MRI. In oblique coronal sections through the posterior half of the anterior commissure, the septum pellucidum (sp), septal veins (v), anterior columns of the fornices (f), and anterior commissure (AC) may take a configuration resembling the Eiffel tower.

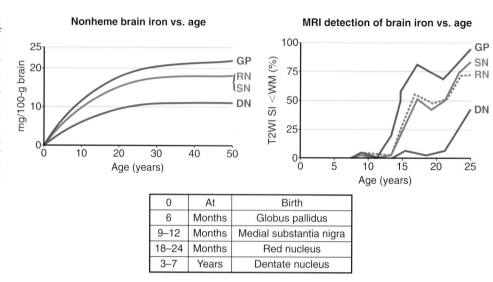

■ **FIGURE 11-31** Iron deposition with age. Diagram of the percentage of patients showing stage III iron deposition using 1.5-T spin-echo imaging (TR = 2000 to 2800 ms; TE 70 to 100 ms). In this study, areas were designated stage III if they showed signal intensity that was both less than gray matter and less than white matter. On MRI, stage III iron deposition appears first in the globi pallidi (GP), next in the substantia nigra (SN) and red nucleus (RN) (nearly simultaneously), and last within the dentate nucleus (DN) of the thalamus. *(From Aoki S, Okada Y, Nishimura K, et al. Normal deposition of brain iron in childhood and adolescence: MR imaging at 1.5 T. Radiology 1989; 172:381-435.)*

0	At	Birth
6	Months	Globus pallidus
9–12	Months	Medial substantia nigra
18–24	Months	Red nucleus
3–7	Years	Dentate nucleus

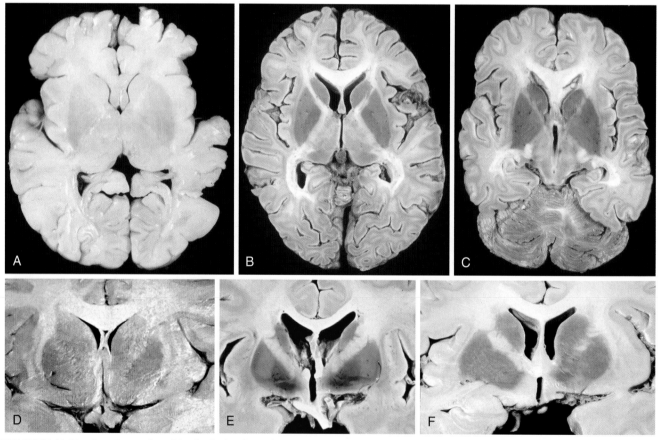

■ **FIGURE 11-32** A to F, Iron deposition in the basal ganglia. Perl ferricyanide stain of formalin-fixed gross anatomic images. A to C, Whole-brain axial sections at ages 3 days (**A**), 21 years (**B**), and 74 years (**C**). D to F, Coned-down coronal plane images through the striatum. Blue coloration signifies deposition of ferric iron within the stained tissue. The amount of ferric iron deposited and the geographic zone affected increase with age. (**A, C,** and **E,** *Courtesy of Dr. Burton P. Drayer, New York.*)

The extent of the signal change varies with the concentration of iron and with the field strength used to image the brain.

Increasingly, diffusion tensor imaging and tractography have been employed to demonstrate fiber pathways within the white matter (see Chapter 12). The same techniques may be applied to trace the connections between the deep gray nuclei and the cerebral cortex (Fig. 11-34).[25]

ANALYSIS
Axial Plane Images (see Figs. 11-4 to 11-8)
Axial sections of the basal ganglia, thalami, and related tracts are best analyzed from superior to inferior, because the relationships of the nuclei to the ventricles are simpler and easier to determine superiorly than inferiorly (see Figs. 11-3 to 11-7).

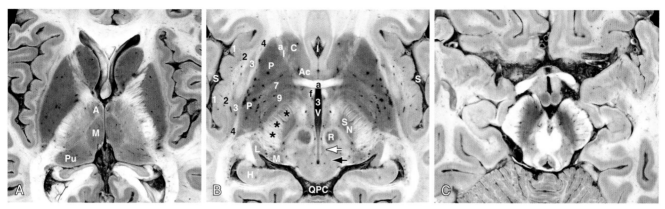

■ **FIGURE 11-33** **A** to **C,** Iron deposition. Magnified axial images after Perl staining. Same specimen as shown in Figure 11-3. The basal ganglia show intense iron stain within the caudate nucleus, putamen, and globus pallidus. The thalami show differential deposition of iron within the anterior nucleus (A), dorsomedial nucleus (M), and pulvinar (Pu) of the thalamus. **B,** Diencephalic-mesencephalic junction. Iron deposition is seen in the red nucleus (R), substantia nigra (SN), and the lateral (7) and medial (9) nuclei of the globi pallidi, with far less iron in the caudate nucleus (C) and putamen (P), and none in the claustrum (3), insular cortex (1), or the medial (M) and lateral (L) geniculate nuclei. H, hippocampus. **C,** The midbrain and hypothalamus show intense staining of the substantia nigra and less intense staining of the mammillary bodies.

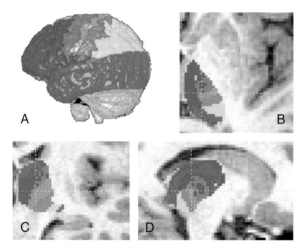

■ **FIGURE 11-34** Connectivity-based segmentation of the thalamus. Behrens and colleagues[28] used probabilistic diffusion tensor tractography to map those thalamic regions with strong reproducible connections to defined areas of the cerebral cortex. **A,** Color-coded parcellation of the cerebral cortex by standard anatomical landmarks. **B** to **D,** Color-coded classification of thalamic voxels based on the probability of their connecting to the defined cortical regions. Note that sagittal image **D** is oriented with anterior to the reader's right, the reverse of the other sagittal images in this chapter. *Anterior, superior medial purple regions* include some of the mediodorsal (dorsomedial) nucleus that receives input from the temporal lobe and parts of the anterior nuclear complex that project to limbic areas in the medial temporal region. *Posterior inferior purple regions* (posterior to the red area shown in **B** and **D**) include parts of the medial and inferior pulvinar that project to the temporal lobe. The *dark blue region* includes some of the mediodorsal nucleus, the ventral anterior nucleus, and portions of the anterior nuclear complex (anterior medial and anterior dorsal nuclei) that project to the prefrontal cortex. The *yellow region* includes anterior portions of the pulvinar that project to posterior parietal cortex. The *pale blue area* includes the lateral posterior and ventral posterolateral nuclei that project to the somatosensory cortices. *The orange area* includes the ventral lateral nucleus (pars posterior [caudalis]) that projects to the primary motor cortex (M1). The *green area* includes the ventral lateral (pars anterior [oralis]) and ventral anterior nuclei that project to premotor areas. The *red regions* include the lateral geniculate nucleus (*visible in the coronal section* **C**), parts of the inferior pulvinar (*most inferior red area visible in sagittal section* **D**), and some of the intralaminar nuclei. These new data confirm the regional interconnections that underlie thalamocortical circuitry. *(From Behrens TEJ, Johansen-Berg H, Woolrich MW, et al. Non-invasive mapping of connections between human thalamus and cortex using diffusion imaging. Nat Neurosci 2003; 6:750-757.)*

1. Identify the upper portions of the lateral ventricles. In this section, the superior lateral angles of the lateral ventricles are composed entirely of white matter. The subependymal veins penetrate this layer of white matter. Just inferior to the lateral angles, the caudate nuclei form long stripes of gray matter along the upper lateral walls of the ventricles. The inferomedial margins of the caudate nuclei abut onto the thalami, forming the caudothalamic grooves. The thalamostriate veins run along these grooves. The heads of the caudate nuclei form bulbous expansions that indent the inferomedial margins of the frontal horns and give them their characteristic "bird wing" shape. This section typically lies superior to the insula, so the extreme capsule, claustrum, and external capsule are not yet visualized.

2. One or two section(s) lower, identify the bulbous heads of the caudate nucleus anteriorly and the tapering bodies of the caudate nuclei posteriorly. The superior portions of the putamina, the caudatolenticular bridges of gray matter, and the intervening internal capsules lie laterally. The uppermost portions of the extreme capsule, claustrum, and external capsule may be seen lateral to the internal capsules. When the patient is canted in the scanner, or the lateral ventricles are asymmetric, the superior portion of the thalamus also may be seen in this section. The lamina affixa covers the superior lateral aspect of the thalamus. The fornices typically overlie the medial portions of the thalamus, with the choroid plexus draped along the lateral borders of the fornices.

3. In the next lower section, identify the paired lateral ventricles, the foramina of Monro, and the third ventricle. Midline structures include the genu of the corpus callosum, the paired leaves of the septum pellucidum, the anterior columns of the fornices, and the third ventricle. The anterior columns form the anteromedial walls of the foramina of Monro. The anterior nuclei of the thalami form the posterolateral walls of the foramina of Monro. Behind the foramina of Monro, the paired thalami form the lateral walls of the third ventricle. The thalami resemble droopy mustaches that have rounded medial borders, are convex toward the midline, and have straighter lateral borders that wing outward, oblique to the midline. The tails of the caudate nuclei arc along the lateral margins of the lateral ventricles just posterolateral to the thalami. Lateral to the caudate heads and thalami, the internal capsules appear as chevrons, open laterally, containing the lenticular nuclei. From lateral to medial, this section displays the sylvian fissure, cistern of the insula, insular cortex,

extreme capsule, claustrum, external capsule, putamen, lateral lamina of the lenticular nucleus, and the lateral nucleus of the globus pallidus (GPe). The caudate nucleus and the putamen show homogeneous density and signal intensity because they are two portions of the same structure. The globus pallidus displays a different density/signal that is closer to white matter. The lateral and medial portions of the thalamus show two different densities/signal intensities, demarcated from each other by the sharp internal medullary lamina.

4. In the next lower section, identify the inferior portions of the atria posteriorly and the midline third ventricle. The anterior commissure forms a prominent white matter bundle in the anterior wall of the third ventricle. The retrocommissural portions of the paired anterior columns of the fornices lie immediately behind the anterior commissure. Together, the midline sections of the anterior commissure and the anterior columns of the fornices characteristically resemble the Greek letter π. This resemblance is a valid landmark for identifying both. Anteriorly, the anterior commissure is related to the heads of the caudate nuclei and the nuclei accumbens. The anterior limbs of the internal capsules just kiss the anterior margins of the anterior commissure. The internal capsules enclose the full widths of the lenticular nuclei. From lateral to medial, this section displays the sylvian fissures, cisterns of the insulae, insular cortices, extreme capsules, claustra, external capsules, putamina, lateral medullary laminae, lateral nuclei of the globus pallidus (GPe), medial medullary laminae, medial nuclei of the globi pallidi (GPi), and internal capsules. The anterior limbs, genus, posterior limbs, and retrolenticular portions of the internal capsules are well shown. This section, or the one below it, usually also displays the upper midbrain. The medial geniculate nuclei form bulges of gray matter along the lateral mesencephalic sulcus. The lateral geniculate nuclei form prominent "carets" of gray matter anterolateral to the medial geniculate nuclei.

5. In the next lower section, identify the transition of basal ganglia to midbrain, the characteristic curvatures of the cerebral peduncles, and, perhaps, the optic tracts encircling the anterior borders of the peduncles. The subthalamic nuclei form paired lenses of gray matter just behind the substantiae nigrae toward the upper strata of the diencephalic-mesencephalic transition. The paired substantiae nigrae also lie immediately posterior to the cerebral peduncles but are most prominent at a level just slightly inferior to the subthalamic nuclei. The substantiae nigrae do not reach to the lateral borders of the midbrain. Instead, the posterior lateral borders of the cerebral peduncles arc backward, lateral to them, sequestering them medially. The paired red nuclei lie behind the substantiae nigrae, just to each side of midline, and resemble "snake eyes." The signal intensities of the substantiae nigrae and red nuclei vary with age and the degree of deposition of ferric iron within them. At this level, dorsally, sections display the aqueduct, the periaqueductal gray matter, and the superior colliculi. It is sometimes helpful to remember that the decussation of the superior cerebellar peduncles lies inferior to the red nuclei and the red nuclei lie slightly inferior to (but overlap with) the subthalamic nuclei.

Coronal Plane Images
Coronal sections of the basal ganglia and thalami are best analyzed from anterior to posterior, beginning in the frontal lobes anterior to the frontal horns and continuing posterior to the pulvinars of the thalami (see Figs. 11-8 to 11-15).

1. Anterior to the frontal horns, the interhemispheric fissure appears as an uninterrupted line of cerebrospinal fluid containing the paired anterior cerebral arteries. The frontal lobe white matter appears as paired masses of white matter, devoid of subependymal veins, ventricles, or gray matter.

2 At the genu of the corpus callosum, the interhemispheric fissure becomes interrupted by the white matter fibers decussating through the genu. Segments of the pericallosal arteries may be seen both inferior to and superior to the genu as they course around the corpus callosum.

3. Immediately posterior to the genu, coronal sections display the septum pellucidum stretched between the body of the corpus callosum above and the rostrum of the corpus callosum below. Anterior to the caudate nuclei, the frontal horns appear as rounded rectangles of cerebrospinal fluid density/signal intensity entirely surrounded by white, not gray, matter. If the anteriormost portions of the caudate heads just protrude into this section, they form small arcs of gray matter along the inferolateral walls of the ventricles.

4. At the levels of the caudate heads and anterior putamina, the white matter fibers radiating from the rostrum diverge laterally and pass under the basal ganglia, forming a layer of white matter that defines the inferior margins of the deep gray nuclei. The septum pellucidum appears as paired parallel septal leaves extending from the undersurface of the body of the corpus callosum to the superior surfaces of the rostrum. The septal veins form small circular flow voids on the septal surface. The heads of the caudate nuclei indent the inferolateral borders of the lateral ventricles. Their subependymal borders appear sharply defined. Their inferolateral borders appear irregular or "ragged" due to the caudatolenticular bridges of gray matter. The gray matter of the caudate nuclei does *not* reach to the superolateral angle of the frontal horns. Instead, the superolateral angles of the frontal horns are entirely surrounded by white matter.

5. Anterior to the foramina of Monro, the nuclei along the inferolateral borders of the lateral ventricles expand substantially. The anterior limbs of the internal capsules enter into the gray matter as wedges of white matter oriented at approximately 45 degrees to the midline. These wedges are wider superolaterally and taper to a point inferomedially. The heads of the caudate nuclei lie superomedial to the wedges. The putamina lie inferolateral to them. In one to two, but not all, sections at this level, the caudate heads are seen to be continuous with the putamina, under the anterior limbs, through portions of the gray matter designated the nuclei accumbens septi. Just lateral to the putamina are the external capsule, claustrum, extreme capsule, and insular cortex. The claustrum is characteristically wider and most easily identified inferiorly where it curves laterally into the temporal lobe.

6. Further posteriorly, the globi pallidi begin to be seen along the inferolateral borders of the internal capsules. Because the globi pallidi are cone shaped with the lateral nuclei larger than the medial nuclei, more anterior sections show only the lateral nuclei of the globi pallidi. More posterior sections show both the medial and the lateral nuclei of the globi pallidi. Far posterior sections again show only the putamen and lateral nucleus.

7. In nearly all coronal sections through the caudate nucleus, the inferolateral edges of the caudate nuclei are connected to the superomedial borders of the putamina by the caudatolenticular bridges of gray matter. The caudatolenticular bridges of gray matter are shorter, thicker, and more numerous anteriorly and longer, thinner, and sparser posteriorly. These bridges mark the site of the internal capsule and establish a landmark for the internal capsule when other landmarks are difficult to discern.

8. The coronal plane through the complete lenticular nucleus (putamen, GPe, and GPi with the intervening laminae) displays the genu of the internal capsule as a crescent of white matter, concave inferiorly, that arches over the lenticular

nuclei. The insula, lenticular nuclei, and associated capsules then resemble a cornucopia composed of alternating bands of gray matter and white matter. For many reasons, it is useful to learn these layers in order from the lateral surface of the brain inward. Thus, from lateral to medial, the structures to be identified are the sylvian fissure, leading to the cistern of the insula, insular cortex, extreme capsule, claustrum, external capsule, putamen, lateral lamina of the lenticular nucleus, lateral nucleus of the globus pallidus (GPe) containing the anterior commissure inferiorly, medial lamina of the lenticular nucleus, medial nucleus of the globus pallidus (GPi) containing the incomplete lamina of the lenticular nucleus within it, and the internal capsule.

9. Further posteriorly, coronal sections display progressively thinner portions of the lenticular nucleus, first the putamen and GPe and then the putamen alone. Posterior to that, the coronal sections pass behind the lenticular nucleus to display the retrolenticular portion of the internal capsule.

10. Posterior to the foramina of Monro, coronal sections begin to display the thalami medial to the posterior limbs of the internal capsules. The thalami appear as large paired masses of gray matter that form, simultaneously, the lateral walls of the third ventricle and the medial floors of the lateral ventricles. The anterior poles of the thalami make up the posterolateral walls of the foramina of Monro. They contain the anterior nuclear groups of the thalami. The mammillothalamic tracts pass upward from the mammillary bodies to the anterior nuclei of the thalami. More posterior sections show the posterior limbs of the internal capsules as paired parentheses of white matter. The major portions of the thalami lie deep to the posterior limbs, within these parentheses. The laminae affixae form thin horizontal layers of white matter that outline and emphasize the superior surfaces of the thalami laterally, just deep to the internal capsules. The density and signal intensity of the ventral/lateral thalamic nuclei differ from those of the medial thalamic nuclei. From lateral to medial, coronal images show the density/signal of the ventral/lateral nuclear groups, a sharp demarcation at their interface along the internal medullary lamina, and a different density/signal intensity within the medial nuclear group. At times, advanced MRI may also resolve the intercalated (intralaminar) nuclei. At present, the identification of specific thalamic nuclei depends on triangulating their location and naming them by location. In one case, the mammillothalamic tract provides additional confirmation for identifying the anterior nuclear group. As yet no specific anatomic criteria have evolved for identifying the other nuclei by their intrinsic features.

11. Posterior to the thalami, the third ventricle, aqueduct, and interpeduncular fossa identify the midline. The perimesencephalic cisterns identify the lateral margins of the midbrain. From superior and lateral, one can trace the posterior limbs of the internal capsules into the cerebral peduncles. The substantiae nigrae lie immediately deep to the peduncles. The red nuclei form paired "snake eyes" just to each side of midline at a level between the third ventricle or aqueduct above and the interpeduncular fossa below. The lens-shaped subthalamic nuclei lie deep to the cerebral peduncles partially lateral to the red nuclei and partially superolateral to them. The widest dimension of the subthalamic nucleus lies at the upper pole of the red nucleus. Just superolateral to the red nuclei, the triangular to flame-shaped zone of white matter density/signal intensity identifies the multiple intermingled fiber tracts of the area tegmentalis (see text and Figs. 11-13B, 11-14, 11-17, 11-18, and 11-20).

12. In coronal images, demonstration of the lateral geniculate nuclei is facilitated by using the posterior commissure/obex (PC-O) line to orient the sections. On sagittal scout images,

draw the PC-O line from the anterior margin of the posterior commissure to the obex. A short series of coronal plane images oriented along the PC-O line from 1 cm anterior to the line to 1 cm posterior to the line will display the lateral geniculate nucleus reproducibly.[15]

Sagittal Images

A number of anatomic relationships establish landmarks for interpreting the sagittal images of the deep gray nuclei and capsules (see Figs. 11-2, 11-19, and 11-20).

1. Interpret the images from the midline outward, because midline structures provide the most secure foundation for starting analysis.

2. Identify the characteristic downward curve of the splenium. Confirm this by noting the tag of the fornix applied to the anterior surface of the splenium.

3. Determine from the density/signal intensity of the splenium (white matter) whether the study depicts white matter as high or low signal intensity.

4. Then follow the curvature of the corpus callosum *backward*: from the splenium, along the body and around the genu to identify the rostrum and the radiations that pass through the rostrum of the corpus callosum. These radiations define the inferior margin of the basal ganglia

5. The gangliothalamic complex and its capsules should resemble a figure-of-eight laid on its side (compare with Fig. 11-2).

6. Recheck the density/signal intensity of the white matter and use that to identify the internal capsule within the figure-of-eight. The shape of the internal capsule varies systematically from medial to lateral (review Figs. 11-19 and 11-20).

7. In three dimensions, the internal capsule resembles a hollow cone, open laterally. Because the cone of the internal capsule is widest laterally and narrowest medially, sagittal sections through the medial portion of the internal capsule show a *narrow* arc of white matter corresponding to the narrow end of the cone. Sagittal sections through the lateral portion of the internal capsule show a *wide* arc of curvature corresponding to the open lateral end of the cone.

8. Far laterally, identify the internal capsule by the caudatolenticular bridges of gray matter that cross the internal capsule between the caudate nucleus superolaterally and the putamen inferomedially. These bridges identify the periphery of the internal capsule reliably when other landmarks are not available.

9. The lenticular nucleus fills the hollow cone of the internal capsule. In all sections through the internal capsule, therefore, identify the gray matter within the arc of the internal capsule as the components of the lenticular nucleus.

10. Because the putamen, GPe, and GPi appear in fixed order from lateral to medial, and because all of these nuclei are oriented obliquely to the midline, medial sagittal sections show the GPe anterior to the GPi, not the GPi alone. Paramedian sections show the putamen, GPe, and GPi in that order from front to back. More lateral sections show the putamen anterior to the GPe, but not GPi, and far lateral sections show the putamen alone.

11. The anterior commissure appears as a round to ovoid white matter structure in all but the most lateral sections. In sequential sagittal images, identify the anterior commissure and trace it from the anterior wall of the third ventricle in the midline, under the anterior limb of the internal capsule, through the inferior portion of the GPe, under the putamen, over the amygdala, and on into the temporal lobe. The position of the anterior commissure helps confirm the identities of the other structures displayed.

12. Identify the gray matter behind the internal capsule as the thalamus. The lateral border of the thalamus wings outward,

oblique to the midline. Therefore, all sagittal sections intersect and display the lateral thalamus before they pass through and display the medial posterior thalamus.

13. The oblique internal medullary lamina roughly parallels the lateral border of the thalamus and provides a sharp interface between the nuclear groups that lie anterolateral to the lamina and those that lie posteromedial to the lamina. In all sagittal sections through the thalamus, therefore, the ventral lateral nuclei of the thalamus lie anterior to and appear sharply demarcated from the medial and pulvinaric nuclei.

14. The sylvian fissure, insula, and all structures situated deep to the insula show a curvature that is convex laterally.

Therefore, the anterior and posterior ends of the cistern of the insula, insular cortex, and subjacent layers of gray and white matter are also convex and curve inward toward the midline. For that reason, *sagittal* sections through these structures display the same layers in the same order from anterior to posterior that *coronal* sections display them from lateral to medial. That is, where the anterior end of the insula curves inward, lateral sagittal sections will display the cistern of the insula, insular cortex, extreme capsule, claustrum, external capsule, and putamen, in that order from anterior to posterior.

A sample report is presented in Box 11-1.

BOX 11-1   Sample Report: MRI of Electrode Placement for Deep Brain Stimulation

PATIENT HISTORY

An immediate postoperative control MR image was obtained in a 75-year-old man with known Parkinson disease returning from the operating room after bilateral placement of deep brain stimulation leads (Fig. 11-35).

COMPARISON STUDY

A preoperative MR image had been obtained immediately before the procedure.

TECHNIQUE

Limited postoperative MRI was performed as axial and coronal plane short tau inversion recovery (STIR) images. No contrast agent was employed.

FINDINGS

Since the preoperative study performed earlier the same morning, two deep brain stimulation leads have been placed into the brain stem. The tips of the electrodes lie in the expected positions of the subthalamic nuclei bilaterally.

Serial images through the whole brain show the postoperative changes in the scalp and skull expected for prior placement of a four-point head holder. The electrodes pass lateral to the ventricular system. There is no evidence of extra-axial or parenchymal hemorrhage and no evidence of excess edema along the tracts. The remaining brain structures appear unchanged.

IMPRESSION

Electrodes were placed into the subthalamic nuclei bilaterally. There is no imaging evidence of hemorrhage, edema, or other complication of the procedure.

KEY POINTS

■ The basal ganglia and their associated fibers may be viewed as a "stained glass window" in which the individual gray nuclei are like the colored pieces of glass, the fibers form laminae and capsules that are like the lead frames that encircle the pieces of glass, and the full composition requires both gray and white matter (glass and leading) to make a meaningful picture.

■ The gray matter and white matter are organized in consistent, reproducible layers that permit the imager to identify one structure within the stack and then count, layer by layer, in any direction, to identify all other layers of the stack.

■ In coronal and axial sections through the midlenticular nucleus, one may name layers from lateral to medial: sylvian fissure, cistern of insula, insular cortex, extreme capsule, claustrum, external capsule, putamen, lateral lamina (of lenticular nucleus), lateral nucleus of the globus pallidus, medial lamina (of the lenticular nucleus), medial nucleus of the globus pallidus containing the intermediate lamina (of the lenticular nucleus), internal capsule, reticular nucleus of the thalamus, lateral medullary lamina of the thalamus, lateral group of thalamic nuclei, internal medullary lamina of the thalamus (containing the intercalated thalamic nuclei), medial group of the thalamic nuclei, and third ventricle in the midline.

■ Because the external surface of the insula is convex laterally, the anterior and posterior ends of the cistern of the insula, the insular cortex, and all the underlying layers also curve toward the midline both anteriorly and posteriorly. Therefore, one can count the same structures in the same order from anterior to posterior on sagittal images that one counted from lateral to medial on axial and coronal images.

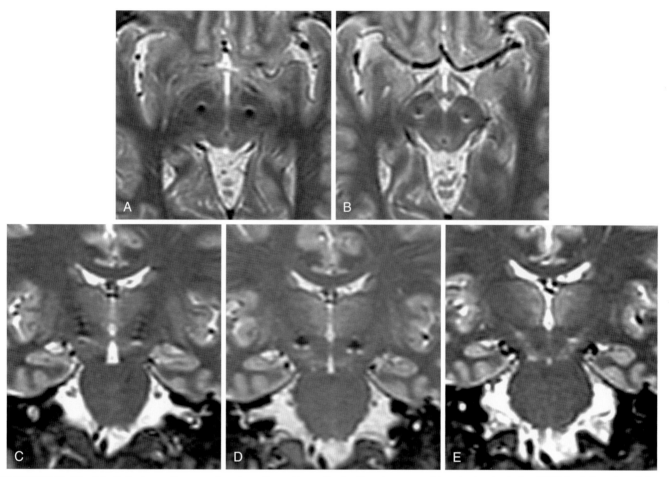

■ **FIGURE 11-35** **A** to **E,** Postoperative control study performed immediately after placement of deep brain stimulation (DBS) leads into the subthalamic nuclei for treatment of Parkinson's disease (see sample report in Box 11-1). Short tau inversion recovery images. **A** and **B,** Axial sections displayed from craniad (**A**) to caudad (**B**), coned to the brain stem. **C** to **E,** Coronal sections displayed from anterior (**C**) through posterior (**E**). Wider areas of the brain are discussed in the report as pertinent negatives but are not illustrated here. See anatomic sections shown in Figure 11-15 (axial) and Figure 11-17 (coronal) for comparison.

SUGGESTED READINGS

Carpenter MB, Sutin J. Human Neuroanatomy, 8th ed. Baltimore, Williams & Wilkins, 1983.

Gilman S, Newman SW. Manter and Gatz' Essentials of Clinical Neuroanatomy and Neurophysiology, 10th ed. Philadelphia, FA Davis, 2003.

Naidich TP, Duvernoy HM, Delman BN, et al. High-field MRI: surface anatomy, internal structure, vascularization and 3D sectional anatomy. In: Duvernoy's Atlas of the Human Brain Stem and Cerebellum. New York, Springer, 2008.

Nieuwenhuys R, Voogd J, van Huijzen C. The Human Central Nervous System, 4th ed. Berlin, Springer, 2008.

Standring S, et al (eds). Gray's Anatomy: The Anatomical Basis of Clinical Practice, 40th ed. Philadelphia, Elsevier, 2008.

Talairach J, Tournoux P. Co-planar Stereotaxic Atlas of the Human Brain. New York, Thieme, 1988.

REFERENCES

1. Daniels DL, Haughton VM, Naidich TP. Cranial and Spinal Magnetic Resonance Imaging: An Atlas and Guide. New York, Raven Press, 1987.

2. Nauta HJW. A Simplified Perspective on the Basal Ganglia and their Relationships to the Limbic System. New York, Raven Press, 1986.

3. Naidich TP, Daniels DL, Haughton VM. Deep cerebral structures. In Daniels DL, Haughton VM, Naidich TP (eds). Cranial and Spinal Magnetic Resonance Imaging: An Atlas and Guide. New York, Raven Press, 1987.

4. Riley HA. An Atlas of the Basal Ganglia, Brain Stem and Spinal Cord. Baltimore, Williams & Wilkins, 1943.

5. Standring S, et al (eds). Gray's Anatomy: The Anatomical Basis of Clinical Practice, 39th ed. Philadelphia, Elsevier, 2005.

6. Standring S, et al (eds). Gray's Anatomy: The Anatomical Basis of Clinical Practice, 40th ed. Philadelphia, Elsevier, 2008.

7. Carpenter MB, Sutin J. Human Neuroanatomy, 8th ed. Baltimore, Williams & Wilkins, 1983.

8. Nieuwenhuys R, Voogd J, van Huijzen C. The Human Central Nervous System. A Synopsis and Atlas, 3rd rev ed. Berlin, Springer, 1988.

9. Nieuwenhuys R, Voogd J, van Huijzen C. The Human Central Nervous System, 4th ed. Berlin, Springer, 2008.

10. Naidich TP, Duvernoy HM, Delman BN, et al. High-field MRI: surface anatomy, internal structure, vascularization and 3D sectional anatomy. In: Duvernoy's Atlas of the Human Brain Stem and Cerebellum. New York, Springer, 2008.

11. Larsen WJ. Human Embryology, 3rd ed. Philadelphia, Churchill Livingstone, 2001.

12. Jain M, Armstrong RJE, Barker RA, Rosser AE. Cellular and molecular aspects of striatal development. Brain Res Bull 2001; 55:533-540.

13. Gilman S, Newman SW. Manter and Gatz' Essentials of Clinical Neuroanatomy and Neurophysiology, 10th ed. Philadelphia, FA Davis, 2003.

14. Naidich TP, Daniels DL, Pech P, et al. Anterior commissure: anatomic-MR correlation and use as a landmark in three orthogonal planes. Radiology 1986; 158:421-429.

15. Tamraz JC, Outin-Tamraz C, Saban R. MR imaging anatomy of the optic pathways. Radiol Clin North Am 37:1-36, 1999.

16. Hikosaka O, Sesack SR, Lecourtier L, et al. Crossroad between the basal ganglia and the limbic system. J Neurosci 2008; 28: 11825-11829.

17. Chakravarthy VS, Joseph D, Bapi RS. What do the basal ganglia do? A modeling perspective. Biol Cybern 2010; 103:237-253.

18. Nakano K, Kayahara T, Tsutsumi T, Ushiro H. Neural circuits and functional organization of the striatum. J Neurol 2000; 247(Suppl 5):V1-V15.

19. Obeso JA, Rodriguez-Oroz MC, Benitez-Temino B, et al. Functional organization of the basal ganglia: therapeutic implications for S548-S559. Mov Disord 2008; 23(Suppl 3):S548-S559.

20. Herrero MT, Barcia C, Navarro JM. Functional anatomy of the thalamus and basal ganglia. Childs Nerv Syst 2002; 18:386-404.

21. Arbuthnott GW, Ingham CA, Wickens JR. Review: dopamine and synaptic plasticity in the neostriatum. J Anat 2000; 196:587-596.

22. Bolam JP, Hanley JJ, Booth PAC, Bevan MD. Review: synaptic organization of the basal ganglia. J Anat 2000; 196:527-542.

23. Li S, Arbuthnott GW, Jutras MJ, et al. Resonant antidromic cortical circuit activation as a consequence of high-frequency subthalamic stimulation. J Neurophysiol 2007; 98:3525-3537.

24. Moss J, Bolam JP. A dopaminergic axon lattice in the striatum and its relationship with cortical and thalamic terminals. J Neurosci 2008; 28:11221-11230.

25. Drayer B, Burger P, Darwin Riederer S, et al. MRI of brain iron. AJR Am J Roentgenol 1986; 147:103-110.

26. Drayer BP. Imaging of the aging brain: I. Normal findings. Radiology 1988;166:785-796.

27. Aoki S, Okada Y, Nishimura K, et al. Normal deposition of brain iron in childhood and adolescence: MR imaging at 1.5T. Radiology 1989; 172:381-385.

28. Behrens TEJ, Johansen-Berg H, Woolrich MW, et al. Non-invasive mapping of connections between human thalamus and cortex using diffusion imaging. Nat Neurosci 2003; 6:750-757.

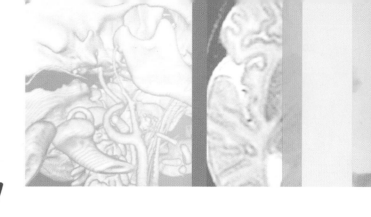

CHAPTER 12

White Matter

Thomas P. Naidich, Niklaus Krayenbühl, Spyros Kollias, Pascal Bou-Haidar, Avraham Y. Bluestone, and David M. Carpenter

The supratentorial white matter is the gross structure formed by the axons that arise from neurons situated within the gray matter (Fig. 12-1).[1-3] The term *white matter* derives from the glistening fatty "white" myelin sheath that surrounds many of the axons. These axons may be heavily myelinated, lightly myelinated or unmyelinated. The proportion of myelinated fibers increases with phylogenetic, embryologic, and developmental growth. From shrews to whales, the composition of the cerebral white matter shifts from compact, slow-conducting unmyelinated axons to large fast-conducting myelinated axons.[4] The fastest of these have conduction times of 1 to 5 ms across the neocortex and less than 1 ms from eye to brain.[4]

Commissural fibers are bihemispheric fibers that cross the midline to interconnect the two cerebral hemispheres. *Homotopic* commissural fibers interconnect corresponding regions of the two hemispheres.[2,3] *Heterotopic* commissural fibers connect one cortical area with noncorresponding areas of the contralateral hemisphere.[2] In many cases, the regions to which heterotopic commissural fibers pass are the same regions to which the contralateral cortex sends association fibers within its own hemisphere.[2]

Projection fibers are unihemispheric fibers that convey impulses from the cortex to subcortical regions such as the basal ganglia, diencephalon, brain stem, and the spinal cord (often after crossing over the midline in the brain stem).[2,3]

Association fibers are unihemispheric fibers that connect diverse regions of the same hemisphere. Short association fibers pass through the deep layers of the cortex and/or the subcortical white matter as short curved U fibers to interconnect adjacent cortical areas.[2] Long association fibers lie more deeply within the white matter and span large distances across a single hemisphere.

Within the white matter, the axons gather into bundles that are classified by their position and function. The nomenclature of fiber bundles is highly variable. On average, rounded bundles of fibers are designated striae, fascicles, and tracts, whereas broad sheets of fibers are designated laminae, capsules, and radiations. These names are broadly descriptive of the size and shape of the fiber bundles but are often used historically or idiosyncratically with little adherence to precise definition.[5] With that understanding, here are some descriptions:

Striae are thin bundles of fibers that pass longitudinally across the brain.

Fascicles are microscopically determinable groups of fibers.[5]

Tracts are groups of axons subserving a similar or corresponding function.[5]

Laminae are relatively thin sheets of axons that proceed in a similar direction.

Capsules are curved sheets of fibers that partially enclose gray matter structures.

Radiations are broad sheets of fibers that arch together to or from one target.

Decussations are crossings of two fiber tracts in the midline. This term has been generalized to signify both the sites at which the fiber tracts cross the midline and the names of the crossing tracts.

ANATOMY
Gross Appearance

Grossly, the white matter of the cerebral hemispheres forms the thick layer between the cortical gray matter of the surface and the deep gray nuclei of the basal ganglia and thalami (Fig. 12-1). Superior to the lateral ventricles the white matter assumes the shape of each hemisphere, so it is designated by the aggregate term *centrum semiovale.* Peripherally, the white matter extends outward into every gyrus to form the central white matter cores (digitations) of the gyri. Centrally, it extends medially, bilaterally, to cross the midline as commissures and decussations and extends craniocaudally to form the corona radiata and the capsules of the hemispheres. Table 12-1 lists some of the fiber tracts discussed in this chapter and summarizes a few of their key connections.[1-8] These will be elaborated on within each section.

The fiber tracts of the brain course through the cerebral hemispheres in multiple directions within multiple overlapping layers. On average, commissural fibers course transversely between the hemispheres. Projection fibers course obliquely craniocaudal within one hemisphere and may extend caudally outside the hemisphere. Long association fibers course obliquely, anteroposteriorly, within one hemisphere. Careful dissection of the brain from the lateral surface, medial surface, and superior surface discloses the major layers of these fibers and their orientation (Figs. 12-2 and 12-3; Box 12-1).[9-11]

Microscopy

Histologic sections of the cerebral white matter demonstrate the orientations and bundling of the axons and their myelin sheaths

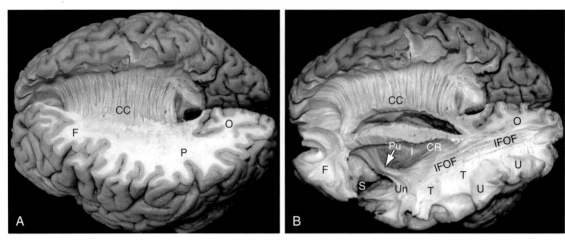

■ **FIGURE 12-1** Gross dissection of the human brain by the Klingler technique (Dr. Nicklaus Krayenbühl). **A,** View from above and the left side. Axial section through the frontal (F), parietal (P), and occipital (O) lobes of the left hemisphere discloses the white matter within the centrum semiovale (F-P-O) and the upper border of the corpus callosum. Klingler dissection of the medial surface of the right hemisphere exposes the multiple, superiorly arching commissural fibers (CC) that extend through the corpus callosum into the medial portion of the opposite hemisphere. **B,** Further dissection of the left hemisphere exposes projection fibers (uncinate fasciculus [Un], internal capsule [I]), short association U fibers (U), and long association fibers (inferior fronto-occipital fasciculus [IFOF]) within the white matter. The uncinate fasciculus (Un) arches over the sylvian fissure (S) to interconnect the temporal lobe (T) with the frontal lobe (F). The inferior fronto-occipital fasciculus extends the length of the hemisphere to interconnect the occipital lobe with the ipsilateral frontal lobe. Its fibers characteristically compact into a narrow bundle (*white arrow*) where the tract traverses the floor of the external capsule just inferolateral to the putamen (Pu). In this position, it courses immediately superior to the fibers of the uncinate fasciculus. The vertical fibers of the corona radiata (CR) converge to form the compact internal capsule (I) that passes medial to the putamen.

TABLE 12-1. Partial Summary of Fiber Tracts Discussed in This Chapter

Fiber Tract	Interconnecting	With
Commissural Fibers		
Corpus callosum	Ipsilateral hemisphere	Contralateral hemisphere
Anterior commissure	Ipsilateral olfactory nuclei and cortex	Contralateral olfactory nuclei and cortex
	Orbitofrontal, temporal, and occipital cortex	Contralateral cortices and possibly the amygdalae
Hippocampal commissure	Ipsilateral hippocampal formation	Contralateral hippocampal formation
Projection Fibers		
Corticospinal tract	Primary motor cortex (BA 4)	Spinal cord
	Premotor cortex (BA 6)	
	Somatosensory cortices (BA 3, 2, 1)	
	Parietal lobe (BA 5)	
Optic radiations	Lateral geniculate nucleus	Primary visual cortex (BA 17) and secondary visual areas
Auditory radiations	Medial geniculate nucleus	Primary auditory cortex (BA 41 and 42) and secondary auditory areas
Fornix	Hippocampal formation	Septal region and mammillary body
		Thalamus?
Short Association Fibers		
U fibers	One gyrus	Adjacent gyrus
Long Association Fibers		
Cingulum bundle	Frontal and parietal lobes	Parahippocampal gyrus and adjacent temporal lobe
Superior longitudinal fasciculus	Frontal lobe (e.g., Broca's area)	Occipital lobe (visual cortex)
		Parietal and temporal lobes (Wernicke's area)
Uncinate fasciculus	Orbital cortices	Entorhinal cortex and hippocampal formation
Extreme capsule	Prefrontal cortex	Temporal cortex
Arcuate fasciculus	Frontal lobe	Temporal and parietal lobes
Superior fronto-occipital fasciculus	Prefrontal cortex	Limbic and paralimbic areas
Inferior fronto-occipital fasciculus	Frontobasal cortex	Temporal and occipital cortices
Inferior longitudinal fasciculus	Temporal lobe and amygdala	Parietal and occipital cortices

BA, Brodmann's area.
Data derived in part from references 1 to 8.

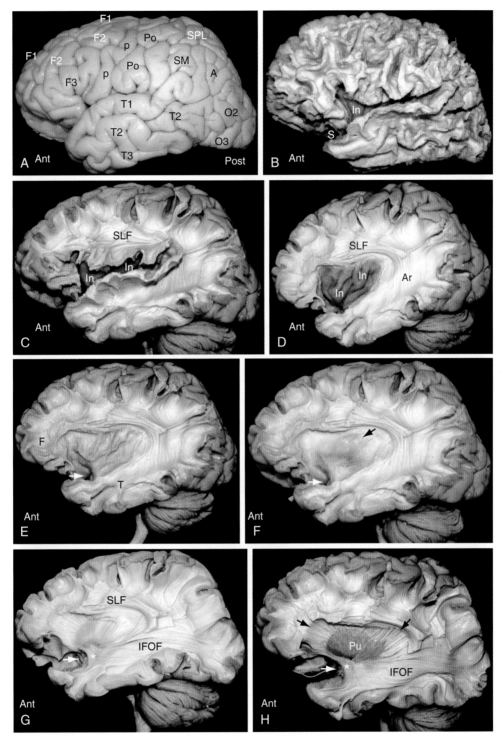

■ **FIGURE 12-2** Dissection of the human brain from the lateral aspect by the Klingler technique (Dr. Nicklaus Krayenbühl). Ant, anterior; Post, posterior. **A,** Lateral surface of the hemisphere. Removal of the leptomeninges and vessels exposes the cortical gray matter. F1, superior frontal gyrus; F2, middle frontal gyrus; F3, inferior frontal gyrus; p, precentral gyrus; Po, postcentral gyrus; SPL, superior parietal lobule; SMG and AG, the supramarginal gyrus and angular gyrus of the inferior parietal lobule; T1, superior temporal gyrus; T2, middle temporal gyrus; T3, inferior temporal gyrus; O2, middle occipital gyrus; O3, inferior occipital gyrus. **B,** Scraping away the cortical gray matter exposes the white matter cores (digitations) of the gyri and the short association U fibers that interconnect them. The insula (In) just becomes visible through the now-wider sylvian fissure. **C,** Resecting the superficial digitations exposes the superior longitudinal fasciculus (SLF) superior to the sylvian fissure and insula (In). Short association U fibers interconnect the adjacent gyri. **D,** Resecting the overhanging margins of the frontal, parietal and temporal opercula exposes the underlying insula (In) and the relationship of the SLF and the arcuate fasciculus (Ar) to the insula (In). **E,** Careful resection of the insular cortex then exposes the thin layer of white matter that makes up the underlying extreme capsule. Fiber tracts passing from the temporal lobe (T) to the frontal lobe (F) must pass deep to the limen insulae (*white arrow*) through the anterior inferior portion of the extreme capsule. **F,** Removal of the extreme capsule exposes the gray matter of the claustrum (*brownish color indicated by the black arrow*). *White arrow* as in **E. G,** Resection of the claustrum exposes the fibers of the external capsule and fibers passing toward the internal capsule (see **H** and **I**). The temporal white matter displays the inferior fronto-occipital fasciculus (IFOF) and the uncinate fasciculus (*asterisk*) (see also Fig. 12-1B). The inferior fronto-occipital fasciculus forms part of the external sagittal stratum lateral to the temporal and occipital horns. *White arrow* as in **E** and **F. H,** Resection of the external capsule exposes the putamen (Pu) and its relationship to the radiating fibers (*black arrows*) converging toward the internal capsule deep to the putamen. The anterior end of the long inferior fronto-occipital fasciculus (IFOF) courses around the deep end (*white arrow*) of the sylvian fissure with and immediately superior to the uncinate fasciculus (*asterisk*).

Continued

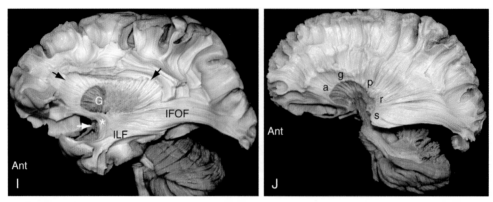

■ FIGURE 12-2, cont'd   **I,** Partial removal of the anterior putamen exposes the medially positioned globus pallidus and the course of the fibers (*black arrows*) converging to the internal capsule deep to both nuclei. *White arrow* as in **E** to **G. J,** Complete resection of the putamen and globus pallidus (lenticular nucleus) and the uncinate fasciculus reveals the radial array of the fibers forming the corona radiata. The curvature of the fibers about the (resected) lenticular nucleus shows the positions of the anterior limb (a), genu (g), posterior limb (p), retrolenticular (r), and sublenticular (s) portions of the internal capsule. Resection of much of the anterior temporal lobe and more lateral portions of the posterior temporal and occipital lobes exposes posterior portions of the optic radiations as they traverse the retrolenticular portion of the internal capsule and then pass posteriorly to the occipital cortex in the external sagittal stratum.

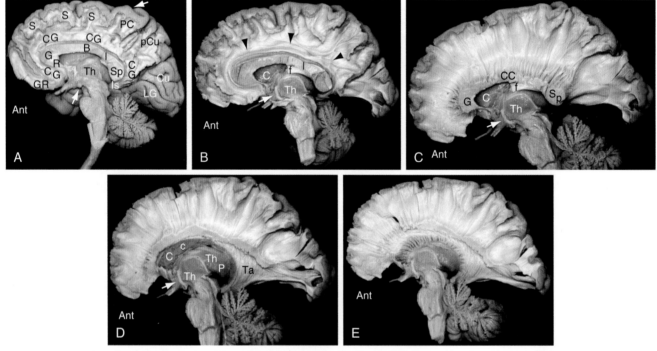

■ FIGURE 12-3   Dissection of the human brain from the medial aspect by the Klingler technique (Dr. Nicklaus Krayenbühl). **A,** Medial surface of the brain after removal of the cortical gray matter of the frontal and parietal lobes exposes the rostrum (R), genu (G), body (B), isthmus (I), and splenium (Sp) of the corpus callosum, the digitations and U fibers of the gyrus rectus (GR), cingulate gyrus (CG), superior frontal gyrus (S), paracentral lobule (PC), precuneus (pCu), and isthmus (Is) of the cingulate gyrus. The cortex of the cuneus (Cu) and lingual gyrus (LG) of the occipital lobe remains in place. The *upper white arrow* indicates the central sulcus on the medial surface. Th, medial surface of the thalamus; *lower white arrow,* mammillary body. **B to E,** The temporal lobe has been resected. **B,** Further dissection reveals the cingulum bundle (*black arrowheads*) coursing through the cingulate gyrus as it arches over the corpus callosum. The midportion of the fornix has been resected to expose the caudate nucleus (C). The posterior portion of the fornix (f) is applied to the undersurface of the corpus callosum at the isthmus (I). The anterior column (*white arrow*) of the fornix extends to the mammillary body (*obscured here but visible in the subsequent images*). The thin curved stria medullaris thalami courses along the medial wall of the thalamus (Th) to interconnect the septal nuclei with the habenular nuclei. The position of the stria medullaris thalami marks the site at which the roof of the third ventricle inserts into the medial surface of the thalamus. Additional portions of the thalamus are just becoming visible posterosuperior to the stria. **C,** Removal of the digitations and U fibers of the medial gyri of the hemisphere exposes the commissural fibers (CC) passing to and from the frontal, parietal, and occipital lobes to form the corpus callosum. Temporal contributions to the corpus callosum are not shown in this specimen. Other labels are as in **A** and **B. D,** Resection of additional portions of the corpus callosum and entry into the lateral ventricle exposes the inner surface of the lateral wall of the ventricle along much of its length. Anteriorly, the head (C) and body (c) of the caudate nucleus form the inferolateral wall of the lateral ventricle. Further posteriorly, the thalamus (Th) forms the floor of the body of the lateral ventricle. The tapetum (Ta) of the corpus callosum forms the lateral wall of the temporal horn, atrium, and occipital horn of the lateral ventricle. A far greater extent of the medial surface of the thalamus is now seen anteroinferior and posterosuperior to the curved stria medullaris thalami. Other labels are as earlier designated. **E,** Further removal of the corpus callosum and removal of much of the caudate nucleus exposes the thalamic peduncles converging/diverging to interconnect the thalamus with all portions of the cortex (see also Fig. 12-14D).

BOX 12-1 Klingler Technique for White Matter Dissection

The Klingler technique and its modifications are methods for dissecting the white matter of the brain. In this method, one starts with a brain specimen obtained at postmortem within 12 hours after death and fixes it in 10% formalin for a minimum of 2 months. The operative microscope is then used to thoroughly remove the leptomeninges and all associated vasculature, thereby exposing the gray matter throughout. This prepared specimen is then subjected to one or more cycles of deep freezing and thawing at −10°C to −15°C to permit formalin ice crystals to expand between and separate the white matter fibers. After thawing, dissection is carried out under the operating microscope at 4 to 10× magnification. The freeze-treated gray matter is readily avulsed to expose the subcortical U fibers. Specially shaped thin wooden spatulas are then used to raise up small numbers of white fibers oriented in specific directions. These fibers are then peeled off *along their length* to expose the next-lower layer. Sequentially, layer by layer, known groups of parallel fibers are peeled away to expose the next-lower, differently oriented groups of fibers. By this serial dissection technique, the specific layers of fibers that form each major fasciculus can be identified, exposed along their length to demonstrate their origins and terminations, and then removed to expose the next-deeper layer. Serial photographs obtained at each stage of dissection document the orientation and extent of each tract.

Data from Klingler J, Gloor P. The connections of the amygdala and of the anterior temporal cortex in the human brain. J Comp Neurol 1960; 115:333-369; Türe U, Yaşargil MG, Friedman AH, Al-Mefty O. Fiber dissection technique: lateral aspect of the brain. Neurosurgery 2000; 47:417-427; and Yasargil MG. Surgical anatomy of supratentorial midline lesions Neurosurg Focus 2005; 18(6b):E1.

(Figs. 12-4 and 12-5). The cerebral white matter contains neuroglial support cells such as oligodendroglia and astrocytes but does not contain neuronal cell bodies.[12] The oligodendroglial cells are moderate-sized cells that extend short branched processes to ensheath adjacent segments of up to 40 neighboring axons (Fig. 12-6).[12] Within each segment, the membrane process of the oligodendroglial cell wraps spirally around the axon and then condenses into a tight myelin sheath of up to 150 layers.[13] The myelin sheath remains continuous with the cell membrane of the oligodendroglial cell but displays a simplified chemical composition. Because each segment of myelin derives from one oligodendroglial cell, the myelin sheath of each axon is composed of multiple different segments supplied by different oligodendroglial cells. These segments are separated from each other by "gaps" designated the nodes of Ranvier. In myelinated axons, nerve impulses "jump" rapidly down the axon from node to node (saltatory conduction), rather than pass slowly along the entire length of the axon.

The astrocytes help to establish and preserve the structure and integrity of the myelin and axons. They stimulate the oligodendroglial cell precursors to proliferate, migrate, and differentiate.[12] They assist in the initial adhesion of the oligodendroglial cell processes to the axons and release growth factors that promote myelination.[12] The astrocytes participate in the conduction of impulses at the nodes of Ranvier and serve to recycle the excitatory neurotransmitter glutamate at synapses.[12] Astrocytes also help to maintain the cerebrospinal fluid-brain and blood-brain barriers. After damage to the white matter, the astrocytes enlarge, proliferate, and accumulate glycogen and filaments, a process designated *gliosis*.[12] The gliosis may occur within a

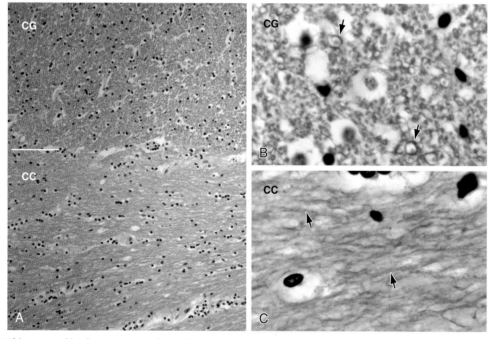

■ FIGURE 12-4 White matter histology. Hematoxylin and eosin (H&E) stain colors the myelin and cytoplasm shades of pink and the nuclei blue. **A,** Coronal section through the interface (*white line*) of the corpus callosum (CC) with the white matter of the cingulate gyrus (CG) (original magnification, ×10). Routine H&E sections resolve the transverse orientation of the callosal fibers (CC) versus the longitudinal orientation of the cingulate white matter (CG) but usually do not distinguish the axon and myelin sheath from the surrounding neuropil. **B** and **C,** Magnified coronal sections of the cingulate gyrus (**B**) and corpus callosum (**C**) (original magnifications, ×60). Higher magnification shows the myelin sheaths (*black arrows*) displaced away from the cytoplasm of the central axon by fixation artifact. In cross section (**B**), the myelin sheaths appear as thin, slightly darker "donut rings" surrounding small slightly lighter dot-like central axons. In longitudinal sections (**C**), the sheaths (*black arrows*) appear as thin dark lines coursing in bundles.

■ **FIGURE 12-5** White matter histology. Axons and myelin. **A** and **B**, Bielschowsky stain for axons (original magnifications, ×4 (**A**) and ×20 (**B**). The Bielschowsky modified silver stain renders axons black and myelin shades of brown. This clearly distinguishes the linear transverse fibers of the corpus callosum (CC) from the dot-like cross sections of the longitudinally oriented cingulate fibers (CG). *Black arrow,* blood vessel. **C** and **D**, Luxol fast blue (LFB) stain for myelin with H&E counterstain (original magnifications, ×4 (**A**) and ×20 (**B**). LFB stains myelin blue. H&E stains myelin and cytoplasm pink and nuclei blue. LFB stains demonstrate the differing orientations of the interwoven fibers, their aggregation into fiber bundles, and the spacing of their myelin sheaths.

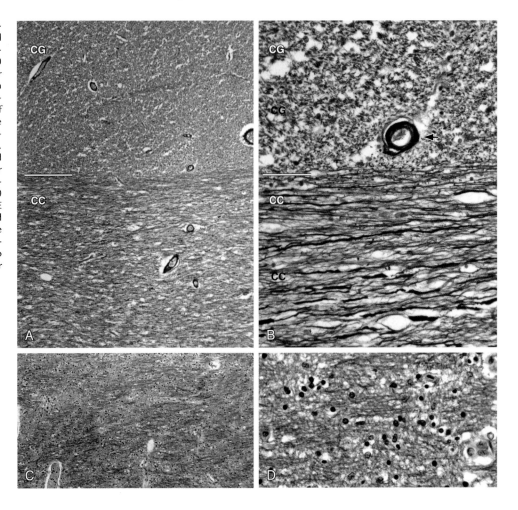

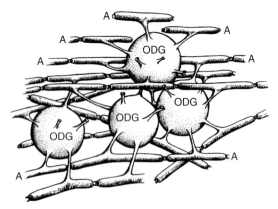

■ **FIGURE 12-6** Each oligodendroglial (ODG) cell extends processes from its cell wall to enwrap segments of multiple adjacent axons (A). These establish the central myelin sheaths. *(Modified from van der Knaap MS, Valk J. Magnetic Resonance of Myelination and Myelin Disorders, 3rd ed. Berlin, Springer, 2005.)*

region of normal or regenerating myelin, or it may be seen to replace all normal tissue as a glial scar.[12] Emery reviews the regulation of oligodendrocyte differentiation and myelination in detail.[14]

Central nervous system (CNS) white matter is approximately half myelin and half protein.[12] It has a lower water content (72%) than gray matter (82%).[12] As a percent of total lipid weight, the lipids of CNS myelin are cholesterol (25% to 28%), galactolipid (27% to 30%), and phospholipids (40% to 45%).[12] No single lipid is unique to myelin, but high concentrations of cerebroside are typical of myelin.[12] In contradistinction to the lipids, most of the myelin proteins are unique to myelin.[12] Sixty to 80 percent of the total myelin protein is proteolipid protein and myelin basic protein.[12] Myelin-associated glycoprotein constitutes about 1% of myelin proteins.[12]

The thickness of the myelin sheath varies from axon to axon. Single oligodendroglial cells that extend processes to axons of differing size establish myelin sheaths of different thicknesses about each axon. The ratio of the outer diameter of the axon to the outer diameter of the combined axon plus sheath, designated the *g ratio,* is stated to be relatively stable at about 0.65.[15] However, the range of g ratios varies considerably across axons within a single fiber tract.[16] Furthermore, the g ratio appears to increase with axon diameter. That is, larger axons have relatively thinner myelin sheaths.[16]

The axonal cytoskeleton contains neurofilaments and microtubules in a ratio of 5 to 10:1.[16] The caliber of the axons is influenced by the number of neurofilaments and their spacing. Neurofilament number is regulated by neurofilament synthesis (gene expression). Neurofilament spacing depends on the lengths of the side arms that extend outward from the filament, perpendicular to the long axis of the filament. Phosphorylation of the side arms increases the length of the side arm and increases the interfilament distance. Such phosphorylation appears to be regulated by myelin-associated glycoprotein synthesized by the oligodendrocytes.

Commissural Fibers

Commissural fibers are fibers that cross the midline to interconnect the two hemispheres. Homotopic commissural fibers interconnect corresponding regions of the two hemispheres.[2] Heterotopic commissural fibers connect a cortical area with noncorresponding areas of the contralateral hemisphere.[2] In humans, the three major supratentorial commissures are the corpus callosum (great commissure), the anterior commissure, and the hippocampal commissure (synonyms: commissure of the fornices, psalterium). The corpus callosum and the major portion of the anterior commissure are formed by crossing axons that arise from the neocortex. A small anterior portion of the anterior commissure designated the basal telencephalic bundle is formed by crossing paleocortical and archicortical fibers. The hippocampal commissure is formed by crossing archicortical fibers (Table 12-2). Other, less prominent commissures include the anterior hypothalamic commissure (of Ganser), dorsal supraoptic commissure (of Meynert), ventral supraoptic commissure (of Gudden), the posterior commissure, the habenular commissure, and the commissures of the superior and inferior colliculi.

In rhesus monkeys, only 2% to 3% of all cortical neurons give rise to axons that cross to the opposite hemisphere.[17] Each commissure carries different numbers of crossing fibers. Because the crossing axons vary in size and in degree of myelination, there is no constant relationship between the cross-sectional area of the commissure and the numbers of crossing fibers. There is no consistent relationship or proportion between the numbers of axons crossing in one tract versus another.[17] Data from rhesus monkeys are provided in Table 12-2 to convey a feeling for the numbers and types of fibers within each commissure of a primate.[17]

Corpus Callosum

The corpus callosum is the largest connective structure in the brain (Fig. 12-7). More than 200 million to 300 million axons interconnect the two cerebral hemispheres over a broad span. Medially, these fibers converge into a thick, compact plate of fibers that arches beneath the interhemispheric fissure. Laterally,

the thick sheet of fibers fans out into wide areas of the two hemispheres. These interhemispheric connections do not simply link all portions of the two hemispheres. Instead, the commissural fibers link *only those areas functionally related to the midline.*[3] In the somatic cortex, commissural fibers through the body predominantly link those cortical areas representing the trunk, rather than those representing the peripheral hands and feet. In the visual cortex, commissural fibers through the splenium interconnect only those cortical areas representing the vertical meridian.[3]

Grossly, the corpus callosum displays a rostrum, genu, body, isthmus, and splenium (Figs. 12-3 and 12-8). The isthmus of the corpus callosum is the point at which the fornix abuts the undersurface of the corpus callosum. Functionally, the isthmus divides the corpus callosum into two portions: (1) a prominent anterior associative segment that carries the commissural fibers of the frontal associative cortex and (2) a smaller posterior splenial

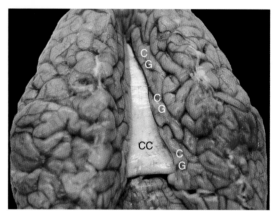

■ **FIGURE 12-7** Fresh unfixed cadaver brain viewed from above and behind. The commissural fibers form transverse ridges on the superior surface of the corpus callosum (CC) as they cross between the two cerebral hemispheres. The cingulate gyri (CG) encircle the corpus callosum on each side.

TABLE 12-2. The Four Major Supratentorial Commissures (Data from Rhesus Monkeys)*

	Commissure			
	Neocortical Corpus Callosum	**Neocortical Anterior Commissure**	**Allocortical Anterior Commissure**	**Allocortical Hippocampal Commissure**
Numbers of Crossing Axons	56.0 m ± 3.8 m	3.15 m ± 0.24 m	193 k ± 28 k	237 k ± 31 k
Percentage of All Commissural Fibers	93%	5.3%	0.3%	0.4%
Predominant Types of Crossing Fibers	Varies with the region	Mostly small and medium myelinated axons; occasional large axon	Mostly small unmyelinated axons; ~20% smallest caliber of myelinated axons (<0.5 μm in diameter)	Mostly medium myelinated axons
Small Unmyelinated Axons	Varies with region: ~6% in regions carrying fibers from primary sensory cortices and ~30% in regions carrying fibers from association cortices	~7%	~80%†	~5%
Regional Variation of Axon Size and Axon Density Within the Commissure	Consistent, region-specific variation along the corpus callosum	None discerned	None discerned	None discerned

*In the rhesus monkey, the neocortex is believed to comprise a slightly smaller percentage of the total cortex than is true for humans.
†This high percentage of unmyelinated fibers is not seen in the other commissures.
k, thousand; m, million.
Data from Lamantia AS, Rakic P. Cytological and quantitative characteristics of four cerebral commissures in the rhesus monkey. J Comp Neurol 1990; 291:520-537.

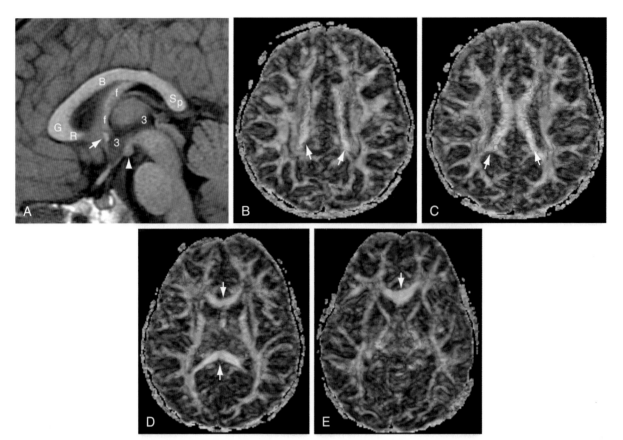

■ **FIGURE 12-8**   Corpus callosum. MR images (1.5 T) from a 4-year-old girl. **A,** Midsagittal T1W MR image for orientation. Because the corpus callosum is curved, axial sections will display the body of the corpus callosum (B) most superiorly, the genu (G) and splenium (Sp) inferior to the body, and the rostrum (R) most inferiorly. The anterior commissure (*white arrow*) lies in the anterior wall of the third ventricle (3) at the junction of the rostrum with the lamina terminalis. The fornix (f) abuts the inferior aspect of the corpus callosum at the isthmus and then curves downward behind the anterior commissure en route to the mammillary body (*white arrowhead*). **B** to **E,** Diffusion tensor imaging (DTI) color maps. **B,** As the commissural fibers converge toward the corpus callosum, they form narrow parasagittal bands (*white arrows*) of inferomedially directed (*pink*) fibers between the sagittally oriented cingulum bundles (*green*) medially and the vertically oriented fibers of the corona radiata (*blue*) laterally. **C,** The commissural fibers cross the midline in the body of the corpus callosum (*red* transversely oriented fibers). **D,** Below the body, the genu and splenium (red fibers, *white arrows*) extend into more inferior sections. **E,** The rostrum (red fibers, *white arrow*) is the lowest portion of the corpus callosum in axial sections.

segment that carries the commissural fibers of the primary visual (calcarine) cortex as well as the more associative posterior parietal and medial occipitotemporal cortices.

The commissural fibers cross through the corpus callosum in defined sequence.

The semi-horizontal rostrum (lamina rostralis, beak) extends anteriorly between the anterior commissure below and the posterior inferior aspect of the genu above. Its fibers have not been studied specifically but are likely to interconnect the frontobasal cortices of the two sides.

The genu (knee) is the thickened anteriormost portion of the corpus callosum. It contains the commissural fibers of the anterior frontal lobe, collectively designated the forceps minor. These fibers interconnect the prefrontal cortex and the anterior cingulate areas. The fibers of the ventromedial prefrontal cortex lie ventrally within the genu. The fibers of the dorsolateral prefrontal cortex lie dorsally within the genu.

The body of the corpus callosum is the horizontal portion that extends from the genu to the isthmus. Laterally, the fibers of the callosal body form the roofs of the two lateral ventricular bodies. These fibers course between the cingulum bundle superiorly and the superior occipitofrontal fasciculi laterally. They pass obliquely across the anterior radiations of the thalamus. The fibers of the body interconnect the precentral cortices (premotor area, supplementary motor area), the adjacent portions of the insulae, and the overlying cingulate gyri.

The isthmus usually appears as a focal narrowing of the corpus callosum at the point where the fornix joins the undersurface of the corpus callosum. As such, it lies between the septum pellucidum anteriorly and the hippocampal commissure posteriorly. The commissural fibers crossing through the isthmus arise from the precentral gyrus (motor strip, M1), the postcentral gyrus (somatosensory strip, S1), and Heschl's gyrus (transverse temporal gyrus, primary auditory cortex, A1).

The splenium is the thickest portion of the corpus callosum in the adult. The splenial fibers form the forceps major and participate in forming the tapetum. These fibers can be subdivided into three groups: (1) the superior group contains the commissural fibers from the posterior parietal cortex; (2) the posterior group carries the commissural fibers of the medial occipital cortex, and (3) the inferior group carries the commissural fibers of the medial temporal cortex.

Histology

The commissural axons arise from neurons located predominantly in the intermediate cortical layers.[18] Callosal fibers that interconnect primary sensorimotor regions are large and heavily myelinated. Callosal fibers that interconnect associative areas are small and poorly myelinated. The highest density of *large* fibers (3 to 5 μm) is found at the isthmus (for motor, somatosensory, and auditory cortex) and in the posterior splenium (for visual cortex). The highest density of *thin* fibers (<0.4 μm) is found in the genu and anterior splenium (high-order prefrontal and temporoparietal associative areas). The largest callosal fibers in humans correspond to fibers interconnecting the primary auditory cortex.[18]

Function

The corpus callosum facilitates interhemispheric interactions for communicating and integrating perceptual, cognitive, learned, and volitional information. It is important for the performance of visual and tactile tasks that require transfer of sensory information between the cerebral hemispheres. Commissural fibers crossing through the anterior portion and body of the corpus callosum are essential to perform temporally independent bimanual finger movements. Commissural fibers passing through the posterior corpus callosum play an important role in visual and visuospatial integration. Callosal fibers are also important for higher-order cognition, including normal social, attentional, and emotional function.[6]

Imaging

From anterior to posterior, fibers cross through the corpus callosum in the same order that their cortices appear on the cerebral surface. Connections of the prefrontal cortex cross through the genu and anterior part of the body. Premotor connections cross within the midbody of the corpus callosum. Then, in order, come the commissural fibers arising in the primary motor strip (M1), the primary sensory strip (S1), and the posterior parietal cortices. Fibers arising in temporal and occipital cortices cross through the splenium of the corpus callosum. Wahl and colleagues showed that the cortical motor fibers connecting defined body representations of M1 cross through circumscribed, somatotopically organized regions of the corpus callosum.[19] Although the callosal fibers cross the midline in a defined order, front to back, they do not appear to be restricted to crossing within specific fractions of the length of the corpus callosum. That is, one cannot say that fibers from any one area consistently cross through, for example, the third sixth of the length of the corpus callosum.[20,21]

Routine sectional CT and MRI display the corpus callosum well in sagittal and coronal planes, but less well in the axial plane (Fig. 12-8). Diffusion tensor tractography (DTT) displays the fibers arching through the corpus callosum in relation to their points of origin (Fig. 12-9). Thus, DTT can document the precise location through which specific fibers cross in one individual, enabling more precise surgical planning.[6,22,23]

The Anterior Commissure

The anterior commissure is a narrow, highly compact fiber bundle that has the shape of bicycle handlebars. Medially, the anterior commissure crosses the midline in the anterior wall of the third ventricle, just rostral to the anterior columns of the fornix (Fig. 12-10; see also Fig. 11-3D).[2,24] From there, on each side, the anterior commissure extends laterally through the basal portions of the caudate and putamen, inferior to the anterior border of the globus pallidus, and then through the temporal stem to reach the temporal and occipital lobes.[25] Anteriorly, the anterior commissure lies medial to and parallels the course of the uncinate fasciculus.[18,26] Posteriorly, the anterior commissure parallels the course of the inferior longitudinal fasciculus.[26] A thin anteroinferior portion of the anterior commissure designated the *basal telencephalic bundle* interconnects non-neocortical (allocortical) portions of the hemispheres including the two olfactory bulbs, the anterior olfactory nuclei, the primary olfactory cortices, and probably the two amygdalae.[2,18,26] A larger posterior neocortical limb of the anterior commissure interconnects portions of the orbitofrontal cortices, portions of the insulae, adjoining limbic portions of the temporopolar cortices, and the inferior temporo-occipital cortices.[26] Studies of fiber degeneration pathways in humans show that the majority of anterior commissural fibers arise from the inferior temporal cortex and distribute to the contralateral hemisphere both homotopically and heterotopically (to the amygdala and possibly the inferior frontal cortex).[25] An additional group of anterior commissural fibers also arises from the inferior and lateral occipital cortices.[25] The anterior commissure probably also links the two nuclei accumbens septi.[3]

Histology

The anterior commissure contains approximately 3 million fibers (see Table 12-2).[17,18] The single macroscopic tract contains two histologically distinguishable fiber bundles separated by a definite glial plane: (1) a small allocortical basal telencephalic bundle courses along the anterior edge of the gross tract and contains small, mostly unmyelinated fibers; and (2) a large, predominant neocortical bundle courses immediately behind the first and contains mostly small myelinated fibers.[18]

Function

The fibers of the thin anterior bundle originate from the anterior olfactory nuclei of one olfactory tract and pass across the midline to the contralateral olfactory bulb.[17] These fibers may act in

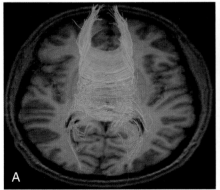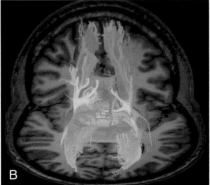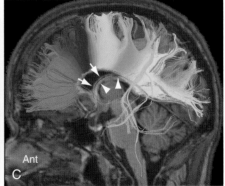

■ **FIGURE 12-9** Corpus callosum. Diffusion tensor MR tractography at 3.0 T. **A,** The red commissural fibers describe a narrow arc of curvature as they extend to and from the cortical areas related to the midline. **B** and **C,** Tractograms of the corpus callosum, color coded from anterior to posterior, display the concordance between the anteroposterior position of the cortical areas of origin and the anteroposterior points at which those fibers cross the midline through the corpus callosum. The precommissural hippocamposeptal portion of the fornix (*white arrow,* blue fibers) and the retrocommissural hippocampomammillary portion of the fornix (*white arrowheads,* green fibers) are also displayed. Other stray fibers remain.

■ **FIGURE 12-10** Anterior commissure. **A,** Axial T2W MR image. The anterior commissure (*white arrows*) has the shape of bicycle handlebars (see also Fig. 12-8A). **B,** Axial DTI. The transversely oriented (predominantly red) fibers of the anterior commissure (*white arrows*) pass posterolaterally through the lenticular nuclei bilaterally. Part of their course parallels the proximal portions of the optic tracts (also red) (*white arrowheads*) and anterior contours of the cerebral peduncles (blue) (*white arrows*).

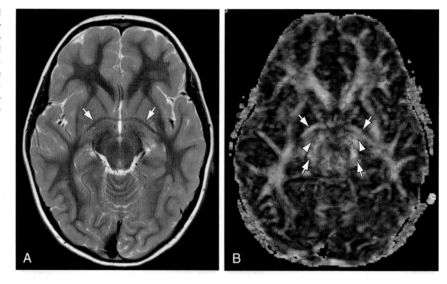

■ **FIGURE 12-11** Anterior commissure. Diffusion tensor MR tractography at 3T. **A to C,** DT tractograms projected onto the axial plane (**A**), midsagittal plane (**B**), and coronal plane (**C**) show the characteristic shapes and positions of the fibers coursing through the anterior commissure (*white arrows*) and the fornices (*black arrows*). **D,** 3D display of the olfactory and nonolfactory components of the anterior commissure. (*D, Reprinted from Kollias S. Parcellation of the white matter using DTI: insights into the functional connectivity of the brain. Neuroradiol J 2009; 22[Suppl I]:45-57.*)

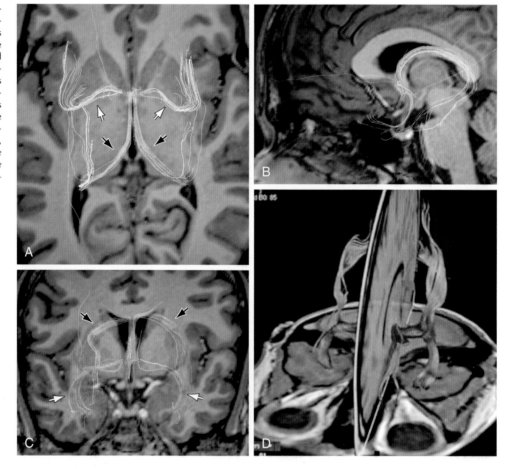

reflex control of activity in the olfactory bulb.[1] The function of the fibers of the large posterior bundle is not well known.

Imaging

The gross anatomy and standard imaging of the anterior commissure are displayed in Figures 11-14 and 11-15. The greatest diameter of the normal anterior commissure never exceeds 6 mm.[18] DTT displays the anterior commissure as arching fibers that pass through the anterior midline toward the inferior frontal regions

and toward the temporo-occipital regions (see Figs. 12-10 and 12-11).

Hippocampal Commissure (Commissure of the Fornices, Psalterium)

Approximately 20% of forniceal fibers cross the midline between the two crura of the fornices to form the hippocampal commissure. Grossly, the hippocampal commissure is a thin triangular sheet of fibers situated between the paired crura of the fornices

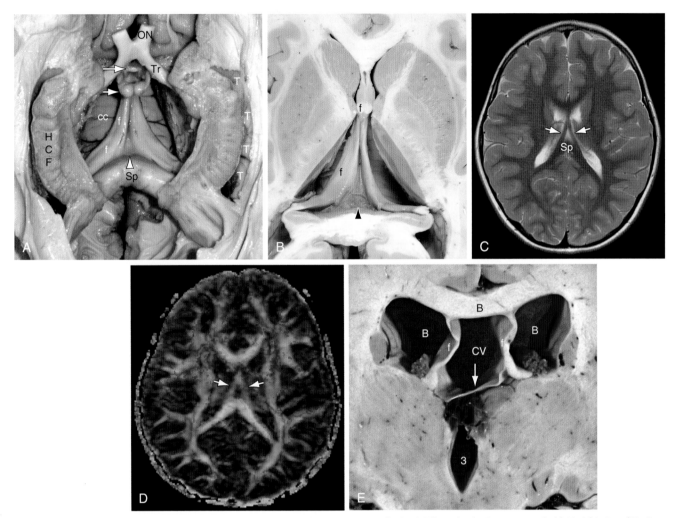

■ FIGURE 12-12 Fornices and forniceal commissure (hippocampal commissure, psalterium) (dissection by Dr. N. Krayenbühl, Zurich). **A** and **B**, Gross dissection of the paired hippocampal formations (HCF) and fornices (f) seen from below. In the triangular region between the two fornices, just anterior to the splenium (Sp) and inferior to the corpus callosum (cc), the commissural fibers of the fornix form a thin sheet of tissue designated the forniceal commissure (hippocampal commissure, psalterium [*arrowhead*]). Anteriorly, the paired anterior columns of the fornices curve downward toward the anterior commissure (*larger white arrow*). Most of the forniceal fibers pass behind the anterior commissure to reach the mammillary bodies (*small white arrow*). A small precommissural contingent passes to the septal region. Also labeled are the optic nerve (ON) and tract (Tr) and the temporal horn (T). **C** and **D**, Axial T2W (**C**) and axial diffusion tensor color map (**D**) at 1.5 T. The fornices (*white arrows*) converge anteriorly (*green*) just inferior to the corpus callosum. The hippocampal commissure lies within the triangle between the fornices and anterior to the splenium (Sp) but is not identifiable individually. **E**, Cavum vergae. Coronal plane gross anatomic section through the bodies of the lateral ventricles (*white* B) and third ventricle (3). The walls of the cavum vergae (CV) are formed by the body of the corpus callosum (*black* B) above, the paired fornices (f, f) laterally, and the commissure of the fornices (*arrow*) inferiorly. At present, routine anatomic imaging resolves the commissure of the fornices only when it is separated from the undersurface of the corpus callosum.

just dorsal to the posterior third ventricle and just ventral to the posterior body of the corpus callosum (Fig. 12-12). The hippocampal commissure contains fibers that interconnect the two medial temporal lobes in both directions. According to Gloor and associates, the human hippocampal commissure interconnects the presubiculum, entorhinal, and parahippocampal cortices of the two sides but not the hippocampi themselves.[18,27]

Histology

In rhesus monkeys, the hippocampal commissure consists mostly of medium-sized myelinated associative fibers and is clearly separated from the splenium of the corpus callosum by a glial plane (see Table 12-2).[17,18]

Function

The function of the hippocampal commissure is very poorly understood.[2]

Imaging

The hippocampal commissure is difficult to resolve by any standard imaging technique. In most cases it merges indistinguishably into the undersurface of the corpus callosum. When a cavum vergae is present, the cavum separates the hippocampal commissure from the corpus callosum, so the hippocampal commissure may be seen as the lower margin of the cavum, overlying the cistern of the velum interpositum (see Fig. 12-12E). In some cases of schizencephaly with absent septum pellucidum, the hippocampal commissure may also be seen free of superimposition by adjoining structures.

Projection Fibers

Projection fibers convey impulses from the cortex to distant sites or from distant sites to the cortex. The afferent and efferent projection fibers are arranged as radiating bundles of fibers that converge to or diverge from the brain stem. Together they form the corona radiata. The most compact portion of the corona radiata situated just cephalic to the brain stem is the internal capsule.

Corona Radiata

The corona radiata is not a specific tract. Instead it is the name given to the broad fan-shaped array of white matter fibers that appear to converge inferiorly into the internal capsule. It is composed of multiple different fiber tracts (see Fig. 12-2J). The fibers of the corona radiata cross between the transversely oriented commissural fibers that converge to the corpus callosum. The coronal fibers lie between the longitudinal fibers of the cingulum bundle and superior fronto-occipital fasciculus medially and the superior longitudinal fasciculus laterally.[3]

Function

The fibers of the corona radiata interconnect the cerebral cortex with the thalamus and brainstem in both directions (Figs. 12-13 and 12-14). From anterior to posterior, they include (1) the thalamic connections to the frontal lobes and the frontopontine motor fibers that pass through the anterior limb of the internal capsule; (2) the thalamic connections to the anterior parietal lobe and the corticonuclear motor projections that pass through the genu; and (3) the thalamic connections to the central parietal and occipitotemporal lobes and corticospinal, corticopontine, and corticotegmental motor fibers that pass through the posterior limb of the internal capsule[2] (see Internal Capsule, later). The thalamic radiations to and from the cortex are grouped into four thalamic peduncles (Fig. 14-D) (Table 12-3).[1]

Imaging

On axial images the corona radiata appears as a nearly uniform region of myelinated white matter (see Figs. 12-13 and 12-14). On diffusion tensor imaging (DTI), the fibers of the corona radiata appear as an open fan of greenish blue mostly craniocaudal fibers that course between the red transversely oriented fibers of the corpus callosum and the green anteroposteriorly oriented long association bundles of the cingulum bundle medially and the superior longitudinal fasciculus laterally.

Internal Capsule

The majority of connections between the cerebral cortex and subcortical structures travel through the internal capsule (Figs. 12-14 and 12-15). Afferent fibers in the internal capsule largely arise from the thalamus and radiate to all parts of the cortex as the thalamocortical radiations.[3] Efferent fibers in the internal capsule arise from cortical neurons and extend widely to specific portions of the thalamus, brain stem, and spinal cord as the corticothalamic, corticopontine, corticobulbar (for medulla oblongata), and corticospinal fibers. The fiber tracts passing through the corona radiata and the internal capsule to interconnect the cortex and the thalamus are designated the *thalamic peduncles* (see Fig. 12-14D and Table 12-3). The anterior, superior, and posterior thalamic peduncles detach from the internal capsule to enter the thalamus dorsally at its rostral and caudal poles.[2] The inferior thalamic peduncle enters the thalamus ventromedially, medial to the posterior limb of the internal capsule.[2] It forms part of the ansa peduncularis.[2]

Function

The topographic organization of tracts within the internal capsule is determined by the anteroposterior position of their *cortical* connections, regardless of whether they are afferent or efferent fibers (see Figs. 12-2J and 12-14A). The *anterior limb* carries ascending thalamic projections from the anterior and medial thalamic nuclei to the frontal lobes and descending frontopontine motor fibers (Fig. 12-16).[3] The *genu* contains anterior portions of the ascending superior thalamic (somaesthetic) radiation to the postcentral gyrus and descending corticobulbar motor projections. The *posterior limb* contains most of the ascending superior thalamic (somaesthetic) radiation to the postcentral gyrus and the descending corticospinal, corticopontine, and corticotegmental motor fibers.[3] The *retrolenticular portion* of the internal capsule conveys the optic radiations from the lateral geniculate nucleus to the calcarine cortex, some of the auditory radiations, and descending parietopontine, occipitopontine, and occipitotectal projections.[2,3] The *sublenticular portion* conveys limited ascending thalamic fibers to the temporal lobe and insula, the auditory radiations from the medial geniculate nucleus to the transverse temporal gyrus of Heschl and the

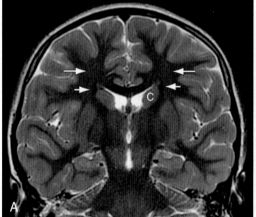
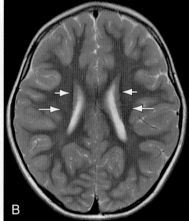
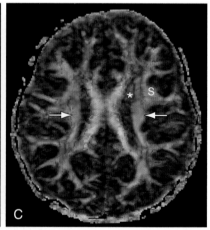

■ **FIGURE 12-13** Corona radiata and superior occipitofrontal fasciculus. **A** and **B,** Coronal (**A**) and axial (**B**) T2W MR images. The small, compact, longitudinally oriented superior occipitofrontal fasciculus (*short white arrows*) appears as a thin, low signal ovoid (coronal plane) or line (axial plane) situated just lateral to the superior portion of the caudate nucleus (c) (see Fig. 12-26). The fibers of the corona radiata (*long white arrows*) lie lateral to this but are difficult to resolve individually on routine sectional imaging. **C,** Axial plane DT color map. The blue craniocaudally oriented fibers (*white arrows*) of the coronal radiata are now identifiable medial to the green longitudinally oriented fibers of the superior longitudinal fasciculus (s). The most medial red fibers are the corpus callosum (see Fig. 12-8). The green longitudinally oriented fibers identified by the *asterisk* could represent a segment of the superior occipitofrontal fasciculus, the more anteriorly directed fibers of the corona radiata (see Fig. 12-14), or a portion of the cingulum bundle sectioned obliquely.

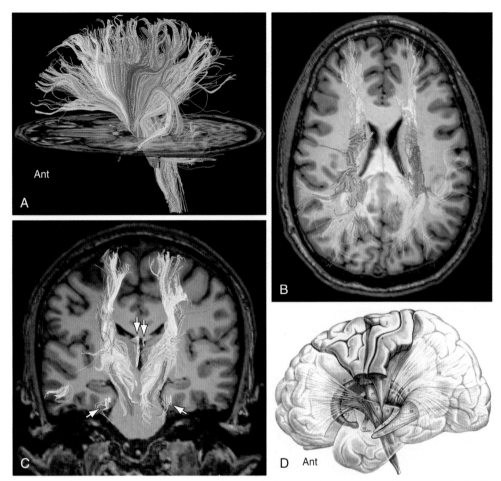

■ **FIGURE 12-14** Diffusion tensor tractography of the corona radiata. Sagittal (**A**), axial (**B**) and coronal (**C**) images display the radiating pattern of fibers for which the corona radiata is named. These fibers converge inferiorly and traverse the internal capsule to reach the thalamus and the brain stem. A few medial forniceal fibers (*arrows*) are seen to pass to the white matter just deep to the entorhinal cortex of the parahippocampal gyrus bilaterally. **D,** Thalamic peduncles. Lateral diagram of the thalamic peduncles and fibers within the internal capsule. The corticospinal and corticopontine fibers have been "resected" to expose the thalamic peduncles (see Table 12-3). The anterior thalamic peduncle (12) runs in the anterior limb of the internal capsule. The superior (7) and posterior (8) thalamic peduncles run in the posterior limb of the internal capsule. The inferior thalamic peduncle (14) passes into the ansa peduncularis (15). Other labeled structures include the following: 1, postcentral gyrus (Brodmann areas 2, 1, 3); 2, precentral gyrus (BA 4); 3, frontal gyri (BA 6, 8); 5, caudate nucleus; 6, pyramidal tract; 9, parietopontine tract; 10, corticotegmental fibers; 11, frontopontine tract; 13, putamen; 16, temporopontine tract in the sublenticular portion of the internal capsule; 17, occipitopontine tract in the retrolenticular portion of the internal capsule; 18, optic radiations; and 19, stratum sagittale. (*D, Modified from Nieuwenhuys R, Voogd J, van Huijzen C. The Human Central Nervous System, 4th ed. Berlin, Springer, 2008.*)

TABLE 12-3. The Thalamic Peduncles

Specific Peduncle	Relation to the Internal Capsule	Interconnects the Cortex	With the Thalamic Nuclei
Anterior (frontal) thalamic peduncle	Via the anterior limb	Prefrontal cortex Orbitofrontal cortex Frontal portion of cingulate cortex	Medial and anterior thalamic nuclei
Superior (central parietal) thalamic peduncle	Via the posterior limb	Central parietal cortex	Ventral tier of thalamic nuclei
Posterior (occipital) thalamic peduncle	Via the posterior limb	Posterior parietal, posterior temporal, and occipital cortex	Caudal portions of the thalamus; this includes the optic radiations.
Inferior (temporal) thalamic peduncle	Medial to the posterior limb	Orbitofrontal cortex, insular cortex, temporal cortex, amygdaloid complex	This includes the auditory radiations.

Data from Carpenter MB, Sutin J. Human Neuroanatomy, 8th ed. Baltimore, Williams & Wilkins, 1983; and Nieuwenhuys R, Voogd J, van Huijzen C. The Human Central Nervous System, 4th ed. Berlin, Springer, 2008.

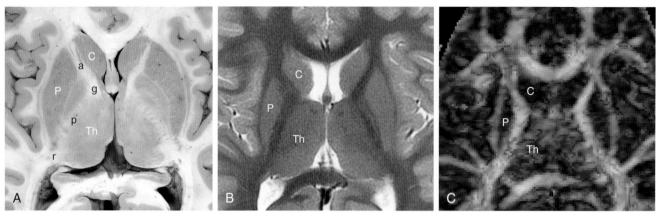

■ **FIGURE 12-15** Internal capsule. Axial anatomic section (**A**), T2W MRI (**B**) and DT color map (**C**). The anterior limb (a), genu (g), posterior limb (p) and retrolenticular (r) portion of the internal capsule course between the caudate nucleus (C) and thalamus (Th) medially and the lenticular nucleus laterally. P, putamen. The more dominant *blue* coloration in the posterior limb indicates that the fibers passing there are oriented more vertically, while the fibers in the anterior limb, genu and retrolenticular portion of the internal capsule course more obliquely, both vertically and longitudinally.

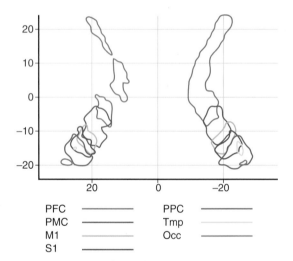

PFC —————	PPC —————
PMC —————	Tmp —————
M1 —————	Occ —————
S1 —————	

■ **FIGURE 12-16** Internal capsule. Topographical distribution of the cortical tracts within the internal capsule. Two-dimensional probabilistic population map from 11 right-handed subjects 23 to 57 years of age. Grouped data. This diagram is color coded to display the fibers related to the prefrontal cortex (PFC), premotor cortex (PMC), primary motor strip of the precentral gyrus (M1), primary sensory strip of the postcentral gyrus (S1), posterior parietal cortex (PPC), temporal cortex (Tmp), and occipital cortex (Occ). The anterior limb and genu of the internal capsule are occupied by prefrontal fibers. The sensorimotor tracts traverse the posterior half of the posterior limb. *(From Zarei M, Johansen-Berg H, Jenkinson M, et al. Two-dimensional population map of cortical connections in the human internal capsule. J Magn Reson Imaging 2007; 25:48-54.)*

superior temporal gyrus, and descending temporopontine and posterior parietal pontine projections.[3]

Imaging

The gross anatomy and standard imaging of the internal capsule are displayed in Figures 11-3 to 11-12. DTT displays the internal capsule as multiple sets of fibers that course predominantly craniocaudally between the caudate nuclei and thalami medially and the lenticular nuclei laterally (see Figs. 12-14 and 12-15).

Corticospinal Tract

The fibers of the corticospinal tract arise from a broad area of the cortical surface.[28] The precise contributions of each cortical area to the tract remain uncertain. According to A. R. Crossman,

only 20% to 30% of corticospinal fibers arise from the primary motor cortex (Brodmann area 4).[3] These "arise from pyramidal cells in layer V and give rise to the largest diameter corticospinal axons."[3] Forty to 60 percent of pyramidal axons arise from the parietal lobe, including Brodmann areas 3 and 5 of the superior operculum and dorsal insula.[3,29] However, according to Ebeling and Reulen, 40% to 60% of corticospinal fibers arise from layer 5 neurons of the primary motor cortex (M1) in the precentral gyrus (Brodmann area 4). About 20% of fibers arise from the somaesthetic cortex of the postcentral gyrus and paracentral lobule (Brodmann areas 3, 2, and 1).[28,30] The remainder arise from the dorsal and ventral premotor areas (Brodmann areas 6 lateral and 8), the supplementary motor area (Brodmann area 6 medial), and the parietal lobe (Brodmann areas 5 and 7).[28,30] Gender and handedness are not associated with consistent difference in the makeup of the left versus right corticospinal tract.[31] A slight asymmetry between left and right corticospinal tracts has been noted in healthy individuals but was not found to be significantly different from zero across individuals.[31]

The corticospinal tract descends obliquely through the posterior limb of the internal capsule.[32-34] If the *posterior* limb of the internal capsule is divided into four equal portions, then the rostral portion of the corticospinal tract crosses through the first or second quarter of the posterior limb while the caudal portion of the corticospinal tract traverses the third quarter or rarely the fourth quarter of the posterior limb (Figs. 12-17 and 12-18).[33] Within the posterior limb of the internal capsule, the fibers of the corticospinal tract are arrayed somatotopically, with individual variation.[35,36] Holodny[35] and Ino[36] found three different arrangements of the corticospinal fibers: (1) the fibers may be arrayed longitudinally from anterior to posterior along the long axis of the posterior limb[35,36]; (2) they may be arrayed transversely across the short axis of the posterior limb; or (3) they may be intermixed without specific localization. Holodny and associates reported that the fibers were arrayed predominantly transversely, from lateral to medial, with the hand fibers lateral and slightly anterior to the leg fibers in 17 of 20 tracts (85%).[35] In 3 of 20 tracts (15%) the fibers were intermixed.[35] Ino and colleagues[36] confirmed that the corticospinal fibers were arrayed transversely as reported by Holodny and associates[35] in four of seven cases (57%). However, the fibers were arrayed longitudinally in the other three cases (43%).[36] In one of these three (14%), the hand fibers lay anteromedial to the foot fibers. In two of the three, the hand fibers lay posterolateral to the foot fibers (29%).[36]

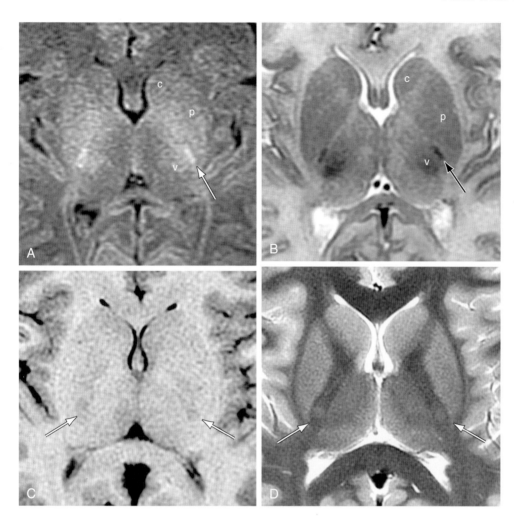

■ **FIGURE 12-17** Corticospinal tracts. Axial MR sections at two ages. The corticospinal tract (*arrow*) descends through the posterior half of the posterior limb of the internal capsule. **A** and **B**, MR images in a newborn girl. Because the corticospinal tract is already myelinated at term, whereas other fiber tracts are not, the corticospinal tract appears as a sharply defined "white" fiber bundle on T1W images (**A**) and sharply defined "black" bundle on T2W images (**B**). It characteristically lies just anterolateral to the also-myelinated ventral posterolateral nucleus of the thalamus (v). c, caudate nucleus; p, putamen. **C** and **D**, MR images from a 9-year-old girl. With maturation and signal change of the adjacent structures, the corticospinal tract comes to show *relatively* low signal on T1W images (**C**) and relatively high signal on T2W (**D**) in older individuals.

Newton and colleagues analyzed the intracerebral courses of the contributions to the corticospinal tracts from each of the dorsal premotor area (PMd), the ventral premotor area (PMv), and the supplementary motor area (SMA).[37]

Fiber connections from the PMd to the cerebral peduncle enter the corona radiata and course caudally, anterior to and overlapping with the corticospinal fibers from the precentral gyrus M1.[37] They then descend through the posterior limb of the internal capsule.[37] Within the internal capsule, the most anterior fibers from the PMd overlap with those from the SMA and the PMv.[37] The most posterior fibers of PMd overlap with those of M1.[37] At the level of the cerebral peduncle, the connections from PMd lie laterally.[37]

Fiber connections arising from the ventral premotor area (PMv) first shift medially to lie anterior to most fibers from the PMd, with some overlap.[37] The PMv fibers then course vertically through the corona radiata and posterior limb of the internal capsule, anterior to most of the M1 and PMd fibers. At the level of the cerebral peduncle, the fibers from the PMv lie less far lateral than those from M1 and the PMd.[37]

Fiber connections arising from the SMA first shift progressively more laterally and posteriorly within the subcortical white matter.[37] The SMA connections then pass through the anterior limb and genu of the internal capsule close to the caudal aspect of the head of the caudate nucleus, before passing over the putamen and descending into the posterior limb of the internal capsule.[37] The fibers from the SMA tend to lie anterior to those of the PMd, PMv, and M1, with some overlap.[37] At the level of

the cerebral peduncle, the SMA fibers lie more ventral and medial than those from the precentral regions.[37]

Histology

The number of corticospinal fibers in one human medullary pyramid has been estimated to be as high as 1.2 million fibers[38] and as low as 100,000 fibers.[39] The largest corticospinal fibers arise from the numerous large Betz cells of the "leg area" of the precentral gyrus and have diameters of about 21 μm. The smallest corticospinal fibers arise from the small sparse Betz cells of the opposite extremity of the motor cortex and have diameters of about 3 μm.

Function

The corticospinal tract is the predominant pathway for the relay of impulses for voluntary skilled movements of the upper extremities, trunk, and lower extremities.[32,36]

Imaging

The corticospinal tract is readily displayed in the posterior limb of the internal capsule as a focal hypointensity on T1W images and a focal hyperintensity on T2W, FLAIR T2W, and diffusion-weighted images (see Fig. 12-17).[40] These signals have been attributed to lower axonal and myelin densities within the corticospinal tract.[41] In the newborn, T2W images display the corticospinal tract as a small very low-signal myelinated tract within the higher signal still-unmyelinated remainder of the posterior limb (see Fig. 12-17).

■ **FIGURE 12-18** Diffusion tensor tractography of the corticospinal tracts. **A** and **B,** Sagittal (**A**) and coronal (**B**) images show the origin of the corticospinal tract (blue) within the precentral and postcentral gyri and its course through the posterior limb of the internal capsule, the cerebral peduncle, and the brain stem. The corticospinal tract characteristically describes an anterior genu within 3 mm of the Talaraich-Tournoux (anterior commissure/posterior commissure) baseline (*red dashes*). **C** to **F,** Projection of the corticospinal tract (*blue*) onto serial axial MR sections displayed from superior (**C**) to inferior (**F**). The corticospinal tract angles from anterosuperior to posteroinferior through the posterior limb of the internal capsule and descends through the midportion of the cerebral peduncle (**F**) into the lower brain stem.

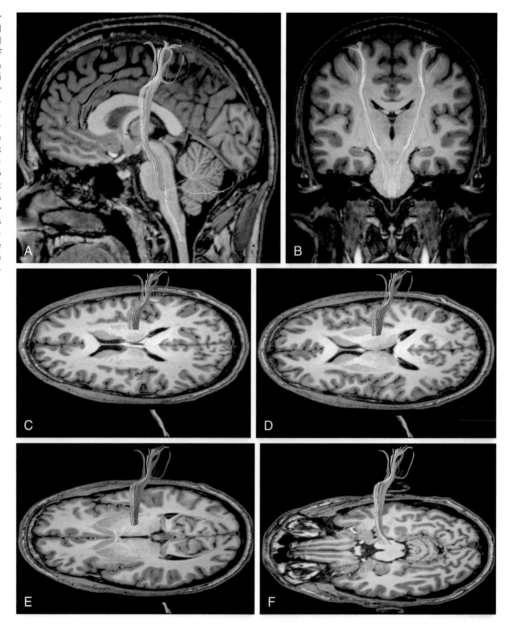

DTT displays the corticospinal tract as a very compact fiber bundle passing craniocaudally from the region of the precentral gyrus through the posterior limb of the internal capsule and the midportion of the cerebral peduncle into the ventral brain stem (Fig. 12-18). If the corticospinal tract is projected onto the midsagittal plane, it typically forms a straight or nearly straight line from the paracentral lobule (mostly anterior to the central sulcus) to the midportion of the Talairach-Tournoux anterior commissure–posterior commissure (AC-PC) baseline.[42] The corticospinal tract passes across the mid fifth of the AC-PC plane in 80% of subjects, posterior to the mid fifth in 17%, and anterior to the mid fifth in only 3% (Fig. 12-18A).[40] It characteristically (98%) displays a bend (genu) within 3 mm of the AC-PC plane, typically just below the AC-PC line. The angle between the projection of the corticospinal tract onto the midsagittal plane and the AC-PC line measures 80° + 4°.[40] Within this portion of the corticospinal tract, the bulbofacial-arm-leg fibers are arrayed somatotopically from anterolateral to posteromedial.[28,30,32,43,44]

Westerhausen and associates showed that consistently left-handed individuals had higher fractional anisotropy values in the posterior limbs of *both* internal capsules as compared with consistently right-handed subjects.[31] They then suggested that handedness was related to overall differences in the architecture of both corticospinal tracts, rather than to asymmetries between the two hemispheres.[31]

Optic Apparatus
Optic Tracts
The optic tracts are the macroscopic fiber tracts that pass posteriorly from the optic chiasm around, and tightly applied to, the cerebral peduncles to reach the anterior ventral aspects of the lateral geniculate nuclei of the metathalamus and the superficial layers of the superior colliculi (Fig. 12-19).[2,45]

Histology
Each tract contains both the uncrossed temporal *retinal* fibers from the ipsilateral eye and the crossed *nasal* retinal fibers from the contralateral eye.[2] Put in terms of the visual fields rather than the retinal fibers themselves, the optic tracts contain the uncrossed fibers of the ipsilateral nasal field and the crossed

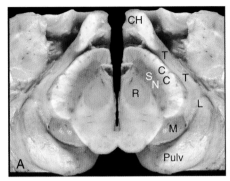 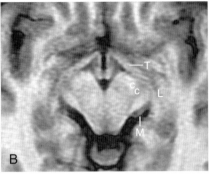 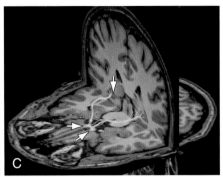

■ **FIGURE 12-19** Optic tracts. **A,** Axial anatomic specimen viewed from below after resection of the obscuring temporal lobes. Composite image. The optic tracts (T) encircle the crus cerebri (CC) as they pass from the optic chiasm (CH) (*disrupted here*) to the lateral geniculate body (L). The medial geniculate body (M) lies at the upper end of the lateral mesencephalic sulcus just behind, below, and medial to the lateral geniculate body and immediately behind the posterolateral edge of the crus cerebri. The pulvinar (Pulv) of the thalamus overhangs both geniculate bodies. R, red nucleus; SN, substantia nigra. **B,** Axial T1W MR image. The optic tracts (T) encircle the crura cerebrorum (CC) en route to the lateral geniculate bodies (L). The upper portion of the medial geniculate body (M) is just seen at the lateral mesencephalic sulcus. **C,** Diffusion tensor tractography viewed from anterior and superior. The intracranial ends of the optic nerves (*white arrows*) partially decussate at the optic chiasm. The optic tracts (*yellow green*) extend around the brain stem from the optic chiasm to the lateral geniculate bodies (*vertical white arrow*).

fibers of the contralateral temporal field. The ipsilateral fibers pass to layers 2, 3, and 5 of the lateral geniculate nucleus, whereas the contralateral fibers pass to layers 1, 4, and 6 of the lateral geniculate nucleus. There is a precise point-to-point (retinotopic) projection from the retina through the lateral geniculate nucleus to the visual cortex.[2]

Function

The optic tracts are simply the retrochiasmatic, postdecussation portions of the retinogeniculate fibers. As such, they mostly convey impulses from the retinal ganglion cells to the lateral geniculate nuclei. Some of the fibers within the tract bypass the lateral geniculate nuclei, enter the brachium of the superior colliculus, and pass to both superior colliculi, the pretectal region, and the terminal nuclei of the optic tract related to the visuo-optic response and the horizontal optokinetic response.[2] In turn, these interconnect with the inferior olivary nuclei of the medulla.[2]

Imaging

The optic tract is well displayed on axial gross anatomic and imaging sections (Fig. 12-19A and B). Routine sectional imaging shows the optic tracts as paired arcs of white matter that hug the lateral aspect of the cerebral peduncles as they course from the chiasm to the lateral geniculate nuclei bilaterally. DTT displays the optic tracts as compact fiber bundles coursing between the optic chiasm and the lateral geniculate nuclei (see Fig. 12-19C).

Geniculocalcarine (Optic) Radiations

The geniculocalcarine fibers (optic radiations) leave the dorsolateral aspect of the lateral geniculate nuclei, traverse the retrolenticular portion of the internal capsule, and then arch around the lateral ventricle to reach the calcarine cortex (primary visual cortex, V1, Brodmann area 17). As these fibers arise from the geniculate nucleus they divide into three bundles[46]: (1) the anterior bundle, called Meyer's loop, first courses laterally and anteriorly over the roof of the temporal horn and then curves posteriorly along the inferolateral aspect of the temporal horn, atrium, and occipital horn to reach the lower bank of the calcarine sulcus. The inferior occipitofrontal fasciculus courses parallel and just superficial to Meyer's loop (see Fig. 12-2J); (2) the central geniculocalcarine bundle passes directly laterally, crosses the roof of the temporal horn, and then courses along the lateral wall and roof of the trigone and occipital horn to the

occipital pole; and (3) the posterior bundle courses directly posteriorly over the roof of the trigone and occipital horn to reach the upper bank of the calcarine sulcus.

In their course, the geniculocalcarine fibers are separated from the ependyma of the ventricle by a thin layer of callosal fibers designated the *tapetum*. The tapetum forms the lateral wall of the ventricle external to the ependyma. It is thicker posteriorly and superiorly. It thins out anteriorly and inferiorly until it becomes indiscernible. The anterior extent of Meyer's loop has surgical importance, lest a surgical procedure cause inadvertent field cut. The anterior tip of Meyer's loop typically lies 27 ± 3.5 mm from the *tip of the temporal lobe* (range, 22 to 37 mm).[46] The anterior edge of Meyer's loop typically lies 5 ± 3.9 mm anterior to the *tip of the temporal horn* (range, 10 mm in front of the tip of the temporal horn to 5 mm posterior to the temporal tip).[46] However, Kier and colleagues[46] suggest that the anterior edge of Meyer's loop may actually run as far forward as 20 mm anterior to the tip of the temporal horn, providing a more restrictive criterion for safe temporal surgery.

Histology

The optic radiations occupy most of the external sagittal stratum. The medial border of the external sagittal stratum lies 2.8 to 4.1 mm lateral to the lateral edge of the ventricle.[47] The stratum itself is 0.9 to 1.4 mm thick (mean, 1.1 mm) and contains large axons with thick myelin sheaths and wide spaces between the axons.[47] It has the lowest axonal density of all the sagittal strata.[47] The histology of the external sagittal stratum is very similar to the histology of the corticospinal tract, so the tracts may be expected to display similar imaging features. The corticotectal tract forms most of the internal sagittal stratum. The axons of the internal sagittal stratum are small, have relatively thin myelin sheaths, and are spaced more closely together.[47] It has the highest axonal density of all the sagittal strata, so it is usually differentiated from the external sagittal stratum.[47]

Function

The fibers relayed from the retina through the geniculate nucleus and onto the occipital cortex are arrayed somatotopically, with specific distributions for each portion of the retina: left versus right eye, nasal versus temporal retina, superior versus inferior retina, and central versus peripheral retina.[2] On each side, the calcarine cortex receives fibers from the *ipsilateral temporal* retina and the *contralateral nasal* retina. Fibers from the inferior retina pass to the inferior bank of the calcarine cortex. Fibers from the superior retina pass to the superior bank of the calcarine cortex. Fibers from the fovea, conveying central vision, pass to a large posterior portion of the calcarine cortex, near to the occipital pole. Fibers from more peripheral portions of the retina, conveying more peripheral *binocular* vision, pass to a smaller more anterior portion of the calcarine cortex. Fibers from the most peripheral portion of the nasal retina, conveying *monocular* peripheral vision, pass to the extreme anterior portion of the calcarine cortex, next to the splenium of the corpus callosum.[2]

Imaging

The optic radiations are well shown by axial T1- and T2-weighted images through the temporal and occipital horns of the lateral ventricles (Fig. 12-20). They appear as one of multiple sagittal layers situated just lateral to the temporal horn, atrium, and occipital horn of the lateral ventricle. From medial to lateral these layers are the (1) tapetum formed by the inferiorly directed fibers of the corpus callosum that descend along the lateral wall of the lateral ventricle, (2) internal sagittal stratum formed by less dense corticofugal fibers passing from the occipital cortex to the superior colliculus and lateral geniculate nucleus, and (3) external sagittal stratum formed by denser, better defined geniculocalcarine fibers and the inferior longitudinal fasciculus.[5] The external sagittal stratum (optic radiations) appears hypointense on routine T1-weighted (T1W) images and hyperintense on routine T2-weighted (T2W) images.[47] However, higher-resolution images and diffusion-weighted imaging (DWI) display additional strata, complicating the imaging interpretation.[48] DTT displays the optic radiations as a broad arch of fibers passing along the superolateral aspects of the temporal horn (Meyer's loop), atria, and occipital horn (Fig. 12-21).

Geniculotemporal (Auditory) Radiations

The geniculotemporal (auditory) radiation arises from the medial geniculate body, traverses the sublenticular portion of the internal capsule, and extends laterally to insert into the transverse temporal gyrus of Heschl) (primary auditory cortex, core, A1, Brodmann area 41).

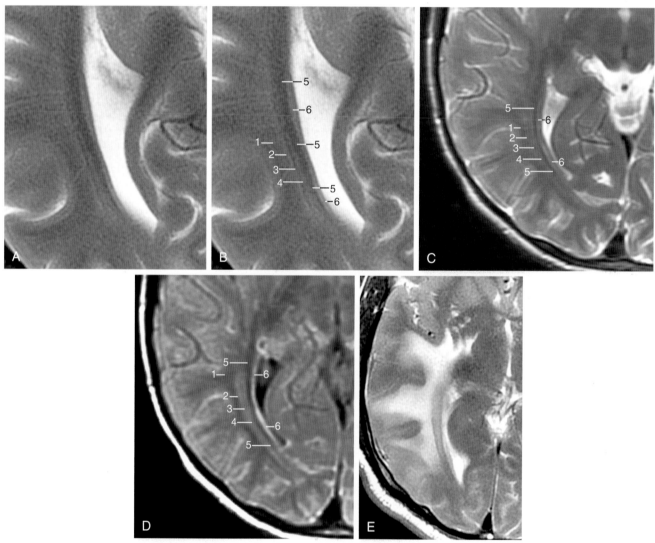

■ **FIGURE 12-20** Sagittal strata. Unlabeled (**A**) and labeled (**B**) axial T2W images from a 26-year-old man. The concentric sagittal strata appear as alternating layers of differing signal intensity. From lateral to medial, these include: 1, the temporo-occipital white matter; 2-4, a triplet formed by a thin sharply defined low signal layer flanked by two broader slightly high signal zones; 5, a broad low signal zone; and 6, a higher signal deep zone. A seventh low signal zone (*unlabeled*) may occupy the immediate periventricular layer. T2W (**C**) and T2-FLAIR (**D**) sequences in a 4-year-old boy closely resemble those in the adult with a thin low signal zone (3) readily visible on the original image. **E,** MR image of a 58-year-old man with temporo-occipital glioma. Thickening and an increased signal intensity within the edematous white lamellae emphasize the stratification.

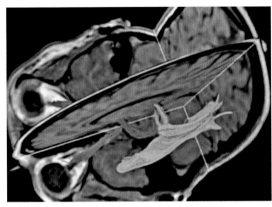

■ **FIGURE 12-21** Human visual pathways. 3D diffusion tensor tractography displays the optic nerves (*blue*), optic tracts (*red*), and optic radiations (*orange*). The anterior ventral bundle of the optic radiations (Meyer's loop) extends far forward into the temporal lobe lateral to the temporal horn. The central and posterior bundles show different trajectories from the lateral geniculate nucleus to the calcarine cortex. *(Reprinted from Kollias S. Parcellation of the white matter using DTI: insights into the functional connectivity of the brain. Neuroradiol J 2009; 22[Suppl I]:45-57.)*

Histology

The auditory fibers ascend from the dorsal and ventral cochlear nuclei to the inferior colliculus, bilaterally but predominantly contralaterally. The auditory data are then relayed from the inferior colliculus to the medial geniculate bodies for analysis of tone and for spatial localization of the sounds.[2]

Function

In humans, the auditory radiations convey the auditory data to the transverse temporal gyrus of Heschl and distribute them, tonotopically, along the length of Heschl's gyrus from posteromedial to anterolateral. Higher frequencies are received predominantly posteromedially. Lower frequencies are received predominantly anterolaterally. From Heschl's gyrus and adjoining areas, a rostral data stream passes to the superior temporal gyrus and inferior prefrontal cortex (Brodmann areas 10, 12, 13, and 45) for identification and recognition of auditory stimuli.[2] A caudal stream passes to the adjacent superior temporal gyrus and the supramarginal gyrus (Brodmann area 40) for spatial localization of auditory stimuli. Additional fibers pass to the middle prefrontal areas (Brodmann areas 8a, 12, and 46), possibly for attaching emotional valence and reward to the auditory stimuli.[2]

Imaging

The auditory radiations are not imaged directly by routine sectional CT and MRI. However, they are known to traverse the sublenticular portion of the internal capsule, so their general location is readily shown on sagittal MRI.

Fornix

The fornix (properly designated the *dorsal* fornix) is the major efferent pathway from the hippocampal formation.[49] It takes the form of a great arching fiber bundle that contains both projection and commissural fibers (see Fig. 12-12). The white matter fibers emerging from the hippocampal formation form the alveus and fimbria of the medial temporal lobes. These fibers gather together, arch posteriorly, and widen into the paired crura of the fornices that form the medial walls of the atria. At the level of the crura, the two fornices commissurate via the hippocampal (forniceal) commissure. The paired crura then continue anteriorly and unite into a single body of the fornix beneath the body of the corpus callosum. Continuing anteriorly, the forniceal fibers again separate into left and right forniceal bundles. At the

level of the anterior commissure, the fibers of each fornix segregate into two bundles: (1) a rather loose *pre*commissural bundle designated the hippocampo-septal tract passes anterior to the anterior commissure, and (2) a highly compact *retro*commissural bundle designated the hippocampo-mammillary tract passes posterior to the anterior commissure. The precommissural hippocampo-septal tract contains the fibers of the hippocampus proper and connects with the lateral septal nucleus. The retrocommissural hippocampo-mammillary tract contains the fibers from the subicular area to the mammillary body. Retrocommissural fibers also pass to the anterior nucleus of the thalamus, both directly as they course past the nucleus and indirectly via the mammillary body and the mammillothalamic tract.

Histology

Overall, approximately 80% of the forniceal fibers pass into the ipsilateral fornix, whereas approximately 20% of fibers cross the midline through the hippocampal commissure to enter the contralateral fornix. In addition, a small number of hippocampal fibers decussate anteriorly to join the contralateral septal area (hippocampal decussation).

Function

The fornix is part of the dorsal limbic system and the Papez circuit. It participates in high-level mental processes relevant to episodic memory and emotion. It also provides the main cholinergic input to the hippocampus.[50]

Imaging

The fornix is readily visualized in gross anatomic specimens (see Fig. 12-13) and standard sectional MRI (see also Figs. 11-3 to 11-5). DTT displays the fornix as a highly arched fiber bundle that first passes posteromedially to reach the anterior surface of the splenium and then reverses course to pass anteromedially along the undersurface of the corpus callosum as far forward as the foramen of Monro (Fig. 12-22). The fornix then curves caudally to form the anterior wall of the foramen of Monro and continues inferiorly to reach the mammillary body.

The Striae

The major supratentorial striae are the olfactory striae, the striae medullares thalamorum, the medial and lateral longitudinal striae, and the striae terminales (semicirculares).

Olfactory Striae

The olfactory tracts pass posteriorly to the posterior edge of the orbital surface of the frontal lobe (see Fig. 9-18). There they divide into the medial, intermediate, and lateral olfactory striae. The medial olfactory striae course medially and superiorly toward the subcallosal and septal regions. The intermediate striae (vestigial in humans) pass directly posteriorly to fan out into the anterior portions of the anterior perforated substance. The lateral olfactory striae take a long "switch-back" path, first passing far laterally along the horizontal portion of the sylvian fissure at the interface of the frontal with temporal lobes, then doubling back medially to reach the rostromedial temporal lobe near the amygdala. The medial and lateral olfactory striae define the anterior border of the anterior perforated substance on each side.

Striae Medullares Thalamorum

The striae medullares thalamorum course along the medial surface of the thalami exactly where the membranous roof of the third ventricle merges into the medial surface of the thalami (see Fig. 12-3). These fibers interconnect (1) the septal regions with the medial habenular nuclei and (2) the lateral preoptic nuclei and the medial nuclei of the globus pallidus (Gpi) with the lateral habenular nuclei (see Fig. 11-25).[51]

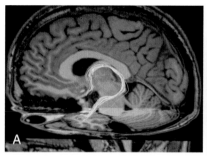
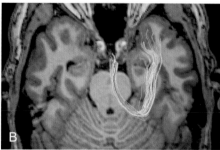
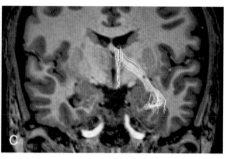

■ **FIGURE 12-22** **A to C,** The fornix arises within the medial temporal lobe and arches upward before passing anteriorly just inferior to the splenium and body of the corpus callosum. At the anterior wall of the foramen of Monro, most fibers curve downward behind the anterior commissure to the mammillary body as the hippocampal-mammillary tract. A smaller contingent (*not shown*) passes anterior to the anterior commissure as the precommissural hippocampal-septal tract.

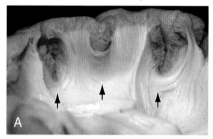
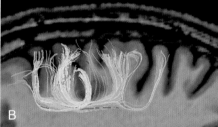
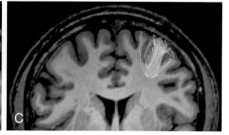

■ **FIGURE 12-23** Short association U fibers. **A,** Klingler dissection (Dr. Nicklaus Krayenbühl). The U fibers (*black arrows*) pass under the sulci to interconnect adjacent gyri through the cortex or through the subcortical white matter. In this specimen the vertical ends of the U fibers are seen to extend into the gray matter. **B** and **C,** Sagittal (**B**) and axial (**C**) diffusion tensor tractography show the U fibers within the middle frontal gyrus.

Medial and Lateral Longitudinal Striae

The dentate gyrus of the hippocampal formation passes posteriorly along the temporal lobe to the level of the splenium. There it morphs into a very thin sheet of gray matter that passes behind and around the splenium and then continues forward along the superior surface of the corpus callosum as the vestigial supracallosal gyrus (indusium griseum). On each side, very narrow white matter tracts designated the *medial and lateral longitudinal striae* are embedded within the indusium griseum. The indusium griseum and the two longitudinal striae course forward toward the genu of the corpus callosum and then curve downward along the external surface of the rostrum to form the paraterminal gyrus. In this portion, on each side, the medial longitudinal striae merge with the lateral longitudinal stria to become the white matter core of the paratemental gyrus. The combined striae then continue medially toward the amygdala and uncus as part of the diagonal band of Broca.[5] The diagonal band of Broca defines the posterior border of the anterior perforated substance.[2]

Striae Terminales (Striae Semicirculares)

The striae terminales are thin threads of white matter that course along the caudothalamic grooves, just where the medial surface of the caudate nucleus meets the thalamus on each side. These fibers originate in the amygdaloid nuclei of the temporal lobe. They arch back and then forward with the caudate nucleus to terminate rostrally in the nuclei of the striae terminales. These nuclei are situated just lateral to the anterior columns of the fornix and dorsal to the anterior commissure. Some fibers pass to the anterior hypothalamus. The striae terminales are one prominent outflow of the amygdaloid complex (especially the corticomedial nuclei of the amygdalae).[1-3]

Association Fibers Overview

Association fibers connect diverse regions of the *same* hemispheres. They are classified into short and long association fibers,

acknowledging that some fiber bundles contain mixed short and long fibers.

Short association fibers course within the cortex or in the most superficial layer of the subjacent white matter to interconnect adjacent gyri of the same or adjacent lobes (Fig. 12-23). As such they resemble the letter U and are designated the subcortical U fibers. U fibers course roughly "perpendicular" to the length of the sulci under which they pass. They are most prominent in the frontal and lateral occipital lobes adjacent to the long association fibers of the superior and inferior longitudinal fasciculi.

Long association fibers interconnect different lobes within the same hemisphere over long distances. They are organized into lengthy compact groupings of fibers, which may be designated bundles, as in the cingulum bundle, or fasciculi as in the uncinate and arcuate fasciculi.

The designation *mixed bundles* is used when long association bundles like the superior longitudinal fasciculus incorporate short association U fibers at multiple points along their course.

Working in nonhuman primates, Schmahmann and colleagues identified 10 long association bundles (Table 12-4).[8] Working in humans, Catani and associates considered the long association fibers in 11 groups (see Table 12-4).[52]

Long Association Fascicles Related to the Cingulate Gyrus
Cingulum Bundle

The cingulum bundle is a mixed association bundle that lies within the cingulate gyrus and forms most of the white matter of that gyrus (see Fig. 12-3B). It contains fibers of differing lengths. The longest of these course around the corpus callosum through the white matter of the cingulate and parahippocampal gyri from the subrostral portions of the frontal lobe into the anterior temporal lobe.[6,8,26] In this way, the cingulum bundle interconnects multiple areas around the corpus callosum, including the orbital surface of the frontal lobe, the subcallosal gyrus, the parolfactory area, the supplementary motor areas, the

TABLE 12-4. Long Association Pathways in Nonhuman Primates* and Humans†

Source of Fibers	Fiber Tract
Cingulate gyrus	Cingulum bundle
Parietal lobe	Superior longitudinal fasciculus (SFL)
	SFL I
	SFL II
	SFL III
Parieto-occipital region	Superior fronto-occipital fasciculus
Temporal-occipital region	Inferior fronto-occipital fasciculus
	Inferior longitudinal fasciculus
Temporal lobe	Uncinate fasciculus
	Extreme capsule
	Arcuate fasciculus

*Data from Schmahmann JD, Pandya DN, Wang R, et al. Association fibre pathways of the brain: parallel observations from diffusion spectrum imaging and autoradiography. Brain 2007; 130:630-653.

‡Data from Catani M, Howard RJ, Pajevic S, Jones DK. Virtual in vivo dissection of white matter fasciculi in the human brain. NeuroImage 2002; 17:77-94.

dorsolateral prefrontal cortex, the caudal inferior parietal lobule, the retrosplenial cortex, the parahippocampal cortex, the entorhinal and perirhinal cortices, and the presubiculum. Shorter fibers that pass into and out from the cingulum bundle connect the medial surface of the superior frontal gyrus, the parietal lobe, and the cingulate, cuneate, lingual and fusiform gyri.[26]

Function

The cingulum bundle is the major component of the dorsal limbic pathway.[6,8] It is involved in a wide range of motivational and emotional aspects of behavior and participates in spatial working memory.[50] It interconnects the hippocampus and parahippocampal gyrus (critical for memory) with the (1) prefrontal areas (important for manipulating information, monitoring behavior and working memory) and (2) rostral cingulate gyrus (involved in motivation and drive).[6] The limbic system is also important for high-level mental processes relevant to memory and emotion. It is part of the Papez circuit that links the hippocampus, parahippocampal gyrus, mammillary bodies, thalamus, and cingulate gyrus. Other structures subsequently integrated into the limbic system include the amygdala, septal region, and olfactory bulb. These structures have been implicated in dementia, epilepsy, and schizophrenia.

Imaging

Standard sectional imaging shows the white matter core of the cingulate gyrus but does not define the cingulum bundle itself (Fig. 12-24). DTT displays the cingulum bundle as a longitudinally oriented fiber bundle that courses around the corpus callosum within the white matter of the cingulate gyrus (Fig. 12-25).

Long Association Fascicles Related to the Parietal Lobe
Superior Longitudinal Fasciculus

The superior longitudinal fasciculus (SLF) is a long arcuate fiber system that lies along the superolateral aspect of the putamen (see Fig. 12-2C and D).[2] In aggregate, the SLF interconnects the frontal lobe with the parietal occipital and temporal lobes. The posterior portion of the SLF displays two arms: a posterior arm that fans out into the parietal, occipital, and posterior temporal lobes and an anterior arm that recurves sharply forward to reach the anterior temporal lobe.[2]

Schmahmann and colleagues[8] and Kollias[6] consider the SLF in three portions, designated SFL I, II, and III (Figs. 12-26 and 12-27). The vertical portion of the arcuate fasciculus is sometimes considered to be a fourth component of the SLF.[53]

The SLF I is the most rostral and medial portion of the SLF. It extends from the medial and dorsal parietal cortex to the medial and dorsal portions of the premotor and prefrontal cortices of the frontal lobe.[8,53] As such, the SLF I courses through the white matter of the superior parietal lobule, the upper precuneus, the upper postcentral and precentral gyri, the supplementary motor area, and the posterior portion of the superior frontal gyrus.[8,53]

The SFL II is the intermediate portion of the SLF. It runs inferior and lateral to SLF I in the white matter of the occipital, inferior parietal, and frontal lobes, It courses from the caudal portion of the inferior parietal lobule deep to the upper shoulder of the sylvian fissure into the white matter deep to the premotor and prefrontal regions. As such, SLF II courses through the white matter within the supramarginal and angular gyri, the mid postcentral and precentral gyri, and the middle frontal gyrus.[53] The *horizontal* portion of the arcuate fasciculus may be inseparable from the SLF II.[53]

The SFL III is the most caudal and lateral portion of the SLF. It runs in the opercular white matter of the parietal and frontal lobes from the rostral inferior parietal lobule to the ventral portion of the premotor and prefrontal cortex. As such, the SLF III courses through the white matter of the supramarginal gyrus, the inferior portions of the postcentral, subcentral, and precentral gyri, and the inferior frontal gyrus (pars opercularis).

Makris and associates consider the vertical portion of the arcuate fasciculus as a fourth component of the SLF. This portion courses through the white matter of the supramarginal gyrus, the posterior portion of the superior temporal gyrus, and the temporo-occipital region[53] (see Figs. 12-34 to 12-36).

Function

The SLF is significant for initiation of motor activity and higher-order control of body-centered action. It connects the superior parietal lobule (important for limb and trunk location in body-centered space) with premotor areas (engaged in higher aspects of motor behavior). The SLF is also significant for spatial attention, because it connects the inferior parietal lobule (concerned with visual spatial information) with the posterior prefrontal cortex (important for perception and awareness). Furthermore, the SLF is relevant to gestural components of language and orofacial working memory, because it connects the supramarginal gyrus (concerned with higher order somatosensory information) with the ventral premotor area (containing mirror neurons for action imitation).

Imaging

The broad regions that contain the SLF are readily shown by routine sectional MRI, but the fasciculus itself is not presently resolved by these studies. DTT shows the SLF as a "spiked crescent" with a smooth concave inferior border that curves around the sylvian fissure and a highly serrated, "multiply-spiked" convex superior border that arches through the frontal, parietal, and temporal lobes (see Figs. 12-26 and 12-27).

Long Association Fascicles Related to the Parietal-Occipital Lobes
Superior Fronto-occipital Fasciculus

Fibers from the dorsal medial occipital lobe and the dorsal, medial, and inferior parietal lobules coalesce at the level of the parieto-occipital junction to form a loosely woven fiber bundle that courses forward, horizontally, to reach the dorsal medial prefrontal and premotor cortices.[54] In coronal plane, the midportion of the superior fronto-occipital fasciculus (SFOF) appears as a triangular fascicle situated within the white matter just superior and lateral to the caudate nucleus, predominantly lateral to the fibers of the corpus callosum and medial to the fibers of the corona radiata and SLF II.[2] The loose weave of the SFOF reflects

■ **FIGURE 12-24** Cingulum bundle. **A** and **B,** Axial T2W MR images. **C** and **D,** Axial DT color maps at comparable levels. The cingulum bundle (*arrows*) forms a parasagittal stripe of white matter that passes longitudinally (*green*) over the corpus callosum (*red,* C) and medial to the commissural fibers (*pink,* C C) that ascend into each hemisphere. Anteriorly and posteriorly, the cingulum bundle arches in front and behind the corpus callosum.

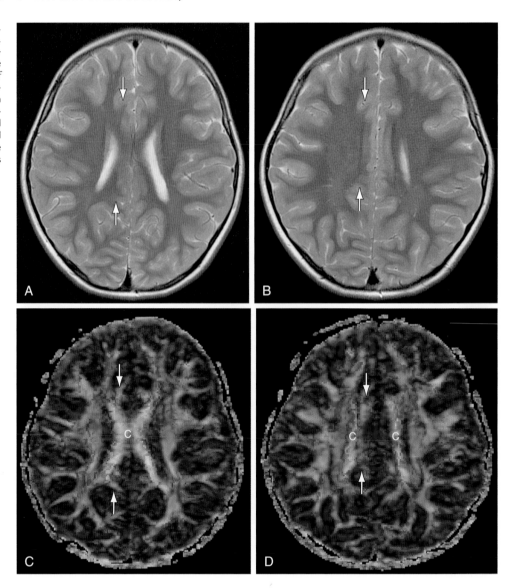

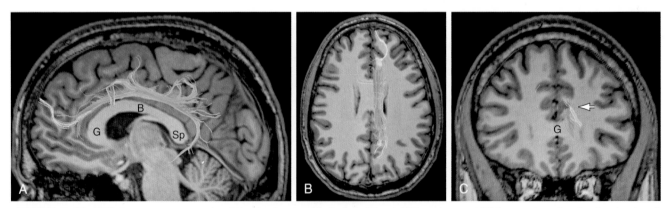

■ **FIGURE 12-25** Diffusion tensor tractography of the cingulum bundle. Sagittal (**A**), axial (**B**), and coronal (**C**) images show that the cingulum bundle (*green*) courses longitudinally through the cingulate gyrus atop the body (B) and around the genu (G) and splenium (Sp) of the corpus callosum. In **C,** the *white arrow* indicates the white matter core of the left cingulate gyrus.

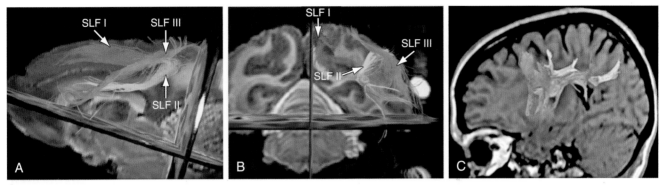

■ **FIGURE 12-26** Superior longitudinal fasciculus (SLF). **A** and **B**, The SLF of the fascicularis monkey. Diffusion spectrum imaging projected onto sagittal (**A**) and coronal (**B**) MR images displays the three components of the SLF (I: *red;* II: *yellow;* III: *blue*). **C,** The SLF of the human brain. 3D diffusion tensor tractography projected onto a sagittal MR image displays the three components of the SLF (I: *yellow;* II: *violet;* III: *blue*). *(A and B, From Schmahmann JD, Pandya DN, Wang R, et al. Association fibre pathways of the brain: parallel observations from diffusion spectrum imaging and autoradiography. Brain 2007; 30:630-653. C, From Kollias S. Parcellation of the white matter using DTI: insights into the functional connectivity of the brain. Neuroradiol J 2009; 22[Suppl I]:45-57.)*

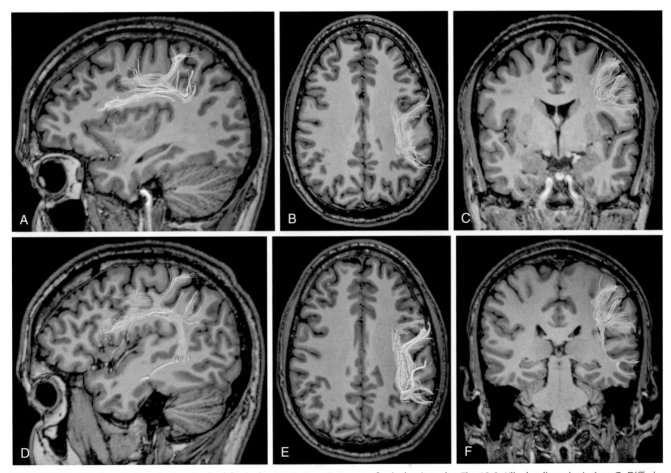

■ **FIGURE 12-27** **A** to **C,** Superior longitudinal fasciculus (SLF). **D** to **F,** Arcuate fasciculus (see also Fig. 12-2, Klingler dissection). **A** to **C,** Diffusion tensor tractography of SLF II and III projected onto the sagittal (**A**), axial (**B**), and coronal (**C**) planes. SLF I is not displayed in these images. **D** to **F,** Addition of the arcuate fasciculus (SLF IV) projected onto the same sagittal (**A**), axial (**B**), and coronal (**C**) plane images shown in **A** to **C** (see also Figs. 12-34 and 12-35).

its need to penetrate between the horizontally arrayed fibers of the corpus callosum medially and the vertically arrayed fibers of the corona radiata laterally (see Figs. 12-13 and 12-27).[8] This bundle is the subject of some debate, because some hold it is a true long association bundle whereas others believe it is only a concatenation of multiple short association U fibers.[55] In their tractography study, Catani and colleagues did not demonstrate occipital connections of the SFOF and have suggested, instead,

that this fasciculus mainly connects the dorsolateral prefrontal cortex with the superior parietal lobule.[26] Makris and associates clearly distinguished this bundle from the closely adjacent subcallosal bundle of Muratoff.[54]

Function

The SFOF is significant for peripheral vision, visual perception of motion, and visual spatial processing. The SFOF connects the

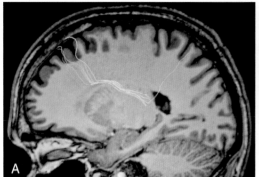
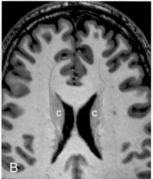
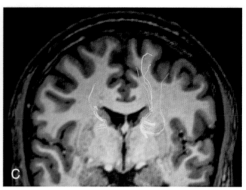

■ **FIGURE 12-28** Superior fronto-occipital fasciculus (SFOF). Diffusion tensor tractography projected onto the sagittal (**A**), axial (**B**), and coronal (**C**) planes. The appearance and position of the SFOF on coronal T2W MRI are shown in Figure 12-13A. On DTT, the SFOF appears as a narrow tract that characteristically passes immediately lateral to the caudate nucleus (c) and displays an undulating sagittal course from the frontal white matter to the parietal white matter.

superior parietal gyrus (parastriate areas important for peripheral vision and visual appreciation of motion) with the dorsolateral prefrontal cortex of the middle and inferior frontal gyri (necessary for attention).

Imaging

The SFOF can be visualized in cross section on coronal T2W images and coronal DTI as a small circular to triangular tract situated just lateral to the caudate nucleus, just inferior to the fibers of the corpus callosum and just medial to the fibers of the corona radiata (see Fig. 12-13). DTT demonstrates the tract as a narrow bundle coursing anteroposteriorly in the same location (Fig. 12-28).

Inferior Fronto-occipital Fasciculus

Fibers from broad regions of the middle and inferior temporal gyri, the fusiform and lingual gyri of the posterior temporal lobe, and the inferior occipital lobe course anteriorly and gather into a narrow bundle that passes upward through the posterior portion of the temporal stem and continues forward along the anterior floor of the external capsule immediately superior to the uncinate fasciculus to reach the frontal lobe (see Fig. 12-1B).[46] There the fasciculus expands into multiple fiber bundles that continue anteriorly to reach the inferolateral and dorsolateral prefrontal cortices.[26] Martino and colleagues identified two components of the inferior fronto-occipital fasciculus (IFOF): (1) a superficial dorsal component that connects the frontal lobe with the superior parietal lobe and the posterior portion of the superior and middle occipital gyri and (2) a deep ventral component that connects the frontal lobe with the posterior portion of the inferior occipital gyrus and the posterior temporobasal area.[56]

Function

This fascicle may be a major component of the ventral subcortical "what" pathway important for object recognition and discrimination. The IFOF most likely also has a significant role in semantic processing, because it interconnects the occipital associative extrastriate cortex with the temporobasal region, two areas important to semantic processing.[56] The IFOF also functions in visuospatial processing and enables the interaction between emotion and cognition.[50]

Imaging

The IFOF is seen on oblique axial T2W MRI as a long swath of white matter passing along the inferior occipitotemporal lobes. It is not yet distinguishable from the adjacent inferior longitudinal fasciculus on routine sections. On sagittal DTT, the IFOF has an asymmetric "bow tie" shape with a characteristic central narrowing or "choke point" along the floor of the extreme capsule (Fig. 12-29).

Inferior Longitudinal Fasciculus

The inferior longitudinal fasciculus (ILF) is a long association fiber tract situated in the external sagittal stratum of the occipital, parietal, and temporal lobes, lateral to and parallel with the lateral walls of the occipital and temporal horns (Fig. 12-30 see also Fig. 12-2G).[2,5,26,46] The ILF has both vertical and horizontal components. Caudally, the vertical portion arises in the extrastriate visual association areas, both medially (cuneus) and laterally (fusiform and lingual gyri). This vertical component lies between, and is distinct from, the tapetum and optic radiations medially and the U fibers of the occipital, parietal, and temporal lobes laterally.[6,8,45] At the ventral aspect of the occipitotemporal lobes, the fibers of the inferior longitudinal fasciculus turn horizontally along the length of the temporal lobe to reach the anterior temporal region, including the lateral temporal cortices of the superior, middle, and inferior temporal gyri; the medial temporal cortices of the uncus and parahippocampal gyrus; and the amygdala.[6] Catani et al found no ILF fibers originating from the calcarine cortex.[45] None of the ILF fibers ascends through the temporal stem to the frontal lobe.

Function

The inferior longitudinal fasciculus has a role in the ventral visual stream for object recognition, discrimination, and memory. It appears to mediate the fast transfer of visual signals to anterior temporal regions and neuromodulatory back-projections from the amygdala to early visual areas. It likely plays a role in linking object representations to their lexical labels.[57] Face recognition probably depends on the ILF, because disruption of the tract has been implicated in associative visual agnosia, prosopagnosia, visual amnesia, and visual hypoemotionality.[6]

Imaging

The ILF is seen on oblique axial T2W MRI as a long swath of white matter passing along the inferior occipitotemporal lobes. It is not yet distinguishable from the adjacent inferior fronto-occipital fasciculus on routine sections. On sagittal DTT, the ILF lies in approximately the same position as the IFOF but it lies slightly more inferiorly and laterally, has a more uniform ribbon shape, lacks the narrow "choke point" seen with the IFOF, and does not ascend through the temporal stem into the frontal lobe (Fig. 12-31). In axial DTT images, the ILF lies more lateral in position and shows a greater lateral convexity, whereas the IFOF lies slightly more medially and shows a prominent lateral concavity at its anterior end (compare Fig. 12-31 with Fig. 12-29).

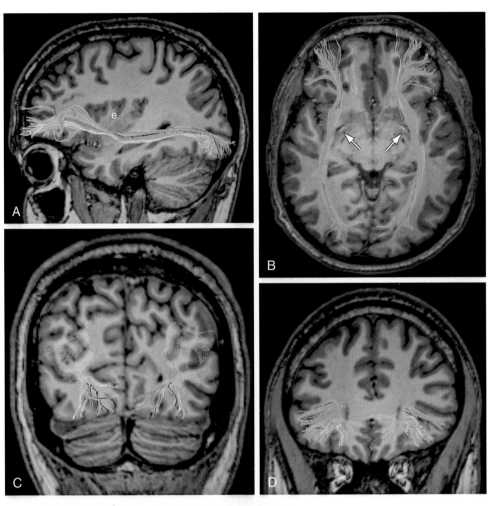

■ **FIGURE 12-29** Inferior fronto-occipital fasciculi (IFOF). Diffusion tensor tractography projected onto the sagittal (**A**), axial (**B**), and coronal (**C** and **D**) planes. From the inferomedial occipital and temporal lobes, the IFOF course forward medial to the inferior longitudinal fasciculi, ascend through the posterior portions of the temporal stems, narrow into compact bundles that traverse the anterior floors of the external capsules (e) immediately superior to the uncinate fasciculi, and then continue forward to the inferolateral and dorsolateral prefrontal cortices. (See composite Fig. 12-33.)

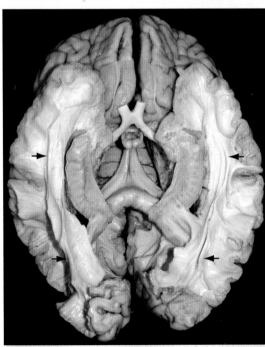

■ **FIGURE 12-30** Inferior longitudinal fasciculus (ILF). Dissection of the human brain from the inferior aspect by the Klingler technique (Dr. Nicklaus Krayenbühl). The inferior longitudinal fasciculi (*arrows*) curves along the inferior aspects of the temporal white matter beneath the fusiform gyri.

Long Association Fascicles Related to the Temporal Lobe

The long association bundles related to the temporal lobe include three curvilinear arched fasciculi, named, from rostral to caudal, the uncinate fasciculus, the extreme capsule, and the arcuate fasciculus.

Uncinate Fasciculus

The uncinate fasciculus is the most rostral of the arcuate long association bundles of the temporal lobe (see Figs. 12-1B and 12-2H).[8] Fibers from the rostral temporal lobe (temporal pole, uncus, hippocampal gyrus, and amygdala) gather lateral to the amygdala and temporal horn and then curve posteriorly, medially, and superiorly through the anterior portion of the temporal stem.[46] They curve along the limen insulae, posterior and then superior to the sylvian fissure and middle cerebral artery, and traverse the inferior portions of the external and extreme capsules immediately inferior to the inferior fronto-occipital fasciculus (Fig. 12-32).[46] From there the uncinate fibers extend into the white matter of the orbitofrontal cortex and may ascend rostrally and medially to reach the ventral prefrontal cortex.[26]

Function

The uncinate fasciculus is a ventral limbic pathway that is critical for processing novel information, for positive/negative valuations of the emotional aspects of data, and for self-regulation.[6] The fibers of the uncinate fasciculus link the rostral superior temporal gyrus (important for sound recognition), the rostral inferior temporal gyrus (important for object recognition), and the medial temporal area (important for recognition memory)

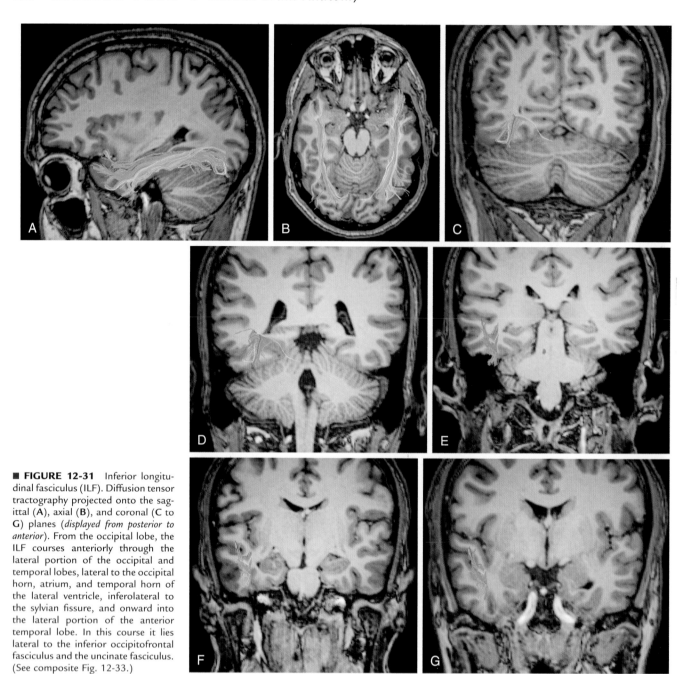

■ FIGURE 12-31 Inferior longitudinal fasciculus (ILF). Diffusion tensor tractography projected onto the sagittal (**A**), axial (**B**), and coronal (**C** to **G**) planes (*displayed from posterior to anterior*). From the occipital lobe, the ILF courses anteriorly through the lateral portion of the occipital and temporal lobes, lateral to the occipital horn, atrium, and temporal horn of the lateral ventricle, inferolateral to the sylvian fissure, and onward into the lateral portion of the anterior temporal lobe. In this course it lies lateral to the inferior occipitofrontal fasciculus and the uncinate fasciculus. (See composite Fig. 12-33.)

with the orbital, medial, and prefrontal cortices (involved in emotion, inhibition, and self-regulation). The uncinate fasciculus may also be critical in visual learning.[6]

Imaging
Routine sectional imaging displays the uncinate fasciculus as a relatively compact fiber bundle situated lateral to the anterior commissure on axial and coronal T2W and DTI images. DTT shows the uncinate fasciculus as a tightly curved fiber tract that arches sharply from the anterior temporal lobe through the temporal stem into the inferior frontal lobe lateral to the lateral end of the anterior commissure (see Fig. 12-32). The three-dimensional relationships of the inferior fronto-occipital fasciculus, the inferior longitudinal fasciculus, and the uncinate fasciculus are best appreciated when all three are seen together in a composite diffusion tensor tractogram (Fig. 12-33).

Extreme Capsule
The extreme capsule is a thin sheet of white matter that lies between the claustrum medially and the insula laterally. It interconnects the midportion of the superior temporal region with the midportion of the ventral and lateral aspects of the prefrontal cortex (see Fig. 12-2E).[8] Within the frontal lobe the extreme capsule divides into two rami. The superior ramus courses within the white matter of the inferior frontal lobe. The inferior ramus passes beneath the claustrum along the floor of the orbital cortex, just medial to the uncinate fasciculus. In sagittal images the extreme capsule lies predominantly above and behind the uncinate fasciculus.

Function
The extreme capsule connects the superior temporal cortex and insula with the orbital and dorsolateral prefrontal cortex, so it

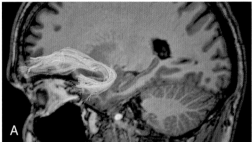
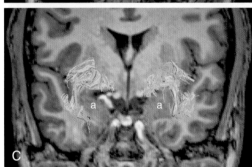
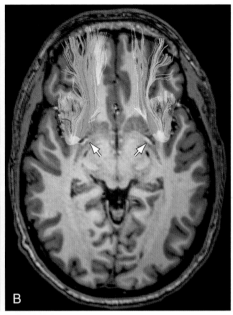

■ **FIGURE 12-32** Uncinate fasciculus. Diffusion tensor tractography projected onto the sagittal (**A**), axial (**B**), and coronal (**C**) planes. The uncinate fasciculi (*blue-green fibers*) arise in the medial portions of the anterior temporal lobes, gather lateral to the amygdalae (a), ascend through the anterior portions of the temporal stems anterolateral to the putamina and to the anterior commissure (*white arrows*), and then recurve sharply anteriorly and medially into the inferior frontal lobe. (See composite Fig. 12-33.)

may function in the linguistic (nonarticulatory) aspects of language communication.[6] The extreme capsule may also relate to sound and language comprehension, because it connects the temporal operculum (auditory association cortices) to the frontal lobe.[6] Functionally, the extreme capsule is distinct from the external capsule, which is a corticostriatal pathway.[6]

Imaging
The extreme capsule is easily appreciated on routine axial, coronal and sagittal T1W, T2W, DTI, and DTT images (see Figs. 12-29 and 12-31). The detailed anatomy of this capsule is presented in Chapter 11.

Arcuate Fasciculus
The arcuate fasciculus consists of both direct and indirect components (Figs. 12-34 to 12-36; see also Fig. 12-2D to F). The direct component interconnects the caudal portion of the superior temporal lobe (Wernicke's area) with the caudal portions of the dorsal premotor and prefrontal cortices of the frontal lobe (Broca's area). This portion of the arcuate fasciculus courses through the frontoparietal white matter dorsal to the external capsule, deep to the upper shoulder of the sylvian fissure and insular cortex, and beneath and adjacent to the fibers of SLF II.[8] The indirect component of the arcuate fasciculus lies lateral to the direct component. It is composed of an anterior segment that connects Broca's area with the inferior parietal lobule and a posterior segment that connects the inferior parietal lobule with Wernicke's territory.[52,57] The arcuate fasciculus also extends between Broca's area and the middle frontal and precentral gyri and between Wernicke's area and the posterior portion of the middle temporal gyrus. The paired arcuate fasciculi show definite left-right asymmetry (lateralization). The arcuate fasciculus is usually larger in the left hemisphere than the right, and the degree of that asymmetry is far greater in males than in females (see Fig. 12-36B).[57] By gender, the arcuate fasciculus shows extreme left lateralization in 85% of males but only 40% of females.[57] Over the whole population, the arcuate fasciculus shows extreme left lateralization in 60% of all individuals, mild left lateralization in 20%, and bilateral symmetry in 20%.[57]

Function
The classical (direct) arcuate fasciculus interconnects Wernicke's receptive, auditory word processing area in the superior temporal lobe with Broca's speech production area in the inferior frontal lobe. This connection provides for the ability to recognize language and respond to it appropriately. Individuals with more symmetric patterns of connection perform better overall on word tasks of semantic association.[58]

Imaging
The arcuate fasciculus shows a smooth concave inferior border and a spiked superior border (see Figs. 12-34 to 12-36). It closely resembles the SLF in position and shape and has been considered by Makris and associates[53] to be a fourth portion of the superior longitudinal fasciculus (SLF IV) (see earlier discussion).

Individual Variability in Fiber Tract Position
Gender and Handedness
Thiebaut de Schotten and colleagues studied the normal variation in fiber tracts in 40 healthy right-handed adults.[59] They confirmed that the long direct component of the arcuate fasciculus is far more asymmetric in males than females.[59] They found a statistically greater volume and number of fibers in the left long direct component of the arcuate fasciculus versus the right and in the right short anterior (frontoparietal) indirect segment of the arcuate fasciculus than the left.[59] They also found a statistically greater volume and number of fibers in the left corticospinal tract and the right inferior fronto-occipital fasciculus.[59]

Specific Type of Tract
Burgel and associates systematically evaluated the size, position, and extensions of individual fiber tracts by postmortem histology in 10 human brains (Table 12-5).[60] Different tracts showed differing degrees of variability. There was relatively little variability in the positions of the corticospinal tracts and the corpus callosum, slightly greater variability in the position of the optic tracts, and greatest variability in the positions of the long association fiber tracts such as the SLF, SFOF, and the IFOF. On average, tracts that begin to myelinate earlier, or that finish myelinating earlier, show less variability in position.[60] Tracts with extremely high density of fibers also show less variation in position. Similarly, "choke points" along tracts, where narrow pathways force multiple fibers into a confined location, show less variation in position than do other points along the same tracts. Thus, there is (1) lower variation in tract position within the internal capsule, close to the lateral geniculate bodies, at the stem of the temporal

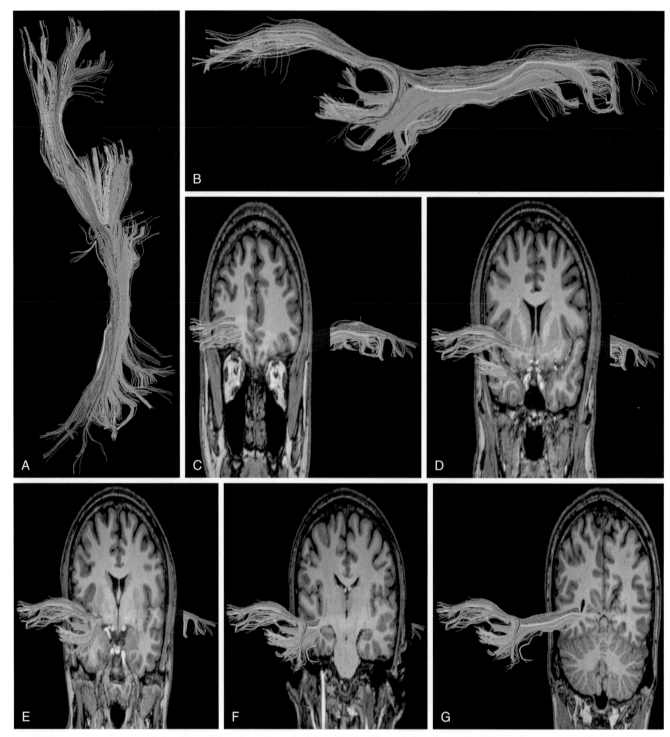

■ **FIGURE 12-33**   Anatomic relationships of the IFOF, ILF, and uncinate fasciculi in a single subject. 3T Diffusion tensor tractography. **A** and **B,** By color coding the IFOF blue, the ILF green, and the uncinate fasciculus red, superimposing them in the same 3D space, and displaying them in the axial (**A**) and sagittal (**B**) planes, it is possible to demonstrate the precise anatomic relationships among these tracts. **C** to **G,** Projecting the tracts onto sequential coronal images displays the relationships of the tracts to the frontal lobe (**C**), the frontal and anterior temporal lobes around the sylvian fissure (**D**), the inferior end of the external/extreme capsules at the temporal stem (**E** and **F**), and (*now viewed from behind*) the lateral border of the atrium-occipital horn (**G**).

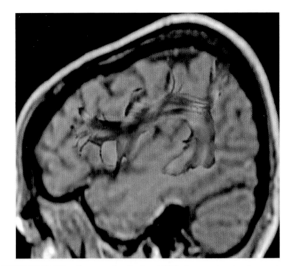

■ **FIGURE 12-34** Arcuate fasciculus. Diffusion tensor tractography projected onto a sagittal MR image. The arcuate fasciculus extends from the posterior portion of the superior and middle temporal gyri to the posterior ventrolateral frontal lobe. (See also Fig. 12-2.) *(From Kollias S. Parcellation of the white matter using DTI: insights into the functional connectivity of the brain. Neuroradiol J 2009; 22[Suppl I]:45-57.)*

lobe, in the central portions of the corpus callosum and in the fornix, and (2) relatively greater variation in tract position away from these narrow zones.[60]

IMAGING
Diffusion Tensor Imaging

Diffusion tensor imaging is an MR technique that relies on the brownian motion (random diffusion) of water molecules to probe the microstructure and three-dimensional macrostructure of the white matter.[61] Within tissue, the random diffusion of water molecules is restricted by the cellular membranes and connective tissues of the local environment. In the CSF, the mobility of the water molecule is restricted equally in all directions. There is no dominant direction of diffusion. Such symmetric diffusion of water molecules is designated *isotropic.* In the white matter, the organized bundles of axons restrict water movement across their membranes significantly more than they do along the length of the fibers. Such asymmetric diffusion of water molecules, greater in one direction than another, is designated anisotropic. Anisotropic diffusion of water within white matter was first observed by Moseley and associates in 1990, using an early MR technique that acquired data in only two different directions of diffusion.[62] Present diffusion techniques acquire diffusion data in 6 or more non-colinear directions, so the data may be modeled mathematically as a tensor.

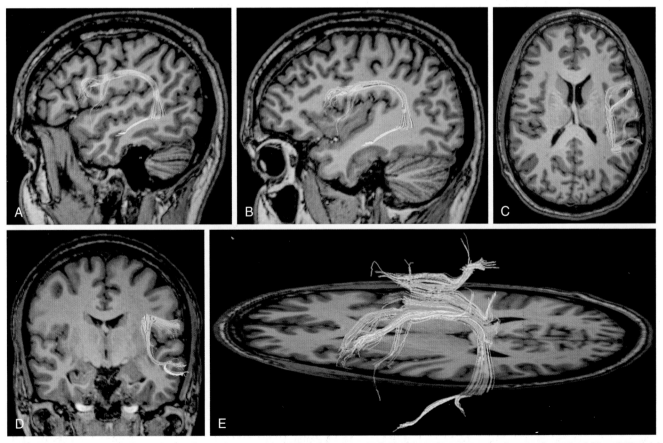

■ **FIGURE 12-35** Arcuate fasciculus. Diffusion tensor tractography of the arcuate fasciculus projected onto sections in the sagittal (**A** and **B**), axial (**C** and **E**), and coronal (**D**) planes. These 3D images demonstrate the relationship of the arcuate fasciculus to the inferior frontal gyrus anteriorly (Broca's area) and to the confluence of the inferior parietal lobule with the superior temporal gyrus posteriorly (Wernicke's area). (See also Fig. 12-27D to F.)

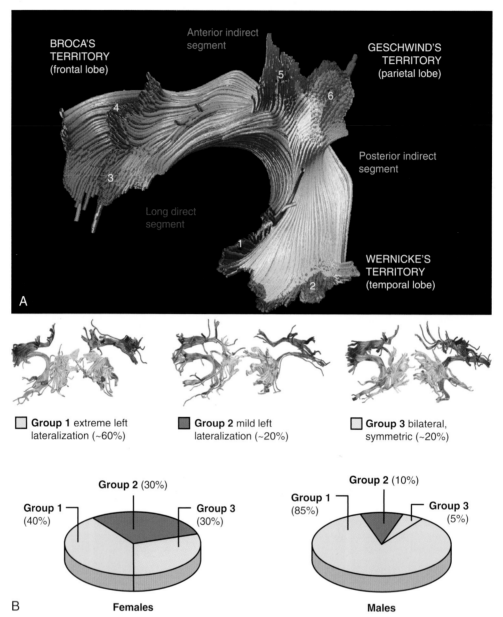

■ FIGURE 12-36 Components and gender asymmetry of the arcuate fasciculus. **A,** Components of the arcuate fasciculus. Detailed diffusion tensor tractography display of the isolated arcuate fasciculus. The long direct segment (*red*) interconnects the caudal portion of the superior temporal lobe (Wernicke's area) with the caudal portion of the dorsal premotor and prefrontal cortices of the frontal lobe (Broca's area). The anterior indirect segment (*green*) interconnects Broca's area with the inferior parietal lobule (Geschwind's area). The posterior indirect segment (*yellow*) interconnects the inferior parietal lobule with Wernicke's area. 1, superior temporal lobe; 2, middle temporal lobe; 3, inferior frontal and precentral gyrus; 4, middle frontal and precentral gyrus; 5, supramarginal gyrus; 6, angular gyrus. **B,** Asymmetry of the arcuate fasciculus by gender. The long segment of the arcuate fasciculus (*red*) shows extreme left lateralization in approximately 60% of the population, mild left lateralization in 20%, and bilateral symmetry in 20%, with a definite tendency toward greater asymmetry in males than females. The anterior indirect segment (*green*) and posterior indirect segments (*yellow*) do not show gender asymmetry. (**A,** *From Catani M, Jones DK, Ffytche DH: Perisylvian language networks of the human brain. Ann Neurol 2005; 57:8-16. **B,** From Catani M, Allin M, Husain M, et al: Symmetries in human brain language pathways predict verbal recall. Proc Natl Acad Sci U S A 2007; 104:17163-17168.*)

The diffusion tensor then provides an estimate of the mobility or restriction of water diffusion in any direction.

Mean Diffusivity, Fractional Anisotropy, and Principal Eigenvectors

Three parameters are used to characterize the diffusion of water within a voxel: the mean diffusivity (MD), the fractional anisotropy (FA) index, and the principal eigenvector (PE) of the tensor[63]:

1. Mean diffusivity is the overall mean-square displacement of molecules within the voxel. It is a measure of the directionally averaged magnitude of the diffusional motion of water.[64]
2. Fractional anisotropy is the degree to which that molecular displacement is directionally dependent, that is, the degree of anisotropy in the diffusional molecular motion.[63,64] Fractional anisotropy is often displayed as a gray scale display of the intensity of the anisotropy at each point in the image (Fig. 12-37). This display is designated the fractional anisotropy map.

TABLE 12-5. Degrees of Variability in the Fiber Tracts in 10 Postmortem Brains*

Name of Tract	Site of Least Variability	Approximate Percent Variability at That Site	Site(s) of Greatest Variability	Approximate Percent Variability at That Site(s)
Corticospinal tract[†]	Within the internal capsule		Immediately below the motor cortex	
Optic radiation[‡]	Near to the lateral geniculate body			
Acoustic radiation	At its ascent into the white matter of Heschl's gyrus	10%	Origin from the medial geniculate body	50-70%
Fornix	Just ventral to the splenium	10-30%	Fimbria and columns of fornix	50-70%
Cingulum	Isthmus of the cingulate gyrus	Near zero	Precallosal region	50-70%
Corpus callosum	Splenium, body and genu	Near zero		
Superior longitudinal fasciculus	Small region between the insula and the corticospinal tract	Near zero		
Superior occipitofrontal fasciculus	Frontally, near the transition of the body to the head of the caudate nucleus		Occipital portion medial to the corticospinal tract	
Inferior occipitofrontal fasciculus	Temporal stem	10-30%		
Uncinate fasciculus				

*Gender did not influence the degree of variability for any tract.
[†]The corticospinal tract was less variable in the left than the right hemisphere.
[‡]The optic radiation was less variable in the right than the left hemisphere.
Data from Bürgel U, et al. White matter fibers tracts of the human brain: three dimensional mapping at microscopic resolution, topography and intersubject variability. NeuroImage 2006; 29:1092-1105.

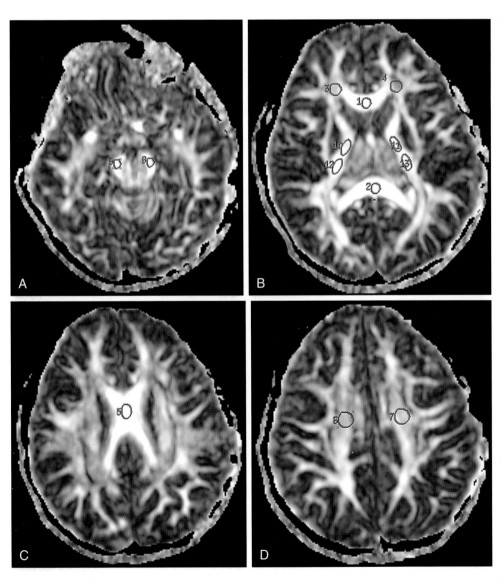

■ **FIGURE 12-37** Maps displayed from caudal to cranial indicate the regions of interest interrogated for the fractional anisotropy index in a 9-year-old girl. **A,** Cerebral peduncles: R, 0.679; L, 0.677. **B,** Frontal white matter: R, 0.392; L, 0.311. Genu: 0.828. Splenium: 0.808. Posterior limb of the internal capsule: anterior half: R, 0.530; L, 0.615; posterior half: R, 0.655; L, 0.601. **C,** Midbody of corpus callosum: 0.676. **D,** Corona radiata: R, 0.349; L, 0.431.

TABLE 12-6. Fractional Anisotropy Index (FA) of the White Matter in Normal Young Adults Ages 21-27 Years

	Mean FA	± Standard Deviation
White Matter Sites		
Genu of corpus callosum	0.78	0.03
Splenium of corpus callosum	0.81	0.03
Anterior limb of internal capsule	0.66	0.05
Posterior limb of internal capsule	0.70	0.03
External capsule	0.51	0.03
Corona radiata	0.62	0.04
Centrum semiovale	0.46	0.05
Subcortical white matter of gyri	0.49	0.06
Gray Matter Sites		
Thalamus	0.33	0.03
Globus pallidus	0.28	0.04
Putamen	0.17	0.02
Caudate nucleus	0.21	0.03
Cortical gray matter	0.18	0.03

Data from Snook L, Paulson L-A, Roy D, et al. Diffusion tensor imaging of neurodevelopment in children and young adults. NeuroImage 2005; 26:1164-1173.

TABLE 12-7. Fractional Anisotropy Index (FA) of the White Matter in Normal Young Adults Ages 20-39 Years

	Right Cerebral Hemisphere		Left Cerebral Hemisphere	
	FA	± SD	FA	± SD
Frontal Lobe				
Superior	0.381	0.043	0.390	0.054
Middle	0.406	0.035	0.390	0.033
Inferior	0.361	0.045	0.384	0.038
Parietal Lobe				
Superior	0.370	0.028	0.364	0.039
Middle	0.402	0.025	0.398	0.030
Inferior	0.519	0.050	0.504	0.063
Temporal Lobe				
Superior	0.539	0.029	0.536	0.044
Inferior	0.419	0.055	0.422	0.040

SD, standard deviation.
Data from Yoshiura T, et al. Age-related structural changes in the young brain shown by magnetic resonance diffusion tensor imaging. Acad Radiol 2005; 12:268-275.

3. The principal eigenvector is the direction of greatest water mobility within each voxel. Thus the PE is a measure of the directionality of the diffusion and corresponds to the predominant orientation of the white matter fibers within that voxel.

Although their biologic bases are still unclear, these three metrics appear to be related to the degree of myelination, integrity of the axonal cell membrane, axon size, and axon density in a complex fashion.[64] Fiber path geometry and the numbers of crossing fibers also influence our present measures of these parameters

The values of fractional anisotropy range from 0 (indicating equal diffusion in all directions with no preferential direction) to 1.0 (indicating perfectly linear diffusion in one single direction).[63] Because diffusion occurs more easily along fibers than across them, the fractional anisotropy of white matter is greater than that of gray matter. Within the *normal* brain as a whole, one may use a fractional anisotropy less than 0.17 to identify gray matter and a fractional anisotropy of > 0.2 to identify white matter and thereby (approximately) distinguish between the two.[64] Within the white matter itself, fractional anisotropy is highest where the white matter is most compact and where the greatest numbers of fibers course in parallel. Thus, in order, the fractional anisotropy of the corpus callosum is greater than the fractional anisotropy of the internal capsule, which is greater than the fractional anisotropy of the centrum semiovale.[63] Tables 12-6 and 12-7 provide values for the fractional anisotropy of normal young adults within the white matter of the major tracts; the white matter of the frontal, parietal, and temporal lobes; and the gray matter.[64,65] Values for infants, children, and teens ages 3 weeks to 19 years are available.[66]

Diffusion Tensor Imaging Color Map
The intensity data from the fractional anisotropy index and the directional data from the principal eigenvectors can be used in multiple ways to display the three-dimensional anatomy of the white matter in vivo.

The first way to combine the fractional anisotropy with the principal eigenvectors is the DTI color map (see Figs. 12-8 and 12-12). The DTI color map is created by assigning one principal color to each of the three orthogonal directions of water diffusion and weighting the intensity of the color at each voxel in

direct proportion to the fractional anisotropy within that voxel. The result is a color map in which red signifies predominant diffusion in the transverse (left-right) direction. Blue signifies predominant diffusion in the superoinferior direction, and green signifies predominant diffusion in the anteroposterior direction. Diffusion in oblique directions is coded by a precisely proportional mixture of the three principal colors.

Diffusion Tensor Tractography
Diffusion tensor tractography attempts to reconstruct a three-dimensional display of axon bundles using the DTI dataset.

Streamline Tractography
One technique for performing DTT is an algorithm called "streamline tractography." A "streamline" or "track" (not tract) is a line through the brain that is generated by the tracking algorithm.[67-69] A true white matter fascicle is indicated by multiple streamlines that group together and follow a coherent curvilinear course through the brain. Streamline tractography begins with the selection of a seed point: a user-defined voxel within the white matter. The principal eigenvector of that seed point determines the direction in which the algorithm will initiate the streamline. From that point the algorithm tracks the principal eigenvectors through the complete diffusion tensor dataset to construct a line that traces out the white matter fibers. The tracking algorithm includes criteria to prevent the algorithm from creating erroneous, anatomically impossible tracks. Thus, the algorithm will terminate the track if the algorithm encounters a sharp change in direction of the principal eigenvector between consecutive voxels. Sharp changes in angle are usually nonanatomic. The algorithm will also terminate the track wherever the principal eigenvector of the subsequent voxel falls below a preset standard, because voxels with low principal eigenvector have no clear directionality. Melham and colleagues provide an excellent overview of the methods and challenges of tractography.[70] Wakana and associates provide a practical and highly readable guide to postprocessing the DTI dataset to generate reproducible tractograms.[7,71,72]

Brute Force Tractography
Streamline tracks can be generated from every white matter voxel and saved for use in a technique called "brute-force tractography."[73] For the brute-force method, streamlines are first

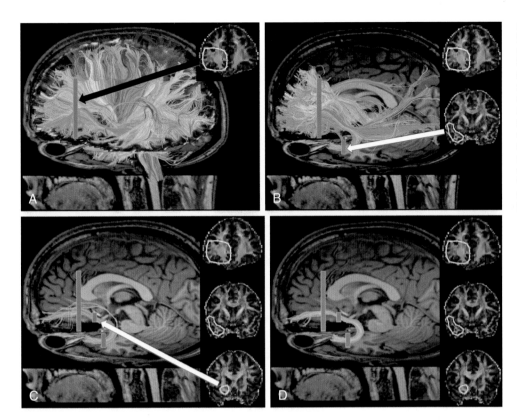

■ **FIGURE 12-38** Refining a brute-force dataset to extract a desired tract. **A,** First select a large region of interest (ROI) through which all fibers of the tract should pass. This generates a reduced dataset that includes the desired tract. **B,** Select a second, smaller distant ROI through which the tract also passes. This restricts the dataset to just those fibers that traverse both ROIs and may be sufficient to select the tract itself. **C,** If necessary, select a third narrow ROI or "choke point" through which only the desired tract passes to generate the final tract. For further details, see text.

generated from every voxel that exceeds a preselected minimum fractional anisotropy and then propagated throughout the entire brain volume (Fig. 12-38). A full brute-force dataset can consist of upwards of one million streamline tracks and includes every fiber bundle from the image. To select a specific fiber bundle from the full brute-force dataset, you apply anatomic knowledge of the course of that bundle to select one slice from the DTI dataset where most of the fibers of the desired bundle are displayed. On that slice, you place a region of interest that encompasses the fibers of the bundle. By "brute force" the computer then displays all of the streamlines that pass through that specific region of interest. The streamlines that do not pass through the selected region of interest are excluded. This brute-force approach generates tractograms of fibers that include the desired fiber bundle plus all other fibers that happen to pass through the specific region of interest selected.

To refine the tractogram, and exclude undesired tracks, one again applies anatomic knowledge to select a second region of interest through which the desired fiber bundle passes but the others do not. One then employs the tracking algorithm to generate only that subset of streamlines that pass through *both* regions of interest.

Occasionally, the tractogram includes a few "stray tracks" that meet the criteria set by the regions of interest but are not part of the tract under investigation. To further refine the image, you select regions of interest traversed only by the stray tracks, not the desired track, and apply a "not" or "delete" instruction to redisplay the fiber bundle excluding all the "stray" tracks that traverse that (negative) region of interest. By careful, knowledgeable selection of each region of interest, one can generate reproducible tractograms of individual fiber bundles.

With increasing experience, the process of track refinement can be condensed and shortened by using standard reproducible sets of anatomic criteria.[71] In a few cases, where a fascicle is known to narrow down into a tightly packed bundle, you can use a "choke point" approach to select the one specific region of interest that will generate the desired bundle (see Fig. 12-38C). Firm knowledge of those regions where given fiber bundles show greater or lesser degrees of normal variation helps you to create tractograms reliably despite human variability (see Table 12-5).

By generating multiple fiber bundles in different colors and then displaying them in a single image, one can begin to discern the small differences in the course of each bundle and learn to select specific regions of interest more precisely (see Fig. 12-33). With increasing expertise, one can even begin to discern the course of the white matter fibers within the gray matter of the cerebral cortex itself (Fig. 12-39).[73] Most usefully, perhaps, tractograms can now be generated from regions of interest defined by functional MRI to map the interconnections among specific functional regions of cortex in each individual. In the future, DTT display of the interconnections among specific functional regions in large populations of individuals will generate atlases of the normal left-right, male-female asymmetries and normal variations in white matter anatomy among diverse populations.[74]

Probabilistic Tracking
Probabilistic tracking algorithms incorporate expected degrees of uncertainty into the tracking algorithm and can be used to produce a connectivity metric for each voxel. These programs focus on the connectivity probabilities rather the actual white matter pathways between voxels. Definition of a "probability density function" allows estimation of the uncertainty of both intravoxel orientation and its propagation. These algorithms have the potential to delineate greater portions of the white matter tracts than do streamline algorithms.[75,76]

■ **FIGURE 12-39** High-resolution postmortem DTI. **A,** Gross specimen. Coronal section through the medial temporal lobe displays the relationships among the parahippocampal gyrus (PHG), subiculum (S), hippocampus (cornu ammonis) (H), and the dentate gyrus (D). The *white dotted lines* approximate the site of the DTI image **B.** (See also Fig. 11-10B.) **B,** Coronal plane DTI at 9.4 Tesla. Within the gray matter of the cortex, the fibers run predominantly perpendicular to the curving surface of the temporal lobe. At their deep ends they curve over to form the short association U fibers that course within the deep portions of the gray matter and the immediately subcortical white matter.

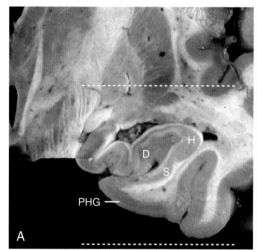
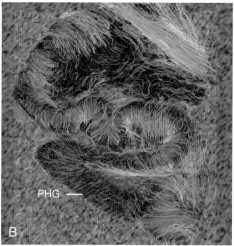

Directional Color Coding

The streamlines generated by the tracking algorithm can be color coded in different ways.

Color Code by Fiber

Each fiber can be coded such that it retains that color throughout its whole course. Coding fibers in this way allows you to trace a single fiber across the brain. Coding multiple adjacent fibers with the same color indicates the course and thickness of a specific tract or fasciculus. Coding adjacent fibers with different colors displays the differences in their courses across the brain.

Color Code by Direction Within Each Voxel

In a second coding system, each fiber can be color coded by the *dominant direction of that fiber within each voxel.* With such coding, single fibers typically display multiple different colors as they weave through the brain. The different colors then signify different directions of fiber orientation, not different tracts. This system is the one used to generate the DTI color maps (see Figs. 12-8 and 12-12). By convention, specific colors signify specific directions of fiber orientation. Red signifies preferential diffusion in the transverse (laterolateral, LL) direction. Blue signifies preferential diffusion in the superoinferior (SI) orientation, and green signifies preferential diffusion in the anteroposterior (AP) direction. Diffusion within tracts coursing at oblique angles is represented by a precisely weighted mix of colors. For example, fibers coursing obliquely between AP and SI (e.g., anterosuperior to posteroinferior, or posterosuperior to anteroinferior) would be represented by cyan, the combination of blue and green. Fibers running obliquely between LL and AP would appear yellow (red plus green), and fibers running obliquely between SI and LL would appear magenta (red plus blue).

Challenges to the Tracking Algorithms

When multiple fiber bundles converge and cross within a voxel, that voxel does not have a clearly dominant direction of diffusion. The *net* principal eigenvector in that voxel may then be significantly different from principal eigenvectors of the individual fiber tracts traversing the voxel. Voxels that contain crossing fibers are poorly modeled with standard DTI. Therefore, tractography through voxels with crossing fibers is an ongoing challenge that requires advanced tracking algorithms and imaging techniques. A newer imaging technique, diffusion spectrum imaging, helps to resolve this difficulty, at least in part, and enables more precise analysis of the origins, courses, and terminations of crossing fiber bundles.[77]

TABLE 12-8. Mean Magnetization Transfer Ratios (MTR) and Analysis of Variance for Cortical and Subcortical Structures

Region	Mean MTR	Standard Error
Corpus callosum	39.33	1.51*
Genu	40.98	0.22
Body	39.52	0.22
Splenium	39.62	0.22
Cingulate gyrus	39.87	1.89*
Anterior cingulate	39.46	0.26
Posterior cingulate	40.09	0.27
Internal capsule	39.80	0.13
White matter	38.61	1.47*
Frontal	38.93	1.51
Parietal	38.87	2.09
Occipital	38.67	1.65
Temporal	38.06	1.47
Brain stem	37.62	1.36*
Subcortical nuclei and gray matter	36.58	1.26*
Thalamus	38.07	0.13
Caudate head	35.22	0.13
Lentiform nucleus	35.11	0.13
Cerebellum	31.93	1.66*

*Indicates standard deviation instead of standard error.
Data from Armstrong CL, Traipe E, Hunter JV, et al. Age-related, regional, hemispheric, and medial-lateral differences in myelin integrity in vivo in the normal adult brain. AJNR Am J Neuroradiol 2004; 25:977-984.

Magnetization Transfer Imaging

Magnetization transfer imaging is a technique sensitive to the exchange of magnetization between a liquid pool of free, mobile protons and a (semi)solid pool of "restricted" protons that are bound to macromolecules. One quantitative measure of the magnetization transfer that occurs between free and bound water molecules is the magnetization transfer ratio (MTR). To obtain this ratio, two sequential MR sequences are obtained, first with and then without the use of a magnetization transfer pulse designed to saturate the restricted (bound) protons (Fig. 12-40). For any region of interest, MTR values are then calculated on a pixel-by-pixel basis from the intensities of the sequential images made with (Im) and without (Io) use of the specific MT pulse. Mathematically,

$$MTR = 100 \ (Io - Im)/Io.$$

White matter has a high concentration of lipids, so the MTR of normal white matter is characteristically higher than the MTR of normal gray matter (Table 12-8).[78]

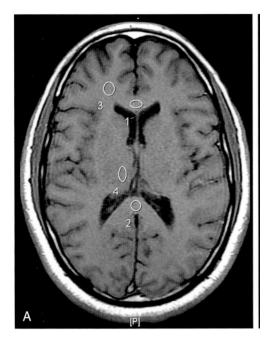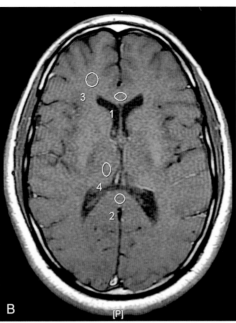

■ **FIGURE 12-40** Magnetization transfer ratio (MTR). T1W MR images before (**A**) and after (**B**) the application of a magnetization transfer pulse permits calculation of the MTR diffusely or at selected regions of interest for comparison with tables of published data (see Tables 12-8 and 12-9). Regions displayed are 1, genu of corpus callosum; 2, splenium of corpus callosum; 3, right frontal white matter; and 4, right thalamus.

Using a gradient-echo technique (fast low angle shot [FLASH]) with and without a magnetization pulse, Armstrong and associates found that whole-brain MTR was normally distributed with a mean of 37.35 (standard deviation: 1.25). The MTR for the whole brain did not correlate with age in healthy individuals aged between 18 and 69 years.[78] There was no significant effect of gender or hand dominance. There was clear hierarchy in the MTRs. The highest values of MTRs were found in the corpus callosum; the subcortical U fibers of the frontal, temporal, parietal, and occipital lobes; the pons; and the subcortical structures that contain myelinated white matter. The subcortical nuclei (i.e., basal ganglia and thalami) have reliably lower MTRs. Of all the cortical and subcortical gray matter, the thalamus showed the highest MTR because of the innumerable myelinated thalamocortical connections.[78]

Using a new magnetization transfer–sensitized balanced steady-state free precession technique that achieves higher spatial resolution images with improved signal to noise, Garcia and colleagues analyzed the MTR values for multiple different regions of white and gray matter and contrasted them to the earlier study of Mehta and associates (Table 12-9).[79-81] Garcia and colleagues found slightly higher values of MTR overall and detected regional differences in the MTR of the white and gray matter not appreciable by the earlier techniques.[79-81] By virtue of their technique, Garcia and colleagues were able to provide additional quantitative metrics for assessing magnetization transfer, including fractional pool size (F), exchange rate (kf), and relaxation times of the protons within the free pool (T1 and T2).[79,80]

Alteration of Imaging Appearance of White Matter by Pathologic Process

Aging of White Matter

Age-related differences in the cerebral white matter reflect both an initial increase in white matter volume due to normal myelin maturation and a later loss of white matter integrity as aging

continues. Overall, white matter volume increases slightly in young adults, reaching a peak in the fourth to fifth decades, and then decreases with age at different rates in different regions.[50,81,82] Yoshiura and associates found a significant increase in the mean fractional anisotropy with age in young adults (20 to 39 years), interpreted as normal maturation of the white matter.[64] Mehta and colleagues reported no statistically significant age-related differences in the MTR of the lobar white matter in adults aged 21 to 78 years whose MR images did not show hyperintensities.[81]

Comparing young adults (age 23 to 40 years) with middle-aged adults (41 to 59 years) and older adults (60 to 81 years), Giorgio and colleagues found different effects of age on the fractional anisotropy and mean diffusivity of the white matter.[82] Within the white matter, fractional anisotropy increased from young to middle-aged adults but not from middle-aged to older adults. Mean diffusivity was stable in young to middle-aged adults and then increased from middle age to old age.[82] That is, the age-related changes in fractional anisotropy preceded those of mean diffusivity. Correlations of total white matter volume, fractional anisotropy, and mean diffusivity with age showed no significant gender difference.[82]

Giorgio and colleagues found no difference in the effect of aging on heavily myelinated fibers (e.g., the corticospinal tracts in the posterior limb of the internal capsule) versus thinly myelinated fibers (e.g., the association fibers of the frontal lobe).[82] Pagani and associates suggested that "cognitive-related" fiber bundles (e.g., the frontoparietal bundles of the corona radiata) show specific vulnerability to aging according to the differing timelines along which they myelinate.[48] Jang and colleagues found a consistent decrease in the fractional anisotropy and number of fibers within the fornix from ages 20 to 78 years, with a consequent increase in mean diffusivity.[83] The precise extent and sites of these age-related changes in the white matter remain controversial. Further details are available elsewhere.[50,81,82,84]

TABLE 12-9. Magnetization Transfer Ratios (MTR) for White Matter and Gray Matter

	Garcia et al.[*] 3D-BSSFP		Mehta et al.[†] 2D T1-SPGR	
	MTR (%)	Δ MTR[‡] (%)	MTR (%)	Δ MTR[‡] (%)
White Matter Structures				
Mean MTR of all white matter	41.8		36.4	
Lobar white matter				
Frontal	43.9 ± 0.2	+5.1	36.6 ± 0.5	+0.6
Parietal	43.2 ± 0.3	+3.4	34.6 ± 0.5	−4.9
Temporal	42.5 ± 0.3	+1.7	38.2 ± 0.3	+5.0
Occipital	41.9 ± 0.2	+0.3	38.2 ± 0.2	+5.0
White matter tracts				
Splenium of corpus callosum	43.8 ± 1.1	+4.8	37.7 ± 0.3	+3.7
Genu of corpus callosum	43.5 ± 2.1	+4.1	40.7 ± 0.3	+11.9
Rostrum of corpus callosum	43.4 ± 1.9	+3.9	NA	NA
Body of corpus callosum	43.2 ± 1.8	+3.4	NA	NA
Posterior limb internal capsule	42.4 ± 0.4	+1.5	38.1 ± 0.3	+4.8
Anterior limb internal capsule	39.2 ± 0.3	−62	34.3 ± 0.3	−5.7
Anterior commissure	37.3 ± 2.7	−10.7	29.9 ± 0.7	−17.8
Cerebral peduncle	37.1 ± 0.5	−11.2	35.4 ± 0.6	−2.7
Gray Matter Structures				
Mean MTR of all gray matter	34.4		27.3	
Lobar gray matter				
Occipital	34.7 ± 0.5	+1.0	27.5 ± 0.2	+0.7
Temporal	33.5 ± 0.3	−2.5	28.4 ± 0.4	+4.0
Parietal	33.2 ± 0.8	−3.4	24.6 ± 0.4	−9.9
Frontal	31.2 ± 0.9	−9.2	25.9 ± 0.2	−5.2
Deep gray matter				
Thalamus	37.9 ± 0.3	+10.3	28.6 ± 0.4	+4.7
Amygdala	36.3 ± 0.2	+5.7	NA	NA
Globus pallidus	36.1 ± 0.5	+5.1	28.4 ± 0.5	+4.0
Hippocampus	34.7 ± 0.2	+1.0	NA	NA
Putamen	34.7 ± 0.2	+1.0	27.4 ± 0.5	+0.3
Mammillary bodies	33.9 ± 0.5	−1.3	NA	NA
Caudate nucleus	31.7 ± 1.0	−7.7	27.7 ± 0.4	−1.4

BSSFP, balanced steady-state free precession; NA, not available; SPGR, spoiled gradient-recalled-echo.

[*]Data from Garcia M, Gloor M, Bieri O, et al. MTR variation in normal adult brain structures using balanced steady-state free precession. Neuroradiology 2011; 53:159-167.

[†]Data from Mehta RC, Pike B, Enzmann DR. Magnetization transfer MR of the normal adult brain. AJNR Am J Neuroradiol 2004; 16:2085-2091.

[‡]Δ signifies the difference from the mean of all white matter structures or the mean of all gray matter structures.

KEY POINTS

■ Commissural fibers are bihemispheric fibers that cross the midline to interconnect the two cerebral hemispheres. They may be homotopic or heterotopic. Prominent commissures include the corpus callosum, the anterior commissure, and the hippocampal commissure.

■ Projection fibers are unihemispheric fibers that convey impulses from the cortex to subcortical regions such as the basal ganglia, diencephalon, brain stem, and the spinal cord (often after crossing over the midline in the brain stem).

■ Prominent projections include the corticospinal tract, thalamic radiations, optic radiations, auditory radiations, and the fornix.

■ Association fibers are unihemispheric fibers that connect diverse regions of the same hemisphere. They may be short U fibers that interconnect adjacent gyri or long tracts that span the hemisphere. Prominent long association bundles include the cingulum bundle, the superior and inferior longitudinal fasciculi, the superior and inferior occipitofrontal fasciculi, the arcuate fasciculus, the uncinate fasciculus, and the extreme capsule.

■ The corpus callosum is composed of commissural fibers that interconnect those regions of the cerebrum that are related to the midline of the body and to coordinated bilateral activity.

The anteroposterior order in which fibers cross through the corpus callosum is determined by the anteroposterior position of the portions of the cortex from which the fibers originate.

■ The corticospinal tract is a projection bundle that arises from a broad region of the cerebral cortex, including the primary motor cortex, the premotor and supplementary motor areas, the primary and secondary sensory cortices, and the superior parietal lobule. As few as 20% to 30% of its fibers may originate in Brodmann area 4 of the primary motor cortex.[3] The corticospinal tract descends through the posterior limb of the internal capsule and the midportion of the cerebral peduncle to reach the medullary pyramids and spinal cord.

■ The fornix is predominantly a projection bundle that arches upward from the hippocampal formation and medial temporal lobe, curves under the corpus callosum, and separates into precommissural and retrocommissural components. The precommissural hippocampo-septal tract interconnects the hippocampus proper with the lateral septal nucleus and adjacent septal structures. The retrocommissural hippocampo-mammillary tract interconnects the subiculum with the mammillary body and the anterior thalamic nucleus. About 20% of forniceal fibers cross the midline as the hippocampal commissure.

ANALYSIS

In routine sectional images, the white matter of the brain is analyzed systematically by comparing the left and right sides in serial sections from vertex to base in axial plane, from anterior to posterior in coronal plane, and from side to side in sagittal plane. In each image, one assesses the thickness, contour, position, density/signal intensity, and homogeneity of the white matter for asymmetry that indicates possible pathology. Level by level, one also makes a mental comparison between the features present and the features expected for patients of similar age to discern more subtle, bilaterally symmetric abnormalities. With knowledge of the fiber tracts, one analyzes the abnormalities detected to determine whether they signify typical vasogenic edema surrounding a lesion, typical cytotoxic edema in a vascular distribution, or a more restricted alteration along the course of a known tract, such as wallerian degeneration of the corticospinal tract or seizure-induced atrophy of the ipsilateral fornix.

In diffusion tensor imaging, one analyzes the images in similar order to detect alterations in fractional anisotropy and alterations in the directionality of known fiber tracts. With diffusion tensor tractography, one analyzes the thickness, contour, and position of the tract as a whole and the cohesiveness versus dispersion of individual fibers within the tract. The degree of (a)symmetry of known tracts can be correlated with differing neurologic function. Such correlations are expected to become increasingly important as large databases become established.

With magnetization transfer imaging, one initially compares the mean magnetization transfer ratios of two cerebral hemispheres as a whole. Then one analyzes the individual regions of the white matter for asymmetry and for deviations from the values expected for age.

All of the abnormalities detected in the white matter are integrated with concurrent abnormalities of the gray matter and the cerebrospinal fluid spaces to construct a coherent concept of the abnormalities present within the brain. These findings are then discussed with the clinicians to see how they contribute to the understanding and management of the case.

A sample report is presented in Box 12-2.

BOX 12-2 Sample Report: MRI of Adrenoleukodystrophy

PATIENT HISTORY

A 7-year-old boy presented with aggressive behavior and impaired hearing.

COMPARISON STUDIES

No prior studies are available for comparison at this institution. It is recommended that any old studies be obtained and submitted for review.

TECHNIQUE

MRI of the head was performed as serial noncontrast sagittal T1W, axial T1W, axial T2W, axial FLAIR T2W, coronal T2W, coronal susceptibility-weighted, and axial diffusion-weighted series with apparent diffusion coefficient maps (Fig. 12-41).

CONTRAST AGENT

No contrast agent was administered.

FINDINGS

There is increased T2 signal within the splenium that extends symmetrically into the forceps major on each side. Increased signal intensity is also present in both lateral lemnisci. No other sites of white matter abnormality are noted. There is no evidence of cyst, cavitation, mass effect, atrophy, hemorrhage, hypervascularity, or hydrocephalus. No congenital malformation is identified. No contrast agent was administered.

In a male child of this age, the combination of increased T2 signal within the forceps major, the splenium, and the lateral lemnisci, bilaterally and symmetrically, strongly suggests a diagnosis of X-linked adrenoleukodystrophy.

IMPRESSION

The findings on this study strongly suggest a diagnosis of X-linked adrenoleukodystrophy. Please correlate clinically. Consideration should be given to performing MR spectroscopy and to obtaining a contrast-enhanced MR study, if these have not already been obtained at another site. Should any previous imaging studies become available, it is recommended that they be submitted for review and comparison with the present study.

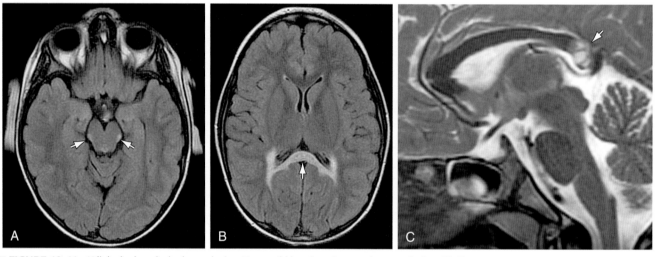

■ **FIGURE 12-41** X-linked adrenoleukodystrophy in a 7-year-old boy (see the sample report in Box 12-2).

SUGGESTED READINGS

Armstrong CL, Traipe E, Hunter JV, et al. Age-related, regional, hemispheric, and medial-lateral differences in myelin integrity in vivo in the normal adult brain. AJNR Am J Neuroradiol 2004; 25:977-984.

Carpenter MB, Sutin J. Human Neuroanatomy, 8th ed. Baltimore, Williams & Wilkins, 1983.

Duvernoy HM, in collaboration with Guyot J, Parratte B, Tatu L, et al. Human Brain Stem Vessels Including the Pineal Gland and Information on Brain Stem Infarction, 2nd ed. New York, Springer, 1999.

Garcia M, Gloor M, Bieri O, et al. MTR variation in normal adult brain structures using balanced steady-state free precession. Neuroradiology 2011; 53:159-167.

Hagmann P, Jonasson L, Maeder P, et al. Understanding diffusion MR imaging techniques: from scalar diffusion-weighted imaging to diffusion tensor imaging and beyond. RadioGraphics 2006; 26(Suppl 1):S205-S223.

Kollias S. Parcellation of the white matter using DTI: insights into the functional connectivity of the brain. Neuroradiol J 2009; 22(Suppl 1):45-57.

Melhem ER, Mori S, Mukundan G, et al. Diffusion tensor MR imaging of the brain and white matter tractography. AJR Am J Roentgenol 2002; 178:3-16.

Nieuwenhuys R, Voogd J, van Huijzen C. The Human Central Nervous System, 4th ed. Berlin, Springer, 2008.

Standring S, et al (eds). Cerebral hemisphere. In: Gray's Anatomy: The Anatomical Basis of Clinical Practice, 40th ed. Philadelphia, Elsevier, 2008.

Wakana S, Caprihan A, Panzenboeck MM, et al. Reproducibility of quantitative tractography methods applied to cerebral white matter. NeuroImage 2007; 36:630-644.

Wakana S, Jiang H, Nagae-Poetscher KM, et al. Fiber tract–based atlas of human white matter anatomy. Radiology 2004; 230:77-87.

REFERENCES

1. Carpenter MB, Sutin J. Human Neuroanatomy, 8th ed. Baltimore, Williams & Wilkins, 1983.
2. Nieuwenhuys R, Voogd J, van Huijzen C. The Human Central Nervous System, 4th ed. Berlin, Springer, 2008.
3. Standring S, et al (eds). Cerebral hemisphere. In: Gray's Anatomy: The Anatomical Basis of Clinical Practice, 40th ed. Philadelphia, Elsevier, 2008.
4. Wang, SS-H, Shultz JR, Burish MJ, et al Functional trade-offs in white matter axonal scaling. J Neurosci 2008; 28:4047-4056.
5. Riley HA. An Atlas of the Basal Ganglia, Brain Stem and Spinal Cord. Baltimore, Williams & Wilkins, 1943.
6. Kollias S. Parcellation of the white matter using DTI: insights into the functional connectivity of the brain. Neuroradiol J 2009; 22(Suppl 1):45-57.
7. Wakana S, Jiang H, Nagae-Poetscher KM, et al. Fiber tract–based atlas of human white matter anatomy. Radiology 2004; 230: 77-87.
8. Schmahmann JD, Pandya DN, Wang R, et al. Association fibre pathways of the brain: parallel observations from diffusion spectrum imaging and autoradiography. Brain 2007; 130:630-653.
9. Klingler J, Gloor P. The connections of the amygdala and of the anterior temporal cortex in the human brain. J Comp Neurol 1960; 115:333-369.
10. Ture U, Yasargil MG, Friedman AH, Al-Mefty O. Fiber dissection technique: lateral aspect of the brain. Neurosurgery 2000; 47:417-427.
11. Yasargil MG. Surgical anatomy of supratentorial midline lesions. Neurosurg Focus 2005; 18(6b):E1.
12. van der Knaap MS, Valk J. Magnetic Resonance of Myelination and Myelin Disorders, 3rd ed. Berlin, Springer, 2005.
13. Fields RD. Change in the brain's white matter. Science 2010; 330:768-769.
14. Emery B. Regulation of oligodendrocyte differentiation and myelination. Science 2010 330:779-782.
15. Rushton WAH. A theory of the effects of fibre size in medullated nerve. J Physiol 1951; 115:101-122.
16. Paus T. Growth of white matter in the adolescent brain: myelin or axon? Brain Cognition 2010; 72:26-35.
17. Lamantia AS, Rakic P, Cytological and quantitative characteristics of four cerebral commissures in the rhesus monkey. J Comp Neurol 1990; 291:520-537.
18. Raybaud C. The corpus callosum, the other great forebrain commissures, and the septum pellucidum: anatomy, development, and malformation. Neuroradiology 2010; 52:447-477.
19. Wahl M, Lauterbach-Soon B, Hattingen E, et al. Human motor corpus callosum: topography, somatotopy, and link between microstructure and function. J Neurosci 2007; 27:12132-12138.
20. Hofer S, Frahm J. Tractography of the human corpus callosum revisited—comprehensive fiber tractography using diffusion tensor magnetic resonance imaging. NeuroImage 2006; 32:989-994.
21. Witelson SF. Hand and sex differences in the isthmus and genu of the human corpus callosum: a postmortem study. Brain 1989; 112:799-835.
22. Melhem ER, Mori S, Mukundan G, et al. Diffusion tensor MR imaging of the brain and white matter tractography. AJR Am J Roentgenol 2002; 178:3-16.
23. Jellison BJ, Field AS, Medow J, et al. Diffusion tensor imaging of cerebral white matter: a pictorial review of physics, fiber tract anatomy, and tumor imaging patterns. AJNR Am J Neuroradiol 2004; 25:356-369.
24. Naidich TP, Daniels DL, Pech P, et al. Anterior commissure: anatomic-MR correlation and use as a landmark in three orthogonal planes. Radiology 1986; 158:421-429.
25. Di Virgilio G, Clarke S, Pizzolato G, Schaffner T. Cortical regions contributing to the anterior commissure in man. Exp Brain Res 1999; 124:1-7.
26. Catani M, Howard RJ, Pajevic S, Jones DK. Virtual in vivo interactive dissection of white matter fasciculi in the human brain. NeuroImage 2002; 17:77-94.
27. Gloor P, Salanova V, Olivier A, Quesney LF. The human dorsal hippocampal commissure: an anatomically identifiable and functional pathway. Brain 1997; 116:1249-1273.
28. Ebeling U, Reulen H-J. Subcortical topography and proportions of the pyramidal tract. Acta Neurochir 1992; 118:164-171.
29. Gilman S, Newman SW. Manter and Gatz's Essentials of Clinical Neuroanatomy and Neurophysiology, 10th ed. Philadelphia, FA Davis, 2003.
30. Ebeling U, Huber P, Reulen HJ. Localization of the precentral gyrus in the CT and its clinical application. J Neurol 1986; 233:73-76.
31. Westerhausen R, Huster RJ, Kreuder F, et al. Corticospinal tract asymmetries at the level of the internal capsule: is there an association with handedness? NeuroImage 2007; 37:379-386.
32. Jang SH, Ahn YH, Kim SH, Chang CH. Corticospinal tract restoration: combined study of diffusion tensor tractography, functional mri, and transcranial magnetic stimulation. J Comp Assist Tomogr 2007; 31:901-904.
33. Ross E. Localization of the pyramidal tract in the internal capsule by whole brain dissection. Neurology 1980; 30:59-64.
34. Kretschmann HJ. Localization of the corticospinal fibers in the internal capsule in man. J Anat 1988; 160:219-225
35. Holodny AI, Gor DM. Watts R, et al. Diffusion-tensor MR tractography of somatotopic organization of corticospinal tracts in the internal capsule: initial anatomic results in contradistinction to prior reports. Radiology 2005; 234:649-653.
36. Ino T, Nakai T, Azuma T, et al. Somatotopy of corticospinal tract in the internal capsule shown by functional MRI and diffusion tensor imaging. NeuroReport 2007; 18:665-668.
37. Newton JM, Ward NS, Parker GJM, et al. Non-invasive mapping of corticofugal fibres from multiple motor areas—relevance to stroke recovery. Brain 2006; 129:1844-1858.
38. Blinkov SM, Glezer II. The Human Brain in Figures and Tables: A Quantitative Handbook. New York, Plenum Press, 1968.
39. Wada A, Goto N, Kawamura N, Matsumoto K. Are there one million nerve fibers in the human medullary pyramid? Okajimas Fol Anat Jpn 2001; 77:221-224.
40. Yamada K, Kizu O, Kobuta T, et al. The pyramidal tract has a predictable course through the centrum semiovale: a diffusion-tensor based tractography study. J Magn Reson Imaging 2007; 26:519-524.
41. Yagishita A, Nakano I, Oda M, Hirano A. Location of the corticospinal tract in the internal capsule at MR imaging. Radiology 1994; 191:455-460.
42. Talairach J, Tournoux P. Co-planar Stereotaxic Atlas of the Human Brain. Stuttgart, Thieme, 1988.
43. Kim JS, Pope A. Somatotopically located motor fibers in corona radiate: evidence from subcortical small infarcts. Neurology 2005; 64:1338-1340.
44. Song Y-M. Somatotopic organization of motor fibers in the corona radiata in monoparetic patients with small subcortical infarct. Stroke 2007; 38:2353-2355.
45. Catani M, Jones DK, Donato R, Ffytche DH. Occipito-temporal connections in the human brain. Brain 2003; 126:2093-2107.
46. Kier EL, Staib LH, Davis LM, Bronen RA. MR imaging of the temporal stem: anatomic dissection tractography of the uncinate fasciculus, inferior occipitofrontal fasciculus, and Meyer's loop of the optic radiation. AJNR Am J Neuroradiol 2004; 25:677-691.
47. Kitajima M, Korogi Y, Takahashi M, Eto K. MR Signal intensity of the optic radiation. AJNR Am J Neuroradiol 1996; 17:1379-1383.
48. Hosoya T, Adachi M, Yamaguchi K, Haku T. MRI anatomy of white matter layers around the trigone of the lateral ventricle. Neuroradiology 1998; 40:477-482.
49. Duvernoy HM, in collaboration with Cattin F, Fatterpekar G, Naidich T, et al. The Human Hippocampus: Anatomy, Vascularization and Serial Sections with MRI, 3rd ed. Berlin, Springer, 2005.
50. Pagani E, Agosta F, Rocca MA, et al. Voxel-based analysis derived from fractional anisotropy images of white matter volume changes with aging. NeuroImage 2008; 41:657-667.
51. Hikosaka O, Sesack SR, Lecourtier L, Shepard PD. Habenula: crossroad between the basal ganglia and the limbic system. J Neurosci 2008; 12:11825-11829.
52. Catani M, Ffytche DH. The rises and falls of disconnection syndromes. Brain 2005; 128:2224-2239.

53. Makris N, Kennedy DN, McInerney S, et al. Segmentation of sub-components within the superior longitudinal fascicle in humans: a quantitative, in vivo, DT-MRI study. Cerebral Cortex 2005; 15:854-869.

54. Makris N, Papadimitriou GM, Sorg S, et al. The occipitofrontal fascicle in humans: a quantitative, in vivo, DT-MRI study. NeuroImage 2007; 37:1100-1111.

55. Ture U, Yasargil MG, Pait TG. Is there a superior occipitofrontal fasciculus? A microsurgical anatomic study. Neurosurgery 1997; 40:1226-1232.

56. Martino J, Brogna C, Robles SG, et al. Anatomic dissection of the inferior fronto-occipital fasciculus revisited in the lights of brain stimulation data. Cortex 2010; 46:691-699.

57. Catani M, Mesulam M. The arcuate fasciculus and the disconnection theme in language and aphasia: history and current state. Cortex 2008; 44:953-961.

58. Catani M, Allin MPG, Husain M, et al. Symmetries in human brain language pathways correlate with verbal recall. Proc Natl Acad Sci U S A 2007; 43:17163-17168.

59. Thiebaut de Schotten M, Ffytche DH, Bizzi A, et al. Atlasing location, asymmetry and inter-subject variablity of white matter tracts in the human brain with MR diffusion tractography. NeuroImage 2011; 54:49-59.

60. Burgel U, Amunts K, Hoemke L, et al. White matter fiber tracts of the human brain: three-dimensional mapping at microscopic resolution, topography, and intersubject variability. NeuroImage 2006; 29:1092-1105.

61. Le Bihan D. Molecular diffusion, tissue microdynamics and microstructure. NMR Biomed 1995;8:375-386.

62. Moseley ME, Cohen Y, Kucharczyk J, et al. Diffusion-weighted MR imaging of anisotropic water diffusion in cat central nervous system. Radiology 1990; 176:439-445.

63. Krejza J, Melhem ER. Quantitative diffusion tensor imaging of the brain in young adults shows age-related structural changes in gray and white matter. Acad Radiol 2005; 12:265-267.

64. Yoshiura T, Mihara F, Tanaka A, et al. Age-related structural changes in the young adult brain shown by magnetic resonance diffusion tensor imaging. Acad Radiol 2005; 12:268-275.

65. Snook L, Paulson L-A, Roy D, et al. Diffusion tensor imaging of neurodevelopment in children and young adults. NeuroImage 2005; 26:1164-1173.

66. Löbel U, Sedlacik J, Gullmar D, et al. Diffusion tensor imaging: the normal evolution of ADC, RA, FA, and eigenvalues studied in multiple anatomical regions of the brain. Neuroradiology 2009; 51:253-263.

67. Basser PJ, Pierpaoli C. Microstructural and physiological features of tissues elucidated by quantitative-diffusion-tensor MRI. J Magn Reson B 1996; 111:209-219.

68. Conturo TE, Lori NF, Cull TS, et al. Tracking neuronal fiber pathways in the living human brain. Proc Natl Acad Sci U S A 1999; 96:10422-10427.

69. Mori S, Crain BJ, Chacko VP, van Zijl PC. Three-dimensional tracking of axonal projections in the brain by magnetic resonance imaging. Ann Neurol 1999; 45:265-269.

70. Melhem ER, Mori S, Mukundan G, et al. Diffusion tensor MR imaging of the brain and white matter tractography. AJR Am J Roentgenol 2002;178:3-16.

71. Wakana S, Caprihan A, Panzenboeck MM, et al. Reproducibility of quantitative tractography methods applied to cerebral white matter. NeuroImage 2007; 36:630-644.

72. Hagmann P, Jonasson L, Maeder P, et al. Understanding diffusion MR imaging techniques: from scalar diffusion-weighted imaging to diffusion tensor imaging and beyond. RadioGraphics 2006; 26(Suppl 1):S205-S223.

73. Huang H, Zhang J, van Zijl PC, Mori S. Analysis of noise effects on DTI-based tractography using the brute-force and multi-ROI approach. Magn Reson Med 2004:52:559-565.

73. Jaermann T, De Zanche N, Staempfli P, et al. Preliminary experience with visualization of intracortical fibers by focused high-resolution diffusion tensor imging. AJNR Am J Neuroradiol 2008; 29:146-150.

74. Tang,CY, Eaves EL, Ng JC, et al. Brain networks for working memory and factors of intelligence assessed in males and females with fMRI and DTI. Intelligence 2010; 38:293-303.

75. Behrens TEJ, Woolrich MW, Jenkinson M, et al. Characterization and propagation of uncertainty in diffusion-weighted MR imaging. Magn Reson Med 2003; 50:1077-1088.

76. Behrens TEJ, Johansen-Berg H, Jbabdi S, et al. Probabilistic diffusion tractography with multiple fibre orientations: what can we gain? NeuroImage 2007; 23:144-155.

77. Wedeen VJ, Hagmann P, Tseng WY, et al. Mapping complex tissue architecture with diffusion spectrum magnetic resonance imaging. Magn Reson Med 2005; 54:1377-1386.

78. Armstrong CL, Traipe E, Hunter JV, et al. Age-related, regional, hemispheric, and medial-lateral differences in myelin integrity in vivo in the normal adult brain. AJNR Am J Neuroradiol 2004; 25:977-984.

79. Garcia M, Gloor M, Bieri O, et al. MTR variation in normal adult brain structures using balanced steady-state free precession. Neuroradiology 2011; 53:159-167.

80. Garcia M, Gloor M, Wetzel SG, et al. Characterization of normal appearing brain structures using high-resolution quantitative magnetization transfer steady-state free precession imaging. NeuroImage 2010; 52:532-537.

81. Mehta RC, Pike B, Enzmann DR. Magnetization transfer MR of the normal adult brain. AJNR Am J Neuroradiol 2004; 16:2085-2091.

82. Giorgio A, Santelli L, Tomassini V, et al. Age-related changes in gray matter and white matter throughout adulthood. NeuroImage 2010; 51:943-951.

83. Jang SH, Cho S-H, Chang MC. Age-related degeneration of the fornix in the human brain: a diffusion tensor imaging study. Int J Neurosci 2011; 121:94-100.

84. Zhang Y, Du A-T, Hayasaka S, et al. Patterns of age-related water diffusion changes in human brain by concordance and discordance analysis. Neurobiol Aging 2010; 31:1991-2001.

CHAPTER 13

Ventricles and Intracranial Subarachnoid Spaces

Jose C. Rios, Merav W. Galper, and Thomas P. Naidich

The brain lies within the skull submerged in a bath of cerebrospinal fluid (CSF). In the adult, the total volume of CSF is approximately 150 mL, of which about 125 mL is intracranial and 25 mL is intraspinal.[1] Within the brain, the CSF fills four hollow spaces designated the *left and right lateral ventricles,* the *third ventricle,* and the *fourth ventricle.* The two lateral ventricles lie off the midline, within the left and right cerebral hemispheres. The third ventricle lies in the midline between the two thalami. The fourth ventricle lies immediately posterior to the brain stem at the center of the cerebellum (Figs. 13-1 to 13-3). In adults, the mean volume of the two lateral ventricles varies from 9 to 27.6 mL and is slightly larger in men than women.[2-5] The mean volumes of the left and right lateral ventricles are estimated individually at 14.4 mL and 13.2 mL, respectively.[3] The combined volume of the third ventricle, aqueduct, and fourth ventricle is estimated at 1.0 to 1.5 mL.[4] Two additional compartments of CSF situated between the leaves of the septum pellucidum (cavum septi pellucidi) and between the fornices (cavum vergae) are occasionally considered to be fifth and sixth ventricles, respectively.

(See also the animations in Videos 13-1 and 13-2 at www. expertconsult.com.)

Outside the brain, CSF within the subarachnoid space bathes the entire surface of the brain, filling the sulci and fissures, and collecting over the surface in large confluent pools designated cisterns. The multiple cisterns are named for the brain structure(s) they overlie. Because each cistern is related to multiple adjacent structures, the cisterns have multiple, overlapping names. In normal individuals, all of the ventricular and cisternal spaces intercommunicate with each other and with the spinal subarachnoid space. On average, CSF flows outward from the ventricular system into the subarachnoid cisterns. Although net CSF flow is outward from the ventricles, the instantaneous direction of CSF flow varies with the phase of the cardiac cycle. Like the tide at the mouth of a river, CSF washes into and out from the ventricles in accord with the systolic-diastolic variation in each heart beat.

ANATOMY
Lateral Ventricles

The lateral ventricles are paired cavities lying to each side of the midline within the cerebral hemispheres (see Figs. 13-1 to 13-5).

They are imperfectly symmetric in most cases and show definite asymmetry in 5% to 12% of neurologically intact patients.[6] The asymmetry does not appear to correlate with handedness, age, gender, or function.[2,6] As seen from the side, each lateral ventricle is roughly C shaped, open anteriorly. Each lateral ventricle shows prominent extensions away from the main body of the ventricle. These extensions are termed *horns.* The anterior extensions into the frontal lobes are the anterior (frontal) horns. The posterior extensions into the occipital lobes are the posterior (occipital) horns. The inferior extensions into the temporal lobes are the inferior (temporal) horns. Posteriorly on each side, the occipital horn and temporal horn unite with the posterior body to form a large, confluent CSF space designated the *atrium (trigone)* of the lateral ventricle.

The *paired frontal horns* are flipper shaped, lie anterior to the foramina of Monro, and contain no choroid plexus. The frontal horns are delimited by the corpus callosum anteriorly, superiorly, and inferiorly, by the ipsilateral leaf of the septum pellucidum medially, and by the heads of the caudate nuclei and adjacent white matter inferolaterally.

The *bodies of the lateral ventricles* extend between the frontal horns anteriorly and the atria of the ventricles posteriorly. They are delimited by the body of the corpus callosum superiorly, the alvei of the fornices medially, and the fimbriae of the fornices and the thalami inferiorly. Laterally, they are delimited by a broad arch of inferiorly directed callosal fibers designated the *tapetum.* The choroid plexi project into the bodies of the lateral ventricles from the choroidal fissure situated along the floor of the ventricles medially.

The *atria* of the lateral ventricles lie immediately posterior and superior to the thalami at the confluence of the posterior bodies, the occipital horns, and the temporal horns. They are delimited by the corpus callosum superiorly, the pulvinars of the thalami anteriorly, and the tapetum laterally. The prominent glomera (singular: glomus) of the choroid plexi project posteriorly into the atria.

The *occipital horns* are the most asymmetric portion of the lateral ventricles and may be absent on one or both sides in normal individuals. They are delimited superiorly by the corpus callosum and the white matter fibers that cross through the splenium (forceps major). They are delimited laterally by the tapetum and medially by the subcortical white matter of the occipital lobes. The deep calcarine and parieto-occipital

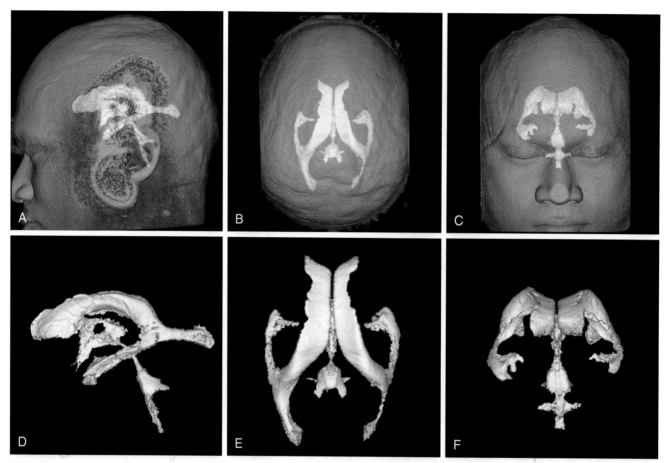

■ **FIGURE 13-1**   Ventricular system. Three-dimensional (3D) computer reformatted volumetric T2W MR images display the ventricles in lateral (**A, D**), superior (**B, E**), and anterior (**C, F**) views. A to C, Orientation of the ventricular system within the head, seen through the partially transparent skin surface. **D to F**, Magnified display of the isolated ventricles in the same orientation.
See also Videos 13-1 and 13-2 at www.expertconsult.com for an interactive rotation.

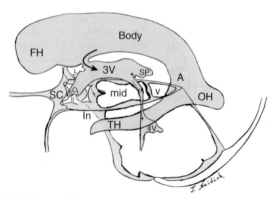

■ **FIGURE 13-2**   Schematic representation of the ventricular system in relation to the suprasellar cistern (SC), optic chiasm (II), incisura (In), midbrain (mid), vermis (v), and subarachnoid cisterns of the posterior fossa. Semilateral view. The lateral ventricle displays the frontal horn (FH), body (Body), atrium (A), occipital horn (OH), and temporal horn (TH). The lateral ventricle leads to the third ventricle through the foramen of Monro (*curved black arrow*). The anterior third ventricle (3V) displays the supraoptic (SO) and infundibular (I) recesses enclosing the optic chiasm (II). The posterior third ventricle displays a large suprapineal recess (SP) and small pineal recess (*black arrowhead*). The aqueduct (*dotted black arrow*) leads into the fourth ventricle (4V). Compare with Figure 13-1A and D.

fissures on the medial surface of the occipital lobe often buckle the subcortical white matter laterally to indent the medial wall of the horn. This creates a variably prominent bulge on the medial surface of the occipital horn designated the *calcar avis*. When particularly large, the calcar avis may (nearly) amputate the posterior portion of the occipital horn. The occipital horns contain no intrinsic choroid plexus but may contain the dependent portion of a pedunculated glomus, unilaterally or bilaterally.

The *temporal horns* of the lateral ventricles extend inferolaterally into the medial temporal lobes. Their mean volume has been estimated to be 0.46 mL in normal subjects.[3] The temporal horns are delimited inferomedially by the hippocampal formations, anterosuperiorly by the amygdalae, and laterally by the tapetum, optic radiations, and other white matter of the temporal lobes.[7] The collateral sulcus on the inferior surface of the temporal lobe often buckles the subcortical white matter upward, into the floor of the temporal horn, to create a characteristic "collateral eminence" along the floor of the temporal horn (see Fig. 13-5) The anterior tips of the temporal horns have no intrinsic choroid plexus. The choroid plexus enters the temporal horns behind the temporal tip through the choroidal fissure along the superior medial wall of the temporal horn.

On each side, the choroid plexus of the body of the lateral ventricle is supplied by the lateral posterior choroidal arteries arising from the posterior cerebral artery. The choroid plexus of the temporal horns is supplied by the anterior choroidal arteries that arise from the supraclinoid internal carotid arteries. The

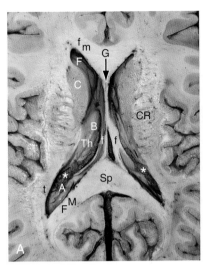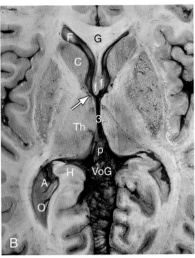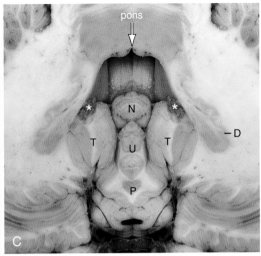

■ **FIGURE 13-3** Ventricular system. Magnified axial plane gross anatomic specimens. **A** and **B,** Supratentorial ventricles. **A,** Slightly asymmetric axial section through the midlateral ventricles. At this level, the frontal horn (F) is delimited anteriorly and medially by the forceps minor (fm) that crosses through the genu (G) of the corpus callosum, delimited medially by the midline septum pellucidum (*black arrow*), laterally by the white matter surrounding the lateral angle of the ventricle, and inferolaterally by the caudate head (C). The body (B) of the lateral ventricle is delimited inferiorly by the superior surface of the thalamus (Th) laterally and by the fornix (f) medially. The atrium (A) is delimited anteriorly by the pulvinar of the thalamus (Th), superiorly and medially by the forceps major (FM) that crosses through the splenium (Sp) of the corpus callosum, and laterally by the tapetum (t). The choroid plexus (*asterisk*) emerges into the lateral ventricle at the lateral edge of the fornix. It forms the glomus of the choroid plexus in the atrium. CR, corona radiata. **B,** Axial section through the frontal horns (F), foramina of Monro (*white arrow*), and third ventricle (3). The anterior columns of the fornices (f) form the anteromedial walls of the foramina of Monro. The anterior nuclei of the thalami (Th) form the posterolateral walls of the foramina of Monro. The medial aspects of the thalami form the lateral walls of the third ventricle. The pineal gland (p) lies at the posterior end of the third ventricle and protrudes backward into the cistern of the vein of Galen (VoG). The occipital horns (O) extend posteriorly from the atria, very often asymmetrically. H, hippocampal formation. **C,** Infratentorial ventricle. In the axial plane, the fourth ventricle (*white arrow*) has the shape of a temple bell. The "top" of the bell is formed by the midline groove (also *white arrow*) in the floor of the fourth ventricle. To each side of midline, the upper curvatures are formed by the paired median eminences. The concave side walls of the fourth ventricle are formed by the superior and inferior cerebellar peduncles. The posterior wall is formed by the nodulus (N) of the vermis in the midline and the paired cerebellar tonsils (T) to each side. Because the midline fastigial recess of the fourth ventricle curves over the nodulus, it is seen in the midline superior to and medial to the paired posterior superior recesses that curve over the paramedial tonsils. The choroid plexus (*white asterisks*) of the fourth ventricle is a paired paramedian structure that lies atop the tonsil on each side and extends symmetrically from there into the foramen of Magendie and the paired foramina of Luschka. The dentate nuclei (D) lie to each side of the fourth ventricle. Also labeled are the uvula (U) and the pyramis (P) of the inferior vermis.

anterior and posterior choroidal supplies meet near the atria of the ventricles and the glomera of the choroid plexus. The choroid plexus of the lateral ventricles is drained by the superior choroidal veins.

Foramina of Monro

The paired foramina of Monro interconnect the two lateral ventricles with the midline third ventricle (see Figs. 13-3 to 13-5; see also Chapter 11). The mean sagittal diameter of each foramen is 2.9 mm, and the mean vertical height is 5.1 mm.[8] The anteromedial walls of the foramina are formed by the two anterior columns of the fornices. The posterolateral walls are formed by the anterior nuclei of the thalami. On each side, the choroid plexus of the lateral ventricle extends through the foramen of Monro to become continuous with the choroid plexus in the roof of the third ventricle.

Third Ventricle

The third ventricle is the midline cavity that connects with the lateral ventricles anterosuperiorly via the foramina of Monro and connects with the fourth ventricle posteroinferiorly via the cerebral aqueduct of Sylvius (Figs. 13-2 and 13-6 to 13-9; see also Chapter 11). It is ellipsoidal and 4 to 11 mm wide.[9] The third ventricle is delimited anteriorly by the lamina terminalis and the anterior commissure; anterosuperiorly by the paired foramina of Monro; superiorly by the velum interpositum (velum transversum) and the habenulae; posteriorly by the pineal gland, the hippocampal commissure, and the posterior commissure; laterally by the thalamus and hypothalamus; and inferiorly by the optic chiasm and hypothalamus. The major hypothalamic

structures related to the third ventricle include the infundibulum, the tuber cinereum, and the paired mammillary bodies. The striae medullares thalamorum course anteroposteriorly along the lateral border of the roof of the third ventricle, just where the roof inserts laterally into the medial walls of the thalami. The lamina terminalis is a thin neuroglial membrane that extends from the rostrum of the corpus callosum and anterior commissure superiorly down to the superior surface of the optic chiasm inferiorly. It is lined on the ventricular surface by ependyma and on the rostral surface by pia-arachnoid. Embryologically, the lamina terminalis is the "top" of the early neural tube and the site of the anterior neuropore. In most cases the cavity of the third ventricle is crossed by the massa intermedia (synonyms: interthalamic connection, interthalamic adhesion). The massa intermedia is composed of thalamic gray matter, not white matter, and varies widely in size from 1×2 mm to 1×2 cm.

The third ventricle exhibits small extensions called *recesses* that project outward from the ventricle (see Figs. 13-2, 13-6, and 13-7). Anteroinferiorly, the supraoptic and infundibular recesses partially enclose the optic chiasm. The supraoptic recess lies between the lamina terminalis and the chiasm and points anteroinferiorly toward the cranial ends of the optic canals. The infundibular recess protrudes into the pituitary stalk (infundibulum) immediately posterior to the optic chiasm and points inferiorly to the pituitary gland. In coronal plane images, the supraoptic recess characteristically has the shape of an Erlenmeyer flask with its base resting on the chiasm. The infundibular recess characteristically has the shape of a long sharp pencil with its point directed inferiorly toward the pituitary gland.[7,10] Behind

Text continued on page 252

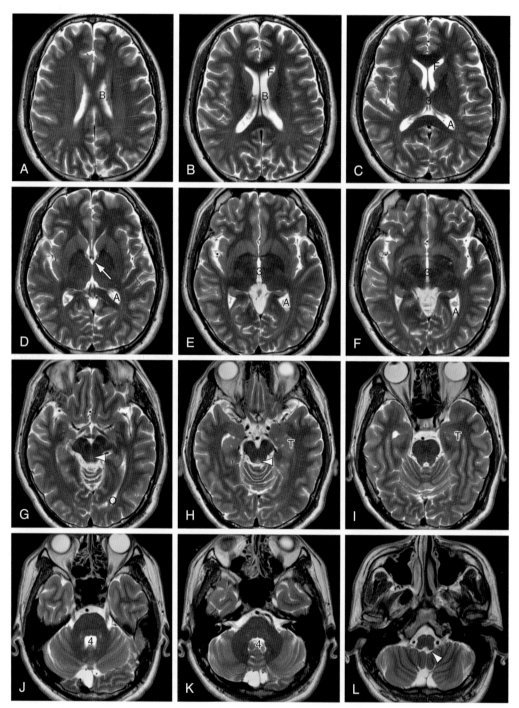

■ **FIGURE 13-4**   Ventricular system. **A** to **L,** Serial axial T2W MR images displayed from superior to inferior. In order from superior to inferior, serial axial sections display the body (B) of the lateral ventricle, then the frontal horns (F), atria (A), superior third ventricle (3), foramina of Monro (*white solid arrow*), mid third ventricle (3), occipital horn (O), aqueduct of Sylvius (*white arrowhead* in **G** and **H**), temporal horn (T), mid fourth ventricle (4), and foramina of Luschka (*white arrowhead* in **L**).

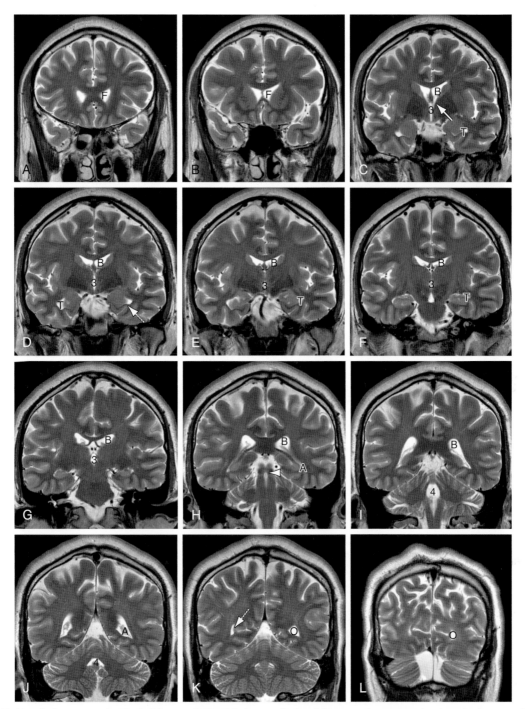

■ **FIGURE 13-5** Ventricular system. **A** to **L,** Serial coronal T2W MR images displayed from anterior to posterior. In order from anterior to posterior, serial coronal sections display the frontal horns (F) of the lateral ventricles, the foramina of Monro (*solid white arrow*), the body (B) of the lateral ventricle, third ventricle (3), temporal horn (T), aqueduct of Sylvius (*white arrowhead*), fourth ventricle (4), atrium (A), and occipital horns (O). The collateral fissure of the temporal lobe buckles inward to indent the floor of the lateral ventricle, raising a prominence designated the collateral eminence (*dotted white arrow* in **D**). The calcarine sulcus and its junction with the parieto-occipital sulcus similarly indent the medial wall of the occipital horn, raising a medial bulge designated the calcar avis (*dotted white arrow* in **K**).

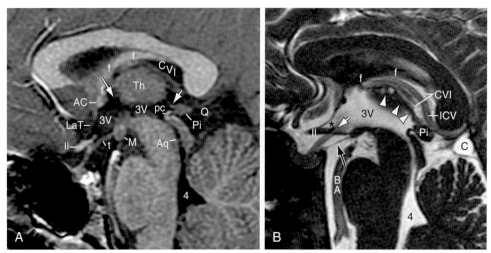

■ **FIGURE 13-6**   Third ventricle. **A,** Midsagittal contrast-enhanced T1W MR image. The walls of the third ventricle (3V) are formed anteriorly by the anterior commissure (AC) and lamina terminalis (LaT); anteroinferiorly by the optic chiasm (II) and anterior recesses of the third ventricle; inferiorly by the tuber cinereum (t), mammillary bodies (M), and midbrain; posteriorly by the posterior commissure (pc), pineal gland (Pi), and habenular commissure (*short white arrow*); laterally by the thalamus (Th); and superiorly by the membranous roof of the third ventricle. Normally, the curvature of the floor of the third ventricle continues smoothly into the aqueduct (Aq) and along the floor of the fourth ventricle (4). The foramen of Monro (*long white arrow*) lies between the anterior column of the fornix (f) and the anterior nucleus of the thalamus (Th) on each side. The cistern of the velum interpositum (CVI) extends forward from the quadrigeminal plate cistern (Q) almost to the foramen of Monro between the fornix (f) above and the roof of the third ventricle below. **B,** Midsagittal T2W FIESTA (fast imaging employing steady-state acquisition) MR image. The supraoptic recess (*asterisk*) lies anteriorly between the lamina terminalis and the upper surface of the chiasm (II). The infundibular recess (*white arrow*) lies farther posteriorly, behind the chiasm, and extends down into the infundibulum. The diencephalic leaf (*black arrow*) of the membrane of Liliequist extends from the dorsum sellae and posterior clinoid processes inferiorly to insert into the mammillary bodies superiorly (20% at the anterior margin of the mammillary bodies, 33% at their apex, and 47% at their posterior edge).[21] This leaf separates the chiasmatic cistern above from the interpeduncular cistern below. Multiple linear defects within the interpeduncular fossa indicate the thalamoperforating branches of the basilar and proximal posterior cerebral arteries. Superiorly, the choroid plexus (*arrowheads*) of the third ventricle gives the roof an irregular contour and presents small choroid plexus cysts. Superior to that, the cistern of the velum interpositum (CVI) shows a well-defined upper margin along the fornix (f) and a well-defined lower margin along the roof of the third ventricle. It contains the internal cerebral vein (ICV). A small loculated arachnoid cyst (C) manifests very high signal intensity when compared with the adjacent subarachnoid fluid.

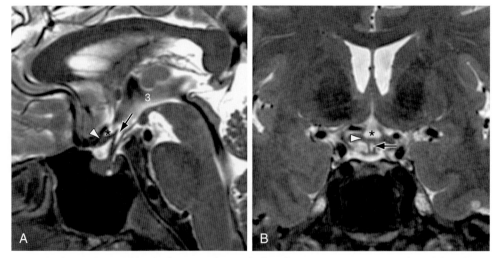

■ **FIGURE 13-7**   Anterior third ventricle. **A,** Midsagittal T2W MR image displays the supraoptic recess (*asterisk*) and the infundibular recesses (*arrow*) of the third ventricle (3) enclosing the optic chiasm (*white arrowhead*). **B,** In coronal section, the supraoptic recess (*asterisk*) resembles an Erlenmeyer flask resting on the chiasm. The infundibular recess (*arrow*) resembles a pencil point directed into the infundibulum and extending inferior to the chiasm (*white arrowhead*). In **A,** the sharp demarcation between the high signal intensity of the CSF of the suprasellar cistern and the low signal pulsation artifacts from the basilar artery also indicates the position of the membrane of Liliequist (see also Fig. 13-6B).

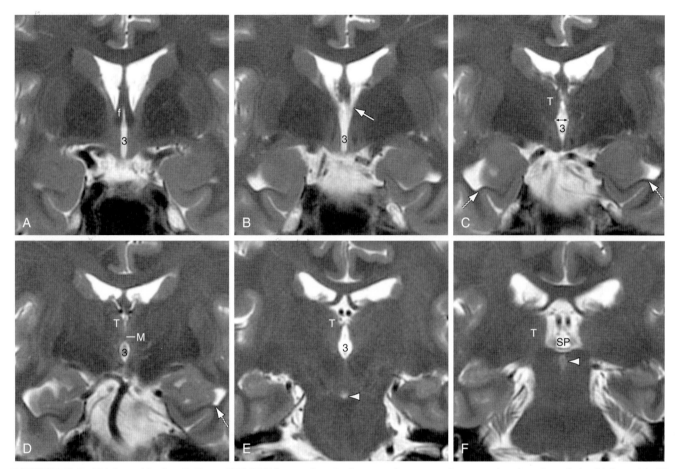

■ **FIGURE 13-8** Third ventricle. **A** to **F,** Coronal T2W MR images. In order from anterior to posterior, coronal sections through the third ventricle (3) display the anterior columns of the fornices (f) that form the anterior walls of the foramina of Monro, the paired foramina themselves (*white arrow in* **B**), the diamond shape of the third ventricle where the hypothalamic sulci (*double-headed black arrow in* **C**) groove, the medial walls of the thalami (T), the constriction of the fluid space where the two thalami unite across the third ventricle at the massa intermedia (M), the re-expansion of the third ventricle behind the massa intermedia, and the posterior extension of the ventricle into the suprapineal recess (SP). The hypothalamic sulci mark the border between the thalami above and the hypothalami below. Also noted are the collateral eminences along the floors of the temporal horns (*dotted white arrows* in **C** and **D**), the interpeduncular fossa (*arrowhead* in **E**), and the aqueduct of Sylvius (*arrowhead* in **F**).

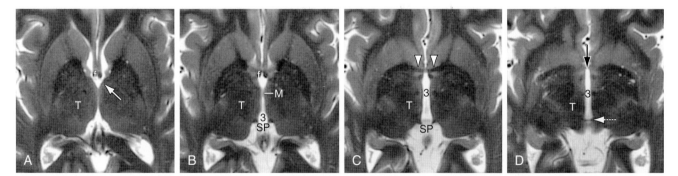

■ **FIGURE 13-9** Third ventricle. **A** to **D,** Axial T2W MR images. In order from superior to inferior, axial images through the third ventricle (3) display the paired thalami (T), foramina of Monro (*white arrow*), massa intermedia (M), suprapineal recess (SP), the anterior commissure (*white arrowheads*) and very thin lamina terminalis (*black arrow* in **D**) that form the anterior wall of the third ventricle, and the habenular commissure (*white dotted arrow*) along the posterior wall of the ventricle. The lateral walls of the third ventricle are normally gently biconcave.

the infundibular recess, a small midline hypothalamic recess extends inferiorly into the floor of the third ventricle.

Posterosuperiorly, the suprapineal recess passes posteriorly into the cistern of the vein of Galen above the pineal gland, and a small pineal recess passes posteriorly into the base of the pineal stalk (see Fig. 13-2). The suprapineal recess varies in length from 1 to 24 mm and in height from 2.5 to 9.0 mm.[11] It is usually larger in young children and smaller in adults. In approximately 2% of patients, especially children, a large suprapineal recess is seen as a normal variation of no pathologic significance.[9] In patients with severe hydrocephalus, the suprapineal recess may enlarge markedly and protrude downward through the incisura into the superior vermian cistern to compress the vermis or rupture into the subarachnoid space to create a free communication between the third ventricle and the quadrigeminal plate cistern (spontaneous ventriculocisternostomy).[9]

The choroid plexus of the third ventricle extends downward into the third ventricle from its roof. It is continuous with the choroid plexus of the lateral ventricles through the foramina of Monro. The choroid plexus is supplied by the paired posterior medial choroidal branches of the posterior cerebral arteries and drains to the deep venous system.

Cerebral Aqueduct

The aqueduct of Sylvius traverses the midbrain to interconnect the third ventricle with the fourth ventricle (see Figs. 13-2, 13-5H, and 13-10). In axial sections, the ventral wall of the aqueduct is pointed where it faces the tegmentum of the midbrain. The dorsal wall of the aqueduct is round where it faces the quadrigeminal plate. The aqueduct is considered in five segments. From anterior to posterior, these are designated the (1) adytum, (2) first constriction, (3) ampulla, (4) second constriction, and (5) egressus. The first and second constrictions correspond to impressions on the roof of the aqueduct by the overlying superior and inferior colliculi, respectively. The ampulla corresponds to the gap between those impressions at the level of the transverse intercollicular sulcus. The first constriction is normally the narrowest point along the aqueduct.[12]

Fourth Ventricle

The fourth ventricle lies in the middle of the posterior fossa (see Figs. 13-1 to 13-5 and 13-11). It connects rostrally with the third ventricle via the aqueduct of Sylvius. It connects caudally with the basal cisterns through three "exit foramina": a midline foramen of Magendie that leads into the cisterna magna and paired lateral foramina of Luschka that lead into the lateral medullary cisterns (low cerebellopontine angle cisterns).[13] The fourth ventricle is delimited anteriorly by the posterior surfaces of the pons and the upper medulla. Thus, the dorsal surface of the brain stem forms the floor of the fourth ventricle. This floor displays a median sulcus, paired paramedian sulci limitantes, transverse striae medullares, paired medial eminences and facial colliculi, and specific depressions (fovea) that mark out the positions of brain stem nuclei (see Chapter 15). The fourth ventricle is delimited anterosuperiorly by the superior vermis and superior (anterior) medullary velum. It is delimited posteroinferiorly by the inferior vermis and inferior (posterior) medullary velum. The fourth ventricle is delimited laterally by the superior and inferior cerebellar peduncles.

Three recesses of the fourth ventricle project into the cerebellum posterosuperiorly (see Figs. 13-1, 13-3C, and 13-11). In the midline, the fastigial recess lies just above the nodulus at the junction of the superior and inferior medullary vela. To each side of midline, and slightly farther caudally, paired posterior superior recesses lie just above the superior poles of the tonsils. Laterally, paired lateral recesses lead from the floor of the fourth ventricle around the brain stem to the cerebellomedullary (lateral medullary) cisterns, where they end as the foramina of Luschka. At the caudal end of the fourth ventricle the paired inferior cerebellar peduncles converge to create an inferior point (the obex) that leads into the central canal of the spinal cord.

Cava Septi Pellucidi et Vergae

Cavum Septi Pellucidi

The septum pellucidum is a thin, vertically oriented structure situated in the midline between the two frontal horns (Figs. 13-12 to 13-14A to C). It is composed of two juxtaposed leaves of tissue. Each leaf is made of an ependymal-lined lateral surface, a thin layer of white matter, a thin layer of gray matter, and a medial (inner) pial layer.[14] Developmentally, the two leaves arise separately and usually merge to form a 1- to 3-mm thick wall before 36 weeks of gestation.[14] On each side, separately, each septal leaf stretches from the undersurface of the corpus callosum to the upper surface of the ipsilateral anterior column of the fornix. Persistent separation of the two septal leaves creates a midline CSF-filled space designated the *cavum septi pellucidi*. The cavum is delimited anteriorly and superiorly by the corpus callosum, laterally by each septal leaf, and inferiorly by the rostrum of the corpus callosum and the anterior columns of the fornices. It contains no choroid plexus.

A cavum septi pellucidi is present in all premature infants/fetuses until 34 weeks' gestation and shows decreasing incidence thereafter. In 108 cranial sonograms of normal newborns, a cavum septi pellucidi was present in 100% of neonates aged 24 to 34 weeks' gestation, 69% at 36 weeks' gestation, 54% at 38 weeks' gestation, and 35% at 40 weeks' gestation.[15] The width, depth, and area of the cavum do not vary with gestational age.[15] In adults, a cavum septi pellucidi is found in 2.0% to 2.5%

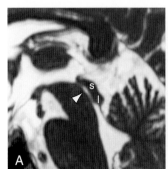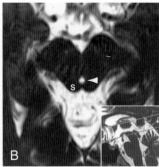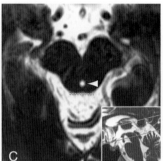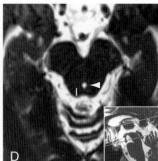

■ **FIGURE 13-10** Cerebral aqueduct. T2W FIESTA MR images in the midsagittal plane (**A**) and an oblique coronal plane (**B** to **D**) perpendicular to the PC-O (posterior commissure-obex) line. In sagittal section, the ventral contour of the aqueduct (*arrowheads*) is smoothly concave along its length from superior to inferior. Anatomically, the dorsal contour shows narrowings at the level of the superior (s) and inferior (i) colliculi with a central expansion at the intercollicular level (*dotted line*). On imaging studies, the apparent caliber of the aqueduct is also affected by CSF pulsations. (See also Fig. 13-11E.)

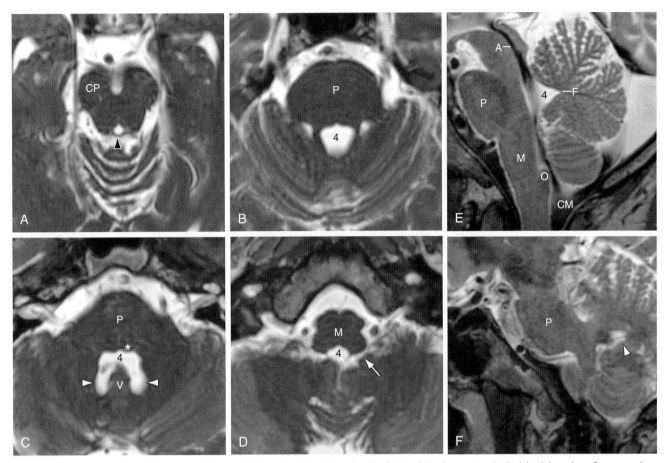

■ **FIGURE 13-11** Fourth ventricle. T2W MR images in the axial (**A** to **D**) and sagittal (**E** and **F**) planes. **A** to **D**, Serial axial sections from superior to inferior show the fourth ventricle (4) expanding from its pointed "aqueductal" contour (*black arrowhead* in **A**) to the full "temple bell" configuration at its height (in **C**) (compare with Fig. 13-3C). **E**, Midsagittal images show the fastigial recess (F) most clearly. The paired posterior superior recesses (*white arrowheads*) are better appreciated in axial (**C**) and parasagittal (**F**) images. The lateral recesses (*white arrow*) pass anterolaterally from the fourth ventricle to the cerebellomedullary (lateral medullary) cisterns. In **E**, low signal flow voids depict the contour of the aqueduct (A) and the preferential flow of CSF from the aqueduct along the floor of the fourth ventricle to the midline foramen of Magendie and the cisterna magna (CM). The dorsal half of the fourth ventricle normally shows little flow effect. Also labeled are the cerebral peduncle (CP), medulla (M), obex (O), pons (P), vermis (V), and facial colliculus (*asterisk* in **C**) at the floor of the fourth ventricle.

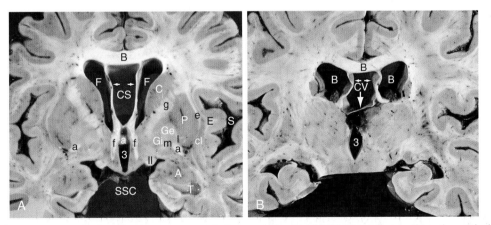

■ **FIGURE 13-12** Large cavum septi pellucidi and cavum vergae. **A,** Cavum septi pellucidi (CS). Coronal anatomic section at the level of the anterior body of the corpus callosum (B), two frontal horns (F), cavum septi pellucidi (CS), anterior columns of the fornices (f), anterior commissure (*white and black* a) and anterior third ventricle (3). The paired leaves of the septum pellucidum (*white arrows*) extend vertically from the undersurface of the corpus callosum (*black* B) to insert onto the ipsilateral fornix (f). The cavum septi pellucidi lies between the corpus callosum above, the two septal leaves laterally, and the fornices inferiorly. The septal veins course within the septal leaves. The suprasellar cistern (SSC) lies inferiorly, the sylvian fissure (S) laterally and the temporal horn (T) and amygdala (A) inferiorly. Also labeled, from lateral to medial, are the extreme capsule (E), claustrum (cl), external capsule (e), putamen (P), lateral medullary lamina of the lenticular nucleus (l), external nucleus of the globus pallidus (Ge), medial medullary lamina (m) of the lenticular nucleus, internal nucleus of the globus pallidus (Gi), the optic tract (II), the caudate nucleus (C), and the genu (g) of the internal capsule. **B,** Cavum vergae (CV). Coronal anatomic section at the level of the posterior body of the corpus callosum (*black* B), bodies of the lateral ventricles (*white* Bs) and third ventricle (3). The cavum vergae (CV) lies inferior to the body of the corpus callosum, between the paired fornices (*horizontal white arrows*), and superior to the inferiorly displaced commissure of the fornices (*vertical white arrow*).

■ **FIGURE 13-13** Small cavum septi pellucidi. Axial (**A**) and coronal (**B**) T2W MR images show a small triangular cavum septi pellucidi situated between the anterior aspects of the paired septal leaves (*white arrowheads*). The cavum septi pellucidi nestles within the curvature of the corpus callosum, delimited anteriorly by the genu (G), superiorly by the body (B), and inferiorly by the rostrum (r) of the corpus callosum.

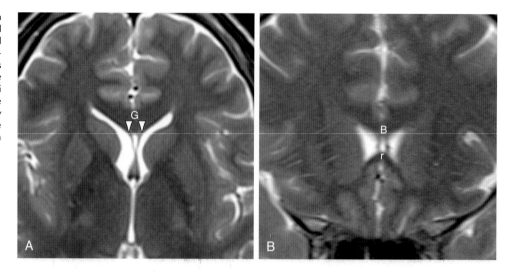

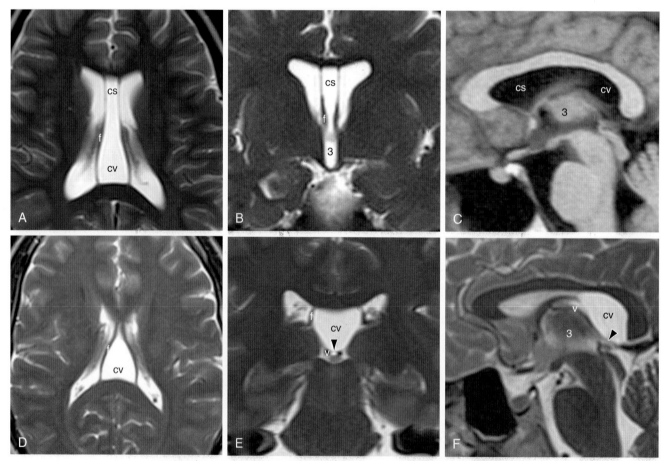

■ **FIGURE 13-14** Cavum septi pellucidi (cs) and cavum vergae (cv). MR images. **A** to **C**, Combined cs and cv. Axial (**A**) and coronal (**B**) T2W MR images and sagittal T1W image (**C**) display the large midline cs between the paired septal leaves and direct extension of that cavity between the two fornices (f), indicating concurrent cv. The undersurface of the posterior body of the corpus callosum is slightly elevated and shows an expanded curvature. The roof of the third ventricle (3) is normal. **D** to **F**, Isolated cavum vergae (cv). Axial (**D**), coronal (**E**), and sagittal (**F**) T2W MR images show expansion of the CSF space between the two fornices (f), increased signal intensity within this space, and similar elevation and fullness of the undersurface of the corpus callosum. In **E** and **F**, a thin layer (*arrowhead*) separates the cv above from the compressed cistern of the velum interpositum below. The paired internal cerebral veins (v) are displaced inferiorly with the velum interpositum.

of normal individuals. The incidence is reported to be higher in patients with mental retardation (15.3%), schizophrenia (23%), and trauma.[16-19]

Cavum Vergae

The paired fornices arch upward from each temporal lobe toward the midline, pass immediately anterior to the splenium and inferior to the body of the corpus callosum, and then arch downward behind the anterior commissure toward the mammillary bodies. Immediately below the posterior body of the corpus callosum, commissural fibers from each fornix cross to the other side, creating a thin flat sheet of commissural fibers designated the forniceal commissure (hippocampal commissure, psalterium). The upper surface of the forniceal commissure is closely applied to the undersurface of the corpus callosum but is not fused to it. Separation of the forniceal commissure from the undersurface of the corpus callosum creates a fluid space designated the cavum vergae (see Fig. 13-14). The cavum vergae is delimited superiorly by the undersurface of the corpus callosum, inferiorly by the upper surface of the forniceal commissure, and laterally by the paired alvei of the fornices. Expansion of the cavum displaces the hippocampal commissure inferiorly, thereby compressing the cistern of the velum interpositum and displacing the internal cerebral veins and posterior choroidal arteries inferiorly. The cavum vergae usually communicates anteriorly with a cavum septi pellucidi (see Fig. 13-14A to C) but may exist alone (see Fig. 13-14 D to F). It contains no choroid plexus.

Subarachnoid Cisterns

The subarachnoid space is the CSF-filled space situated between the outer arachnoid membrane (superficially) and the pia mater (deeply). The arteries, veins, and cranial nerves traverse these cisterns as they course between the skull and the brain.[20]

The subarachnoid fluid spaces form one confluent sea of fluid that extends over the complete surface of the brain (Figs. 13-15 to 13-17). For convenience, the spaces are classically divided into supratentorial (see Fig. 13-16) and infratentorial (see Fig. 13-17) compartments, with the understanding that these compartments interconnect with each other through the incisura. In both compartments, arachnoid septa and trabeculae partially subdivide the subarachnoid space into smaller, (in)constant compartments called *cisterns*.[20] These cisterns may be single midline spaces or paired bilateral spaces. The arachnoid

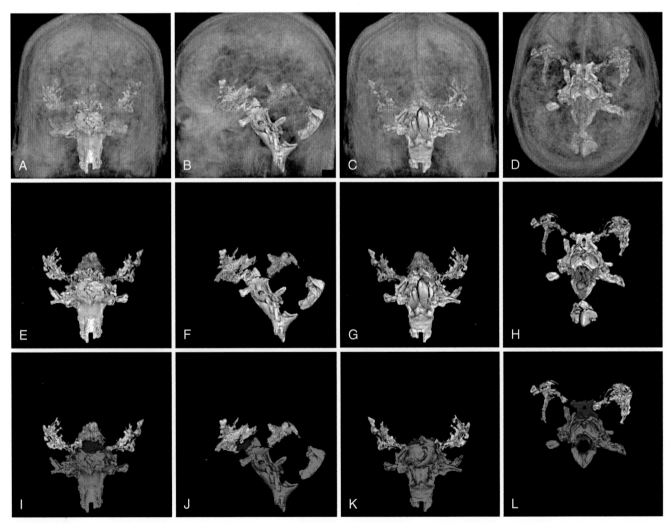

■ **FIGURE 13-15**   Overview of the subarachnoid cisterns. **A** to **D,** 3D reformatted MR images of the subarachnoid cisterns seen through a semitransparent scalp, skull, and brain. Anterior (**A**) lateral (**B**), posterior (**C**), and superior (**D**) views. **E** to **H,** Corresponding isolated subarachnoid cisterns oriented as **A** to **D. I** to **L,** Color coding of the cisterns displayed in **A** to **H**: *silver,* sylvian cisterns; *blue,* suprasellar cistern; *red,* the group of cisterns surrounding the brain stem; *green,* cisterna magna; and *gold,* superior vermian and quadrigeminal plate cisterns. In **K** and **L,** the cisterna magna (*green*) and superior vermian-quadrigeminal plate cisterns (*gold*) have been deleted to permit unobscured display of the other cisterns. Compare with the displays of the individual cisterns in Figures 13-16 and 13-17.

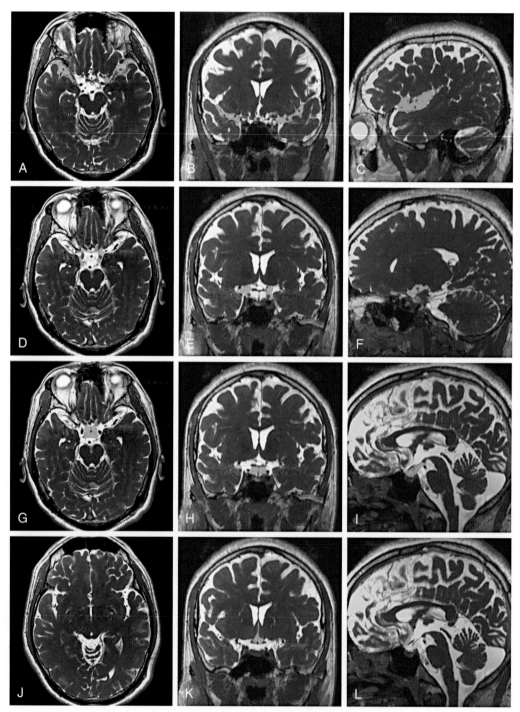

■ FIGURE 13-16 Supratentorial subarachnoid cisterns. FIESTA MR images color coded to provide a visual approximation to the borders of the individually named supratentorial cisterns. These images are arrayed so that each row depicts a single cistern in the axial plane (column 1), coronal plane (column 2), and sagittal plane (column 3). It must be understood that this montage is intended to indicate the general location for each cistern within the sea of multiple confluent CSF spaces around the brain. See text for more detailed information. **A** to **C,** Paired sylvian cisterns. **D** to **F,** Paired carotid cisterns. **G** to **I,** Midline chiasmatic cistern. **J** to **L,** Midline cistern of the lamina terminalis.

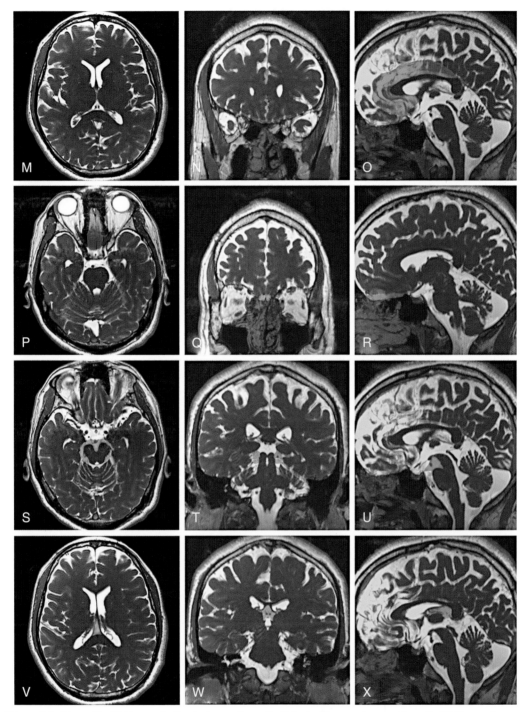

■ **FIGURE 13-16, cont'd** M to O, Midline pericallosal cistern. P to R, Paired olfactory cisterns, S to U, Midline perimesencephalic cistern. V to X, Cistern of the velum interpositum. The perimesencephalic cistern is often considered in four portions (S to U): midventral interpeduncular fossa (*red*), paired anterolateral crural cisterns (*green*), paired posterolateral ambient cisterns (*blue*), and middorsal quadrigeminal plate (vein of Galen) cistern (*yellow*).

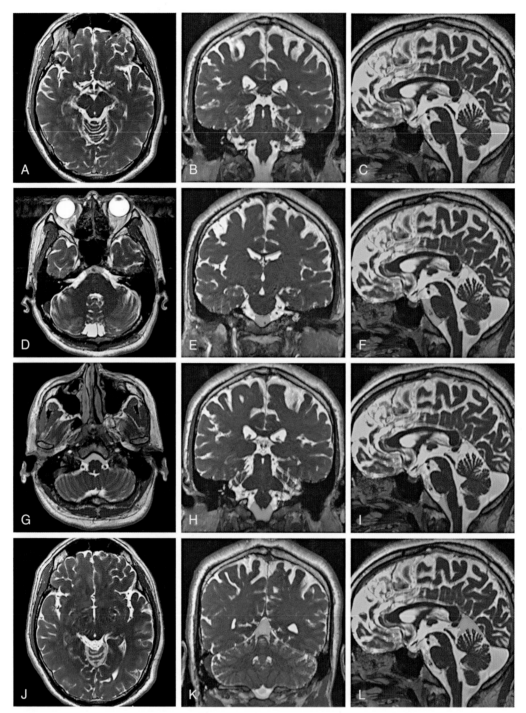

■ **FIGURE 13-17** Infratentorial subarachnoid cisterns. FIESTA MR images color coded to provide a visual approximation to the borders of the individually named infratentorial cisterns. These images are arrayed so that each row depicts a single cistern in axial plane (column 1), coronal plane (column 2), and sagittal plane (column 3) images. It must be understood that this montage is intended to indicate the general location for each cistern within the sea of multiple confluent CSF spaces around the brain. See text for more detailed information. **A to C,** Midline quadrigeminal plate (vein of Galen) cistern (*yellow*). **D to F,** Midline prepontine cistern. **G to I,** Midline premedullary cistern. **J to L,** Midline superior vermian cistern.

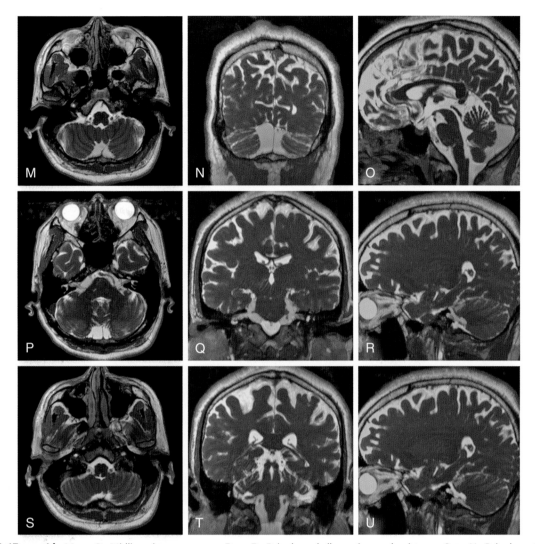

■ **FIGURE 13-17, cont'd** M to O, Midline cisterna magna. **P to R**, Paired cerebellopontine angle cisterns. **S to U**, Paired cerebellomedullary cisterns.

trabeculae that partition the cisterns have been given names to facilitate discussion. However, even the named supratentorial membranes are actually found at dissection in only 73% to 100% of hemispheres and are variably complete when found.[20] For these reasons, the "boundaries" given for specific cisterns, and any indications that specific membranes "separate" one cistern from another, must be understood as general concepts, not as documentation of constant watertight barriers between isolated spaces.

Further, over the years, the same cisterns have been renamed for each of the many adjacent structures that form its walls or lie within it. Therefore, different speakers may use different names for the same fluid space and the name used at any one moment may depend on which aspect of the cistern is considered to be most significant for that specific discussion. Thus, the same broad zone of CSF may be referred to as the subsplenial cistern, the vein of Galen cistern, the peripineal cistern, or the quadrigeminal plate cistern, depending on the focus of the discussant.

Supratentorial Cisterns
Paired Sylvian Cisterns (Fissures)
The sylvian cisterns have two compartments on each side, designated the anterior (horizontal) and posterior (vertical) compartments (see Fig. 13-16A to C).[21] The anterior compartment is

also known as the "sphenoidal compartment" because it borders the sphenoid ridge. The anterior compartment extends from the origin of the middle cerebral artery to the limen insulae. Its roof is formed by the orbital gyri of the frontal lobe and the anterior perforated substance. Its floor is the superior surface of the anterior temporal lobe (planum polare).[21] The thin proximal sylvian membrane separates the sylvian fissure laterally from the carotid cistern medially. The middle cerebral artery arises in the carotid cistern, penetrates the proximal sylvian membrane, and then courses laterally in the anterior compartment of the sylvian cistern. The lenticulostriate arteries originate from this portion of the middle cerebral artery. The distal portion of the recurrent artery of Heubner also traverses the anterior compartment. The posterior compartment extends from just beyond the limen insulae into the space between the insula and the overlying opercula and continues farther laterally between the opercula to reach the outer surface of the brain.[21] The M2 and M3 segments of the middle cerebral artery course through the posterior compartment to reach the lateral surface of the hemisphere. A lateral sylvian membrane extends vertically between the upper and lower opercula near the lateral edge of the sylvian fissure. The superficial sylvian veins pass along the posterior compartment superficial to the lateral sylvian membrane to reach the spheno-parietal sinus at the posterior inferior margin of the lesser wing of the sphenoid.[21]

Paired Carotid Cisterns

The carotid cisterns are found between the lateral edges of the optic chiasm medially and the medial surfaces of the unci laterally (see Fig. 13-16D to F).[21] The lateral walls of the carotid cisterns are the medial surfaces of the temporal lobes and the arachnoid overlying the anterior clinoid processes.[21] The medial walls are the paired medial carotid membranes that extend from the undersurface of the optic chiasm to the lateral surface of the sella on each side. The superior walls are the anterior perforated substance. The inferior walls are the arachnoid overlying the posterior clinoid process and the cavernous sinus. The carotid cisterns face the sylvian cisterns laterally, the chiasmatic cisterns medially, the interpeduncular cisterns posteromedially, the cistern of the lamina terminalis superomedially, and the crural cisterns posteriorly. In many cases, no membrane separates the carotid, interpeduncular, and crural cisterns, leading to a large confluent pool of CSF in this region.[21] On each side, the internal carotid arteries emerge from the cavernous sinus, penetrate the outer arachnoid membrane, and pass upward into the carotid cistern as the supraclinoid segments of the internal carotid arteries. The ophthalmic arteries arise from the initial intra-arachnoid segments of the internal carotid arteries. The anterior choroidal and posterior cerebral/posterior communicating arteries arise from the internal carotid arteries within the carotid cistern and pass posteriorly to enter the crural cistern. The anterior and middle cerebral arteries arise within the carotid cistern as the two terminal branches of the distal internal carotid artery (forming the carotid T). Dense trabeculae connect the internal carotid arteries and their branches to the inferior surface of the optic chiasm and tract.[21]

Midline Suprasellar (Suprachiasmatic) Cistern

The chiasmatic cistern surrounds the optic nerves and chiasm. It is bounded laterally by the medial carotid membrane, which separates the chiasmatic from the carotid cisterns; anteroinferiorly by the outer arachnoid membrane that overlies the tuberculum and diaphragma sellae; and posteriorly by the diencephalic leaf of the membrane of Liliequist. This leaf arises from the outer arachnoid overlying the posterior clinoid processes and dorsum sellae and arches upward between the oculomotor nerves to insert into the hypothalamus at the mammillary bodies.[21] The chiasmatic cistern faces the cistern of the lamina terminalis superomedially, the carotid cisterns laterally, and the interpeduncular cistern posteriorly (see Fig. 13-16G to I). It communicates anterolaterally with the subarachnoid spaces that surround the optic nerves in the optic canals. The chiasmatic cistern contains the optic nerves, optic chiasm, pituitary stalk, and branches of the internal carotid artery that penetrate the medial carotid membrane to supply these structures.[7,21]

Midline Cistern of the Lamina Terminalis

The cistern of the lamina terminalis lies immediately superior to the optic chiasm and directly anterior to the lamina terminalis (anterior wall) of the third ventricle (see Fig. 13-16J to L).[7,21] It is bordered anteriorly by the posterior ends of the gyri recti, the medial lamina terminalis membrane that stretches between the posteromedial ends of the gyri recti, and the paraterminal gyri. The cistern is bounded laterally by the paired lateral lamina terminalis membranes that stretch between the posterolateral edges of the gyri recti and the upper lateral edges of the optic chiasm. The cistern of the lamina terminalis borders onto the pericallosal cistern of the interhemispheric fissure anteriorly and superiorly, the chiasmatic cistern posteroinferiorly, the carotid cisterns laterally and the olfactory cisterns anterolaterally. It contains portions of both anterior cerebral arteries, including the distal A1 segments, the anterior communicating artery, and the proximal A2 segments.[21]

Midline Pericallosal Cistern

The pericallosal cistern is located in the interhemispheric fissure along the outer surface of the corpus callosum (see Fig. 13-16M to O). It may be considered to have three (inferior, anterior, and superior) components. The inferior compartment lies superior to the cistern of the lamina terminalis, inferior to the rostrum of the corpus callosum and medial to the apposing surfaces of the cerebral hemispheres. The anterior compartment lies anterior to the genu of the corpus callosum, so it is bordered anteriorly by the outer arachnoid membrane, posteriorly by the genu of the corpus callosum, and laterally by the cingulate gyri. The superior compartment lies external to the body of the corpus callosum and deep to the outer arachnoid membrane. It narrows posteriorly and ends along the superior surface of the splenium. The pericallosal cistern contains the paired anterior cerebral arteries and their branches. The inferior compartment contains the origins of the frontopolar branches of both anterior cerebral arteries. The anterior compartment contains the internal frontal branches of the anterior cerebral arteries. The superior compartment contains the paracentral artery and the superior and inferior internal parietal branches of the anterior cerebral arteries.[21]

Paired Olfactory Cisterns

The olfactory cisterns lie beneath and within the olfactory sulci between the gyri recti medially, the posterior orbital gyri laterally, and the outer arachnoid membrane inferior to the olfactory tracts. They border on the sylvian cisterns laterally, the carotid cisterns posteriorly, and the cistern of the lamina terminalis medially (see Fig. 13-16P to R). They contain the olfactory nerves and the orbitofrontal branches of the anterior cerebral arteries that enter the cistern from the lamina terminalis cistern.[21]

Midline Perimesencephalic (Circummesencephalic) Cistern

The perimesencephalic cistern surrounds the midbrain at the incisura (see Fig. 13-16S to U). The nomenclature related to this cistern is used differently by differing authors and therefore is particularly complex. In one terminology, the entire perimesencephalic cistern is designated the ambient cistern. More commonly, the perimesencephalic cistern is considered to have four confluent zones along the circumference of the midbrain, one of which is named the ambient cistern. The more precise terminology, from anterior to posterior, is used in the following paragraphs.

The midline interpeduncular cistern (interpeduncular fossa) lies between the two cerebral peduncles, bordered superiorly by the diencephalic leaf of the membrane of Liliequist and inferiorly by the mesencephalic leaf of this membrane.[21] The *diencephalic leaf* stretches from the posterior clinoid processes and dorsum sellae inferiorly to the mammillary bodies superiorly (see Figs. 13-6B and 13-7A). This leaf separates the chiasmatic cistern above from the interpeduncular cistern below. The *mesencephalic leaf* of the membrane of Liliequist stretches from the posterior clinoid processes and dorsum sellae anteriorly to the pontomesencephalic junction posteriorly and to the oculomotor nerves and adjacent arachnoid of the temporal and posterior fossae on each side.[21] This horizontal, crescentic membrane partially separates the interpeduncular cistern above from the prepontine cistern below.[21] The basilar artery ascends into the upper interpeduncular fossa behind the posterior free margin of the crescentic mesencephalic leaf (see also Figs. 14-5 and 14-6 in Chapter 14).[22] The interpeduncular cistern also contains the origins of the paired posterior cerebral arteries, the thalamoperforating arteries, the proximal portion of the anterior pontomesencephalic vein, and the proximal portions of the oculomotor nerves (CN III).

The paired crural cisterns lie between the posterior borders of the unci and the cerebral peduncles on each side. They are bordered superiorly by the optic tracts and inferiorly by the lateral pontomesencephalic membranes on each side. These membranes extend from the surface of the brain stem at the pontomesencephalic junction to the outer arachnoid near to the free edges of the tentorium.[21] The crural cisterns border on the carotid cisterns anteriorly, the interpeduncular cistern anteromedially, the ambient cisterns posteriorly, and the cerebellopontine angle cistern inferiorly.[21] The crural cisterns contain the anterior choroidal arteries, proximal (P1) segments of the posterior cerebral arteries, the proximal portion of the posterior medial choroidal arteries, portions of the basal veins of Rosenthal, and the trochlear nerves (CN IV).

The paired ambient cisterns lie between the parahippocampal and dentate gyri of the temporal lobes laterally and the lateral surface of the midbrain behind the cerebral peduncles medially.[21] The ambient cisterns border on the crural cisterns anteriorly, the quadrigeminal plate cistern posteriorly, and the cerebellopontine angle cisterns inferiorly. They are bordered by the optic tracts, lateral geniculate bodies, and pulvinars on each side. Like the crural cisterns, they are bordered inferiorly by the lateral pontomesencephalic membranes. The ambient cisterns contain the P2 segments of the posterior cerebral arteries and portions of the trochlear nerves.[21]

The midline quadrigeminal plate cistern (vein of Galen cistern, peripineal cistern) lies posterior to the pineal gland and midbrain, inferior to the splenium of the corpus callosum, and medial to the pulvinar of the thalamus and the adjacent medial occipital cortex on each side. The cistern merges into the ambient cisterns anteriorly, the pericallosal cistern superiorly, and the superior vermian cistern posteriorly. The quadrigeminal plate cistern contains the pineal gland, the P3 segments of the posterior cerebral arteries, portions of the medial and lateral posterior choroidal arteries, and the confluence of the basal veins of Rosenthal with the internal cerebral veins to form the vein of Galen. The tentorium crosses the plane of the midbrain, usually at the level of the intercollicular groove between the superior colliculi supratentorially and the inferior colliculi infratentorially. For that reason, the quadrigeminal plate cistern is often considered with both the supratentorial and the infratentorial cisterns, depending on the text and the medical needs of the analysis.

Cistern of the Velum Interpositum (Velum Transversum)
The velum interpositum is a horizontally oriented double fold of pia and arachnoid[23] that is interposed between the fornix superiorly and the roof of the third ventricle inferiorly (see Fig. 13-16V to X). The space between the upper and lower folds of the velum is the cistern of the velum interpositum. This cistern is delimited anteriorly by the foramen of Monro and laterally by the choroidal fissures of the lateral ventricles. Superiorly, it faces onto the undersurface of the fornices. Inferiorly, it faces onto the membranous roof of the third ventricle. Posteriorly, it opens into the quadrigeminal plate cistern. This cistern contains the paired internal cerebral veins that drain the deep brain, the paired medial posterior choroidal arteries that supply the choroid plexus of the third ventricle, and the paired posterior lateral choroidal arteries that supply the choroid plexus of the posterior portions of both lateral ventricles. Expansion of this space is designated a cavum veli interpositi.

Infratentorial Cisterns
Midline Quadrigeminal Plate Cistern
In addition to the features of this cistern discussed as part of the perimesencephalic cistern earlier, the paired trochlear nerves arise from the dorsal surface of the brain stem immediately inferior to the inferior colliculi and course around the midbrain through the infratentorial portion of the quadrigeminal plate cistern to reach the side walls of the cavernous sinuses (see

Fig. 13-17A to C). The distal portions of the superior cerebellar arteries, superior vermian veins, and precentral cerebellar vein also traverse this cistern.

Midline Prepontine Cistern
The prepontine cistern lies between the arachnoid mater overlying the upper clivus and the anterior surface of the pons (see Fig. 13-17D to F). It is separated from the interpeduncular cistern superior to it by the mesencephalic leaf of Liliequist's membrane. Its lower border is the pontomedullary sulcus, where thick arachnoid trabeculae about the vertebrobasilar arterial junction form a less well-defined medial pontomedullary membrane.[20] On each side, the lateral border of the prepontine cistern is the anterior pontine membrane that extends vertically from the third nerve above to the *medial aspect* of the sixth nerve below.[20] This membrane is better defined superiorly, attenuates caudally, and may be absent along the lower pons.[20] The prepontine cistern contains the basilar artery, the origins and proximal portions of the anterior inferior cerebellar arteries, the pontine portion of the anterior pontomesencephalic vein, and the proximal portions of the transverse pontine veins. Because the anterior pontine membranes lie along the medial aspects of the abducens nerves, the anterior pontine cistern contains no cranial nerves.[20]

Midline Premedullary Cistern
The premedullary cistern lies between the arachnoid mater overlying the lower clivus and the anterior surface of the medulla oblongata (see Fig. 13-17G to I). It is delimited laterally along the dorsal surface of the inferior olive, anterior to cranial nerves IX, X, and XI.[20] It is separated from the prepontine cistern above by the medial pontomedullary membrane. Inferiorly, the premedullary cistern is directly confluent with the anterior spinal subarachnoid space through the foramen magnum. The premedullary cistern contains the vertebral arteries, the anterior spinal arteries that arise from them, and the rootlets of CN XII.[20]

Midline Superior Vermian Cistern
The superior vermian cistern lies between the arachnoid mater immediately inferior to the midline tentorium and the superior surface of the vermis beneath it (see Fig. 13-17J to L). It is confluent with the quadrigeminal plate cistern rostrally and the paired superior cerebellar cisterns laterally. It is variably confluent with the upper portion of the inferior vermian cistern caudally. It contains the superior vermian arteries and veins.

Midline Cisterna Magna
The cisterna magna is the largest subarachnoid cistern, containing from 3 to 10 mL of CSF. It lies posterior to the medulla, the inferior vermis, and the adjacent medial portions of the cerebellar hemispheres (see Fig. 13-17M to O). It lies ventral to the occipital dura and any falx cerebelli present. The cisterna magna is enclosed within a triangular membrane that resembles a wind-filled spinnaker sail. It may be narrower or wider depending on the variable lateral attachments of that membrane to the cerebellum. Very wide attachments lead to a "mega cisterna magna." The cisterna magna is confluent inferiorly with the dorsal spinal subarachnoid space through the foramen magnum and confluent anteriorly with the cerebellomedullary and premedullary cisterns surrounding the medulla. Usually, the cisterna magna is isolated from the superior vermian cistern above and from the retrocerebellar cisterns lateral to it by tight adherence of the membrane to the cerebellum. When those attachments are incomplete, the cisterna magna may communicate with the superior vermian cistern above and/or the retrocerebellar cisterns laterally. The cisterna magna is partially subdivided by mesh-like arachnoid trabeculae that extend from the cerebellar tonsils to the medulla and the margin of the foramen of

Magendie.[20] It may be bisected into paired sagittal halves by a median sheet of arachnoid. The cisterna magna contains the medial branches of the posterior inferior cerebellar arteries, including the inferior vermian arteries and the inferior vermian veins.

Paired Cerebellopontine Angle (CP Angle) Cisterns

The CP angle cisterns lie between the arachnoid overlying the posterior surfaces of the petrous pyramids and the anterolateral surfaces of the pons and cerebellum (see Fig. 13-17P to R).[20] On each side, they extend from the level of the tentorium above to the level of the pontomedullary junction below and from the *medial border* of CN VI (abducens nerve) medially to the edge of the cerebellum that overhangs the pons (quadrangular lip) laterally.[20] Superiorly, the CP angle cisterns are separated from the ambient cisterns by the lateral pontomesencephalic membranes that extend across the cisterns between the posterior cerebral arteries above and the superior cerebellar arteries below. Inferiorly, the CP angle cisterns are separated from the cerebellomedullary (lateral medullary) cisterns by the lateral pontomedullary membranes that extend across the subarachnoid space between CNs VIII (vestibulocochlear nerves) above and CNs IX (glossopharyngeal nerves) below. Medially, the CP angle cisterns are separated from the prepontine cistern by the paired vertical anterior pontine membranes. Laterally, the CP angle cisterns extend into the internal auditory canals to enclose intracanalicular segments of CNs VII and VIII.[20] The CP angle cisterns contain the superior cerebellar arteries, the distal ends of the AICAs that extend toward the internal auditory canals, the petrosal veins, and CN V, VI, VII, and VIII (trigeminal, abducens, facial, and vestibulocochlear nerves).[20]

Paired Cerebellomedullary (Lateral Medullary) Cisterns

The cerebellomedullary cisterns lie along the lateral surfaces of the medulla oblongata, dorsal to the olives and inferior to the lower margins of the cerebellopontine cisterns (see Fig. 13-17S to U).[20] Laterally, they extend around the medulla to the biventral lobules of the cerebellum.[20] They are confluent with the cisterna magna posteriorly. They are partially separated from the cerebellopontine cisterns by incomplete lateral pontomedullary membranes. They are partially separated from the premedullary cistern by arachnoid trabeculae that lie anterior to CN IX, X, and XI (glossopharyngeal, vagus, and spinal accessory nerves). They contain the lateral recesses of the fourth ventricle, the tufts of choroid plexus that protrude through the recesses into the cisterns and CN IX, X, and XI.[20]

Cerebrospinal Fluid

CSF is a secretion of the choroid plexus admixed with interstitial fluid elaborated in the brain. It has a density of 1.003 to 1.008 g/cm[3].[24] Its composition is similar to that of brain interstitial fluid. As compared with plasma, CSF shows lower levels of sodium, potassium, calcium, and bicarbonate but higher levels of magnesium and chloride.[25]

In an adult, the total volume of CSF ranges from 150 to 270 mL—25% within the ventricles and 75% within the intracranial and spinal subarachnoid space.[26] In a child, the total CSF volume is proportionately smaller and varies with head size. The total daily production of CSF is approximately 600 mL, so the total CSF volume turns over approximately three to four times per day.[27] Classically it has been thought that 40% to 90% of total CSF was produced by the choroid plexi[25-27] and the rest by extrachoroidal mechanisms.[26] This CSF production shows circadian variation: minimum in the afternoon and peaking after midnight.[28]

The choroid plexi elaborate CSF at a rate of 0.35 to 0.4 mL/min.[1,25-27] This high rate of production is supported by a rich blood supply from the choroidal arteries, a large number of mitochondria in the epithelial cells to supply the adenosine triphosphate needed for CSF secretion, and a large surface area for exchange of fluid between the blood vessels at the base of the choroidal cells and the microvilli on their apical (ventricular) surface.[26,27,29] The blood supply to the choroid plexus is 3 mL/min per gram of choroid plexus, a rate higher than any other secretory epithelium[25-27] and four to seven times greater than the blood flow to the brain itself. Chapter 49 presents recent concepts of CSF production. In an adult in lateral recumbent position, CSF pressure is 100 to 200 mm H_2O.[27] Over broad ranges, the rate of CSF production appears to be independent of the intracranial pressure, so CSF production may continue despite rising intracranial pressure, until the intracranial pressure exceeds arterial perfusion pressure (brain death), at which point it stops. With age and disease, the rate of CSF formation can decrease by 50% or more.[27]

Choroid Plexi

The choroid plexi are paired paramedian structures with a total mass of approximately 2 g in the adult and a total surface area of approximately 200 cm[2].[24,26,29] Embryologically, the choroid plexus appears first in the fourth ventricle, then in the two lateral ventricles, and last in the third ventricle.[30,31] The aqueduct has no intrinsic choroid plexus. Anatomically, the choroid plexi are protrusions of capillaries into the lumina of the ventricles. These protrusions enter the ventricles via the choroidal fissures and expand within the ventricles to their full mushroom shapes. Their deep surfaces become covered by a simple cuboidal epithelium derived from the ependymal cells lining the ventricle. The choroid plexus of the lateral ventricles is relatively thin. The choroid plexus of the third ventricle has intermediate thickness, and the choroid plexus of the fourth ventricle is thick, highly lobulated, and more complex.[32]

Anatomy of the Plexi

Lateral Ventricles

The choroid plexi of the lateral ventricles are C shaped, extending backward from each foramen of Monro around the pulvinar of the thalamus into the temporal horns (Figs. 13-18 and 13-19). At the atria, the choroid plexi form distinct thickenings designated *glomera* (singular: *glomus*) of the choroid plexus. The glomera may appear as broad thickenings, sessile grape-like structures, or balls of choroid suspended on long vascular pedicles (Fig. 13-20). Pedunculated glomera may migrate from the posterior body of the ventricle to the atrium to the back of the occipital horn with changes in body position. No choroid plexus is found within the frontal horns or within the most anterior portion of the temporal horns. The choroid plexus of the lateral ventricles is supplied by the paired anterior choroidal arteries and paired posterior lateral choroidal arteries (Fig. 13-21).

Third Ventricle

The choroid plexi of the third ventricle are continuous with the choroid plexi of the lateral ventricles at the foramina of Monro (see Fig. 13-18A). They continue posteriorly along the roof to the back of the third ventricle (see Fig. 13-18B). The choroid plexus of the third ventricle is supplied by the paired posterior medial choroidal arteries.

Fourth Ventricle

On each side, the choroid plexus of the fourth ventricle overlies the superior pole of the tonsil and, from there, angles anteroinferolaterally to pass along the lateral recess, exit the ventricle through the foramen of Luschka into the cerebellomedullary cistern, and form a tuft of choroid plexus within the cistern. Portions of the choroid may also extend inferomedially into the foramen of Magendie and even protrude through it into the vallecula. The major upper portion of the choroid plexus of the

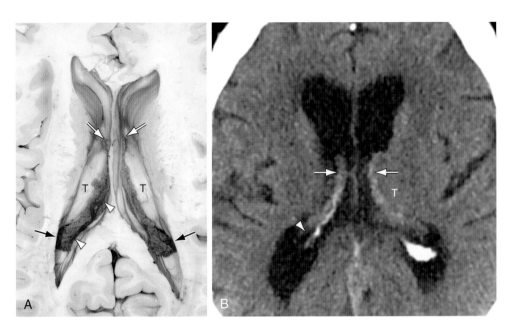

■ **FIGURE 13-18** Choroid plexus of the lateral ventricle and superior choroidal vein. **A,** Gross anatomic specimen. Axial section through the lateral ventricles shows the choroid plexus extending over the thalami (T) from the foramina of Monro (*white arrows*) to the atria of the ventricles (*black arrows*). The superior choroidal vein (*white arrowheads*) undulates over the superior surface of the choroid plexi on both sides but is better filled and more easily appreciated on the reader's left. **B,** Comparable, noncontrast axial CT scan shows the curved course of the calcified choroid plexus (*white arrows*) over the thalami (T) and the thinner more medial superior choroidal vein (*arrowhead*).

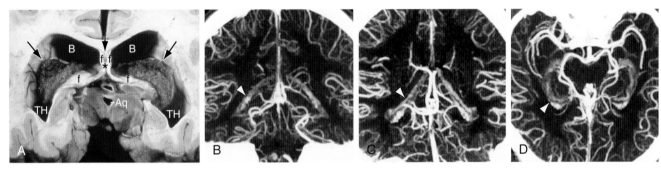

■ **FIGURE 13-19** Choroid plexus and choroidal blush. **A,** Coronal section through the atria of a hydrocephalic brain. Posterior view. On each side, the choroid plexus (*black arrows*) lies along the floor of the body (B) of the lateral ventricle at the lateral edge of the fornix (f) and curves behind the pulvinar of the thalamus (obscured by the plexus) into the temporal horn (TH). A small cavum vergae (*short black arrow*) is bordered by the corpus callosum above, the fornices (f) to each side, and the commissure of the fornices (*asterisk*) inferiorly. **B** to **D,** Reformatted maximum intensity projection (MIP) images from a contrast-enhanced CT angiogram presented as coronal (**B**), upper oblique axial (**C**) and lower oblique axial (**D**) sections. The choroidal blush (*white arrowheads*) and the prominent choroidal veins demonstrate the position and configuration of the choroid plexus within the ventricles.

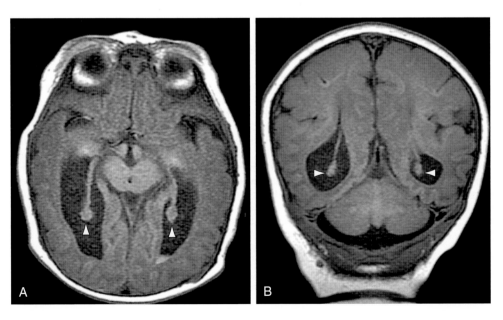

■ **FIGURE 13-20** Pedunculated choroid plexus. Axial (**A**) and coronal (**B**) T1W MR images of a child with callosal dysgenesis and mild intraventricular hemorrhage. The round glomera (*white arrowheads*) of the choroid plexus hang downward into the atria.

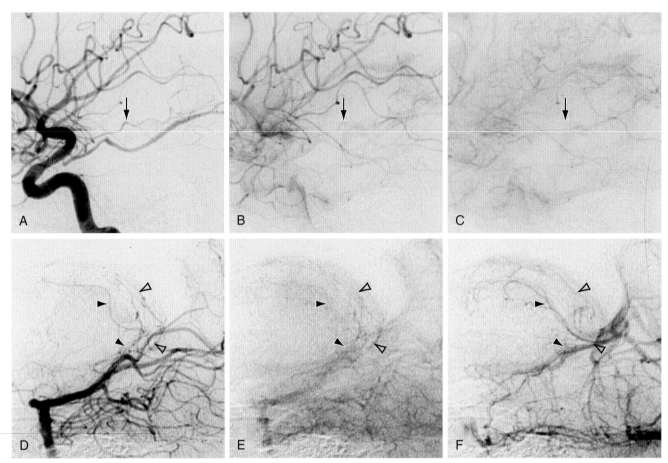

■ **FIGURE 13-21** Vascular supply of the choroid plexus. **A** to **C,** Lateral projection internal carotid angiogram. **A,** Arterial phase. The anterior choroidal artery (*arrow*) supplies the choroid plexus of the temporal horn and a variable portion of the glomus. **B** and **C,** Late arterial and early venous phases show early blush of the choroid plexus within the temporal horn and atrium. The position of the arrows is unchanged from that in **A. D** to **F,** Lateral projection vertebral arteriogram. **D,** Arterial phase. The posterior medial choroidal artery (*closed black arrowheads*) supplies the choroid plexus in the roof of the third ventricle as far forward as the foramen of Monro. It displays a characteristic "figure of 3" configuration. The posterior lateral choroidal artery (*open black arrowheads*) supplies the choroid plexus of the atrium and body of the lateral ventricle as far forward as the foramen of Monro. Because the choroid plexus encircles the thalamus, the posterior lateral choroidal artery displays a rounder configuration and normally lies posterior and superior to the posterior medial choroidal artery. **E** and **F,** Late arterial and early venous phases show the blush of the choroid plexus and the appearance of the choroidal veins. The position of the arrowheads is unchanged from that in **E.** The choroid plexus of the lateral ventricle is continuous with the choroid plexus of the third ventricle through the foramen of Monro.

fourth ventricle is supplied by choroidal branches of the posterior inferior cerebellar arteries.[33] The portions of the choroid plexus within the lateral recess and the cerebellomedullary cistern are supplied by choroidal branches of the anterior inferior cerebellar artery.[34]

Additional Functions of the Plexi

The choroid plexi have functions beyond secretion of CSF. Tight junctions between adjacent epithelial cells form a physical barrier between the blood and the CSF (the blood-CSF barrier). Transporters in the apical membrane of the choroid plexus epithelium actively remove organic anions and other toxins.[27] The choroid plexi secrete neuropeptides, growth factors, nutrients, and cytokines.[26] These include transthyretin, which binds beta amyloid peptide (Aβ) to prevent the toxicity that may occur if beta amyloid peptide (Aβ) forms oligomers.[27] The choroid plexi transport glucose, folate, and vitamins B_6, B_{12}, C, and probably E from the blood into the CSF.[25]

CSF Flow

CSF pulses to and fro. It washes into and out from the ventricular system with every cardiac cycle, like the tide at the mouth of a river (Figs. 13-22 and 13-23).[35-39] Over multiple cycles, there is net outward flow from the lateral ventricles through the foramina of Monro into the third ventricle, from the third ventricle through the aqueduct of Sylvius into the fourth ventricle, and from the fourth ventricle through the midline foramen of Magendie and the paired lateral foramina of Luschka into the cerebellomedullary (lateral medullary) cisterns and the cisterna magna at the skull base. From there, CSF circulates both downward through the foramen magnum into the spinal subarachnoid space surrounding the spinal cord and upward around the cerebellum and brain stem, through the incisura, and along the sylvian fissures, convexity cisterns, and interhemispheric fissure to reach the arachnoid granulations for resorption.[26] This directional flow is maintained by the beating of ependymal cilia that propel CSF forward, by systolic-diastolic variations in vascular pulsations transmitted to the CSF and the choroid plexi with each heart beat, and by a downhill pressure gradient between the subarachnoid space and the dural venous sinuses.[4]

CSF flow velocity is typically highest along the floor of the fourth ventricle, then through the aqueduct and the foramen of Monro (see Fig. 13-22).[24] Children show higher CSF peak velocities through the foramen magnum than do control adults aged 21 to 61 years.[37] From age 21 to 61 years the flow rate appears

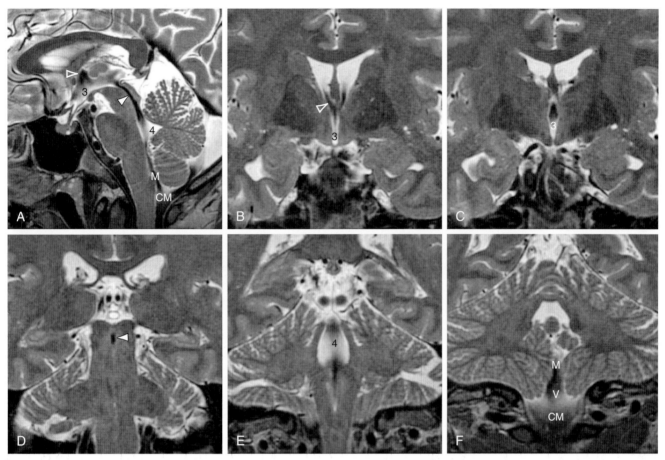

■ FIGURE 13-22 Normal CSF flow voids. Sagittal (**A**) and coronal (**B** to **F**) T2W MR images show the low signal flow voids where CSF jets through the foramen of Monro (*open white arrowhead*), within the third ventricle (3), along the aqueduct (*closed white arrowhead*) and the floor of the fourth ventricle (4), to pass outward through the foramen of Magendie (M) into the vallecula (V) and cisterna magna (CM).

relatively constant.[37] With circadian variation, the CSF flow is twice as great at night as during the day.[27,40]

The instantaneous direction of CSF flow—caudal or cranial—depends on the stage of the cardiac cycle, the distance of the specific CSF compartment from the heart, and respiration.[27] With cardiac systole, a pressure and volume pulse is ejected from the heart. It travels via the carotid and vertebral arteries to the skull base, enters the head, and ascends along the vascular trees into the higher and deeper portions of the brain. The pressure/volume pulse first expands the arteries in the subarachnoid cisterns. As it passes downstream into the arterioles and capillaries, the pulse then expands the choroid plexus and the brain itself.

Because the skull base is inclined, the posterior fossa lies slightly closer to the heart than does the supratentorial space. In health, the flow rate within the vertebral and carotid arteries is nearly equal, so the pulse of volume and pressure that passes through the vertebral arteries reaches the closer posterior fossa before the same pulse passes through the carotid arteries to reach the more distant supratentorial compartment. This difference in anatomic position creates a key, temporal offset between the earlier arrival time of the cardiac pulse to the nearer posterior fossa and the later arrival time of the cardiac pulse to the more distant supratentorial space. The same temporal offset is then maintained as the cardiac pulse passes distally. The pulse ascends the vertebrobasilar tree earlier than the carotid tree, reaches the choroid plexus of the fourth ventricle before the choroid plexi of the third and lateral ventricles, expands the cerebellum before expanding the cerebral hemispheres, and

then fades out within the posterior fossa before it fades out within the cerebrum as systole passes into diastole.

In adults with closed sutures and fixed intracranial volume, the incoming pulse of volume and pressure must be accommodated by corresponding egress of venous blood and CSF from the head (Monro-Kellie doctrine[27]). The instantaneous egress of venous blood and CSF damp the cardiac volume and pressure pulse. Because cardiac systole causes CSF to flow out of the head, the descending caudal flow of CSF from the head into the spinal canal is designated *CSF systole*. The opposite, ascending cranial flow of CSF into the head is designated *CSF diastole*.

The cyclic nature of CSF pulsations also depends on three other anatomic features: (1) The bony walls and tentorium give the posterior fossa the shape of a funnel with its spout directed toward the foramen magnum. This directs pulsations and motion toward the foramen magnum. (2) In the skull, the meningeal dura and the periosteal dura form a single layer abutting directly on the skull. There is no normal cranial epidural space. In the spine, however, the meningeal dura separates from the periosteal dura at the foramen magnum. The meningeal dura forms the thecal sac and is separated from the periosteal dura by the compressible epidural fat and epidural venous plexus. (3) The epidural venous plexus is directly continuous with the paraspinal veins via valveless radicular communications, creating Batson's plexus.

During the cardiac cycle, the cardiac pulse that enters the head causes CSF to move caudally through foramen magnum into the thecal sac. That distends the thecal sac, compresses the epidural fat and veins, and drives intraspinal blood into the

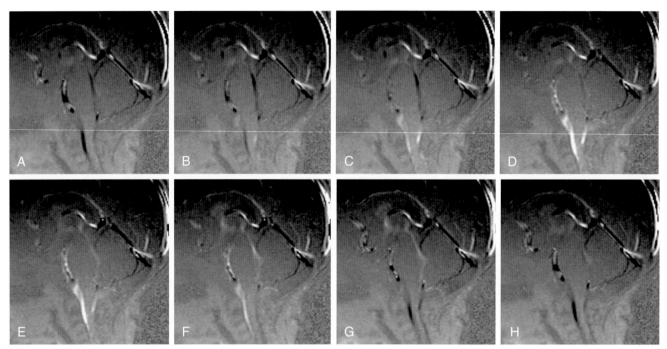

■ **FIGURE 13-23** Cardiac-gated phase contrast MRI sensitized to motion in the superoinferior directions with velocity encoding at 8.0 cm/s. The MR sequence partitions the flow data into 16 phases of the cardiac cycle and displays them in a pseudo-cine loop as if each phase were acquired sequentially. In this sequence, *white* signifies CSF systole, when CSF pulsations pass caudally toward the spinal canal in response the systolic expansion of intracranial blood volume and pressure. *Black* signifies CSF diastole, when CSF returns cranially in response to the waning of the systolic pressure-volume pulse. **A,** Analysis proceeds most easily from complete CSF diastole, when all CSF motion is directed cranially and all cisterns appear black. **B,** As CSF systole begins, CSF first moves caudally through foramen magnum posterior to the cord (CSF *white*), even as CSF still ascends (*black*) at other sites. **C,** Caudal motion of CSF through foramen magnum increases behind the cord and now begins anterior to the cord. **D,** Caudal motion of CSF through foramen magnum peaks behind and anterior to the cord just as the ascending cranial motion of CSF is diminishing or pausing in the aqueduct and fourth ventricle. **E,** Caudal motion of CSF through foramen magnum begins to diminish (*less white*). CSF now begins to move caudally through the aqueduct and fourth ventricle. The fraction of the cardiac cycle in which CSF moves caudally at all sites is designated complete CSF systole. **F,** CSF diastole begins as spinal recoil reverses CSF motion posterior to the cord. At this instant, the caudal motion of CSF continues anterior to the cord but is less forceful than in **E.** Caudal motion of CSF increases in the aqueduct and fourth ventricle. **G,** As CSF diastole progresses, cranial motion of CSF increases behind the cord and first appears anterior to the cord, even as CSF continues to move caudally through the aqueduct and fourth ventricle. **H,** CSF motion has decreased at all sites, with reduced ascent around the cord, reduced descent through the aqueduct and fourth ventricle, and the first faint appearance of ascending black CSF flow along the floor of the fourth ventricle. This instantly transitions directly into **A,** above, as the cycle continues. These stages may be summarized in the chant: "Down behind the cord. Down in front of the cord. Down through the aqueduct. Up behind the cord. Up in front of the cord. Up through the aqueduct," repeated for every cardiac cycle.

paraspinal veins. As the cardiac pulse passes, the intraspinal veins refill. The epidural fat re-expands, and the spinal theca becomes less distended. This "spinal recoil" causes the flow of CSF to reverse direction and ascend back into the posterior fossa.

Because of the temporal offset between the earlier peak of posterior fossa pressure and the later peak of supratentorial pressure, the ascending flow of spinal CSF into cisterna magna occurs just as the supratentorial space expands and pushes supratentorial CSF downward through the third ventricle, aqueduct, and fourth ventricle into cisterna magna. The ascending spinal flow and descending aqueductal-fourth ventricular flow converge at the cisterna magna. The large size of cisterna magna may reflect the need for a mixing chamber and relief valve to accommodate these convergent CSF flows.

Video 13-3 (available at www.expertconsult.com) shows the rhythmic flow of CSF as depicted in 16 partitions of the cardiac cycle, beginning at CSF diastole. Figure 13-23 illustrates half of these to show the temporal sequence of CSF pulsations.

CSF Clearance

Arachnoid *villi* are microscopic structures that may be found within the superior sagittal sinus of fetuses and newborns.[1] Arachnoid *granulations* (pacchionian granulations) are larger, more complex protrusions of the arachnoid membrane and subarachnoid space into the dural venous sinus, usually at points where the veins enter the sinuses.[1,41]

The relationship between the arachnoid granulations and CSF reabsorption is unclear. Not all arachnoid projections are associated with veins. Arachnoid granulations do not exist before birth. They only start to become visible in the dura at birth, then increase in number with age.[42] In animal models, a substantial portion of CSF is cleared via the olfactory and optic nerves, nasal submucosa, and cervical lymphatics.[24,27,43] In rodents and sheep, for example, the lymphatic pathway clears 40% to 50% of CSF.[43] Chapter 49 presents a discussion of recent concepts of CSF production and reabsorption.

Circumventricular Organs

The circumventricular organs are a set of chemosensory and neurosecretory structures situated at specific sites along the walls of the third and fourth ventricles to monitor the microenvironment at the blood-CSF interface. Histologically, they are characterized by (1) networks of fenestrated, leaky capillaries that form a partial, leaky blood-brain barrier and (2) a specialized layer of ependymal cells, the tanycytes, which form a partial, leaky CSF-brain barrier. The circumventricular organs related to the third ventricle include the subfornical organ, organum vasculosum of the lamina terminalis, the median eminence, the neurohypophysis, the pineal gland, and the subcommissural organ.[44] The subfornical organ lies along the anterior wall of the third ventricle between the two foramina of Monro. It is rich in receptors for the peptide hormone angiotensin II and has widespread connections to the hypothalamus. When hypovolemic thirst increases circulating levels of angiotensin II, neurons of the subforniceal organ stimulate responses that maintain blood pressure and replace fluid volume.[45] The organum vasculosum extends along the lamina terminalis from the anterior commissure superiorly down to anterior edge of the optic chiasm.[44] It is also rich in receptors for angiotensin II and appears to be especially sensitive to hyperosmolarity of the blood, another stimulus of thirst.[44,45] The neurohypophysis receives neurosecretory projections from the hypothalamus. Vasopressin from the supraoptic nucleus and oxytocin from the paraventricular nucleus are released into the capillary bed of the neurohypophysis from which they disperse to the general circulation.[1] The median eminence receives neurosecretory projections from the hypothalamus. Peptides released from these projecting axons control the hormonal secretions of the anterior pituitary gland via the hypothalamic-pituitary portal system.[1] The subcommissural organ covers the anterior and inferior surfaces of the posterior commissure just above the opening of the cerebral aqueduct.[44] Alone among the circumventricular organs, the subcommissural organ lacks fenestrated capillaries and is impermeable to the bloodstream.

The circumventricular organ of the fourth ventricle is the area postrema, a bilateral, paired organ situated along the floor of the fourth ventricle just rostral to the obex.[44] The area postrema is known to induce nausea and vomiting in response to emetics circulating in the blood.[45] It may also serve as a chemoreceptive trigger zone for regulating water and energy balance and cardiovascular function.[45] Recent data suggest that the circumventricular organs express specific filament proteins (nestin, vimentin, GFAP) and transcription factors (Sox2) that mark out progenitor cell pathways, suggesting a possible stem cell role for the circumventricular organs.[46,47]

IMAGING

The sizes, positions, and configurations of the ventricles and cisterns are displayed well by CT and MRI (see Figs. 13-1 and 13-15 to 13-17). CSF appears uniformly dense on CT scans, of uniformly high signal on T2-weighted (T2W) MR images, and of uniformly low signal on T1-weighted (T1W) and fluid-suppressed inversion recovery (FLAIR) T2W MR images (away from areas of flow void). On sectional images, the configurations of the CSF spaces vary with the planes of section (see Figs. 13-4 and 13-5). On 3D-reformatted images, the full contours of the spaces may be displayed from any vantage point and rotated through multiple axes to depict any particular point of anatomy (see Videos 13-1 and 13-2). With appropriate software, the CSF volume may also be determined and even parcellated into ventricular and cisternal contributions.[48-52]

Calcifications and Cysts of the Choroid Plexus
Calcifications
Normal, physiologic calcifications of the choroid plexi have been found in approximately 51% of 1000 CT brain scans (see Fig. 13-18B).[53] Their incidence and extent increase with age from 0.5% in the first decade to 86% in the eighth decade. In 2877 CT scans of the brain, specific analysis of calcifications of the glomus of the choroid plexus showed no calcifications in children younger than the age of 9 years, an increasing incidence of calcification from 10 to 39 years of age, a subsequent decrease in incidence, and a terminal peak after age 80 years (Table 13-1). A special form of ring-like calcifications of the glomus, designated "string of pearls," correlates with mucoid degeneration of the glomus (Fig. 13-24). Myxoid cysts arise when choroid epithelium degenerates or desquamates, leading to lipid accumulation within vacuoles.[54]

Cysts
Choroid plexus cysts are non-neoplastic, epithelial-lined structures most often found incidentally in fetuses, neonates, and

TABLE 13-1. Frequency of Calcification of the Glomus of the Choroid Plexus by Age in 2877 CT Scans of the Brain

Age Range	Frequency of Calcification
0-9 yr	None
10-14 yr	5.9%
15-19 yr	17.4%
30-39 yr	51.5%
All patients > 20 yr	64.7%
All patients > 50 yr	70.7%
All patients > 79 yr	74.4%

From Kwak R, Takeuchi F, Yamamoto N, et al. [Intracranial physiological calcification on computed tomography: II. Calcification in the choroid plexus of the lateral ventricles]. No To Shinkei 1988; 40:707-711. In Japanese.

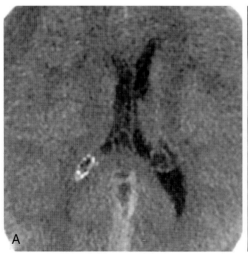
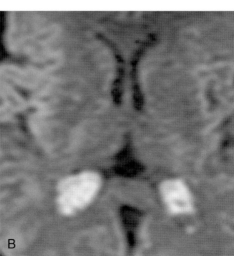

■ **FIGURE 13-24** Myxoid degeneration of the glomera of the choroid plexus. **A**, On axial noncontrast CT sections myxoid degeneration appears as a ring of small calcifications designated the "string of pearls." **B**, On axial diffusion-weighted MR images, the same degeneration appears as regions of very high signal within the choroid plexi.

■ **FIGURE 13-25** Choroidal cysts. Axial T2W MR image (**A**) and contrast-enhanced axial T1W MR image (**B**) show prominent bilateral choroid plexus cysts (*arrows*) that expand the posterior bodies and atria of both lateral ventricles, displacing the choroidal veins.

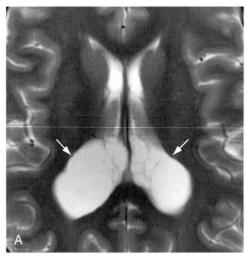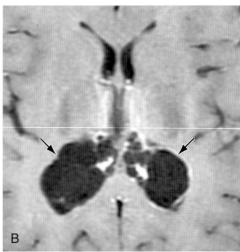

older adults. They have been detected by obstetric ultrasound as early as 18 to 20 weeks of gestation in 0.7% to 2.3% of fetuses.[55,56] They tend to be smaller in normal fetuses and larger in fetuses with abnormal karyotypes (4.5 vs. 7.3 mm).[56] There is a definite correlation of choroidal cysts with hypoplastic left heart syndrome.[57]

In adults, cysts of the choroid plexus are found in up to 50% of autopsy cases and are the most common of all intracranial cysts (Fig. 13-25).[54] Most are bilateral and located in the glomera of the choroid plexi at the atria. They appear as nodular, yellowish gray masses within the glomus. Most measure from 2 to 8 mm in diameter; cysts greater than 2 cm are rare.[54] (See also the sample report in Box 13-1.)

Compartment Formation

On CT, the uniformly low density of normal CSF reflects its low protein concentration. With stagnation of flow, as in a cyst or an obstructed ventricle, the protein concentration of the fluid often increases, causing the space to appear brighter than normal CSF. Such differential density may permit CT detection of non-communicating spaces adjoining the CSF pathways.

On MR images, the same increase in protein concentration causes isolated compartments to show higher signal intensity on both T1W and T2W images. In MRI, however, the signal returned from CSF also varies with CSF motion. Normally moving CSF shows signal dispersion and returns only partial CSF signal. Stagnant, nonpulsatile fluid returns a full MR signal, so it appears brighter than "normal" CSF on T2W images (see Fig. 13-6B).

CSF Flow Patterns and Velocities

CSF flow causes loss of signal intensity that manifests as variably prominent flow voids (see Fig. 13-22). In phase-contrast MRI, gradations in the flow rate help to assess the rhythmic motion of CSF with each cardiac cycle (see Fig. 13-23). CSF flow can also be assessed as the "stroke volume" of CSF associated with each cardiac cycle. CSF stroke volumes can be quantified at the aqueduct of Sylvius[35,36] and at the foramen magnum.[37,39] Hyperdynamic CSF flow may be associated with disease states such as normal pressure hydrocephalus.[36,58] Peak CSF flow velocity through the aqueduct has been measured as 3.8 to 24.7 mm/s in normal individuals but 6.6 to 65.7 mm/s in patients with NPH.[58] Defining aqueductal CSF stroke volume as the average volume of CSF moving caudally during systole and cranially during diastole, it is proposed that aqueductal stroke volumes greater than 42 mm³ suggest that NPH patients will benefit from shunting (positive predictive value: 100%), whereas volumes less than 42 mm³ suggest that they will have less benefit from the procedure (negative predictive value: 50%).[36]

BOX 13-1   Sample Report: MRI of Transincisural Mass

PATIENT HISTORY

A 57-year-old man presented with occipital headache of 4 years' duration. He had known sensorineural hearing loss with negative prior imaging 8 years previously.

COMPARISON STUDY

Noncontrast MRI was performed 8 years previously.

TECHNIQUE

MRI of the brain was performed as a multiplanar multi-sequence study including noncontrast sagittal, axial, and coronal T1W and T2W series (Fig. 13-26), gradient-recalled-echo susceptibility series, and axial diffusion-weighted series with apparent diffusion coefficient (ADC) map. Additional contrast-enhanced T1W series were then obtained in axial, sagittal, and coronal planes.

CONTRAST AGENT

Gadolinium-chelate was administered intravenously in a dose of 1 mMol per kilogram of body weight.

FINDINGS

Since the prior study eight years earlier there is interval appearance of a lobulated, transincisural CSF-intensity mass that expands the left cerebellopontine cistern, expands the left crural cistern, and encroaches on the interpeduncular cistern, chiasmatic cistern, and left carotid cistern. The mass deviates the left trigeminal nerve and left free margin of the tentorium laterally. It invaginates into the anterolateral left pons, deviates the left cerebral peduncle posteriorly, and invaginates into the medial aspect of the left uncus and hippocampus.

The walls of the lesion are thin, smooth, and devoid of nodules. There is homogeneously increased signal intensity that is greater than the surrounding cisternal CSF. There is no evidence of hypervascularity, hemorrhage, fluid level within the lesion, or edema within the displaced brain tissue. There is no restriction of diffusion on diffusion-weighted images or ADC maps, and no contrast enhancement after gadolinium administration.

IMPRESSION

There is an interval appearance of a left-sided transincisural mass. The imaging characteristics strongly suggest a diagnosis of arachnoid cyst.

Special Procedures

Gadolinium ventriculography and cisternography are analogous to CT ventriculography and cisternography but use injection of dilute gadolinium-chelate into the ventricles and cisterns to assess patency of CSF communication and to detect pathologic processes within the CSF flowways.[59-61]

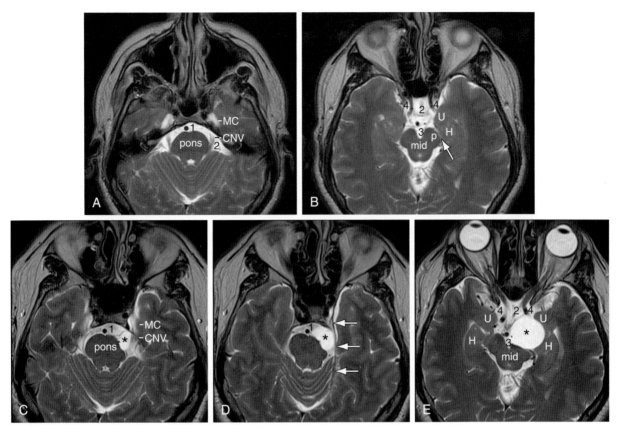

■ **FIGURE 13-26** Arachnoid cyst developing within the left crural cistern. **A** and **B,** Axial spin-echo T2W MR images obtained 8 years earlier are normal. The pons (pons) and midbrain (mid) show normal contours. The basilar artery traverses the prepontine cistern (1). The trigeminal nerve (CNV) traverses the upper pontocerebellar cistern (2 in **A**) en route to Meckel's cave (MC). The cerebral peduncle (p) abuts the posterior face of the uncus (U) and the hippocampus (H) across the crural cistern (*white arrow*). The chiasmatic cistern (2 in **B**) and carotid cisterns (4) are normal. **C** to **E,** Axial propeller fast spin-echo T2W MR images. A well-circumscribed, broadly lobulated mass (*asterisk*) expands within the left cerebellomedullary and crural cisterns and bulges through the incisura to encroach on the interpeduncular (3) and left carotid cisterns (4). It invaginates the anterolateral surfaces of the pons (pons) and midbrain (mid), deviates the trigeminal nerve (CNV), and the free margin of the tentorium (*white arrows*) laterally, and invaginates the medial surface of the uncus (U) and hippocampus (H). The lesion is homogeneously hyperintense with greater signal intensity than the surrounding cisternal CSF. The lesion had low signal intensity on diffusion-weighted images (not shown). Final pathological diagnosis was arachnoid cyst.

KEY POINTS

■ The brain contains four ventricles: two lateral ventricles, a midline third ventricle, and a midline fourth ventricle. The cavum septi pellucidi and cavum vergae are sometimes designated the fifth and sixth ventricles, respectively.

■ The lateral ventricles exhibit paired frontal horns, bodies, atria, occipital horns, and temporal horns. All but the occipital horns are nearly symmetric. The occipital horns may be markedly asymmetric in normal individuals.

■ The third ventricle exhibits anterior recesses that project anterior to (supraoptic) and behind (infundibular) the optic chiasm and posterior recesses that project posteriorly above (suprapineal) and into (pineal) the pineal gland.

■ The fourth ventricle exhibits two lateral recesses that lead to the foramina of Luschka and three posterior recesses: one midline fastigial recess superior to the nodulus and paired paramedian posterior superior recesses above the tonsils.

■ The cavum septi pellucidi lies within the curvature of the anterior corpus callosum between the separated leaves of the septum pellucidum. It is found in 2.0% to 2.5% of normal adults.

■ The cavum vergae lies inferior to the corpus callosum, between the left and the right fornix, and superior to the hippocampal commissure. The cavum veli interpositi lies between the fornices above and the roof of the third ventricle below.

■ In an adult, the total CSF volume is 150 to 250 mL: 25% within the ventricles and 75% within the intracranial and intraspinal subarachnoid space. Intraventricular volumes are estimated at 28 mL within the lateral ventricles and 1.0 to 1.5 mL in the third ventricle, aqueduct, and fourth ventricle, combined.

■ The subarachnoid cisterns are all confluent with each other but are partially subdivided by local condensations of the arachnoid designated membranes. Those membranes that are found more commonly are given specific names, for example, membrane of Liliequist (see Fig. 13-6B).

■ The choroid plexi are bilaterally symmetric structures in each of the ventricles. There is no choroid plexus present in the frontal horns or the anterior tips of the temporal horns. The occipital horns have no intrinsic choroid plexus but harbor the dependent ends of pedunculated glomera.

■ CSF flow is "tidal." Over multiple cardiac cycles, net CSF flow passes from the lateral ventricles via the foramina of Monro into the third ventricle, then from the third ventricle via the aqueduct to the fourth ventricle, and then from the fourth ventricle via the foramina of Luschka and Magendie into the cisterna magna and other subarachnoid cisterns.

■ The direction of instantaneous CSF flow varies with the cardiac cycle and follows a rhythmic pattern, passing caudally as CSF systole and cranially as CSF diastole.

SUGGESTED READINGS

Inoue K, Seker A, Osawa S, et al. Microsurgical and endoscopic anatomy of the supratentorial arachnoidal membranes and cisterns. Neurosurgery 2009; 65:644-664; discussion 665.

Rhoton AL Jr. The posterior fossa cisterns. Neurosurgery 2000; 47(3 Suppl):S287-S297.

Standring S (ed). Gray's Anatomy: The Anatomical Basis of Clinical Practice, 40th ed. Philadelphia, Elsevier, 2008.

REFERENCES

1. Standring S (ed). Gray's Anatomy: The Anatomical Basis of Clinical Practice, 40th ed. Philadelphia, Elsevier, 2008.
2. Allen JS, Damasio H, Grabowski TJ. Normal neuroanatomical variation in the human brain: an MRI-volumetric study. Am J Phys Anthropol 2002; 118:341.
3. Giesel FL, Hahn HK, Thomann PA, et al. Temporal horn index and volume of medial temporal lobe atrophy using a new semiautomated method for rapid and precise assessment. AJNR Am J Neuroradiol 2006; 27:1454.
4. Naidich TP, Altman NR, Gonzalez-Arias SM. Phase contrast cine magnetic resonance imaging: normal cerebrospinal fluid oscillation and applications to hydrocephalus. Neurosurg Clin North Am 1993; 4:677.
5. Zhu DC, Xenos M, Linninger AA, et al. Dynamics of lateral ventricle and cerebrospinal fluid in normal and hydrocephalic brains. J Magn Reson Imaging 2006; 24:756.
6. Kiroglu Y, Karabulut N, Oncel C, et al. Cerebral lateral ventricular asymmetry on CT: how much asymmetry is representing pathology? Surg Radiol Anat 2008; 30:249.
7. Newton TH, Potts DG. Radiology of the Skull and Brain. St. Louis, Mosby, 1978.
8. Rohde V, Gilsbach JM. Anomalies and variants of the endoscopic anatomy for third ventriculostomy. Minim Invasive Neurosurg 2000; 43:111.
9. Krokfors G, Katila O, Taalas J. Enlarged suprapineal recess of the third ventricle. Acta Neurol Scand 1967; 43:607.
10. Corrales M, Torrealba G. The third ventricle: normal anatomy and changes in some pathological conditions. Neuroradiology 1976; 11:271.
11. Andy OJ, Browne JS. Suprapineal recess. Surg Forum 1957; 7:544.
12. Longatti P, Fiorindi A, Perin A, et al. Endoscopic anatomy of the cerebral aqueduct. Neurosurgery 2007; 61:1.
13. Rhoton AL Jr. Cerebellum and fourth ventricle. Neurosurgery 2000; 47:S7.
14. Griffiths PD, Batty R, Reeves MJ, et al. Imaging the corpus callosum, septum pellucidum and fornix in children: normal anatomy and variations of normality. Neuroradiology 2009; 51:337.
15. Mott SH, Bodensteiner JB, Allan WC. The cavum septi pellucidi in term and preterm newborn infants. J Child Neurol 1992; 7:35.
16. Bodensteiner JB, Schaefer GB, Craft JM. Cavum septi pellucidi and cavum vergae in normal and developmentally delayed populations. J Child Neurol 1998; 13:120.
17. Degreef G, Lantos G, Bogerts B, et al. Abnormalities of the septum pellucidum on MR scans in first-episode schizophrenic patients. AJNR Am J Neuroradiol 1992; 13:835.
18. Greitz D, Greitz T, Hindmarsh T. A new view on the CSF-circulation with the potential for pharmacological treatment of childhood hydrocephalus. Acta Paediatr 1997; 86:125.
19. Schwidde JT. Incidence of cavum septi pellucidi and cavum vergae in 1,032 human brains. AMA Arch Neurol Psychiatry 1952; 67:625.
20. Rhoton AL Jr: The posterior fossa cisterns. Neurosurgery 2000; 47:S287.
21. Inoue K, Seker A, Osawa S, et al: Microsurgical and endoscopic anatomy of the supratentorial arachnoidal membranes and cisterns. Neurosurgery 2009; 65:644.
22. Froelich SC, Abdel Aziz KM, Cohen PD, et al. Microsurgical and endoscopic anatomy of Liliequist's membrane: a complex and variable structure of the basal cisterns. Neurosurgery 2008; 63:ONS1.
23. Tubbs RS, Louis RG Jr, Wartmann CT, et al. The velum interpositum revisited and redefined. Surg Radiol Anat 2008; 30:131.

24. Brodbelt A, Stoodley M: CSF pathways: a review. Br J Neurosurg 2007; 21:510.
25. Serot JM, Bene MC, Faure GC: Choroid plexus, aging of the brain, and Alzheimer's disease. Front Biosci 2003; 8:s515.
26. Redzic ZB, Segal MB. The structure of the choroid plexus and the physiology of the choroid plexus epithelium. Adv Drug Deliv Rev 2004; 56:1695.
27. Johanson CE, Duncan JA 3rd, Klinge PM, et al. Multiplicity of cerebrospinal fluid functions: new challenges in health and disease. Cerebrospinal Fluid Res 2008; 5:10.
28. Nilsson C, Stahlberg F, Thomsen C, et al. Circadian variation in human cerebrospinal fluid production measured by magnetic resonance imaging. Am J Physiol 1992; 262:R20.
29. Praetorius J. Water and solute secretion by the choroid plexus. Pflugers Arch 2007; 454:1.
30. Dziegielewska KM, Ek J, Habgood MD, et al. Development of the choroid plexus. Microsc Res Tech 2001; 52:5.
31. Redzic ZB, Preston JE, Duncan JA, et al. The choroid plexus–cerebrospinal fluid system: from development to aging. Curr Top Dev Biol 2005; 71:1.
32. Strazielle N, Ghersi-Egea JF. Choroid plexus in the central nervous system: biology and physiopathology. J Neuropathol Exp Neurol 2000; 59:561.
33. Kumar AJ, Naidich TP, George AE, et al. The choroidal artery to the fourth ventricle and its radiological significance. Radiology 1978; 126:431.
34. Naidich TP, Kricheff II, George AE, et al. The normal anterior inferior cerebellar artery: anatomic-radiographic correlation with emphasis on the lateral projection. Radiology 1976; 119:355.
35. Bradley WG Jr. Diagnostic tools in hydrocephalus. Neurosurg Clin North Am 2001; 12:661.
36. Bradley WG Jr, Scalzo D, Queralt J, et al. Normal-pressure hydrocephalus: evaluation with cerebrospinal fluid flow measurements at MR imaging. Radiology 1996; 198:523.
37. Iskandar BJ, Haughton V. Age-related variations in peak cerebrospinal fluid velocities in the foramen magnum. J Neurosurg 2005; 103:508.
38. Quencer RM, Post MJ, Hinks RS. Cine MR in the evaluation of normal and abnormal CSF flow: intracranial and intraspinal studies. Neuroradiology 1990; 32:371.
39. Quigley MF, Iskandar B, Quigley ME, et al. Cerebrospinal fluid flow in foramen magnum: temporal and spatial patterns at MR imaging in volunteers and in patients with Chiari I malformation. Radiology 2004; 232:229.
40. Nilsson C, Stahlberg F, Gideon P, et al. The nocturnal increase in human cerebrospinal fluid production is inhibited by a beta 1-receptor antagonist. Am J Physiol 1994; 267:R1445.
41. Grzybowski DM, Herderick EE, Kapoor KG, et al. Human arachnoid granulations: I. A technique for quantifying area and distribution on the superior surface of the cerebral cortex. Cerebrospinal Fluid Res 2007; 4:6.
42. Johnston M, Papaiconomou C. Cerebrospinal fluid transport: a lymphatic perspective. News Physiol Sci 2002; 17:227.
43. Kapoor KG, Katz SE, Grzybowski DM, et al. Cerebrospinal fluid outflow: an evolving perspective. Brain Res Bull 2008; 77:327.
44. Duvernoy HM, Risold PY. The circumventricular organs: an atlas of comparative anatomy and vascularization. Brain Res Rev 2007; 56:119.
45. Nieuwenhuys R, Voogd J, Huijzen C. The Human Central Nervous System, 4th ed. New York, Springer, 2008.

46. Bennett L, Yang M, Enikolopov G, et al. Circumventricular organs: a novel site of neural stem cells in the adult brain. Mol Cell Neurosci 2009; 41:337.
47. Johansson CB, Momma S, Clarke DL, et al. Identification of a neural stem cell in the adult mammalian central nervous system. Cell 1999; 96:25.
48. Harris GJ, Rhew EH, Noga T, et al. User-friendly method for rapid brain and CSF volume calculation using transaxial MRI images. Psychiatry Res 1991; 40:61.
49. Pitiot A, Delingette H, Thompson PM, et al. Expert knowledge-guided segmentation system for brain MRI. NeuroImage 2004; 23(Suppl 1):S85.
50. Jernigan TL, Zatz LM, Moses JA Jr, et al. Computed tomography in schizophrenics and normal volunteers: I. Fluid volume. Arch Gen Psychiatry 1982; 39:765.
51. Shenton ME, Kikinis R, McCarley RW, et al. Application of automated MRI volumetric measurement techniques to the ventricular system in schizophrenics and normal controls. Schizophr Res 1991; 5:103.
52. Barra V, Frenoux E, Boire JY. Automatic volumetric measurement of lateral ventricles on magnetic resonance images with correction of partial volume effects. J Magn Reson Imaging 2002; 15:16.
53. Modic MT, Weinstein MA, Rothner AD, et al. Calcification of the choroid plexus visualized by computed tomography. Radiology 1980; 135:369.
54. Osborn AG, Preece MT. Intracranial cysts: radiologic-pathologic correlation and imaging approach. Radiology 2006; 239:650.
55. Furness ME. Reporting obstetric ultrasound. Lancet 1987; 1:675.
56. Perpignano MC, Cohen HL, Klein VR, et al. Fetal choroid plexus cysts: beware the smaller cyst. Radiology 1992; 182:715.
57. Glauser TA, Rorke LB, Weinberg PM, et al. Congenital brain anomalies associated with the hypoplastic left heart syndrome. Pediatrics 1990; 85:984.
58. Sharma AK, Gaikwad S, Gupta V, et al. Measurement of peak CSF flow velocity at cerebral aqueduct, before and after lumbar CSF drainage, by use of phase-contrast MRI: utility in the management of idiopathic normal pressure hydrocephalus. Clin Neurol Neurosurg 2008; 110:363.
59. Munoz A, Hinojosa J, Esparza J. Cisternography and ventriculography gadopentate dimeglumine-enhanced MR imaging in pediatric patients: preliminary report. AJNR Am J Neuroradiol 2007; 28:889.
60. Siebner HR, Grafin von Einsiedel H, Conrad B. Magnetic resonance ventriculography with gadolinium DTPA: report of two cases. Neuroradiology 1997; 39:418.
61. Tali ET, Ercan N, Krumina G, et al. Intrathecal gadolinium (gadopentetate dimeglumine) enhanced magnetic resonance myelography and cisternography: results of a multicenter study. Invest Radiol 2002; 37:152.

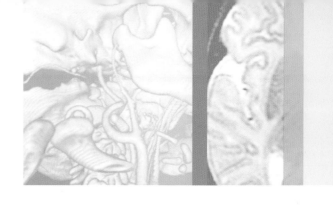

CHAPTER 14

Sella Turcica and Pituitary Gland

Vinodkumar Velayudhan, Michael D. Luttrull, and Thomas P. Naidich

The *sellar* and *parasellar regions* comprise the sella turcica, the pituitary gland, and the adjoining soft tissues and bone. The parasellar structures include the sphenoidal sinus and adjoining central skull base, the paired cavernous sinuses and adjoining venous sinuses, the cavernous and supraclinoid segments of the internal carotid arteries, the circle of Willis, the optic nerves and chiasm, the infundibulum and hypothalamus, the anterior recesses of the third ventricle, and the suprasellar subarachnoid space (suprasellar cistern). The sellar/parasellar region is an important junction for neurovascular, ophthalmologic, and endocrinologic structures.

The sella turcica (L., "Turkish saddle") forms as a spherical depression within the dorsal surface of the sphenoid bone. The sella and pituitary gland are related superiorly to the suprasellar cistern, the supraclinoid segments of the internal carotid arteries and circle of Willis, the pituitary stalk (infundibulum), the hypothalamus and anterior recesses of the third ventricle, the optic nerves, the optic chiasm, and the optic tracts. The sella is related laterally, on each side, to the paired cavernous sinuses, the cavernous segments of the internal carotid arteries, and cranial nerves (CN) III, IV, V1 and V2, and VI). It is related posteriorly to the basilar artery in the prepontine and interpeduncular cisterns and posteroinferolaterally to Meckel's cave, CN V, and the trigeminal ganglion. Directly inferiorly, the sella and pituitary gland are related to the sphenoidal sinus and, through that, to the nasopharynx. Dural reflections from the diaphragma sellae overlie the sella and the walls of the cavernous sinuses laterally.[1-3] Surgical access to the sella is limited by the surrounding vital structures, making the preferred surgical routes to sellar lesions the transsphenoidal approach through the sphenoidal sinus and the subfrontal approach along the floor of the anterior cranial fossa.[4,5] Familiarity with the anatomy and surgical landmarks of this region will permit proper display and appreciation of regional pathologic processes to facilitate diagnosis and medical/surgical management of sellar-parasellar disease.

ANATOMY
Gross Anatomy
Sphenoid Bone, Sphenoidal Sinus,
and Anatomic Relationships
Sphenoid Bone
The sphenoid bone lies within the central skull base. When viewed anteriorly, it displays a central body and numerous

projections, like a bat with outstretched wings (Figs. 14-1 to 14-3). Two lesser wings of the sphenoid bone project upward from the superolateral surfaces of the body on each side. Two greater wings of the sphenoid bone originate from the inferior portion of the sphenoid body and also project superolaterally, inferior to the lesser wings. Paired gaps between the lesser wings above and the greater wings below are designated the superior orbital fissures. Paired pterygoid processes arise from the undersurface of the sphenoid body on each side, project inferiorly, and flare outward as paired medial and lateral pterygoid plates. Cranial nerves (CN) III, IV, V1, and VI pass through the superior orbital fissure (Fig. 14-4). The posterior frontal lobes, olfactory tracts, and gyri recti rest on the smooth dorsal surfaces of the lesser sphenoid wings and planum sphenoidale. The lateral margin of each lesser wing forms the sphenoid ridge. On each side, the sphenoid ridges project upward into the sylvian fissure between the undersurface of the frontal lobe and the superior surface of the temporal lobe. The basilar artery and brain stem lie posterior to the clivus (Figs. 14-5 and 14-6).

The cavernous segments of the internal carotid arteries form paired grooves (carotid sulci) along the lateral surfaces of the upper sphenoid bone. The carotid sulci bulge into the lateral sinus wall in 32% to 71% of patients.[5] The bony wall between the carotid artery and the sphenoidal sinus varies from 0.4 to 1.7 mm in thickness and is 0.5 mm or less in approximately 90% of patients (Fig. 14-7). It is absent in 4%, leaving only mucosa between the sinus and the artery.[4] The bony wall becomes thinner as one moves anteriorly along the sphenoid and is thinnest in the region of the tuberculum sella.

The intracarotid distance between the two internal carotid arteries is variable along the course of the cavernous and supraclinoid segments of the artery. In some patients the medial wall of the internal carotid artery (ICA) lies as little as 4 mm from the midline, limiting surgical access. Such medially positioned carotid arteries may flatten or indent the pituitary gland.[5]

The superior surface of the sphenoidal sinus is a bony plate designated the planum sphenoidale (see Figs. 14-1 to 14-3). Posterior to the planum sphenoidale, the superior surface of the sphenoid bone displays a bony ridge (the limbus), a transverse groove (the chiasmatic sulcus), and a second ridge (the tuberculum sella). The tuberculum sella is the anterior lip of the sella turcica. The contours of these ridges and grooves are always gently rounded, not angular.

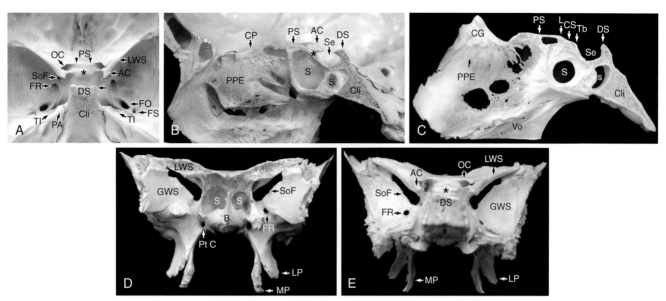

■ **FIGURE 14-1** Gross anatomy of the skull base and sphenoid bone. Three specimens of dried skulls. **A,** Specimen 1. View of the sella turcica (Se) from above and behind. **B** and **C,** Specimen 2. Sagittal sections through the sella and parasellar region. **D** and **E,** Specimen 3. Anterior surface (**D**) and posterior surface (**E**) of an isolated sphenoid bone. The sphenoid bone contains the pneumatized sphenoidal sinus (S) and gives rise to multiple bony processes. These include the lesser (L) and greater (G) sphenoid wings (SW), the anterior clinoid processes (AC) at the medial ends of the lesser wings, the posterior clinoid processes (PC, *horizontal arrow* in **A**) projecting forward from the dorsum sellae (DS), and the lateral (L) and the medial (M) ptery-goid (P) plates projecting inferiorly. Parasellar foramina include the foramen rotundum (FR), foramen ovale (FO), foramen spinosum (FS), optic canals (OC), superior orbital fissure (SoF), and pterygoid (vidian) canals (Pt C). From anterior to posterior, note the relationships of the crista galli (CG), planum sphenoidale (PS), limbus (L), chiasmatic sulcus (CS), tuberculum sellae (TS), sella turcica (Se), dorsum sellae (DS), and the clivus (Cli). In **A,** the chiasmatic sulcus lies between the intracranial ends of the two optic canals (OC) laterally, the limbus (*paired arrowheads*) anteriorly, and the tuber-culum sellae (*asterisk*) behind. It has been left unlabeled to show its full contour. The petrous apices (PA) lie just posterolateral to the clivus and posterior clinoid processes. They display prominent trigeminal impressions (TI) on their anterior surfaces where the fifth cranial nerve (CN V) passes over the petrous apex to reach Meckel's cave. Also labeled are the perpendicular plate of the ethmoid bone (PPE) and the vomer (Vo), which together form the nasal septum, and the cribriform plate (CP), which overlies the ethmoid labyrinth.

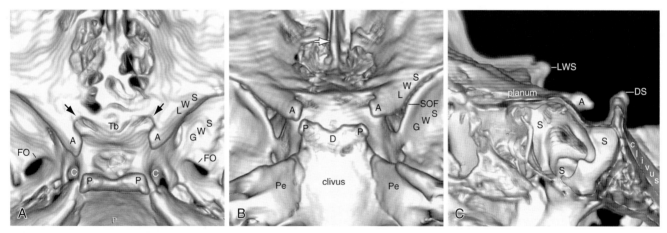

■ **FIGURE 14-2** **A** to **C,** Three-dimensional (3D) surface reformatted images of the sella turcica. **A,** Top view. **B,** Posterosuperior view. **C,** Cut-plane midsagittal section of the 3D reformatted image, with anterior to the reader's left. Compare with the dried bone specimens of Figure 14-1. A, anterior clinoid process; C, carotid groove; D, dorsum sellae; FO, foramen ovale; GWS, greater wing of the sphenoid; LWS, lesser wing of the sphenoid; Pe, petrous apex; S, sphenoid air cells; SOF, superior orbital fissure; Tb, tuberculum sellae. *Black arrows* show intracranial ends of the optic canals. *White arrow* in **B** indicates the crista galli.

See www.expertconsult.com for 3D surface-rendered videos of the sella with rotation in the horizontal, vertical, and multiaxial planes, respectively. These renderings provide a frame of reference regarding the spatial relationships of the sella, orbits, and skull base structures described throughout this chapter that are hard to capture on conventional 2D images.

■ **FIGURE 14-3** CT of the sella turcica and parasellar structures—bone algorithm images in axial plane (A to D), coronal reformatted sections (E to J), and sagittal reformatted sections (K to L). A to D, Axial images presented from superior to inferior demonstrate the normal anatomy of the sphenoid bone (S), anterior clinoid (AC) processes, and dorsum sellae (DS). The optic canals (*black arrows*) align with the optic nerves and pass toward the sella turcica immediately medial to the anterior clinoid processes. In B, the position of the sella turcica is indicated by the *asterisk*. The posterior clinoid processes form paired projections extending anteriorly from the dorsum. The partially ossified petroclinoid ligaments extend posterolaterally from the dorsum. The superior orbital fissure (SOF) appears to align with the medial walls of the orbit. In C and D, the bony grooves (*horizontal white arrows*) for the internal carotid arteries mold the lateral contours of the sella. Cli, clivus. E to H, Coronal images displayed from anterior to posterior. The body of the sphenoid contains asymmetric sphenoidal air cells (S) of diverse size. The planum sphenoidale (PS) forms the roof of the sphenoidal sinus anteriorly. The superior orbital fissure (SO) lies between the lesser wing of the sphenoid (LW) above and the greater wing of the sphenoid (GW) below. The anterior clinoid processes (AC) project posteriorly from the medial edges of the lesser wings. The optic canals (OC) lie between the body of sphenoid medially, the optic struts superiorly and inferiorly, and the anterior clinoid processes (AC) laterally. The inferior optic strut separates them from the superior orbital fissure (SOF). The floor of the optic canal extends further posterior than the roof, so sections through its intracranial end of the optic canals (G) show thinning to absence of the roof but a robust floor. The medial (MP) and lateral (LP) pterygoid plates project inferiorly from the body of the sphenoid. The lateral plate is larger and extends further posterior, so it is depicted in multiple adjacent posterior sections. The inferior surface of the sphenoid has a "keel" shape designated the rostrum. The vaginal processes of the vomer insert onto the inferior surface of the rostrum, just to each side of midline. The foramen rotundum passes anteriorly at the side of the sphenoid, so it is always seen best on coronal sections. The vidian canals (pterygoid canals) (VC) pass through the body of the sphenoid just above the pterygoid processes.

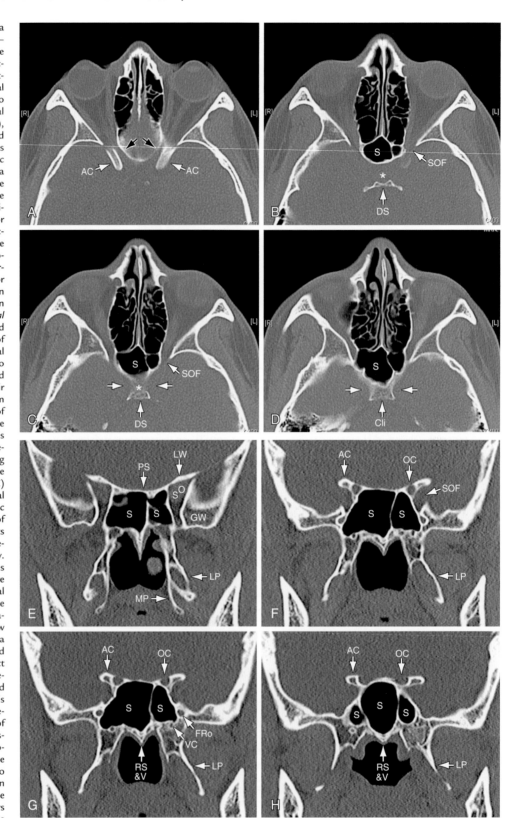

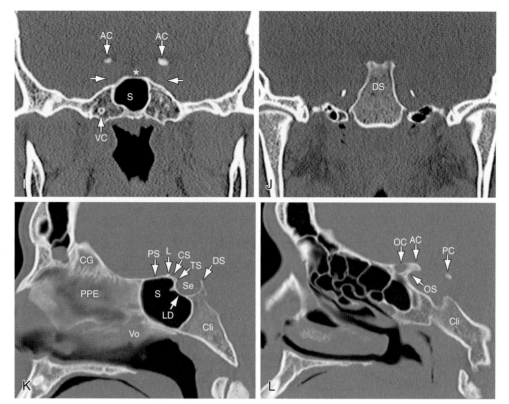

■ FIGURE 14-3, cont'd   I and J, Coronal images continued. **I,** Coronal section through the mid sella turcica (*asterisk*) shows the thin floor of the sella above the sphenoidal sinus (S), the carotid grooves (*white arrows*) molding the walls of the sphenoid laterally, and the posteriormost ends of the anterior clinoid processes. **J,** Immediately posteriorly, the dorsum sellae (DS) forms the posterior wall of the sella turcica. Nubbins of the posterior clinoid processes are seen at the top of the dorsum. Short ossified segments of the petroclinoid ligaments lie laterally. **K** and **L,** Sagittal images. **K,** Midsagittal section shows the crista galli (CG), perpendicular plate of the ethmoid bone (PPE), and the vomer (Vo) anteriorly, and the sphenoid sinus (S) and sella turcica (Se) posteriorly. In order from anterior to posterior, the parasellar bony structures are the planum sphenoidale (PS), limbus (L), chiasmatic sulcus (CS), tuberculum sellae (TS), lamina dura (LD), and the dorsum sellae (DS). The cortical bone of the floor of the sella turcica (lamina dura, LD) is thicker and more easily seen where it overlies the aerated sphenoid sinus. It is thinner and less easily appreciated where it overlies the cancellous basi-sphenoid bone. **L,** Off midline, parasagittal section shows portions of the anterior (AC) and posterior (PC) clinoid processes, the optic canal (OC), and the optic strut (OS).

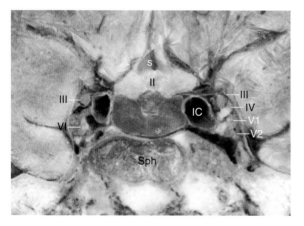

■ FIGURE 14-4   Gross anatomy of the sella and pituitary gland. Coronal cryomicrotome section through the sella turcica. The sphenoid bone (Sph) forms the bony floor of the sella turcica. The purplish pituitary gland (unlabeled) rests on the floor of the sella between the paired cavernous segments of the internal carotid arteries (IC). The optic chiasm (II) and flask-shaped supraoptic recess (s) of the third ventricle lie above the gland. Cranial nerve VI courses through the cavernous sinus immediately lateral to the internal carotid artery on each side. Cranial nerves III, IV, V1, and V2 course within the lateral wall of the cavernous sinus in strict order from superior to inferior. The deep freezing required for the cryomicrotome technique causes water-containing structures to expand, producing artifactual expansion and crowding of the anatomy. (*Courtesy of Dr. V. M. Haughton, Madison, WI.*)

The intracranial ends of the optic canals lie at the lateral ends of the chiasmatic sulcus (see Figs. 14-1 to 14-3). The paired anterior clinoid processes form the superolateral margins of the optic canals and give rise to the optic struts that form the lateral walls and floor of each optic canal, separating them from the superior orbital fissure below. The bony wall of the optic canal is less than 5 mm thick in 80% of patients. The wall may be dehiscent, leaving no bony separation between the sinus mucosa and the optic nerve sheath.[4]

Three bony foramina lie along the floor of the middle cranial fossa medially, at the junction of the body and greater wing of the sphenoid. From anterior to posterior, these are the foramen rotundum (transmitting V2), foramen ovale (transmitting V_3), and the foramen spinosum (transmitting the middle meningeal artery). Paired pterygoid (vidian) canals transmit the vidian arteries (arteries of the pterygoid canal) and vidian nerves (nerves of the vidian canal) through the sphenoid bones just where the

pterygoid processes arise from the sphenoid body (see Fig. 14-1D and E).

Sphenoidal Sinus

The sphenoidal sinus lies within the body of the sphenoid bone and displays wide variation in size, shape, and degree of pneumatization (Fig. 14-8).[6] The sinus is present in rudimentary form at birth as small paired cavities with an intervening septum. The sinus enlarges and expands into the sphenoid bone at least into

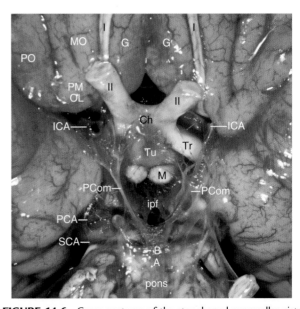

■ **FIGURE 14-6** Gross anatomy of the star-shaped suprasellar cistern as seen from the skull base, looking upward. Unfixed anatomic specimen after partial resection of the arachnoid septations. The paired CN I course along the olfactory sulci between the paired gyri recti (G) medially and the medial orbital gyri (MO) laterally. The posterior orbital gyrus (PO) merges with the medial orbital gyrus (MO) to form the posteromedial orbital lobule (PMOL) that makes up the anterolateral border of the suprasellar cistern on each side. The intracranial segments of the optic nerves (CN II) (II) converge to form the optic chiasm (Ch) in the anterior half of the suprasellar cistern. The optic tracts (Tr) diverge laterally in the posterior half of the suprasellar cistern. The mammillary bodies (M) and tuber cinereum (Tu) form the floor of the hypothalamus just behind the chiasm. The supraclinoid segments of the internal carotid arteries (ICA) lie laterally. The points of the suprasellar star arise where the suprasellar cistern merges into the interhemispheric fissure (anterior point), sylvian fissures (paired anterolateral points), perimesencephalic cistern (paired posterolateral points), and interpeduncular fossa (ipf) (posterior point). Posteriorly, the distal basilar artery (BA) gives rise to the paired superior cerebellar arteries (SCA) and paired posterior cerebral arteries (PCA). The posterior communicating arteries (PCom) pass from the PCAs to the ICAs in the lateral portions of the suprasellar cistern.

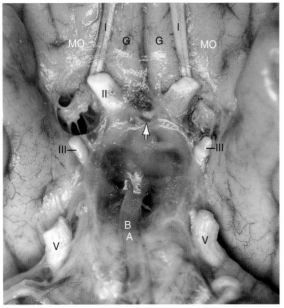

■ **FIGURE 14-5** Gross anatomy of the suprasellar cistern as seen from below with many arachnoid septations preserved. Unfixed anatomic specimen. The olfactory nerves (CN I) (I) pass posteriorly along the olfactory sulci between the paired gyri recti (G) and the paired medial orbital gyri (MO). Arachnoid trabeculae enclose the intracranial ends of the optic nerves (CN II) (II), the oculomotor nerves (CN III) (III) and the trigeminal nerves (CN V) (V). The pituitary stalk (*arrow*) passes immediately behind the optic chiasm and descends through the trabeculae en route to the neurohypophysis. The basilar artery (BA) ascends along the belly of the pons to enter the suprasellar cistern.

■ **FIGURE 14-7** Thin wall of the carotid groove. Coronal (**A**) and axial (**B**) noncontrast CT images through the sphenoidal sinus demonstrate very thin walls between the internal carotid arteries and the aerated sphenoidal sinus (*arrows*).

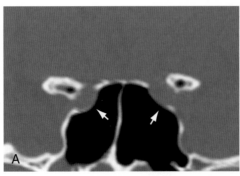

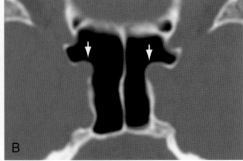

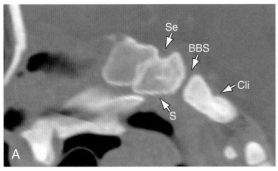
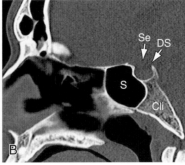
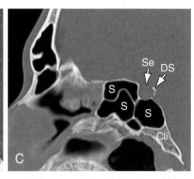

■ FIGURE 14-8 Sphenoidal sinus aeration. Reformatted midsagittal scan. **A,** Conchal pattern. This newborn exhibits no aeration of the sphenoid bone (S). The sella turcica (Se) is entirely surrounded by cancellous bone. The basi-sphenoidal/basi-occipital synchondrosis (BBS) separates the basi-sphenoid of the upper clivus from the basi-occiput of the lower clivus (Cli). **B,** Sellar pattern. Adult with partial pneumatization of the sphenoid bone, reaching to and partially underlying the sellar floor. **C,** Sellar pattern. Adult with extensive pneumatization of the sphenoid bone extending below the sella and dorsum sellae to reach the posterior cortex of the clivus (Cli). Multiple intrasphenoid septa create air cells of diverse size.

TABLE 14-1. Patterns of Sphenoidal Sinus Aeration, Septation, and Grooving

Pattern	Percentage
Conchal type pneumatization	~2
Presellar type pneumatization	21-24
Sellar type pneumatization	76-78
Sphenoid wing pneumatization	16
Dorsum sella pneumatization	14
No major septum	28
Single major septum	68 (48 off midline)
Two major septa	4
Septum terminating on carotid groove	32-40
Carotid artery bulging into sinus	71 (4% have no bony separation)

Data from Rhoton AL Jr. The sellar region. Neurosurgery 2002; 51(4 Suppl):S335-S374; Renn WH, Rhoton AL Jr. Microsurgical anatomy of the sellar region. J Neurosurg 1975; 43:288-298; and Hamid O, et al. Anatomic variations of the sphenoid sinus and their impact on transsphenoid pituitary surgery. Skull Base 2008; 18:9-15.

adolescence and is said to be mature by 14 years of age.[6] Nonetheless, some investigators have found that sphenoidal sinus development may continue until the third decade of life.[7] The pace of sinus expansion is determined, in part, by the fusion of the sphenoid synchondroses. The adult sphenoid bone forms from multiple individual ossification centers separated by synchondroses. Pneumatization does not cross an intact synchondrosis, so the sphenoidal sinus does not expand into new portions of the sphenoid until the intervening synchondroses have fused.

Rhoton[4] described three patterns of sphenoidal sinus aeration: conchal, presellar, and sellar (Table 14-1).

1. In the conchal pattern, the sphenoid bone inferior to the sella is formed by solid, nonaerated bone (<2%). The conchal pattern is encountered frequently in children prior to complete sphenoidal sinus pneumatization but is less common in adults.
2. In the presellar pattern (24%), pneumatization stops at the anterior wall of the sella turcica.
3. In the sellar pattern (76%), pneumatization extends below the sella turcica, sometimes as far posteriorly as the clivus (see Fig. 14-8).[4,8]

Expansion of the sphenoidal sinus laterally into the greater sphenoid wings, either symmetrically or asymmetrically, is designated lateralization (16%).[8] Expansion inferiorly into the pterygoid processes and pterygoid plates creates asymmetric pterygoid

recesses of the sphenoidal sinus. The sphenoidal sinus may also extend into the vomer, the hard palate, the ethmoid bone, and the basi-occiput, which forms the lower clivus. These variations are generally asymptomatic.[9]

The degree of pneumatization and the depth of the sphenoidal sinus become important considerations when choosing instrument length for transsphenoidal surgery. During transsphenoidal surgery, the sella turcica appears as a prominent bulge in the roof of the well-aerated sphenoidal sinus. This sellar bulge is an important surgical landmark for the sellar floor.[10,11] The sphenoidal sinus depth is defined as the anteroposterior distance from the sphenoidal sinus ostium to the most anterior portion of the sella turcica.[4,10] The average depth of the sphenoidal sinus is 15 to 17 mm (range: 11 to 23 mm).[4,10] In adults, the instruments used for transsphenoidal surgery must first pass inward along the approach for 11 to 12 cm before encountering the anterior sellar wall. They must then be long enough to reach into the sella and to pass above the sella turcica if additional suprasellar tumor is present.[4] In the conchal pattern of sphenoidal sinus aeration, the nonpneumatized sinus is believed to make the transsphenoidal approach less favorable, especially for larger tumors.[4,8,12]

The septations within the sphenoidal sinus vary widely in size, number, location, orientation, thickness, completeness, and relation to the sellar floor. Sixty-eight to 80 percent of patients show one major septum. The majority of these are situated *asymmetrically* and may lie several millimeters lateral to the midline. Approximately 28% of patients have no single major septum. Some 4% manifest two major septa. The major sphenoidal sinus septa are typically accompanied by smaller minor septa that may be oriented in any direction, dividing the sinus cavity into multiple smaller cavities. The orientation of these septa and their relationships to the sellar floor and the carotid grooves become important considerations in determining the precise surgical approach to sellar lesions. In 32% to 40% of patients, the major sinus septa terminate on a carotid groove; thus, following the wrong septum at surgery may lead to the artery not the pituitary gland. Further, major septa must be at least partially resected anteriorly to gain access to the sella. Fracture of a septum into the carotid groove may cause inadvertent hemorrhage if such relationships are not identified.[5,8,10,13]

Sella Turcica and Pituitary Gland
Bony Fossa
The sella turcica has three major components:

1. The tuberculum sella forms the anterior boundary of the sella.

2. The pituitary fossa (hypophysial fossa) is the bony depression that houses the pituitary gland. The floor of the pituitary fossa displays a well-corticated bony wall designated the lamina dura. This lamina is less than 1 mm thick in approximately 82% of cases.[5] It is most conspicuous where the sellar floor overlies the aerated sphenoidal sinus and is subtler where the floor overlies cancellous bone.

3. The dorsum sellae forms the posterior wall of the sella. It is continuous inferiorly with the upper portion of the clivus (L., "slope") that derives from the sphenoid bone (basi-sphenoid).

Sellar Size

The shape and linear dimensions of the sella turcica are highly variable (Fig. 14-9).[14] The depth of the sella is measured as the greatest distance perpendicular to a line connecting the tip of

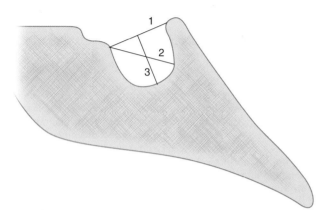

■ **FIGURE 14-9** Schematic representation of measurements made to assess sellar size. Line 1 is drawn from the tuberculum sellae to the tip of the dorsum sellae. Line 2 is the anteroposterior diameter of the sella, which is taken as the line drawn from the tuberculum sellae to the farthest point on the posterior sellar wall. Line 3 indicates the depth of the sella, which is taken as the length of the perpendicular line drawn from line 1 to the deepest portion of the sella turcica.

the dorsum sellae to the tuberculum sellae. That line corresponds to the plane of the diaphragma sellae. The anteroposterior diameter of the sella has been defined as a line connecting the tuberculum with the farthest portion of the posterior sella wall. Sellar width is defined as the width of the sellar floor between the two carotid sulci. The normal upper limits for these metrics are 17 mm in greatest anteroposterior length, 13 mm in depth, and 15 mm in width. The sellar volume has proved to be a more useful metric than any one linear measure. Total sellar volume is estimated using the equation for the volume of an ellipsoid: 0.5 (length × width × depth in mm)/1000. Total sellar volume should not exceed 1100 mm³.[4,5,15]

The length and diameter of the sella turcica increase with age. The growth rate is rapid in the first few years of life, decreases later in childhood, increases again substantially at puberty, and then ceases during late adolescence to early adulthood.[14,16,17] The growth rate is greatest during puberty when the pituitary gland undergoes physiologic hypertrophy. Females reach puberty at an earlier age than males, so they show sellar enlargement approximately 2 years earlier than males. After puberty, and into early adulthood, males and females show nearly equal sellar size (except in females during pregnancy).[18,19]

Clinoid Processes and Dural Reflections/Ligaments

Three pairs of clinoid processes arise in relation to the sella turcica (see Figs. 14-1 to 14-3). Anteriorly, the paired anterior clinoid processes arise from the medial aspects of the lesser sphenoid wings and project laterally to each side of the sella turcica.[20] Paired middle clinoid processes form tiny bony elevations along the anterolateral margins of the sellar floor. Posteriorly, the posterior clinoid processes arise at the lateral margins of the dorsum sella and project anteriorly. The transverse distance between the anterior clinoid processes is greater than the transverse distance between the posterior clinoid processes.

The clinoid processes give attachment to important dural reflections (Fig. 14-10) (see also Chapter 8). The free medial margins of the tentorium sweep anteriorly, pass lateral to the posterior clinoid processes, and insert into the anterior clinoid processes on each side. The lateral margins of the tentorium pass

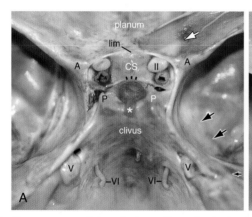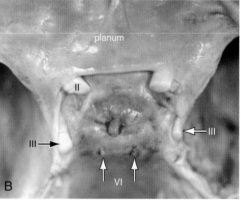

■ **FIGURE 14-10** Gross anatomy of the sellar/parasellar region in situ. Two unfixed cadaver specimens seen from above. **A,** The dural cover of the right orbital roof has been deflected medially to show the optic canal (*white arrow*) beneath its thin bony roof. The optic nerves (II) enter the intracranial space medial to the anterior clinoid processes (A) and anterosuperior to the internal carotid arteries. The pituitary gland lies within the sella turcica between the tuberculum sellae (*three black dashes*) anteriorly and the dorsum sellae posteriorly. The cut end of the pituitary stalk (infundibulum) (*asterisk*) joins the superior surface of the pituitary gland by passing through the hiatus in the thin glistening diaphagma sellae. The transverse dimension between the two anterior clinoid processes (A-A) is wider than the transverse distance between the two posterior clinoid processes (P-P). The petroclinoid ligaments pass anteromedially from the petrous apices to insert into the posterior clinoid processes, forming the superior margins of the ostia through which the trigeminal nerves (V) enter into Meckel's cave (*black arrows*). The abducens nerves (VI) pass into the clivus and traverse Dorello's canal to enter the cavernous sinuses. Also labeled are the chiasmatic sulcus (CS), limbus (lim), and planum sphenoidale (planum). **B,** More nearly direct suprasellar view shows the diaphragma forming the roof of the sella turcica. The oculomotor nerves (CN III) (III) pass into the upper lateral wall of the cavernous sinus bilaterally. The abducens nerve (CN VI) (VI) enters the dorsal surface of the clivus bilaterally. The greenish cast to the image signifies patient jaundice.

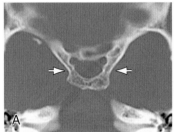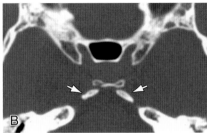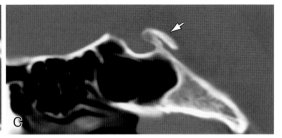

■ **FIGURE 14-11** Calcification of parasellar dural reflections. **A,** Bridged sella. Axial noncontrast CT shows ossification of the dural reflections (*arrows*) between the anterior and posterior clinoid processes bilaterally, "bridging over" the sella. **B** and **C,** Calcified/ossified petroclinoid ligaments (*arrows*) extending from the petrous apices to the dorsum/posterior clinoid processes. These ligaments may ossify completely or only segmentally (as here).

medially along the superior petrous ridges, become the petroclinoid ligaments, pass medially below the free margins of the tentorium, and insert into the posterior clinoid processes. The petroclinoid ligaments are the superior margins of the ostia into Meckel's caves. The cavernous segments of the internal carotid arteries transition into the supraclinoid segments by passing immediately medial to the anterior clinoid processes. They are maintained in position, in part, by the caroticoclinoid ligaments that extend between the anterior and middle clinoid processes to enclose the arteries. The diaphragma sellae is the dural covering of the sella turcica. It merges with the dura of the cavernous sinuses, laterally, and extends farther into the dural folds surrounding the anterior and posterior clinoid processes.[3,4,13]

The dural reflections commonly ossify. Ossification of the dura stretched between the anterior and posterior clinoid processes produces a "bridged" sella (Fig. 14-11A). Ossification of the caroticoclinoid ligament between the anterior and middle clinoid processes produces a caroticoclinoid canal. Ossification of the petroclinoid ligament forms a linear density that angles posteroinferolaterally from the dorsum (see Figs. 14-3B and 14-11). In sagittal view, the dorsum and the calcified ligaments give an appearance classically likened to the winged helmet of Mercury.

Dura and Cisternal Relationships

The margins of the sella turcica are covered by dura. The diaphragma sellae forms the roof of the sella turcica and the pituitary gland (see Fig. 14-10). The diaphragma lies in a plane inferior to the level of the anterior clinoid processes. It is typically rectangular and shows a concave or flat superior border in 96% of cases. The diaphragma is usually very thin. However, it is as thick as a single layer of dura in something less than 40% of cases and can form a tenacious barrier during transsphenoidal hypophysectomy. A small central opening in the diaphragma sella, termed the *diaphragmatic hiatus,* provides passage for the infundibulum. The diaphragmatic hiatus is typically round to oval. It is 5 mm or larger in nearly 60% of cases. The arachnoid of the suprasellar cistern may protrude through the hiatus into the sella in up to half of cases. Such arachnoid diverticula may be the origin of the empty sella syndrome and may become a source of cerebrospinal fluid (CSF) leak, either spontaneously, or after surgery (Fig. 14-12).[4,21,22]

The suprasellar cistern lies above the diaphragma sellae and contains the circle of Willis, optic chiasm and nerves, the floor of the third ventricle, the inferior hypothalamus, and the infundibulum (Figs. 14-11 to 14-16). The suprasellar cistern corresponds roughly to an area lying between the free edges of the tentorial incisura and the ventral midbrain. It is bound by the interhemispheric fissure anteriorly, the sylvian fissures anterolaterally, the perimesencephalic cisterns between the uncus and brain stem posterolaterally, and the cerebral peduncles and interpeduncular cistern posteriorly. The cisternal segments of the oculomotor nerves pass anteriorly from the interpeduncular

cistern toward the cavernous sinuses through the lateral portions of the suprasellar cisterns, inferior to the inferior surface of the uncus. The chiasmatic cistern surrounds the optic chiasm and is continuous into the cistern of the lamina terminalis anteriorly. The membrane of Liliequist stretches from the mammillary bodies to the dorsum sellae, separating the chiasmatic cistern from the interpeduncular cistern (see Fig. 14-16).[23,24]

Pituitary Stalk (Infundibulum)

The pituitary stalk (infundibulum) projects downward and anteriorly from the median eminence of the hypothalamus. It passes through the hiatus in the diaphragma sellae and inserts into the pituitary gland between the anterior and posterior lobes (see Fig. 14-10). The infundibulum is widest superiorly and tapers inferiorly. In adults, the upper limits for normal infundibular thickness are 3.5 mm at the median eminence, 2.9 mm at the midportion, and 1.9 mm at its insertion into the gland. The lower limit of normal thickness is 1 mm.[25] On CT examinations, assessment of the infundibulum can be made by comparing the diameter of the pituitary stalk to that of the basilar artery at a similar level. In normal patients, the pituitary stalk-to-basilar artery ratio should be less than 1. Ratios equal to or greater than 1 can be compared against normal reference ranges of infundibular size based on age and sex of the patient. An abnormally large infundibulum may warrant further evaluation for an underlying pathologic process such as hypothalamic tumors, Langerhans cell histiocytosis, or sarcoidosis.[26]

Pituitary Gland

The pituitary gland has two dominant lobes: the larger anterior lobe (adenohypophysis) and the smaller posterior lobe (neurohypophysis) (see Figs. 14-11 and 14-13 to 14-17). The anterior and posterior lobes are closely related anatomically but are distinct embryologically and functionally. During fetal development, the anterior lobe arises by upward evagination of Rathke's pouch from the nasopharynx, whereas the posterior lobe arises by inferior extension of the median eminence of the hypothalamus.

On surgical inspection from above, the anterior lobe fills the anterior and central portions of the pituitary fossa and has two wings that project posteriorly toward the dorsum sellae. The superior surface of the anterior lobe is darker than the superior surface of the posterior lobe. The anterior lobe has a firmer consistency and is more easily separable from the bony wall of the sella turcica. The posterior lobe of the pituitary gland is nearly always found in the midline, has a more gelatinous texture, and is generally more densely adherent to the adjacent sellar wall.

The anterior lobe occupies up to 90% of the total volume of the sella turcica. It is composed of a pars distalis, forming most of the anterior lobe; a pars tuberalis, formed as an upward extension of the anterior gland that wraps around the lower

Text continued on page 285

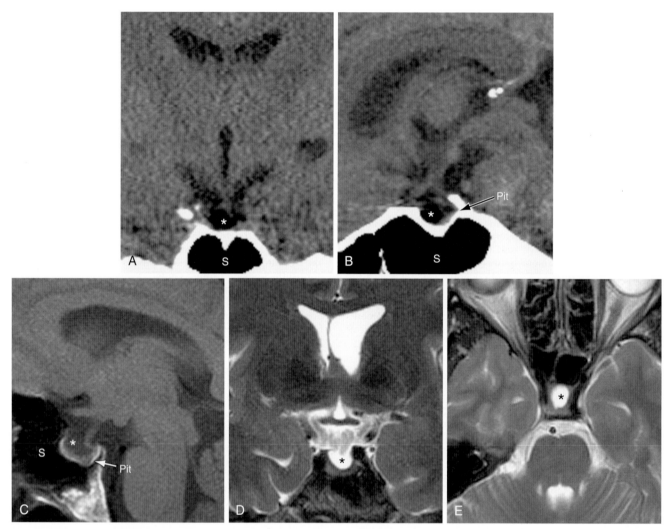

■ **FIGURE 14-12** Empty sella. Coronal (**A**) and sagittal (**B**) reformatted CT images demonstrate prominent cerebrospinal fluid attenuation within the sella (*asterisk*) and a thin sliver of pituitary gland (Pit) along the floor of the sella posteriorly. **C**, Midsagittal T1W image through the sella shows low signal cerebrospinal fluid (*asterisk*) and a thin rim of pituitary tissue (Pit) along the sellar floor posteriorly. Coronal (**D**) and axial (**E**) T2W images show bright fluid signal throughout the sella (*asterisks*).

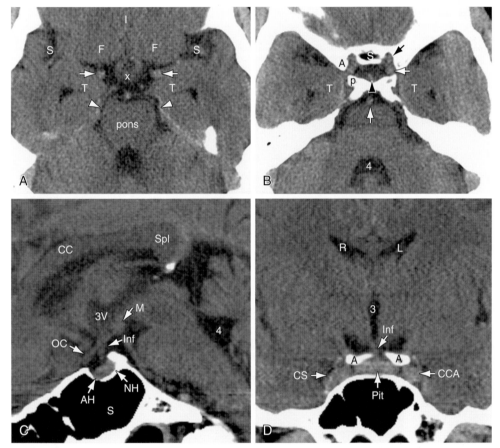

■ **FIGURE 14-13** Noncontrast CT of sella turcica for soft tissue. **A,** On axial noncontrast CT scans the suprasellar cistern is characteristically "star shaped." The anterior point is the intersection with the interhemispheric fissure (I). The paired anterolateral points are the intersections with the sylvian fissures (S, S). The paired posterolateral points are the intersections with the perimesencephalic or peripontine cisterns (*white arrowheads*). The posterior point is the shallow midpontine groove or the deeper interpeduncular fossa, depending on the level and angle of the section. The borders of the suprasellar cistern are normally convex toward the cistern, owing to the rounded surfaces of the frontal lobes (F, F), medial temporal lobes (T, T) and brain stem (here, pons). The optic chiasm (x), supraclinoid internal carotid arteries (*white arrows*), and basilar artery (*unlabeled*) are seen at this level. **B,** Further inferiorly, the infundibulum (*black arrowhead*) appears as a central "dot" within the posterior sella. The optic nerves (*black arrow*) emerge into the intracranial space medial to the anterior clinoid processes (A) and anterosuperior to the internal carotid arteries (*horizontal white arrow*). The basilar artery (*vertical white arrow*) is seen between the dorsum sellae and the brain stem. An aerated portion of the sphenoidal sinus (S) is seen in the midline anteriorly. p, posterior clinoid process. **C,** Midsagittal CT reformatted image shows the adenohypophysis (AH), the neurohypophysis (NH), and the infundibulum (Inf). In this patient, the optic chiasm lies close to the chiasmatic sulcus over the anterior sella turcica. The mammillary body (M) forms a prominent bulge posterior to the infundibulum. Other prominent midline structures include the body (CC) and splenium (Spl) of the corpus callosum, the brain stem, and the fourth ventricle (4). **D,** Reformatted coronal plane CT shows the midline third ventricle (3), infundibulum (Inf) and pituitary gland (Pit), the paired anterior clinoid processes (A, A), and the paired left (L) and right (R) lateral ventricles (LV). On each side, the cavernous sinus (CS) forms the lateral wall of the sella turcica and gives passage to the cavernous segment of the internal carotid artery (CCA).

■ **FIGURE 14-14** CT of sella turcica with contrast enhancement. **A** and **B,** The infundibulum (Inf) and cavernous sinuses (CS) enhance after administration of a contrast agent. The intracranial vessels are more readily identified, including the anterior cerebral arteries (ACA), basilar artery (BA), and internal carotid arteries (ICA). Also labeled are the anterior clinoid process (A), the dorsum sellae (D), and the pons. **C** and **D,** Reformatted sagittal (**C**) and coronal (**D**) plane images. On both of these planes, arrows indicate the vessel identifications. The pituitary gland (Pit) and infundibulum (Inf) show diffuse enhancement. Also labeled are the vein of Galen (G), internal cerebral vein (ICV), the partially calcified pineal gland (Pin), the middle cerebral artery (MCA), and the aerated sphenoidal sinus (S).

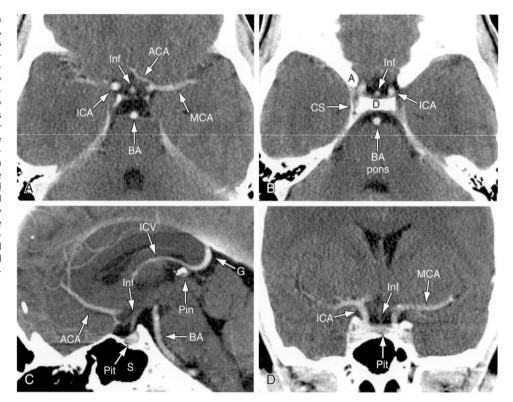

■ **FIGURE 14-15** Axial MR images of the sella turcica displayed from superior to inferior. **A** to **D,** T1W contrast-enhanced MR images. **E** to **G,** T2W images. **A** and **E,** Superior portion of the suprasellar cistern. The anterior recesses (*asterisk*) of the third ventricle, hypothalamus (H), and mammillary bodies (M) protrude into the star-shaped cistern from above. The interpeduncular fossa (i) lies between the two cerebral peduncles (p). The optic tracts (OT) diverge posterolaterally along the anterolateral borders of the cerebral peduncles (p), along the anterior border of the midbrain (mid) in the upper portion of the suprasellar cistern. **B, C,** and **F,** Midportion of the suprasellar cistern. The optic nerves (CN II) (II) and optic chiasm (OCh) lie within the anterior half of the suprasellar cistern. The contrast-enhancing infundibulum (Inf) descends to the pituitary gland immediately behind the chiasm, forming a small "dot" in axial sections. The supraclinoid internal carotid arteries (ICA, flow voids) lie anterolaterally. The posterior communicating artery (PCom) lies laterally, and the basilar artery (BA) lies posteriorly. **D** and **G,** The pituitary gland (Pit) lies within the sella turcica, just anterior to the dorsum sellae (D).

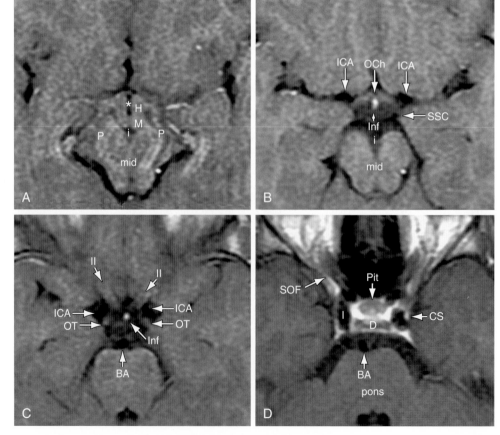

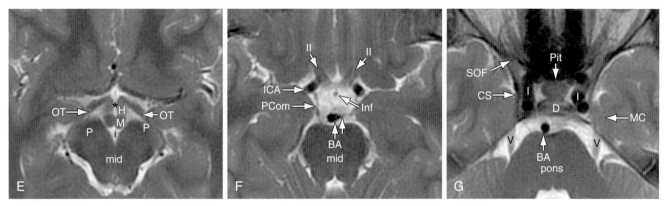

■ **FIGURE 14-15, cont'd**   E to G, T2W images. The paired cavernous sinuses (CS) and the internal carotid arteries (i, ICA) form the side walls of the sella turcica. The superior orbital fissures (SOF) are related to the anterior ends of the cavernous sinuses. The paired trigeminal nerves (V) enter Meckel's caves (MC) just posterior, inferior, and lateral to the cavernous sinuses (CS). The infundibulum joins the upper surface of the pituitary gland (Pit). The pons is also labeled.

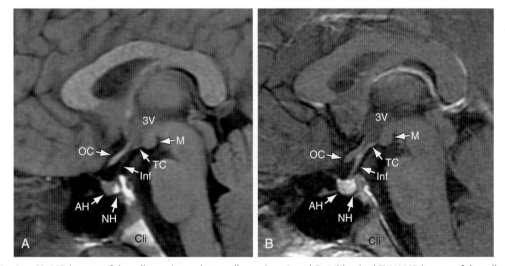

■ **FIGURE 14-16**   A to H, MR images of the sella turcica and parasellar region. A and B, Midsagittal T1W MR images of the sella turcica before (A) and after (B) contrast enhancement demonstrate a normal pituitary gland with the adenohypophysis (AH) anteriorly and the "bright spot" of the neurohypophysis (NH) posteriorly. The pituitary gland and infundibulum show uniform contrast enhancement in B. In this patient, the optic chiasm lies directly superior to the pituitary gland. The tuber cinereum (TC) and mammillary bodies (M) of the hypothalamus form the inferior wall of the third ventricle (3V) behind the infundibulum and chiasm. The clivus (Cli) is noted at the inferior aspect of both images.

Continued

■ **FIGURE 14-16, cont'd** C to H, Coronal images through the sella turcica. C to F, T1W images after enhancement with a contrast agent. G and H, T2W images displayed from anterior to posterior. The optic nerves (CN II) enter the intracranial space just anterior and superior to the internal carotid arteries (see Fig. 14-10), converge posteromedially, partially decussate at the optic chiasm (OCh), and then diverge posterolaterally as the optic tracts (OT). The pituitary stalk (infundibulum) (Inf) passes just behind the optic chiasm as it descends to the contrast-enhancing pituitary gland (Pit). The nonenhancing dorsum sella (DS) lies just behind the pituitary gland. The cavernous sinuses (CS) and the cavernous (c, C) and supraclinoid (s, S) segments of the internal carotid artery (I, ICA) lie lateral to the pituitary gland. The suprasellar cistern (SC) lies above the gland. The oculomotor nerve (CN III) is seen in the upper lateral wall of the cavernous sinus. The anterior cerebral (ACA) and middle cerebral arteries (MCA) are also labeled.

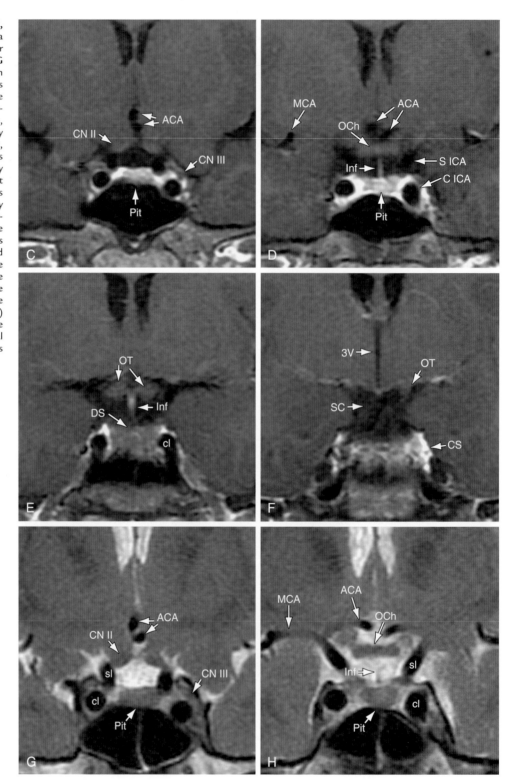

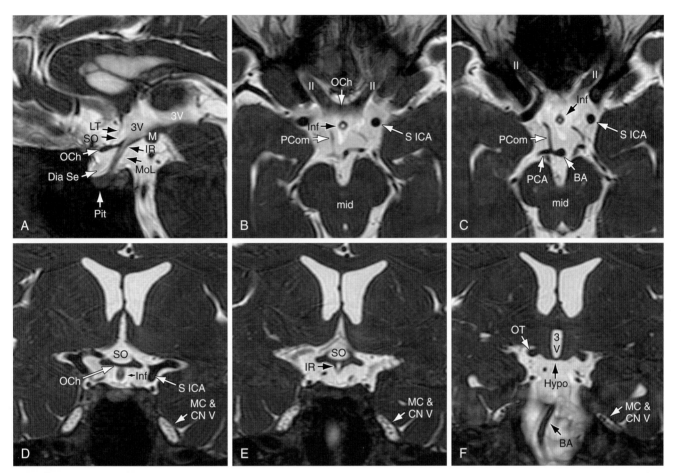

■ **FIGURE 14-17**   T2W high-resolution images of the suprasellar/parasellar region using the FIESTA (fast imaging employing steady-state acquisition) series (GE, Milwaukee, WI). **A,** Midsagittal section shows the supraoptic recess (SO) and infundibular recess (IR) of the anterior third ventricle (3V) enclosing the optic chiasm (OCh) between them. A thin diaphragma sellae (Dia Se) overlies the pituitary gland (Pit). The lamina terminalis (LT) forms the anterior wall of the third ventricle (3V). The membrane of Liliequist (MoL) is seen faintly behind the infundibulum. **B** and **C,** Axial sections demonstrate the paired optic nerves (II), optic chiasm (OCh), infundibulum (Inf), supraclinoid ICA (S ICA), basilar artery and tip (BA), posterior communicating artery (PCom), and posterior cerebral artery (PCA). **D** to **F,** Coronal sections demonstrate the flask shape of the supraoptic recess (SO), the pencil shape of the infundibular (IR) recess, and the relationships of the optic chiasm (OCh) and optic tracts (OT) to the third ventricle (3V). Inferolaterally, the rootlets of the trigeminal nerve (CN V) traverse the predominantly CSF-filled Meckel's caves (MC). Other labels include the hypothalamus (hypo) and midbrain (mid).

infundibulum; and a pars intermedia. The pars intermedia is present in lower animals and in human fetal life but later becomes dispersed into the anterior lobe. In human adults it is either not present or may remain as a small nonfunctional cystic remnant (pars intermedia cyst) (Fig. 14-18).[4,27] These elements are believed to produce the prohormone pro-opiomelanocortin (POMC).

The anterior lobe synthesizes a number of hormones under the regulatory control of the hypothalamus. These are made by five different cell types, defined by the hormone they produce and secrete. Somatotropes secrete growth hormone (GH). Lactotropes make prolactin. Corticotropes secrete adrenocorticotropic hormone (ACTH), which regulates adrenal function via proteolysis of POMC. Thyrotropes produce thyroid-stimulating hormone (TSH) and regulate growth and hormone function of the thyroid gland. Gonadotropes secrete follicle-stimulating hormone (FSH) and luteinizing hormone (LH) that regulate gonadal function. These cell types show topographic organization within the adenohypophysis.[28] Prolactin- and GH-secreting cells are found mostly in the lateral portions of the gland. Thyrotropes, corticotropes, and gonadotropes are usually located more centrally. Histologically, the hormone-secreting cells have been divided into different populations, including basophilic (FSH, LH, ACTH, and TSH) and acidophilic/eosinophilic (prolac-

tin and GH) cells. However, these histologic types do not correlate well with cell function.

The anterior lobe receives chemical messengers from the median eminence of the hypothalamus via the hypothalamic-hypophysial portal system. Regulatory hormones released into the portal system pass to the capillary bed of the anterior lobe, regulating the secretion of hormones from the adenohypophysis. Transmission of messenger hormones via the portal system has been termed the *parvocellular pathway.*

The posterior pituitary lobe consists mainly of the pars nervosa. The posterior lobe develops as a direct extension of the median eminence of the hypothalamus and remains connected to it by the pituitary stalk. The posterior lobe contains pituicytes, axonal projections from hypothalamic neurons, and the axonal terminals (Herring bodies) that serve as reservoirs for the hormones. Axons derived from the supraoptic nucleus (SON) convey vesicles containing antidiuretic hormone (ADH) down the stalk for storage in the Herring bodies. Axons derived from the paraventricular nucleus (PVN) similarly convey vesicles containing oxytocin down the stalk to the Herring bodies. Transmission of hormones in this fashion has been termed the *magnocellular pathway.*[29]

The height and volume of the pituitary gland vary during life. In both males and females, gland size increases significantly with

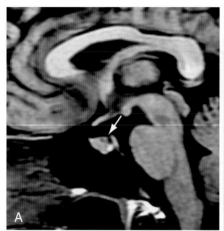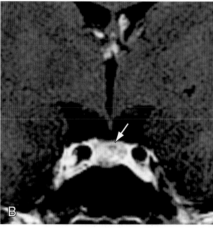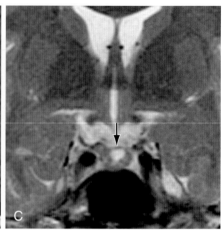

■ **FIGURE 14-18**   Pars intermedia cyst. **A,** Sagittal T1W noncontrast MR image. **B,** Coronal T1W contrast-enhanced image. **C,** Coronal T2W image. A small cyst (*arrow*) in the middle of the pituitary gland is largest in its transverse dimension, is uniformly hypointense on the noncontrast T1W image, is uniformly hyperintense on the T2W images, and displays no contrast enhancement. These imaging features are typical of a pars intermedia cyst but do overlap with the imaging features of Rathke's cleft cysts.

the onset of puberty. The increase is larger in females. The volume of the normal, young adult pituitary gland is smaller (586 mg) in males than in females (655 mg), most likely reflecting differing hormonal activity during menses.[30] The volume of the pituitary gland increases progressively during pregnancy, reaching a peak of approximately 847 (±110) mg in the first few days post partum owing to hormonal influence.[31]

The inferior surface of the pituitary gland usually conforms to the shape of the bony sellar floor. The lateral and superior surfaces have more variable contour, because these margins abut on more pliable soft tissue structures. The superior surface varies in shape depending on patient age, gender, and hormonal status. The lateral surface may be molded by the adjacent cavernous internal carotid arteries.[4,32,33]

Vascular Supply of the Pituitary Gland

The anterior and posterior pituitary lobes have separate arterial blood supplies owing to their distinct embryologic origins.[29,34,35] The anterior lobe is supplied mainly by the hypophysial portal venous system. This lies on the surface of the infundibulum and receives blood from the median eminence, which is in turn supplied via the superior hypophysial arteries. In addition, up to one third of the anterior lobe supply comes through short portal veins draining venous blood from the posterior to the anterior lobes. Peripheral portions of the anterior lobe may receive direct supply from the inferior hypophysial artery, a branch of the precavernous ICA. The posterior lobe receives its major supply from the inferior hypophysial artery. The upper surface of the pituitary gland, the median eminence, portions of the infundibulum, and the optic chiasm are supplied by the superior hypophysial artery. This artery arises from the supraclinoid ICA or the posterior communicating artery. Within the pituitary gland, the vascular supply is distributed through a loosely organized network lined by fenestrated capillaries.[36]

The venous drainage from the anterior and posterior lobes passes through the cavernous sinus into the petrosal sinuses. Each side of the gland usually drains preferentially into the ipsilateral cavernous and petrosal sinuses, so sampling the hormonal concentrations of inferior petrosal blood may help to lateralize an otherwise occult, hormonally active pituitary lesion.[29,37]

Optic Apparatus

The intracanalicular segments of the optic nerves emerge from the optic canals at each side of the chiasmatic sulcus, just medial to the anterior clinoid processes. In this location, the prechiasmal optic nerves lie anterior and superior to the cavernous carotid arteries and cross the arteries from lateral to medial as they converge toward the chiasm (see Figs. 14-6, 14-10, and 14-15 to 14-17). The lengths of the intracranial segments of the optic nerves are variable, so the chiasm may lie close to the optic canals (prefixed chiasm), directly above the sella turcica, or unusually far posteriorly, overlying the dorsum sella (postfixed chiasm). According to Rhoton,[4] the chiasm lies directly above the diaphragma sellae in 70% of patients (see Fig. 14-16), is prefixed in 15%, and is postfixed in 15%. The pituitary stalk lies immediately behind the chiasm, so the position of the stalk varies with the position of the chiasm. These relationships determine, in part, the specific neuro-ophthalmologic symptoms observed in patients with pituitary tumors. These relationships also determine how easily the pituitary fossa can be exposed through a subfrontal approach.[4]

Cavernous Sinuses and Contents

The cavernous sinuses are dural-covered venous sinuses that form the lateral boundaries of the sella turcica. They extend along each side of the sphenoidal sinus, sella turcica, and pituitary gland from the superior orbital fissures anteriorly to the petrous apices posteriorly (see Figs. 14-13 to 14-17). The cavernous sinuses contain small endothelial-lined sinusoids that drain the pituitary gland and also receive inflow from other venous structures, including the ophthalmic and middle cerebral veins and the sphenoparietal sinuses. The cavernous sinuses then drain posteriorly into the superior and inferior petrosal veins, which drain into the transverse sinus and sigmoid sinus, respectively. The cavernous sinuses are compartmentalized structures, not freely confluent spaces, so different portions of the sinuses may receive blood from, and drain to, separate structures. Carotid-cavernous fistulas, for example, may drain just anteriorly, just posteriorly, or in both directions. Because the ophthalmic vein drains into the cavernous sinuses, pathologic processes that result in venous congestion of the cavernous sinuses may produce proptosis and conjunctival ecchymoses.[19,29]

Intercavernous venous connections connect the two cavernous sinuses along the edges of the diaphragma sellae and around the pituitary gland. These connections are named for their relationship to the gland. The largest intercavernous connection is the basilar sinus. The basilar sinus connects both cavernous sinuses posteriorly, passes along the upper clivus and dorsum sellae, and joins with the greater and lesser petrosal sinuses. Anterior, posterior, and inferior intercavernous sinuses may pass anterior, posterior, and inferior to the pituitary gland in different individuals. When both anterior and posterior intercavernous sinuses are present, the combination has been termed a *circular sinus.*[4]

Cavernous Segment of Internal Carotid Artery

The cavernous segment of the ICA is the most medial structure within the cavernous sinus. It is fixed in place by the dural/bony ring formed by the anterior and middle clinoid processes and the (sometimes ossified) caroticoclinoid ligament.[4] The cavernous segment of the internal carotid artery begins at the superior margin of the petroclinoid ligament, just lateral to the posterior clinoid process, where the artery turns sharply forward. The horizontal segment of the ICA extends anteriorly and superiorly for approximately 2 cm before perforating the roof of the cavernous sinus along the medial edge of the anterior clinoid process to transition into the supraclinoid ICA (see Figs. 14-10 and 14-14 to 14-17). The cavernous ICA usually lies 1 to 7 mm lateral to the lateral surface of the pituitary gland. In approximately one in four cases, however, the ICA forms a deep carotid groove that abuts upon or indents the pituitary gland, molding its contour. The lateral surface of the pituitary gland may then wrap over the superior and inferior margins of the ICA. In these cases, it may prove impossible to resect a pituitary lesion completely via a transsphenoidal approach.

The intracavernous segment of the ICA gives rise to two major branches that supply sellar structures.[4] The larger branch is the meningohypophysial trunk. The smaller is McDonnell's capsular artery. The meningohypophysial trunk arises from the cavernous carotid artery at the level of the dorsum sella and gives rise to the inferior hypophysial artery. The inferior hypophysial artery supplies the posterior pituitary capsule, posterior lobe of the pituitary gland, and the dura of the sellar floor before anastomosing with the contralateral inferior hypophysial artery. McDonnell's artery is an inconsistent vessel that arises from the medial aspect of the intracavernous ICA to supply the pituitary capsule and the dura lining the anterior floor of the sella.[4]

Cranial Nerves

Cranial nerves (CN) III, IV, V1, V2, and VI bear close anatomic relationships to the cavernous sinuses (see Figs. 14-4 to 14-6 and 14-15 to 14-17). The abducens nerve (CN VI) is the only cranial nerve that actually courses within the cavernous sinus. It penetrates the dura along the posterior surface of the clivus and traverses Dorello's canal to enter the cavernous sinus at the lower aspect of its posterior wall. CN VI then courses anteriorly along the lateral surface of the intracavernous ICA before exiting the sinus via the superior orbital fissure. CN VI may traverse the sinus as a single nerve bundle, or it may separate into as many as five rootlets that traverse the sinus before reassembling into a single bundle that exits the sinus via the superior orbital fissure.

The other cranial nerves course within the lateral wall of the cavernous sinus, between the two dural leaves of the wall, not through the sinus cavity itself. They are arrayed in strict order from superior to inferior as CN III, CN IV, CN V1, and CN V2. CN III (oculomotor nerve) enters the cavernous sinus just anterolateral to the dorsum sella and nearly superior to the meningohypophysial trunk. It exits the sinus via the superior orbital fissure. CN IV (trochlear nerve) enters the roof of the cavernous sinus posterior and lateral to CN III. It exits the sinus via the superior orbital fissure. The ophthalmic division of the trigeminal nerve (CN V1) courses through the inferior portion of the lateral wall of the cavernous sinus, ascends, and eventually exits the sinus wall through the superior orbital fissure. The maxillary division of the trigeminal nerve (CN V2) is the inferiormost cranial nerve within the lateral wall of the cavernous sinus. It exits the skull via the foramen rotundum (see Figs. 14-1

to 14-3). The relationships of the cranial nerves are detailed in Chapter 17.

Meckel's Cave

Meckel's cave is a CSF-containing space situated inferior and lateral to the sella turcica and cavernous sinus. It houses the sensory trigeminal ganglion (gasserian ganglion), its central processes, and the motor root of the trigeminal nerve (see Figs. 14-4, 14-10, 14-14, 14-15G, and 14-17). Meckel's cave is bounded laterally by a dural reflection and medially by the trigeminal impression on the anterior surface of the petrous apex. It abuts directly onto the posterolateral aspect of the cavernous sinus and communicates with the basilar cisterns via an ostium situated immediately inferior to the petroclinoid ligament.[19]

Light Microscopy

The divisions of the pituitary gland can be readily discerned on histologic evaluation. The adenohypophysis contains a heterogeneous population of cells that are displayed on standard Hematoxylin and Eosin (H&E)–stained sections as eosinophilic (pink) acidophils, dark purple basophils, and pale chromophobes. The neurohypophysis contains a more homogeneous population of cells that appear similar to nervous tissue. The pars intermedia is situated between the adenohypophysis and neurohypophysis and can contain cystic elements filled with eosinophilic material.[38]

IMAGING

Computed Tomography

Pituitary Gland

The size of the pituitary gland has been studied by both linear and volumetric measures.[30] For linear measurements, normal gland size is reported to be 10 to 15 mm (width), 7 to 11 mm (anteroposterior length), and 4 to 7 mm (height).[39] The width of the gland is usually the largest of these three dimensions, but gland height is easier to determine accurately and is usually taken as the most useful single linear metric for pituitary size. Owing to variations in gland shape, however, simple linear measurements of gland height are less accurate than measures of gland volume.[15] Gland volume may be estimated on imaging studies by summing the volumes on individual slices in a single plane (usually sagittal) or by averaging the results from two to three planes. At puberty, the gland increases in size markedly and may reach approximately 10 mm in height in females and up to 8 mm in height in males.[31,40-42] Pituitary height increases progressively during the course of pregnancy and reaches up to 12 mm in height immediately post partum.[30]

Pituitary Gland Maturation

Glands of preterm infants are greater in height than those of term infants. This is thought to result from elevated growth hormone and reduced insulin-like growth factor levels in preterm infants.[34] During the first 2 years of life, the *height* of the gland remains relatively constant but the gland increases in size in the other dimensions. Prepubertal pituitary volumes increase linearly with age, independent of gender, up to approximately 5 years of age. Boys continue this pattern of linear pituitary growth with a slight increase in rate at puberty and into the late second decade. After age 5 years, girls demonstrate an increased rate of pituitary growth that exceeds the rate in boys and that peaks near puberty, followed by a return to the rate previously seen before age 5 years.[29,30] In adulthood, pituitary height is greatest during the third to fifth decades of life.[39] Pituitary glands are slightly larger in adult females than adult males, with this pattern persisting into later life.

Kato and coworkers studied the shape of the pituitary gland in young teenagers.[39] In the early teenage years (age 10-14), the pituitary glands of females first become convex superiorly, followed by a gradual increase in gland height that peaks approximately 10 years later. This is accompanied by an increase in intrasellar volume. In Kato and coworkers' study, superior convexity of the gland was present in more than 30% of females younger than age 10 and more than 50% of young females aged 10 to 14 years. After this peak, there is a decline in percentage of female pituitary glands with superior convexity, with 25% to 30% demonstrating a convex superior margin at ages 20 to 49 and 15% at age 50 and above. In contrast to females, superior convexity of the gland was not present in any of the males younger than the age of 20. Instead, the superior margin of the gland was relatively flat in 88% of males younger than 20 years of age. After age 20, the percentage of male pituitary glands with superior convexity was similar to that seen in females. Later in adulthood, the superior surface of the gland became more concave and gland height diminished in both genders, likely owing to ischemic degeneration of the anterior lobe of the pituitary gland.

Takano and colleagues[30] performed volumetric measurements of the posterior pituitary region in children and adolescents. They observed gradual growth in the posterior pituitary region over time, with no abrupt growth spurt in either sex. Boys demonstrated a more significant contribution of the posterior pituitary lobe to overall gland growth during the first 5 years, followed later by more balanced growth of both lobes. Alternatively, the contribution from the posterior pituitary lobe to overall gland volume in girls is less than that seen in boys. This is largely secondary to the rapid growth spurt of the anterior pituitary gland in young females during puberty. Surprisingly, however, the actual size of the posterior pituitary glands is smaller in young girls than in young boys, particularly in the age range from 5 to 9 years. One theory for this finding is that posterior gland growth is hindered by that of the more rapidly enlarging anterior gland in young females.[30]

For imaging the pituitary gland, CT has largely been replaced by MRI (Figs. 14-3, 14-11, and 14-13). However, CT remains useful for characterizing the bony anatomy in and around the sella turcica and central skull base as well as for detecting calcifications. Because the anatomy of the osseous structures is important for surgical planning, CT is useful for assessing the thickness of the bony sellar floor, the degree of pneumatization of the sphenoid bone, the attachments of the major sinus septa, the sphenoidal sinus depth, and the other surgical landmarks.

MRI (Standard, Perfusion/Diffusion, f-MRI, DTI)

At birth, the normal pituitary gland appears diffusely hyperintense on T1-weighted (T1W) images. The anterior and posterior lobes are indistinguishable. This uniform high T1 signal is believed to reflect the influence of residual maternal hormones. By age 8 to 10 weeks, the signal in the anterior gland begins to resemble the adult gland and becomes nearly isointense on all pulse sequences (Fig. 14-19).

On noncontrast T1W images, the signal intensity of the anterior lobe should be isointense to the posterior pons. However, the posterior lobe typically demonstrates high signal, the pituitary "bright spot," on noncontrast T1W images (see Fig. 14-16A and 14-19). The high signal is believed to be due to neurophysin, a carrier protein associated with vasopressin.[29] The bright spot most likely represents the more posterior aspect of the neurohypophysis, where there is a greater concentration of neurosecretory granules, so the size of the bright spot underestimates the true size of the posterior gland. Patients with diabetes insipidus often lack the posterior pituitary "bright" spot (Fig. 14-20). However, absence of the bright spot may be seen in normal patients, depending on the state of their hydration. Ectopic location of the bright spot suggests ectopic location of the posterior pituitary lobe (Fig. 14-21) but may be mimicked by a tuber cinereum lipoma (Fig. 14-22).[29] On T2-weighted (T2W) images, the posterior gland is typically hypointense.

The pituitary gland is highly vascular and lies outside the blood-brain barrier. Therefore, the anterior lobe, infundibulum, and pituitary stalk all enhance rapidly after contrast administration (see Figs. 14-14 and 14-15). Because of the special portal vascular supply to the anterior lobe, the enhancement starts at the infundibulum and spreads outward from there into the gland in a centrifugal pattern (Fig. 14-23). Enhancement is more difficult to assess in the posterior lobe, because the posterior lobe enhances more modestly, and the signal is already high on the precontrast T1W images. Areas of decreased enhancement within the anterior lobe of the pituitary gland should be regarded with suspicion, because they may represent pituitary adenomas.

The morphology of the pituitary gland changes with age and patient hormonal status in a complex fashion. Some indication of these variations has been detailed previously. Upward convexity of the superior surface of the gland may be seen in normal newborns and in early infancy owing to the effects of maternal

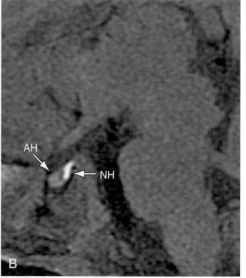

■ **FIGURE 14-19** Variable hyperintensity of the pituitary gland in the newborn. Sagittal T1W MR images. **A,** Neonate, age 4 days. The adenohypophysis (AH) is homogeneously hyperintense when compared with the posterior pons. **B,** Neonate, age 11 weeks. The adenohypophysis has become isointense to the posterior pons. In both patients, the neurohypophysis (NH) appears as a small posterior pituitary "bright" spot.

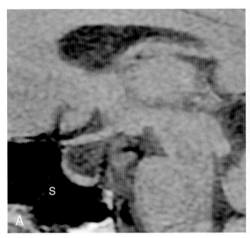

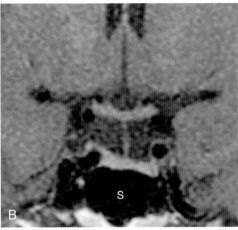

■ **FIGURE 14-20** Diabetes insipidus. Sagittal (**A**) and coronal (**B**) noncontrast T1W images through the pituitary gland in a patient with known diabetes insipidus show no normal posterior pituitary "bright" spots. The sphenoid sinus (S) shows the sellar pattern of aeration.

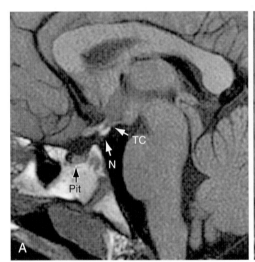

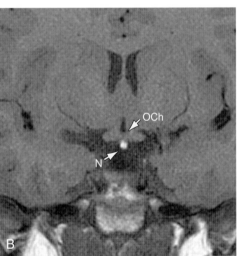

■ **FIGURE 14-21** Ectopic neurohypophysis in a young patient with growth hormone deficiency. **A,** Sagittal noncontrast T1W image through the sella turcica and pituitary gland (Pit) shows no posterior pituitary "bright spot" and no evidence of a pituitary stalk. Instead, there is a hyperintense nodule (N) immediately posterior to the thin tuber cinereum (TC). **B,** Coronal noncontrast T1W image shows the hyperintense nodule (N) just inferior to the optic chiasm (OCh).

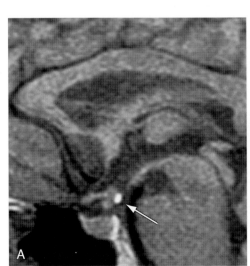

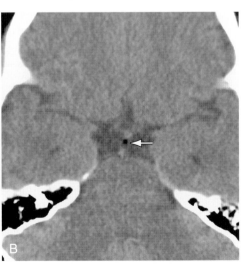

■ **FIGURE 14-22** Lipoma of the tuber cinereum mimicking an ectopic neurohypophysis. **A,** Noncontrast sagittal T1W image of the sella shows a hyperintense bright lesion immediately posterior to the tuber cinereum (*arrow*), a finding that can be seen with an ectopic neurohypophysis. **B,** Axial noncontrast CT demonstrates fat attenuation within the lesion (*arrow*), suggesting a diagnosis of lipoma of the tuber cinereum.

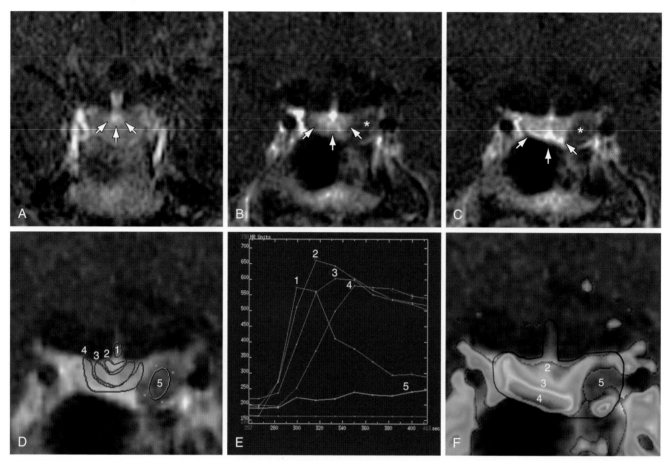

■ **FIGURE 14-23** Pituitary perfusion. **A** to **C**, Coronal contrast-enhanced T1W MR images. In sequential stages, the perfusion of the pituitary gland (*arrows*): **A**, descends the stalk to the upper central portion of the gland; **B**, passes circumferentially into the gland, and **C**, reaches to the periphery of the gland. The adenoma (*asterisk*) shows no early perfusion. **D**, Dynamic perfusion study of the pituitary gland with numbered regions of interest (1-4) drawn from the infundibulum (1) in small segments extending outward to the periphery of the normal-appearing pituitary gland (4). An additional region of interest has been placed over a nonenhancing pituitary adenoma (5). **E**, A "time-intensity curve" generated from these regions of interest demonstrates the normal, expected perfusion pattern of the pituitary gland with early enhancement of the infundibulum (1) followed by sequential enhancement of the remainder of the pituitary gland in a centrifugal pattern (2-4). The pituitary adenoma (5) shows almost no enhancement. **F**, Color map of the "mean time to enhancement" generated from the same dataset provides an alternate display of the same data. Areas in *dark blue* represent structures that enhance early (2), whereas structures that enhance after a greater delay are colored *light blue* (3), *green, yellow, orange,* and finally *red* (4). The nonenhancing pituitary adenoma shows no color, because the intensity of its enhancement falls below the threshold of detection. (*Courtesy of B. Delman, MD.*)

hormones. Upward convexity may be expected in pubertal and pregnant females but is less common in pubertal males. The normal gland may have an asymmetric shape, so it is not uncommon for coronal images to demonstrate asymmetric superior contour of the gland and eccentric insertion of the infundibulum just to one side of the midline.

When evaluating the pituitary gland, it is important to note that incidental lesions of the pituitary gland are commonly observed in asymptomatic patients. In a series of 1000 pituitary autopsies, Teramato and associates found that approximately 18% of the studied glands had incidental lesions and approximately 6% of pituitaries contained lesions larger than 2 mm, that is, large enough to visualize on imaging studies.[43] Approximately 5% of autopsied glands contained pituitary microadenomas or nodular hyperplasia, of which nearly half (2%) were larger than 2 mm. Rathke cleft cysts were found in approximately 11% of specimens, with 4% being larger than 2 mm. Other lesions, such as pituitary hemorrhage and infarcts, were less frequently encountered (Table 14-2).

The suprasellar cistern typically has the shape of a six-pointed star at the level of the cerebral peduncles and of a five-pointed star at the level of the pons (see Figs. 14-4, 14-5, 14-14, and 14-15). It contains the pituitary infundibulum centrally, the optic

TABLE 14-2. Incidental Pituitary Lesions Found at Autopsy in 1000 Pituitary Glands

Lesion Found	Total No. Found (%)	>2 mm (%)
Pituitary adenoma	31 (3.1)	18 (1.8)
Pituitary hyperplasia	20 (2)	2 (0.2)
Rathke cleft cyst	113 (11.3)	37 (3.7)
Infarct of anterior gland	6 (0.06)	2 (0.2)
Hemorrhage	6 (0.06)	2 (0.2)
Granular cell myoblastoma	1 (0.01)	unk
Nodular lymphocytic infiltration	1 (0.01)	unk

Adapted from Teramoto A, Hirakawa K, Sanno N, Osamura Y. Incidental pituitary lesions in 1,000 unselected autopsy specimens. Radiology 1994; 193:161-164.

chiasm and paired optic nerves, the cisternal portions of cranial nerves III to VI, the circle of Willis, and the inferior portion of the hypothalamus (see Figs. 14-14 to 14-16). The signal intensity of the cisterns should follow that of CSF with low signal on T1W images and high signal on T2W images. Vascular pulsations transmitted to the CSF may create areas of signal loss within these cisterns (pulsation-induced artifact). These are most apparent near areas of greatest turbulence, especially in relation to the tip of the basilar artery. Fast spin-echo sequences are more susceptible to this artifact than routine spin-echo sequences. Specific sequences may be used to display cisternal anatomy in fine detail (see Fig. 14-16). These include steady-state free precession sequences such as fast imaging employing steady-state acquisition (FIESTA) and constructive interference in steady-state (CISS) sequences.

The infundibulum should be seen to taper from its origin to its insertion into the pituitary gland and should pass immediately behind the optic chiasm in the midline (see Figs. 14-16A, B and 14-17A). On noncontrast T1W images, the stalk appears isointense to gray matter and is conspicuous as a higher signal soft tissue structure within the lower signal CSF of the cistern. The infundibulum is isointense to hypointense to brain on T2W images but is still conspicuous against the higher signal CSF within the suprasellar cistern. After administration of a contrast agent, the infundibulum enhances avidly (see Figs. 14-14 and 14-15).

The supraoptic and infundibular recesses of the third ventricle project downward into the suprasellar cistern, immediately anterior and posterior to the optic chiasm (see Fig. 14-17). In sagittal images, each recess appears as an angular, inferiorly directed extension of the third ventricle, enclosing the chiasm between them. In coronal images, the supraoptic recess takes the shape of an Erlenmeyer flask seated on the optic chiasm while the infundibular recess resembles a very sharp pencil point extending into the infundibulum just behind the chiasm. On axial images, the infundibular recess can appear as a dot or column of CSF signal situated centrally within the infundibulum (see Fig. 14-17).

The optic chiasm is situated anterior to the pituitary stalk within the anterior half of the suprasellar cistern. In axial plane, the converging prechiasmal optic nerves, the chiasm, and the diverging optic tracts take the shape of the letter X (Roman X for "deca"-ssation) (see Figs. 14-15 and 14-17). The chiasm itself may lie directly above the sella, closer to the chiasmatic sulcus (prefixed chiasm), or above the dorsum sella (postfixed chiasm). The optic tracts pass posterolaterally, hugging the anterior surfaces of the cerebral peduncles to reach the lateral geniculate nuclei (see Chapter 12). The optic nerves, chiasm, and tracts should appear isointense to white matter on T1W and T2W images and should not enhance significantly on postcontrast images. The chiasm should be smooth, sharply marginated, and biconvex in sagittal images, with the superior surface slightly more convex than the inferior surface. In coronal images the chiasm commonly appears biconcave due to the supraoptic recess above it.

Cavernous Sinuses

The cavernous sinuses should appear isointense on T1W images and mildly hyperintense on T2W images. The lateral dural wall should be concave laterally and sharply delineated from the adjacent CSF of the middle cranial fossa. The medial dural margin abuts upon the pituitary gland and is poorly resolved by MRI. The largest and most conspicuous structures within the cavernous sinuses are the cavernous segments of the internal carotid arteries. These should demonstrate the typical signal void of rapidly flowing arterial blood (see Figs. 14-13 to 14-17). The cavernous sinuses typically enhance avidly after administration of a contrast medium on both MRI and CT, allowing for better visualization of their content. On high-resolution coronal studies, the cranial nerves can often be delineated as low signal structures within the lateral walls of the cavernous sinuses.

Meckel's Cave

Meckel's cave lies just lateral to the posterior aspect of the cavernous sinus. It contains the CSF of the trigeminal cistern, the trigeminal (semilunar, gasserian) ganglion, and the central processes that arise from the ganglion. MRI displays the sensory and motor roots of the trigeminal nerve as they emerge from the lateral border of the pons, cross through the lateral pontine cistern, and pass over the petrous apex and then under the petroclinoid ligament to enter Meckel's cave (see Figs. 14-10, 14-15G, and 14-17). The large sensory root courses through Meckel's cave to form the semilunar ganglion at the inferolateral aspect of the cave. The small motor root of the trigeminal nerve passes with V$_3$ into the foramen ovale directly below Meckel's cave. The dural margins of Meckel's cave enhance on postcontrast T1W images.

BOX 14-1 Sample Report: MRI of Sella Turcica and Parasellar Region

PATIENT HISTORY

A 7-year-old boy presented with growth hormone deficiency.

COMPARISON STUDIES

No prior studies are available for comparison.

TECHNIQUE

MRI of the sella and parasellar region was performed using high-resolution noncontrast axial, sagittal, and coronal T1W and T2W pulse sequences (see Fig. 14-21). After intravenous injection of gadolinium-chelate in a dose of 0.1 mMol/kg for a total of 5 mL, contrast-enhanced T1W series were obtained in axial, coronal, and sagittal planes. Additionally, large field axial T2W and postcontrast axial T1W sequences were obtained through the whole head to display the anatomy of the brain.

FINDINGS

There is no evidence of a mass within the sella or parasellar regions. The sella turcica is hypoplastic. The pituitary gland measures 5 × 4 × 3 mm.

The pituitary stalk is not visualized. No posterior pituitary bright spot is demonstrated on the sagittal T1W sequence. A 4 × 4-mm hyperintense structure is visualized posterior to the tuber cinereum on the sagittal T1W sequence. This is compatible with an ectopic neurohypophysis. The hypothalamus is otherwise unremarkable.

The pituitary gland shows homogeneous enhancement after gadolinium administration. There is no evidence of a focal hypoenhancing mass to suggest an adenoma. The optic chiasm, carotid arteries, and anterior cerebral arteries are unremarkable. The posterior third ventricle and pineal gland are normal.

Survey of the remaining brain structures demonstrates that the ventricles and sulci are normal in size, position, and configuration for the patient's stated age. No parenchymal mass is noted. Gray and white matter appear normal. The brain stem, cerebellum, and other structures of the posterior fossa appear normal.

The visualized portions of the orbits are unremarkable.

IMPRESSION

Findings are compatible with an ectopic neurohypophysis.

KEY POINTS

- The pituitary gland lies within the sella turcica, a bony fossa situated within the sphenoid bone at the central skull base.
- CT is highly useful to display the variable pneumatization and septation of the sphenoidal sinus for presurgical planning.
- MRI displays the complex relationships of the pituitary gland, cavernous sinus, cavernous-supraclinoid segments of the internal carotid artery, and the optic apparatus for selection of surgical approach and specific presurgical planning.
- Cranial nerve VI (abducens) courses through the cavernous sinus in direct relation to the lateral wall of the cavernous carotid artery and is the only cranial nerve to run *within* the cavernous sinus.
- Cranial nerves III, IV, V1 and V2 course through the lateral wall of the cavernous sinus, not the cavity of the sinus. They are arrayed in strict order, from superior to inferior, as CN III, CN IV, CN V1, and CN V2.
- The anterior lobe of the pituitary gland occupies approximately 90% of the sellar volume. It receives its major blood supply via the hypophysial portal system, but up to one third of its supply may come through short portal veins draining from the posterior lobe. The periphery of the anterior lobe may be supplied by the inferior hypophysial artery.
- The posterior lobe is supplied by the inferior hypophysial artery.
- The veins of the anterior lobe drain into the ipsilateral cavernous sinus and petrosal veins, so detection of asymmetric concentrations of pituitary hormones in petrosal venous samples may help to lateralize otherwise-occult functioning adenomas.
- Contrast-enhanced MRI is the modality of choice for evaluating the sella turcica, the pituitary gland, and the adjoining parasellar structures.

SUGGESTED READINGS

Delman BN. Imaging of pediatric pituitary abnormalities. Endocrinol Metab Clin North Am 2009; 38:673-698.

Ghandhi CD, Christiano LD, Eloy JA, et al. The historical evolution of transsphenoidal surgery: facilitation by technological advances. Neurosurg Focus 2009; 27:E8.

Mazumdar A. Imaging of the pituitary and sella turcica. Expert Rev Anticancer Ther 2006; 6(9 Suppl):S15-S22.

Pisaneschi M, Kapoor G. Imaging of the sella and parasellar region. Neuroimaging Clin North Am 2005; 15:203-219.

Rhoton AL Jr. The sellar region. Neurosurgery 2002; 51(4 Suppl):S335-S374.

Ruscalleda J. Imaging of parasellar lesions. Eur Radiol 2005; 15:549-559.

Swallow CE, Osborn AG. Imaging of the sella and parasellar disease. Semin Ultrasound CT MRI 1998; 19:257-271.

REFERENCES

1. Tang YC, Zhao ZM, Lin XT, et al. The thin sectional anatomy of the sellar region with MRI correlation. Surg Radiol Anat 2010; 32:573-580.
2. Rennert J, Doerfler A. Imaging of sellar and parasellar lesions. Clin Neurol Neurosurg 2007; 109:111-124.
3. Destrieux C, Kakou MK, Velut S, et al. Microanatomy of the hypophysial fossa boundaries. J Neurosurg 1998; 88:743-752.
4. Rhoton AL Jr. The sellar region. Neurosurgery 2002; 51(4 Suppl):S335-S374.
5. Renn WH, Rhoton AL Jr. Microsurgical anatomy of the sellar region. J Neurosurg 1975; 43:288-298.
6. Scuderi AJ, Harnsberger HR, Boyer RS. Pneumatization of the paranasal sinuses: normal features of importance to the accurate interpretation of CT scans and MR images. AJR Am J Roentgenol 1993; 160:1101-1104.
7. Yonetsu K, Watanabe M, Nakamura T. Age-related expansion and reduction in aeration of the sphenoid sinus: volume assessment by helical CT scanning. AJNR Am J Neuroradiol 2000; 21:179-182.
8. Hamid O, El Fiky L, Hassan O, et al. Anatomic variations of the sphenoid sinus and their impact on trans-sphenoid pituitary surgery. Skull Base 2008; 18:9-15.
9. Fujioka M, Young LW. The sphenoidal sinuses: radiographic patterns of normal development and abnormal findings in infants and children. Radiology 1978; 129:133.
10. Sethi DS, Stanley RE, Pillay PK. Endoscopic anatomy of the sphenoid sinus and sella turcica. J Laryngol Otol 1995; 109:951-955.
11. Romano A, Zuccarello M, van Loveren HR, Keller JT. Expanding the boundaries of the transsphenoidal approach: a microanatomic study. Clin Anat 2001; 14:1-9.
12. Massoud AF, et al. Transsphenoidal surgery for pituitary tumours. Arch Dis Child 1997; 76:398-404.
13. Abdullah BJ, Arasaratnam S, Kumar G, Gopala K. The sphenoid sinuses: computed tomographic assessment of septation, relationship to the internal carotid. J Hong Kong Coll Radiol 2001; 4:185-188.
14. Axelsson S, Storhaug K, Kjaer I. Post-natal size and morphology of the sella turcica: longitudinal cephalometric standards for Norwegians between 6 and 21 years of age. Eur J Orthodont 2004; 26:597-604.
15. Di Chiro G, Nelson KB. The volume of the sella turcica. Am J Roentgenol Radium Ther Nucl Med 1962; 87:989-1008.
16. Melsen B. The cranial base: the postnatal development of the cranial base studied historically on human autopsy material. Acta Odontol Scand 1974; 32(Suppl 62):57-71.
17. Choi WJ, Hwang EH, Lee SR. The study of shape and size of normal sella turcica in cephalometric radiographs. Korean J Oral Maxillofac Radiol 2001; 31:43-49.
18. Israel H. Continuing growth in sella turcica with age. Am J Roentgenol Radium Ther Nucl Med 1970; 108:516-527.
19. Pisaneschi M, Kapoor G. Imaging of the sella and parasellar region. Neuroimaging Clin North Am 2005; 15:203-219.
20. Huynh-Le P, Natori Y, Sasaki T. Surgical anatomy of the anterior clinoid process. J Clin Neurosci 2004; 11:283-287.
21. Laws ER Jr, Kern EB: Complications of trans-sphenoidal surgery. Clin Neurosurg 1976; 23:401-416.
22. Rozario R, Hammerschlag SB, Post KD, et al. Diagnosis of empty sella with CT scan. Neuroradiology 1977; 13:85-88.
23. Snell RS. Clinical Anatomy for Medical Students, 3rd ed. Boston, Little, Brown, 1986.

24. Osborn AG. Diagnostic neuroradiology. St. Louis, Mosby–Year Book, 1994.

25. Rupp D, Molitch M. Pituitary stalk lesions. Curr Opin Endocrinol Diabetes Obes 2008; 15:339-345.

26. Seidel FG, Towbin R, Kaufman RA. Normal pituitary stalk size in children: CT study. Am J Roentgenol 1985; 145:1297-1302.

27. Horvath E, Kovacs K, Lloyd RV. Pars intermedia of the human pituitary revisited: morphologic aspects and frequency of hyperplasia of POMC-peptide immunoreactive cells. Endocr Pathol 1999; 10:55-64.

28. Treier M, Rosenfeld MG. The hypothalamic-pituitary axis; co-development of two organs. Curr Opin Cell Biol 1996; 8:833-843.

29. Delman BN. Imaging of pediatric pituitary abnormalities. Endocrinol Metab Clin North Am. 2009; 38:673-698.

30. Takano K, Utsunomiya H, Ono H, et al. Normal development of the pituitary gland: assessment with three-dimensional MR volumetry. AJNR Am J Neuroradiol 1999; 20:312-315.

31. Dinc H, Esen F, Demirci A, et al. Pituitary dimensions and volume measurements in pregnancy and post partum: MR assessment. Acta Radiol 1998; 39:64-69.

32. Rhoton AL Jr. Microsurgical anatomy of the region of the third ventricle. In Apuzzo MLJ (ed). Surgery of the Third Ventricle. Baltimore, Williams & Wilkins, 1987, pp 92-166.

33. Rhoton AL Jr: Anatomy of the pituitary gland and sellar region. In Thapar K, Kovacs K, Scheithauer BW, Lloyd RV (eds). Diagnosis and Management of Pituitary Tumors. Totowa, NJ, Humana Press, 2000, pp 13-40.

34. Kiortsis D, Xydis V, Drougia AG, et al. The height of the pituitary in preterm infants during the first 2 years of life: an MRI study. Neuroradiology 2004; 46:224-226.

35. Makulski DD, Taber KH, Chiou-Tan FY. Neuroimaging in posttraumatic hypopituitarism. J Comput Assist Tomogr 2008; 32:324-328.

36. Okado N, Yokota N. Axoglial synaptoid contacts in the neural lobe of the human fetus, Anat Rec 1982; 202:117-124.

37. Jehle S, Walsh JE, Freda PU, Post KD. Selective use of bilateral inferior petrosal sinus sampling in patients with adrenocorticotropin-dependent Cushing's syndrome prior to transsphenoidal surgery. J Clin Endocrinol Metab 2008; 93:4624-4632.

38. Young B, Heath JW. Wheater's Functional Histology, 4th ed. Philadelphia, Elsevier–Churchill Livingstone, 2000.

39. Kato K, et al. Morphological changes on MR imaging of the normal pituitary gland related to age and sex: main emphasis on pubescent females. J Clin Neurosci 2002; 9:53-56.

40. Elster AD, Chen MY, Williams DW, Key LL. Pituitary gland: MR imaging of physiologic hypertrophy in adolescence. Radiology 1990; 174:681-685.

41. Konishi Y, Kuriyama M, Sudo M, et al. Growth patterns of the normal pituitary gland and in pituitary adenoma. Dev Med Child Neurol 1990; 32:69-73.

42. Doraiswamy PM, Potts JM, Figiel GS, et al. MR imaging of physiologic pituitary gland hypertrophy in adolescence. Radiology 1991; 178:284-285.

43. Teramoto A, Hirakawa K, Sanno N, Osamura Y. Incidental pituitary lesions in 1,000 unselected autopsy specimens. Radiology 1994; 193:161-164.

Infratentorial Brain

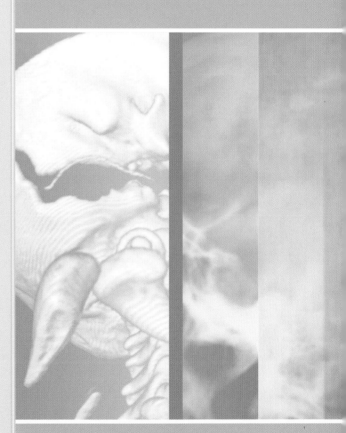

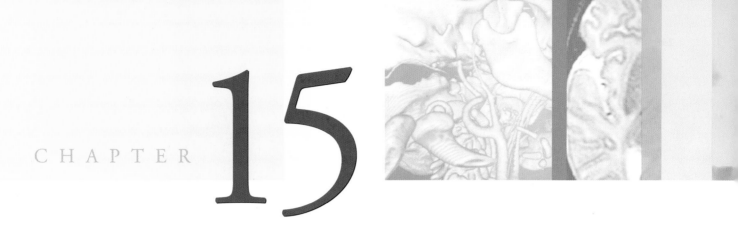

CHAPTER 15

Brain Stem

Thomas P. Naidich, Bradley N. Delman, Mary Elizabeth Fowkes, Mark E. Smethurst, Jonathan D. Steinberger, Amish H. Doshi, Cheuk Ying Tang, and Pedro Pasik

The brain stem is the narrow length of tissue that interconnects the spinal cord caudally with the brain rostrally.[1-8] As such it extends from the transverse plane just caudal to the pyramidal decussation to the transverse plane just rostral to the superior colliculi.

Common terms and synonyms used throughout this discussion include the following:

Basis: the most ventral lamina of the full brain stem
  Basis medullae: the pyramids of the medulla
  Basis pontis: the portion of the pons ventral to the medial lemnisci
  Basis mesencephali: the portion of the mesencephalon ventral to the anterior border of the substantia nigra (i.e., the paired crura cerebrorum)
Brain: the portion of the central nervous system rostral to the midbrain (i.e., the diencephalon and telencephalon)
Cerebellar peduncles
  Inferior cerebellar peduncle (restiform body): the interconnection of the medulla with the cerebellum
  Middle cerebellar peduncle (brachium pontis): the interconnection of the pons with the cerebellum
  Superior cerebellar peduncle (brachium conjunctivum): the interconnection of the midbrain with the diencephalon and the cerebellum
Cerebral peduncles: Classically, the terms *left and right cerebral peduncles* signify all of the midbrain ventral to the cerebral aqueduct. On each side, a curved line drawn along the anterior surface of the substantia nigra subdivides the cerebral peduncle into a ventral crus cerebrorum and a dorsal tegmentum. As a consequence, the two crura cerebrorum form paired structures situated to each side of the interpeduncular fossa, while the tegmentum of the midbrain forms a single, bilaterally symmetric structure situated dorsal to the crura and ventral to the aqueduct. Presently, the term *cerebral peduncle* is most often used to indicate the crus cerebri.
Comb system: the bundles of striatal and pallidal fibers passing through the internal capsule
Corticobulbar: This term refers to fibers that descend from the cerebral cortex to any portion of the brain stem (not just the medulla). It derives from the old term *bulb* previously used to indicate the entire brain stem.

Crus (crura) cerebrorum: the most ventral portion of the midbrain ventral to the anterior border of the substantia nigra and lateral to the interpeduncular fossa
Lemniscal arc: This term is used to describe the group of ascending axons that, in aggregate, form the paired, transverse arches of white matter in the upper pons and midbrain. The structures of the lemniscal arc include the paired medial lemnisci medially, the paired lateral lemnisci laterally, and the paired spinothalamic tracts (spinal lemnisci) that angle over from lateral to medial as they ascend through the brain stem.
Sensory neurons: primary and secondary (relay). Each primary sensory neuron has (1) a peripheral process that extends to peripherally situated sensory endings, (2) a cell body that lies within the dorsal root ganglion or sensory ganglion related to a cranial nerve, and (3) a central process that enters the central nervous system via spinal or cranial nerves to synapse on second order neurons within the CNS. Secondary sensory (relay) neurons then receive the sensory data from the primary neuron and convey it onward to tertiary neurons and beyond.[8]
Tectum: the dorsal lamina of the midbrain situated dorsal to the aqueduct
Tegmentum: the middle lamina of the full brain stem situated between the basis ventrally and the aqueduct-fourth ventricle dorsally
Trapezoid body: the bundle of transverse fibers in the tegmentum of the pons that conveys auditory information bilaterally

ANATOMY
Longitudinal Divisions
From caudal to cranial, the brain stem is divided into three parts: the medulla oblongata inferiorly, the pons varolii in the middle, and the mesencephalon (midbrain) rostrally (Figs. 15-1 to 15-4). The caudal border of the medulla is a transverse plane situated just caudal to the decussation of the pyramids.[4] The rostral border of the medulla and caudal border of the pons is the pontomedullary sulcus (ventrally) and the striae medullares at the floor of the fourth ventricle (dorsally). The rostral border of the pons and caudal border of the midbrain is the pontomesencephalic sulcus ventrally and a line drawn just inferior to the inferior colliculi dorsally. The rostral border of the mesencephalon and caudal border of the diencephalon

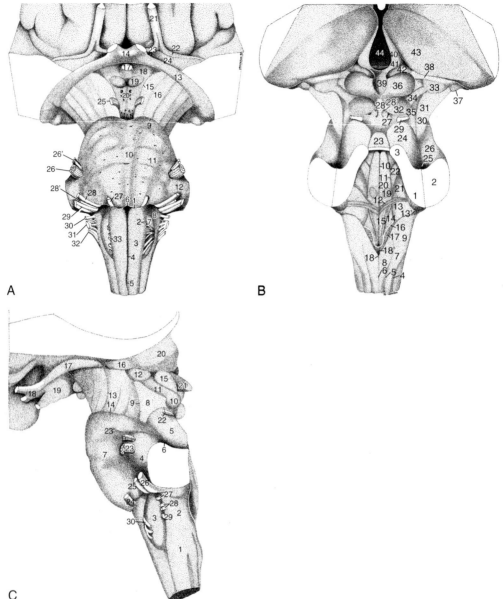

■ **FIGURE 15-1** Surface of the brain stem and cranial nerves. Diagrammatic representations. **A,** Ventral view. **B,** Dorsal view, **C,** Lateral view with anterior to the reader's left. **A,** Ventrally, the medulla is separated from the pons by the pontomedullary sulcus (1). The anterior median medullary sulcus (4) ascends between the paired medullary pyramids (3) to end superiorly at the foramen cecum (midline portion (6) of pontomedullary sulcus). Inferiorly, the anterior median sulcus shows a deflection (5) that indicates the site of the decussation of the pyramids. Laterally, the image displays the pyramids of the medulla (3), the preolivary sulcus (2) with the emerging rootlets of the hypoglossal nerve (CN XII), the olive (7), the supraolivary fossette (8), and the retro-olivary sulcus with the emerging rootlets of the glossopharyngeal, vagus and accessory nerves (CN IX, X, and medullary portion of XI). The pons is delimited inferiorly by the pontomedullary sulcus (1) and superiorly by the pontomesencephalic sulcus (9). The ventral aspect of the pons displays the median pontine sulcus (10), the transversely ridged "belly" of the pons (11), and the ventral aspect of the middle cerebellar peduncle (brachium pontis) (12). The abducens nerves (CN VI) (27) emerge from the pontomedullary sulcus 1 to 2 cm lateral to the midline. The facial and vestibulocochlear nerves (CN VII and VIII) (28 and 29) and the nervus intermedius (28') emerge from the lateral aspect of the supraolivary fossette just inferior to the middle cerebellar peduncles. The smaller motor (26') and larger sensory (26) roots of the trigeminal nerve emerge from the lateral aspect of the mid pons. The midbrain (mesencephalon) is delimited inferiorly by the pontomesencephalic sulcus (9) and superiorly by the inferior borders of the optic tract (13) and chiasm (14) and by the medial mesencephalic sulcus (15). The ventral aspect of the midbrain displays the crus cerebri (16) to each side of the interpeduncular fossa, and the oculomotor nerves (CN III) (25) emerging into the interpeduncular fossa from the medial aspects of each crus cerebri. The pituitary stalk (17), tuber cinereum (18), and mammillary bodies (19), of the hypothalamus of the diencephalon project inferiorly into the interpeduncular fossa but are not part of the brain stem. Laterally, the medial and lateral geniculate bodies project ventrolaterally from the thalamus (33 and 37 in **B**). **B,** Dorsally, the brain stem shows the rhomboid (diamond) shape of the fourth ventricle and the transversely oriented striae medullares (12) that subdivide that diamond into an inferior medullary triangle and a superior pontine triangle. The floor of the fourth ventricle shows the vertical median sulcus and the paired paramedian sulci limitantes (10 and 11) that flank the midline. The obex (18) lies at the inferior point of the fourth ventricle. The superior medullary velum forms the roof of the upper triangle. The lateral walls of the inferior fourth ventricle are formed by the inferior cerebellar peduncles (9). The lateral walls of the superior triangle are formed by the superior cerebellar peduncles (3). The middle cerebellar peduncles lie lateral to both the inferior and the superior cerebellar peduncles and do not contribute directly to the walls of the fourth ventricle. Further laterally, the groove (depression) between the superior and middle cerebellar peduncles is the parabrachial recess (25). *Medulla.* The medulla displays a "closed" portion situated inferior to the fourth ventricle and an "open" portion underlying the lower, medullary triangle of the fourth ventricle. The dorsal surface of the closed medulla shows the posterior median medullary sulcus (6), the paired posterior intermediate medullary sulci (5) and the posterolateral medullary sulci (4). The

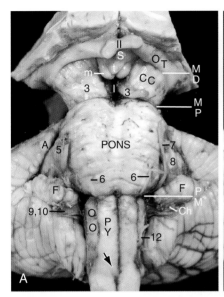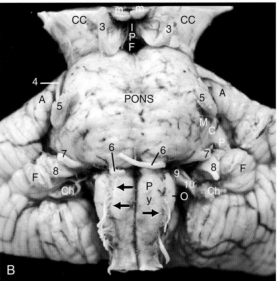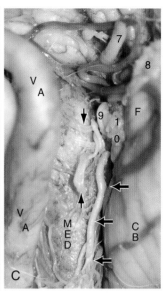

■ **FIGURE 15-2** Surface of the brain stem and cranial nerves. Three specimens. **A** and **B,** Ventral surfaces of two gross specimens after removal of the arachnoid and blood vessels. Ventrally, the mesodiencephalic junction (MD) is the lower margin of the optic chiasm and optic tract. The mesopontine junction (MP) is the curved pontomesencephalic sulcus. The pontomedullary junction (PM) is the curved pontomedullary sulcus. *Midbrain.* The midbrain gives rise to two cranial nerves. CN III (3) exits the brain surface at the medial aspect of the crus cerebri (CC) and traverses the interpeduncular fossa (I, IPF) en route to the lateral dural wall of the cavernous sinus. CN IV (4) exits the brain surface contralateral to its nucleus of origin, emerges just inferior to the inferior colliculus (see Fig. 15-3B), and courses around the midbrain to enter the lateral dural wall of the cavernous sinus immediately inferior to CN III. In this specimen, the cut anterior end of CN IV has fallen over the upper pons and trigeminal nerve (5). m, paired mammillary bodies. *Pons.* The pons gives rise to four cranial nerves. CN V (5) crosses the dorsal brain surface at the upper lateral pons just anterior, inferior and medial to the overhanging anterior angle (A) of the cerebellum. CN VI (6) exits the brain surface at the pontomedullary sulcus, 1 to 2 cm lateral to the midline, courses anteriorly, superiorly, and slightly laterally to exit the skull via Dorello's canal through the clivus. The arrow indicates the decussation of the pyramids. In **B,** the cut ends of CN VI have fallen to overlie the pontomedullary sulcus. CN VII (7) and CN VIII (8) cross the brain surface within the supraolivary fossette just superior to the upper pole of the inferior olive (O), just inferior to the middle cerebellar peduncle (MCP), and just ventromedial to the flocculus (F). These nerves exit the skull through the internal auditory canals. *Medulla.* The medulla gives rise to four cranial nerves. Cranial nerve IX (9) and cranial nerve X (10) cross the brain surface at the retro-olivary sulcus, dorsal to the olive (O), and traverse the jugular fossa to their distal innervations. CN XI (not labeled) crosses the brain surface at the medulla (medullary root) and at the lateral surface of the cervical spinal cord (spinal accessory root) and traverses the jugular fossa to its distal innervations. The rootlets (12, *black arrows* in **B**) of cranial nerve XII cross the brain surface at the preolivary sulcus, ventral to the olive (O), and exit the skull base via the hypoglossal canal. **C,** Coned-down lateral view. From ventral to dorsal, the vertebral artery (VA), medulla (MED), and the cerebellum (CB) form parallel vertical columns. The spinal accessory nerve (CN XI) (*horizontal black arrows*) ascends along the lateral surface of the medulla caudal to, and in line with, the rootlets of the glossopharyngeal (9) and vagal (10) nerves. The rootlets of the hypoglossal nerve (*vertical black arrows*) lie ventrally. The intervening olive is largely obscured by the nerve roots. As in **A,** the facial (CN VII) (7) and vestibulocochlear (CN VIII) (8) nerves emerge from the supraolivary fossette just below the middle cerebellar peduncle and just superior and ventral to the flocculus (F).

fasciculus gracilis ascends to the nucleus gracilis (8) just to each side of the median sulcus. The dorsal bulge caused by the gracile nucleus is designated the clava. The fasciculus cuneatus ascends to the nucleus cuneatus (7) between the posterior intermediate and posterolateral medullary sulci just lateral to the fasciculus and nucleus gracilis on each side. The dorsal surface of the rostral open medulla displays the hypoglossal trigone (15) medially, the vagal trigone (14) more centrally, and the medullary vestibular area (13) laterally. *Pons.* The dorsal surface of the pons forms the upper triangle of the floor of the fourth ventricle. Medially, it displays the median eminence (20) and the facial colliculus (19) that marks the site where the fibers of the facial nerve (CN VII) curve dorsal to the nucleus for the abducens nerve (CN VI). Superolaterally the trigeminal fovea (superior fovea) (22) marks the site of the underlying principal sensory and motor nuclei of the trigeminal nerve. The pontine vestibular area (21) lies far laterally at the lateral angle of the diamond. The dorsal cochlear nucleus (13') forms the acoustic tubercle (13') at the dorsal aspect of the inferior cerebellar peduncle. *Midbrain.* The superior (36) and inferior (32) colliculi take the shape of a butterfly with wider upper than lower wings. The cruciate sulcus is formed by a vertical arm that runs in the midline between the left and right colliculi and a horizontal arm that runs transversely between the superior and the inferior colliculi. The infracollicular sulcus delimits the inferior borders of the inferior colliculi. Inferior to the inferior colliculi, the frenulum veli acts as a midline suspensory ligament to elevate the superior medullary velum (23) over the fourth ventricle. Laterally, on each side, the brachium (34) of the inferior colliculus ascends to the medial geniculate body (33). The brachium (38) of the superior colliculus ascends over the medial geniculate body to connect with the optic tract, bypassing the lateral geniculate body (37). The lateral mesencephalic sulcus (30) delimits the dorsal edge of the crus cerebri (31). The trochlear nerves (CN IV) (29) emerge from the dorsal surface of the midbrain just inferior to the inferior colliculi, to each side of the frenulum veli. The pretectum (42), the pineal gland, the habenular trigones (41), and the striae medullares thalami (40) lie superior to the superior colliculi. **C,** Laterally, the medulla displays the lateral aspect of the pyramid ventrally, the hypoglossal rootlets (30) emerging from the pre-olivary sulcus, the olive (3), the rootlets of CN IX, X, and medullary XI (27, 28, and 29) emerging from the retro-olivary sulcus, the inferior cerebellar peduncle (2), and the lateral medullary funiculus (1). The rootlets of the abducens nerve (CN VI) (24), the facial nerve (CN VII) (25) and the vestibulocochlear nerve (CN VIII) (26) emerge along the pontomedullary sulcus in a line from paramedian (CN VI) into the supraolivary fossette (CN VII and VIII). The pons displays the profile of the belly of the pons, the rootlets of the motor (23') and sensory (23) fibers of CN V, the middle cerebellar peduncle (4), the parabrachial recess (6), and the superior cerebellar peduncle (5). The midbrain displays the lateral aspect of the crus cerebri (13), the lateral mesencephalic sulcus (9), the lateral aspect of the midbrain (8) behind the crus, the superior cerebellar peduncle (5), the lateral aspects of the inferior colliculus (10) and its brachium (11), the superior colliculus (15), and the rootlets of CN IV (22) passing from the infracollicular groove around the lateral aspect of the mesencephalon. The optic chiasm (18), optic tract (17), lateral geniculate body (16), medial geniculate body (12), pineal gland (21), and thalamus (20) overhang the midbrain. *(Modified from Naidich TP, Duvernoy HM, Delman BN, et al. Duvernoy's Atlas of the Human Brain Stem and Cerebellum: High-Field MRI, Surface Anatomy, Internal Structure, Vascularization and 3D Sectional Anatomy. New York, Springer, 2008.)*

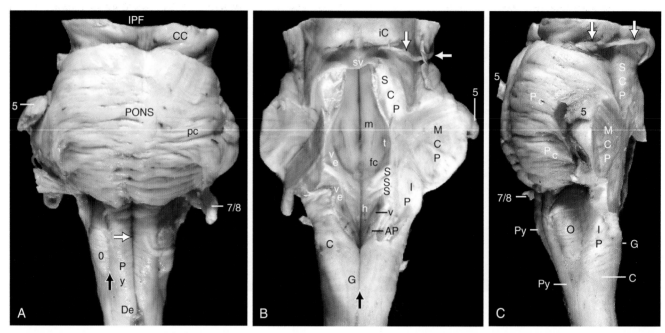

■ **FIGURE 15-3** Gross anatomy of the brain stem. Cleaned ventral (**A**), dorsal (**B**) and lateral (**C**) surfaces of the medulla, pons, and inferior portion of midbrain, after removal of the arachnoid and blood vessels. The cerebellum was resected by sectioning the inferior (IP), middle (MCP), and superior (SCP) cerebellar peduncles. **A,** The ventral surface displays the anterior median medullary sulcus (*white arrow*), the paired medullary pyramids (Py) that flank the sulcus, the decussation (De) of the pyramids, the preolivary sulcus (*black arrow*), the olive (O), and the transversely oriented pontocerebellar fibers (pc) that give the pons its corrugated appearance. The facial (CN VII) (7) and vestibulocochlear (CN III) (8) nerves arise from the lateral portion of the pontomedullary junction. The trigeminal nerves (CN V) (5) arise from the lateral surface of the upper pons. A very small segment of the upper midbrain is seen superiorly, including parts of the crura cerebrorum (CC) and the interpeduncular fossa (IPF). **B,** The dorsal surface displays the rhomboid (diamond) shape of the fourth ventricle, the prominent midline median sulcus, and the transversely oriented striae medullares (S,S,S). The striae divide the floor of the fourth ventricle into a lower medullary triangle situated inferior to the striae and an upper pontine triangle situated superior to the striae. The lateral walls of the lower fourth ventricle are formed by the inferior cerebellar peduncles (IP). The lateral walls of the upper fourth ventricle are formed by the superior cerebellar peduncles (SCP). The middle cerebellar peduncles (MCP) lie lateral to both the ICP and the SCP, so they do not form part of lateral walls of the fourth ventricle. The medulla displays two portions: a closed lower portion of the medulla situated inferior to the fourth ventricle and an open upper portion of the medulla situated ventral to the medullary triangle of the fourth ventricle. The posterior median medullary sulcus (*vertical black arrow*) and the flanking fasciculi and nuclei graciles (G) terminate at the lower margin of the fourth ventricle medially. The paired fasciculi and nuclei cuneati (C) lie lateral to the gracilis, so they must ascend higher to terminate at the lower lateral border of the fourth ventricle. The floor of the medullary triangle displays a median sulcus, paired inferomedial hypoglossal trigones (h) marking the hypoglossal nuclei, and paired superolateral vagal trigones (v) marking the dorsal vagal nuclei. The area postrema (AP) lies caudal to the vagal trigone. At the pontine triangle, the floor of the fourth ventricle displays the paired medullary eminences (m) to each side of the median sulcus, the prominent hillocks of the facial colliculi (fc), at the lower ends of the medullary eminences, and the slight depressions of the foveae trigeminales (t) that mark the motor and principal sensory trigeminal nuclei on each side. The lateral angles of the fourth ventricle are occupied by broad vestibular areas (ve) that extend through both the medullary and the pontine triangles. **C,** The lateral surface of the brain stem is oriented with the ventral side to the reader's left. The medulla shows the pyramids (Py) ventrally, the olive (O) laterally, and the inferior cerebellar peduncle (IP), fasciculus cuneatus (C), and fasciculus gracilis (G) dorsally. Cranial nerves VII and VIII (7/8), V (5), and IV (*white arrows* in **B** and **C**), the middle cerebellar peduncle (MCP), and the superior cerebellar peduncle (SCP) are also labeled.

■ **FIGURE 15-4** Posterior superior view of the midbrain and diencephalon. The quadrigeminal plate (tectum) of the midbrain displays the "butterfly" pattern of the paired superior colliculi (sC) extending farther laterally than do the inferior colliculi (iC). The lateral lemnisci (LL) form the lateral border of the midbrain as they ascend to the inferior colliculi. The brachium of the inferior colliculus (bi) courses to the medial geniculate body (MG). The brachium of the superior colliculus (bs) leads over the medial geniculate body to carry fibers from the optic tract directly to the superior colliculus, bypassing the lateral geniculate body (LG). The frenulum veli (*black arrow*) originates between the two inferior colliculi and inserts like a suspensory ligament into the upper surface of the superior medullary velum. The trochlear nerves (avulsed from this specimen) emerge (*thin white arrow*) from the superior medullary velum just inferior to the inferior colliculi and just lateral to the frenulum veli. The pineal gland (P) overlies the vertical groove between the two superior colliculi. The habenular trigones (H) lie to each side of the posterior third ventricle (3) just anterior to the pineal gland. The large white arrow indicates the posterolateral margin of the crus cerebri.

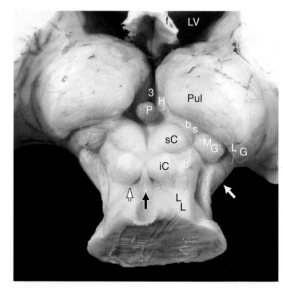

is the line drawn along the medial mesencephalic sulcus and the inferior margins of the optic chiasm and tract (ventrally) and the posterior commissure (dorsally).[4]

Anteroposterior Divisions

From ventral to dorsal, the brain stem is also divided into three major layers (laminae, lamellae): the basis, the tegmentum, and the tectum.

The *basis* is the most ventral lamina of the brain stem and runs its full length (see Figs. 15-1 and 15-5).[7] The basis mesencephali is the portion of midbrain ventral to the substantia nigra (i.e., the paired crura cerebrorum). The basis pontis is the portion of the pons ventral to the medial lemnisci. The basis medullae is the portion of the medulla formed by the pyramids.

The *tegmentum* is the middle lamina of the brain stem and also runs its full length. The tegmentum is situated between the basis ventrally and the aqueduct and fourth ventricle dorsally. The tegmentum of the midbrain is defined as the portion of the midbrain between the crura cerebrorum ventrally and the aqueduct dorsally. The tegmentum of the pons is defined as the portion of the pons situated between the medial lemnisci ventrally and the floor of the fourth ventricle. The tegmentum of the medulla is taken to be all of the medulla situated dorsal to the pyramids. The tegmental layer is further subdivided into ventral and dorsal sublaminae. The ventral sublamina contains the supplementary motor nuclei, including the red nuclei and substantia nigra of the midbrain and the inferior olivary nuclei of the medulla. The dorsal sublamina contains multiple cranial nerve nuclei, with the special visceral efferent nuclei situated more ventrally and the general somatic motor and sensory nuclei situated more dorsally (Fig. 15-6). The ventral and lateral portions of the tegmentum also contain the sensory tracts (lemnisci) that ascend to the thalami. The remainder of the tegmentum is occupied by the reticular formation and chemically defined cell groups that produce acetylcholine, norepinephrine, serotonin, and dopamine.

The *tectum* is the dorsal lamina of the midbrain situated dorsal to the aqueduct. This lamina does *not* extend the full length of the brain stem. As such, the term *tectum* is most often used as a synonym for *quadrigeminal plate* and refers only to the paired superior and inferior colliculi of the midbrain.

Surface Anatomy
Medulla
Ventral Surface

From medial to lateral on each side, the ventral surface of the medulla displays the anterior median medullary sulcus in the midline, the paired pyramids that flank that sulcus, the paired anterolateral (preolivary) medullary sulci from which the hypoglossal (CN XII) nerve fascicles emerge, the ventral surfaces of the two olives, the paired retro-olivary sulci (lateral fossae of the medulla) from which the fascicles of the glossopharyngeal, vagal, and accessory (CN IX, X, and medullary portion of the XI) nerves emerge, and the ventral surfaces of the two inferior cerebellar peduncles (see Figs. 15-1, 15-2A, and 15-3A).

Lateral Surfaces

From ventral to dorsal on each side, the lateral surface of the medulla displays the lateral aspect of the pyramid, the fascicles of the hypoglossal nerves emerging at the preolivary sulcus, the olive, the retro-olivary sulcus (lateral fossa of the medulla), the supraolivary fossette immediately rostral to the olive and inferior to the middle cerebellar peduncle, the fascicles of CN IX, X, and XI emerging at the retro-olivary sulcus, and the inferior cerebellar peduncle. The lateral funiculus of the spinal cord ascends to join the medulla just behind the olive (see Figs. 15-1, 15-2B, and 15-3C).

Dorsal Surface

The dorsal surface of the medulla is divided into a caudal "closed" portion in which the central canal is covered over as it is in the spinal cord, and a rostral "open" portion in which the central canal opens out into the floor of the fourth ventricle. In the caudal closed portion of the medulla, from medial to lateral on each side, the dorsal surface displays the posterior median medullary sulcus, the paired fasciculi graciles that terminate in the paired gracile tubercles (clavae), the paired posterior intermediate medullary sulci, the fasciculi cuneati that terminate superiorly in the paired cuneate tubercles, the paired posterolateral medullary sulci, and the dorsal surfaces of the two inferior cerebellar peduncles. In the open rostral portion of the medulla, from medial to lateral, the dorsal surface displays the median sulcus, the paired hypoglossal trigones, the paired sulci limitantes, the paired dorsal vagal trigones, the medullary vestibular areas containing portions of the medial and inferior vestibular nuclei,[4] and the dorsal aspects of the inferior cerebellar peduncles. The area postrema lies just inferior to the vagal trigone on each side. At the caudal point of the fourth ventricle, the two inferior cerebellar peduncles converge together, creating a shape descriptively termed *calamus scriptorius* for its resemblance to the sharp cut end of an antique goose quill pen. At this point, the obex of the fourth ventricle leads into the cephalic end of the central canal of the closed portion of the medulla (see Figs. 15-1 and 15-3B).

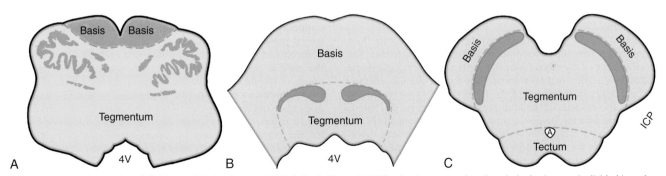

■ **FIGURE 15-5** Ventrodorsal divisions of the brainstem. **A,** Medulla. **B,** Pons. **C,** Midbrain. From ventral to dorsal, the brain stem is divided into three laminae: the basis, the tegmentum, and the tectum. The demarcation between the basis and the tegmentum is the dorsal border of the pyramids (*red*) in the medulla, the ventral surface of the medial lemnisci (*red*) in the pons, and the ventral surface of the substantia nigra (*red*) in the midbrain. The line of demarcation between the tegmentum and the tectum is the ventral aspect of the aqueduct of Sylvius in the midbrain. The medulla and pons have no tectum. 4V, fourth ventricle. In **A,** the inferior and dorsal accessory olivary nuclei are drawn in to give the tegmentum perspective.

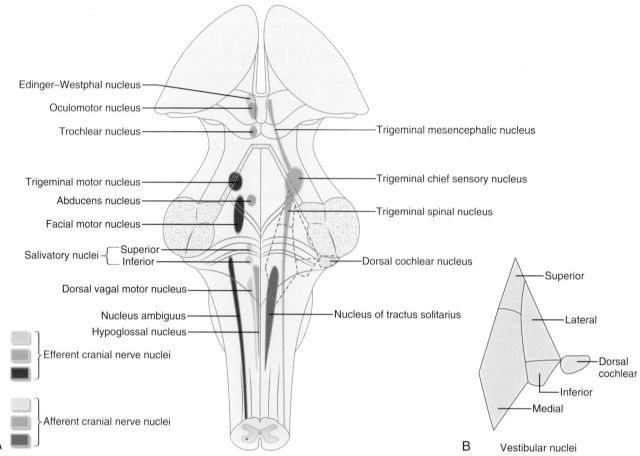

■ **FIGURE 15-6**   Cranial nerve nuclei of the brain stem. Projection of the nuclei onto a dorsal schematic of the brain stem. *(From Standring S [ed]. Gray's Anatomy: The Anatomical Basis of Clinical Practice, 40th ed. Philadelphia, Elsevier, 2008.)*

Pons

Ventrolateral Surface

The curved anterolateral surface of the pons has no distinct ventral or lateral border, so these surfaces are considered together. From medial to lateral on each side, the ventrolateral surface of the pons displays the shallow median pontine sulcus, the horizontally ridged belly of the pons leading directly into the middle cerebellar peduncles, the fascicles of the abducens (CN VI) nerve that exit at the pontomedullary sulcus 1 to 2 cm lateral to the median sulcus, and the fascicles of the facial (CN VII) and vestibulocochlear (CN VIII) nerves that arise at the lateral aspect of the pontomedullary sulcus in the supraolivary fossette (see Figs. 15-1 to 15-3).

Dorsal Surface

The dorsal surface of the pons forms the rostral half of the floor of the fourth ventricle. From medial to lateral on each side, the dorsal surface of the pons (floor of fourth ventricle) displays the median sulcus; the medial eminence; the facial colliculus formed by the passage of the fibers of the facial (CN VII) nerve around and over the nucleus of the abducens (CN VI) nerve; the sulcus limitans; the pontine vestibular area that contains portions of the medial, lateral, and superior vestibular nuclei; the acoustic tubercle that marks the site of the dorsal cochlear nucleus; the trigeminal trigone that marks the site of the principal sensory and motor nuclei of the trigeminal nerve; the dorsal surface of the superior cerebellar peduncle; the parabrachial recess situated between the superior and middle cerebellar peduncles; and the middle cerebellar peduncle most laterally (see Figs. 15-1 and 15-3B).

Mesencephalon (Midbrain)

Ventral Surface

From medial to lateral on each side, the ventral surface of the midbrain displays the median interpeduncular fossa, the fascicles of the oculomotor (CN III) nerve that emerge into the interpeduncular fossa from the medial aspect of each crus cerebri, and the flanking crura cerebrorum. Diencephalic structures seen between the two crura include the paired mammillary bodies, the tuber cinereum, and the pituitary stalk. These hang down into the interpeduncular fossa, but, anatomically, lie outside the confines of the midbrain (see Fig. 15-1).

Lateral Surface

From ventral to dorsal on each side, the lateral surface of the midbrain displays the lateral surface of the crus cerebri, the lateral mesencephalic sulcus, the lateral aspect of the inferior colliculus, the brachium of the inferior colliculus that leads to the medial geniculate body, the superior colliculus, the brachium of the superior colliculus that carries fibers from the optic tract directly to the superior colliculus, bypassing the lateral geniculate nucleus, the exit of the trochlear (CN IV) nerve from the superior medullary velum just caudal to the inferior colliculus, the frenulum veli, and the superior cerebellar peduncle. The pineal gland of the diencephalon overhangs the superior colliculi (see Fig. 15-1).

Dorsal Surface

The dorsal surface of the mesencephalon displays the vertical and horizontal portions of the cruciate intercollicular sulcus, the horizontal infracollicular sulcus caudal to the paired inferior colliculi, the median frenulum veli, the paired superior colliculi, the brachia of the superior colliculi that convey fibers of the optic tract around the lateral geniculate bodies to reach the superior colliculi, the paired inferior colliculi, the brachia of the inferior colliculi that extend to the medial geniculate bodies, the exits of the trochlear (CN IV) nerves just inferior to each inferior colliculus and lateral to the frenulum veli, and the paired lateral mesencephalic sulci (see Figs. 15-1 and 15-4).

Midsagittal Section through the Brain Stem

The midsagittal section through the brain stem displays the central anatomy of the brain stem and the relationship of the brain stem to the cerebellum dorsally and the diencephalon rostrally (see Figs. 15-1 and 15-7). The ventral surface of the brain stem displays the gentle, ventrally directed convexity of the medulla, the inscription point or "notch" at the pontomedullary sulcus, the prominent rounded "belly" of the pons, and the characteristic "7" shape of the interpeduncular fossa of the midbrain. The mammillary bodies of the hypothalamus hang downward into the uppermost portion of the interpeduncular fossa.

Farther dorsally, the smooth dorsal convexity of the aqueduct leads downward, along the gentle dorsal concavity of the floor of the fourth ventricle, to the obex, and, via the obex, into the central canal of the closed portion of the medulla. Most dorsally, the superior and inferior colliculi form the roof (tectum) of the midbrain. The fasciculus gracilis of the medulla terminates superiorly at the nucleus gracilis (clava) just behind the obex.

In parasagittal sections, the medulla displays the pyramid and the start of the pyramidal decussation (see Figs. 15-1 and 15-7). The pons displays the pontine nuclei, the medial lemnisci, the median longitudinal fasciculus, and the penetrating paramedian perforating vessels. The midbrain displays the decussation of the superior cerebellar peduncles and the upper portion of the medial longitudinal fasciculus.

Selected Gross Axial Sections

Gross axial sections display the changing contours of the brain stem, the changing proportions of the basis, tegmentum, and tectum in each portion, and the gross features of the major ascending and descending fiber tracts, gray nuclei, and cranial

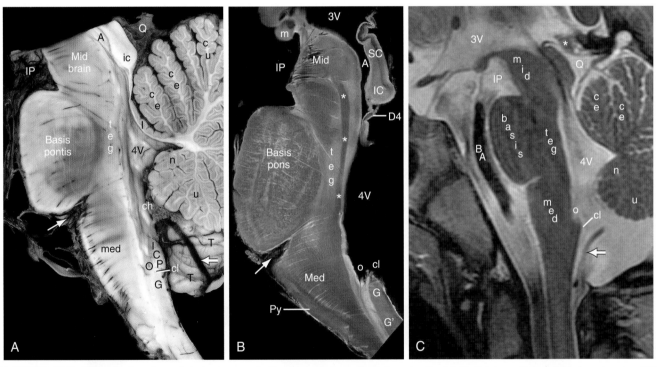

■ **FIGURE 15-7** Midsagittal sections of the brain stem. **A,** Gross anatomic specimen (see also Fig. 16-4). **B,** Intermediate-weighted postmortem MR image of the brain stem at 9.4 T (composite image). **C,** Clinical image at 1.5 T. Note the oblique, curved course of the multiple small vessels that penetrate the ventral aspect of the brain stem. BA, basilar artery traversing the prepontine cistern. *Midbrain.* The midbrain (mid) shows the characteristic shape of the interpeduncular fossa (IP) ventrally, the aqueduct (A) more dorsally, the superior colliculus (sc) and inferior colliculus (ic) of the quadrigeminal plate (tectum) at the dorsal surface of the brain stem, the quadrigeminal plate cistern (Q) behind the colliculi, and the pineal gland (*asterisk* in C) that projects into the quadrigeminal plate cistern. In **B,** the decussation (D4) of the trochlear nerve fascicles appears as a well-defined low signal fiber bundle in the superior medullary velum of the fourth ventricle. The mammillary bodies (m) of the hypothalamus overhang the interpeduncular fossa, contributing to its shape. 3V, third ventricle. *Pons.* The pons shows the prominent ovoid "belly" formed by the basis pontis, the tegmentum (teg) of the pons situated between the basis pontis and the floor of the upper portion of the fourth ventricle (4V), and the well-defined upper portion of the medial longitudinal fasciculus (*white asterisks* in **B**) that extends between the abducens (CN VI) and oculomotor (CN III) nerve nuclei. *Medulla.* The curved pontomedullary sulcus (*oblique white arrow* in **A** and **B**) delimits the pons from the medulla. The prominent ventral bulge of the basis pontis ("belly" of the pons) is formed by the transversely oriented pontocerebellar fibers. The gently convex curvature of the basis medullae is formed by the pyramids (Py). The dorsal surface of the upper medulla forms the lower half of the floor of the fourth ventricle as far inferiorly as the obex (o). The dorsal surface of the lower closed medulla lies inferior to the fourth ventricle. The fasciculus gracilis (G') ascends along the dorsal surface of the lower medulla to terminate at the nucleus gracilis (G). The upper pole of the nucleus gracilis forms a dorsal eminence designated the clava (cl). The inferior cerebellar peduncle (ICP) forms the lateral wall of the lower fourth ventricle as it passes superiorly and laterally into the cerebellum. *Cerebellum.* Behind the brain stem lie the choroid plexus (ch) of the fourth ventricle; the lingula (l) of the vermis attached to the superior medullary velum; the central lobule (ce) and culmen (cu) of the superior vermis; the nodulus (n) and uvula (u) of the inferior vermis; the tonsil (T) and the posterior inferior cerebellar artery (PICA) (*thicker horizontal white arrow* in **A** and **C**). 4V, fourth ventricle. (**B** *Modified from Naidich TP, Duvernoy HM, Delman BN, et al. Duvernoy's Atlas of the Human Brain Stem and Cerebellum: High-Field MRI, Surface Anatomy, Internal Structure, Vascularization and 3D Sectional Anatomy. New York, Springer, 2008.*)

nerves. These gross anatomic features are illustrated and described in Figures 15-8 to 15-10.

Selected Axial Histologic Sections
Lower Medulla
Axial sections through the caudal (closed) medulla (Fig. 15-11A and B) display the central canal and the central gray matter surrounding the canal. From ventral to dorsal on each side, the central gray matter contains the nuclei of the hypoglossal nerve (CN XII), the dorsal motor nucleus for the vagus nerve (CN X), and the nucleus of the solitary tract. From medial to lateral, the dorsal quadrant displays the fasciculus and nucleus gracilis, the fasciculus and nucleus cuneatus, and the spinal trigeminal tract and nucleus. In this plane, the spinal trigeminal tract lies at the lateral surface of the medulla. Continuing around the curvature, from lateral to medial, the anterior quadrant of the lower medulla displays the site of the anterolateral fasciculus and the pyramidal tract. At the caudal medullary level, the anterolateral fasciculus contains the dorsal and ventral spinocerebellar tracts at the surface and the spinothalamic tract just deep to those. A rubrospinal tract is seen within the anterolateral fasciculus in other species but is rudimentary in humans.

Mid Medulla
Axial sections through the upper end of the closed portion of the medulla (see Fig. 15-11C) display anatomy similar to that just described. Centrally, however, the secondary relay (internal arcuate) fibers arise from the dorsal nuclei gracilis and cuneatus

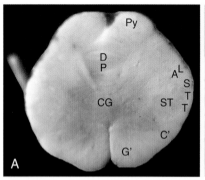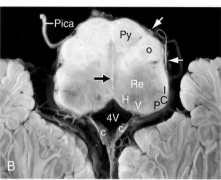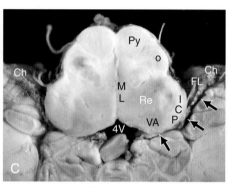

■ **FIGURE 15-8** **A to C,** Gross axial sections of the medulla displayed from caudal to cranial. Each section is oriented with ventral toward the top of the image. **A,** Closed far caudal medulla. This section displays the midline ventral sulcus between the two pyramids (Py), the decussation of the pyramids (DP), and the central gray matter (CG). Dorsally and laterally one sees the fasciculi gracilis (G') and cuneatus (C'), the superficial position of the spinal trigeminal tract (STT), and the spinal trigeminal nucleus (ST) immediately medial to the spinal trigeminal tract. Just ventral to the spinal trigeminal tract, a grouping of ascending and descending fibers forms a composite structure designated the anterolateral fasciculus (AL), which includes the ascending ventral and dorsal spinocerebellar tracts, the ascending spinothalamic tract, and the descending rubrospinal tract. **B,** Open mid medulla. This section displays the median sulcus and paired pyramids ventrally, the inferior olivary nucleus (O) with ventral preolivary and dorsal retro-olivary sulci (*white arrows*) laterally, and a thin caudal portion of the inferior cerebellar peduncle (ICP) dorsolaterally. At this level, the floor of the fourth ventricle (4V) shows a narrow transverse dimension with hypoglossal and dorsal vagal eminences that indicate the sites of the underlying hypoglossal (H) and dorsal vagal (V) nuclei. The roof of the inferior fourth ventricle (inferior medullary velum) partially tents over the floor, enclosing the paired choroid plexi (c,c). The median raphe (*black arrow*), reticular substance (Re), and a branch of the posterior inferior cerebellar artery (PICA) are also indicated. **C,** Open high medulla. The transverse dimension of the fourth ventricle (4V) is now wider and leads directly into the lateral recesses (*three black arrows*) of the fourth ventricle on each side. The choroid plexi (Ch) extend the full length of the lateral recesses to emerge from the foramina of Luschka (FL) into the cerebellopontine angle cisterns. The medullary vestibular areas (VA) form the floor of the fourth ventricle at the widest portion of the medullary triangle. In the medulla, the medial lemnisci take the form of paramedian columns of white matter just to each side of the median raphe. Other labels as in **A** and **B**.

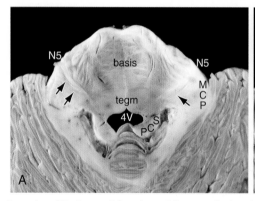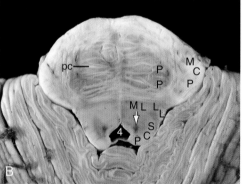

■ **FIGURE 15-9** Pons. **A** and **B,** Gross axial sections of the pons displayed from caudal to cranial. Each section is oriented with ventral toward the top of the image. The pons displays an ovoid contour with a gentle ventral median sulcus, a broad lateral extension, and rounded lateral edges. The medial lemniscus (ML) and lateral lemniscus (LL) define the two ends of a lemniscal arc. The ventral surface of this arc marks the interface between the basis pontis (basis) ventrally and the pontine tegmentum (tegm) dorsally. The pontocerebellar fibers (pc) course transversely between the pontine nuclei (p), cross the midline, and gather into the contralateral middle cerebellar peduncles (MCP). The fibers (*black arrows*) of the trigeminal nerves (N5) penetrate the brain surface in the upper lateral pons and cross through the middle cerebellar peduncles to reach the secondary (relay) trigeminal nuclei in the dorsolateral pons. The superior cerebellar peduncles (SCP) form the lateral wall of the upper fourth ventricle (in **A**) and then migrate medially into the tegmentum (in **B**) as they converge to their decussation in the midbrain. On each side, the locus ceruleus (*white arrow* in **B**) forms a vertical bluish black column of melanin-containing cells. In cut cross section, these columns appear as small pigmented circles in the dorsal tegmentum.

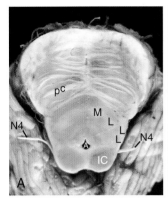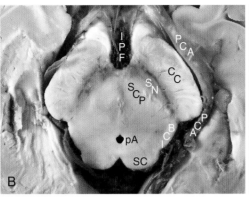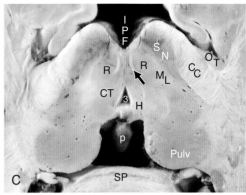

■ **FIGURE 15-10** Midbrain into thalamus. **A** to **C,** Gross axial sections from the midbrain into the thalamus displayed from caudal to cranial. Each section is oriented with ventral toward the top of the image. **A,** Caudal midbrain—upper pons. The caudal midbrain shows a narrow transverse extension and gently rounded contours. In the tegmentum, the lateral lemnisci (LL) contribute to the capsule of white matter surrounding the inferior colliculi (IC). The trochlear nerves (N4) emerge from the dorsal surface (not seen) and then normally course ventrally around the low midbrain. In this image, the cut ends of the two trochlear (N4) nerves pass artifactually far laterally. The ventral aspect of the lemniscal arc (ML-LL) divides the basis ventrally from the rest of the tegmentum dorsally. **B,** Mid midbrain. The mid midbrain shows a wider transverse dimension, more angular contours, and a deep interpeduncular fossa (IPF) containing multiple posterior thalamoperforating vessels. The anterior border of the substantia nigra (SN) separates the crura cerebrorum (CC) ventrally from the tegmentum of the midbrain dorsally. The aqueduct (unlabeled) separates the tegmentum ventrally from the tectum dorsally. The uppermost portions of the superior cerebellar peduncles (SCP) are still visible within the tegmentum and will decussate one level more superiorly. The brachium of the inferior colliculus (BCI) passes ventral to the superior colliculus (SC) en route to the medial geniculate body. The posterior cerebral artery (PCA) encircles the midbrain. pA, periaqueductal gray matter. **C,** Upper midbrain. The optic tract (OT) encircles the crus cerebri (CC) on each side. The tegmentum displays the substantia nigra (SN), the paired red nuclei (R), the central tegmental tracts (CT) at the dorsomedial aspects of the red nuclei, and the medial lemnisci (ML) at the dorsolateral aspects of the red nuclei. The paired habenulointerpeduncular tracts (fasciculi retroflexi) (*black arrow*) pass ventrally from the habenular trigones (H) at the posterior third ventricle through the medial aspects of the red nuclei to reach the interpeduncular nuclei. Other structures labeled include the third ventricle (3), pineal gland (P), pulvinar (pulv), and splenium (Sp).

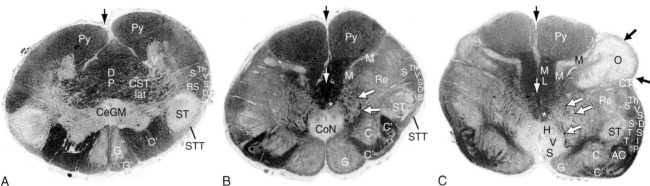

■ **FIGURE 15-11** **A** to **C,** Axial histologic sections of the lower medulla. Figures 15-11 to 15-13 are histologic sections displayed in ascending order from caudal to rostral. Each section is oriented with ventral toward the top of the image. Klüver-Barrera stain for myelin (*blue*) and gray matter nuclei *purplish*). The inferior medulla lies caudal to the fourth ventricle. Far caudally (**A**), the medullary gray matter resembles the spinal cord with the central gray matter (CeGM) surrounding the closed central canal, and ventral gray matter (*white V*) reminiscent of ventral horns far laterally. Farther rostrally (**B**), the central gray matter contains the commissural nucleus (CoN) through which the caudal ends of the paired nuclei of the solitary tracts unite in the midline. Near the top of the closed medulla (**C**), the central gray matter moves dorsally and displays a vertical alignment of nuclei, with the darker-stained more myelinated hypoglossal nucleus (H) situated ventrally, the lighter less myelinated dorsal nucleus of the vagus (V) situated centrally, and the light nucleus of the solitary tract (S) situated most dorsally. *Dorsally,* the dorsal sensory fasciculi gracilis (G′) and cuneatus (C′) ascend to their relay nuclei gracilis (G) and cuneatus (C). From these nuclei, secondary relay fibers designated the internal arcuate fibers (*white arrows*) curve ventrally around the central gray nuclei, cross the midline ventrally as the lemniscal (great sensory) decussation (*thin vertical white arrows*), and emerge on the contralateral side to form the paired medial lemnisci (ML). In the lower and mid medulla, the medial lemnisci form paired paramedian columns of white matter. The accessory cuneate nucleus (AC) first appears as small islands of gray matter within the upper fasciculus cuneatus (also seen, unlabeled, between the two C′ in **B**). In more rostral sections (**C** and above), the accessory cuneate nucleus becomes a substantial nucleus lying rostrolateral to the cuneate nucleus. The medial longitudinal fasciculi (*white asterisk*) form a vertically oriented fiber system that courses in the general area ventral to the central gray matter and dorsal to the medial lemnisci (ML). *Ventrally,* the corticospinal tracts descend within the paired paramedian pyramids (Py) to each side of the anterior median medullary sulcus (*thin vertical black arrow*). They decussate (DP) in the lower medulla and then course posteroinferolaterally (CST lat) toward the posterior aspect of the lateral columns of the cord (*caudal to the sections shown*). *Laterally,* the descending fibers of the spinal trigeminal tract (STT) present at the surface of the medulla inferiorly (**A** and **B**) but become buried deep to the inferior cerebellar peduncle (IP) more rostrally. The large spinal trigeminal nucleus (ST) runs vertically directly medial to the spinal trigeminal tract. The dorsal spinocerebellar tract (DS) and ventral spinocerebellar tract (VS) lie adjacent to each other as they ascend into the low medulla (**A**). However, the dorsal spinocerebellar tract then separates from the ventral spinocerebellar tract and curves dorsally as it ascends to enter the inferior cerebellar peduncle (IP) at more rostral levels (**B** and **C**). Just anterolateral to the spinal trigeminal system, multiple fiber systems course vertically in a combined anterolateral fasciculus. These anterolateral fibers include the ascending ventral spinocerebellar tract (VS) and the ascending spinothalamic tract (STh). The inferior olivary nucleus (O) and its capsule (the amiculum, *two black arrows*) form the gross bulge designated the olive. Between the inferior olivary nucleus and the medial lemniscus, the medial accessory olivary nucleus (M) forms a vertical column of gray with a ventral horizontal wing oriented at right angles to the vertical dorsal wing. Also indicated are the accessory cuneate nucleus (AC) and the reticular formation of the medulla (one portion of which is labeled Re).

and pass ventrally around the central gray matter to decussate in the ventral midline. The decussated fibers assemble into compact fiber bundles just to each side of the midline and are renamed the medial lemnisci. Dorsally, the accessory cuneate nucleus now appears lateral to the cuneate nucleus. Laterally, the dorsal spinocerebellar tract has moved dorsally in preparation to enter the inferior cerebellar peduncle more rostrally. As a result, the spinal trigeminal tract and nucleus now lie deep to the dorsal spinocerebellar tract and the anterolateral fasciculus now contains the ventral spinocerebellar tract and the spinothalamic tract but not the dorsal spinocerebellar tract. The medial accessory olivary nucleus may be seen within the ventral quadrant.

Upper Medulla

Axial sections through the rostral (open) medulla (Fig. 15-12) display the lower half of the fourth ventricle. The central gray matter that surrounded the central canal more caudally now opens dorsally and folds outward, so the previously ventral nuclei now lie medially and the previously dorsal nuclei now lie laterally. From medial to lateral, therefore, the medullary portion of the floor of the fourth ventricle displays the hypoglossal nucleus at the hypoglossal trigone, the dorsal nucleus of the vagus at the vagal trigone, and the nucleus of the solitary tract lateral to the vagal nucleus and extending deeply to surround

the solitary tract. The medullary vestibular area containing the medial and inferior vestibular nuclei lies at the lateral end of the floor of the fourth ventricle. The ventral surface of the rostral medulla displays the paired paramedian pyramids carrying the corticospinal tracts, the preolivary sulci at which the hypoglossal (CN XII) nerve roots emerge, the olives formed by the underlying inferior olivary nuclei, and the retro-olivary sulci at which the fibers of the glossopharyngeal, vagus, and accessory nerves (CN IX, X, and XI) transit into and out from the stem. The dorsal quadrant displays the nucleus ambiguus and the inferior cerebellar peduncle (restiform body) that now contains the ipsilateral dorsal spinocerebellar fibers and the olivocerebellar fibers that arise from the contralateral inferior olivary nucleus. The anterolateral fasciculus lies along the surface of the upper medulla just ventral to the inferior cerebellar peduncle. The ventral quadrant displays the C-shaped, markedly folded inferior olivary nucleus and the medial accessory and dorsal accessory olivary nuclei. Just to each side of the midline, from dorsal to ventral, rostral medullary sections display the paired medial longitudinal fasciculi and the paired medial lemnisci.

Lower Pons

Axial MRI through the caudal pons (Fig. 15-13A) will display the upper half of the fourth ventricle. The width of the fourth ventricle tapers progressively toward the aqueduct. From medial to

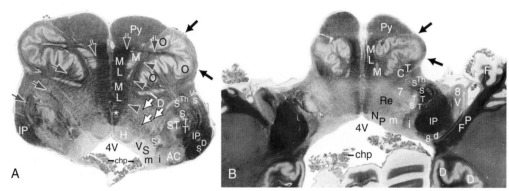

■ **FIGURE 15-12** A and B, Axial histologic sections of the upper medulla. Figures 15-11 to 15-13 are histologic sections displayed in ascending order from caudal to rostral. Each section is oriented with ventral toward the top of the image. Klüver-Barrera stain for myelin (*blue*) and gray matter nuclei (*purplish*). The rostral medulla displays the lower half of the open fourth ventricle (inferior medullary triangle of the rhombencephalic ventricle) (4V). **A,** The central canal opens dorsally, so the gray matter nuclei that were situated dorsally in the low medulla come to lie laterally in the upper medulla. *Dorsally,* along the floor of the open fourth ventricle, the hypoglossal nuclei (H) lie medially and bulge into the floor of the ventricle at the hypoglossal trigones. The more lightly myelinated dorsal vagal nuclei (V) lie lateral to these and bulge into the floor of the fourth ventricle at the vagal trigones. The nuclei (*black* S) of the solitary tract lie lateral to the vagal nuclei and extend ventrolaterally to surround the myelinated solitary tracts (s). The vestibular nuclei form the vestibular areas at the lateral aspects of the fourth ventricle. In this section, these include the medial (*black* m) and the inferior (i) vestibular nuclei. The spinal trigeminal nucleus (ST) and tract (STT) occupy nearly the same location but at this level are buried deeply by the expansion of the inferior cerebellar peduncle (IP). Internal arcuate fibers (*white arrows*) continue to course from the nuclei gracilis and cuneatus across the midline into the contralateral medial lemnisci. *Ventrally,* the paired pyramids (Py) lie to each side of the anterior median medullary sulcus. *Laterally,* the dorsal spinocerebellar tract has moved farther into the inferior cerebellar peduncle (IP). The ascending ventral spinocerebellar tract (VS) and the ascending spinothalamic tract (STh) maintain their positions within the anterolateral fasciculus. The inferior olivary nucleus (O) and its capsule (amiculum, *black arrows*) bulge laterally, creating the preolivary sulcus and retro-olivary sulcus. Large numbers of olivocerebellar fibers (*red arrows*) emerge from the hilum of one olive, pass medially to cross the midline, and then turn dorsally and laterally to enter the contralateral inferior cerebellar peduncle (IP). In their course, they cross directly through all intervening structures, including the medial accessory olive (*white* M) and dorsal accessory olive (D) and the spinal trigeminal tract. *Centrally,* vertically oriented fibers form paired paramedian columns of myelinated white matter, with the medial longitudinal fasciculi (MLF) (*white asterisk*) situated centrally deep to the hypoglossal nuclei (H) and the medial lemnisci situated ventral to the MLF. The intramedullary fibers of the hypoglossal nerve (CN XII) (*red arrowheads*) course ventrally from the hypoglossal nucleus, pass lateral to the medial lemnisci (ML), pass between the medial accessory olivary nucleus (*white* M) and the inferior olivary nucleus (O), and emerge at the preolivary sulcus. Also indicated are the choroid plexus (chp) and accessory cuneate nucleus (AC). **B,** Upper medulla. The fourth ventricle (4V) is widely open. *Dorsally,* the positions occupied by the hypoglossal nuclei in the low medulla are now occupied by the nuclei prepositus hypoglossi (NP). The medial (m) and inferior (i) vestibular nuclei lie laterally. The external aspect of the inferior cerebellar peduncle (IP) is covered by the ventral (8V) and dorsal (8D) cochlear nuclei. The flocculus (F) and floccular peduncle (FP) lie posterolateral to the inferior cerebellar peduncle. *Ventrally,* the pyramids (Py) lie to each side of the anterior median medullary sulcus. *Laterally,* the spinal trigeminal nucleus (ST) and tract (STT) and the structures of the anterolateral fasciculus maintain their positions. The central tegmental tract (CT) is now seen contributing to the capsule (amiculum, *black arrows*) of the inferior olivary nucleus (O). The facial nucleus (7) lies ventrolaterally, anteromedial to the spinal trigeminal system and medial to the anterolateral fasciculus. Other structures shown are the choroid plexus (chp), portions of the dentate nuclei of the cerebellum (D), medial accessory olivary nucleus (M), reticular substance (Re), and spinothalamic tract (STh). The ventral spinocerebellar tract is also present but not labeled.

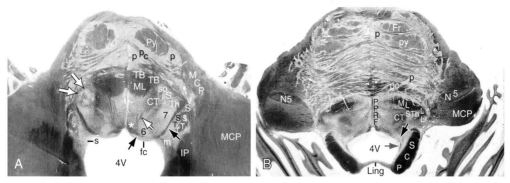

■ **FIGURE 15-13** **A** and **B,** Axial histologic sections of the pons. Figures 15-11 to 15-13 are histologic sections displayed in ascending order from caudal to rostral. Each section is oriented with ventral toward the top of the image. Klüver-Barrera stain for myelin (*blue*) and gray matter nuclei (*purplish*). **A,** Lower pons. The fourth ventricle (4V) is widely open. *Dorsally,* the facial colliculi (fc) form prominent paired paramedian eminences that bulge into the floor of the fourth ventricle (4V). The abducens fibers (*thinner white arrow*) arise from the medial aspects of the abducens nuclei (6) and course ventrally, slightly laterally, and slightly caudally through all intervening structures, ultimately reaching the pontomedullary sulcus. The facial nerve fibers (*black arrows*) arise from the facial nuclei (7) and form a diffuse spread of fibers that course medially and superiorly around the medial aspect and upper pole of the abducens nucleus. These proximal fibers are not visualized. The facial fibers then coalesce into a prominent bundle (*medial black arrow*) that recurves ventrally and laterally (*lateral black arrow*) between its own nucleus of origin (7) and the spinal trigeminal nucleus (ST). The superior vestibular nuclei (s) form the lateral aspect of the floor of the fourth ventricle at this level. The inferior cerebellar peduncle (IP) and middle cerebellar peduncle (MCP) lie far laterally. *Ventrally,* the basis pontis contains the pontocerebellar fibers (pc), the pontine nuclei (p), and the descending pyramidal tracts (Py). Within the tegmentum, the medial lemnisci (ML) now appear as ovoid tracts of medially placed ascending fibers. The trapezoid body (TB) appears as a horizontal tract of transverse fibers interwoven with the vertical medial lemniscal fibers. The spinothalamic tract (STh) and ventral spinocerebellar tract (VS) lie farther laterally. At this level, the superior olivary nuclear complex (so) lies in the ventral pontine tegmentum and is particularly well seen on the contralateral side (*two thick white arrows*). The well-named central tegmental tract (CT) forms a prominent centrally located bundle of vertical fibers. Also indicated are the medial longitudinal fasciculus (*white asterisk*) and medial vestibular nucleus (m). **B,** Upper pons. The fourth ventricle (4V) is now narrowing. The lateral walls of the fourth ventricle are formed by the obliquely oriented, nearly rectangular superior cerebellar peduncles (SCP). The roof of the fourth ventricle is formed by the superior medullary velum. The lingula (Ling) of the vermis forms the thin sheet of cerebellar cortex applied directly onto the posterior (external) surface of the superior medullary velum. The locus ceruleus (*black arrow*) and the mesencephalic tract of the trigeminal nerve (*red arrow*) lie at the ventral lateral angle of the upper fourth ventricle on each side. *Dorsally,* the medial longitudinal fasciculi (*white asterisk* in **A**) form vertically oriented, paired paramedian fiber tracts. The paramedian pontine reticular formation (PPRF) lies along the median raphe just ventral to the medial longitudinal fasciculi. *Ventrally,* the basis pontis contains the pontine nuclei (p), the pontocerebellar fibers (pc), and the descending pyramidal tracts (Py). Most of the pontocerebellar fibers arise from one side, pass medially to cross the midline, continue laterally across the opposite half basis pontis, and then gather together to form the middle cerebellar peduncle (MCP) on the side opposite their origin. *Centrally,* the medial lemnisci (ML), the spinothalamic tract (STh) (synonym: spinal lemniscus), and lateral lemnisci (LL) mark out a prominent transverse "lemniscal arc." The paired lateral lemnisci (LL) arise from the superior olivary nuclear complexes, so they are seen only in sections superior to **A.** The central tegmental tract (CT) forms the prominent vertical fiber bundle in the central tegmentum. Fr, frontopontine fibers; N5, trigeminal nerve fibers crossing the MCP.

lateral, the pontine portion of the fourth ventricle displays the ventral median sulcus, the median eminences with the median longitudinal fasciculi and facial colliculi, the paired sulci limitantes, and the pontine vestibular areas containing the medial, superior and lateral vestibular nuclei. On each side, the fibers of the abducens nerve (CN VI) emerge from the ventral medial aspect of the abducens nucleus. The fibers of the facial nerve (CN VII) arise from the facial nucleus ventral, lateral and caudal to the abducens nucleus. The facial fibers ascend to the medial aspect of the abducens nucleus, turn over the dorsal dome of the abducens nucleus from medial to lateral, recurve ventrally, and descend between the facial nucleus and the spinal trigeminal nucleus to emerge from the brain stem just inferior to the middle cerebellar peduncle. The facial fibers turning over the abducens nucleus produce the characteristic facial colliculus on the floor of the fourth ventricle. Within the diverging arms of the abducens and facial fibers, low pontine sections display the facial nucleus, the superior olivary nuclear complex, the central tegmental tract, and the lateral lemniscus.

At this level, the ascending fibers of the medial lemniscus assemble into an ovoid bundle that separates the basis pontis ventrally from the rest of the pontine tegmentum dorsally. The trapezoid body forms an elongated bundle of transversely directed fibers that cross the ventral pontine tegmentum and interweave with the ascending fibers of the medial lemniscus. The basis pontis contains the pontine nuclei, the transversely oriented pontocerebellar fibers that pass contralaterally to form the contralateral middle cerebellar peduncles, and the longitudinally oriented frontopontine, corticospinal, and

parietotemporo-occipitopontine fibers. Far dorsally, the superior cerebellar peduncles form the inclined dorsolateral walls of the fourth ventricle.

Upper Pons

Axial sections through the rostral pons (see Fig. 15-13B) display a smaller cross section of the fourth ventricle. On each side, the ventral contour of the upper pons is formed by the pontine nuclei and the pontocerebellar fibers that arise on the contralateral side, cross the midline, and then converge laterally to form the middle cerebellar peduncle. At this level, the ascending fibers of the medial lemnisci assemble into a curved, nearly transverse bundle that demarcates the basis pontis ventrally from the pontine tegmentum dorsally. Within the dorsal tegmentum, the floor of the fourth ventricle shows the paired median longitudinal fasciculi just to each side of the median raphe and the paired trigeminal complexes at the trigeminal trigones laterally. Within the ventral tegmentum, from medial to lateral, the spinothalamic tract and lateral lemniscus extend the arc of the medial lemnisci dorsally and laterally. Together they define a broad "lemniscal arc." Far laterally, at the trigeminal trigones on each side, the motor nucleus of CN V lies medial to the principal sensory nucleus of CN V (see Fig 15-24B and C). Fascicles of the trigeminal nerve course dorsomedially through the middle cerebellar peduncles to pass between the motor and principal sensory nuclei of CN V. The basis pontis contains the pontine nuclei, the transverse pontocerebellar fibers, and the descending corticopontine, corticobulbar, and corticospinal fibers.

Pontomesencephalic Junction and Lower Midbrain

Axial sections through the pontomesencephalic junction and low midbrain (Figs. 15-14 and 15-15) display a small cross section of the uppermost fourth ventricle. The ventral contour is formed by the median interpeduncular fossa and the flanking crura cerebrorum. The lateral contour displays a prominent lateral mesencephalic sulcus. The dorsal contour is formed by the median intercollicular groove and the flanking inferior colliculi. The basis mesencephali ventrally is demarcated from the tegmentum dorsally by a curved line drawn along the anterior border of the substantiae nigra. Within the basis, from medial to lateral on each side, the crus cerebri conveys the descending frontopontine, corticobulbar, corticospinal, and parietotemporo-occipitopontine fibers. The frontopontine fibers occupy the anteromedial one sixth of the arc of white matter.[8] The corticobulbar and corticospinal fibers occupy the middle two thirds of the arc of the crus cerebri.[8] The parietotemporo-occipitopontine fibers occupy approximately the posterolateral one sixth of the arc of white matter.[8] The substantiae nigra abut the inner aspects of the crura cerebrorum and are divided into two portions. Ventrally and interdigitating with the fibers of the crus cerebri is the γ-aminobutyric acid (GABA)-ergic pars reticulata of the substantia nigra (SNr). Immediately dorsal to the SNr is the dopaminergic pars compacta (SNc) of the substantia nigra. In the ventral tegmentum, just dorsal to the substantia nigra, the decussation of the superior cerebellar peduncle forms a prominent midline ovoid of white matter. Lateral to this, the broad arc of white matter is formed by the medial lemniscus, the trigeminothalamic tract, the spinothalamic tract, and the lateral lemniscus. Dorsally,

the aqueduct of Sylvius is surrounded by a circle of periaqueductal gray matter. The paired paramedian trochlear nuclei (CN IV) lie at the ventral aspect of the periaqueductal gray matter. The fibers of the medial longitudinal fasciculi partially enclose the ventral borders of the trochlear nuclei. The central tegmental tracts lie laterally within the tegmentum.

Upper Midbrain

Axial sections through the upper midbrain and mesencephalic-diencephalic junction (Fig. 15-15) display the aqueduct of Sylvius. The dorsal contour is formed by the midline vertical arm of the cruciate (intercollicular) sulcus and the flanking superior colliculi. The ventral contour is again formed by the median interpeduncular fossa and the flanking crura cerebrorum. The fascicles of the oculomotor nerve (CN III) emerge into the interpeduncular fossa through the medial walls of the crura cerebrorum. The lateral contour displays a prominent lateral mesencephalic sulcus. Depending on section angulation, this section may also display the inferior pole of the medial geniculate nucleus at the superior end of the lateral mesencephalic sulcus. From medial to lateral on each side, the basis mesencephali contains the frontopontine, corticobulbar and corticospinal fibers, and parietotemporo-occipitopontine fibers. The substantia nigra lies immediately dorsal to the crus cerebri. In the ventral tegmentum, just dorsal to the substantia nigra, the paired paramedian red nuclei replace the decussation of the superior cerebellar peduncle. Crossed fibers from the contralateral superior cerebellar peduncle pass through or around the red nucleus en route to the thalamus. The ascending fibers of the

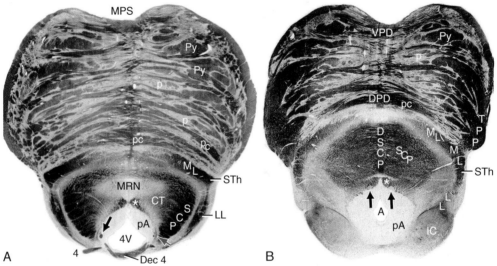

■ **FIGURE 15-14** Pontomesencephalic junction. At this transition, the uppermost fourth ventricle (4V) narrows into the cerebral aqueduct (A). *Dorsally,* the inferior colliculi (IC) show a relatively narrow transverse dimension. The superior cerebellar peduncles (SCP) that formed the well-defined oblique, nearly rectangular walls of the fourth ventricle in the prior figure now migrate medially to form thick arcs of white matter (in A). The lateral walls of these arcs remain sharply defined. The medial walls become blurred as the fibers ascend medially toward their decussation. Further superiorly (in B), the fibers of the medially positioned superior cerebellar peduncles (SCP) form a prominent ovoid and decussate (DSCP) in the midline. The central tegmental tracts (CT) form distinct fiber bundles medial to the superior cerebellar peduncles (SCP) in A but become difficult to distinguish from the superior cerebellar peduncles in **B**. The trochlear nuclei (*paired black arrows in B*) give rise to fibers (*black arrow in A*) that curve posterolaterally and caudally at the lateral aspects of the ipsilateral periaqueductal gray matter (pA). These fibers decussate (Dec 4) slightly farther caudally in the superior medullary velum of the fourth ventricle, to emerge as the fully decussated trochlear nerves (4) on the dorsal surface of the caudal midbrain just inferior to the inferior colliculi. The paired medial longitudinal fasciculi (*white asterisk*) maintain their paramedian position and lie generally ventral to the trochlear nuclei. The median raphe nuclei (MRN) form a prominent central ovoid of gray matter ventral to the medial longitudinal fasciculi. The mesencephalic nucleus and tract (*red arrow*) of the trigeminal nerve course vertically at the lateral edge of the periaqueductal gray matter. *Ventrally,* the shallow medial pontine sulcus (MPS) deepens superiorly as it approaches the interpeduncular fossa of the midbrain (see Fig. 15-15). *Laterally,* the medial lemnisci (ML) form thin, coronally oriented bundles of ascending fibers. The lateral lemnisci (LL) now form prominent horns that arch dorsally, lateral to the medially migrating superior cerebellar peduncles (in A), and ascend to form the capsules of the inferior colliculi (IC) (in B). The spinothalamic tract (STh) lies laterally along the horizontal portion of the lemniscal arc, between the medial and lateral lemnisci. The temporoparietopontine fibers (TPP) of the crus cerebri descend into this section laterally (see Fig. 15-15A). Other structures labeled include the dorsal and ventral pontine decussations (DPD and VPD), the pontine nuclei (p), pontocerebellar fibers (pc), pyramidal tract (PY) and the temporoparietopontine fibers (TPP).

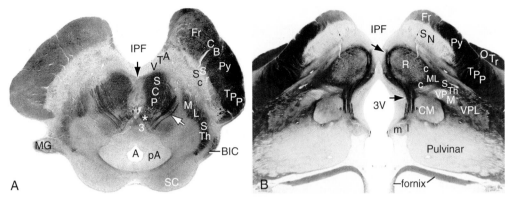

■ **FIGURE 15-15** Upper midbrain. **A,** *Dorsally,* the superior colliculi (SC) lie relatively far apart (wide transverse dimension). The aqueduct (A), periaqueductal gray matter (pA), and sinuous oculomotor fibers (*white arrow*) form a characteristic shape resembling an inverted jellyfish with tentacles. The groups of oculomotor nuclei (3) lie at the ventral median aspect of the periaqueductal gray matter with the medial longitudinal fasciculi (*white asterisk*) immediately ventral to the nuclei. The oculomotor fibers (*white arrow*) initially pass ventrolaterally before recurving ventromedially to emerge at the medial aspects of the crura cerebrorum (see Fig. 15-2B). *Ventrally,* the crura cerebrorum form very prominent arcs of white matter containing, from ventromedial to dorsolateral, the frontopontine fibers (Fr), the corticobulbar fibers (CB), the corticospinal fibers (Py), and the temporoparieto-occipitopontine fibers (TPP). Just dorsomedial to the crus cerebri, the substantia nigra (SN) forms arcs of tissue co-curvilinear with the crus. The GABAergic pars reticulata of the substantia nigra (SNr) lies immediately dorsomedial to the cerebral peduncles and interdigitates between its fibers. The dopaminergic pars compacta of the substantia nigra (SNc) lies immediately dorsomedial to the pars reticulata. The decussation of the rubrospinal tracts (*black arrow*) and the ventral tegmental areas (VTA) lie ventromedially. *Laterally,* the lemniscal arc contains the medial lemniscus (ML) and spinothalamic tract (STh). The lateral lemniscal ended at the inferior colliculi. The brachium of the inferior colliculus (BIC) conveys auditory data from the inferior colliculus to the ipsilateral medial geniculate body. In this slightly oblique section, the upper pole of the medial geniculate body (MG) is just visible on the contralateral side. **B,** Mesodiencephalic transition. Ventrally, the optic tract (OTr) curves posteriorly around the external surface of the cerebral peduncle. The red nuclei (R) form prominent ovoids ventromedial to the substantiae nigrae. At the dorsal aspect of the third ventricle (3V), the medial and lateral habenular nuclei (m, l) give rise to the ipsilateral habenulointerpeduncular tracts (fasciculi retroflexi) (*black arrows*) that curve through the medial portion of the red nuclei en route to the interpeduncular nuclei and other sites (see Chapter 11). The red nuclei give rise to both the rubrospinal tracts that cross the midline to the opposite side in the ventral tegmental decussation (see **A**) and the central tegmental tracts (c) that descend ipsilaterally to the inferior olivary nuclei. At this level, the medial lemnisci (ML) and spinothalamic tracts (STh) pass just dorsolateral to the red nuclei as they converge toward the ventral posterolateral (VPL) nuclei of the thalamus. The fornices and the pulvinars, centromedian nuclei (CM), and ventral posteromedial (VPM) nuclei of thalamus are also labeled.

medial lemniscus and the spinothalamic tract converge dorsolateral to the red nuclei as they approach the ventral posteromedial and ventral posterolateral nuclei of the thalamus. The structures of the lemniscal arc lie lateral to the red nuclei. However, the arc no longer includes the lateral lemniscus, which terminated more caudally in the inferior colliculus. Dorsally, the aqueduct of Sylvius is surrounded by the periaqueductal gray matter. The paired paramedian oculomotor nuclei (CN III) lie at the ventral aspect of the periaqueductal gray matter. The parasympathetic Edinger-Westphal nuclei appear as paired paramedian structures along the rostromedial contours of the oculomotor nuclei. The fibers of the medial longitudinal fasciculi partially enclose the ventral contours of the oculomotor nuclei.

Functional Divisions
Nuclei of the Brain Stem
The structures of the brain stem are illustrated anatomically in Figures 15-11 to 15-15. These should be compared with their appearance in the clinical 1.5- and 3-T MR images (Figs. 15-16 to 15-21) and the 9.4-T postmortem MR images (Figs. 15-22 to 15-26).

Olivary Complex
Inferior Olivary Nuclei
The olives on the lateral surfaces of the medulla are formed by the underlying paired inferior olivary nuclei (see Figs. 15-8, 15-11, and 15-12). These nuclei display a highly pleated convex outer surface and a medially directed hilum. The descending fibers of the ipsilateral central tegmental tract pass into the capsule (amiculum) on the external aspect of each inferior olivary nucleus. Each inferior olivary nucleus then gives rise to prominent olivocerebellar fibers that emerge from the hilum medially, pass transversely across the full width of the brain

stem, enter the contralateral inferior cerebellar peduncle, and traverse that peduncle to reach the deep nuclei and cortex of the cerebellum contralateral to the nucleus from which they originated.

Medial Accessory Olivary Nuclei
The medial accessory olivary nuclei of the medulla (see Figs. 15-11 and 15-12) form long columns of gray matter medial to the inferior olivary nuclei and lateral to the medial lemnisci. In axial sections, the medial accessory olivary nuclei resemble a right angle, with a ventral leg that is oriented transversely and a dorsal leg that is oriented sagittally.

Dorsal Accessory Olivary Nuclei
The dorsal accessory olivary nuclei of the medulla (see Fig. 15-12A) form thin laminae of gray matter situated just dorsal to and aligned along the vertical axis of the inferior olivary nuclei.[4]

Superior Olivary Complex
The superior olivary complex contains the superior olivary nuclei and the trapezoid body (see Fig. 15-13A). Fibers of the ventral acoustic stria and secondary fibers arising from the superior olivary complex form the large, transversely oriented fiber bundle designated the trapezoid body.[4] In their course, the transverse fibers of the trapezoid body interweave with the ascending fibers of the medial lemniscus.

The relationships of the olivary nuclei to the cerebellum are discussed in Chapter 16.

Substantia Nigra
The substantia nigra (see Figs. 15-10B and 15-15) is a crescentic zone of gray matter situated just dorsomedial to the

Text continued on page 320

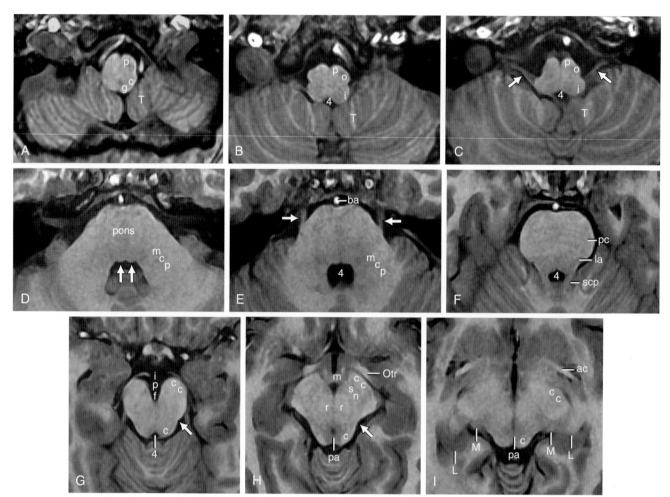

■ **FIGURE 15-16** Serial axial 3-T T1W MR images of the brain stem of a 33-year-old man displayed in ascending order from caudal to rostral. **A** to **C,** Medulla. T1W images of the caudal closed medulla (**A**) and rostral open medulla (**B** and **C**) display the progressive widening of the fourth ventricle (4) and the characteristic changes in the shapes and positions of the dorsal columns (g, c), pyramids (p), olives (o), and inferior cerebellar peduncles (i) as the sections ascend rostrally. The slightly lower signal intensity seen along the floor of the fourth ventricle identifies the gray matter of hypoglossal and dorsal vagal nuclei (*not labeled*). The rootlets of CN IX and CN X (*white arrows* in **C**) pass from the retro-olivary sulcus to the jugular foramina bilaterally. c, cuneatus; g, gracilis; T, cerebellar tonsils. **D** to **F,** Pons. The basilar artery (ba) lies just anterior to the shallow median pontine sulcus. The fourth ventricle (4) tapers progressively superiorly. The curved lemniscal arc (la) and differences in signal intensity separate the brighter basis pontis ventrally from the lower signal pontine tegmentum dorsally. Transverse pontocerebellar fibers (pc) "stripe" the basis pontis. A faint midsagittal interface marks the median raphe. Paired paramedian eminences that bulge into the floor of the fourth ventricle identify the facial colliculi (*white arrows* in **D**). More caudally, the broad middle cerebellar peduncles (mcp) pass posterolaterally from the pons into the cerebellum. More rostrally, the narrow superior cerebellar peduncles (scp) form the lateral walls of the upper fourth ventricle. **G** to **I,** Midbrain. **G,** Lower midbrain. The lower midbrain exhibits a narrow transverse dimension, rounded contours, and a transition in the shape of the CSF as the fourth ventricle merges into the aqueduct. The crura cerebrorum (cc) form the ventral contours to each side of the interpeduncular fossa (ipf). The paired inferior colliculi (c) form the dorsal contours. The lateral mesencephalic sulci (*white arrow* in **G** and **H**) groove the sides of the midbrain. The interpeduncular fossa passes directly anteriorly into the suprasellar cistern. The mammillary bodies do not project into this section. **H,** Mid-upper midbrain. The broad transverse dimension, more angular contours, narrow cerebral aqueduct, presence of mammillary bodies (m) in the interpeduncular fossa, and the encircling optic tracts (Otr) identify the more rostral midbrain. Lower signal intensity of gray matter localizes the periaqueductal (pa) and the substantia nigra (sn). The red nuclei (r, r) lie centrally. Other labels as above. **I,** Mesodiencephalic junction. The "ghost-like" shape of the upper midbrain can still be discerned as it widens out and fades into the diencephalon. The medial geniculate bodies (M) lie at the cephalic ends of the lateral mesencephalic sulci (compare with **H**). The lateral geniculate bodies (L) lie just lateral to them. The contours of the anterior commissure (ac) mirror those of the crura cerebrorum (cc).

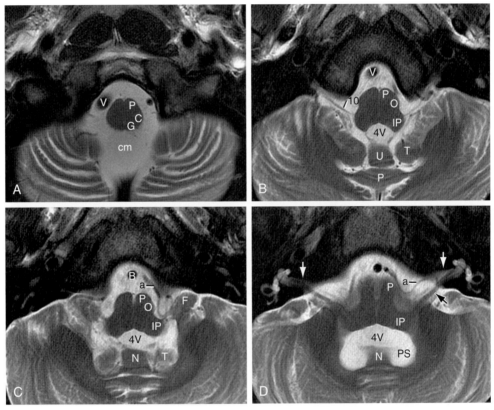

■ **FIGURE 15-17** Serial axial 3-T T2W MR images of the medulla. Figures 15-17 to 15-19 are serial axial 3-T T2W images from a 26-year-old man displayed in ascending order from caudal to rostral. **A,** The caudal closed portion of the medulla displays the curves of the sensory columns gracilis (G) and cuneatus (C) dorsally and the curves of the pyramids (P) ventrally. cm, cisterna magna; V, dominant right vertebral artery. **B to D,** The upper open portion of the medulla shows progressive widening of the floor of the fourth ventricle (4V) rostrally and progressive thickening and lateral expansion of the inferior cerebellar peduncles (IP). The paired inferior olivary nuclei (O) bulge laterally, creating a ventral preolivary groove and a dorsal retro-olivary groove. The cisternal fibers of the vagus (10) arise from the retro-olivary sulcus and exit at the jugular foramina. The cisternal fibers of the vestibulocochlear nerve (*black arrow* in **D**) arise immediately inferior to the inferior cerebellar peduncle and pass to the internal auditory canal (*white arrows* in **D**). The anterior inferior cerebellar artery (a) arises from the basilar artery (B) and passes laterally across the brain stem and along the vestibulocochlear nerve to form a meatal loop near to or within the internal auditory canal. Other labeled structures are the flocculus (F), nodulus (N), posterior superior recess (PS) of the fourth ventricle that lies atop the tonsil (T), the pyramid (P), and the uvula (U) that lies between the two tonsils.

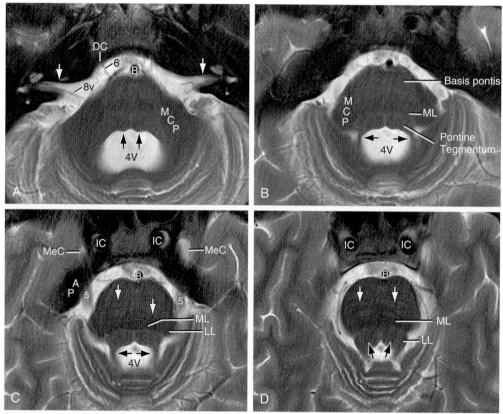

■ **FIGURE 15-18**   Serial axial 3-T T2W MR images of the pons. Figures 15-17 to 15-19 are serial axial 3-T T2W images from a 26-year-old man displayed in ascending order from caudal to rostral. **A**, Low pons. The facial colliculi (*black arrows*) form paired paramedian eminences on the floor of the fourth ventricle (4V). The cisternal segments of the abducens nerves (6) angle anterosuperolaterally from the pontomedullary junction to Dorello's canal (DC) through the clivus. The vestibular division of the vestibulocochlear nerve (CN VIII) (8v) passes into the posterior portion of the internal auditory canal (*white arrows*). The middle cerebellar peduncle (MCP) carries afferent pontocerebellar fibers to the deep cerebellar nuclei and cortex. **B** to **D**, In the mid-upper pons, the medial lemnisci (ML) are oriented in a near coronal plane that demarcates the basis pontis ventrally from the pontine tegmentum dorsally. The basis pontis displays the transversely oriented low signal pontocerebellar fibers (*small white arrows*) and the interspersed higher signal gray pontine nuclei (*unlabeled*). The trigeminal nerves (5) enter/exit the upper pons laterally and pass across the apex of the petrous pyramids (AP) to enter Meckel's caves (MeC) on each side. The superior cerebellar peduncles (*paired black arrows*) form the side walls of the upper fourth ventricle and then migrate medially as they ascend through the upper pontine tegmentum to their decussation in the low midbrain (see Fig. 15-14A). The lateral lemnisci (LL) lie lateral to the medial lemnisci and contribute to the coronally oriented "lemniscal arc" in the mid-upper pons, The lateral lemnisci then arch sharply dorsally, lateral to the medially migrating superior cerebellar peduncles, to enter the inferior colliculi (see Fig. 15-14B). The two internal carotid (IC) arteries are also shown.

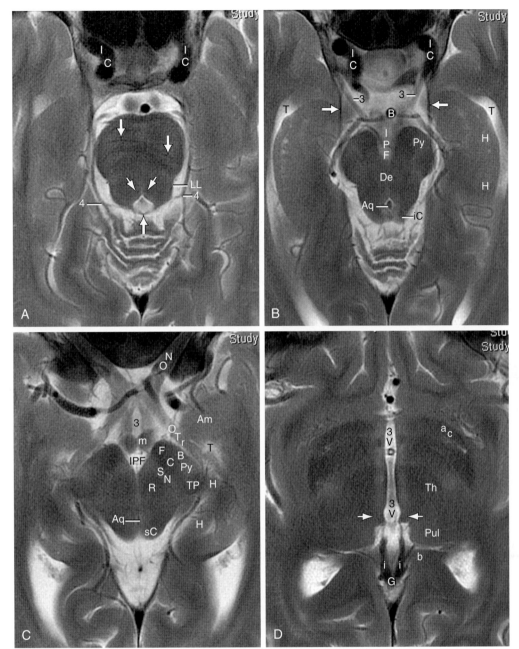

■ **FIGURE 15-19** Serial axial 3-T T2W MR images of the upper brain stem. Figures 15-17 to 15-19 are serial axial 3-T T2W images from a 26-year-old man displayed in ascending order from caudal to rostral. **A,** *Dorsally,* the uppermost pons displays the proximal cisternal segments of the trochlear nerves (4). The lateral lemnisci (LL) form the lateral borders of the uppermost pons en route to the inferior colliculi. The paired medial longitudinal fasciculi (*thin white arrows*) lie to each side of midline along the floor of the fourth ventricle. *Ventrally,* the pontocerebellar fibers (*thicker white arrows*) pass transversely across the pons toward the middle cerebellar peduncles (see next lower sections Fig. 15-18). The two internal carotid (IC) are also shown. **B,** Lower midbrain. The inferior midbrain shows narrow, rounded contours. Dorsally, the inferior colliculi (iC) lie close together with a narrow transverse dimension. The aqueduct (Aq) identifies the site of the periaqueductal gray matter. The decussating fibers (De) of the superior cerebellar peduncles form a prominent, transversely oriented ovoid in the mid brain stem. The fibers of the corticospinal tract display a relatively high T2 signal intensity compared with the other fibers in the crura cerebrorum. The deep interpeduncular fossa (IPF) does not show mammillary bodies. The oculomotor nerves (CN III) (3, 3) pass to the upper lateral wall of the cavernous sinus. IC indicates the intercavernous segments of the two internal carotid arteries. The free margins of the tentorium (*paired horizontal arrows*) mark the incisura. The dark lines formed by the free medial edges of the tentorium may be confused with cisternal segments of cranial nerves. **C,** Upper midbrain. The upper midbrain shows more angular contours and expands farther laterally than the lower midbrain. The superior colliculi (sC) extend farther laterally than do the inferior colliculi (see Fig. 15-4). The crura cerebrorum appear more angular and pass further laterally at the upper midbrain than in the lower midbrain. The center of the upper midbrain displays paired paramedian red nuclei (R) rather than the midline ovoid of the decussating fibers of the superior cerebellar peduncle seen in the lower midbrain. The interpeduncular fossa shows the paired paramedian mammillary bodies (m) and the third ventricle (3) entering this section from the hypothalamus above. The optic apparatus includes the prechiasmal optic nerves (ON), the chiasm (*not labeled*), and the optic tracts (OTr) that encircle the upper crura cerebrorum. Ventrolaterally, from superficial to deep, these structures form sequential strata: (1) optic tract; (2) cerebral peduncle conveying the frontopontine fibers (F), corticobulbar fibers (CB), corticospinal fibers (Py) and temporoparietal pontine fibers (TP); (3) substantia nigra with the GABAergic pars reticularis superficial to the dopaminergic pars compacta; and (4) the red nuclei (R). Lateral to the midbrain, the curving contour of the temporal lobe shows the amygdala (Am) anterior to the temporal horn (T) and the hippocampal formations (H) medial to the temporal horn (T). **D,** Thalamus. The paired thalami (Th) lie to each side of the third ventricle (3V). The paired habenular nuclei (*white arrows*) lie just to each side of the posterior third ventricle. The pulvinars (Pul) of the thalami bulge posterior to the habenular nuclei. Other structures labeled include the anterior commissure (ac), the posterior ends of both the basal vein of Rosenthal (b) and the internal cerebral veins (i), and the vein of Galen (G).

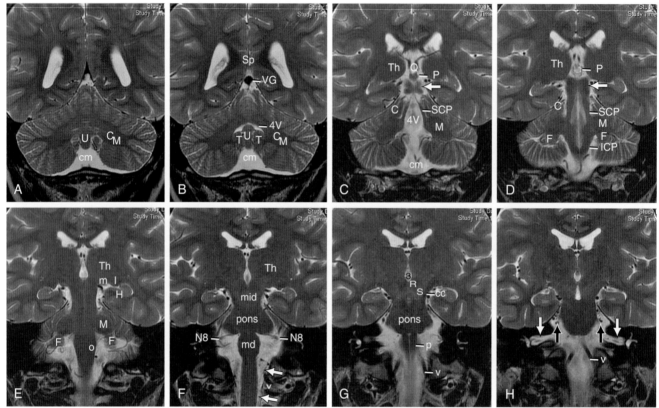

■ **FIGURE 15-20**   Serial coronal 3-T T2W images of the brain stem in a 10-year-old boy displayed in order from dorsal to ventral (same study as in Fig. 15-7C). **A** and **B,** Posterior to the brain stem, coronal sections demonstrate the cisterna magna (cm), the uvula (U) situated between the two tonsils (T), the posterior portion of the fourth ventricle (4V), and the white matter of the cerebellar hemispheres (corpora medullares [CM]). The splenium (Sp) and vein of Galen (VG) overhang the vermis. **C** and **D,** Farther ventrally, the quadrigeminal (tectal) plate of the midbrain (*horizontal white arrow*) resembles a "butterfly" situated just inferior to the pineal gland (P) and the quadrigeminal plate cistern (Q). The fourth ventricle (4V) displays a diamond (rhomboid) shape, with the upper lateral walls formed by the superior cerebellar peduncles (SCP) and the inferior lateral walls formed by the inferior cerebellar peduncles (ICP). The median sulcus on the floor of the fourth ventricle appears as a vertical white line that bisects the rhomboid in **D.** The middle cerebellar peduncles (M) transition into the corpora medullares (CM) in these sections. The superior cerebellar peduncles are separated from the adjacent portions of the cerebellar hemispheres (C) on each side by paired narrow cisterns. The flocculi (F) form the centers of the anterior faces of the cerebellar hemispheres (see also **E**). The posterior portions of the thalami (Th) overhang the upper brain stem. **E** and **F,** Sections along the length of the brain stem display the symmetric undulant contours of the midbrain (mid), pons, and medulla (md), the lateral flaring of the white matter at the middle cerebellar peduncles (M), and the prominent lateral bulges of the medulla at the inferior olivary nuclei (o). In **F,** inferiorly, MRI identifies the point at which the vertebral artery (v) penetrates the arachnoid at C1; the vertical course of the spinal accessory nerve (CN XI) (*dual white arrows*) that passes just medial to the vertebral artery at that point; the paired vestibulocochlear nerves (N8) that emerge at the pontomedullary junction and course laterally just inferior to the middle cerebellar peduncles (M); and the anterior edge of the cerebellum that overhangs the middle cerebellar peduncle. Superiorly, the medial (m) and lateral (l) geniculate bodies form an undulating contour along the inferior lateral border of the thalamus (Th) immediately superior and medial to the hippocampal formations (H) of the temporal lobe. **G** and **H,** At the ventral aspect of the brain stem, MRI displays the paired vertebral arteries (v); the belly of the pons (basis pontis); the paired pyramids (p) of the medulla; and the alternating signal intensities of the crura cerebrorum (cc), the substantia nigra (S), and red nucleus (R) in relation to the third ventricle (3) and the interpeduncular fossa. The trigeminal nerves (CN V) (*paired black arrows*) appear dot-like as they course anteriorly through the lateral pontine cistern toward their entry into Meckel's caves (in adjacent anterior sections). Portions of the cochlear and vestibular division of CN VIII course through the internal auditory canals (*dual white arrows*).

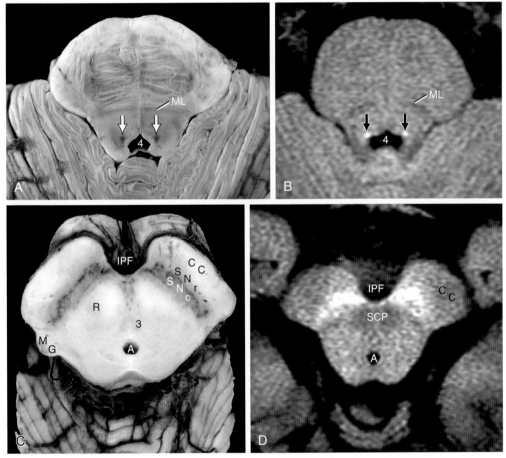

■ FIGURE 15-21 Neuromelanin. Gross axial section (**A**) and axial 3-T T1W (**B**) MR images through the high pons display the paired pigmented loci cerulei (*arrows*) as well-defined foci of high signal intensity within the dorsal tegmentum. Gross axial section (**C**) and axial 3-T T1W (**D**) MR images through the midbrain display the paired substantiae nigrae (SN) as well-defined swaths of high signal intensity within the ventral tegmentum. Other labeled structures include the aqueduct (A), crus cerebri (CC), interpeduncular fossa (IPF), red nucleus (R), substantia nigra pars compacta (SNc), substantia nigra pars reticulata (SNr), and medial geniculate body (MG). (***B** and **D**, courtesy of Drs. Eri Shibata and Makoto Sasaki, Iwate Medical University School of Medicine, Uchimaru, Morioka, Japan.*)

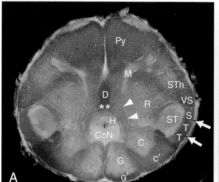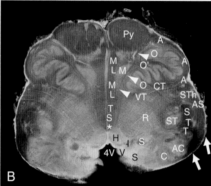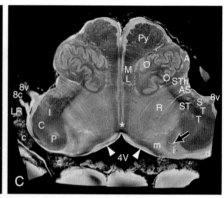

■ **FIGURE 15-22**   High-resolution postmortem intermediate-weighted MR images of the axial medulla at 9.4 T. Original resolution: 40 to 60 μm in plane and 500 μm thick. Representative axial sections displayed from caudal to rostral. Compare with histologic preparations (see Figs. 15-11 and 15-12) and with clinical MRI (see Fig. 15-17). **A,** Lower (closed portion of) medulla. MRI displays the dorsal sensory columns with fasciculus gracilis (G'), nucleus gracilis (G), fasciculus cuneatus (C'), and nucleus cuneatus (C). The spinal trigeminal nucleus (ST) lies immediately medial to the spinal trigeminal tract (STT). The components of the anterolateral fasciculus lie at an approximate 3 o'clock position ventral to the spinal trigeminal system. At this level the dorsal spinocerebellar tract (*white arrows*) covers over the spinal trigeminal tract as it moves posteriorly toward the inferior cerebellar peduncle (see next images). The anterolateral fasciculus contains the ventral spinocerebellar tract (VS) and the spinothalamic tract (STh). The paired pyramids (Py) form the ventral border of the medulla. Centrally, the hypoglossal nucleus (H) lies ventrally and shows lower signal. The nuclei that are paired separate structures at higher levels converge caudally into the single midline commissural nucleus (CoN) seen at this level. On each side, the internal arcuate (secondary relay) fibers (*white arrowheads*) from the nuclei gracilis and cuneatus arch around the central gray matter, decussate in the midline (D), and emerge on the opposite side as the contralateral medial lemniscus. The medial longitudinal fasciculi (*white asterisks*) characteristically lie just off midline, immediately ventral to the central gray matter. The medial accessory olivary nucleus (M) forms a characteristic chevron of gray matter with a transverse ventral arm and a sagittally oriented dorsal arm. R indicates some of the reticular nuclei present at this level. **B,** Mid medulla, just as the fourth ventricle starts to open. As the fourth ventricle (4V) opens, the deep gray nuclei come to occupy the middorsal surface of the medulla to each side of the midline. Because the dorsal nuclei rotate outward, they come to lie farther laterally, while the ventral nuclei remain in paramedian position. Thus, the floor of the fourth ventricle shows a consistent medial to lateral array of the lower signal hypoglossal nucleus (H), the thin nucleus intercalatus, and the higher signal dorsal vagal nucleus (V). The nucleus of the solitary tract (*black S*) lies farthest laterally and extends deeply to surround the low signal solitary tract (*white S*). This section passes superior to the nucleus gracilis, so the lateral portion of the dorsal surface displays the fasciculus and nucleus cuneatus (C) and the accessory cuneate nucleus (AC). The spinal trigeminal tract (STT) and its nucleus (ST) maintain their position. The dorsal spinocerebellar tract (*white arrows*) continues to move posteriorly into the inferior cerebellar peduncle. The structures of the anterolateral fasciculus remain little changed. Centrally, the medial longitudinal fasciculus (*white asterisk*), tectospinal tract (TS), and medial lemniscus (ML) form a sagittal column of vertically directed fibers just to each side of the median raphe. The intramedullary fibers of the hypoglossal nerve (*white arrowheads*) pass ventrally between the medial accessory olive (M) and the inferior olivary nucleus (O) toward their exit at the preolivary sulcus. The inferior olivary nucleus (O) and its capsule (amiculum [A]) begin to bulge laterally, forming the surface eminence designated the olive. The central tegmental tract (CT) descends from the red nucleus to the inferior olivary nucleus, contributing to the amiculum. Other labeled structures include the ventral trigeminothalamic tract (VT), which lies dorsal to the inferior olivary nucleus and lateral to the medial lemnisci at this level, and a portion of the medullary reticular substance (R). **C,** Upper medulla. The medullary striae (*white arrowheads*) lie at the upper end of the medullary triangle, so they mark the cephalic extent of the open medulla. At this level, the fourth ventricle (4V) flares outward, forming the lateral angles of the fourth ventricle and giving rise to the lateral recesses (LR) of the fourth ventricle. The choroid plexus (c) traverses the lateral recesses to enter the cerebellopontine angle cisterns. The four (superior, inferior, medial, and lateral) vestibular nuclei form the floor of the fourth ventricle laterally. This section displays the medial (m) and inferior (i) vestibular nucleus. The descending myelinated fibers of the vestibular nerve pass to the inferior vestibular nucleus, causing characteristic stippling and low signal intensity (*arrow*). The inferior cerebellar peduncle (ICP) is now well developed and conveys dorsal spinocerebellar and olivocerebellar fibers into the cerebellum. The dorsal cochlear nucleus (d) forms the acoustic tubercle atop the dorsal surface of the inferior cerebellar peduncle. The cochlear (8c) and vestibular (8v) divisions of CN VIII are seen laterally. *(Modified from Naidich TP, Duvernoy HM, Delman BN, et al. Duvernoy's Atlas of the Human Brain Stem and Cerebellum: High-Field MRI, Surface Anatomy, Internal Structure, Vascularization and 3D Sectional Anatomy. New York, Springer, 2008.)*

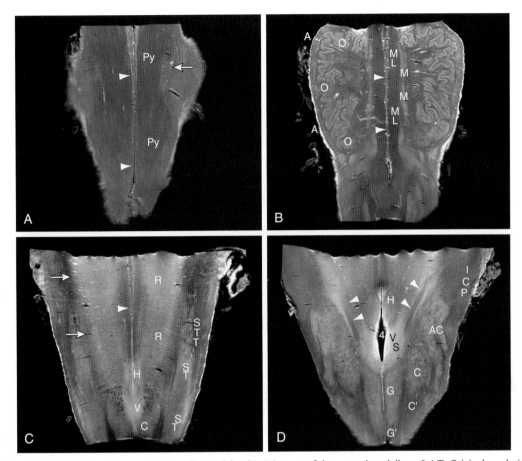

■ **FIGURE 15-23** High-resolution postmortem intermediate-weighted MR images of the coronal medulla at 9.4 T. Original resolution: 40 to 60 μm in plane and 500 μm thick. Representative coronal sections are displayed from anterior to posterior (compare with the clinical MR image in Fig. 15-20). **A,** Ventrally, the pyramids (Py) lie to each side of the median sulcus. Midline dots indicate the entry points (*white arrowheads*) for the paramedian perforating vessels that supply the anteromedial arterial compartment. Anterolateral dots (*white arrows*) indicate the entry points for the short circumflex vessels that supply the anterolateral arterial compartment. **B,** The paired paramedian columns of the medial lemnisci (ML) lie to each side to the median raphe (*white arrowheads*). The paramedian perforating vessels entering the anteromedial arterial compartment form a median column of "dots." The inferior olivary nucleus (O) displays a highly folded ("crenated") lamina of gray matter, a well-defined low signal capsule (the amiculum [A]), and a well-defined hilum that is directed medially. The medial accessory olivary nuclei (M) form symmetric vertical columns of gray matter interposed between the medial lemnisci and the inferior olivary nuclei. **C,** The central gray matter forms a vertical column that contains the low-signal hypoglossal (H) and higher signal dorsal vagal (V) nuclei. The remaining structures incline outward in conformity with the widening lateral walls of the medulla. The spinal trigeminal tract (STT) lies at the surface of the medulla caudally but becomes covered by the inferior cerebellar peduncle rostrally. The spinal trigeminal nucleus (ST) is a large obliquely oriented vertical column of secondary relay nuclei that lie immediately deep to the spinal trigeminal tract. The nucleus cuneatus (C) is seen inferiorly. The medullary reticular substance (R) forms very substantial columns of gray matter. The anteromedial entry line (*white arrowhead*) remains in the midline as the anterolateral entry line (*white arrows*) mirrors the changing width of the brain stem. **D,** Dorsally, the fasciculus gracilis (G′), nucleus gracilis (G), fasciculus cuneatus (C′), and nucleus cuneatus (C) form the dorsal surface medially. From medial to lateral, on each side, the nuclei gracilis (G), cuneatus (C), and accessory cuneatus (AC) ascend progressively more superiorly to reach the lateral wall of the rhomboid fourth ventricle. The paired solitary tracts (*white arrowheads*) angle superolaterally, resembling narrow antelope horns. The hypoglossal (H) and dorsal vagal (v) nuclei maintain their relationships to the midline and each other. The nucleus (S) of the solitary tract lies farther laterally and extends superiorly to surround the solitary tracts. Note that the spinal trigeminal nucleus (seen in **C**) is thick and lies wholly medial to the thick spinal trigeminal tract while the nucleus of the solitary tract is thinner and extends deeply to surround the thin solitary tracts. The inferior cerebellar peduncle (ICP) forms a prominent low-density band of white matter superolaterally. *(Modified from Naidich TP, Duvernoy HM, Delman BN, et al. Duvernoy's Atlas of the Human Brain Stem and Cerebellum: High-Field MRI, Surface Anatomy, Internal Structure, Vascularization and 3D Sectional Anatomy. New York, Springer, 2008.)*

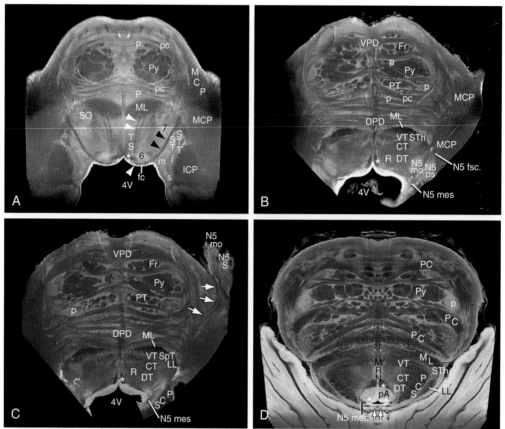

■ **FIGURE 15-24** High-resolution postmortem intermediate-weighted MR sections of the axial pons at 9.4 T. Original resolution: 40 to 60 μm in plane and 500 μm thick (compare with histologic appearance in Fig. 15-13 and with clinical MRI in Fig. 15-18). **A,** Lower pons (composite image). The fourth ventricle (4V) is widely open. *Dorsally,* the paired facial colliculi (fc) bulge into the floor of the fourth ventricle. Abducens nerve fibers (*dual white arrowheads*) emerge from the medial aspects of the mildly hyperintense abducens nuclei (6) and course ventrally, slightly laterally and slightly caudally through all intervening structures to reach the pontomedullary sulcus. Facial nerve fibers arise from the facial nuclei (7) as a diffuse, indetectable spread of fibers. These fibers course medially and superiorly around the medial and dorsal aspects of the abducens nucleus. The facial nerve fibers first become visible where they coalesce into a prominent low signal bundle (*white arrowhead*) overlying the abducens nucleus. The facial nerve bundle (*dual black arrowheads*) then recurves ventrally and laterally between its own nucleus of origin (7) and the spinal trigeminal nucleus (ST) and tract (STT). At this level, the medial (m), inferior (i), and superior (s) vestibular nuclei form the vestibular area at the lateral aspect of the floor of the fourth ventricle, deep to the inferior cerebellar peduncle (ICP). The middle cerebellar peduncle (MCP) lies far laterally. *Ventrally,* the basis pontis contains the pontocerebellar fibers (pc), the pontine nuclei (p), and the descending pyramidal tracts (Py). The coronally oriented lemniscal arcs contain the medial lemnisci (ML) medially, the trapezoid bodies more centrally, and the spinothalamic tracts (STh) laterally. The superior olivary nuclei (SO) lie along the dorsal aspect of the lemniscal arc within the pontine tegmentum. The medial longitudinal fasciculus (*white asterisk*) and tectospinal tract (TS) are seen in paramedian location dorsally. **B** and **C,** Mid pons. The motor (N5 mo) and sensory (N5 S) roots of the trigeminal nerve cross the surface of the pons at this level. The fascicles (N5 fsc, *white arrows* in **C**) traverse the middle cerebellar peduncle (MCP) to reach the dorsolateral pontine tegmentum. There they pass between the principal sensory nucleus (N5 ps) of the trigeminal nerve laterally and the motor nucleus (N5 mo) of the trigeminal nerve medially, giving the construct a faint resemblance to a Foley balloon catheter. The mesencephalic nucleus and tract of the trigeminal nerve (N5 mes) lie dorsolaterally. The superior olivary nucleus (SO) and trapezoid body seen in **A** send fibers to the lateral lemnisci (LL), which, in these sections, ascend along the lateral edge of the lemniscal arc to reach the inferior colliculi (see Fig. 15-25). Other structures labeled include the descending frontopontine (Fr) and pyramidal (Py) fibers, the ventral (VPD) and dorsal (DPD) pontine decussations, the central tegmental tract (CT), the spinothalamic tract (SpT), the ventral (VT) and dorsal (DT) trigeminothalamic tracts, the medial longitudinal fasciculus (*asterisk*), the superior cerebellar peduncle (SCP), and others already specified in **A**. **D,** Upper pons (composite image). The fourth ventricle has narrowed to the aqueduct. The fascicles of the trochlear nerves (*dual white arrowheads*) course posteriorly through the outer portion of the periaqueductal gray matter (pA) and then decussate (*dual white arrows*) in the superior medullary velum. The mesencephalic tracts (N5 mes) of the trigeminal nerves form crescent-shaped vertical columns of white matter at the margins of the periaqueductal gray matter. The superior cerebellar peduncles (SCP) are migrating medially toward their decussation, so they display medial position, sharp lateral borders, and feathered medial borders that encroach upon the central tegmental tracts (CT). The lateral lemnisci now migrate dorsally and ascend toward the inferior colliculi *external* to the superior cerebellar peduncles. In this position, the lateral lemnisci (LL) form characteristic, well-defined, sharply pointed arcs (horns) of white matter that extend the curvature of the lemniscal arc dorsomedially (see histologic appearance in Fig. 15-14A). *(Modified from Naidich TP, Duvernoy HM, Delman BN, et al. Duvernoy's Atlas of the Human Brain Stem and Cerebellum: High-Field MRI, Surface Anatomy, Internal Structure, Vascularization and 3D Sectional Anatomy. New York, Springer, 2008.)*

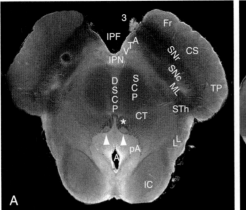
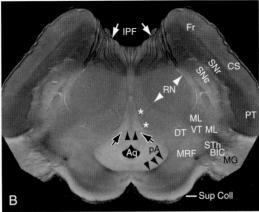

■ **FIGURE 15-25** High-resolution postmortem intermediate-weighted MR images of the midbrain at 9.4 T. Original resolution: 40 to 60 μm in plane and 500 μm thick. High-resolution, intermediate-weighted MR images at 9.4 T (compare with histologic appearance in Fig. 15-14B and 15-15A and with clinical MR images in Fig. 15-19). **A,** Lower midbrain. The dorsal surface of the lower midbrain is formed by the paired inferior colliculi (IC). More ventrally, the aqueduct (A) is surrounded by periaqueductal gray matter (pA). The paired trochlear nuclei (*white arrowheads*) lie just ventral to the peri-aqueductal gray matter, with the paired medial longitudinal fasciculi (*white asterisk*) just ventral to the nuclei. The fibers of the superior cerebellar peduncles (SCP) now form a central ovoid of low signal white matter and decussate (DSCP) in the midline. The paired central tegmental tracts (CT) lie dorsolaterally. Ventrolaterally, each crus cerebri contains the frontopontine tracts (Fr) medially, the corticobulbar and corticospinal (CS) tracts centrally, and the temporoparieto-occipitopontine tracts (TP) laterally. The GABAergic substantia nigra pars reticulata (SNr) lies posterior to and interdigitates with the fascicles of the crura cerebrorum. The dopaminergic substantia nigra pars compacta (SNc) lies posteromedial to the pars reticulata. The medial lemniscus (ML) now lies between the SNc and the superior cerebellar peduncles. The spinothalamic tract (STh) maintains its position within the tegmentum. The lateral lemnisci (LL) extend dorsally to form the capsules of the inferior colliculi. In the midline ventrally, the oculomotor rootlets (3) emerge into the interpeduncular fossa (IPF) from the medial walls of the cerebral peduncles. The interpeduncular nucleus (IPN) and the ventral tegmental area (VTA) lie within the deep gray matter walls of the interpeduncular fossa. **B,** Upper midbrain. The dorsal surface of the upper midbrain is formed by the paired superior colliculi (Sup Coll). The superior colliculi display a thin superficial layer designated the stratum zonale. Deep to this layer, the superior colliculi display distinct lamellar organization with three gray strata and three white strata. The oculomotor complex forms a roughly triangular collection of nuclei at the ventral aspect of the periaqueductal gray matter (pA). The paired parasympathetic nuclei of Edinger-Westphal (*dual black arrowheads*) lie dorsal to the remainder of the oculomotor complex (*black arrows*). The medial longitudinal fasciculi (*white asterisks*) course just ventral to the oculomotor complex. The oculomotor fascicles follow a sinuous course medial to and through the red nuclei (RN) to emerge (*white arrows*) in the interpeduncular fossa (IPF). The paired red nuclei (RN) and their capsules (*white arrowheads*) form prominent ovoids of gray matter in the tegmentum. Other labeled structures include the brachium of the inferior colliculus (BIC) leading to the medial geniculate nucleus (MG), the mesencephalic reticular formation (MRF) and the marginal fibers of the periaqueductal gray matter (*three black arrowheads*). The remaining labels are as in **A.** *(Modified from Naidich TP, Duvernoy HM, Delman BN, et al. Duvernoy's Atlas of the Human Brain Stem and Cerebellum: High-Field MRI, Surface Anatomy, Internal Structure, Vascularization and 3D Sectional Anatomy. New York, Springer, 2008.)*

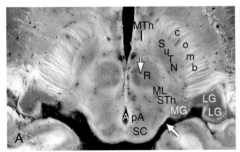
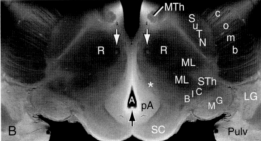

■ **FIGURE 15-26** Mesencephalic-diencephalic junction. **A,** Gross specimen. **B,** Postmortem high-resolution postmortem intermediate-weighted MR image of the mesencephalic-diencephalic junction of a different specimen at 9.4 T. Original resolution: 40 to 60 μm in plane and 500 μm thick. The dorsal surface of the midbrain displays the superior colliculi (SC), the aqueduct (A), the periaqueductal gray matter (pA), and the subcommissural organ (*midline black arrow* in **B**) that indents the aqueduct. The medial lemnisci (ML) and spinothalamic tracts (STh) converge dorsolateral to the red nuclei (R) as they ascend to the thalamus. The habenulointerpeduncular tracts (fasciculi retroflexi) (*white arrows*) curve medial to the paired red nuclei (R). The mammillothalamic tracts lie anteriorly in the hypothalami. The multiple striatal and pallidal fibers passing through the internal capsule form a highly striated appearance designated the comb system (Comb). The subthalamic nuclei (SuTN) appear as lens-shaped structures just deep to the comb system. Other structures labeled include the brachium of the inferior colliculus (*short thick white arrow* in **A**, BIC in **B**) leading to the medial geniculate body (MG), the lateral geniculate body (LG), and the pulvinar of the thalamus (Pulv). The low-signal capsule of the medial geniculate body is well seen in **B** but is not specifically labeled. *(Modified from Naidich TP, Duvernoy HM, Delman BN, et al. Duvernoy's Atlas of the Human Brain Stem and Cerebellum: High-Field MRI, Surface Anatomy, Internal Structure, Vascularization and 3D Sectional Anatomy. New York, Springer, 2008.)*

crus cerebri on each side. It contains two "layers" of gray matter: the pars reticulata (SNr) and the pars compacta (SNc). Tongues of SNr extend ventrally between the fibers of the crus cerebri. Functionally, the SNr should be considered with the globus pallidus pars interna (GPi). Together, they constitute one major output nucleus for the basal ganglia (see Chapter 11). The SNc is the major dopaminergic nucleus of the brain stem. It sends fibers widely to the basal ganglia, particularly the striatum.

Ventral Tegmental Area

The ventral tegmental area is a dopaminergic cell group situated medial to the substantia nigra. It innervates the limbic system and the cerebral cortex.

Red Nucleus and Triangle of Guillain-Mollaret

The paired red nuclei lie within the upper midbrain rostral to the decussation of the superior cerebellar peduncles (see Figs. 15-10C and 15-15B; see also Fig. 15-25). On each side, the parvocellular division of the red nucleus gives rise to rubro-olivary fibers that descend ipsilaterally within the central tegmental tract to enter the capsule (amiculum) of the inferior olivary nucleus. From that olive, olivocerebellar fibers cross the midline and traverse the contralateral inferior cerebellar peduncle to reach the cerebellar cortex and dentate nucleus contralateral to the side of the original red nucleus. The dentate nucleus then gives rise to dentatorubral fibers that ascend through the superior cerebellar peduncle, cross the midline in the decussation of the superior cerebellar peduncles, and "return" to the original red nucleus. This three-legged pathway is designated the "triangle of Guillain-Mollaret."[1,2] Clinically, disruption of the triangle leads to palatal myoclonus.

Locus Ceruleus

The locus ceruleus (see Figs. 15-9A and 15-13B) is a compact, longitudinal column of pigmented, noradrenergic cells situated in the dorsolateral pons and midbrain on each side. It lies just ventrolateral to the floor of the fourth ventricle and the periaqueductal gray matter and just ventromedial to the mesencephalic nucleus and tract of the trigeminal nerve. Noradrenergic fibers of the locus ceruleus extend widely through the diencephalon and cerebrum and extend to other brain stem nuclei. Fibers also descend into the ipsilateral anterolateral funiculus of the spinal cord to synapse on cells within both the dorsal and the ventral horns.[2] The name *locus ceruleus* derives from the dark melanin visible as a bluish coloration (i.e., cerulean) on gross specimens.

Tracts Traversing the Brain Stem

The brain stem conveys large fiber tracts between the cerebrum and thalami superiorly and the spinal cord inferiorly. These may be characterized as (predominantly) descending or (predominantly) ascending tracts, as below. However, many of these tracts convey important fibers in both directions.

Descending Tracts
Corticospinal Tracts

The corticospinal tracts descend through the posterior half of the posterior limb of the internal capsule, the midportion of the crus cerebri, the midportion of the basis pontis, and the paired pyramids of the medulla to reach the spinomedullary junction (see Figs. 15-8 to 15-15). At this junction, approximately 80% of corticospinal fibers decussate and descend within the *posterior* portions of the contralateral lateral spinal columns as the crossed lateral corticospinal tracts. Crossed corticospinal fibers for the digits of the hand extend predominantly to the alpha motor neurons of the spinal cord that innervate the distal musculature of the extremities. Crossed corticospinal fibers for other areas

terminate within the intermediate networks of neurons in the spinal gray matter. Approximately 10% of corticospinal fibers continue directly inferiorly from the pyramids into the ipsilateral anterior columns of the spinal cord just to each side of the anterior median fissure. These fibers decussate caudally, within the spinal cord itself, to reach the contralateral ventral horn. Ultimately, therefore, these fibers do cross the midline to terminate within the contralateral anterior horn.

Corticopontine and Corticobulbar Tracts

Other fibers descend from the cerebral cortex to terminate within the brain stem (see Figs. 15-13 to 15-15). Frontopontine fibers descend through the medial portion of the crus cerebri medial to the corticospinal tracts and continue inferiorly through the ventral basis pontis, anterior to the corticospinal tracts, to innervate ipsilateral pontine nuclei. Parietotemporo-occipito-pontine fibers traverse the crus cerebri posterolateral to the corticospinal tracts, continue inferiorly through the basis pontis dorsolateral to the corticospinal tracts, and terminate on ipsilateral pontine nuclei. The corticomedullary (corticobulbar) tracts descend similarly through the pontine and medullary tegmentum to terminate ipsilaterally in networks that activate cranial nerve motor nuclei.

Central Tegmental Tract

The central tegmental tracts (see Figs. 15-12 to 15-14) convey at least three sets of important fibers: (1) Fibers from the red nucleus descend through the dorsal pons within the central tegmental tract to the capsule (amiculum) of the ipsilateral inferior olivary nucleus. These descending fibers form one arm of the triangle of Guillain-Mollaret.[1,2] (2) Special visceral afferent (SVA) fibers for taste reach the cephalic portion of the nucleus of the solitary tract (gustatory nucleus) via the nervus intermedius (anterior two thirds of the tongue), the glossopharyngeal nerve (posterior one third of the tongue), and the vagus (epiglottis). They synapse there within the gustatory nucleus. Secondary relay fibers from the gustatory nucleus then ascend within (or near) the central tegmental tract to the ventral posteromedial nucleus of the thalamus and higher centers.[4] (3) Projection fibers from the reticular formation of the brain stem ascend to the thalami and hypothalami through the central tegmental tracts.

Ascending Tracts
Lemnisci

Paired Medial Lemnisci. Secondary sensory fibers from the nuclei gracilis and cuneatus form the ascending fiber tract designated the medial lemniscus (see Figs. 15-8 to 15-15).[1-6] It arises as follows. The somatosensory fibers from the dorsal columns of the spinal cord ascend to the medulla. The fibers of the fasciculus gracilis and cuneatus synapse somatotopically over the lengths of the corresponding nuclei gracilis and cuneatus. From these nuclei, secondary relay fibers designated the internal arcuate fibers pass circumferentially around the central gray matter of the lower medulla and decussate in the midline of the low medulla ventral to the central gray matter. As the fibers emerge on the contralateral side of midline they form a fiber bundle now designated the medial lemniscus. In the lower medulla, the paired medial lemnisci form sagittally oriented paramedian columns of fibers just to each side of the midline. They lie dorsal to the pyramids, ventral to the medial longitudinal fasciculi and hypoglossal nuclei, lateral to the midline, and medial to the medial accessory olivary nuclei. In this portion of the medial lemniscus, fibers from the most distal somatosensory receptors lie farthest anteriorly within the medial lemnisci. Additional fibers conveying data from progressively ascending spinal levels then "fill in" the medial lemniscus from ventral to dorsal. As the medial lemnisci ascend through the caudal pons,[4] the most ventral portion of each medial lemniscus gradually slides laterally, so the medial lemnisci come to lie horizontally in the upper pons. Therefore, the somatosensory fibers from the most distal extremity that lie anteriorly in the caudal portion of the medial lemniscus come to lie at the lateral end of each, now-horizontal upper portion of the medial lemniscus. Farther cephalically, the medial lemnisci ascend past the dorsolateral aspect of the red nucleus to reach the ventroposterolateral nuclei of the thalami.

In sagittal sections, the medial lemnisci form arches of fibers that appear concave ventrally as they curve upward through the pons. In this portion the medial lemniscus "mirrors" the convex contour of the belly of the pons, together forming an ovoid. In the uppermost pons, the medial lemnisci recurve dorsally and ascend dorsolateral to the red nucleus of the midbrain to reach the ventral posterolateral nuclei of the thalami. Within the pons the medial lemnisci mark the border between the basis pontis ventrally and the pontine tegmentum dorsally.

Paired Lateral Lemnisci. Secondary auditory fibers of the ipsilateral and contralateral cochlear nuclei ascend through the dorsolateral pons and low midbrain as the lateral lemnisci (see Figs. 15-9, 15-10, 15-13, and 15-14). Additional fibers from relays in and traversing the supraolivary complex and trapezoid body (see Fig. 15-13A) contribute significantly to the lateral lemnisci. The lateral lemnisci form the lateral surface of the high pons and low midbrain at the acoustic (lemniscal) trigone, pass superficial to (external to) the superior cerebellar peduncles, and synapse within the inferior colliculi.[4] In axial images through the high pons, the medial and the lateral lemnisci anchor the two ends of the broad lemniscal arc.

Spinothalamic Tracts (Spinal Lemnisci). Secondary sensory fibers for pain, temperature, and coarse (nondiscriminative) touch arise from neurons of the spinal cord, decussate in the ventral white commissure of the cord, and ascend to the brain stem in two streams.[8] (1) The secondary pain and temperature fibers form the lateral spinothalamic tract that ascends within the lateral funiculus, deep to the ventral spinocerebellar tract. At the lower brain stem, these axons continue upward in the anterolateral funiculus as the spinal lemniscus.[8] (2) The secondary coarse tactile fibers form the ventral spinothalamic tract that ascends within the anterior funiculus medial to the exit of the ventral roots. At the lower brain stem, these axons join the medial lemniscus.[8] In humans, both spinothalamic tracts terminate predominantly within the ventral posterolateral nuclei of the thalamus.

Trigeminothalamic Tracts

Ventral Trigeminothalamic Tract. Secondary relay fibers originating in the rostral and middle thirds of the spinal trigeminal nucleus cross the midline and enter the ventral trigeminothalamic tract. Secondary sensory fibers from the ventral portion of the principal sensory nucleus of CN V also cross the midline to the contralateral ventral trigeminothalamic tract and ascend with the crossed secondary fibers of the spinal trigeminal nucleus. Both sets of fibers reach the ventral posteromedial nucleus of the contralateral thalamus.

Dorsal Trigeminothalamic Tract. Secondary fibers of the *caudal* one third of the spinal trigeminal nucleus pass to the ipsilateral dorsal trigeminothalamic tract and ascend in the anterolateral fasciculus of the ventrolateral medulla with the spinothalamic tract.[4] This tract migrates dorsally into the dorsolateral pons, where it is joined by secondary fibers of the dorsomedial portion of the principal sensory nucleus of CN V. Together, these dorsal trigeminothalamic tract fibers ascend through the dorsal tegmentum of the pons and lower midbrain, turn ventrally, and converge toward the ventral trigeminothalamic tract in the upper midbrain. The crossed fibers of the ventral trigeminothalamic tract and the uncrossed fibers of the dorsal trigeminothalamic tract both reach the ventral posteromedial nucleus of each thalamus.[4]

Medial Longitudinal Fasciculus

The medial longitudinal fasciculus coordinates eye movements and integrates them with head and body movements.[2] Within the brain stem, a well-defined portion of this fasciculus ascends through the tegmentum immediately ventral to the abducens, trochlear and oculomotor (CN VI, IV, and III) nuclei, partially enclosing their ventral borders (see Figs. 15-7B and Figs. 15-11 to 15-15). This ascending portion is responsible for conjugate gaze and helps to maintain gaze fixation despite movements of the head and body.[2] Fibers from the medial vestibular nucleus to the abducens nuclei help mediate horizontal eye movements in response to stimulation of the horizontal semicircular canals.[2] Fibers from the superior vestibular nucleus to the oculomotor nuclei help mediate vertical eye movements in response to stimulation of the lateral and posterior semicircular canals.[2] Inferior to the abducens nuclei a less well-defined portion of the medial longitudinal fasciculus descends into the upper thoracic spinal cord.[2] The medial and inferior vestibular nuclei send medial vestibulospinal fibers into the descending portion of the fasciculus bilaterally.[2]

Spinocerebellar Tracts

Dorsal (Posterior) Spinocerebellar Tract. Somatosensory data from muscle spindles, cutaneous touch receptors, and joint receptors for the lower extremities and trunk pass to the spinal cord and synapse in the ipsilateral dorsal nucleus (dorsal column) of Clarke situated in the intermediate gray matter of the spinal cord (Rexed lamina VII) from approximately L3 to C8. Sensory data from segments caudal to L3 first ascend in the fasciculus gracilis and then pass to the caudal end of Clarke's column where they synapse. Sensory data from segments L3 to C8 enter with the segmental dorsal roots and pass directly to Clarke's column. From L3 through C8, first-order efferent fibers from Clarke's column form the dorsal spinocerebellar tract that ascends ipsilaterally along the length of the spinal cord to reach the brain stem (see Fig. 15-11).[4] Within the brain stem, the dorsal spinocerebellar tract ascends along the lateral surface of the low medulla, just anterior to the spinal trigeminal tract. It then passes posteriorly external to and covering the spinal trigeminal tract to enter the ipsilateral inferior cerebellar peduncle.[4]

Ventral (Anterior) Spinocerebellar Tract. Somatosensory data for proprioception, pain, and pressure from the lumbar and some sacral levels enter the dorsal horns of the spinal cord to synapse with neurons in the intermediate gray matter and base of the dorsal horns (Rexed laminae V to VII). Most relay fibers then cross the midline through the ventral white commissure of the spinal cord and ascend as the primarily crossed ventral spinocerebellar tract to reach the brain stem (see Figs. 15-11 to 15-13).[4] Within the brain stem, the ventral spinocerebellar tract ascends in the anterolateral fasciculus with the spinothalamic tract. Further rostrally, the ventral spinocerebellar tract curves posterolaterally and spreads out into a thin lamina that ascends along the external surface of the superior cerebellar peduncle of the midbrain. From there, the fibers recurve ventrally and medially to enter the superior aspect of the cerebellum medial (deep) to the superior cerebellar peduncle.[4] Other ventral spinocerebellar fibers ascend to the cerebellum ipsilaterally.[1]

Cuneocerebellar Tract for the Upper Extremities. Somatosensory data from muscle spindles, cutaneous touch receptors, and joint receptors in the upper extremities enter the dorsal horns of the spinal cord and ascend in the lateral portion of the ipsilateral fasciculus cuneatus to synapse somatotopically in the ipsilateral accessory cuneate nucleus and the adjacent lateral portion of the cuneate nucleus.[8] Together, these nuclei serve as the upper extremity counterpart of the dorsal nucleus of Clarke. From these nuclei, secondary relay (external arcuate) fibers pass to the cerebellum through the inferior cerebellar peduncle as the cuneocerebellar tract.[1,8]

Transverse Tracts
Pontocerebellar Fibers
Pontine nuclei within the basis pontis give rise to pontocerebellar fibers (see Figs. 15-9, 15-10, 14-15, and 15-14). These (predominantly) cross the midline, pass posterolaterally across the contralateral half pons, and enter the middle cerebellar peduncle opposite to their side of origin.

Olivocerebellar Tracts
Fibers from the inferior olivary nucleus and the medial accessory olivary nucleus pass medially, cross the midline, traverse the full thickness of the contralateral brain stem, enter the contralateral inferior cerebellar peduncle, and through that peduncle pass into the cerebellum (see Fig. 15-12). In their course, these olivocerebellar fibers pass directly through all intervening structures, penetrating white matter tracts and nuclear complexes, without deviation.

Trapezoid Body
The trapezoid body (see Fig. 15-13A) is a complex, transversely oriented fiber stream that carries secondary auditory fibers from the cochlear and related nuclei to the lateral lemnisci bilaterally. Its course intersects and weaves through the vertically directed fibers of the medial lemniscus.[4]

Arterial Supply of the Brain Stem
The arterial territories of the brain stem are best considered in two ways: (1) the parent vessels of supply/drainage for the region and (2) the intrinsic vascular compartment within the brain stem.

The Parent Vessels
Multiple large arteries bring blood supply to the brain stem. These include the two vertebral arteries, the basilar artery, and their four major branches: the paired anterior spinal arteries, paired posterior inferior cerebellar arteries (PICA), paired anterior inferior cerebellar arteries (AICA), and paired superior cerebellar arteries (SCA). In addition, smaller branches of these arteries supply limited extents of the surface and deep structures of the brain stem. The precise arrangement of these vessels is highly variable, with substantial left-right asymmetry and highly variable size of the PICA, AICA, and SCA in different individuals. This variability is indicated by terms such as dominant left (or right) vertebral artery, hypoplastic left (or right) PICA, and combined AICA-PICA trunks. The courses of these major arteries are reviewed in Chapters 15 and 18.

The Intrinsic Vascular Compartments
Duvernoy[4] has shown that the medulla, pons, and midbrain have relatively fixed intrinsic vascular compartments (Figs. 15-27 and 15-28). No matter which (variable) parent vessel brings supply to the surface of the brain stem, at the surface the smaller intrinsic vessels of the brain stem reliably supply four distinct anteromedial, anterolateral, lateral, and posterior vascular compartments (see Fig. 15-27):

1. The anteromedial compartments are fed by small intrinsic paramedian perforating vessels. These enter the brain stem along the median raphe, forming a vertical midline series of "vascular entry points" (see Fig. 15-23). Each paramedian perforating vessel supplies its own side of the stem.

2. The anterolateral compartments are fed by short circumflex branches of the vertebral and basilar arteries or by small side branches of PICA, AICA, or SCA. These vessels enter the anterolateral compartments of the brain stem at fixed anterolateral entry points that align with the convex lateral curvature of the brain stem on each side.

3. The lateral compartments of the brain stem are fed by long circumflex vessels or small side branches of PICA, AICA or SCA that enter the brain stem at fixed dorsolateral entry

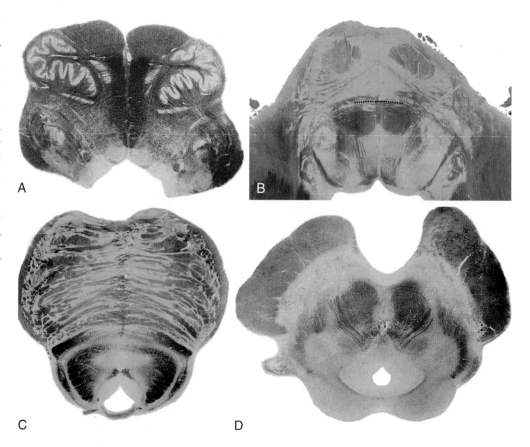

■ **FIGURE 15-27** Intrinsic arterial compartments of the brain stem. The medulla (**A**), lower pons (**B**), upper pons (**C**), and midbrain (**D**) each display intrinsic anteromedial (*green*), anterolateral (*blue*), lateral (*pink*), and posterior (*purple*) arterial compartments. The vessels vascularizing these compartments enter the brain stem at defined entry points that align vertically along the length of the brain stem. The intrinsic venous compartments are similar but not identical. *(Modified from Naidich TP, Duvernoy HM, Delman BN, et al. Duvernoy's Atlas of the Human Brain Stem and Cerebellum: High-Field MRI, Surface Anatomy, Internal Structure, Vascularization and 3D Sectional Anatomy. New York, Springer, 2008.)*

A   B

C   D

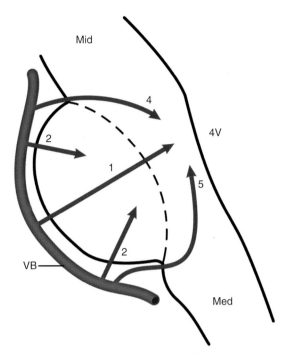

■ FIGURE 15-28 Schematic representation of the vascularization of the tegmentum of the pons. The vertebrobasilar arteries (VB) vascularize the basis pontis (*ventral to the dashed line*) and the pontine tegmentum (*dorsal to the dashed line*). At the mid pons, the paramedian perforating arteries for the anteromedial compartment (1) extend directly through the pons into the tegmentum. At the upper and lower pons, the paramedian perforators (2) vascularize just the basis pontis. The pontine tegmentum is supplied, instead, by vessels that enter the brain stem at the interpeduncular fossa (4) and the pontomedullary sulcus (5) and arch over the basis to reach the high (4) and low (5) pontine tegmentum. Other structures labeled include the fourth ventricle (4V), medulla (Med), and midbrain (Mid). (*Modified from Naidich TP, Duvernoy HM, Delman BN, et al. Duvernoy's Atlas of the Human Brain Stem and Cerebellum: High-Field MRI, Surface Anatomy, Internal Structure, Vascularization and 3D Sectional Anatomy. New York, Springer, 2008.*)

points. These also align with the convex lateral curvature of the brain stem on each side.[4]

4. The posterior compartments of the brain stem are only present at the medulla and mesencephalon, because the dorsal aspect of the pons is the floor of the fourth ventricle. The posterior compartments are fed by small branches of any vessel passing dorsal to the stem. In similar fashion, the brain stem exhibits four major intrinsic venous drainage compartments that closely resemble the arterial compartments in size and position.[4]

In sagittal sections, the paramedian perforating vessels that supply the anteromedial compartment form multiple co-curvilinear stripes that arch gently superiorly as they curve through the basal stem into the tegmentum (see Fig. 15-7). As a special case, the pontine tegmentum is fed by three different sets of vessels (see Fig. 15-28). At the midpontine level, the paramedian feeders to the anteromedial compartment extend through the full thickness of the basis pontis to supply the pontine tegmentum directly. Farther caudally, the lower pontine tegmentum is supplied, instead, by vessels that enter the brain stem at the pontomedullary sulcus and then arch upward into the lower pontine tegmentum. Superiorly, the upper pontine tegmentum is supplied by vessels that enter the brain stem at the interpeduncular fossa and then arch downward to supply the upper pontine tegmentum.

FUNCTION

Brain stem function is a deeply complex subject. Smith and DeMyer present one concise discussion of the anatomy behind brain stem function.[7] Gaze was reviewed by Fernández-Gil and colleagues,[9] and the anatomy and clinical sequelae of brain stem stroke have been reviewed by Burger and associates.[10]

IMAGING

Ultrasonography and CT have limited value for displaying brain stem anatomy, so these images are not illustrated here. MRI is the modality of choice for depicting and evaluating the anatomy and pathologic processes of the brain stem (see Figs. 15-16 to 15-20). The 3-T fast spin-echo (FSE) T2-weighted (T2W) techniques such as FSE T2 with "propeller" show the surface contours and myelinated structures of the brain stem very well. High (spatial) resolution series such as fast imaging employing steady-state acquisition (FIESTA) or constructive interference in steady state (CISS) are useful for depicting fine surface detail, the cisternal segments of the cranial nerves (see Chapter 17), and any membranes or septations within the cisterns. On average, intermediate-weighted conventional spin-echo sequences utilizing long repetition times and short echo times remain the best way to depict the gray matter structures of the brain stem. Spoiled gradient-recalled-echo (SPGR) series capture much of the gray matter anatomy, so they too are useful for imaging the brain stem. T2W fluid-attenuated inversion recovery (FLAIR) sequences are not recommended for the brain stem, because they produce images with lower contrast between normal structures and lower conspicuity of pathologic processes.

Heavily T1-weighted (T1W) series at 3 T successfully depict neuromelanin within the substantia nigra and locus ceruleus (see Figs. 15-16 to 15-21).[11,12] Using this technique, Sasaki and Shibata displayed the increased signal intensity of neuromelanin within the locus ceruleus and used differences in the signal intensity to help identify patients with Parkinson's disease, major depression, and schizophrenia.[11,12] Keren and colleagues[13] reported that the T1 signal intensity within the locus ceruleus correlates with the numbers of locus ceruleus cells present and with patient age. Younger individuals showed the greatest signal intensity in the rostral portion of the locus ceruleus, whereas older adults showed greatest signal within the caudal portion of the locus ceruleus.

Double inversion recovery sequences suppress the signal from gray matter and from white matter in two separate inversion recovery acquisitions, which, when combined, are very sensitive to changes in T1 signal intensity. Raff and coworkers,[14] Hutchinson and Raff,[15] and Minati and associates[16] showed the utility of this technique for evaluating the substantia nigra in patients with Parkinson's disease. Combined with fully automated analyses of the T1 signal of tissue (the spin lattice distribution index), this technique may prove increasingly useful in the future.[15]

High field strength clinical scanners operating at 4 T and 7 T are beginning to resolve the fine anatomy of the brain stem in vivo. Susceptibility-weighted imaging[16-18] depicts the iron-containing substantia nigra and red nuclei, the nigropallidal and pallidonigral fibers within the comb system, and the venous anatomy of the brain stem especially beautifully. Intermediate weighted 9.4-T images of postmortem specimens display brain stem anatomy with "near-histological" detail and provide an MR "template" for appreciating this anatomy on clinical images with lower resolution (see Figs. 15-22 to 15-26).[4]

Diffusion tensor imaging (DTI) and tractography (DTT) demonstrate the location and direction of the white matter tracts and help to distinguish among adjacent tracts with differing connections and function (Fig. 15-29).[4,20,21] Alvarez-Linera[22] has reviewed a variety of sophisticated techniques for MRI depiction of brain stem anatomy and pathology.

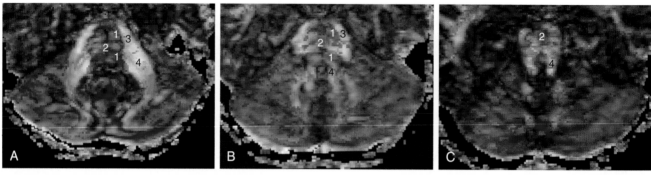

■ **FIGURE 15-29** Diffusion tensor imaging (DTI) of the brain stem at 1.5 T. Serial axial colormaps displayed from caudal to cranial. In this series, *blue* signifies the vector directed superior to inferior, *red* the vector directed left to right, and *green* the vector directed anterior to posterior. Regions with predominant oblique directionality show mixing of the prime colors in exact proportion to the vectors directed in each of the cardinal directions (see also Chapter 12). **A,** Pons. The pontocerebellar fibers (2) course transversely (*red*) across the pons, turn dorsolaterally (*green*) in the lateral pons (3), and continue back to form the middle cerebellar peduncles (4) that pass into the cerebellum. The corticobulbar and corticospinal tracts (1) course longitudinally (*blue*) between the transverse fibers. **B,** Pontomesencephalic junction. **C,** Midbrain. The superior cerebellar peduncles (4) form light blue bands as they course superiorly and anteriorly toward their decussation.

Qualitative Versus Quantitative Imaging

Early works by Han and associates[23] and Flannigan and colleagues[24] and later studies by Naidich and coworkers[4] give qualitative descriptions of the imaging anatomy of the brain stem. Recent work has begun to provide quantitative data on some of the MR features of the brain stem.

Signal Intensities

Asao and associates[25] compared the contrast-to-noise ratio of the pontine tegmentum to the basis pontis at the upper, mid, and lower pons in adults and children. This ratio was significantly higher in the pontine tegmentum at each level, leading them to conclude that the pontine tegmentum normally displayed higher signal intensity than the basis pontis.

Ngai and colleagues[26] compared the signal intensity of the middle cerebellar peduncles to the signal intensities of the adjacent pons and cerebellar white matter on T2W FLAIR images in 122 patients aged 15 to 78 years. They found broad zones of higher signal extending across the full thickness of the middle cerebellar peduncle in 14% of normal individuals. The high signal intensity had no significant correlation with patient age.

Lengths

By taking the apex of the dome of each colliculus as the point of measurement, then:

The transverse distance between the left and right *inferior* colliculi measured 9.1 to 14.3 mm (mean + standard deviation: 11.4 mm + 1.3 mm.[27]
The transverse distance between the left and right *superior* colliculi measured 9.6 to 17.4 mm (mean + standard deviation: 13.3 mm + 1.8 mm.[27]

Somatotopy

Hong and associates[28] used diffusion tensor imaging to analyze the somatotopy of the hand and leg fibers within the pontine portion of the corticospinal tract. They found that hand fibers descended through the anteromedial portion of the pons and that leg fibers descended through the pons posterolateral to the hand fibers.[28]

Kwon and colleagues[29] similarly analyzed the somatotopy of the hand and leg in the medullary pyramids. They found that the hand fibers descended in the medial portion of the medullary pyramid, whereas the leg fibers descended in the lateral portion of the medullary pyramid.

ANALYSIS

Illustrated Approach

One useful approach to identifying lesions of the brain stem is as follows:

1. Determine whether the lesion is:
   - Intra-axial (intrinsic to the brain stem) *or*
   - Extra-axial (extrinsic to the brain stem)
2. Determine whether the lesion is unifocal, multifocal, or diffuse.
3. For each intrinsic lesion, localize the site of the pathologic process on a three-dimensional grid:
   - *Longitudinal:* medulla versus pons versus midbrain
   - *Transverse:* unilateral versus bilateral
   - Medial versus lateral
   - *Ventral-dorsal:* basis versus tegmentum versus tectum
4. Identify the density/signal intensity of each lesion.
5. Determine whether there is mass or atrophy.
6. Analyze the adjacent arteries and veins for clues to the diagnosis:
   - Vessel *structure:* normal versus anomalous
   - Normal versus acquired stenoses/dilations/mural thickenings
   - *Vessel location:* normal versus displaced
   - *Vessel flow:* normal versus reduced (atretic, thrombosed) versus increased (hypervascular lesions)
7. Determine whether lesion location and shape conform to:
   - Specific vascular territory
   - Specific tracts
   - Specific nuclei
   - Diffuse distribution
8. Review prior studies to assist in determining lesion:
   - *Acuity:* new versus subacute versus chronic
   - *Trajectory:* interval progression versus static versus regression
9. Utilize patient age and gender as a quick guide to formulating likely differential diagnoses.
10. Review the clinical history as a guide to selecting the most probable diagnosis from this group of possible differential diagnoses.

Examples

Hypertrophic olivary degeneration affects the inferior olivary nucleus of the medulla as a consequence of disruption of the triangle of Guillain-Mollaret (Fig. 15-30).[30] Anteromedial pontine infarction affects a medial wedge of the basis pontis abutting on the median raphe (Fig. 15-31).

A sample report is shown in Box 15-1.

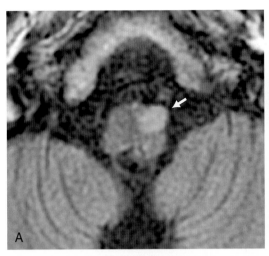

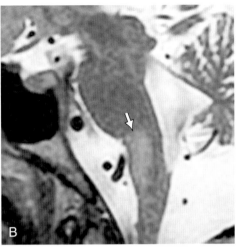

■ FIGURE 15-30 Hypertrophic olivary degeneration in a 48-year-old man. **A,** Axial T2W FLAIR image. **B,** Sagittal T2W fast spin-echo image. The lesion (*arrows*) is intrinsic to the brain stem, unifocal, unilateral, and situated in the medulla, ventrally and laterally. Its position and shape conform to the inferior olivary nucleus. The nucleus is expanded, indicating a mass. The adjacent arteries are normal with no anomaly, no stenosis, and no hypervascularity.

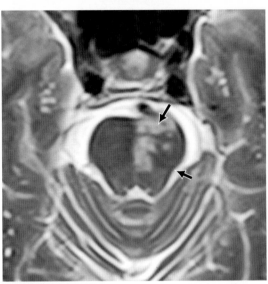

■ FIGURE 15-31 Anteromedial pontine infarction in a 61-year-old man. The lateral pontine sulcus (*short arrow*) marks the approximate interface between the higher signal pontine tegmentum and lower signal basis pontis. The high signal lesion (*long arrow*) has a geographic shape suggesting a vascular territory. The lesion extends from the basis pontis into the pontine tegmentum, is delimited medially by the median raphe, and shows a wider transverse dimension ventrally than dorsally. This conforms to the unilateral anteromedial pontine compartment irrigated by left paramedian perforating arteries.

BOX 15-1   Sample Report: MRI of Wallerian Degeneration

PATIENT HISTORY

A 49-year-old man presented with trauma, acute right hemiparesis, and subsequent coma 3 months before this study.

COMPARISON STUDIES

No prior studies were available for comparison at this institution. It is recommended that any old studies be obtained and submitted for review.

TECHNIQUE

MRI of the head was performed first as serial noncontrast sagittal T1W, axial T1W, axial T2W, axial FLAIR T2W, coronal T2W, coronal susceptibility-weighted, and axial diffusion-weighted series with apparent diffusion coefficient maps (Fig. 15-32). The diffusion-weighted images were postprocessed offline to generate diffusion tensor tractograms of the corticospinal tracts.

CONTRAST AGENT

No contrast agent was administered.

FINDINGS

There is evidence of prior left craniotomy, left cerebral atrophy with asymmetric dilatation of the left lateral ventricle, and an elongated left hemosiderin cleft extending through the striatum, posterior limb of the internal capsule, and corona radiata. There is reduced size of the left cerebral peduncle with a broad zone of increased T2 signal intensity encompassing the left crus cerebri and left substantia nigra at the sites of the corticospinal and corticobulbar fibers. The abnormal high signal extends inferiorly through the left basis pontis along the course of the descending corticospinal and corticobulbar tracts. In the low medulla, the abnormally increased T2 signal conforms precisely to the site of the left medullary pyramid. In subsequent images, the abnormal T2 signal first passes posteriorly, inferiorly, and medially along the expected course of the decussation of the pyramid. It then continues inferiorly on the contralateral right side at the expected site of the crossed lateral corticospinal tract. At that level, the left hemicord is smaller than the right. These imaging features conform to those expected for Wallerian degeneration along the corticospinal and corticobulbar tracts caudal to the left cerebral, capsular, and ganglionic hemorrhage. Diffusion tensor tractography confirms that the hemorrhage has disrupted the left corticospinal fibers, so only a thin remnant of the left corticospinal tract descends through the brain stem.

There is no associated mass effect, no hypervascularity, and no sign of venous occlusion. There is no imaging evidence of additional hemorrhage within the brain stem inferior to the major gangliocapsular hemorrhage.

IMPRESSION

There is a prior left cerebral and gangliocapsular hemorrhage with residual long hemosiderin cleft, a prior left craniotomy, residual left cerebral atrophy, and Wallerian degeneration within the left corticospinal and corticobulbar tracts caudal to the site of the cerebral hemorrhage. If there is clinical concern as to the caudal level of the Wallerian degeneration, dedicated MR studies of the cervical and thoracic spine may be obtained.

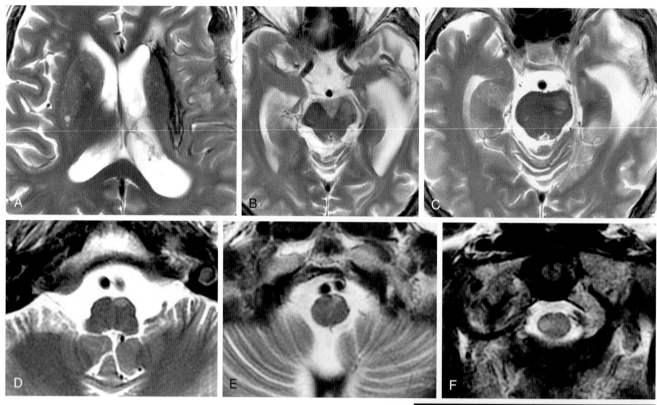

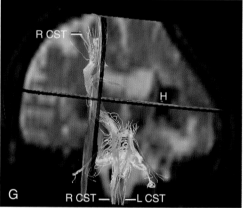

■ **FIGURE 15-32** Wallerian degeneration along the corticospinal tract in a 49-year-old man with prior traumatic hemorrhage into the left lenticular nucleus and posterior limb of the left internal capsule. Sequential axial T2W MR images at the levels of the cerebral hemispheres (**A**), midbrain (**B**), pons (**C**), medulla (**D**), cervicomedullary junction (**E**), and upper cervical spinal cord (**F**). The high signal intensity descends ipsilaterally along the corticospinal and corticobulbar tracts to the midbrain, pons, and medulla, passes posteromedially at the decussation of the pyramids (**E**), and continues inferiorly as the crossed lateral corticospinal tract in the posterior portion of the contralateral lateral funiculus (**F**). **G**, Diffusion tensor tractography of the left and right corticospinal tracts (CST) projected onto a coronal plane MR image. H, hemorrhage.

KEY POINTS

■ The brain stem shows three craniocaudal divisions: the medulla inferiorly, the pons in the middle, and the midbrain superiorly.

■ The brain stem shows three ventral dorsal divisions: the basis most ventrally, the tegmentum in the middle, and the tectum dorsally.

■ The midbrain has two cranial nerves, CN III and IV; the pons has four cranial nerves, CN V, VI, VII, and VIII; and the medulla has four cranial nerves, CN IX, X, XI, and XII.

■ The locations of brain stem structures and lesions may be simplified by applying a three-dimensional grid and specifying the following:
  ● Rostrocaudal location as midbrain, pons or medulla
  ● Ventrodorsal location as basis, tegmentum, or tectum
  ● Mediolateral location as, first, left, right or bilateral, and, second, as paramedian, intermediate or lateral. Thus, a lesion might first be characterized involving the paramedian pontine tegmentum.

■ Such initial localizations may then be refined by specifying the relationship of the brain stem structure or lesion to specific external landmarks, to brain stem nuclei, and to fiber tracts within the brain stem. Thus, the same lesion might be further characterized as a small focus of abnormal signal intensity in the medial left pontine tegmentum involving the facial colliculus.

■ Comparison of lesion shape and extent with known intrinsic anteromedial, anterolateral, lateral, and dorsal arterial compartments will usually help to diagnosis brain stem infarctions.

■ Correlation of all the imaging features with clinical history and neurologic examination will then determine whether the imaging findings support the initial clinical diagnoses or, instead, suggest the need to explore other differential possibilities.

SUGGESTED READINGS

Carpenter MB, Sutin J. Human Neuroanatomy, 8th ed. Baltimore, Williams & Wilkins, 1983.

Gilman S, Newman SW. Manter and Gatz' Essentials of Clinical Neuroanatomy and Neurophysiology, 10th ed. Philadelphia, FA Davis, 2003.

Miller RA, Burack E. Atlas of the Central Nervous System in Man, 3rd ed. Baltimore, Williams & Wilkins, 1981.

Naidich TP, Duvernoy HM, Delman BN, et al. Duvernoy's Atlas of the Human Brain Stem and Cerebellum: High-Field MRI: Surface Anatomy, Internal Structure, Vascularization and 3D Sectional Anatomy. New York, Springer, 2008.

Nieuwenhuys R, Voogd J, van Huijzen C. The Human Central Nervous System, 4th ed. Berlin, Springer, 2008.

Riley HA. An Atlas of the Basal Ganglia, Brainstem and Spinal Cord. Baltimore, Williams & Wilkins, 1943.

Smith LH, DeMyer WE. Anatomy of the Brainstem. Semin Pediatr Neurol 2003; 10:235-240.

Standring S (ed). Gray's Anatomy: The Anatomical Basis of Clinical Practice, 40th ed. Philadelphia, Elsevier, 2008.

REFERENCES

1. Carpenter MB, Sutin J. Human Neuroanatomy, 8th ed. Baltimore, Williams & Wilkins, 1983.
2. Gilman S, Newman SW. Manter and Gatz' Essentials of Clinical Neuroanatomy and Neurophysiology, 10th ed. Philadelphia, FA Davis, 2003.
3. Miller RA, Burack E. Atlas of the Central Nervous System in Man., 3rd ed. Baltimore, Williams & Wilkins, 1981.
4. Naidich TP, Duvernoy HM, Delman BN, et al. Duvernoy's Atlas of the Human Brain Stem and Cerebellum: High-Field MRI: Surface Anatomy, Internal Structure, Vascularization and 3D Sectional Anatomy. New York, Springer, 2008.
5. Nieuwenhuys R, Voogd J, van Huijzen C. The Human Central Nervous System, 4th ed. Berlin, Springer, 2008.
6. Riley HA. An Atlas of the Basal Ganglia, Brainstem and Spinal Cord. Baltimore, Williams & Wilkins, 1943.
7. Smith LH, DeMyer WE. Anatomy of the Brainstem. Semin Pediatr Neurol 2003; 10:235-240.
8. Standring S (ed). Gray's Anatomy: The Anatomical Basis of Clinical Practice, 39th ed. Edinburgh, Elsevier Churchill Livingstone, 2005.
9. Fernández-Gil MA, Palacios-Bote R, Leo-Barahona M, Mora-Escinas JP. Anatomy of the brainstem: a gaze into the stem of life. Semin Ultrasound CT MRI 2010; 31:196-219.
10. Burger KM, Tuhrim S, Naidich TP. Brainstem vascular stroke anatomy. Neuroimaging Clin North Am 2005; 15:297-324.
11. Sasaki M, Shibata E, Tohyama K, et al. Neuromelanin magnetic resonance imaging of locus ceruleus and substantia nigra in Parkinson's disease. NeuroReport 2006; 17:1215-1218.
12. Shibata E, Sasaki M, Tohyama K, et al. Age-related changes in locus ceruleus on neuromelanin magnetic resonance imaging at 3 Tesla. Magn Reson Med Sci 2006; 5:197-200.
13. Keren NI, Lozar CT, Harris KC, et al. In vivo mapping of the human locus coeruleus. NeuroImage 2009; 47:1261-1267.
14. Raff U, Hutchinson M, Rojas GM, Huete I. Inversion recovery MRI in idiopathic Parkinson's disease is a sensitive tool to assess neurodegeneration in the substantia nigra: preliminary investigation. Acad Radiol 2006; 13:721-727.
15. Hutchinson M, Raff U. Detection of Parkinson's disease by MRI: spin-lattice distribution imaging. Movement Disord 2008; 23:1991-1997.
16. Minati L, Grisoli M, Carella F, et al. Imaging degeneration in the substantia nigra in Parkinson disease with inversion recovery MRI. AJNR Am J Neuroradiol 2007; 28:309-313.
17. Haacke EM, Xu Y, Cheng YN, et al. Susceptibility-weighted imaging (SWI). Magn Reson Med 2004; 52:612-618.
18. Haacke EM, Cheng NY, House MJ, et al. Imaging iron stores in the brain using magnetic resonance imaging. Magn Reson Imaging 2005; 23:1-25.
19. Manova ES, Habib CA, Boikov AS, et al. Characterizing the mesencephalon using susceptibility-weighted imaging. AJNR Am J Neuroradiol 2009; 30:569-574.
20. Nagae-Poetscher LM, Jiang H, Wakana S, et al. High-resolution diffusion tensor imaging of the brain stem at 3 T. AJNR Am J Neuroradiol 2004; 25:1325-1330.
21. Salamon N, Sicotte N, Alger J, et al. Analysis of the brain-stem white-matter tracts with diffusion tensor imaging. Neuroradiology 2005; 47:895-902.
22. Alvarez-Linera J. Magnetic resonance techniques for the brainstem. Semin Ultrasound CT MRI 2010; 31:230-245.
23. Han JS, Bonstelle CT, Kaufman B, et al. Magnetic resonance imaging in the evaluation of the brainstem. Radiology 1984; 150:705-712.
24. Flannigan BD, Bradley WG Jr, Mazziotta JC, et al. Magnetic resonance imaging of the brainstem: normal structure and basic functional anatomy. Radiology 1985; 154:375-383.
25. Asao C, Hirai T, Imuta M, et al. Signal intensity of the normal pontine tegmentum on T2-weighted MR imaging. Neuroradiology 2006; 48:166-170.
26. Ngai S, Tang YM, Du L, Stuckey S. Hyperintensity of the middle cerebellar peduncles on fluid-attenuated inversion recovery imaging: variation with age and implications for the diagnosis of multiple system atrophy. AJNR Am J Neuroradiol 2006; 27:2146-2148.
27. Columbano L, Stieglitz LH, Wrede KH, et al. Anatomic study of the quadrigeminal cistern in patients with 3-dimensional magnetic resonance cisternography. Neurosurgery 2010; 66:991-998.
28. Hong J, Son SM, Jang SH; Somatotopic location of the corticospinal tract at pons in human brain: a diffusion tensor tractography study. NeuroImage 2010; 51:952-955.
29. Kwon HG, Hong JH, Kwon YH, Jang SH. Somatotopic arrangement of the corticospinal tract at the medullary pyramid in the human brain. Eur Neurol 2011; 65:46-49.
30. Goyal M, Versnick E, Tuite P, et al. Hypertrophic olivary degeneration: metaanalysis of the temporal evolution of MR findings. AJNR Am J Neuroradiol 2000; 21:1073-1077.

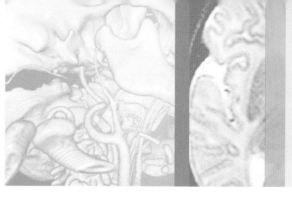

CHAPTER 16

Cerebellum

Thomas P. Naidich, Evan G. Stein, Patrick A. Lento, George M. Kleinman, Mary Elizabeth Fowkes, and David M. Carpenter

The cerebellum (little brain) is the dorsal portion of the metencephalon situated within the posterior fossa. It is composed of three lobes: the anterior lobe, posterior lobe, and flocculonodular lobe.

ANATOMY

Grossly, the cerebellum is a small structure situated posterior and inferior to the bulk of the cerebrum (Fig. 16-1). It constitutes approximately 10% of the brain by weight but contains about half as many neurons as the cerebral hemispheres. The three lobes of the cerebellum contain nine lobules, distributed with three lobules in the anterior lobe, five in the posterior lobe, and one in the flocculonodular lobe. In most cases, the lobules of the vermis merge laterally with the lobules of the hemispheres. Along the posterior surface of the cerebellum, however, there is a slight offset in the alignment of the medial vermal lobules with the corresponding lateral hemispheric lobules (Fig. 16-2). The lobes and lobules have been classified in many ways. For the purposes of comparative anatomy, the Larsell classification is most specific.[1] For clear medical communication, the common

names are more useful. These are both provided, with synonyms, in Table 16-1.

Cerebellar Surfaces

The cerebellum has three major surfaces: (1) a superior surface that faces the tentorium, (2) a posterior surface that faces the occipital bone, and (3) an anterior surface that faces the petrous pyramids (see Fig. 16-2). These surfaces may also be designated the tentorial, occipital, and petrous surfaces of the cerebellum, respectively. Each surface displays multiple thin folia separated by variably deep fissures.

Superior (Tentorial) Surface

The superior surface is roughly triangular, with notches anteriorly and posteriorly (see Figs. 16-2A and B). In the midline anteriorly, the superior surface is recessed to accommodate the brain stem. In the midline posteriorly, the superior surface is recessed at the vermis, leaving a posterior indentation designated the posterior cerebellar notch. The paired cerebellar hemispheres project forward to each side of the midbrain and

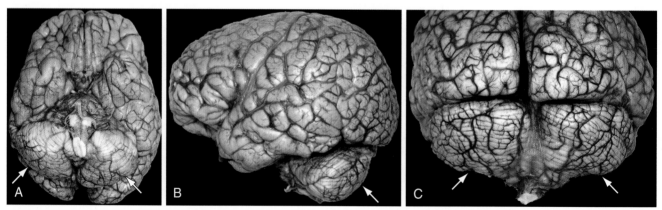

■ **FIGURE 16-1** Relationships of the cerebrum to the cerebellum. Formalin-fixed human brain. **A,** Base view. **B,** Lateral view. **C,** Posterior view. The dural folds of the falx and tentorium have been removed. The cerebellum (little brain) (*white arrows*) lies posteroinferior to the cerebrum in relation to the inferior surfaces of the posterior temporal and occipital lobes. The thin "parallel" folia and fissures of the cerebellum are distinctly different from the swirling gyri and sulci of the cerebrum. The large vessels of the cerebellar surface course nearly perpendicular to the lines of folia and fissures. In **C,** the glistening arachnoid marks the posterior wall of cisterna magna. The posterior cerebellar notch of the cerebellum often does not align perfectly with the interhemispheric fissure above.

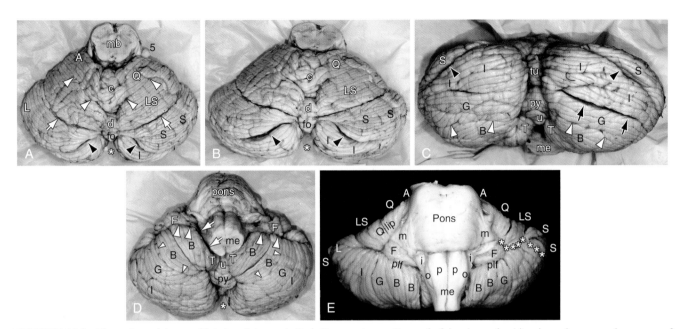

■ **FIGURE 16-2** The surfaces, lobes, and lobules of the cerebellum. Two specimens. Removal of the pia-arachnoid and vessels exposes the pattern of the folia, fissures, and lobules. The major fissures have been opened by blunt finger dissection to emphasize their position and configuration. **A** to **D**, Specimen 1. **A** and **B**, The superior (tentorial) surface seen from directly above (**A**) and from above and behind (**B**). The superior surface has an overall butterfly shape, with a midline vermis situated between flanking cerebellar hemispheres. The back of the midbrain (mb) is enclosed by the anterior cerebellum. The anterior angles (A) mark the anteriormost extent of the cerebellum and lie just above and behind the sites at which CN V (trigeminal nerve) (5) enters the pons. The lateral angles (L) mark the lateral extremes of the hemispheres. The anterolateral and posterolateral margins separate the superior surface from the anterior and posterior surfaces. The posterior surface of the vermis is recessed within the posterior cerebellar notch (*asterisk*) between the two overhanging hemispheres. The primary fissure (*white arrowheads*) has a distinct trapezoidal shape, oblique within the hemispheres and horizontal within the vermis. The primary fissure separates the anterior lobe from the posterior lobe of the cerebellum. The posterior superior fissure (*white arrows*) is far rounder and just "kisses" the deepest portion of the posterior cerebellar notch. The medialmost portions of the great horizontal fissures (*black arrowheads*) are exposed on the superior surface far posteriorly. Laterally the great horizontal fissures pass onto the posterior (occipital) surfaces to separate the superior semilunar lobules (S) from the inferior semilunar lobules (I). The superior semilunar lobules lie between the posterior superior and the great horizontal fissures. They resemble sections of an orange, lain on their sides. The superior semilunar lobules form the lateral angles and most of the posterolateral margins of the hemispheres. In the vermis, from anterior to posterior: c, culmen; d, declive; fo, folium; tu, tuber. In the hemispheres: Q, (anterior) quadrangular lobule; LS, lobulus simplex; S, superior semilunar lobule; I, inferior semilunar lobule. **C** and **D**, The posterior (**C**) and posteroinferior surfaces (**D**) show deeper, better-defined paravermian grooves. The great horizontal fissures (*black arrowheads*) extend to the lateral edges of the posterior surface, pass approximately 1 cm inferior to the lateral angles, and, from there, cross onto the anterior (petrous) surfaces of the hemispheres (see **E**). The inferior semilunar lobules (I) form prominent crescents just inferior to the horizontal fissures. The ansoparamedian fissures (*black arrows*) separate the inferior semilunar lobules above from the gracile lobules (G) below. The gracile (G) and biventral (B) lobules form the rest of the posteroinferior cerebellar surface. The pyramis (py) of the vermis has a characteristic quadrifoil shape. The uvula (u) is narrow and lies ventral to the pyramis along the curving surface of the vermis. The paired cerebellar tonsils (T, T) flank the uvula to each side and lie half behind and half alongside the medulla oblongata (me). The tonsils and the biventral lobules are separated from the medulla by the cerebellomedullary fissures (*thin white arrows* in **D**). In **D**, the paired flocculi (F) are visible, projecting forward from the anterior (petrous) surfaces of the hemispheres. *Small white arrowheads* indicate the prebiventral fissures. *Large white arrowheads* indicate the posterolateral fissures that separate the posterior lobe from the flocculonodular lobe of the cerebellum. The intrabiventral fissures are visible between the two Bs but are not specifically labeled. **E**, Specimen 2. Anterior (petrous) surface of the brain stem and cerebellum. The pons (pons), medulla (me), pontomedullary sulcus, paired pyramids (p) of the medulla, and inferior olives (o) are seen along the midline. The inferior cerebellar peduncles (i) arise from the medulla and angle posterolaterally into the cerebellum. The middle cerebellar peduncles (m) arise from the lateral aspects of the pons and angle posteroinferiorly into the cerebellar hemispheres. The anterior angles (A), anterolateral margins, and lateral angles (L) define the border between the anterior and superior surfaces of the hemisphere. No defined landmark separates the posterior from the anterior surface. The strip of cerebellum formed by the anterior surfaces of the quadrangular lobule (Q) and lobulus simplex (LS) is designated the quadrangular lip. This lip borders directly on the upper surfaces of the middle cerebellar peduncles (brachium pontis) (m) on each side. The paired flocculi (F, F) border directly on the posterior inferior surface of the middle cerebellar peduncle. The posterolateral fissures (plf) form the posterior borders of the flocculi, between the flocculi anteriorly and the lobulus gracilis (G) and biventral lobules (B) behind. The inferior medial border of the biventral lobule is the biventral ridge. This flanks the medulla bilaterally, and is separated from it by the cerebellomedullary fissure. The great horizontal fissures (*row of asterisks*) extend onto the anterior surfaces of the cerebellum toward and then superolateral to the flocculi (F). o, olive; p, pyramid.

backward to each side of the posterior cerebellar notch. The most anterior point on the cerebellum is the anterior angle. The anterior angles overlie the origins of the trigeminal nerves from the pons and may serve as a landmark for them. The most lateral point on the cerebellum is the lateral angle. The lateral edge of the superior surface between the anterior angle and the lateral angle is designated the anterolateral margin. The posterior edge of the superior surface between the lateral angle and the posterior cerebellar notch is the posterolateral margin. The superior surface rises far higher in the midline than laterally (Fig. 16-3).

The most superior portion of the cerebellum lies in the midline just behind the midbrain and corresponds to the culmen of the vermis.

The superior surface shows three large lobules delimited by three fissures. From anterior to posterior, these are the primary fissure, the posterior superior fissure, and the medial portion of the great horizontal fissure. The anteriormost (primary) fissure is trapezoidal and lies between the culmen/quadrangular lobule in front and the declive/lobulus simplex behind. It separates the anterior from the posterior lobe of the cerebellum and is the

TABLE 16-1. Lobes and Lobules of the Cerebellum

Classical 3 lobes	Yasargil 4 lobes	Larsell 10 divisions	Vermis 9 lobules	Hemispheres 10 lobules	Intervening fissure 10 fissures
			Anterior medullary velum		
		I	Lingula	Vinculum	
					Precentral fissure
Anterior lobe	Anterior lobe	II, III	Central	Wing of central	
					Preculminate fissure
		IV, V	Culmen	Anterior quadrangular	
					Primary fissure
	Middle lobe	VI	Declive	Lobulus simplex	
					Posterior superior fissure
		VII	Folium	Superior semilunar	
					Great horizontal fissure
				Inferior semilunar	
Posterior lobe		VII	Tuber		Fissura ansoparamedianus
		Prepyramidal fissure		Lobulus gracilis	
					Prebiventral fissure
				Biventral lobule	
					Intrabiventral fissure
	Posterior lobe	VIII	Pyramis	Biventral lobule	
					Secondary fissure
		IX	Uvula	Tonsil	
					Posterolateral fissure
Flocculo-nodular lobe	Flocculo-nodular lobe	X	Nodulus	Flocculus	
			Posterior medullary velum		

deepest fissure in the vermis.[2] The next most posterior fissure is the rounder posterior superior (postclival) fissure. It has a rounded shape and just "kisses" the anterior edge of the posterior cerebellar notch in the midline. This posterior superior fissure separates the declive/lobulus simplex anteriorly from the folium/superior semilunar lobule posteriorly. Two small oblique fissures arise in the posterior cerebellar notch and extend posterolaterally for a short distance. These are the small, medial portions of the great horizontal fissures that become very much larger on the posterior surface. The great horizontal fissures separate the folium/superior semilunar lobules anteriorly from the tuber/inferior semilunar lobules posteriorly. On the superior surface, the midline vermis is delimited laterally by two shallow paramedian grooves and by the abrupt angulations made by the cerebellar fissures as they pass from the hemispheres laterally to the vermis medially.

Along the superior surface, the anterior angle is formed by the quadrangular lobule. The anterolateral margin is formed, from anterior to posterior, by the quadrangular lobule, the lobulus simplex, and the superior semilunar lobule. The lateral angle and the entire posterolateral margin are formed by the superior semilunar lobule.

Posterior (Occipital) Surface
The posterior surface is round with an undulant lateral border (see Figs. 16-1C and 16-2C). The superior edge of the posterior surface is the posterolateral margin that is formed by the superior semilunar lobule. This margin is highest in the midline and slopes gently downward as it passes laterally. The inferior edge of the posterior surface is the biventral ridge, formed by the

inferior margin of the biventral lobule. The lateral border of the posterior surface is sinuous, convex laterally more superiorly and convex medially most inferiorly. On the posterior surface, the medial border of each hemisphere is largely convex medially. The posterior surfaces of the hemispheres are clearly demarcated from the vermis by deep paravermian grooves/fissures.

Up to seven variably large fissures are seen along the posterior and inferior surfaces of the cerebellum (see Table 16-1). The most superior, deepest, and most prominent fissure on each side is the *great horizontal fissure*. This starts on the superior surface near the midline, passes inferolaterally onto the posterior surface, and then continues inferolaterally across the entire posterior surface of the hemisphere. It passes approximately 1 cm inferior to the lateral angle of the cerebellum and then swings onto the anterior (petrosal) surface of the cerebellum. The great horizontal fissure separates the folium/superior semilunar lobule above from the tuber/inferior semilunar lobule below (Fig. 16-2).

Farther inferiorly, the vermian fissures and lobules are offset from the cerebellar fissures and lobules. Medially, restricted to the vermis only, the *prepyramidal fissure* separates the tuber above from the pyramis below. Laterally to each side, and restricted to the hemispheres only, the *ansoparamedian fissures* separate the inferior semilunar lobules from the gracile lobules, the *prebiventral fissures* separate the gracile from the biventral lobules, and the *intrabiventral fissures* partially subdivide the biventral lobules.

Inferior to this point, the vermian and hemispheric structures realign with each other and curve onto the undersurface of the cerebellum, like a dog with its tail between its legs. Tucked deeply into the posterior surface (and not readily visible on the

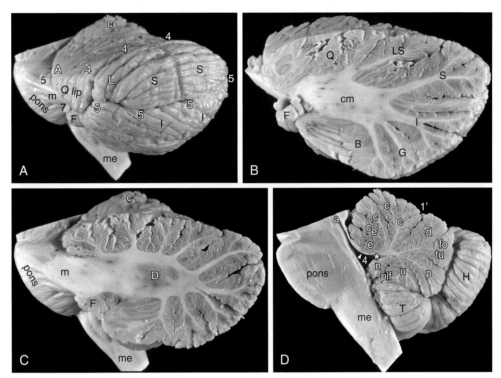

■ FIGURE 16-3 Lateral surface and sagittal sections of the cerebellum. Formalin-fixed postmortem specimen after removal of the vessels and pia-arachnoid. **A,** Lateral view. The cerebellum has a characteristic undulant contour. The highest point on the cerebellum is the culmen (c) of the vermis. The anterior angle (A), lateral angle (L), and anterolateral margin are well seen. The posterior superior fissure (4) and the great horizontal fissure (5) define the superior semilunar lobule (S). They meet at the lateral aspect of the anterior surface and angle together toward and then superior to the floc-culus (F). The middle cerebellar peduncle (m) passes laterally from the pons (pons) into the cerebellar hemisphere. me, medulla; 5, CN V (trigeminal nerve); 7, CN VII (facial nerve). **B,** Sagittal section through the flocculus (F) and the lateral portion of the hemisphere shows the central body of cerebellar white matter (corpus medullare) (cm) extending outward into each lobule of the vermis in a characteristic branching pattern. Note the quadrangular lobule (Q), lobulus simplex (LS), superior semilunar lobule (S), inferior semilunar lobule (I), lobulus gracilis (G), and the biventral lobule (B). **C,** Lateral sagittal section through the middle cerebellar peduncle (m). The peduncle arises from the pons and passes into the corpus medullare. The dentate nucleus (D) lies centrally surrounded by the corpus medullare. **D,** Midsagittal section through the lowermost midbrain, pons (pons), medulla (me), aqueduct (a), and fourth ventricle (4). Midsagittal section through the cerebellum displays the midline vermis, the posterior cerebellar notch behind the vermis, and the medial surfaces of the *opposite* tonsil (T) and cerebellar hemisphere (H). The white matter of the vermis has a characteristic, spokewheel pattern designated the arbor vitae. There are nine lobules of the vermis. In order from cranial to caudal: the lingua (*arrowhead*) is closely applied to the superior medullary velum. The central lobule (ce) shows paired fronds that face the posterior surface of the midbrain and upper pons. The culmen (c) forms the apex of the vermis and typically displays a vertically oriented spike of white matter. In this specimen, the anteriormost part of the culmen more closely resembles a third frond of the central lobule (see Fig. 16-4A). The declive (d), folium (fo), and tuber (tu) appear to arise from a common spike of white matter that is oriented nearly perpendicular to the floor of the fourth ventricle (i.e., the posterior surface of the brain stem). The angle formed by the floor of the fourth ventricle and the central spike normally measures more than 90 degrees (see precise definition in text). The pyramis (p) forms the posteroinferior curvature of the vermis, typically diametrically opposite the apex of the culmen. The midline uvula (u) lies directly atop and between the two tonsils, giving it its name. The nodulus (n) indents the posterior medullary velum, giving it its characteristic shape. The fastigial recess (*asterisk*) of the fourth ventricle (4) is the midline angle of the fourth ventricle between the superior and the inferior medullary vela. The primary fissure (1') sepa-rates the anterior from the posterior lobes of the cerebellum. The vermian portion of the primary fissure lies between the culmen and the declive. The posterolateral fissure (plf) separates the posterior from the flocculonodular lobes. The vermian portion of the posterolateral fissure separates the uvula from the nodulus. Note that the white matter of the vermis has a "spokewheel" configuration, whereas the folia and fissures of the tonsil (T) are oriented parallel to each other, perpendicular to the posterior surface of the medulla. The choroid plexus passes inferiorly along the floor of the fourth ventricle toward the midline foramen of Magendie.

posterior surface), the *postpyramidal (secondary) fissure* sepa-rates the pyramis/biventral lobule above from the uvula/tonsils below. The *posterolateral fissure* separates the uvula/tonsils behind from the nodulus/flocculus in front. The relationships of the pyramis, uvula, and nodulus are best appreciated on midsag-ittal sections, rather than by surface inspection (see Figs. 16-3B and C). Along the posterior surface, two deep paravermian grooves delimit the lateral borders of the inferior vermis, incom-pletely separating the vermis from the cerebellar hemispheres lateral to it.

Anterior (Petrous) Surface
The anterior surface of the cerebellum is largely obscured by the brain stem (see Fig. 16-2E). The paired middle cerebellar

peduncles arise from the lateral borders of the pons and dive deeply into the cerebellar hemispheres, enclosed by a superior and inferior rim of cerebellum. On each side, the superolateral rim and the upper edge of the anterior surface is the antero-lateral margin. The small band of tissue that lies between the anterolateral margin and the brain stem itself is designated the quadrangular lip. The lip is formed, from medial to lateral, by the quadrangular lobule, the lobulus simplex, and the superior semilunar lobule. The band of cerebellum inferior to the middle cerebellar peduncle and lateral to the medulla is composed of the flocculus immediately inferior to the peduncle and (from lateral to medial) by the inferior semilunar, gracile, and biventral lobules more peripherally. On each side, the margin of the hemisphere situated immediately lateral to the medulla is the biventral ridge. The cerebellomedullary fissures separate the biventral ridges from the medulla on each side.

Lateral Surface

The lateral surface is really a different perspective on the combined superior, posterior, and anterior surfaces already described (see Fig. 16-3A). These surfaces show a constantly changing undulant contour that peaks at the culmen of the vermis in the midline.

Sectional Anatomy of the Cerebellum

Midline sections of the brain stem and cerebellum (see Figs. 16-3B and D) display the midbrain, pons, and medulla of the brain stem anterior to the aqueduct and fourth ventricle. The roof of the fourth ventricle is formed by the anterior (superior) medullary velum and the posterior (inferior) medullary velum. These meet at a sharp angle called the fastigial recess of the fourth ventricle. Behind the fourth ventricle lies the vermis. The vermis has a variable shape, sometimes trilobed like a three-leaf clover and at other times very smoothly rounded like a "Pacman" character. The nodulus of the vermis indents the fourth ventricle in the midline, along the posterior medullary velum, immediately inferior to the fastigial recess. It is the upper border of the nodulus that creates the curved midline contour of the posterior medullary velum. The paired cerebellar tonsils lie just off the midline to each side. They are ovoid and appear to align parallel with the long axis of the medulla. The upper poles of the tonsils indent the posterior wall of the fourth ventricle just to each side of midline, forming the paired posterior superior recesses of the fourth ventricle. It is the upper poles of the tonsils that create the curved contours of the posterior fourth ventricle laterally on each side. In midline sections, the upper pole of the tonsil is obscured by the midline vermis while the lower pole extends caudal to the vermis. The vermis and the tonsil show very different relations to the fourth ventricle and very different folial patterns. The folia and fissures of the vermis appear to radiate

outward from the fastigial recess of the fourth ventricle like a spokewheel. The folia and fissures of the tonsils align perpendicular to the long axis of the medulla.

The three lobes and nine lobules of the cerebellum are readily seen in the vermis. Clockwise, from rostral to caudal the three lobes are the anterior, posterior, and flocculonodular lobes. Clockwise, from rostral to caudal, the nine lobules are the lingula, central lobule, and culmen of the anterior lobe; the declive, folium, tuber, pyramis, and uvula of the posterior lobe; and the nodulus of the flocculonodular lobe. The individual lobules are delimited by well-defined fissures (see Figs. 16-3D and 16-4). The primary fissure separates the anterior from the posterior lobe. The posterolateral fissure separates the posterior from the flocculonodular lobe.

The white matter of the vermis forms a prominent branching pattern (the arbor vitae) that appears to radiate out from the fastigial recess of the fourth ventricle like a spokewheel (Fig. 16-4). The cerebellar white matter of each hemisphere extends across the midline, forming a cerebellar commissure. This commissure passes forward into the superior medullary velum. The choroid plexus of the fourth ventricle lies on the intraventricular side of the posterior medullary velum. It is a paired paramedian structure, not a midline structure. On each side the choroid plexus overlies the upper pole of the tonsil and extends both inferomedially toward Magendie and anterolaterally through the lateral recess of the fourth ventricle to emerge into the cerebellopontine angle through the foramen of Luschka.

Serial sections through the cerebellum display this anatomy in detail (Figs. 16-5 and 16-6).

Finer Architecture of the Cerebellum
Cerebellar Cortex

The cortex of the cerebellum is composed of three layers.[1] From superficial to deep, these are the superficial cell-poor molecular layer, a middle one-cell-thick Purkinje cell layer, and the deep granule cell layer (Fig. 16-7).[1] The Purkinje cell layer

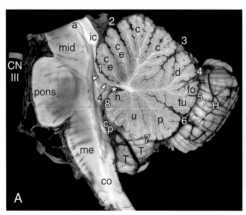
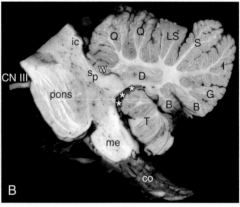

■ **FIGURE 16-4** Midline (**A**) and parasagittal (**B**) sections of the cerebellum. Formalin-fixed specimen with vessels and pia-arachnoid intact. **A,** The lobules of the vermis are labeled as in Figure 16-3D. The fissures associated with these lobules are marked with white numbers: precentral fissure (1), preculminate fissure (2), primary fissure (3), posterior superior fissure (4), great horizontal fissure (5), prepyramidal fissure (6), secondary fissure (7) and posterolateral fissure (8). The posterior superior fissure just "kisses" the depth of the posterior cerebellar notch, so it appears to lie very posterior with respect to the vermis but shows the expected location with respect to the hemisphere (H). This specimen displays the typical configuration of the culmen, with a single near-vertical spike of white matter leading to the apex, posterior to two fronds of the central lobule. The lingula (*arrowheads*) lies directly upon the superior medullary velum. The nodulus (n) indents the posterior wall of the fourth ventricle in the midline, creating the fastigial recess (*asterisk*). The orientation of the paramedian perforating vessels to the brain stem is particularly well shown in this specimen. Other labels indicate the inferior colliculus (ic) of the midbrain, the choroid plexus of the fourth ventricle (cp), and the spinal cord (co). **B,** The upper pole of each tonsil indents the posterior wall of the fourth ventricle, off midline, forming a paramedian, posterosuperior recess of the fourth ventricle. As a result, the posterior surface of the fourth ventricle displays three recesses: a midline fastigial recess that lies more anterior and superior and paired paramedian posterior superior recesses (*three asterisks*) that lie more posterior and inferior. The choroid plexus (*same asterisks*) of the fourth ventricle lies along the posterior superior recesses atop the two tonsils. The choroid also extends laterally through the lateral recesses into the cerebellopontine angles and caudally toward or through the midline foramen of Magendie. The dentate nucleus (D) lies within the cerebellar white matter and contributes efferent fibers to the superior cerebellar peduncle (sp). This more lateral sagittal section shows the wing of the central lobule (w), quadrangular lobule (Q), lobulus simplex (LS), superior (S) and inferior (I) semilunar lobules, lobulus gracilis (G), and biventral lobule (B).

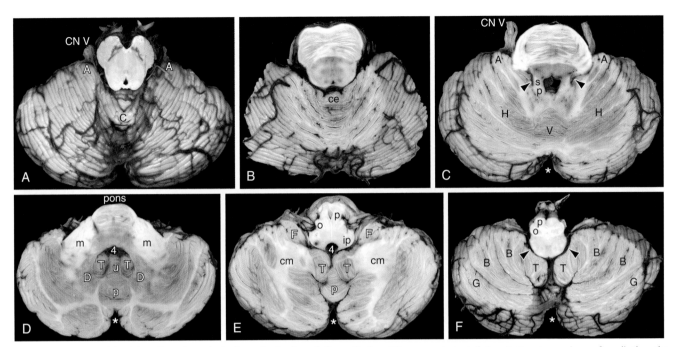

■ FIGURE 16-5 Serial axial sections through the formalin-fixed cerebellum, displayed from superior to inferior. **A,** Uncut superior surface displays the typical relationships among the midbrain, culmen of vermis (c), anterior angles of the cerebellum overlying the origins of CN V (trigeminal nerve), array of cerebellar folia co-curvilinear "parallel" with the posterolateral margin and each other, and the course of the blood vessels approximately perpendicular to that folial pattern. **B,** Section through the pontomesencephalic junction and the upper cerebellum. The folia are continuous from one hemisphere across the vermis to the other side. Their course angles sharply at the paravermian boundary, from oblique to horizontal to oblique again, giving the folia a characteristic trapezoidal configuration. The central lobule (ce) of the vermis faces the tectal plate at this level. This section lies above the posterior cerebellar notch, so the posterior contour of the section is convex. **C,** Section through the pons, upper fourth ventricle (4), vermis (V), and hemispheres (H). The anterior angles (A) overlie the entries of CNV into the lateral pons on each side. The superior cerebellar peduncles (sp) that form the lateral walls of the upper fourth ventricle appear as thin plates of white matter interposed between the fourth ventricle medially and the ambient cisterns (*arrowheads*) laterally. *Asterisk* indicates the posterior cerebellar notch. **D,** Section through the midpons and fourth ventricle (4) at level of the upper poles of the tonsils (T). The thick middle cerebellar peduncles (m) pass obliquely from the lateral aspects of the pons into the central white matter (corpus medullare) of each cerebellar hemisphere. The paired dentate nuclei (D) form pleated crescents to each side of the fourth ventricle. The paired tonsils (T) flank the uvula (u) of the vermis. **E,** Section through the medulla, low fourth ventricle (4), flocculi (F), and pyramis (*white* p) of the vermis. The medulla shows the characteristic curvatures of the medullary pyramids (*black* p), olives (o), and inferior cerebellar peduncles (ip). The flocculi (F) form fronds that extend laterally along the anterior surface of the cerebellum. The paired tonsils protrude toward the midline from the medial borders of each hemisphere. The pyramis of the vermis displays its characteristic bulbous quadrifoil shape at the depth of the posterior cerebellar notch (*asterisk*). This section displays the lowest portion of the cerebellar white matter (cm). A tiny hemorrhage is seen in the right inferior cerebellar peduncle. **F,** Section through the medulla, tonsils, and biventral lobules inferior to the cerebellar white matter and vermis. The pyramids (p) and olives (o) of the medulla are well shown. The paired tonsils (T) lie half behind and half alongside the medulla. The portions of the tonsils situated behind the medulla are convex medially. The portions situated lateral to the medulla are concave medially. The cerebellomedullary fissures (*black arrowheads*) separate the tonsils and biventral lobules from the medulla on each side. The folia and fissures of the biventral lobule appear co-curvilinear with the lateral border of the hemispheres. *Asterisk* indicates posterior cerebellar notch.

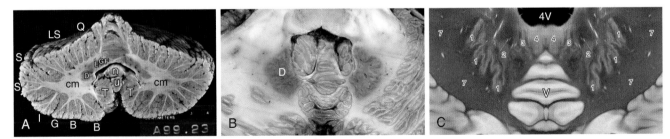

■ FIGURE 16-6 Cerebellar nuclei. Two formalin-fixed human cerebella. **A,** Unstained coronal section through the fourth ventricle, corpora medullare (cm) of the two hemispheres, the paired tonsils (T), the nodulus (n), and the uvula (u). The deep cerebellar nuclei (roof nuclei) are arrayed symmetrically around the roof of the fourth ventricle. In order from medial to lateral, these roof nuclei are the paired fastigial (F), globose (G), emboliform (E), and dentate (D) nuclei. In the coronal plane, the surface fissures and the central spikes of white matter for each lobule localize and identify the quadrangular lobule (Q), lobulus simplex (LS), superior (S) and inferior (I) semilunar lobules, lobulus gracilis (G), and biventral lobule (B). **B,** Perl (ferricyanide) stain of an axial section comparable to the section shown in Figure 16-5D. Blue coloration of the dentate nuclei (D) indicates the presence of ferric (Fe^{3+}) iron. Peripheral blue-green coloration is an artifact of prolonged formalin fixation. **C,** Composite image of postmortem specimen. Oblique 9.4-T MR image demonstrates the roof nuclei arrayed about the fourth ventricle (4V) within the cerebellar white matter (7). From medial to lateral these are the fastigial (4), globose (3), emboliform (2), and dentate (1) nuclei. C, Cerebellar hemisphere; V, vermis. (**C,** *Modified from Naidich TP, Duvernoy HM, Delman BN, et al (eds). Duvernoy's Atlas of the Human Brainstem and Cerebellum. New York, Springer-Verlag, 2009.*)

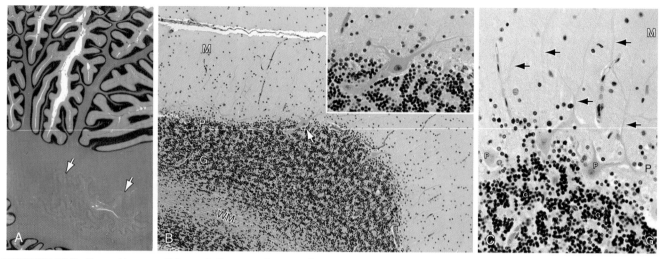

■ **FIGURE 16-7** Cytoarchitecture of the cerebellar cortex (hematoxylin & eosin stain). **A,** Cerebellar folia (original magnification, ×3). The cerebellar folia resemble the fronds of a fern leaf. The dentate nucleus (*white arrows*) is seen faintly within the white matter. **B,** The cerebellar cortex has three layers resting on a white matter (WM) base: the outer cell-sparse molecular layer (M), the middle single-cell-thick Purkinje cell (P) layer, and the inner densely cellular granule cell layer (G) (original magnification, ×100). *Inset,* Magnified view of the single Purkinje cell indicated by the *white arrow* (×250). **C,** Purkinje cells and their processes. The goblet-shaped Purkinje cells (P) extend their dendritic processes (*black arrows*) outward into the molecular layer (M), perpendicular to the surface of the cerebellum and perpendicular to the parallel fibers (original magnification, ×250). The numerous granule cells (G) lie deep to the Purkinje cell layer.

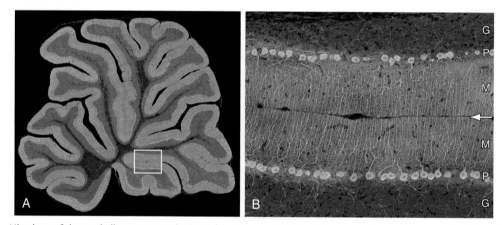

■ **FIGURE 16-8** Histology of the cerebellar cortex: rat brain. Dual-photon multicolored fluorescent laser microscopy. In this specimen, the Purkinje cell neurons have been rendered light blue with green processes, the Bergmann glial cells and their processes red, and DNA-containing cell nuclei blue by use of three differently colored fluorescent dyes (fluorescein, rhodamine, and Hoechst 33342). **A,** Cross section of the whole cerebellum. The *white box* indicates the area and orientation of part B. **B,** Magnified view of two cortical layers apposed across the cerebellar fissure (*white arrow*). The myriad nuclei within the highly cellular granule cell layer (G) give the granule cell layer a blue coloration. The one-cell-thick Purkinje cell layer (P) stains bluish green. The Purkinje cells send their processes far out into the molecular layer (M). *(Images courtesy of Thomas Deerinck and Mark Ellisman, The National Center for Microscopy and Imaging Research, University of California, San Diego.)*

gives rise to the efferent, output fibers from the cerebellum. The granule and molecular layers contain processes of the Purkinje cells and multiple interneuron (Fig. 16-8).[1]

The cerebellar white matter contains afferent mossy fibers, afferent climbing fibers, and Purkinje cell axons en route to the cerebellar/vestibular nuclei.[1] The mossy fibers originate in the spinocerebellar tracts ascending from the spinal cord, in the cuneocerebellar tracts ascending from the medulla, and in the vestibular nuclei, reticular nuclei, and pontine nuclei of the brain stem. They terminate on dendrites of granule cells to form islands of synaptic complexes (glomeruli) within the granule cell layer. Climbing fibers originate exclusively from the contralateral olivary complex. They terminate on Purkinje cell dendrites in the molecular layer.

Within the cerebellar white matter, the fibers are highly organized into mutually perpendicular systems formed by long parallel fibers that course parallel to the cerebellar surfaces and perpendicular fibers that are restricted to specific narrow parasagittal compartments (stripes) aligned perpendicular to the cerebellar surfaces (Figs. 16-9 to 16-11).

Parallel Fibers

The "parallel fibers" are the long axons of the granule cells. These ascend into the molecular layer and bifurcate into long fibers that course parallel to the cerebellar surface over great distances, intersecting multiple parasagittal stripes as they go (Fig. 16-9).

Perpendicular Fibers

The perpendicular fibers arborize solely within narrow parasagittal compartments called stripes. They have two sources. (1) The dendritic trees of the Purkinje cells extend superficially into the molecular layer to intersect the parallel fibers at right angles (Fig. 16-9). The axons of the Purkinje cells in each stripe then project to a specific cerebellar or vestibular nucleus, creating a highly

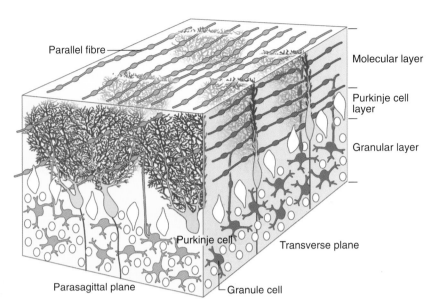

Parallel fibre

Molecular layer

Purkinje cell layer

Granular layer

Purkinje cell

Transverse plane

Parasagittal plane

Granule cell

■ FIGURE 16-9 Perpendicular array of the Purkinje and granule cell processes within the cortex. The axons of the granule cells ascend through the Purkinje cell layer into the molecular layer where they bifurcate to form long fibers that course parallel to the surface of the cerebellum. The dendritic trees of the Purkinje cells arborize into the molecular layer in parasagittal stripes that are perpendicular to the surface of the cerebellum and perpendicular to the parallel fibers of the granule cells. The climbing fibers (not shown) ascend in parasagittal stripes like, and very closely related to, the Purkinje cells. *(Modified from Nieuwenhuys R, Voogd J, van Huijzen C. Cerebellum. In The Human Central Nervous System, 4th ed. Berlin, Springer-Verlag, 2008, pp 807-839.)*

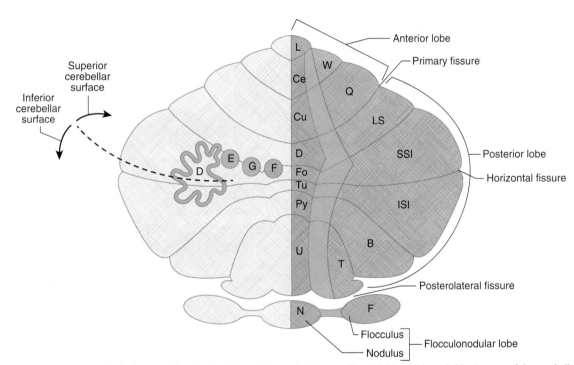

■ FIGURE 16-10 Diagrammatic depiction of the relationships of the medial, intermediate (pink), and lateral (blue) zones of the cerebellar cortex to the deep cerebellar nuclei. *Vermis:* from cranial to caudal, the vermian lobules are the lingua (L), central (Ce), culmen (Cu), declive (D), folium (Fo), tuber (Tu), pyramis (Py), uvula (U), and nodulus (N). *Hemispheres:* from cranial to caudal, the hemispheric lobules are the wing (W) of the central lobule, quadrangular lobule (Q), lobulus simplex (LS), superior semilunar lobule (SSl), inferior semilunar lobule (ISl), biventral lobule (B), tonsil (T), and flocculus (F). Gracile lobule not shown. *Nuclei:* from medial to lateral, the four major deep cerebellar nuclei are the fastigial (F), globose (G), emboliform (E), and dentate (D). As the color code shows, on each side, the medial vermian zone relates to the ipsilateral fastigial nucleus. The intermediate zone relates to the ipsilateral globose and emboliform nuclei (together designated the interposed nuclei), and the lateral zone relates to the ipsilateral dentate nucleus. This diagram does not include the interstitial cell group or the lateral vestibular nucleus. See Figure 16-11 and text.

modular signaling system (see Fig. 16-11). (2) Climbing fibers arise solely in the nuclei of the contralateral olivary complex and extend into the cerebellar cortex within the same narrow stripes as the Purkinje cell dendrites. By virtue of this anatomic arrangement, each Purkinje cell forms more than 100,000 synapses with those parallel fibers that intersect its dendritic tree.[1]

Cerebellar Zones

The cerebellum is best conceptualized as having three zones: a midline vermian zone, paired intermediate (paravermian) zones,

and paired lateral (hemispheric) zones (Fig. 16-10). These zones, and specific "stripes" within them, identify functional units that project to defined cerebellar nuclei and receive input from specific olivary nuclei (Fig. 6-11).

Specific Cerebellar Stripes

The parallel stripes of the cortex are oriented vertically, perpendicular to the folia and fissures of the cerebellar surface.[1] Each stripe is designated by an upper case letter (Figs. 16-10 and 16-11). Some stripes extend along the full rostrocaudal

■ **FIGURE 16-11** Relationship of specific cerebellar cortical stripes to the deep cerebellar nuclei: fastigial (Fast), globose (Glob), emboliform (Emb), dentate, interstitial cell group (LCG), and the dorsal portion (LV) of the lateral vestibular nucleus (Vest). *(Modified from Nieuwenhuys R, Voogd J, van Huijzen C. Cerebellum. In The Human Central Nervous System, 4th ed. Berlin, Springer-Verlag, 2008, pp 807-839.)*

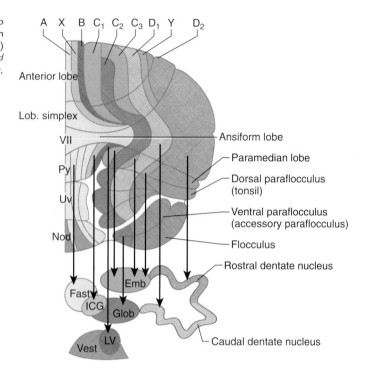

circumference of the hemisphere. Others show more limited rostrocaudal extent. The different stripes appear to use different neurotransmitters.

The cerebellar stripes fall naturally into three groups of three major stripes each: three vermian, three intermediate, and three lateral (hemispheric) stripes. Each stripe projects to a specific cerebellar nucleus and receives climbing fibers from a specific portion of the inferior olivary complex of the medulla.

Vermian Stripes
Three medial stripes situated within the cerebellar vermis are considered vermian stripes:

The most medial *stripe A* extends over the full length of the vermis, projects to the fastigial nucleus, and receives climbing fibers from the caudal medial accessory olive.
The middle *stripe X* is limited to the vermis of the anterior lobe, the declive, and a small portion of pyramis. It projects to the interstitial cell group and receives climbing fibers from a separate portion of the caudal medial accessory olive.
The lateral *stripe B* has limited geographic extent similar to the X stripe, projects to the lateral vestibular nucleus of Deiters, and receives climbing fibers from the caudal half of the dorsal accessory olive.

Intermediate Stripes
Three stripes situated in the paravermian region are considered intermediate stripes:

Stripes C1 and C3 are limited to the same craniocaudal extent as the vermal stripes X and B and are found in the anterior lobe, the lobulus simplex, the lobulus gracilis, and the biventral lobe. They project to the anterior interposed (emboliform) nucleus of the cerebellum and receive a somatotopically organized climbing fiber projection from the rostral half of the dorsal accessory olive.

The *C2 stripe* extends over nearly the full length of the cerebellum and projects to the dorsal interposed (globose) nucleus. It receives climbing fiber afferents from the rostral portion of the medial accessory olivary nucleus.

Hemispheric Stripes
Three stripes situated farther laterally within the cerebellar hemisphere are considered lateral (hemispheric) stripes:

The *D1 and D2 stripes* extend over most of the length of the cerebellum and project to the dentate nucleus of the cerebellum. D1 receives climbing fibers from the ventral lamina of the inferior olivary nucleus and projects to the caudal portion of the dentate nucleus. D2 receives climbing fibers from the dorsal lamina of the inferior olivary nucleus and projects to the rostral portion of the dentate nucleus. D1 makes up the bulk of the cerebellar cortex in primates.
The *Y stripe* lies between D1 and D2 in anterior and posterior portions of the cerebellum. Its connections are similar to those of C1 and C3.

Cerebellar Nuclei
Four major cerebellar nuclei lie within the white matter of the cerebellar hemispheres on each side. From posteromedial to anterolateral, these are the paired fastigial, globose, emboliform, and dentate nuclei (FGED) (see Figs. 16-6, 16-10, and 16-11). Because the globose and emboliform nuclei lie between the fastigial and dentate nuclei, they are sometimes grouped together as the "interposed nuclei" and designated, separately, as the posterior interposed (globose) nucleus and the anterior interposed (emboliform) nucleus. Recent analyses indicate that a fifth cerebellar nucleus, designated the interstitial cell group, lies between the fastigial and globose nuclei in nonhuman primates. Furthermore, a portion of the lateral vestibular nucleus (of Deiters) is better considered to be a sixth cerebellar nucleus, rather than a vestibular nucleus, because it does not receive direct root fibers of the vestibular nerve, it does not receive

Purkinje cell afferents from the cerebellum, it does receive ascending climbing fibers from the olivary complex, and it gives rise to the paired lateral vestibulospinal tracts (see Fig. 16-11).[1] The large dentate nucleus is now considered to be composed of two different portions that interact with different cerebellar stripes and that function in different pathways, at least in nonhuman primates.

Fastigial Nuclei

Grossly, the fastigial nuclei lie most superiorly and medially, just to each side of midline, overlying the fastigial recess of the fourth ventricle (see Fig. 16-6). They receive Purkinje cell axons from the A stripe of the cerebellar vermis. The major efferents from the rostral fastigial nuclei pass medially and decussate within the cerebellar commissure to form the uncinate fasciculus (crossed fastigiobulbar tract).[1] This tract loops over (dorsal to) the superior cerebellar peduncle and passes into the inferior cerebellar peduncle. Additional uncrossed fastigiobulbar fibers course ventrally in the lateral wall of the fourth ventricle to join the ipsilateral juxtarestiform body. These direct (ipsilateral) and crossed (contralateral) fastigial fibers synapse in the medial and descending (inferior) vestibular nuclei and traverse these nuclei to synapse in the medial reticular formation.

Other projections from the fastigial nucleus cross the midline in the uncinate fasciculus and then ascend on the contralateral side to reach the horizontal gaze center in the paramedian pontine reticular formation, the vertical gaze center in the rostral interstitial nucleus of the medial longitudinal fasciculus, the interstitial nucleus of Cajal, the superior colliculi bilaterally, the pontine nuclei, and the nucleus reticularis tegmenti pontis.

Emboliform Nuclei

The emboliform (anterior interposed) nuclei (see Fig. 16-6) receive Purkinje cell axons from the C1, C3, and Y stripes of the cerebellar cortex. Their efferent fibers pass through the superior cerebellar peduncle, decussate in the midbrain, and innervate the contralateral nucleus reticularis tegmenti pontis, red nucleus, and thalamus.[1] The emboliform projections to the ventral lateral thalamus are then relayed to the primary motor cortex (M1).

Globose Nuclei

The globose (posterior interposed) nuclei (see Fig. 16-6) receive Purkinje cell axons from the C2 stripes of the cerebellar cortex. The efferent fibers from the globose nuclei pass through the superior cerebellar peduncle, decussate in the midbrain, and ascend to innervate the periaqueductal gray matter, superior colliculus, and the nucleus of Darkschewitsch.[1] Efferent globose projections also pass to the intralaminar nuclei of the thalamus for relay to the striatum and the ventrolateral nucleus of the thalamus for relay to the cerebrum.[1]

Dentate Nuclei

The paired dentate nuclei (see Fig. 16-6) form large pleated sheets of tissue that closely resemble the folds of the inferior olivary nuclei. Purkinje cells of the D1 stripe of the cerebellar cortex project to the caudolateral dentate nucleus for relay to the eye fields and the parietal lobes.[1] Purkinje cells of the D2 stripe project to the rostrodorsal portion of the dentate nucleus for relay to the contralateral red nucleus and the ventral lateral thalamic nucleus. The red nucleus gives rise to the central tegmental tract that descends through the brain stem to the ipsilateral inferior olivary nucleus. The red nucleus and central tegmental tract form part of the dentatorubro-olivary circuit (triangle of Guillain-Mollaret).[1] This circuit (triangle) passes from one red nucleus down the central tegmental tract to the ipsilateral inferior olivary nucleus, from that inferior olivary nucleus via the olivocerebellar tract to the contralateral dentate nucleus, from that dentate nucleus, via the superior cerebellar peduncle

and its decussation, back across the midline to the original red nucleus.

Cerebellar Peduncles

The brain stem connects to the cerebellum through three cerebellar peduncles. From rostral to caudal, the paired superior cerebellar peduncles connect the midbrain with the cerebellum on each side. The paired middle cerebellar peduncles connect the pons with the cerebellum on each side, and the paired inferior cerebellar peduncles connect the medulla with the cerebellum on each side.

Superior Cerebellar Peduncle (Brachium Conjunctivum)

The paired superior cerebellar peduncles (see Fig. 16-5C) form thin, tile-like structures that angle obliquely from the medial aspects of the upper cerebellum to the midbrain. They are bounded medially by the upper fourth ventricle and laterally by the ambient (perimesencephalic) cisterns at the surface of the midbrain superiorly and the middle cerebellar peduncles within the white matter of the cerebellum inferiorly.[1] The two superior cerebellar peduncles decussate at the lower border of the midbrain. Fibers emerging from the globose, emboliform, and dentate nuclei traverse the superior cerebellar peduncles en route to synapse in the contralateral red nucleus and thalamus.[2] A small contingent of fibers from the fastigial nuclei also ascends in the superior cerebellar peduncle.

Some fibers of the paired anterior (ventral) spinocerebellar tracts ascend from the spinal cord through the brain stem, form a thin sheet of myelinated fibers on the external surface of the superior cerebellar peduncles, arch medially over the upper margins of the superior cerebellar peduncles, and then descend into the cerebellar hemispheres deep to the peduncles to join the spinocerebellar fibers that enter via the inferior cerebellar peduncle.[2]

Middle Cerebellar Peduncle (Brachium Pontis)

The paired middle cerebellar peduncles (see Fig. 16-5D) are the largest and most lateral of the three cerebellar peduncles. They are purely afferent and constitute the largest afferent system to the cerebellum. More than 90% of the fibers in the middle cerebellar peduncle are part of the corticopontocerebellar pathway.[2] In this pathway, corticopontine fibers from the cerebral hemispheres synapse onto ipsilateral pontine nuclei, which relay the data onward, across the midline and through the contralateral middle cerebellar peduncles, to reach the cerebellar hemisphere opposite the initiating cerebral hemisphere. Fibers related to the frontal lobe traverse the medial portion of the middle cerebellar peduncle. Fibers related to the parietal, occipital, and temporal lobes traverse the lateral portion of the middle cerebellar peduncle.

Inferior Cerebellar Peduncles (Restiform Bodies)

The inferior cerebellar peduncles (see Fig. 16-5E) lie inferomedial to the middle cerebellar peduncle. They consist of an outer compact fiber tract designated the restiform body and an inner, medial set of fibers designated the justarestiform body.[2] The restiform body is a purely afferent pathway.[1,2] It carries the ipsilateral dorsal spinocerebellar tract from the spinal cord, the olivocerebellar fibers from the contralateral inferior olivary nuclei, the cuneocerebellar and trigeminocerebellar tracts from the medulla oblongata, and the external arcuate fibers from the ipsilateral reticular nuclei. The restiform body enters the cerebellum deep to the middle cerebellar peduncle and dorsal to the cerebellar nuclei. The juxtarestiform body is mainly an efferent system that carries to the vestibular nuclei (1) axons from the Purkinje cells in the cortex of the vestibulocerebellum and (2) the uncrossed fastigiobulbar tract from the fastigial nuclei to the ipsilateral vestibular nuclei (especially the medial vestibular nucleus). The juxtarestiform body also carries primary afferent fibers descending within the vestibular nerve and secondary afferent fibers from the vestibular nuclei.[2] The uncinate fasciculus carries crossed fastigiobulbar fibers from the fastigial nucleus to the contralateral vestibular nuclei. It passes dorsal to the superior cerebellar peduncle and then curves inferiorly to enter the brain stem at the border between the restiform and juxtarestiform bodies.[2]

Vascularization
Arterial Supply
The cerebellum is supplied by three major pairs of arteries.

The posterior inferior cerebellar arteries (PICAs) typically arise from the intracranial segments of the vertebral arteries, course around the brain stem to reach the dorsal surface of the stem, circumnavigate the tonsils (tonsillar loops), and then ramify on the posterior (occipital) surface of the cerebellum (Fig. 16-12A and B). Notably, the PICA branches supply the posterior cerebellum from medial to lateral and from inferior to superior. That is, the first major branch of each PICA is the inferior vermian artery that ascends within the paravermian groove toward the

superior surface of the cerebellum. Thereafter, the PICAs give off, in order, ascending cerebellar branches to the medial and then the middle and lateral portions of the posterior surface of the cerebellum. Each branch ascends along the surface perpendicular to the horizontally oriented folia and fissures of the hemisphere, so occlusions of branch vessels will devascularize a narrow strip of tissue perpendicular to and crossing multiple folia and fissures. The most superior extent of the PICA branches is variable. They may terminate at the great horizontal fissure on the posterior surface. They may pass farther superiorly, over the posterolateral margin of the hemisphere and onto the superior surface as far forward as the posterior superior fissure. Their full extent varies inversely with the extents of the superior cerebellar and anterior inferior cerebellar arteries (reciprocal territories of supply).

The *superior cerebellar arteries* (SCAs) arise from the upper basilar artery, immediately proximal to the origins of the posterior cerebral arteries, at the ventral aspect of the upper pons or low midbrain. The SCAs then course around the brain stem to enter the ambient cistern between the dorsolateral surface of the brain stem and the anterior surface of the cerebellum. Within

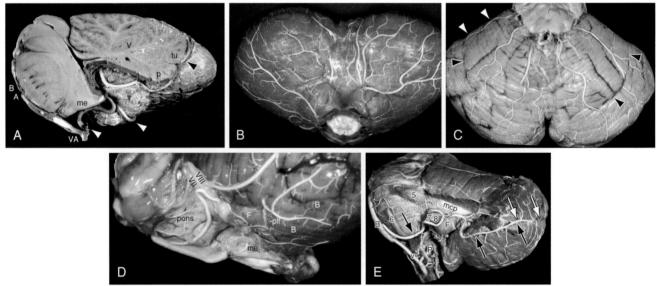

■ **FIGURE 16-12** Arterial supply to the cerebellum. Human cerebella with microbarium injection of vessels prior to formalin fixation. **A,** Origin and proximal portions of posterior inferior cerebellar artery (PICA). The lower medulla has been resected to expose the portion of PICA passing lateral to it. The PICA arises (*lower white arrowhead*) from the vertebral artery (VA), passes lateral to the resected portion of the low medulla (*upper white arrowhead*), circumnavigates the tonsil (T) to form the tonsillar loop, and gives off the inferior vermian branch (*black arrowhead*) posterior to the tonsil. This branch hooks under the pyramis (p) of vermis (V) to ascend along the posterior surface of the vermis. The apex of the curve around the pyramis is the pyramidal point. The branch of the PICA to the choroid plexus of the fourth ventricle arises from the tonsillar segment, usually near the junction of the retromedullary and supratonsillar segments. The hemispheric branches (partially visible) arise distal to the inferior vermian branch. BA, basilar artery; me, upper medulla. **B,** The hemispheric branches of PICA ascend over the posterior surface of the cerebellum nearly perpendicular to the folia and fissures. Proximal branches supply more medial portions of the hemisphere along the paravermian grooves. More distal branches supply progressively more lateral portions of the hemispheres. The faint translucency overlying the vermis and the medial hemisphere is the posterior arachnoid wall of cisterna magna. **C,** The branches of the superior cerebellar artery (SCA) arise within the ambient cistern. The most proximal branch courses along the cerebellar margin (marginal artery) (*white arrowheads*). Progressively more distal hemispheric branches supply progressively more medial portions of the superior surface, until the last, most medial superior vermian branch courses in the paravermian groove. Some SCA branches terminate in the depths of the posterior superior fissure (*black arrowheads*). Others extend over the posterolateral margin onto the posterior surface of the hemisphere. **D,** The anterior inferior cerebellar artery (AICA) arises from the basilar artery, crosses the belly of the pons, ascends toward the internal auditory canal (IAC) along the anterior margin of CN VII, abruptly reverses course to create a hairpin turn at its closest approach to the IAC (meatal loop of AICA), and then descends along CN VIII to reach the middle cerebellar peduncle. The AICA then passes over the top of the flocculus (F) and loops behind it into the posterolateral fissure (plf), forming a flocccular loop. From there AICA supplies the anterior inferior surface of the cerebellum, including the biventral lobule (B). AICA may also ascend into the great horizontal fissure to supply the lateral angle and adjoining posterior and superior surfaces of the cerebellum. **E,** In this specimen, the lateral portion of the superior surface has been resected to uncover the middle cerebellar peduncle (mcp). A small posterior inferior cerebellar artery (PICA [P]) arises from the vertebral artery (V). The large anterior inferior cerebellar artery (AICA) (*black arrows*) arises from the basilar artery (B), follows the typical course over CNVI (6), out toward the internal auditory canal on CN VII (7), back to the middle cerebellar peduncle (mcp) on CN VIII (8), and then back along the middle cerebellar peduncle (mcp) to pass over and behind the flocculus (F). The AICA then ascends within the great horizontal fissure (*white arrows*) on the posterior surface of the hemisphere to supply the superior and inferior semilunar lobules. The distal end of this AICA anastomosed directly, end-to-end, with ascending hemispheric branches of the small PICA.

the ambient cistern, the first (marginal) SCA branch recurves laterally, reaches the anterior angle of the cerebellum, and then courses on or near to the anterolateral margin to supply the adjoining portions of the anterior and superior surfaces of the cerebellum (see Fig. 16-12C). The next SCA branch, the superior vermian artery, arises within the ambient cistern and courses over the superior surface roughly parallel to the anterolateral margin but farther medially and superiorly. Sequentially, additional SCA branches arise within the ambient cistern to supply progressively more medial strips of the superior surface until the last SCA branch takes a paramedian course, along the paravermian groove, to supply the medialmost portion of the superior surface. The distal end of the superior vermian branch often anastomoses, end to end, with the distal end of the inferior vermian branch of PICA to complete a paravermian vascular loop. Because the superior surface of the cerebellum angles upward toward the midline like a steep roof, more medial branches are also more superior in position. Like the PICA, the SCA branches course perpendicular to the folia and fissures of the cerebellar surface, so occlusions of branch vessels will devascularize a narrow strip of tissue, perpendicular to and crossing multiple folia and fissures. The SCA supplies the superior surface of the cerebellar hemisphere from lateral to medial, unlike the PICA that supplies the posterior surface of the hemisphere from medial to lateral.

The *anterior inferior cerebellar arteries* (AICAs) arise from the first or second thirds of the basilar artery, course laterally across the belly of the pons, extend outward along CN VII toward the internal auditory canal, reverse course to form a sharp (meatal) loop within or near to the internal auditory canal, and then descend along CN VIII toward the middle cerebellar peduncle (see Fig. 16-12D). From there the AICA passes in two directions—above and behind the flocculus, ascending posteriorly within the great horizontal fissure to supply the lateral angles of the cerebellar hemispheres, and behind and below the flocculus within the posterolateral fissure to supply the adjacent anterior surfaces of the cerebellar hemispheres. In this course, the AICA supplies the anterior inferior surface of the cerebellar hemispheres. In reciprocity with the ipsilateral PICA and SCA, the AICA may remain confined to the anterior (petrosal) surface of the cerebellum or may ascend high into the great horizontal fissure to supply lateral portions of the dorsal and superior surfaces of the cerebellar hemisphere (see Fig. 16-12E). In its course, the AICA supplies the cerebellum from anteromedial toward posterolateral, filling in progressively more posterior, lateral and superior portions of the anterior surface, until it crosses the margins onto the dorsal and superior surfaces.

Venous Drainage

The surface veins of the cerebellum are also oriented primarily perpendicular to the folia and fissures (see Fig. 16-1C). They gather into major outflow channels that pass to the adjacent dural venous sinuses. The veins situated near the midline of the superior and anterior surfaces join to form the precentral cerebellar vein and the superior vermian vein, among others. These pass to the vein of Galen as the superior or galenic group of cerebellar veins. The veins along the posterior surface and the lateral portions of the superior surface pass to the transverse sinuses as the posterior (occipital) draining group. The veins along lateral portions of the anterior surface may drain to the sigmoid sinuses or, via the petrosal veins, to the superior petrosal sinuses. These form the anterior or petrosal draining group.

FUNCTIONAL CONSIDERATIONS

Functionally, the cerebellum may be considered as three major systems: an oculomotor cerebellum (synonym: vestibulocerebellum), a spinocerebellum, and a (cerebro)pontine cerebellum.[3]

Oculomotor Cerebellum (Vestibulocerebellum)

Anatomically, this division of the cerebellum includes the nodulus and the adjacent anterior face of the uvula, the flocculus, the tonsils, and the ansiform lobe composed of the folium/superior semilunar lobule and tuber/inferior semilunar lobule (lobule VII of Larsell).[1] In this system, primary fibers of the vestibular nerve pass directly to the nodulus and uvula. Mossy fiber afferents from the vestibular nuclei pass to the nodulus, the uvula, the flocculi, and the bottoms of the deep transverse fissures. Climbing fiber afferents from the optokinetic subnuclei of the inferior olive pass to the flocculus. The efferent fibers of the nodulus/uvula pass mainly to the vestibular nuclei.

Spinocerebellum

Anatomically, this division of the cerebellum includes the declive and lobulus simplex in the anterior lobe and the lobulus gracilis and medial belly of the biventral lobule in the posterior lobe.[1] In this system, mossy fiber afferents arise from the vestibular nuclei, the spinocerebellar tracts, the lateral reticular nucleus, the trigeminal nuclei, pontine nuclei relaying data from the sensorimotor cortex, and the nucleus reticularis tegmenti pontis. The spinocerebellar fibers pass to more superficial sites along the apices of the anterior lobe, the base of the lobulus simplex, and the pyramis. The major spinocerebellar stripes of the cortex are the A, X, and B stripes of the vermis with their spinal connections; the C1 and C3 stripes of the intermediate zones, which connect to the red nucleus and the primary motor cortex; and the D2 stripes of the hemispheres with their somatotopically organized connections to the dentate nucleus and the motor and premotor cortices.

(Cerebro)pontine Cerebellum

Anatomically, this division of the cerebellum includes portions of all lobules except the nodulus and the flocculus. In this system, the dorsolateral prefrontal cortex and limited portions of the parietal and occipital lobes send out corticopontine fibers that synapse on pontine nuclei ipsilateral to the cerebral hemisphere from which they arise.[1] In turn, the pontine nuclei give rise to pontocerebellar fibers that relay the data across the midline to the contralateral cerebellar hemisphere. These pontocerebellar fibers pass to large portions of both cerebellar hemispheres, except the flocculus and nodulus. They terminate in the apical portions of the anterior lobe and pyramid and more extensive portions of the rest of the cerebellum, especially the folium and tuber, the uvula, and the lateral portions of the hemispheres. Purkinje cells of the D1 stripe of the cerebellar cortex project to the caudolateral dentate nucleus for relay to the eye fields and the parietal lobes. Purkinje cells of the D2 stripe project to the rostrodorsal portion of the dentate nucleus for relay to the contralateral red nucleus and the ventral lateral thalamic nucleus. Interruption of the dentatorubro-olivary circuit (triangle of Guillain-Mollaret) is associated with a rhythmic vertical palatal motion designated *palatal myoclonus*.

Cognitive Cerebellum

Recent studies indicate that a cognitive region lies within the lateral hemispheric portion of the posterior lobe and an affective region lies in the medial (vermal) portion of the posterior lobe of the cerebellum.[4,5]

Lesions and Malfunction

Classic anatomic and physiologic studies demonstrate that there is a primary sensorimotor region within the anterior lobe of the cerebellum and a secondary sensorimotor region within the medial aspect of the posterior lobe of the cerebellum.[2,6] Therefore, lesions of the cerebellum cause loss of motor coordination (cerebellar ataxia). Muscle tone is altered, often manifesting as hypotonia. Imprecise muscle contractions cause motions toward a target to overshoot or undershoot the target (dysmetria). A tremor may manifest on action, not rest, and may increase in amplitude as the target is approached (intention tremor). Vermian injuries may lead to truncal ataxia, where patients cannot sit or stand alone without falling.[2] Unilateral hemispheric lesions produce symptoms ipsilateral to the lesion, because the relevant fiber tracts decussate twice—once at the superior cerebellar peduncle as they ascend from the cerebellum to the cortex and again at the medullary pyramids where the corticospinal tracts cross. Alternating hand motions are slow and clumsy (dysdiadochokinesia).[2] Eye movements are uncoordinated, leading to a nystagmus that is worse when the eyes turn to the side of the lesion.[2] Bilateral hemispheric lesions cause dysarthria with long drawn-out syllables and poor phrasing (scanning speech).[2] They also cause wide-based gait.[2,4]

Lesions of the posterior cerebellum may manifest as the cerebellar cognitive affective syndrome (CCAS).[4] When such lesions affect the lateral hemispheric portion of the posterior lobe, the CCAS is characterized by impairments in executive function (planning, set shifting, verbal fluency, abstract reasoning, working memory), spatial cognition (visuospatial organization and memory), and linguistic processing (agrammatism and dysprodia).[4] When such lesions encroach on the limbic cerebellum (vermis and fastigial nucleus), the CCAS includes dysregulation of affect.[4,5]

IMAGING

CT displays the cerebellar surfaces, the patterns of folia and fissures, the position and configuration of the pericerebellar cerebrospinal fluid (CSF) cisterns, the fourth ventricle within the cerebellum, portions of the cerebellar peduncles, and some of the branching pattern of the white matter. Portions of the normal dentate nuclei may also be discerned (Fig. 16-13). The fourth ventricle lies in the midline with a complex undulant shape sometimes designated the "temple bell" or "Kaiser Wilhelm's helmet." The cisterna magna contains lucent CSF, and the pericerebellar cisterns show nearly symmetric shape and density.

MRI displays the same structures and much finer detail of the cerebellar white matter. Midsagittal T1- and T2-weighted (T1W and T2W) images show the lobes and lobules of the vermis and hemispheres and the branching pattern of the cerebellar white matter in fine detail (Fig. 16-14). Axial (Figs. 16-15 and 16-16) and coronal (Fig. 16-17) MR images display nearly all of the anatomy shown in the axial and coronal anatomic sections (see

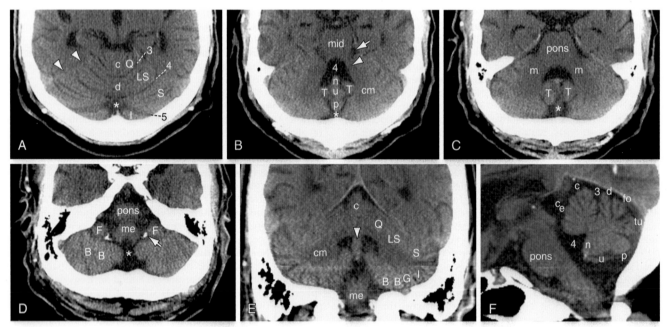

■ **FIGURE 16-13** Noncontrast CT scans of the cerebellum and brain stem in direct axial (**A** to **D**), reformatted coronal (**E**), and reformatted sagittal (**F**) planes. **A,** Superior cerebellum. The trapezoid-shaped primary fissure (3) separates the culmen-quadrangular lobule (c, Q) from the declive-lobulus simplex (d, LS), while the rounded posterior superior fissure separates the declive-lobulus simplex from the superior semilunar lobule (S, folium not seen in this image). The medial portion of the great horizontal fissure (5) separates the superior semilunar lobule from the small medial portion of the inferior semilunar lobule (I) that is visible on the superior surface. The posterior superior fissure just "kisses" the deepest portion of the posterior cerebellar notch (*asterisk*). *Arrowheads* indicate the tentorium. **B and C,** Midcerebellum. The fourth ventricle (4) lies centrally within the cerebellum and has the shape of a "temple bell" or military helmet. The midbrain (mid) and pons (pons) form the floor of the fourth ventricle anteriorly. The median sulcus of the fourth ventricle creates the midline point of the bell or helmet. The superior (*white arrowhead*) and middle (m) cerebellar peduncles help form the concave lateral walls of the fourth ventricle. The nodulus (n) and tonsils (T) indent the posterior wall of the fourth ventricle, giving it a three-lobed appearance. The nodulus indents the fourth ventricle in the midline, creating the fastigial recess. The paired tonsils indent the fourth ventricle off midline to each side, creating paired paramedian posterior superior recesses. The uvula (u) lies between the two tonsils. The pyramis (p) forms the posterior inferior wall of the vermis, indenting the posterior cerebellar notch (*asterisk*). The large areas of cerebellar white matter are the corpora medullare (cm). The ambient cisterns (*white arrow*) outline the posterolateral midbrain, lateral surface of the superior cerebellar peduncle, and the anterior medial surface of the cerebellum. **D,** CT sections through the inferior cerebellum traverse ventral portions of the pons (pons), medulla (me), and biventral lobules (B) obliquely. The paired flocculi (F) project forward from the anterior surface of the cerebellum. In this patient, calcified portions (*white arrow*) of the choroid plexus are seen within the lateral recesses of the fourth ventricle. **E and F,** Reformatted coronal (**E**) and sagittal (**F**) images display the characteristic shape and central position of the fourth ventricle (4), indentation of the midline posterior wall by the nodulus (n, *white arrowhead*), and the culmen (c) at the apex of the vermis. The lobules of the hemispheres are arrayed circumferentially around the fourth ventricle and corpus medullare, from superior to inferior: quadrangular lobule (Q), lobulus simplex (LS), superior (S) and inferior (I) semilunar lobule, gracile (G), and biventral (B) lobules. The lobules of the vermis are arrayed circumferentially around the fourth ventricle, from cranial to caudal: central (ce), culmen (c), declive (d), folium (fo), tuber (tu), pyramis (p), uvula (u), and nodulus (n). The primary fissure (3) separates the anterior lobe from the posterior lobe of the cerebellum. The declive, folium, and tuber appear slightly full in the image, because the reformatted view angles just slightly off midline.

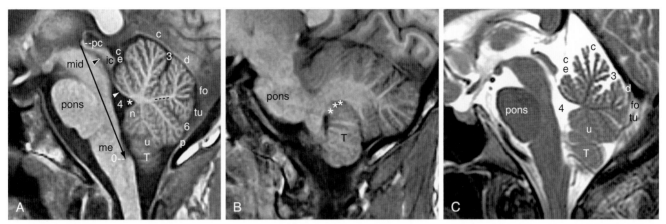

■ **FIGURE 16-14** Sagittal MRI. Two patients. **A** and **B,** First patient. Sagittal T1W MR image to compare with Figure 16-4. **A,** Midsagittal section comparable to Figure 16-4A. The midbrain (mid), pons, and medulla (me) lie ventral to the aqueduct (*black arrowhead*) and fourth ventricle (4). The nine lobules of the vermis encircle the fourth ventricle. The lingua (*white arrowhead*) forms a thin, barely visible "ripple" of tissue applied to the superior medullary velum. The central lobule (ce), culmen (c), declive (d), folium (fo), tuber (tu), pyramis (p), uvula (u), and nodulus (n) follow in order, clockwise. In this image, the nodulus is labeled on the tissue itself but the other lobules are labeled just peripheral to the tissue to afford clearest demonstration. The primary fissure (3) separates the anterior from the posterior lobe. The prepyramidal fissure (6) is restricted to the vermis, separating the tuber (tu) from the pyramis (p). In the midline, the white matter of the vermis forms a branching pattern centered on the fastigial recess (*asterisk*). A line drawn from the most anterior portion of the posterior commissure to the obex (PC-O line of Tamraz) provides one standard approximation to alignment of the brain stem (floor of the fourth ventricle). The central spike of white matter that passes to the declive, folium, and tuber (*dft line* [dotted line]) normally forms an angle greater than 90 degrees to the PC-O line (average 107 degrees). **B,** Second patient. Parasagittal section comparable to Figure 16-4B. The posterior superior recess (*asterisks*) of the fourth ventricle lies atop the tonsil (T). **C,** Midsagittal T2W MR image displays the same anatomy as labeled in **A.**

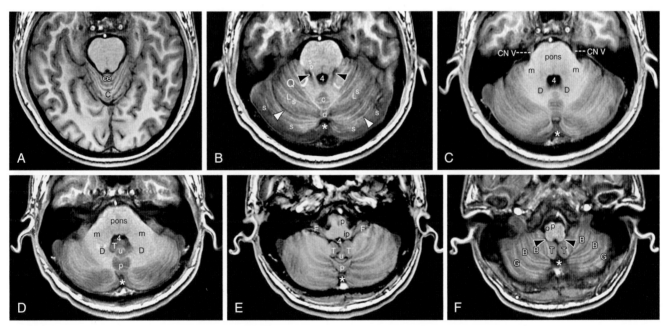

■ **FIGURE 16-15** Axial T1W MR images. Serial axial sections displayed from superior to inferior to compare with Figure 16-5. **A** and **B,** The upper two sections display, medially, the low midbrain, the central lobule (ce), and the culmen (c) of vermis extending upward into incisura, the thin plate-like superior cerebellar peduncles (sp) situated between the upper fourth ventricle (4), and the ambient cistern (*black arrowheads*) and the declive of the vermis (d). Laterally, they show the lobules of the upper cerebellar hemisphere: quadrangular lobule (Q), lobulus simplex (LS), and superior semilunar lobule (S). The posterior superior fissure (*white arrowheads*) separates the lobulus simplex from the superior semilunar lobule. **C** and **D,** The middle two sections display, medially, the pons, cranial nerves V (trigeminal nerves) (CN V), the middle cerebellar peduncles (m) extending into the central white matter (corpus medullare) of the cerebellum, the fourth ventricle (4), the paired dentate nuclei (D) seen faintly to each side of the fourth ventricle, the uvula (u) and pyramis (p) of the vermis, and the posterior cerebellar notch (*asterisk*). **E** and **F,** The lower two sections display, medially, the pyramid (*black p*), olive (o), and inferior cerebellar peduncle (ip) of the medulla, the cerebellomedullary fissures (*black arrowheads*), the low fourth ventricle (4), the paired tonsils (T) flanking the uvula (u), the pyramis (*white p*), and the posterior cerebellar notch (*asterisk*). Laterally, they show the paired flocculi (F) on the anterior face of the cerebellum, the gracile lobules (G) and biventral (B) lobules of the hemispheres. The choroid plexus that emerges through the foramen of Luschka into the cerebellopontine angle overlies the flocculi, so images at this level often show components of both together.

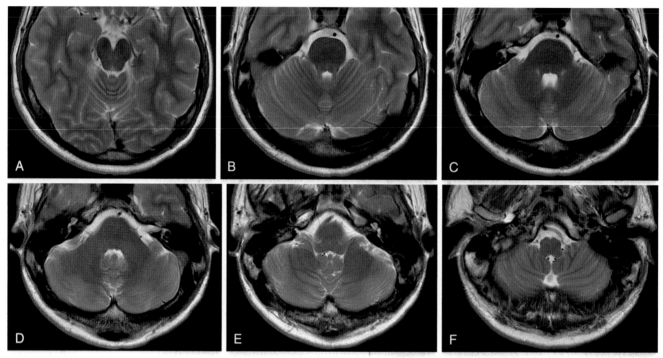

■ **FIGURE 16-16** Axial T2W MR images. Serial axial sections displayed from superior to inferior to compare with Figures 16-5 and 16-9.

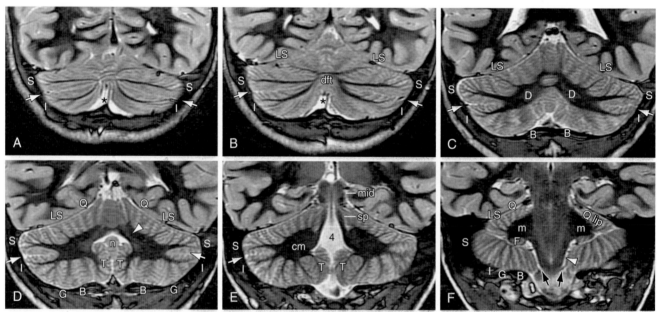

■ **FIGURE 16-17** Serial coronal inversion recovery MR images displayed from posterior toward anterior. **A** and **B,** Analysis of the central spikes of white matter to each lobule ("cat's whiskers") from posterior to anterior helps to identify the lobules. Most posteriorly, the nearly horizontal spike that passes approximately 1 cm inferior to the lateral margin of each hemisphere defines the superior semilunar lobule (S). The next lower oblique spike that is convex medially defines the inferior semilunar lobule (I). The great horizontal fissures (*white arrows*) form thin white lines between these lobules. The flat "dft line" in **B** is the central spike of white matter to the declive (d), folium (f), and tuber (t) in the vermis. The white spikes angling superolaterally from this line define the lobulus simplex (LS) on each side. Within each lobule, the folia and fissures of each lobule appear to radiate off these central white matter spikes. *Asterisk* indicates the posterior cerebellar notch. **C,** Farther anteriorly, the spikes of each lobule converge at the central white matter of the hemispheres. The dentate nuclei (D) are seen faintly within the white matter. B, biventral lobule. **D,** Section through the back of the fourth ventricle shows the deep cerebellar nuclei (*white arrowhead*) flanking the fourth ventricle, the nodulus (n) indenting the posterior medullary velum, and the paired tonsils protruding from the medial surface of the hemispheres. The major spikes to the superior (S) and inferior (I) semilunar lobules defines those structures. At this level, the white matter of the two sides may be likened to the outstretched wings of an eagle. Tracing the white matter spikes from image to image permits identification of the other lobules as well. **E,** Section through the anterior fourth ventricle (4) shows the symmetrical undulant "temple bell" shape of the ventricle, a vertical signal void within the fourth ventricle corresponding to the jet of CSF from the aqueduct, the central white matter of each hemisphere (corpora medullares) (cm), and the thin plate-like superior cerebellar peduncles (sp) passing toward the midbrain (mid). **F,** Section through the brain stem and the anterior surface of the cerebellum. The anterior surfaces of the quadrangular lobule (Q) and the lobulus simplex (LS) form a quadrangular lip (Q lip) that lies immediately superior to the middle cerebellar peduncle (m). The paired flocculi (F) lie inferior to the middle cerebellar peduncles (m). The biventral lobules (B) form an inferior medial margin of each hemisphere designated the biventral ridge (*white arrowhead*). The cerebellomedullary fissures (*black arrows*) lie between the medulla medially and the flanking biventral ridges. The folia and fissures of the anterior surface of the hemispheres align perpendicular to both the outer surface of the hemisphere at each point and the middle cerebellar peduncle.

Figs. 16-5 and 16-6). Fortunate CT and MR sections may display specific anatomic structures especially well (Fig. 16-18).

The dentate nuclei are usually displayed well, but the smaller fastigial, globose, and emboliform nuclei are rarely seen (Fig. 16-19). Beginning in the early teens, and increasingly after age 20 years, deposition of iron within the dentate nuclei changes the signal intensity with age.[7] On T1W, T2W, and gradient-recalled T2* (susceptibility) images, the dentate nuclei are typically brighter than the surrounding cerebellar white matter in children and show progressively lower signal intensity with increasing age (see Fig. 16-19). The degree of iron deposition is always less than in the basal ganglia, so the dentate nuclei should not exhibit as low signal as the basal ganglia in any one patient.

Contrast-enhanced CT and MRI display the arteries and veins that supply the cerebellum and the configuration of the enhancing choroid plexus of the fourth ventricle. MR and CT arteriography and venography display many of the vessels along the brain surface (Fig. 16-20) but do not yet depict the anatomy that can be shown by transfemoral catheter angiography.

Cerebellar White Matter

When axial, coronal, and sagittal CT and MR images are viewed systematically, from end to end, the branching pattern of the white matter displays a characteristic progression that helps to identify the individual lobules of the posterior vermis and hemispheres (see Figs. 16-14 to 16-17).[8-10] Diffusion tensor imaging (Fig. 16-21) and tractography (Figs. 16-22 and 16-23) now display the cerebellar white matter in greater detail, depicting the coherence and directionality of the fibers that form the white matter fascicles and tracts (see Chapter 12).

Diffusion Tensor Imaging and Tractography

Diffusion tensor imaging (see Fig. 16-21) and tractography (see Figs. 16-22 and 16-23) now display many of the cerebellar fiber pathways that form the white matter fascicles and tracts. Diffusion tensor imaging uses the diffusion of water molecules (brownian motion) in the white matter as an endogenous probe to reveal the microstructure of the white matter, including the predominant orientation of the fibers within each voxel. Diffusion tensor tractography then applies a streamline tracking

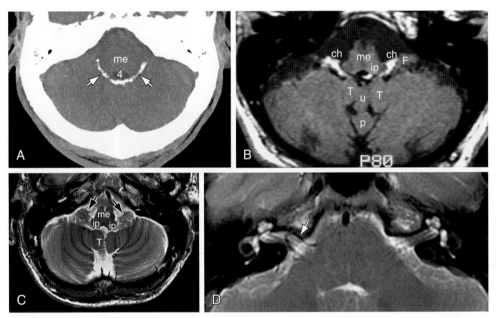

■ **FIGURE 16-18** Cerebellopontine angle. **A,** Noncontrast axial CT. There is dense calcification (*arrows*) of the choroid plexus of the fourth ventricle extending into both lateral recesses. **B,** Contrast-enhanced axial T1W MR image shows the medulla (me), the inferior cerebellar peduncle (ip), and the enhancing choroids plexus (ch) passing through the lateral recesses of the fourth ventricle to emerge at the foramina of Luschka immediately anteroinferior to and partially covering the flocculi (F). Also labeled are the pyramis (p), uvula (u), and tonsil (T). **C,** Axial T2W noncontrast MR image shows the paired flocculi (*arrows*) in relation to the inferior cerebellar peduncles (ip) of the medulla (me), the lateral recesses of the fourth ventricle, and the cerebellopontine angle cisterns. There is a double falx cerebelli. T, tonsils. **D,** Axial T2W MR image. The anterior inferior cerebellar artery (AICA) makes a hairpin turn (the meatal loop) at its closest approach to the internal auditory canal, here within the canal itself (*arrow*).

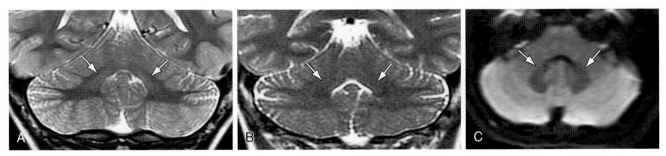

■ **FIGURE 16-19** Dentate nucleus (*white arrows*). **A** and **B,** T2W coronal MR images. **A,** At age 3 years the crenellated structure of the dentate nucleus is brighter than the surrounding myelinated white matter of the corpus medullare. **B,** At age 55 years, the dentate nucleus has just slightly lower signal than the myelinated white matter. At later ages, the dentate nucleus has far lower signal intensity than the white matter. **C,** Axial diffusion-weighted MR image at age 35 years. The dentate nuclei are displayed especially well. Compare with the Perl stain of the dentate nuclei in Figure 16-6B.

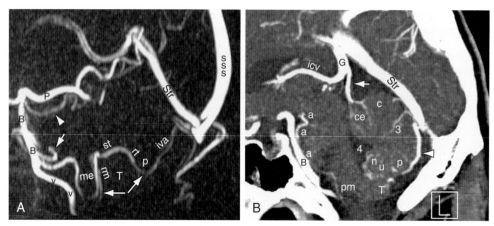

■ **FIGURE 16-20**   Cerebellar vascularity. Two patients. **A,** MR time-resolved, phase-contrast MR angiogram. Sagittal maximum intensity projection. The PICA (*two white arrows*) arises from the vertebral artery (V) ventral to the brain stem and arcs around the medulla (me) to form the retromedullary segment (rm) along the dorsal surface of the medulla. From there, the PICA arches over the cerebellar tonsil (T) (supratonsillar segment [st]) and posterior to the tonsil (retrotonsillar segment [rt]) to reach the pyramis (p) of the vermis. The inferior vermian branch of the PICA hooks under the pyramis (p) to ascend along the posterior surface of the vermis as the inferior vermian artery (iva). The AICA (*single white arrow*) arises from the proximal basilar artery (B) and arches along the ventral surface of the pons and CN VII to reach its apex near to, at, or within the internal auditory canal. The superior cerebellar artery (*arrowhead*) arises from the distal basilar artery and arches around the lateral surface of the high pons to the ambient cistern. sss, superior sagittal sinus; Str, straight sinus; P, posterior cerebral artery. **B,** Contrast-enhanced CT angiogram. Midsagittal section. The basilar artery (B), anterior pontomesencephalic vein (a), and premedullary vein (pm) outline the ventral brain stem. Venous tributaries from the central lobule (ce) of vermis drain through the precentral cerebellar vein (*white arrow*) to the vein of Galen (G) and straight sinus (Str). The inferior vermian vein (*white arrowhead*) outlines the posterior surface of the vermis. Also labeled are a vein within the primary fissure (3), fourth ventricle (4), culmen (c), internal cerebral vein (icv), nodulus (n) covered anteriorly by the enhancing choroid plexus, pyramis (p), tonsil (T), and uvula (u).

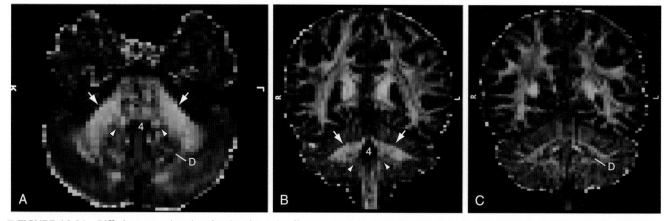

■ **FIGURE 16-21**   Diffusion tensor imaging showing the major fiber tracts of the cerebellum. In these images, the color signifies the direction of the fibers at the point imaged: blue for craniocaudal, green for anteroposterior, and red for transverse (left-right). Fibers coursing in intermediate directions display a color directly proportional to the color mix of their vectors in each of the three orthogonal primary directions. **A,** Axial image at the fourth ventricle (4) and midcerebellum shows the inferior cerebellar peduncles (*blue, paired white arrowheads*) ascending into the cerebellum, the middle cerebellar peduncles (*green, paired white arrows*) turning posterolaterally into the cerebellar hemispheres, and the multicolored paired dentate nuclei (D) arrayed symmetrically about the fourth ventricle. **B** and **C,** Coronal images at (**B**) and behind (**C**) the fourth ventricle (4) show the coronal orientation of the inferior cerebellar peduncles (*blue, white arrowheads*), central white matter of the cerebellum (*green, white arrows*), and the central location of the dentate nuclei (*multicolored,* **D**) within the white matter. The radial orientation of the white matter cores of each lobule is reflected by the broad spectrum of starburst colors.

algorithm to follow the orientation of those fibers from voxel to voxel, throughout the image, and links the related voxels to display the paths of the neural fiber bundles across the brain. Chapter 12, White Matter, discusses diffusion tensor tractography more fully.

ANALYSIS

Modern CT scanners now provide "automatic" triplanar reconstructions; thus, CT and MR studies can be analyzed in much the same way. However, analysis of CT images usually begins with axial images, whereas analysis of the MR images usually starts with the sagittal plane.

CT

1. First evaluate the overlying scalp for edema, mass, tracts, and so on.
2. Then analyze the bony posterior fossa for hyperostosis, erosion, permeation, fracture, and other signs of disease.
3. Next look at the CSF spaces in and around the cerebellum. Check the foramen magnum for any evidence of tonsillar herniation. Then check that the cisterna magna is visible and contains lucent CSF. Inability to visualize a cisterna magna suggests possible Chiari I malformation, meningeal-filling processes such as blood, pus, or tumor, or compression of the cistern by mass effect. The cisterna magna is often

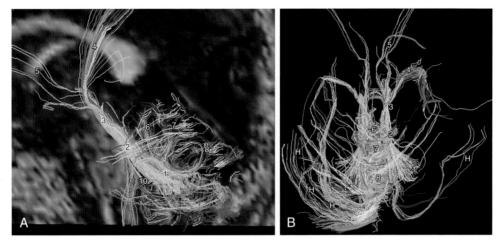

■ **FIGURE 16-22** Diffusion tensor tractography. A 7 T MR DT tractograph in vivo. Lateral (**A**) and posterosuperior (**B**) views of tracts related to the superior cerebellar peduncle and vermis. Seed placed within the superior cerebellar peduncle. For these images the standard colors signify the direction of the tract *at the midpoint of the path shown.* Colors in these images do not reflect the direction within each voxel as is done in other tractography techniques. Fibers (1) from the dentate and adjacent nuclei on each side ascend through the superior cerebellar peduncles (2), decussate within the midbrain, and continue (3) to the red nucleus and thalamus for relay onto the striatum (5) and cerebrum (4). Fibers from the spinal cord ascend into the cerebellum via the inferior cerebellar peduncle (10). Fibers to the central lobule (6), culmen (7), declive (8), and other vermian lobules course radially through the centers of the lobules and appear to course transversely at the apices of the vermian lobules. Other fibers (H) appear to course more circumferentially within the lobules of the hemispheres.

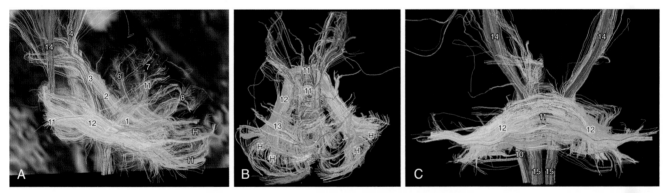

■ **FIGURE 16-23** Diffusion tensor tractography. A 7 T MR DT tractograph in vivo. Additional fiber tracts added to Figure 6-22 above. **A,** Sagittal projection. **B,** Posterosuperior projection. **C,** Anterior projection. The pontocerebellar fibers arise within the pons (11) and sweep posterolaterally within the middle cerebellar peduncles (12) to the cerebellar white matter (13) for distribution to the cerebellar lobules, Most of the pontocerebellar fibers pass medially and immediately cross to the opposite middle cerebellar peduncle for distribution to the contralateral cerebellar hemisphere. Some pass ipsilaterally. The corticospinal fibers (14) descend through the pons en route to the pyramids.

asymmetric normally. Asymmetry can aid in diagnosis and localization of pathology but is not sufficient to diagnose a pathologic process. Analyze the fourth ventricle for size, midline position, and undulant "temple bell" contour. Straightening of the undulant contours is abnormal. Then check that the aqueduct of Sylvius is normal in size, position, and configuration.

4. Analyze the vessels within the CSF for size, density, and configuration. Increased density may signify thrombosis or embolism. Increased size and contour may signify high flow, as to a vascular malformation.

5. Analyze the presence, contours, and symmetry of the folia and fissures of the vermis and hemispheres. Failure to detect fissures raises the question of edema with a mass or a meningeal-filling process. Enlargement of the fissures suggests cerebellar atrophy or, perhaps, communicating hydrocephalus.

6. Evaluate the superficial gray matter/white matter junctions for preservation of gray/white distinction, symmetry, mass, edema, or other pathologic condition.

7. Evaluate the (a)symmetry of the branching pattern of the cerebellar white matter. The spikes of white matter within the folia should be nearly symmetric. The corpus medullare on each side should fan out to resemble outstretched "eagle wings," especially in coronal sections.

8. Specifically review the inferior, middle, and superior cerebellar peduncles for size, position, configuration, and density.

9. Analyze the gray matter of the dentate and other cerebellar nuclei within the white matter for density, position, and symmetry.

10. Review the supratentorial brain for associated features that may assist the analysis of posterior fossa findings.

11. After administration of a contrast agent, evaluate the structures that normally enhance (i.e., the arteries, veins, and choroid plexus). Then evaluate the images for any abnormal contrast enhancement.

12. When triplanar images are available, deliberately review all of the coronal and sagittal images for things that might have been missed on axial images. The sagittal images may be

especially useful for the ventricular system and for the skull base, especially the clivus. Specific attention to the brain surface and the adjacent bone/dura may detect superficial lesions like small meningiomas that are not appreciable in other planes.

13. Specifically review any older imaging studies for interval changes that help to understand the temporal evolution of any pathologic process discerned.

MRI

Analyze the MR images for the same features analyzed for CT, usually starting with the sagittal series. The greater sensitivity of

MRI may disclose pathologic processes in regions that appear normal on CT.

In addition, the analysis should include those imaging features unique to MRI:

14. Review the diffusion-weighted series for restriction of diffusion by infarction, infection, and some tumors.
15. Review the T2* images for abnormal magnetic susceptibility.
16. Review the diffusion tensor images for directionality and integrity of white matter tracts.

A sample report is presented in Box 16-1.

BOX 16-1   Sample Report: Distortion of Normal Anatomy

PATIENT HISTORY

This 14-year-old boy who had a small bowel transplant 7 years prior was recently placed on therapy with metronidazole (Flagyl) for *Salmonella* and *Clostridium difficile* enteritis.

TECHNIQUE

Noncontrast MRI of the head was performed in three orthogonal planes using multiple pulse sequences, including sagittal T1W, axial T1W, T2W, FLAIR T2W, coronal T2W and T2*W, and axial diffusion-weighted series (Fig. 16-24).

FINDINGS

Within the posterior fossa, the dentate nuclei show slight fullness and marked, bilaterally symmetric increase in T2 signal intensity with no

alteration of their intrinsic architecture. There is no alteration in T1 signal intensity and no restriction of diffusion (not shown in Fig. 16-24). There is no significant mass effect. The brain stem, fourth ventricle, middle cerebellar peduncles, and folia and fissures of the vermis and hemispheres appear normal. The surrounding CSF cisterns are normal. The supratentorial compartment is normal. Specifically, the ventricles are normal in size, position, and configuration. There is no midline shift, mass, hemorrhage, or confluent ischemic infarction. The gray and white matter of the cerebral hemispheres, the basal ganglia, and the thalami show no abnormality.

IMPRESSION

Symmetric increase in the signal intensity of the dentate nuclei is consistent with metronidazole toxicity.[11] Follow-up MRI is recommended.

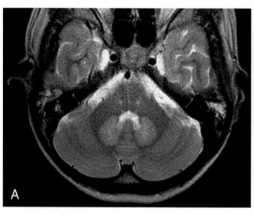
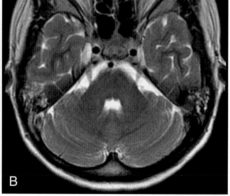

■ **FIGURE 16-24** A 14-year-old boy presented after a small bowel transplant with a compromised immune system and bacterial enteritis that was treated with metronidazole (Flagyl). **A,** Noncontrast T2W axial MR image shows fullness and increased T2 signal of the dentate nuclei bilaterally and symmetrically without loss of dentate architecture. Adjoining structures are grossly normal. **B,** Noncontrast MR image 6 days after cessation of Flagyl therapy shows complete resolution of the dentate signal changes. (Compare with Figs. 16-5D and 16-6B.)

KEY POINTS

- In many ways, the cerebellum conforms to a *"rule of three."* That is, there are:
  - 3 Components: midline vermis and paired cerebellar hemispheres
  - 3 Surfaces (superior, posterior, and anterior)
  - 3 Major arteries on each side, one supplying each surface:
    - Superior cerebellar artery (SCA) for the superior surface
    - Posterior inferior cerebellar artery (PICA) for the posterior surface
    - Anterior inferior cerebellar artery (AICA) for the anterior surface
  - 3 Major venous drainages: superior (galenic), posterior (transverse sinus), and anterior (petrosal)
  - 3 Lobes (anterior, posterior, and flocculonodular)
  - 3^2 (= 9) Lobules (see Table 16-1)
  - 3 Peduncles on each side, one from each division of the brain stem:

  - Superior cerebellar peduncle from the midbrain
  - Middle cerebellar peduncle from the pons
  - Inferior cerebellar peduncle from the medulla oblongata
  - 3 Anatomic-functional zones:
    - Medial vermian zone
    - Intermediate paravermian zone
    - Lateral hemispheric zone
  - 3^2 (= 9) Vertical "alphabetical" stripes:
    - 3 medial vermian stripes (A, X, B)
    - 3 intermediate stripes (C1, C2, C3)
    - 3 lateral hemispheric stripes (D1, Y, D2)
  - 3 Layers of the cerebellar cortex, from superficial to deep: the molecular, Purkinje, and granule cell layers. Of these only the Purkinje cells provide efferent outflow from the cerebellum.
  - 3 Broad functional divisions: the oculomotor cerebellum, the spinocerebellum, and the pontocerebellum

---

KEY POINTS—cont'd

■ There are four major pairs of cerebellar nuclei, designated from medial to lateral: fastigial, globose, emboliform and dentate nuclei. The globose and emboliform are often grouped as the interposed nuclei. The acronym *FGED* may help you remember not to *FGED* them. However, a fifth pair of cerebellar nuclei designated the interstitial cell group lies between the fastigial and the globose nuclei on each side. The lateral vestibular nuclei of Deiters are best regarded as a sixth pair of cerebellar nuclei, so there are really 3 × 2 = 6 cerebellar nuclei per side. That is, the "rule of three" holds.

■ The cerebellar white matter displays a characteristic branching pattern. In midsagittal plane, the white matter of the vermis resembles a spokewheel, with the fastigial recess of the fourth ventricle as the hub of the wheel. The white spike to the culmen is approximately vertical. The central white matter spike to the declive, folium, and tuber ("dft line") is normally oriented at an obtuse angle (>90 degrees) to the line drawn from the posterior commissure to the obex (PCO line).[12]

■ In coronal plane images viewed from posterior to anterior, the branching pattern of the white matter displays a characteristic progression that helps to identify the individual lobules of the posterior vermis and hemispheres.[8]

SUGGESTED READINGS

Courchesne E, Press GA, Murakami J, et al. The cerebellum in sagittal plane—anatomic MR correlation: 1. The vermis. AJR Am J Roentgenol 1989; 153:829-835.

Heaney CJ, Campeau N, Lindell EP. MR imaging and diffusion-weighted imaging changes in metronidazole (Flagyl)-induced cerebellar toxicity. AJNR Am J Neuroradiol 2003; 24:1615-1617.

Press GA, Murakami J, Courchesne E. The cerebellum in sagittal plane—anatomic MR correlation: 2. The cerebellar hemispheres. AJR Am J Roentgenol 1989; 153:837-846.

Press GA, Murakami J, Courchesne E, et al. The cerebellum: 3. Anatomic-MR correlation in the coronal plane. AJNR Am J Neuroradiol 1990; 11:41-50.

REFERENCES

1. Nieuwenhuys R, Voogd J, van Huijzen C. The human central nervous system. In Cerebellum. Berlin, Springer-Verlag, 2008, pp 807-839.

2. Standring S (ed). Gray's Anatomy: The Anatomical Basis of Clinical Practice, 40th ed. Philadelphia, Elsevier Churchill Livingstone, 2008, p 1576.

3. Gilman S, et al (eds). Manter and Gatz's Essentials of Clinical Neuroanatomy and Neurophysiology, 10th ed. Philadelphia, FA Davis, 1996.

4. Schmahmann JD, Caplan D. Cognition, emotion and the cerebellum. Brain 2006; 129(pt 2):290-292.

5. Schmahmann JD, Weilburg JB, Sherman JC. The neuropsychiatry of the cerebellum—insights from the clinic. Cerebellum 2007; 6(3):254-267.

6. Carpenter M, Sutin J. The cerebellum. In Human Neuroanatomy. Baltimore, Williams & Wilkins, 1983, pp 454-492.

7. Aoki S, Okada Y, Nishimura K, et al. Normal deposition of brain iron in childhood and adolescence: MR imaging at 1.5 T. Radiology 1989; 172:381-385.

8. Courchesne E, Press GA, Murakami J, et al. The cerebellum in sagittal plane—anatomic-MR correlation: 1. The vermis. AJR Am J Roentgenol 1989; 153:829-835.

9. Press GA, Murakami J, Courchesne E, et al. The cerebellum in sagittal plane—anatomic-MR correlation: 2. The cerebellar hemispheres. AJR Am J Roentgenol 1989; 153:837-846.

10. Press GA, Murakami JW, Courchesne E, et al. The cerebellum: 3. Anatomic-MR correlation in the coronal plane. AJNR Am J Neuroradiol 1990; 11:41-50.

11. Heaney CJ, Campeau NG, Lindell EP. MR imaging and diffusion-weighted imaging changes in metronidazole (Flagyl)-induced cerebellar toxicity. AJNR Am J Neuroradiol 2003; 24:1615-1617.

12. Tamraz J, Saban R, Reperant J, Cabanis EA. A new cephalic reference plane for use with magnetic resonance imaging: the chiasmato-commissural plane. Surg Radiol Anat 1991; 13:197-201.

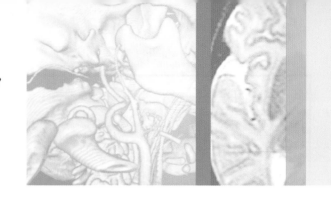

17

Cranial Nerves

Jennifer Linn

The twelve cranial nerves consist of the olfactory (I), optic (II), oculomotor (III), trochlear (IV), trigeminal (V), abducens (VI), facial (VII), vestibulocochlear (VIII), glossopharyngeal (IX), vagus (X), accessory (XI), and hypoglossal (XII) nerves. Each nerve has an intra-axial, cisternal, dural, osseous, and extracranial segment. This chapter addresses the anatomy and function of the cranial nerves and the different imaging techniques preferred for depicting each segment of the cranial nerves.

GROSS ANATOMY

From cranial to caudal, cranial nerves II to XII can be grouped by their origin from the brain stem:

- CN II originates from the diencephalon.
- CN III and IV originate from the mesencephalon.
- CN V through VIII originate from the pons.
- CN IX through XII originate from the medulla oblongata.

CN I: Olfactory Nerve, Bulb, and Tract

The olfactory nerve consists of a collection of sensory nerve fibers (the olfactory filiae), which represent the axons of the olfactory receptor neurons, located in the olfactory mucosa of the nasal cavity. The olfactory filiae enter the anterior cranial fossa via the cribriform plate of the ethmoid bone (Fig. 17-1) and terminate in the olfactory bulbs, which lie in bony grooves formed by the cribriform plate (see Figs. 17-1 and 17-2). The olfactory bulbs constitute the primary olfactory cortices. In the olfactory bulbs, the primary axons form synapses with the secondary neurons of the olfactory system. The axons of the secondary neurons leave the olfactory bulb in the olfactory tract, which runs inferior to the olfactory sulcus (see Fig. 17-2) to reach the posterior aspect of the orbital surface of the forebrain. At the rostral border of the anterior perforated substance the olfactory tract divides into three olfactory striae: (1) the medial olfactory stria, which curves medially and upward to the septal region, (2) the lateral olfactory stria, which first curves far laterally along the sylvian fissure and then recurves medially to reach the medial surface of the temporal lobe, and (3) the vestigial intermediate olfactory stria, which continues onto the anterior perforated substance and ends at the olfactory tubercle. The striae and tubercle constitute the olfactory trigone. Areas that receive direct projections from the olfactory tract consist of the anterior olfactory nucleus, the olfactory tubercle, the piriform cortex, the anterior cortical nucleus of the amygdala, the periamygdaloid cortex, and a small anteromedial portion of the entorhinal cortex. These constitute the secondary olfactory cortices.

CN II: Optic Nerve, Chiasm, and Tract

The optic nerve emerges from the posterior pole of the ocular globe, extends posteriorly through the orbit, and leaves the orbit via the optic canal to reach the anterior cranial fossa (Fig. 17-3). Intracranially, both optic nerves join to form the optic chiasm within the suprasellar cistern. At the chiasm the nasal fibers of each optic nerve cross the midline (decussate) to join with the uncrossed temporal fibers of the opposite optic nerve, forming the optic tracts (see Fig. 17-3). From the optic chiasm, the paired optic tracts curve posteriorly around the cerebral peduncles to terminate in the lateral geniculate bodies (see Fig. 17-3). From the lateral geniculate bodies the optic radiations curve toward the primary visual cortices (Brodmann areas 17) at the medial aspect of the occipital lobes, along the calcarine and anterior calcarine fissures.

CN III: Oculomotor Nerve

The nuclear complex of the third nerve is located in the midbrain at the level of the superior colliculi immediately dorsal to the medial longitudinal fasciculus (MLF) and just ventral to the periaqueductal gray matter (Fig. 17-4). The parasympathetic motor fibers originate in the Edinger-Westphal nucleus situated at the dorsal-rostral aspect of the oculomotor nuclear complex. The fascicles of CN III curve ventrally through the midbrain at the level of the red nucleus and exit the brain stem along the ventromedial aspect of the cerebral peduncle within the interpeduncular fossa (see Fig. 17-4). The cisternal segment of CN III courses through the interpeduncular and the perimesencephalic cisterns, passing between the P1 segment of the posterior cerebral artery (PCA) above and the superior cerebellar artery (SCA) below (see Fig. 17-4). CN III then enters the lateral dural wall of the cavernous sinus and courses superiorly and laterally within it (Fig. 17-5) to enter the orbital cavity via the superior orbital fissure within the annulus of Zinn (the common tendinous ring of the extraocular muscles).

CN IV: Trochlear Nerve

The nucleus of CN IV is located in the midbrain at the level of the inferior colliculus, caudal to the nuclear complex of CN III,

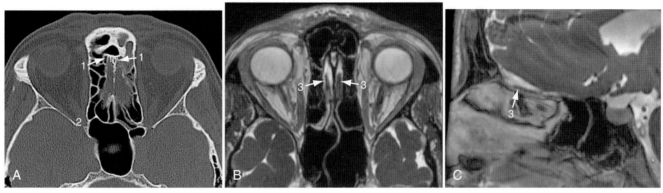

■ **FIGURE 17-1** Axial (**A, B**) and sagittal (**C**) scans through the olfactory groove. **A,** CT. **B** and **C,** MR FIESTA sequence. 1, ethmoid plate; 2, inferior orbital fissure; 3, olfactory bulb.

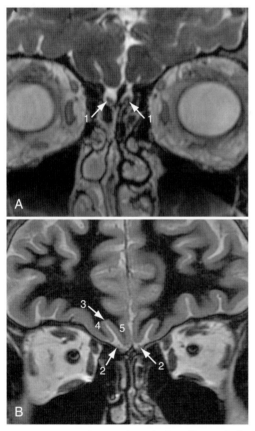

■ **FIGURE 17-2** Coronal scans through the olfactory bulb (**A**) and olfactory tract (**B**). **A,** MR FIESTA sequence; **B,** Inversion-recovery sequence. 1, olfactory bulb; 2, olfactory tract; 3, olfactory sulcus; 4, medial orbitofrontal gyrus; 5, gyrus rectus.

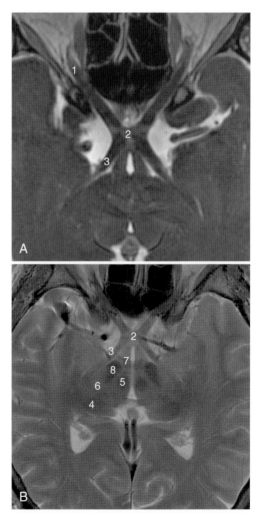

■ **FIGURE 17-3** Axial scans at the level of the optic nerve, chiasm, and tract. **A,** MR FIESTA sequence; **B,** T2W MR image. 1, optic nerve; 2, optic chiasm; 3, optic tract; 4, lateral geniculate body; 5, red nucleus; 6, cerebral peduncle; 7, mammillary body; 8, substantia nigra.

immediately dorsal to the medial longitudinal fasciculus (MLF), and just ventral to the periaqueductal gray matter (Fig. 17-6). The nerve fascicles pass posteriorly and caudally within the periaqueductal gray matter and then decussate within the superior medullary velum before emerging at the dorsal surface of the midbrain just inferior to the contralateral inferior colliculus (see Fig. 17-6). CN IV is the sole cranial nerve to exit the brain stem dorsally and on the side opposite its nucleus. CN IV then courses ventrally and laterally through the quadrigeminal and ambient cisterns to reach the free margin of the tentorium cerebelli, where it typically runs just inferior and lateral to the free

margin of the tentorium cerebelli (see Fig. 17-6).[1] The trochlear nerve enters the cavernous sinus just inferior to the petroclinoid ligament and passes anteriorly in the lateral dural wall of the cavernous sinus, inferior to the third nerve and superior to the ophthalmic division of the fifth cranial nerve (see Fig.

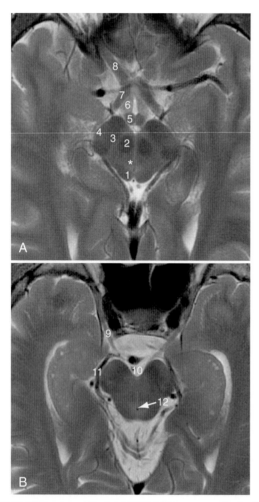

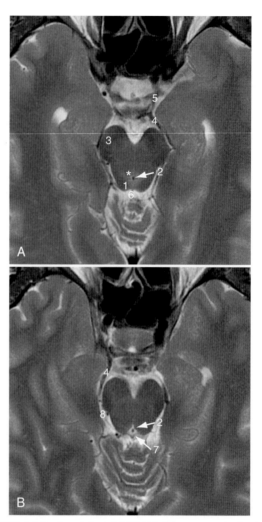

■ **FIGURE 17-4   A** and **B,** Axial T2W MR images at the level of the midbrain. 1, superior colliculus; 2, red nucleus; 3, substantia nigra; 4, cerebral peduncle; 5, mammillary body; 6, fornix; 7, optic chiasm; 8, optic nerve; 9, oculomotor nerve; 10, interpeduncular fossa; 11, posterior cerebral artery; 12, cerebral aqueduct. *Asterisk* is on the oculomotor nucleus.

■ **FIGURE 17-6   A** and **B,** Axial T2W MR images at the level of the inferior colliculi. *Asterisk,* trochlear nucleus; 1, inferior colliculus; 2, cerebral aqueduct; 3, cerebral peduncle; 4, posterior cerebral artery; 5, posterior communicating artery; 6, quadrigeminal cistern; 7, superior medullary velum; 8, ambient cistern.

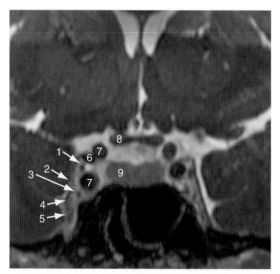

■ **FIGURE 17-5**   Coronal scan through the cavernous sinus. MR contrast-enhanced FIESTA sequence. 1, oculomotor nerve; 2, trochlear nerve; 3, abducens nerve; 4, ophthalmic nerve; 5, maxillary nerve; 6, optic nerve; 7, internal cerebral artery, cavernous segment; 8, optic chiasm; 9, pituitary gland.

17-5). After passing the cavernous sinus, it enters the orbital apex via the superior orbital fissure external to the annulus of Zinn to innervate the contralateral superior oblique muscle.

CN V: Trigeminal Nerve

CN V consists of preganglionic roots, a large sensory root and one to three smaller motor roots,[2] as well as three postganglionic branches: the ophthalmic nerve (CN V_1), the maxillary nerve (CN V_2), and the mandibular nerve (CN V_3).

The four main trigeminal nuclei extend over a long distance from the upper cervical medulla (level of C3) up to the midbrain. They consist of the spinal nucleus of CN V (located posterolaterally in the upper cervical medulla and the lower brain stem), the principal sensory nucleus of CN V (located in the mid pons and providing discriminative tactile information), the motor nucleus of CN V (located in the mid pons medial to principal sensory nucleus), and the mesencephalic nucleus (located posterolaterally in the midbrain and providing proprioception for muscles of mastication).

The trigeminal ganglion (also called the semilunar or gasserian ganglion) is situated along the anterior inferior lateral wall of Meckel's cave. Meckel's cave itself is formed by the meningeal

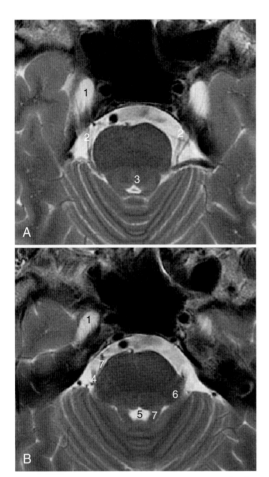

■ **FIGURE 17-7** **A** and **B**, Axial T2W MR images at the level of the superior cerebellar peduncles. 1, Meckel's cave; 2, trigeminal nerve roots; 3, medial longitudinal fasciculus; 4, point of exit/entry of trigeminal nerve roots; 5, fourth ventricle; 6, middle cerebellar peduncle (brachium pontis); 7, superior cerebellar peduncle (brachium conjunctivum); 8, anterior inferior cerebellar artery (AICA).

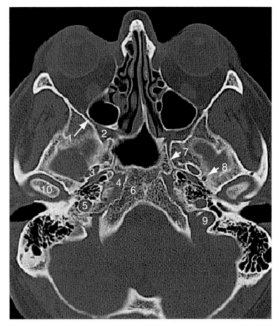

■ **FIGURE 17-8** Axial CT scan at the level of the inferior orbital fissure. 1, inferior orbital fissure; 2, foramen rotundum; 3, foramen ovale; 4, foramen lacerum; 5, carotid canal, vertical portion; 6, basioccipital portion of clivus; 7, vidian canal; 8, foramen spinosum; 9, jugular foramen, pars vascularis; 10, mandibular condyle.

layer of the dura and is located within the middle cranial fossa posteroinferolateral to the cavernous sinus. It is largely filled with cerebrospinal fluid and houses the trigeminal ganglion at its inferior aspect (Fig. 17-7).

The trigeminal sensory nerve root emerges from the concave portion of the trigeminal ganglion as several small sensory rootlets that pass posteriorly to enter the brain stem at the level of the lateral pons (see Fig. 17-7). The motor nerve roots of CN V exit the pons just anterosuperomedial to the entry point of the sensory root.[2] All CN V nerve roots traverse the prepontine cistern in close relationship to the superior cerebellar artery (see Fig. 17-7) and the anterior inferior cerebellar artery (AICA). The motor root of CN V passes through Meckel's cave inferior to the trigeminal ganglion and is adherent to the basal wall of the cave in its distal portion.[3]

The postganglionic branches of CN V (CN V₁-V₃) emerge from the convex portion of the trigeminal ganglion. CN V₁ and CN V₂ run through the lateral wall of the cavernous sinus inferior to CN IV (see Fig. 17-5).[4] The ophthalmic nerve (CN V₁) then enters the orbit via the superior orbital fissure together with CN III, CN IV, and CN VI and the superior ophthalmic vein. The nasociliary branch of CN V₁ passes through the annulus of Zinn, while the lacrimal and frontal branches of CN V₁ enter the orbit outside the annulus of Zinn. CN V₂ leaves the skull base through the foramen rotundum (Fig. 17-8) and crosses the pterygopalatine fossa. The nerve then courses laterally, enters the orbit via the inferior orbital fissure (see Fig. 17-8), and passes through (or

beneath) the orbit within the infraorbital groove/canal to reach the face via the infraorbital foramen.

The third division of CN V, the mandibular nerve, consists of the inferior division of the sensory root and the motor root. These nerve roots leave the skull base through the foramen ovale (see Fig. 17-8), unite, and run through the infratemporal fossa. Within the infratemporal fossa, CN V₃ gives off some branches and then divides into an anterior and a posterior division, both of which give off multiple branches (e.g., to the muscles of mastication, the otic ganglion, the skin of the temporal region, the auricle, and the buccal mucosa).

CN VI: Abducens Nerve

The nucleus of the abducens nerve lies just beneath the floor of the fourth ventricle in the dorsal pons, close to the medial longitudinal fasciculus (MLF). The fascicles of the seventh nerve course around the abducens nucleus, first medial, then dorsal, then lateral to it, forming a protuberance that bulges into the fourth ventricle as the facial colliculus (Fig. 17-9). The abducens fibers course ventrally, caudally, and slightly laterally to exit the brain stem at the pontomedullary sulcus (or the caudalmost pons). The cisternal segment of CN VI recurves anteriorly, laterally, and rostrally; approaches the upper clivus; and passes through a dural channel within the basilar venous plexus (Dorello's canal)[5] to enter the cavernous sinus (see Fig. 17-5). Within the cavernous sinus, CN VI courses along the lateral aspect of the internal carotid artery and its surrounding sympathetic plexus (see Fig. 17-5). CN VI is the only cranial nerve to actually course through the central venous portion of the cavernous sinus. CN III, CN IV, CN V₁, and CN V₂ all course in the lateral dural wall of the cavernous sinus, not within the central venous portion. CN VI then enters the orbit via the superior orbital fissure within the annulus of Zinn.

CN VII: Facial Nerve

CN VII consists of two portions: (1) CN VII proper, a pure motor nerve, and (2) the intermediate nerve (nervus intermedius),

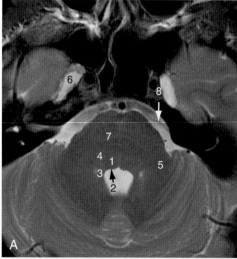

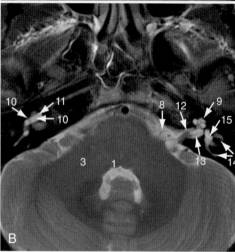

■ **FIGURE 17-9** **A** and **B**, Axial T2W MR images at the level of the facial colliculi. 1, abducens nucleus; 2, facial colliculus (genu of facial nerve); 3, superior cerebellar peduncle (brachium conjunctivum); 4, facial nucleus; 5, middle cerebellar peduncle (brachium pontis); 6, Meckel's cave; 7, pontocerebellar fibers; 8, anterior inferior cerebellar artery (AICA); 9, second turn of cochlea; 10, basal turn of the cochlea, scala vestibuli; 10′, basal turn of the cochlea, scala tympani; 11, osseous spiral lamina; 12, cochlear nerve; 13, inferior vestibular nerve; 14, lateral and posterior semicircular canals; 15, vestibule.

which contains both sensory and parasympathetic motor fibers (see later). Both portions merge at the geniculate ganglion (see later).

The motor nucleus of CN VII is located in the lower portion of the pons, ventral, lateral and slightly caudal to the nucleus of CN VI (see Fig. 17-9). On each side, the motor fasciculi of CN VII course dorsally and cranially and pass medial to the abducens nucleus, and then dorsal to it, between the floor of the fourth ventricle and the abducens nucleus to form the facial colliculus along the floor of the fourth ventricle (see Fig. 17-9). The fascicles of CN VII then curve ventrally and laterally to exit the ventral brain stem at the lower border of the pons in the lateral portion of the pontomedullary sulcus (medial to CN VIII). CN VII traverses the cerebellopontine angle cistern to enter the petrous portion of the temporal bone via the internal acoustic meatus (see Fig. 17-9 for details on the intrameatal course and see the later section on CN VIII).

CN VII runs through the petrous bone within the *facial canal,* which extends from the internal acoustic meatus to the

stylomastoid foramen (Fig. 17-8).[6] Three portions of CN VII can be distinguished within the facial canal:

1. The first segment (*labyrinthine* portion) begins in the internal acoustic meatus and runs perpendicular to the long axis of the petrous bone, directed anteriorly and laterally.
2. The second segment (*tympanic* portion) begins at the geniculate ganglion and curves dorsally and slightly caudally, between the lateral semicircular canal (superiorly) and the oval window (inferiorly).
3. The third segment (*mastoid* portion) runs vertically toward the stylomastoid foramen (see Fig. 17-14).

After exiting the skull base via the stylomastoid foramen, the main trunk of CN VII passes through the parotid gland, where it divides into five major branches.

The geniculate ganglion is located at the distal end of the labyrinthine portion. The cell bodies of the afferent fibers of the intermediate nerve are located within this ganglion. These afferent fibers originate from receptors within the first two thirds of the tongue. They first course with the lingual nerve (CN V) to reach the geniculate ganglion via the chorda tympani (see later). They then run with the intermediate nerve through the internal acoustic meatus and the cerebellopontine angle cistern (Fig. 17-10) to terminate in the upper pole of the nucleus of the solitary tract (designated the gustatory nucleus).

The parasympathetic fibers of the intermediate nerve originate in the superior salivatory nucleus. They bypass the geniculate ganglion without forming synapses and run with the greater petrosal nerve. Both the superficial greater petrosal nerve and the lesser petrosal nerve emerge from CN VII at the level of the geniculate ganglion. These nerves leave the temporal bone via the hiatus of the canal for the greater petrosal nerve and the hiatus of the canal for the lesser petrosal nerve. The superficial greater petrosal nerve merges with the deep greater petrosal nerve (from CN IX) and provides preganglionic, parasympathetic fibers for the lacrimal gland and the connective tissue of mouth, nose, and pharynx. As the so-called pterygoid nerve it runs toward the pterygopalatine ganglion located within the pterygopalatine fossa, where it synapses. The postsynaptic fibers then run with the maxillary nerve.

The superficial lesser petrosal nerve joins the deep lesser petrosal nerve (from CN IX) and leaves the skull base via the canal of the otic ganglion to reach the otic ganglion.

From the mastoid segment of CN VII two nerves emerge. The nerve of the stapedius muscle passes to the stapedius muscle, and the chorda tympani connects CN VII with the lingual nerve. It courses between the malleus and the stapes and leaves the temporal bone through the petrotympanic fissure to reach the infratemporal fossa. It joins the lingual nerve and runs toward the submandibular ganglion.

CN VIII: Vestibulocochlear Nerve
CN VIII consists of two components: the cochlear (or auditory) nerve and the vestibular nerve.

The cochlear nerve is formed by the axons of the bipolar cells of the spiral ganglia, located within the spiral organ of Corti. The dendrites of these cells terminate at the inner hair cells.

The vestibular ganglion is located within the internal acoustic meatus. The axons of its nerve cells constitute the superior and the inferior vestibular nerves, whereas their peripheral dendrites terminate in the receptor organs of the membranous labyrinth (saccule, utricle, and semicircular canals).

The cochlear and the vestibular nerves traverse the internal acoustic meatus to reach the cerebellopontine angle cistern. Within the internal acoustic meatus, CN VII, the superior and the inferior vestibular nerve, as well as the cochlear nerve run parallel to each other, with CN VII anterosuperior, the superior vestibular nerve posterosuperior, the cochlear nerve anteroinferior, and the inferior vestibular nerve posteroinferior (see Fig. 17-10).

After traversing the cerebellopontine angle cistern, CN VIII enters the brain stem at the lateral aspects of the pontomedullary sulci at the level of the inferior cerebellar peduncles. The dorsal and ventral cochlear nuclei and the four vestibular nuclei are located in the dorsolateral pons in relation to the lateral angles of the floor of the fourth ventricle (see later).

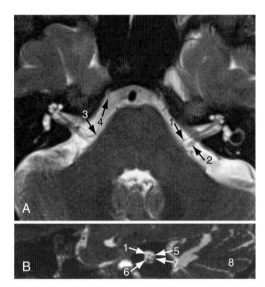

■ **FIGURE 17-10** Axial (**A**) and sagittal (**B**) scans though the internal acoustic meatus. **A,** MR T2W image. **B,** MR FIESTA sequence. 1, Facial nerve; 2, vestibulocochlear nerve; 3, anterior inferior cerebellar artery (AICA); 4, abducens nerve; 5, superior vestibular nerve; 6, cochlear nerve; 7, inferior vestibular nerve; 8, cerebellum.

CN IX: Glossopharyngeal Nerve

The motor fibers of CN IX originate in the nucleus ambiguus. The parasympathetic fibers originate in the inferior salivary nucleus. The sensory fibers of CN IX project to the solitary nucleus and the spinal nucleus of the trigeminal nerve. These nuclei all reside in the medulla oblongata. CN IX emerges from the medulla oblongata as 10 to 20 rootlets along the upper third of the postolivary sulcus.[7,8] These rootlets form the cisternal segment of CN IX and traverse the lateral cerebellomedullary cistern (Fig. 17-11) to enter the jugular foramen through the glossopharyngeal meatus (see Fig. 17-11). Within the jugular foramen, CN IX forms a superior and an inferior ganglion. The superior ganglion is located immediately below the external opening of the cochlear aqueduct, and the inferior ganglion is located immediately caudal to the superior one.[8]

At the inferior ganglion, CN IX gives off its tympanic branch (Jacobson's nerve), which traverses the tympanic canaliculus to enter the tympanic cavity.[8]

After leaving the skull base via the jugular foramen, CN IX runs first between the internal carotid artery and the jugular vein and then between the stylopharyngeal and the styloglossal muscles to reach the base of the tongue. En route, CN IX crosses the ascending palatine artery and the inferior portion of the tonsil and gives off several branches.

CN X: Vagus Nerve

The motor fibers of CN X emerge from the base of the nucleus ambiguus and from the dorsal nucleus of the vagus (i.e., the upper portion of the spinal nucleus of the vagus). Both nuclei are located in the medulla oblongata, where the dorsal nuclei of CN X form the "vagal trigone" at the caudal aspect of the floor of the fourth ventricle (Fig. 17-11). The CN X rootlets emerge from the brain stem along the upper third of the postolivary sulcus, slightly caudal to CN IX, and typically form two nerve bundles (the upper and lower CN X nerve root bundles).[8,9] These traverse the lateral cerebellomedullary cistern and enter the

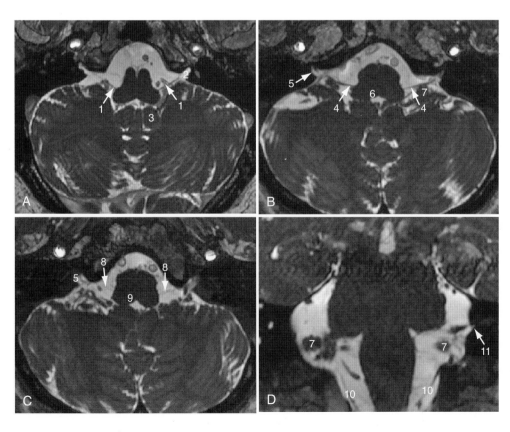

■ **FIGURE 17-11** Axial (**A-C**) and coronal (**D**) images at the level of the medulla oblongata. MR FIESTA sequence. 1, Glossopharyngeal nerve; 2, glossopharyngeal meatus; 3, cerebellar tonsil; 4, vagus nerve; 5, vagal meatus; 6, vagal trigone; 7, flocculus; 8, cranial nerve roots of the accessory nerve; 9, hypoglossal trigone; 10, spinal root of the accessory nerve; 11, external opening of the cochlear aqueduct.

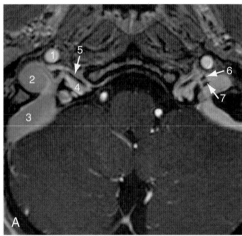

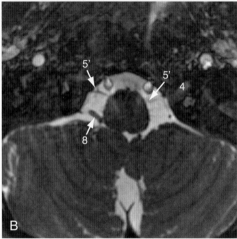

■ **FIGURE 17-12** Axial scans at the level of the hypoglossal canal. **A,** T1W contrast-enhanced MR image. **B,** MR FIESTA sequence. 1, Internal carotid artery; 2, jugular bulb within the venous portion of jugular foramen; 3, sigmoid sinus; 4, hypoglossal canal; 5, hypoglossal nerve, canalicular segment; 5′, hypoglossal nerve, cisternal segment; 6, glossopharyngeal nerve, jugular foramen portion; 7, vagus nerve, jugular foramen portion; 8, posterior inferior cerebellar artery (PICA).

jugular foramen via the vagal meatus (see Fig. 17-11), which is located immediately inferior to the glossopharyngeal meatus. CN X forms a superior ganglion at the level of the intracranial orifice of the jugular foramen. This extends below the extracranial orifice of the jugular foramen. The auricular branch of CN X (Arnold's nerve) emerges from CN X at this ganglion. CN X traverses the jugular foramen in the immediate vicinity of CN XI and posteromedial to CN IX (Fig. 17-12). Just below the jugular foramen, CN X forms the inferior vagal ganglion and runs in close relationship to CN XII, which courses medially to CN X.[7]

After leaving the skull base, CN X descends vertically over a long distance together with the carotid artery. It traverses the neck within the retrostyloid space and enters the upper mediastinum via the superior thoracic hiatus. Here, the right CN X crosses the subclavian artery, while the left one courses anterior to the aorta. Both give off the recurrent laryngeal nerves and reach the esophagus dorsally (right CN X) and ventrally (left CN X) to form the esophageal plexus. The nerves enter the abdominal cavity via the esophageal hiatus.

CN XI: Spinal Accessory Nerve

CN XI is traditionally considered to have both a cranial root (crCN XI) and a spinal root (spCN XI). However, the existence of the cranial roots of CN XI is controversial. Some authors assign the "traditional" crCN XI rootlets to the vagus nerve, because there is evidence that these rootlets originate in the caudal portion of the nucleus ambiguus and the dorsal nucleus of the vagus nerve. Thus they are functionally vagal rootlets.[10,11] Six to 16 of these so-called crCN XI rootlets emerge from the medulla oblongata in the retro-olivary sulcus, just caudal to the vagal nerve bundles (see Fig. 17-11).

The spCN XI consists of 6 to 7 spinal rootlets, which emerge from the upper cervical spinal cord segments C1 to C6, ventral to the posterior cervical roots. spCN XI ascends vertically within the spinal canal, between the posterior cervical roots (dorsally) and the denticulate ligament (ventrally). The spinal rootlets coalesce into a single spCN XI trunk that courses upward through the foramen magnum to reach the posterior cranial fossa (see Fig. 17-11).

The crCN XI and spCN XI nerve roots enter the jugular foramen together with CN X, via the vagal meatus (see Fig. 17-11).[7] Within the jugular foramen, the crCN XI nerve roots blend into the vagus nerve at the level of the superior vagal ganglion. The spCN XI exits the jugular foramen and descends obliquely laterally between the internal carotid artery and internal jugular vein. It traverses the posterior subparotid space and reaches the posterior aspect of the sternocleidomastoid muscle and finally the trapezius muscle.

CN XII: Hypoglossal Nerve

The nucleus of CN XII is located at the posterior aspect of the medulla oblongata, where it raises a focal protrusion on the floor of the fourth ventricle, the so-called hypoglossal trigone (see Fig. 17-11). The fascicles of CN XII emerge from the ventral aspect of the nucleus, pass ventrally and laterally, just medial to the inferior olivary nucleus, and exit from the medulla oblongata as 10 to 15 nerve roots in the anterolateral or preolivary sulcus, between the olive and the pyramid. The nerve roots traverse the premedullary cistern in close relationship to the vertebral artery and the posterior inferior cerebellar artery and coalesce to form one or two hypoglossal trunks (Fig. 17-12). These trunks perforate the dura mater and leave the skull base via the hypoglossal canal (canalicular segment of CN XII[8,12]; see Fig. 17-12). Then, CN XII joins CN X and XI inferior to the jugular foramen just below the skull and runs with them in the carotid sheath adjacent to CN X. CN XII descends between the internal carotid artery and the internal jugular vein in the retrostyloid and the carotid space and reaches the genioglossus muscle via the submandibular and sublingual areas.

FUNCTIONAL DIVISIONS

The functions of the different cranial nerves are as follows:

- CN I transmits olfactory information from the olfactory receptor neurons within the nasal mucosa to the olfactory bulb.
- CN II transmits the visual information from the retina to the brain.
- CN III innervates the superior, medial, and inferior rectus muscles, the inferior oblique muscle, as well as the levator palpebrae superioris of the upper eyelid. Furthermore, it supplies the ciliary ganglion with parasympathetic fibers.
- CN IV is a pure motor nerve that innervates the superior oblique muscle.
- CN V's sensory territories cover the skin of the forehead and nose (CN V_1), the cheek (CN V_2), the jaw (CN V_3), the sinuses, the mucosal membranes of the nasal cavity, the meninges, and the tympanic membrane (external surface). Furthermore, its third division (CN V_3) provides sensory and motor supply to the muscles of mastication (temporalis muscle, masseter muscle, pterygoid muscles, digastric muscle (anterior belly), mylohyoid muscle, tensor veli palatine, and tensor tympani muscles).

- CN VI innervates the ipsilateral lateral rectus muscle, resulting in an abduction of the globe.
- CN VII provides motor fibers to the stapedius muscle, stylohyoid muscle, facial muscles, buccinator muscle, posterior belly of the digastric muscle, and the platysma. Its parasympathetic fibers innervate the lacrimal, submandibular, and parotid glands. It transmits sensory information (taste) from the anterior two thirds of the tongue (via the chorda tympani) and from the periauricular skin and the external surface of the tympanic membrane (via the auricular branch of CN X).
- CN VIII is a pure sensory nerve with two components: the cochlear (or auditory nerve), which is responsible for the sense of hearing, and the vestibular nerve, which is responsible for equilibrium.
- CN IX contains motor fibers (innervating the stylopharyngeus muscle), parasympathetic fibers (to the parotid gland via the otic ganglion), and sensory fibers from the posterior third of the tongue, the pharynx, the tonsils, the carotid body, and the tympanic membrane (internal surface).
- CN X's motor component innervates the muscles of the pharynx and larynx. It transmits parasympathetic fibers to and receives sensory fibers from the pharynx, the larynx, and the thoracic and abdominal visceral organs.
- CN XI is a motor nerve that supplies the sternocleidomastoid muscle and the upper portion of the trapezius muscle.
- CN XII provides the motor innervation to the tongue.

IMAGING
Ultrasonography

In general, ultrasound is of very limited use in the evaluation of cranial nerve lesions. A possible application is the evaluation of infrahyoid cervical masses.[13]

CT

High-resolution CT (HRCT) of the bone plays an important role in evaluating the intraosseous segments of the cranial nerves and in characterizing neural lesions situated near bony structures such as the skull base, the orbit, or the mandible. Although CT is inferior to MRI in the depiction of the cranial nerves themselves, the information provided by both modalities is often complementary.

HRCT of the bone is indicated for the evaluation of the following structures:

- The nasal vault, the sinuses, and the cribriform plate (CN I; see Fig. 17-1)
- The orbital apex, the optic canal, the inferior and the superior orbital fissure (CN II, III, IV, and VI; see Figs. 17-1 and 17-13)
- The sella turcica and the medial sphenoid bone (CN III, IV, V, and VI)
- The clivus and Dorello's canal (CN VI)
- The mandible (CN V$_3$)
- The temporal bone including the internal acoustic meatus, facial canal, and osseous labyrinth (CN VII, CN VIII[14]; Fig. 17-14)
- The bony components of the jugular foramen: the occipital and temporal bones with their intrajugular processes (CN IX, CN X, CN XI; see Fig. 17-8)
- The hypoglossal canal (CN XII; see Fig. 17-13)

For the evaluation of the distal portion of CN X, contrast-enhanced CT of the thorax is recommended (Fig. 17-15).

MRI

MRI is the gold standard for the evaluation of the cranial nerves. In general, lesions can affect the cranial nerves throughout their

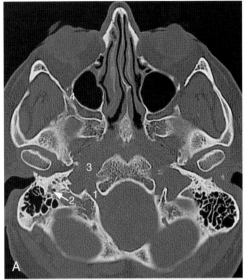
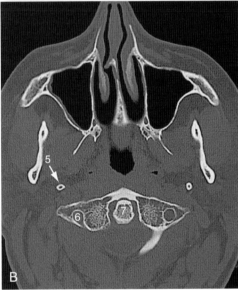

■ **FIGURE 17-13** Axial CT scans through the skull base (**A**) and through the atlas (**B**). 1, Hypoglossal canal; 2, stylomastoid foramen; 3, nasopharyngeal carotid space; 4, inferior orbital fissure; 5, styloid process of the temporal bone; 6, vertebral canal; 7, dens axis.

entire course from the brain stem to beyond the skull base; thus, imaging should cover the entire region. Nevertheless, imaging often must focus on the clinically suspected segment of the nerve in order to take best advantage of the improved resolution provided by new MR sequences and techniques.

Three-dimensional, heavily T2-weighted (T2W) steady-state sequences (e.g., constructive interference in steady-state sequence [CISS], fast-imaging employing steady-state acquisition sequence [FIESTA], and driven equilibrium radiofrequency reset pulse sequence [DRIVE]) are valuable for depicting the cranial nerves, especially their cisternal segments.[15-18] In the following, FIESTA or CISS images are used to exemplify this technique.

The MRI appearance of CN I and CN II is treated separately, whereas the imaging anatomy of CN III to CN XII is presented together with respect to their different segments:

- The brain stem nuclei and intra-axial segments
- Cisternal segments

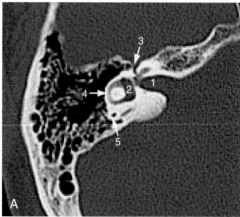

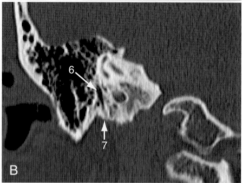

■ **FIGURE 17-14** Axial CT scan (**A**) and coronal reconstruction (**B**) through the right temporal bone. 1, Internal acoustic meatus; 2, vestibule; 3, tympanic segment of facial canal; 4, lateral semicircular canal; 5, posterior semicircular canal; 6, mastoid segment of facial canal; 7, stylomastoid foramen.

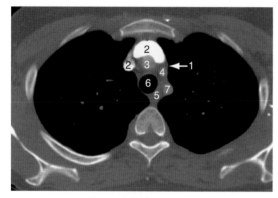

■ **FIGURE 17-15** Axial contrast-enhanced CT scan through the upper mediastinum. 1, Left vagus nerve; 2, brachiocephalic veins; 3, brachiocephalic artery; 4, left common carotid artery; 5, esophagus; 6, trachea; 7, left subclavian artery.

- Intradural or interdural segments (where applicable)
- Intraosseous segments
- Extracranial segments

CN I

The actual olfactory nerves—namely the olfactory filiae—still cannot be depicted by clinical MR scanners. Thin (3-mm) coronal and axial T2W images and/or a FIESTA sequence should be used to visualize the olfactory bulbs, tracts, and striae. On consecutive

FIESTA or T2W images (from anterior to posterior), the olfactory bulb is visualized as an oval-to-round structure on the first slices through the anterior cribriform plate (see Fig. 17-2). Behind it the olfactory tract is depicted as a triangular structure that lies in or just below the olfactory sulcus, bordered medially by the gyrus rectus and laterally by the medial orbital gyrus (see Fig. 17-2). Axial 3D-FIESTA images, reconstructed parallel to the course of the olfactory bulb and tract, depict the olfactory bulb (see Fig. 17-1) and the lateral and medial olfactory striae, which emerge immediately rostral to the anterior perforated substance.

CN II

The optic nerve and chiasm are best depicted on thin axial and coronal fat-saturated T2W imaging, noncontrast T1-weighted (T1W) imaging, and fat-saturated contrast-enhanced T1W imaging.[19] Axial FIESTA and T2W images depict (1) the intraorbital segment of the optic nerve with the surrounding subarachnoid space, (2) the intracanalicular and (3) the intracranial segment of CN II, as well as the optic chiasm within the suprasellar cistern (see Fig. 17-3). The optic tracts also are best depicted on axial slices as they course around the cerebral peduncles to reach the lateral geniculate bodies (see Fig. 17-3).

CN III to CN XII

Brain Stem Nuclei and Intra-axial Segments of CN III to CN XII
With regard to clinical MRI, the brain stem is best evaluated on thin (3-mm) axial proton density–weighted images and/or T2W imaging. In general, the brain stem nuclei of the cranial nerves cannot be visualized directly on conventional, clinical MR sequences. Nevertheless, their anatomic location can be estimated by identifying appropriate anatomic landmarks (*marked in italics throughout the next paragraphs*).

Consecutive T2W axial slices covering the whole brain stem from the midbrain to the medulla oblongata are presented from rostral to caudal. The first slice demonstrates the midbrain at the level of the *superior colliculi* (see Fig. 17-4). The paired paramedian nuclear complex of CN III is located anterior to the aqueduct, partially embedded within the *periaqueductal gray matter*. The parasympathetic Edinger-Westphal nuclei are also found within the periaqueductal gray matter. The CN III fascicles curve ventrally through the midbrain at the level of the *red nuclei* (see Fig. 17-4) to reach the *interpeduncular fossa*, where CN III exits the brain stem (see Fig. 17-4).

On the next-lower slice through the *inferior colliculi*, the CN IV nuclei are found in the paramedian midbrain, ventral to the periaqueductal gray matter and inferior to the oculomotor nerve (CN III) complex (see Fig. 17-6). The trochlear fascicles decussate within the *superior medullary velum* to exit the brain stem dorsally immediately inferior to *the inferior colliculi* (see Fig. 17-6). This section also contains the cephalic portion of the mesencephalic nucleus of CN V just anterolateral to the aqueduct.

The next-lower axial slice is located at the level of the upper pons (including the *facial colliculi* and the *middle cerebellar peduncles* (see Fig. 17-9). The facial colliculi are paramedian elevations of the floor of the fourth ventricle, which are caused by the axons of CN VII as they loop around the abducens nerve nuclei. The facial nerve nuclei (motor nuclei of CN VII), the superior salivatory nuclei, and the nuclei of the solitary tract nucleus) are also located at this level in the ventrolateral pontine tegmentum. In order, the motor nucleus of CN VII is located most anteriorly and medially, followed by the salivatory nucleus further posterolaterally, and the nucleus of the solitary tract most dorsolaterally at the border with the middle cerebellar peduncle. The abducens nerve nuclei are located near the midline, just anterior to the fourth ventricle and immediately ventral to the *facial colliculi* (see Fig. 17-9). Furthermore, the principal sensory

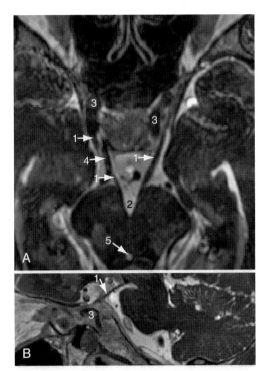

■ **FIGURE 17-16** Axial (**A**) and sagittal (**B**) reconstructions parallel to the cisternal course of the oculomotor nerve. MR FIESTA sequence. 1, Oculomotor nerve; 2, interpeduncular fossa; 3, internal carotid artery, cavernous segment; 4, posterior cerebral artery, embryonal variant; 5, cerebral aqueduct.

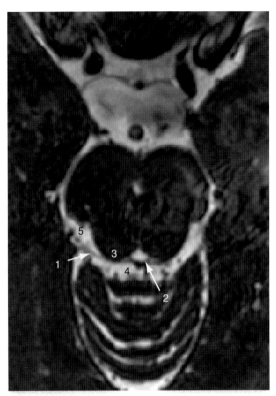

■ **FIGURE 17-17** Axial scan through the inferior colliculi. MR FIESTA sequence. 1, Right trochlear nerve; 2, superior medullary velum; 3, inferior colliculi; 4, quadrigeminal cistern; 5, ambient cistern.

nucleus (dorsolateral) and the motor nucleus (anteromedial) of CN V are found within the pontine tegmentum anterolateral to the facial colliculi.

The consecutive axial slice goes through the lower pons at the level of the *inferior cerebellar peduncles* and *the entry/exit points of CN VII and CN VIII.* Here, the dorsal and ventral cochlear nuclei and the four vestibular nuclei (CN VIII) are located in the dorsolateral pons, anteromedial to the *lateral recess of the fourth ventricle.*

The next-lower slice through the upper medulla oblongata, at the level of the *inferior olive,* and the *vagal trigone,* shows a bulge in the floor of the fourth ventricle, caused by the dorsal vagal nucleus (see Fig. 17-11). The inferior salivatory nucleus is located in the immediate vicinity of the dorsal vagal nucleus. The nucleus ambiguus (motor fibers of CN IX and X), the medullary portion of the nucleus of the solitary tract (in which the taste fibers from the posterior third of the tongue terminate), as well as the spinal nucleus of CN V extend through the upper medulla oblongata.

Although the brain stem nuclei and the intra-axial segments of the cranial nerves are typically not visualized on standard MRI, recent developments and advanced MRI techniques, such as diffusion tensor imaging[20] as well as PROPELLER-diffusion MRI[21] promise to improve the visualization of brain stem structures in vivo. Ex-vivo MRI performed on ultra-high-field scanners (9.4 T; "MR microscopy") already depict the brain stem nuclei and the nerve fascicles in high detail, but these scanners are not yet available for clinical use in patients.[22]

Cisternal Segments of CN III to CN XI

The cisternal segments of the cranial nerves are best depicted on a FIESTA sequence, which is then reconstructed in planes parallel to the specific cisternal course of each cranial nerve to be displayed.[1,2,5,15-18,23] CN III exits the brain stem in the interpe-

duncular fossa (Fig. 17-16) and traverses the peduncular cistern to enter the cavernous sinus (see Fig. 17-5). CN IV exits the brain stem dorsally, caudal to the inferior colliculi (Fig. 17-17), crosses the quadrigeminal and the ambient cisterns (see Fig. 17-17), and passes forward inferior to and just lateral to the free margin of the tentorium to enter the cavernous sinus at its posterolateral angle. The CN V nerve roots exit (or enter, respectively) the lateral pons and traverse the prepontine cistern in an anterosuperior direction (Fig. 17-18) to enter Meckel's cave. The cisternal segment of the abducens nerve emerges from the pontomedullary sulcus and ascends through the prepontine cistern in a strongly anterosuperior and slightly lateral direction toward the high clivus (Fig. 17-19). CN VII and CN VIII exit the brain stem at the level of the pontomedullary junction and traverse the cerebellopontine angle cistern to enter the internal acoustic meatus, with CN VII emerging from the brain stem ventral to CN VIII (Figs. 17-19 and 17-20).

CN IX, CN X, and crCN XI exit the brain stem close to each other within the postolivary sulcus, with CN IX (see Fig. 17-11) emerging most cranially, followed caudally first by the CN X rootlets (see Fig. 17-11) and then by the crCN XI rootlets (see Fig. 17-11). They traverse the perimedullary cistern to enter the glossopharyngeal (CN IX) and the vagal (CN X, and crCN XI) meatus, respectively (see Fig. 17-11). The spCN XI rootlets exit the upper cervical spinal cord and coalesce into a single spCN XI trunk. This trunk runs through the spinal canal in close relationship with the vertebral artery (see Fig. 17-11), ascends through the foramen magnum, and enters the vagal meatus together with CN X and crCN XI.[8]

The CN XII rootlets exit the brain stem via the preolivary sulcus at the level of the hypoglossal trigone, course through the perimedullary cistern, and enter the hypoglossal canal (see Fig. 17-12).

■ **FIGURE 17-18** Axial (**A**) and sagittal (**B**) reconstructions parallel to the cisternal course of the trigeminal nerve, as well as coronal reconstructions (**C, D**) perpendicular to its cisternal course. MR FIESTA sequence. 1, Trigeminal nerve, sensory nerve root; 2, Meckel's cave; 3, trigeminal nerve, motor nerve root; 4, trigeminal ganglion, located at the anteroinferior wall of Meckel's cave; 5, sensory rootlets arising from the trigeminal ganglion.

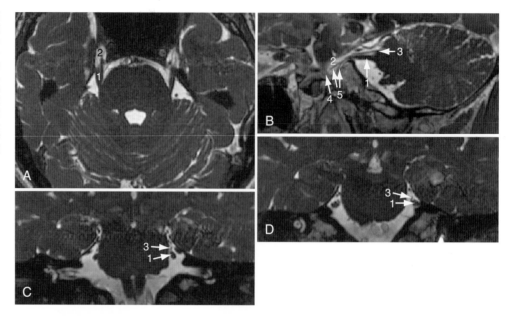

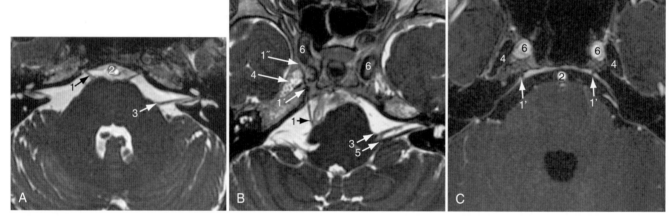

■ **FIGURE 17-19** Axial reconstructions parallel to the cisternal course of the abducens nerve (**A, B**) as well as perpendicular to the Dorello canal (**C**). **A** and **B,** MR FIESTA images. **C,** Contrast-enhanced T1W image. 1, Abducens nerve, cisternal segment, 1′, abducens nerve within Dorello canal, 1″, abducens nerve, cavernous segment; 2, basilar artery; 3, facial nerve; 4, Meckel's cave with sensory rootlets of the trigeminal nerve; 5, vestibulocochlear nerve; 6, internal carotid artery, cavernous segment.

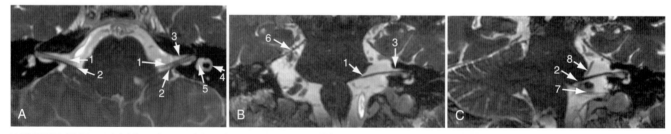

■ **FIGURE 17-20** Axial (**A**) and coronal (**B, C**) reconstructions parallel to the cisternal course of the facial nerve and the vestibulocochlear nerve, respectively. MR FIESTA sequence. 1, Facial nerve; 2, vestibulocochlear nerve; 3, internal acoustic meatus; 4, horizontal semicircular canal; 5, vestibule; 6, tentorium cerebelli; 7, glossopharyngeal nerve; 8, anterior inferior cerebellar artery (AICA).

Intradural Segments of CN V
CN V within Meckel's Cave

The structures of Meckel's cave are best evaluated by thin-section coronal and sagittal T2W imaging or—as a gold standard—a 3D-FIESTA sequence.[3] The FIESTA images demonstrate the trigeminal divisions V_1 to V_3 as they emerge from the anterior convex surface of the ganglion (see Fig. 17-18).

Cavernous Sinus

Imaging of the cavernous sinus must cover the whole extent of the cavernous sinus from the superior orbital fissure anteriorly to the petrous apex posteriorly. The cavernous sinus is best visualized on thin-section contrast-enhanced T1W coronal and axial slices, on a contrast-enhanced 3D-FIESTA sequence, or on a contrast-enhanced high-resolution MR angiography.[4]

Consecutive coronal slices from anterior to posterior depict the cavernous venous plexus itself, its lateral dural borders, the cavernous segment of the internal carotid artery, and the cavernous segments of CN III, CN IV, CN V$_1$, CN V$_2$, and CN VI. CN VI is the only cranial nerve that traverses the venous portion of the cavernous sinus. The other cranial nerves course through its lateral dural wall with CN III located most cranially, followed by CN IV, CN V$_1$, and then CN V$_2$, which is located most caudally within the cavernous sinus (see Fig. 17-5).[24]

Interdural Segment of CN VI—Dorello's Canal
Dorello's canal is a channel that is formed by two layers of dura and is located within the basilar venous plexus. The segment of CN VI within Dorello's canal is best visualized on thin-section, contrast-enhanced T1W imaging or on contrast-enhanced FIESTA images (see Fig. 17-19).[1,4]

Intratemporal Segments of CN VII and CN VIII
Thin-section T2W or 3D-FIESTA images display CN VII and CN VIII within the internal acoustic meatus and clearly demonstrate the membranous labyrinth of the inner ear, including the cochlea, vestibule, and the three semicircular canals (see Figs. 17-9 and 17-10).[15] Pathology affecting the intratemporal course of the CN VII is best displayed by contrast-enhanced thin-section fat-saturated axial and coronal T1W images (see later). High-resolution bone CT is also essential for the evaluation of CN VII within the facial canal (see Fig. 17-14).[14]

Intraosseous Segments (at the Skull Base)
The jugular foramen segments of CN IX to CN XI and the intra-canalicular segment of CN XII within the hypoglossal canal are best visualized on thin-section, contrast-enhanced T1W images (see Fig. 17-12),[12] or on a contrast-enhanced high-resolution MR angiography.[8]

Extracranial Segments
Extracranial pathologic processes that result in cranial nerve palsies are best studied by axial and coronal fat-saturated T2W, axial T1W and T2W, and fat-saturated axial and coronal contrast-enhanced T1W imaging covering the entire course of the cranial nerve in question. For a lesion of the distal vagus nerve, contrast-enhanced CT is the modality of choice (see Fig. 17-15). Imaging of CN XI and CN XII must cover the neck as far caudally as the trapezius muscle (CN XI) and the hyoid bone (CN XII), respectively (Fig. 17-21).

Surface Coils and Parallel Imaging
The use of small surface coils as well as the introduction of parallel imaging techniques can further improve the imaging of the cranial nerves, especially with regard to the thinner nerve branches.[25-27]

Time-of-Flight MR Angiography
Time-of-flight MRA before and after the administration of an intravenous contrast agent is valuable in the evaluation of neurovascular contacts.[12,13,27]

Special Procedures
To date, conventional, digital subtraction angiography (DSA) is no longer routinely used in the imaging of pathologic processes of the cranial nerves.

Nevertheless, it can be indicated if, for example, an aneurysm may be the underlying cause of a cranial nerve palsy. DSA is still the gold standard for pretherapeutic imaging in patients with intracranial aneurysms. Further applications of DSA might be the evaluation of (1) highly vascular tumors and (2) dural arteriovenous fistulas.

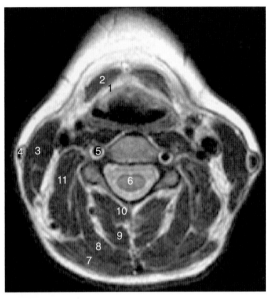

■ **FIGURE 17-21** Axial T2W MR image at the level of the hyoid bone. 1, Hyoid bone; 2, digastric muscle; 3, sternocleidomastoid muscle; 4, external jugular vein; 5, vertebral artery; 6, cervical spinal cord; 7, trapezoid muscle; 8, splenius capitis muscle; 9, semispinalis capitis muscle; 10, semispinalis cervicis muscle; 11, levator scapulae muscle.

HOW PATHOLOGY ALTERS NORMAL APPEARANCE
A wide variety of pathologic processes can involve the cranial nerves. It is necessary to differentiate between primary lesions that affect the nerve itself and secondary nerve dysfunction that reflects the presence of neighboring disease. Furthermore, one must distinguish a central (supranuclear) pathologic process from a peripheral (infranuclear) process. Supranuclear palsy can be caused by ischemic or hemorrhagic infarctions, vascular malformations, trauma, demyelinating disease, neoplasm, or inflammatory/infectious diseases. Peripheral cranial nerve palsies may result from infection, inflammation, postinfectious diseases, primary or secondary neoplasms, neurovascular compression syndromes, aneurysms, direct physical or chemical damage, and congenital lesions.[13,28,29]

Neoplasms
Primary cranial nerve tumors should be distinguished from neoplasms affecting the nerves secondarily.

Primary Neoplasms
Primary neoplasms include schwannomas, neurofibromas, and several rarer tumors such as hemangiomas, paragangliomas, and hamartomas.[29,30]

Schwannomas (also called neurinomas) constitute the most common primary cranial nerve tumors. They arise from the neural sheath, usually at the transition zone where the central myelin derived from oligodendroglia gives way to the peripheral myelin derived from Schwann cells. CN VIII (especially the inferior division of the vestibular nerve) is most often involved (Figs. 17-22 and 17-23), followed by CN V, CN X, CN XII, and CN VII (Fig. 17-24). Neurofibromatosis type 2 typically presents as multiple schwannomas. The imaging appearance of schwannomas varies with their size. Small tumors are typically solid and show homogeneous contrast enhancement (see Fig. 17-23). Larger schwannomas are usually more heterogeneous, with one or more cystic zones and areas of intratumoral hemorrhage (see Fig. 17-22).

■ **FIGURE 17-22** Large vestibulo-cochlear schwannoma of the left CN VIII in a 51-year-old man. Axial proton density–weighted (**A**), T2W (**B**), and axial (**C**) and coronal (**D**) contrast-enhanced T1W MR images. *Arrows,* extrameatal portion of the schwannoma; *asterisks,* intrameatal portion of the schwannoma. The schwannomas shows a heterogeneous signal on T2W and a strong contrast enhancement.

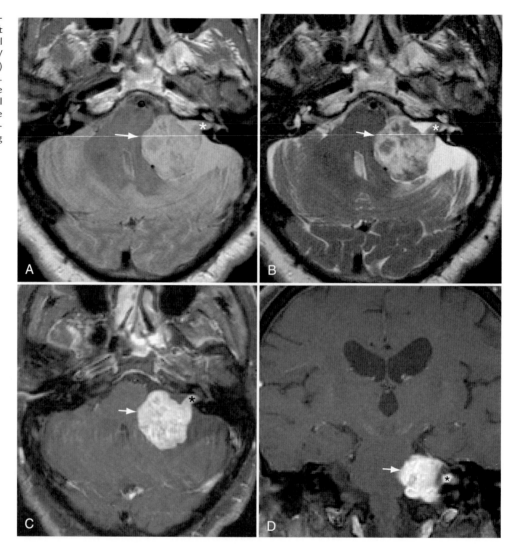

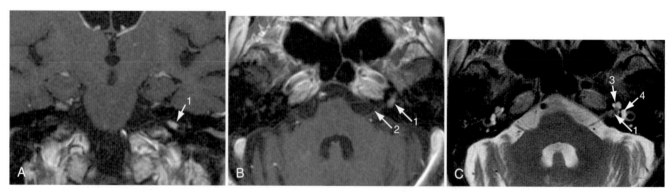

■ **FIGURE 17-23** Small intrameatal schwannoma of the left CN VIII in a 70-year-old woman. Coronal (**A**) and axial (**B**) contrast-enhanced T1W and axial T2W (**C**) MR images. 1, Intrameatal schwannoma; 2, cisternal segment of left CN VIII; 3, cochlea; 4, vestibule. The schwannomas show a strong, homogeneous contrast enhancement on T1W images and are relatively hypointense on the T2W image.

Neurofibromas may arise from Schwann cells or from other perineural cells and fibroblasts. In contrast to schwannomas, the neurofibromas are more typically found extracranially. They are associated with neurofibromatosis type 1 and can show malignant transformation. On imaging studies, benign neurofibromas appear well-defined, enhance moderately, and can present with calcifications. Cystic areas and intratumoral hemorrhages are less common than with schwannomas.[29]

Paragangliomas may also be called glomus tumors (e.g., glomus jugulare and glomus tympanicum). These lesions are tumors of the paraganglionic cells that are found around the cranial nerves and their branches, with a predilection for CN X and CN IX. They are characteristically hypervascular, resulting in strong contrast enhancement (Fig. 17-25) with a "salt-and-pepper" pattern created by the flow voids interspersed within the enhancing tumor. Bone erosion can be demonstrated on HRCT.

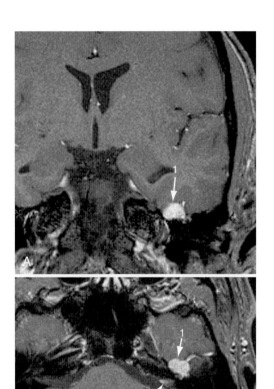

■ **FIGURE 17-24** Facial nerve schwannoma of the left CN VII in the region of the geniculate ganglion in a 56-year-old woman. Coronal (**A**) and axial (**B**) contrast-enhanced T1W MR images. 1, Facial schwannoma in the region of the geniculate ganglion; 2, intrameatal portion of the schwannoma. The schwannoma presents as a homogeneously contrast-enhancing mass.

Secondary Neoplasms

The cranial nerves can be involved secondarily by any intra-axial masses (gliomas), solid extra-axial masses (meningiomas [Fig. 17-26], pituitary adenomas, craniopharyngiomas [Fig. 17-27]), intracranial metastases, leptomeningeal carcinomatosis (Fig. 17-28), or lymphomatous and leukemic infiltrates of the meninges.

Trauma

Because of their long courses and their close relationship to the skull base, the cranial nerves are commonly affected by accidental or iatrogenic trauma. Traumatic injury can result in an (often reversible) edema and/or hematoma of the nerve or in a disruption of the nerve. HRCT of the bone is the modality of choice for depicting skull base fractures and any involvement of the neurovascular foramina. MRI, especially T2*W weighting, helps to display the nerve itself and any intraneural edema or hemorrhage.[31] If the nerve sheath is not disrupted, cranial nerve injury may be missed on MRI. CN III is the nerve most commonly affected by trauma. A traumatic lesion of CN I is often accompanied by contusion of the overlying basal frontal lobe. CN II is often injured in conjunction with orbital fractures, whereas CN VII can be injured by temporal bone fractures. CN IV is particularly vulnerable to injury because of its long cisternal course and close relation to the edge of the tentorium. Trauma is the most common cause of unilateral or bilateral isolated CN IV palsy.[13]

Ischemia

Small pontine or midbrain infarctions can cause isolated cranial nerve palsies. CN III and VI are affected most commonly, followed by CN IV, CN V, CN VII, and CN VIII. Brain stem infarctions are the principal cause of nontraumatic cranial nerve palsies in the elderly population.[32] Acute ischemic lesions are best visualized on diffusion-weighted images, whereas subacute and old infarctions are best shown by thin-sectioned T2W and FLAIR sequences (Fig. 17-29).

Neurovascular Compression Syndromes

With aging, the intracranial arteries elongate and form loops that may displace and compress the cisternal segments of the cranial nerves. These neurovascular contacts may cause a wide variety of neurovascular compression syndromes, including trigeminal and glossopharyngeal neuralgia (CN V and CN IX, respectively [Fig. 17-30]), vestibular paroxysms (CN VIII), superior oblique myokymia (CN IV), and hemifacial spasm (CN VII).[1,28,29] Neurovascular compression has also been proposed as a possible pathogenesis of essential hypertension (CN X) and spasmodic torticollis (CN XI). These contacts or compressions can occur anywhere along the cisternal course of a cranial nerve. Nevertheless, only neurovascular contacts at the so-called root entry/exit zones are widely believed to be responsible for neurovascular compression syndromes. Although there are some discrepancies in the anatomic and clinical literature concerning the definition of the root entry/exit zones, most authors define it as the transition zone between central and peripheral myelin. The issue is further complicated by the fact that neurovascular contact has low specificity for predicting clinical symptomatology and has been observed in patients with no symptoms at all. At present, therefore, neurovascular contact should be evaluated only in the context of a specific clinical presentation.[23]

Demyelinating Disorders

Multiple sclerosis (MS) is the most important demyelinating disorder to affect the cranial nerves. Isolated cranial nerve palsies have been described as rare symptoms in patients with multiple sclerosis, occurring in about 1.5% of all MS patients (Fig. 17-31).[33] Although MRI is the most sensitive imaging method for the demonstration of MS lesions, it may fail to depict lesions that correspond to the clinical symptom of an isolated cranial nerve palsy,[23] even in cases when electrophysiological tests demonstrate brain stem dysfunction at the appropriate level. Acute demyelinating optic neuritis is a common manifestation of MS, found in nearly 50% of MS patients. Recent developments in MRI including measurements of magnetization transfer ratio and diffusivity in the optic nerve have increased the sensitivity of MRI in the detection of demyelinating lesions of the optic nerve.

Aneurysms

Aneurysms of the intracranial arteries might cause a direct physical compression of neighboring cranial nerves, causing palsy of that cranial nerve. Typical locations of aneurysms that present with a cranial nerve palsy are the cavernous segment of the internal carotid artery or the posterior circulation (PCA or SCA; CN IV and CN III; Fig. 17-32). Rare aneurysms of the petrous segment of the internal carotid artery and the extracranial segment of the internal carotid artery (CN IX and CN XII) may also cause cranial nerve palsies.

Infections and Inflammatory Diseases

Viral, bacterial, fungal, and parasitic infections as well as granulomatous diseases can affect the cranial nerves. Of these, the most common are the viral diseases, especially herpes simplex, varicella zoster, cytomegalovirus, and human immunodeficiency virus.[13]

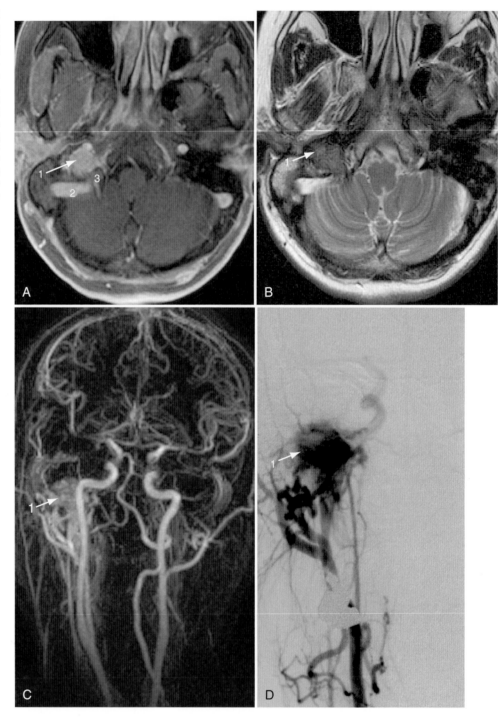

■ **FIGURE 17-25** Right-sided paraganglioma (glomus jugulare tumor) in a 35-year-old man. Axial contrast-enhanced T1W (**A**) and T2W (**B**) MR images, MR angiography (**C**), and digital subtraction angiography (DSA, **D**) images. 1, Paraganglioma in the region of the right jugular foramen; 2, sigmoid sinus; 3, hypoglossal canal. The paraganglioma shows a strong contrast enhancement and a "salt-and-pepper" appearance on the T2W image due to prominent flow voids within the tumor. MR angiography and DSA also clearly demonstrate the hypervascularized tumor.

CN VII is most frequently affected by reactivation of the herpes simplex virus (causing Bell's palsy) followed by herpes zoster infection causing the Ramsay Hunt syndrome. Ramsay Hunt syndrome most commonly involves CN VII and CN VIII and often causes pathologic contrast enhancement within the nerves.

Bacterial infections of the cranial nerves are now rare, except in immunocompromised patients. When present, they often first involve the middle ear or the paranasal sinus, which then leads to secondary infection of the petrous apex and the skull base (Fig. 17-33).

Fungal infections can either affect both immunocompetent and immunocompromised patients (e.g., *Cryptococcus neoformans*) or mostly immunocompromised patients (e.g., *Aspergillus*). These infections often begin in the paranasal sinuses and secondarily affect the adjacent soft tissues and the intracranial compartments.

Noninfectious inflammatory diseases include sarcoidosis, tuberculosis, Wegener's granulomatosis, Behçet's disease, Tolosa-Hunt syndrome, and ophthalmoplegic migraine (Fig. 17-34). They typically present as a thickening of the meninges that shows diffuse or nodular contrast enhancement. The meninges

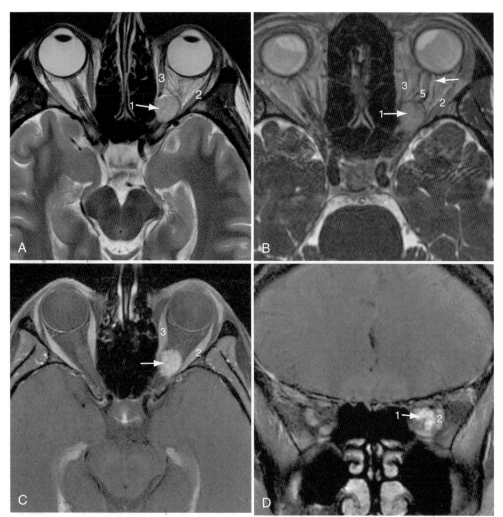

■ **FIGURE 17-26** Intraorbital meningioma in a 46-year-old woman. Axial T2W (**A**) and FIESTA MR (**B**) images as well as axial (**C**) and coronal (**D**) contrast-enhanced T1W MR images. 1, Meningioma in the left orbital apex; 2, lateral rectus muscle; 3, medial rectus muscle; 4, optic nerve sheath; 5, optic nerve surrounded by cerebrospinal fluid. The meningioma is relatively hypointense on T2W images and shows a strong contrast enhancement.

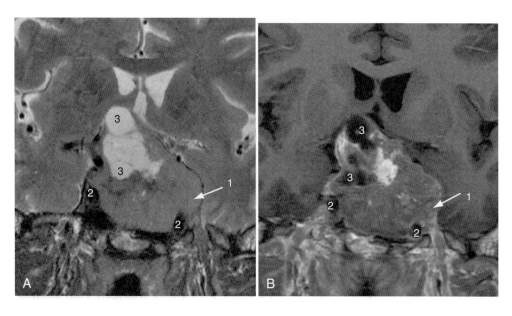

■ **FIGURE 17-27** Intrasellar and suprasellar craniopharyngioma in a 25-year-old man. Coronal T2W (**A**) and contrast-enhanced T1W (**B**) MR images. 1, Tumor infiltration of the left cavernous sinus; 2, internal carotid artery, cavernous segment; 3, cystic area of the tumor.

■ **FIGURE 17-28** Leptomeningeal carcinomatosis in a 74-year-old woman with breast cancer. Axial contrast-enhanced T1W (**A-C**) and T2W (**D**) MR images. 1, Leptomeningeal contrast enhancement in basal cisterns; 2, contrast-enhancing abducens nerves; 3, contrast-enhancing glossopharyngeal nerves; 4, hyperintense brain stem lesions.

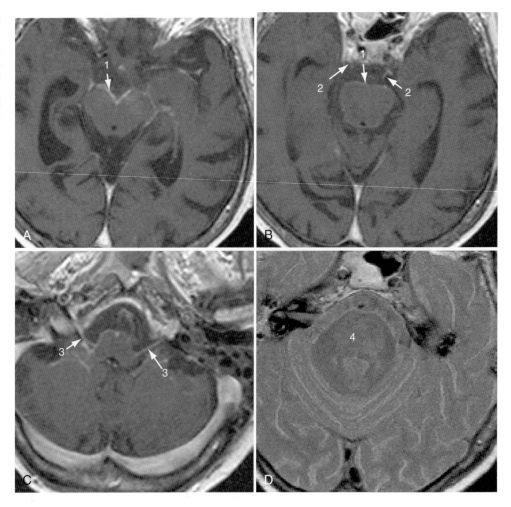

■ **FIGURE 17-29** Acute ischemic lesion (*arrows*) in the anteromedial medulla oblongata in a 76-year-old man with hypoglossus paresis. Axial T2W (**A**), and diffusion-weighted (**B**) MR images.

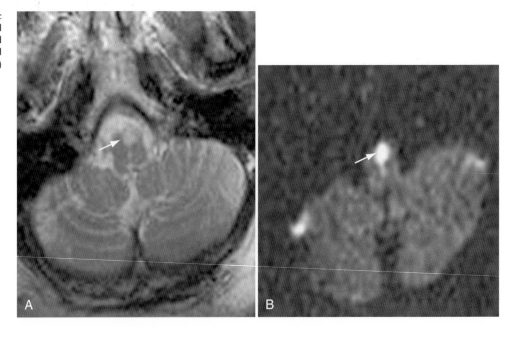

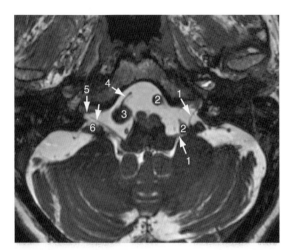

■ **FIGURE 17-30** Glossopharyngeal neuralgia in a 56-year-old woman due to neurovascular contact between the left CN IX and the vertebral artery. Axial MR FIESTA image. 1, Glossopharyngeal nerves; 2, vertebral artery; 3, incidental finding of an aneurysm of the right posterior inferior cerebellar artery; 4, right posterior inferior cerebellar artery; 5, glossopharyngeal meatus; 6, flocculus.

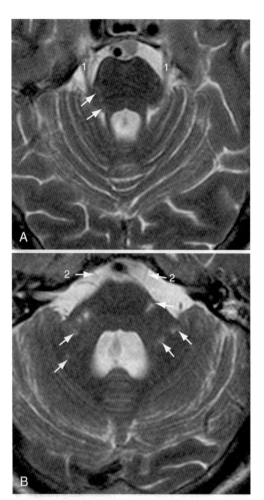

■ **FIGURE 17-31** Multiple sclerosis lesions (*arrows*) in the pons and the middle cerebellar peduncles in a 32-year-old man. Axial T2W MR images. 1, Trigeminal nerves; 2, abducens nerves.

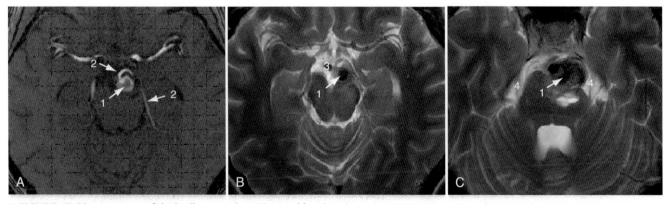

■ **FIGURE 17-32** Aneurysm of the basilar artery in a 67-year-old patient (*arrows*). 3D TOF MR angiography (**A**) and axial T2W MR images (**B, C**). 1, Aneurysm; 2, left posterior cerebral artery; 3, basilar artery; 4, trigeminal nerves.

■ **FIGURE 17-33** Intracranial empyema in a 46-year-old patient secondary to infection of the paranasal sinuses. Coronal (**A, B**) and sagittal (**C, D**) contrast-enhanced T1W MR images show pathologic enhancement (*arrows*).

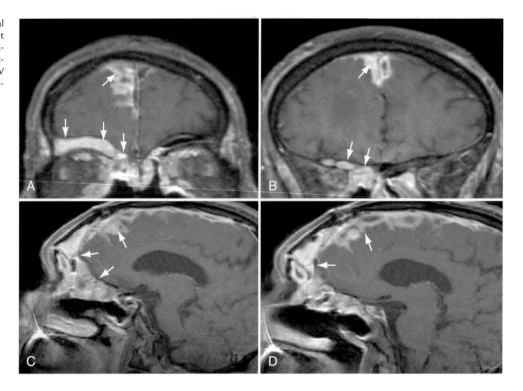

■ **FIGURE 17-34** Ophthalmoplegic migraine of the left oculomotor nerve in a 38-year-old woman. Axial contrast-enhanced T1W (**A**) and T2W (**B**) images. The contrast-enhanced T1W image depicts a strong and homogeneous contrast-enhancing lesion of the left oculomotor nerve. On the T2W image the lesion is barely recognizable as a circumscribed enlargement of the cisternal segment of the nerve.

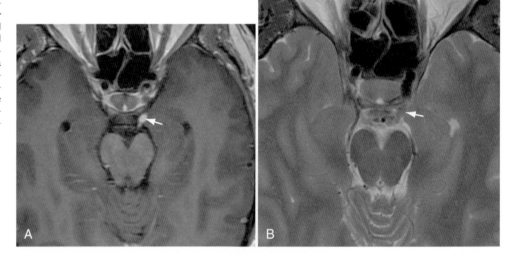

of the basal and suprasellar cisterns are most commonly involved.

ANALYSIS

Because cranial nerves may be damaged throughout their course, the clinical history of the patient is essential for planning and interpreting an MRI study of the cranial nerves. Involvement of multiple cranial nerves in combination suggests specific anatomic sites:

>*Cavernous sinus:* CN III, CN IV, CN V$_1$, CN V$_2$ and/or CN VI (see Fig. 17-5).

>*Sellar region:* CN II chiasm
>*Orbit:* CN II, CN III, CN IV, and/or CN VI
>*Cerebellopontine angle* or *internal acoustic meatus:* CN VII and CN VIII
>*Jugular foramen:* CN IX to CN XI (see Fig. 17-12).

If symptoms have a paroxysmal character, and a neurovascular compression syndrome is suspected, imaging should focus on the cisternal segment of the respective cranial nerve using 3D-FIESTA (or equivalent), 3D-TOF before and after administration of gadolinium contrast agent, and thin-section T2W imaging through the brain stem. A sample report is presented in Box 17-1.

BOX 17-1   Sample Report

PATIENT HISTORY

This 38-year-old woman presented with intermittent attacks of migrainous headache, which lasted for several days and started in the left frontal area. She also suffered from nausea and vomiting. After 3 days, the headache also involved the retrobulbar region of the left eye and was accompanied by horizontal double vision and left eyelid droop. The patient reported having two to three similar attacks per year for the last 6 years.

TECHNIQUE

MRI was performed on a 3-T MR scanner using axial diffusion-weighted MRI, axial 5-mm FLAIR images, axial 3-mm T2W imaging covering the brain stem and the cerebellum, axial 3-mm T1W imaging before and after contrast administration, coronal 3-mm contrast-enhanced T1W imaging, and a FIESTA sequence (acquired axially, slice thickness of 0.6 mm). Gadobenate dimeglumine, 0.1 mmol/kg (0.2 mL/kg), was administered intravenously.

FINDINGS

The diffusion-weighted sequence showed no acute ischemic infarction. The brain stem was unremarkable. The FIESTA and thin-section T2W images demonstrated a circumscribed enlargement of the cisternal segment of the left CN III. Contrast-enhanced T1W imaging showed an approximately 4 × 6-mm lesion with marked homogeneous enhancement (see Fig. 17-34). The cavernous sinus and sellar/suprasellar region were unremarkable.

IMPRESSION

The lesion was a granulomatous inflammatory process, consistent with ophthalmoplegic migraine of the oculomotor nerve.

KEY POINTS

- MRI is the gold standard for the evaluation of the cranial nerves.
- Bone CT is a valuable tool for the assessment of the intraosseous segments of the cranial nerves and areas adjacent to the skull base.
- A wide variety of pathologic processes can affect the cranial nerves throughout their entire courses.

- Evaluation of the cranial nerves must address both the intracranial and the extracranial segments.
- Precise clinical information enables the radiologist to focus high-resolution MR techniques on the affected segment of the cranial nerve to obtain diagnostic images within a reasonable time frame.

SUGGESTED READINGS

Aviv RI, Casselman J. Orbital imaging: portion 1. Normal anatomy. Clin Radiol 2005; 60:279-287.

Borges A. Trigeminal neuralgia and facial nerve paralysis. Eur Radiol 2005; 15:511-533.

Borges A, Casselman J. Imaging the cranial nerves: portion I. Methodology, infectious and inflammatory, traumatic and congenital lesions. Eur Radiol 2007; 17:2112-2125.

Borges A, Casselman J. Imaging the cranial nerves: portion II. Primary and secondary neoplastic conditions and neurovascular conflicts. Eur Radiol. 2007; 17:2332-2344.

Castillo M. Imaging of the upper cranial nerves I, III-VIII, and the cavernous sinuses. Magn Reson Imaging Clin North Am. 2002; 10:415-431.

Gunny R, Yousry TA. Imaging anatomy of the vestibular and visual systems. Curr Opin Neurol. 2007; 20:3-11.

Laine FJ, Underhill T. Imaging of the lower cranial nerves. Magn Reson Imaging Clin North Am 2002; 10:433-449.

Larson TC 3rd, Aulino JM, Laine FJ. Imaging of the glossopharyngeal, vagus, and accessory nerves. Semin Ultrasound CT MR 2002; 23:238-255.

Monstad P. Microvascular decompression as a treatment for cranial nerve hyperactive dysfunction—a critical view. Acta Neurol Scand Suppl 2007; 187:30-33.

Wichmann W, Müller-Forell W. Anatomy of the visual system. Eur J Radiol 2004; 49:8-30.

REFERENCES

1. Yousry I, Moriggl B, Dieterich M, et al. MR anatomy of the proximal cisternal segment of the trochlear nerve: neurovascular relationships and landmarks. Radiology 2002; 223:31-38.
2. Yousry I, Moriggl B, Schmid U, et al. Detailed anatomy of the motor and sensory roots of the trigeminal nerve and their neurovascular relationships. J Neurosurg 2004; 101:427-434.
3. Yousry I, Moriggl B, Schmid UD, et al. Trigeminal ganglion and its divisions: detailed anatomic MR imaging with contrast-enhanced 3D constructive interference in the steady state sequences. AJNR Am J Neuroradiol. 2005; 26:1128-1135.
4. Linn J, Peters F, Lummel N, et al. Detailed imaging of the normal anatomy and pathologic conditions of the cavernous region at 3 Tesla using a contrast-enhanced MR angiography. Neuroradiology 2011; 53:947-654.
5. Yousry I, Camelio S, Wiesmann M, et al. Detailed magnetic resonance imaging anatomy of the cisternal segment of the abducent nerve: Dorello's canal, neurovascular relationships and landmarks. J Neurosurg 1999; 91:276-283.
6. Phillips CD, Bubash LA. The facial nerve: anatomy and common pathology. Semin Ultrasound CT MR 2002; 23:202-217.
7. Özveren MF, Türe U, Özek MM, Pamir MN. Anatomic landmarks of the glossopharyngeal nerve: a microsurgical anatomic study. Neurosurgery 2003; 52:1400-1410.
8. Linn J, Peters F, Moriggl B, et al. The jugular foramen: imaging strategy and detailed anatomy at 3T. AJNR Am J Neuroradiol 2009; 30:34-41.
9. Rhoton AL; Buza R. Microsurgical anatomy of the jugular foramen. Neurosurg 1975; 42:541-550.
10. Wiles CCR, Wrigley B, Greene JRT. Re-examination of the medullary rootlets of the accessory and vagus nerves. Clin Anat 2007; 20:19-22.
11. Lachman N, Acland RD, Rosse C. Anatomical evidence for the absence of a morphologically distinct cranial root of the accessory nerve in man. Clin Anat 2002; 15:4-10.
12. Yousry I, Moriggl B, Schmid UD, et al. Detailed anatomy of the intracranial segment of the hypoglossal nerve: neurovascular rela-

tionships and landmarks on magnetic resonance imaging sequences. J Neurosurg 2002; 96:1113-1133.

13. Borges A, Casselman J. Imaging the cranial nerves: portion I. Methodology, infectious and inflammatory, traumatic and congenital lesions. Eur Radiol 2007; 17:2112-2125.
14. Fatterpekar GM, Doshi AH, Dugar M, et al. Role of 3D CT in the evaluation of the temporal bone. Radiographics 2006; 26(Suppl 1): S117-S132.
15. Casselman JW, Kuhweide R, Deimling M, et al. Constructive interference in steady state-3DFT MR imaging of the inner ear and cerebellopontine angle. AJNR Am J Neuroradiol 1993; 14:47-57.
16. Yousry I, Camelio S, Schmid UD, et al. Visualization of cranial nerves I-XII: value of 3D-CISS and T2-weighted FSE sequences. Eur Radiol 2000; 10:1061-1067.
17. Mikami T, Minamida Y, Yamaki T, et al. Cranial nerve assessment in posterior fossa tumors with fast imaging employing steady-state acquisition (FIESTA). Neurosurg Rev 2005; 28:261-266.
18. Jung NY, Moon WJ, Lee MH, Chung EC. Magnetic resonance cisternography: comparison between 3-dimensional driven equilibrium with sensitivity encoding and 3-dimensional balanced fast-field echo sequences with sensitivity encoding. J Comput Assist Tomogr 2007; 31:588-591.
19. Gunny R, Yousry TA. Imaging anatomy of the vestibular and visual systems. Curr Opin Neurol 2007; 20:3-11.
20. Salamon N, Sicotte N, Alger J, et al. Analysis of the brain-stem white-matter tracts with diffusion tensor imaging. Neuroradiology 2005; 47:895-902.
21. Adachi M, Kabasawa H, Kawaguchi E. Depiction of the cranial nerves within the brainstem with use of PROPELLER multishot diffusion-weighted imaging. AJNR Am J Neuroradiol 2008 [Epub ahead of print].
22. Fatterpekar GM, Naidich TP, Delman BN, et al. Cytoarchitecture of the human cerebral cortex: MR microscopy of excised specimens at 9.4 Tesla. AJNR Am J Neuroradiol 2002; 23:1313-1321.
23. Linn J, Moriggl B, Schwarz F. Cisternal segments of the glossopharyngeal, vagus, and accessory nerves: detailed magnetic resonance imaging demonstrated anatomy and neurovascular relationships. J Neurosurg 2009; 110:1026-1041.
24. Yagi A, Sato N, Taketomi A, et al. Normal cranial nerves in the cavernous sinuses: contrast-enhanced three-dimensional constructive interference in the steady state MR imaging. AJNR Am J Neuroradiol 2005; 26:946-950.
25. Wichmann W. Reflections about imaging technique and examination protocol 2. MR examination protocol. Eur J Radiol 2004; 49:6-7.
26. Stone JA, Chakeres DW, Schmalbrock P. High-resolution MR imaging of the auditory pathway. MRI Clin North Am 1998; 6:195-219.
27. Held P, Fellner C, Fellner F, et al. MRI of the inner ear and facial nerve pathology using 3D MP-RAGE and 3DCISS sequences. Br J Radiol 1997; 70:558-556.
28. Yousry I, Dieterich M, Naidich TP, et al. Superior oblique myokymia: magnetic resonance imaging support for the neurovascular compression hypothesis. Ann Neurol 2002; 51:361-368.
29. Borges A, Casselman J. Imaging the cranial nerves: portion II. Primary and secondary neoplastic conditions and neurovascular conflicts. Eur Radiol 2007; 17:2332-2344.
30. Mrugala MM, Batchelor TT, Plotkin SR. Peripheral and cranial nerve sheath tumors. Curr Opin Neurol 2005; 18:604-610.
31. Mariak Z, Mariak Z, Stankiewicz A. Cranial nerve II-VII injuries in fatal closed head trauma. Eur J Ophthalmol 1997; 7:68-72.
32. Thömke F, Gutmann L, Stoeter P, Hopf HC. Cerebrovascular brain-stem diseases with isolated cranial nerve palsies. Cerebrovasc Dis 2002; 13:147-155.
33. Thömke F, Lensch E, Ringel K, Hopf HC. Isolated cranial nerve palsies in multiple sclerosis. J Neurol Neurosurg Psychiatry 1997; 63:682-685.

Cerebrovascular Anatomy and Disease

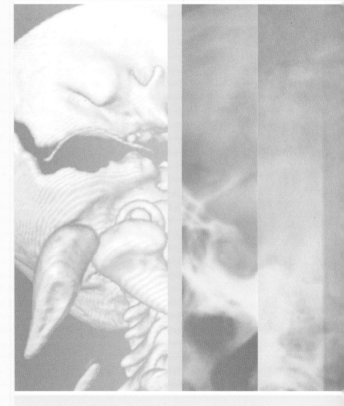

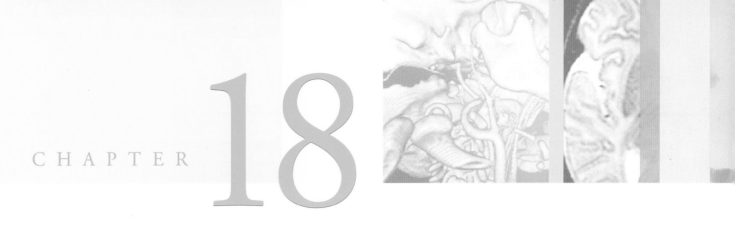

CHAPTER 18

Normal Vascular Anatomy

Amish H. Doshi, Amit Aggarwal, and Aman B. Patel

EMBRYOGENESIS OF INTRACRANIAL VASCULATURE

Normal Fetal Development

The aortic arch, great vessels, and their branches approach their adult configuration by the eighth week of gestation.[1] These vessels arise from paired embryonic aortic arches, which connect the aortic sac with the dorsal aorta. The initial embryonic arterial circulation is symmetric and consists of paired aortic arches connecting to paired dorsal aortae. As segments of the paired arches and dorsal aortae selectively persist or involute, the aorta and its branches take their adult form.[2]

Involution of the first and second aortic arches occurs by day 29 of gestation. The third, fourth, and sixth arches persist and eventually give rise to the aortic arch, pulmonary arteries, subclavian arteries, common carotid, and proximal internal carotid arteries (ICAs).[3] The fifth arches may give rise to rudimentary vessels that eventually degenerate or may fail to develop.[4]

Dorsally, the vertebral arteries arise from paired plexiform longitudinal anastomoses that interconnect the six cervical intersegmental arteries. The basilar artery arises from paired plexiform arterial arcades designated the *dorsal longitudinal neural arteries.* The two dorsal longitudinal neural arteries eventually fuse to form the single basilar artery, so, in the adult, the two vertebral arteries unite to form one basilar artery.[5]

Internal Carotid Arteries

The cervical portions of the ICAs arise from the third aortic arch. The intracranial portions of the ICAs develop as an extension of the dorsal aortae.[3]

During embryologic development, the distal ICAs consist of cranial and caudal divisions. The paired cranial divisions initially terminate as the primitive olfactory arteries. These arteries give origin to the anterior cerebral arteries (ACAs), the anterior choroidal arteries, and the middle cerebral arteries (MCAs).[6] The caudal divisions of the ICAs initially anastomose with the paired dorsal longitudinal neural arteries to form temporary connections between the vertebrobasilar circulation and the ICA. Portions of the caudal divisions anastomose with the cranial ends of the dorsal longitudinal neural arteries to give rise to the posterior communicating arteries (PCoAs). The remaining portions typically regress and disappear.[2] On occasion, other portions of these caudal anastomoses persist into adulthood, giving rise to a group of unusual primitive carotid-basilar anastomoses.

Anterior Cerebral Arteries

At days 41 to 48 of gestation, the primitive olfactory artery gives off two branches, one directed toward the nasal fossa and the other directed medially. The medially directed vessel gives rise to the ACA. By the sixth week of gestation, both ACAs course toward the midline and connect to each other through a plexiform anastomosis.[7] This plexus ultimately forms the anterior communicating artery (ACoA). The medial lenticulostriate arteries and the recurrent artery of Huebner are thought to arise from the primitive olfactory artery or the anastomosis between this artery and the primitive ACAs.[6]

Middle Cerebral Arteries

The MCAs develop from the primitive ICAs proximal to the ACAs. Branches of the MCAs extend over the cerebral hemispheres during days 47 to 48 of gestation. Initially, the MCA branches ascend almost vertically over the lateral surfaces of the early hemispheres. As the brain matures, and the opercula fold progressively over the insula, the MCA branches are constrained to fold with the brain, creating the looping adult course of the MCA across the insula, along the inner wall of the opercula, and then upward around the frontal and parietal opercula and downward over the temporal operculum.[1]

Posterior Cerebral Artery

The posterior cerebral arteries (PCAs) develop as continuations of the PCoAs. After the caudal divisions of the ICAs anastomose with the cranial ends of the dorsal longitudinal neural arteries, both regress to form the early PCoAs. Embryonic vessels arise from the caudal end of these PCoAs and then coalesce into the proximal segments of the PCAs. Over time, concurrent with the development of the vertebrobasilar system, the early PCoAs involute into the small adult PCoAs.[1,3] In 20% to 30% of individuals, the PCoAs do not regress, so the posterior cerebral circulation continues to be supplied from the ICAs rather than from the vertebrobasilar system.[8] In these cases, the PCoAs remain large in caliber and are designated "persistent fetal PCAs."

Vertebrobasilar System

A series of longitudinal anastomoses connect six cervical intersegmental arteries, eventually giving rise to the vertebral arteries. Proximal connections to the dorsal aortae regress, except for the paired sixth intersegmental arteries.[9] The sixth intersegmental arteries give rise to the subclavian arteries.[9] Distally, the paired VAs supply the paired longitudinal neural arteries, which ultimately coalesce to form the single definitive basilar artery.

Connections between the carotid and basilar system exist in early fetal development. These connections are named for the cranial nerves with which they course and include the trigeminal artery, otic artery, and hypoglossal artery. An additional proatlantal intersegmental artery also connects the carotid with the vertebral arteries.[10] In normal fetal development, these connections involute after the PCoAs form from the caudal ICAs.[1]

The branches of the vertebrobasilar system develop relatively late compared with the normal cerebral vasculature. The major cerebellar branches develop "top down," first the superior cerebellar arteries (SCAs), then the anterior inferior cerebellar arteries (AICAs), and last the posterior inferior cerebellar arteries (PICAs). The vascular plexus supplying the primitive hindbrain persists late into embryologic development, allowing them time to develop a broad range of final vascular configurations.[11]

ARTERIAL SYSTEM
Anterior Arterial Circulation
Internal Carotid Artery

The ICAs originate at the bifurcation of the common carotid arteries in the neck, most commonly at the C3-4 or C4-5 level. Variability in the level of bifurcation of the common carotid arteries has been described, ranging from C1 to T2.[12] The ICAs course upward through the anterior neck to the skull base and ascend through carotid canals within the petrous temporal bones to enter the intracranial space. The ICAs then pass forward over the intracranial surface of the foramen lacerum, course lateral to the sphenoid bone and sella turcica, ascend medial to the anterior clinoid processes, and enter the subarachnoid space just superior to the anterior clinoid processes. The ICAs terminate in the suprasellar cistern by bifurcating into the ACAs and MCAs. The long course of the ICA is typically subdivided into seven anatomic segments (Table 18-1 and Fig. 18-1).[13]

C1

The cervical segment of the ICA (C1) extends from the origin of the ICA to its entry into the skull base. C1 can be further subdivided into the proximal carotid bulb and the ascending segment distal to the bulb. The carotid bulb is a focal dilatation at the origin of the ICA. It commonly demonstrates turbulent flow dynamics at angiography.[14] The ascending portion of C1 passes superiorly through the carotid space, accompanied, for parts of its course, by the external carotid artery (ECA), internal jugular vein, and cranial (CN) nerves IX, X, XI, and XII to the level of the skull base. No consistent anatomic branches arise from the ascending cervical segment of the ICA, although anomalous vessels have occasionally been reported to arise there. The ascending cervical ICA arises posterolateral to the ECA but gradually passes medial to the ECA as it ascends superiorly.

Variations in the origin and course of the ICA may occur, including medial origin of the ICA relative to the ECA, direct origin of the ICA from the aortic arch, and idiopathic tortuosity and kinking of the ascending portion. Congenital anomalies of the cervical ICA are exceedingly uncommon, but include hypoplasia and aplasia, duplication and fenestration, anomalous origin and branches, and persistent primitive carotid-basilar anastomoses.

C2

The petrous segment of the ICA (C2) spans the course of the artery through the carotid canal of the petrous temporal bone. Initially, the petrous ICA ascends vertically within the canal (vertical portion of C2). It then turns anteriorly, medially, and

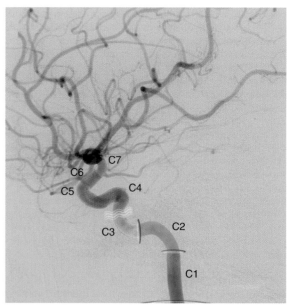

■ **FIGURE 18-1** Lateral view of a carotid artery angiogram showing the seven segments of the internal carotid artery (ICA) from its origin to the bifurcation of the anterior and middle cerebral arteries. The cervical segment (C1) extends from the origin of the ICA to the petrous bone. As the ICA enters the petrous bone and carotid canal (*horizontal oval*) it becomes the petrous segment (C2). The artery then exits the carotid canal (*vertical oval*) and travels superior to the foramen lacerum as the lacerum segment (C3) extending to the level of the petrolingual ligament (*curved lines*). At the superior aspect of the ligament the ICA becomes the cavernous segment (C4). This segment has two vertical segments with an intervening horizontal segment. As the ICA courses through the dural reflections at the level of the anterior clinoid process it is termed the clinoid segment (C5). The distal portion of the dural reflection at the anterior clinoid gives rise to the ophthalmic segment (C6), which extends to the level just proximal to the origin of the posterior communicating artery. The communicating segment (C7) extends from the origin of the posterior communicating artery and terminates at the bifurcation of the ICA.

TABLE 18-1. Internal Carotid Artery Segments

Segment	Course
C1 (cervical)	Extends from the origin of the internal carotid artery to its entry into the skull base
C2 (petrous)	Portion of the artery within the carotid canal of the petrous temporal bone Initially, ascends vertically within the canal (vertical portion) and then turns anteriorly, medially, and superiorly within the canal (genu) and continues horizontally (horizontal portion) toward the petrous apex, where it exits the temporal bone
C3 (lacerum)	Begins where the internal carotid artery exits from the carotid canal and extends up to the level of the petroclinoid ligament
C4 (cavernous)	Begins at the superior aspect of the petroclinoid ligament and includes the portion of the internal carotid artery that courses through the cavernous sinus
C5 (clinoid)	Short segment; courses through the dural reflections related to the anterior clinoid process
C6 (ophthalmic)	Begins at the distal dural reflection around the anterior clinoid process and extends to the level of the posterior communicating artery
C7 (communicating)	Begins just proximal to the origin of the posterior communicating artery and terminates where the internal carotid artery bifurcates into the anterior and middle cerebral arteries

superiorly within the canal (genu) and continues horizontally (horizontal portion) toward the petrous apex, where it exits the temporal bone.[15] The petrous segment of the ICA lies just anterior and inferior, to the tympanic cavity and cochlea, separated only by a thin bony plate.[16,17] The vidian artery and caroticotympanic artery may (variably) arise from the petrous ICA and may provide collateral flow from the ECA in cases of more proximal ICA occlusion.[18]

An aberrant petrous ICA segment may reflect a defect during embryogenesis. Abnormal involution or underdevelopment of the petrous ICA, and consequent collateral flow between the caroticotympanic artery and an augmented inferior tympanic artery, may establish an aberrant course of the ICA through the middle ear.[19] Such an aberrant ICA may be confused with a vascular tumor, particularly a glomus tympanicum tumor.[19,20] A persistent stapedial artery may arise from the vertical portion of the petrous ICA as an uncommon anomalous branch. The stapedial artery passes into the middle ear, courses across the footplate of the stapes, and terminates as the middle meningeal artery. The stapedial artery is typically *not* identified at digital angiography but may be seen on CT angiography as a focal defect in the lateral wall of the carotid canal, an enlarged geniculate fossa, and irregularity of the anterior epitympanic recess. An additional, indirect sign is hypoplasia or absence of the ipsilateral foramen spinosum.[21,22]

C3

The lacerum segment of the ICA (C3) begins where the ICA exits from the carotid canal. It includes the portion of the ICA superior to the foramen lacerum and extends up to the level of the petroclinoid ligament that extends from the petrous apex to the posterior clinoid process of the sphenoid bone. No named branches arise from this segment of the ICA.

C4

The cavernous segment of the ICA (C4) begins at the superior aspect of the petroclinoid ligament and includes the sinuous portion that courses through the cavernous sinus. C4 initially ascends into the cavernous sinus (first vertical segment), where it lies medially. It then turns (first genu) to course horizontally within the cavernous sinus (horizontal segment), turns upward (second genu), and ascends as a shorter more lateral ascending vertical segment (second ascending segment).[13] The posterior genu characteristically lies medial to the anterior genu. The cavernous portion of the ICA lies in close proximity to numerous anatomic structures. The sella turcica and sphenoidal sinus lie medial and inferomedial to the cavernous segment of the ICA. CN VI courses forward through the cavernous sinus along the lateral wall of C4, so it is often the first cranial nerve affected by aneurysms of the cavernous carotid artery. CN III, IV, V1, and V2 course within the lateral wall of the cavernous sinus lateral to C4. Meckel's cave and the trigeminal ganglion lie just inferolateral to the cavernous sinus.[23]

Several important branches originate from the cavernous segment of the ICA. The meningohypophysial artery, also called the posterior trunk, arises from the posterior genu of C4 and gives rise to three major branches: the inferior hypophysial artery, the marginal tentorial artery, and the dorsal clival (meningeal) artery.[24] The inferolateral trunk commonly arises from the horizontal portion of C4 and courses laterally to supply CN III, IV, and VI in addition to the trigeminal ganglion and the dura covering the cavernous sinus (Fig. 18-2).[25] The inferolateral trunk also arises from C4. It gives off branches that anastomose with branches from the external carotid circulation, so the inferolateral trunk provides a route for collateral ECA-to-ICA flow around stenoses/occlusions of the cervical ICA.[26]

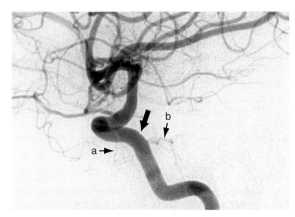

■ **FIGURE 18-2** Lateral view of a carotid artery angiogram shows the branches of the cavernous portion of the internal carotid artery (*large arrow*), inferolateral trunk (a), and meningohypophysial trunk (b).

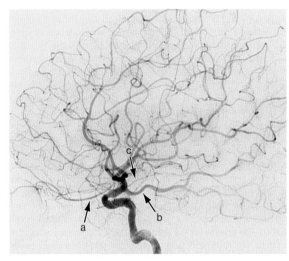

■ **FIGURE 18-3** Lateral view from an internal carotid artery (ICA) angiogram shows three major branches of the distal ICA. The ophthalmic artery (a) is the first major branch that arises from the C6 or ophthalmic segment of the ICA. The communicating or C7 segment of the ICA gives rise to the posterior communicating artery (b) and anterior choroidal artery (c).

C5

The very short clinoid segment of the ICA (C5) courses through the dural reflections related to the anterior clinoid process. It does not give rise to consistent named branches.

C6

The ophthalmic segment of the ICA (C6) begins at the distal dural reflection about the anterior clinoid process and extends to the level of the PCoA. The major branches arising from the C6 segment include the ophthalmic artery and the superior hypophysial artery. The ophthalmic artery typically arises from the medial aspect of the C6 segment and courses with the optic nerve through the optic canal into the orbit (Fig. 18-3).[27] Occasionally, the ophthalmic artery may arise, instead, from the C5 segment of the ICA or from the middle meningeal artery.[1] The ophthalmic artery gives rise to multiple ocular, orbital, and extraorbital branches. The ocular branches include the central retinal artery and ciliary arteries. The orbital branches include the lacrimal artery and muscular branches. The recurrent meningeal artery is a small branch of the lacrimal artery, which courses through the superior orbital fissure to anastomose with branches of the middle meningeal artery.[28] The extraorbital branches include the supraorbital, anterior, and posterior ethmoidal, dorsal nasal, palpebral, medial frontal, and supratrochlear arteries.[27] These generally anastomose with branches of the ECA, providing another route for collateral flow from the ECA to the ICA. The C6 segment also gives rise to the superior hypophysial artery. This artery arises from the medial aspect of C6, anastomoses with its contralateral counterpart, and forms a vascular plexus about the pituitary stalk. This plexus supplies the anterior pituitary gland, tuber cinereum, optic nerve, and optic chiasm.[28]

C7

The communicating segment of the ICA (C7) begins just proximal to the origin of the PCoA and terminates where the ICA bifurcates into the MCAs and ACAs. The first major branch of C7 is the PCoA. This arises from the posterior wall of the ICA and courses posteriorly through the suprasellar cistern to anastomose with the PCA (see Fig. 18-3). The size of the PCoA varies widely from aplastic to hypoplastic to enlarged. Large size suggests that the PCoA directly supplies the PCA territory as a persistent fetal PCA (Fig. 18-4).[8] The origin of the PCoA often exhibits a focal enlargement, designated the infundibulum. To be considered an infundibulum, rather than an aneurysm, the focal dilatation must lie precisely at the origin of the PCoA, must be widest at its base, must not measure greater than 3 mm at its base, and must give rise to the rest of the vessel exactly at its apex (Fig. 18-5).[29] CN III courses through the suprasellar cistern close to the PCoA, so it is often affected by aneurysms of the PCoA. The anterior thalamoperforating arteries arise from the PCoAs and course superiorly to supply portions of the medial hypothalamus, thalamus, and lateral aspect of the third ventricle.[1]

The second major branch of C7 is the anterior choroidal artery. This arises from the posterior aspect of C7 just above the PCoA and proximal to the bifurcation of the ICA (see Fig. 18-3). Its long course is divided into three segments. The anterior choroidal artery first courses through the suprasellar cistern just medial to the uncus of the temporal lobe (cisternal segment). It then turns laterally and passes through the choroidal fissure to enter the temporal horn of the lateral ventricle. Within the ventricle, the anterior choroidal artery supplies the choroid plexus and courses posterosuperiorly with the choroid plexus up to and around the pulvinar of the thalamus. The point at which the

anterior choroidal artery enters the choroid fissure is termed the *plexal point.* The segment of the artery distal to the plexal point is termed the *plexal segment.* The plexal segment is typically associated with the vascular blush of the choroid plexus on angiography.[12] In its course, the anterior choroidal artery supplies the medial temporal lobe, the optic tract and lateral geniculate body, the dorsal globus pallidus, the inferior half of the posterior limb of the internal capsule, the lateral aspect of the cerebral peduncle, the tail of the caudate nucleus, and the choroid plexus.[28]

The circle of Willis is a vascular "ring" at the base of the brain, interconnecting segments from multiple individual vessels. When complete, it is made up of the two ICAs (C7 segments), the two precommunicating A1 segments of the ACAs, the ACoA, the two PCoAs, the two precommunicating (P1) segments of the PCAs, and the distal segment of the basilar artery (Fig. 18-6). The

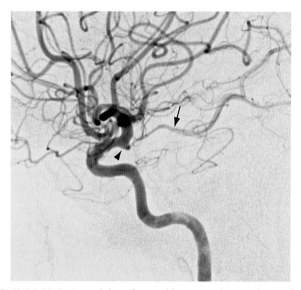

■ **FIGURE 18-5** Lateral view of a carotid artery angiogram shows a focal conical dilatation (*arrowhead*) at the origin of the posterior communicating artery (*arrow*) representing an infundibulum.

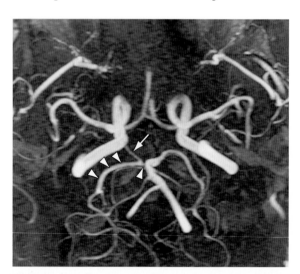

■ **FIGURE 18-4** Collapsed maximal intensity projection (MIP) of a time-resolved contrast-enhanced MR angiogram. The right posterior communicating artery (*arrow*) is shown to provide dominant blood supply to the right P2 segment of the posterior cerebral artery (*triple arrowheads*). The P1 segment is hypoplastic (*single arrowhead*).

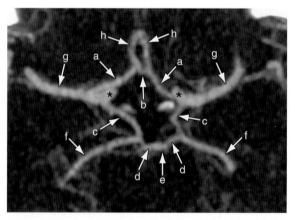

■ **FIGURE 18-6** Axial maximum intensity projection image from a CT angiogram shows a complete circle of Willis, which interconnects segments from multiple individual arteries at the base of the brain. A complete circle of Willis is formed by two internal carotid arteries (*asterisk*), the two precommunicating A1 segments of the anterior cerebral arteries (a), the anterior communicating artery (b), the two posterior communicating arteries (c), the two precommunicating (P1) segments of the posterior cerebral arteries (d), and the basilar artery (e). The posterior cerebral (f), middle cerebral (g), and anterior cerebral (h) arteries are shown.

circle of Willis is complete in approximately 70% of patients and exhibits numerous anatomic variants of variable clinical significance.

The ICA terminates at its bifurcation into the ACA and MCA, just inferior to the anterior perforated substance.

Anterior Cerebral Artery

The ACA is typically divided anatomically into three segments: the horizontal or precommunicating segment (A1), the vertical or postcommunicating segment (A2), and the more distal cortical branches (A3). The A1 segment follows an anteromedial, relatively horizontal course toward the midline interhemispheric fissure. It typically passes very close to the superior surface of the optic chiasm and/or the prechiasmal optic nerves. In the midline, A1 anastomoses with the ACoA. Distal to the ACoA, the A2 segment ascends through the cistern of the lamina terminalis and the interhemispheric fissure and gives rise to the pericallosal artery, callosomarginal artery, and distal branches (Table 18-2).

Perforating Branches

The ACA gives rise to numerous named perforating branches. Small branches from the ACoA supply the optic chiasm, infundibulum, hypothalamus, corpus callosum, septum pellucidum, and fornix.[30] The medial lenticulostriate arteries arise from the A1 segment and pass superiorly into the brain via the anterior perforated substance. The recurrent artery of Huebner arises variably from A1, ACoA, or A2 and passes laterally and superiorly to enter the anterior perforated substance.[31] As a group, the perforating branches of the ACA supply the head of the caudate nucleus, portions of the basal ganglia, and the anterior limb of the internal capsule. Additional perforating branches of the pericallosal artery supply portions of the corpus callosum.

Cortical Branches

The A2 segment gives rise to numerous cortical branches (Table 18-3). The orbitofrontal artery is the first cortical branch of the pericallosal artery. It supplies the undersurface of the frontal lobe, including the gyrus rectus, medial orbital gyrus, and olfac-

tory bulb and tract. The frontopolar artery is the next cortical branch of the pericallosal artery. It supplies the anterior portion of the medial and lateral aspects of the superior frontal gyrus. The branching pattern of the more distal ACA is highly variable, with multiple different patterns of pericallosal and callosomarginal segments. In general, the pericallosal artery courses anterior to the lamina terminalis within the interhemispheric fissure to the level of the genu of the corpus callosum and continues posteriorly within the pericallosal cistern to the splenium, where it anastomoses with the posterior pericallosal branches of the posterior circulation.[28] The pericallosal artery supplies cortical branches to the medial surface and convexities of the frontal and parietal lobes. Perforating branches arising from the pericallosal artery give blood supply to the corpus callosum, septum pellucidum, and fornix.

A callosomarginal artery is seen in approximately 50% of cerebral angiograms and passes posteriorly along the cingulate sulcus.[1] It provides numerous cortical branches to the medial surfaces of the frontal and parietal lobes with variable extension onto the superior convexities.[28]

The ACA territory is substantial and typically includes at least the anterior two thirds of the medial interhemispheric cortex, in addition to a variable distribution along the cerebral convexities (Fig. 18-7).[1,28]

The ACA shows multiple anatomic variations. The A1 segment may be absent or hypoplastic. In such cases, the contralateral ACA provides blood supply to both hemispheres via two A2 segments (Fig. 18-8). Uncommonly, the ACA may arise from the C6 (ophthalmic) segment of the ICA and pass beneath, not above, the optic nerve. This infraoptic origin of the ACA has been associated with an increased incidence of intracranial aneurysms.[32,33] The A2 segment may be hypoplastic or absent, with the single contralateral A2 supplying both A2 vascular distributions. Azygos ACA is seen in 0.2% to 3.7% of humans. The azygos portion of the ACA may run as a short or long trunk, with the short trunk bifurcating at the genu of the corpus callosum and the long trunk coursing nearly the entire extent of the corpus callosum.[34] A completely azygous ACA is a single midline vessel supplying the ACA distributions bilaterally.[35] This may be seen in association with holoprosencephaly and in association with aneurysmal dilatation of the azygous artery within a callosal lipoma.[1,28,36]

TABLE 18-2. Anterior Cerebral Artery Segments

Segment	Course
A1 (precommunicating)	From the internal carotid artery bifurcation to the anastomosis of the anterior communicating artery
A2 (postcommunicating)	From anastomosis of the anterior communicating artery to termination into cortical branches
A3 (cortical branches)	Terminal cortical branches

TABLE 18-3. Cortical Branches of the Anterior Cerebral Artery

Division	Gives Supply to:
Orbitofrontal artery	Undersurface of frontal lobe—gyrus rectus, medial orbital gyrus, and olfactory bulb and tract
Frontopolar artery	Anterior portion of the medial and lateral aspects of the superior frontal gyrus
Terminal pericallosal and callosomarginal artery branches	Variable; supply cortical branches to the medial surface and convexities of the frontal and parietal lobes

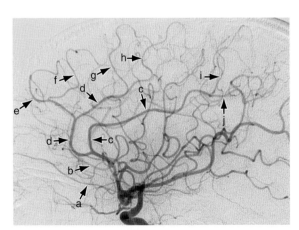

■ **FIGURE 18-7** Lateral view of a carotid artery angiogram shows branches of the anterior cerebral artery (ACA). The orbitofrontal (a), frontopolar (b), pericallosal (c), callosomarginal (d), anterior internal frontal (e), middle internal frontal (f), posterior internal frontal (g), paracentral lobule artery (h), superior internal parietal (i), and inferior internal parietal (j) branches of the ACA are seen.

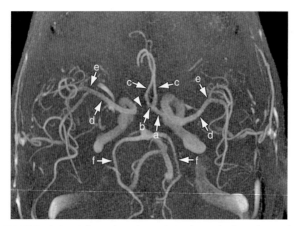

■ FIGURE 18-8 Collapsed maximum intensity projection of a 3D time-of-flight MR angiogram. The right A1 segment of the anterior cerebral artery (ACA) is absent (*arrowhead*). The left A1 segment of the ACA (a) is the only blood supply to the bilateral A2 segments (c) via an anterior communicating artery (b). Also shown are the M1 segments of the middle cerebral artery (d) and its bifurcation (e). The posterior circulation including the posterior cerebral arteries (f) is demonstrated.

TABLE 18-4. Middle Cerebral Artery Segments

Segment	Course
M1 (horizontal)	From the internal carotid artery bifurcation to the genu, where it turns superiorly within the sylvian fissure
M2 (insular)	From the genu to the superior limiting sulcus
M3 (opercular)	From the superior limiting sulcus, to egress from the lateral cerebral fissure
M4 (cortical)	Ramify over the lateral cerebral convexity as multiple cortical branches

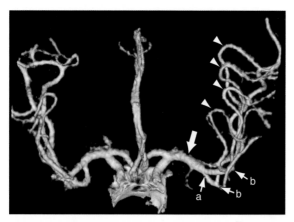

■ FIGURE 18-9 3D Volume-rendered CT angiogram of the anterior intracranial circulation shows the M1 segment (*large arrow*) of the middle cerebral artery (MCA) and its branches. After the MCA bifurcates (a), the artery forms a genu (b). The M2 segments consist of arteries from the genu to the superior aspect of the insula, where the arteries form another bend (*arrowheads*) to continue as the M3 segments along the operculum.

Middle Cerebral Artery

The MCA is the larger of the two terminal branches of the ICA and, consequently, the most frequent site of vascular complications. The MCA is typically divided into four segments, including the horizontal segment (M1), the insular segment (M2), the opercular segment (M3), and the cortical segment (M4) (Table 18-4 and Fig. 18-9).

M1

The initial M1 segment courses horizontally and laterally from the bifurcation of the ICA to the genu, where the MCA turns superiorly within the sylvian fissure. This initial course is gently convex anteriorly and superiorly. The division of the MCA into the major insular branches usually occurs within the M1 segment, so M1 includes both prebifurcation and postbifurcation portions of the MCA.[37] The point of bifurcation of the MCA typically lies greater than 10 mm from the origin of the MCA, so an MCA bifurcation that occurs less than 10 mm from the origin is called an early bifurcation.[1] The first inferiorly directed branch of M1 is the anterior temporal artery. This passes anteriorly and inferiorly over the temporal pole to supply the temporal pole and adjacent portions of the anterior and lateral aspects of the superior, middle, and inferior temporal gyri. The first superiorly directed branches of M1 are the lateral lenticulostriate arteries. These arise as a narrow group of six to nine vessels that ascend through the anterior perforating substance to supply the basal ganglia.[28,31]

M2

Distal to the genu, the three arterial trunks that arose at the M1 trifurcation course posterosuperiorly over the insula to the superior and inferior limits of the peri-insular sulcus. The point at which the most superior and medial M2 branch loops back to exit the sylvian fissure is designated the *sylvian point.*

M3

At the outer limits of the insula, the MCA branches are reflected back along the inner surfaces of the opercula as M3 segments. These course along the inner cortex of the opercula, to emerge at the lateral cerebral fissure. The inflections of the arteries where they reverse course at the top of the insula give rise to a line of vascular loops, convex superiorly, that defines the upper margin of the insula.

M4

From the lateral fissure, the *ascending* opercular (frontal and parietal) branches and the *descending* opercular (temporal) branches continue over the convexity surface of the hemisphere as the M4 cortical vessels. At its posterior superior end of the insula, where the lateral cerebral fissure becomes shallow, the last insular branch may suffer little deflection by the parietal operculum or even ascend directly onto the cortical surface. That artery is typically the angular artery.

The M4 segments include numerous named cortical branches, classified as anterior, central, and posterior groups (Table 18-5 and Fig. 18-10).[28]

The angiographic sylvian triangle is the triangular configuration of the M2 and M3 branches in relation to the insula. It is appreciated most easily on lateral projection/section arteriograms (Fig. 18-11). A triangle is defined by three points and the lines that connect them. The anterior superior point of the sylvian triangle is taken as the top of the first loop of an ascending frontal opercular artery where the vessel transitions from the M2 into the M3 segment. The posterior superior (sylvian) point of the triangle is taken as the last MCA loop on the insula. This is often a very shallow loop. The superior border of the triangle is then taken as the line drawn tangent to the superior aspects of the multiple M2 loops where they are deflected downward at the superior limiting sulcus. The anterior inferior point of the triangle is taken as the most anterior point of the anterior convexity of the M1 segment. Connecting the three points defines the borders of the sylvian triangle. The two sylvian triangles typically show the normal asymmetry associated with cerebral hemispheric dominance and petalia. Significant asymmetry or deformity of the sylvian triangle may indicate the presence of intracranial mass effect, from various causes.[1,28] Anomalies of the

MCA such as hypoplasia and aplasia, are very infrequent.[38] The M1 segment of the MCA may be "duplicated," in which case an additional large MCA vessel arises from the C7 segment of the ICA just proximal to the terminal bifurcation. This duplicated MCA courses laterally, just inferior to the true M1 segment, to supply the anterior temporal lobe.[39] Occasionally, an accessory MCA may originate from the ACA and course laterally adjacent to M1. The accessory MCA gives blood supply to the anteroinferior frontal lobe. An accessory MCA may be mistaken for a prominent recurrent artery of Heubner.[1,38,40,41]

Posterior Arterial Circulation

Vertebral Arteries

The vertebral arteries most commonly arise from the subclavian arteries but may arise directly from the aortic arch (in approximately 5% of angiograms).[36] The left vertebral artery arises directly from the aortic arch in 2.4% to 5.8% of cases.[42] The right

vertebral artery may arise anomalously from the right common carotid artery or the aortic arch in less than 1% of cases.[43] The vertebral arteries typically ascend for a short distance anterior to the cervical spine along the longus coli muscle and then enter the transverse foramen at C6 (93%). Less commonly, the vertebral arteries enter the foramen transversarium at C7 (<1%), C5 (5%), C4 (1%), or C3 (0.2%).[44] The two vertebral arteries are commonly asymmetric in size, with the larger one designated the dominant vertebral artery, most commonly the left.[1]

The course of the vertebral artery is typically divided into four segments, including the extraosseous segment (V1), the foraminal segment (V2), the extraspinal segment (V3), and the intradural segment (V4). The V1 segment courses posteriorly and superiorly from its origin and most commonly enters the C6 foramen transversarium. The V2 segment ascends within successive transverse foramina from its entry up through the transverse foramen of C1. It gives off multiple small muscular and spinal

TABLE 18-5. Cortical Branches of the Middle Cerebral Artery

Division	Gives Supply to the:
Anterior Branches	
Orbitofrontal artery	Inferior frontal lobe
Prefrontal artery	Inferior and middle frontal gyri
Central Branches	
Precentral artery	Posterior aspect of inferior and middle frontal gyri and inferior portion of precentral gyrus
Central (rolandic artery)	Precentral and postcentral gyri
Postcentral artery (anterior parietal artery)	Ascending parietal gyrus, superior portion of the central sulcus, and anterior aspect of inferior parietal lobule
Posterior Branches	
Posterior parietal artery	Inferior parietal lobule and supramarginal gyrus
Angular artery	Supramarginal gyrus and superior portion of the occipital lobe
Temporo-occipital artery	Superior temporal gyrus, lateral occipital lobe
Temporal arteries (posterior, medial)	Temporal lobe

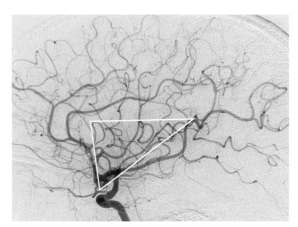

■ **FIGURE 18-11** Lateral view from a carotid artery angiogram showing the sylvian triangle. Middle cerebral arteries overlying the insular cortex are contained within the sylvian triangle. Asymmetry or deformity of the triangle may indicate an intracranial mass effect.

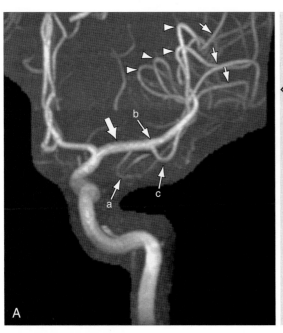

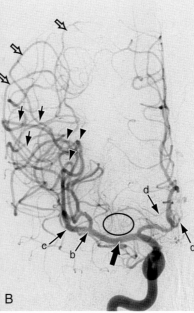

■ **FIGURE 18-10** Maximum intensity projection of a 3D time-of-flight MR angiogram (**A**) and anteroposterior image of an internal carotid artery angiogram (**B**) of the internal carotid artery and its branches. Both show the M1 segment (*large arrow*) of the middle cerebral artery (MCA). The anterior temporal artery (a) arises from the main MCA trunk usually before the bifurcation (b). The M1 segment gives rise to multiple lateral lenticulostriate arteries (*circle*). The medial lenticulostriate arteries (d) arise from the anterior cerebral artery. The M2 segment of the MCA begins at the genu (c) where the artery bends and courses superiorly within the sylvian fissure. The MCA turns again at the level of the superior limiting sulcus (*arrowheads*), continuing as the M3 segment (*small arrows*) along the operculum. Once the MCA branches exit the sylvian fissure, they turn superiorly and travel over the cortex as the M4 branches (*open arrows*).

branches as it ascends. The anterior and posterior meningeal artery branches of the vertebral artery also arise from V2. The V3 segment begins at the artery's egress from the C1 transverse foramen. The V3 segment passes posteromedially around the atlanto-occipital joints toward the midline and then courses anterosuperiorly to reach the dura at the foramen magnum. The occipital artery that is usually a branch of the external carotid artery may arise aberrantly from the V3 segment.[12] The intradural V4 segment then courses cephalically for a short distance along the clivus to unite with its counterpart to form the basilar artery at the level of the pontomedullary sulcus (Fig. 18-12).[1,45]

Branches of V4

The V4 segments give rise to multiple important branches.

Spinal Arteries

The anterior spinal arteries arise from V4 as small paired arteries that usually unite to form the top of the anterior spinal axis. The anterior spinal axis courses inferiorly in the midline along the anterior medulla and spinal cord to the tip of the conus medullaris.[45] Paired posterior spinal arteries also arise from the V4 segments of the vertebral arteries, or from the posterior inferior cerebellar arteries. The posterior spinal arteries pass to the posterior aspect of the medulla and spinal cord where they form a variably complete pair of longitudinal vessels on the posterolateral aspect of the cord.[1]

Posterior Inferior Cerebellar Artery

The PICAs most commonly arise from the V4 segments.[46] Occasionally, they originate instead from the foraminal (V2) segment of the vertebral artery or as a common AICA-PICA trunk from the basilar artery.[47] From its origin anterior to the medulla, the PICA initially courses around the medulla to reach its posterior surface. It then turns superiorly, anteriorly, and slightly medially to ascend along the posterior surface of the medulla as the retromedullary segment of the PICA. Because the tonsil lies immediately posterior to this portion of the medulla, the retromedullary segment is, simultaneously, an anterior tonsillar segment. PICA then turns posteriorly to loop over and behind the tonsil (supratonsillar and retrotonsillar segments), forming the tonsillar loop of PICA. Choroidal branches arise from the supratonsillar or retrotonsillar segments to supply the choroid plexus of the fourth ventricle.[1,48,49] Distal to the tonsillar loop, the PICA gives off the inferior vermian artery that loops under the pyramis of the vermis before ascending in the paravermian groove as the inferior vermian artery. The PICA then gives off sequential hemispheric branches to the posterior inferior surface of the cerebellum (Fig. 18-13).[45]

Basilar Artery

The basilar artery arises from the confluence of the vertebral arteries along the posterior aspect of the clivus and terminates within the interpeduncular fossa as the PCAs. The normal basilar artery often follows a tortuous, S-shaped path as it ascends within the prepontine cistern, typically with the proximal basilar artery concave toward the dominant vertebral artery.[12]

The basilar artery gives rise to numerous branches (Fig. 18-14). Pontine perforating vessels arise as median and transverse (lateral) pontine branches to supply the pons and brachium pontis. The AICAs and SCAs arise from the basilar artery to supply anterolateral portions of the brain stem and the cerebellar hemispheres. The AICAs arise from the first or second thirds of the basilar artery and course laterally across the pons and along CN VII (facial nerve) to approach or enter the internal auditory canal. They then reverse course sharply (meatal loop) and return to the brain stem along CN VIII (vestibulocochlear nerve).[50] From there the AICAs circumnavigate the flocculus (floccular loop) and extend onto the anteroinferior (petrous) surfaces of the cerebellar hemispheres (see Fig. 18-13).[1,45,49,51] The SCAs arise from the distal third of the basilar artery as one,

■ **FIGURE 18-12**   3D Volume-rendered images from a CT angiogram of the neck show the course of the vertebral artery (*depicted in red*). The V1 or extraosseous segment of the vertebral artery originates directly from the subclavian artery. The artery extends superiorly through the transverse foramina (*arrowheads*) as the V2 or foraminal segment. Once the vertebral artery exits the transverse foramina it travels posteromedially around the atlanto-occipital joint (*black arrow*) as the V3 or extraspinal segment. The artery courses superiorly and enters the foramen magnum and travels a short distance along the clivus as the V4 or intradural segment before uniting with the contralateral artery to form the basilar artery (V4 not shown).

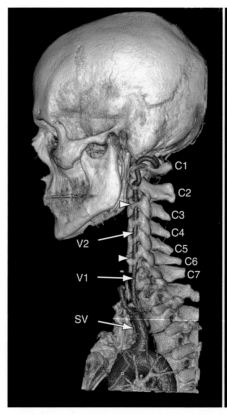
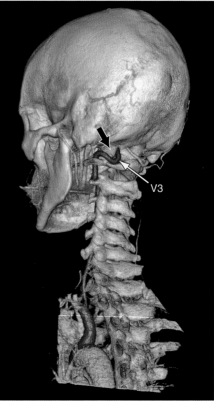

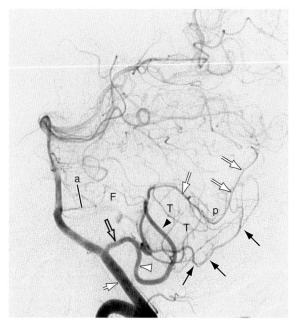

■ **FIGURE 18-13** Left vertebral artery angiogram. Lateral projection. The vertebral artery (*short black arrow*) gives rise to the posterior inferior cerebellar artery (PICA) (*open arrow*). The PICA courses around the medulla (*white arrowhead*) and then turns upward along the posterior surface of the medulla as the posterior medullary segment (*black arrowhead*). This segment gives off the inferior vermian artery (*small white arrows*) that passes over and behind the tonsil as the supratonsillar and retrotonsillar segments of the tonsillar loop (T) and then recurves under the pyramis (p) of the vermis to ascend along the posterior margin of the vermis. The retromedullary segment of PICA also gives rise to the hemispheric branches of PICA (*small black arrows*). The anterior inferior cerebellar artery (AICA) (a) arises from the basilar artery. The AICA circumnavigates the flocculus (F) as the floccular loop and extends onto the anteroinferior surface of the cerebellar hemisphere.

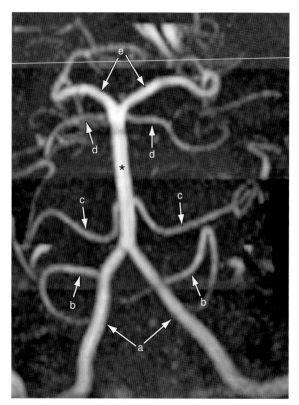

■ **FIGURE 18-14** Maximum intensity projection of a 3D time-of-flight MR angiogram of the posterior circulation. The bilateral vertebral arteries (a) join to form the basilar artery (*asterisk*). The posterior inferior cerebellar arteries (b) originate from the distal vertebral arteries. The basilar artery gives rise to the anterior inferior cerebellar arteries more proximally (c) and the superior cerebellar arteries more distally (d). The basilar artery bifurcates giving rise to the P1 segments of the posterior cerebral arteries (e).

two, or three superior cerebellar branches on one or both sides. The SCAs pass laterally around the upper pons or lower midbrain to the dorsal surface of the brain stem, giving off small branches to supply the upper pons and midbrain, including the tectum. The SCAs then enter the ambient cistern between the brain stem and cerebellum and, from there, give off sequential hemispheric branches to the superior surface of the cerebellum and vermis (Fig. 18-15). The labyrinthine arteries arise variably from the basilar artery, SCAs, or AICAs and course within the internal acoustic meatus.[50] The cerebellar circulation is highly interconnected, with multiple vascular anastomoses among the PICAs, AICAs, and SCAs.

Posterior Cerebral Arteries

The PCAs arise at the bifurcation of the basilar artery within the interpeduncular cistern and course posterolaterally around the brain stem, just superior to the tentorium. The course of the PCA is divided into four segments, including the precommunicating/mesencephalic segment (P1), the ambient segment (P2), the quadrigeminal segment (P3), and the calcarine segment (P4) (Table 18-6). The P1 segment arises from the bifurcation of the basilar artery within the interpeduncular cistern and courses posterolaterally along the anterior surface of the brain stem, terminating at the junction of the PCA with the PCoA.[1,45] The posterior thalamoperforating arteries arise from P1 and the terminal portion of the basilar artery. They ascend through the interpeduncular fossa, enter the posterior perforated substance, and continue through the midbrain to the posterior inferior thalamus. In their course, they supply the midbrain, posterior inferior thalamus, and posterior internal capsule.[45,52,53] The P2 segment begins just distal to the PCoA and extends along the ambient cistern to the posterior surface of the midbrain. P2 gives off branches to supply the brain stem, the ventricle, the choroid plexus, and the cerebral cortex. The thalamogeniculate arteries most commonly arise from the P2 segment to supply portions of the thalamus (including the pulvinar and lateral geniculate nucleus) and portions of the subthalamus. Peduncular perforating arteries arising from P2 supply portions of the midbrain. The medial posterior choroidal artery passes around the brain stem and through the cistern of the velum interpositum to supply the choroid plexus along the roof of the third ventricle. It then courses through the foramen of Monro to supply the choroid plexus of the ipsilateral lateral ventricle.[54] The lateral posterior choroidal branches enter the choroid fissure near their origins from the PCA and display two branches. The anterior branch gives supply to the choroid plexus of the anterior temporal horn. The posterior branch passes over the thalamus and along the floor of the lateral ventricle, terminating within the choroid plexus of the trigone and tela choroidea. The branches of the posterior chorioidal arteries anastomose with the anterior choroidal artery.[45] The anterior temporal artery arises from P2 to supply the anteroinferior aspect of the temporal lobe. It anastomoses with corresponding anterior temporal branches of the MCA. The posterior temporal artery arises from P2 to supply the posteroinferior temporal lobe and the anterior occipital lobe.[55]

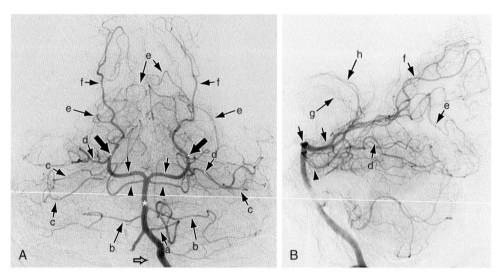

■ **FIGURE 18-15**   Anteroposterior (**A**) and lateral (**B**) projections from a left vertebral artery (posterior circulation) angiogram. The angiogram shows the posterior inferior cerebellar artery (a) arising from the distal left vertebral artery. The basilar artery (*asterisk*) gives rise to multiple branches that supply the brain stem and two larger arteries that supply the cerebellum: the anterior inferior cerebellar arteries (b), and the superior cerebellar arteries (*arrowheads*). The hemispheric branches of the SCAs are shown (c) on the anteroposterior projection. The basilar artery bifurcates into the P1 segments (*small arrows*) of the posterior cerebral arteries. The P1 segment extends from the level of the basilar artery bifurcation to the posterior communicating artery anastomosis (not seen here). The P2 segments (*large arrows*) of the posterior cerebral arteries arise distal to the posterior communicating artery anastomosis and extend to the posterior midbrain. This segment gives rise to the posterior temporal arteries (c), which supply the posteroinferior temporal lobes and anterior occipital lobes. The medial (g) and lateral (h) posterior choroidal arteries are best seen on the lateral view and supply portions of the ventricles and choroid plexus. Terminal branches of the PCAs include the calcarine arteries (e) and parieto-occipital arteries (f). The anterior spinal artery (*open arrow* in **A**) is also seen arising from the distal vertebral arteries.

TABLE 18-6.   Posterior Cerebral Artery Segments

Segment	Course
P1 (precommunicating/ mesencephalic)	From the basilar artery bifurcation to the junction with the posterior communicating artery
P2 (ambient)	Begins just distal to the posterior communicating artery and extends along the ambient cistern to the posterior surface of the midbrain
P3 (quadrigeminal)	Short portion of the posterior cerebral artery between the quadrigeminal plate and the calcarine fissure
P4 (calcarine)	Terminal division of the posterior cerebral artery into major cortical branches

The P3 segment is a short portion of the PCA between the quadrigeminal plate and the calcarine fissure.[45] The thalamogeniculate arteries may arise from the P3 segment of the PCA in 20% of cases.[1]

The PCA terminates by dividing into two major cortical branches (P4), at or just proximal to the level of the calcarine fissure. The medial occipital artery gives rise to the parieto-occipital and calcarine arteries. The parieto-occipital artery travels within the parieto-occipital sulcus to supply the medial parietal and occipital lobes. Posterior pericallosal branches of the parieto-occipital artery course posterosuperiorly around the splenium of the corpus callosum to anastomose with the pericallosal artery of the ACA.[45,55] The calcarine artery travels within the calcarine fissure to supply the occipital lobe, particularly the visual cortex. The lateral occipital artery gives rise to multiple temporal branches that supply the inferior aspect of the temporal lobe (see Fig. 18-15).[56] The proximal PCA segments are best appreciated on anteroposterior view of submentovertex angiographic projections. The more distal segments and their branches are best appreciated on lateral angiographic projections. A "fetal

origin" of the PCA is noted in approximately 20% of cases and is associated with hypoplasia of the P1 segment (see Fig. 18-4).[57]

Variability of the Intracranial Circulation

The circle of Willis maintains collateral blood flow within the intracranial circulation through connections between the anterior (carotid) and posterior (vertebrobasilar) circulations and through connections between the circulations of the left and right sides. Variations in the anatomy of the circle of Willis are common. A complete circle of Willis is seen in less than 50% of the population. The most common variation is hypoplasia or aplasia of the PCoA, unilaterally or bilaterally. Other common variations include hypoplasia of the A1 segment of the ACA, a fetal origin of the PCA with hypoplasia of the P1 segment, and absence of the AComm artery.[58] The frequencies of these variations in multiple studies of large populations are summarized in the bar graph in Figure 18-16.

In addition to the variability of the circle of Willis, the territory and volume of brain supplied by the major ACA, MCA, and PCA branches also vary widely within and between individuals.[59-63] One ACA may supply portions of the contralateral cerebral hemisphere in 12% to 25% of brains.[61-63] The area of supply to the contralateral hemisphere is usually small, but in 4% to 7% of brains there is a major contralateral supply.[61-63] Postmortem study of the territory irrigated by the ACA, MCA, and PCA in 25 brains showed that each of the brains had asymmetric vascular supply; none showed symmetric arterial supply to the two hemispheres.[59,60] The ACA could supply 18% to 35% of any one hemisphere; the MCA 34% to 64% of the same hemisphere, and the PCA 9% to 40% of that hemisphere.[59,60] Furthermore, the range of variation among the 25 brains was so large, that no dominant or modal pattern of supply could be discerned for any of the vessels or sides.[59,60] However, the *relative* volumes of brain irrigated by the ACA, MCA, and PCA in an individual could be determined by comparing the diameters of the A1, M1, and P1 segments of their vessels.[59,60] The differences in the diameters of these arteries is thought to reflect variations in the intracranial

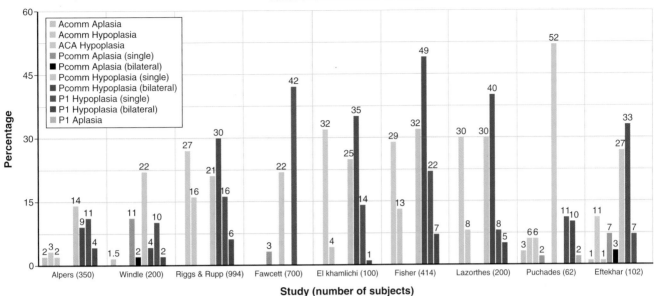

■ **FIGURE 18-16** Variability in circle of Willis from multiple studies. Numbers cited are percentages. *(Data from Eftekhar B, Dadmehr M, Ansari S, et al. Are the distributions of variations of circle of Willis different in different populations? Results of an anatomical study and review of literature. BMC Neurol 2006; 6:22.)*

hemodynamics.[59,60] This variability correlates with the differing patterns of infarct volumes involving the ACA, PCA, ACA-PCA, and triple ACA-PCA-MCA territories.[64,65]

Anterior-Posterior Circulation Communications

Persistent primitive carotid-basilar anastomoses arise when primitive embryonic carotid-hindbrain connections fail to involute. These primitive anastomoses include the persistent trigeminal artery, persistent hypoglossal artery, persistent otic artery, and proatlantal intersegmental artery. These persistent primitive communications are uncommon to rare. The PCoAs are the only common persistent carotid-basilar anastomoses.

The persistent trigeminal artery is the most common of the primitive carotid-basilar anastomoses. When present, it arises from the cavernous (C4) portion of the ICA and courses either lateral to or directly through the dorsum sellae to anastomose with the basilar artery. It supplies the distal basilar artery territory, including the PCAs. Because the more proximal segment of the basilar artery then supplies only the brain stem and cerebellum, the caliber of the proximal basilar artery may appear very reduced. In these patients, the PCoA shows variable hypoplasia/aplasia. The persistent trigeminal artery is associated with an increased incidence of intracranial aneurysms (Fig. 18-17).[66]

A persistent hypoglossal artery is the next most common persistent carotid-basilar anastomosis. This arterial communication typically arises from the cervical ICA at approximately the C1 or C2 level and courses posteriorly via a prominent hypoglossal canal to anastomose with the basilar artery. The ipsilateral vertebral artery is typically hypoplastic. Both PCoAs may also be aplastic.[67-69]

A proatlantal intersegmental artery is an additional persistent carotid-basilar anastomosis, typically arising from the cervical ICA at the C2-3 level. It runs superiorly to the level of the occipitoatlantal space, enters the foramen magnum, and gives rise to the ipsilateral vertebral artery.[70,71]

Meningeal Arteries

The meningohypophysial branch of the ICA (synonym: posterior trunk) provides vascular supply to the tentorium via the marginal tentorial artery.[1] The ophthalmic branch of the ICA gives rise to the anterior ethmoidal artery that, in turn, gives rise to the anterior falcine artery (anterior meningeal artery). This supplies the anterior falx and a portion of the dural convexity.[28]

The anterior and posterior meningeal branches of the vertebral artery arise from the V2 segment. The anterior meningeal artery characteristically arises at the C2 level and courses anterosuperiorly to supply the dura overlying the anterior lip of the foramen magnum and the adjacent lower clivus. The posterior meningeal artery characteristically arises at the C1 level, between the posterior arch of C1 and the foramen magnum. It courses posteriorly and superiorly through the foramen magnum to supply the falx cerebelli, the posterior portion of the falx cerebri (via a medial branch), and medial portions of the convexity dura adjoining the falx (via a lateral branch).[45]

Intracranial Venous System

The intracranial venous circulation can be divided into superficial and deep systems. These two systems have numerous interconnections and are not independent entities.

Supratentorial Veins

Superficial Venous System

The superficial venous system is quite variable with the superficial middle cerebral vein (SMCV) and superior and inferior anastomotic channels (veins of Trolard and Labbé, respectively) seen most commonly.[1] The SMCV overlies the lateral cerebral fissure and drains regions of the operculum. The SMCV may be single or duplicated. It may drain into the cavernous sinus, sphenoparietal sinus, or pterygoid venous plexus.[72] The superior anastomotic vein of Trolard (also called the frontoparietal vein) runs posteriorly and superiorly from the sylvian fissure to the superior sagittal sinus. It serves as an anastomosis between the SMCV and the sagittal sinus (Fig. 18-18). The inferior anastomotic vein of Labbé (also referred to as the occipitotemporal vein) courses posteriorly over the occipitotemporal sulcus to interconnect the superficial middle cerebral vein with the transverse sinus (Fig. 18-19).[1] The superficial venous system is best appreciated on the venous phase of lateral angiographic projections. The inferior and superior anastomotic veins often demonstrate an inverse

■ **FIGURE 18-17** Anteroposterior (**A**) and lateral (**B**) views from a carotid artery angiogram and anteroposterior (**C**) and superior (**D**) views from a maximum intensity projection of a 3D time-of-flight MR angiogram. An abnormal connection (*long arrow*) is noted between the cavernous (C4) segment of the internal carotid artery (*short arrows*) and the basilar artery (*arrowheads*). This connection represents a persistent trigeminal artery.

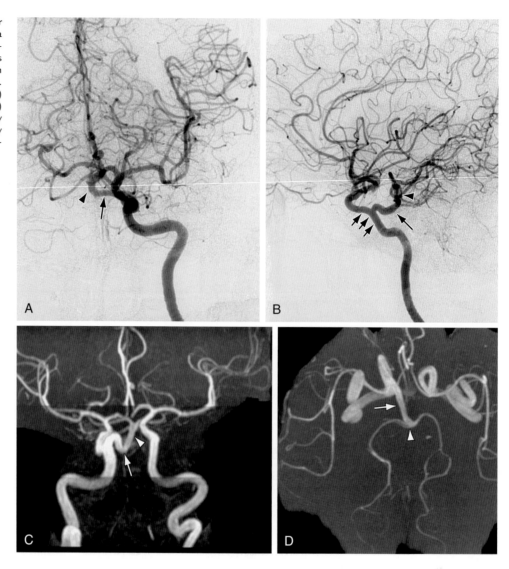

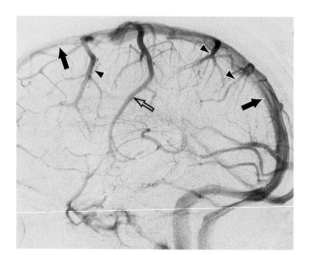

■ **FIGURE 18-18** Lateral view of the venous phase of an internal carotid artery angiogram. The superior anastomotic vein of Trolard (*open arrow*) is seen. It anastomoses the superficial middle cerebral vein to the superior sagittal sinus (*large arrows*). Some cortical veins (*arrowheads*) are seen to drain directly into the superior sagittal sinus.

relationship in size, depending on which is dominant in particular individuals.[1]

Deep Venous System
The deep cerebral white matter and basal ganglia are variably drained by the deep cerebral veins. Compared with the superficial system, the deep cerebral veins are far more constant in their distribution and patterns of drainage. The medullary veins arise in the subcortical white matter, drain medially toward the ventricles, and coalesce to form the subependymal veins at the walls of the lateral ventricles.[73] The septal veins initially course within the frontal horns of the lateral ventricles and subsequently run medially along the septum pellucidum, ultimately joining the thalamostriate veins to form the internal cerebral veins. They may extend farther posteriorly to merge with the internal cerebral veins directly or even pass directly to the vein of Galen. The internal cerebral veins arise by the union of the septal with the thalamostriate veins just posterior to the foramen of Monro. They course posteriorly through the cistern of the velum interpositum, just above the roof of the third ventricle, to the quadrigeminal plate cistern, where they usually coalesce with the basal veins of Rosenthal to form the vein of Galen.[74] The vein of

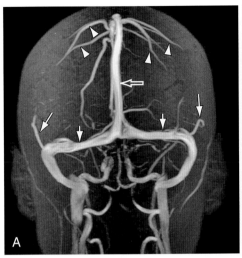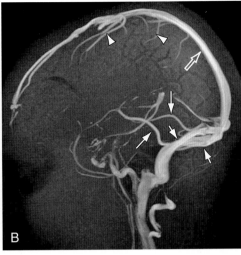

■ **FIGURE 18-19** Phase-contrast MR venogram maximum intensity projection in the anteroposterior (**A**) and lateral (**B**) projections demonstrate the superficial intracranial venous system. Multiple cortical veins (*arrowheads*) drain directly into the superior sagittal sinus (*open arrows*). The inferior anastomotic vein of Labbé (*long arrows*) anastomoses the superficial middle cerebral vein to the transverse sinus (*short arrows*).

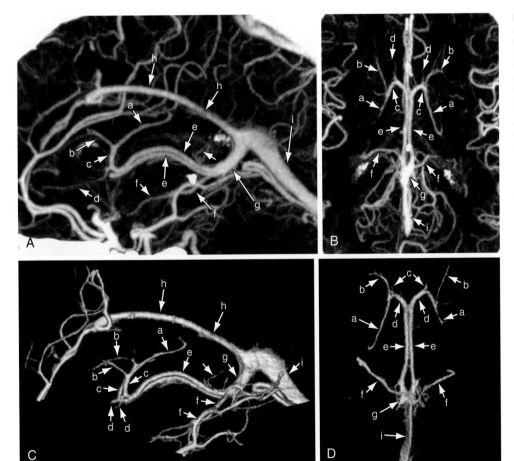

■ **FIGURE 18-20** Sagittal (**A**) and axial (**B**) maximum intensity projection and lateral (**C**) and superior (**D**) 3D volume-rendered images from a CT angiogram show the veins of the deep venous system. The terminal veins (a) and anterior caudate veins (b) drain into the thalamostriate veins (c), which join the septal veins (d) to form the internal cerebral veins (e). These veins run along the roof of the third ventricle and travel posteriorly, receiving venous drainage from the thalamus and lateral ventricles. Medial atrial veins draining the lateral ventricles are shown (*unlabeled white arrow* in **A** and **C**). The internal cerebral veins terminate at the quadrigeminal plate cistern by coalescing with the basal vein of Rosenthal (f) to form the vein of Galen (g). The vein of Galen passes superiorly and posteriorly to join the inferior sagittal sinus (h in **A** and **C**) to form the straight sinus (i). The straight sinus drains directly into the torcular Herophili (sinus confluence) in most cases (not shown).

Galen (also referred to as the great cerebral vein) passes posteriorly and superiorly behind the splenium of the corpus callosum and joins the anterior end of the inferior sagittal sinus to form the straight sinus (Fig. 18-20).

Infratentorial Veins
The infratentorial veins are made up of multiple groups including the superior (galenic) draining group and the inferior and anterior groups. The superior (Galenic) draining group is made

up of multiple veins, the most noteworthy of which include the precentral cerebellar vein, superior vermian vein, and anterior pontomesencephalic vein. The most important of the inferior group are the inferior vermian veins. The anterior group includes the petrosal veins. The infratentorial veins primarily drain posterior fossa structures, including the brain stem and cerebellum.

ANALYSIS
Sample reports are presented in Boxes 18-1 to 18-3.

BOX 18-1 Sample Report: CT Angiography of the Head

PATIENT HISTORY

A 30-year-old woman presented with aphasia and right arm weakness.

TECHNIQUE

CT angiography of the head was performed during bolus intravenous infusion of 50 mL Isovue 370. Study was coordinated using CT fluoroscopy trigger. Angiography was then performed with thin-section overlapping images. Data were interpreted through source images, maximal intensity projection reformatted images, and surface renderings.

FINDINGS

There is no evidence of significant aneurysmal dilatation in either the anterior or posterior circulation. The visualized ICAs are patent. The bilateral ACAs and MCAs are patent as are their visualized distal branches. The visualized bilateral vertebral arteries, basilar artery, and PCAs and their branches are patent. No significant stenosis or occlusion is identified.

Grossly, the visualized brain parenchyma is normal in configuration. No significant mass effect or midline shift is seen. The ventricles are normal in size.

Bone windows demonstrate no evidence of fracture or focal lytic or blastic lesion.

IMPRESSION

Unremarkable CTA of the head.

BOX 18-2 Sample Report: MR Angiography of the Head

PATIENT HISTORY

A 37-year-old man presented with weakness and lethargy.

COMPARISON STUDIES

There were no prior studies available for comparison.

TECHNIQUE

MR angiography was performed using a 3D time-of-flight sequence (see Fig. 18-17, C and D). Source images and maximal intensity projection reconstructions projected over the circle of Willis were reviewed.

FINDINGS

There is normal symmetric flow-related enhancement of the ICAs, MCAs, and ACAs. There is no evidence of aneurysm, vascular malformation, or flow-limiting stenosis.

There is an abnormal arterial connection between the right cavernous portion of the ICA and the distal portion of the basilar artery. The vertebral arteries are not seen on this study. There is no evidence of aneurysm associated with this abnormal connection.

There is normal flow-related enhancement in the distal basilar artery and both PCAs. There is no evidence of aneurysm, vascular malformation, or flow-limiting stenosis.

Evaluation of the parenchyma demonstrates no gross abnormality.

IMPRESSION

Findings are compatible with a persistent trigeminal artery on the right. There is no evidence of aneurysm and no evidence of a vascular malformation or flow-limiting stenosis.

BOX 18-3 Sample Report: Cerebral Angiogram

PATIENT HISTORY

A 50-year-old man presented to the emergency department with a severe headache. The patient underwent CT examination of the head, which revealed a subarachnoid hemorrhage. A diagnostic cerebral angiogram was requested. The patient had no additional past medical history.

Informed consent was obtained after explaining the risks and benefits of the procedure.

TECHNIQUE AND FINDINGS

The patient was transferred to the angiography suite where he was sedated using fentanyl and midazolam (Versed).

The bilateral groins were sterilely prepped and draped in the usual fashion. A 19-gauge single wall puncture needle was used to enter into the right femoral artery. The Seldinger technique was then used to pass a No. 5 French sheath into the right femoral artery. This was then attached to a continuous flush drip.

A No. 5 French Terumo angled glide catheter was first used to catheterize the right common carotid artery. Anteroposterior and lateral angiograms of the cervical region and cervical carotid artery were then obtained. These angiograms show that there is no evidence of stenosis of the common carotid artery bifurcation or within the cervical segments of the ICA. The external carotid artery branches in the cervical region are unremarkable.

The catheter was then advanced under fluoroscopic guidance into the right ICA. Anteroposterior lateral and oblique angiograms of the cerebral right ICA were then obtained. These angiograms show that the distal cervical, petrous, cavernous, and supraclinoid portions of the ICA are unremarkable without any evidence of stenosis, aneurysms, or vascular malformations. The ACAs and MCAs are unremarkable without any evidence of aneurysms or vascular malformations or stenoses. The venous phases of the angiogram show that the dural venous sinuses and the deep venous system are patent.

The catheter was then withdrawn under fluoroscopic guidance and advanced into the right external carotid artery. Anteroposterior and lateral angiograms of the right external carotid artery show that the external carotid artery branches are unremarkable.

At this point the catheter was withdrawn and then passed into the right subclavian artery. Under fluoroscopic guidance the catheter was then advanced into the origin of the right vertebral artery. Anteroposterior and lateral angiograms of the right vertebral artery were then obtained. These angiograms show that the right vertebral artery fills normally into the intracranial space without any evidence of stenosis, aneurysms, or vascular malformations. The origin of the right PICA is visualized, and there is no evidence of aneurysm at that location. The basilar apex is unremarkable without any evidence of aneurysm. The PCAs and SCAs are unremarkable. The venous phases of the angiogram are unremarkable.

At this point the catheter was withdrawn and then passed into the left common carotid artery. Anteroposterior and lateral angiograms of the cervical region were then obtained. These angiograms show that there is no evidence of stenosis of the common carotid artery bifurcation or within the cervical segments of the ICA. The external carotid artery branches in the cervical region are unremarkable.

The catheter was then advanced into the left ICA. Anteroposterior, lateral, and oblique angiograms of the left ICA of the cerebral circulation were then obtained. These angiograms show that the distal cervical, cavernous, petrous, and supraclinoid portions of the ICA are unremarkable without any evidence of aneurysms, vascular malformations, or stenoses. The ACAs and MCAs are normal without any evidence of aneurysms, vascular malformations, or stenoses. The venous phases of the angiogram showed the dural venous sinuses and the deep venous system are patent.

The catheter was then withdrawn and then passed into the left external carotid artery. Anteroposterior and lateral angiograms of the left external carotid artery show that these vessels are unremarkable.

The catheter was then withdrawn and then passed into the left vertebral artery. Anteroposterior and lateral angiograms of the posterior circulation were then obtained. These angiograms show that the left vertebral artery is normal without any evidence of stenosis. There are no aneurysms or vascular malformations seen within the posterior fossa. The distal basilar artery and its branches were normal. The venous phases of the angiogram were unremarkable.

At this point the Terumo angled glide catheter was removed. An anteroposterior image of the femoral sheath was obtained confirming that the puncture site was on the common femoral artery. Therefore, the puncture site was closed using a closure device.

The patient was then transferred to the recovery room. There were no complications during the procedure.

IMPRESSION

The cerebral angiogram is normal. There is no evidence of an intracranial aneurysm, vascular malformation, or intracranial stenosis.

REFERENCES

1. Osborn AG. Diagnostic Cerebral Angiography, 2nd ed. St. Louis, Mosby, 1999.
2. Mavroudis C, Backer CL. Pediatric Cardiac Surgery, 3rd ed. Philadelphia, Mosby, 2003.
3. Larsen WJ. Human embryology, 2nd ed. New York, Churchill Livingstone, 1997.
4. Gerlis LM, Dickinson DF, Wilson N, Gibbs JL. Persistent fifth aortic arch: a report of two new cases and a review of the literature. Int J Cardiol 1987; 16:185.
5. Truwit CL. Embryology of the cerebral vasculature. Neuroimaging Clin North Am 1994; 4:663-689.
6. Okahara M, Kiyosue H, Mori H, et al. Anatomic variations of the cerebral arteries and their embryology: a pictorial review. Eur Radiol 2002; 12:2548-2561.
7. Padget D. The development of the cranial arteries in the human embryo. Contrib Embryol 1948; 32:205-261.
8. Bisaria KK. Anomalies of the posterior communicating artery and their potential clinical significance. J Neurosurg 1984; 60:572-576.
9. Siclari F, Burger IM, Fasel JH, Gailloud P. Developmental anatomy of the distal vertebral artery in relationship to variants of the posterior and lateral spinal arterial systems. AJNR Am J Neuroradiol 2007; 28:1185-1190.
10. Caldemeyer KS, Carrico JB, Mathews VP. The radiology and embryology of anomalous arteries of the head and neck. AJR Am J Roentgenol 1998; 170:197-203.
11. Keir E. Development of cerebral vessels. In Newton TH, Potts DG (eds). Radiology of the Skull and Brain. St. Louis, Mosby, 1974, pp 1089-1141.
12. Newton TH, Potts DG. Radiology of the Skull and Brain. St. Louis, Mosby, 1974.
13. Bouthillier A, van Loveren HR, Keller JT. Segments of the internal carotid artery: a new classification. Neurosurgery 1996; 38:425-432; discussion 432-433.
14. Kerber CW, Heilman CB. Flow dynamics in the human carotid artery: I. Preliminary observations using a transparent elastic model. AJNR Am J Neuroradiol 1992; 13:173-180.
15. Paullus WS, Pait TG, Rhoton AI. Microsurgical exposure of the petrous portion of the carotid artery. J Neurosurg 1977; 47:713-726.
16. Osborn AG. The vidian artery: normal and pathologic anatomy. Radiology 1980; 136:373-378.
17. Sekhar LN, Schramm VL Jr, Jones NF, et al. Operative exposure and management of the petrous and upper cervical internal carotid artery. Neurosurgery 1986; 19:967-982.
18. Quisling RG. Intrapetrous carotid artery branches: pathological application. Radiology 1980;134:109-113.
19. Lo WW, Solti-Bohman LG, McElveen JT Jr. Aberrant carotid artery: radiologic diagnosis with emphasis on high-resolution computed tomography. RadioGraphics 1985; 5:985-993.
20. Glasscock ME 3rd, Seshul M, Seshul MB Sr. Bilateral aberrant internal carotid artery case presentation. Arch Otolaryngol Head Neck Surg 1993; 119:335-339.
21. Pahor AL, Hussain SS. Persistent stapedial artery. J Laryngol Otol 1992; 106:254-257.
22. Petrus LV, Lo WW. The anterior epitympanic recess: CT anatomy and pathology. AJNR Am J Neuroradiol 1997;18:1109-1114.
23. Fujii K, Chambers SM, Rhoton AL. Neurovascular relationships of the sphenoid sinus: a microsurgical study. J Neurosurg 1979; 50:31-39.
24. Tran-Dinh H. Cavernous branches of the internal carotid artery: anatomy and nomenclature. Neurosurgery 1987; 20:205-210.
25. Krisht A, Barnett DW, Barrow DL, Bonner G. The blood supply of the intracavernous cranial nerves: an anatomic study. Neurosurgery 1994; 34:275-279.
26. Yamaki T, Tanabe S, Hashi K. Prominent development of the inferolateral trunk of the internal carotid artery as a collateral pathway to the external carotid system. AJNR Am J Neuroradiol 1989; 10:206.
27. Lang J, Kageyama I. The ophthalmic artery and its branches, measurements and clinical importance. Surg Radiol Anat 1990; 12:83-90.
28. Takahashi M, Atlas of Carotid Angiography. Tokyo, Igaku Shoin, 1977.
29. Marshman LA, Ward PJ, Walter PH, Dossetor RS. The progression of an infundibulum to aneurysm formation and rupture: case report and literature review. Neurosurgery 1998; 43:1445-1448.
30. Ghika JA, Bogousslavsky J, Regli F. Deep perforators from the carotid system: template of the vascular territories. Arch Neurol 1990; 47:1097-1100.
31. Marinkovic S, Gibo H, Milisavljevic M. The surgical anatomy of the relationships between the perforating and the leptomeningeal arteries. Neurosurgery 1996; 39:72-83.
32. Mercier P, Velut S, Fournier D, et al. A rare embryologic variation: carotid-anterior cerebral artery anastomosis or infraoptic course of the anterior cerebral artery. Surg Radiol Anat 1989; 11:73-77.
33. Odake G. Carotid-anterior cerebral artery anastomosis with aneurysm: case report and review of the literature. Neurosurgery 1988; 23:654-658.
34. Vasovic LP. Fetal azygos pericallosal artery. Clin Anat 2006; 19:327-331.
35. Cinnamon J, et al. Aneurysm of the azygos pericallosal artery: diagnosis by MR imaging and MR angiography. AJNR Am J Neuroradiol 1992; 13:280-282.
36. Wolpert SM, Carter BL, Ferris EJ. Lipomas of the corpus callosum: an angiographic analysis. Am J Roentgenol Radium Ther Nucl Med 1972; 115:92-99.
37. Gibo H, Carver CC, Rhoton AL Jr, et al. Microsurgical anatomy of the middle cerebral artery. J Neurosurg 1981; 54:151-169.
38. Han DH, Gwak HS, Chung CK. Aneurysm at the origin of accessory middle cerebral artery associated with middle cerebral artery aplasia: case report. Surg Neurol 1994; 42:388-391.
39. Komiyama M, et al. Middle cerebral artery variations: duplicated and accessory arteries. AJNR Am J Neuroradiol 1998; 19:45-49.
40. Takahashi S, Hoshino F, Uemura K, et al. Accessory middle cerebral artery: is it a variant form of the recurrent artery of Heubner? AJNR Am J Neuroradiol 1989; 10:563-568.
41. Takahashi T, Suzuki S, Ohkuma H, Iwabuchi T. Aneurysm at a duplication of the middle cerebral artery. AJNR Am J Neuroradiol 1994; 15:1166-1168.
42. Adachi B. Das Arteriensystem der Japaner. Kyoto and Tokyo, Kaiserlich-Japanische Universitat zu Kyoto, 1928.
43. Maisel H. Some anomalies of the origin of the left vertebral artery. S Afr Med J 1958;32:1141-1142.
44. Bruneau M, Cornelius JF, Marneffe V, et al. Anatomical variations of the V2 segment of the vertebral artery. Neurosurgery 2006; 59(1 Suppl 1):ONS20-ONS24; discussion ONS20-ONS24.
45. Takahashi M. Atlas of Vertebral Angiography. Tokyo, Bunkyo-ku, 1974.
46. Friedman DP. Abnormalities of the posterior inferior cerebellar artery: MR imaging findings. AJR Am J Roentgenol 1993; 160:1257-1263.
47. Salas E, Ziyal IM, Bank WO, et al. Extradural origin of the posteroinferior cerebellar artery: an anatomic study with histological and radiographic correlation. Neurosurgery 1998; 42:1326-1331.
48. Kumar AJ, Naidich TP, George AE, et al. The choroidal artery to the fourth ventricle and its radiological significance. Radiology 1978; 126:431-439.
49. Naidich TP, Kricheff II, George AE, Lin JP. The normal anterior inferior cerebellar artery: anatomic-radiographic correlation with emphasis on the lateral projection. Radiology 1976; 119:355-373.
50. Brunsteins DB, Ferreri AJ. Microsurgical anatomy of VII and VIII cranial nerves and related arteries in the cerebellopontine angle. Surg Radiol Anat 1990; 12:259-265.
51. Martin RG, Grant JL, Peace D, et al. Microsurgical relationships of the anterior inferior cerebellar artery and the facial-vestibulocochlear nerve complex. Neurosurgery 1980; 6:483-507.
52. Barkhof F, Valk J. "Top of the basilar" syndrome: a comparison of clinical and MR findings. Neuroradiology 1988; 30:293-298.
53. George AE, Raybaud C, Salamon G, Kricheff II. Anatomy of the thalamoperforating arteries with special emphasis on arteriography of the third ventricle: I. Am J Roentgenol Radium Ther Nucl Med 1975; 124:220-230.
54. Zeal AA, Rhoton AL. Microsurgical anatomy of the posterior cerebral artery. J Neurosurg 1978; 48:534-559.

55. Margolis MT, Newton TH, Hoyt WF. Cortical branches of the posterior cerebral artery: anatomic-radiologic correlation. Neuroradiology 1971; 2:127-135.

56. Gloger S, Gloger A, Vogt H, Kretschmann HJ. Computer-assisted 3D reconstruction of the terminal branches of the cerebral arteries: II. Middle cerebral artery. Neuroradiology 1994; 36:181-187.

57. Saeki N, Rhoton AL. Microsurgical anatomy of the upper basilar artery and the posterior circle of Willis. J Neurosurg 1977; 46: 563-578.

58. Eftekhar B, Dadmehr M, Ansari S, et al. Are the distributions of variations of circle of Willis different in different populations? Results of an anatomical study and review of literature. BMC Neurol 2006; 6:22.

59. van der Zwan A, Hillen B. Review of the variability of the territories of the major cerebral arteries. Stroke 1991; 22: 1078-1084.

60. van der Zwan A, Hillen B, Tulleken CA, Dujovny M. A quantitative investigation of the variability of the major cerebral arterial territories. Stroke 1993; 24:1951-1959.

61. Baptista AG. Studies on the arteries of the brain: II. The anterior cerebral artery: some anatomic features and their clinical implications. Neurology 1963; 13:825-835.

62. Moniz E. Die Cerebral Arteriographie und Phlebographie. Berlin, SpringerVerlag, 1949.

63. Perlmutter D, Rhoton AL Jr. Microsurgical anatomy of the distal anterior cerebral artery. J Neurosurg 1978; 49:204-228.

64. Naidich TP, Brightbill TC. Vascular territories and watersheds: a zonal frequency analysis of the gyral and sulcal extent of cerebral infarcts: I. The anatomic template. Neuroradiology 2003; 45: 536-540.

65. Naidich TP, Firestone MI, Blum JT, Abrams KJ. Zonal frequency analysis of the gyral and sulcal extent of cerebral infarcts: III: Middle cerebral artery and watershed infarcts. Neuroradiology 2003; 45:785-792.

66. O'Uchi E, O'Uchi T. Persistent primitive trigeminal arteries (PTA) and its variant (PTAV): analysis of 103 cases detected in 16,415 cases of MRA over 3 years. Neuroradiology 2010; 52:1111-1119.

67. Brismar J. Persistent hypoglossal artery, diagnostic criteria: report of a case. Acta Radiol Diagn (Stockh) 1976; 17:160-166.

68. Terayama R, Toyokuni Y, Nakagawa S, et al. Persistent hypoglossal artery with hypoplasia of the vertebral and posterior communicating arteries. Anat Sci Int 2011; 86:58-61.

69. Wardwell GA, Goree JA, Jimenez JP. The hypoglossal artery and hypoglossal canal. Am J Roentgenol Radium Ther Nucl Med 1973; 118:528-533.

70. Bahsi YZ, Uysal H, Peker S, Yurdakul M. Persistent primitive proatlantal intersegmental artery (proatlantal artery I) results in 'top of the basilar' syndrome. Stroke 1993; 24:2114-2117.

71. Vasović L, Mojsilović M, Andelković Z, et al. Proatlantal intersegmental artery: a review of normal and pathological features. Childs Nerv Syst 2009; 25:411-421.

72. Galligioni F, Bernardi R, Pellone M, Iraci G. The superficial sylvian vein in normal and pathologic cerebral angiography. Am J Roentgenol Radium Ther Nucl Med 1969; 107:565-578.

73. Friedman DP. Abnormalities of the deep medullary white matter veins: MR imaging findings. AJR Am J Roentgenol 1997; 168: 1103-1108.

74. Ture U, Yasargil MG, Al-Mefty O. The transcallosal-transforaminal approach to the third ventricle with regard to the venous variations in this region. J Neurosurg 1997; 87:706-715.

Intracranial Hemorrhage

Robert D. Zimmerman and Austin D. Jou

Intracranial hemorrhage is defined as a pathologic distribution of hemorrhage within the calvaria. It is subdivided into extra-axial and intra-axial/intracerebral hemorrhage. Extra-axial hemorrhage includes blood in the epidural, subdural, and subarachnoid spaces. Intra-axial/intracerebral hemorrhage includes blood in the intraparenchymal and intraventricular spaces.

The focus of this chapter is on nontraumatic causes of intracranial hemorrhage. Traumatic causes of hemorrhage are discussed separately elsewhere in this text.

EPIDEMIOLOGY

Subarachnoid Hemorrhage

The worldwide incidence of nontraumatic subarachnoid hemorrhage (SAH) is estimated to be about 6 cases per 100,000 patient-years.[1] SAH is seen predominantly in patients younger than 60 years of age. The principal causes of spontaneous SAH are ruptured aneurysms (85%), benign nonaneurysmal perimesencephalic (pretruncal) hemorrhage (10%), and rare causes (5%). Gender, race, and geographic region affect the incidence of SAH. Women have a 1.6 times greater risk of developing SAH than men. Black individuals have a 2.1 times greater risk than whites. The highest incidences of SAH occur in Japan (23 cases per 100,000 patient-years) and Finland (22 cases per 100,000 patient-years). The most important *nonmodifiable* risk factor for developing SAH is having a first-degree relative with SAH (increase in relative risk 6.6). Important *modifiable* risk factors are heavy alcohol consumption (relative risk 4.7), hypertension (relative risk 2.8), and smoking (relative risk 1.9).[1]

Intraparenchymal Hemorrhage

Intracranial hemorrhage is believed to occur in 10% to 30% of all strokes and is predominantly intraparenchymal in such cases. The exact incidence may be higher or lower, with more recent sources reporting a much lower incidence.[2] Hypertension is the most common cause underlying most nontraumatic intracerebral hemorrhage (50%-60%). Hemorrhages associated with hyperten-

sion increase in frequency with age. Cerebral amyloid angiopathy (CAA) is the second most common cause of nontraumatic intraparenchymal hemorrhage and is responsible for 10% to 12% of all hemorrhagic strokes. As with hypertensive hemorrhage, the incidence of CAA-related hemorrhage increases with age. It is rarely encountered in patients younger than 70 years of age. Parenchymal hemorrhage may occur as a result of venous thrombosis, underlying neoplasm, vascular lesion, and inflammatory lesion. Hemorrhagic neoplasms include high-grade gliomas, vascular metastases, and extra-axial masses such as pituitary adenomas and (rarely) meningiomas. Underlying vascular lesions include arteriovenous malformations (AVMs), cavernous malformations, and, less commonly, telangiectatic AVMs, developmental venous anomalies (DVAs), and dural arteriovenous fistulas (DAVFs). Hemorrhagic inflammatory lesions include herpes simplex virus type 1 and angioinvasive fungal infections such as aspergillosis and mucormycosis.

CLINICAL PRESENTATION

Given the myriad locations in which intracranial hemorrhage can occur and the diversity of potential causes of hemorrhage, the associated clinical presentations are varied. No single criterion is specific for intracranial hemorrhage. Instead, diagnosis depends on the presence of appropriate signs and symptoms, the pertinent patient history (hypertension, prior hemorrhage, drug use, anticoagulation, trauma) and appropriate diagnostic imaging.

Classically, nontraumatic SAH presents as an acute severe "thunderclap" headache, which patients may characterize as "the worst headache of their life." Although only 1 in 10 patients presenting with thunderclap headache actually has SAH, headache remains the most common presenting complaint for SAH. It may be the sole presenting symptom in 25% to 33% of patients with SAH. The remainder of patients with acute severe headaches may suffer instead from symptoms of migraine or tension headache, viral meningitis, and so on. SAH also causes meningeal irritation that mimics meningitis, with meningismus, photophobia, prominent neck or upper back pain, seizures, and obtundation. Because the symptoms and signs of SAH are nonspecific, SAH is misdiagnosed clinically in 12% to 51% of cases.[3] Failure to detect acute aneurysmal SAH has serious consequences, because (1) the rate of recurrent SAH from an untreated ruptured aneurysm is 50% in the first year and (2) recurrent hemorrhage predicts a poorer outcome.

Spontaneous parenchymal hemorrhage also presents as signs and symptoms that depend on the location and extent of the hemorrhage. Common presenting symptoms include nausea and vomiting, headache, seizure activity, altered mentation, and/or focal neurologic deficits referable to the affected region. When the volume of hemorrhage is large, clinical sequelae often reflect the local mass effect, any associated herniation (transfalcine, transtentorial, and tonsillar), hydrocephalus, diffuse intraventricular extension, and/or diffuse increase in intracranial pressure. These symptoms include asymmetric pupil dilatation, increased systemic blood pressure, respiratory depression, and decorticate/decerebrate posturing.

Isolated nontraumatic subdural hemorrhage is rare (but may be seen with bleeding diatheses, aneurysmal SAH, venous sinus thrombosis, osseous metastases, and intracranial hypotension). When present, nontraumatic subdural hemorrhage may cause nonspecific clinical findings such as headache, altered mentation, nausea or vomiting, lethargy, dysarthria, and ataxia. Focal neurologic deficits are not common. Large subdural hemorrhages can cause pupillary abnormalities such as ipsilateral pupillary dilatation and the inability to react to light. Chronic subdural hemorrhage is often more insidious in its clinical presentation. Generalized weakness, ataxia, global cognitive decline, memory dysfunction, and headache can be present in varying severity. In the setting of a chronically debilitated or elderly patient, these nondescript symptoms may be overlooked, especially if they are subacute in onset.

PATHOPHYSIOLOGY

The vast majority of nontraumatic SAH results from rupture of cerebral aneurysms. Most aneurysms are now believed to arise from degenerative injury to the vessel wall that accumulates over time as a result of hemodynamic stress, perhaps with congenital predisposition. Aneurysms are rarely encountered in children and young adults and when present have a different distribution and configuration than the typical "berry aneurysm" of older patients. The formation of aneurysms at characteristic locations is the result of the turbulent flow common to these locations rather than the result of any inherited defects in the arterial walls. Congenital aneurysms do arise in association with specific genetic conditions such as polycystic kidney disease and connective tissue disorders (e.g., Marfan's syndrome) but are uncommon. Infective aneurysms arise secondary to septic emboli, most often in the setting of bacterial endocarditis. Aneurysms may rarely result from vasculopathies such as fibromuscular dysplasia and inflammatory arteritis. Atherosclerosis may lead to aneurysmal enlargement of the involved vessel, most often the vertebral basilar arteries. Aneurysms and their causes are discussed elsewhere in this text.

Nontraumatic, nonaneurysmal causes for SAH include arteriovenous malformations (AVM), infectious arteriopathies, and extension of intraparenchymal hemorrhage into the subarachnoid space. When SAH occurs in isolation anterior to the midbrain, the most likely cause is perimesencephalic (pretruncal)

nonaneurysmal SAH. This entity most likely results from rupture of posterior fossa veins and occurs most commonly after sexual intercourse. It is regarded as benign, because recurrent hemorrhage is rare and the usual complications of SAH such as hydrocephalus and vasospasm are uncommon and/or mild.[4]

Intraparenchymal hemorrhage is most often the sequel of chronic systemic hypertension. Chronic arterial hypertension is believed to induce changes in small fragile vessels arising from the major proximal intracranial arteries. Fisher showed that chronic arterial hypertension causes histologic disorganization of the walls of small vessels and termed that pathology *lipohyalinosis*.[5] Since then, lipohyalinosis has been understood to be either fibrinoid change or collagenous fibrosis, depending on which element predominates.[6] Lipohyalinosis diminishes the integrity of the vessel wall, predisposes the patient to rupture of penetrating arterioles within the brain, and leads to hemorrhagic stroke. Hypertensive hemorrhage may also result from Charcot-Bouchard aneurysms, although these are less common than initially suspected. Hypertensive hemorrhages most commonly involve the basal ganglia and thalami of the deep supratentorial gray matter, the pons and midbrain of the brain stem, and the cerebellum. In common, all of these regions are supplied by small perforating arteries that arise from proximal intracranial arteries (e.g., proximal middle cerebral arteries and the basilar artery) and are therefore the sites most exposed to the deleterious effects of chronic systemic hypertension.

Cerebral amyloid angiopathy (CAA) is the second most important cause of intraparenchymal hemorrhage. It is clinically distinct from systemic amyloidosis and is caused by progressive deposition of β-amyloid protein in the media and adventitia of small to medium-sized vessels, resulting in the formation of twisted β-pleated sheet fibrils in the vessel walls.[7] Histologic examination demonstrates staining with Congo red and deposition of crystals that appear birefringent under polarizing light microscopy. The abnormal protein weakens the structure of the vessel wall, causing fibrinoid necrosis, microaneurysms, and increased likelihood of hemorrhage. Recently, additional factors, such as the presence of apolipoprotein E4, have been shown to hasten the development of intraparenchymal hemorrhage in patients with CAA.[8,9]

CAA is most frequently seen in the subcortical vessels, so the resultant hemorrhages typically occur in or adjacent to the cortex, not within the deep gray matter, brain stem, and cerebellum, which are more commonly affected by hypertensive hemorrhage. CAA is also characterized by recurrent hemorrhages in the same location and multiple small focal asymptomatic hemorrhages (microbleeds) in other cortical regions. Recurrent hemorrhage leads to complex hematomas with acute and subacute elements and vasogenic edema that together may mimic the appearance of neoplastic hemorrhage on gross inspection and imaging.

Intraparenchymal hemorrhage can also result from reperfusion injury with acute hemorrhagic transformation of previously bland embolic arterial infarctions. After a clot occludes a vessel to cause infarction, naturally occurring fibrinolytic enzymes or thrombolytic therapy with tissue plasminogen activator (tPA) can cause lysis of the clot and restoration of blood flow to the damaged endothelial bed. The details underlying reperfusion damage have yet to be completely elucidated. However, a combination of oxidative radicals and metalloproteinases produced during reperfusion, and the thrombolytic agents themselves, can damage the endothelial cells, injure the basal lamina, and thereby open the blood-brain barrier, destroying the integrity of the cerebrovascular system.[10,11] Increased vascular permeability then allows red blood cells to migrate into the surrounding extravascular space. Embolic infarctions typically undergo subacute mild hemorrhagic conversion. Revascularization of infarcted regions begins at 3 to 5 days after occlusion. Ingrowth of new immature vessels leads to extravasation of small amounts of blood into the infarcted brain.

Other causes of parenchymal hemorrhage include venous thrombosis and hemorrhage secondary to underlying vascular, neoplastic, or rarely inflammatory lesions. Hemorrhage associated with AVMs is typically parenchymal. Intraventricular, subarachnoid, and subdural hemorrhage also occur in conjunction with AVMs, but isolated hemorrhages in these locations are uncommon. Other vascular anomalies including cavernous malformations, DVAs, and DAVFs may present as parenchymal hemorrhage that partially or completely (rare) obscures the underlying malformation, at least temporarily.

High-grade gliomas are the most common hemorrhagic neoplasm. Small amounts of hemorrhage are present in virtually all grade IV astrocytomas. Extensive hemorrhage into a necrotic glioma may partially obscure the underlying mass. The most commonly encountered hemorrhagic metastases are melanoma (a common lesion that often bleeds), lung and breast carcinomas (extremely common lesions that bleed occasionally), renal and thyroid carcinomas (uncommon lesions that frequently bleed), and choriocarcinoma (rare lesion that bleeds in most cases). Hemorrhagic metastases are typically small solid masses that are perched on the margin of a large parenchymal hematoma.

Herpes simplex virus type 1 encephalitis is a hemorrhagic infective process, but the hemorrhage is typically microscopic and may not be detectable on CT or MRI. Angioinvasive fungi and tuberculosis may also produce hemorrhagic masses in the brain, particularly in immunocompromised individuals.

The common causes for intraparenchymal hemorrhage are summarized in Table 19-1. Other less common causes of intraparenchymal hemorrhage include congenital bleeding diatheses (e.g., hemophilia, protein C and S deficiencies, von Willebrand factor deficiency), acquired coagulopathies (e.g., disseminated intravascular coagulopathy), and vasculitides.

Lastly, intraventricular hemorrhage (IVH) most often results from direct intraventricular extension of primary subarachnoid or intraparenchymal hemorrhage. Isolated IVH is rare. The most likely cause is hypertensive hemorrhage adjacent to the ventricle with spontaneous evacuation of the hemorrhage into the ventricle. Vascular malformations and/or aneurysms of the choroid plexus may lead to isolated IVH.

IMAGING

CT

CT is often the first diagnostic modality employed to assess intracranial hemorrhage. The CT appearance of hemorrhage is largely determined by the degree of attenuation of radiation by the globin fraction of the hemoglobin molecule, not the iron bound by the hemoglobin. The concentration of hemoglobin has a linear relationship with the degree of attenuation. Therefore, factors such as severe anemia that affect the integrity of the hemoglobin molecule or the concentration of hemoglobin alter the appearance of hemorrhage on CT. In general, acute intracerebral hemorrhage appears hyperdense in all patients with hemoglobin concentrations greater than 9 g/dL.

Acute hemorrhage can measure anywhere from 55 to 80 Hounsfield units (HU), higher than both normal gray matter (30-40 HU) and normal white matter (20-30 HU). In the clinical setting of severe anemia, acute hemorrhage can have a considerably lower attenuation and appear isodense to the brain. Although red blood cells begin to lose their integrity within hours of extravasation, complete cell lysis does not occur until later during the subacute stage of hemorrhage. In the first 12 hours after acute hemorrhage, the density of the blood often increases, because the hemoglobin becomes concentrated through clot formation and retraction. During the hyperacute period, the small amount of acellular serum expressed from the retracting clot forms a thin hypodense layer at the periphery of the hematoma (Fig. 19-1). Over the next 3 to 5 days, the brain surrounding the hemorrhage shows increasing lucency as proteases derived from the red cells induce vasogenic and cytotoxic edema and as an inflammatory response to the blood products disrupts the blood-brain barrier.

During the following weeks, the blood clot decreases in density as the red blood cells lyse and hemoglobin is removed. The cellular debris, including breakdown products of hemoglobin, is absorbed by macrophages and further degraded. Typically, the progressive decrease in attenuation starts at the periphery of the blood clot and then moves centrally. This appearance has been likened to a "melting ice cube" (Fig. 19-2). Eventually the hematoma may become isodense or hypodense, even though blood products persist. In such cases, MRI is often a useful way to display residual hemorrhage. Complete resolution of an uncomplicated hematoma usually occurs within weeks to months (depending on hematoma size). Clot resolution often leaves little evidence of the preceding parenchymal clot except for a narrow cleft-like scar with mildly hyperdense margins (hemosiderin cleft).

Contrast-enhanced CT (CECT) is not routinely used for uncomplicated acute hemorrhage. However, in cases in which an underlying malignancy, vascular malformation, or aneurysm is suspected, CECT can provide valuable data on an underlying etiology. Early enhancement within the center of a hematoma is a sign of active, ongoing hemorrhage, often correlates with later increase in clot size, and implies a likelihood of poor outcome. Irregular peripheral nodular enhancement or rim enhancement at the time of presentation may indicate the presence of an underlying neoplasm. Relatively smooth-walled marginal (rim)

TABLE 19-1. Common Causes of Nontraumatic Intraparenchymal Hemorrhage

Hypertension
Infarction
   Arterial infarction with hemorrhagic transformation
   Venous infarction
Cerebral amyloid angiopathy
Vascular malformations
   Arteriovenous malformations
   Developmental venous anomaly
   Cavernous angioma ("cavernoma")
Neoplastic hemorrhage
   High-grade gliomas
   Metastases (e.g., melanoma, lung, breast, renal, thyroid, choriocarcinoma)
Drugs
   Amphetamines
   Cocaine
Medication-related bleeding diatheses
   Warfarin
   Heparin

■ **FIGURE 19-1** Acute hemorrhage evident on CT images as a thin hypodense rim corresponding to acellular serum.

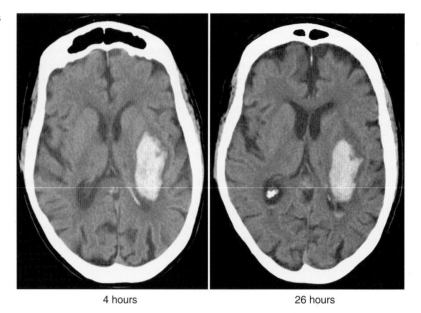

4 hours   26 hours

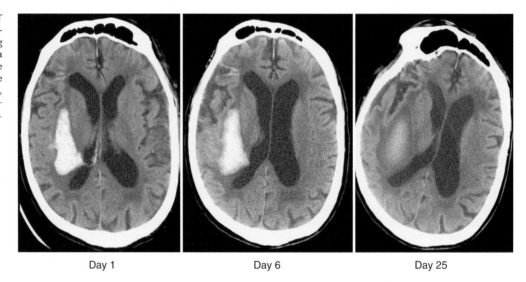

■ **FIGURE 19-2** Serial CT imaging of intraparenchymal hemorrhage illustrating the "melting ice cube" effect, as a hematoma becomes progressively more hypodense, starting from the periphery. *(From Yousem DM, Zimmerman RD, Grossman RI: Neuroradiology, 3rd ed. The Requisites. Philadelphia: Mosby, 2010.)*

Day 1   Day 6   Day 25

enhancement may be seen as early as 4 days after hemorrhage and is commonly observed during the subacute period (7-14 days). It results from (1) breakdown of the blood-brain barrier at the margin of the hematoma due to local compression and ischemia of the surrounding tissue and (2) inflammation induced by blood products. Ingrowth of new vessels leads to contrast enhancement that may persist for several weeks. Over time, the radius of enhancement gradually contracts toward the center of the hematoma.[12] Hemorrhage secondary to cerebral amyloid angiopathy may demonstrate irregular enhancement during the acute phase (under 3 days) mimicking the appearance of neoplastic hemorrhage. This results from reaction to a pre-existent subclinical subacute hemorrhage at the site of the acute hemorrhage.

Recent studies have documented decreased perfusion surrounding acute intraparenchymal hematomas. The prognostic significance and clinical utility of this information has yet to be determined.

Determination of the cause of the hematoma is very important, often more important than detecting the hemorrhage itself.

Table 19-2 summarizes common patterns of nontraumatic intracranial hemorrhage.

SAH produces hyperdensity within the cisterns at the base of the brain, the fissures, and the superficial sulci overlying more superior portions of the brain. Typically, SAH remains in liquid form, so it takes on the contour of the affected cerebrospinal fluid (CSF) spaces without causing mass effect. Clot usually does not form because CSF contains anticlotting factors and mechanically dilutes the hemorrhage. However, particularly brisk bleeding may form a subarachnoid hematoma with local mass effect. Sensitivity of CT for detecting aneurysmal SAH is 95% for the first 48 hours and decreases to less than 50% by day 5 as the blood is diluted and "washed away" by the CSF (to be reabsorbed within the pacchionian granulations). Isodense SAH may be seen when patients with SAH present in delayed fashion, more than 48 hours after onset of symptoms, or when the initial hemorrhage is small ("sentinel" bleed). In these circumstances correct diagnosis may be difficult. Key imaging findings include nonvisualization of normal CSF spaces around the brain (suprasellar cistern, cistern of the lamina terminalis, interhemispheric fissure

TABLE 19-2. Major Patterns of Non-traumatic Intracranial Hemorrhage

Type of Hemorrhage	Pattern of Distribution
Subarachnoid hemorrhage (aneurysmal)	Basilar cisterns, as well as in the region of the insula (particularly important in cases of aneurysmal hemorrhage)
	Convexities, often conforming to sulci
	Can be associated with intraventricular hemorrhage (mostly in cases of trauma)
Perimesencephalic or pretruncal subarachnoid hemorrhage (nonaneurysmal)	Isolated SAH anterior to the brainstem
Hypertensive hemorrhage	Deep cerebrum (putamen and thalamus)—majority (60%)
	Cerebral hemispheres (20%)
	Cerebellum and pons
Cerebral amyloid angiopathy (CAA)	Often lobar hemorrhages that are peripherally located
	Deep cerebral involvement is atypical, distinguishing CAA from hypertensive hemorrhage
Hemorrhagic transformation of an arterial infarct	Most typically unilateral and along a single vascular distribution
Hemorrhagic parenchymal venous infarction	Bilateral hemorrhages in a nonarterial vascular distribution
	Commonly found in the parasagittal regions when the superior sagittal sinus is thrombosed

and sylvian fissure) on good-quality thin-section CT scans (section thickness ≤5 mm). Unusually prominent visualization of the temporal horns and a mildly prominent anterior third ventricle are also suggestive of isodense SAH. The mild hydrocephalus and the absence of normal CSF density in the adjacent cisterns make the CSF within the temporal horns and third ventricle "jump out" on the images. It is useful to carefully evaluate the occipital horns of the lateral ventricles for small amounts of hemorrhage, which can accumulate in the dependent portions of the ventricles, because SAH washing into the ventricles and layering in the dependent occipital horns can confirm the diagnosis of subtle SAH. When the clinical suspicion of SAH is strong, a normal CT scan is not adequate evidence to exclude a diagnosis of SAH. Spinal tap and/or fluid attenuated inversion recovery (FLAIR) MR may be used to further search for SAH.

Subdural and epidural hematomas are most often the result of trauma and are discussed in greater detail elsewhere in this text. In brief, subdural hematomas are typically diffuse crescent-shaped lesions but may show loculation when repeat hemorrhage leads to acute-on-chronic subdural hemorrhage. Epidural hematomas are typically focal lentiform hematomas that are nearly always associated with skull fractures and subcutaneous hematomas. If an epidural hematoma occurs in the absence of documented trauma or fracture, an underlying epidural hemorrhagic mass is likely to be present.

MRI

MRI is superior to CT for evaluating most acute neurologic disorders, particularly acute infarction. Because hemorrhage is a frequent concern and complicating factor in the setting of acute infarction, radiologists need to understand the complex imaging appearances of hemorrhage and the biochemical and physical bases of these MR features.

Structure and Oxidation States of Hemoglobin

The signal intensity of hemorrhage on each pulse sequence is determined by multiple factors, especially the structure and oxi-

dation states of hemoglobin. The most common form of hemoglobin in the adult human is hemoglobin A. This is a tetramer composed of four covalently bound globular protein subunits: two α and two β subunits. Each protein subunit is associated with a nonprotein heme group containing a porphyrin ring and a charged iron ion. The iron ion in the heme group can exist in either the ferrous (Fe^{2+}) or ferric (Fe^{3+}) state. However, only the ferrous state can bind oxygen.

In the systemic circulation, hemoglobin usually exists in the *ferrous* state as either oxyhemoglobin or deoxyhemoglobin. When oxygen is bound to the hemoglobin, the iron ion is *diamagnetic*, that is, it possesses no unpaired electrons. In oxyhemoglobin, four electrons are bound in the same plane with four nitrogens at the center of the porphyrin ring. A fifth electron is bound to the imidazole ring of the F8 histidine below the porphyrin ring, and a sixth electron is reversibly bound to the oxygen. In deoxyhemoglobin, no oxygen is bound to the hemoglobin. When no oxygen is bound to the hemoglobin, the iron ion is paramagnetic. Absence of the oxygen induces a change in the conformation of the hemoglobin. This change leads to unpairing of the four electrons on the heme iron, making the heme iron ion *paramagnetic*.

Oxidation of deoxyhemoglobin forms methemoglobin. Methemoglobin possesses a heme group in the ferric (Fe^{3+}) state that cannot bind oxygen. Within the vascular system, the relatively high oxygen tension and reactivation of the hemoglobin by the enzyme NADH methemoglobin reductase prevents the formation of methemoglobin. When blood extravasates into the extravascular space, however, the mechanisms to reactivate methemoglobin are rendered inactive, so methemoglobin accumulates progressively. In methemoglobin, the ferric from of the heme group has five unpaired electrons, making it *paramagnetic*.

Chronic hemorrhage is characterized by lysis of the red blood cells, movement of the hemoglobin products into the extracellular space, and continued oxidative denaturation of the methemoglobin. This degradation initially creates low-spin breakdown products of methemoglobin known as ferric hemichromes.[15] The ferric hemichromes are *diamagnetic*. The diamagnetic ferric hemichromes are later absorbed by macrophages and further broken down into hemosiderin and ferritin, which are *superparamagnetic*.

Paramagnetic Effects of Hemorrhage

The structure and oxidation states of hemoglobin produce paramagnetic effects that cause T1 and T2 shortening. All paramagnetic substances have unpaired spins (protons, electrons, and even neutrons). Because of these unpaired spins paramagnetic molecules have the property of becoming magnetic when placed in an external magnetic field. Paramagnetic substances like deoxyhemoglobin and methemoglobin possess unpaired electrons and become magnetized in the magnetic field. Two properties of paramagnetic compounds affect hematoma intensity: (1) dipole-dipole interactions that shorten T1 and (2) susceptibility effects that shorten T2.

Dipole-Dipole Interactions (T1 Shortening)

The dipole-dipole effect is the result of the interaction between the magnetic field generated around unpaired electrons and the unpaired hydrogen protons. Because the electric field generated around the electrons is highly localized, it can occur only when the unpaired electrons and the water protons approach within

3 Å of each other. Under these conditions, T1 recovery of the water protons is facilitated and T1 shortening occurs. This is the same mechanism that underlies the action of gadolinium-based MR contrast agents. Among the heme proteins only methemoglobin significantly shortens the T1 relaxation time in an aqueous solution. This difference results from the different configurations of the methemoglobin molecule and the deoxyhemoglobin molecule that permit dipole-dipole interactions to occur, or not, respectively. Oxyhemoglobin and the low-spin derivatives of methemoglobin also do not significantly shorten T1 because they are diamagnetic.

Susceptibility Effects (T2* Shortening)

The susceptibility effect of paramagnetic substances is caused by the disturbances that they generate in the local magnetic field. Each paramagnetic molecule generates a local internal magnetic field when placed in the external magnetic field of the MR scanner. If the paramagnetic molecules are homogeneously distributed, the field will be homogeneous and proton dephasing within the sample will not be affected. That is, on balance all protons will experience the same magnetic field strength during the duration of the MR sequence acquisition. If the paramagnetic molecules are heterogeneously distributed, however, the internal magnetic field will also be heterogeneous, so individual water protons are subject to marked variation in the magnetic field they "experience" during the MR acquisition. This heterogeneity causes variations in their precessional rates, which lead to rapid signal decay that is independent of the "true" T2 of the sample (T2* effect, susceptibility effect). Heterogeneous distribution of paramagnetic heme proteins occurs when the hemoglobin is sequestered within intact red cells. Thus, the marked T2 hypointensity seen in acute and early subacute hemorrhage occurs as a result of the presence of deoxyhemoglobin or methemoglobin within intact red cells. When the red cell lyse, the paramagnetic substances within them become homogeneously distributed, so the susceptibility effects are eliminated. The signal of the hematoma then depends on the "true T2," not the T2*. The magnitude of T2* effects increases with field strength. T2* effects are small at extremely low field strengths (<0.3 T). At higher field strengths (>1.0 T) nonparamagnetic sources of T2 shortening may contribute more to the signal intensity. At the field strengths used in most current clinical MR scanners (>0.7 T), small differences in the base magnetic field strength (b_0) cause no appreciable T2* differences in the appearance of hematomas. Because gradient-recalled-echo (GRE) and echoplanar (EPI) sequences are most sensitive to susceptibility effects, these sequences display small hemorrhages particularly well.

Nonparamagnetic Effects on Hematoma Intensity

Although the paramagnetic effects on T1 and T2 relaxation dominate hematoma intensity, other factors also affect the signal of blood. The globin molecules exert an effect on T1 relaxation independent of the paramagnetic effects of the heme iron. The free or unbound water found in CSF has an extremely long T1 relaxation time owing to its high precessional frequency relative to the Larmor frequency. For that reason CSF appears hypointense on T1-weighted (T1W) images. The addition of a protein such as hemoglobin causes water molecules to bind to the charged side groups of the protein to form a hydration layer.[13] This slows the free precession of the water molecules, allows their rotational frequency to approximate the Larmor frequency more closely, and thereby shortens the T1 relaxation time. To a lesser degree, water bound in fluids with a high protein concentration also shows shortening of T2 relaxation times. As the hematoma ages, clot formation and retraction initially decrease the amount of free water within a hematoma, causing true T2 shortening. As the hematoma evolves further, the water content within the hematoma increases, prolonging the T2 relaxation time.

Evolution of an Intraparenchymal Hematoma

Stages of Hemorrhage

The evolution of an intraparenchymal hematoma can be divided into five stages: hyperacute, acute, early subacute, late subacute, and chronic. Each stage features unique MR signal intensities (Table 19-3). It is important to bear in mind that although the evolution of an intraparenchymal hematoma is presented as an orderly progression, these stages are often superimposed, because differing portions of the clot proceed through each stage at different times.

Hyperacute (<6 hours) (Fig. 19-3)

The appearance of hyperacute hemorrhage is similar to that of normal intravascular blood. Blood is a proteinaceous, cellular high-water-content fluid. The proteins shorten the T1 relaxation time relative to CSF, and the high water content prolongs the T2 relaxation time. These signal intensities are not normally encountered in vivo, because the signal intensities of flowing intravascular blood are dominated by flow effects. In situations of slow flow (e.g., giant aneurysms) these intensities may be appreciated. Hyperacute hemorrhage is composed of intact red blood cells and high protein fluid (serum). Oxyhemoglobin predominates, resulting in a clot that is isointense to mildly hyperintense with respect to the surrounding brain parenchyma on

TABLE 19-3. Evolution of Intraparenchymal Hemorrhage on Magnetic Resonance

Stage	Time Course	Hemoglobin Type	Oxidation State and Location	Intensity of Hemorrhage Relative to Normal Brain Parenchyma		
				T1WI	T2WI	GRE
Hyperacute	<6 hours	Oxyhemoglobin	Intracellular	iso/↓	↑	↓
Acute	6-72 hours	Deoxyhemoglobin	Intracellular	iso/↓	↓↓	↓↓
Early Subacute	3-10 days	Methemoglobin	Intracellular	↑↑	↓↓	↓/↓↓ centrally ↓↓ peripherally
Late Subacute	1 week-months	Methemoglobin	Extracellular	↑↑	↑↑ centrally ↓ peripherally	Iso/↑ centrally ↓↓ peripherally
Chronic	Months-years	Hemosiderin and ferritin	Mostly intracellular within the macrophages	↓/↓↓	↓↓	↓

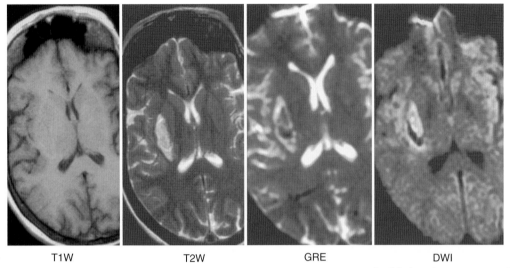

■ **FIGURE 19-3** Hyperacute hemorrhage. The hemorrhage is isointense on T1W MR sequences and mildly hyperintense on T2W images. Gradient-recalled echo and echoplanar DWI images are centrally hyperintense with curvilinear hypointensity posteriorly.

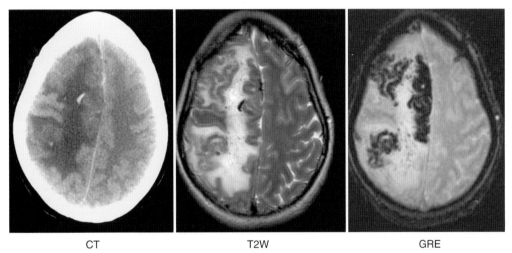

■ **FIGURE 19-4** Hyperacute hemorrhage and gradient-recalled-echo sequences. Profound cortical hypointensity is seen on the gradient-recalled-echo image, indicating a much greater burden of hyperacute hemorrhage than would be suspected on the accompanying CT and T2W images. Although hypointensity is present on T2W images, these signal abnormalities are the result of hemorrhage that has already progressed to the acute stage. The hyperacute cortical hemorrhage is much less conspicuous.

T1W imaging. On T2-weighted (T2W) imaging the hematoma is hyperintense, reflecting the high water content and lack of T2 shortening by the diamagnetic oxyhemoglobin. The imaging features of hyperacute hemorrhage are therefore relatively nonspecific. *The key finding is the presence of hypointensity on GRE sequences (and other "susceptibility weighted" sequences such as echoplanar imaging) because such hypointensity is not seen in other focal brain lesions. As the result of early formation of deoxyhemoglobin at the margin of the hematoma and bulk susceptibility effects between the hematoma and the adjacent brain, GRE sequences are more sensitive than other MR sequences or CT for detecting hyperacute and acute hemorrhage* (Fig. 19-4).

Acute (6-72 hours) (Fig. 19-5)
During the acute stage, red blood cells are intact but isolated from the vascular supply. With decreasing oxygen tension and

accumulation of metabolic wastes, the oxygen dissociates from the hemoglobin, leaving deoxyhemoglobin. Although deoxyhemoglobin is paramagnetic, the structure of the molecule prevents water molecules from associating closely with the unpaired electrons of the iron ion. This separation impedes T1 shortening due to dipole-dipole effects. Acute hematomas are typically mildly hypointense on T1W images owing to the effects of T2 shortening. On T2W images they show pronounced hypointensity, beginning at the periphery of the clot. The T2 shortening results from many factors, especially the susceptibility effect of intracellular deoxyhemoglobin. Local field inhomogeneity generated by intracellular deoxyhemoglobin leads to rapid dephasing of water molecules. Each molecule of water diffuses in and around the red cell so each experiences a markedly different and unique magnetic field. Clot formation and retraction further decreases water content within the hematoma, contributing to T2 shortening, particularly at lower field strengths.[14]

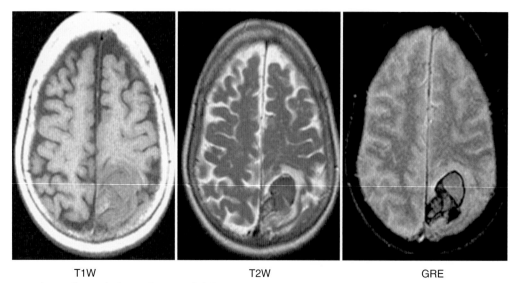

T1W   T2W   GRE

■ **FIGURE 19-5** Acute hemorrhage. The hemorrhage is mildly hypointense on T1W sequences and hypointense on T2W sequences. A rim of susceptibility effect is already present on the gradient-recalled-echo sequence.

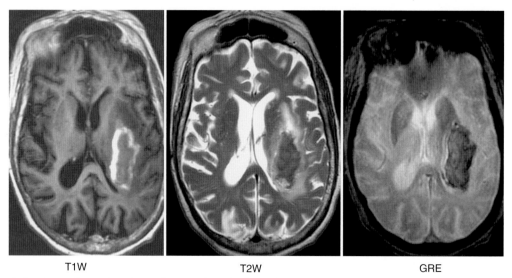

T1W   T2W   GRE

■ **FIGURE 19-6** Early subacute hemorrhage in a patient at 4 days. The hemorrhage is hyperintense beginning at the periphery on T1W sequences and initially hypointense on T2W sequences.

Early Subacute (3-7 days) (Fig. 19-6)

In the early subacute phase, the red blood cells typically remain intact. Intracellular deoxyhemoglobin is converted to methemoglobin, causing marked shortening of the T1 relaxation times via the dipole-dipole interactions between hemoglobin and water molecules. The clot appears hyperintense on T1W imaging, first at the periphery of the clot and then progressively closer to its center. T2 hypointensity is present initially. However, as the red cells lyse, the heme proteins become homogeneously distributed within the hemorrhage. The signal loss related to T2* resolves progressively and the hematoma becomes isointense. On GRE sequences the central portion of the hematoma slowly becomes less hypointense. The periphery of the hematoma becomes more hypointense because the heme proteins degrade further into paramagnetic hemosiderin that is sequestered in macrophages, which migrate to the evolving capsule of the hematoma.

Late Subacute (1 week-months) (Fig. 19-7)

In the late subacute phase of hemorrhage, red blood cells have undergone lysis, releasing methemoglobin into the extracellular space. The hemorrhage remains hyperintense on T1W imaging, because extracellular methemoglobin exerts the same effect on T1 relaxation time as intracellular methemoglobin. However, late subacute hemorrhage appears bright on T2W imaging, because lysis of the red cells disperses the methemoglobin homogeneously throughout the liquid hematoma, eliminating the local field inhomogeneities that previously caused low T2 signal. Furthermore, red blood cell lysis increases the free fluid/water content in the hematoma, thereby lengthening the T2 relaxation time. Meanwhile, at the periphery of the clot, paramagnetic hemosiderin and ferritin accumulate in macrophages, producing marked hypointensity along the rim.

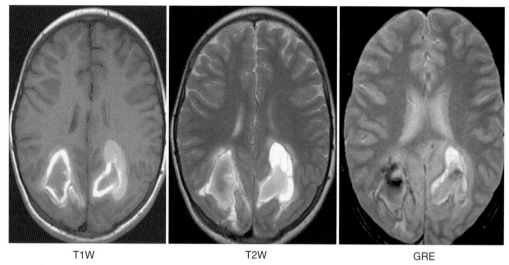

| T1W | T2W | GRE |

■ **FIGURE 19-7** Late subacute hemorrhage in a patient at 7 days. This patient demonstrates hemorrhages of varying ages; however, the left parasagittal parietal hemorrhage is late subacute in age. The hemorrhage is largely hyperintense on both T1W and T2W sequences. A thin peripheral rim of hypointensity is present on the gradient-recalled-echo sequence.

Chronic (months-years) (Fig. 19-8)

As hemorrhage enters the chronic stage, the size of the clot diminishes progressively. Hemosiderin and ferritin become the principal hemoglobin breakdown products and are largely contained within macrophages along the margin of the hemorrhage. Owing to increasing concentrations of superparamagnetic hemosiderin and ferritin, magnetic susceptibility effects predominate and generate low signal intensity on all sequences. These effects are most pronounced on susceptibility-weighted sequences such as GRE, EPI, and (susceptibility-weighted imaging) SWI sequences. Therefore, chronic hemorrhage appears mildly hypointense on T1W images and hypointense on T2W images. Once resorption of the hemorrhage is nearly complete, there may be little residual parenchymal change to mark the site of the hemorrhage, except for a small cleft lined by hemosiderin-laden macrophages, often detectable only on GRE, SWI, and the b_0 image of the DWI sequence.

Microhemorrhages

Multifocal microhemorrhages ("microbleeds") are a common finding in patients with prior ischemic or hemorrhagic stroke and, with lesser frequency, in healthy elderly patients.[15,16] In contrast to larger hemorrhagic strokes, microbleeds are often clinically silent. On T2*-GRE images, microbleeds appear as foci of marked signal hypointensity, reflecting the pronounced susceptibility effects of residual hemosiderin (Fig. 19-9). They are typically not detected on other (nonsusceptibility) sequences (T2W, FLAIR, or b_0 DWI). Microbleeds most commonly occur in elderly patients, in chronic hypertension, and in CAA. In patients with hypertension, microhemorrhages are often found in the deep gray matter, brain stem, and subcortical regions, whereas in CAA the microbleeds are typically confined to the subcortical portions of the cerebral hemispheres. The number of microhemorrhages increases in parallel to the severity of the hypertension-related ischemic white matter disease.[17] A growing body of evidence now suggests that microhemorrhages are both a marker of microangiopathy and a predictor of future hemorrhagic events, including hemorrhagic transformation after acute infarction.[18]

Subarachnoid Hemorrhage

On MRI, the appearance of SAH differs from that of other hemorrhages, because the admixture of blood with CSF dilutes the hemorrhage and because factors in the CSF prevent or impede clot formation. Subarachnoid CSF has a relatively high oxygen content, so SAH has a lower concentration of deoxyhemoglobin than is seen in parenchymal hemorrhage. Therefore, hyperacute and acute SAH typically do not cause the marked T2 and T2* hypointensity seen in other hematomas. Dilute unclotted blood is quickly absorbed and often does not have time to become hyperintense on T1W imaging. For these reasons SAH may be difficult to detect on routine T1W and T2W images. The presence of red blood cells produces moderate decrease in T1, leading to a mild hyperintensity on T1W imaging. The hemorrhage renders the CSF isointense to brain on proton density–weighted imaging ("dirty CSF sign"), but these subtle changes are easy to overlook. Because SAH is difficult to detect on routine MR series, it was thought that MR could not be used for primary screening of acute neurologic emergencies. However, FLAIR sequences now detect SAH with exquisite sensitivity. The modest change in T1 induced by red cells and by blood serum protein is sufficient to prevent fluid suppression. The intrinsic T2 hyperintensity of CSF is "unmasked," and CSF appears extremely hyperintense (Fig. 19-10). FLAIR is actually more sensitive than CT in detecting acute SAH and can be used when CT is equivocal or when clinical suspicion of SAH is high.

CT remains the imaging tool of choice in suspected aneurysmal SAH, because CT can be performed in conjunction with CT angiography to provide critical information on the source of the SAH. MRI and MR angiography do provide this information, but the MR examinations take longer and the anatomic detail is less precise with MR angiography than CT angiography. In addition, the FLAIR changes are not specific for SAH. CSF may also appear hyperintense on FLAIR images owing to inflammatory and neoplastic meningeal disease or to artifact. Pulsatile CSF motion in the basal cisterns anterior to the brain stem often appears hyperintense because of failed fluid suppression. This can mimic and obscure basal SAH such as may be seen in benign perimesencephalic SAH. In addition, metal structures such as dental braces may interfere

■ **FIGURE 19-8** Chronic hemorrhage. **A** to **C**, These images demonstrate the temporal evolution of a clot from the late subacute phase (3 weeks [**A**]) into the chronic phase (6 [**B**] and 12 [**C**] weeks). At 6 weeks, the hematoma remains bright centrally on T2W imaging as a result of extracellular methemoglobin. However, by 12 weeks, hemosiderin and ferritin predominate, resulting in a hypointense appearance on both T1W and T2W imaging.

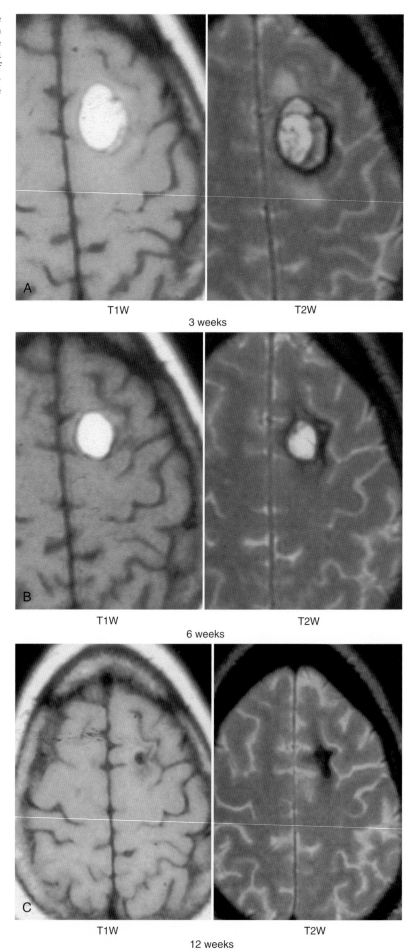

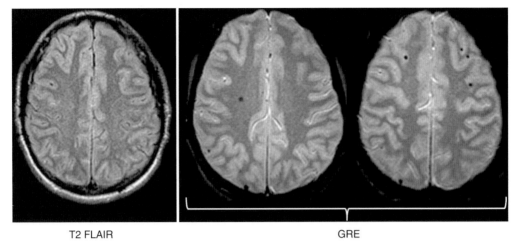

T2 FLAIR   GRE

■ **FIGURE 19-9** Microhemorrhages. Multiple foci of susceptibility effect are present primarily in the subcortical regions on the gradient-recalled-echo sequence. However, these foci are much less conspicuous on the accompanying T2W FLAIR sequence.

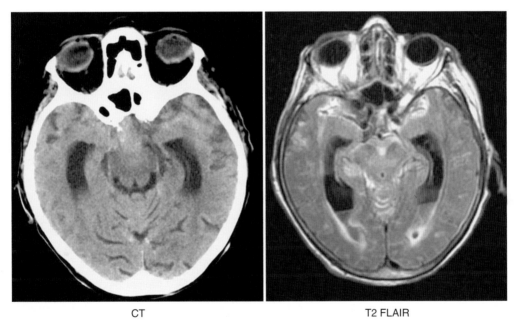

CT   T2 FLAIR

■ **FIGURE 19-10** Subarachnoid hemorrhage demonstrated on CT and T2W FLAIR sequence. Subtle hyperdensity is present in the basilar and suprasellar cisterns on the CT. However, this acute hemorrhage is much more apparent on the T2W FLAIR sequence where there is prominent hyperintensity in the basilar and suprasellar cisterns. Intraventricular hemorrhage is also more conspicuous on the FLAIR image.

with fluid suppression, producing sulcal hyperintensity. Finally, administration of oxygen during MR examinations produces sulcal hyperintensity because of the T1 shortening effect of the gas.

When SAH is particularly brisk, the blood may form a solid clot. In this circumstance, the intensity of the hemorrhage will evolve in a manner similar to that seen with parenchymal hemorrhage. Because focal clot often forms immediately adjacent to the site of hemorrhage, MRI may prove valuable for assessing the specific source of hemorrhage when angiographic studies fail to demonstrate an aneurysm. In the acute and early subacute phases the T2 hypointense hemorrhage may be obscured by normal hypointense CSF. In these cases, T2W images are best for detecting SAH.

ANALYSIS

A sample report is presented in Box 19-1.

BOX 19-1   Sample Report: MRI of Brain for Intracranial Hemorrhage

PATIENT HISTORY

The patient presented with uncontrolled hypertension after sudden onset of left hemiplegia and obtundation.

TECHNIQUE

An MRI of the brain was performed utilizing axial T1W, axial T2W, axial T2W FLAIR, axial GRE, axial diffusion-weighted (DWI), and sagittal T1W sequences without the use of intravenous gadolinium.

FINDINGS

There is a lesion in the right basal ganglia that demonstrates isointensity on T1W sequences, hyperintensity on T2W sequences, and hypointensity on susceptibility images. On DWI the lesion is predominantly hyperintense centrally with regions of curvilinear hypointensity posteriorly. There is no edema, but the lesion itself exerts minimal mass effect. This constellation of findings is typical for hyperacute hemorrhage (<6 hours). An underlying mass or vascular lesion is not excluded on the basis of this examination but is unlikely.

The ventricles and sulci are normal in size and configuration for age. No acute infarction is identified.

IMPRESSION

Hyperacute hemorrhage is evident in the right basal ganglia. Given the patient's clinical history, these findings are typical for hypertensive cerebrovascular disease.

KEY POINTS: DIFFERENTIAL DIAGNOSIS

■ CT is the imaging modality of choice for the assessment of suspected aneurysmal subarachnoid hemorrhage.

■ Gradient sequences are the most sensitive for detecting acute hemorrhage and should be part of any MR protocol in patients with acute neurologic dysfunction.

■ T2 hypointensity is the hallmark of acute parenchymal hemorrhage on MRI.

■ T1 hyperintensity is the hallmark of subacute parenchymal hemorrhage on MRI.

SUGGESTED READINGS

Bradley WG. MR Appearance of hemorrhage in the brain. Radiology 1993; 189:15-26.

Chao CP, Kotsenas AL, Broderick DF. Cerebral amyloid angiopathy: CT and MR imaging findings. RadioGraphics 2006; 26:1517-1531.

van Gijn J, Kerr RS, Rinkel GJ. Subarachnoid hemorrhage. Lancet 2007; 369:306-318.

REFERENCES

1. van Gijn J, Rinkel GJE. Subarachnoid hemorrhage: diagnosis, causes and management. Brain 2001; 124:249-278.
2. Mullins ME, Lev MH, Schellingerhout D, et al. Intracranial hemorrhage complicating acute stroke: how common is hemorrhagic stroke on initial head CT scan and how often is initial clinical diagnosis of acute stroke eventually confirmed? Am J Neuroradiol 2005; 26:2207-2212.
3. Kowalski RG, Claassen J, Kreiter KT, et al. Initial misdiagnosis and outcome after subarachnoid hemorrhage. JAMA 2004; 291:866-869.
4. van Gijn J, Van Dongen KJ, Vermeulen M, Hijdra A. Perimesencephalic hemorrhage: a nonaneurismal and benign form of subarachnoid hemorrhage. Neurology 1985; 35:493-497.
5. Fisher CM. The arterial lesion underlying lacunes. Acta Neuropathol 1969; 12:1-15.
6. Graham DI, Lantos PL (eds). Greenfield's Neuropathology, 7th ed. London, Arnold, 2002.
7. Vinters HV. Cerebral amyloid angiopathy: a critical review. Stroke 1987; 18:311-324.
8. Greenberg SM, Rebeck GW, Vonsattel JPV, et al. Apolipoprotein E e4 and cerebral hemorrhage associated with amyloid angiopathy. Ann Neurol 1995; 38:254-259.
9. Greenberg SM, Briggs ME, Hyman BT, et al. Apolipoprotein E e4 is associated with the presence and earlier onset of hemorrhage in cerebral amyloid angiopathy. Stroke 1996; 27:1333-1337.
10. Nelson CW, Wei EP, Povlishock JT, et al. Oxygen radicals in cerebral ischemia. Am J Physiol 1992; 263:H1356-H1362.
11. Lapchak PA, Chapman DF, Zivin JA. Metalloproteinase inhibition reduces thrombolytic (tissue plasminogen activator)-induced hemorrhage after thromboembolic stroke. Stroke 2000; 31:3034-3040.
12. Takasugi S, Ueda S, Matsumoto K. Chronological changes in spontaneous intracerebral hematoma: an experimental and clinical study. Stroke 1985; 16:651-658.
13. Bradley WG. MR appearance of hemorrhage in the brain. Radiology 1993; 189:15-26.
14. Clark RA, Watanabe AT, Bradley WG, Roberts JD. Acute hematomas: effects of deoxyhemoglobin, hematocrit, and fibrin clot formation and retraction on T2 shortening. Radiology 1990; 174:201-206.
15. Roob G, Schmidt R, Kapeller P, et al. MRI evidence of past cerebral microbleeds in a healthy elderly population. Neurology 1999; 52:991-994.
16. Tsushima Y, Tanizaki Y, Aoki J, Endo K. MR detection of microhemorrhages in neurologically healthy adults. Neuroradiology 2002; 44:31-36.
17. Tsushima Y, Aoki J, Endo K. Brain microhemorrhages detected on T2*-weighted gradient-echo MR images. AJNR Am J Neuroradiol 2003; 24:88-96.
18. Nighoghossian N, Hermier M, Adeleine P, et al. Old microbleeds are a potential risk factor for cerebral bleeding after ischemic stroke: a gradient-echo T2*-weighted brain MR study. Stroke 2002; 33:735-742.

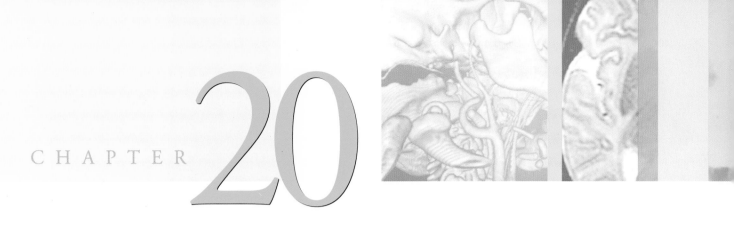

CHAPTER 20

Atherosclerosis and the Chronology of Infarction

Richard Ivan Aviv, Richard Bitar, Laurent Létourneau-Guillon, Robert Yeung, Sean P. Symons, and Allan J. Fox

DOLICHOECTASIA

Dolichoectasia is broadly defined as increased tortuosity of intracranial arteries due to elongation and dilatation of the vessel. It is also referred to as *dilative arteriopathy*.

Epidemiology

Dolichoectasia is found in fewer than 10% of patients. Its etiology is unknown but appears to be related to aberrant vascular remodeling. It is associated with traditional cardiovascular risk factors including hypertension, old age, and male sex, but also nonatherosclerotic diseases.[1] Genetic associations are common in younger patients and include Marfan syndrome, Ehlers-Danlos syndrome, human immunodeficiency virus, Fabry's disease, sickle cell disease, and α-glucosidase deficiency.

Clinical Presentation

The vertebrobasilar arteries are affected most often, with less frequent involvement of the terminal internal carotid artery (ICA) and proximal middle cerebral artery (MCA). Dolichoectasia may also be associated with parenchymal mass effect, neurovascular impingement syndromes including trigeminal neuralgia and tinnitus, aneurysm formation, subarachnoid hemorrhage, and hydrocephalus. Supraclinoid lesions may impinge locally on the optic nerves and chiasm (Fig. 20-1). Focal fusiform aneurysmal dilatations are not uncommon. In older patients, dolichoectasia has been associated with severe small vessel ischemic change, lacunar infarcts, and état criblé but not carotid atherosclerosis.[1a] It is unclear as to what extent dolichoectasia contributes to white matter change or whether it is part of a more widespread vasculopathy affecting small and large intracranial vessels.

Pathology

Gross pathologic examination reveals dilated and redundant vasculature. Thick atherosclerotic plaques may encroach on the vessel lumen.

Microscopically, there is fibrosis of the vessel wall, attenuation of the muscularis and internal elastic lamina, calcification, and formation of intraluminal thrombus. Angulation of the tortuous vessel segment may reduce perforator flow with resultant ischemia. There is a generalized reduction in antegrade flow, with to and fro blood flow reported. Intravascular thrombus may result from aberrant flow patterns and stagnation.

Imaging
Ultrasonography
Transcranial Doppler ultrasonography may reveal the aberrant flow pattern with reduced mean flow velocities but preserved peak velocities.

CT and MRI
Both CT and MRI reveal tortuous dilated vessels, which often impinge on and mold the medulla and pons (Fig. 20-2). Loss of signal void may be apparent on standard MRI. Intravascular contrast enhancement may be seen after contrast agent administration for the same reason (Fig. 20-3). Smoker's criteria for basilar dolichoectasia includes artery diameter, laterality of basilar trunk, and height of basilar bifurcation.[1]

Special Procedures
Conventional angiography is seldom required for diagnosis. CT angiography (CTA) and MR angiography (MRA) can confirm vessel redundancy and the presence of aneurysmal dilatation. Loss of signal void may be evident on time-of-flight (TOF) MRA secondary to stagnation and altered flow to which TOF is susceptible.

Analysis
A sample report on the MRI evaluation of dolichoectasia is shown in Box 20-1.

NEUROVASCULAR COMPRESSION SYNDROMES
The prototypes of neurovascular compression syndromes actually are aneurysms and pulsating masses that can directly affect cranial nerves. For example, optic nerve dysfunction can be caused by aneurysms of the cavernous and ophthalmic regions.

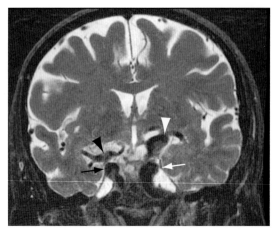

■ **FIGURE 20-1** Coronal fat-saturated T2W MR image. There is marked dolichoectasia and aneurysmal dilatation of the bilateral cavernous (*arrows*) and terminal carotid arteries (*arrowheads*). Note the distortion of the bilateral cavernous sinuses, chiasm, and left basal ganglia.

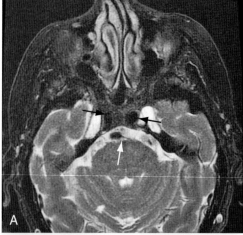

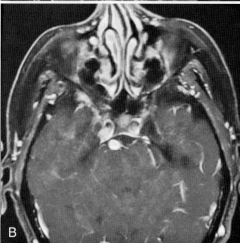

■ **FIGURE 20-3** Fat-saturated axial T2W (**A**) and postcontrast T1W (**B**) MR images (same case as Figs. 20-1 and 20-2). Note the dilated bilateral cavernous carotid segments and vertebral artery (*arrows*). There is a conspicuous absence of flow voids after contrast agent administration owing to hemodynamic disturbances.

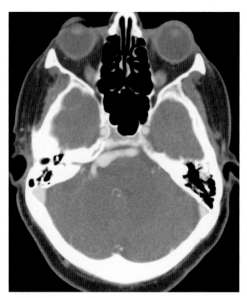

■ **FIGURE 20-2** Enhanced axial CT at the level of the pons. There is a dolichoectatic right vertebral artery demonstrating variable dilatation that is distorting the pons.

Aneurysms, arteriovenous malformations, and tumors are, however, found as the cause for neurovascular syndromes in only 2% of cases.

The diagnosis, management, and even existence of neurovascular compression syndromes are controversial. Central to all conditions within this group is a clinically driven diagnosis of neurovascular impingement. Clinical impingement syndromes are commonly described for the facial nerve (hemifacial spasm), trigeminal nerve (trigeminal neuralgia), and glossopharyngeal nerve (glossopharyngeal neuralgia). Compression of the brain stem by a dolichoectatic vertebral artery has also been implicated in essential hypertension.

The success reported in several case series provides compelling evidence for the existence of neurovascular compression and for patient improvement after treatment.[2,3] However, there is extreme variation of both the arterial and venous structures within the posterior fossa. Up to one third of asymptomatic patients may have imaging findings suggestive of cranial nerve/vascular contact.[4] Therefore, imaging criteria have evolved to permit more specific diagnosis of symptomatic neurovascular

---

BOX 20-1 Sample Report: MRI of Orbits

PATIENT HISTORY

The patient has a 2-year history of visual blurring and reduced acuity.

TECHNIQUE

MRI was performed with multiple multiplanar pulse sequences including noncontrast sagittal T1-weighted (T1W) fluid-attenuated inversion recovery (FLAIR), axial T2-weighted (T2W) FLAIR, coronal T1W and T2W fat-saturated sequences and gadolinium-enhanced axial, coronal, and sagittal oblique T1W fat saturation of the orbits. No previous study is available for comparison.

FINDINGS

There are notable dolichoectatic changes of the vertebrobasilar arteries, with secondary distortion of the contour of the brain stem without signal alteration.

The brain shows mild diffuse atrophic change. A few scattered hyperintensities are seen in the deep subcortical white matter of both cerebral hemispheres, compatible with minimal microangiopathic change. There is no suggestion of an intra-axial mass, hemorrhage, or hydrocephalus.

IMPRESSION

Marked dolichoectasia of the vertebrobasilar artery is evident.

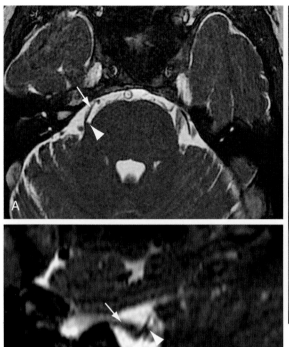

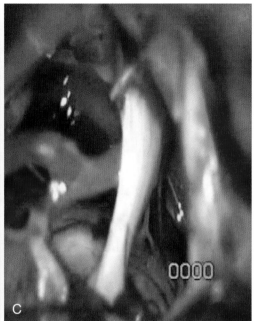

■ FIGURE 20-4 A, Axial FIESTA with **(B)** oblique sagittal reformat centered on the trigeminal level. There is attenuation and distortion of the right trigeminal nerve (*white arrow*) by the right superior cerebellar artery (*white arrowhead*), which passes perpendicularly across the nerve entry zone. **C,** Operative microscopic image demonstrating attenuation and pallor of the cisternal portion of the trigeminal nerve. A vascular structure crosses the nerve inferiorly. (*C, Courtesy of Milan Spaic, MD, Military Medical Academy, Serbia.*)

compression. These include the distortion of the appropriate cranial nerve by a vessel passing perpendicular to it at the nerve root entry/exit zone.[5] No prospective studies exist to assess the reliability of MRI for the diagnosis of neurovascular compression syndromes. Sensitivities and specificities for case series range from 44% to 100% and 50% to 100%, respectively. The lack of randomized trials with comparative outcomes (and for the patterns of treated normal anatomic variations) adds further uncertainty as to which patients should be submitted to surgery based on imaging.

Trigeminal Neuralgia

The International Association for the Study of Pain defines *trigeminal neuralgia* as a sudden, usually unilateral, severe, brief stabbing recurrent pain in the distribution of one or more branches of the fifth cranial nerve. This is also known as tic douloureux.

Epidemiology

Trigeminal neuralgia occurs in 4.5/100,000 patients. Middle-aged and elderly patients are affected most often, but younger patients have also been described.

Clinical Presentation

Patients present with a lancinating, shock-like, recurrent pain within the distribution of one or more trigeminal nerve branches. Attacks are often provoked by touching trigger points, talking, chewing, or brushing teeth.

Pathophysiology

The pathogenesis is thought to be secondary to aberrant impulses, ephaptic cross talk, and conduction block secondary to neural injury. Neurovascular compression is implicated in the

majority of cases (Fig. 20-4), but primary demyelination, tumor infiltration, amyloid, infarction, cavernous malformations, and idiopathic causes are also implicated. Familial cases have been described.

Pathology

Histopathologically, demyelination extending less than 2 mm from the zone of vascular contact is reported.[6] Demyelinated axons are in close apposition with no intervening glial processes. Electron microscopy demonstrates a combination of demyelination and remyelination. The trigeminal ganglion may show degenerative hypermyelination and microneuromas.

Imaging

Trigeminal neuralgia remains a clinical diagnosis. Microvascular compression is considered to be the major cause, so decompressive surgery is the mainstay of therapy. Other procedures to ablate the affected root of the fifth nerve, such as partial rhizotomy, radiofrequency thermocoagulation, stereotactic radiosurgery, and glycerol gangliolysis, are also performed.[7] Pharmacotherapy is a further option. Imaging studies are indicated to exclude other lesions, such as aneurysm, arteriovenous lesion, schwannoma, meningioma, or other structural lesions in the cerebellopontine angle or Meckel's cave. A vascular study may have little influence on management decisions,[4] but MRI with a volumetric study and MRA with or without gadolinium are used. Diffusion tensor imaging has also emerged as a promising tool in assessing nerve integrity, showing decreased fractional anisotropy on the affected side.[7a]

Other Neurovascular Syndromes

A number of other syndromes have been attributed to neurovascular compression, including superior oblique myokymia

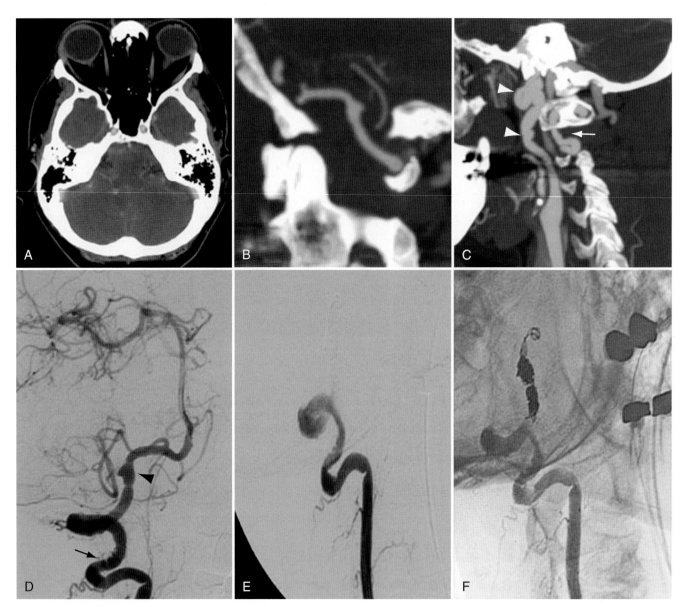

■ **FIGURE 20-5** Rupture of a dissecting aneurysm secondary to fibromuscular dysplasia. **A** to **C,** Postcontrast CT and CTA rotational and sagittal maximal intensity projection images demonstrate subarachnoid hemorrhage from a dissecting aneurysm of the vertebral artery. Vertebral artery irregularity is present between C1 and C2 (*arrow*). The distal internal carotid artery demonstrates marked redundancy and beaded irregularity secondary to fibromuscular dysplasia (*arrowheads*). **D** to **F,** Cerebral angiography confirms cervical vertebral artery beading (*arrow*), a concentric band of narrowing within the cisternal vertebral segment, and a dissecting aneurysm inferior to the posterior inferior cerebellar artery origin (*arrowhead*). The patient was treated by ipsilateral vertebral artery coil occlusion across the level of the dissection. She had full recovery with no neurologic deficit on 1-year follow-up.

(trochlear nerve), geniculate neuralgia (nervus intermedius), vestibular paroxysmia (vestibulocochlear nerve), spontaneous gagging (vagus nerve), and spasmodic torticollis (accessory nerve).

FIBROMUSCULAR DYSPLASIA

Fibromuscular dysplasia (FMD) is a disorder of unknown etiology characterized by systemic arterial wall abnormality, including beading and tubular stenosis.

Epidemiology

This uncommon disorder of the arterial wall is present in 0.02% to 1% of the population. Women are affected three to four times more often than men. Patients typically present in the fourth to fifth decades of life.

Clinical Presentation

Fibromuscular dysplasia is often asymptomatic. However, patients are predisposed to dissection and aneurysm formation with rupture (Fig. 20-5). Up to 15% of cervical artery dissections are secondary to fibromuscular dysplasia, but the risk of dissection in FMD patients is unknown.[7b] Vessel tortuosity and wall thickening may impair flow, resulting in transient ischemia attack (TIA) or ischemic stroke. Although the natural history is unknown, progression is reported in up to 25% of patients.

The extracranial ICAs are involved in 95% of cases. Bilateral disease occurs in 60% to 80%. The carotid bifurcation and proximal ICA are frequently spared, distinguishing fibromuscular dysplasia from atherosclerotic disease (Fig. 20-6). The vertebral arteries are affected at the level of C2 in 12% to 43% of cases with sparing of the origins and proximal portions of the vessels.

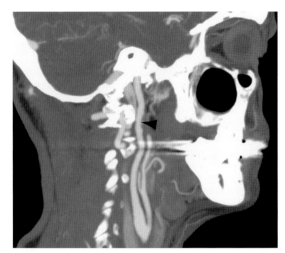

■ **FIGURE 20-6** Rotational sagittal maximal intensity projection. The upper carotid artery shows irregularity of the wall with alternating dilatation and narrowing consistent with beading. There is greater involvement of the anterior wall, where diverticulation can be appreciated (*arrowhead*). The carotid bifurcation is normal.

Intracranial involvement is rare and most often from extracranial disease extension, although isolated intracranial FMD has been reported. Systemic vessels affected include renal, subclavian, iliac, and mesenteric arteries.

Pathophysiology

The etiology is unknown, but aneurysm formation and dissection are associated, indicating a presumptive underlying disorder of connective tissue. This is further supported by the association of fibromuscular dysplasia with collagen mutation, cutis laxa, and α_1-antitrypsin deficiency. The majority of cases are sporadic, but familial cases have been reported.

Pathology

Fibromuscular dysplasia is subdivided according to medial, intimal, or adventitial involvement. Three distinct histologic types of medial dysplasia are described. Medial fibroplasia is most common (80%). Perimedial fibrosis occurs in 10% of patients, usually in younger women. The characteristic gross pathologic appearance is that of beading, although the beads are fewer in perimedial fibrosis. Regions of focal dilatation may be larger than the original luminal diameter. Medial hyperplasia is least common, resembling intimal fibroplasia. Intimal fibroplasia occurs in 10% of cases. Discrete bands of narrowing or tubular stenosis may occur (Fig. 20-7). Adventitial fibroplasia occurs in less than 1% of cases.

Histopathologically, concentric rings of fibrous proliferation and smooth muscle hyperplasia are present, resulting in elastic lamina destruction. The media is affected in 90% to 95% of cases followed by the intima in about 5% of cases. Adventitial dysplasia is rare.

Imaging
Ultrasonography

Involvement of high cervical and vertebral arteries usually precludes assessment by transcranial Doppler ultrasonography.

MRI

A T1-weighted (T1W), fat-saturated study is helpful to detect the presence of mural blood products in dissections that complicate fibromuscular dysplasia.

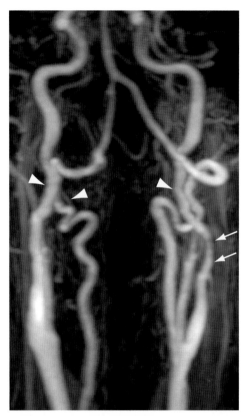

■ **FIGURE 20-7** Rotational maximum intensity projection contrast-enhanced MRA. There is marked bilateral carotid and vertebral artery irregularity with subtle beaded appearance and modest redundancy (*arrowheads*). The left carotid artery demonstrates tubular narrowing above the carotid bifurcation (*arrows*).

CTA and MRA

CTA and MRA have evolved as cross-sectional techniques and routinely detect arterial changes consistent with fibromuscular dysplasia (see Figs. 20-6 and 20-7). No published comparisons of noninvasive techniques for the diagnosis of fibromuscular dysplasia are found. Comparisons from the renal literature demonstrate higher accuracy for CTA and MRA than for transcranial Doppler ultrasonography. It can be inferred from experience with carotid atherosclerotic disease that conventional angiography may be reserved for cases in which CTA and MRA are equivocal or prior to transluminal intervention.

Special Procedures

Conventional angiography remains the gold standard. Angiographic appearances are typical, with 80% to 90% demonstrating alternating dilatation and narrowing producing a "string of beads" or "concertina" appearance (type 1 lesion) (see Figs. 20-5 and 20-6). Diffuse tubular narrowing is seen in 5% to 10% of cases (type 2 lesion) (see Fig, 20-7). The appearances may be difficult to distinguish from dissection, especially because dissection frequently coexists in fibromuscular dysplasia. Rarely, unilateral vessel wall involvement is seen. These lesions resemble diverticula (see Fig. 20-6), may be difficult to distinguish from atherosclerotic disease, and may be a source of thomboembolism.[8] A web-like defect at the origin of the internal carotid artery is also rarely described (more commonly in black patients) and thought to be related to intimal FMD.[7b]

Analysis

A sample report of CTA for fibromuscular dysplasia is shown in Box 20-2.

BOX 20-2   Sample Report: CTA for Fibromuscular Dysplasia

PATIENT HISTORY

A 55-year-old female patient with amaurosis fugax.

TECHNIQUE

CTA before and after contrast CT of the head with multiplanar reformatted angiographic images.

FINDINGS

The brain and ventricles are unremarkable. CTA demonstrates incidental beading both within vertebral artery at the C2-3 junction and between C7 and T1. Similar irregularity and lumen expansion is present in both internal carotid arteries at the skull base. This appearance is most consistent with fibromuscular dysplasia.

IMPRESSION

Incidental bilateral fibromuscular dysplasia is present.

ATHEROSCLEROTIC DISEASE

Epidemiology

Atherosclerotic disease accounts for approximately one third of all cases of cerebral infarcts. Ten percent of such cases are caused by carotid stenosis that is amenable to revascularization. Carotid stenosis of more than 50% is found in 10% to 15% of patients with ipsilateral ischemic stroke and TIA, respectively.[9,10] Imaging is, therefore, central to the prevention and treatment of stroke. Symptomatic disease is commonly secondary to atheroembolus and less commonly secondary to distal hypoperfusion caused by stenosis. The risk of atherosclerotic lesion progression is 9.3%. Numerous imaging-detectable risk factors impact on the annual stroke risk and should be actively sought. The two most important factors are degree of stenosis and symptom status. North American Symptomatic Carotid Endarterectomy Trial (NASCET) reported a threefold annual risk of stroke for symptomatic stenosis greater than or equal to 90% compared with 70% to 79% (11% and 35%, respectively). The stroke risk for near occlusion, however, is low (11%). Absence of symptoms decreases the risk significantly. Asymptomatic annualized stroke risk is 1.0% to 2.4% for 60% to 99% stenosis. The Asymptomatic Carotid Surgery Trial also found no increased stroke risk with increasing severity of stenosis. Imaging-detectable risk factors include plaque morphology, prior silent stroke, the presence of contralateral or intracranial disease, and intracranial collateral status.

Clinical Presentation

Presentation of patients with cervical and cranial atherosclerosis is variable and depends on disease burden and distribution. Most frequently, patients are asymptomatic. Disease may be detected incidentally during investigations for other disease processes. Symptomatic presentations may be attributable to disease elsewhere, including myocardial infarction or peripheral claudication. Symptomatic cerebrovascular and cervical vascular disease most commonly presents acutely with TIAs and stroke or chronically with cognitive impairment and vascular dementia.

Pathophysiology

Atherosclerosis is a complex disease with a multifactorial pathogenesis. It is believed to result from the interaction among endothelial cell injury, lipid accumulation, smooth muscle proliferation, plaque formation, inflammatory cell recruitment, matrix synthesis, and intimal neovascularization.[11-14] Savory[15] first noted an association between carotid artery disease and strokes in 1856. Subsequent pathologic series confirmed the presence of intracranial carotid atheroembolic material in stroke patients.[16]

Fisher,[17] evaluating carotid arteries pathologically, concluded that intraplaque hemorrhage, plaque ulceration, and luminal thrombosis were the main substrates for cerebral embolism.

Pathology

Atherosclerosis is the most common pattern of arteriosclerosis. It affects arteries of medium-to-large caliber.[18] Other patterns are Mönckeberg medial calcific sclerosis and arteriolosclerosis.[18] Mönckeberg medial calcific sclerosis refers to calcific arterial deposits usually in people aged 50 years or older. Arteriolosclerosis affects small arteries and arterioles with arteriolar wall thickening usually associated with diabetic and hypertensive patients.

The components of atherosclerotic plaques can be divided into four categories[19]: (1) lipids (including crystalline cholesterol, phospholipids, and cholesteryl esters), (2) connective tissue matrix components (including collagen, proteoglycans, and fibronectin), (3) cellular components (e.g., monocytes, macrophages, T lymphocytes, and smooth muscle cells), and (4) thrombotic materials (platelets and fibrin). The components are present in varying proportions throughout the life of the plaque. The specific composition of atherosclerotic plaques forms the basis for a variety of classification schemes for plaques.

The American Heart Association (AHA) Committee on Vascular Lesions classification, or Stary classification, is the most widely used scheme. It attempts to correlate histologic lesion appearance with imaging appearance.[20-23] Plaque histologic/histochemical composition and cellular/matrix components form the basis for classification. Eight plaque categories (types I-VIII) make up this classification.[20,22] Type I to III lesions may regress to a normal phenotype. Type IV to VIII plaques that progress to lesions are termed *atheromas* or advanced atherosclerotic lesions. Up to type V, remodeling of the arterial wall[24] occurs with outward displacement of the wall in response to increased atheroma. Initially, an eccentric pattern of remodeling occurs.[24] Subsequently, collagen layer formation limits outward displacement, resulting in luminal narrowing, hemorrhage and ulceration (type VI), calcification (type VII), and fibrosis (type VIII). The scheme has been criticized for not including plaque features such as plaque erosion and thin-cap fibroatheroma, features that are addressed by other schemes beyond the scope of this text.[19,25]

Imaging

Ultrasonography

Ultrasound assesses vessel wall morphology and luminal flow by employing B mode and Doppler ultrasound. Color-encoded and power Doppler imaging facilitate velocity measurements by demonstrating directionality and detecting trickle flow.

B mode imaging may detect plaque irregularity, ulceration, and echogenicity, which are markers of stroke risk. Hyperechoic areas are shown to represent plaque fibrosis/microcalcifications. Hypoechoic areas are associated with hemorrhage, thrombosis, and/or lipids in the vessel wall.[26,27] Intimal thickness has been used as a marker of atherosclerosis. However, an increased intimal thickness does not differentiate between atherosclerotic disease and other processes such as intimal or medial infiltration/hypertrophy, which might increase this measurement.[28,29] Intravascular ultrasound enables high spatial resolution imaging of the arterial wall (100-250 μm); however, low sensitivities for thrombus and lipid-rich lesion detection have been reported.[30]

Numerous diagnostic criteria exist for the diagnosis of carotid stenosis. A consensus group recommended that the peak systolic velocity (PSV) should be the main determining parameter. In the presence of tandem lesions, contralateral high-grade stenosis, and hyperdynamic or hypodynamic cardiac pulsation, the PSV may be inaccurate. Under such conditions ICA/common carotid artery (CCA) PSV and ICA end-diastolic volume (EDV) may be helpful.[31] A PSV, ICA/CCA PSV ratio, and EDV less than 125 cm/s,

2 cm/s, and 40 cm/s, respectively, is considered normal. PSV, ICA/CCA PSV ratio, and EDV of 125 to 230 cm/s, 2 to 4 cm/s, and 40 to 100 cm/s, respectively, is consistent with 50% to 69% stenosis. A 70% and greater stenosis is diagnosed when PSV, ICA/CCA PSV ratio, and EDV are greater than 230 cm/s, 4 cm/s, and 100 cm/s, respectively. In all cases the PSV is the primary parameter and the ICA/CCA PSV ratio and EDV are additional parameters.[31] Applying different thresholds, the sensitivity of Doppler ultrasonography in diagnosing a stenosis greater than or equal to 70% relative to conventional angiography is reported as 77% to 98% in a study of 1006 carotid arteries. Specificity is 53% to 82%. Agreement with conventional angiography for stenosis of greater than or equal to 70% is 96%. However, agreement with conventional angiography for less severe stenosis is poor (45%).[32] Cervical artery examination may be supplemented by transcranial ultrasound to screen for intracranial atherosclerosis and to assess for hemodynamic changes resulting from hemodynamically significant extracranial stenosis. Embolic signal detection by transcranial examination appears to predict stroke risk in acute stroke, in symptomatic carotid stenosis, and post-operatively following carotid endarterectomy.[32a]

The main limitation of ultrasonography is wide variation in agreement of parameters that are indicative of carotid stenosis. The well-known high interoperator dependence and variation between machines and manufacturers result in a lower reproducibility.[28] Heavily calcified plaques, tortuous vessels, hairline residual lumen, and high carotid tandem lesions may not be assessable. Only the cervical portion of the ICA is evaluated if the study is not supplemented by transcranial ultrasound. Contralateral carotid occlusion may increase peak systolic velocity and may lead to stenosis overestimation. Despite these limitations, ultrasonography remains the most widely used modality for screening of carotid disease. Although it is often the only examination performed, several studies confirm the benefit of a combination of noninvasive tests.[33,34] One study compared ultrasonography and MRA to conventional angiography, reporting a misclassification rate of 28% and 18% for ultrasonography and MRA, respectively. Misclassification is reduced to 6% to 11% when two noninvasive modalities are combined.[33,35] We recommend the use of ultrasonography for screening with a second noninvasive confirmatory test. Our preference is CTA. In the case of agreement, no further investigation is required. Disagreement necessitates conventional angiography rather than a third noninvasive test.

CTA

CTA is performed by injecting a contrast bolus followed by saline chaser. The injection is usually triggered by a bolus tracking technique. The contrast bolus is then tracked over the required field of view, usually from the arch to vertex, in seconds. The result is multiple submillimeter axial slices with near isotropic spatial resolution enabling thin slab maximum intensity projection or volumetric reconstructions and multiplanar reformatting. Similar to conventional angiography, the technique is limited by the total safe dose of iodinated contrast material and ionizing radiation. However, the procedure is fast, safe, cost effective, and widely available. The addition of proprietary software packages enables automated assessment of cross-sectional or percent stenosis without the requirement for a high level of experience in stenosis measurement.

The performance of CTA compared with digital subtraction angiography (DSA), MRA, and ultrasonography has been studied in multiple small series. A meta-analysis[36] of studies prior to 2003, including only single-slice scanners, found a sensitivity and specificity for detection of 70% to 99% stenosis of 85% and 93%, respectively. For occlusion, values of 97% and 99% are reported. A recent small study utilizing a four-slice scanner showed sensitivity, specificity, and accuracy of 95%, 93%, and 94%,

respectively, for stenosis of 50% or more. There have been rapid technologic software and hardware advances since these studies, and now 64- and 320-slice multidetector scanners are in routine clinical use. These scanners have higher through-plane resolution because of smaller detector size. Together with reduced scan times, the extent of coverage is improved and there is less venous contamination. Reversal of scan direction may further limit venous contamination, but in our experience this is seldom a problem.[37] A recent study utilizing an 8-slice scanner found that CTA underestimated the degree of stenosis relative to DSA but achieved a high correlation of 0.95. Interobserver agreement was 3.9% for DSA and 5.8% to 5.9% for CTA using manual or automated measures, respectively.[38] In practice, non-invasive cross-sectional imaging has replaced conventional angiography for this purpose. It is unlikely that a large study comparing newer generations of multidetector CTs to DSA will ever be published.

In the acute setting, the differentiation of near occlusion (string sign) from a total occlusion is of importance because a very high-grade stenosis can be addressed with either surgical or endovascular procedures, whereas a total occlusion cannot unless occluded with fresh thrombus. CTA appears almost as accurate as DSA for differentiating carotid occlusion from near occlusion, and significantly superior to carotid Doppler ultrasound.[38a] In this setting, a major caveat of CTA is the possibility of nonopacification of the distal ICA secondary to very slow flow, therefore mimicking a carotid occlusion. This problem can be overcome by delayed CTA acquisition.[38b] Furthermore, in near occlusion, the distal carotid artery will collapse secondary to severely reduced poststenotic arterial pressure. This may lead to underestimation of the stenosis when using NASCET-style measurements unless this pitfall is recognized.[38c]

The method of data reconstruction significantly alters the performance of both CTA and MRA.[39] In our experience, axial source images are the most accurate and reproducible method for stenosis measurement. Although calcium complicates measurement on axial imaging, a wider window (WW 900, WL 275) is usually sufficient to overcome this. Multiplanar reconstructions (MPR) and especially maximum intensity projection (MIP) techniques are less reliable in the presence of calcification. Dual energy CT is a novel approach to remove calcified plaques from the CTA images.[39a,39b] A thorough review of different processing techniques is described elsewhere.[39] With proper attention to detail we have found that axial source images are equivalent to axial oblique images (performed tangential to the vessel lumen). We use a combination of MPR and axial source images to understand the position and course of the lumen through the axial plane before stenosis measurement are made on axial images (Fig. 20-8). An advantage of cross-sectional imaging is that NASCET style measurements are no longer needed. Stenosis can be described as a cross-sectional area or single proximal measurement. There is an excellent agreement for a single proximal measurement with a NASCET style measure[40] and cross-sectional area.[41]

Multidetector CT has been used to image atherosclerotic plaques in the coronary and carotid arterial circulations.[42,43] Plaques may be classified as fatty (Fig. 20-9), mixed or calcified, and stratified by Hounsfield unit (HU) attenuation.[42,44] In vitro and in vivo studies have produced mixed results for CTA plaque characterization,[45-47] favoring MRI for this application.

MRI

Advances in MRI sequences, coils, and higher gradient scanners have resulted in improved contrast and spatial and temporal resolution. Whereas TOF studies dominated the earlier literature, increasingly contrast-enhanced MRA is performed. Reflected in these changes is the improved performance of MRA when compared with DSA. A meta-analysis of MRA studies between 1990 and 1999 reported that MRA appeared accurate but that

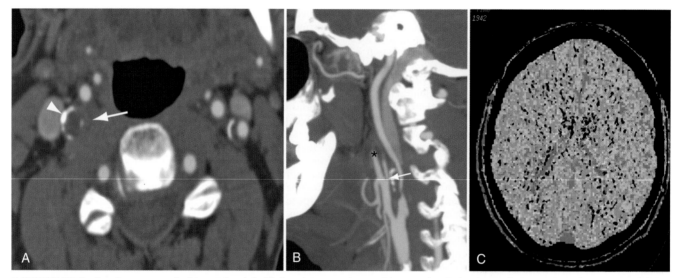

■ **FIGURE 20-8** A patient presented with transient left-sided weakness consistent with a transient ischemic attack. Reconstructed 0.63-mm axial CTA (**A**) and sagittal MIP (**B**) images demonstrate bilateral carotid bifurcation atherosclerotic changes. Low-density atheroma and peripheral calcification (*arrowhead*) surround both vessels. The residual right lumen measures 0.1 mm (*white arrow*). The distal carotid is reduced relative to the contralateral carotid, although it is larger than the ipsilateral external carotid artery (*asterisk*). The appearances are consistent with a high-grade stenosis. **C,** Mean transit time map demonstrates prolongation of transit time within the distribution of the right carotid artery.

interpretation was hampered by study heterogeneity. More recent studies report high sensitivity, specificity, and accuracy for both 3D TOF MRA and contrast-enhanced MRA.[48]

A recent study comparing TOF MRA and contrast-enhanced MRA with conventional angiography and 3D DSA in 98 carotid arteries found high agreement for all techniques.[49] The sensitivity/specificity for contrast-enhanced MRA and TOF MRA using rotational angiography as a reference standard was 100%/90% and 95.5%/87%, respectively. The specificity was lower when compared with conventional angiography because of the inherent underestimation of this technique relative to DSA. TOF sequences are longer than contrast-enhanced MRA and suffer from dephasing secondary to in-plane flow and flow-related artifacts such as turbulence and patient movement. Contrast-enhanced MRA overcomes many of these limitations with rapid scan times, greater coverage, and improved contrast to noise. Administration of contrast agents such as gadobenate dimeglumine with higher T1 relaxivity and signal intensity enhancement further improves contrast resolution.

Similar to CT, MRA data may be displayed in a variety of ways, influencing the test performance. In general, review of source data together with other reformatted images is the best approach, with MPR demonstrating higher concordance than MIP images.[39] We routinely acquire a venous-phase CT after CTA, which allows distinction of near occlusion from total occlusion. In our experience, acute carotid occlusion will often show peripheral enhancement of the carotid, the lumen being filled with nonenhancing thrombus. Advantages of MRI are noninvasiveness, high contrast resolution, and lack of ionizing radiation. However, MRI is still not widely available, is expensive, and requires a longer study time than CT. The administration of gadolinium compounds should be avoided in patients with acute renal failure or in renal dialysis patients because of the association with nephrogenic systemic fibrosis.[50] Six to 10 percent of patients are unable to undergo MRI studies.[51] MRI contraindications including metallic implants and clips and patient claustrophobia are the most common reasons.

Recent advances in MRI have made it an emerging modality for assessment of atherosclerotic carotid plaques (Fig. 20-10).[52-55] The development of carotid phase-array coils has allowed increasing signal-to-noise and contrast-to-noise ratios and submillimeter voxel-size imaging of carotid atherosclerotic plaques.[54,56-60] Plaque composition is an important factor influencing plaque rupture.[61,62] Good correlation between MRI and ex vivo histopathology specimens is reported.[53,54,63-66] Imaging of the vessel wall area has also been shown to be feasible with high-resolution carotid plaque imaging. Both 2D[67] and 3D[68-70] sequences have been described. A recent study by Mani and coworkers[71] demonstrated good correlation between black-blood MRI carotid imaging and intimal thickness for the detection of carotid wall area, wall thickness, and plaque index. Contrast-enhanced studies have also been very useful in assessing plaque inflammation, with the degree of enhancement seen in the fibrous regions of the plaque correlating with the amount of neovasculature present in the plaque.[72] The two most important features of a vulnerable plaque that can be identified by MR are adventitial enhancement and intraplaque hemorrhage.[72a]

Special Procedures

Angiography is considered the reference standard against which noninvasive modalities are compared. Angiography assesses the vessel's luminal diameter and is dependent on a view tangential to the tightest stenosis. In the presence of the typical eccentric stenosis two projections are insufficient to achieve this goal. It is unsurprising, therefore, that compared with 3D DSA, conventional DSA is repeatedly shown to underestimate luminal stenosis.[49,73] In the absence of calibration methods, expression of stenosis severity is limited to a percent stenosis relative to the distal ICA. The NASCET measure has been adopted as the technique of choice. The technique of stenosis measurement is well described.[74] The tightest luminal diameter at the stenosis site is measured (a). The normal distal ICA is measured at a site where the walls are parallel (b). The percentage stenosis is calculated by the equation $1 - (a/b)$. Assessment of plaque morphology including ulceration is poor, with a reported sensitivity of 46%. Nonetheless, angiography is very sensitive to calcifications and/or luminal thrombosis.[28] Limitations include the risk of permanent or transient neurologic deficit (0.5%-0.9%, respectively) use of ionizing radiation, and use of iodinated contrast media.

Angiography may underestimate stenosis where diffuse atherosclerosis narrows the entire arterial lumen and in early atherosclerosis where outward displacement of the vessel wall occurs.[24] The measurement of near occlusion will underestimate stenosis using the NASCET ratio. For this reason and those

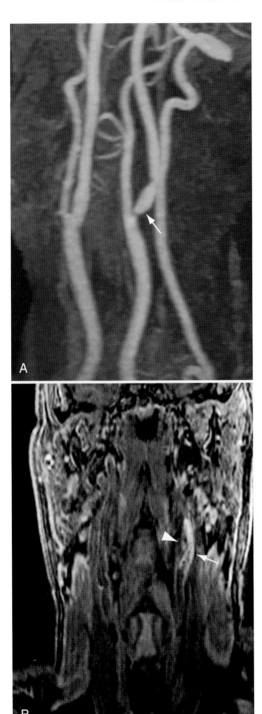

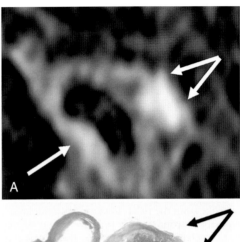

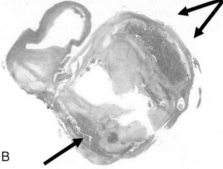

■ **FIGURE 20-10** MRI (3D T1W fat suppressed spoiled gradient echo sequence) of intraplaque hemorrhage in a 74-year-old man with symptomatic high-grade carotid stenosis. **A,** MR image at the level of the carotid bifurcation. Intraplaque hemorrhage is seen as high-signal (*arrows*) in the carotid wall. **B,** Corresponding H&E-stained section of carotid endarterectomy specimen confirms the presence of intraplaque hemorrhage (*arrows*).

■ **FIGURE 20-9** A and **B,** Magnified rotational maximum intensity projection contrast-enhanced MRA to illustrate cervical findings. There is a high-grade left ICA stenosis. A flow void at the stenosis site makes a direct measurement impossible (*arrow*). A gradient coronal 3D T1W spoiled gradient with fat saturation confirms the presence of a complicated or hemorrhagic plaque (*arrowhead*).

outlined earlier, the exclusion of near occlusion is important. Angiographic features include ipsilateral carotid artery smaller than contralateral ICA, smaller or equal to ipsilateral external carotid artery (ECA), and delayed filling relative to the ipsilateral superficial temporal artery.

A variety of radiopharmaceuticals have been designed to image atherosclerotic plaques. These include labeling of lipoproteins (e.g., low-density lipoprotein [LDL]), as well as antibodies

against cells (macrophages) or cell surface proteins (e.g., intercellular adhesion molecule-1 [ICAM-1]) with agents such as technetium (^{99m}Tc) and indium (^{111}In, ^{123}In). Experimental models of atherosclerosis have shown promising results, but the technique is limited by poor signal-to-noise ratios and prolonged clearance of the radiopharmaceuticals.[75]

Fluorodeoxyglucose-labeled positron emission tomography (FDG-PET) is a promising technique. There is a fast clearance rate and better contrast-to-noise compared with other radiotracers.[76] Macrophages have high FDG uptake and are shown to be good markers of plaque inflammation. FDG thus has good potential to evaluate macrophage density in plaques.[77,78]

Treatment
Treatment of Carotid Disease
Carotid endarterectomy (CEA) is the primary treatment for atherosclerotic carotid artery disease, so the use of this surgical technique has steadily increased during the past decades.[79] Its increased use is in part due to many randomized, controlled clinical trials where both symptomatic and asymptomatic carotid stenosis were studied. The two major trials assessing benefit from carotid endarterectomy in patients with symptomatic carotid artery stenosis are the NASCET[80] and the European Carotid Surgery Trial (ECST).[81]

By demonstrating relative and absolute risk reductions in those patients randomized to surgical treatment compared with those who were randomized to the best medical treatment available, these two trials firmly established the benefits of carotid endarterectomy among patients with symptomatic high-grade (>70%) carotid artery stenosis. The NASCET trial was stopped after 18 months because of the significant benefit found from carotid endarterectomy.

For patients with symptomatic moderate carotid stenosis (50%-69%), the benefits are less than for high-grade stenosis. NASCET demonstrated some benefit, but no significant benefit was seen in ECST. Patients with low-grade stenosis (<50% stenosis) did not benefit in either study.

The 2011 U.S. guidelines endorsed by multiple societies, including the American Heart Association (AHA), recommend carotid endarterectomy for patients with symptomatic stenosis between 70% and 99% within 6 months of a TIA or ischemic stroke provided that the periprocedural morbidity and mortality is lower than 6%. They recommend that carotid endarterectomy should be considered in moderate carotid artery stenosis, depending on associated comorbidities, but not in patients with low-grade carotid artery stenosis.[82-84a]

The presence of asymptomatic carotid artery stenosis is a risk factor for strokes, but the risk is lower when compared with that of symptomatic carotid artery stenosis.[12] The Asymptomatic Carotid Atherosclerosis Study (ACAS) is the largest randomized controlled trial evaluating the effects of carotid endarterectomy on asymptomatic patients with carotid artery stenosis.[85] In this trial, patients with asymptomatic 60% to 99% carotid stenosis were randomized to receive either medical treatment or carotid endarterectomy. The latter was found to be more beneficial than medical treatment; however, the ACAS reported a smaller absolute risk reduction when compared with the trials in symptomatic patients.

Benefit from carotid endarterectomy is greatest when the presentation is stroke, followed by TIA and retinal events. There is also a trend to greater benefit in patients with irregular plaques.[86] Men have a greater benefit from carotid endarterectomy with lower rates of perioperative complications compared with women. The indications of carotid endarterectomy for asymptomatic patients with carotid artery stenosis are less clear. The guidelines from the American Heart Association and the National Stroke Association (U.S.) recommend that carotid endarterectomy should be considered in patients younger than 80 years old with asymptomatic carotid stenosis greater than 60%. Surgery should be offered by experienced surgeons with low complication rates. Patient comorbidities, life expectancy, and patient preference should also be considered.[82-84]

Carotid Angioplasty and Stenting

Endovascular treatment of carotid stenosis is less invasive than carotid endarterectomy. Stent deployment is favored over angioplasty alone. Advantages of endovascular treatment include ability to perform the procedure under local rather than general anesthesia. Surgery requires a neck dissection, which increases the risk of cranial nerve injury and wound sepsis. Complications related to carotid artery stenting (CAS) are secondary to periprocedural ischemic events, arterial puncture, and iodinated contrast administration. Periprocedural TIAs and strokes are largely the result of atheroembolus at the time of angioplasty or stenting. Filter devices, occlusion balloons, and basket devices have been developed in an attempt to minimize these occurrences. These devices appear to work. A systematic review of the literature reported combined stroke and death rate for symptomatic and asymptomatic patients of 1.8% versus 5.5% with and without cerebral protection devices, respectively. Minor stroke accounted for the majority of events (3.7% vs. 0.5% with protection).[87] Stroke reduction with cerebral protection devices is indeed confirmed in the recent, prematurely terminated study. A protection device was utilized in 78% and 27% of patients in the EVA-3S and SPACE trials, respectively. SPACE found no difference in the primary outcome measures in patients with and without cerebral protection devices. A stroke reduction was reported in EVA-3S. However, the magnitude of reduction was not sufficient to demonstrate any benefit of carotid artery surgery over carotid endarterectomy. Furthermore, diffusion-weighted imaging (DWI)

studies performed after stenting have shown significant difference in the incidence of silent infarcts in patients with and without cerebral protection. The clinical significance of these subclinical infarcts, however, is not known.

Studies of both carotid angioplasty and stenting have demonstrated varying results. Earlier studies, including CAVATAS,[88] Wallstent, SAPPHIRE,[89] SPACE,[90] and EVA-3S,[91] have failed to demonstrate benefit over carotid endarterectomy. CREST, the most recent and largest study to date, has provided support for carotid stenting, showing similar long-term outcome between CAS and CEA in symptomatic and asymptomatic patients.[91a] Differences in periprocedural (<30 days) complications remain the major focus of current studies and are a leading consideration in selection of the most appropriate procedure. The Carotid Stent Trialists Collaboration (CSTC) meta-analyzed data from EVA-3S, SPACE, and ICSS (3433 patients) and showed that the 30-day rate of stroke or death was significantly higher after CAS (7.7%) versus CEA (4.4%); risk ratio for CAS relative to CEA 1.74 (1.32 to 2.30, $p = 0.0001$)[91b] The CREST trial showed similar findings, including higher periprocedural (30-day) stroke rate for CAS (4.1%) versus 2.3% for CEA ($p = 0.01$). Conversely, periprocedural myocardial infarctions were higher for CEA (2.3%) than for CAS (1.1%, $p = 0.03$) in the CREST study. Another important observation from CREST was that CAS provided slightly better outcomes in younger (<70-year-old) patients compared to CEA. In conclusion, there is increasing evidence to support the use of carotid stenting. Selected patients with age younger than 70; cardiac comorbidities, including congestive heart failure, recent unstable angina, or myocardial infarction; surgically inaccessible lesions; prior endarterectomy; or neck irradiation may benefit from endovascular treatment.

INTRACRANIAL ATHEROSCLEROSIS

Intracranial atherosclerosis is defined as mural atherosclerotic changes of intracranial arteries, including the portions of the ICA and vertebrobasilar artery systems contained within the dura. Other names include intracranial stenosis, middle cerebral atherosclerosis, and MCA stenosis.

Epidemiology

Intracranial atherosclerosis accounts for 8% to 12% of all ischemic strokes,[92] corresponding to 70,000 cases per year in the United States.[93] Much attention has been paid to the extracranial carotid arteries as a source of ischemic cerebrovascular disease since Fisher's 1951 report. Furthermore, NASCET has emphasized measurements of extracranial carotid stenosis to stratify patients into treatment regimens. Disease in the intracranial circulation was often attributed to spread from more proximal disease, such as emboli. However, in the Joint Study of Extracranial Arterial Occlusion, 6.1% of patients had isolated intracranial disease, which was independently and highly associated with stroke.[94]

The incidence varies widely among populations. Asians, blacks, and Hispanics have a much higher incidence of intracranial atherosclerosis than whites. Conversely, whites have a much higher incidence of extracranial carotid atherosclerosis. In China, intracranial disease accounts for one third of ischemic strokes.[92] The reason for this variation is not yet known. In the Northern Manhattan Stroke Study intracranial atherosclerosis was found in 11% of Hispanic, 6% of black, and 1% of white stroke patients.[95] The stroke risk factors of diabetes and hypercholesterolemia were also determinants of intracranial atherosclerotic disease. In the United States there is a fourfold higher incidence of MCA disease in Chinese-American stroke patients than whites.[96] Conversely, whites with strokes had a fivefold higher incidence of severe extracranial carotid disease. Pathologic data from deceased Hong Kong Chinese[97] showed a 31% incidence of atherosclerosis in the intracranial arteries. In symptomatic patients enrolled in the Extracranial/Intracranial Bypass Study, 58% of Asians, 34% of blacks, and only 18% of whites had MCA disease.[98]

Older age, hypertension, ischemic heart disease, hypercholesterolemia, cigarette smoking, and diabetes are factors associated with MCA stenosis. Among asymptomatic Asian patients with vascular risk factors (hypertension, diabetes, or hyperlipidemia) the prevalence of MCA stenosis increases with the number of risk factors present (7.2% for one, 10.6% for two, 20.4% for three, 29.6% for four, and 12.6% overall incidence for any risk factors).[99] Vascular risk factors alone do not entirely explain MCA stenosis, because Western whites have similar risk factors but a much lower incidence of disease. Interestingly, obesity (as measured by body mass index) is inversely associated with MCA stenosis. The reason is uncertain but does correspond to a Japanese study that found low body mass index (<18) was associated with a higher risk of total stroke and intraparenchymal hemorrhage.[100]

Atherosclerosis is a systemic process, with disease in one vascular system predictive that others may also be affected. The presence of plaques in the aorta is associated with coronary artery disease and thickening of the extracranial carotid artery. Aortic plaques are also an independent predictor of intracranial atherosclerotic disease.[101]

Clinical Presentation

Patients with intracranial atherosclerotic disease are at high risk for stroke. Stroke incidence varies with degree of stenosis and presence of symptoms. Patients with at least 30% intracranial stenosis have an annual ipsilateral stroke and death rate of 3.1% to 8.1% and 4.7% to 17.2%, respectively.[102,103] Highest stroke rates occur with MCA occlusion.[92] Symptomatic patients with more than 50% stenosis had a recurrent stroke rate of 32% over a 6-month period[92] whereas 61% of those with more than one stenotic artery had a recurrent stroke in the same period. The Standford Stroke Centre study reported an annual stroke or death rate of 45% in patients with intracranial stenosis failing medical therapy. These mostly occurred within the first 36 days.[104] The Groupe d'Étude des Stenoses Intra-Craniennes Atheromateuses Symptomatiques (GESICA) study assessed the natural history of symptomatic patients on medical treatment with 50% to 99% stenosis.[105] After a 23-month follow-up, 38.2% had either an ipsilateral stroke (13.7%) or TIA (24.5%), with a median of 2 months between the initial and recurrent event. Those with hemodynamically significant stenosis had a 60.7% incidence of a recurrent stroke or TIA. Stenoses were classified as hemodynamically significant if symptoms related to the stenosis occurred during a change in position, on effort, or if there was an introduction or increase of an antihypertensive medication.

The risk of stroke associated with posterior circulation intracranial disease (vertebral, basilar, posterior cerebral artery [PCA], or posterior inferior cerebellar artery [PICA]) is 2.5% to 5.5% per year.[106] As a subset of the Warfarin-Aspirin Symptomatic Intracranial Disease trial,[107] 22% of patients with symptomatic posterior circulation disease greater than 50% had an ipsilateral stroke after 13.8 months. Patients with basilar or vertebral artery disease and greater degrees of stenosis had the highest stroke rates.[106] Patients with more than 50% stenosis of the distal vertebral artery or basilar artery had an 18% incidence of stroke over 6.1 years (11.4% in the same territory as the stenotic lesion). Distal vertebral disease had a higher stroke or TIA rate than proximal disease.

Pathophysiology

Atherosclerotic disease is a dynamic process that can progress, regress, or remain stable over time. Serial angiographic follow-up of intracranial disease has shown that up to 80% remain stable or progress over 26.7 months while the remaining 20% regress.[102] The ICA is the most frequent site of intracranial stenosis (50% of cases).[102] The morphology of the plaque is important in determining plaque stability. Plaque morphology can be either white or yellow.[103] White plaques have thicker fibrous caps and lower distensibility, giving them more stability. Yellow plaques are often found in acute coronary syndromes and tend to have a thinner fibrous cap, lipid-rich core, and higher distensibility, resulting in more vulnerability and instability. As yellow plaques heal over time, they tend to become white.

The presence of atherosclerotic disease in the intracranial arteries can lead to stroke via one of three mechanisms: (1) reduced perfusion; (2) thromboembolism, and (3) penetrating artery occlusion.[103] The first two are similar to the pathophysiology of extracranial carotid disease whereas the third is unique to the intracranial circulation. Perfusion failure occurs when the stenosis causes a reduction in flow that cannot be compensated by collateral circulation. The brain maintains metabolism by reflex autodilatation and increased oxygen extraction. When both mechanisms reach their limit, a further decrease in perfusion leads to cell death. The subgroup of patients with perfusion failure may benefit from endovascular therapy. Intracranial atherosclerosis can also lead to and occurs when there is occlusion of the origin of small penetrating arteries resulting in strokes in the deep structures or brain stem.

Imaging

Ultrasonography

Transcranial Doppler (TCD) is a noninvasive and portable modality for assessing the intracranial vessels. A 2-MHz transducer is typically used through the temporal window with the patient supine. A depth of 50 to 60 mm is typically used for the MCA. The main application of TCD is in velocity measurements. The greater the degree of stenosis, the higher the velocity of blood flow through the narrowing. There have been various studies attempting to correlate measured velocities with degree of stenosis. One study comparing transcranial Doppler imaging to MRA found an optimal PSV cutoff of 140 cm/s defined MCA stenosis of more than 50% with a sensitivity of 91.4% and specificity of 82.7%. The optimal cutoff for stenosis greater than 75% was 180 cm/s.[108]

The Stroke Outcomes and Neuroimaging (SONIA) trial[109] attempted to define velocities on transcranial Doppler imaging that would identify 50% to 99% M1 stenosis with an 80% positive predictive value (PPV) and exclude stenosis with a 90% negative predictive value (NPV). They found that more than 100 cm/s at M1 had a 36% PPV and 86% NPV for identifying greater than 50% M1 stenosis. To maximize PPV at 55% (with 83% NPV), velocity measurements required were 240 cm/s for MCA, 120 cm/s for ICA, 110 cm/s for vertebral artery, and 130 cm/s for basilar artery. Transcranial Doppler imaging was good for ruling out intracranial stenosis but not accurate at quantifying it when present. A difference greater than 30 cm/s compared to the opposite side suggests vessel disease even if the absolute velocities are within normal limits.[110]

Intracranial atherosclerosis is a dynamic process because luminal diameter varies with disease stage. Imaging soon after a stroke may demonstrate greater narrowing from plaque rupture and thrombosis. Imaging during the asymptomatic phase may show a remodeled and stable lumen. Overall, in the best hands recognition of vessels and sampling of velocities is good on transcranial Doppler imaging, although the lack of anatomic imaging of intracranial vessels as in CTA or DSA has some inherent pitfalls.

CTA and MRA

CTA and digital subtraction angiography (DSA) are low-risk, less invasive, and faster alternatives to angiography. CTA has the

TABLE 20-1. Diagnostic Performance of CTA and MRA for Intracranial Stenosis and Occlusion

Abnormality	Modality	No.	Sensitivity	Specificity	PPV	NPV
Stenosis (50%-99%)	CTA (single 4 slice)*	28	98%	99%	93%	100%
	CTA† (8-16 slice)	41	97.1%	99.5%		
	TOF-1.5T MRA*	28	70%	97%	65%	98%
	3D TOF 3T MRA‡	39	82%	95%	77%	96%
Occlusion	CTA (single 4 slice)*	28	100%	100%	100%	100%
	CTA† (8-16 slice)	41	100%	100%		
	TOF-1.5T MRA*	28	87%	98%	59%	99.5%
	3D TOF 3T MRA‡	39	100%	99%	87%	100%

PPV, Positive predictive value; NPV, negative predictive value.

*Data from Bash S, Villablanca JP, Jahan R, et al. Intracranial vascular stenosis and occlusive disease: evaluation with CT angiography, MR angiography, and digital subtraction angiography. AJNR 2005; 26:1012-1021.

†Data from Nguyen-Huynh MN, Wintermark M, English J, et al. How accurate is CT angiography in evaluating intracranial atherosclerotic disease? Stroke 2008; 39:1184-1188.

‡Data from Choi CG, Lee DH, Lee JH, et al. Detection of intracranial atherosclerotic steno-occlusive disease with 3D time-of-flight magnetic resonance angiography with sensitivity encoding at 3T. AJNR Am J Neuroradiol 2007; 28:439-446.

advantage of higher spatial resolution over MRA. MRA is more expensive but does not involve radiation. Noncontrast MRA protocols are generally limited by longer acquisition times and are prone to flow-related artifacts. These problems are averted with contrast-enhanced MRA techniques. CTA and MRA diagnostic accuracy using DSA as a reference standard is illustrated in Table 20-1.[111] CTA is higher in all performance measures and also in interobserver reliability. CTA can also detect low-flow states distal to a tight stenosis in the posterior circulation that may appear occluded on angiography. This may be related to the difference in acquisition times because CTA images are acquired over a longer period, allowing contrast agent to percolate past a tight stenosis. Differentiating a tight stenosis from occlusion is critical for treatment decisions. A tight stenosis may benefit from aggressive antithrombotic or endovascular therapy whereas an occluded vessel may not.

The SONIA trial also showed that MRA measurements of stenosis greater than 50% or presence of a flow gap had a 59% PPV and 91% NPV in detecting stenosis greater than 50% on DSA. To maximize PPV, an MRA measurement of more than 80% stenosis was needed to detect stenosis of more than 50% on DSA with 66% PPV and 87% NPV.

Sensitivity encoding at 3 T has been used to improve performance of 3D-TOF MRA in detecting high grade (50%-99%) intracranial stenosis.[112] The overall diagnostic accuracy is given in Table 20-1.[112] 3D-TOF MRA can overestimate stenoses particularly at the cavernous ICA, ICA bifurcation, and MCA bifurcation, where there is turbulent flow and differential flow velocities. The higher field strength at 3T increases signal-to-noise linearly and increases T1 relaxation times for brain and fat more than blood, making background suppression more effective. Sensitivity encoding reduces the acquisition time by reducing the number of phase-encoding steps. Overall, there is improvement in the image quality and shorter study times.

In summary, MRA is excellent at excluding intracranial stenosis but fares less well at characterizing stenosis when present.[109] CTA achieves higher spatial resolution in a faster time frame but suffers from the usual limitations of radiation dose and contrast injection.

Special Procedures

Digital subtraction angiography remains the reference standard in assessment of the intracranial vessels, mainly for its high spatial resolution and ability to assess flow dynamics. However, its main drawbacks are its invasiveness, length of time for study, complications, expertise requirements, and cost. Transcranial Doppler ultrasonography is a portable and noninvasive alternative. In recent years, CTA and MRA have developed into powerful and relatively low-risk modalities.

The key characteristics of the intracranial arteries are the luminal diameter, wall features, and flow dynamics. In quantifying luminal narrowing, the NACSET method for extracranial carotid disease is used:

$$\text{Percentage stenosis (\%)} = [1 - (\text{narrowest ICA diameter})/ \\ \text{diameter of normal distal vessel}] \\ \times 100\%.$$

The diameter of the normal vessel is typically chosen distal to the stenosis, but some studies have utilized the proximal vessel. There is currently no consensus on stenosis grading, but many agree that narrowing between 50% and 99% is high grade and significant.

Treatment

There is still much debate as to the appropriate management of acute strokes resulting from intracranial disease. Treatment regimens fall into one of three categories: risk modification, antithrombotics/antiplatelets, and endovascular therapies.

Medical therapy is currently the first-line treatment for intracranial atherosclerosis. This includes antiplatelet or anticoagulation drugs and risk factor control. Anticoagulation was first used to treat intracranial arterial stenosis by Millikan in 1955.[113] Subsequent retrospective studies suggested that warfarin may be more effective than aspirin.[104] The WASID study prospectively compared the outcomes of symptomatic patients with intracranial atherosclerosis (50%-99%) treated with either aspirin or warfarin. The study was stopped because of higher rates of adverse events (9.7% vs. 4.3%), major hemorrhage (8.3% vs. 3.2%), and myocardial infarction (7.3% vs. 2.9%) in patients on warfarin, which did not provide any benefit over aspirin.[93] The retrospective component of the study revealed a 50% decrease in stroke incidence but higher incidence of hemorrhage in patients with posterior circulation stenosis treated with warfarin as compared with aspirin.[106] Ischemic stroke, brain hemorrhage, or death from other vascular causes occurred in 22% of patients on either high-dose aspirin (1300 mg/day) or warfarin over 1.8 years. Hence, symptomatic intracranial atherosclerotic stenosis is a marker of aggressive vascular disease.

The Fraxiparine in Ischemic Stroke Study (FISS)[114] found that symptomatic Asian patients receiving high-dose low molecular weight heparin (LMWH) within 48 hours of symptom onset had less occurrence of death or functional dependence after 6 months than those given placebo. They hypothesized that LMWH may reduce the volume of the infarct by limiting the extension of the thrombus to the ischemic penumbra. However, the larger Faxiparine in Ischaemic Stroke Study (FISS-bis) trial could not reproduce these results.[114a] Similarly, the Tinzaparin in Acute Ischemic Stroke Trial (TAIST) showed that low molecular weight heparin did not improve functional outcome in acute stroke patients at 6 months when compared with aspirin.[115]

The multicenter U.S. Trial of ORG 10172 in Acute Stroke Treatment of Intracranial Atherosclerosis trial (TOAST) showed a very favorable outcome in symptomatic patients given intravenous heparinoid after 7 days but no difference after 3 months as compared with placebo.[116] The subset with large vessel intracranial atherosclerosis treated with heparinoid did show a significant increase in favorable and very favorable outcome at 3 months. The results of FISS and TOAST suggest that strokes from intracranial atherosclerosis may respond differently to heparin than strokes caused by extracranial disease. Because Asians have a much higher incidence of intracranial atherosclerotic disease (one third to one half of ischemic strokes in Asia), various studies have assessed the efficacy of heparin specifically in this population. Comparison of subcutaneous low molecular weight heparin with aspirin in acute stroke patients in Hong Kong with large artery occlusive disease[117] showed only a slightly higher incidence of good outcomes in the heparin group at 6 months. The overall consensus was that the results were somewhat neutral and did not have significant benefit. The occurrence of hemorrhagic transformation and adverse events was not different between the two treatment arms.

The National Institutes of Health (NIH)–funded international Extra- to Intracranial Bypass Study randomized symptomatic patients with ICA occlusions, ICA stenosis not accessible to endarterectomy, MCA trunk occlusion, and MCA trunk stenosis. The trial had scrupulous follow-up to completion, and no patient was lost to follow-up. In all four categories there was failure to show benefit of revascularization. In fact, one category, MCA stenosis, was associated with a worse outcome of stroke or death for patients undergoing revascularization. It is postulated that an increase in pressure in peripheral MCA branches after surgery removed the pressure gradient across the MCA trunk stenosis. Subsequently, MCA trunk thrombosis resulted, occluding the adjacent perforator supply with it. This resulted in serious basal ganglia and internal capsule infarctions.

Many microvascular surgeons were upset with the results, and many letters and editorials were written denouncing the Bypass Study as flawed because it scientifically showed the lack of value for the intuitively logical operation. The Carotid Occlusion Surgery Study (COSS), which compared EC-IC bypass to medical management in recently symptomatic atherosclerotic internal carotid occlusions,[117a] attempted to resolve the controversy. The study included extracranial and intracranial carotid occlusions and utilized PET to select patients based on increased oxygen extraction, a marker of hemodynamic ischemia. Despite imaging-based patient selection, the study failed to demonstrate benefits from the surgical procedure. There was no difference in the risk of ipsilateral stroke at 2 years but a significantly increased number of periprocedural strokes in the EC-IC bypass group. Results of the Japanese EC-IC Bypass (JET) Trial are pending. Advances in surgical procedures and imaging technique may improve patient selection and stimulate future studies on this controversial topic. The use of CT and MRI perfusion techniques, and perhaps assessment of cerebrovascular reactivity, may help better identify candidates for revascularization procedures.

Endovascular management for intracranial atherosclerosis is a relatively new approach. This is typically reserved for high-risk stroke patients who have failed maximal medical therapy. The earliest percutaneous transluminal angioplasty (PTA) for intracranial stenosis was reported in 1980 by Sundt and associates.[118] The results of PTA alone have been suboptimal, with high complication rates. In 2000, Gomez and colleagues[119] first reported the addition of selective stenting to PTA in MCA stenosis. It was thought that stents can address some of the complications of PTA alone, which include arterial thrombosis, distal embolization, vessel recoil, dissection, rupture, vasospasm, and perforator stroke. Studies comparing PTA alone with PTA plus stenting for treating petrous and cavernous ICA stenosis showed that the addition of a stent resulted in increased initial luminal dilatation and less restenosis after 6 months.[120] Vessel dissection and recoil of stenosis can be diminished by stent placement, but the intraluminal thrombus and vessel rupture risks still remain.

Results of stenting of symptomatic intracranial stenoses vary. Jiang and coworkers[121] reported a technical success rate of 97.6%, whereas Kim and associates had 85.7% success.[122] The morbidity and mortality rates of the former study were 10% and 2.5%, respectively, and for the latter study 33.3% and 8.3%, respectively. The better outcome in Jiang's patients may partially be accounted for by individualizing therapy based on location, morphology, and access of the M1 lesions. The study showed that all three factors impacted on technical success and clinical outcome.

Complication rates can be reduced by undersizing the balloon and inflating it slowly. If it is undersized too much, stents may migrate and not be completely accommodated in different vessel diameters. Stenting of Symptomatic Atherosclerotic Lesions in the Vertebral or Intracranial Arteries (SSYLVIA)[123] is a prospective study of Neurolink (Guidant, California), a balloon and stent designed specifically for the intracranial arteries. A technical and procedural success rate of 95% was reported. The incidence of postprocedural stroke was 6.6% at 30 days and 13.1% at 1 year. Restenosis occurred in 35% of patients, but 61% of these were asymptomatic. Risk factors for restenosis were diabetes, small pretreatment vessel diameter, and postprocedural stenosis greater than 30%. The investigators described neointimal proliferation after stent insertion conferring a lower risk of thromboembolism than atherosclerosis. Other studies of intracranial stents report 0% incidence of 50% or greater restenosis up to 5 months. Gomez and associates reported a restenosis rate of 10.7%.[119]

One of the unique risks to the intracranial circulation is perforator stroke. These include the lenticulostriate arteries arising from the MCA, the thalamogeniculate arteries arising from the PCA, and the median perforating and circumferential arteries arising from the basilar artery. Displacement of debris by the stent into the ostia of small perforating vessels (referred to as "snowplowing") is one potential cause. Jiang and coworkers[124] report a 3% incidence of perforator strokes after balloon-expandable stent insertion in symptomatic patients with intracranial stenosis. Patients with a preoperative infarct in the territory of a perforator vessel arising from the stenotic segment had a significantly higher frequency of a postprocedural perforator stroke (8.2%) than those without (0.8%). Most occurred during the procedure and reached maximum intensity immediately. All had good functional outcome and reached functional independence by 12 months.

Earlier stents used in intracranial stenosis were balloon-expandable coronary stents, because these were the only ones available.[125] Unlike the coronary arteries, the intracranial vessels lack a thick adventitia, making them vulnerable to injury at the typical 6 to 8 atm of pressure required to inflate a balloon.[125] This can potentially result in the forceful displacement of atheromatous material into branch vessels. High-pressure angioplasty of recently symptomatic plaques can lead to intimal dissection or further plaque displacement and emboli. Some centers use a newer approach termed *submaximal angioplasty* that separates the procedure into two stages. In the first phase, the patient undergoes submaximal angioplasty with a balloon sized to two thirds the parent vessel diameter. The patient returns 4 to 6 weeks later for insertion of a self-expandable stent if the stenosis

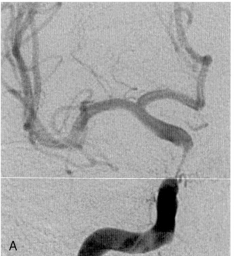
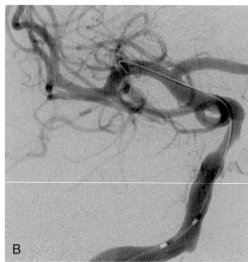

is more than 50%. During the weeks after the initial angioplasty, the damaged vessel has time to undergo intimal fibrosis and remodeling, potentially preventing plaque rupture from later stent insertion. Comparison of periprocedural complications between direct conventional stent placement with that of staged placement in the basilar artery show a lower rate of complication for the staged stent placement.[126]

One main disadvantage of balloon-expandable stents is the limited flexibility of the system. Self-expandable stents are advantageous because they are highly flexible, making them suitable for placement in tortuous vessels such as the distal ICA and MCA.[127] The Wingspan (Boston Scientific) is a new self-expanding stent with initial reports of 98% technical and procedural success. The death and ipsilateral stroke rate was 4.5% at 30 days and 7.0% at 6 months.[128]

Several stents have been given humanitarian device exemption approval by the U.S. Food and Drug Administration (FDA) to treat symptomatic or high-risk patients who have failed medical therapy. Recently, however, the SAMMPRIS trial, a randomized controlled study, was stopped prematurely because of a higher incidence of poor outcome in patients undergoing intracranial stenting. The study evaluated symptomatic stenosis ranging from 70% to 99% and allocated patients to either aggressive medical management alone or in combination with endovascular treatment using the self-expanding Wingspan stent. There was a higher-than-expected 30-day rate of stroke and stroke-related mortality (14.7%) after stenting compared to a lower-than-expected stroke and mortality rate (5.8%, $p = 0.002$) in the medical management arm.[128a] Long-term results and detailed analyses are pending, but this study is expected to significantly alter the use of intracranial stenting for atherosclerosis. Better patient and interventionalist selection and timing of intervention may eventually identify subsets of patients who can benefit from this procedure. In the meantime, endovascular therapies remain an option for carefully selected patients refractory to maximal medical therapy if performed by skilled operators and preferably in the setting of a research protocol.

DISSECTIONS

An arterial dissection is a defect in the intima through which blood dissects into the wall of the vessel. The intramural blood can narrow the true vessel lumen, reducing or obstructing flow, weaken the wall leading to rupture or pseudoaneurysm, or expose the wall to the bloodstream, leading to aggregation of platelets and other products that may subsequently embolize to the distal circulation. These lesions are also referred to as intimal tear, pseudoaneurysm, and dissecting hematoma.

Epidemiology

Dissections can be either traumatic or spontaneous. They can be related to an underlying vascular abnormality such as fibromuscular dysplasia, Marfan syndrome, cystic medial necrosis, and Ehlers-Danlos syndrome type IV. Even fairly minor trauma has been implicated. Predisposition to dissection is reported with hypertension, migraine headaches, oral contraceptives, syphilis, pharyngeal infections, drug abuse (primarily sympathomimetic drugs), physical activity, and smoking.[129] A seasonal variation is described with peak presentation said to occur in the month of October.[130] Pseudoaneurysms are more common in children. Previous dissection or a family history of dissection increases the risk.[131]

Clinical Presentation

Presentation may be determined by the type of dissection. Most dissections are subintimal, with hemorrhage between the intima and media. Less commonly, subadventitial dissection directs the hemorrhage between the media and adventitia[132] and leads to pseudoaneurysm. The intramural thrombus can embolize and lead to a TIA or infarction. Overall, approximately 2% of stroke is caused by dissection. This is higher in younger cohorts. Patients can also develop Horner's syndrome, headache, neck pain, pulsatile tinnitus, or orbital pain. Arterial dissections cause 20% to 30% of ischemic infarctions of the medulla, rarely cause pontine strokes, and account for 5% of ischemic infarctions of the midbrain.[133]

Cranial nerve palsies occur rarely. They involve cranial nerve (CN) XII most often but also affect CN IX, X, and XI. Pseudoaneurysms can enlarge and cause local mass effect or hemorrhage and can act as a emboli source of emboli.

The natural history of stroke risk with dissection is uncertain and has been the subject of some small series. It is reported that 15% to 25% of patients have persistent severe stenosis after dissection.[134] The remaining patients demonstrate recanalization/remodeling over weeks to months. In a retrospective study of a cohort of 71 patients with cervical vessel dissection, 42 (59%) harbored pseudoaneurysms. One third of lesions were asymptomatic. No ischemic complications occurred during a mean 3-year follow-up. A further study of 92 patients with persistent stenosis reported an ipsilateral stroke risk of 0.7%.[134]

Treatment is generally supportive. Antiplatelets or anticoagulation is used despite the lack of evidence for optimal

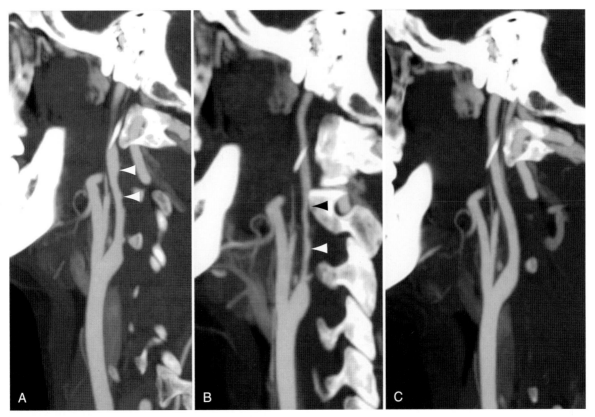

■ FIGURE 20-12 A 35-year-old man presented with right ICA irregularity and narrowing on sagittal CTA MIP image (**A,** *arrowheads*) arising above the carotid bifurcation and extending to the C1-2 level after traumatic ICA dissection. The patient was treated with anticoagulants prophylactically. **B,** Four weeks later there is interval worsening without a change of clinical status (*arrowheads*). **C,** Three months later the condition has nearly completely resolved. Minor irregularity is visible within the mid-carotid segment but distal vessel caliber has returned to normal.

management. Remodeling occurs in many lesions, so often no further treatment is required (Fig. 20-12). Some cases progress to pseudoaneurysm (Fig. 20-13) or become symptomatic from hemodynamic or thromboembolic causes. In patients with carotid or vertebral artery dissection who experience recurrent ischemia despite medical therapy, endovascular procedure (stenting) or surgery may be considered.[84a]

Pathology

Soft tissue injury to the neck can be seen with traumatic dissections. Skull fracture or vertebral column fracture can be seen with traumatic dissections. It is not uncommon for dissection to occur when a cervical fracture crosses a transverse foramen. Intracranial dissections can lead to subarachnoid hemorrhage. The intimal flap can be evident. Hemorrhage can be seen in the divided wall. Thrombus formation can be seen at the site of the intimal tear.

Pathologic findings in dissection are similar to those of any vessel injury. A defect in the endothelium and platelet aggregation may be present. Ultimately a hemostatic plug forms, composed of an amorphous platelet mass and trapped red cells in a mesh of fibrin.[135] The dissection cleft can be seen between the intima and subadventitia, filled with evolving hematoma. Microscopic pathology can also demonstrate the vessel changes consistent with a predisposing arteriopathy such as fibromuscular dysplasia, Marfan syndrome, or Ehlers-Danlos syndrome. Volker and colleagues performed superficial temporal artery biopsies on patients with spontaneous cervical artery dissections. The majority demonstrated pathologic changes, including a zone of connective tissue weakening with fissuring between the tunica media and tunica adventitia, erythrocytes, and other cellular debris in the wall in various stages of degradation, occasional immune cells, and smooth muscle vacuolation.[136]

Imaging

Dissections of the internal carotid and vertebral arteries most commonly occur near the skull base at the C2 region.[137] Vertebral artery dissection can rarely be seen at the vertebral artery origin in the context of iatrogenic injury. Cervical trauma may affect the midvertebral segment. Carotid artery dissections can also be seen just above the bifurcation. Extracranial dissections can extend superiorly but usually terminate at the skull base. Intracranial dissections most commonly occur in the posterior circulation.[138] In the anterior circulation, dissection can occur in the anterior cerebral artery where it crosses under the falx, with pseudoaneurysm formation. In the setting of blunt cervical injury, the modified Denver criteria are used to screen patients for cervical artery dissection.[138a]

Ultrasonography

Ultrasonography can display narrowing or occlusion of the vessel lumen and mixed echogenic material in the wall of the vessel. The intimal flap can be seen. However, it is less sensitive than MRI, CT, or angiography.[139] Generally, patients should go on to a more definitive test if the ultrasound study is negative.[140] Transcranial Doppler imaging can be used to detect embolic hits as a result of a dissection.

CT and CTA

Noncontrast CT is often normal. Sometimes a hyperdense crescent can be seen in the vessel, representing intramural thrombus. If the vessel is completely occluded, a completely

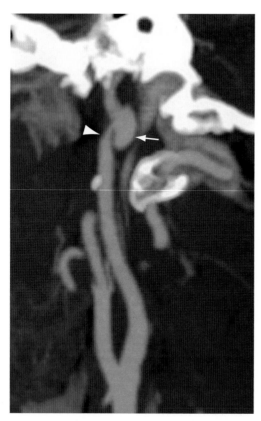

■ **FIGURE 20-13** Sagittal CTA MIP image in a patient with spontaneous dissection demonstrating a pseudoaneurysm at the atlanto-occipital level (*arrow*). There is a characteristic narrowing of the ICA proximal to the pseudoaneurysm (*arrowhead*). The remaining ICA is unremarkable.

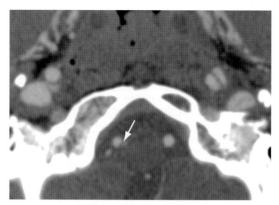

■ **FIGURE 20-14** Axial CTA MIP image demonstrating a dissection flap (*arrow*) and patency of both native and false lumen.

hyperdense lumen can be seen. CTA is very helpful in detecting dissections.[141,142] CTA will demonstrate vessel narrowing or pseudoaneurysm (Fig. 20-13) and occasionally an intimal flap (Fig. 20-14). The false lumen is usually thrombosed. Occasionally (approximately 10% of cases), the false lumen can be seen to fill. Most carotid dissections will terminate at the skull base. The brain should be imaged to detect secondary infarcts. Intracranial dissections can cause subarachnoid hemorrhage, usually detectable by CT.

Dental artifacts may mimic or mask dissections. Where possible, the artifact may be displaced by altering the degree of neck flexion or extension.

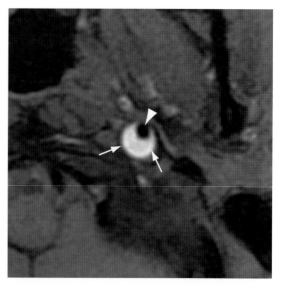

■ **FIGURE 20-15** Axial fat-saturated T1W MR image. There is crescentic T1 hyperintensity, consistent with methemoglobin, expanding the outer ICA luminal diameter (*arrows*) with lesser inner luminal narrowing (*arrowhead*). The appearance is characteristic of a thrombosed false channel.

MRI and MRA

Routine MRI sequences will demonstrate loss of the normal flow void within part of or the entire affected vessel. The intramural thrombus will be bright on T1-weighted (T1W) imaging in the acute to subacute phase (methemoglobin). This is best imaged with a fat-saturated T1W study (Fig. 20-15). MRA will demonstrate luminal narrowing or occlusion.[143] MRI at 3 T provides even greater detail of cervical dissections.[144] Occasionally an intimal flap will be seen. As with CTA, the false lumen will usually be thrombosed but occasionally does show filling. There are numerous potential pitfalls, including false positives secondary to altered flow, poor fat saturation, or slice entry phenomenon, and false negatives may arise from exclusion of arterial segments from the study or lack of methemoglobin in acute intramural hematoma.[144a] Diffusion-weighted imaging can detect the ischemic sequelae of dissections.

Special Procedures

With advanced MRI and CT, angiography is rarely required for dissection diagnosis, although it is still considered the reference standard. Angiography will demonstrate similar findings as MRA and CTA. Luminal narrowing and vessel wall irregularity can be seen. The vessel can be occluded with a tapering "rat tail" appearance. Pseudoaneurysms may be present. The most important current application of angiography is in the treatment of dissections that have failed medical treatment. Extracranial and intracranial stenting is reported, but endovascular vessel occlusion is sometimes required.[145,146] Pseudoaneurysms may be occluded by coils or covered stents.

Analysis

A sample report for MRI and MRA evaluation of a dissection is presented in Box 20-3.

CEREBRAL ISCHEMIA AND INFARCTION

The World Health Organization defines *stroke* as a clinical syndrome of rapid onset of focal cerebral deficit secondary to a vascular etiology lasting 24 hours or resulting in death. The definition includes acute deficits from both ischemic and hemorrhage categories, including global deficit from subarachnoid or intracerebral hemorrhage

TABLE 20-2.   Oxford Classification

Classification	Description
Lacunar infarct (LACI)	Pure motor or sensory stroke, sensorimotor stroke, or ataxic hemiparesis
Total anterior circulation infarct (TACI)	Combination of higher cerebral dysfunction including dysphasia, dyscalculia, visuospatial disorder; homonymous hemianopia and ipsilateral motor and/or sensory deficit of at least two areas of the face, arm, and leg
Partial anterior circulation infarct (PACI)	Two of the three components described above, including higher cerebral dysfunction alone or with a motor/sensory deficit less than LACI
Posterior circulation infarct (POCI)	Ipsilateral cranial nerve palsy with contralateral motor and/or sensory deficit, bilateral motor and/or sensory deficit, disorder of conjugate eye movement; cerebellar dysfunction without ipsilateral long-tract deficit (i.e., ataxic hemiparesis) or isolated homonymous visual field defect

Epidemiology

Stroke is the third most common cause of death globally. It is the second most common cause in the United States in people older than 60 years and the fifth leading cause of death in people 15 to 59 years of age.[147] There are more than 700,000 strokes per year in the United States. Approximately 50% of stroke survivors have disability, with 20% requiring transfer to skilled nursing facilities.[148] Survivors are at greater risk for recurrent stroke, resulting in significant morbidity and co-contributing to other morbidity, such as falls, seizure, dementia, and depression.

Imaging is central to the prevention and treatment of stroke. Carotid stenosis greater than or equal to 50% is found in 10% to 15% of patients with ipsilateral ischemic stroke and TIA, respectively.[9,10]

Clinical Presentation

Classification of Stroke

Differing classifications of stroke etiology are based on the mechanism of ischemia, type of vascular injury, or territorial localization. In the United States, ischemic stroke accounts for approximately 80% of all strokes, intracerebral hemorrhage (ICH) for 15%, and subarachnoid hemorrhage (SAH) for 5%. Approximately 50% of ischemic infarction is secondary to larger artery-to-artery atherosclerotic embolization from the extracranial circulation. Intracranial stenosis contributes less in the Western nations but is a major cause in Asia.[149] Cardioembolism accounts for 20%, small vessel disease for 25%, and rarer causes, including dissection, vasculitis, hypercoagulable states, venous occlusion, and undefined causes, for the remainder.[150-152] Incidence of stroke subtypes varies geographically and with patient age. ICH, for example, occurs more commonly as a cause of stroke in Asia, where the incidence is 20% to 44% of stroke presentations.[153] Stroke prognosis, recurrence risk, and management options are dependent on stroke subtype. When assessing a patient with stroke, therefore, it is crucial to attempt to categorize stroke etiology. A commonly used classification scheme is the TOAST criteria (Trial of ORG 1072 in Acute Treatment of Intracranial Atherosclerosis).[152] There are five categories: (1) large artery atherosclerosis including large artery thrombosis with artery to artery atheroembolus, (2) cardioembolism, (3) small artery occlusion, (4) stroke of other determined cause (OC), and (5) stroke of indeterminate cause (UND).

A further approach for infarct classification is the Oxford classification, which distinguishes geographic location (anterior vs. posterior circulation) and severity based on clustering of clinical symptoms (Table 20-2).[154]

A study using acute multimodal imaging including DWI and perfusion-weighted imaging found that the highest agreement between clinical assessment of infarct location and confirmatory presence on imaging was for total anterior circulation territory infarct (TACI). A partial anterior circulation infarct had much lower accuracy for location prediction.[155]

Risk Factors

Despite the heterogeneity of stroke subtype, the risk factors for stroke remain similar to those for vascular disease and include age, hypertension, cigarette smoking, diabetes mellitus, hypercholesterolemia, and obesity.[156] However, hypertension appears more closely associated with stroke than ischemic heart disease.[157] There is growing interest in genetic factors and inflammatory and infective causes that may accelerate the atherosclerotic process.[158-160] Numerous single gene disorders are now described that are associated with ischemic stoke by virtue of accelerated atherosclerosis,[161] predisposition to dissection (Marfan syndrome, Ehler-Danlos syndrome), small vessel arteriopathy,[162] disorders of coagulation (sickle cell disease), and metabolic processes (mitochondrial encephalopathy, lactic acidosis, and stroke-like episodes [MELAS]).

Pathophysiology

Infarction occurs when cerebral perfusion is unable to meet the metabolic demands of the tissue it is supplying. Cerebral autoregulation maintains constant cerebral blood flow (CBF) over a wide range of systemic pressure. After vascular occlusion, CBF is maintained by capillary vasodilatation of the distal microcirculation with a resultant increase in cerebral blood volume (CBV) and prolongation of the arterial transit time.[163] The extent to which the collateral circulation contributes effective perfusion depends on the severity of proximal vascular occlusion. Pathophysiologic studies demonstrate that *functional disturbances* occur when the CBF drops below 15 to 25 mL/100 g/min (30%-40% of normal), but *irrecoverable neuronal damage* occurs only when CBF falls below the critical threshold of 10 to 15 mL/100 g/min (<20% of normal). The brain's ability to tolerate such reductions in CBF is dependent on the duration and severity of ischemia[164-166] and the inherent vulnerability of affected tissue. The greater the severity of ischemia, the more rapid is the transition from symptom onset to infarction. Less severe reductions in CBF may be tolerated for long periods of time with viable penumbral tissue reported beyond 48 hours.[167-169] When inadequate perfusion leads to failure of the adenosine triphosphate pump, there is a shift of water from

TABLE 20-3. Evolution of Stroke on CT

Hyperacute (<6 hr)
Noncontrast CT
  Normal
  Early ischemic signs
  Hyperdense middle cerebral artery sign
  Primary intracranial or subarachnoid hemorrhage
CTA
  Occlusion/stenosis
  Collateral assessment
CTA-SI
  Hypodensity
CTP
  Perfusion abnormality

Acute (<24 hr)
Loss of gray-white differentiation
Sulcal effacement
Intra-arterial enhancement

Subacute (<1 wk)
Edema, mass effect (peaks 3-4 days)
Shift
Gyral and meningeal enhancement
Hemorrhagic transformation

Subacute to Chronic (1 wk to 2 mo)
Edema/mass effect resolution
Parenchymal enhancement
CT fogging

Chronic (>2 mo)
Encephalomalacia, gliosis
Sulcal and ventricular enlargement/parenchymal volume loss
Wallerian degeneration

TABLE 20-4. Evolution of Stroke on MRI

Hyperacute (<6 hr)
Conventional MRI, FLAIR, and DWI
  Hypointense MCA sign
  Loss of flow voids
  Slow intravascular flow
  DWI restriction
  Intravascular contrast enhancement
MRP
  Perfusion abnormality

Acute (<24 hr)
Blurring of gray matter/white matter interface
T2 hyperintensity cortex
Gyral swelling and sulcal effacement
Intravascular/meningeal enhancement

Subacute (<1 wk)
T1 hypointensity and T2 hyperintensity
Peak edema and mass
Shift
Hemorrhagic transformation

Subacute to Chronic (1 wk to 2 mo)
Edema/mass effect resolution
Meningeal enhancement
Parenchymal enhancement
MR fogging

Chronic (>2 mo)
Encephalomalacia, gliosis
Sulcal and ventricular enlargement/parenchymal volume loss
Wallerian degeneration

the extracellular to intracellular compartment, resulting in cell swelling. Fifteen to 30 minutes[170,171] after infarction, there is a net increase in tissue water that may be mediated through the osmotic effect of a shrinking extracellular space and ingress of water from the adjacent vasculature.[172,173]

The region of hypoperfusion contains three distinct zones. The *central zone* is the infarct core, where failure of the ion pump and depolarization of the cell membrane result in shift of water from extracellular to intracellular compartments (cytotoxic edema) and inevitable cell death. In about half of all acute stroke patients, a *penumbral zone* of electrically inactive but viable neurons surrounds the core.[174] Tissue within this zone may remain viable for up to 48 hours, so the penumbral tissue is the target for therapeutic thombolysis.[167,168] Peripherally, there is an *outer zone* of oligemia, in which mildly hypoperfused tissue is unlikely to proceed to infarction, unless there is an additional insult, such as progressive reduction of perfusion pressure from vasogenic edema or metabolic derangements such as hyperglycemia. The sites and extents of these three zones may be defined on CT and MRI by using published threshold values for the absolute and relative values of CBF, CBV, and mean transit time (MTT) (see Table 20-6).[175-177] The infarction may progress and enlarge from the core into penumbra over hours to days. Hyperglycemia, advanced age, and hypoxia frequently accelerate this process.[178,179] Many cellular processes are implicated in infarct growth into the penumbra, including progression of cytotoxic edema, apoptosis, late energy failure, reperfusion injury, mechanical compression, and microvascular congestion.[169,180,181]

Imaging

Stroke is a dynamic process that is best divided into the hyperacute, acute, subacute, and chronic time periods. The specific imaging findings vary with the period after infarction and with the modality used for imaging (Tables 20-3 and 20-4).

In the hyperacute period, imaging is used to determine the subtype of the stroke, to select patients who may be eligible for thrombolytic or neuroprotective treatment, to exclude patients in whom such treatment is contraindicated, and to identify those patients in whom other conditions mimic strokes. The two major questions to be addressed in the hyperacute stroke patient are (1) is there hemorrhage and (2) what is the extent of the ischemic change. Beyond that, advanced imaging attempts to predict final infarct size,[182,183] distinguish the infarct core from the penumbral tissue at risk,[175-177] identify special risks to performing antithrombotic/thrombolytic therapy,[184,185] localize the site(s) of vessel occlusion, and characterize the morphology of the carotid plaque. MRI and CT are the modalities most widely used for these purposes. Which of the two is employed is determined largely by local resources and specific clinical information required. Their relative roles are discussed next.

CT

Acute Imaging

CT is the most widely available, affordable, and effective modality for the investigation and diagnosis of acute stroke patients. A typical CT protocol includes noncontrast CT, CTA (arch to vertex, and increasingly cardiac apex to vertex), contrast-enhanced CT, and CT perfusion (CTP).

After the noncontrast CT acquisition an arterial phase contrast-enhanced CT or CTA study is performed from arch to vertex. A typical CT sequence is acquired with 1.25-mm thick slices reconstructed to 0.6 mm. A kVp of 80 is commonly employed, because this kVp is close to the k-edge for iodinated contrast agents,[186] permitting a twofold to threefold dose reduction versus conventional values of 120 to 140 kVp. The volume of contrast agent injected varies between 50 and 80 mL. The acquisition is usually triggered by a bolus tracking technique or alternatively initiated after a preset 5- to 10-second delay. Venous contamination is common but may be reduced by beginning the study further cranially (to image the arteries before there has been significant venous return) or by scanning in the reverse direction from the vertex downward.[37] The region of interest will determine the direction or starting point of the CTA

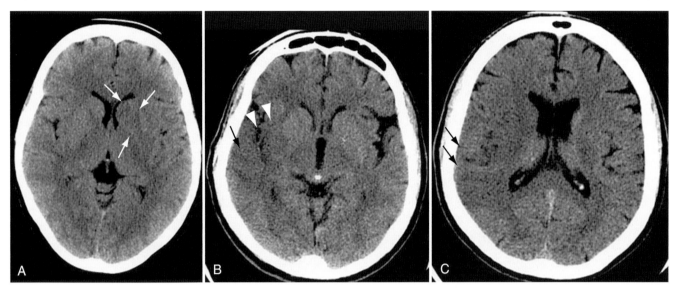

■ **FIGURE 20-16**   Noncontrast CT studies of early ischemic signs. All represent loss of gray matter density. **A,** Loss of the left caudate head and putamen (*arrows*). **B,** Right insular and posterior putaminal loss (*arrowheads*). Temporal operculum has lost gray matter/white matter differentiation (*arrow*). **C,** Right caudate head and body and parietal gray matter density loss with frontoparietal sulcal effacement (*arrows*).

acquisition. For carotid imaging an arch-up approach is used. For intracranial vasculature the acquisition may be started at C5-6 or at the vertex.

CT perfusion is acquired using a cine mode with rapid temporal sampling of a 2- to 4-cm volume after the intravenous injection of a contrast agent. The length of dynamic acquisition varies typically between 45 and 60 seconds. Obtaining clinically useful perfusion maps requires a balance between the temporal scan interval and volume of contrast bolus administered. The minimum scan interval is important in determining the best strategies to increase spatial coverage.[186] The perfusion study can be extended and biphasic with a reduced frequency of temporal sampling in the second portion of the scan to acquire permeability data simultaneously.

Acute and Subacute Infarct Detection—Noncontrast CT
Subtle infarctions can be difficult to detect by noncontrast CT. However, this difficulty poses no clinical limitation, because the intended targets for thrombolysis are precisely those patients with no evidence of gross infarction on CT. Extensive infarctions are less difficult to detect and must be appreciated, because patients with extensive infarction are more likely to suffer complications with thrombolysis. The criteria for diagnosing an extensive infarction are controversial.

Infarcts become visible on noncontrast CT when failure to perfuse the tissue leads to failure to maintain fluid homeostasis within the cell. Fluid then shifts from the extracellular compartment into the intracellular compartment. Such fluid shifts do not change the net tissue water, so they are not, themselves, enough to permit detection of the infarction. There must also be a net increase in the total volume of fluid present. The mechanism by which additional water accumulates is not known for certain, but it is thought that shifting fluid into the intracellular space changes the osmolality of the extracellular space and thereby creates a gradient for fluid to pass across the adjacent capillaries into the injured tissue.[173] Each 1% gain in tissue water is associated with a 1.5- to 2.4-HU change in tissue density.[187,188] The minimum change in tissue water needed to detect an infarction on noncontrast CT is 2% to 3%, corresponding to a density change of about 4 HU.[189] The edema fluid accumulates preferentially within the gray matter, lowering the density of the gray matter so that it becomes nearly equal to the density

of the white matter. This phenomenon is called "loss of gray matter/white matter distinction or differentiation" or early ischemic signs.

Noncontrast CT may detect ischemic change as soon as 45 minutes after infarction.[190] Within 6 hours of an acute infarction, noncontrast CT may show hypodensity of the gray matter. Early alterations in the normal unenhanced CT appearance are called early ischemic signs and usually indicate irreversible ischemia. The early ischemic signs include hypoattenuation, loss of gray matter/white matter distinction, blurring/loss of basal ganglia outline,[191] loss of the insular ribbon,[192] loss of the caudate stripe, cerebral swelling,[193] and cortical sulcal effacement (Fig. 20-16). All but the last two signs are simply specific instances of the reduced density of gray matter with loss of gray matter/white matter distinction. Two methods are used to quantify the extent of early ischemic signs: (1) The 1/3 MCA rule arose from the first European Cooperative Acute Stroke Study (ECASS I)[194] but was not clearly defined until more than 6 years later,[195] resulting in variable interobserver agreement.[196,197] The Alberta Program Early CT Score (ASPECTS) is a 10-point score of the MCA territory. One point is assigned to each of the caudate, putamen, internal capsule, insula, and six cortical regions. For each ASPECT region showing low density, 1 point is subtracted from the best possible score of 10. An infarction of the basal ganglia causing lucency in the caudate, putamen, and internal capsule would receive an Aspect sore of 10 − 3 = 7 (Fig. 20-17).

The score has the advantage of high interobserver and intraobserver agreement[198-200] and is easy to apply. Early results indicated a sharp cutoff at a threshold of 7, with scores lower than 7 predictive of higher risk of hemorrhage and poor outcome. Retrospective application to several intravenous and intra-arterial thrombolytic trials, however,[201-204] demonstrated a more gradual worsening in outcome with score reduction.

A meta-analysis of 15 eligible studies and 3468 patients[205] found that the positive early ischemic symptoms were associated with a threefold higher risk of poor outcome. Symptoms affecting more than a third of the MCA territory in the ECASS I study[194] were associated with a trend to increased mortality with recombinant tissue plasminogen activator (tPA) treatment. This finding could not be confirmed in ECASS II nor in the National Institute of Neurological Disorders and Stroke (NINDS) dataset.[206,207] Despite a lack of treatment interaction with thrombolysis, the

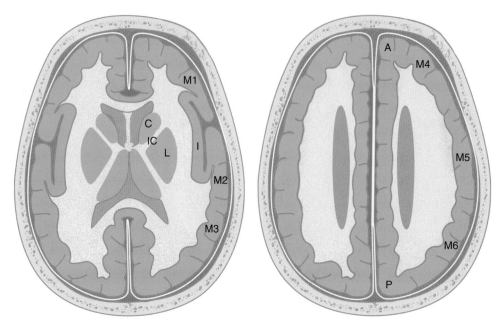

■ **FIGURE 20-17**   ASPECTS study form. A, Anterior circulation; P, posterior circulation; C, caudate; L, lentiform; IC, internal capsule; I, insular ribbon; MCA, middle cerebral artery; M1, frontal cortex; M2, temporal operculum; M3, temporo-occipital MCA cortex; M4, M5, and M6 are anterior, middle, and posterior MCA territories immediately superior to MI, M2, and M3, rostral to basal ganglia. Subcortical structures are allotted 3 points (C, L, and IC). MCA cortex is allotted 7 points (insular cortex, M1, M2, M3, M4, M5, and M6). *(From Barber PA, Demchuk AM, Zhang J, et al. Validity and reliability of a quantitative computed tomography score in predicting outcome of hyperacute stroke before thrombolytic therapy. Lancet 2000; 355:1670-1674.)*

■ **FIGURE 20-18**   Noncontrast CT with standard (**A**: WW 80, WL 40) and stroke (**B**: WW 35, WL 35) windows. There is subtle loss of right corpus striatum that is more easily appreciated with the narrower stroke window (*arrows*).

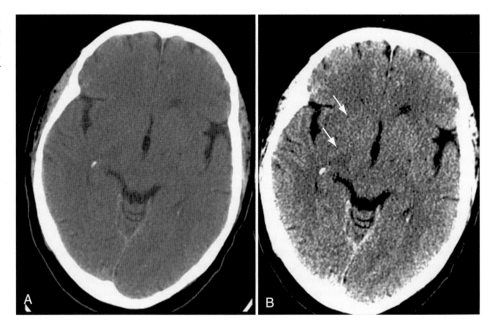

presence of hypodensity is associated with a worse clinical outcome and higher risk of hemorrhage.[208,209] The detection of early ischemic symptoms therefore remains key to the correct diagnosis of stroke, and the extent may determine whether a patient receives thrombolysis treatment.

Unfortunately, early ischemic symptoms are poorly recognized, with a reported sensitivity of 30% within 3 hours[206] and 60% within 6 hours after infarction.[208] Meta-analysis of 15 studies showed that the mean sensitivity and specificity for detecting early ischemic symptoms on noncontrast CT were 66% (range, 20%-87%) and 87% (range, 56%-100%), respectively.[205] Use of a narrow "stroke window" (window width and level of 35 HU)

improves sensitivity by increasing the distinction between gray and white matter density (Fig. 20-18). Knowledge of infarction side does not appear to improve detection[210-212]; increasing reader experience does.[213] Overall, noncontrast CT may be negative in 40% to 60% of cases within 3 hours. Non-neuroradiologists are reported to have a low interobserver agreement for detecting early ischemic symptoms on unenhanced CT (0.14 to 0.78).[205] In the period 2 to 3 weeks after ictus, the density of the ischemic infarction changes from hypodensity to isodensity, rendering the infarct very difficult to appreciate. The obscuration effect is called "CT fogging." The etiology of the change is uncertain. A similar finding may be seen at MRI.

Acute and Subacute Detection: CTA

CTA displays the intracranial vessels. It provides valuable information on vessel occlusion, helps define the degree of collateralization, and improves infarct detection.[214,215] The 0.6- to 1.25-mm thick axial source data slices require reconstruction to thicker slices, usually 3 mm, because otherwise excessive noise precludes easy infarct visualization. Gray matter normally has a higher CBF and a larger CBV than white matter. Because injected contrast material partitions in proportion to the CBF and CBV of the tissue, contrast-enhanced studies can depict ischemic infarctions as regions of altered CBF and CBV. The sensitivity and specificity of MCA infarct detection, excluding small lacunar lesions, is 75% to 95% and 80% to 90%, respectively.[216] Hypodensity visible on CTA source images (CTA-SI) signifies a reduction in whole brain blood volume (CBV)[214,217] and therefore represents a different physiologic process distinct from the cytotoxic edema visualized on noncontrast CT. The volume of infarct detected on CTA-SI significantly correlates with the abnormality seen in DWI and is an independent predictor of final infarct volume in patients presenting within 6 hours of infarct.[214] The sharper definition between gray and white matter also displays the geographic extent of the infarction more clearly (Fig. 20-19) and facilitates ASPECT scoring,[209] particularly by less experienced readers.[216]

Hemorrhage Detection

For patients with acute stroke, the single most important function of noncontrast CT is the exclusion of hemorrhage. Intracranial hemorrhage is a contraindication to thrombolysis. The imaging features of intraparenchymal hemorrhage of differing ages are well described.[218-221] In diagnosing acute hemorrhage, however, one must always consider the patient's hematocrit/hemoglobin, to allow for the lower density of acute hemorrhage in severely anemic patients.[222] The diagnostic performance of CT and MRI for detecting hemorrhage remains controversial. CT has long been considered the reference standard based on level 3 evidence. However, the study cited analyzed the detection of subarachnoid not parenchymal blood[223] and the features of the two clearly differ. Detection of hemorrhage depends on the time interval since ictus. CT sensitivity falls from 98% to 100% within 12 hours after ictus to 93% to 95% within 24 hours and 74% to 84% after 2 days.[223,224]

Vascular Assessment: Noncontrast CT

Flowing blood has a density range of 35 to 60 HU. Thrombus has a higher density range of 70 to 90 HU, owing to the exclusion of serum from the clot and consequently increased electron density of the coagulum.[225] Therefore, an additional noncontrast CT sign of hyperacute stroke is hyperdensity within the intracranial vasculature: the hyperdense vessel sign.[226] This was first described in the MCA as the hyperdense MCA sign (Fig. 20-20), which is present in 35% to 50% of such patients. It is defined as hyperdensity of the affected M1 segment versus another vessel of similar size (e.g., the contralateral MCA). This definition excludes the pseudohyperdense sign caused by atherosclerosis, calcification, and raised hematocrit, which produces bilateral and variably symmetrical hyperdensity (Fig. 20-20).[227] Atherosclerosis and calcification may usually be distinguished from thrombosis by their higher attenuation (120-320 HU). Hyperdensity can occur in any vessel or branch, including the M2 and M3 segments of the MCA ("sylvian dot sign") (Fig. 20-21),[228] the PCA,[229] and the basilar artery[230] but is less commonly observed in the ACA. Conventional angiography has confirmed that thrombotic occlusion of the MCA is the cause of the hyperdense MCA sign.[231,232] The presence of a proximal thrombus is associated with poorer outcome, lower thrombolytic response,[233] and variable mortality of 5% to 45%. The sign is easily detected with high interobserver agreement and has a reasonable sensitivity of 72%

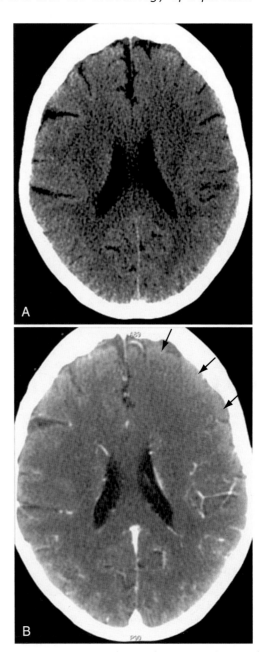

■ **FIGURE 20-19** Noncontrast CT and CTA source images. The noncontrast image appears normal, but the concurrent CTA source image demonstrates a reduction of gray matter attenuation within the left frontal lobe (*arrows*).

and specificity and accuracy of 93% and 91%, respectively. The density and the thrombus burden measured on thin-slice (<2.5 mm) non-contrast CT is reported to predict the likelihood of recanalization.[233a] Knowledge of likelihood of recanalization for a given thrombus may be a useful guide to determine the most appropriate modality of reperfusion therapy.[233b] Recently a hypodense MCA sign was reported with fat embolism.[234] Calcific emboli are rarely visible on noncontrast CT but when seen usually embolize from the heart valves. Other reported cases include post–coronary catheterization putatively from calcific aortic stenosis and spontaneous brachicephalic embolus in a patient with heavily calcified vessel after breast irradiation for carcinoma.

Vascular Assessment: CTA

The primary purpose of CTA is to determine the nature, site, and extent of vessel disease and to assess the collateral circulation. The site of vascular occlusion is of major importance, because it determines the probability of recanalization,[235,236] infarct progression, and outcome.[237-239] Different treatment approaches may be utilized according to the site of occlusion (Fig. 20-22). Intravenous thrombolysis is associated with a low recanalization rate for terminal ICA occlusion (15%-20%),[240] increasing to 26% to 40% for proximal MCA and 40% to 100% for distal MCA occlusions. Intra-arterial or mechanical approaches are associated with higher rates of proximal vessel recanalization. ICA terminus and proximal

MCA recanalization is achievable in 60% to 65% of cases.[235,241] Vascular imaging may also provide prognostic information relating to the degree of recanalization. This is important because patients with greatest patency restoration are most likely to achieve good clinical outcomes[242] and apparent diffusion coefficient (ADC) normalization.[243] Modern CTA has a spatial resolution of 0.5 to 0.7 mm, providing isotropic data for multiplanar reconstruction. Several techniques are available for vascular assessment including volume rendering, surface shaded display, maximum intensity projection (MIP), and multiplanar reconstruction (MPR). Discussion of individual techniques is beyond the scope of this chapter and the reader is referred elsewhere.[244] Individual use is often predicated by preference; however, we find the use of a thin-slab MIP the most useful technique, allowing rapid assessment for site of occlusion or other vascular abnormality without the need for bone subtraction algorithms. The MIP thickness may be selected according to the size of the vessel being imaged. We use a 7-mm thickness to demonstrate both intracranial and extracranial vasculature from arch to vertex. Limitations include vessel, bone, or calcium superimposition, which seldom present a problem when viewed in the thin-slab format. The sensitivity and specificity for proximal sites of vessel occlusion are 83% to 100% and 99% to 100%, respectively, based on conventional angiographic comparisons, but is lower for more distal occlusions.[245,246]

CTA source images (CTA-SI) are shown to be more sensitive and accurate in the detection and delineation of early ischemic changes compared to unenhanced CT.[246a-246c] CTA-SIs provide assessment of the whole brain compared to the often limited volume of acquisition achievable by the more prevalent 64-slice CTP protocols. Hypodensity seen on CTA-SI was previously shown to correspond to CBV,[38a] a surrogate marker of infarct core. However these studies were performed on slower, earlier generation CT scanners resulting in postcontrast image acquisition during the steady state, which allowed contrast to reach the blood vessels in the ischemic/infarct region associated with prolonged transit time. Newer scanners permit rapid image acquisition, and hypodensity now mainly reflects CBF,[246d,246e] or tissue at risk. An important proviso is that no prior contrast injection has been given (e.g., perfusion CT). The role of CTA in acute stroke remains the delineation of vascular anatomy, including site of occlusion and presence of collaterals. CTA protocols should be optimized for vascular, not parenchymal, imaging. Estimation of infarct volume on CTA-SI was useful when CT perfusion (CTP) was not widely available but should not be relied upon with modern scanners. CTP provides outstanding estimates of core and tissue at risk and is preferred. For centers where CTP is unavailable, postcontrast CT (PCT), performed after CTA, demonstrates hypodensity that closely estimates core.

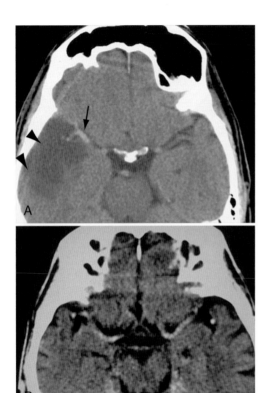

■ **FIGURE 20-20**   **A,** Noncontrast CT in a patient with increased vessel density within the right middle cerebral artery (MCA) relative to the left (*arrow*). There is an established right temporal lobe infarct (*arrowheads*). Findings are consistent with a hyperdense sign and M1 and M2 segment MCA thrombus. **B,** Pseudohyperdense sign. Bilateral increased vessel density is appreciated.

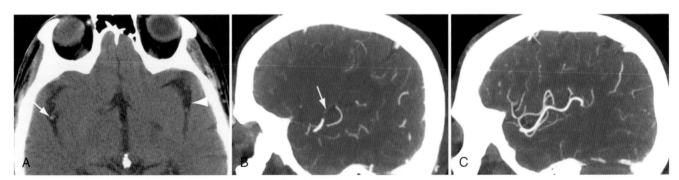

■ **FIGURE 20-21**   **A,** Noncontrast CT demonstrating hyperdensity within the right sylvian fissure consistent with the sylvian dot sign (*arrow*). Note the increased density of the M2 segment relative to the contralateral M2 vessel (*arrowhead*). **B,** Parasagittal CT angiogram on the affected side demonstrates abrupt termination of the MCA with lesser density seen peripheral to this (*arrow*). **C,** The normal contralateral side is given for comparison.

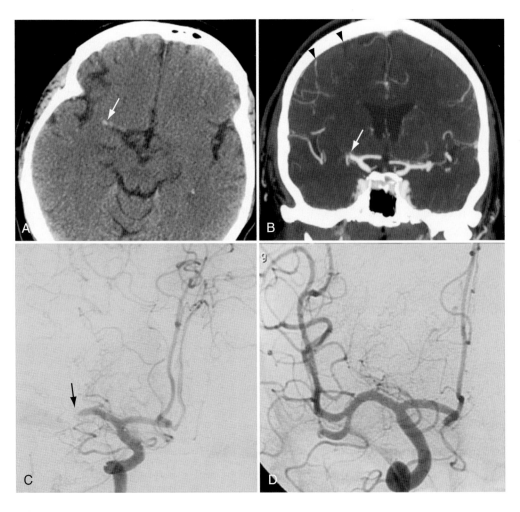

■ **FIGURE 20-22** A 52-year-old woman presented within 45 minutes of a left hemiplegia. **A,** Noncontrast CT demonstrates a hyperdense right middle cerebral artery (MCA) sign (*arrow*), confirmed to represent occlusion of the M1 segment of the right MCA on coronal MIP CTA (*arrow*, **B**). Good collaterals are seen over the brain surface (*arrowheads*). The presence of proximal MCA occlusion facilitated the decision to treat aggressively with a combination of intravenous and intra-arterial tPA. **C,** Initial anteroposterior cerebral angiogram confirmed MCA occlusion (*arrow*). **D,** Final angiogram confirms restoration of vessel patency (TIMI 3).

PCT can be obtained at lower dose than a CTP and in those institutions where CTP is not available.

Finally, CTA provides information on the degree of leptomeningeal collateralization. In large vessel involvement, such as carotid termination or proximal MCA occlusion, the identification of collateral flow may be an important consideration when selecting therapeutic options. The absence of collateral vessels is associated with a poor outcome in the absence of reperfusion, while the presence of good collateral flow correlates with smaller final infarct size and better clinical outcome.[246f-246h]

Role of Contrast

Contrast enhancement has improved stroke visualization and determination of stroke extent by CT. The use of contrast in stroke has historically been controversial. Early studies reported neurotoxicity from using hyperosmolar contrast agents in animal[247] and human[248,249] studies. One large case series showed that stroke patients receiving contrast agents did worse than those who did not. However, there was no prescribed CT or contrast agent administration protocol for stroke investigation at that time. The usual practice was to administer contrast medium only in patients exhibiting signs of mass effect in order to exclude intracranial tumors. This approach introduced selection bias, because patients with worse infarcts and poorer outcomes received the contrast agent. A further study, using high doses of hyperosmolar contrast media for acute stroke,[249] showed frank hemorrhage on delayed scanning in cases with infarction associated with contrast leakage. We now know these findings are consistent with increased permeability in tissue with advanced blood-brain barrier breakdown (Fig. 20-23). Although the author

presented the technique as a predictive test for hemorrhagic transformation, there were detractors who claimed that the use of double contrast was the cause rather than marker of hemorrhage. The use of contrast agents in stroke fell into disrepute. New studies using low or iso-osmolar contrast agents reported no adverse effect of contrast use on cerebral ischemic infarctions.[250]

The administration of contrast media, a prerequisite to these advanced CT techniques, may theoretically increase the risk of contrast-induced nephropathy. Multiple studies have now demonstrated the overall good safety profile of iodinated contrast administration in the acute stroke population.[250a-250e] In patients at high risk of contrast-induced nephropathy, preventive measures, including the use of low-osmolar contrast agents and hydration, are recommended.

CT Perfusion

The literature on CT perfusion (CTP) is scarce compared with that for MRI, but the same principles underlie both techniques. CTP is a feasible and inexpensive[251] addition to stroke imaging.[252-254] Studies comparing MR perfusion (MRP) and CTP are limited but show good correlation, so clinical applications are likely to be similar.[183] CTP has a higher spatial resolution (1.5 × 1.5 × 5 cm) than MRP but is limited by spatial coverage, ionizing radiation, and iodinated contrast injection. The extended coverage provided by 64-slice scanners combined with the table toggle technique[255] or reduced scan acquisition and repeat injection may allow for greater coverage.[256] Clinical information is essential to maximize the accuracy of CTP so that the zone of acquisition may be positioned correctly, for example, over the

■ **FIGURE 20-23** A 52-year-old, right-handed woman presented with left hemiplegia that was successfully treated with intra-arterial thrombolysis. **A,** Immediate postprocedural noncontrast CT demonstrates generalized increased striatal density with more focal posterior putaminal density (*arrow*). The follow-up study at 24 hours (not shown) was unremarkable. Appearances are most consistent with contrast enhancement rather than extravasation. **B,** Gradient-recalled-echo MR image performed 1 week later demonstrates hemorrhagic transformation (hemorrhagic infarct type 1 [HT1]) within the region of most intense enhancement on the prior study (*arrow*).

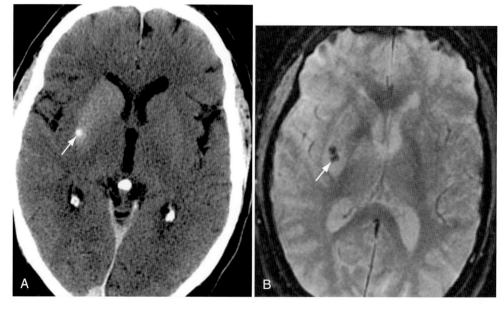

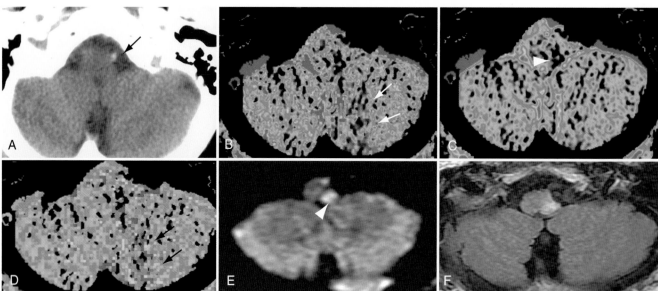

■ **FIGURE 20-24** A 48-year-old man presented with acute onset of clinically suspected Wallenberg's syndrome (lateral medullary syndrome). **A,** Noncontrast CT demonstrates left vertebral artery hyperdensity consistent with thrombus (*arrow*). **B to D,** Cerebral blood flow, cerebral blood volume, and mean transit time were centered on the region of interest. Maps confirm an inferior cerebellar peduncle infarct (*arrowhead*) with ischemia within the ipsilateral PICA territory (*arrows*). Patient received tPA. DWI (**E**) and FLAIR imaging (**F**) 24 hours later confirmed inferior cerebellar penduncular infarct (*arrowhead*) and resolution of cerebellar.

posterior fossa for a suspected brain stem lesion (Fig. 20-24). Compared to noncontrast CT or a combination of noncontrast CT and CTA-source images, the addition of CTP improves the accuracy and interobserver and intraobserver variability for acute stroke detection.[246b,256a] The accuracy of CTP for stroke detection and determination of extent is 72% to 86%. Sensitivities and specificities lie between 78% and 95%, respectively. False-negative results are usually due to inadequate spatial coverage, lacunar infarcts, or failure to detect multiple small emboli (Fig. 20-25).[257] The radiation dose associated with CTP depends on the scan parameters set, but under normal circumstances with careful attention to scan parameters[186] a 2-cm coverage can be achieved with an effective dose less than a standard noncontrast CT.[258] In contradistinction to MRI there is a linear relationship between iodinated contrast concentration and attenuation,

and quantitative measures of blood flow, blood volume, and transit time are possible. Integrity of the blood-brain barrier may be assessed by prolonging the CTP acquisition with reduced temporal resolution to restrict radiation dose delivery. Permeability imaging is a promising way to predict both hemorrhagic transformation and malignant edema.[258a,258b]

Clinical studies have reported mixed results regarding penumbral-based decision. One recent retrospective study of delayed endovascular recanalization (>8 hours) demonstrated encouraging results in carefully selected patients based on CTP mismatch.[258c] Other encouraging MR-based phase II studies, such as DIAS, EPITHET, and DEDAS, have also stimulated the interest in perfusion imaging. Despite these promising first steps, the largest prospective randomized trial using penumbral-based patient selection, DIAS-2, failed to show a benefit in the treated

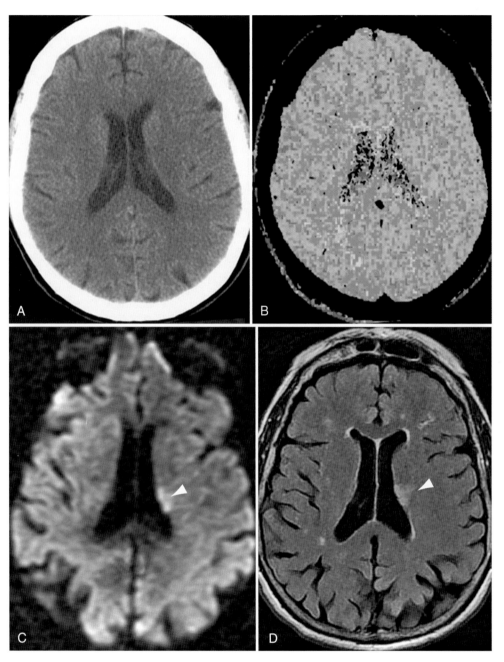

■ **FIGURE 20-25** Noncontrast CT (**A**) and mean transit time map (**B**) in a 60-year-old woman with acute-onset right hemiplegia reveals no abnormality. DWI (**C**) and FLAIR imaging (**D**) reveal corona radiata infarct (*arrowheads*) and other non-specific white matter hyperintensities consistent with microangiopathic change.

arm.[258d] This trial was mainly based on MRI DWI-PWI mismatch, although CTP was used in approximately 20% of the cases. Several limitations to this study have been identified and may explain the negative results in the face of this conceptually pleasing technique.[258e] Another recent retrospective study also failed to demonstrate an improvement in short-term favorable clinical outcome when CTP-guided endovascular treatment was used.[258f] Further technical refinements as well as better standardization and validation of CTP are needed before its benefit can be proved in clinical trials. To better achieve these goals, technical recommendations for stroke imaging were published for both CT and MR.[258g]

MRI

Technique

The MRI environment challenges physicians caring for the acutely ill stroke patient. It takes time just to place a new patient into the MR scanner. Checks are needed to verify the safety of the patient. Monitoring equipment must be MRI compatible. Medical personnel should be available during the scan. MR protocols may be streamlined to 5 to 10 minutes of scan time for acute stroke, but others require 45 minutes or more to compete. Furthermore, each portion of the study requires the elderly and perhaps confused patient to remain quiet for minutes at a time. Twenty to 30% of patients with stroke may be ineligible for MRI because of contraindications or medical instability.[259,260] Lastly, MRI may not be available in local general hospitals where the majority of stroke patients are treated.[261] For these reasons, stroke studies typically use CT to screen the acute patient for possible thrombolytic therapy. Frequently, the therapy with tPA commences after CT and continues during a subsequent MRI study.

MRI remains the most accurate modality for acute stroke detection largely because of the sensitivity of DWI to early

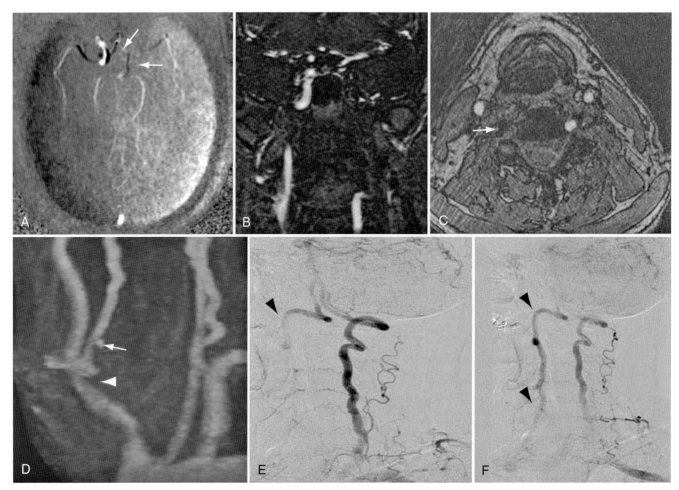

■ **FIGURE 20-26**　A 50-year-old male patient presented with subclavian steal syndrome. **A,** Phase-contrast view demonstrates left cavernous ICA occlusion with reversal of flow within the left A1 and posterior communicating artery (*arrows*). **B,** Contrast-enhanced MRI confirms occlusion of the left ICA. **C,** Time-of-flight source data demonstrate apparent absence of the right vertebral artery (*arrow*), which is clearly seen to be patent on contrast-enhanced MRA (*arrows* in **D**). The application of a superior saturation band eliminates flow signal from the retrograde right vertebral artery flow demonstrated on early (**E**) and delayed (**F**) cerebral angiography (*arrowheads*). Proximal brachiocephalic/subclavian artery occlusion is noted in **D** (*arrowhead*).

infarction.[262] A typical MRI protocol includes DWI; gradient-recalled-echo (GRE)/T2*-weighted (T2*W) imaging or suscepti-bility-weighted imaging (SWI); perfusion-weighted imaging (PWI, T2* echoplanar imaging [EPI]); and a vascular study that may be a postcontrast TOF study of the intracranial vessels or contrast-enhanced MRA of the neck and head from arch to vertex. The scan time is about 10 minutes. Rapid imaging techniques are exploited to reduce scan time. DWI is the single most important sequence with high sensitivity, specificity, and interobserver agreement for infarct detection. A GRE (or SWI) sequence is sensitive to the presence of blood breakdown products and may detect CT occult microbleeds, intravascular thrombus, and acute or remote parenchymal hemorrhage. CT remains superior, however, for acute subarachnoid hemorrhage assessment.[263] Both TOF and contrast-enhanced MRA techniques are utilized for vascular assessment. Approaches differ as to whether full arch to vertex coverage or intracranial vasculature alone is visualized. Contrast-enhanced MRA achieves higher spatial resolution than TOF with the advantage of arch to vertex coverage. The disadvantage of this technique is the necessity for a repeat contrast pump injection for subsequent perfusion-weighted study. Postcontrast T1W imaging is a useful but not essential adjunct to the imaging protocol. Infarct enhancement or contrast leakage may be identified. A coronal gradient T1W fat-saturated sequence provides useful information regarding plaque morphology (Fig. 20-9). A phase-contrast study of the circle of Willis provides useful information of collateral vessels (Fig. 20-26).

Acute and Subacute Infarct Detection

The sensitivity of conventional MRI for infarct detection under 3 hours is less than 50%.[264] T2W or T1W imaging is often normal for the first 8 and 16 hours, respectively.[265] However, the majority of T2W images and approximately half the T1W studies will be abnormal within 24 hours. By 48 hours, a conventional MRI will show the presence of an infarction as well as DWI.[266] Acute infarction is characterized by blurring of the gray matter/white matter interface[267] and progressive T2 hyperintensity best appreciated in the cortex. The distribution of free and bound water within the intracellular and extracellular environment and the rate of exchange between them determine the T2 of tissue.[268] An increase in free water increases the T2 of tissue (Fig. 20-27). Gyral swelling and sulcal effacement are best appreciated beyond 24 hours and become more conspicuous between the acute to subacute stages at 3 to 4 days when vasogenic edema peaks.[269] Loss of flow voids may be evident on T1W and T2W imaging consistent with intravascular stasis. FLAIR imaging exploits a 180-degree inversion pulse and 90-degree refocusing pulse. By suppressing the cerebrospinal fluid (CSF) signal that may interfere with the detection of subtle cortical T2 hyperintensity, improved sensitivity from that of conventional sequences is achieved.[270,271] Engorged, slow-flowing pial vessels may also be

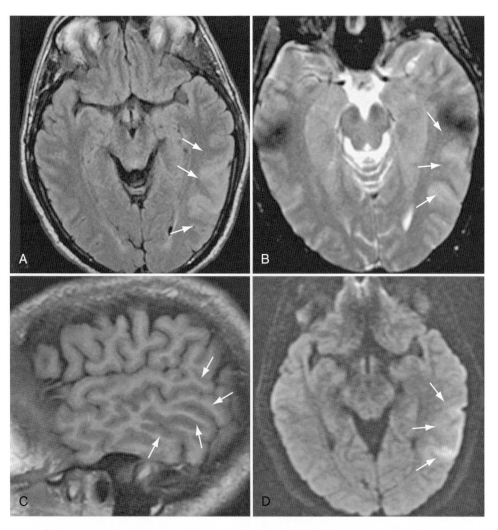

■ **FIGURE 20-27** Axial FLAIR (**A**), gradient-recalled-echo T2W (**B**), DWI (**C**), and sagittal T1W FLAIR (**D**) images within 24 hours of acute right-sided hemiplegia demonstrate early left temporo-occipital gyral swelling and sulcal effacement (*arrows*). Restricted diffusion is present on DWI consistent with acute infarct (*arrows*).

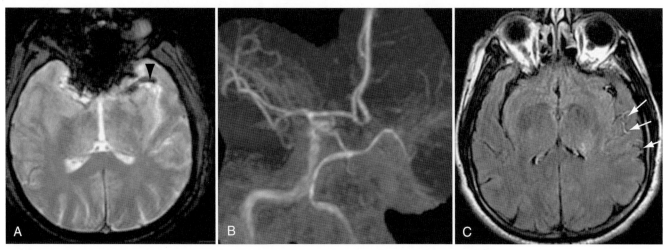

■ **FIGURE 20-28 A,** Axial MPGR demonstrating a left hypointense MCA sign in a 69-year-old man (*arrowhead*). **B,** Contrast-enhanced MRA demonstrates right vertebral and left internal carotid artery and middle cerebral artery occlusion. **C,** FLAIR demonstrates prominent intravascular hyperintensity consistent with slow flow (*arrows*).

seen in the subarachnoid space in the context of proximal vessel occlusion akin to flow alterations on T1W and T2W imaging described above (Fig. 20-28). These findings have been reported in the presence of DWI negative studies that subsequently proceeded to infarction.[272] However, FLAIR requires close scrutiny and knowledge of common artifacts and remains inferior to DWI

for stroke detection.[266] A recently described phenomenon coined HARM (hyperintense acute reperfusion marker) has been observed. This refers to FLAIR hyperintensity within the subarachnoid space. It occurs with a prevalence of about 33% and is thought to represent blood-brain barrier breakdown, allowing leakage of contrast agent into the subarachnoid space. It has been described as a marker of worse outcome and is associated with reperfusion, hemorrhagic transformation, and use of thrombolytics.[273]

MR fogging is an important cause for false-negative MRI studies in the subacute period.[274,275] Initially described on CT,[276] a period of pseudonormalization occurs at 2 to 3 weeks. The mechanism is uncertain. The progressive reduction in the extent of edema, occurrence of microhemorrhages, ischemia-related demyelination, and/or macrophage infiltration have all been suggested as explanations for the MR features observed. Because fogging may lead to misdiagnosis, imaging of patients with possible subacute infarctions should be delayed beyond this 2- to 3-week period to avoid misinterpretation. Alternatively, a contrast agent may be administered to identify these lesions.[277] Another important feature on both MRI and CT is intracranial shift and different patterns of intracranial herniation. These are described in detail elsewhere.

DWI

DWI is a technique for assessing the freedom with which water molecules may move (diffuse) within the voxel. Technically, DWI relies on the application of two temporally spaced (~40 ms) gradient pulses of equal strength but opposite direction. If the water molecules within the image volume remain stationary for the interval between pulses, there is complete recovery of the signal. If, however, small amounts of water change position during that interval, there is incomplete recovery of signal with consequent signal attenuation. The exact mechanism of DWI restriction in cerebral infarction is uncertain but extracellular to intracellular water shift is considered the main mechanism.[278] However, the relative contribution of the intracellular or extracellular spaces to the DWI restriction remains uncertain.[279,280]

DWI detects ischemic change within minutes after infarction[281,282] and displays the abnormality as easily recognizable hyperintensity. DWI is consistently more sensitive for detecting early infarction than noncontrast CT and conventional MRI with higher sensitivity (88%-100%), specificity (95%-100%), and good interobserver agreement even when less experienced individuals are assessed.[283-286] Perhaps the most compelling characteristic of DWI—unmatched by CT—is the ability of MR to detect small acute embolic infarcts and acute lacunar infarcts within a background of microangiopathic change (Fig. 20-29).[287] The clinical significance for such distinction in the hyperacute phase is

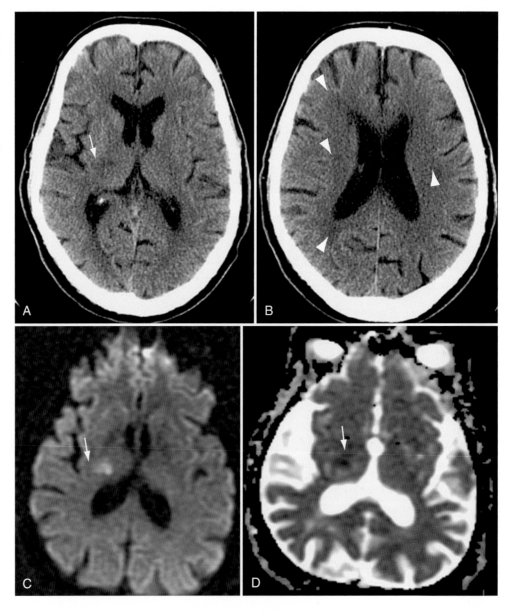

■ **FIGURE 20-29 A** and **B,** Non-contrast CT at two levels demonstrating patchy foci of hypodensity consistent with microangiopathic change (*arrowheads*). Patient presented with left-sided weakness. Subtle hypodensity is seen within the right posterior internal capsule, but appearances are of indeterminant age (*arrow*). **C** and **D,** DWI and ADC map confirm the acute nature of the lenticulostriate territory infarct (*arrows*).

doubtful, although the finding certainly impacts on initiation of secondary preventive treatments. DWI lesion size correlated with final infarct size and acute and follow-up National Institutes of Health Stroke Scale (NIHSS) scores.[288,289] The extent and severity of reduction may also predict ischemic progression or recovery. Absolute and apparent diffusion coefficient (ADC) values of infarct core lie below 580×10^{-6} mm^2/s and 0.62, respectively. Penumbral values are 580×10^{-6} mm^2/s to 860×10^{-6} mm^2/s or 0.89 to 0.91, respectively.[290,291] ADC values between 300 and 520×10^{-6} mm^2/s may predict an increased risk of hemorrhagic transformation.[292,293] DWI has also been reported to help distinguish stroke subtype. The presence of multiple peripheral regions of restricted diffusion within different vascular territories, for example, suggests a cardioembolic source (Fig. 20-30).[155,294] Negative DWI helps to exclude acute infarct as the cause for neurologic decline in a patient with intercurrent illness. It should be noted that 19% to 40%[243,295,296] of early DWI changes may be reversible, although histopathologically these regions may demonstrate neuronal reduction in animal models,

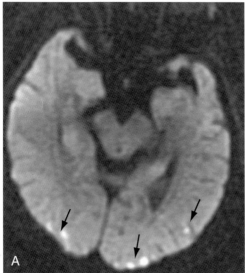
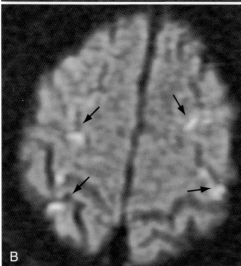

■ **FIGURE 20-30** A and B, Multi-territorial, peripheral foci of DWI restriction (*arrows*) consistent with a cardioembolic cause in an 80-year-old woman with newly diagnosed paroxysmal atrial fibrillation. Noncontrast CT (not shown) at presentation was normal. DWI prompted early cardiac investigation.

suggesting subclinical cellular damage. This is further supported by reappearance of delayed DWI abnormality.[296]

DWI images should always be evaluated in the context of an ADC map. The DWI is a composite of both T2 and diffusion effects. The ADC map, however, is purely a representation of diffusion with no competing T2 effects. The interaction between T2 and diffusion in DWI is important and accounts for the prolonged visualization of hyperintensity on the DWI map after infarct. This prolonged signal increase due to T2 effects is designated "T2 shine-through."[281] As the degree of diffusion restriction diminishes and vasogenic edema increases, the DWI may remain bright due to T2 shine-through. The baseline B0 images should always be examined to assess the magnitude of contribution of T2 hyperintensity on DWI. The hyperintensity on DWI may persist for months, but with infarct maturation and tissue boundary disruption the increased T2 signal is "washed out," becoming isointense to hypointense. With acute infarctions, the acute hypointensity is seen on the ADC map for 2 to 5 days. The hypointensity of the ADC map "pseudonormalizes" between days 5 and 10. Thereafter, the ADC map appears hyperintense.[297-299] The evaluation of DWI and ADC changes may therefore facilitate the timing of infarcts.

Up to 20% of infarctions have been reported to be DWI negative within 24 hours of symptom onset.[300,301] In one series, 31% of posterior fossa infarcts had no detectable DWI change compared with 2% of anterior circulation infarcts.[302] Although the mechanism is uncertain, explanations for these findings include (1) lesions that are too small for detection, (2) less severe reduction in blood flow so it remains above a threshold that manifests cytotoxic edema, (3) reperfusion with resolution of DWI defect, (4) posterior fossa susceptibility artifacts obscuring detail or resulting in inferior signal to noise or, least likely, (5) a second subsequent infarct in the same distribution.[302] In one study, the sensitivity of DWI for detecting hyperacute infarctions was improved by increasing the b value used for the diffusion study.[303] This does not appear to have any benefit in the acute[304] and subacute[305] period. False-positive DWI studies may be seen in acute[306] and subacute encephalitis,[307,308] seizures,[309] abscess,[310] Creutzfeldt-Jakob disease,[310a,310b] and cellular tumors.

Hemorrhage Detection

A variety of MRI techniques help to identify blood products, including T2*-GRE sequences, gradient EPI series, and SWI. Overall, T2*-GRE studies detect chronic hemorrhage more sensitively than do gradient EPI sequences. GRE has a higher spatial (256 vs. 128) and contrast resolution, greater signal-to-noise ratio (SNR), and less distortion at air/bone interfaces. In one study, GRE detected more lesions at the gray matter/white matter junction and within the infratentorial space, where the greater susceptibility artifact of EPI sequences limited visualization. However, EPI sequence may still be useful in uncooperative or pediatric patients when faster scan time is important. The study concluded that spin-echo (SE) EPI should not be used.[311] Unlike CT, the ability of GRE to detect recurrent hemorrhage and accurately distinguish between calcification and blood remains uncertain.

FLAIR is useful for detecting subarachnoid blood (Fig. 20-31). On FLAIR images, however, CSF hyperintensity is not specific and is also found with raised protein,[312] CSF pulsation and susceptibility artifacts,[313] high inspired oxygen tension,[314] and patient movement.[315] MRI may detect parenchymal hemorrhage as early as 23 minutes.[220] Sensitivity, specificity, and accuracy for MRI hemorrhage detection in expert and trainee readers have been shown to be high (95%-100%). In a comparative study,[263] MRI and CT were found to be concordant in 96% of cases for acute hemorrhage detection. MRI, however, remains superior to CT in the detection of microbleeds and hemorrhagic transformation of infarctions (Fig. 20-32).[218]

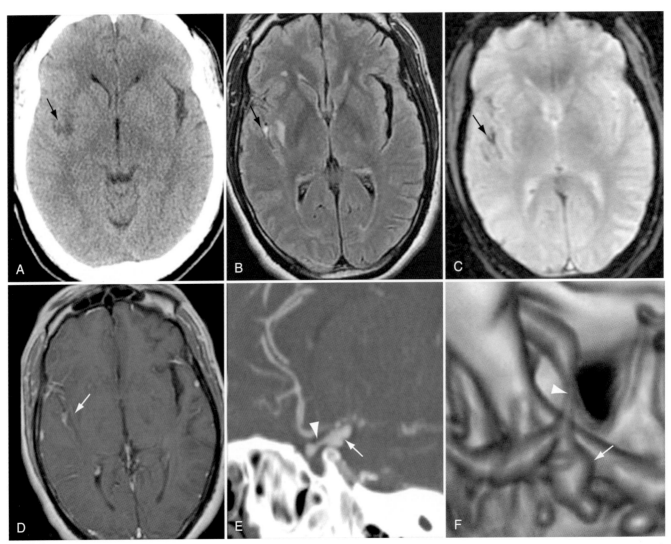

■ FIGURE 20-31 A 45-year-old Afro-Caribbean man with a past history of cocaine use presented with left-sided stroke a week after drug use associated with acute-onset headache. **A,** Noncontrast CT demonstrates insular and subinsular subacute infarct (*arrow*). **B** and **C,** FLAIR and MPGR demonstrate sylvian blood products not detected on noncontrast CT (*arrow*). **D,** Postcontrast T1 demonstrates shortening from subarachnoid blood in addition to overlying meningeal and subtle parenchymal enhancement (*arrow*). The finding of subarachnoid hemorrhage prompted a search for the source of bleeding. Parasagittal MIP (**E**) and volume-rendered CTA (**F**) demonstrate a multilobular posterior communicating artery aneurysm (*arrow*) with severe supraclinoid vasospasm (*arrowhead*) implicated in the stroke etiology.

Hemorrhagic transformation is seen in up to 43% of CT studies but is more prevalent in autopsy studies (70%),[316,317] suggesting a lower sensitivity of CT to hemorrhagic transformation. Although hemorrhagic transformation is often considered to be a complication of thrombolytic therapy, it is also seen in the natural evolution of cerebral infarct. The major thrombolytic trials have used varying definitions of hemorrhagic transformation that is (1) symptomatic (based on deterioration in the NIHSS score of 4 points or more) and (2) contemporary (within a 24- to 36-hour window of treatment).[318,319] The ECASS investigators utilized a radiologic classification that divides hemorrhage into hemorrhagic infarct when the hemorrhagic transformation is petechial without mass effect (Fig. 20-23) and parenchymal hematoma when the hemorrhage is associated with mass effect. Parenchymal hemorrhage is further subclassified as type 1 if the transformation involves less than 30% and type 2 if it involves equal to or more than 30% of the ischemic region.[194,320] The clinical significance of hemorrhagic transformation is contested.[321-323] A strong argument is offered that hemorrhage indicates revascularization of the infarct territory, which itself is an independent predictor for outcome. Early hemorrhagic infarct (<48 hr) is associated with early revascularization at a time when there has been less disruption of the blood-brain barrier. Parenchymal hemorrhage is associated with late revascularization (>48 hr), greater disruption of the blood-brain barrier, larger infarct size, and worse outcome (see Fig. 20-23).[324]

Vascular Assessment

Conventional MRI very commonly shows vascular abnormalities in hyperacute infarctions. These include flow-related abnormalities such as arterial enhancement, absence of flow voids, and loss of flow-related enhancement on MRA.[265,272] The absence of flow voids should be carefully sought and is not uncommonly missed when present at the skull base. The skull base should be carefully studied to avoid missing "absent" flow voids, signs of dissection, or other vascular compromise. On T2*-GRE or EPI gradient sequences, the hypointense MCA sign is the MRI equivalent of hyperdense vessel sign of CT.[325-327] Hypointense blooming results from deoxyhemoglobin within the clot (see Fig. 20-28). Susceptibility artifact from sinuses and surrounding bone may mask the presence of distal intracranial ICA clot.

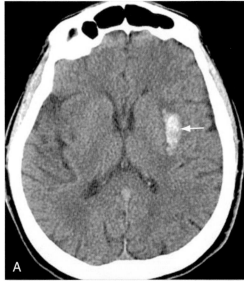

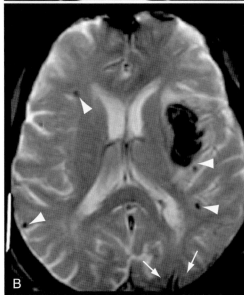

■ FIGURE 20-32 Noncontrast CT (**A**) and axial MPGR (**B**) in an 80-year-old man with lateral putaminal and subinsular hemorrhage. CT reveals a subinsular hematoma (*arrows*) with minor perihematomal edema and periventricular and deep white matter microangiopathic changes. MPGR confirms CT findings but demonstrates numerous peripherally located microhemorrhages (*arrowheads*) and occipital pial siderosis. MRI facilitated a presumptive diagnosis of amyloid angiopathy (*arrow*).

MRA

Most stroke protocols use 3D TOF MRA to assess the vessels. This sequence adequately assesses the proximal vasculature and permits assignment of patients to appropriate management according to the site of vessel occlusion. Comparative studies with DSA reveal sensitivities of 85% to 90% and specificity of 90% to 97% for proximal intracranial disease.[328,329] There are, however, numerous limitations to this sequence. Artifacts are common in the carotid siphon due to spin dephasing or turbulent flow. There is poor visualization of the distal vasculature because of limitations of spatial resolution and spin saturation. Scan duration is longer than CTA and motion artifact may cause problems. Insertion of a superior saturation band limits the detection of a subclavian steal syndrome (see Fig. 20-26). Contrast-enhanced MRA has superior SNR and spatial resolution but necessitates a further gadolinium injection.

Role of Contrast

MRI demonstrates a variable degree of contrast enhancement depending on the adequacy of collateral circulation. Meningeal enhancement is present in 30% of patients with hyperacute infarction. Intravascular enhancement is seen in approximately 80% of these patients. It precedes any T1 or T2 alteration, gradually decreases to approximately 30% at 1 week, and disappears by the second week.[330] In the absence of collateral circulation, parenchymal enhancement follows an opposite pattern, because the contrast agent is unable to reach the infarct site. Under these conditions enhancement is seldom present in the first week. If cortical collaterals are present, the frequency of enhancement increases from 30% to 100% at 1 week (Fig. 20-33).[331] Parenchymal enhancement may persist for up to 2 months. A reduction in mass effect after the first week and the appearance of peak parenchymal enhancement after the first week help to distinguish infarction from other processes, such as neoplasm. Large cerebral infarcts may show meningeal enhancement at the end of the first week.[332]

MR Perfusion (MRP)

Paramagnetic contrast agents cause a low signal intensity due to T2* effects. Perfusion measurement uses this low signal to assess the vacularity within a region. When a bolus of paramagnetic contrast passes through a region of interest, the bolus will cause a transient drop in signal intensity. The time course of signal change during the bolus passage gives information about the region's vasculature. That is, MRI can exploit the initial time of bolus arrival, the time to the peak of the bolus, the width of the bolus peak (narrow = rapid passage, wide = slow passage), and the total volume of the bolus (blood volume) to characterize the vascularization of the region. A drop of approximately 25% is induced by local susceptibility differences between the vessels and surrounding tissues. A sequence rapid enough to detect the T2* reduction is required. The two most commonly used sequences are GRE-EPI and SE-EPI. Gradient sequences have a higher SNR but suffer from more susceptibility artifact, which can generally be overcome by reduced slice thickness. GRE reflects changes in larger vessels compared with SE sequence changes, which reflect the microvasculature (<5 μm). Multiple factors affect the integrity of the perfusion map, including patient motion, delayed or poor contrast bolus arrival, and contrast leakage associated with blood-brain barrier disruption. These are reviewed in detail elsewhere.[333] Another emerging technique is arterial spin labeling (ASL), which does not require gadolinium injection but uses tagging of endogenous arterial spins. However, ASL has not had the widespread appeal of contrast-based perfusion protocols and is largely limited to large research centers at present.

Ischemic infarctions are thought to have three zones: an inner core of infarction, a penumbra of ischemic tissue at risk for infarction, and an outer ring of benign oligemia. Initially, the zone of restricted diffusion was considered to define an irreversibly infarcted core. The zone of reduced perfusion was considered to define the penumbra of underperfused tissue at risk for infarction but potentially salvageable by reperfusion. The outer ring of benign oligemia was considered to represent a region of sustainable levels of mild underperfusion. The term *perfusion-diffusion mismatch* signified that (1) a smaller zone of restricted diffusion lay within a larger zone of reduced perfusion and (2) the larger outer zone signified the presence of a salvageable rim of ischemic penumbra. Concordance of the zone of restricted diffusion with the zone of impaired perfusion signified that there was a completed infarction with no residual penumbra of salvageable tissue.

Experience with MRI and recognition of DWI reversibility has resulted in a revision of the core-penumbra hypothesis. The penumbral tissue is now considered to be a combination

■ **FIGURE 20-33** DWI (**A**) and postcontrast T1W MR image (**B**) 1 day after anterior cerebral artery territory infarct demonstrates corpus striatum (*arrowheads*) and gyriform restriction (*arrows*) consistent with an acute infarct. Meningeal and intravascular enhancement is present around the interhemispheric fissure (*arrows*) with early parenchymal enhancement within the striatum (*arrowheads*). **C,** Postcontrast study 9 days after presentation shows extension of parenchymal enhancement, which decreases at 40 days (**D**).

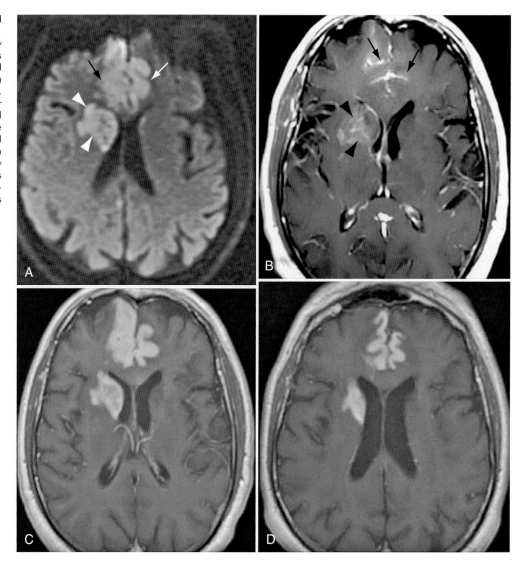

of both a peripheral rim of the zone of DWI restriction and the inner rim of the perfusion abnormality. The outer rim of the perfusion abnormality is termed *benign oligemia* because of the low rate of conversion to infarction even when untreated.[334]

MRI has provided mixed results regarding the validity of the mismatch model. Large perfusion-diffusion mismatches signify substantial zones of penumbra that may become infarcted if perfusion fails further. The greatest expansions of the zones of restriction (i.e., the greatest increases in the infarct core) are observed in patients who have the largest perfusion abnormalities (greatest mismatches).[169,181] Expansion of DWI abnormality into the surrounding penumbral tissue may be prevented by early reperfusion.[335] In patients with large diffusion-perfusion mismatches, there may still be time to salvage the ischemic penumbra, even if the patients present for treatment outside the traditional 0- to 3-hour window for instituting thrombolytic therapy. The Diffusion and Perfusion Imaging Evaluation for Understanding Stroke Evolution (DEFUSE) Echoplanar Imaging Thrombolytic Evaluation Trial, and Desmoteplase in Acute Ischemic Stroke Trial (DIAS) studies both utilized MRI to select patients with a diffusion-perfusion mismatch beyond the traditional time frame. Both demonstrate benefit in targeted groups of patients with penumbral tissue.[336-338] However, as described above, DIAS-2, the phase III, double-blinded study of desmopletase using penumbral selection criteria failed to demonstrate a benefit of this plasminogen activator compared to placebo. This was the largest study including perfusion imaging as a selection criteria and included acute stroke 3 to 9 hours after symptom onset with DWI-PWI mismatch. A small proportion (20%) of patients were selected using CTP.[258d] It is likely that advances in image analysis may confirm the utility of MR perfusion. For example, after re-analysis of the EPITHET data using co-registration of the DWI and PWI maps to determine the presence of a mismatch, alteplase was found to significantly reduce infarct growth.[338a] Introduction of automated MRI analysis software (RAPID) might also be beneficial in assessing penumbra and will likely be included in future acute stroke studies.[338b]

The Blood-Brain Barrier and Contrast Enhancement

More than 20 years ago, disruption of the blood-brain barrier was implicated in the enhancement/extravasation of contrast media seen after high doses of contrast media were administered to patients with stroke. Four of seven patients with infarct enhancement developed confluent hemorrhagic transformation versus none of the patients with nonenhancing studies (see Fig. 20-23).[249,339] It has been postulated that contrast enhancement and contrast extravasation may reflect varying degrees of severity of disruption of microcirculatory integrity analogous to hemorrhagic infarct and parenchymal hemorrhage. The blood-brain barrier comprises tight interendothelial junctions and a basal lamina constructed of type IV collagen and laminin. The latter is the main barrier to red cell extravasation.[340,341] Experience from CT and arterial angiography suggests that contrast enhancement may be due to the gradual accumulation of contrast agent associated with larger volumes of contrast injection over a prolonged period of time. The presumptive mechanism is disruption of endothelial tight junctions.[342] Extravasation, on the other hand, may indicate more severe disruption of the blood-brain barrier involving the basal lamina, accounting for the higher risk of parenchymal hemorrhage. The contribution of contrast agent,[343] thrombolytics,[344] and exogenous plasminogen activators[340] to disruption of the blood-brain barrier remains unresolved. Irrespective of causation there may be a selective vulnerability of basal ganglia blood-brain barrier because of the presence of multiple end-arterial supply.[345]

A more recent publication[342] clarified the distinction between enhancement from extravasation and studied the effect on hemorrhagic outcome after intra-arterial thrombolysis with urokinase in 62 patients. Extravasation was defined as hyperdensity on the initial post-thrombolysis noncontrast CT that persisted on the 24-hour noncontrast CT study with a density greater than 90 HU. Enhancement similarly was hyperdense on postprocedure noncontrast CT but dissipated at 24 hours. Hemorrhage was distinguished from contrast extravasation by the persistence of hyperdensity at 24 hours less than 90 HU. Enhancement and extravasation were present in 22.6% and 11.3% of patients, respectively. In this study patients with both contrast enhancement and extravasation had a trend to more proximal occlusions and lower recanalization than treated patients without these signs. Patients with both enhancement and extravasation showed statistically higher risks of hemorrhagic transformation, although only extravasation was significantly associated with symptomatic hemorrhage and poor outcome (defined as modified Rankin scale > 3) (see Fig. 20-23). These findings would be consistent with extravasation signifying greater injury to the blood-brain barrier than enhancement. The distinction of these two entities is currently useful at predicting hemorrhage after intra-arterial thrombolysis. It would be advantageous, however, to incorporate blood-brain barrier status into the decision-making process before thrombolysis treatment.

One recent report used dynamic contrast-enhanced MRI with kinetic modeling[184] to demonstrate the feasibility of measuring blood-brain barrier disruption at infarct presentation in 10 patients, 3 of whom progressed to hemorrhagic transformation within 48 hours. All three patients demonstrated elevated blood-brain barrier permeability measured by permeability surface product (PS), compared with contralateral normal white matter. The region of blood-brain barrier disruption predictably occurred in areas of lowest ADC, confirming the association between extent of ischemia and blood-brain barrier disturbance. Only one of the three patients had clear enhancement on delayed imaging. PS showed that the enhancement was due to extravasation and not increased CBV. These findings support a rethinking of the infarct model and the concept of a "core within the core,"[334] that is, an area of more advanced infarct within the DWI-positive core. As described earlier, CT permeability techniques are available, as shown in animal tumor models and a small human case series.[346] In our own series we utilized a dual-phase CT perfusion protocol, which acquires both CTP and permeability measurements through a single injection. This process has the advantage over MRP of requiring only a single contrast injection rather than two separate injections. Using this protocol we imaged 41 patients with acute ischemic stroke within 3 hours. Hemorrhagic transformation (HT) was assessed on follow-up MR or CT at 3 to 5 days. HT developed in 23 patients (56%) who had a higher National Institute of Health Stroke Scale (NIHSS) score ($p = 0.005$) and a poorer outcome ($p = 0.001$), and who were more likely to have received TPA ($p = 0.005$) than those without HT. Baseline blood flow ($p = 0.17$), blood volume defects ($p = 0.11$), and extent of flow reduction ($p = 0.27$) were comparable between patient groups. Permeability surface area product (PS) of HT patients (0.49 ± 0.3 ml$^{-1} \cdot$ min$^{-1} \cdot$ (100 g)$^{-1}$) was significantly higher than that of non-HT patients (0.09 ± 0.10 ml$^{-1} \cdot$ min$^{-1} \cdot$ (100 g)$^{-1}$) ($p < 0.0001$). PS was associated with HT according to a stepwise multivariate analysis (OR 3.5; 95% CI 1.7-7.1, $p = 0.0007$). The area under the ROC curve was 0.92 ± 0.05 (95% CI of 82.8%-100%). A PS threshold of ≥ 0.23 ml$^{-1} \cdot$ min$^{-1} \cdot$ (100 g)$^{-1}$ had a sensitivity, specificity, accuracy, and positive and negative predictive value of 77%, 94%, 87%, 94% and 75%, respectively, for HT.[346a] Thus far, the clinical application of permeability imaging has met with mixed results and large series are yet to be published (Fig. 20-34).

Interpreting the Pattern of Perfusion Abnormality
Correlative MRI and CT perfusion studies show fair to excellent correlation between CBV and DWI[183,347] and excellent prediction

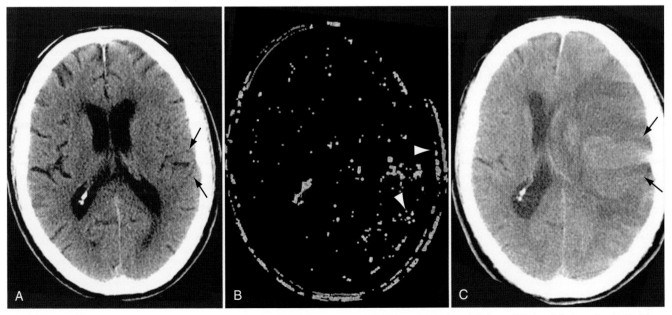

■ **FIGURE 20-34** Noncontrast CT (**A**) and CT permeability map (**B**) in an 85-year-old man presenting with dense right hemiplegia and aphasia. There is subtle sulcal effacement and loss of gray matter/white matter differentiation within the left MCA territory (*arrows*). Increased permeability (*arrowheads*) indicates the site of future parenchymal hematoma. There is marked mass effect and subfalcine herniation (**C**, *arrows*).

of final infarct size.[348] In the presence of recanalization the CBV/DWI abnormality most closely predicts final infarct size.[349] The penumbra is represented by the abnormalities of the CBF and MTT outside the infarct core and predicts the final infarct size if no recanalization occurs.[349] MTT has a lower specificity for final infarct size, because MTT is also influenced by compensated chronic vessel occlusion in the absence of acute ischemia.

Four different PWI patterns are seen in the context of a suspected acute stroke. These patterns guide further management and are listed in Table 20-5.

1. If there is no abnormality of the DWI or CT CBV/perfusion study, then a TIA or stroke mimic should be considered. Stroke mimics account for up to 30% of acute stroke-like presentations[350] to the emergency department. Conditions mimicking a stroke include seizures, demyelination, hypoglycemia, posterior reversible encephalopathy syndrome (PRES), subdural hemorrhage, and tumor.[351]
2. Occasionally, no penumbra is identified in a patient with focal infarction consistent with auto-recanalization.[352]
3. The definition of perfusion-diffusion mismatch is arbitrary. A definition often used in clinical trials is a perfusion abnormality exceeding the infarct core by 20% or more. These patients were thought to be ideal targets for thrombolytic treatment and account for 50% to 70% of stroke patients seen within 6 hours.[174,353] However, increasingly larger ratios of mismatch are being considered to be more optimal for patient selection. Smaller mismatches may still be a proper target for treatment if the region of perfusion abnormality is clinically significant (e.g., Broca's region). Utilizing this model there is a growing body of evidence supporting the treatment of patients beyond the conventional time windows based on CT- or MRI-defined perfusion mismatch. One study using an MRI perfusion protocol treated patients up to 9 hours after

infarction and resulted in excellent clinical outcome and low risk of hemorrhage.[336] However, these results were not confirmed in the phase III DIAS study or DEDAS. Patients with infarcts of more than 100 mL have a worse prognosis and higher risk of hemorrhage.[354] In a recent study in patients treated within 3 to 6 hours, lesions greater than 100 mL on DWI or Tmax >8 seconds were considered malignant because of their high propensity for intracranial hemorrhage and poor outcome. A pooled analysis of the EPITHET and DEFUSE further suggested that this malignant pattern could be predicted by a similar threshold value of 100 mL using a Tmax >8 seconds on PWI.[354a]

The same study found that patients with a matched defect did not benefit from treatment.[337] Other studies have, however, shown some reduction in final infarct size, suggesting benefit.[243,355] The treatment of these patients is controversial, and it is thought that these patients may do well irrespective of treatment.

Several investigators have proposed that quantitative thresholds or ratios for CTP and MRP be used to define infarction, penumbra that proceeds to infarction, and penumbra that recovers. However, widely adopted definitions for these thresholds are still lacking for both CTP and MRP.[355a] Normal CBF and CBV values for gray matter are 60 mL/100 g/min and 4 mL/100 g/min, respectively. For white matter these values are approximately 25 mL/100 g/min and 2 mL/100 g/min. Previously, authors have relied on mean values of regions of interest that incorporate both gray and white matter; however, independent thresholds for gray and white matter have been recently calculated.[176] These values are summarized in Table 20-6.

Several historical studies are summarized in Table 20-7. These are provided only as a guide because the data are dependent on many factors, including the scan acquisition parameters, data postprocessing method, duration of ischemia, presence of collaterals, and recanalization status.

CHRONIC INFARCT

After the reduction of edema and mass effect in the first week there is progressive evolution to parenchymal volume loss with atrophic/ex vacuo dilatation of adjacent ventricles and overlying sulci. Contrast enhancement may persist for the first 2 months. Histopathologically, gliosis and encephalomalacia dominate. The underlying white matter may demonstrate CT hypodensity, T1 hypointensity, and T2 hyperintensity. The cortex may appear thin and of heterogeneous signal, reflecting varying degrees of gliosis, vacuolation, and residual gray matter integrity (Fig. 20-35). Laminar necrosis is histopathologically confined to layers 3, 5, and 6 of the cerebral cortex. Serial MRI identifies these lesions at about 2 weeks. They may persist indefinitely.[357,358] T1W MRI demonstrates ribbon-like cortical hyperintensity (Fig. 20-36). T2 signal varies from hypointense to hyperintense. The

---

TABLE 20-5. Patterns of Perfusion Abnormality in Suspected Acute Stroke

1. No perfusion or CBV/DWI abnormality
   TIA
   Stroke mimic
   Lacunar infarct beyond spatial resolution or DWI negative
   Infarct outside spatial coverage of scan (CT)
2. CBV/DWI abnormality with normal or increased perfusion
   Spontaneous recanalization. No treatment
3. Diffusion/perfusion mismatch
   Target mismatch
   Vessel location proximal: intra-arterial thrombolysis
   Vessel location distal: intravenous thrombolysis
   Malignant mismatch (>100 mL core or Tmax > 8 s): no treatment[337]
4. Matched PWI abnormality
   Probably no thrombolysis

TABLE 20-6. Published Thresholds of Cerebral Blood Flow (CBF) and Volume (CBV) for White and Gray Matter Defining Infarction, Penumbra that Proceeds to Infarction and Benign Oligemia, or Penumbra Proceeding to Recovery

	Penumbra Proceeding to Recovery (MRP)	Penumbra Proceeding to Infarct (MRP)	Penumbra Proceeding to Recovery (CTP)	Penumbra Proceeding to Infarct (CTP)
Gray CBF	27.2 ± 9.7	17.2 ± 8.7*	25.0 ± 3.8	13.3 ± 3.7†
White CBF	14.1 ± 7.6	10.1 ± 4.8*	12.3 ± 1.98	7.56 ± 2.02‡
Gray CBV	3.9 ± 0.6	3.5 ± 1.3*	2.15 ± 0.4	1.12 ± 0.4†
White CBV	2.3 ± 0.9	2.6 ± 1.4*	1.12 ± 0.25	0.66 ± 0.24‡

*Data from Schaefer PW, et al. First-pass quantitative CT perfusion identifies thresholds for salvageable penumbra in acute stroke patients treated with intra-arterial therapy. AJNR Am J Neuroradiol 2006; 27:20-25.
†Data from Murphy BD, et al. Identification of penumbra and infarct in acute ischemic stroke using computed tomography perfusion-derived blood flow and blood volume measurements. Stroke 2006; 37:1771-1777.
‡Data from Murphy BD, et al. White matter thresholds for ischemic penumbra and infarct core in patients with acute stroke: CT perfusion study. Radiology 2008; 247:818-825.
CTP, CT perfusion; MRP, MR perfusion.

TABLE 20-7. Published Thresholds of Whole-Brain Cerebral Blood Flow (CBF) and Volume (CBV) Defining Infarction, Penumbra that Proceeds to Infarction and Benign Oligemia or Penumbra Proceeding to Recovery

	Penumbra Proceeding to Recovery	Penumbra Proceeding to Infarct	Infarct Core	Cut-off Infarct vs. Recovery	Sensitivity	Specificity
CBF Thresholds						
MRP	0.62	0.42	0.26 11 mL/100 g/m	0.59	91%	73%[289]
MRP	0.69		0.39[291]			
MRP		0.37 18.5 mL/100 g/m	0.12[286] 6 mL/100 g/m			
CTP	0.62		0.34	0.48	76%	73%[356]
CTP	0.46 ± 0.1 17.9 ± 4 mL/100 g/m	0.34 ± 0.1 16.1 ± 6 mL/100 g/m	0.19 ± 0.1 8.9 ± 2.3 mL/100 g/m	0.44[176]		
CBV Thresholds						
MRP	0.94	0.84	0.55	0.85[289]		
MRP	0.78		0.43	0.6	90%	86.5%[356]
MRP		<0.7[290]				
CTP	0.96 ± 0.2 2.94 ± 0.5 mL/100 g	0.84 ± 0.2 2.83 ± 0.7 mL/100 g	0.48 ± 0.1 1.47 ± 0.4 mL/100 g[176]			
CTP	2.15 ± 0.4 mL/100 g		1.12 ± 0.4 mL/100 g[177]			

*Values are ratios compared to normal contralateral tissue unless unit given, implying absolute value.

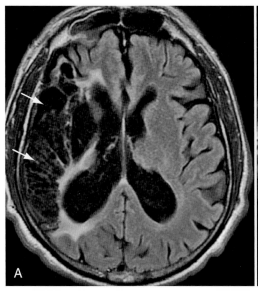
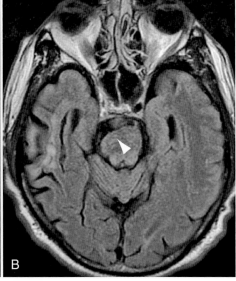

■ **FIGURE 20-35** Axial FLAIR sequence in a 65-year-old man with a past history of extensive right MCA territory infarct. **A,** There is encephalomalacia (*arrows*) and ex vacuo dilatation of the right lateral ventricle. Peripheral high signal and linear stranding within the infarct core suggest gliosis. **B,** The right cerebral peduncle is reduced in size without signal alteration, consistent with wallerian degeneration (*arrowhead*).

etiology is uncertain; petechial hemorrhage, demyelination, lipid-laden macrophages, and calcification have been suggested. Calcification is best seen in chronic infarcts on CT but is infrequent (Fig. 20-37). Wallerian degeneration is the anterograde degeneration of axons and myelin sheaths caused by more proximal axonal or neuronal damage. Its presence predicts persistent hemiparesis and a poor long-term neurologic outcome. First described in peripheral nerves by Waller in 1850, four stages are described. Stage 3 degeneration, consistent with edema and lipid breakdown, is the first change detectable by conventional MRI and appears around 4 weeks after infarction. CT can only detect stage 4 changes or atrophy. On MRI, T2 hyperintensity is present within the affected fiber tracts. These findings may persist for up to 6 months, after which volume loss is commonly seen (Fig. 20-35). DWI and diffusion tensor imaging detect changes earlier than conventional MRI, even as early as 2 days.[359,360]

Thrombolysis

FDA approval for the use of intravenous thrombolysis was based on the National Institute of Neurological Disorders and Stroke (NINDS) rt-PA Stroke Study Group study.[207] Of 624 patients, half achieved an excellent outcome compared with 38% of controls.

Symptomatic hemorrhage was 10 times more common in the thrombolysis group (6.4%). There was no significant mortality difference in the two groups at 3 months. Subsequently, similar findings have been reported in other trials and confirmed with meta-analyses.[361,362] The NINDS study created a ceiling of 3 hours for treatment accepted by the American Heart Association guidelines,[363] despite a meta-analysis demonstrating benefit for intravenous thrombolysis up to 4.5 hours.[361] ECASS-3 subsequently confirmed a benefit of intravenous alteplase administered between 3 and 4.5 hours after the onset of symptoms and led to the adoption of the current 4.5-hour limit for IV thrombolysis.[363a] Attempts to increase the time window of chemical thrombolysis through the arterial or combined intravenous/arterial route[235,364,365] and mechanical interventional strategies continue. However, only the MERCI clot retrieval and Penumbra system devices have received FDA approval.[241] The number of patients receiving any form of thrombolysis remains low (~5%), largely because of inability to meet the tight time constraint of 3 hours.[366,367] Increasing recognition that the penumbra persists beyond the 3-hour time constraint discussed earlier has stimulated a shift to using the penumbra rather than the time after infarction to determine management.[368] The DEFUSE/EPITHET, DIAS/DEDAS,

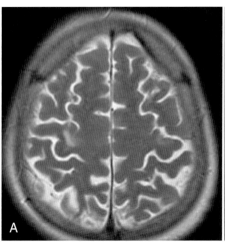
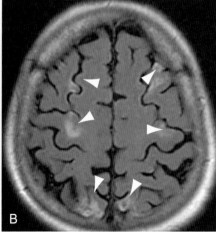
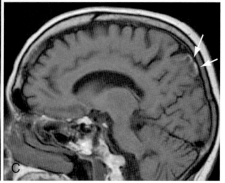

■ **FIGURE 20-36**   Axial T2W (**A**), FLAIR (**B**), and sagittal T1W (**C**) images in a 58-year-old woman with new-onset atrial fibrillation. Multiple cortical border zone embolic infarcts are seen between the ACA, MCA, and PCA territories (*arrowheads*). Sagittal T1W image demonstrates laminar necrosis of the superior parietal lobule cortex (*arrows*).

and other studies[369] suggest that patients may be selected on the basis of an ischemic penumbra, receive treatment beyond the conventional 3-hour time window, and achieve results consistent with earlier studies that were limited to 3 hours. Although DIAS-2 could not prove the usefulness of penumbral imaging, further studies incorporating refinement of perfusion techniques are under way.

Special Procedures

Conventional angiography is not routinely performed for the diagnosis of infarct. It is, however, central to intra-arterial directed stroke therapies. Conventional angiography is critical for determining the location, extent, and severity of cerebrovascular occlusion. It provides additional functional data on the circle of Willis and pial collateral networks. Angiographic findings in acute stroke include vessel occlusion, reduced intravascular flow proximal to the occlusion, regions of hypoperfusion on capillary phase, and retrograde/collateral flow patterns. In subacute infarct, mass effect and luxury perfusion may be demonstrated. Intra-arterial techniques of vascular recanalization include intra-arterial thrombolytic injection through clot, catheter and wire clot disruption, device-assisted clot removal (MERCI or Penumbra), angioplasty, and stenting. Further discussion of these techniques is beyond the scope of this chapter. Arteriovenous shunting of contrast agent during thrombolysis is an important sign, reported to predict a significantly increased risk of hemorrhagic transformation and poor outcome.

Microbleeds, Thrombolysis, and Antiplatelets

Microbleeds or microhemorrhages are punctate, homogeneous regions of susceptibility, remote from the sulcal regions, visible as T2 hypointensity only on gradient T2*W or susceptibility-weighted imaging (SWI) studies (see Fig. 20-32). Initially, these lesions were defined as 2 to 5 mm. Although some studies have included larger lesions, more than 80% conform to a threshold below 10 mm.[370] T2* susceptibility, however, is a nonspecific finding that may also be seen with intracranial air, cavernous malformation, mineralization, septic embolus, metastasis, and vascular flow voids. In a clinicopathologic study of 11 patients the T2* signal loss was attributed to hemosiderin deposits.[371] Parenchymal hemosiderin deposition is seen in a number of conditions, including cerebral amyloid angiopathy, hypertension, disseminated intravascular coagulation, and diffuse axonal injury. The prevalence of microbleeds in the normal population is 4% to 8%.[370] Microbleeds are found with increased frequency in patients with severe white matter disease (57%), intracranial

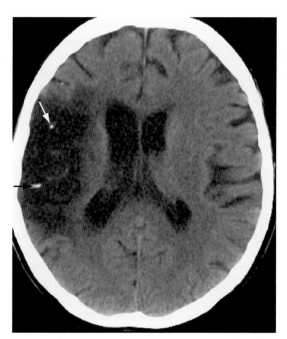

■ **FIGURE 20-37**   Noncontrast CT of chronic right MCA territory infarct demonstrating encephalomalacia, ex vacuo dilatation, and linear and punctate calcification (*arrows*).

hemorrhage (47%-80%), cerebral autosomal dominant arteriopathy with subcortical infarcts and leukoencephalopathy (CADASIL) (31%-78%), and cerebral amyloid angiopathy (69%-100%).[370]

Whether microbleeds are a risk factor for antithrombotic- or thrombolysis-related hemorrhage remains controversial.[296,372] The results of several studies highlight the controversy. The number of microbleeds in patients on antithrombotic agents in these studies was similar, increased, or decreased. However, microbleeds do appear more prevalent in patients presenting with intracranial hemorrhage on antithrombotics than those who are not. A limited literature exists demonstrating mixed results. There are currently insufficient data to exclude such patients from thrombolytic therapy.[370]

Transient Ischemic Attack (TIA) Imaging

TIA is clinically and arbitrarily defined as a transient neurologic deficit lasting less than 24 hours. This definition is favored because it can be consistently applied for epidemiologic purposes but does not take into account restricted diffusion seen in up to 50% of such patients. The distinction between TIA and stroke may not be so important because they have a common pathogenesis and common approach to secondary prevention. The overlap is acknowledged in a recent proposal for a new definition of TIA as a "brief episode of neurologic dysfunction caused by a focal disturbance of brain or retinal ischemia, with clinical symptoms typically lasting less than 1 hour, and without evidence of infarction."[373]

This definition has not been widely accepted, however, because implicit to it is the requirement for similar imaging resources worldwide.[374] Although TIAs are often considered benign, patients with TIA have a 10% to 20% risk of infarction in the first 90 days, with half the infarcts occurring at 24 to 48 hours.[375] The TIA patients with the highest risk of subsequent stroke are those who (1) manifest a speech or motor deficit (9%-12%; 30-day risk), (2) have a large vessel atheroembolic etiology (19%; 90-day risk), or (3) have cardiac causes for the TIA (12%; 90-day risk). The potential for preventing cerebral ischemia or recurrent infarction makes TIA a clinical condition that requires early diagnosis, investigation, and treatment. The proposal of a new TIA definition discussed above also underscores the important role of imaging in these patients.

At a minimum, TIA patients should undergo CT to exclude a stroke mimic such as subdural hemorrhage. However, MRI may help to identify a subset of patients at higher risk for recurrent infarct. CT is insensitive to the typical small focal abnormalities seen on DWI in 20% to 50% of patients. Patients with DWI abnormality on MRI are associated with a 2.6 times higher risk of infarction than those without DWI change. However, one study showed that patients with CT evidence of infarction do worse despite clinical improvement.[376]

Patients should have early carotid Doppler ultrasound, CTA, or MRA to exclude cervical atherosclerotic disease. In a large meta-analysis, this group accounted for only 14% of all TIAs but 37% with recurrent stroke.[9] Carotid endarterectomy has also been shown to be of benefit in symptomatic patients within 2 to 4 weeks of a hemispheric, nondisabling carotid artery ischemic event and a 70% to 99% carotid stenosis. Time to endarterectomy influences efficacy, with the number needed to treat increasing from 5 at 2 weeks to 125 beyond 3 months. Some patients with TIA and 50% to 69% carotid stenosis may also benefit when the perioperative complication rate is less than 6%.[377]

SMALL VESSEL ISCHEMIA

Small vessel ischemia signifies a spectrum of histopathologic findings commonly seen in aging patients. These appear on CT as small bilateral multifocal regions of nonspecific white matter lucency and on MRI as similar regions of T2 hyperintensity.

Initially called leukoaraiosis,[378] this condition is now designated by multiple synonyms, including small vessel change, small vessel ischemia, microangiopathic change, white matter hyperintensities,[379] and age-related white matter change.[380]

Epidemiology

White matter changes are often seen in patients with vascular risk factors, cerebrovascular disease, and cognitive impairment.[381] The prevalence of these changes is 11% to 20% in normal middle-aged individuals, increasing to 100% at age 90 years.[381] Similar findings are reported in 48% to 100% of dementia patients. The extent of white matter abnormality predicts risk of subsequent stroke, especially lacunar infarction.[382,383]

Pathophysiology

The pathogenesis of white matter change is poorly understood. There is good basis to suggest an underlying vascular etiology given the frequent association with increasing age, hypertension, stroke, and markers of cellular ischemia.[379,384,385] Impaired cerebral autoregulation, hypoperfusion, CSF flow disturbances, and blood-brain barrier disruption have also been implicated.[384] The frequent periventricular distribution of this disease and the absence of juxtacortical involvement agree with known patterns of white matter vascular supply. Centripetally directed penetrating vessels arise from the superficial pial network and supply discrete white matter units. Centrifugal supply to the periventricular white matter from ependymal vessels is controversial. In either case the periventricular white matter is particularly vulnerable either as a watershed zone or as a zone dependent on terminal arteriole supply (Fig. 20-38). Conversely, the juxtacortical white matter shares numerous anastomoses, making it more resistant to ischemic change (see Fig. 20-38). This difference in the vascular anatomy may also account for why deep and periventricular white matter changes appear to be caused by different pathophysiologic processes.[386] It is suggested that periventricular lesions may be secondary to fluid accumulation through reduction of ependymal integrity and increased transependymal flow or due to impaired CSF/venous drainage.[385]

Pathology

Histopathologic correlates of small vessel ischemia include loss of ependyma with gliosis, glial swelling, demyelination, and dilated perivascular spaces; lacunar infarcts; spongiosis; arteriolar hyalinosis; amyloid angiopathy; and cystic formation.[387-389] The walls of penetrating arterioles show replacement of smooth muscle cells by fibrohyaline material. The wall thickening and luminal attenuation that results are referred to as arteriosclerosis.[390]

Imaging

CT

White matter abnormality is frequently detected on CT as bilateral, imperfectly symmetric, patchy to confluent, periventricular, deep and subcortical hypodensity.

MRI

MRI reveals foci of T2 hyperintensity not easily appreciable on T1W images. The signal characteristics are nonspecific with a broad differential diagnosis: perivascular spaces are found in characteristic locations and have a signal intensity that follows CSF on all sequences. Ependymitis granularis and terminal zones of myelination are excluded by their characteristic location and their orientation around the frontal horns and peritrigonal regions, respectively (Fig. 20-39). In addition, the hyperintensity found in the terminal zones of myelination usually does not exceed the intensity of gray matter on T2W imaging. Vertical periventricular lesion orientation and callosal and juxtacortical white matter involvement are important discriminators of ischemic change from demyelination. Temporal lobe white matter ischemic involvement is unusual except in the context of Cerebral Autosomal Dominant Arteriopathy with Subcortical Infarcts and Leukoencephalopathy (CADASIL). Primary central nervous system lymphoma commonly shows contrast enhancement, whereas small vessel ischemia does not. Primary and secondary vasculitides and metabolic disorders are also in the differential diagnosis but are discussed elsewhere. Patients with migraine are at increased risk of deep white matter lesion load when compared with control subjects. This increases with hypertension and a history of smoking.

The small vessel ischemic changes of the white matter are often associated with large vessel ischemic injury but may be found as isolated lesions. Several rating scales exist to provide some quantification of disease burden. The Age-Related White Matter Change (ARWMC) scale[391] can be applied to both CT and MRI and has recently been recommended to standardize

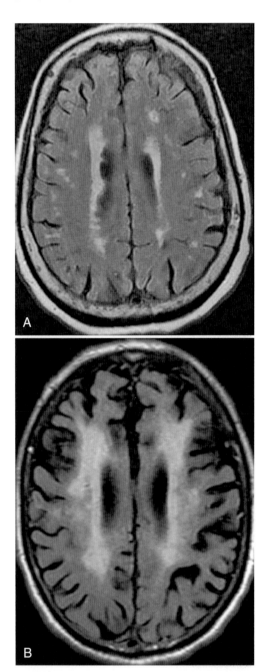

■ **FIGURE 20-38**   Axial FLAIR sequence at the level of the lateral ventricles in two patients with white matter disease. **A,** Confluent periventricular and patchy deep and subcortical white matter change is present. **B,** The periventricular, deep and subcortical white matter changes are confluent with sparing of the juxtacortical region.

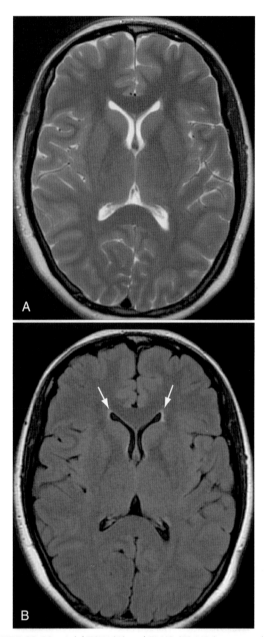

■ **FIGURE 20-39**   Axial T2W (**A**) and FLAIR (**B**) MR images at the level of the frontal horns demonstrating subtle periventricular hyperintensity consistent with ependymitis granularis (*arrows*). The typical location discriminates the findings from white matter changes.

nomenclature for imaging of vascular cognitive impairment.[392] Visual scores perform best in cross-sectional cohort studies, but interrater variability remains a concern. Performance in longitudinal studies is limited by a ceiling effect inherent to such visual scores.

LACUNAR INFARCTS

The word "lacune" means lake in French and describes small cavitations secondary to infarction. These are commonly found in the brain stem and deep cerebral white and gray matter. Multiple extensive basal ganglia lacunes are designated as a "lacunar state" ("état lacunaire"). Although the term was coined for

cavitated deep infarctions, small deep noncavitary infarctions in the same locations have similar etiology, so they will be discussed together.

Epidemiology

Lacunar infarcts account for up to 25% of all ischemic strokes. They are reported more frequently in men, with an increased incidence in African-American and Chinese patients.

Clinical Presentation

Lacunar infarction is a recognized stroke subtype. There are four distinct clinical lacunar syndromes. The most common is a pure motor hemiparesis followed by ataxic hemiparesis. Pure sensory and mixed motor sensory stroke are also described. Patients with lacunar infarction have better survival (75%-97%) and lower

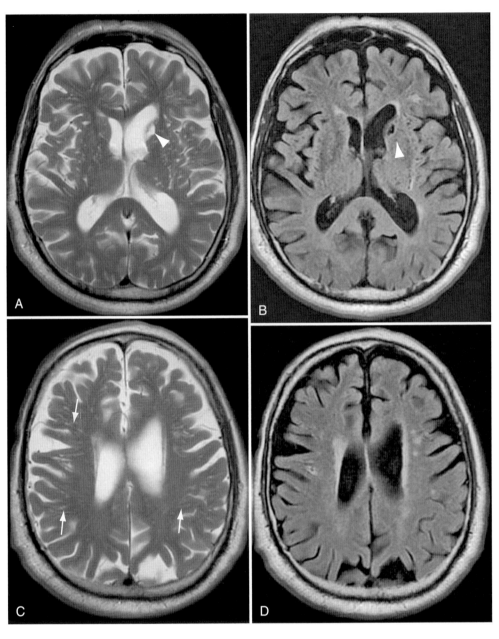

■ **FIGURE 20-40** Axial T2W and FLAIR imaging at the level of the basal ganglia and lateral ventricles. **A,** Numerous small linear hyperintensities are present throughout the corpus striatum, subinsular region, and left thalamus. **B,** On FLAIR the majority are not associated with signal alteration. The linear course and characteristic location confirms multiple perivascular spaces producing a cribriform state. A larger left caudate head lesion (*arrowheads*) is present with surrounding hyperintensity on T2W (**A**) and FLAIR (**B**) imaging. Location and size suggest caudate lacunar infarct. **C, D,** There is a background of periventricular and patchy deep white matter hyperintensities most consistent with white matter disease along with moderate generalized atrophy. Numerous linear T2 hyperintensities are consistent with Virchow-Robin perivascular spaces (VRS) (*arrows*).

levels of disability (20%-30%) than do patients with other stroke subtypes.

Pathophysiology

The etiology of lacunar infarction remains controversial.[393] Many appear to result from penetrating artery lipohyalinosis or microatheroma, because there is a higher risk of recurrent lacunar infarctions (rather than embolic infarctions) in patients presenting with lacunar infarct. There is a strong association with white matter ischemic change and microhemorrhage. Nevertheless, an embolic origin of lacunar infarction is thought to account for 10% to 15% of cases.[394] The finding of multiple cortical and deep lesions in patients presenting with a lacunar syndrome suggests an embolic etiology.[395] Recent work suggests that endothelial dysfunction and increased permeability lead to vessel wall damage and subsequent infarction.[393]

Imaging

MRI

Lacunar infarcts are well-defined lesions that are hypodense on CT, hypointense on T1W imaging, and hyperintense on T2W imaging. Because they are small, acute lacunar infarcts are challenging to identify on CT and conventional MRI, especially in the presence of other white matter change (Fig. 20-40). DWI successfully demonstrates the acute small symptomatic lesions and the chronic asymptomatic lesions that coexist with them[396] or that appear on subsequent studies.[397] The volume of a lacune is usually smaller than 1.8×10 mm^3 or 15 mm in diameter, assuming a spherical shape.[398] Lesion size does not really distinguish between lacunar infarcts and striatocapsular infarcts or enlarged Virchow-Robin perivascular spaces (VRS). Striatocapsular infarcts arise secondary to transient MCA branch occlusions and subsequent clot fragmentation and migration. It is suggested that PWI may distinguish striatocapsular infarcts from lacunae by demonstrating a small penumbra around the striatocapsular infarcts.

VRS are pial-lined interstitial spaces that accompany a penetrating vessel into the brain substance. They are usually smaller than lacunae (<2-5 mm), but larger VRS are described, some exceeding 1 cm. Their signal follows CSF on all pulse sequences. VRS usually show no surrounding signal abnormality, but larger VRS may show peripheral signal change.[399] VRS do not enhance, whereas subacute lacunar infarcts may show contrast enhancement. Most important, VRS are characteristically located within the inferior third of the basal ganglia centered on the anterior commissure.[400] Occasionally, more extensive basal ganglial involvement produces a cribriform appearance called état criblé (see Fig. 20-40).[401] VRS may also be seen within the deep white matter on MRI as linear T2 hyperintensities radiating toward the ventricular margins, corresponding to the centripetal course of penetrating cortical arterioles (Fig. 20-40, C and D). Other locations include the subinsular region, substantia nigra of midbrain, cerebellum, and dentate nuclei.

WATERSHED INFARCTION

Watershed infarcts are infarcts that occur at the junctions of two vascular territories, either at the cortical border zone or at the internal border zone. They are also referred to as border zone infarct, watershed territory infarct, external and internal border zones, cortical border zone, and internal border zone.

Epidemiology

Border zone infarcts account for 5% to 10% of all cerebral infarctions.[311] Carotid stenosis or occlusion and cardiac bypass surgery/ cardiac arrest are two potential causes of border zone infarction. The incidence of infarcts in patients undergoing cardiac surgery is about 9%[402] with up to half of these due to watershed ischemia.

Pathophysiology

Cortical border zone infarcts are infarcts of the superficial cerebral hemispheres occurring at the junctions between two main vascular territories such as the ACA and the MCA (see Figs. 20-36 and 20-41). Internal border zone infarcts occur at the junction between the deep perforating branches of a single major artery such as the border zone between the lenticulostriate branches and deep cortical perforators of the MCA (Figs. 20-41 and 20-42).[403] The mechanism of infarct is controversial. The etiology may be embolic, hypotensive, or both in combination.[404] One study found that three fourths of patients with internal border zone infarcts had evidence of hemodynamic compromise secondary to ICA stenosis or MCA occlusion. Cortical border zone infarcts were associated with other evidence of cortical emboli in 65% of cases compared with 30% for internal border zone infarcts. The apparently greater association of hemodynamic

compromise with internal border zone infarcts is supported by the greater susceptibility of periventricular white matter to ischemia (see earlier). The duration of hypotension may further influence internal border zone lesions. Brief reductions in blood pressure may lead to the rosary pattern of border zone infarction, whereas sustained reductions may lead to confluent border zone infarctions (Fig. 20-42).[405] Internal border zone infarcts should be regarded as markers of reduced cerebral perfusion reserve. Concomitant misery perfusion within the overlying cerebral cortex and more widespread hemodynamic impairment support this supposition.[406]

Imaging

Ultrasonography, MRI, and CT

CTA, MRA, or Doppler ultrasonography may demonstrate carotid stenosis. Circle of Willis collaterals are assessed by CTA, MRA, and transcranial carotid Doppler sonography. Absence of both anterior and posterior communicating artery supply in the presence of an ICA stenosis is associated with higher risk of watershed infarcts. The locations of cortical border zone infarcts on CT and MRI depend on the normal vascular variation (Fig. 20-41) and the organization of the circle of Willis. Cortical border zone infarctions are commonly seen as wedge-shaped infarcts affecting gray and white matter. They occur most commonly between the ACA and MCA territories (Fig. 20-36). Internal border zone infarcts are seen within the deep and periventricular white matter. Confluent (linear, chain) or rosary-like CT hypodensity or T2 hyperintensity is present within the centrum semiovale and corona radiata (see Fig. 20-42). Watershed infarction secondary to hypoperfusion may have a higher propensity for hemorrhagic transformation and early enhancement. This may result from vascular occlusion and infarction of a hypotensive etiology followed by early reperfusion of the infarcted tissue. In patients with cardiac arrest or complications of hypotension during bypass surgery bilateral corpus striatum infarction may also be evident.

Special Procedures

Perfusion imaging has contributed to our understanding of pathophysiology in ICA stenosis. PET, SPECT, xenon CTP, and MRP have been performed. The details are beyond the scope of this chapter but well covered elsewhere.

KEY POINTS: DIFFERENTIAL DIAGNOSIS

Dolichoectasia
■ Dilated redundant vasculature is evident.
■ There is an association with mass effect, aneurysm formation, and white matter change.

Trigeminal Neuralgia
■ Vascular studies have little influence on management decisions.
■ Neurovascular conflict is best defined when there is distortion of the affected nerve by a vessel passing perpendicular to the nerve precisely at the nerve root entry/exit zone.

Fibromuscular Dysplasia
■ The histologic subtype determines the macroscopic appearance.
■ A beaded appearance is characteristic.
■ The upper cervical vasculature is involved.
■ There is systemic vascular involvement of the renal, subclavian, iliac, and mesenteric arteries.

Atherosclerotic Disease
■ Ultrasonography is the most effective screening tool for carotid stenosis.
■ CTA and MRA should be performed to verify suspected abnormal cases.

■ Conventional angiography may be required if there is disagreement between modalities.
■ Near occlusion has a different natural history than high-grade stenosis and must be distinguished from it.
■ Carotid artery stenting has become an alternative to endarterectomy in selected patients.

Intracranial Atherosclerosis
■ Intracranial atherosclerosis accounts for up to 10% of strokes.
■ Asians, blacks, and Hispanics have a much higher incidence of intracranial atherosclerosis.
■ CTA and MRA are useful for intracranial stenosis detection, but conventional angiography remains the reference standard.
■ Management remains controversial; aggressive medical therapy is the mainstay of treatment, while endovascular procedures should be reserved for refractory cases and performed by experienced operators.
■ Angioplasty and stenting have been used with high technical success, but risk-benefit is finely balanced by rate of periprocedural complications.

Dissection
■ Dissection accounts for 2% of all strokes and may be either traumatic or spontaneous.

ACA

MCA

PCA

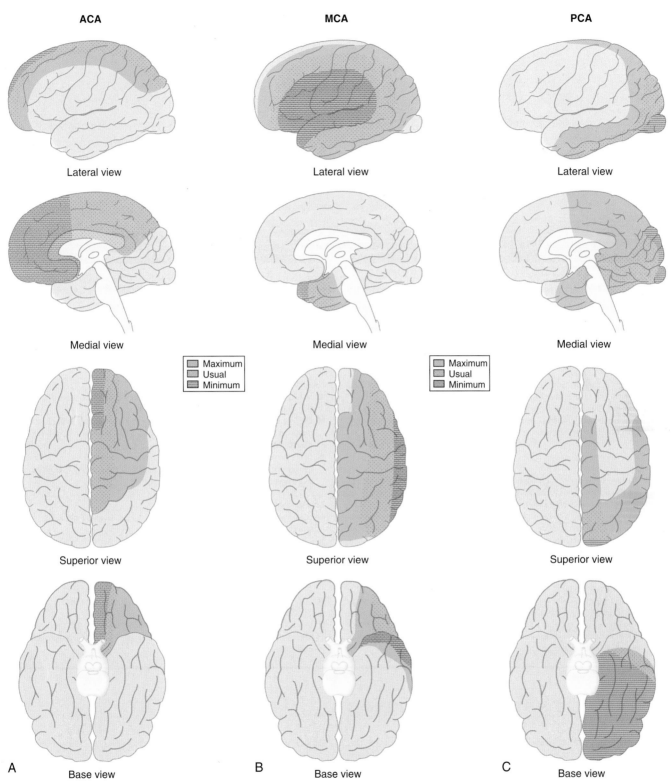

Lateral view

Lateral view

Lateral view

Medial view

Medial view

Medial view

	Maximum
	Usual
	Minimum

	Maximum
	Usual
	Minimum

Superior view

Superior view

Superior view

A

Base view

B

Base view

C

Base view

■ **FIGURE 20-41** **A,** Vascular territories of the cortical (hemispheric) ACA branches with the maximum, usual, and minimum distributions as delineated by van der Zwan.[403] **B** and **C** show the similar distributions for MCA and PCA cortical branches, respectively. *(Redrawn from Osborn AG: Diagnostic Neuroradiology. Philadelphia, Mosby, 1994.)*

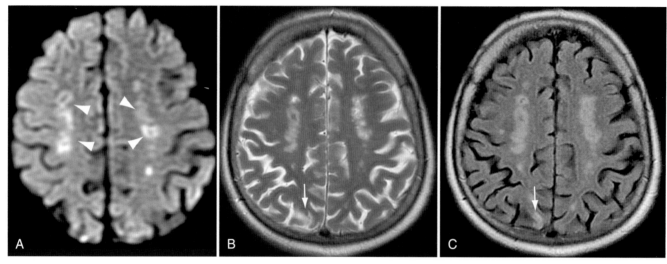

■ **FIGURE 20-42** Axial DWI (**A**), T2W (**B**), and FLAIR (**C**) images demonstrate centrum infarcts in a rosary configuration consistent with internal border zone infarcts in a patient with hypotension. Note right superior parietal lobule infarct in the expected location of the MCA/PCA cortical border zone (*arrow*).

KEY POINTS: DIFFERENTIAL DIAGNOSIS—cont'd

- Internal carotid and vertebral arteries are most commonly involved around the C2 region.
- Imaging findings are usually nonspecific, but MRI may be useful in demonstrating T1 crescentic periluminal hematoma, which has high diagnostic specificity.

Infarct
- Failure to visualize the infarction on noncontrast CT is not necessarily a clinical limitation because patients without CT signs of infarction are the intended target for thrombolysis.
- Although acute hemorrhage usually appears hyperdense on noncontrast CT, patients with severe anemia may show acute hemorrhage with significantly lower density.
- Primary care physicians sometimes refer patients for noncontrast CT at some delay after their infarction. Such patients are best studied more than 2 to 3 weeks after the infarction to avoid misinterpretation due to fogging.
- Infarctions typically show progressive decrease in mass effect starting late in the first week and increasing contrast enhancement peaking in the second week, whereas patients with other processes such as neoplasm usually show progressive mass effect and immediate peak enhancement (absent steroid therapy).

Small Vessel Ischemia
- White matter hyperintensities are nonspecific with a broad differential diagnosis.
- Differences in the distribution of white matter lesions reflect variations in the anatomic vascular supply, with periventricular white matter being the most vulnerable.
- Juxtacortical and temporal white matter involvement is uncommon in ischemic change and should suggest demyelination. CADASIL is the exception to temporal involvement.

Lacunar Infarcts
- Lacunar infarcts are associated with higher rates of disability-free survival than other stroke subtypes.
- The etiology of lacunar infarction is uncertain. Arterial lipohyalinosis or microatheroma accounts for the majority of cases, whereas thromboembolus accounts for 10% to 15% of lacunae.
- DWI can identify the acute lacunar infarct and differentiate it from chronic lacunes, Virchow-Robin spaces, and other mimics.
- Size is a poor discriminator between lacunar infarcts and enlarged Virchow-Robin/perivascular spaces.
- Virchow-Robin/perivascular spaces follow CSF on all sequences and occur in typical locations, especially around the anterior commissure.

SUGGESTED READINGS

Ecker RD, Levy EI, Sauvageau E, et al. Current concepts in the management of intracranial atherosclerotic disease. Neurosurgery 2006; 59(5 Suppl 3):S210-S218; discussion S3-S13.

Ederle J, Brown MM. The evidence for medicine versus surgery for carotid stenosis. Eur J Radiol 2006; 60:3-7. Epub 2006; Aug 21.

Fayad P. Endarterectomy and stenting for asymptomatic carotid stenosis: a race at breakneck speed. Stroke 2007; 38(2 Suppl):707-714.

Flis CM, Pager HR, Sidhu PS. Carotid and vertebral artery dissections: clinical aspects, imaging features and endovascular treatment. Eur Radiol 2007; 17:820-834.

Inzitari D. Leukoaraiosis: an independent risk factor for stroke? Stroke 2003; 34:2067-2071.

Levine RL, Turski PA, Grist TM. Basilar artery dolichoectasia: review of the literature and six patients studied with magnetic resonance angiography. J Neuroimaging 1995; 5:164-170.

Leys D, Lucas C, Gobert M, et al. Cervical artery dissections. Eur Neurol 1997; 37:3-12.

Mokri B, Sundt TMJ, Houser OW, et al. Spontaneous dissection of the cervical internal carotid artery. Ann Neurol 1986; 19: 126-138.

Momjian-Mayor I, Baron J-C. The pathophysiology of watershed infarction in internal carotid artery disease: review of cerebral perfusion studies. Stroke 2005; 36:567-577.

Munoz DG. Leukoaraiosis and ischemia: beyond the myth. Stroke 2006; 37:1348-1349.

Nighoghossian N, Derex L, Douek P. The vulnerable carotid artery plaque: current imaging methods and new perspectives. Stroke 2005; 36:2764-2772. Epub 2005; Nov 10.

Norrving B. Long-term prognosis after lacunar infarction. Lancet Neurol 2003; 2:238-245.

Olin JW. Recognizing and managing fibromuscular dysplasia. Cleve Clin J Med 2007; 4:273-274; discussion 277-282.

Provenzale JW. Dissection of the internal carotid and vertebral arteries: imaging features. AJR Am J Roentgenol 1995; 165:1099-1104.

Qureshi AI. Carotid angioplasty and stent placement after EVA-3S trial. Stroke 2007; 38:1993-1996. Epub 2007; Apr 26.

Taschner CA, Leclerc X, Lucas C, Pruvo JP. Computed tomography angiography for the evaluation of carotid artery dissection. Front Neurol Neurosci 2005; 20:119-128.

van Gijn J. Leukoaraiosis and vascular dementia. Neurology 1998; 51(3 Suppl 3):S3-S8.

Virmani R, Ladich ER, Burke AP, Kolodgie FD. Histopathology of carotid atherosclerotic disease. Neurosurgery 2006; 59(5 Suppl 3): S219-S227; discussion S3-S13.

Wardlaw JM, Sandercock PA, Dennis MS, Starr J. Is breakdown of the blood-brain barrier responsible for lacunar stroke, leukoaraiosis, and dementia? Stroke 2003; 34:806-812.

REFERENCES

1. Gutierrez J, et al. Dolichoectasia—an evolving arterial disease. Nat Rev Neurol 2011; 7:41-50.

1a. Pico F, et al. Intracranial arterial dolichoectasia and small-vessel disease in stroke patients. Ann Neurol 2005; 57:472-479.

2. Barker FG 2nd, et al. Microvascular decompression for hemifacial spasm. J Neurosurg 1995; 82:201-210.

3. Meaney JF, et al. Demonstration of neurovascular compression in trigeminal neuralgia with magnetic resonance imaging: comparison with surgical findings in 52 consecutive operative cases. J Neurosurg 1995; 83:799-805.

4. Hutchins LG, et al. Trigeminal neuralgia (tic douloureux): MR imaging assessment. Radiology 1990; 175:837-841.

5. Tash R, et al. Hemifacial spasm: MR imaging features. AJNR Am J Neuroradiol 1991; 12:839-842.

6. Love S, Coakham HB. Trigeminal neuralgia: pathology and pathogenesis. Brain 2001; 124:2347-2360.

7. Nurmikko TJ, Eldridge PR. Trigeminal neuralgia—pathophysiology, diagnosis and current treatment. Br J Anaesth 2001; 87:117-132.

7a. Lutz J, et al. Trigeminal neuralgia due to neurovascular compression: high-spatial-resolution diffusion-tensor imaging reveals microstructural neural changes. Radiology 2011; 258:524-530.

7b. Touzé E, et al. Fibromuscular dysplasia of cervical and intracranial arteries. Int J Stroke 2010; 5:296-305.

8. Furie D, Tien R. Fibromuscular dysplasia of arteries of the head and neck: imaging findings. AJR Am J Roentgenol 1994; 162: 1205-1209.

9. Lovett JK, Coull AJ, Rothwell PM. Early risk of recurrence by subtype of ischemic stroke in population-based incidence studies. Neurology 2004; 62:569-573.

10. Fairhead JF, Mehta Z, Rothwell PM. Population-based study of delays in carotid imaging and surgery and the risk of recurrent stroke. Neurology 2005; 65:371-375.

11. Jeziorska M, Woolley DE. Local neovascularization and cellular composition within vulnerable regions of atherosclerotic plaques of human carotid arteries. J Pathol 1999; 188:189-196.

12. Sacco RL. Clinical practice: extracranial carotid stenosis. N Engl J Med 2001; 345:1113-1118.

13. Ross R, Glomset JA. The pathogenesis of atherosclerosis: II. N Engl J Med 1976; 295:420-425.

14. Ross R, Glomset JA. The pathogenesis of atherosclerosis: I. N Engl J Med 1976; 295:369-377.

15. Savory WS. Case of a young woman in whom the arteries of both upper extremities and of the left side of the neck were throughout completely obliterated. Med-Chir Trans London 1856; 39:205-219.

16. Chiari H. Uber das Verhalten des Teilingsungswinkels der Carotis communis bei der Endarteritis chronica deformans. Verh Dtsch Pathol Ges 1905; 9:326-339.

17. Fisher CM. Occlusion of the internal carotid artery. Arch Neurol Psychiatry 1951; 65:346-377.

18. Kumar V, Abbas A, Fausto N (eds). Robbins and Cotran Pathologic Basis of Disease, 7th ed. Philadelphia, Elsevier Saunders, 2005, p 1525.

19. Fuster V, et al. Atherothrombosis and high-risk plaque: I. Evolving concepts. J Am Coll Cardiol 2005; 46:937-954.

20. Stary HC. Natural history and histological classification of atherosclerotic lesions: an update. Arterioscler Thromb Vasc Biol 2000; 20:1177-1178.

21. Stary HC, et al. A definition of the intima of human arteries and of its atherosclerosis-prone regions. A report from the Committee on Vascular Lesions of the Council on Arteriosclerosis, American Heart Association. Arterioscler Thromb 1992; 12:120-134.

22. Stary HC, et al. A definition of advanced types of atherosclerotic lesions and a histological classification of atherosclerosis. A report from the Committee on Vascular Lesions of the Council on Arteriosclerosis, American Heart Association. Arterioscler Thromb Vasc Biol 1995; 15:1512-1531.

23. Stary HC, et al. A definition of initial, fatty streak, and intermediate lesions of atherosclerosis. A report from the Committee on Vascular Lesions of the Council on Arteriosclerosis, American Heart Association. Circulation 1994; 89:2462-2478.

24. Glagov S, et al. Compensatory enlargement of human atherosclerotic coronary arteries. N Engl J Med 1987; 316:1371-1375.

25. Virmani R, et al. Lessons from sudden coronary death: a comprehensive morphological classification scheme for atherosclerotic lesions. Arterioscler Thromb Vasc Biol 2000; 20:1262-1275.

26. Nissen SE, Yock P. Intravascular ultrasound: novel pathophysiological insights and current clinical applications. Circulation 2001; 103:604-616.

27. Cohen A, et al. Aortic plaque morphology and vascular events: a follow-up study in patients with ischemic stroke. FAPS Investigators. French Study of Aortic Plaques in Stroke. Circulation 1997; 96:3838-3841.

28. Fayad ZA, Fuster V. Clinical imaging of the high-risk or vulnerable atherosclerotic plaque. Circ Res 2001; 89:305-316.

29. Pignoli P, et al. Intimal plus medial thickness of the arterial wall: a direct measurement with ultrasound imaging. Circulation 1986; 74:1399-1406.

30. Franzen D, Sechtem U, Hopp HW. Comparison of angioscopic, intravascular ultrasonic, and angiographic detection of thrombus in coronary stenosis. Am J Cardiol 1998; 82:1273-1275.

31. Grant EG, et al. Carotid artery stenosis: gray-scale and Doppler US diagnosis—Society of Radiologists in Ultrasound Consensus Conference. Radiology 2003; 229:340-346.

32. Sabeti S, et al. Quantification of internal carotid artery stenosis with duplex US: comparative analysis of different flow velocity criteria. Radiology 2004; 232:431-439.

32a. King A, Markus HS. Doppler embolic signals in cerebrovascular disease and prediction of stroke risk: a systematic review and meta-analysis. Stroke 2009; 40:3711-3717.

33. Johnston DCC, Goldstein LB. Clinical carotid endarterectomy decision making: noninvasive vascular imaging versus angiography. Neurology 2001; 56:1009-1015.

34. Borisch I, et al. Preoperative evaluation of carotid artery stenosis: comparison of contrast-enhanced MR angiography and duplex sonography with digital subtraction angiography. AJNR Am J Neuroradiol 2003; 24:1117-1122.

35. Patel SG, et al. Outcome, observer reliability, and patient preferences if CTA, MRA, or Doppler ultrasound were used, individually or together, instead of digital subtraction angiography before carotid endarterectomy. J Neurol Neurosurg Psychiatry 2002; 73:21-28.

36. Koelemay MJW, et al. Systematic review of computed tomographic angiography for assessment of carotid artery disease. Stroke 2004; 35:2306-2312.

37. de Monye C, et al. Optimization of CT angiography of the carotid artery with a 16-MDCT scanner: craniocaudal scan direction

reduces contrast material-related perivenous artifacts. AJR Am J Roentgenol 2006; 186:1737-1745.

38. Silvennoinen HM, et al. CT angiographic analysis of carotid artery stenosis: comparison of manual assessment, semiautomatic vessel analysis, and digital subtraction angiography. AJNR Am J Neuroradiol 2007; 28:97-103.

38a. Latchaw RE, et al. Recommendations for imaging of acute ischemic stroke: a scientific statement from the American Heart Association. Stroke 2009; 40:3646-3678.

38b. Lev MH, et al. Total occlusion versus hairline residual lumen of the internal carotid arteries: accuracy of single section helical CT angiography. AJNR Am J Neuroradiol 2003; 24:1123-1129.

38c. Bartlett ES, et al. Diagnosing carotid stenosis near-occlusion by using CT angiography. AJNR Am J Neuroradiol 2006; 27:632-637.

39. Lell M, et al. Evaluation of carotid artery stenosis with multisection CT and MR imaging: influence of imaging modality and post-processing. AJNR Am J Neuroradiol 2007; 28:104-110.

39a. Uotani K, et al. Dual-energy CT head bone and hard plaque removal for quantification of calcified carotid stenosis: utility and comparison with digital subtraction angiography. Eur Radiol 2009; 19:2060-2065.

39b. Thomas C, et al. Automatic lumen segmentation in calcified plaques: dual-energy CT versus standard reconstructions in comparison with digital subtraction angiography. AJR Am J Roentgenol 2010; 194:1590-1595.

40. Bartlett ES, et al. Quantification of carotid stenosis on CT angiography. AJNR Am J Neuroradiol 2006; 27:13-19.

41. Bartlett ES, Symons SP, Fox AJ. Correlation of carotid stenosis diameter and cross-sectional areas with CT angiography. AJNR Am J Neuroradiol 2006; 27:638-642.

42. de Weert TT, et al. In vitro characterization of atherosclerotic carotid plaque with multidetector computed tomography and histopathological correlation. Eur Radiol 2005; 15:1906-1914.

43. Carrascosa PM, et al. Characterization of coronary atherosclerotic plaques by multidetector computed tomography. Am J Cardiol 2006; 97:598-602.

44. Schroeder S, et al. Noninvasive detection and evaluation of atherosclerotic coronary plaques with multislice computed tomography. J Am Coll Cardiol 2001; 37:1430-1435.

45. Viles-Gonzalez JF, et al. In vivo 16-slice, multidetector-row computed tomography for the assessment of experimental atherosclerosis: comparison with magnetic resonance imaging and histopathology. Circulation 2004; 110:1467-1472.

46. Oliver TB, Lammie GA, Wright AR, et al. Atherosclerotic plaque at the carotid bifurcation: CT angiographic appearance with histopathologic. AJNR Am J Neuroradiol 1999; 20:897-901.

47. Walker LJ, et al. Computed tomography angiography for the evaluation of carotid atherosclerotic plaque: correlation with histopathology of endarterectomy specimens. Stroke 2002; 33:977-981.

48. Nederkoorn PJ, et al. Carotid artery stenosis: accuracy of contrast-enhanced mr angiography for diagnosis. Radiology 2003; 228:677-682.

49. Anzalone N, et al. Carotid artery stenosis: intraindividual correlations of 3D time-of-flight MR angiography, contrast-enhanced MR angiography, conventional DSA, and rotational angiography for detection and grading. Radiology 2005; 236:204-213.

50. Broome DR, et al. Gadodiamide-associated nephrogenic systemic fibrosis: why radiologists should be concerned. AJR Am J Roentgenol 2007; 188:586-592.

51. Nederkoorn PJ, et al. Preoperative diagnosis of carotid artery stenosis: accuracy of noninvasive testing. Stroke 2002; 33:2003-2008.

52. Yuan C, Hatsukami TS, O'Brien KD. High-resolution magnetic resonance imaging of normal and atherosclerotic human coronary arteries ex vivo: discrimination of plaque tissue components. J Invest Med 2001; 49:491-499.

53. Moody AR, et al. Characterization of complicated carotid plaque with magnetic resonance direct thrombus imaging in patients with cerebral ischemia. Circulation 2003; 107:3047-3052.

54. Bitar R, et al. In vivo high-resolution volumetric imaging of carotid complicated plaque: 3-dimensional high-resolution magnetic resonance direct thrombus imaging (hiresMRDTI). Presented before the 14th Scientific Meeting of the International Society of Magnetic Resonance in Medicine (ISMRM). Seattle, 2006.

55. Wasserman BA, et al. Carotid artery atherosclerosis: in vivo morphologic characterization with gadolinium-enhanced double-oblique MR imaging initial results. Radiology 2002; 223:566-573.

56. Cappendijk VC, et al. In vivo detection of hemorrhage in human atherosclerotic plaques with magnetic resonance imaging. J Magn Reson Imaging 2004; 20:105-110.

57. Yuan C, et al. Identification of fibrous cap rupture with magnetic resonance imaging is highly associated with recent transient ischemic attack or stroke. Circulation 2002; 105:181-185.

58. Yuan C, et al. Phased-array magnetic resonance imaging of the carotid artery bifurcation: preliminary results in healthy volunteers and a patient with atherosclerotic disease. J Magn Reson Imaging 1995; 5:561-565.

59. Ouhlous M, et al. Evaluation of a dedicated dual phased-array surface coil using a black-blood FSE sequence for high resolution MRI of the carotid vessel wall. J Magn Reson Imaging 2002; 15:344-351.

60. Mani V, et al. Comparison of gated and non-gated fast multislice black-blood carotid imaging using rapid extended coverage and inflow/outflow saturation techniques. J Magn Reson Imaging 2005; 22:628-633.

61. Libby P. What have we learned about the biology of atherosclerosis? The role of inflammation. Am J Cardiol 2001; 88:3J-6J.

62. Falk E, Shah PK, Fuster V. Coronary plaque disruption. Circulation 1995; 92:657-671.

63. Yuan C, et al. In vitro and in situ magnetic resonance imaging signal features of atherosclerotic plaque-associated lipids. Arterioscler Thromb Vasc Biol 1997; 17:1496-1503.

64. Chu B, et al. Hemorrhage in the atherosclerotic carotid plaque: a high-resolution MRI study. Stroke 2004; 35:1079-1084.

65. Morrisett J, et al. Discrimination of components in atherosclerotic plaques from human carotid endarterectomy specimens by magnetic resonance imaging ex vivo. Magn Reson Imaging 2003; 21:465-474.

66. Coombs BD, et al. Structure of plaque at carotid bifurcation: high-resolution MRI with histological correlation. Stroke 2001; 32:2516-2521.

67. Zhang S, et al. Comparison of carotid vessel wall area measurements using three different contrast-weighted black blood MR imaging techniques. Magn Reson Imaging 2001; 19:795-802.

68. Crowe LA, et al. Elimination of residual blood flow-related signal in 3D volume-selective TSE arterial wall imaging using velocity-sensitive phase reconstruction. J Magn Reson Imaging 2006; 23:416-421.

69. Crowe LA, et al. 3D volume-selective turbo spin echo for carotid artery wall imaging with navigator detection of swallowing. J Magn Reson Imaging 2005; 22:583-588.

70. Crowe LA, et al. Volume-selective 3D turbo spin echo imaging for vascular wall imaging and distensibility measurement. J Magn Reson Imaging 2003; 17:572-580.

71. Mani V, et al. Carotid black blood MRI burden of atherosclerotic disease assessment correlates with ultrasound intima-media thickness. J Cardiovasc Magn Reson 2006; 8:529-534.

72. Kerwin W, et al. Quantitative magnetic resonance imaging analysis of neovasculature volume in carotid atherosclerotic plaque. Circulation 2003; 107:851-856.

72a. Qiao Y, et al. Carotid plaque neovascularization and hemorrhage detected by MR imaging are associated with recent cerebrovascular ischemic events. AJNR Am J Neuroradiol 2012; 33:755-760.

73. Berg M, et al. Multi-detector row CT angiography in the assessment of carotid artery disease in symptomatic patients: comparison with rotational angiography and digital subtraction angiography. AJNR Am J Neuroradiol 2005; 26:1022-1034.

74. Fox AJ. How to measure carotid stenosis. Radiology 1993; 186:316-318.

75. Loscalzo J, Rocco TP. Imaging arterial thrombi: an elusive goal. Circulation 1992; 85:382-385.

76. Vallabhajosula S, et al. Radiotracers for low density lipoprotein biodistribution studies in vivo: technetium-99m low density lipoprotein versus radioiodinated low density lipoprotein preparations. J Nucl Med 1988; 29:1237-1245.

77. Zhang Z, et al. Non-invasive imaging of atherosclerotic plaque macrophage in a rabbit model with F-18 FDG PET: a histopathological correlation. BMC Nucl Med 2006; 6:3.

78. Davies JR, et al. Identification of culprit lesions after transient ischemic attack by combined 18F fluorodeoxyglucose positron-emission tomography and high-resolution magnetic resonance imaging. Stroke 2005; 36:2642-2647.

79. Faries PL, et al. Current management of extracranial carotid artery disease. Vasc Endovascular Surg 2006; 40:165-175.

80. Beneficial effect of carotid endarterectomy in symptomatic patients with high-grade carotid stenosis. North American Symptomatic Carotid Endarterectomy Trial Collaborators. N Engl J Med 1991; 325:445-453.

81. MRC European Carotid Surgery Trial: interim results for symptomatic patients with severe (70-99%) or with mild (0-29%) carotid stenosis. European Carotid Surgery Trialists' Collaborative Group. Lancet 1991; 337:1235-1243.

82. Goldstein LB, et al. Primary prevention of ischemic stroke: A statement for healthcare professionals from the Stroke Council of the American Heart Association. Circulation 2001; 103:163-182.

83. Gorelick PB, et al. Prevention of a first stroke: a review of guidelines and a multidisciplinary consensus statement from the National Stroke Association. JAMA 1999; 281:1112-1120.

84. Albers GW, et al. AHA Scientific Statement. Supplement to the guidelines for the management of transient ischemic attacks: A statement from the Ad Hoc Committee on Guidelines for the Management of Transient Ischemic Attacks, Stroke Council, American Heart Association. Stroke 1999; 30:2502-2511.

84a. Furie KL, et al. Guidelines for the prevention of stroke in patients with stroke or transient ischemic attack: a guideline for healthcare professionals from the American Heart Association/American Stroke Association. Stroke 2011; 42:227-276.

85. Endarterectomy for asymptomatic carotid artery stenosis. Executive Committee for the Asymptomatic Carotid Atherosclerosis Study. JAMA 1995; 273:1421-1428.

86. Rothwell PM, et al. Endarterectomy for symptomatic carotid stenosis in relation to clinical subgroups and timing of surgery. Lancet 2004; 363:915-924.

87. Kastrup A, et al. Early outcome of carotid angioplasty and stenting with and without cerebral protection devices: a systematic review of the literature. Stroke 2003; 34:813-819.

88. Endovascular versus surgical treatment in patients with carotid stenosis in the Carotid and Vertebral Artery Transluminal Angioplasty Study (CAVATAS): a randomised trial. Lancet 2001; 357:1729-1737.

89. Yadav JS, et al. Protected carotid-artery stenting versus endarterectomy in high-risk patients. N Engl J Med 2004; 351:1493-1501.

90. Ringleb PA, et al. 30 Day results from the SPACE trial of stent-protected angioplasty versus carotid endarterectomy in symptomatic patients: a randomised non-inferiority trial. Lancet 2006; 368: 1239-1247.

91. Mas J-L, et al. Endarterectomy versus stenting in patients with symptomatic severe carotid stenosis. N Engl J Med 2006; 355: 1660-1671.

91a. Mantese VA, et al. The Carotid Revascularization Endarterectomy versus Stenting Trial (CREST): stenting versus carotid endarterectomy for carotid disease. Stroke 2010; 41(10 Suppl):S31-S34.

91b. Bonati LH, et al. Short-term outcome after stenting versus endarterectomy for symptomatic carotid stenosis: a preplanned meta-analysis of individual patient data. Lancet 2010; 376:1062-1073.

92. Asil T, Balci K, Ilkay U, et al. Six-month follow-up study in patients with symptomatic intracranial arterial stenosis. J Clin Neurosci 2006; 12:913-916.

93. Chimowitz MI, Lynn MJ, Howlett-Smith H, et al. Comparison of warfarin and aspirin for symptomatic intracranial arterial stenosis. N Engl J Med 2005; 352:1305-1316.

94. Hass WK, Field WS, North RR, et al. Joint study of extracranial arterial occlusion: II. Arteriography, techniques, sites, and complications. JAMA 1986; 203:961-968.

95. Sacco RL, Kargman DE, Gu Q, Zamanillo C. Race-ethnicity and determinants of intracranial atherosclerotic cerebral infarction: The Northern Manhattan Stroke Study. Stroke 1995; 26:14-20.

96. Feldmann E, Daneault N, Kwan E, et al. Chinese-white differences in the distribution of occlusive cerebrovascular disease. Neurology 1990; 40:1541-1545.

97. Leung SY, Ng TH, Yuen ST, et al. Pattern of cerebral atherosclerosis in Hong Kong Chinese: Severity in intracranial and extracranial vessels. Stroke 1993; 24:779-786.

98. Bogousslavsky J, Barnett HJM, Fox AJ, et al. Atherosclerotic disease of the middle cerebral artery. Stroke 1986; 17:1112-1120.

99. Wong KS, Ng PW, Tang A, et al. Prevalence of asymptomatic intracranial atherosclerosis in high-risk patients. Neurology 2007; 68:2035-2038.

100. Cui R, Iso H, Toyoshima H. Body mass index and mortality from cardiovascular disease among Japanese men and women: the JACC study. Stroke 2005; 36:1377-1382.

101. Nam HS, Han SW, Lee JY, et al. Association of aortic plaque with intracranial atherosclerosis in patients with stroke. Neurology 2006; 67:1184-1188.

102. Akins PT, Pilgrim TK, Cross DT III, Moran CJ. Natural history of stenosis from intracranial atherosclerosis by serial angiography. Stroke 1998; 29:433-438.

103. Komotar RJ, Mocco J, Wilson DA, et al. The natural history of intracranial carotid artery atherosclerosis. Neurosurg Focus 2005; 18(1):E4.

104. Thijs VN, Albers GW. Symptomatic intracranial atherosclerosis. Neurology 2000; 55:490-498.

105. Mazighi M, Tanasescu R, Ducrocq X, et al. Prospective study of symptomatic atherothrombotic intracranial stenoses: The GESICA study. Neurology 2006; 66:1187-1191.

106. Chimowitz MI, Strong J, et al. Prognosis of patients with symptomatic vertebral or basilar artery stenosis. Stroke 1998; 29:1389-1392.

107. Moufarrij NA, Little JR, Furlan AJ, et al. Basilar and distal vertebral artery stenosis: Long-term follow-up. Stroke 1986; 17:938-942.

108. Gao S, Lam WWM, Chan YL, et al. Optimal values of flow velocity on transcranial Doppler in grading middle cerebral artery stenosis in comparison with magnetic resonance angiography. J Neuroimaging 2002; 12:213-219.

109. Feldmann E, Wilterdink JL, Kosinski A, et al. The Stroke Outcomes and Neuroimaging of Intracranial Atherosclerosis (SONIA) trial. Neurology 2007; 68:2099-2105.

110. Arenillas JF, Molina CA, Montaner J, et al. Progression and clinical recurrence of symptomatic middle cerebral artery stenosis: a long-term follow-up transcranial Doppler ultrasound study. Stroke 2001; 32:2898-2904.

111. Bash S, Villablanca JP, Jahan R, et al. Intracranial vascular stenosis and occlusive disease: evaluation with CT angiography, MR angiography, and digital subtraction angiography. AJNR 2005; 26:1012-1021.

112. Choi CG, Lee DH, Lee JH, et al. Detection of intracranial atherosclerotic steno-occlusive disease with 3D time-of-flight magnetic resonance angiography with sensitivity encoding at 3T. AJNR Am J Neuroradiol 2007; 28:439-446.

113. Millikan CH, Siekert RG, Shick RM. Studies in cerebrovascular disease: III: The use of anticoagulant drugs in the treatment of insufficiency or thrombosis within the basilar arterial system. Proc Staff Meet Mayo Clin 1955; 30:116-126.

114. Kay R, Wong KS, Yu YL, et al. Low-molecular-weight heparin for the treatment of acute ischemic stroke. N Engl J Med 1995; 333:1588-1593.

114a. Kay R, Wong KS, Yu YL, et al. Low-molecular weight heparin for the treatment of acute ischemic stroke. N Engl J Med 1995; 95(333):1588–1593.

115. Bath PMW, Lindenstrom E, Boysen G, et al. Tinzaparin in acute ischemic stroke (TAIST): a randomized aspirin-controlled trial. Lancet 2001; 358:702-710.

116. Bendixen BH, Adams HP, Davis H, et al. Low molecular weight heparinoid, ORG 10172 (Danaparoid), and outcome after acute ischemic stroke. JAMA 1998; 279:1265-1272.

117. Wong KS, Chen C, Ng PW, et al. Low-molecular-weight heparin compared with aspirin for the treatment of acute ischaemic stroke in Asian patients with large artery occlusive disease: a randomised study. Neurology 2007; 6:407-413.

117a. Powers WJ, et al. Extracranial-intracranial bypass surgery for stroke prevention in hemodynamic cerebral ischemia: the Carotid Occlusion Surgery Study randomized trial. JAMA 2011; 306:1983-1992.

118. Sundt TM Jr, Smith HC, Campbell JK, et al: Transluminal angioplasty for basilar artery stenosis. Mayo Clin Proc 1980; 55:673-680.

119. Gomez CR, Mistra VK, Campbell MS, Soto RD. Elective stenting of symptomatic middle cerebral artery stenosis. AJNR Am J Neuroradiol 2000; 21:971-973.

120. Terada T, Tsuura M, Matsumoto H, et al. Endovascular therapy for stenosis of the pterous or cavernous portion of the internal carotid artery: percutaneous transluminal angioplasty compared with stent placement. J Neurosurg 2003; 98:491-497.

121. Jiang WJ, Wang YJ, Du B, et al. Stenting of symptomatic M1 stenosis of middle cerebral artery: an initial experience of 40 patients. Stroke 2004; 35:1375-1380.

122. Kim JK, Ahn JY, Lee BH, et al. Elective stenting for symptomatic middle cerebral artery stenosis presenting as transient ischaemic deficits or stroke attacks: short term arteriographical and clinical outcome. J Neurol Neurosurg Psychiatry 2004; 75:847-851.

123. Helmi LL, Barnwell S, Mawad M, et al. Stenting of symptomatic atherosclerotic lesions in the vertebral or intracranial arteries (SSYLVIA): study results. Stroke 2004; 35:1388-1392.

124. Jiang WJ, Srivastaba T, Gao F, et al. Perforator stroke after elective stenting of symptomatic intracranial stenosis. Neurology 2006; 66:1868-1872.

125. Levy EI, Chaturvedi S. Perforator stroke following intracranial stenting: a sacrifice for the greater good? Neurology 2006; 66: 1803-1804.

126. Levy EI, Hanel RA, Bendok BR, et al. Comparison of periprocedure complications resulting from direct stent placement compared with those due to conventional and staged stent placement in the basilar artery. J Neurosurg 2003; 99:653-660.

127. Hartmann M, Jansen O. Angioplasty and stenting of intracranial stenosis. Curr Opin Neurol 2005; 18:39-45.

128. Bose A, Hartmann M, Henkes H, et al. A novel, self-expanding, nitinol stent in medically refractory intracranial atherosclerotic stenoses—the Wingspan study. Stroke 2007; 38;1531-1537.

128a. Chimowitz MI, et al. Stenting versus aggressive medical therapy for intracranial arterial stenosis. N Engl J Med 2011; 365:993-1003.

129. Sue DE, Brant-Zawadzki MN, Chana J. Dissection of cranial arteries in the neck: correlation of MRI and arteriography. Neuroradiology 1992; 34:273-278.

130. Schievink WI, Wijdicks EFM, Kuiper JD. Seasonal pattern of spontaneous cervical artery dissection. J Neurosurg 1998; 46:101-103.

131. Schievink WI, Mokri B, Piepgras DG, et al. Recurrent spontaneous arterial dissections: risk in familial and nonfamilial disease. Stroke 1996; 27:622-624.

132. Kalimo H, Kaste M, Haltia M. Vascular diseases. In Gram DI, Lantos PL (eds). Greenfield's Neuropathology, 6th ed. London, Arnold, 1997, pp 315-396.

133. Burger KM, Tuhrim S, Naidich TP. Brainstem vascular stroke anatomy. Neuroimaging Clin North Am 2005; 15:297-324.

134. Kremer C, et al. Carotid dissection with permanent and transient occlusion or severe stenosis: long-term outcome. Neurology 2003; 60:271-275.

135. Cotran RS, Kumar V, Robbins SL. Fluid and hemodynamic derangements. In Cotran RS, Kumar V, Robbins SL (eds). Robbins Pathologic Basis of Disease, 4th ed. Philadelphia, WB Saunders, 1989, pp 87-120.

136. Volker W, Besselmann M, Dittrich R, et al. Generalized arteriopathy in patients with cervical artery dissection. Neurology 2005; 64:1508-1513.

137. Fraser AR, Zimbler SM. Hindbrain stroke in children caused by extracranial vertebral artery trauma. Stroke 1975; 6:153-159.

138. Mizutani T, Aruga T, Kirino T, et al. Recurrent subarachnoid hemorrhage from untreated ruptured vertebrobasilar dissecting aneurysms. Neurosurgery 1995; 36:905-911.

138a. Eastman AL, et al. CTA-based screening reduces time to diagnosis and stroke rate in blunt cervical vascular injury. J Trauma 2009; 67:551-556; discussion 555-556.

139. Benninger DH, Baumgartner RW. Ultrasound diagnosis of cervical artery dissection. Front Neurol Neurosci 2006; 21:70-84.

140. Dittrich R, Dziewas R, Ritter MA, et al. Negative ultrasound findings in patients with cervical artery dissection. J Neurol 2006; 253:424-433.

141. Elijovich L, Kazmi K, Gauvrit JY, Law M. The emerging role of multidector row CT angiography in the diagnosis of cervical arterial dissection: preliminary study. Neuroradiology 2006; 48:606-612.

142. Leclerc X, Lucas C, Godfrey O, et al. Helical CT for the follow-up of cervical internal artery dissections. Am J Neuroradiol 1998; 19:831-837.

143. Rizzo L, Crasto SG, Savio D, et al. Dissection of the cervicocephalic arteries: early diagnosis and follow-up with magnetic resonance imaging. Emerg Radiol 2006; 12:254-265.

144. Bachmann R, Nassenstein I, Kooijman H, et al. High-resolution magnetic resonance imaging (MRI) at 3.0 Tesla in the short-term follow-up of patients with proven cervical artery dissection. Invest Radiol 2007; 42:460-466.

144a. Provenzale JM, et al. Causes of misinterpretation of cross-sectional imaging studies for dissection of the craniocervical arteries. AJR Am J Roentgenol 2011; 196:45-52.

145. Halbach VV, Higashida RT, Dowd CF, et al. Endovascular treatment of vertebral artery dissections and pseudoaneurysms. J Neurosurg 1993; 79:183-191.

146. Lempert TE, Halback VV, Higashida RT, et al. Endovascular treatment of pseudoaneurysms with electrolytically detachable coils. Am J Neuroradiol 1998; 19:907-911.

147. Mackay J, Mensah GA. The Atlas of Heart Disease and Stroke. Geneva, World Health Organization and Centers for Disease Control, 2004.

148. Public health and aging: hospitalizations for stroke among adults aged ≥65 years—United States, 2000. MMWR Morbid Mortal Wkly Rep 2003; 52:586-589.

149. Leung SY, et al. Pattern of cerebral atherosclerosis in Hong Kong Chinese. Severity in intracranial and extracranial vessels. Stroke 1993; 24:779-786.

150. Bamford J, et al. A prospective study of acute cerebrovascular disease in the community: the Oxfordshire Community Stroke Project 1981-86. I. Methodology, demography and incident cases of first-ever stroke. J Neurol Neurosurg Psychiatry 1988; 51:1373-1380.

151. Grau AJ, et al. Risk factors, outcome, and treatment in subtypes of ischemic stroke: The German Stroke Data Bank. Stroke 2001; 32:2559-2566.

152. Adams HP Jr, et al. Classification of subtype of acute ischemic stroke: Definitions for use in a multicenter clinical trial. TOAST. Trial of Org 10172 in Acute Stroke Treatment. Stroke 1993; 24:35-41.

153. Li SC, et al. Cerebrovascular disease in the People's Republic of China: epidemiologic and clinical features. Neurology 1985; 35:1708-1713.

154. Bamford J, et al. Classification and natural history of clinically identifiable subtypes of cerebral infarction. Lancet 1991; 337: 1521-1526.

155. Allder SJ, et al. Differences in the diagnostic accuracy of acute stroke clinical subtypes defined by multimodal magnetic resonance imaging. J Neurol Neurosurg Psychiatry 2003; 74: 886-888.

156. Kannel WB, et al. The Framingham Study: Its 50-year legacy and future promise. J Atheroscler Thromb 2000; 6:60-66.

157. Lewington S, et al. Age-specific relevance of usual blood pressure to vascular mortality: a meta-analysis of individual data for one million adults in 61 prospective studies. Lancet 2002; 360: 1903-1913.

158. Ridker PM. Inflammatory biomarkers, statins, and the risk of stroke: cracking a clinical conundrum. Circulation 2002; 105:2583-2585.

159. Goldstein LB, et al. Novel risk factors for stroke: homocysteine, inflammation, and infection. Curr Atheroscler Rep 2000; 2:110-114.

160. Hassan A, Markus HS. Genetics and ischemic stroke. Brain 2000; 123:1784-1812.

161. Mudd SH, et al. The natural history of homocystinuria due to cystathionine beta-synthase deficiency. Am J Hum Genet 1985; 37:1-31.

162. Kalaria RN, et al. The pathogenesis of CADASIL: an update. J Neurol Sci 2004; 226:35-39.

163. Powers WJ. Cerebral hemodynamics in ischemic cerebrovascular disease. Ann Neurol 1991; 29:231-240.

164. Astrup J, Siesjo BK, Symon L. Thresholds in cerebral ischemia—the ischemic penumbra. Stroke 1981; 12:723-725.

165. Heiss WD, Rosner G. Functional recovery of cortical neurons as related to degree and duration of ischemia. Ann Neurol 1983; 14:294-301.

166. Hossmann KA. Viability thresholds and the penumbra of focal ischemia. Ann Neurol 1994; 36:557-565.

167. Heiss WD, et al. Dynamic penumbra demonstrated by sequential multitracer PET after middle cerebral artery occlusion in cats. J Cereb Blood Flow Metab 1994; 14:892-902.

168. Furlan M, et al. Spontaneous neurological recovery after stroke and the fate of the ischemic penumbra. Ann Neurol 1996; 40:216-226.

169. Baird AE, et al. Enlargement of human cerebral ischemic lesion volumes measured by diffusion-weighted magnetic resonance imaging. Ann Neurol 1997; 41:581-589.

170. Kato H, et al. Characterization of experimental ischemic brain edema utilizing proton nuclear magnetic resonance imaging. J Cereb Blood Flow Metab 1986; 6:212-221.

171. Mellergard P, et al. Time course of early brain edema following reversible forebrain ischemia in rats. Stroke 1989; 20:1565-1570.

172. Young W, et al. Regional brain sodium, potassium, and water changes in the rat middle cerebral artery occlusion model of ischemia. Stroke 1987; 18:751-759.

173. Hatashita S, Hoff JT, Salamat SM. Ischemic brain edema and the osmotic gradient between blood and brain. J Cereb Blood Flow Metab 1988; 8:552-559.

174. Perkins CJ, et al. Fluid-attenuated inversion recovery and diffusion- and perfusion-weighted mri abnormalities in 117 consecutive patients with stroke symptoms [Editorial Comment]. Stroke 2001; 32:2774-2781.

175. Wintermark M, et al. Perfusion-CT assessment of infarct core and penumbra: receiver operating characteristic curve analysis in 130 patients suspected of acute hemispheric stroke. Stroke 2006; 37:979-985.

176. Schaefer PW, et al. First-pass quantitative CT perfusion identifies thresholds for salvageable penumbra in acute stroke patients treated with intra-arterial therapy. AJNR Am J Neuroradiol 2006; 27:20-25.

177. Murphy BD, et al. Identification of penumbra and infarct in acute ischemic stroke using computed tomography perfusion-derived blood flow and blood volume measurements. Stroke 2006; 37:1771-1777.

178. Baird TA, et al. Persistent poststroke hyperglycemia is independently associated with infarct expansion and worse clinical outcome. Stroke 2003; 34:2208-2214.

179. Ay H, et al. Conversion of ischemic brain tissue into infarction increases with age. Stroke 2005; 36:2632-2636.

180. Beaulieu C, et al. Longitudinal magnetic resonance imaging study of perfusion and diffusion in stroke: evolution of lesion volume and correlation with clinical outcome. Ann Neurol 1999; 46:568-578.

181. Barber PA, et al. Prediction of stroke outcome with echoplanar perfusion- and diffusion-weighted MRI. Neurology 1998; 51:418-426.

182. Schaefer PW, et al. Predicting cerebral ischemic infarct volume with diffusion and perfusion MR imaging. AJNR Am J Neuroradiol 2002; 23:1785-1794.

183. Wintermark M, et al. Comparison of admission perfusion computed tomography and qualitative diffusion- and perfusion-weighted magnetic resonance imaging in acute stroke patients. Stroke 2002; 33:2025-2031.

184. Kassner A, et al. Prediction of hemorrhage in acute ischemic stroke using permeability MR imaging. AJNR Am J Neuroradiol 2005; 26:2213-2217.

185. Chalela JA, Kang DW, Warach S. Multiple cerebral microbleeds: MRI marker of a diffuse hemorrhage-prone state. J Neuroimaging 2004; 14:54-57.

186. Wintermark M, et al. Using 80 kVp versus 120 kVp in perfusion CT measurement of regional cerebral blood flow. AJNR Am J Neuroradiol 2000; 21:1881-1884.

187. Kucinski T, et al. Correlation of apparent diffusion coefficient and computed tomography density in acute ischemic stroke. Stroke 2002; 33:1786-1791.

188. Unger E, Littlefield J, Gado M. Water content and water structure in CT and MR signal changes: possible influence in detection of early stroke. AJNR Am J Neuroradiol 1988; 9:687-691.

189. von Kummer R, Weber J. Brain and vascular imaging in acute ischemic stroke: the potential of computed tomography. Neurology 1997; 49(5 Suppl 4):S52-S55.

190. Kucinski T, et al. The predictive value of early CT and angiography for fatal hemispheric swelling in acute stroke. AJNR Am J Neuroradiol 1998; 19:839-846.

191. Tomura N, et al. Early CT finding in cerebral infarction: obscuration of the lentiform nucleus. Radiology 1988; 168:463-467.

192. Truwit CL, et al. Loss of the insular ribbon: another early CT sign of acute middle cerebral artery infarction. Radiology 1990; 176:801-806.

193. Na DG, et al. CT sign of brain swelling without concomitant parenchymal hypoattenuation: comparison with diffusion- and perfusion-weighted MR imaging. Radiology 2005; 235:992-948.

194. Hacke W, et al. Intravenous thrombolysis with recombinant tissue plasminogen activator for acute hemispheric stroke. The European Cooperative Acute Stroke Study (ECASS). JAMA 1995; 274:1017-1025.

195. Silver B, et al. Improved outcomes in stroke thrombolysis with pre-specified imaging criteria. Can J Neurol Sci 2001; 28:113-119.

196. Schriger DL, et al. Cranial computed tomography interpretation in acute stroke: physician accuracy in determining eligibility for thrombolytic therapy. JAMA 1998; 279:1293-1297.

197. Grotta JC, et al. Agreement and variability in the interpretation of early CT changes in stroke patients qualifying for intravenous rtPA therapy. Stroke 1999; 30:1528-1533.

198. Coutts SB, et al. Interobserver variation of ASPECTS in real time. Stroke 2004; 35:e103-e105.

199. Pexman JH, et al. Use of the Alberta Stroke Program Early CT Score (ASPECTS) for assessing CT scans in patients with acute stroke. AJNR Am J Neuroradiol 2001; 22:1534-1542.

200. Barber PA, et al. Validity and reliability of a quantitative computed tomography score in predicting outcome of hyperacute stroke before thrombolytic therapy. ASPECTS Study Group. Alberta Stroke Programme Early CT Score. Lancet 2000; 355:1670-1674.

201. Demchuk AM, et al. Importance of early ischemic computed tomography changes using ASPECTS in NINDS rtPA stroke study. Stroke 2005; 36:2110-2115.

202. Dzialowski I, et al. Extent of early ischemic changes on computed tomography (CT) before thrombolysis: prognostic value of the Alberta Stroke Program Early CT Score in ECASS II. Stroke 2006; 37:973-978.

203. Hill MD, et al. Selection of acute ischemic stroke patients for intra-arterial thrombolysis with pro-urokinase by using ASPECTS. Stroke 2003; 34:1925-1931.

204. Demchuk AM, et al. Importance of early ischemic computed tomography changes using ASPECTS in NINDS rtPA stroke study. Stroke 2005; 36:2110-2115.

205. Wardlaw JM, Mielke O. Early signs of brain infarction at CT: observer reliability and outcome after thrombolytic treatment—systematic review. Radiology 2005; 235:444-453.

206. Patel SC, et al. Lack of clinical significance of early ischemic changes on computed tomography in acute stroke. JAMA 2001; 286:2830-2838.

207. The National Institute of Neurological Disorders and Stroke rt-PA Stroke Study Group, Tissue Plasminogen Activator for Acute Ischemic Stroke. N Engl J Med 1995; 333:1581-1588.

208. von Kummer R, et al. Early prediction of irreversible brain damage after ischemic stroke at CT. Radiology 2001; 219:95-100.

209. Coutts SB, et al. ASPECTS on CTA source images versus unenhanced CT: added value in predicting final infarct extent and clinical outcome. Stroke 2004; 35:2472-2476.

210. Tomsick TA, et al. Hyperdense middle cerebral artery sign on CT: efficacy in detecting middle cerebral artery thrombosis. AJNR Am J Neuroradiol 1990; 11:473-477.

211. von Kummer R, et al. Interobserver agreement in assessing early CT signs of middle cerebral artery infarction. AJNR Am J Neuroradiol 1996; 17:1743-1748.

212. Wardlaw JM, et al. Can stroke physicians and neuroradiologists identify signs of early cerebral infarction on CT? J Neurol Neurosurg Psychiatry 1999; 67:651-653.

213. von Kummer R. Effect of training in reading CT scans on patient selection for ECASS II. Neurology 1998; 51(3 Suppl 3):S50-S52.

214. Schramm P, et al. Comparison of CT and CT angiography source images with diffusion-weighted imaging in patients with acute stroke within 6 hours after onset. Stroke 2002; 33:2426-2432.

215. Ezzeddine MA, et al. CT angiography with whole brain perfused blood volume imaging: added clinical value in the assessment of acute stroke. Stroke 2002; 33:959-966.

216. Aviv RI, et al. Early stroke detection and extent: impact of experience and the role of computed tomography angiography source images. Clin Radiol 2007; 62:447-452.

217. Hamberg LM, et al. Measurement of cerebral blood volume with subtraction three-dimensional functional CT. AJNR Am J Neuroradiol 1996; 17:1861-1869.

218. Arnould M-C, et al. Comparison of CT and three MR sequences for detecting and categorizing early (48 hours) hemorrhagic transformation in hyperacute ischemic stroke. AJNR Am J Neuroradiol 2004; 25:939-944.

219. Hackney DB, et al. Subacute intracranial hemorrhage: contribution of spin density to appearance on spin-echo MR images: mechanisms of MR signal alteration by acute intracerebral blood: old concepts and new theories. Radiology 1987; 165:199-202.

220. Linfante I, et al. MRI features of intracerebral hemorrhage within 2 hours from symptom onset. Stroke 1999; 30:2263-2267.

221. Bergstrom M, et al. Variation with time of the attenuation values of intracranial hematomas. J Comput Assist Tomogr 1977; 1:57-63.

222. Smith WP Jr, Batnitzky S, Rengachary SS. Acute isodense subdural hematomas: a problem in anemic patients. AJR Am J Roentgenol 1981; 136:543-546.

223. van der Wee N, et al. Detection of subarachnoid haemorrhage on early CT: is lumbar puncture still needed after a negative scan? J Neurol Neurosurg Psychiatry 1995; 58:357-359.

224. Adams HP Jr, et al. CT and clinical correlations in recent aneurysmal subarachnoid hemorrhage: a preliminary report of the Cooperative Aneurysm Study. Neurology 1983; 33:981-988.

225. New PF, Aronow S. Attenuation measurements of whole blood and blood fractions in computed tomography. Radiology 1976; 121:635-640.

226. Gacs G, et al. CT visualization of intracranial arterial thromboembolism. Stroke 1983; 14:756-762.

227. Rauch RA, et al. Hyperdense middle cerebral arteries identified on CT as a false sign of vascular occlusion. AJNR Am J Neuroradiol 1993; 14:669-673.

228. Barber PA, et al. Hyperdense sylvian fissure MCA "dot" sign: a CT marker of acute ischemia. Stroke 2001; 32:84-88.

229. Krings T, et al. The hyperdense posterior cerebral artery sign: a computed tomography marker of acute ischemia in the posterior cerebral artery territory. Stroke 2006; 37:399-403.

230. Ehsan T, et al. Hyperdense basilar artery: an early computed tomography sign of thrombosis. J Neuroimaging 1994; 4:200-205.

231. Bastianello S, et al. Hyperdense middle cerebral artery CT sign: comparison with angiography in the acute phase of ischemic supratentorial infarction. Neuroradiology 1991; 33:207-211.

232. Leary MC, et al. Validation of computed tomographic middle cerebral artery "dot" sign: an angiographic correlation study. Stroke 2003; 34:2636-2640.

233. Tomsick TA, et al. Hyperdense middle cerebral artery: incidence and quantitative significance. Neuroradiology 1989; 31:312-315.

233a. Puig J, et al. Quantification of thrombus Hounsfield units on noncontrast CT predicts stroke subtype and early recanalization after intravenous recombinant tissue plasminogen activator. AJNR Am J Neuroradiol 2012; 33:90-96.

233b. Riedel CH, et al. Assessment of thrombus in acute middle cerebral artery occlusion using thin-slice nonenhanced computed tomography reconstructions. Stroke 2010; 41:1659-1664.

234. Lee TC, et al. The hypodense artery sign. AJNR Am J Neuroradiol 2005; 26:2027-2029.

235. Furlan A, et al. Intra-arterial prourokinase for acute ischemic stroke. The PROACT II study: a randomized controlled trial. Prolyse in Acute Cerebral Thromboembolism. JAMA 1999; 282:2003-2011.

236. Georgiadis D, et al. Does acute occlusion of the carotid T invariably have a poor outcome? Neurology 2004; 63:22-26.

237. Rother J, et al. Effect of intravenous thrombolysis on MRI parameters and functional outcome in acute stroke <6 hours. Stroke 2002; 33:2438-2445.

238. Schellinger PD, et al. Monitoring intravenous recombinant tissue plasminogen activator thrombolysis for acute ischemic stroke with diffusion and perfusion MRI. Stroke 2000; 31:1318-1328.

239. von Kummer R, et al. Does arterial recanalization improve outcome in carotid territory stroke? Stroke 1995; 26:581-587.

240. Jansen O, et al. Thrombolytic therapy in acute occlusion of the intracranial internal carotid artery bifurcation. AJNR Am J Neuroradiol 1995; 16:1977-1986.

241. Smith WS, et al. Safety and efficacy of mechanical embolectomy in acute ischemic stroke: results of the MERCI trial. Stroke 2005; 36:1432-1438.

242. Rother J, et al. Hemodynamic assessment of acute stroke using dynamic single-slice computed tomographic perfusion imaging. Arch Neurol 2000; 57:1161-1166.

243. Fiehler J, et al. Predictors of apparent diffusion coefficient normalization in stroke patients. Stroke 2004; 35:514-519.

244. Lell MM, et al. New techniques in CT angiography. RadioGraphics 2006; 26(Suppl 1):S45-S62.

245. Shrier D, et al. CT angiography in the evaluation of acute stroke. AJNR Am J Neuroradiol 1997; 18:1011-1020.

246. Knauth M, et al. Potential of CT angiography in acute ischemic stroke. AJNR Am J Neuroradiol 1997; 18:1001-1010.

246a. Camargo ECS, et al. Acute brain infarct: detection and delineation with CT angiographic source images versus nonenhanced CT scans. Radiology 2007; 244:541-548.

246b. Hopyan J, et al. Certainty of stroke diagnosis: incremental benefit with CT perfusion over noncontrast CT and CT angiography. Radiology 2010; 255:142-153.

246c. Bhatia R, et al. CT angiographic source images predict outcome and final infarct volume better than noncontrast CT in proximal vascular occlusions. Stroke 2011; 42:1575-1580.

246d. Sharma M, et al. CT angiographic source images: flow- or volume-weighted? AJNR Am J Neuroradiol 2011; 32:359-364.

246e. Yoo AJ, et al. CT angiography source images acquired with a fast-acquisition protocol overestimate infarct core on diffusion weighted images in acute ischemic stroke. J Neuroimaging 2011; doi: 10.1111/j.1552-6569.2011.00627.x. (E pub ahead of print).

246f. Tan IY, et al. CT angiography clot burden score and collateral score: correlation with clinical and radiologic outcomes in acute middle cerebral artery infarct. AJNR Am J Neuroradiol 2009; 30:525-531.

246g. Maas MB, et al. Collateral vessels on CT angiography predict outcome in acute ischemic stroke. Stroke 2009; 40:3001-3005.

246h. Lima FO, et al. The pattern of leptomeningeal collaterals on CT angiography is a strong predictor of long-term functional outcome in stroke patients with large vessel intracranial occlusion. Stroke 2010; 41: 2316-2322.

247. Fox AJ, et al. The effect of angiography on the electrophysiological state of the spinal cord: a study in control and traumatized cats. Radiology 1976; 118:343-350.

248. Kendall BE, Pullicino P. Intravascular contrast injection in ischemic lesions: II. Effect on prognosis. Neuroradiology 1980; 19:241-243.

249. Hayman LA, et al. Delayed high dose contrast CT: identifying patients at risk of massive hemorrhagic infarction. AJR Am J Roentgenol 1981; 136:1151-1159.

250. Doerfler A, et al. Are iodinated contrast agents detrimental in acute cerebral ischemia? An experimental study in rats. Radiology 1998; 206:211-217.

250a. Krol AL, et al. Incidence of radiocontrast nephropathy in patients undergoing acute stroke computed tomography angiography. Stroke 2007; 38: 2364-2366.

250b. Dittrich R, et al. Low rate of contrast-induced nephropathy after CT perfusion and CT angiography in acute stroke patients. J Neurol 2007; 254:1491-1497.

250c. Lima FO, et al. Functional contrast-enhanced CT for evaluation of acute ischemic stroke does not increase the risk of contrast-induced nephropathy. AJNR Am J Neuroradiol 2010; 31:817-821.

250d. Langner S, et al. No increased risk for contrast-induced nephropathy after multiple CT perfusion studies of the brain with a nonionic, dimeric, iso-osmolal contrast medium. AJNR Am J Neuroradiol 2008; 29:1525-1529.

250e. Hopyan JJ, et al. Safety of contrast-induced CT angiography and perfusion imaging in the emergency evaluation of acute stroke. AJNR Am J Neuroradiol 2008; 29:1826-1830.

251. Gleason S, et al. Potential influence of acute CT on inpatient costs in patients with ischemic stroke. Acad Radiol 2001; 8:955-964.

252. Wintermark M, et al. Prognostic accuracy of cerebral blood flow measurement by perfusion computed tomography, at the time of emergency room admission, in acute stroke patients. Ann Neurol 2002; 51:417-432.

253. Mayer TE, et al. Dynamic CT perfusion imaging of acute stroke. AJNR Am J Neuroradiol 2000; 21:1441-1449.

254. Eastwood JD, et al. CT perfusion scanning with deconvolution analysis: pilot study in patients with acute middle cerebral artery stroke. Radiology 2002; 222:227-236.

255. Roberts HC, et al. Multisection dynamic CT perfusion for acute cerebral ischemia: the "toggling-table" technique. AJNR Am J Neuroradiol 2001; 22:1077-1080.

256. Wintermark M, et al. Dynamic perfusion CT: optimizing the temporal resolution and contrast volume for calculation of perfusion CT parameters in stroke patients. AJNR Am J Neuroradiol 2004; 25:720-729.

256a. Scharf J, et al. Improvement of sensitivity and interrater reliability to detect acute stroke by dynamic perfusion computed tomography and computed tomography angiography. J Comput Assist Tomogr 2006; 30:105-110.

257. Wintermark M, et al. Accuracy of dynamic perfusion CT with deconvolution in detecting acute hemispheric stroke. AJNR Am J Neuroradiol 2005; 26:104-112.

258. Cohnen M, et al. Radiation exposure of patients in comprehensive computed tomography of the head in acute stroke. AJNR Am J Neuroradiol 2006; 27:1741-1745.

258a. Aviv RI, et al. Hemorrhagic transformation of ischemic stroke: prediction with CT perfusion. Radiology 2009; 250:867-877.

258b. Hom J, et al. Blood-brain barrier permeability assessed by perfusion CT predicts symptomatic hemorrhagic transformation and malignant edema in acute ischemic stroke. AJNR Am J Neuroradiol 2010; 32:41-48.

258c. Natarajan SK, et al. Safety and effectiveness of endovascular therapy after 8 hours of acute ischemic stroke onset and wake-up strokes. Stroke 2009; 40:3269-3274.

258d. Hacke W, et al. Intravenous desmoteplase in patients with acute ischaemic stroke selected by MRI perfusion-diffusion weighted imaging or perfusion CT (DIAS-2): a prospective, randomised, double-blind, placebo-controlled study. Lancet Neurol 2009; 8:141-150.

258e. Donnan GA, et al. Penumbral selection of patients for trials of acute stroke therapy. Lancet Neurol 2009; 8:261-269.

258f. Hassan AE, et al. A comparison of computed tomography perfusion-guided and time-guided endovascular treatments for patients with acute ischemic stroke. Stroke 2010; 41:1673-1678.

258g. Wintermark M, et al. Acute stroke imaging research roadmap. AJNR Am J Neuroradiol 2008; 29:e23-e30.

259. Hand PJ, et al. Magnetic resonance brain imaging in patients with acute stroke: feasibility and patient related difficulties. J Neurol Neurosurg Psychiatry 2005; 76:1525-1527.

260. Singer OC, et al. Practical limitations of acute stroke MRI due to patient-related problems. Neurology 2004; 62:1848-1849.

261. Handschu R, et al. Acute stroke management in the local general hospital. Stroke 2001; 32:866-870.

262. Buckley BT, et al. Audit of a policy of magnetic resonance imaging with diffusion-weighted imaging as first-line neuroimaging for in-patients with clinically suspected acute stroke. Clin Radiol 2003; 58:234-237.

263. Kidwell CS, et al. Comparison of MRI and CT for detection of acute intracerebral hemorrhage. JAMA 2004; 292:1823-1830.

264. Mohr JP, et al. Magnetic resonance versus computed tomographic imaging in acute stroke. Stroke 1995; 26:807-812.

265. Yuh WT, et al. MR imaging of cerebral ischemia: findings in the first 24 hours. AJNR Am J Neuroradiol 1991; 12:621-629.

266. Ricci PE, et al. A comparison of fast spin-echo, fluid-attenuated inversion-recovery, and diffusion-weighted MR imaging in the first 10 days after cerebral infarction. AJNR Am J Neuroradiol 1999; 20:1535-1542.

267. Castillo M, et al. Postmortem MR imaging of lobar cerebral infarction with pathologic and in vivo correlation. RadioGraphics 1996; 16:241-250.

268. Knight RA, et al. Temporal evolution of ischemic damage in rat brain measured by proton nuclear magnetic resonance imaging. Stroke 1991; 22:802-808.

269. Schwamm LH, et al. Time course of lesion development in patients with acute stroke: serial diffusion- and hemodynamic-weighted magnetic resonance imaging. Stroke 1998; 29:2268-2276.

270. Brant-Zawadzki M, et al. Fluid-attenuated inversion recovery (FLAIR) for assessment of cerebral infarction: initial clinical experience in 50 patients. Stroke 1996; 27:1187-1191.

271. Lutsep HL, et al. Clinical utility of diffusion-weighted magnetic resonance imaging in the assessment of ischemic stroke. Ann Neurol 1997; 41:574-580.

272. Maeda M, et al. Arterial hyperintensity on fast fluid-attenuated inversion recovery images: a subtle finding for hyperacute stroke undetected by diffusion-weighted MR imaging. AJNR Am J Neuroradiol 2001; 22:632-636.

273. Warach S, Latour LL. Evidence of reperfusion injury, exacerbated by thrombolytic therapy, in human focal brain ischemia using a novel imaging marker of early blood-brain barrier disruption. Stroke 2004; 35(11 Suppl 1):2659-2661.

274. Pereira AC, et al. Case reports. The transient disappearance of cerebral infarction on T(2) weighted MRI. Clin Radiol 2000; 55:725-727.

275. Asato R, Okumura R, Konishi J. "Fogging effect" in MR of cerebral infarct. J Comput Assist Tomogr 1991; 15:160-162.

276. Skriver EB, Olsen TS. Transient disappearance of cerebral infarcts on CT scan, the so-called fogging effect. Neuroradiology 1981; 22:61-65.

277. Uchino A, et al. Report of fogging effect on fast FLAIR magnetic resonance images of cerebral infarctions. Neuroradiology 2004; 46:40-43.

278. Moseley M, et al. Diffusion-weighted MR imaging of acute stroke: correlation with T2- weighted and magnetic susceptibility-enhanced MR imaging in cats. AJNR Am J Neuroradiol 1990; 11:423-429.

279. Duong TQ, et al. Evaluation of extra- and intracellular apparent diffusion in normal and globally ischemic rat brain via 19F NMR. Magn Reson Med 1998; 40:1-13.

280. van der Toorn A, et al. Dynamic changes in water ADC, energy metabolism, extracellular space volume, and tortuosity in neonatal rat brain during global ischemia. Magn Reson Med 1996; 36:52-60.

281. Conturo TE, et al. Diffusion MRI: precision, accuracy and flow effects. NMR Biomed 1995; 8:307-332.

282. Provenzale J, Sorensen A. Diffusion-weighted MR imaging in acute stroke: theoretic considerations and clinical applications. AJR Am J Roentgenol 1999; 173:1459-1467.

283. Fiebach JB, et al. CT and diffusion-weighted MR imaging in randomized order: diffusion-weighted imaging results in higher accuracy and lower interrater variability in the diagnosis of hyperacute ischemic stroke. Stroke 2002; 33:2206-2210.

284. Lee LJ, et al. Impact on stroke subtype diagnosis of early diffusion-weighted magnetic resonance imaging and magnetic resonance angiography. Stroke 2000; 31:1081-1089.

285. Saur D, et al. Sensitivity and interrater agreement of CT and diffusion-weighted MR imaging in hyperacute stroke. AJNR Am J Neuroradiol 2003; 24:878-885.

286. Keir SL, Wardlaw JM. Systematic review of diffusion and perfusion imaging in acute ischemic stroke. Stroke 2000; 31:2723-2731.

287. Geijer B, et al. Radiological diagnosis of acute stroke: comparison of conventional MR imaging, echo-planar diffusion-weighted imaging, and spin-echo diffusion-weighted imaging. Acta Radiol 1999; 40:255-262.

288. van Everdingen KJ, et al. Diffusion-weighted magnetic resonance imaging in acute stroke. Stroke 1998; 29:1783-1790.

289. Lovblad KO, et al. Ischemic lesion volumes in acute stroke by diffusion-weighted magnetic resonance imaging correlate with clinical outcome. Ann Neurol 1997; 42:164-170.

290. Rohl L, et al. Viability thresholds of ischemic penumbra of hyperacute stroke defined by perfusion-weighted MRI and apparent diffusion coefficient. Stroke 2001; 32:1140-1146.

291. Hatazawa J, et al. Cerebral blood volume in acute brain infarction: a combined study with dynamic susceptibility contrast MRI and 99mTc-HMPAO-SPECT. Stroke 1999; 30:800-806.

292. Selim M, et al. Predictors of hemorrhagic transformation after intravenous recombinant tissue plasminogen activator: prognostic value of the initial apparent diffusion coefficient and diffusion-weighted lesion. Stroke 2002; 33:2047-2052.

293. Oppenheim C, et al. DWI prediction of symptomatic hemorrhagic transformation in acute MCA infarct. J Neuroradiol 2002; 29:6-13.

294. Roh J-K, et al. Significance of acute multiple brain infarction on diffusion-weighted imaging. Stroke 2000; 31:688-694.

295. Schaefer PW, et al. Characterization and evolution of diffusion MR imaging abnormalities in stroke patients undergoing intra-arterial thrombolysis. AJNR Am J Neuroradiol 2004; 25:951-957.

296. Kidwell CS, et al. Late secondary ischemic injury in patients receiving intraarterial thrombolysis. Ann Neurol 2002; 52:698-703.

297. Welch KMA, et al. A model to predict the histopathology of human stroke using diffusion and T2-weighted magnetic resonance imaging. Stroke 1995; 26:1983-1989.

298. Schlaug G, et al. Time course of the apparent diffusion coefficient (ADC) abnormality in human stroke. Neurology 1997; 49: 113-119.

299. Chien D, et al. MR diffusion imaging of cerebral infarction in humans. AJNR Am J Neuroradiol 1992; 13:1097-1102; discussion 1103-1105.

300. Lefkowitz D, et al. Hyperacute ischemic stroke missed by diffusion-weighted imaging. AJNR Am J Neuroradiol 1999; 20:1871-1875.

301. Wang PY-K, et al. Diffusion-negative stroke: a report of two cases. AJNR Am J Neuroradiol 1999; 20:1876-1880.

302. Oppenheim C, et al. False-negative diffusion-weighted MR findings in acute ischemic stroke. AJNR Am J Neuroradiol 2000; 21: 1434-1440.

303. Kim HJ, et al. High b-value diffusion-weighted MR imaging of hyperacute ischemic stroke at 1.5T. AJNR Am J Neuroradiol 2005; 26:208-215.

304. Meyer JR, et al. High b-value diffusion-weighted MR imaging of suspected brain infarction. AJNR Am J Neuroradiol 2000; 21: 1821-1829.

305. Burdette JH, Elster AD. Diffusion-weighted imaging of cerebral infarctions: are higher B values better? J Comput Assist Tomogr 2002; 26:622-627.

306. Sener RN. Herpes simplex encephalitis: diffusion MR imaging findings. Comput Med Imaging Graph 2001; 25:391-397.

307. Lin YR, et al. Creutzfeldt-Jakob disease involvement of rolandic cortex: a quantitative apparent diffusion coefficient evaluation. AJNR Am J Neuroradiol 2006; 27:1755-1759.

308. Kallenberg K, et al. Creutzfeldt-Jakob disease: comparative analysis of MR imaging sequences. AJNR Am J Neuroradiol 2006; 27:1459-1462.

309. Chu K, et al. Diffusion-weighted magnetic resonance imaging in nonconvulsive status epilepticus. Arch Neurol 2001; 58:993-998.

310. Reddy JS, Mishra AM, Behari S, et al. The role of diffusion-weighted imaging in the differential diagnosis of intracranial cystic mass lesions: a report of 147 lesions. Surg Neurol 2006; 66:246-250.

310a. Shiga Y, et al. Diffusion-weighted MRI abnormalities as an early diagnostic marker for Creutzfeldt-Jakob disease. Neurology 2004; 63:443-449.

310b. Kallenberg K, et al. Creutzfeldt-Jakob disease: comparative analysis of MR imaging sequences. AJNR Am J Neuroradiol 2006; 27:1459-1462.

311. Liang L, et al. Detection of intracranial hemorrhage with susceptibility-weighted MR sequences. AJNR Am J Neuroradiol 1999; 20:1527-1534.

312. Singer M, Atlas S, Drayer B. Subarachnoid space disease: diagnosis with fluid-attenuated inversion-recovery MR imaging and comparison with gadolinium-enhanced spin-echo MR imaging—blinded reader study. Radiology 1998; 208:417-422.

313. Bakshi R, et al. Intraventricular CSF pulsation artifact on fast fluid-attenuated inversion-recovery MR images: analysis of 100 consecutive normal studies. AJNR Am J Neuroradiol 2000; 21: 503-508.

314. Braga FT, et al. Relationship between the concentration of supplemental oxygen and signal intensity of CSF depicted by fluid-attenuated inversion recovery imaging. AJNR Am J Neuroradiol 2003; 24:1863-1868.

315. Cianfoni A, et al. Artifact simulating subarachnoid and intraventricular hemorrhage on single-shot, fast spin-echo fluid-attenuated inversion recovery images caused by head movement: a trap for the unwary. AJNR Am J Neuroradiol 2006; 27:843-849.

316. Fisher M, Adams RD. Observations on brain embolism with special reference to the mechanism of hemorrhagic infarction. J Neuropathol Exp Neurol 1951; 10:92-94.

317. Jorgensen L, Torvik A. Ischemic cerebrovascular diseases in an autopsy series. 2. Prevalence, location, pathogenesis, and clinical course of cerebral infarcts. J Neurol Sci 1969; 9:285-320.

318. Intracerebral hemorrhage after intravenous t-PA therapy for ischemic stroke. The NINDS t-PA Stroke Study Group. Stroke 1997; 28:2109-2118.

319. Hill MD, Buchan AM. Thrombolysis for acute ischemic stroke: results of the Canadian Alteplase for Stroke Effectiveness Study. Can Med Assoc J 2005; 172:1307-1312.

320. Larrue V, et al. Hemorrhagic transformation in acute ischemic stroke: potential contributing factors in the European Cooperative Acute Stroke Study. Stroke 1997; 28:957-960.

321. von Kummer R. Brain hemorrhage after thrombolysis: good or bad? Stroke 2002; 33:1446-1447.

322. Kent DM, et al. In acute ischemic stroke, are asymptomatic intracranial hemorrhages clinically innocuous? Stroke 2004; 35: 1141-1146.

323. Dzialowski I, et al. Asymptomatic hemorrhage after thrombolysis may not be benign: prognosis by hemorrhage type in the Canadian Alteplase for Stroke Effectiveness Study Registry. Stroke 2007; 38:75-79.

324. Molina CA, et al. Thrombolysis-related hemorrhagic infarction: a marker of early reperfusion, reduced infarct size, and improved outcome in patients with proximal middle cerebral artery occlusion. Stroke 2002; 33:1551-1556.

325. Chalela JA, et al. The hypointense MCA sign. Neurology 2002; 58: 1470.

326. Rovira A, et al. Hyperacute ischemic stroke: middle cerebral artery susceptibility sign at echo-planar gradient-echo MR imaging. Radiology 2004; 232:466-473.

327. Flacke S, et al. Middle cerebral artery (MCA) susceptibility sign at susceptibility-based perfusion MR imaging: clinical importance and comparison with hyperdense MCA sign at CT. Radiology 2000; 215:476-482.

328. Stock KW, et al. Intracranial arteries: prospective blinded comparative study of MR angiography and DSA in 50 patients. Radiology 1995; 195:451-456.

329. Korogi Y, et al. Intracranial vascular stenosis and occlusion: diagnostic accuracy of three-dimensional, Fourier transform, time-of-flight MR angiography. Radiology 1994; 193:187-193.

330. Crain MR, et al. Cerebral ischemia: evaluation with contrast-enhanced MR imaging. AJNR Am J Neuroradiol 1991; 12:631-639.

331. Karonen JO, et al. Evolution of MR contrast enhancement patterns during the first week after acute ischemic stroke. AJNR Am J Neuroradiol 2001; 22:103-111.

332. Elster AD, Moody DM. Early cerebral infarction: gadopentetate dimeglumine enhancement. Radiology 1990; 177:627-632.

333. Wu O, Ostergaard L, Sorensen AG. Technical aspects of perfusion-weighted imaging. Neuroimaging Clin North Am 2005; 15: 623-637.

334. Kidwell CS, Alger JR, Saver JL. Beyond mismatch: evolving paradigms in imaging the ischemic penumbra with multimodal magnetic resonance imaging. Stroke 2003; 34:2729-2735.

335. Parsons MW, Barber PA, Chalk J, et al. Diffusion- and perfusion-weighted MRI response to thrombolysis in stroke. Ann Neurol 2002; 51:28-37.

336. Hacke W, et al. The Desmoteplase in Acute Ischemic Stroke Trial (DIAS): a phase II MRI-based 9-hour window acute stroke thrombolysis trial with intravenous desmoteplase. Stroke 2005; 36: 66-73.

337. Albers GW, Thijs VN, Wechsler L, et al., for the DEFUSE Investigators. Magnetic resonance imaging profiles predict clinical response to early reperfusion: the Diffusion and Perfusion Imaging Evaluation for Understanding Stroke Evolution (DEFUSE) study. Ann Neurol 2006; 60:508-517.

338. Schlaug G, et al. The ischemic penumbra: operationally defined by diffusion and perfusion MRI. Neurology 1999; 53:1528.

338a. Nagakane Y, et al. EPITHET: positive result after reanalysis using baseline diffusion-weighted imaging/perfusion-weighted imaging co-registration. Stroke 2011; 42:59-64.

338b. Lansberg MG, et al. RAPID automated patient selection for reperfusion therapy: a pooled analysis of the Echoplanar Imaging Thrombolytic Evaluation Trial (EPITHET) and the Diffusion and Perfusion Imaging Evaluation for Understanding Stroke Evolution (DEFUSE) Study. Stroke 2011; 42:1608-1614.

339. Hornig CR, Dorndorf W, Agnoli AL. Hemorrhagic cerebral infarction—a prospective study. Stroke 1986; 17:179-185.

340. Del Zoppo GJ, Von Kummer R, Hamann GF. Ischemic damage of brain microvessels: inherent risks for thrombolytic treatment in stroke. J Neurol Neurosurg Psychiatry 1998; 65:1-9.

341. Hamann GF, Okada Y, del Zoppo GJ. Hemorrhagic transformation and microvascular integrity during focal cerebral ischemia/reperfusion. J Cereb Blood Flow Metab 1996; 16:1373-1378.

342. Yoon W, et al. Contrast enhancement and contrast extravasation on computed tomography after intra-arterial thrombolysis in patients with acute ischemic stroke. Stroke 2004; 35:876-881.

343. Wilcox J, et al. A comparison of blood-brain barrier disruption by intracarotid iohexol and iodixanol in the rabbit. AJNR Am J Neuroradiol 1987; 8:769-772.

344. Lo EH, Broderick JP, Moskowitz MA. tPA and proteolysis in the neurovascular unit. Stroke 2004; 35:354-356.

345. Komiyama M, et al. Extravasation of contrast medium from the lenticulostriate artery following local intracarotid fibrinolysis. Surg Neurol 1993; 39:315-319.

346. Roberts HC, et al. Dynamic, contrast-enhanced CT of human brain tumors: quantitative assessment of blood volume, blood flow, and microvascular permeability: report of two cases. AJNR Am J Neuroradiol 2002; 23:828-832.

346a. Aviv R. Radiology 2009; 250:1–11.

347. Eastwood JD, et al. Correlation of early dynamic CT perfusion imaging with whole-brain MR diffusion and perfusion imaging in acute hemispheric stroke. AJNR Am J Neuroradiol 2003; 24:1869-1875.

348. Ueda T, et al. Outcome of acute ischemic lesions evaluated by diffusion and perfusion MR Imaging. AJNR Am J Neuroradiol 1999; 20:983-989.

349. Parsons MW, et al. Perfusion computed tomography: prediction of final infarct extent and stroke outcome. Ann Neurol 2005; 58:672-679.

350. Kothari RU, et al. Emergency physicians: accuracy in the diagnosis of stroke. Stroke 1995; 26:2238-2241.

351. Libman RB, et al. Conditions that mimic stroke in the emergency department: implications for acute stroke trials. Arch Neurol 1995; 52:1119-1122.

352. Kidwell CS, et al. Diffusion-perfusion MRI characterization of post-recanalization hyperperfusion in humans. Neurology 2001; 57:2015-2021.

353. Barber PA, et al. Absent middle cerebral artery flow predicts the presence and evolution of the ischemic penumbra. Neurology 1999; 52:1125.

354. Lev MH, et al. Utility of perfusion-weighted CT imaging in acute middle cerebral artery stroke treated with intra-arterial thrombolysis: prediction of final infarct volume and clinical outcome. Stroke 2001; 32:2021-2028.

354a. Mlynash M, et al. Refining the definition of the malignant profile: insights from the DEFUSE-EPITHET pooled data set. Stroke 2011; 42:1270-1275.

355. Intracerebral hemorrhage after intravenous t-PA therapy for ischemic stroke. The NINDS t-PA Stroke Study Group. Stroke 1997; 28:2109-2118.

355a. Dani KA, et al. Computed tomography and magnetic resonance perfusion imaging in ischemic stroke: definitions and thresholds. Ann Neurol 2011; 70:384-401.

356. Koenig M. Quantitative assessment of the ischemic brain by means of perfusion-related parameters derived from perfusion CT. Stroke 2001; 32:431-437.

357. Siskas N, et al. Cortical laminar necrosis in brain infarcts: serial MRI. Neuroradiology 2003; 45:283-288.

358. Takahashi S, et al. Hypoxic brain damage: cortical laminar necrosis and delayed changes in white matter at sequential MR imaging. Radiology 1993; 189:449-456.

359. Mazumdar A, et al. Diffusion-weighted imaging of acute corticospinal tract injury preceding wallerian degeneration in the maturing human brain. AJNR Am J Neuroradiol 2003; 24:1057-1066.

360. Thomalla G, et al. Time course of wallerian degeneration after ischemic stroke revealed by diffusion tensor imaging. J Neurol Neurosurg Psychiatry 2005; 76:266-268.

361. Hacke W, et al. Association of outcome with early stroke treatment: pooled analysis of ATLANTIS, ECASS, and NINDS rt-PA stroke trials. Lancet 2004; 363:768-774.

362. Wardlaw JM. Overview of Cochrane thrombolysis meta-analysis. Neurology 2001; 57(9002):69S-76S.

363. Adams HP Jr, et al. Guidelines for the early management of patients with ischemic stroke: a scientific statement from the Stroke Council of the American Stroke Association. Stroke 2003; 34:1056-1083.

363a. Hacke W, et al. Thrombolysis with alteplase 3 to 4.5 hours after acute ischemic stroke. N Engl J Med 2008; 359:1317-1329.

364. del Zoppo GJ, et al. PROACT: a phase II randomized trial of recombinant pro-urokinase by direct arterial delivery in acute middle cerebral artery stroke. PROACT Investigators. Prolyse in Acute Cerebral Thromboembolism. Stroke 1998; 29:4-11.

365. Combined intravenous and intra-arterial recanalization for acute ischemic stroke: the Interventional Management of Stroke Study. Stroke 2004; 35:904-911.

366. Katzan IL, et al. Use of tissue-type plasminogen activator for acute ischemic stroke: the Cleveland area experience. JAMA 2000; 283:1151-1158.

367. Kleindorfer D, et al. Eligibility for recombinant tissue plasminogen activator in acute ischemic stroke: a population-based study. Stroke 2004; 35:27e-29e.

368. Gonzalez RG. Imaging-guided acute ischemic stroke therapy: from "time is brain" to "physiology is brain." AJNR Am J Neuroradiol 2006; 27:728-735.

369. Ribo M, et al. Safety and efficacy of intravenous tissue plasminogen activator stroke treatment in the 3- to 6-hour window using multi-modal transcranial Doppler/MRI selection protocol. Stroke 2005; 36:602-606.

370. Koennecke H-C. Cerebral microbleeds on MRI: prevalence, associations, and potential clinical implications. Neurology 2006; 66:165-171.

371. Fazekas F, et al. Histopathologic analysis of foci of signal loss on gradient-echo t2*-weighted MR images in patients with spontaneous intracerebral hemorrhage: evidence of microangiopathy-related microbleeds. AJNR Am J Neuroradiol 1999; 20:637-642.

372. Kakuda W, et al. Clinical importance of microbleeds in patients receiving IV thrombolysis. Neurology 2005; 65:1175-1178.

373. Albers GW, et al. Transient ischemic attack—proposal for a new definition. N Engl J Med 2002; 347:1713-1716.

374. Warlow C, et al. Stroke. Lancet 2003; 362:1211-1224.

375. Gladstone DJ, et al. Management and outcomes of transient ischemic attacks in Ontario. Can Med Assoc J 2004; 170:1099-1104.

376. Douglas VC, et al. Head computed tomography findings predict short-term stroke risk after transient ischemic attack. Stroke 2003; 34:2894-2898.

377. Johnston SC, et al. National Stroke Association guidelines for the management of transient ischemic attacks. Ann Neurol 2006; 60:301-313.

378. Hachinski VC, Potter P, Merskey H. Leuko-araiosis. Arch Neurol 1987; 44:21-23.

379. Murray AD, et al. Brain white matter hyperintensities: relative importance of vascular risk factors in nondemented elderly people. Radiology 2005; 237:251-257.

380. Pantoni L, et al. Visual rating scales for age-related white matter changes (leukoaraiosis): can the heterogeneity be reduced? Stroke 2002; 33:2827-2833.

381. Breteler MM, et al. Cerebral white matter lesions, vascular risk factors, and cognitive function in a population-based study: the Rotterdam study. Neurology 1994; 44:1246-1252.

382. Kuller LH, et al. White matter hyperintensity on cranial magnetic resonance imaging: a predictor of stroke. Stroke 2004; 35:1821-1825.

383. El-Saed A, et al. Factors associated with geographic variations in stroke incidence among older populations in four US communities. Stroke 2006; 37:1980-1985.

384. Pantoni L, Garcia JH. The significance of cerebral white matter abnormalities 100 years after Binswanger's report: a review. Stroke 1995; 26:1293-1301.

385. Fernando MS, et al. White matter lesions in an unselected cohort of the elderly: molecular pathology suggests origin from chronic hypoperfusion injury. Stroke 2006; 37:1391-1398.

386. Fazekas F, et al. MR signal abnormalities at 1.5 T in Alzheimer's dementia and normal aging. AJR Am J Roentgenol 1987; 149:351-356.

387. Inzitari D, et al. Histopathological correlates of leuko-araiosis in patients with ischemic stroke. Eur Neurol 1989; 29(Suppl 2):23-26.

388. Scarpelli M, et al. MRI and pathological examination of post-mortem brains: the problem of white matter high signal areas. Neuroradiology 1994; 36:393-398.

389. Janota I, et al. Neuropathologic correlates of leuko-araiosis. Arch Neurol 1989; 46:1124-1128.

390. Fazekas F, et al. Pathologic correlates of incidental MRI white matter signal hyperintensities. Neurology 1993; 43:1683-1689.

391. Wahlund LO, et al. A new rating scale for age-related white matter changes applicable to MRI and CT. Stroke 2001; 32:1318-1322.

392. Hachinski V, et al. National Institute of Neurological Disorders and Stroke-Canadian Stroke Network Vascular Cognitive Impairment Harmonization Standards. Stroke 2006; 37:2220-2241.

393. Wardlaw JM. What causes lacunar stroke? J Neurol Neurosurg Psychiatry 2005; 76:617-619.

394. Ay H, et al: Diffusion-weighted imaging identifies a subset of lacunar infarction associated with embolic source. Stroke 1999; 30:2644-2650.

395. Gerraty RP, et al. Examining lacunar hypothesis with diffusion and perfusion magnetic resonance imaging. Stroke 2002; 33:2019-2024.

396. Chowdhury D, Wardlaw JM, Dennis MS. Are multiple acute small subcortical infarctions caused by embolic mechanisms? J Neurol Neurosurg Psychiatry 2004; 75:1416-1420.

397. O'Sullivan M, et al. Frequency of subclinical lacunar infarcts in ischemic leukoaraiosis and cerebral autosomal dominant arteriopathy with subcortical infarcts and leukoencephalopathy. AJNR Am J Neuroradiol 2003; 24:1348-1354.

398. Donnan GA, Norrving B, Bamford JM, Bogousslavsky J. Subcortical infarction: classification and terminology. Cerebrovasc Dis 1993; 3:248-251.

399. Salzman KL, et al. Giant tumefactive perivascular spaces. AJNR Am J Neuroradiol 2005; 26:298-305.

400. Jungreis CA, et al. Normal perivascular spaces mimicking lacunar infarction: MR imaging. Radiology 1988; 169:101-104.

401. Poirier J, Derouesne C: [The concept of cerebral lacunae from 1838 to the present.] Rev Neurol (Paris) 1985; 141:3-17.

402. McKhann GM, et al. Stroke and encephalopathy after cardiac surgery: an update. Stroke 2006; 37:562-571.

403. van der Zwan A, Hillen B, Tulleken CAF, et al: Variability of the major cerebral arteries. J Neurosurg 1992; 77:927-940.

404. Caplan LR, Hennerici M. Impaired clearance of emboli (washout) is an important link between hypoperfusion, embolism, and ischemic stroke. Arch Neurol 1998; 55:1475-1482.

405. Krapf H, Widder B, Skalej M. Small rosary-like infarctions in the centrum ovale suggest hemodynamic failure. AJNR Am J Neuroradiol 1998; 19:1479-1484.

406. Arakawa S, et al. Topographic distribution of misery perfusion in relation to internal and superficial borderzones. AJNR Am J Neuroradiol 2003; 24:427-435.

CHAPTER 21

Other Arteriopathies

Richard Ivan Aviv, Laurent Létourneau-Guillon, Sean P. Symons, and Allan J. Fox

CEREBRAL AUTOSOMAL DOMINANT ARTERIOPATHY WITH SUBCORTICAL INFARCTS AND LEUKOENCEPHALOPATHY

Cerebral autosomal dominant arteriopathy with subcortical infarcts and leukoencephalopathy (CADASIL) describes a widespread small vessel arteriopathy that also affects the intracranial circulation. CADASIL has also previously been called chronic familial vascular encephalopathy, autosomal dominant syndrome with stroke-like episodes and leukoencephalopathy, and hereditary multi-infarct dementia.

Epidemiology

The prevalence of CADASIL is reported as 2 to 4 per 100,000 population. It usually presents in the fourth to sixth decades. The mean age at death is 59 to 65 years.[1]

Clinical Presentation

Patients may experience prodromes of neuropsychiatric symptoms, migraine with aura, and seizure. Recurrent stroke occurs in middle-aged adults often in the absence of vascular risk factors. Patients may manifest pseudobulbar palsy that progresses to subcortical dementia.

Pathophysiology

CADASIL is a monogenic abnormality isolated to the *NOTCH3* gene, a 33-exon gene encoded on the long arm of chromosome 19 and expressed in smooth muscle cells. Over 60% of mutations occur on exons 3 and 4. There is wide variation of phenotypic expression despite complete disease penetrance.

Pathology

Histopathologically, electron-dense granular material is deposited within the media of the walls of small and medium-sized leptomeningeal arteries, causing concentric thickening of the wall, splitting of the internal elastic lamina, duplication, hyalinosis, and fibrosis of the adventitia with loss of vascular smooth muscle cells.[2]

Imaging
MRI

The radiologic spectrum of MRI findings in CADASIL includes white matter hyperintensity, subcortical lacunar lesions, lacunar infarcts, and microbleeds (Fig. 21-1). The white matter T2 hyperintensities are found in both symptomatic and asymptomatic patients. The subcortical lacunar lesions are formed by dilated perivascular spaces and adjacent spongiform change. These lesions are linearly arrayed, well circumscribed, and rounded with signal intensity identical to cerebrospinal fluid (CSF). They are identified by their location at the gray matter/white matter junctions in the anterior temporal, frontal, and parietal lobes.[3]

The lesions of CADASIL show typical temporal evolution.[4] The T2 hyperintensity has a predilection for the subcortical white matter of the temporal pole in the third decade, with progressive extension to involve the internal/external capsules, posterior temporal, frontal, and parietal lobe white matter, basal ganglia, and thalamus by the fourth decade. Callosal or infratentorial involvement is rare.[5] Increasing confluence of periventricular and subcortical white matter signal abnormality continues in the fourth decade. Although all patients manifested signal change within the temporal pole in one study,[4] another study found that one third of patients in the third decade had no signal abnormality in this location.[5] Lacunar infarcts are present in 75% of patients in the fourth decade, increasing to 94% in the fifth decade. Subcortical perivascular spaces are seen in the fourth decade, increasing to 56% in the fifth decade. Microbleeds are present in 20% of patients in the fifth decade. By the sixth decade all patients show these features. Recently, white matter scores, diffusion tensor imaging (DTI) histograms, and T1-weighted (T1W) lesion volumes have been correlated with clinical measures.[1,5,6] Cerebral angiography carries increased risk of neurologic complications in patients with CADASIL (32% transient and 11% permanent).[7] These complications are attributed to a combination of vessel wall abnormality and possible functional alterations.[7] The imaging differential diagnosis of CADASIL includes small vessel ischemia (despite the absence of risk factors), primary and secondary vasculitis, leukodystrophy, Fabry's disease, and mitochondrial disorders. The predominance of temporal pole disease and paucity of callosal involvement help to distinguish CADASIL from multiple sclerosis.

FABRY'S DISEASE

Fabry's disease is an X-linked disorder secondary to deficiency of the lysosomal hydrolase α-galactosidase A. It is also known as Anderson-Fabry disease.

■ **FIGURE 21-1** Axial T2W and FLAIR images at the level of temporal poles (**A, B**) and corona radiata (**C,D**) in a 63-year-old man with CADASIL. There is widespread T2 signal abnormality throughout the periventricular, deep, and subcortical white matter. Moderate cerebral volume loss is present. Notable is the extensive temporal pole involvement (*arrows*) and subcortical lacunar lesions (*arrowheads*). No microhemorrhages were present.

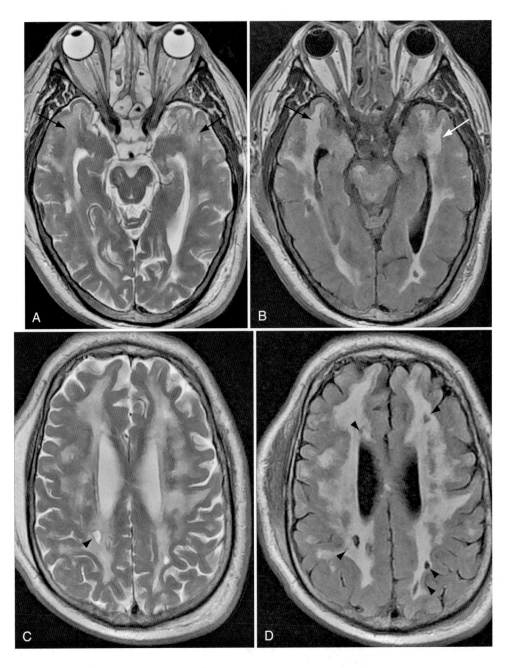

Epidemiology

Men are more severely affected. Heterozygous women may show variably reduced levels of α-galactosidase A activity secondary to random X chromosome inactivation. White matter lesions are more common with male gender and increasing age.

Clinical Presentation

Fabry's disease is reported to account for 4% of strokes in patients younger than 55 years of age.[8] Clinical features include corneal inclusions and cataracts, acroparesthesia, and neuropathic pain. Mortality is secondary to cardiac, renal, or cerebrovascular complications. There is no definite evidence that enzyme replacement therapy benefits patients with cerebral infarcts, but cerebral perfusion and renal function are improved with a reduction in glycosphingolipid deposition. Vasculopathy manifests as dolichoectasia and small vessel ischemic change. Large vessel infarcts are uncommon but may be increased with vertebrobasilar dolichoectasia. Infarcts are distributed within the territory of the posterior circulation in two thirds of patients. Cardioembolic infarcts are secondary to premature cardiac infarcts, valvular thickening, and arrhythmias. Parenchymal and subarachnoid hemorrhage is described. The ischemic infarcts are frequently asymptomatic.

Pathophysiology

Globotriaosylceramide (ceramide trihexoside), a glycosphingolipid, accumulates in the lysosomes of endothelial and smooth muscle cells, renal and cardiac parenchymal cells, and the central nervous system. Lipid deposition results in vascular dysfunction, occlusion, and ischemia. The exact mechanism of stroke is uncertain. Altered flow hemodynamics, wall thickening, and alterations in blood constituents, including concentrations of leukocyte adhesion molecules and homocysteine, may all contribute to the vasculopathy. Hyperperfusion with selective regional vulnerability has been implicated in the etiology of white matter abnormality in Fabry's disease, in contradistinction to leukoaraiosis.

Pathology

Lipid staining is found within central autonomic nuclei, including brain stem and dorsal motor nuclei, sensory neurons of dorsal root ganglia, and autonomic ganglia. The choroid plexus, leptomeninges, hypothalamic nuclei, entorhinal cortex, amygdala, and nucleus of the median eminence are particularly affected. Small and medium-sized vessels are thickened with luminal narrowing. Large vessel dolichoectasia is hypothesized to be secondary to reduction in extracellular matrix proteins, collagen, elastin, glycosaminoglycans, and proteoglycans.[9]

Imaging

CT

Coarse calcification is frequently seen in the striatopallidal nuclei. Finer or more granular calcification is seen within the thalami. Calcification may also be seen in subcortical white matter and cerebellar corticomedullary junction.

MRI

White matter hypodensity on CT corresponds to nonspecific T2 hyperintensity within periventricular white matter, deep white matter, and gray matter on MRI. Although white matter abnormality is increasingly frequent with increasing age, it has also been described in affected children. Two recent studies comprising approximately 100 patients reported lateral pulvinar T1 hyperintensity with increasing frequency over the age of 30 years (23%-70%).[10] The etiology of this finding was speculative and frequently associated with calcification on CT in the larger study. There was no signal alteration on fat saturation to suggest lipid deposition. T2 was reported as reduced in one study and normal in the other. Susceptibility-weighted imaging demonstrated proportional loss of signal depending on the extent of mineralization on CT. Milder cases were not associated with any T2* signal abnormality, eliminating blood products as a cause for T1 shortening. Increased posterior fossa perfusion was shown in one study. The authors concluded that increased perfusion may induce dystrophic calcification with selective vulnerability of the pulvinar. Both authors suggested that the lateral pulvinar T1 hyperintensity may be a specific sign for Fabry's disease (Fig. 21-2). Diffusion-weighted imaging (DWI) and DTI demonstrate changes that may not be apparent on conventional imaging. Increased white matter diffusion without differences in fractional anisotropy is described.[11] The basilar artery diameter is previously described as the best discriminator between patients with Fabry's disease and age-matched controls. This measurement has been suggested as a means of early detection and monitoring of brain involvement in Fabry's disease. This measurement was superior to white matter lesion load and white matter diffusivity assessed by diffusion tensor imaging.[11a]

Analysis

A sample imaging report is shown in Box 21-1.

MOYAMOYA

Moyamoya syndrome is a slowly progressing vasculopathy that results in narrowing of the distal internal carotid artery and proximal circle of Willis. Moyamoya *disease* implies no underlying cause. When a secondary cause is implicated, the term *phenomenon* is used.

Epidemiology

Moyamoya can occur in both children and adults. The majority of cases present before the age of 20 years (70%) and half occur before the age of 10 years.[12] Children present with stroke symptoms and progressive neurologic impairment. Adults tend to present with parenchymal, intraventricular, or, less commonly, subarachnoid hemorrhage.[13] Females are affected twice as often as males. Familial inheritance occurs in approximately 10% of

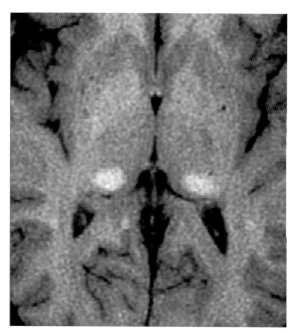

■ **FIGURE 21-2** T1-weighted MR image showing pulvinar hyperintensity in Fabry's disease. This abnormality is seen in about 30% of patients with the disease. *(From Moore DF, Kaneski CR, Askari H, Schiffmann R: The cerebral vasculopathy of Fabry disease. J Neurol Sci 2007; 257:258-263.)*

BOX 21-1 Sample Report: Imaging Evaluation for Fabry's Disease

HISTORY

Fabry's disease, with recent episode of transient right arm weakness.

FINDINGS

There is extensive periventricular and deep white matter hyperintensity consistent with microangiopathic change. No evidence of acute infarct is shown on DWI. T1 hyperintensity is present within the bilateral pulvinar region without associated T2 change. Foci of susceptibility are present within the subcortical white matter in the frontal and parietal region consistent with calcification present on noncontrast CT. There is marked dolichoectasia of the vertebrobasilar system with pontine distortion but no signal abnormality.

IMPRESSION

Findings are consistent with known Fabry's disease.

---

cases. Related chromosomal defects include 17q25, 12p, and 3p24.2-p26. Numerous genetic disorders are associated, including Down syndrome, sickle cell disease, tuberous sclerosis, glycogen storage disease type 1a, neurofibromatosis type 1, progeria, hereditary spherocytosis, and morning glory syndrome. Skull base, pituitary, or suprasellar tumors are causative either idiopathically or secondary to radiation treatment. Infectious causes include basal meningitis, particularly tuberculosis, leptospirosis, and complicated tonsillitis or otitis media. Vasculitis-induced vessel occlusions may be secondary to systemic lupus erythematosus, anticardiolipin syndrome, neuro-Behçet's syndrome, polyarteritis nodosa, collagen vascular diseases, Kawasaki disease, and factor V Leiden. There is increased association of moyamoya with aneurysms, arteriovenous malformations, fenestrations, and congenital heart disease.

Pathophysiology

Arterial stenosis and occlusion is seen as a result of fibrocellular concentric intimal thickening with a dense array of smooth

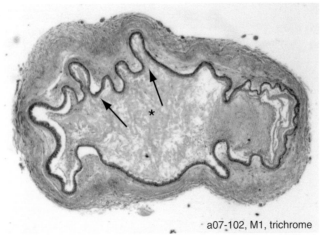

a07-102, M1, trichrome

■ **FIGURE 21-3** Trichrome stain of cross-section through M1 segment reveals a profuse fibrosis of intima with obliteration of the lumen (*asterisk*); a folded, wavy, internal elastic lamina (*arrow*); and media thinning. *(Courtesy of Dr. Juan Bilbao, Neuropathologist, Sunnybrook Health Sciences Centre.)*

muscle cells, multilayered elastic lamina, and few lipid deposits. Folds are seen in the internal elastic lamina. The external diameter of the vessel shrinks, and there is thinning of the media (Fig. 21-3).[14-16]

Pathology

Skull thickening can be seen in etiologies that result in chronic anemia.

Gross examination of the brain reveals increased lenticulostriate, thalamostriate, and extraconal/intraconal collaterals. Saccular aneurysms can be seen. Areas of infarction and hemorrhage of various ages can be visualized.

Imaging
Ultrasonography

Ultrasound has a limited role in diagnosis or monitoring. Transcranial Doppler and power Doppler imaging can demonstrate the stenoses.

CT

Atrophy and infarcts occur in the distribution of the anterior circulation. Noncontrast CT shows acute intraparenchymal and subarachnoid hemorrhage. Dilated lenticulostriate and thalamoperforate collaterals appear as punctate and linear contrast enhancement within the basal ganglia (Fig. 21-4). CTA confirms

■ **FIGURE 21-4** Patient with moyamoya disease. Axial CTA 0.625-mm reconstruction (**A**) and 7-mm Cor MIP (**B**) images demonstrate bilateral basal ganglia perforator enlargement (*arrowheads*) and ICA and proximal ACA and MCA occlusion. Numerous anterior cranial fossa collaterals are seen within the subarachnoid space. **C,** MTT CTP confirms prolongation of transit time within the bilateral frontal lobes and left MCA territory posteriorly. **D,** Anteroposterior DSA with left ICA selective injection confirms terminal carotid, proximal ACA, and MCA occlusion. Numerous lenticulostriate perforator and leptomeningeal collaterals are evident that showed retrograde distal left MCA filling (*arrowheads*).

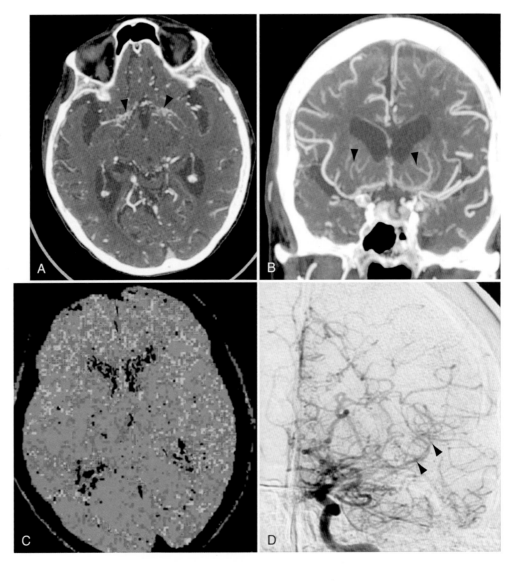

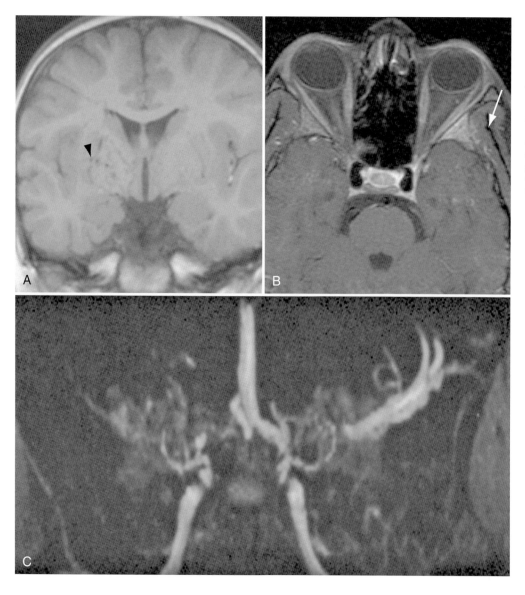

■ **FIGURE 21-5** Coronal T1W (**A**), fat-saturated T1W postcontrast (**B**), and TOF MRA MIP (**C**) images demonstrating multiple flow voids within the basal ganglia that are greater on the right (*arrowhead*). Bilateral terminal carotid and right MCA occlusion with collateral enlargement producing the characteristic "puff of smoke" appearance. There is enhancement within the left greater wing of the sphenoid consistent with bone infarction (*arrow*).

these findings and assesses the severity of any stenoses of the distal internal carotid arteries (ICAs), proximal middle cerebral arteries (MCAs), and proximal anterior cerebral arteries (ACAs) (Fig. 21-4). Saccular aneurysms involving the basilar artery and lenticulostriate vessels are seen. CT perfusion may assist in highlighting regions at increased risk for infarction and assess the outcome of surgical treatment (see Fig. 21-4).[17]

MRI

MRI shows generalized atrophy in the distribution of anterior circulation. Prior infarcts or hemorrhage are well seen on fluid-attenuated inversion recovery (FLAIR) or gradient-recalled-echo (GRE) imaging. DWI will detect acute infarcts. Flow voids in the distal ICAs and proximal ACAs/MCAs may be absent or diminished. Flow voids are increased in the basal ganglia, consistent with dilation of the lenticulostriate collateral circulation (Fig. 21-5). These enhance after administration of gadolinium.[18,19] Slow flow through enlarged pial collaterals and arachnoid thickening results in intravascular signal or enhancement coined the "ivy sign." This is best detected with FLAIR and contrast-enhanced T1W images.[20] This sign appears to correlate with reduced cerebrovascular reactivity.[20a] Perfusion MRI may also assist in highlighting regions at increased risk for infarction, in assessing the outcome of surgical treatment.[21] It is uniquely

challenging for MR-based methods. Quantitative mapping of cerebral blood flow, cerebral blood volume, and mean transit time (MTT) requires temporal knowledge of the input concentration of the administered contrast agent or tracer for each of the major vascular territories. These concentration time curves are usually measured empirically by positioning a region of interest over the major vessel input to a vascular territory. This information is then compared with the concentration time curves derived from the microcirculation in the tissue fed by this vessel, and a quantitative flow map for the whole brain is generated. Unfortunately, it is not accurate to apply the concentration time curve from a diseased input vessel to the microcirculation fed by an entirely different diseased input vessel. The flow map will be accurate for the territory supplied by the vessel in which the input function was measured, but not for those tissues fed by other vessels. Positron emission tomography (PET) avoids this problem because arterial sampling of the tracer concentration over time is performed, providing knowledge of the arterial input to all brain vessels. Single photon emission CT (SPECT) is also somewhat immune to this problem because single pass tracers are used, but the information is weighted toward tracer delivery/deposition. The resulting perfusion map is proportional, but not equivalent, to blood flow.

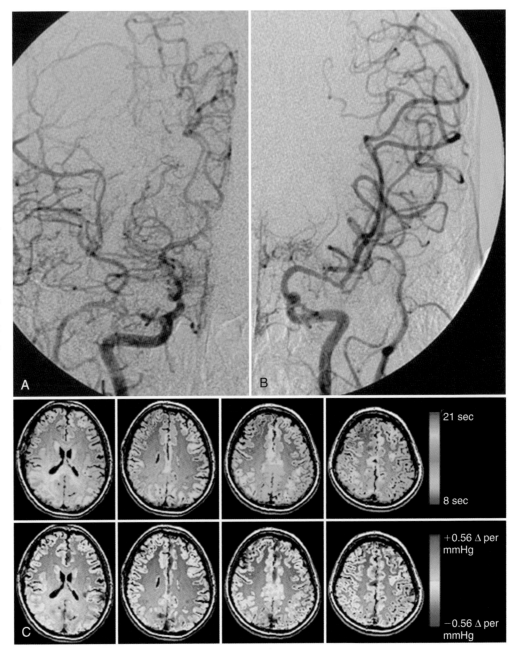

■ **FIGURE 21-6** **A,** Angiogram in a patient with moyamoya disease shows severe narrowing of the proximal right ACA and MCA vessels at the bifurcation of the internal carotid artery. **B,** The left ACA does not fill and there is stenosis of the left MCA. **C,** The images in the top row are from a dynamic gadolinium bolus perfusion study in this patient. Because selection of a vessel for placement of a region of interest to measure flow was ambiguous, an input function independent time to bolus peak was generated from the gadolinium bolus (*scale is in seconds*). The lower row shows CVR data (*scale shows the percentage of BOLD signal change per mm Hg of end-tidal CO$_2$*). *Blue* shows decreased BOLD signal with increases in end-tidal CO$_2$ indicating a paradoxical effect (i.e., steal phenomenon). Note the precision in mapping the territory of the steal, indicating maximum impairment in flow physiology not as clearly outlined by the time to peak map. *(Courtesy of Dr. David Mikulis.)*

It can be argued that measurement of cerebrovascular reactivity (CVR), which is defined as a change in blood flow per unit change in stimulus such as carbon dioxide, is a more accurate indicator of the physiologic impact of vascular stenosis. Because the brain can locally control perfusion through arteriolar vascular tone, flow compensation is possible in the setting of vascular stenosis. Relaxation of vascular tone can lead to normalization of blood flow. Conventional CBF maps can therefore be normal, although CBV and MTT maps usually show increases. However, the use of PET, CT, DSC MRI, and SPECT for this purpose is cumbersome because two measurement sessions, one with baseline and one with post-stimulus (CO$_2$ or acetazolamide) acquisitions are necessary. Furthermore, DSCE MRI and CT suffer from the input function problem, especially in those patients with multiple-vessel disease.

A technique has been developed using blood oxygenation level dependent contrast (BOLD) MRI that circumvents all of these issues.[22,23] This technique is quantitative, is input function independent, and clearly outlines tissues, not only where CVR is exhausted but also where there is "paradoxical" reactivity, that is, vascular steal. It can be performed on all MRI systems with echoplanar capability using a 12-minute acquisition at 1.5 T and a 6-minute acquisition at 3 T. The only requirement is the need to precisely cycle end-tidal CO$_2$ between periods of normocapnia and hypercapnia during the MR acquisition. It has been determined that the BOLD signal normally increases during hypercapnia owing to washout of deoxyhemoglobin. In tissues with complete relaxation of vascular tone due to proximal stenosis, the BOLD signal decreases because of shift of blood flow toward tissue still capable of lowering its vascular resistance in response to CO$_2$. This vascular steal phenomenon is an extreme physiologic condition but is easily mapped as the BOLD signal becomes negative relative to the baseline. BOLD CVR is especially well suited for mapping patients with moyamoya because they have complex multiple-vessel compromise and are quite difficult to assess using conventional blood flow imaging techniques (Fig. 21-6). Extracranial-intracranial bypass has been shown to reverse preprocedural CVR defects in Moyamoya patients.[23a]

Special Procedures

Angiography demonstrates narrowing of the distal ICAs and the proximal MCAs and ACAs. Prominent lenticulostriate and thalamoperforate collaterals give rise to a vascular blush designated the "puff of smoke" (moyamoya) (Fig. 21-4).[24] In late stages, transdural and transosseous extraconal/intraconal collaterals will be seen.[24,25] Similar findings can be visualized on both MRI[26] and CTA. Dilation and abnormal branching of the anterior choroidal and posterior communicating arteries have been shown to be strong predictors of hemorrhagic events in adults with moyamoya.[27]

SPECT imaging, like perfusion MRI, can demonstrate regions at risk for infarction as well as monitor the benefits of treatment.[28]

Analysis

A sample MRI report is shown in Box 21-2.

VASCULITIS

Vasculitis is an umbrella term that includes multiple different diseases with the common feature of vessel stenosis. So defined, vasculitis is responsible for up to 5% of strokes in young patients and remains an elusive diagnosis. The demographic distribution, pathology, and presentation are heterogeneous depending on the etiology and will be dealt with under each vasculitis subtype. Vasculitis is classified as *primary vasculitis* when it is confined to the central or peripheral nervous system (Fig. 21-7). It is classified as *secondary vasculitis* when the nervous system is affected as one aspect of a primary systemic vasculitis or of systemic disorders associated with inflammatory vasculopathy such as infection and collagen vascular disorders (Fig. 21-8). Secondary vasculitis may itself be subclassified as primary systemic vasculitis when no preceding or accompanying disease is present and as secondary when it is associated with other disease processes. However, no accepted classification or diagnostic criteria exist.[29,30] Some of the primary systemic vasculitides are even known to be associated with infectious agents. Some of the more common causes of vasculitis are listed in Table 21-1.

Primary Vasculitis

Primary angiitis of the central nervous system (PACNS) is the preferred term for a primary CNS vasculitis. Other names include granulomatous angiitis (GANS), granulomatous giant cell angiitis, noninfectious granulomatous angiitis, and isolated angiitis.

Epidemiology

PACNS is rare, occurs in the fourth to sixth decades of life, shows a predilection for small arteries 200 to 300 μm in diameter, and occasionally involves medium-sized (500 μm)

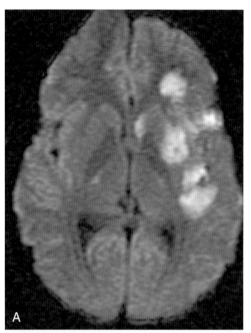

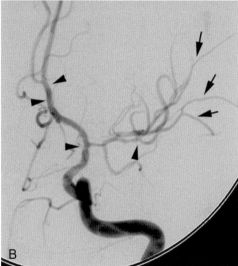

■ **FIGURE 21-7** **A,** DWI demonstrates multiple basal ganglia and subinsular and cortical regions of restriction consistent with acute infarct. **B,** Multiple regions of stenosis are present on DSA. Beaded appearance is present within terminal ICA, proximal ACA, and distal M2 (*arrowheads*). Fine alterations in caliber are present within the M3 branches (*arrows*).

vessels. Leptomeningeal and cortical arteries are commonly involved. Veins are affected less often.

Clinical Presentation

The clinical presentation is heterogeneous. Early biopsy-proven cases were reported to have a male predilection and be uniformly fatal. Subsequently, increasing numbers of cases have been diagnosed solely on the basis of digital subtraction angiography (DSA). These cases have demonstrated important differences from the biopsy-proven cases. They appeared to have a female predilection, present with headache and focal signs rather than progressive encephalopathy, have a benign CSF profile, and carry a better prognosis. The term *benign angiopathy* (BACNS) was coined to identify this subgroup.[31] It appears there is a spectrum of disease severity under the banner of PACNS.

■ **FIGURE 21-8** A 65-year-old woman with an idiopathic rheumatologic condition, elevated antinuclear antigen, and prior skin biopsy showing subacute lupus presented with acute subarachnoid hemorrhage on noncontrast CT (**A**). **B,** Coronal 7-mm MIP CTA demonstrated 90% supraclinoid ICA stenosis (*arrow*). Circumferential filling defects were seen within the first genu of the cavernous ICA (*arrowhead*). **C,** High-resolution postcontrast T1W MR image through the cavernous region demonstrates wall thickening and enhancement suggesting vasculopathy (*arrowheads*). **D,** DSA revealed alternating narrowing and dilatation of the supraclinoid carotid (*arrows*). She subsequently developed a palpable purpuric rash in the left leg that was sampled. A leukocytoclastic vasculitis was diagnosed but no specific cause was found.

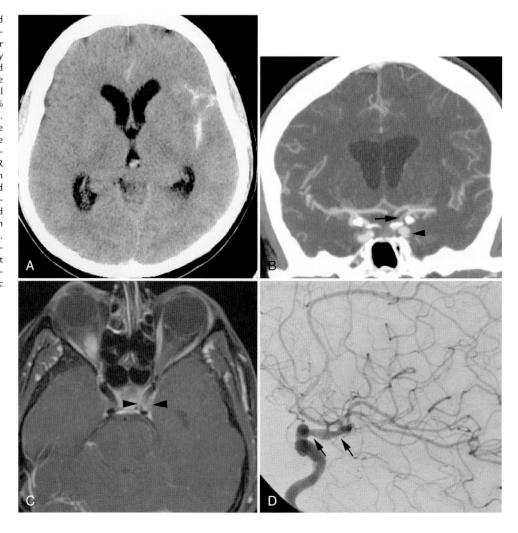

Pathology

Histopathologically there is focal and segmental inflammatory infiltrate of giant cells, plasma cells, and lymphocytes accompanied by vessel wall necrosis with or without perivascular parenchymal granuloma formation, myelin loss, and axonal degeneration. The heterogeneity of disease distribution accounts for negative brain or meningeal biopsy in about 25% of patients.

Imaging
CT

The imaging features of vasculitis are nonspecific. The diagnostic sensitivity of CT is lower than that of MRI. CT may be normal or demonstrate focal hemorrhage or low density ischemic lesions.[32] Medium and large vessel changes are described under Special Procedures (see later). CTA is able to consistently identify cortical arterial branches with significant stenoses. Interpretation, however, remains limited by a 0.5-mm spatial resolution that is below the threshold for detecting small vessel vasculitides.

MRI

MRI is the modality of choice for assessing brain parenchymal change, but MRI does not have the spatial resolution to detect small vessel abnormalities. MRI-negative studies are described in patients with angiographically proven disease, but the majority of these MR studies did not use FLAIR or DWI,[33,34] which accounts

for the varying reported sensitivity of 50% to 100%. In comparison, the sensitivity of CSF analysis is 50% to 90%. The specificity of both tests, however, is low (~36%). We and other authors reported MRI abnormalities in all patients with vasculitis, including some with normal initial angiography.[35-37] Current MRA techniques may show large intracranial vessel stenosis but do not show smaller stenoses consistently. Abnormalities include bilateral, multiple, supratentorial white matter T2-weighted (T2W) hyperintensities, although basal ganglia and cortical lesions also occur (see Fig. 21-7). Infratentorial disease is uncommon in the absence of supratentorial involvement. Contrast enhancement of the lesions, meninges, and perivascular spaces is also described. Mass lesions may be seen in 15% of patients. Parenchymal hemorrhage and subarachnoid hemorrhage are uncommon (see Fig. 21-8) and occur in 10% of patients. DWI may facilitate the identification of new lesions against a background of white matter hyperintensities, and FLAIR might help detect cortical or periventricular lesions. A negative CSF and negative MRI are strong negative predictors of CNS vasculitis.[38] High resolution imaging of the vessel wall is an emerging technique aimed at characterizing disease processes involving the intracranial circulation. This technique uses optimized T1 black blood precontrast and postcontrast to evaluate for the presence and pattern of enhancement. Although limited experience is available with this technique, early data suggest that the enhancement pattern

TABLE 21-1. Types of Vasculitis

Primary Systemic Vasculitis
Granulomatous
    Large vessel: giant cell arteritis
    Takayasu's arteritis
    Small vessel: Wegener's granulomatosis
    Churg-Strauss syndrome
Nongranulomatous
    Medium vessel: polyarteritis nodosa
    Kawasaki disease
    Small vessel: microscopic polyangiitis

Secondary Systemic Vasculitis
Collagen vascular disorders
    Systemic lupus erythematosus
    Rheumatoid arthritis
    Scleroderma
    Sjögren's syndrome
Infectious
    Virus
    Herpes virus (varicella zoster virus/herpes simplex virus)
    Human immunodeficiency virus
    Cytomegalovirus
    Bacteria
    Purulent meningitis (meningococcus, *Haemophilus influenzae,*
      pneumococcus)
    Tuberculosis (*Mycobacterium tuberculosis*)
    Syphilis (*Treponema pallidum*)
    Lyme disease (*Borrelia burgdorferi*)
    Fungi
    Tuberculosis type: histoplasmosis, actinomycosis, cryptococcosis,
      nocardiosis
    Hyphal type: aspergillosis, mucormycosis

Other
Lymphoproliferative disease
Paraneoplastic
Neuro-Behçet's syndrome
Sarcoid

Vasculitis Mimics
Drug abuse
Radiation

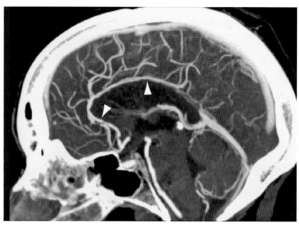

■ FIGURE 21-9 A 75-year-old hypertensive patient with type 2 diabetes and hypercholesterolemia presented with TIA. There are multiple regions of focal A2 and pericallosal stenoses (*arrowheads*). Appearances are nonspecific but consistent with atherosclerotic disease.

BOX 21-3   Sample Report: MRI of Vasculitis

HISTORY

A 45-year-old man with right-sided weakness and no known infarcts.

FINDINGS

Multiple T2 hyperintensities are present within the deep and subcortical white matter. There is acute restriction within the left basal ganglia and frontal cortex consistent with acute infarct. No microhemorrhages are noted. Contrast-enhanced MRA demonstrates beading of the bilateral proximal M1 MCA segment. There is subtle M2 and M3 caliber alteration in addition. No aneurysms are present.

    The appearances are nonspecific. The white matter findings are nonspecific but, combined with abnormal intracranial vasculature, should raise suspicion for vasculitis.

---

may differentiate between vasculitis, atherosclerosis, and intracranial dissections.[38a,38b]

Special Procedures

In patients with PACNS, conventional angiography demonstrates abnormality in about 83% of cases. Yet, clinically, it is most common for clinically suspected arteritis to be negative even on angiography (40%-60%). Biopsy remains the reference standard for diagnosis and is frequently positive in the presence of negative vascular imaging. The classic findings of segmental narrowing and dilatation or beaded appearance may be seen in 20% to 65% of patients (see Fig. 21-7). Rarely, small presumed vasculitic aneurysms are present. The angiography may appear normal in up to 20% to 40% of cases, because the small vessels affected fall below the spatial resolution of the technique.[39] The current spatial resolution of MRA and CTA also precludes assessment of small vessel changes less than 500 µm. However, medium-sized vessel involvement is within the spatial resolution of these modalities. Our experience in children shows that whereas MRA detected fewer lesions than did conventional angiography, the diagnosis is unaltered because of the multiplicity of lesions. The ability of MRA to accurately quantify the degree of stenosis is important because angiographic features are used to assess the response to treatment. Our and others' experience show 78% to 100% sensitivity for stenosis greater than 50%.[40,41] MRA overestimates the degree of stenosis due to dephasing and in-plane flow artifacts. CTA may be better, but significant limitations remain in attempting to discern small changes in the luminal diameter of 1- to 2-mm intracranial vessels.

Patients with BACNS manifest a different appearance on angiography. In BACNS, angiography reveals multiple, bilateral, symmetric smooth narrowings of cerebral vessels, often with post-stenotic dilatation.[42]

There is a wide differential diagnosis for the nonspecific angiographic appearances described. Atherosclerosis (Fig. 21-9), radiation vasculopathy, angiocentric lymphoma, intravascular neoplasia (angioendotheliomatosis, intravascular lymphoma), thrombotic thrombocytopenic purpura, hypercoagulable states, vasospasm secondary to migraine, reversible vasoconstriction syndrome[42a] (Fig. 21-10), and subarachnoid hemorrhage may all produce similar findings.

Analysis

A sample report for primary vasculitis is presented in Box 21-3.

Secondary Vasculitis

Giant Cell Arteritis and Takayasu's Arteritis

Giant cell arteritis (GCA) and *Takayasu's arteritis* are large vessel vasculitides that share similarities in terms of vessels affected, ischemic complications, corticosteroid responsiveness, and presumed cell-mediated etiology.

Epidemiology

GCA usually affects the superficial temporal artery but like Takayasu's arteritis may involve the vertebral artery and the aorta and its main branches. Takayasu's arteritis is limited to the aorta, its proximal major branches, and the pulmonary arteries.

■ **FIGURE 21-10** A 50-year-old woman who presented with acute onset of the worst headache of her life was evaluated for subarachnoid hemorrhage. Initial noncontrast CT and lumbar puncture demonstrated no abnormality or blood. **A,** DSA was unremarkable. **B,** TOF MRA performed 1 day later because of new neurologic deficit demonstrates multiple stenoses within the M2 segments of the left MCA not present on DSA (*arrowheads*). **C,** Repeat contrast-enhanced MRA 3 months later demonstrates resolution. Patient was diagnosed as having thunderclap headache with reversible vasoconstriction syndrome. Appearances mimic vasculitis.

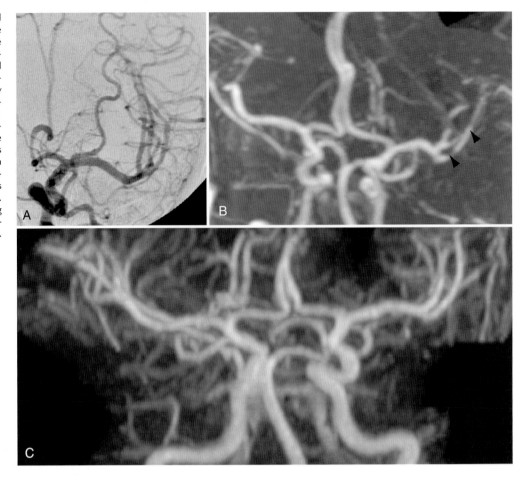

Clinical Presentation

Visual disturbances are present in one third of GCA patients and progress to blindness if untreated. Patients with aortic aneurysms have a significant reduction in life expectancy.[43] Patients with Takayasu's arteritis have hypertension. Multiple absent pulses are seen in one third of patients. Chest radiography demonstrates cardiomegaly, vessel calcification, scalloped rib margins, notched aortic arch, and pulmonary arterial pruning.

Pathophysiology

GCA is most common in older patients (>50 years) often with a history of polymyalgia rheumatica. Takayasu's arteritis preferentially affects young Asian women. The etiology of Takayasu's arteritis is uncertain, but autoantibodies against aortic endothelial cells are present in most patients. The role of elevated cytokines is unclear, but these may be a useful marker of disease activity.[44]

Pathology

Histopathologically, GCA manifests a granulomatous panarteritis with inflammatory infiltrate. Superficial temporal artery biopsy is positive in 10% to 20% of cases, reflecting the segmental nature of involvement.

Imaging

MRI

MRI may show enhancement of the wall of the affected vessel and serve as a surrogate marker for Takayasu's disease activity. A segmented k-space inversion recovery, GRE sequence can be used to obtain delayed postcontrast imaging. Thickening and enhancement of the aortic wall may be demonstrated even in some patients without clinical evidence of disease. One study

suggested there was an increased degree of arterial enhancement in patients with elevated inflammatory markers, but the sample size was small.[45] A similar approach can be adopted for the superficial temporal arteries using 3-T MRI.[46]

Special Procedures

In GCA, cerebral angiography reveals irregularity of the superficial temporal, meningeal, and cerebral arteries with focal and diffuse stenosis and dilatation. Aneurysm formation is also described.[47] Panarteritis occurs in approximately two thirds of patients with Takayasu's arteritis. In the remaining one third the arteritis is limited to the thoracic aorta. Patients are classified angiographically, as shown below, according to segment of aorta and the branches involved[48]:

Type 1: Aortic arch branches only
Type 2: Thoracic aorta and branches only
Type 3: Abdominal aorta and branches only
Type 4: Whole length of aorta and branches

Stenosis is the most common finding, followed by dilatation, occlusion, and aneurysm formation. Conventional angiography, however, cannot distinguish active from chronic inflammation.

PET labeled with fluorodeoxyglucose (FDG) appears to be more sensitive than MRI for demonstrating the early stages of Takayasu's arteritis. Increased uptake is seen within the vessel wall in active disease and regresses on treatment.[44]

Polyarteritis Nodosa

The definition of polyarteritis nodosa (PAN) has changed over the past 15 years. Different subsets of patients are now included under the PAN label, such as patients with associated hepatitis

B virus (HBV-PAN). Microscopic polyangiitis (MPA) may be distinguished from PAN, but there is controversy regarding the correct criteria for differential diagnosis. One definition limits PAN to medium and small vessels, sparing arterioles and capillaries, whereas MPA mainly affects small vessels of the order spared in PAN (even if it also affects medium-sized vessels). MPA also manifests an antineutrophil cytoplasmic antibody (ANCA).[49] Presently, MPA should be considered an ANCA-associated small vessel vasculitis that shares some similarities with Churg-Strauss and Wegener's diseases.

Epidemiology
PAN is rare, with an estimated incidence of 2 to 3/100,000. It presents in the fifth to seventh decades of life with weight loss, fever, and malaise.

Clinical Presentation
The peripheral nervous system is affected in 70% of cases, so patients present with a mononeuropathy or polyneuropathy. Multiple visceral aneurysms are present, especially in the kidney, liver, and intestine. CNS involvement is seen in 20% to 40% of cases, primarily in the brain but also in the spine. Patients present with encephalopathy, focal neurologic deficit, and seizures.

Imaging
CT and MRI reveal cortical and subcortical infarcts. Angiography reveals segmental nonspecific narrowing and dilatation, with predilection for branch points, consistent with vasculitis.[50] Catheter angiography may be normal, despite clinical evidence of CNS involvement. Intracranial aneurysms, subarachnoid hemorrhage, and parenchymal hemorrhage are reported but rare.

Kawasaki Disease
Kawasaki disease is a necrotizing vasculitis of medium-sized vessels.

Epidemiology
In contrast to PAN, Kawasaki disease affects children younger than 5 years of age.

Clinical Presentation
Patients present with a mucocutaneous syndrome that includes fever, rash, limb edema, conjunctivitis, oromucosal erythema, and lymphadenopathy. Coronary artery aneurysms are present in up to 25% of patients and account for 1% to 2% of Kawasaki-related deaths. CNS involvement occurs in approximately 1%. Irritability, lethargy, aseptic meningitis, encephalopathy, seizures, and infarction are described. Lower facial nerve palsy involvement is a rare additional finding.

Churg-Strauss Syndrome
Churg-Strauss syndrome is a small vessel necrotizing vasculitis characterized by eosinophilic infiltrate and granuloma formation in patients with a history of asthma and allergic rhinitis. It is also called allergic granulomatosis.

Epidemiology
The incidence ranges from 0.5 to 7/100,000.

Clinical Presentation
The peripheral nervous system is involved in 50% to 80% of cases, so patients present with a mononeuritis multiplex. CNS involvement is reported in 10% to 30% of patients and manifests as seizures, stroke, and encephalopathy. Subarachnoid and intraventricular hemorrhages are described. Gastrointestinal, skin, and renal disease are common. The prognosis is good, with a 5-year survival exceeding 90%.[51] Cardiac involvement is the predominant cause of death.

Pathophysiology
The exact pathogenesis of Churg-Strauss syndrome remains unclear. Eosinophilia, ANCA positivity, cytokines, and the presence of anti-myeloperoxidase are contributory. ANCA is present in 30% to 50% of cases. ANCA-negative patients are less likely to manifest vasculitis but appear at higher risk for cardiac involvement.

Pathology
Vasculitis may be granulomatous or nongranulomatous involving arteries and systemic veins. Small vessel angiitis and extravascular necrotizing granulomas are characteristic. Cutaneous biopsies are often not helpful and demonstrate only nonspecific inflammation. Muscle and nerve biopsies, however, are often useful.

Imaging
MRI
Imaging of the CNS is often noncontributory. Infarct and hemorrhage have the typical imaging appearances described above. Granulomatous involvement of the meninges and choroid plexus is described. Lesions are nonspecific but are hypointense on T2W imaging and enhance uniformly. These appearances are suggestive of granulomatous processes. Similar findings are described in other granulomatous diseases such as Wegener's, sarcoid, and tuberculosis.

Special Procedures
There are few studies describing aneurysmal subarachnoid hemorrhage in association with vasculitic changes attributed to Churg-Strauss syndrome.

Wegener's Arteritis
Like Churg-Strauss syndrome and microscopic polyangiitis (MPA), Wegener's arteritis is a necrotizing small vessel vasculitis. The terms *necrotizing granulomatosis with polyangiitis* or *necrotizing granulomatosis* may be preferred to *Wegener's granulomatosis,* owing to the questionable involvement of Wegener with the Nazi party during World War II.[43]

Epidemiology
Wegener's arteritis is a rare disease with a prevalence of 112/million. The proteinase 3–antineutrophil cytoplasmic autoantibody (PR3-ANCA) associated form predominates in whites in the Northern hemisphere whereas the myeloperoxidase (MPO)-ANCA associated form is predominant in whites and nonwhites in the Southern hemisphere. Cocaine use and silica exposure are presumptive environmental factors, especially in patients in whom the airway is affected.

Clinical Presentation
Necrotizing granulomatosis affects the upper and lower respiratory tract, orbit, and kidney. Peripheral nervous system signs and symptoms are seen in approximately 50% of patients. CNS disease is usually a later manifestation of the disease in fewer than 20% of patients. CNS manifestations arise via contiguous sino-orbital spread, CNS vasculitis, or, least commonly, granulomatous intracerebral lesions and include headache, encephalopathy, stroke, seizure, cranial neuropathy, and visual impairment. Pituitary or suprasellar involvement may manifest as pituitary dysfunction.

Pathophysiology
There is some evidence that Churg-Strauss syndrome is a variant of Wegener's arteritis or MPA. ANCA is found in all patients with Wegener's arteritis. ANCA is implicated in the pathogenesis by activating primed neutrophils. Lytic enzymes are released, damaging endothelial cells. Cocaine use and silica exposure are

implicated as etiologic environmental factors, whereas smoking may be protective. Genetic associations include increased functional polymorphism of tyrosine phosphatase.

Pathology

Typical appearances include necrotizing granulomatous pachymeningitis comprising multinucleate giant cell infiltrates. Vessels demonstrate transmural granulomatous necrotizing inflammation consistent with small vessel vasculitis.

Imaging
MRI

Meningeal involvement is reported in up to 6% of patients and manifests as nonspecific meningeal thickening with enhancement. The differential diagnosis includes benign tumors (meningioma, plasma cell tumor), malignant tumors (metastatic carcinoma, lymphoma), infectious (tuberculosis) and inflammatory (sarcoid) conditions, intracranial hypotension, and idiopathic conditions. Spinal involvement is rare. Arterial and venous sinus occlusion and aneurysmal subarachnoid hemorrhage are demonstrated by MRA or CTA. Orbital and nasal involvement are nonspecific. Bone destruction is best visualized on CT but is reported in less than half of patients. Granuloma formation may be seen in either location. Early on, edema elevates the T2 signal intensity. In later stages, the signal intensity is characteristically low on both T1W and T2W images. Distinction from inflammatory sinus disease is then not possible. Other differential diagnostic considerations are squamous cell carcinoma, lymphoma, and melanoma. Orbital disease may be contiguous with sinus disease or may appear as a discrete intraconal or extraconal lesion. Enhancement may be either homogeneous or heterogeneous. The differential diagnoses of orbital lesions include lymphoma, idiopathic orbital inflammation, sarcoid, idiopathic midline granuloma, and metastases.

Special Procedures

The diagnostic yield of cerebral angiography is low because of inability to accurately visualize small vessel disease.

Systemic Lupus Erythematosus

Systemic lupus erythematosus (SLE) is a diverse autoimmune disease with widespread systemic involvement.

Epidemiology

The CNS is affected in about 20% of cases, although involvement in up to 70% is described. CNS disease accounts for 5% to 7% of SLE-related mortality.

Clinical Presentation

Cutaneous lesions are the most common clinical expression of vasculitis, including erythematous lesions of the palms and fingertips, purpura, urticarial and nodular lesions, and ischemia. Systemic vasculitis also affects gastrointestinal, pulmonary, and cardiac regions. Neurologic presentation includes cerebral hemorrhage, infarction, transient ischemic attacks, transverse myelitis, neurocognitive impairment, and neuropsychiatric symptoms. Mononeuritis multiplex occurs when the peripheral nervous system is involved. CNS complications resulting from the treatment of SLE should also be considered, including posterior reversible encephalopathy syndrome (PRES), drug toxicity, and infection.

Pathophysiology

The etiology of CNS disease is multifactorial and includes cardioembolism from left-sided valvular disease, thrombosis, antiphospholipid (aPL) antibody, thrombotic thrombocytopenic purpura (TTP), antibody-mediated injury, and vasculitis or a combination. Although vasculitis is one of the most common processes involved in the systemic expression of this multisystem disorder, it is an uncommon cause of CNS disease (~7% of patients). Primary systemic vasculitides such as polyarteritis nodosa, cryoglobulinemia, and other vasculitides may coexist in up to 40% of SLE cases.[52] Cardioembolism remains the predominant cause of cerebrovascular events. Medium-size vessel involvement, although uncommon, is an important cause of mononeuritis multiplex. aPL is strongly associated with transient ischemic attacks, ischemic stroke, and venous thrombosis. The recognition of aPL is important, because patients are treated with anticoagulation rather than corticosteroids.

Pathology

Gross vessel changes include intimal proliferation and thickening of the vessel wall. Small vessel occlusion and infarct ensue.

Vessels are most commonly affected by an arteriopathy and platelet-fibrin intracranial vessel occlusion. Hyalinization, perivascular lymphocytosis, and endothelial proliferation are seen. Fewer than 10% of cases present with a true vasculitis comprising inflammatory infiltrate and fibrinoid necrosis.

Imaging
MRI

In approximately half of patients imaged, MRI demonstrates multiple T2 hyperintensities in the deep and subcortical frontoparietal white matter. Periventricular hyperintensities are particularly associated with aPL. These T2 signal abnormalities are presumed to represent small vessel ischemic injury suggestive of an underlying vasculopathy. The sensitivity and specificity of MRI for assessing neuropsychiatric SLE remain poor. The appearances are nonspecific, and the differential diagnosis includes multiple sclerosis, Sjögren's syndrome, migraine, Behcet's disease, sarcoidosis, and human immunodeficiency virus (HIV) encephalopathy. Although apparently asymptomatic, patients harboring T2 hyperintensities commonly demonstrate subclinical cognitive impairment when specifically tested.[53] Large vessel infarction is most commonly a result of cardioembolism in association with bland endocarditis. Medium and large vessel occlusions are rarely reported (see Fig. 21-8). Bilateral middle cerebellar peduncle infarcts have been reported as a presenting feature of SLE.[54] Both magnetization transfer imaging (MTI) and magnetic resonance spectroscopy (mRS) have been applied. In chronic disease, MTI demonstrates MT ratio reduction indicative of subclinical damage. Active SLE demonstrates reductions in N-acetyl-aspartate (NAA) to creatine and choline ratios and absolute NAA values. Reduction may be seen in acute and chronic states and reflects neuronal loss. Choline and myoinositol are increased in the acute and chronic stages, probably reflecting ongoing inflammation.[55]

Special Procedures

Conventional angiography may be abnormal in as few as 5% to 10% of cases, because only small-caliber vessels are affected. Nonspecific small vessel occlusion may be seen. Symptomatic large vessel occlusion is unusual in SLE and appears only several years after diagnosis. Large vessel occlusion is often associated with active disease and is a rare cause of moyamoya disease. This pattern of involvement is associated with poor outcome and a 13% recurrent stroke risk. Carotid branch occlusion, focal ectasia, and intracranial aneurysm formation are also reported.[48]

Infectious Vasculitides
Varicella-Zoster Virus Vasculitis

Varicella-zoster virus (VZV) is a human herpesvirus that causes chickenpox. Secondary reactivation of dormant virus from cranial nerve ganglia causes shingles or central and peripheral nervous system complications such as myelitis and

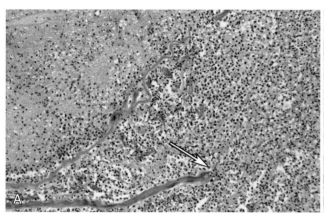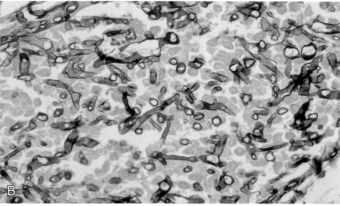

■ **FIGURE 21-11** A, LFB-H&E and (B), silver methenamine stains demonstrating disruption of the internal elastic lamina by an acute diffuse inflammatory infiltrate. B, Multiple mucormycosis hyphae are demonstrated consistent with a ruptured mycotic aneurysm. *(Courtesy of Dr. Juan Bilbao, Neuropathologist, Sunnybrook Health Sciences Centre.)*

encephalitis. VZV encephalitis is now considered secondary to a vasculopathy. It is the most common CNS complication of VZV in immunocompromised patients. The size of vessels affected depends on the patient's immune status. Encephalitis is frequently preceded by a remote herpetic rash.

MRI appearances of small vessel encephalitis are consistent with those of other encephalitides and demonstrate gray matter hyperintensity, swelling, and superimposed cortical and subcortical white matter ischemic foci or hemorrhage. The CSF shows features consistent with viral meningitis and yield VZV DNA or antibody. Treatment is empirical with acyclovir. Large vessel involvement occurs in immunocompetent individuals. The carotid terminus and proximal ACA and MCA are affected. Large vessel and lenticulostriate perforator territory infarcts are common. One study showed that the most common pattern of arterial involvement was large and small arteries in combination (50%) followed by only small arteries (37%) or large arteries in 13%. Negative angiographic studies were reported in 30 % of cases.[55a] Viral DNA may be detected in the vessel walls using polymerase chain reaction techniques. Imaging reveals bilaterally symmetric segmental stenosis and/or occlusion of proximal vessels, frequently with a corrugated appearance.[56]

HIV Vasculitis

HIV vasculitis may affect the CNS (encephalitis, myelitis, and infarction) and the peripheral nervous system (peripheral neuropathy). Concomitant VZV, cytomegalovirus infection, syphilis, and *Toxoplasma* vasculitis should also be considered.

Bacterial Vasculitis

Bacterial infection may cause vascular injury by direct extension from an adjacent sinusitis or mastoiditis with or without associated osteomyelitis or by extension from cerebritis, abscess, empyema, or septic embolus. Vessel irregularity, narrowing, occlusion, or fusiform aneurysm formation is described. The basal vessels including the cavernous carotid arteries are most commonly affected. Peripheral vessels may also be involved, in combination with basal disease or less commonly in isolation. The latter finding is rare in tuberculous meningitis.[48]

Tuberculous Vasculitis

The CNS manifestations of CNS tuberculosis are described elsewhere. Tuberculous vasculitis is most commonly found along the base of the brain, in the terminal carotid, proximal MCA, ACA, posterior cerebral artery, and basilar artery. Vascular irregularity and narrowing are reported to involve the inferior aspect of the affected vessels. Vasculitis may be limited to the region surrounding a tuberculoma.[48]

Fungal Vasculitis

An uncommon form of vasculitis, fungal infections may be divided into two patterns (see Table 21-1). The tuberculous type has a presentation indistinguishable from tuberculosis. The hyphal type produces hyphal elements that are angioinvasive. Hyphal elements impact within vessels, promoting thrombosis and inflammation. Therefore, these patients may present with hemorrhagic infarction, abscess, and mycotic aneurysm formation (Fig. 21-11).

Neuro-Behçet's Disease

Neuro-Behçet's disease is a multisystem autoimmune condition usually preceded by a classic systemic triad of uveitis and genital and oral ulceration.

Epidemiology

Neuro-Behçet's disease is common in the Mediterranean region (190/100,000) and follows the "silk road," with an increased incidence in Japan. The etiology is uncertain, but viral, autoimmune, and human leukocyte antigen (HLA)-related predispositions are suggested.

Clinical Presentation

CNS involvement of Neuro-Behçet's disease occurs in 4% to 50% of affected patients. Neuro-Behçet's disease is usually preceded by the classic systemic triad of uveitis and genital and oral ulceration. CNS involvement has a protean onset, with manifestations and progression mimicking the patterns seen in multiple sclerosis. More than half of patients with CNS disease are moderately to severely disabled after 10 years. Peripheral nervous system involvement is rare.

Pathophysiology

The etiology is uncertain, but viral, autoimmune, and HLA-related predispositions are suggested.

Pathology

Pathologically, a mononuclear vascular and perivascular infiltrate involves both arteries and veins. The intima and medial layers are absent, and the internal elastic lamina is disrupted. Fibrinoid necrosis and immune complex deposition are present within the vessel wall. Vascular involvement includes occlusion, aneurysm formation, and thrombophlebitis/thrombosis.

Imaging
MRI and Angiography

CNS involvement takes two forms: vascular Behçet's, in which sinovenous thrombosis occurs, and neuro-Behçet's, in which the cerebral parenchyma is involved. The two forms seldom coexist. Neuro-Behçet's occurs in approximately three fourths of cases and has a worse prognosis.[57] A recent large MRI series of acute and subacute neuro-Behçet's cases describes lesion distribution.[58] Asymmetric T2 hyperintensity is most common at the mesencephalic-thalamic junction. Pontobulbar extension spares the red nucleus but involves the tegmentum, superior cerebellar peduncle, and corticospinal tracts. Twenty percent show T2 hyperintensity in the anterior and posterior limbs of the internal capsule, lentiform nucleus, and external capsule. Fewer than 10% show asymmetric periventricular, deep white matter, and subcortical white matter hyperintensity. The prevalence of tel-encephalic involvement may be higher in chronic disease, probably reflecting secondary demyelination or wallerian degeneration. Large vessel angiographic involvement includes stenosis and occlusion. The aorta, aortic arch and major branches, and ilio-femoral vessels are affected. Extensive occlusion may mimic Takayasu's arteritis and cause multiple absent pulses. However, coronary involvement is rare. True or pseudoaneurysm formation and recurrent aneurysm formation are described, including aneurysms of the aorta and major aortic branches. Vessel thrombosis occurs more commonly in veins (80%) than in arteries (20%). Widespread involvement includes the superior vena cava, the subclavian veins, and the jugular veins. The appearances are nonspecific and are seen overall in approximately 30% of patients.[58]

DRUG-INDUCED VASCULOPATHY

Numerous drugs are associated with CNS complications. These include cocaine, heroin, amphetamines, phencyclidine (PCP), lysergic acid diethylamide (LSD), and ephedrine. The mechanisms of CNS complications are protean, including cerebral emboli secondary to dysrhythmias, infective endocarditis, dilated cardiomyopathy, and injected foreign particulate material, drug-induced vasospasm, malignant hypertension, subarachnoid hemorrhage, and vasculitis. Patients may present with seizures and hemorrhage (intraparenchymal, intraventricular, and subarachnoid), ischemic stroke, transient ischemic attacks, anoxic encephalopathy, movement disorders, encephalopathy, and transverse myelitis. Peripheral neuropathy and rhabdomyolysis may also occur. Hemorrhage may be primary due to the sympathomimetic effects or vasculitis-induced drug effects or may be secondary to rupture of underlying vascular malformations or aneurysm. The presence of a primary hemorrhage within the basal ganglia in a young patient is highly suggestive of drug-induced infarction but can also result from hypertension of another cause.[59]

RADIATION-INDUCED VASCULOPATHY

Radiation-induced vasculopathy may develop months to years after radiotherapy. The majority of patients present a year or more after treatment. Hyperlipidemia, hypertension, and diabetes may be additional risk factors for radiation-induced vascular injury. Small and medium vessel damage primarily affects the endothelial cells and basal lamina with hyalinization, intimal proliferation, intimal and subintimal fibrinoid necrosis, obliteration of the vasa vasorum, and mural accumulation of lipid-laden macrophages. Radiation injury to large vessels is a rare but well-known complication of prior radiotherapy for intracranial tumors (including lymphoma/leukemia, pituitary tumors, craniopharyngioma, and optic glioma), vascular malformations, and head and neck tumors. Involvement of the carotid bifurcations and terminal carotid arteries bilaterally is described. Experimental evidence demonstrates foam cell accumulation and myointimal proliferation indistinguishable from atherosclerosis. Patients may present with ischemic or thromboembolic complications or consequences of aneurysm growth and rupture. The spectrum of findings include angiographic irregularity, steno-occlusive

disease, and intracranial aneurysm formation.[60] Appreciation that the distribution of injury is limited to the radiation field may help in differential diagnosis. CT may demonstrate mineralization. MRI findings include thickening and enhancement of the walls of the terminal internal carotid arteries with luminal narrowing. Radiation-induced vasculopathy typically narrows the vessel lumen but preserves the vessel diameter, whereas idiopathic moyamoya disease typically reduces the vessel diameter.[61]

HYPERTENSIVE ENCEPHALOPATHY

Hypertensive encephalopathy is a syndrome characterized by loss of cerebrovascular autoregulation usually due to elevated blood pressure.[62] This results in preferential hyperperfusion, arteriolar leakiness, and vasogenic edema in the posterior portion of the cerebrum. Other names include posterior reversible encephalopathy syndrome (PRES), reversible posterior leukoencephalopathy syndrome (RPLS), reversible posterior edema syndrome, and reversible occipitoparietal encephalopathy.

Epidemiology

PRES is usually seen in the setting of severe, uncontrolled hypertension and usually associated with very rapid rise in the blood pressure. Typically there is frank hypertension, but PRES can be seen with normotensive pressures that are elevated for the specific individual. PRES can be the result of preeclampsia or eclampsia. Drug-induced causes include cyclosporine, OKT3, cisplatin, L-asparaginase, RAF kinase inhibitor BAY 43-9006, and tacrolimus (FK506).[63-70] Renal failure with uremia, overhydration and fluid retention, hemolytic-uremic syndrome, thrombotic thrombocytopenic purpura, and, rarely, systemic lupus erythematosus may also cause PRES.[71,72] Children are rarely affected in the absence of precipitating drugs or systemic illnesses.[73]

Clinical Presentation

Symptoms include headache, change in level of consciousness and cognition, nausea, vomiting, seizures, and visual disturbances such as blindness, homonymous hemianopia, and visual blurring.[74] The syndrome is typically reversible once the inciting cause is corrected.

Pathophysiology

Elevated blood pressure results in passive overdistention of intracranial vessels. The elevated pressure and/or direct endothelial toxic effects blunt the myogenic autoregulatory response. Posterior circulation sympathetic innervation is reduced relative to the anterior circulation. As a result, the posterior circulation is more susceptible to hyperperfusion and increased pressure. Blood-brain barrier disruption and vasogenic edema ensue. Endothelins (ET 1-3) that increase endothelial permeability have been implicated in PRES.[75] Higher levels of these are seen in preeclampsia than in normal pregnancies,[76] and increased levels are induced by tacrolimus and cyclosporine in cultured endothelial cells.[77]

Pathology

The lesions consist of cortical and subcortical vasogenic edema. Severe cases may also manifest as cytotoxic edema representing infarction as well as petechial hemorrhage in both the cortex and the white matter. The lesions are generally situated in the posterior brain, primarily the parietal and occipital lobes. However, the posterior cerebellum, basal ganglia, and internal/external capsules may become involved with increased severity.

Microscopy demonstrates edematous cortex and white matter. Microinfarcts can be seen in severe cases. Fibrinoid necrosis is found in the walls of small arteries and arterioles. A fibrinous exudate can be seen around the affected vessels. With time there can be a perivascular lymphocytic infiltrate. Changes

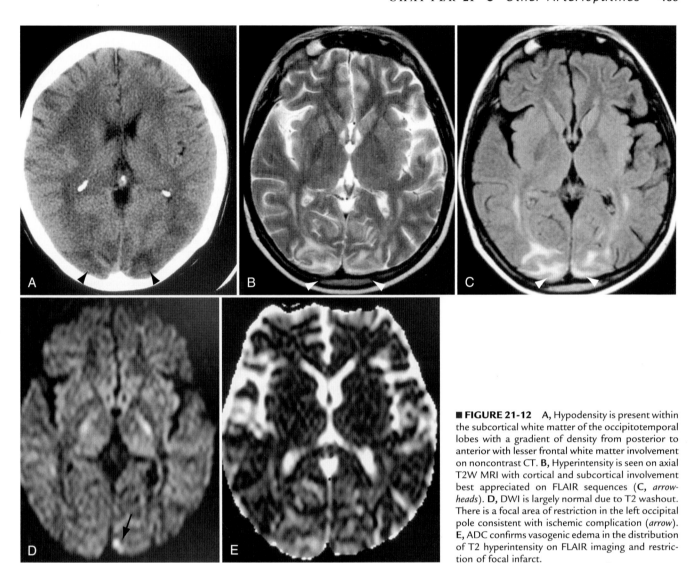

■ **FIGURE 21-12** **A,** Hypodensity is present within the subcortical white matter of the occipitotemporal lobes with a gradient of density from posterior to anterior with lesser frontal white matter involvement on noncontrast CT. **B,** Hyperintensity is seen on axial T2W MRI with cortical and subcortical involvement best appreciated on FLAIR sequences (**C,** *arrowheads*). **D,** DWI is largely normal due to T2 washout. There is a focal area of restriction in the left occipital pole consistent with ischemic complication (*arrow*). **E,** ADC confirms vasogenic edema in the distribution of T2 hyperintensity on FLAIR imaging and restriction of focal infarct.

related to chronic hypertension can also be evident, including arteriolar deposition of collagen, fibronectin, and laminin. Mural thickening can be seen. With treatment, recovery is usually complete with no residual microscopic changes.[78]

Imaging

CT

Regions of patchy hypodensity are seen in the posterior brain, particularly in the parietal and occipital lobes. The lesions are generally bilateral and symmetric. Importantly, the distribution does not conform to a vascular territory. The lesions involve cortex and subcortical white matter.[79] Occasionally, minor patchy enhancement can be seen. CT perfusion has demonstrated increased CBV and CBF with decreased MTT, consistent with hyperperfusion.[80]

MRI

T1W hypointense and T2W/FLAIR hyperintense cortical and subcortical lesions are seen in the posterior brain bilaterally and symmetrically. Basal ganglia,[81] frontal, and brain stem involvement is reported. The gradient of severity is consistently from posterior to anterior (Fig. 21-12). FLAIR consistently shows early disease most clearly owing to the absence of confounding CSF hyperintensity.[82] Petechial hemorrhage is best detected on T1W or GRE sequences. Hemorrhage has been reported in 7% to 15% of cases and include microhemorrhages, convexity, subarachnoid hemorrhage, and intraparenchymal hematoma.[82a] Contrast enhancement is very unusual, but patchy enhancement is occasionally seen. Subtle mass effect and sulcal effacement may be demonstrated. DWI intensity is usually normal or reduced. Signal intensity on DWI is a combination of diffusion effects and T2 prolongation effects ("T2 shine-through"). Vasogenic edema is hyperintense on T2W imaging and negated ("T2 washout") by the increased diffusion, resulting in isointensity. The apparent diffusion coefficient (ADC) is typically elevated consistent with vasogenic edema.[83] The combination of DWI and ADC gives useful prognostic information. Without reference to the ADC it may be unclear whether the hyperintensity on DWI is indicative of restriction (infarction) or a T2 shine-through. When there is restricted diffusion, the ADC values are normal or slightly reduced. This so-called pseudo-normalization results from intravoxel averaging of cytotoxic and vasogenic edema and

BOX 21-4 Sample Report: MRI for Suggested Hypertensive Encephalopathy

HISTORY

Headache and reduced level of consciousness in a 50-year-old famale patient with a history of SLE.

TECHNIQUE

Sagittal T1W, axial fast spin-echo T2W, axial FLAIR, axial DWI, axial T1W, axial T1W post contrast, and coronal T1W post contrast images were obtained.

FINGINGS

There are patches of increased T2W and FLAIR signal within the posterior aspects of the occipital and parietal lobes in a nonvascular distribution. The lesions involve both cortex and underlying subcortical white matter. Diffusion is increased on ADC with a normal-appearing DWI. No enhancement or hemorrhage is seen. The intracranial vessels are patent.

IMPRESSION

There is vasogenic edema with a posterior to anterior gradient of distribution. With the known history of hypertension, the findings are consistent with hypertensive encephalopathy.

---

represents an early sign of nonreversibility in PRES, heralding conversion to infarction.[84] Quantitative ADC measurements confirm a posterior to anterior gradient, reinforcing the presence of a selective vulnerability of the posterior circulation. Areas of infarction tend to occur in areas with the most severe ADC abnormality. MR changes are reversible with treatment except where infarction has occurred.[85] MR perfusion changes are variable. Normal, increased, and decreased perfusion has been reported.[86,87] MR spectroscopy demonstrates decreased NAA. Lactate is present where infarction has occurred.[88]

Special Procedures

Angiography has demonstrated peripheral vascular constriction but is rarely performed.

Analysis

A sample report is shown in Box 21-4.

ACKNOWLEDGMENT

The authors would like to acknowledge the assistance of Dr. David Mikulis, Professor of Neuroradiology at Toronto Western Hospital, in the preparation of portions of the discussion of moyamoya disease.

KEY POINTS: DIFFERENTIAL DIAGNOSIS

CADASIL
- Temporal lobe subcortical hyperintensity in young patients with no vascular risk factors is highly suggestive of CADASIL.
- One third of younger patients may have no temporal involvement.

Fabry's Disease
- Widespread dystrophic calcification in the presence of white matter disease should raise suspicion for Fabry's disease.
- Lateral pulvinar T1 hyperintensity is reported as a specific sign for Fabry's disease but has not been replicated in all studies.

Moyamoya
- The absence of a cause for terminal ICA occlusive disease is referred to as moyamoya disease.
- Moyamoya phenomenon has an identical appearance but is associated with an underlying condition.

Primary Angiitis
- Vasculitis has nonspecific imaging features, requires a high index of suspicion, and is a diagnosis of exclusion.
- Heterogeneous distribution of disease accounts for heterogeneous distribution of imaging features and high negative biopsy rates.
- Cerebral angiography remains a reference standard for small vessel involvement on the order of 250 to 500 μm. CTA and MRA detect medium and larger vessel involvement.

Takayasu's Arteritis and Giant Cell Arteritis
- These disorders affect large vessels.
- GCA is more common in elderly patients with a history of polymyalgia rheumatica.
- Takayasu's arteritis preferentially affects young Asian women.

Polyarteritis Nodosa
- This medium vessel vasculitis affects the peripheral nervous system more than the CNS.
- Imaging shows nonspecific features consistent with vasculitis.

Kawasaki Disease
- This nonspecific medium vessel vasculitis affects children younger than age 5.
- It presents as a mucocutaneous syndrome.
- Coronary artery aneurysms are a significant cause of death.

Churg-Strauss Syndrome
- Eosinophilia in patients with asthma and allergic rhinitis is highly suggestive of this nonspecific small vessel angiitis.

Wegener's Arteritis
- This is a systemic small vessel granulomatous vasculitis with sino-orbital involvement.
- Hypointense granulomas are not specific but are suggestive.

Systemic Lupus Erythematosus
- This is a nonspecific small vessel vasculitis.
- Widespread systemic effects are present with variable CNS involvement.
- CNS complications of treating SLE include posterior reversible encephalopathy syndrome, opportunistic infection, and drug toxicity.

Neuro-Behçet's Disease
- This clinical triad includes uveitis and genital and oral ulceration.
- Midbrain and internal and external capsular involvement characterizes neuro-Behçet's disease.
- Vascular involvement is protean and includes arterial and venous occlusion, thrombosis, and aneurysm formation.

Drug-Induced Vasculopathy
- Primary basal ganglia intracranial hemorrhage in a young patient should raise the suspicion for drug-induced hemorrhage (rule out hypertension).

Hypertensive Encephalopathy
- Posterior reversible encephalopathy syndrome has an anterior to posterior gradient.
- Symmetry and nonconformity to vascular territories are important discriminators.
- DWI signal is normal or reduced in contrast to infarction.
- Progressive multifocal leukoencephalopathy can look similar to hypertensive encephalopathy on imaging. Mass effect, hemorrhage, and enhancement are all described. Gray matter involvement and history of slower onset of symptoms may be helpful discriminators.

SUGGESTED READINGS

Alpagut U, Ugurlucan M, Dayioglu E. Major arterial involvement and review of Behçet's disease. Ann Vasc Surg 2007; 21:232-239.

Andrews J, Mason JC. Takayasu's arteritis—recent advances in imaging offer promise. Rheumatology 2007; 46:6-15.

Bartlett E, Mikulis DJ. Chasing "chasing the dragon" with MRI: leukoencephalopathy in drug abuse. Br J Radiol 2005; 78:997-1004.

Benseler S, Schneider R. Central nervous system vasculitis in children. Curr Opin Rheumatol 2004; 16:43-50.

Burns JC, Glode MP. Kawasaki syndrome. Lancet 2004; 364:533-544.

Burns TM, Schaublin GA, Dyck PJ. Vasculitic neuropathies. Neurol Clin 2007; 25:89-113.

Carolei A, Sacco S. Central nervous system vasculitis. Neurol Sci 2003; 24(Suppl 1):S8-S10.

Cuellar ML. Drug-induced vasculitis. Curr Rheumatol Rep 2002; 4:55-59.

Dichgans M. Cerebral autosomal dominant arteriopathy with subcortical infarcts and leukoencephalopathy: phenotypic and mutational spectrum. J Neurol Sci 2002; 15:203-204.

Falcini F. Kawasaki disease. Curr Opin Rheumatol 2006; 18:33-38.

Fam AG, et al. Cranial pachymeningitis: an unusual manifestation of Wegener's granulomatosis. J Rheumatol 2003; 30:2070-2074.

Fellgiebel A, Muller MJ, Ginsberg L. CNS manifestations of Fabry's disease. Lancet Neurol 2006; 5:791-795.

Gottschlich S, et al. Head and neck manifestations of Wegener's granulomatosis. Rhinology 2006; 44:227-233.

Gotway MB, Araoz PA, Macedo TA, et al. Imaging findings in Takayasu's arteritis. AJR Am J Roentgenol 2005; 184:1945-1950.

Guillevin L, Lhote F, Gherardi R. The spectrum and treatment of virus-associated vasculitides. Curr Opin Rheumatol 1997; 9:31-36.

Jeong YJ, Kim KI, Seo IJ, et al. Eosinophilic lung diseases: a clinical, radiologic, and pathologic overview. RadioGraphics 2007; 27:617-637; discussion 637-639.

Kalaria RN, Viitanen M, Kalimo H, et al. CADASIL Group of Vas-Cog. The pathogenesis of CADASIL: an update. J Neurol Sci 2004; 226:35-39.

Kissin EY, Merkel PA. Diagnostic imaging in Takayasu arteritis. Curr Opin Rheumatol 2004; 16:31-37.

Lamy C, Oppenheim C, Meder JF, Mas JL. Neuroimaging in posterior reversible encephalopathy syndrome. J Neuroimaging 2004; 14:89-96.

Lebovics RS. Sinonasal complications of vasculitic diseases. Cleve Clin J Med 2002; 69(Suppl 2):SII152-154.

Mitsias P, Levine SR. Large cerebral vessel occlusive disease in systemic lupus erythematosus. Neurology 1994; 44:385-393.

Nastri MV, Baptista LP, Baroni RH, et al. Gadolinium-enhanced three-dimensional MR angiography of Takayasu arteritis. RadioGraphics 2004; 24:773-786.

Pagnoux C, Cohen P, Guillevin L. Vasculitides secondary to infections. Clin Exp Rheumatol 2006; 24(2 Suppl 41):S71-S81.

Ringelstein EB, Nabavi DG. Cerebral small vessel diseases: cerebral microangiopathies. Curr Opin Neurol 2005; 18:179-188.

Rodriguez-Pla A, Stone JH. Vasculitis and systemic infections. Curr Opin Rheumatol 2006; 18:39-47.

Roman GC, Erkinjuntti T, Wallin A, et al. Subcortical ischaemic vascular dementia. Lancet Neurol 2002; 1:426-436.

Said G, Lacroix C. Primary and secondary vasculitic neuropathy. J Neurol 2005; 252:633-641.

Sanna G, Bertolaccini ML, Mathieu A: Central nervous system lupus: a clinical approach to therapy. Lupus 2003; 12:935-942.

Segelmark M, Selga D. The challenge of managing patients with polyarteritis nodosa. Curr Opin Rheumatol 2007; 19:33-38.

Seror R, et al. Central nervous system involvement in Wegener granulomatosis. Medicine (Baltimore) 2006; 85:54-65.

Siva A. Vasculitis of the nervous system. J Neurol 2001; 248:451-468.

Steeds RP, Mohiaddin R. Takayasu arteritis: role of cardiovascular magnetic imaging. Int J Cardiol 2006; 109:1-6.

Stott VL, Hurrell MA, Anderson TJ. Reversible posterior leukoencephalopathy syndrome: a misnomer reviewed. Intern Med J 2005; 111:e7-e11.

Treadwell SD, Robinson TG. Cocaine use and stroke. Postgrad Med J 2007; 83:389-394.

West SG. Central nervous system vasculitis. Curr Rheumatol Rep 2003; 5:116-127.

REFERENCES

1. Yousry TA, et al. Characteristic MR lesion pattern and correlation of T1 and T2 lesion volume with neurologic and neuropsychological findings in cerebral autosomal dominant arteriopathy with subcortical infarcts and leukoencephalopathy (CADASIL). AJNR Am J Neuroradiol 1999; 20:91-100.

2. Baudrimont M, et al. Autosomal dominant leukoencephalopathy and subcortical ischemic stroke: a clinicopathological study. Stroke 1993; 24:122-125.

3. van den Boom R, et al. Subcortical lacunar lesions: An MR imaging finding in patients with cerebral autosomal dominant arteriopathy with subcortical infarcts and leukoencephalopathy. Radiology 2002; 224:791-796.

4. van den Boom R, et al. Cerebral autosomal dominant arteriopathy with subcortical infarcts and leukoencephalopathy: MR imaging findings at different ages—3rd-6th decades. Radiology 2003; 229:683-690.

5. Singhal S, Rich P, Markus HS. The spatial distribution of MR imaging abnormalities in cerebral autosomal dominant arteriopathy with subcortical infarcts and leukoencephalopathy and their relationship to age and clinical features. AJNR Am J Neuroradiol 2005; 26:2481-2487.

6. Holtmannspotter M, et al. Diffusion magnetic resonance histograms as a surrogate marker and predictor of disease progression in CADASIL: a two-year follow-up study. Stroke 2005; 36:2559-2565.

7. Dichgans M. CADASIL. Lancet 1997; 349:776-777.

8. Mitsias P, Levine SR. Cerebrovascular complications of Fabry's disease. Ann Neurol 1996; 40:8-17.

9. Rolfs A, et al: Prevalence of Fabry disease in patients with cryptogenic stroke: a prospective study. Lancet 2005; 366:1794-1796.

10. Moore DF, et al. Increased signal intensity in the pulvinar on T1-weighted images: a pathognomonic MR imaging sign of Fabry disease. AJNR Am J Neuroradiol 2003; 24:1096-1101.

11. Albrecht J, et al. Voxel-based analyses of diffusion-tensor imaging in Fabry disease. J Neurol Neurosurg Psychiatry 2007; 78:964-969.

11a. Fellgiebel A, et al. Diagnostic utility of different MRI and MR angiography measures in Fabry disease. Neurology 2009; 72:63-68.

12. Harwood-Nash DC, Fitz CR. Neuroradiology in Infants and Children. St. Louis, Mosby, 1976, vol 3, pp 920-964.

13. Suzuki J, Kodama N. Moyamoya disease: a review. Stroke 1983; 14:104-109.

14. Haltia M, Iivanainen M, Majuri, Puranen M. Spontaneous occlusion of the circle of Willis (moyamoya syndrome). Clin Neuropathol 1982; 1:11-22.

15. Takebayashi S, Matsuo K, Kaneko M. Ultrastructural studies of cerebral arteries and collateral vessels in moyamoya disease. Stroke 1984; 15:728-732.

16. Yamashita M, Oka K, Tanaka K. Histopathology of the brain vascular network in moyamoya disease. Stroke 1983; 14:50-58.

17. Sakamoto S, Ohba S, Shibukawa M, et al. CT perfusion imaging for childhood moyamoya disease before and after surgical revascularization. Acta Neurochir (Wien) 2006; 148:77-81.

18. Fujisawa I, Asato R, Nishiura K, et al. Moyamoya disease: MR imaging. Radiology 1987; 164:103-105.

19. Brown WD, Graves VB, Chun RW, Turski PA. Moyamoya disease: MR findings. J Comput Assist Tomogr 1989; 13:770-771.

20. Yoon HK, Shin HJ, Chang YW. "Ivy sign" in childhood moyamoya disease: depiction on FLAIR and contrast-enhanced T1-weighted MR images. Radiology 2002; 223:384-389.

20a. Mori N, et al. The leptomeningeal "ivy sign" on fluid-attenuated inversion recovery MR imaging in Moyamoya disease: a sign of decreased cerebral vascular reserve? AJNR Am J Neuroradiol 2009; 30:930-935.

21. Calamante F, Ganesan V, Kirkham FJ, et al. MR perfusion imaging in moyamoya syndrome: potential implications for clinical evaluation of occlusive cerebrovascular disease. Stroke 2001; 32:2810-2816.

22. Vesely A, Sasano H, Volgyesi G, et al. MRI mapping of cerebrovascular reactivity using square wave changes in end tidal PCO_2. Magn Reson Med 2001; 45:1011-1013.

23. Mikulis DJ, Krolczyk G, Desal H, et al. Pre-operative and post-operative mapping of cerebrovascular reactivity in moyamoya disease using BOLD MRI. J Neurosurg 2005; 103:347-355.

23a. Han JS, et al. Impact of extracranial-intracranial bypass on cerebrovascular reactivity and clinical outcome in patients with symptomatic moyamoya vasculopathy. Stroke 2011; 42:3047-3054.

24. Kudo T. Juvenile occlusion of the circle of Willis. Clin Neurol 1956; 5:607-611.

25. Hasuo K, Tamura S, Kudo S, et al. Moyamoya disease: the use of digital subtraction angiography in its diagnosis. Radiology 1985; 157:107-111.

26. Yamada I, Matsushima Y, Suzuki S: Moyamoya disease: diagnosis with three-dimensional time-of-flight angiography. Radiology 1992; 184:773-778.

27. Morioka M, Hamada J-I, Kawano T, et al. Angiographic dilatation and Branco extension of the anterior choroidal and posterior communicating arteries are predictors of hemorrhage in adult moyamoya patients. Stroke 2003; 34:90-95.

28. So Y, Lee HY, Kim SK, et al. Prediction of the clinical outcome of pediatric moyamoya disease with postoperative basal/acetazolamide stress brain perfusion SPECT after revascularization surgery. Stroke 2005; 36:1485-1489.

29. Lightfoot RW Jr, et al. The American College of Rheumatology 1990 criteria for the classification of polyarteritis nodosa. Arthritis Rheum 1990; 33:1088-1093.

30. Jennette JC, et al. Nomenclature of systemic vasculitides: proposal of an international consensus conference. Arthritis Rheum 1994; 37:187-192.

31. Calabrese LH, Gragg LA, Furlan AJ. Benign angiopathy: a distinct subset of angiographically defined primary angiitis of the central nervous system. J Rheumatol 1993; 20:2046-2050.

32. Panda K, et al. Primary angiitis of CNS: Neuropathological study of three autopsied cases with brief review of literature. Neurol India 2000; 48:149-154.

33. Alhalabi M, Moore PM. Serial angiography in isolated angiitis of the central nervous system. Neurology 1994; 44:1221-1226.

34. Imbesi SG. Diffuse cerebral vasculitis with normal results on brain MR imaging. AJR Am J Roentgenol 1999; 173:1494-1496.

35. Harris KG, et al. Diagnosing intracranial vasculitis: the roles of MR and angiography. AJNR Am J Neuroradiol 1994; 15:317-330.

36. Greenan TJ, Grossman RI, Goldberg HI. Cerebral vasculitis: MR imaging and angiographic correlation. Radiology 1992; 182:65-72.

37. Aviv RI, et al. MR imaging and angiography of primary CNS vasculitis of childhood. AJNR Am J Neuroradiol 2006; 27:192-199.

38. Stone JH, et al. Sensitivities of noninvasive tests for central nervous system vasculitis: a comparison of lumbar puncture, computed tomography, and magnetic resonance imaging. J Rheumatol 1994; 21:1277-1282.

38a. Kuker W, et al. Vessel wall contrast enhancement: a diagnostic sign of cerebral vasculitis. Cerebrovasc Dis 2008; 26:23-29.

38b. Swartz RH, et al. Intracranial arterial wall imaging using high-resolution 3-tesla contrast-enhanced MRI. Neurology 2009; 72:627-634.

39. Calabrese LH, Mallek JA. Primary angiitis of the central nervous system: report of 8 new cases, review of the literature and proposal for diagnostic criteria. Medicine 1987; 67:20-39.

40. Korogi Y, et al. Intracranial vascular stenosis and occlusion: diagnostic accuracy of three-dimensional, Fourier transform, time-of-flight MR angiography. Radiology 1994; 193:187-193.

41. Aviv RI, et al. Angiography of primary central nervous system angiitis of childhood: conventional angiography versus magnetic resonance angiography at presentation. AJNR Am J Neuroradiol 2007; 28:9-15.

42. Hajj-Ali RA, et al. Benign angiopathy of the central nervous system: cohort of 16 patients with clinical course and long-term followup. Arthritis Rheum 2002; 47:662-669.

42a. Singhal AB, et al. Reversible cerebral vasoconstriction syndromes: analysis of 139 cases. Arch Neurol 2011; 68:1005-1012.

43. Jennette JC, Falk RJ. Nosology of primary vasculitis. Curr Opin Rheumatol 2007; 19:10-16.

44. Seko Y. Giant cell and Takayasu arteritis. Curr Opin Rheumatol 2007; 19:39-43.

45. Desai MY, et al. Delayed contrast-Enhanced MRI of the aortic wall in Takayasu's arteritis: initial experience. AJR Am J Roentgenol 2005; 184:1427-1431.

46. Bley TA, et al. Assessment of the cranial involvement pattern of giant cell arteritis with 3T magnetic resonance imaging. Arthritis Rheum 2005; 52:2470-2477.

47. Yamato M, et al. Takayasu arteritis: radiographic and angiographic findings in 59 patients. Radiology 1986; 161:329-334.

48. Ferris EJ, Levine HL. Cerebral arteritis: classification. Radiology 1973; 109:327-341.

49. Segelmark M, Selga D. The challenge of managing patients with polyarteritis nodosa. Curr Opin Rheumatol 2007; 19:33-38.

50. Provenzale J, Allen N. Neuroradiologic findings in polyarteritis nodosa. AJNR Am J Neuroradiol 1996; 17:1119-1126.

51. Pagnoux C, Guilpain P, Guillevin L. Churg-Strauss syndrome. Curr Opin Rheumatol 2007; 19:25-32.

52. Ramos-Casals M, et al. Vasculitis in systemic lupus erythematosus: prevalence and clinical characteristics in 670 patients. Medicine (Baltimore) 2006; 85:95-104.

53. Sabbadini MG, et al. Central nervous system involvement in systemic lupus erythematosus patients without overt neuropsychiatric manifestations. Lupus 1999; 8:11-19.

54. Okamoto K, et al. MR features of diseases involving bilateral middle cerebellar peduncles. AJNR Am J Neuroradiol 2003; 24:1946-1954.

55. Peterson PL, et al. Quantitative magnetic resonance imaging in neuropsychiatric systemic lupus erythematosus. Lupus 2003; 12:897-902.

55a. Nagel MA, et al. The varicella zoster virus vasculopathies: clinical, CSF, imaging, and virologic features. Neurology 2008; 70:853-860.

56. Gilden DH, et al. Neurologic complications of the reactivation of varicella-zoster virus. N Engl J Med 2000; 342:635-645.

57. Siva A. Vasculitis of the nervous system. J Neurol 2001; 248:451-468.

58. Kocer N, et al. CNS involvement in neuro-Behçet syndrome: an MR study. AJNR Am J Neuroradiol 1999; 20:1015-1024.

59. Neiman J, Haapaniemi HM, Hillbom M. Neurological complications of drug abuse: pathophysiological mechanisms. Eur J Neurol 2000; 7:595-606.

60. Ghoshhajra BB, McLean GK. Radiation-induced cerebral aneurysms. J Vasc Interv Radiol 2006; 17:1891-1896.

61. Aoki S, et al. Radiation-induced arteritis: thickened wall with prominent enhancement on cranial MR images—report of five cases and comparison with 18 cases of moyamoya disease. Radiology 2002; 223:683-688.

62. Port JD, Beauchamp NJ. Reversible intracerebral pathologic entities mediated by vascular autoregulatory dysfunction. RadioGraphics 1998; 18:353-367.

63. Appignani BA, Bhadelia RA, Blacklow SC, et al. Neuroimaging findings in patients on immunosuppressive therapy: experience with tacrolimus toxicity. AJR Am J Roentgenol 1996; 168:683-688.

64. Govindarajan R, Adusumilli J, Baxter DL, et al. Reversible posterior leukoencephalopathy syndrome induced by RAF kinase inhibitor BAY 43-9006. J Clin Oncol 2006; 24:48.

65. Tomura N, Kurosawa R, Kato K, et al. Transient neurotoxicity associated with FK506: MR findings. J Comput Assist Tomogr 1998; 22:505-507.

66. Cooney MJ, Bradley WG, Symko S, et al. Hypertensive encephalopathy: complication in children treated for myeloproliferative disorders—report of three cases. Radiology 2000; 214:711-716.

67. Ebner F, Ranner G, Slavc I, et al. MR findings in methotrexate-induced CNS abnormalities. AJR Am J Roentgenol 1989; 13:761-776.

68. Ito Y, Arahata Y, Goto Y, et al. Cisplatin neurotoxicity presenting as reversible posterior leukoencephalopathy syndrome. AJNR Am J Neuroradiol 1998; 19:415-417.

69. Parizel PM, Snoeck H, van den Hauwe L, et al. Cerebral complications of murine monoclonal CD3 antibody (OKT3): CT and MR findings. AJNR Am J Neuroradiol 1997; 18:1935-1938.

70. Schwartz RB, Bravo SM, Klufas RA, et al. Cyclosporine neurotoxi-city and its relationship to hypertensive encephalopathy: CT and MR findings in 16 cases. AJR Am J Roentgenol 1995; 165:627-631.

71. Sherwood JW, Wagle WA. Hemolytic uremic syndrome: MR findings of CNS complications. AJNR 1991; 12:703-704.

72. Cunningham S, Conway EE. Systemic lupus erythematosus presenting as an intracranial bleed. Ann Emerg Med 1991; 20:810-812.

73. Jones BV, Egelhoff JC, Patterson RJ. Hypertensive encephalopathy in children. AJNR Am J Neuroradiol 1997; 18:101-106.

74. Hinchey J, Chaves C, Appignani B, et al. A reversible posterior leukoencephalopathy syndrome. N Engl J Med 1996; 334: 494-500.

75. Stanimirovic D, Bertrand N, McCarron R, et al. Arachidonic acid release and permeability changes induced by endothelins in human cerebromicrovascular endothelium. Acta Neurochir 1994; 60:71-31.

76. Taylor RN, de Groot CJM, Cho YK, Lim KH. Circulating factors as markers and mediators of endothelial cell dysfunction in pre-eclampsia. Semin Reprod Endocrinol 1998; 16:17-31.

77. Bunchman TE, Bookshire CA. Cyclosporin-induced synthesis of endothelin by cultured human endothelial cells. J Clin Invest 1991; 88:310-314.

78. Chester EM, et al. Hypertensive encephalopathy: a clinicopathologic study of 20 cases. Neurology 1978; 28:928.

79. Schwartz RB, Jones KM, Kalina P, et al. Hypertensive encephalopathy: findings on CT, MR imaging, and SPECT imaging in 14 cases. AJR Am J Roentgenol 1992; 159:379-383.

80. Wartenberg KE, Parra A. CT and CT-perfusion findings of reversible leukoencephalopathy during triple-H therapy for symptomatic subarachnoid hemorrhage-related vasospasm. J Neuroimaging 2006; 16:170-175.

81. Sanders TG, Clayman DA, Sanchez-Ramos L, et al. Brain in eclampsia: MR imaging with clinical correlation. Radiology 1991; 180:475-478.

82. Casey SO, Sampaio RC, Michel E, Truwit CL. Posterior reversible encephalopathy syndrome: utility of fluid-attenuated inversion recovery MR imaging in the detection of cortical and subcortical lesions. Am J Neuroradiol 2000; 21:1199-1206.

82a. Cuvinciuc V, et al. *Isolated acute nontraumatic cortical subarachnoid hemorrhage*. AJNR Am J Neuroradiol 2010; 31:1355-1362.

83. Schwartz RB, Mulkern RV, Gudbjartsson H, et al. Diffusion-weighted MR imaging in hypertensive encephalopathy: clues to pathogenesis. AJNR Am J Neuroradiol 1998; 19:859-862.

84. Covarrubias DJ, Leutmer PH, Campeau NG. Posterior reversible encephalopathy syndrome: prognostic utility of quantitative diffusion-weighted MR images. AJNR Am J Neuroradiol 2002; 23:1038-1048.

85. Provenzale JM, Petrella JR, Cruz LCH Jr, et al. Quantitative assessment of diffusion abnormalities in posterior reversible encephalopathy syndrome. AJNR Am J Neuroradiol 2001; 22:1455-1461.

86. Engelter ST, Petrella JR, Alberts MJ, et al. Assessment of cerebral microcirculation in a patient with hypertensive encephalopathy using MR perfusion imaging. AJR Am J Roentgenol 1999; 173:1491-1493.

87. Sundgren PC, Edvardsson B, Holtas S. Serial investigation of perfusion disturbances and vasogenic oedema in hypertensive encephalopathy by diffusion and perfusion weighted imaging. Neuroradiology 2002; 44:299-304.

88. Senger AR, Gupta RK, Dhanuka AK, et al. MR imaging, MR angiography, and MR spectroscopy of the brain in eclampsia. AJNR Am J Neuroradiol 1997; 18:1485-1490.

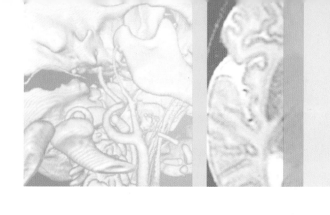

CHAPTER 22

Venous Occlusive Disease

Edward D. Greenberg and Robert D. Zimmerman

The term *cerebral venous occlusive disease* signifies partial to complete occlusion of one or more of the dural venous sinuses, deep cerebral veins, or superficial cerebral veins on an acute, subacute, or chronic basis. Other names include cerebral venous thrombosis (CVT), dural sinus thrombosis (DST), deep cerebral venous thrombosis (DCVT), and superficial cerebral venous thrombosis (SCVT).

EPIDEMIOLOGY

The annual incidence of cerebral venous occlusive disease may be as low as two to seven cases per million in the general population.[1,2] Autopsy series estimate the prevalence of CVT from less than 1% to as high as 9% of patients dying of stroke.[3] CVT tends to affect women more than men and has a younger age distribution than arterial thrombosis, with a particularly high incidence in neonates. Most patients have underlying congenital or acquired hypercoagulable states, but the disease may result from local vascular compression or be idiopathic. The prognosis for recovery is better than that for arterial infarction.

CLINICAL PRESENTATION

The signs and symptoms of CVT are highly variable, depending on the acuity of thrombosis, its location and extent, and the availability of collateral pathways. Clot propagation and spontaneous thrombolysis occur simultaneously in as many as 70% of patients,[4] complicating the clinical picture. Overall, CVT presents acutely in approximately 30% of cases (<2 days from onset of symptoms), subacutely in approximately 50% of patients (from 2 to 30 days), and chronically in 20% of patients (>30 days).[5] The acute presentation may be abrupt or rapidly progressive. Because of this variation, venous thrombosis may mimic the temporal course of acute cerebral infarction or subarachnoid hemorrhage (abrupt onset), acute encephalitis (rapidly progressive over 1 to 3 days), brain abscess (progressive abnormalities developing over 1 to 2 weeks), or brain tumor and neurodegenerative disease (slow progression over months to years). Therefore, CVT is often underdiagnosed or misdiagnosed.

The symptoms of CVT can be nonfocal or focal. Nonfocal findings typically result from DST, secondary venous hypertension, and raised intracranial pressure. Headache is reported by 74% to 90% of patients and is typically the first manifestation of

CVT. The headache can develop gradually or suddenly and can mimic the typical "thunderclap" presentation of subarachnoid hemorrhage.[6] Other nonfocal findings include papilledema (45%), seizures with possible Todd paresis (29%), confusion and coma (26%), as well as nausea, vomiting, visual changes, and cranial nerve palsies.[2,3] Overall, 20% to 40% of patients with CVT present with signs and symptoms of intracranial hypertension, so the possibility of CVT should be considered in any patient with raised intracranial pressure.[2] Idiopathic intracranial hypertension must be considered only as a diagnosis of exclusion.

Focal signs and symptoms usually result from SCVT or DCVT with focal hemorrhage or edema (with or without venous infarction). The specific focal signs depend on the precise location of the lesion.

In most cases, the thrombus is formed within the sinus and subsequently extends retrograde into adjacent deep or cortical veins. Isolated thrombosis within a deep or superficial vein without sinus thrombosis is uncommon. In DST, focal deficits such as hemiplegia, dysphasia, paresthesias, and cranial nerve palsies may occur in conjunction with the nonfocal symptoms of intracranial hypertension. Focal or generalized seizures, followed by hemiparesis, aphasia, hemianopia, or other focal deficits occur without the signs of intracranial hypertension typically seen with DST.[7] In cavernous sinus thrombosis, presenting symptoms include headache, periorbital edema, proptosis, chemosis, and abnormalities of eye movements secondary to compromise of nerves that run through the cavernous sinus (oculomotor, trochlear, and abducens). Patients with isolated SCVT present with focal neurologic deficits dependent on the location of the occlusion. Patients with DCVT often present with altered consciousness and signs referable to the corticospinal tract and other long white-matter tracts. They may have a more rapidly declining clinical course with poor outcomes more common, including death and long-term morbidity.[8] Symptoms secondary to severe dysfunction of the diencephalon, such as coma and abnormalities of eye movements and reflexes, are more common.[8] In one small series, five of seven patients with DCVT presented with headache, nausea, vomiting, and altered level of consciousness.[9] However, clinical findings and outcome in DCVT are variable. On occasion, presentation can be relatively mild with headache and no disturbance of consciousness. If deep venous thrombosis is rapidly reversed (by spontaneous or therapeutic clot lysis), patients may have complete recovery.

In contrast to arterial ischemic stroke, relief of venous obstruction, even if delayed, has been shown to yield dramatic clinical improvement in particular with regard to signs and symptoms of increased intracranial pressure. The median time from the onset of symptoms to the correct diagnosis of CVT is reported to be as much as 7 days.[10] Shortening the time from symptom onset to diagnosis has important prognostic implications because early diagnosis and treatment (anticoagulation and/or endovascular thrombolysis) can lead to recovery with surprisingly few sequelae. Resolution of edema in patients with CVT with normalization of the apparent diffusion coefficient has been reported after treatment.[11]

PATHOPHYSIOLOGY

There are many causes of CVT (Table 22-1). These are subclassified into local processes such as infection, which hinder local blood flow, and systemic processes such as pregnancy and the

TABLE 22-1. Etiology of Cerebral Venous Thrombosis

Systemic Causes
Hypercoagulable States
Pregnancy/puerperium
Oral contraception
Primary coagulopathy: protein C deficiency, protein S deficiency, antithrombin III deficiency, hyperhomocysteinemia, antiphospholipid syndrome
Dehydration
Inflammatory bowel disease
Collagen vascular disease: systemic lupus erythematosus, Behçet's disease, rheumatoid arthritis
Polycythemia
Nephrotic syndrome
Sarcoidosis
Postoperative state
Malignancy
Red blood cell disorder: polycythemia, sickle cell disease, paroxysmal nocturnal hemoglobinuria

Medications
Chemotherapeutic agents (L-asparaginase)
Oral contraceptives

Metabolic
Thyrotoxicosis

Infection, Systemic
Bacteremia
Viral: measles, hepatitis
Parasitic: malaria, trichinosis
Fungal: aspergillosis

Local Causes
Infection
Meningitis/encephalitis
Osteomyelitis
Otitis
Sinusitis
Mastoiditis
Orbital infection

Neoplasm
Solid extra-axial tumors: both primary (meningioma) hematopoietic and metastatic

Trauma
Venous epidural hematoma dural sinus rupture or compression
Iatrogenic
   External—neurosurgery
   Internal (secondary to catheter manipulation within the jugular vein or sinus itself)
   Lumbar puncture

Idiopathic

puerperium, oral contraceptives, coagulopathies, and inflammatory bowel disease, which lead to hypercoagulable states.[12] Approximately 25% of patients with CVT have detectable genetic bases for their hypercoagulable state. Inherited hypercoagulability should be suspected if a patient has recurrent CVT, is younger than 45 years of age, has a family history of venous thrombosis, or has no acquired risk factors. The most common genetic risk factor for CVT is factor V Leiden, followed by the prothrombin gene mutation G20210A. Other less common inherited causes of CVT are deficiencies of protein S, protein C, and antithrombin III.[13] In as many as 33% of patients, no cause can be identified.[12]

CVT does not occur in an even distribution throughout the cerebral venous system. In a large study of 624 patients the distribution frequency of CVT was superior sagittal sinus, 62%; left and right transverse sinuses, 44.7% and 41.2%, respectively; straight sinus, 18%; isolated cortical veins, 17.1%; deep venous system, 10.9%; cavernous sinus, 1.3%; and cerebellar veins, 0.3%.[10] Multifocal thromboses, particularly in the contiguous transverse and sigmoid sinuses, are present in as many as 33% of patients.[2] Thirty to 40 percent of patients with DST have concurrent thrombosis of adjacent cerebral veins.[14]

Thrombus typically begins within the dural sinuses with subsequent retrograde extension into the cortical veins that drain into that sinus. A four-step process has been described in a pig model of superior sagittal sinus thrombosis. Nonocclusive thrombus forms within the dural sinus, leading to eventual occlusion. Subsequently, there is extension of thrombus into the cortical veins. It is hypothesized that the extension into cortical veins is the key event leading to pathologic changes in the brain parenchyma secondary to lack of sufficient collateral drainage.[15,16] The pathophysiology described in this model likely applies to humans as well. In many cases, isolated sinus thrombosis is tolerated until secondary involvement of cortical and medullary veins causes more substantial impairment of cerebral venous drainage and more significant clinical signs and symptoms. This model may also explain why the extent of the sinus thrombus does not always correlate with the extent of the resulting lesion, because extension into feeding veins is more important in determining the severity of the parenchymal lesion.[17]

Regardless of the location of the thrombosis, the pathophysiology that transpires once CVT occurs is not completely understood. Two mechanisms have been proposed: (1) local effects from the occlusion of cerebral veins and (2) more global effects secondary to major sinus occlusion and resultant intracranial hypertension. In most cases, both mechanisms are at play because sinus thrombosis is commonly associated with thrombosis of adjacent superficial or deep veins.

Local effects secondary to occlusion of cerebral veins include focal edema, hemorrhage, and venous infarction. The acute phase of occlusion is marked by venous engorgement and prominence of collateral veins. If venous drainage cannot be adequately supplied by these collateral vessels, venous pressure rises, leading to breakdown of the blood-brain barrier and leakage of blood serum into the interstitial space (vasogenic edema). As pressures continue to increase, tearing of thin-walled medullary veins results in hemorrhage. Hemorrhage occurs most commonly in the parenchymal subcortical white matter near the thrombosed sinus. Hematoma formation leads to mass effect on adjacent brain parenchyma and rupture of neural pathways. Less commonly, hemorrhage occurs in the subarachnoid and subdural spaces, presumably due to rupture of cortical and bridging veins as they course through these spaces. This pathophysiology has been validated by studies correlating pressure measurements within a thrombosed sinus and the presence of edema and hemorrhage. Hemorrhage was present with intrasinus pressures higher than 42 mm Hg, whereas lower pressures produced edema without hemorrhage.[18] Increased venous pressure may also lead to decreased arterial regional cerebral blood flow (rCBF) that, when severe or prolonged, produces ischemia with resultant ion-pump failure, cytotoxic edema, and cell death (venous infarction). MRI has demonstrated restricted diffusion in brain lesions resulting from CVT, and it has been estimated that venous infarction occurs in about 50% of patients with CVT.[10]

Global cerebral effects become relevant in CVT when the major dural sinuses are involved. Occlusion of a large dural sinus, such as the superior sagittal sinus or the dominant transverse sinus, causes decreased absorption of cerebrospinal fluid secondary to impaired function of arachnoid granulations within the affected sinus. Because the increased pressure is transmitted to both the subarachnoid space as well as the ventricles there is no pressure gradient between the two regions of cerebrospinal fluid and hydrocephalus does not generally result. Even sinus stenosis without thrombosis can lead to increased intracranial pressure that can be reversed with stenting of the sinus.

After thrombus formation and sinus occlusion, thrombus breakdown can lead to spontaneous partial or complete recanalization. This recanalization process tends to occur earlier rather than later, with one study at 3 weeks after CVT demonstrating 40% complete recanalization and 20% partial recanalization.[19] After 4 months of anticoagulation therapy, there is typically no further resolution.[19] Recanalization after anticoagulation therapy occurs more often with thrombosis of the superior sagittal and straight sinuses as opposed to thrombosis of the transverse and sigmoid sinuses.[19] Complete recanalization is not necessary for clinical recovery, and the extent of recanalization may not correlate closely with the clinical outcome.[19] This is likely secondary to the numerous venous collateral pathways that form after sinus thrombosis, which typically include dural collaterals that surround the occluded sinus, cortical venous collaterals that drain into other patent sinuses, and diploic, emissary, and meningeal collaterals as well.[2]

An interesting yet poorly understood aspect of the pathophysiology of chronic CVT is related to the formation of dural arteriovenous fistulas (AVFs). Arterial growth into the wall of the occluded vein leads to recanalization of chronic CVT with formation of AVFs. Dural AVFs may produce hemorrhage or infarction if venous pressure is high and cortical veins are dilated. Chronic venous hypertension may present as cognitive decline that mimics neurodegenerative disease. This is a rare but well-established long-term complication of CVT and should be sought in patients with CVT who undergo subsequent imaging studies.[20]

PATHOLOGY

Acute thrombus in the superior sagittal sinus is identical to other thrombi, with fresh clot rich in red blood cells and fibrin. The fresh clot is eventually replaced with fibrous tissue. The vessel may recanalize. The affected brain shows subcortical hemorrhage, infarction, and edema. Histologic analysis reveals hemorrhage or hemorrhagic infarction. Typically, *venous* infarctions show more pronounced leukocyte infiltrations than do *arterial* infarctions, because the patent artery allows inflow of white cells.[21] In protracted cases with chronic VST, venous hypertension causes marked fibrous thickening and hyalinization of the walls of the veins draining into the sinus.[22]

The venous anatomy of the brain is variable and complex. This variability underlies the wide range of clinical and imaging features of CVT. In considering this anatomy, one can divide the system into three components: (1) superficial venous drainage, (2) deep venous drainage, and (3) dural venous sinuses (Figs. 22-1 to 22-3).

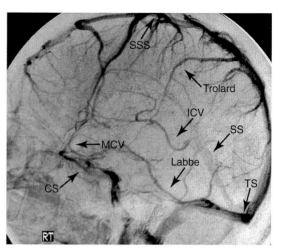

■ **FIGURE 22-1**   Normal venous anatomy as seen on lateral projection DSA. CS, Cavernous sinus; SSS, superior sagittal sinus; MCV, middle cerebral vein; ICV, internal cerebral vein; TS, transverse sinus.

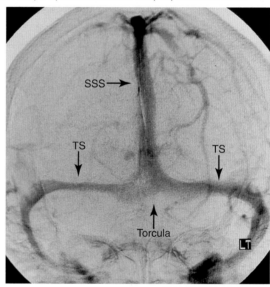

■ **FIGURE 22-2**   Normal venous anatomy as seen on anteroposterior projection DSA. SSS, superior sagittal sinus; TS, transverse sinus.

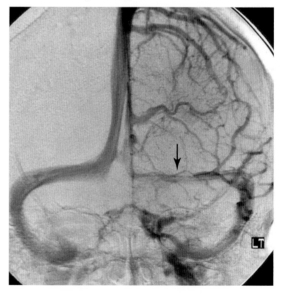

■ **FIGURE 22-3**   Atretic left transverse sinus (*arrow*), a common normal variant, seen on DSA.

Superficial Drainage

The superficial cerebral veins drain the cerebral cortex and the adjacent white matter into the dural venous sinuses. The superficial veins are subclassified by their location and by the dural sinus into which they most often drain: (1) superior group draining predominantly into the superior sagittal sinus; (2) sphenoidal group draining predominantly into the sphenoparietal then cavernous sinuses; (3) tentorial group draining predominantly into the transverse sinus, and (4) the falcine veins, which drain predominantly to the deep and midline drainage system.[23]

The superior sagittal group includes veins from the superior part of the medial and lateral surfaces of the frontal, parietal, and occipital lobes and from the anterior portion of the orbital surface of the frontal lobe. These veins drain predominantly into the superior sagittal sinus. The cortical veins of the convexity are highly variable; there is usually a dominant frontoparietal vein draining superiorly into the superior sagittal sinus designated the vein of Trolard.

The sphenoidal group drains the region of the sylvian fissure and deep sylvian veins into the sphenoparietal sinus, which then empties into the cavernous sinus.

The tentorial group drains the lateral surface of the temporal lobe and the basal surfaces of the temporal and occipital lobes into the transverse sinus. This group includes the descending veins from the lateral surface of the temporal lobe (including the anastomotic vein of Labbé) and the temporobasal-occipitobasal veins of the inferior surface. These veins generally drain into the lateral tentorial sinus, which feeds into the transverse sinus. The vein of Labbé drains directly into the transverse sinus.

The falcine group is composed of veins that drain into the deep venous system, including the internal cerebral veins, the basal veins of Rosenthal, and the great vein of Galen. Cortical areas drained by the falcine group correspond to the limbic system and include the parahippocampal, cingulate, paraterminal, parolfactory gyri, and the uncus. The venous drainage from the region of the sylvian fissure deserves special mention. Drainage occurs via the superficial sylvian vein into the sphenoparietal sinus along the sphenoid ridge, as well as the veins of Trolard and Labbé. Because these veins communicate with each other, their relative caliber is inversely proportional.[23]

Deep Drainage

The deep venous system consists of the internal cerebral, vein, the basal vein of Rosenthal, and the vein of Galen and their respective tributaries. The deep system drains the deep white and gray matter around the ventricles and structures around the basal cisterns. It can be divided into a ventricular group that drains the walls of the ventricles and a cisternal group that drains the structures around the cisterns.[23] In forming the ventricular group, subependymal and thalamostriate veins course along the walls of the ventricles and converge on the internal cerebral, basal, and great veins. Veins draining the frontal horn and the body of the lateral ventricle generally drain into the internal cerebral vein, whereas veins originating from the temporal horn generally drain into the basal vein. Veins from the ventricular atrium drain into all three veins. The cisternal group of deep veins drains the area beginning just anterior to the third ventricle and extending laterally and posteriorly to the sylvian fissure and quadrigeminal plate cistern. The main structures drained by the deep system include the inferior frontal lobe; most of the deep white matter of the frontal, temporal, and parietal lobes; the corpus callosum; the upper brain stem; the basal ganglia; the choroid plexus; the hippocampus; the cortical areas of the limbic lobe (cingulate and parahippocampal gyri); the visual cortex; parts of the cerebellum; and the thalamus. Knowledge of these drainage patterns is important in accurately diagnosing deep venous obstruction. As a direct result of this anatomy, deep venous obstruction spares the subcortical white matter of the cerebral convexities; cortical involvement is limited to the inferior frontal, limbic lobe, and visual cortex.[23,24]

The basal vein of Rosenthal is an important component of the deep venous system. It arises near the uncus by the confluence of the anterior and deep middle cerebral veins. Although the basal vein drains into the vein of Galen, it communicates with the superior petrosal sinus (via the lateral mesencephalic vein), with the cavernous sinus and pterygoid plexus in adults (via the deep and superficial sylvian veins), and on occasion with the straight or transverse sinus. Communications between the basal vein and the vein of Galen through choroidal, thalamic, and striate anastomoses can divert outflow from the deep system in the case of vein of Galen occlusion. Because of these anastomotic interconnections, only simultaneous obstruction of the vein of Galen and the basal vein of Rosenthal effectively obstructs deep venous outflow.[8] This situation most commonly arises near their confluence, in the posterior aspect of the tentorial incisura. Any lesion that causes sufficient mass effect on the midbrain may cause such venous obstruction. Complete obstruction of the great vein of Galen and basal veins leads to rapid death. Incomplete obstruction leads to various degrees of injury within areas drained by these deep veins.[25]

Dural Sinuses

The dural sinuses are endothelium-lined channels that run between the inner meningeal and outer periosteal layers of dura. They collect blood from the cerebral and meningeal veins and form important communications with the extracranial circulation via emissary veins that traverse the skull and provide collateral pathways in the event of sinus occlusion.

The superior sagittal sinus drains the anterior part of the inferior surface of the frontal lobe and the superior portions of the lateral and medial surfaces of the frontal, parietal, and occipital lobes. The anterior portion of the superior sagittal sinus is small and may be absent anterior to the coronal suture. The superior sagittal sinus increases in caliber as it arches posteriorly and receives increasing numbers of tributaries. It eventually joins the straight and transverse sinuses at the torcular. The drainage pattern of the superior sagittal sinus is characteristically asymmetric, with the majority of blood flowing into the right transverse sinus. If present anteriorly, the superior sagittal sinus communicates with the extracranial circulation via the facial and nasal veins. Absence of the anterior superior sagittal sinus is often accompanied by prominent paired cortical veins that course posteriorly to enter the sinus near the bregma. These should not be confused with collateral drainage around a CVT. The internal surface of the superior sagittal sinus contains septa that help to maintain laminar flow and prevent reflux into cortical veins. The vessels surrounding the superior sagittal sinus include scalp veins, intermediate veins (diploic, emissary, and meningeal), and cortical veins. Cortical veins may drain directly into the sinus or may first drain into meningeal sinuses that receive drainage from several cortical veins and subsequently drain into the superior sagittal sinus. Cavernous spaces located within the dura surrounding the sagittal sinus lack an endothelial lining but can provide collateral venous drainage in the case of thrombosis. Congestion of these spaces produces the empty delta sign and the extensive irregular falcine enhancement seen in sinus thrombosis on CT.[26]

A group of enlarged venous spaces, termed *lacunae,* are found adjacent to the superior sagittal sinus. They drain the meningeal veins and contain the arachnoid or pacchionian granulations, which play a major role in the resorption of cerebrospinal fluid. Arachnoid granulations are found within all of the dural sinuses and can protrude into the sinus lumen, mimicking sinus thrombosis. In some cases, large arachnoid granulations can actually cause venous obstruction.[2]

The inferior sagittal sinus is small and variably present. It courses in the free inferior edge of the falx cerebri from the middle third of the falx to its junction with the vein of Galen. It receives drainage from the adjacent veins of the falx, corpus callosum, and cingulate gyrus, with its largest tributaries generally being the anterior pericallosal veins. Because of the small size of the inferior sagittal sinus and ample collateral drainage, symptomatic thrombosis is rare.

The transverse sinuses run within the lateral attachments of the tentorium to the calvaria and drain blood from the inferolateral portions of the occipital and temporal lobes as well as the cerebellum. They are often asymmetric or hypoplastic. The right transverse sinus is typically larger than the left, which may be small or absent.[5] In 20% to 30% of patients, stenotic segments can be seen within the nondominant transverse sinus.[14] After receiving drainage from the superior petrosal sinus, the transverse sinus turns inferomedially and becomes the sigmoid sinus. The right transverse sinus, sigmoid sinus, and internal jugular vein system receive drainage mainly from the superior sagittal sinus (mostly superficial system drainage), whereas the left transverse sinus, sigmoid sinus, and internal jugular vein system primarily drain the straight sinus or deep system. Thus, blockage of an internal jugular vein may cause different symptoms, depending on the side obstructed.

The straight sinus runs from the vein of Galen toward the torcular within the falcotentorial junction and usually drains into the left transverse sinus. The confluence of the sinuses (torcular Herophili) is formed by the union of the superior sagittal sinus, straight sinus, transverse sinuses and occipital sinus. Asymmetry of the transverse sinuses is often associated with asymmetry of the torcular, which deviates to the side of the larger transverse sinus.

A small, variably present occipital sinus lies in the midline at the attachment of the falx cerebelli, extending from the foramen magnum upward to the torcular. Medial and lateral tentorial sinuses are usually present in each half of the tentorium, although they are rarely symmetric. The medial tentorial sinuses receive drainage from the superior surface of the cerebellum and drain into the straight sinus or the junction of the straight and transverse sinuses. The lateral tentorial sinuses receive drainage from the basal and lateral surfaces of the temporal and occipital lobes and drain into the transverse sinus.

The cavernous sinuses sit on either side of the sella turcica and communicate freely with each other and with a number of important venous structures. Anteriorly, they communicate with the sphenoparietal sinus and the ophthalmic veins, laterally with the pterygoid plexus via the foramina spinosum and ovale, and posteriorly with the basilar sinus, the superior and inferior petrosal sinuses, and thence by extension with the transverse and sigmoid sinuses.

Posterior Fossa

Posterior fossa venous drainage is divided into three groups. Anteriorly, drainage occurs via the petrosal sinus, superiorly via the vein of Galen, and posteriorly via the transverse sinuses and torcular. Within the posterior fossa, vertebral plexuses at the skull base can provide alternative drainage in the case of internal jugular vein occlusion.

IMAGING
CT

Noncontrast head CT is usually the first imaging test performed in patients ultimately diagnosed with CVT. Because acute thrombi are hyperdense on CT, a direct sign of acute CVT is high density within a dural sinus or cerebral vein. High-density clot within the wedge-shaped dural sinus is referred to as the dense triangle sign (Fig. 22-4). The cord sign refers to the presence of a thrombosed hyperdense cortical vein (Fig. 22-5). The

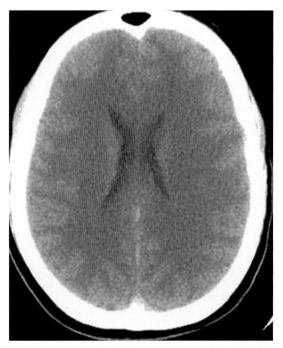

■ **FIGURE 22-4**   Dense triangle sign. Noncontrast CT with high-density, wedge-shaped, posterior sagittal sinus indicative of clot.

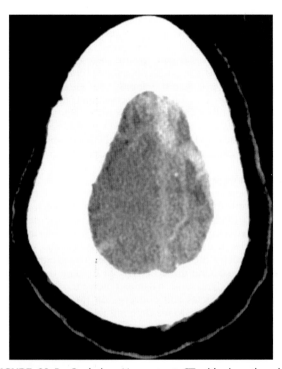

■ **FIGURE 22-5**   Cord sign. Noncontrast CT with sinus thrombosis extending into a left cortical vein.

thrombosed sinus and cortical veins are often enlarged and irregular. Although these features are characteristic of CVT, they are detected in only 20% of cases of thrombosis.[26] Furthermore, hyperdensity within a sinus is not pathognomonic of CVT. Patent hyperdense dural sinuses may be seen with elevated hematocrit, such as may occur with severe dehydration and polycythemia. Therefore, the density of the venous structure in

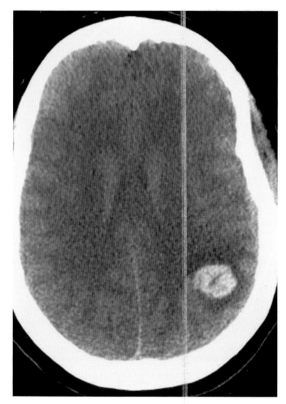

■ **FIGURE 22-6** Parenchymal hematoma with surrounding edema secondary to venous thrombosis.

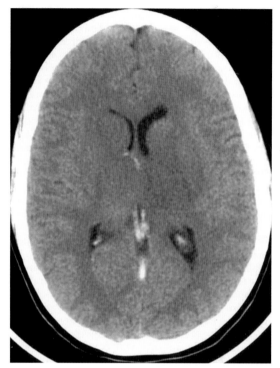

■ **FIGURE 22-7** Hyperdense deep cerebral veins (internal cerebral veins and vein of Galen) consistent with thrombosis with resultant hypodensity within the bilateral basal ganglia indicative of edema.

question should be compared with the density of other vascular structures (e.g., middle cerebral arteries). The dural sinuses typically appear hyperdense in neonates owing to the normal relative hypodensity of the unmyelinated brain and the physiologic polycythemia of newborns. Furthermore, dural sinuses often appear large due to transient increased intracranial pressure associated with childbirth and/or minimal hemorrhage along dural surfaces. Therefore, the diagnosis of DVT in newborns is difficult and additional imaging studies are needed to confirm or exclude this diagnosis. Focal or partial thrombosis may not be detected because no images perpendicular to the occluded portion of the sinus are obtained (e.g., transverse sinus thrombosis). Beam-hardening artifact from adjacent bone can obscure thrombus within the sinus or vein, and anemic patients may never develop hyperdense clot, further confounding the diagnosis. In subacute and chronic thrombosis the density of the sinuses will be normal, because the hyperdensity resolves within 1 to 2 weeks.

The pathologic consequences of CVT leading to indirect imaging signs of its presence include brain edema, hemorrhage, and infarction. These features can be appreciated on noncontrast CT, although MRI is more sensitive and specific in most cases. In patients with CVT, focal edema without hemorrhage is seen in up to 10% of patients, whereas hemorrhage and edema are seen on noncontrast CT in approximately one third of patients (Fig. 22-6).[2] Bilateral parasagittal subcortical hemorrhage or edema near the vertex suggests superior sagittal sinus thrombosis, whereas ipsilateral temporo-occipital and/or cerebellar hemorrhages suggest transverse sinus thrombosis. DCVT typically causes bilateral thalamic edema and hemorrhage (76%),[2] whereas structures adjacent to the thalami, including the basal ganglia and the mesencephalon, are affected in one third of patients with DCVT (Fig. 22-7).[5] In CVT, an isolated zone of cortical hemorrhage with subcortical extension can be seen in 38% of patients. In cases of isolated subcortical hemorrhage it is

important to look for an associated dilated hyperdense cortical vein (cord sign) because this may suggest CVT as the etiology.[27,28] Isolated subarachnoid hemorrhage[29] and subdural hematomas or effusion are occasionally seen secondary to CVT, but these are nonspecific findings.

In the majority of cases, unenhanced CT must be supplemented with a contrast-enhanced CT examination to make or confirm the diagnosis of CVT. The major diagnostic finding on standard contrast-enhanced CT is a filling defect within the dural sinus that is surrounded by intense enhancement in the wall of the dural sinus (empty delta sign). The empty delta sign is appreciated most easily on scans perpendicular to the thrombosed dural sinus and is therefore most often seen in the superior sagittal sinus torcular and sigmoid sinus. It may not be appreciated when there is short segment thrombosis. It is not seen in the transverse sinus, which is oriented parallel to the axial scanning plane. In a minority of cases, a linear filling defect is seen in the transverse sinus when a scan is fortuitously obtained directly through the thin sinus. The empty delta sign is seen in only 30% of cases of dural sinus thrombosis.[2,26] Over time, organized thrombus enhances and the empty delta sign is no longer apparent.

Indirect signs of CVT on contrast-enhanced CT include visualization of prominent cortical veins, indicative of venous congestion. Collateral veins within the dura cause thick and irregular enhancement of the falx and/or tentorium. Transcortical medullary veins can become sources of collateral blood drainage. Subsequent dilatation of these vessels causes them to be visible on contrast-enhanced CT.[26]

CT venography (CTV) uses techniques developed for CT angiography to provide high-resolution multiplanar and 3D images of the entire intracranial venous system. The acquisition of thin-section CT slices after a time-optimized bolus of intravenous contrast agent results in peak venous enhancement. Axial source images as well as 2D multiplanar reformatted images are created, with the quality of the reformatted images equivalent to that of the axial source images with isotropic data acquisition. Further evaluation can also be undertaken with different types of post-processing software that allows for production of excellent 3D images of the venous anatomy. CTV allows for accurate detection of filling defects in the dural sinuses and cortical veins.[5]

Several studies have shown that CTV is comparable in its sensitivity and specificity to MR venography (MRV) and catheter angiography in detecting CVT.[30,31] A large filling defect within a dural sinus or cortical vein is the most reliable sign of CVT. False-negative CTV examinations can be caused by hyperdense acute thrombus, which can mimic a normally enhancing sinus. This problem can be avoided by careful attention to the unenhanced portion of the scan to distinguish hyperdensity in the sinus from contrast agent enhancement. Chronic thrombus can demonstrate contrast enhancement and mimic a patent sinus filling with contrast. Arachnoid granulations within the dural sinuses can produce focal filling defects that mimic sinus clot and partial thrombosis.

Advantages of CTV when compared with MRV include its resistance to motion artifact; its ease of acquisition after noncontrast CT, and the accessibility and cost-effectiveness of CT in general. There is better spatial resolution compared with MRV, and there are no flow-related artifacts. CTV better depicts venous anatomy than time-of-flight MRV and detects thrombosis with equal accuracy. When compared with digital subtraction angiography (DSA), CTV may be better at demonstrating the cavernous sinus, inferior sagittal sinus, and the basal vein of Rosenthal.[31] New CT protocols allow for visualization of the arterial and venous systems with one contrast bolus, which is a possible advantage in the emergent setting or when the diagnosis is uncertain.[30] Drawbacks of CTV are the ionizing radiation dose and the risks/contraindications of intravenous contrast media. Streak artifact secondary to the presence of metal adjacent to the sinus can obscure evaluation. Creation of maximum-intensity projection (MIP) images can be time consuming, and it is difficult to remove all the bone from the image without removing some of the sinus as well. Matched mask bone elimination technique has helped improve the quality of MIP images in this regard.[32] Of course, the diagnosis of CVT must be entertained before CTV can be performed.

MRI
Direct Signs of CVT
Normal Sinus/Vein Signal

To accurately diagnose CVT on MRI, one must recognize the normal MR characteristics of patent sinuses and veins and understand the appearance of clotted blood as it evolves over time. Flow-related signal is variable and depends on multiple factors, including pulse sequence, orientation of imaging plane relative to flow direction, slice thickness, and specific acquisition parameters. On spin-echo sequences, flowing blood is most commonly characterized by a flow void, or dark signal, on both T1- (T1W) and T2-weighted (T2W) images (Figs. 22-8 to 22-10). Flowing blood exits the imaging plane in the interval between the 90- and 180-degree pulses of the spin-echo sequence and therefore fails to contribute to the intraluminal signal. Flow voids therefore are signs of vascular patency. This effect is most pronounced with rapid flow and with flow perpendicular to the imaging plane. When flow is slow or occurs parallel to the imaging plane, the intrinsic signal from blood may be captured, producing variable hyperintensity within the vessel on T2W imaging sequences. On T1W sequences, perpendicular flow may produce hyperintensity due to entry of blood into the imaging plane that has not been exposed to prior radiofrequency pulses. This flow-related enhancement is the basis of time-of-flight (TOF) MR angiographic sequences. On both T1W and T2W sequences, the signal from flowing blood may be captured but spatially misregistered. A

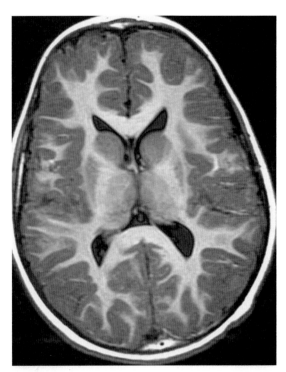

■ **FIGURE 22-8** FLAIR MR sequence depicts a normal flow void within the posterior superior sagittal sinus and high signal in an adjacent vein (*just left of the sinus*) indicative of slow flow within that vein.

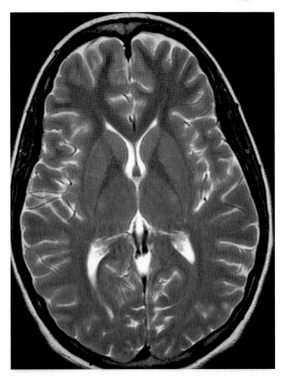

■ **FIGURE 22-9** T2W MR image shows a normal flow void in the superior sagittal sinus.

ghost or smear artifact extending across an MR image with the same configuration as that of a dural sinus seen on the same image is a reliable sign of venous patency. These ghost artifacts are particularly prominent on enhanced T1W images. On gradient-recalled-echo (GRE) sequences that do not incorporate a rephasing pulse, blood flowing into the plane of imaging section

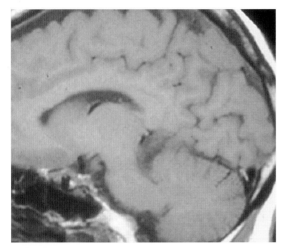

■ **FIGURE 22-10** T1W MR image shows a normal flow void in the superior sagittal sinus as well as in the transverse sinus.

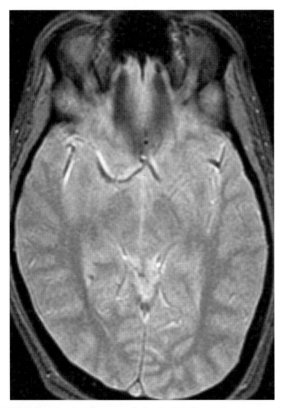

■ **FIGURE 22-11** Gradient-recalled-echo MR image shows normal high signal within the superior sagittal sinus.

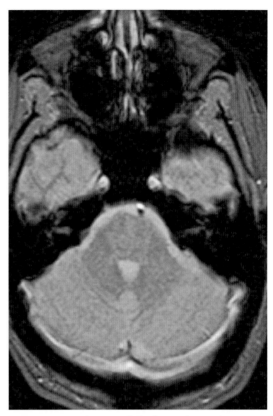

■ **FIGURE 22-12** Gradient-recalled-echo MR image shows normal high signal within the transverse sinuses.

appears bright (Figs. 22-11 and 22-12). This is in marked contrast to the dramatic hypointensity seen in acute thrombus due to susceptibility effects of deoxyhemoglobin (see later). Therefore, when evaluating for sinus thrombosis on unenhanced spin-echo and GRE sequences, one looks for absence of the normal flow void and absence of hyperintensity within the sinus on GRE sequences to suggest the diagnosis. As a general rule of thumb, the presence of hyperintensity within the dural sinus on GRE sequences in conjunction with hypointensity on T2W sequences is indicative of venous patency.

Acute CVT

Acute cerebral venous thrombus (days 1-5) is mostly composed of intracellular deoxyhemoglobin, a paramagnetic substance that appears isointense to mildly hyperintense on T1W images. Isointensity or hyperintensity within the sinus represents a change from the normal hypointense flow void seen when the sinus is patent. (On T1W images intraluminal hypointensity and/or inconsistent hyperintensity are good and isointensity is bad [Figs. 22-13 and 22-14].) The paramagnetic properties of deoxyhemoglobin cause proton dephasing and shortening of the T2 relaxation time with resultant hypointensity on T2W images. This leads to a potential source of confusion in the diagnosis of CVT, because both flowing blood and acute thrombus within the sinus are hypointense on T2W images. Susceptibility-weighted (T2*) GRE sequences are particularly useful in the acute setting. The marked dephasing effect characteristic of this sequence produces marked hypointensity within and hypointense blooming artifact adjacent to the thrombosed vessel, representing a significant change from the appearance of a normal hyperintense patent sinus (Fig. 22-15). This feature of T2* sequences makes them critical in the detection of acute thrombus.[33] Diffusion-weighted sequences are mostly utilized for evaluation of the brain parenchyma in the setting of CVT. However, the acute thrombus itself demonstrates restricted diffusion in approximately 40% of patients, a finding associated with less frequent recanalization and a longer duration of clinical symptoms in one study.[34] When diagnosis is in doubt or to determine the extent of thrombosis, MRV and contrast-enhanced MR images can be performed to improve diagnostic accuracy.

Subacute CVT

SCVT (4 to 15 days) is characterized first by the presence of intracellular methemoglobin and later by red cell lysis. The

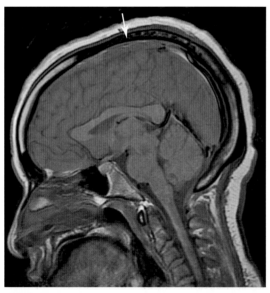

■ **FIGURE 22-13** T1W sagittal MR image with isointense signal within the superior sagittal sinus consistent with acute thrombosis (*arrow*).

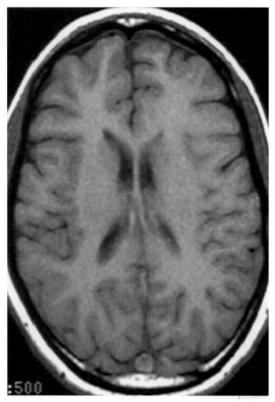

■ **FIGURE 22-14** T1W axial MR image with isointense signal within the superior sagittal sinus consistent with acute thrombosis.

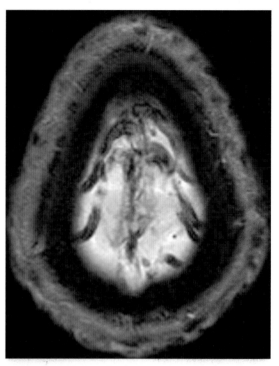

■ **FIGURE 22-15** Gradient-recalled-echo axial MR image with marked low signal within the superior sagittal sinus and adjacent draining veins consistent with acute thrombosis.

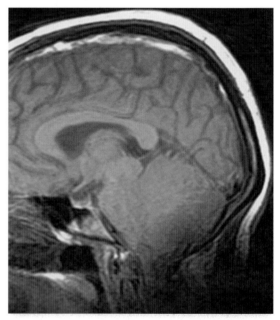

■ **FIGURE 22-16** T1W sagittal MR image with high signal within the superior sagittal sinus consistent with subacute thrombosis.

paramagnetic properties of methemoglobin, as well as its ability to participate in proton-electron dipole-dipole interactions with water molecules, allow marked T1 shortening and resultant high signal on T1W images (Fig. 22-16). On T2W images, the nonuniformity in the distribution of intracellular methemoglobin during the early subacute phase causes dephasing of water protons and resultant hypointensity. Red cell lysis markedly decreases this dephasing effect, and late subacute thrombus will appear hyperintense on T2W images. SCVT therefore transitions from bright on T1W and dark on T2W images in the early phase to bright on both T1W and T2W images in the late phase. The subacute phase is the easiest stage to detect on conventional MR sequences, and a confident diagnosis may not require additional sequences.

Chronic CVT

Chronic venous sinus thrombosis (>15 days) may present a diagnostic dilemma on MRI. Breakdown and evolution of the subacute thrombus leads to a decrease in its signal intensity on T1W and T2W sequences. Chronic thrombus tends to appear

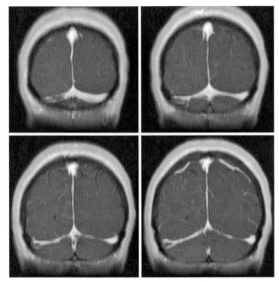

■ **FIGURE 22-17** Gadolinium-enhanced, spoiled gradient recalled acquisition in steady state (GRASS) MR sequence showing the empty delta sign consistent with right transverse sinus thrombosis.

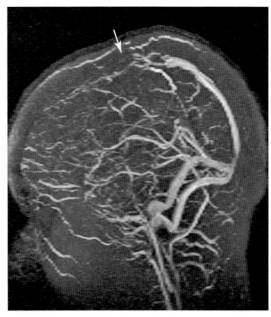

■ **FIGURE 22-18** MRV image showing cutoff of the superior sagittal sinus consistent with thrombosis (*arrow*).

isointense or slightly hyperintense on T2W imaging and isointense on T1W imaging. Partial recanalization leads to flow-related signal effects that, when combined with the varying proportions of different blood products remaining within the thrombus, result in a variable MRI appearance that is similar to that of slow-flowing blood.

The bottom line in MRI is that a perceived abnormality on one sequence, or in one plane, must be confirmed with other planes and sequences. Signal from thrombus should remain consistent no matter what the plane of section or sequence, allowing differentiation of artifact or flow from real thrombosis.

Contrast MRI and MRV

Contrast-enhanced MRI sequences may be utilized in precisely the same manner as contrast-enhanced CT in the evaluation of CVT. The empty delta sign, originally described on CT, can also be seen on gadolinium-enhanced MRI (Fig. 22-17). As with contrast-enhanced CT, organized subacute to chronic thrombus can enhance and the enhancement of collateral dural vessels along the sinus can mimic the appearance of a patent sinus.[2] An advantage of MRI when compared with CT is that multiplanar enhanced sequences are typically acquired, allowing for more accurate detection of the filling defects in the transverse sinuses, which are seen to better advantage on coronal and sagittal images. Contrast-enhanced images acquired with 3D isotropic GRE T1W techniques (similar to those used for MR angiography) allow for image quality and manipulation comparable to that obtained with CTV.

2D TOF MRV is the most common method utilized for diagnosis of CVT (Fig. 22-18). A thrombus that is stationary within the plane of imaging will appear as a dark filling defect, with the patent sinus appearing bright (owing to flow-related enhancement). The susceptibility effects of acute clot enhance the hypointensity of the clot (MRV sequences utilize GRE techniques). Effects of in-plane and turbulent flow may produce flow gaps that may mimic thrombosis. Flow gaps typically occur where the sinuses and veins turn into the plane of the coronal imaging. Therefore, the most problematic areas include the posterior aspect of the sagittal sinus and parts of the transverse and sigmoid sinuses. Despite these drawbacks, 2D TOF techniques have been shown to reliably diagnose CVT.[35]

2D phase-contrast (PC) MRV may also prove useful. In this technique the change in phase of flowing blood during image acquisition produces intraluminal hyperintensity relative to stationary spins in the adjacent brain. Phase-contrast flow techniques are sensitive to different rates of flow. Therefore, on PC MR images it is possible to select for venous flow alone. 2D PC sequences are extremely rapid and can be performed in three orthogonal planes in less than 1 minute. These sequences are not plagued by flow effects seen on TOF studies. They allow for detection of dural sinus thrombosis but without sufficient resolution for evaluation of cortical veins. During the subacute phase of sinus thrombosis when thrombus is hyperintense on T1W images, clot may mimic hyperintense flow on TOF MRV. This does not occur with PC MRV in which high intensity of stationary spins (e.g., clot or fat) does not occur.

Newer techniques in MRV include gadolinium-enhanced sequences, such as the auto-triggered elliptic centric-ordered sequence. This technique has demonstrated greater success than traditional 2D TOF in both identifying intracranial veins and dural sinuses and in diagnosing CVT, including the more difficult cases of chronic sinus thrombosis. The presence of intravenous gadolinium shortens the T1 of blood and results in high signal within the venous structures. This also allows for a shorter repetition time and greater background suppression. Unlike traditional 2D TOF, no flow artifacts are seen and the depiction of vessels becomes flow-independent. Vessels are adequately imaged using this technique provided contrast agent is present within the vessel at the time of signal acquisition and the caliber of the vessel is greater than the spatial resolution limitations of the sequence. The timing of the image acquisition is an important factor in the diagnosis of CVT, because it has been shown that first-pass venous imaging is able to demonstrate the filling defect within a sinus before a chronic thrombus enhances.[36]

Indirect Signs of CVT

Parenchymal signal abnormalities are appreciated on MRI in approximately 57% of patients with CVT. In 25% of patients cerebral edema is seen without evidence of hemorrhage, and 32% of patients demonstrate a combination of hemorrhage and edema.[2] Mass effect with diffuse parenchymal swelling, sulcal and cisternal effacement, and decreased ventricular size may

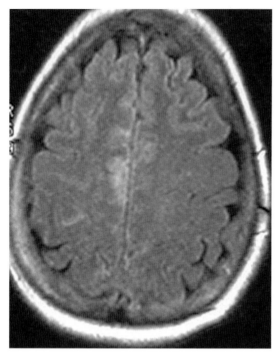

■ **FIGURE 22-19** FLAIR MR image showing high signal mostly in the right vertex, consistent with edema from superior sagittal sinus thrombosis. On diffusion-weighted sequences there was no restricted diffusion.

occur in up to 40% of patients without focal signal abnormality.[2] Subcortical hematomas and/or small petechial microhemorrhages, are common. These are hypointense on T2 and markedly hypointense on GRE images. Focal regions of T2 hyperintensity are seen in white matter, gray matter, or both owing to cytotoxic and/or vasogenic edema (Fig. 22-19). Diffusion-weighted sequences are useful in distinguishing these two types of edema. It has been observed that most foci of T2 hyperintensity are isointense on diffusion-weighted images and demonstrate increased apparent diffusion coefficient (ADC) values on ADC maps. These lesions are the result of vasogenic edema and typically resolve with treatment or time. Lesions with restricted diffusion are hyperintense on diffusion-weighted imaging and have low ADC values. These lesions likely represent foci of cytotoxic edema from venous infarction and typically represent regions of permanent brain injury. Some of these lesions resolve without imaging or clinical evidence of permanent brain injury. Although the pathophysiology is not yet fully delineated, there is the suggestion in the literature that mildly restricted diffusion occurs early in the time course of some cases of CVT. Subsequent resolution of the diffusion abnormality may have to do with early collateralization and rescue of ischemic brain tissue.[11,37] Other indirect signs of CVT include prominent patent cortical veins as well as dilated medullary veins that represent collateral

venous drainage. Medullary veins are visible on GRE sequences at 3.0 T. Parenchymal contrast enhancement may occur secondary to breakdown of the blood-brain barrier. Enhancement secondary to collateral flow can be seen in the dura, as well as in the form of prominent cortical veins. The thrombus may enhance in the late subacute to chronic phase, a feature that can confuse diagnosis on contrast-enhanced scans.

MR Perfusion (MRP) and MR Spectroscopy (MRS)
Because the pathophysiology of CVT involves venous congestion and decreased cerebral blood flow, abnormalities on MRP and MRS studies are expected, although little published data exist at present. As in the case of arterial stroke, the main goal of perfusion imaging is quantification of salvageable brain in and around a given lesion. Reports exist of parenchymal lesions from CVT that demonstrate initially increased mean transit times, with normalization after treatment. On MRS, small lactate peaks have been observed within parenchymal lesions caused by CVT.[38,39]

Advantages/Pitfalls of MRI
The major advantage of MRI when compared with CT is that the diagnosis can be made on routine unenhanced images of the brain in the majority of cases, whereas on CT, contrast-enhanced studies are required in most cases. Given the protean clinical manifestations of CVT, there is often little or no clinical suspicion of CVT at the time of the routine "emergent" unenhanced study (be it CT or MRI). The correct diagnosis is more likely to be made and appropriate additional imaging studies performed when the initial examination is MRI rather than CT. It is certainly true that an understanding of normal flow-related signal on multiple sequences and an appreciation of the appearance of blood at various stages of clot evolution are necessary to make the diagnosis. The level of expertise required to make the diagnosis of CVT is therefore high but well within the reach of practitioners who routinely use MRI in emergent situations. With CT, on the other hand, there are many cases where no amount of expertise will allow for correct diagnosis. Other advantages of MRI include lack of radiation exposure, the relative safety of gadolinium contrast, and the better depiction of parenchymal abnormalities when compared with CT.[40] This is particularly true for identification of diffuse and/or focal edema and differentiation between reversible vasogenic edema and irreversible cytotoxic edema (venous infarction). Aside from the need for some expertise in the detection of CVT on unenhanced MRI, the major drawbacks of MRI are logistical. The examinations take longer to perform than CT, and MR scanners are not always available on an emergent basis.

Special Procedures
Digital subtraction angiography (DSA) was the gold standard for the diagnosis of CVT before the advent of MR and noninvasive vascular imaging; it is now generally performed only for treatment of CVT, not for diagnosis.

ANALYSIS
A sample report is presented in Box 22-1.

BOX 22-1   Sample Report: MRI and MRV for Cortical Vein Thrombosis[41]

PATIENT HISTORY

The patient is a 25-year-old woman with sickle cell trait who is 1 week post partum. She had epidural anesthesia during delivery. Soon after delivery she developed a severe occipital headache that improved on lying down. The headache was assumed to be secondary to intracranial hypotension, and the patient was treated with a blood patch. The headache worsened in the few days after the blood patch, and the patient then presented to the emergency department with a chief complaint of headache. She described the magnitude as 8/10 in the occipital region, with no associated symptoms of nausea, vomiting, fevers, or chills.

TECHNIQUE

MRI and MRV of the brain were performed in the emergency department using the following sequences: sagittal and axial T1W, axial T2W, axial fluid-attenuated inversion recovery (FLAIR), axial gradient-recalled-echo (GRE), diffusion-weighted sequences, 2D TOF, and 2D PC. Gadolinium was not administered.

FINDINGS
MRI

The middle and anterior segments of the superior sagittal sinus demonstrate loss of flow voids with isointense signal on the T1W sequence best seen on the sagittal image (see Fig. 22-13). The GRE images demonstrate susceptibility artifact in the same area of the superior sagittal sinus with extension into the superficial cortical draining veins (see Fig. 22-15).

MRV

The middle and anterior segments of the superior sagittal sinus and associated superficial cortical draining veins demonstrate loss of signal consistent with thrombosis (see Fig. 22-18).

IMPRESSION

The findings are consistent with superior sagittal sinus thrombosis at its middle and anterior segments with associated superior cortical vein thrombosis.

COMMENT

The patient was admitted to neurology and put on anticoagulation (heparin drip with partial thromboplastin time titrated to 60 to 80). The interventional neuroradiology service offered the option of endovascular treatment in the setting of clinical worsening despite anticoagulation. The patient's clinical condition improved, and she was discharged a few days later.

KEY POINTS

- CVT is manifested by a wide range of clinical signs and symptoms that include the broad categories of raised intracranial pressure, usually due to large dural sinus occlusion, and focal deficits, likely caused by deep or superficial cerebral vein occlusion and resultant edema/hemorrhage.
- Normal anatomic variation in the cerebral venous anatomy contributes to the wide range of clinical and imaging manifestations of CVT.
- Imaging findings of CVT on CT include direct signs such as the dense triangle sign and the cord sign. The empty delta sign is seen on postcontrast images. Indirect signs include foci of edema or hemorrhage.

- Imaging findings of CVT on MRI include complex abnormalities of signal within the sinus secondary to loss of the normal flow void and the presence of thrombus. Gradient-recalled-echo sequences are critical in the detection of acute venous thrombosis because normal sinuses are hyperintense and thrombosed sinuses have dramatic hypointensity and blooming artifact. Indirect signs include areas of edema or hemorrhage with or without areas of restricted diffusion.
- The diagnosis of CVT is of critical importance because treatment, even long after initial thrombus, can have a positive effect on outcome.

SUGGESTED READINGS

Ameri A, Bousser M-G. Cerebral venous thrombosis. Neurol Clin 1992; 10:87-111.

Connor SEJ, Jarosz JM. Magnetic resonance imaging of cerebral venous sinus thrombosis. Clin Radiol 2002; 57:449-461.

Lasjaunias P, Berenstein A, terBrugge KG, et al. Intracranial venous system. In Lasjaunias P, Berenstein A, terBrugge KG (eds). Surgical Neuroangiography, 2nd ed. Berlin, Springer Verlag, 2001, pp 631-695.

Leach JL, Fortuna RB, Jones BV, Gaskill-Shipley MF. Imaging of cerebral venous thrombosis: current techniques, spectrum of findings, and diagnostic pitfalls. RadioGraphics 2006; 26(Suppl 1):S19-S41.

Rhoton A. The cerebral veins. Neurosurgery 2002; 51(Suppl 1): S159-S205.

Stam J. Thrombosis of the cerebral veins and sinuses. N Engl J Med 2005; 352:1791-1798.

REFERENCES

1. Bogousslavsky J, Pierre P. Ischaemic stroke in patients under age 45. Neurol Clin 1992; 10:113-124.
2. Leach JL, Fortuna RB, Jones BV, Gaskill-Shipley MF. Imaging of cerebral venous thrombosis: current techniques, spectrum of findings, and diagnostic pitfalls. RadioGraphics 2006; 26(Suppl 1):S19-S41.
3. Bousser M-G, Chiras J, Bories J, Castaigne P. Cerebral venous thrombosis—a review of 38 cases. Stroke 1985; 16:199-213.
4. Masuhr F, Mehraein S, Einhaupl K. Cerebral venous and sinus thrombosis. J Neurol 2004; 251:11-23.
5. Rodallec MH, Krainik A, Feydy A, et al. Cerebral venous thrombosis and multidetector CT angiography: tips and tricks. RadioGraphics 2006; 26(Suppl 1):S5-S18.
6. de Bruijn SF, Stam J, Kappelle LJ. Thunderclap headache as first symptom of cerebral venous sinus thrombosis. Lancet 1996; 348:1623-1625.
7. Jacobs K, Moulin T, Bogousslavsky J, et al. The stroke syndrome of cortical vein thrombosis. Neurology 1996; 47:376-382.
8. van den Bergh W, van der Schaaf I, van Gijn J. The spectrum of presentations caused by venous infarction caused by deep cerebral vein thrombosis. Neurology 2005; 65:192-196.
9. Crawford SC, Digre KB, Palmer CA, et al. Thrombosis of the deep venous drainage of the brain in adults: analysis of seven cases with review of the literature. Arch Neurol 1995; 52:1101-1108.

10. Ferro J, Canhão P, Stam J, et al. Prognosis of cerebral vein and dural sinus thrombosis: results of the International Study on Cerebral Vein and Dural Sinus Thrombosis (ISCVT). Stroke 2004; 35:664-670.

11. Ducreux D, Oppenheim C, Vandamme X, et al. Diffusion-weighted imaging patterns of brain damage associated with cerebral venous thrombosis. AJNR Am J Neuroradiol 2001; 22:261-268.

12. Saw VPJ, Kollar C, Johnston IH. Dural sinus thrombosis: a mechanism-based classification and review of 42 cases. J Clin Neurosci 1999; 6:480-487.

13. Ahmad A. Genetics of cerebral venous thrombosis. J Pak Med Assoc 2006; 56:488-490.

14. Renowden S. Cerebral venous sinus thrombosis. Eur Radiol 2004; 14:215-226.

15. Fries G, Wallenfang T, Hennen J, et al. Occlusion of the pig superior sagittal sinus, bridging and cortical veins: multistep evolution of sinus-vein thrombosis. J Neurosurg 1992; 77:127-133.

16. Nakase H, Heimann A, Kempski O. Alterations of regional cerebral blood flow and oxygen saturation in a rat sinus-vein thrombosis model. Stroke 1996; 27:720-728.

17. Bergui M, Bradac G, Daniele D. Brain lesions due to cerebral venous thrombosis do not correlate with sinus involvement. Neuroradiology 1999; 41:419-424.

18. Tsai FY, Wang AM, Matovich VB, et al. MR staging of acute dural sinus thrombosis: correlation with venous pressure measurements and implications for treatment and prognosis. AJNR Am J Neuroradiol 1995; 16:1021-1029.

19. Stolz E, Trittmacher S, Rahimi A, et al. Influence of recanalization on outcome in dural sinus thrombosis: a prospective study. Stroke 2004; 35:544-547.

20. Preter M, Tzourio C, Ameri A, Bousser MG. Long-term prognosis in cerebral venous thrombosis: follow-up of 77 patients. Stroke 1996; 27:243-246.

21. Kalimo H, Kaste M, Haltia M. Vascular diseases. In Graham DI, Lantos PL (eds). Greenfield's Neuropathology, 7th ed. New York, Oxford University Press, 2002, pp 281-355.

22. Shintaku M, Yasui N. Chronic superior sagittal sinus thrombosis with phlebosclerotic changes of the subarachnoid and intracerebral veins. Neuropathology 2006; 26:323-328.

23. Rhoton A. The cerebral veins. Neurosurgery 2002; 51(Suppl 1): S159-S205.

24. Andeweg J. Consequences of the anatomy of deep venous outflow from the brain. Neuroradiology 1999; 41:233-241.

25. Rhoton A. The posterior cranial fossa: microsurgical anatomy & surgical approaches. Neurosurgery 2000; 47(Suppl):S131-S153

26. Virapongse C, Cazenave C, Quisling R, et al. The empty delta sign: frequency and significance in 76 cases of dural sinus thrombosis. Radiology 1987; 162:779-785.

27. Leach JL, Bulas RV, Ernst RJ, Cornelius RS. MR imaging of isolated cortical vein thrombosis: the hyperintense vein sign. J Neurovasc Dis 1996; 1:1-7.

28. Derdeyn CP, Powers WJ. Isolated cortical venous thrombosis and ulcerative colitis. AJNR Am J Neuroradiol 1998; 19:488-490.

29. Lin JH, Kwan SY, Wu D. Cerebral venous thrombosis initially presenting with acute subarachnoid hemorrhage. J Chin Med Assoc 2006; 69:282-285.

30. Linn J, Ertl-Wagner B, Seelos KC, et al. Diagnostic value of multidetector-row CT angiography in the evaluation of thrombosis of the cerebral venous sinuses. Am J Neuroradiol 2007; 28:946-952.

31. Wetzel S, Kirsch E, Stock K, et al. Cerebral veins: comparative study of CT venography with intraarterial digital subtraction angiography. Am J Neuroradiol 1999; 20:249-255.

32. Majoie CB, van Straten M, Venema HW, den Heeten GJ. Multisection CT venography of the dural sinuses and cerebral veins by using matched mask bone elimination. Am J Neuroradiol 2004; 25:787-791.

33. Idbaih A, Boukobza M, Crassard I, et al. MRI of clot in cerebral venous thrombosis: high diagnostic value of susceptibility-weighted images. Stroke 2006; 37:991-995.

34. Favrole P, Guichard J, Crassard I, et al. Diffusion-weighted imaging of intravascular clots in cerebral venous thrombosis. Stroke 2004; 35:99-103.

35. Ayanzen RH, Bird CR, Keller PJ, et al. Cerebral MR venography: normal anatomy and potential diagnostic pitfalls. AJNR Am J Neuroradiol 2000; 21:74-78.

36. Farb RI, Scott JN, Willinsky RA, et al. Intracranial venous system: gadolinium-enhanced three-dimensional MR venography with autotriggered elliptic centric-ordered sequence—initial experience. Radiology 2003; 226:203-209.

37. Mullins ME, Grant PE, Wang B, et al. Parenchymal abnormalities associated with cerebral venous sinus thrombosis: assessment with diffusion-weighted MR imaging. AJNR Am J Neuroradiol 2004; 25:1666-1675.

38. Doege CA, Tavakolian R, Kerskens C, et al. Perfusion and diffusion magnetic resonance imaging in human cerebral venous thrombosis. J Neurol 2001; 248:564-571.

39. Li-Chi Hsu, Jiing-Feng Lirng, Jong-Ling Fuh, et al. Proton magnetic resonance spectroscopy in deep cerebral venous thrombosis. Clin Neurol Neurosurg 1998; 100:27-30.

40. Connor SEJ, Jarosz JM. Magnetic resonance imaging of cerebral venous sinus thrombosis. Clin Radiol 2002; 57:449-461.

41. Rau C-S, Lui C-C, Liang C-L, et al. Superior sagittal sinus thrombosis induced by thyrotoxicosis: case report. J Neurosurg 2001; 94:130-132.

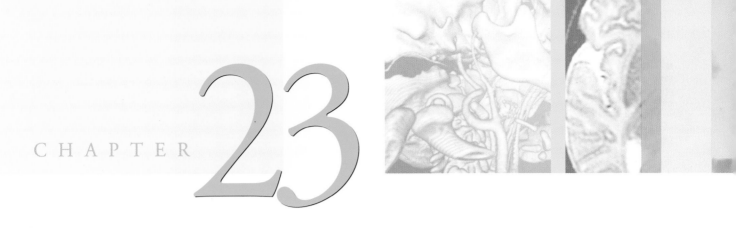

CHAPTER 23

Aneurysms

Timo Krings, Sasikhan Geibprasert, Vitor M. Pereira, Pakorn Jiarakongmun, Sirintara Pongpech, and Pierre L. Lasjaunias

Aneurysms are focal abnormal dilatations of an artery. In 1997, Schievink proposed that "intracranial arterial aneurysms are acquired lesions that are most commonly located at the branching points of the major cerebral arteries coursing through the subarachnoid space at the base of the brain." He pointed out that "intracranial arteries have an attenuated tunica media and a lack of external elastica lamina" and that "intracranial arterial aneurysms have a thin tunica media or none, and the internal elastica lamina is either absent or severely fragmented." These observations are generally correct but do not attempt to distinguish among the diverse diseases that give rise to arterial aneurysms. The concept that the arterial bloodstream first "expands" and then "bursts" an "aneurysmal herniation of the wall" is now considered too simple to explain the complex features of arterial aneurysms. Different classification schemes have been based on aneurysm size (small vs. large vs. giant), location (posterior circulation vs. anterior circulation), clinical presentation (ruptured vs. unruptured), morphology (saccular vs. fusiform), or etiology (false or traumatic aneurysms, dissecting aneurysms, flow-related aneurysms, infectious aneurysms). Each of these classifications has advantages, but we will use the etiologic classification in this chapter because therapeutic decision-making can be improved by a better understanding and recognition of the many different lesions grouped together as aneurysms (Fig. 23-1).

EPIDEMIOLOGY

The prevalence of arterial aneurysms is reported to be 3% to 5% in Western populations, which is approximately 10 times higher than the frequency of arteriovenous malformations (AVMs) in the same group. At autopsy, the overall frequency of aneurysms in the general population ranges from 0.4% to 10%. The recent meta-analysis by Rinkel and colleagues found a prevalence of 2.3% in adults. More than 50% of aneurysms identified at postmortem examination are asymptomatic. In Western countries, the average annual incidence of subarachnoid hemorrhage (SAH) is approximately 10 cases per 100,000 people per year. In both autopsy and clinical series, the incidence of arterial aneurysms and of arterial aneurysm–associated SAH increases with age from the third decade, peaking at the sixth decade. The incidence of arterial aneurysms in children is very low, even in familial arterial aneurysms or associated diseases. Intracranial aneurysms are more common in adult women than adult men but more frequent in boys than girls. The relative frequency of females increases systematically with age, so that the male-to-female ratio

changes from 3:1 in children up to 8 years of age to 1.2:1 in the 10- to 20-year-old age group, reverses in the 5th decade (male to female: 0.9:1), and reaches 1:3 in the seventh decade of life.

Multiplicity

The incidence of multiple intracranial aneurysms appears to be extremely variable, depending in part on the patient population; whether the series included surgical, radiologic, or autopsy findings; and whether the aneurysms were ruptured or unruptured. The prevalence of multiple intracranial aneurysms varies between 25% and 31% in autopsy series and 12% to 26% in larger clinical series. Female patients account for 60% to 81% of patients with multiple aneurysms. The internal carotid artery (ICA) and middle cerebral artery (MCA) are most prone to form multiple aneurysms.

Mirror-Image or Twin Aneurysms

A special subgroup of multiple aneurysms is the "mirror-like" or "twin" aneurysms at symmetric sites on each side. Twin aneurysms occur in 5% to 10% of all aneurysm patients but in as many as 36% of all multiple aneurysm patients. They are found on all intracranial vessels but are most common in the MCA. Twin aneurysms may be discovered in the same clinical context as "classic" saccular aneurysms (e.g., during SAH), but their origin is likely to be different. The occurrence of mirror-like aneurysms, their association with familial disease, and their tendency to rupture earlier in life than "classic" aneurysms suggests that congenital weakness of the vessel wall may be an underlying cause (Fig. 23-2).

The intracranial vascular system is composed of multiple different vascular segments. Each segment may have a unique "segmental identity" that carries with it selective vulnerability to specific triggers. During cephalic vasculogenesis, a defect in migrating cells might be transmitted to the next generation of cells, resulting in a clonal distribution of the defect. The synchronous occurrence of mirror-like aneurysms suggests that these aneurysms develop in segments that share the same defective characteristics. For those reasons, "twin" aneurysms might be a better term than "mirror-like" aneurysms.

Familial Forms and Screening

Intracranial aneurysms are found approximately twice as often in first-degree relatives of patients with aneurysmal SAH than in

■ **FIGURE 23-1** Same morphologic type of aneurysm (fusiform aneurysm) depicted in four different patients. The term *fusiform aneurysm* corresponds to an enlargement of the entire vessel circumference over a segment of the artery and is a morphologic description rather than a pathomechanism. Although these aneurysms look similar, their pathomechanisms are completely different, inferring different treatment strategies. The four different underlying etiologies are aneurysm in the presence of atrial myxoma most likely resembling a neoplastic aneurysm (**A**), acute transmural dissection with subarachnoid hemorrhage (**B**), aneurysmal dilatation present in familial candidasis (**C**), and fusiform lumen of a partially thrombosed aneurysm following a healed dissecting process (**D**).

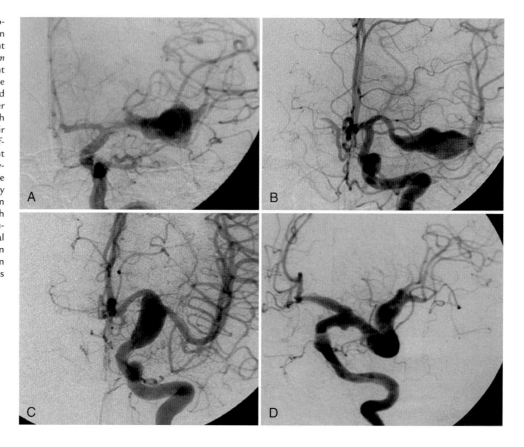

the general population. Within families, the greater the number of members affected, the greater the risk that any one member will have an aneurysm, up to four times the incidence in the general population. Females predominate (54% to 70%) in familial SAH. In males, the SAH occurs 7 to 10 years earlier in familial forms of aneurysms than in nonfamilial forms. Sibling pairs with arterial aneurysms tend to bleed within the same decade. Most familial arterial aneurysms arise in the MCA territory (50%), especially on the right side, and tend to bleed at relatively small arterial aneurysm size (<6 mm at rupture). The rate of multiplicity is not higher in familial arterial aneurysms, but collected data suggest that fewer arterial aneurysms remain asymptomatic in SAH families.

It is *not* recommended to screen the general population or to screen families with only one affected family member (relative risk, 1.8), because the resulting slight increase in life expectancy does not offset the risk of postoperative sequelae. However, screening programs should be implemented for first-degree relatives of patients with familial forms of SAH because these individuals are four times more likely to experience a SAH than the general population.

PATHOPHYSIOLOGY

Aneurysms that present with similar features, such as SAH, may result from entirely different disease processes, including bacterial or viral infections and inflammations, connective tissue diseases, traumatic or spontaneous dissections, neoplasms, radiation therapy, and high-flow cerebral AVMs. Therefore, in this chapter we will differentiate among "classic saccular," dissecting, infectious, and traumatic aneurysms and will discuss their individual pathophysiologies in specific subdivisions.

SACCULAR ANEURYSMS

Saccular aneurysms are the most frequently encountered form of aneurysms (70%-80%). They typically arise at arterial bifurca-

tions and resemble berry-like outpouchings of the vessel wall. Their etiology and pathophysiology are complex and poorly understood. Genetic factors contribute to their development as underlined by (1) the familial form of aneurysms described previously and (2) the many genetic diseases that manifest with aneurysmal dilatation. Endogenous factors such as aging, elevated blood pressure, vessel wall shear stresses, and anatomic variations of the circle of Willis as well as exogenous risk factors such as cigarette smoking are thought to contribute to the formation and/or rupture of an aneurysm. In addition to these "offensive" factors, there may also be "defective defense mechanisms," such as improper spontaneous self-repair of a vessel wall. The roles of these different factors in a given individual are unknown. Therefore, the concept of individual host response must be considered when assessing the etiology of an aneurysm in a given patient. This individual host response is dependent on the individual life span and the regeneration capacity of arteries in normal or in pathologic circumstances, at their branching or nonbranching portions.

Aging, hypertension, and/or smoking are thought to lead to general thickening of the intima of arteries, which is most pronounced distal and proximal to branching sites. These thickened intimal "pads" are inelastic and lead to an increased strain on more elastic parts of the vessel wall adjacent to these pads. Increased strain on the vessel leads to an increased activity of metalloproteinases and other extracellular matrix-degrading proteins, culminating in aneurysmal outpouching of the vessel wall. A vicious circle may then ensue as turbulent flow against the outpouching increases the strain on the vessel wall. Such hemodynamic stress may be especially significant at sites of congenital weakness of the vessel wall. For example, aneurysms often form in the vicinity of anatomic variations such as incomplete fusion of the basilar artery or unilateral absence of the horizontal segment of an anterior cerebral artery (A1) (Fig. 23-3). However, these theories are not able to explain why certain patients

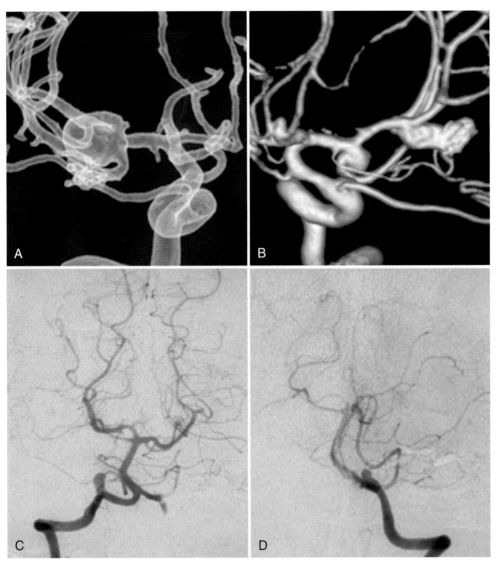

■ **FIGURE 23-2** A to D, Multiple mirror aneurysms in a single patient who harbored bilateral symmetric MCA aneurysms, bilateral symmetric PICA aneurysms, and an anterior communicating artery aneurysm. The multiplicity and the mirror or twin occurrence suggest a congenital predisposition to be more likely than degenerative causes alone for the appearance of these aneurysms.

develop aneurysms and others with similar "offensive exposures" do not. Therefore, individual defects in host response (e.g., a missing defensive line) may be present that finally lead to the formation of an aneurysm.

The construction and maintenance of blood vessels are the result of complex biologic factors and events that involve repetitive steps and feedback to the vascular tree. The structural integrity of arteries is maintained and modified according to hemodynamic or metabolic demands (e.g., shear stress forces), which are genetically programmed and controlled. Vascular remodeling is an active and adaptive process of structural alteration and includes changes in cellular processes such as cell growth, cell death, cell migration, and production or degradation of the extracellular matrix. Shear stress forces activate specific (genetically programmed) steps that alter the balance of the mediators of remodeling (e.g., metalloproteinases, nitric oxide synthase, platelet-derived growth factor [PDGF], and transforming growth factor β1). Aging decreases the capacity of the vessel wall to adapt to variations in the hemodynamic parameters or to compensate for stressful events. This progressive aging process is an acquired vulnerability of the vessel wall, which will differ in males and females and with patient age. Congenital alterations in these programs could well result in a variant, defective, or

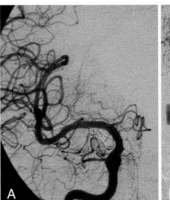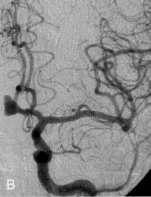

■ **FIGURE 23-3** A and B, In the absence of a contralateral A1 segment, aneurysms tend to form more often on the ipsilateral anterior communicating ramus. Whether this is due to increased hemodynamic shear stress forces or to a relative immaturity (and therefore increased fragility) of the vascular system is unclear.

absent reconstruction of the vessel wall. Similarly, we believe that the association of arterial variants with arterial aneurysms points to an incomplete maturation process of the arterial wall. The lack of cell selection that such a pattern implies may preserve "weaker," that is, less mature endothelial cells that will later develop arterial aneurysms when subject to secondary triggers such as hemodynamic stress.

In the individual patient there is a complex interplay between the aggressive "offensive" factors and the host response. Formation of an aneurysm, therefore, indicates failure of the repair system at a given period in time and/or the persistence of the abnormal triggering factors responsible for the failure of the remodeling processes. Therapy can then be targeted either toward augmenting the host's defensive system (not yet possible) or toward ameliorating local, aggressive "offensive" factors leading to the aneurysm. The ultimate goal is to stimulate the vascular remodeling system to repair the local injury to the vessel wall triggered by the offensive insult. Spontaneous resolution of berry-like aneurysms, seen after correction of abnormal flow dynamics, holds the promise of such therapy in the future (Fig. 23-4).

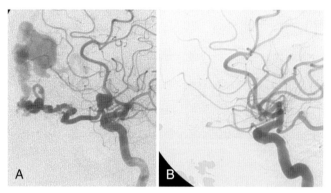

■ **FIGURE 23-4** **A** and **B,** Spontaneous resolution of an ophthalmic artery aneurysm that was associated with a high-flow shunting lesion of the ophthalmic artery that spontaneously regressed after occlusion of the shunt. This example testifies for the repair system of the vascular system after removing locally aggressive factors.

Clinical Presentation

Most saccular aneurysms of the intracranial circulation remain undetected until they rupture and present as SAH. Arterial aneurysms are the most important cause of primary nontraumatic SAH and account for 65% to 85% of all SAH (Fig. 23-5). After acute SAH, recurrent hemorrhage from the aneurysm poses continued serious threat to the patient, with an estimated risk of re-rupture of more than 20% at 2 weeks and 40% at 6 months. Therefore, treatment of ruptured aneurysms is mandatory.

Patients typically complain about a history of abrupt onset of the "worst headache of their life." Loss of consciousness, meningismus, focal neurologic deficits, and nausea may be present. Many patients report earlier, milder headaches over the days preceding the acute event, most likely representing small "sentinel bleeds" from an unstable aneurysm. In a large series of ruptured intracranial saccular aneurysm, a significantly higher rate of rebleeding was found in patients with poor overall clinical status compared with those with good clinical status.

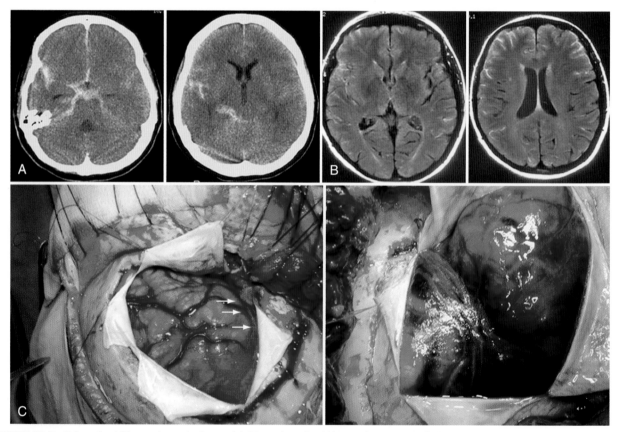

■ **FIGURE 23-5** Subarachnoid hemorrhage. **A,** On cranial CT, a subarachnoid hemorrhage is typically hyperdense and fills the subarachnoid spaces. **B,** On FLAIR-weighted images, blood in the subarachnoid space fails to suppress like usual CSF and is therefore bright as well. The distribution of blood may shed light on the location of the aneurysm, which may be of special importance in the presence of multiple aneurysms. **C,** Intraoperative photos following opening of the dura, with extensive blood in the subarachnoid space and brain swelling ("angry brain").

TABLE 23-1. Five-Year Cumulative Percentage Risk of Rupture of Previously Unruptured Aneurysms According to the ISUIA Study

Aneurysm Size vs. Localization	<7 mm*	7-12 mm	13-24 mm	>24 mm
Intracavernous ICA	0	0	3.0%	6.4%
Other ICA, MCA, ACA	0 (1.5%)	2.6%	14.5%	40.0%
Posterior circulation and posterior communicating artery	2.5% (3.4%)	14.5%	18.4%	50.0%

*The numbers in parentheses denote the cumulative risk if a previous subarachnoid hemorrhage has occurred from a different aneurysm.

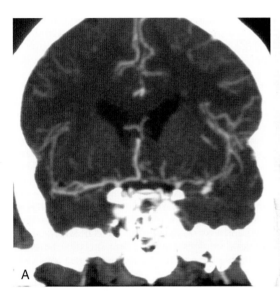 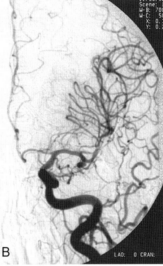

■ **FIGURE 23-6** CTA (**A**) and DSA (**B**) in the detection of a small MCA aneurysm. The major advantages of CTA over other angiographic methods is its added information about the surrounding bony structures, the possible detection of associated calcifications close to the aneurysm neck, the depiction of extraluminal parts of the aneurysms (such as present in partially thrombosed aneurysms), and the accurate 3D demonstration of the aneurysm and its neck. Because CTA is widely available and CT is the first diagnostic choice to detect subarachnoid hemorrhage, many centers perform CTA immediately after CT detection of a subarachnoid hemorrhage for subsequent treatment planning.

The clinical consequences of SAH are so severe that emphasis should be placed on the prevention of rupture once the aneurysms are detected incidentally. Therefore, it is useful to identify factors that stabilize or destabilize the aneurysm. Factors known to predict increased risk of future hemorrhage include prior SAH from a different aneurysm, large aneurysm size, and location in the posterior circulation, as shown by the International Study of Unruptured Intracranial Aneurysms (ISUIA) study (Table 23-1). Additional factors suggesting increased risk of rupture include familial SAH, smoking, specific aneurysm morphology (e.g., multilobulated berry aneurysms with "daughter" aneurysms or aneurysmal "blebs"), multiplicity of aneurysms, and the presence of arterial variations in the vicinity of an aneurysm (pointing toward an incomplete maturation that may preserve "weaker" cells that may be more prone to rupture).

Despite the known risk of complications from an intracranial aneurysm, the decision not to intervene should certainly be considered in the appropriate clinical circumstances. Once treatment is considered, the choice of treatment should consider first the patient's needs and, second, the quality of the treatment available at a given center. One should therefore avoid quoting results reported in the literature that may not reflect the individual physician's experience. Treatment options include surgical clipping and endovascular therapies (e.g., coiling). Depending on the configuration of the aneurysm, additional endovascular techniques such as the balloon remodeling technique or stenting have been proposed. Over the course of the last years, especially since the results of the International Subarachnoid Aneurysm Trial (ISAT) have been published, the endovascular treatment of cerebral aneurysms has gained more and more importance, not only in those aneurysms that are difficult to access surgically (i.e., those in the posterior circulation) but also in uncomplicated aneurysms of the anterior circulation. It was found that patients harboring ruptured aneurysms that were rated by both the neurosurgeon and the interventional neuroradiologist as possible candidates for their respective therapies had better outcomes concerning morbidity, dependency, and mortality when being treated endovascularly at the 2- and 12-month follow-up evaluations. However, the risk of aneurysm recurrence and even rebleeding is higher in coiled aneurysms than in clipped ones, requiring follow-up imaging in specific intervals. Whether this increased risk is counterbalanced by the better immediate outcome after endovascular treatment remains a matter of debate.

Imaging
CT and CTA
CT is a widely available, noninvasive method to detect aneurysms and their major associated complications such as SAH, intraparenchymal hemorrhage, and acute hydrocephalus. CT angiography (CTA) is extremely fast, relatively free from motion artifact, and particularly suitable for an emergency situation with an unstable patient. It is not painful, requires little to no sedation to obtain a diagnostic study, and typically uses limited numbers of personnel, who are usually already in place within the hospital at the time required.

Multislice CT (MSCT) is a technique in which scanning is performed continuously as the CT table is drawn through the gantry (helical or spiral scanning). At least two rows of detector elements (and, at present, as many as 320 rows of detector elements) are employed in the z-axis to create almost isotropic voxels. Although there is no standard protocol, the technique typically entails injection of high-concentration (300 to 400 mg/mL) iodinated contrast media at a dose of 1 to 2 mL/kg. Injection is made through an antecubital vein at a flow of 3 to 5 mL/s up to a total of 60 to 100 mL. The scanned region extends from the C1 vertebra to the vertex. What slice thickness is possible depends on scanner performance (Fig. 23-6). Generally, slice thickness ranges from 0.5 to 1.25 mm, with a reconstruction interval of up to 0.6 mm. In many centers, a scan is started using a triggering technique to optimize acquisition of early arterial phase images. After real-time CT bolus tracking, the region of interest is placed at the internal carotid artery, and scanning is started automatically when the contrast agent in the ICA reaches 80 Hounsfield units (HU). With the use of triggering and real-time CT the increased attenuation of acute subarachnoid blood has no effect on the ability to define the vessels during 3D reconstruction, because it remains lower than the attenuation of the enhanced vessels in all cases. With this technique even small vascular structures can be imaged. The CT data can then be reconstructed to produce maximum intensity projection (MIP) or 3D representations employing shaded surface displays (SSD) or volume rendering techniques (VRT). The main drawback of the MIP images is vessel superposition, which may impair appreciation of vessel relationships. Multiplanar reconstructions of variable thickness may overcome superposition problems. The VRT allows direct 3D analysis; however, bone or venous superposition in the cavernous sinus region may render carotid siphon or posterior communicating artery aneurysms difficult to appreciate. Compared with single-slice CT, the concurrent acquisition of multiple slices and the superior resolution in z-axis in MSCT allows for a dramatic reduction of scanning time and an improvement of visualization of aneurysms.

All studies that compare CTA with digital subtraction angiography (DSA)—the current gold standard for aneurysm detection—have found that the sensitivity for detecting aneurysms is strongly dependent on the size and location of the aneurysms. Large and medium-sized aneurysms are detected by MSCT in nearly 100% of cases. Small and even medium-sized aneurysms that arise from the intracavernous or supraclinoid carotid artery may be obscured by bony structures or the cavernous sinus and are detected less often. Detection rates vary from 75% to 98% according to different sources. Although further advances with new generation CTs can be anticipated, some aneurysms smaller than 3 mm and close to the carotid siphon near the clinoid processes may still be missed even with the latest CTA technology. Therefore, the negative predictive value is still inadequate, so patients with clinical suspicion but negative CT angiograms will still go on to DSA. DSA can also disclose uncommon causes of SAH, such as dural arteriovenous fistulas, vasculitis, small and micro AVMs, and transmural dissections, which can be missed by CTA. Positive CTA findings, however, show a high specificity and may provide sufficient information to plan therapy, obviating DSA. In our opinion, CTA is the method of choice for studying acutely ruptured aneurysms since it provides immediate triage in the emergency setting.

MRI and MRA

MR pulse sequences can exploit blood motion to visualize vascular structures directly and without the use of intravascular contrast material. However, MRI and MR angiography (MRA) are seldom used in the setting of acutely ruptured aneurysms because patient monitoring may be difficult, imaging time is typically more extended compared with CT, the field of view is often limited, and specific MR artifacts (discussed later) are likely to result in a lower sensitivity and specificity of aneurysm detection. Although T2-weighted (T2W) fluid-attenuated inversion recovery (FLAIR) sequences are supposed to detect SAH (see Fig. 23-5), artifacts in the perimesencephalic cistern are often present that make identification of true SAH difficult. Nonetheless, MRA may still be useful for screening and follow-up of previously detected aneurysms, because it is noninvasive, uses no ionizing radiation, and requires no iodinated contrast media.

As with any imaging technique, MRA has its own artifacts and problems, which must be recognized to avoid misdiagnosis. MRA usually displays normal anatomy accurately. In the presence of vascular disease, especially aneurysms, however, techni-cal shortcomings may cause inaccurate depiction of aneurysm size, configuration, and neck morphology, all of which are important characteristics for choosing the appropriate therapy.

Three different MRA techniques may be employed to detect cerebral aneurysms: time-of-flight (TOF) MRA, phase-contrast (PC) MRA, and 3D contrast-enhanced (CE) MRA.

TOF MRA is usually performed using a flow-compensated gradient-refocused sequence to "saturate" stationary tissues, causing them to show only low signal intensity. Blood upstream of the imaging volume, however, is "unsaturated." When the unsaturated blood flows into the imaging volume, it is bright compared with the saturated stationary background tissues.

PC MRA creates images by depicting the shifts induced in the phases of moving spins as the blood flows in the presence of "flow-encoding" gradients. Using phase difference images, the signal intensity of the phase shift is proportional to the vector velocity of flow perpendicular to the image plane and stationary background tissue is suppressed. The flow-encoding gradients can be applied in any or multiple directions depending on the desired flow sensitivity.

Although both PC MRA and TOF MRA can visualize normal vessel anatomy, there are intrinsic problems that may degrade MRA quality, especially for aneurysm detection. These problems are complex flow, slow flow, flow stasis and recirculation, and thrombus visualization. These artifacts are more pronounced in small aneurysms (<5 mm). Complex flow due to turbulence, eddy currents, and nonlaminar or vortex flow result in intravoxel phase dispersion and loss of signal on both TOF MRA and PC MRA. PC sequences are sensitive only to a specified range of velocities. Within the aneurysm dome, turbulence causes a broad spectrum of rapidly changing velocities, which, in turn, causes intravoxel phase dispersion and signal loss. The signal loss can potentially lead to misjudgment of the size of the aneurysm. 3D TOF is less affected by complex flow signal loss because of small voxel size and shorter echo time. Concerning slow flow, it is known that flow near the aneurysm dome is often significantly reduced. Recirculation or even flow stasis may occur. The reduced velocities cause increased saturation effects within the imaging volume and decreased signal intensity within the vessel lumen. Intraluminal signal may even become imperceptible and, therefore, lead to a misjudgment in the size of the aneurysm. Flow stasis and recirculation result in signal loss due to saturation effects and intravoxel dephasing. Slow-flow signal loss is particularly a problem with 3D TOF imaging of vessels deep within the imaging volume. The MIP processing technique contributes to the problem because it ignores signal intensities that fall below a certain threshold. With PC techniques, normally effective arterial velocity encoding factors may fail to image slow flow within an aneurysm. Thrombus and tissues with short T1 relaxation times such as fat or blood degradation products can interfere with vascular imaging. Methemoglobin within thrombus has a short T1 relaxation time and generates high signal on TOF images, simulating intraluminal flow, therefore overestimating the size of the aneurysm lumen. Both TOF MRA and PC MRA are subject to signal loss from the magnetic susceptibility effects of deoxyhemoglobin and hemosiderin/ferritin. The patent lumen of the aneurysm may be obscured or the margins of the residual lumen may appear indistinct. Likewise, other tissues with short T1 relaxation times (i.e., fat) may mimic flow on TOF MRA.

Many of these problems can be overcome with CE MRA, which is performed in a manner analogous to conventional contrast angiography. Instead of relying on blood motion to create intravascular signal, a contrast agent is introduced to change the T1 relaxation of blood. Blood can be directly imaged regardless of flow, which alleviates many of the problems inherent to TOF and PC angiography. Contrast medium can reduce spin saturation due to its T1 shortening effect. Shorter echo time then diminishes phase dispersion. Therefore, sensitivity to turbulence is dramatically reduced and in-plane saturation effects are eliminated. The technique allows a small number of slices oriented in the plane of the vessels of interest to image an extensive region of vascular anatomy (equal to the field of view) in a short period of time. At present the major shortcoming of CE MRA is its limited spatial resolution. Small aneurysms are likely to remain undetected using this technique. With the different MR angiographies, sensitivities and specificities of 50% to 100% have been reported depending on the cited source, the technique used, the reconstruction algorithm used, and the employed field strength.

In our practice, we use TOF techniques for screening and evaluating unruptured aneurysms for neck morphology and aneurysm configuration. We especially rely on the raw TOF MRA data. For the follow-up of treated aneurysms both TOF and contrast-enhanced MRA techniques may be helpful.

DSA and 3D DSA

Despite recent advances in noninvasive diagnostic vascular neuroimaging by CTA and MRA, diagnostic cerebral angiography combined with 3D rotational angiography remains the "gold standard" for evaluating patients presenting with SAH and suspected intracranial aneurysms. DSA and 3D DSA have the highest temporal and spatial resolution and provide the most precise depictions of intracranial vessel morphology and hemodynamic analysis.

In SAH, the aim of diagnostic angiography is to demonstrate or to confirm the presence of an aneurysm and to provide detailed anatomic and hemodynamic information for planning of endovascular or surgical treatment, including precise morphology and size of the aneurysm neck and dome and the presence and location of any perforating vessels arising in relation to the aneurysm. These techniques also demonstrate any concurrent vasospasm, additional aneurysms, or associated vascular lesions. Should the studies prove negative for aneurysm, they must then address vasculitis, cranial dural arteriovenous fistulas, and sinus thrombosis as possible alternate causes for hemorrhage.

Diagnostic angiography after SAH typically requires injections into each of the four major vessels: both internal carotid arteries and both vertebral arteries. However, if injection of a single vertebral artery opacifies the contralateral vertebral artery sufficiently by retrograde filling, with excellent depiction of the intradural segments of the opposite vertebral and the posteroinferior cerebellar arteries, then three-vessel injection may be sufficient. Conversely, if no aneurysm has been detected by four-vessel angiography, the study must be extended to depict both external carotid arteries (six-vessel study) to rule out a dural arteriovenous shunt as the possible cause of the SAH. The global vessel examination usually begins with biplane anteroposterior and lateral acquisitions, using a field of view large enough to cover the intradural arteries and draining sinuses. For aneurysmal detection and pretherapeutic planning, additional 3D angiography is considered the gold standard. If it is not available, additional oblique views with magnification should be obtained for aneurysm detection and detailed pretherapeutic morphologic analysis. The volume of contrast medium injected should be adapted to the vessel caliber and the hemodynamic conditions and may be 9 mL with a flow of 3 mL/s for the internal carotid artery and 12 mL with a flow of 4 mL/s for a large-caliber vertebral artery, allowing reflux in the opposite intracranial vertebral segment. Films are typically acquired at a rate of three frames per second for the arterial phase and may be decreased for the venous phase. Flat panel technology allows for nondistorted high-quality images and a reduced radiation dose. For 3D rotational angiography, an angiographic C-arm rotation around the patient's head is necessary. Typically, this rotation covers a total angular range of 200 degrees at a speed of 40 degrees/s. A "mask" rotation is performed first to provide a subtraction mask, after which 15 to 20 mL of contrast medium is injected selectively in the studied artery throughout the second rotation. These subtracted images are transferred for further evaluation to a workstation in which volume renderings, surface renderings, and virtual endoscopic views can be generated using dedicated software. This technique provides a precise delineation of the aneurysm in relation to the parent vessel and possible perforators and an optimal analysis of its neck and dome characteristics. Because each 3D projection is defined in space by two angles that appear on the computer screen, the optimal working view for endovascular treatment can be determined. Some artifacts may degrade 3D rotational angiography. Patient movements during rotational acquisition will degrade 3D reconstruction. Metallic objects such as previously placed aneurysm coils may render appreciation of the truly filled aneurysmal lumen difficult. Large aneurysms may fill only partially during rotational acquisition, resulting in incomplete reconstruction and underestimation of lumen size on 3D angiography. Less often, an anterior communicating artery aneurysm may not be visualized clearly on 3D angiography because of flow competition phenomenon from the contralateral A1. Finally, windowing may artificially enlarge or reduce the size of an aneurysm or its neck.

The high diagnostic accuracy of DSA, however, must be weighed against the risk of permanent or transient neurologic deficits, silent microemboli, or potential non-neurologic risks as a direct result of performing the DSA. Non-neurologic risks are mainly hematomas at the puncture site. Most of these are minor hematomas. However, hematomas necessitating blood transfusion or surgery, peripheral emboli, and arteriovenous fistulas may also happen. Other general risks include risks related to iodinated contrast media, especially allergy and nephrotoxicity, and concerns about the radiation dose. The most important risks are neurologic complications related to the angiography. Rates are reported to be as high as 1.8% for angiographies performed for diagnostic workup of SAH and 0.3% for angiographies performed for the diagnostic workup of unruptured aneurysms. Patients with associated atherosclerotic cerebrovascular disease have a higher risk of stroke or silent microemboli from diagnostic cerebral angiography that may be related to difficulties in probing the vessels (elongation of vessels), the presence of fragile arteriosclerotic plaques that might be scraped off the vessel wall (especially during the inversion maneuver when using a Simmons catheter), and the instability of fresh thrombus within ulcerating plaques, which might embolize during the contrast agent injection. Dissections by the catheter or the guidewire may also account for the just-mentioned neurologic deficits.

Despite these considerable risks, in our practice we use DSA and 3D DSA for the workup of all intracranial aneurysms to get the most precise structural and hemodynamic information before an endovascular or neurosurgical procedure. The best working position and the exact aneurysm dimensions can be evaluated, and potential complications of the SAH (vasospasm) or associated vascular diseases can be evaluated.

Differential Diagnosis

Aneurysm Distribution

Aneurysms typically arise at branch points on the parent artery. The branch point may be formed by the origin of a side branch from the parent artery (e.g., posterior communicating artery) or by subdivision of a main arterial trunk into two trunks (e.g., MCA or terminal ICA bifurcation, tip of the basilar trunk). Sidewall aneurysms are rare and if present usually arise at a turn or curve in the artery and point in the direction that the blood would have gone if the curve was not present. At both the branch points and the curves, local alterations in intravascular hemodynamics are present that exert high shear stress forces on those regions that receive the greatest force of the pulse wave. Therefore, the aneurysm dome typically points in the direction of the maximal hemodynamic thrust in the pre-aneurysmal segment of the parent artery. Aneurysms that are encountered on a straight, nonbranching segment of an intracranial artery should raise the suspicion of a dissecting process, because saccular aneurysms are infrequently encountered at these sites. More than 90% of all saccular intracranial aneurysms are located at one of the following five sites:

● Internal carotid artery at the origin of the posterior communicating artery
● Junction of the anterior cerebral artery (ACA) and anterior communicating artery
● Proximal bifurcation of the MCA
● Terminal bifurcation of the basilar artery into posterior cerebral arteries
● Terminal bifurcation of the carotid artery into the ACA and MCA

In the anterior circulation, other common sites of aneurysms are the origins of the ophthalmic, superior hypophysial, and anterior choroidal arteries. In the posterior circulation the origin of the posterior inferior cerebellar artery (PICA), anterior inferior cerebellar artery (AICA), and the superior cerebellar artery (SCA) and the junction of the basilar and vertebral arteries are likely sites of aneurysm formation.

The size, configuration, and neck morphology of the aneurysm and the location of adjacent perforating arteries are important determinants in the decision whether to treat by neurosurgical approaches (e.g., clipping of the aneurysm) or by endovascular techniques (e.g., coiling) and, if endovascular, what kinds of devices and techniques to employ for the procedure. Therefore, the size, configuration, and neck morphology of the aneurysm and the location of adjacent perforating arteries should be described meticulously in the report.

Supraclinoid Segment of the Internal Carotid Artery
Aneurysms most commonly form along the supraclinoid segment of the ICA immediately distal to the origins of each large branch. Overall, 35% of all intracranial aneurysms arise at five sites along the supraclinoid segment of the ICA:

● The upper surface of the ICA at the origin of the ophthalmic artery (supraophthalmic aneurysms) (~5%)
● The medial wall of the ICA at the origin of the superior hypophysial artery (hypophysial artery aneurysms) (~1%)
● The posterior wall of the ICA superolateral to the origin of the posterior communicating artery (posterior communicating aneurysms) (~25%)
● The posterior wall of the ICA immediately superior to the origin of the anterior choroidal artery (anterior choroidal artery aneurysms) (~5%)
● The apex of the terminal ICA bifurcation into the ACA and MCA (carotid bifurcation aneurysms) (~5%)

Supraophthalmic Artery and Superior Hypophysial Artery Aneurysms
Aneurysms arising from the ICA close to the ophthalmic artery constitute about 5% of all intracranial aneurysms and are more frequent in women than men. They typically arise from the superior wall of the carotid artery at the distal edge of the origin of the ophthalmic artery close to the roof of the cavernous sinus (Figs. 23-7 to 23-9). At this point, the ICA changes direction from superior toward posterior, so the maximal hemodynamic force is directed toward the superior wall of the carotid artery just distal to the ophthalmic artery. Therefore, these aneurysms project upward toward the optic nerve. Supraophthalmic aneurysms are easily approached endovascularly but may be complicated to expose surgically, because the ophthalmic artery has a variable origin and course and because multiple folds of the dura enclose the region of the optic foramen and clinoid process. Supraophthalmic aneurysms are often large with complex, multilobulated shape. Many are wide-necked aneurysms that may require remodeling techniques. Unruptured aneurysms may become symptomatic due to headaches or compression of cranial nerves.

Superior hypophysial artery aneurysms arise just distal to the origin of the superior hypophysial artery from the medial or posterior wall of the ICA where the curvature of the ICA is convex medially (Fig. 23-10). In this location they lie lateral to the pituitary stalk and point medially under the optic chiasm. Medial expansion of the aneurysm may compromise the perforating arteries to the floor of the third ventricle, the optic nerves, the chiasm, the pituitary stalk, and the hypophysial vascular supply.

Posterior Communicating and Anterior Choroidal Artery Aneurysms
The posterior communicating and anterior choroidal arteries arise from the posterior wall of the ICA, where the ICA forms a posteriorly convex curve as it ascends to its terminal bifurcation under the anterior perforated substance. The most frequent ICA aneurysm is the posterior communicating artery aneurysm, which constitutes about 25% of all intracranial aneurysms (Figs. 23-11 to 23-14). These aneurysms arise near the apex of the posteriorly convex turn, immediately superior to the distal edge of the origin of the posterior communicating artery. They point downward and posteriorly toward the oculomotor nerve, so the posterior communicating artery is usually found inferomedial to the neck of the aneurysm and the anterior choroidal artery is found superior or superolateral to the neck of the aneurysm. The oculomotor nerve enters the dural roof of the cavernous sinus lateral to the posterior clinoid process and medial to a dural band that runs between the tentorium cerebelli and the anterior clinoid process. Posterior communicating artery aneurysms larger than 4 to 5 mm may compress the oculomotor nerve at its entrance into the dural roof, causing ophthalmoplegia.

Should the posteriorly convex curve of the supraclinoid ICA form its apex at the level of the anterior choroidal artery the hemodynamic force is shifted distally from the origin of the posterior communicating artery to the origin of the anterior choroidal artery. The anterior choroidal aneurysms form just distal, superior, or superolateral to the origin of the anterior choroidal artery and account for about 5% of all intracranial aneurysms (Fig. 23-15). Similar to posterior communicating artery aneurysms, anterior choroidal artery aneurysms also point posterior or posterolaterally but are usually well above the oculomotor nerve. Aneurysms arising from the choroidal segment commonly have more perforating branches stretched around their neck than those arising from the communicating or ophthalmic segment, because the choroidal segment has a greater number of perforating branches arising from it and the majority arise from the posterior wall, where the neck of the aneurysm is situated.

Carotid Bifurcation Aneurysms
Aneurysms of the carotid bifurcation are the second most common supraclinoid ICA aneurysm and account for about 5% of all intracranial aneurysms. They arise at the apex of the T-shaped bifurcation and point superiorly in the direction of the long axis of the pre-bifurcation segment of the artery. As they grow, they lie lateral to the optic chiasm and may indent the

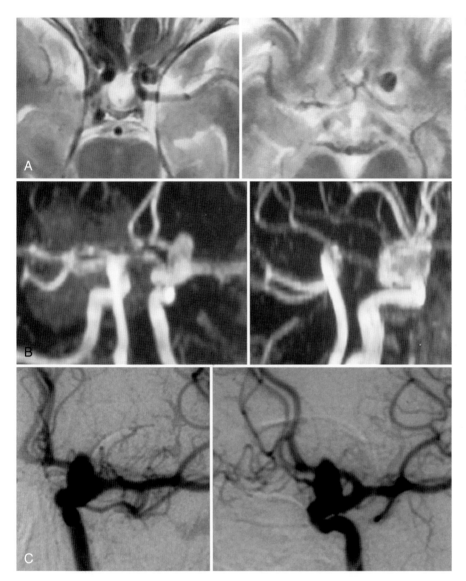

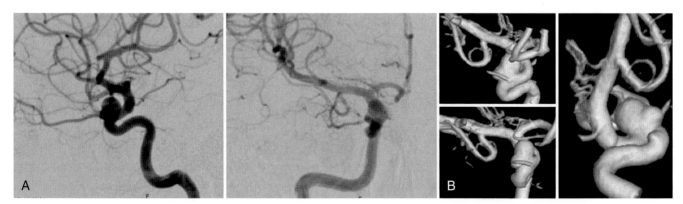

■ **FIGURE 23-8** **A,** Supraophthalmic ICA aneurysms are often broad based and typically large. The origin of the ophthalmic artery has to be specially considered to avoid erratic emboli entering the artery during endovascular therapies. **B,** Most often, 3D rotational angiography is necessary to determine the exact localization of the artery in relation to the neck of the aneurysm.

■ **FIGURE 23-9** A to D, Small-necked large aneurysm of the ICA at the origin of the ophthalmic artery. Typically these aneurysms point superiorly owing to the hemodynamic thrust in this vessel segment.

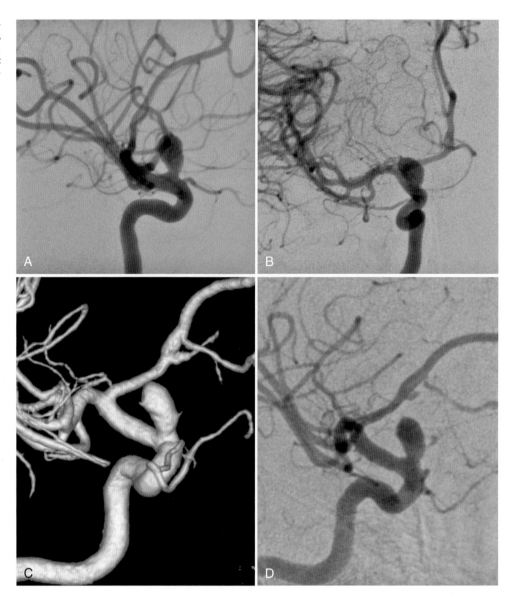

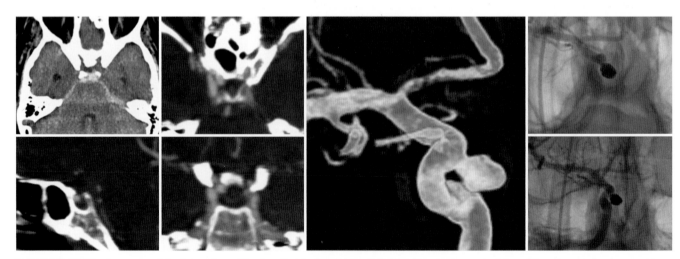

■ **FIGURE 23-10** Aneurysm of the internal carotid artery that is directed medially into the superior part of the sella and most closely resembles a superior hypophysial artery aneurysm that in this patient led to a circumscribed subarachnoid hemorrhage, because the superior aspect of the aneurysm is not completely extradural but points toward the dural fold surrounding the cavernous sinus. CTA is especially helpful to detect the close spatial relationship between the aneurysm and the bone, whereas 3D rotational angiography can plan the subsequent endovascular treatment that was carried out with a complete and dense coil packing in this patient.

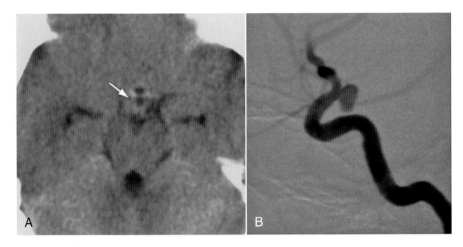

■ **FIGURE 23-11** This patient had a sudden oculomotor nerve palsy on the right side. **A,** Nonenhanced CTA demonstrated a dense structure within the subarachnoid spaces within the pentagon of the basal cisterns (*arrow*). Because of the clinical presentation and this suspicious CT finding, DSA was performed that demonstrated a typical posterior communicating artery aneurysm (**B**), that, owing to its downward and posterior direction, had led to irritation of the third cranial nerve.

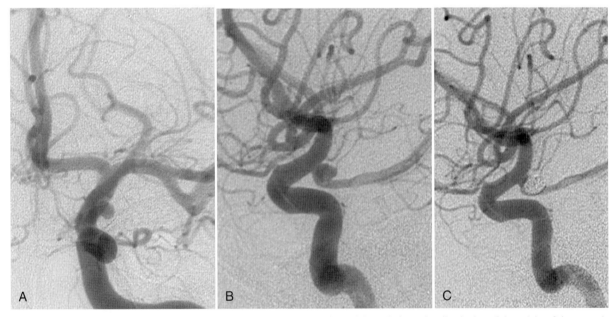

■ **FIGURE 23-12** A to C, Classic posterior communicating artery aneurysm that originated above the distal edge of the origin of the posterior communicating artery that is found inferomedial to the aneurysm. Endovascular therapy was performed that resulted in complete occlusion of the aneurysm with preservation of the parent artery.

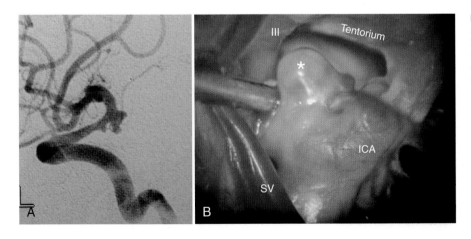

■ **FIGURE 23-13** DSA (**A**) and corresponding surgical aspect (**B**) of a posterior communicating artery aneurysm (*asterisk*) and its close spatial relationship to the oculomotor nerve (III) and the tentorium cerebelli. ICA, internal carotid artery; SV, sylvian vein.

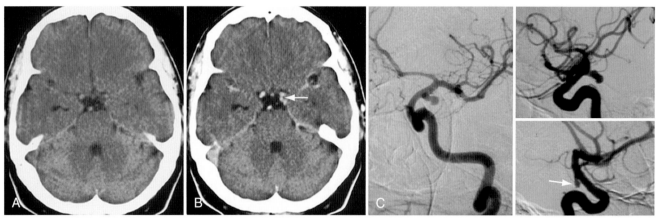

■ **FIGURE 23-14**   Unenhanced (**A**) and enhanced (**B**) cranial CT images in a patient with a spontaneous oculomotor nerve palsy on the left side demonstrating an "additional" vessel within the pentagon of the basal cisterns (*arrow* in B) that was found to be a classic posterior communicating artery aneurysm on DSA (**C**). Of note is a mirror or "twin" aneurysm on the contralateral side at exactly the same location (*arrow* in C).

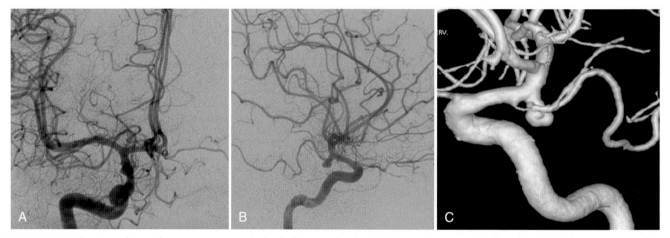

■ **FIGURE 23-15**   Internal carotid artery aneurysm at the level of the anterior choroidal artery that may arise when the posteriorly convex curve of the supraclinoid ICA is located at the level of the origin of the anterior choroidal artery, which shifts the hemodynamic force distally from the level of origin of the posterior communicating artery to that of the anterior choroidal artery. Aneurysms located at this site are just distal, superior, or superolateral to the origin of the anterior choroidal artery.

undersurface of the anterior perforated substance (Figs. 23-16 to 23-19). The perforating branches arising from the choroidal segment of the internal carotid and the proximal segments of the anterior and middle cerebral arteries are stretched around the posterior aspect of the neck and wall of the aneurysm.

Anterior Cerebral Artery Aneurysms

Aneurysms of the ACA typically form close to the anterior communicating artery complex. They constitute about 30% of all intracranial aneurysms and are considered one of the most common types of aneurysm (Figs. 23-20 to 23-26). They are frequently associated with variants of anatomy. The segment of the ACA between the ICA and the anterior communicating artery is referred to as the A1 segment. The segment between the anterior communicating artery and the rostrum of the corpus callosum is referred to as the A2 segment. Aneurysms often occur when one A1 segment is hypoplastic and the dominant A1 gives rise to both A2s. In such case, the aneurysm arises at the level of the anterior communicating artery at the point where the dominant A1 segment bifurcates to give rise to both the left and right A2 segments. The direction in which the dome of the aneurysm points is determined by the course of the dominant A1 segment proximal to its junction with the anterior com-

municating artery. Thus, these aneurysms usually point away from the dominant segment toward the opposite side. When the A1 segment is tortuous, they may also project in other directions. Approaches to anterior communicating artery aneurysms must ensure that the anterior communicating artery and the adjacent recurrent artery of Heubner remain patent. The anterior communicating artery gives rise to small perforating branches for the dorsal surface of the optic chiasm and suprachiasmatic area that perfuse the fornix, corpus callosum, and septal region. Occlusion of the anterior communicating artery may lead to personality disorders, even if both A2 segments are perfused from their respective A1 segments. The recurrent artery of Heubner arises, variably, from the distal A1, the proximal A2, or the frontopolar branch of the ACA. The artery then pursues a long, redundant path, looping forward on the gyrus rectus or the posterior part of the orbital surface of the frontal lobe and then passing back over the carotid bifurcation to accompany the MCA and enter the anterior perforating substance. Occlusion of the recurrent artery of Heubner may cause hemiparesis or aphasia.

The second most common aneurysm of the ACA is the so-called pericallosal aneurysm, which arises at the origin of the callosomarginal artery from the pericallosal artery, usually in close proximity to the anterior portion of the corpus callosum,

Text continued on page 500

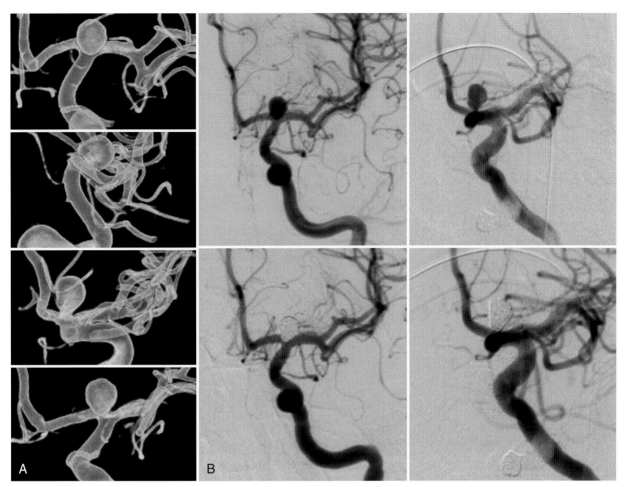

■ **FIGURE 23-16** **A** and **B,** A 21-year-old woman complained about persistent headaches and was referred for MRI, which demonstrated a 7-mm, small-necked, round aneurysm of the bifurcation of the carotid artery. The gender, the young age, the easy accessibility, and the fact that the patient was a rather heavy smoker prompted endovascular intervention that was performed without complications and with complete and stable occlusion of the aneurysm. The 3D reconstruction allows for the best endovascular view for subsequent treatment. These aneurysms are typically directed upward and anterior.

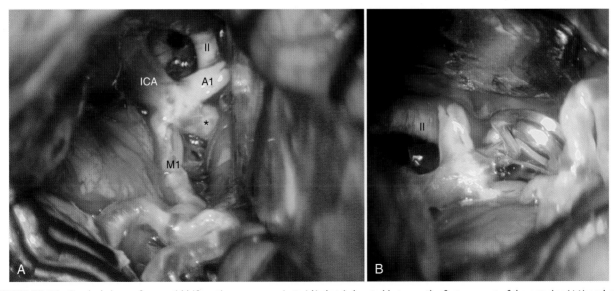

■ **FIGURE 23-17** Surgical views of a carotid bifurcation aneurysm (*asterisk*) that is located between the first segment of the anterior (A1) and middle cerebral artery (M1). The symbol II indicates the optic nerve both before (**A**) and after (**B**) surgical clipping with complete and stable occlusion of the aneurysm.

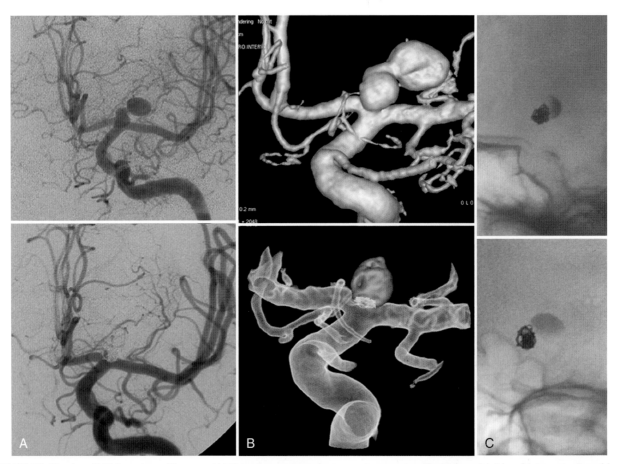

■ **FIGURE 23-18** **A to C,** This patient with a carotid bifurcation aneurysm became symptomatic with a subarachnoid and intraparenchymal hemorrhage. On angiography an aneurysm can be seen that is associated with a bleb-like secondary, or daughter, aneurysm. In most instances, these daughter
aneurysms represent the site of rupture and have a highly vulnerable wall. In some instances they may even represent false aneurysms, and endovascular
procedures aimed at coiling this segment should be avoided because they carry a high risk of periprocedural re-rupture. Instead, the parent aneurysm
should be treated with a very dense packing of the coils, as demonstrated in this example that led to occlusion of both the aneurysm and the false sac
associated with the aneurysm. The fluoroscopy after completion of the endovascular procedure demonstrates contrast material stasis within the false
sac suggestive that subsequent thrombosis will occur here. No rebleeding occurred and the patient was stable at 12-month follow-up with no aneurysm
recurrence.

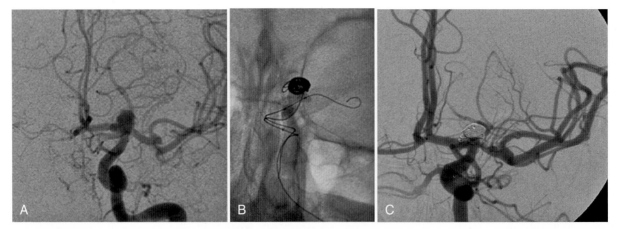

■ **FIGURE 23-19** **A to F,** Some carotid bifurcation aneurysms may have an unfavorable neck-to-dome ratio that necessitates balloon remodeling
techniques, as demonstrated in this example: The balloon is advanced via a J-shaped guidewire (which is less aggressive and less prone to distal perforations than a straight guidewire) and inflated during the coiling procedure, which enables stable position of the coils and the microcatheter within the
aneurysm during coiling.

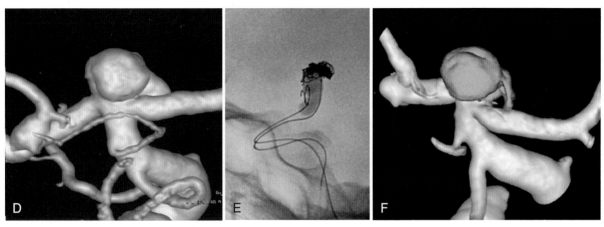

■ FIGURE 23-19, cont'd For legend see opposite page.

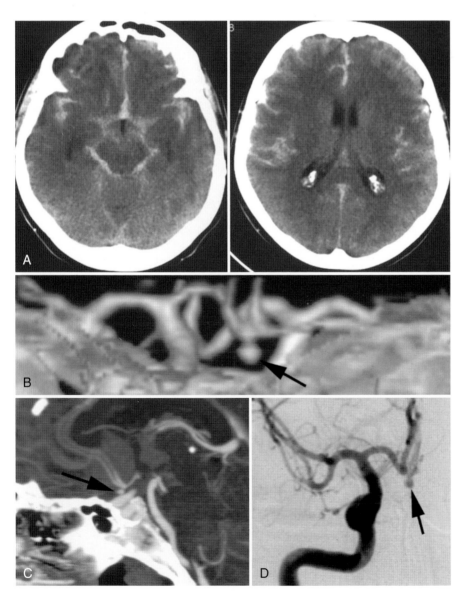

■ FIGURE 23-20 A to D, Ruptured anterior communicating artery aneurysm. CT typically displays a bilaterally symmetric distribution of blood, with blood along the interhemispheric fissure and along the corpus callosum. CTA demonstrates both in the 3D and sagittal 2D reconstructions the aneurysm with a defined neck that is pointed downward and anterior (*arrow*, **D**).

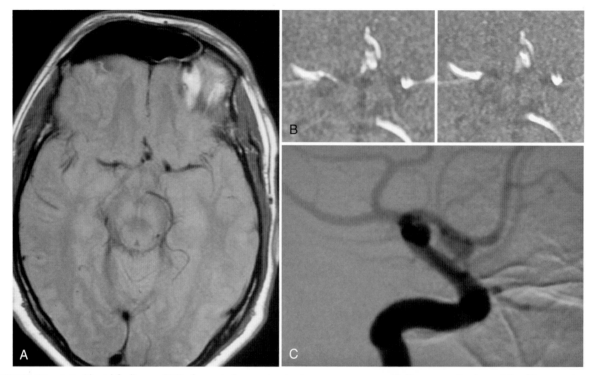

■ **FIGURE 23-21** **A,** Incidental finding on MRI of an anterior communicating artery aneurysm. **B,** On proton density–weighted images, the aneurysm can be seen as a flow void between both A2 segments that is well appreciated on the raw data of the TOF MRA and confirmed during angiography (**C**).

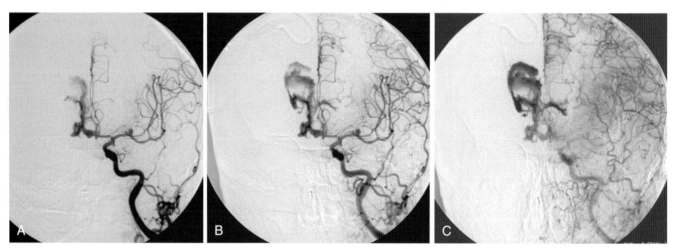

■ **FIGURE 23-22** A to C, Acute rupture of an anterior communicating artery aneurysm during angiography. Before endovascular therapy could be done this patient with an acute subarachnoid hemorrhage suddenly demonstrated increased intracranial pressure. Angiography demonstrated active extravasation of contrast material into the subarachnoid spaces, suggesting acute rupture of this aneurysm.

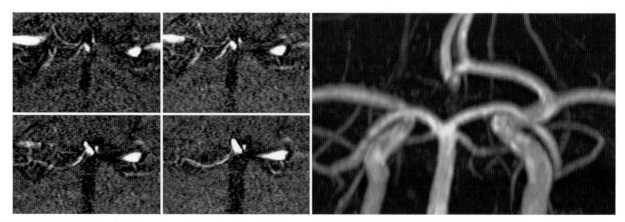

■ **FIGURE 23-23** Incidental finding of a small unruptured anterior communicating artery aneurysm in the presence of a hypoplastic A1 on the right side that predisposes for aneurysms of the anterior communicating artery complex. Although therapy is not indicated at this time because of the small size, controls with MRA are scheduled for this patient. Whenever this variant of anatomy is found, aneurysms should be specifically sought.

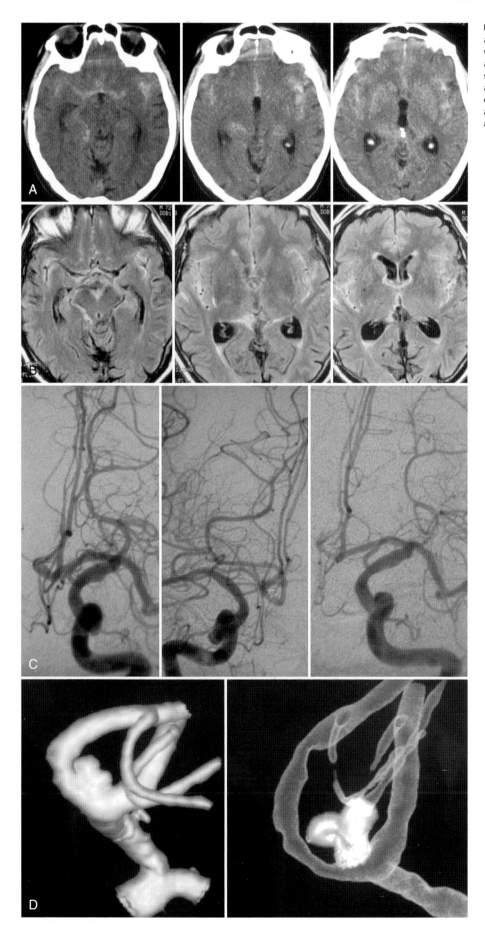

■ **FIGURE 23-24** Acutely ruptured small anterior communicating artery aneurysm with typical blood distribution on CT (**A**) and FLAIR (**B**) imaging. On DSA (**C**), a small, bilobulated anterior communicating artery aneurysm was found whose two lobules could be coiled despite the small size of the aneurysm (1.6 × 1.8 mm). **D,** 3D DSA before and after coiling.

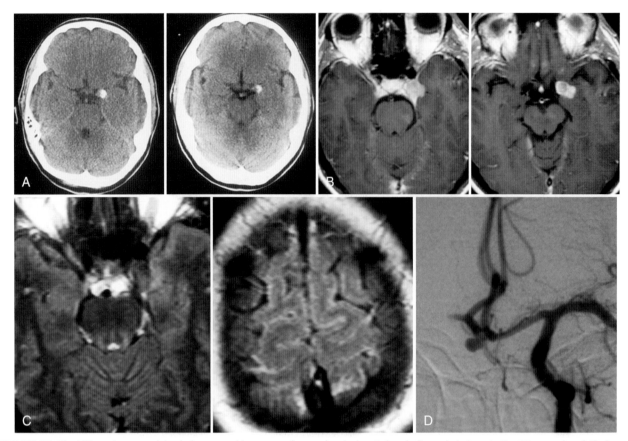

■ **FIGURE 23-25** This patient complained about a sudden onset of severe headaches 6 days before admission. **A,** On CT, a partly calcified mass of the left cavernous sinus was seen, suggesting a meningioma. Because the clinical presentation was suggestive of hemorrhage, MRI (**B** and **C**) was performed that demonstrated on FLAIR-weighted images unsuppressed CSF in the peripontine cistern and the apical subarachnoid spaces and also confirmed the diagnosis of a cavernous sinus meningioma. **D,** However, DSA was performed to rule out an aneurysm as the source of hemorrhage, which could be found in the anterior communicating artery. This case demonstrates that the clinical findings should always guide the examination.

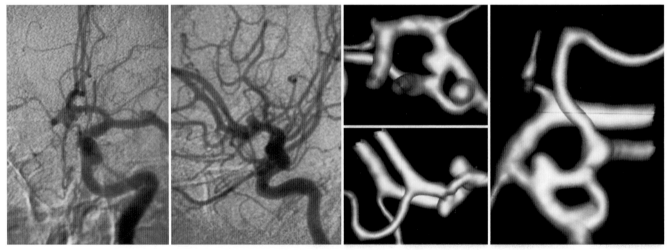

■ **FIGURE 23-26** Complex nonfusion of the anterior cerebral artery in the A1 segment with apparent duplication of the anterior communicating ramus and two associated aneurysms in statu nascendi. Anatomic variations such as these may point toward an immature vessel wall that may be more prone to aneurysm formation or to increased local shear stress forces on the vessels.

near the point where the genu of the ACA has its greatest angulation (Figs. 23-27 and 23-28). Pericallosal aneurysms account for approximately 3% of all intracranial aneurysms. They point distally into the window between the junction of the pericallosal and callosomarginal arteries.

Middle Cerebral Artery Aneurysms

Approximately 15% of all saccular aneurysms arise from the MCA. Typically they originate at the level of the first major bifurcation or trifurcation of the artery and point laterally in the direction of the long axis of the pre-bifurcation segment of the

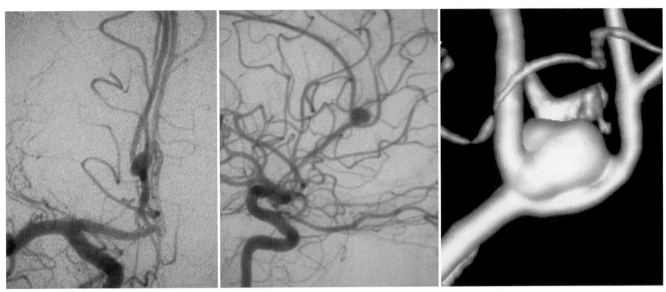

■ **FIGURE 23-27** "Pericallosal" aneurysms are aneurysms located at the origin of the callosomarginal artery from the pericallosal artery, usually in close proximity to the anterior part of the corpus callosum, near the point of greatest angulation of the artery at the genu.

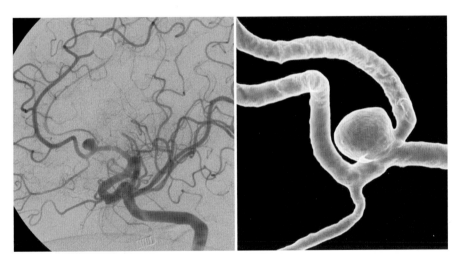

■ **FIGURE 23-28** Pericallosal aneurysm at the bifurcation of the callosomarginal and pericallosal artery. A broad neck is often encountered in these aneurysms.

MCA (Figs. 23-29 to 23-33). When unruptured, these aneurysms are typically clinically silent. The MCA branches to the anterior perforated substance are called the lenticulostriate arteries. They typically arise from the pre-bifurcation M1 segment of the MCA in three distinct groups: (1) the medial or straight group, (2) the intermediate or candelabra group (named for their complex branching pattern as they approach the anterior perforated substance), and (3) the lateral or S-shaped group (named for their curved course). Aneurysms at these sites are exceedingly rare (Fig. 23-34) and when present tend to point upward toward the anterior perforated substance. The more proximal the bifurcation, the greater the number of lenticulostriate branches arising distal to the bifurcation that may be stretched around the neck of the MCA aneurysm. Because of the many different branches present close to an MCA aneurysm, endovascular treatment in the pre-3D rotational angiography era has been considered to be rather difficult.

MCA aneurysms may also arise from the temporopolar branch of the M1 segment. When present, these tend to point inferiorly. Aneurysms distal to the MCA bifurcation are rare and are typically encountered in the setting of infectious diseases.

Vertebrobasilar System

Approximately 15% of saccular aneurysms occur in the vertebrobasilar system, the majority of which (63%) arise at the basilar bifurcation. The incidence of basilar artery aneurysms increases when the basilar system shows anomalous or variant architecture, including basilar nonfusion (fenestration), asymmetric or caudal fusion of the caudal divisions of the fetal ICA, hypoplastic communicating artery, or fetal (persistent carotid) origin of the posterior cerebral artery. Saccular aneurysms of the vertebral and basilar arteries also arise at the branch points near to the apex of a curve, point in the direction the blood would have followed were there no curve, and are surrounded by a set of constant perforating branches.

Posterior Inferior Cerebellar Artery Aneurysms

Most aneurysms of the vertebral artery take origin at the posterior inferior cerebellar artery (PICA), especially when the origin of the PICA falls at the apex of a superiorly directed curve of the vertebral artery (Fig. 23-35). These aneurysms almost invariably point upward and usually communicate widely with the PICA. The size of the territory supplied by the PICA varies widely, and

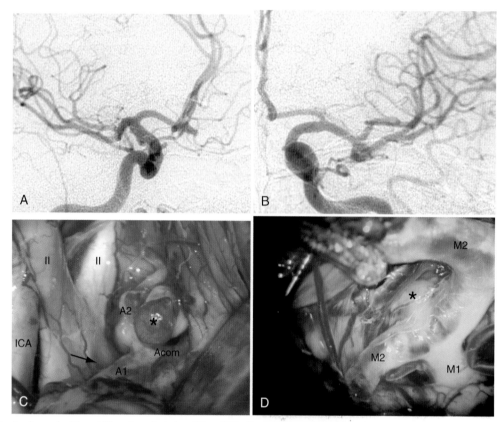

■ **FIGURE 23-29**   Angiography (**A** and **B**) and surgical views (**C** and **D**) of an acutely ruptured anterior communicating artery aneurysm and an unruptured MCA aneurysm. It is our policy that when there is a second unruptured aneurysm in the surgical path to a ruptured aneurysm that is amenable to surgery that the surgical option is preferred over the endovascular option. II indicates the optic nerve (the *arrow* points toward the chiasm). A1 and A2 denote the left first and second segment of the anterior cerebral artery whereas M1 and M2 denote the first (pre-bifurcational) segment of the MCA and the second (post-bifurcational) segments, respectively. The blood blister on the anterior communicating artery at the point of rupture can be seen both on angiography and in the surgical view, whereas the MCA bifurcation aneurysm does not have any surrounding blood.

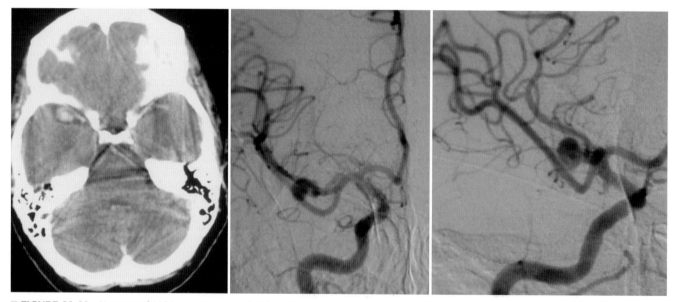

■ **FIGURE 23-30**   Unruptured MCA aneurysm as an incidental finding on contrast-enhanced CT that demonstrates an outpouching of the MCA that points laterally in the direction of the long axis of the pre-bifurcation segment of the main trunk of the MCA.

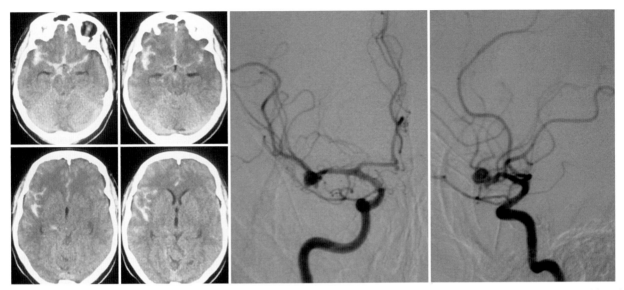

■ **FIGURE 23-31** Ruptured MCA aneurysm with typical distribution of blood within the basal cisterns and the subarachnoid spaces with a classic asymmetry within the sylvian fissure. The aneurysm arises at the level of the first major bifurcation or trifurcation of the artery and points directly laterally.

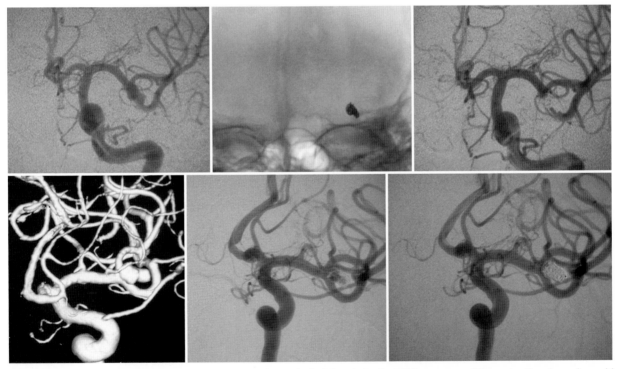

■ **FIGURE 23-32** Although surgical therapies may constitute the method of first choice for MCA aneurysms, 3D rotational angiography enables the exact depiction of the aneurysm neck and helps thereby in choosing the optimal plane of treatment that allowed for a complete occlusion in this aneurysm. As can be seen in this case, the aneurysm is directed with its long axis typically along the long axis of the pre-bifurcational M1 segment.

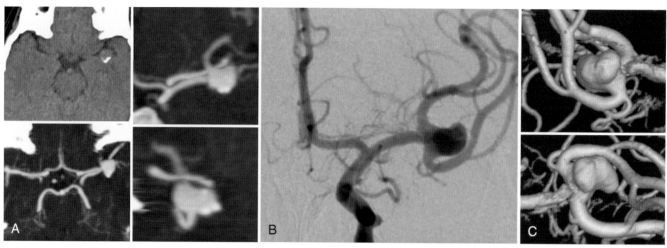

■ **FIGURE 23-33**   A to C, Incidental finding of a large, partially calcified MCA bifurcation aneurysm in a psychiatric patient demonstrating the useful-ness of CTA in depicting the exact localization of the calcification in relation to the neck, which is of utmost importance for the neurosurgeon. If a cal-cification is located close to the neck that needs to be clipped, there is a risk of tearing the vessel during clip placement. The solely luminal view of DSA is unable to demonstrate these findings.

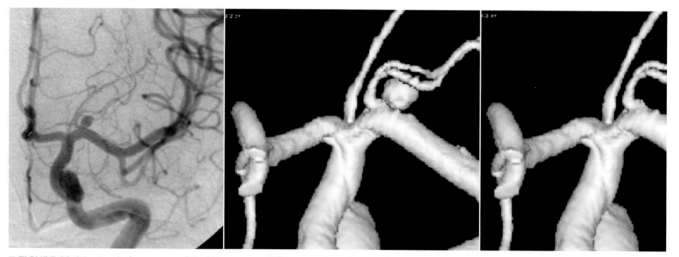

■ **FIGURE 23-34**   Atypical aneurysm of the M1 segment of the MCA arising close to the medial or straight group of the lenticulostriate arteries before and after endovascular occlusion of the aneurysm.

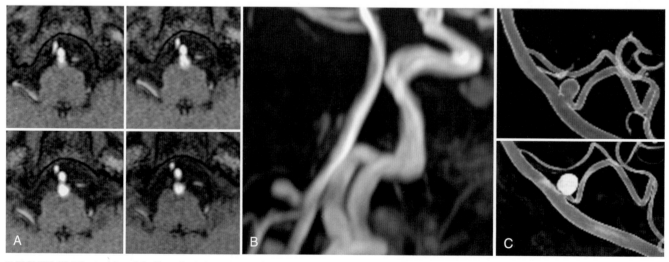

■ **FIGURE 23-35**   Incidental finding of a PICA aneurysm in a 34-year-old woman. The raw data (**A**) and the 3D reconstruction (**B**) of the TOF MRA demonstrate the aneurysm is located at the midline pointing into the medulla oblongata, which is why we opted for treatment in this young patient. 3D angiography both before (**C**, *top*) and after (**C**, *bottom*) coiling demonstrates the close relationship to the PICA and the typical aspect with a rather large communication of the aneurysm with the PICA at its origin.

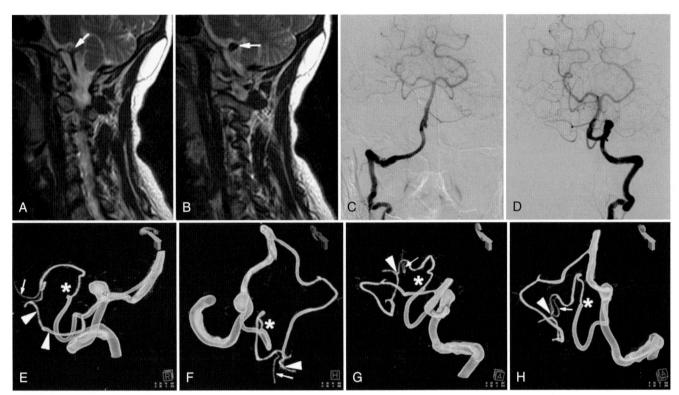

■ FIGURE 23-36 **A to H,** During diagnostic workup for radiculopathies, cervical MRI was performed in this 47-year-old woman demonstrating, on T2W sagittal images, a flow void of 8 mm in the PICA territory. 3D rotational angiography revealed a solitary left-sided PICA aneurysm with broad communication to the left PICA, and injection of the right vertebral artery revealed no right-sided PICA. The posterior view of the left vertebral artery on 3D DSA demonstrated that the right supratonsillar PICA, after reaching the apex of its course in the choroidal point (*asterisk*), bifurcated into lateral hemispheric branches and medial branches to the vermis. Here the medial branch not only gave rise to the (unpaired) vermian artery (*arrow*), but also continued to cross the midline along the dorsal aspect of the vermis to anastomose with a dominant right-sided AICA (*arrowhead*). Because of the huge variations of the PICA territory, its course has to be determined before treatment is planned.

will influence the best approach to aneurysm therapy. Phylogenetically, the PICA is a recent vessel with acquisition of highly variable cerebellar territories. Embryologically, the proximal PICA is best regarded as a hypertrophied radiculopial artery, while the distal PICA supplies a secondary territory that may vary. Common anatomic variants associated with the vertebral artery include unilateral agenesis/hypoplasia, double (duplicated, fenestrated) origin, and extracranial or epidural origin. There are close reciprocal inverse relationships among the sizes of the hemispheric territories supplied by the PICA, AICA, and SCA. Any one may annex (part of) the territory of the adjacent vessel, commonly leading to variations such as the AICA-PICA trunk. PICA supply to both cerebellar hemispheres is very uncommon but does occur and must be appreciated prior to endovascular procedures (Fig. 23-36).

Proximal Basilar Artery Aneurysms
Proximal nondissecting basilar artery aneurysms are rare and typically arise in patients with failure to form a single basilar artery during embryologic development (Fig. 23-37). The single basilar artery normally develops by union of paired longitudinal neural arteries that fuse together by about the fifth fetal week (when the embryo is 9 mm long). Each of the longitudinal neural arteries gives rise to the perforating arteries for its own side of the brain stem. Failed fusion of the neural arteries is often associated with aneurysms at the proximal portion of the nonfused artery. The lateral walls of the unfused arteries have normal intrinsic architecture. At the base of the medial wall, however, the media is absent, the elastic is discontinuous, and the subendothelium is thinned. Moreover, the presence of arterial variants

such as incomplete fusion indicates that (1) the arterial wall may not have matured completely, and (2) lack of cell selection may have preserved "weaker," less mature endothelial cells in that segment. These segments are more likely to develop arterial aneurysms when subject to secondary "offensive" triggers such as hemodynamic stress. The surgical treatment of these aneurysms is difficult due to their relationship to the cranium, lower cranial nerves, and the complex surgical approaches to this region. Endovascular embolization of aneurysms at an unfused basilar artery is an alternative to surgery. However, it must be recognized that both limbs of the unfused basilar artery have to be preserved, that the neck of such aneurysms is often broad, and that the aneurysm may regrow due to the unfavorable hemodynamics at the site of an unfused segment.

Anterior Inferior Cerebellar Artery Aneurysms
The aneurysm located at the origin of the AICA commonly arises from the convex side of the curve in the basilar artery and points in the direction of the long axis of the basilar segment immediately proximal to the aneurysm.

Superior Cerebellar Artery Aneurysms
Basilar artery aneurysms at the level of the SCA often arise where the upper basilar artery curves and tilts, so the hemodynamic thrust created by flow along the basilar artery impacts just above the origin of the SCA rather than at the basilar apex (Fig. 23-38). SCA aneurysms often have a broad connection with the SCA, a rather large neck, and a neck-to-dome ratio that makes endovascular therapy demanding. Endovascular therapy must attempt to preserve this artery, because this is the major vessel to supply

■ **FIGURE 23-37** A and B, Proximal nondissecting aneurysms of the basilar artery are rare and almost invariably associated with a segmental basilar artery nonfusion, as present in this case. They may be of the mirror type with one aneurysm pointing anterior and the other aneurysm pointing posteriorly. Neither of the two basilar artery channels may be occluded because the nonfusion of the basilar artery leads to a lateralized supply to the medulla oblongata and pons for both channels. Often, there is a broad-based communication between the aneurysm and the parent vessel.

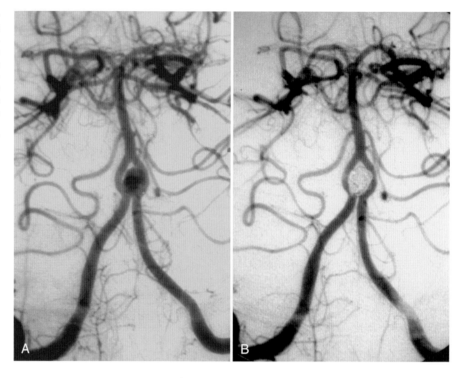

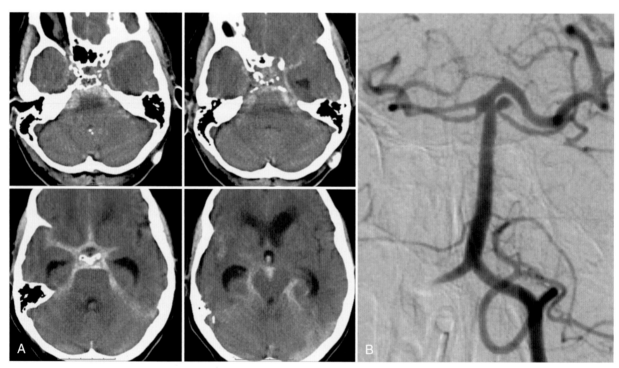

■ **FIGURE 23-38** Subarachnoid hemorrhage with a midline distribution and with the main amount of blood in the interpeduncular and ambient cistern raises the suspicion of a hemorrhage of the posterior circulation. A typical superior cerebellar artery aneurysm was found in this patient that is often associated with an asymmetric fusion of the basilar tip. A broad connection with the superior cerebellar artery is often encountered, but preservation of this artery is of utmost importance because this is the only vessel to supply the deep nuclei of the cerebellum.

the deep nuclei of the cerebellum. Large SCA aneurysms may cause oculomotor nerve palsies by direct impression on the oculomotor nerve as it courses through the interpeduncular cistern just cranial to the SCA.

Top of the Basilar Artery Aneurysms

Basilar apex aneurysms arise where the posterior cerebral arteries branch off from the tip of the basilar artery. At the aneurysm site the blood flow changes from vertical to nearly horizontal, so these aneurysms project upward in the direction of the long axis of the basilar artery (Figs. 23-39 to 23-41). The majority of patients with basilar tip aneurysms display a relatively short basilar artery (caudal fusion disposition) with the tip of the basilar artery near the caudal end of the interpeduncular fossa. The neck of the basilar aneurysm is preferentially implanted on the caudal part of the fusion. The largest and most important perforators to arise from the basilar tip are the posterior thalamoperforate arteries (retromammillary arteries). These originate from the basilar tip and P1, enter the brain through the posterior perforated substance in the interpeduncular fossa medial to the cerebral peduncles, and ascend through the midbrain to the thalamus. On occasion, one P1 may not give rise to a thalamoperforate artery, in which case a well-developed (dominant) thalamoperforate branch on the contralateral side will supply the area normally perfused by the branches of both P1s. Typically, the caudal portions of P1 each supply their own sides, whereas the cranial segments of P1 may supply bilateral territories. In patients with caudal fusions of the basilar artery, the posterior communicating artery flows caudally and is likely to supply diencephalic-mesencephalic territories. In patients with cranial fusion of the basilar artery, there is likely to be a basilar contribution to the supply of this area. The risks from occlusion of these vital perforating vessels include visual loss, paralysis,

somesthetic disturbances, weakness, memory deficits, autonomic and endocrine imbalance, abnormal movements, diplopia, and depression of consciousness. Endovascular approaches have been widely adopted to treat basilar apex aneurysms, because the surgical approach is associated with a higher morbidity. This is especially true for the more posterior basilar tip aneurysms, because greater numbers of vital thalamoperforators are affected as the aneurysm enlarges and projects more deeply into the interpeduncular fossa. Posterior cerebral artery aneurysms (Fig. 23-42) are most often dissecting aneurysms and will therefore be discussed in the next section.

DISSECTING ANEURYSMS

Intradural spontaneous dissections differ from cervical or extradural spontaneous dissections, although they may be associated with the same underlying diseases. Spontaneous hemorrhagic intracranial dissection is an uncommon disease but has been increasingly recognized as a cause for SAH with an unfavorable prognosis and a high rebleeding rate. One percent to 10% of all intracranial nontraumatic SAH is thought to result from ruptured intracranial dissections. This rate may rise to 5% to 20% in young patients. There is no gender dominance. The majority of hemorrhagic intracranial dissections are located in the posterior circulation, where histologic studies have shown that the intradural vertebral artery has a thin media and adventitia with fewer elastic fibers, so dissections of the intradural vertebral artery are more likely to result in SAH in contrast to dissections of other vessel segments.

Epidemiology and Pathogenesis

Although some arterial dissections result from specific diseases such as syphilis, fibromuscular dysplasia, and collagen disease, most dissections remain idiopathic, with no clear cause

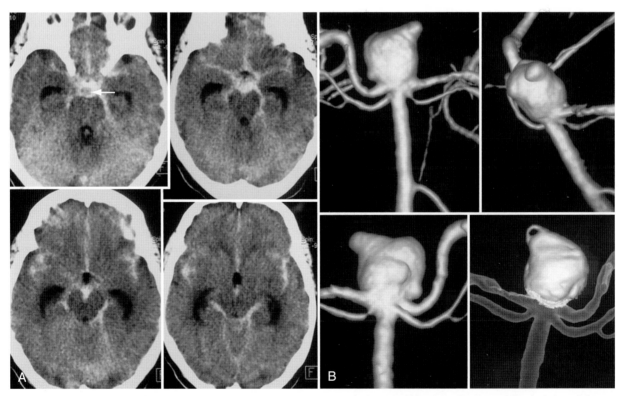

■ **FIGURE 23-39** **A,** Subarachnoid hemorrhage in a large basilar tip aneurysm with the typical blood distribution and the depiction of the aneurysm on nonenhanced CT as a faint area of sparing of subarachnoid blood in the interpeduncular cistern indicative of an aneurysm ("ghost sign," *arrow* in **A**). **B,** 3D rotational angiography both before and after coiling shows the large aneurysm with the broad communication to the posterior cerebral arteries and a daughter aneurysm on the tip that most likely resembles the site of bleeding and that should be spared during coiling. A dense packing is in our opinion necessary to ensure stable results in these kinds of large aneurysms.

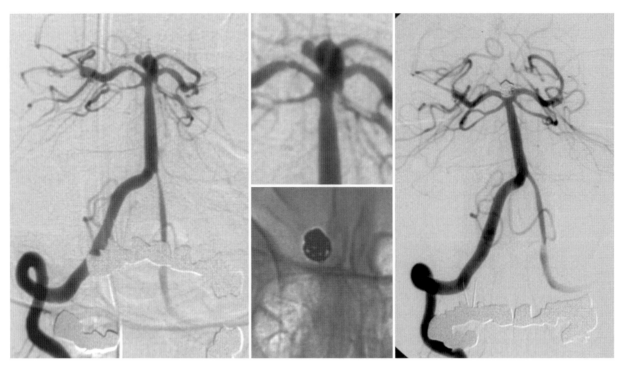

■ **FIGURE 23-40** Small basilar tip aneurysm with a small satellite aneurysm as the presumed site of bleeding and with a broad communication with the left posterior cerebral artery.

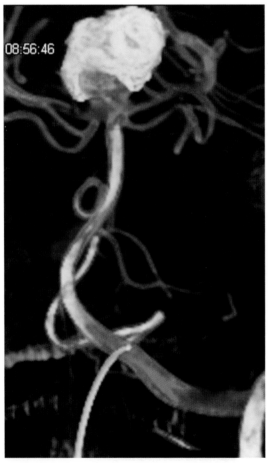

■ **FIGURE 23-41** 3D reconstruction of a typical compaction of a large coiled basilar tip aneurysm with a remnant in the midst of the coils.

identified. Pathologically, sudden disruption of the internal elastic lamina with subsequent penetration of circulating blood into the media is the primary mechanism underlying the development of cerebral dissecting aneurysms (Fig. 29-43). Histopathology shows no evidence of inflammatory infiltration within the vessel wall. However, the elastic lamina is destroyed and only rare elastic fragments remain. The dissection typically appears between the media and the adventitia, with a rupture site at the level of the adventitia. The internal elastica lamina can be disrupted. The media shows degenerative changes. Neovascularization and subadventitial dissecting hemorrhage are present at the site of rupture. On occasion, the entire arterial wall is disrupted. Depending on the number of layers of the vessel wall affected, an aneurysm might develop; alternatively, the blood clot within the vessel wall can push against the vessel lumen, leading to narrowing or occlusion of the vessel. Therefore, the neuroimaging features are variable. The most frequent angiographic demonstration is regular or irregular fusiform dilatation (Figs. 23-44 and 23-45). However, ruptured dissections may not have an obvious "aneurysmal" dilatation, and stenotic vessel segments may cause hemorrhage. That is why the term *hemorrhagic dissection* describes the present disease better than *hemorrhagic dissecting aneurysm.*

Natural History

The choice of treatment and its timing continue to be controversial. Acutely ruptured dissections are unstable. Up to 70% of cases rebleed, often soon after the initial hemorrhage, with a mortality rate from rebleeding as high as 50% (Fig. 23-46). After SAH, 70% of rebleeding occurs within the first 24 hours, with 80% occurring within the first week. The rebleeding rate decreases considerably beyond the first week after initial hemorrhage, and only 10% of rebleeding occurs more than 1 month after the initial hemorrhage. Overall, however, patients with poor clinical status on admission tend to rebleed more often.

A ruptured dissecting aneurysm begins to heal approximately 1 month after the initial SAH. The precise nature and timing of

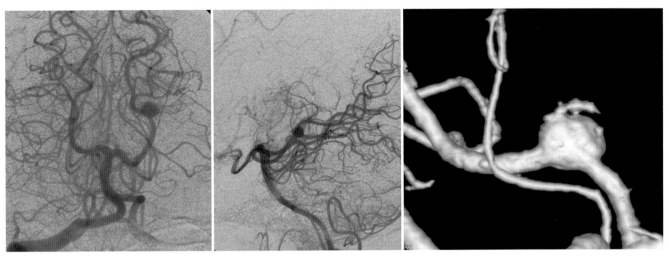

■ **FIGURE 23-42** Distal posterior cerebral artery aneurysm. These aneurysms are most likely dissecting in nature. They typically appear at the junction between the P2 and P3 segments, where the PCA crosses the tentorium. The aneurysms are often fusiform.

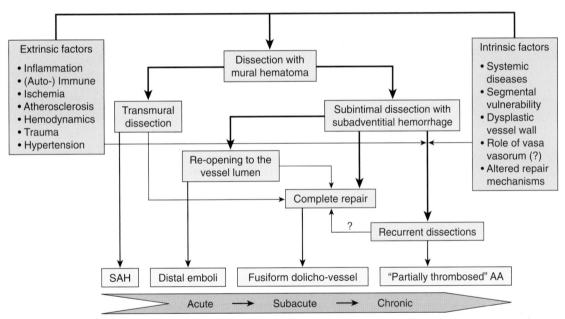

■ **FIGURE 23-43** Arterial dissections may generate a wide range of intracranial arterial aneurysms depending on the impact of extrinsic factors (e.g., inflammation, hemodynamic forces), the vessel wall integrity, and the intrinsic repair systems, as depicted in this schematic representation. A complete transmural dissection involves all vessel wall layers and will lead to an acute subarachnoid hemorrhage. This pathomechanism is present in the hemorrhagic dissections that most commonly present in the intradural vertebral artery segment but may also be seen in other vessels (see Figs. 23-44 to 23-55). A subintimal dissection that reopens itself to the distal vessel lumen may result in distal emboli due to intramural clotting of the subadventitial hematoma and subsequent migration of the clot to the distal vasculature. Whereas a repaired dissection will have a fusiform (or dolicho-) aspect (see Fig. 23-56), recurrent dissections will lead to what is called partially thrombosed aneurysms (see Figs. 23-57 to 23-61).

the healing response are presently unpredictable. In general, the healing response consists of formation of a neointima, which arises from the disrupted ends of the media at the edge of the gap and extends inward to cover the entire area of the disrupted arterial wall. The healing mechanism may be delayed when the defect in the wall is extensive (i.e., large aneurysms), when the media is completely separated from the adventitia, and when there is abundant thrombus in the ruptured portion (because neointima appears in synchrony with retraction of the thrombus). Late recurrence of dissection usually does not occur at the

same site, so the disease of hemorrhagic dissection appears to represent an acute injury that can undergo efficient spontaneous healing/repair of the vessel wall. Potential bilateral or isochronic dissections point to focal failures following systemic triggers (infectious or immune).

Patients with spontaneous dissections may have an underlying systemic vessel wall disease and harbor multiple dissections. In this situation, increased hemodynamic stress after unilateral vessel occlusion can result in the development of de novo dissections.

■ **FIGURE 23-44** **A** to **D,** Acute dissecting MCA aneurysm with subarachnoid hemorrhage. Although the blood distribution is common for an MCA aneurysm, the angiography demonstrates a fusiform dilatation of the artery with no identifiable aneurysm neck or solitary outpouching of the vessel wall. The infarction present in the lenticulostriate perforator territory suggests an underlying dissection with occlusion of perforators due to mural hematoma.

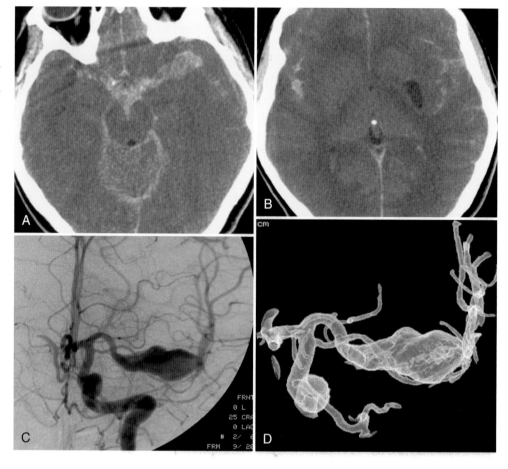

Diagnosis

The diagnosis of a true dissection is challenging. Angiographic criteria for spontaneous dissections are the stagnation of the contrast medium in an aneurysmal pouch, the presence of stenotic segments proximal and/or distal to the ectasia, and a fusiform appearance of the aneurysm (Figs. 23-47 to 23-56). T1-weighted (T1W) MRI can sometimes demonstrate increased signal intensity within the vessel wall indicating the intramural hematoma (see Fig. 23-51). On contrast-enhanced MRI, most cases show thick ring-like or railroad-like enhancement that includes the entire vessel wall, with a central or eccentric signal flow void. In other instances, the enhancement within the wall is confined to a mural bulge. This enhancement is thought to correspond to increased permeability of contrast material from the dissected false lumen to the vessel wall. The thick, dense enhancement disappears at approximately the same time as the dissecting arterial aneurysm disappears on the angiograms. Patients with dissections may show repeated episodes of ischemia thought to be due to reopening of the mural hematoma into the true lumen leading to distal emboli from the thrombosed hematoma. Furthermore, the dissection may lead to an extensive mural hematoma that may compress perforating arteries close to the site of dissection. Finally, a dissection can cause critical stenosis, leading to hemodynamic infarcts in the distal territory.

Treatment should be targeted at excluding the damaged vessel wall segment from the circulation, either endovascularly or via surgical approaches.

PARTIALLY THROMBOSED ANEURYSMS

Neuroimaging techniques successfully differentiate large and giant aneurysms that are completely patent from those that are partially thrombosed, by either directly comparing the outer contour of the mass with the perfused lumen on the cross-sectional images or comparing the measured diameter of the mass shown on cross-sectional images with the diameter of the lumen opacified by DSA. If the outer contour of the mass is significantly larger than the (measured) diameter of the lumen, then the aneurysm is at least partly thrombosed.

Partially thrombosed aneurysms are not simply large saccular aneurysms with some clot along the wall. Partially thrombosed aneurysms typically present with mass effect and show imaging features of thrombus of different ages in an onionskin fashion surrounding a smaller patent lumen. Regardless of their size when detected, partially thrombosed aneurysms usually continue to grow. They probably grow by a special form of "dissection" in which recurrent subacute, intramural (not transmural) dissections and repeated subadventitial bleeding from the vasa vasorum enlarge the aneurysm progressively. Thus, the pathogenesis of partially thrombosed aneurysms is likely distinct from the classic saccular aneurysms that develop in response to shear stress (flow, turbulences, jet effects) and therefore may require different approaches to therapy.

Clinical Presentation

Partially thrombosed aneurysms typically present with progressive symptoms due to mass effect and seldom present with SAH. If there is SAH with this type of aneurysm, it usually arises at the neck of the aneurysm, presumably due to a transmural dissection at this site.

Imaging

Neuroimaging studies of partially thrombosed aneurysms show evidence for intramural hemorrhage of different ages. Typically,

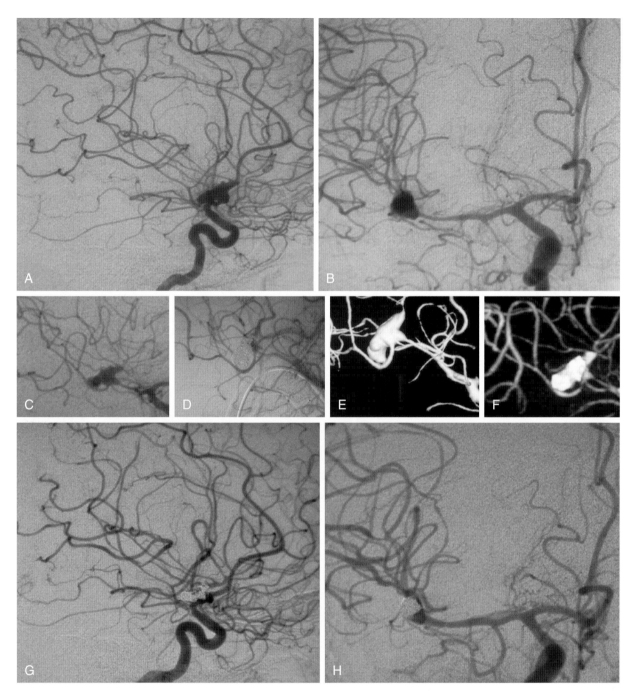

■ **FIGURE 23-45** **A to F,** Acute dissecting MCA aneurysm with subarachnoid hemorrhage in a 42-year-old woman who presented with sudden loss of consciousness preceded by acute and severe headaches. On angiography, a fusiform aneurysm of the MCA bifurcation can be seen that involves various M2 branches. The irregular aspect, the fusiform involvement of distal branches, and the stenosis proximal to the aneurysm suggest a dissecting process, with the stenosis being secondary to an extension of a subadventitial intramural hemorrhage compressing the parent vessel. Because of the anticipated severe infarction a careful coil deposition in the aneurysmal sac was performed to prevent rebleeding and to allow for spontaneous healing of the dissection. On control angiography 3 months after the acute hemorrhage (**G, H**), the stenosis has resolved and there is only a small residual ectasia of the origin of the preserved M2 branch.

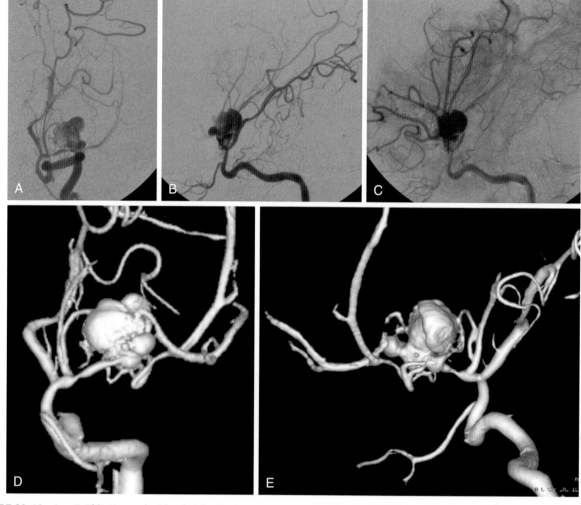

■ **FIGURE 23-46** A to E, This 13-month-old male infant had recurrent subarachnoid and intraparenchymal hemorrhages at a 2-week interval with an acute dissection involving the MCA. The stenosis preceding the aneurysmal ectasia, the fusiform aspect involving the circumference of the artery without a defined lumen, the contrast stagnation within the aneurysm, and the age of the patient are indicators for a dissecting process that is further suggested by the 3D aspect.

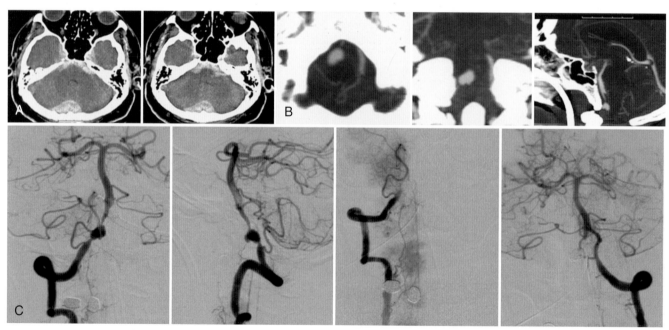

■ **FIGURE 23-47** Acute hemorrhagic vertebral artery dissection. **A,** On CCT the blood distribution with the major focus in the peripontine and perimedullary cistern and an atypical subarachnoid blood collection within the retrocerebellar and infravermian cistern suggest a posterior fossa origin of the hemorrhage. **B,** On CTA, the diagnosis can be easily made by the irregular contour and the fusiform ectasia of the aneurysm that involves the circumference of the vertebral artery. **C,** DSA confirms the diagnosis and is able to demonstrate the location of the dissection in relation to the PICA, the brain stem perforators, and the anterior spinal artery supply. Based on this information the site where to exclude the parent artery can be chosen.

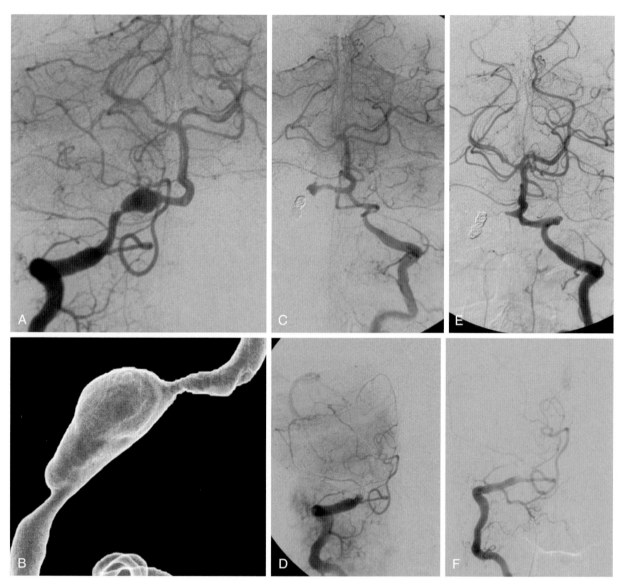

■ **FIGURE 23-48** **A** and **B**, Acute hemorrhagic vertebral artery dissection. The fusiform aspect and the stenosis proximal to the ectasia are indicators of the dissecting nature of this aneurysm. The location at the intradural segment of the vertebral artery is also typical. Directly after the intervention with a proximal coil occlusion of the parent vessel a residual flow into the dissection is visible (**C**, **D**) that remodeled completely in the 3 months as shown by control angiography (**E**, **F**).

CT and MRI show fresh clot at the periphery of the thrombosed portion of the aneurysm, with no apparent connection between the clot and the patent lumen of the aneurysm. The oldest thrombus is present close to the patent lumen, indicating that the aneurysm has grown from the periphery. There is surrounding edema in nearly all cases. Contrast-enhanced studies may show a crescent-shaped zone or complete ring of contrast enhancement at the periphery of the aneurysm. The aneurysm wall is vascularized by a dense network of vasa vasorum and intramural hemorrhages are the main factor for the observed growth (Figs. 23-57 to 23-60). Macroscopic inspection during surgery further supports the proposed pathogenesis of partially thrombosed intracranial aneurysms, because surgical exposure has disclosed a vast network of fine vessels covering the aneurysm, most likely representing the vasa vasorum. Markedly developed vasa vasorum can also be recognized on the parent artery and neck of the aneurysm.

In patients with thrombosed giant aneurysms, serial neuroimaging often demonstrates stable size of the aneurysm lumen but growth of the thrombosed portion due to hemorrhage into the thrombus and/or wall. In these cases, new intramural hemorrhage is seen distal to the patent lumen but close to the periphery of the aneurysm, suggestive of dissection between the layers of the aneurysm wall at the periphery of the thrombus. Partially thrombosed aneurysms may continue to grow, even when the lumen of the aneurysm is completely occluded or thrombosed, confirming that they grow by hemorrhages from the vasa vasorum not the lumen. It is known that after aneurysmal wall rupture a protective layer of collagen is formed and capillaries begin to proliferate to form a neomembrane. A vicious circle may then start in which minimal trauma (or other triggering events such as inflammatory responses) might induce bleeding into the neomembrane and this hemorrhage might then induce further proliferation of neomembranes. The more peripheral layers of the thrombus therefore represent the more recent clots leading to progressive growth of the aneurysm.

Text continued on page 518

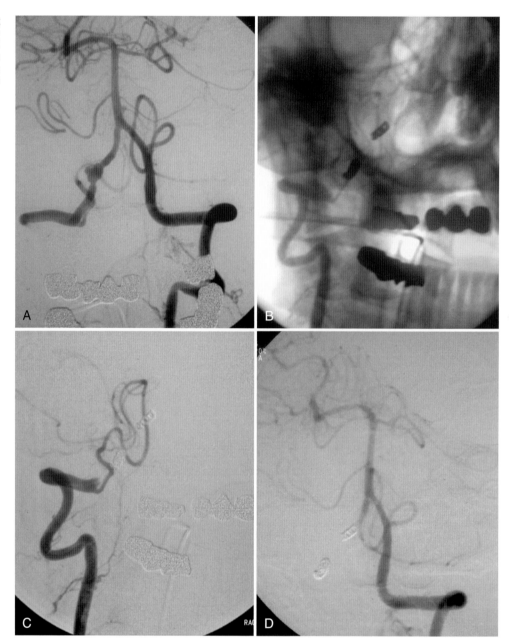

■ **FIGURE 23-49** A to D, Trapping of an acute vertebral artery hemorrhagic dissection with dense coil packing both proximal and distal to the dissected vessel segment with preservation of the PICA and the anterior spinal artery supply.

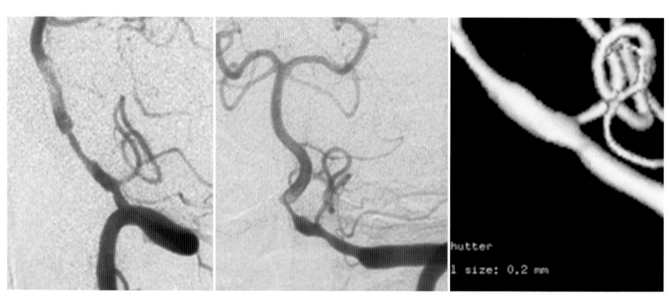

■ **FIGURE 23-50** This patient presented with a subarachnoid hemorrhage. Although no aneurysm was found, the irregular aspect of the vertebral artery and the fusiform mild enlargement of the vertebral artery with stenosis both proximal and distal were believed to indicate the site of dissection. This example demonstrates that, although not typical, hemorrhagic dissections can present solely as a stenosis.

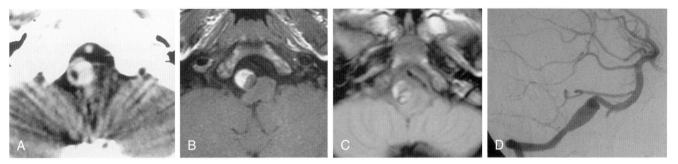

■ **FIGURE 23-51** Contrast-enhanced CT (**A**) and MRI (**B**) in an acute dissection demonstrate contrast enhancement of the mural hematoma that is brightly hyperintense on T1W MRI (**C**) indicative of blood in the methemoglobin stage within the hematoma. **D**, DSA confirms the fusiform aspect of the dissection.

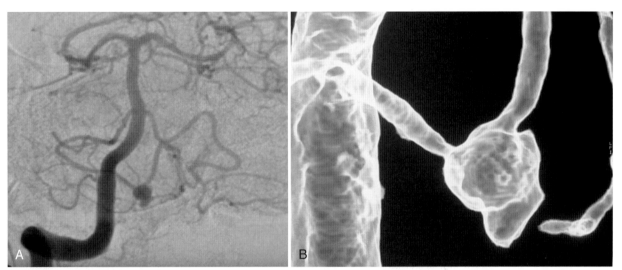

■ **FIGURE 23-52** Dissecting PICA aneurysm. Although vertebral artery aneurysms are the most commonly observed dissecting aneurysms, the fusiform ectasias located on distal cerebellar branches are most likely dissecting in nature, too, as evidenced by the proximal stenosis and the irregular involvement of the whole circumference of the vessel.

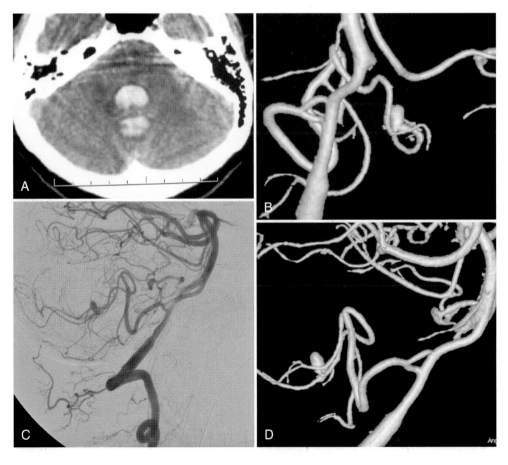

■ **FIGURE 23-53** A to D, Distal hemorrhagic AICA aneurysm. The aneurysm most likely represents a false sac, which is why an occlusion of this sac with intraluminal deposition of coils may harbor a high risk of periprocedural re-rupture. It is our policy to perform a proximal parent vessel occlusion of the aneurysm to prevent rebleeding.

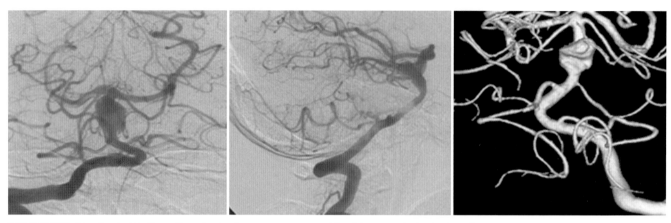

■ **FIGURE 23-54** Atypical fusiform dissecting basilar artery aneurysm with a false sac pointing backward.

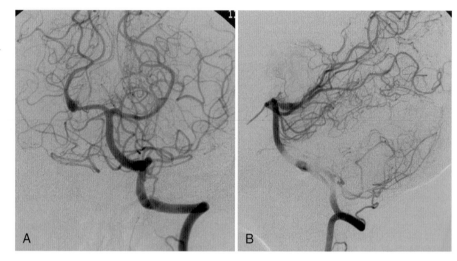

■ **FIGURE 23-55** A and B, Dissecting posterior cerebral artery aneurysm in a 42-year-old man with acute subarachnoid hemorrhage. The P2 segment at the point where the posterior cerebral artery crosses the tentorium within the ambient cistern is the second most common site for a dissection in the posterior circulation and is presumably due to microtrauma of the vessel along the tentorium. As in all dissections, closure of the parent artery seems to be necessary to prevent rebleeding.

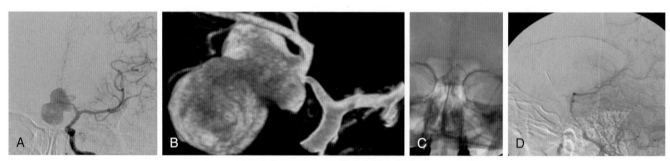

■ **FIGURE 23-56** A to D, Atypical giant anterior communicating artery aneurysm in a 37-year-old woman who presented with recurrent episodes of severe headaches. Angiography and 3D angiography demonstrate a large aneurysm with a fusiform involvement of the A1 and A2 segments of the left side. To plan treatment in this patient a balloon test occlusion was done in the right A1 segment while injection into the vertebral artery was performed, which demonstrated sufficient collateral flow via the posterior pericallosal artery with subsequent filling of the callosomarginal artery via the anterior pericallosal artery.

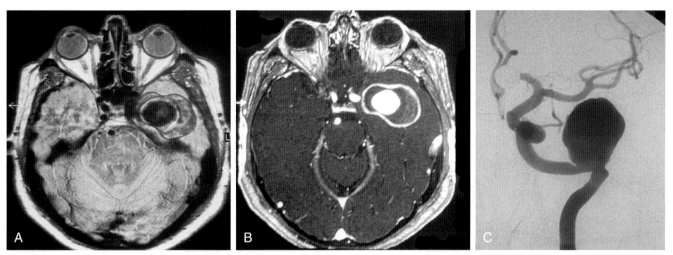

■ **FIGURE 23-57** A and B, MRI in a patient with a giant partially thrombosed aneurysm demonstrates onion-skin appearance of the thrombus and dense rim enhancement of the aneurysm wall. C, Cathether angiography reveals only the perfused part of the aneurysm.

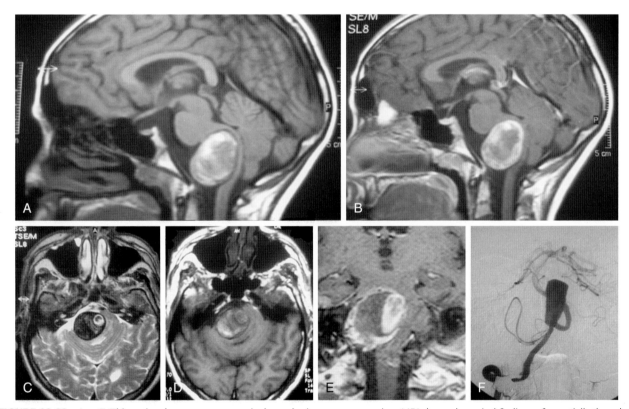

■ **FIGURE 23-58** A to F, This patient became symptomatic due to brain stem compression. MRI shows the typical findings of a partially thrombosed aneurysm of the V4 segment. Methemoglobin (T1 hyperintense on precontrast images) as a sign for an acute bleeding is present at the rim of the aneurysm far from the perfused part that is, in this case, located medially. T2W images show perifocal edema and the onion-skin layer of mural thrombus of different ages.

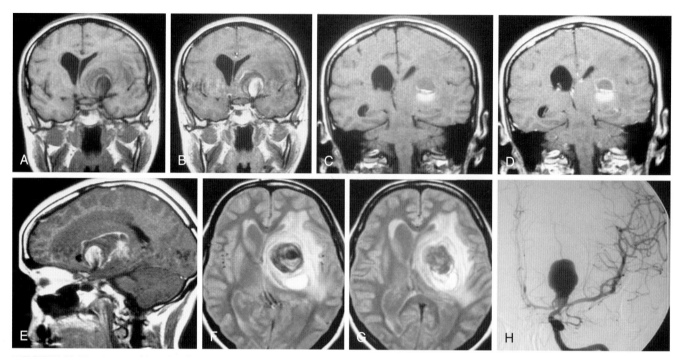

■ **FIGURE 23-59** A to H, This patient became symptomatic with intraparenchymal bleeding that was observed posterior and superior to a mass lesion in the left basal ganglia. The mass lesion extended to the basal cisterns and could be identified as a partially thrombosed carotid bifurcation aneurysm. T1W images before and after contrast administration demonstrate that the site of the bleeding is distant from the perfused part of the aneurysm that is located more anterior and inferior. There is partial rim enhancement, and T2W images demonstrate an extensive perifocal edema. The angiography demonstrates only the perfused lumen but not the full extent of the aneurysm.

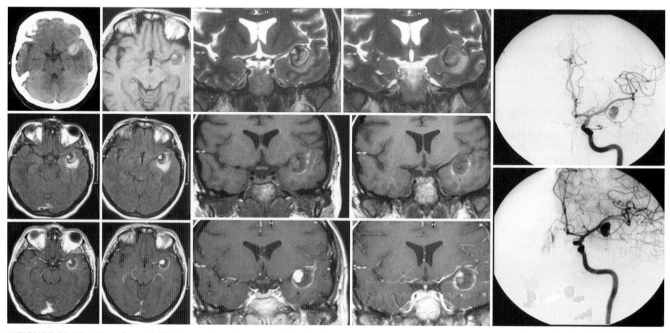

■ **FIGURE 23-60** Nonenhanced CT shows a hyperdense mass lesion in the MCA cistern with perifocal edema. On T1W nonenhanced images a crescent-shaped hyperintensity on the lateral wall of the lesion suggesting intramural hemorrhage can be seen. The source of the bleeding is not close but distant to the perfused aneurysm (demonstrated on T1W images after contrast). There is clot/intramural hematoma between the site of the bleeding and the aneurysm lumen. After contrast administration, a contrast-enhancing ring surrounding the aneurysm can be seen.

The salient imaging features to be searched for in assessing partially thrombosed aneurysms are peripheral hemorrhage within the "thrombosed part" of the aneurysm far from the patent lumen, a strongly enhancing rim, and an edematous reaction (or abluminal inflammatory activity) of the adjacent brain parenchyma.

Pathophysiology

Histologic examination of thrombosed giant aneurysms demonstrates more recent hemorrhage layered between old thrombus and the aneurysm wall, with clefts of fresh blood indicating dissection of the aneurysm wall by blood flow. Intrathrombotic vascular channels can be seen, some of which manifest endothelial

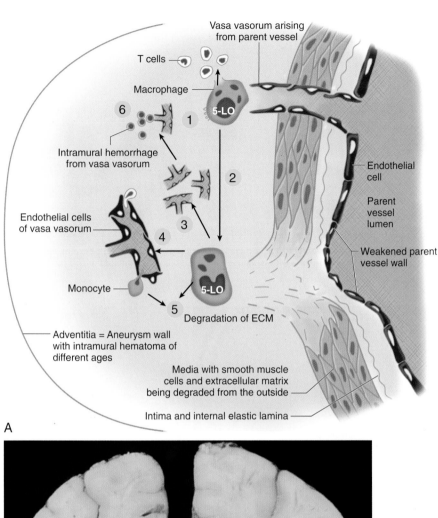

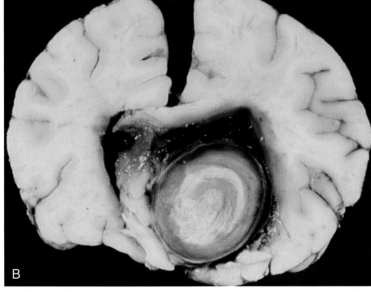

■ **FIGURE 23-61** **A,** Model of the vasa vasorum and the 5-lipoxygenase pathway participation in leukocyte recruitment, arterial remodeling, and, finally, intracerebral arterial giant aneurysm formation. Macrophages reach the adventitia via the vasa vasorum that arises from the parent vessel. These adventitial macrophages express 5-lipoxygenase and subsequently generate leukotrienes, which in turn activate (1) T cells, (2) other macrophages, (3) proliferation of the vasa vasorum, and (4) monocytes, and lead to an increased extravasation of leukocytes from the vasa vasorum to the adventitia. These activated leukocytes release proinflammatory factors (e.g., metalloproteinases) that damage the media by degradation of the extracellular matrix (ECM) and the elastic lamina that leads to a focally weakened parent vessel wall from which subsequently the aneurysmal lumen may form (5). We complement this biologic cascade with the traditional clinical observation of subadventitial hematomas in so-called partially thrombosed aneurysms. **B,** Pathology specimen. Fresh intracerebral hemorrhage from a partly calcified giant atherosclerotic aneurysm of the anterior communicating artery which had become embedded in the brain. Repeated subadventitial bleeding from the vasa vasorum (6 in A) leads to onion-skin intramural hematomas of different ages, as shown on this macroscopic pathologic image where the bleeding of a thrombosed aneurysm actually was seen to occur away from the patent lumen. (**B,** *Courtesy of John Deck, MD.*)

lining and proliferating smooth muscle cells. Macrophages are present in the aneurysm wall, especially near the periphery of the thrombus. The role of inflammation in the formation of giant aneurysms has recently been further underlined. Macrophages positive for a key enzyme in the inflammatory pathway (i.e., 5-lipoxygenase) are localized to the adventitia of diseased mouse and human arteries in areas of neoangiogenesis. These cells constitute a main component of aneurysms. 5-Lipoxygenase generates different forms of leukotrienes that are potent mediators of inflammation by further activating macrophages and recruiting monocytes and T cells. One of the leukotrienes, LTD4, binds to

endothelial cells of the newly formed vascular channels, leading in turn to an increase of leukocyte extravasation. This adventitial inflammation weakens the media by release of proinflammatory factors that invade the media and lead to dilation and aneurysm formation. Inflammation of the vessel wall by a chemokine intermediary route can thereby be linked to weakening of the vessel wall due to degradation of the extracellular matrix and the elastic lamina with subsequent aneurysm formation. A possible inflammatory component might be deduced from the extensive rim enhancement of the aneurysm wall seen in some patients and from the concomitant edema that is often present (Fig. 23-61).

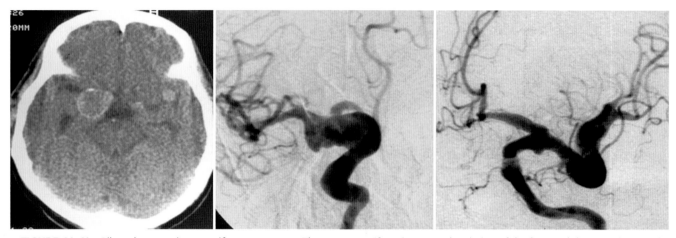

■ **FIGURE 23-62**   Bilateral symmetric serpentiforme aneurysms. The term *serpentiforme* is a mere description of the form and does not describe the underlying pathomechanism, which is most likely due to a chronic dissecting process with a segmental vulnerability, as exhibited in this patient with a mirror aspect of these peculiar aneurysms.

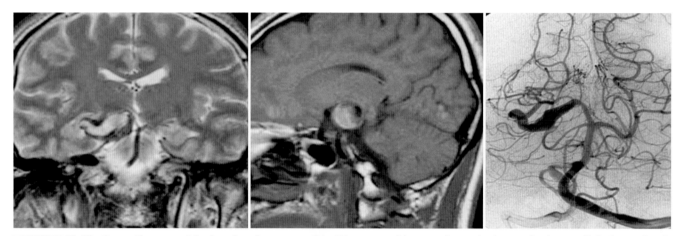

■ **FIGURE 23-63**   Serpentiforme, partially thrombosed aneurysm of the P2 segment of the posterior cerebral artery that is most likely due to chronic and repetitive subadventitial hemorrhages due to microtrauma along the tentorial edge.

Therapeutic Implications

For the reasons given earlier, the term *partially thrombosed aneurysm* is misleading and might mistakenly imply that the thrombus is located within the aneurysm lumen. Because neuroimaging, surgery, and histology all indicate there is clot of different ages within the vessel wall, not lumen, we prefer the term *aneurysm with intramural hematoma*. Furthermore, we believe that there is a real inflammatory component to these aneurysms. Therefore, aneurysms with intramural hematoma can be regarded as a proliferative disease of the vessel wall with growth induced by extravascular (partly inflammatory) activity. Mural thrombosis might act as a chronic trigger for perivascular growth factors, which then stimulate further proliferation of vessels both within the clot and within the vessel wall. Because the mechanism proposed for aneurysms with mural thrombus is markedly different from that proposed for nonthrombosed or saccular aneurysms, even saccular aneurysms larger than 2 cm, aneurysms with mural thrombus should be regarded as a separate clinical and pathologic entity.

Given the specific histologic considerations discussed earlier, we do not think that endovascular repair of these aneurysms by coils is an appropriate treatment option. In fact, clinical observations of such aneurysms treated with coils shows aneurysm regrowth over time, maybe owing to compaction of the coil mass or to the fact that the pathologic process continues to function in the vessel wall. Occlusion of the parent vessel might be a treatment option, because (especially in the ICA territory) the vasa vasorum arise from the ICA itself and are thus occluded. However, for these kinds of aneurysms, the results of parent vessel occlusion are not predictable and it has been shown that aneurysms can continue to grow even after their parent vessels have been sacrificed. Again, we presume that this is due to persistence of vessel wall disease.

The ideal treatment should be complete surgical excision of the lesion, but this procedure might be possible only after distal and proximal vessel wall occlusion (trapping). Apart from medical, that is, anti-inflammatory, treatment (e.g., corticosteroids), one might also consider, in the future, a treatment regimen that is able to cross the vessel wall to reach the newly formed vascular channels and the most peripheral parts of the aneurysm wall.

GIANT SERPENTINE OR FUSIFORM ANEURYSMS

Giant serpentine or fusiform aneurysms are subtypes of the partially thrombosed giant aneurysms and are differentiated from them purely on morphologic grounds. These aneurysms are characterized by an irregular (serpentine-like) vascular channel through the aneurysm or perforators/cortical branches coming from the aneurysmal sac. They account for approximately 0.6% of all aneurysms and about 20% of all giant aneurysms (Figs. 23-62 and 23-63). Their main clinical presentations are mass effect, ischemia, and hemorrhage, although SAH may occur in

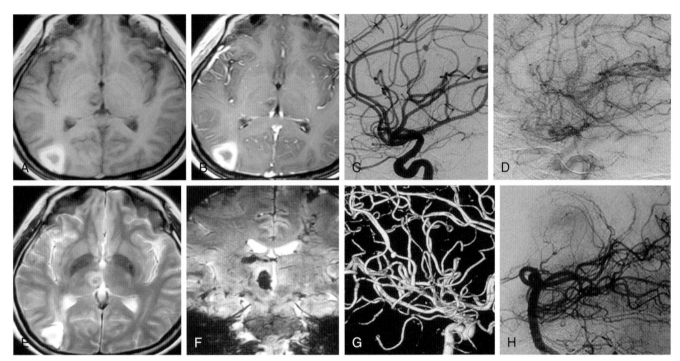

■ **FIGURE 23-64** A to H, This patient complained about headaches and low-grade fever in the afternoon for the last months. MRI was performed after an acute onset of headaches. Nonenhanced T1W MRI revealed a hyperintensity in the parieto-occipital region with edema on T2. A second focus of edematous changes was found in the right thalamus; on gradient-recalled-echo images, microbleedings in various brain areas could be seen and there was diffuse leptomeningeal contrast enhancement. Angiography revealed multiple distal small aneurysm-like ectasias on the peripheral vessels that were read as infectious or "mycotic" aneurysms. Blood cultures revealed gram-positive cocci as the underlying infectious agents. In these kinds of aneurysms the direct infectious involvement of the arterial wall with the infectious agent is the most likely cause for the occurrence of aneurysms, with the infectious process progressing from the lumen to the extravascular space. As the infectious agent circulates during septicemia, endothelial impact occurs in vulnerable vessel zones where there is turbulence or at the level of preexisting atheromatous plaques.

one fourth of cases. Giant serpentine or fusiform aneurysms occur more frequently in males with a mean age of approximately 40 years (range: 5 to 69 years) and with no history of hypertension or atherosclerosis. The MCA territory is most often affected, followed by the ICA, the PCA, and the basilar and vertebral arteries; other locations are exceptional. CT demonstrates calcification in the wall, whereas MRI shows the intramural thrombus at various stages. Postmortem microscopic studies demonstrate that the aneurysmal wall consists of fibrous tissue with calcification, loss or almost complete loss of internal elastic lamina and muscularis, and a number of small vessels within the wall. The sac contains thrombi of various ages, occasionally with calcification and hemorrhage. The tiny channels that end blindly in the thrombus show no endothelial lining.

Congenital defects of the arterial wall combined with a dissection process, as discussed earlier, are the possible underlying causes of giant fusiform or serpentine aneurysms because these lesions occur in all age groups and their gross appearance (and MR images) are similar to that of intracranial dissections. If not treated, these aneurysms may grow over time. Proximal occlusion of the parent vessel almost invariably causes complete thrombosis of the aneurysm; the safety of the outcome depends on the collateral circulation in both the deep and superficial territories. Spontaneous occlusion can occur and is usually associated clinically with severe headaches and neurologic deficit, often related to an increase in size.

Differential diagnoses of these aneurysms are dysplastic pseudoaneurysmal segments that are elongated into a dolichodysplastic segment, fusiform ectasias seen in the context of acutely ruptured dissecting aneurysms, fusiform vessel ectasias seen after healed dissections, infectious aneurysms seen in HIV infection, and fusiform aneurysms seen in connective tissue diseases.

MRI demonstrating thrombus in different ages and the patient's history should be sufficient to make these differentiations.

INFECTIOUS ANEURYSMS

The term *mycotic arterial aneurysm* was proposed in 1901 to describe those intracranial aneurysms seen during bacterial endocarditis. The designation has been kept to identify aneurysms associated with an infectious state. Today the term *infectious arterial aneurysm* seems more appropriate. Although they can be caused by fungal infections, they are most often of bacterial origin and account for 1.5% to 9% of all intracranial aneurysms (pediatric and adult). The most common organism is *Staphylococcus aureus,* followed by *Streptococcus viridans* and then gram-negative organisms. Blood and CSF cultures will show the suspected causative agent in two thirds of patients, but no infectious agent can be identified in the other third of cases. The exact pathophysiology of infectious arterial aneurysm is unclear. The direct infectious involvement of the arterial wall is the mechanism most often advocated (Fig. 23-64). In distal small arteries, an infectious process is suspected to progress from the lumen to the extravascular space. As the infectious agent circulates during septicemia, it impacts against the endothelium at specific sites where turbulence or preexisting atheromatous plaques make the vessel vulnerable. A different mechanism is present when larger arteries are affected. Here the infection typically extends from the outside toward the lumen and may be caused by involvement of infectious emboli originating from the vasa vasorum. In such cases, the primary effect is on the adventitia, with infection of the media and intima secondarily (Fig. 23-65). Most infectious aneurysms are either dissected or false arterial aneurysms. The lumen communicates with the endothelialized cavity within the hematoma, with peripheral

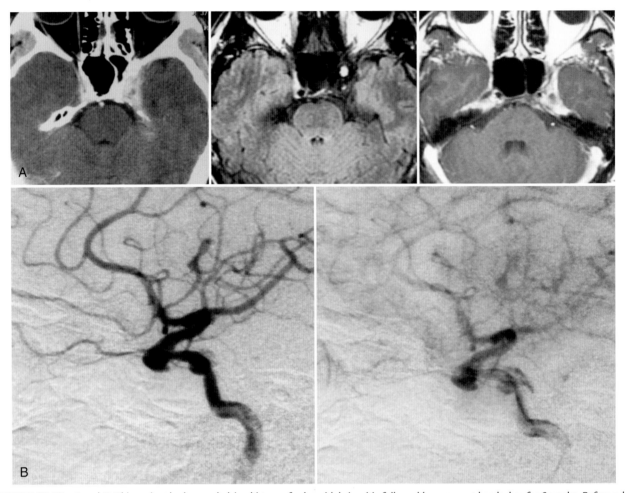

■ **FIGURE 23-65** **A** and **B,** This patient had an underlying history of sphenoidal sinusitis followed by recurrent headaches for 2 weeks. Before admission he suffered from an acute onset of ophthalmoplegia. On contrast-enhanced CCT, there is intense and prominent enhancement of the left cavernous sinus. The carotid artery shows a fusiform ectasia of the infraophthalmic portion. In large vessel mycotic aneurysms, the infection typically extends from the outside toward the lumen and may be caused by involvement of infectious emboli originating from the vasa vasorum.

fibrous changes constituting the "wall" of the aneurysm. Infectious aneurysms are typically located distal on the arterial tree in the MCA or less frequently in the PCA territories. In 20% of cases, infectious arterial aneurysms are multiple, especially in immunodeficient patients and those (partially) treated with inappropriate antibiotics or cytotoxic drugs. Infectious arterial aneurysms typically present as ICH. In rare cases, focal SAH may be the presenting event. These aneurysms are often small, extend into the hematoma, and may have a fusiform appearance with no neck, because they involve the full thickness of the vessel wall as a focal dissection. Alternatively, an extremely small neck may be visualized with a large false aneurysm representing small vessel rupture (the "neck" being in fact the remnant of the ruptured vessel while the "aneurysm" constitutes the hematoma cavity). Proximal infectious aneurysms may involve the intracavernous ICA by contiguity, following severe sphenoidal sinus infections with osteomyelitis and cavernous sinus thrombophlebitis. These aneurysms are often bilateral, occur more frequently in children, and in half the cases increase in size on follow-up angiography.

Infectious aneurysms require antibiotic treatment for a minimum of 4, and preferably 6, weeks. Mortality is reported to be as high as 80% for ruptured aneurysms and 30% for unruptured aneurysms. Early endovascular management is sometimes mandatory for ruptured infectious arterial aneurysms responding poorly or not at all to treatment. Endovascular management may require sacrifice of the involved arterial segment, even in eloquent areas, after assessing the leptomeningeal anastomotic circulation, because preservation of the artery is usually not possible. New infectious aneurysms will appear in more than 10% of patients, underlining the importance for repeated cerebral angiography at short intervals. MRI and MRA are not sufficient for this purpose, because they may fail to detect new small distal aneurysms.

HIV-RELATED ANEURYSMS

Aneurysms associated with HIV infection exhibit some specific features. These aneurysms are multifocal, typically fusiform, and located proximally on the arterial intracranial tree (M1 segment). They develop over a short period of time, and symptoms often include ischemic strokes (Fig. 23-66). Because the vasculopathy is often concomitant with a severe immunodeficiency, an infectious cause has been suspected, although the agent is seldom detected. Occasionally, a major HIV transmembrane glycoprotein (gp41) is found in the aneurysmal artery, suggesting a direct cause of the HIV in the formation of the arterial dilatations. Alternatively, they may be seen in the course of an opportunistic infection such as *Mycobacterium,* cytomegalovirus, or herpes zoster virus infection. However, because most histologic and bacteriologic analyses of these lesions have failed to detect the presence of an infectious agent and patients did not improve despite proper medical treatment it was recently suggested that

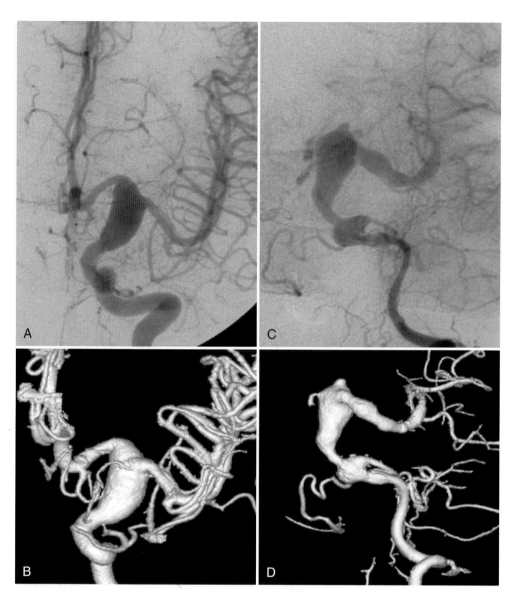

■ **FIGURE 23-66** A to D, This patient suffered from chronic mucocutaneous candidasis, a familial immune deficiency that leads to aneurysms that are not distinguishable from those seen in HIV vasculopathy. These aneurysms are typically multiple, subarachnoid, and fusiform and involve the proximal arteries of the base of the brain, preferentially the supraclinoid part of the internal carotid artery.

the aneurysmal dilatations were in fact due to a panarteritis, resulting in the destruction of the lamina elastica with subintimal fibrosis due to ischemia of the arterial wall. Such an inflammatory, noninfectious mechanism accords well with the fact that these lesions do not regress despite medical therapy, An active biologic response of the vessel wall to an inflammatory trigger leading to the formation of aneurysms can also be encountered in certain other forms of transmural angiitis (e.g., systemic lupus erythematosus, polyarteritis nodosa, or giant cell arteritis).

ANEURYSMS RELATED TO OTHER IMMUNE DEFICIENCIES

There are striking similarities between the aneurysms seen in the acquired immunodeficiency syndrome (AIDS) and those observed in chronic mucocutaneous candidiasis (CMCC) (see Fig. 23-66). CMCC is a rare familial disorder of unknown etiology, characterized by recurrent infections of the mucous membranes, nails, and skin with *Candida albicans* due to immune deficiency. The intracranial aneurysms seen in CMCC are typically multiple, subarachnoid, and fusiform and involve the proxi-

mal arteries of the base of the brain, preferentially the supraclinoid part of the internal carotid artery. These neurovascular manifestations have a very similar neuroradiologic aspect compared with those aneurysms encountered in patients with AIDS and raise the suspicion about a similar pathomechanism.

NEOPLASTIC ANEURYSMS

Neoplastic aneurysms are rare aneurysms most often seen with atrial myxomas (Fig. 23-67). They are believed to arise from cerebral embolization of neoplastic cells and consequent infiltration of the vessel wall. Atrial myxomas are neoplasms thought to arise from pluripotential subendocardial mesenchymal cells. They are more common in women and have no familial preponderance. Emboli composed of tumor, blood clot, or both lodge in cerebral vessels and cause cerebral infarction. They may manifest as arterial filling defects or as focal dilatations that may increase in size even after removal of the cardiac tumor. Histologically, the myxomatous tissue invades the vessel wall, proliferates there, and replaces the wall, leading to dilatation. These aneurysms are therefore the result of tumor material that lodges and grows in situ, invading the intima and media of the vessel wall.

■ **FIGURE 23-67** **A** and **B,** Two patients with MCA aneurysms in whom an atrial myxoma was found. These neoplastic aneurysms are focal dilatations that may increase in size even after removal of the cardiac tumor. Histologically, vessel wall invasion and proliferation of the myxomatous tissue replacing the vessel wall of a dilated artery are present.

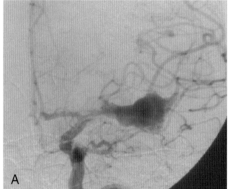
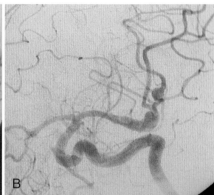

■ **FIGURE 23-68** A 23-year-old man had severe head trauma due to an accident at work resulting in a frontal impression fracture. One day after the accident he showed a sudden decrease in consciousness. **A,** Emergency CCT demonstrated a severe subarachnoid hemorrhage. **B,** 3D angiography demonstrated this multilobulated aneurysm without a discernible neck that most likely represents a false sac with a disruption of the arterial wall.

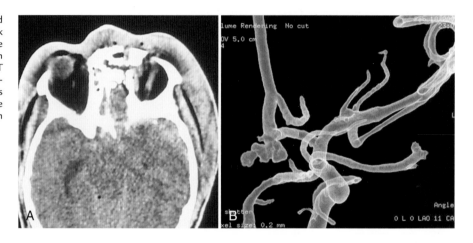

The simultaneous occurrence of a cerebral arterial aneurysm and a brain tumor is rare, so the coexistence of both is usually random. In neurofibromatosis, however, tumor and the aneurysm both arise from a common genetic defect, so they concur commonly. Patients with neurofibromatosis have a 12% risk of harboring a brain tumor and an increased risk of aneurysms. Metastatic disease from different primary locations such as choriocarcinoma or bronchogenic carcinomas may be associated with arterial aneurysms exceptionally. Metastatic tumoral colonization of the cerebral vessel wall is often implicated but remains mostly unproven.

TRAUMATIC ANEURYSMS

Intradural traumatic aneurysms most commonly involve the internal carotid and vertebral arteries at their transdural portions. Traumatic aneurysms may result from penetrating injuries such as a stabbing accident, a high-velocity gunshot wound, or iatrogenic trauma (e.g., third ventriculostomy). These injuries result in a false sac or pseudoaneurysm, which is produced by disruption of the arterial wall (Fig. 23-68). An extravascular hematoma communicates with the arterial lumen (Fig. 23-69). The fibrotic reaction produced in the surrounding tissues forms the wall of the false aneurysm. Other intradural traumatic aneurysms include the fusiform aneurysms of the posterior cerebral artery, in which microtrauma along the tentorium is believed to produce subacute or chronic dissection. Similarly, traumatic arterial aneurysms have been described as involving the ACA along the falx and the tentorium, either following major head injuries or as part of the shaken baby syndrome.

Extradural false aneurysms are by far more often encountered and usually result from gunshot or stabbing wounds. In the pediatric population, an additional type of carotid injury may occur as a result of intraoral trauma. After a fall onto an object that enters the mouth or a fall with an object already in the mouth, an injury is produced in the tonsillar region; these so-called pencil injuries have a mortality of about 30%.

False carotid aneurysms may also occur after tracheostomy, mastoidectomy, carotid endarterectomy, infections associated with carotid surgery, or disintegration of silk sutures. Another mechanism of vessel injury is blunt trauma, which may affect the vessel wall in a manner similar to penetrating injuries. This may occur after the application of force to the angle of the mandible, which is then transmitted to the carotid wall. If the mandible is fractured, a bony fragment may lacerate the ICA (or the ascending pharyngeal artery), producing a pseudoaneurysm. Ingested foreign bodies also have been reported to cause pseudoaneurysms of the ICA. A false aneurysm of the cervical ICA protruding into the posterior pharyngeal wall may be misdiagnosed as a peritonsillar abscess.

FAMILIAL SYNDROMES WITH ANEURYSMS
Polycystic Kidney Disease

Polycystic kidney disease (PKD) is an autosomal dominant disease that is associated with intracranial aneurysms in the adult age group but rarely in children, despite its familial character. PKD is genetically heterogeneous, and two chromosomal loci have been identified to account for the disease. PKD1 is associated with a mutation on the short arm of chromosome 16 (near to the gene associated with tuberous sclerosis). PKD1 codes for polycystin, a membrane protein that is involved in interactions between cells or between cells and the extracellular matrix. The prevalence of the disease is as high as 1/400 to 1000 and accounts for 2% to 7% of all patients with intracranial aneurysms that are

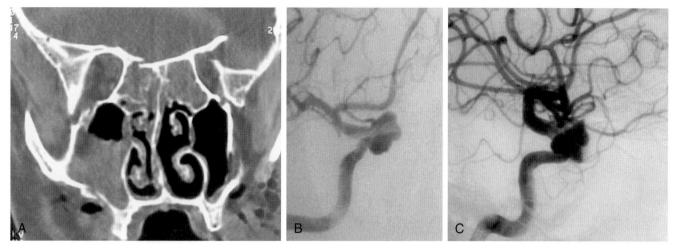

■ **FIGURE 23-69** A to C, Traumatic aneurysm of the internal carotid artery after severe head trauma with multiple fractures of the skull base and frontal viscerocranium. Two days later, the patient had life-threatening epistaxis that was controlled with dense packing of the nasal cavities. Angiography revealed a medially directed ICA aneurysm that was directed into the sphenoidal sinus and that represents an extravascular hematoma communicating with the arterial lumen. Attempts to coil these kinds of aneurysms are therefore useless and will lead to coil migration into the nasal cavity and recurrent bleeding.

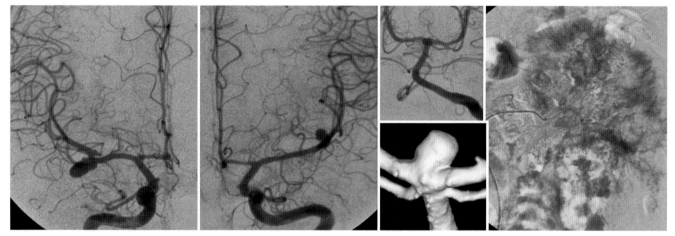

■ **FIGURE 23-70** Multiple aneurysms in a case of polycystic kidney disease with mirror localizations on the MCA and a small broad-based basilar tip aneurysm. The capillary phase of the renal artery injections shows multiple cysts.

usually of the saccular type. Histology in aortic dissections and dolichoectatic arteries in patients with PKD1 revealed immunostaining for polycystin in smooth muscle cells and myofibroblasts, along with disruption of the elastic laminae. PKD2 is associated with a gene defect on chromosome 4. The gene codes for a transmembranous ion channel. PKD2 patients show only a mild phenotype, and aneurysms are rarely present.

The frequency of SAH in the PKD population is about 1 in 2000 affected persons per year, about five times higher than the general population. There is no sex dominance. The mean age at aneurysm rupture is approximately 40 years (range: 6 to 69 years), which is close to the value of the familial forms of intracranial aneurysms without PKD but 10 years earlier than the sporadic forms. Autopsy reveals unruptured arterial aneurysms in 25% of PKD patients in whom the cause of death was not a ruptured aneurysm. The most frequent location of aneurysms is supratentorial (91%), with 50% of these on the MCA (Fig. 23-70). Multiple aneurysms are present in about 30%. The only risk factor clearly associated with aneurysmal rupture in PKD is a positive family history of aneurysm, which is five times more common in patients with an SAH than in a control group without SAH.

Ehlers-Danlos Syndrome

Ehlers-Danlos syndrome type IV is an autosomal dominant disease caused by a mutation in the gene for the type III procollagen (*COL3A1*). As a result, these patients synthesize abnormal type III collagen, leading to weak vascular walls. Multiple different mutations are described, but no relation has been found between the specific genotype and the phenotype. The prevalence is estimated at 1/50,000. The clinical diagnosis of Ehlers-Danlos syndrome type IV is established on two of four criteria: thin translucent skin; arterial, intestinal, or uterine rupture; easy bruising; and facial appearance. In this syndrome the arterial disease progresses in severity, so the occurrence of an arterial rupture signifies also the likelihood of further ruptures to come. Screening patients in their 30s for intradural arterial aneurysm is recommended, and careful preventive endovascular approaches by highly experienced teams should be offered.

The classic neurovascular manifestations include recurrent bilateral spontaneous high-flow carotid-cavernous fistulas due to rupture of the ICA within the cavernous sinus, dissection of the ICA, and arterial aneurysms (Fig. 23-71). Most of the arterial ruptures involve the large vessels, the extradural ICA, or the vertebral artery. The external carotid artery is not affected. The

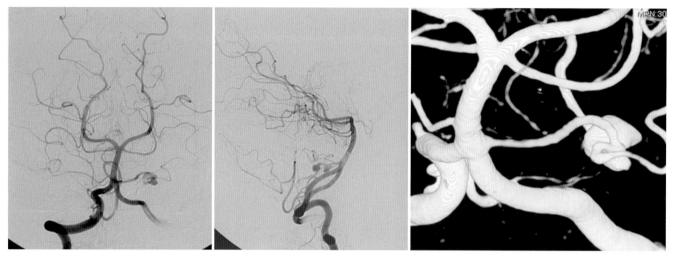

■ **FIGURE 23-71** Distal AICA aneurysm in a patient with Ehlers-Danlos disease. Although carotid-cavernous fistulas are the typical finding of Ehlers-Danlos disease, aneurysms that may be berry type, or, like in this patient, dissecting may also be present. Extreme caution must be taken during angiography in these patients because vessel wall dissections can easily be produced by catheter maneuvers.

arterial wall is very fragile, so arterial rupture is associated with high mortality and extreme danger with surgery and endovascular therapy in these patients.

As with all familial arterial aneurysms, the lesions of Ehlers-Danlos syndrome are often multiple and spread out along the arterial tree in the same general locations as berry aneurysms. They may be saccular or fusiform. They are not confined to a single metameric location but can involve noncontiguous zones. The natural history of these arterial aneurysms is unknown, but the risk of SAH in unruptured arterial aneurysms will be high. Up to 15% of deaths in Ehlers-Danlos syndrome are due to ruptured aneurysms. SAH occurs at a mean age of 33 years. Cervical aneurysms and dissections are frequent and may involve the entire ICA, from a few millimeters beyond the bifurcation up to the ophthalmic artery origin. Segmental dysplastic changes can be observed on the ICA or the vertebral artery. In our experience, the rupture is located at the junction of the abnormal and the apparently normal segment cranially. Sacrifice of the ruptured vessel is most often needed at the neck or skull base, despite the risk of recurrence on the opposite side. There is high risk that the dissecting process will extend intracranially after lengthy and traumatic endovascular maneuvers.

Neurofibromatosis Type 1

Neurofibromatosis type 1 (NF1) can be associated with arterial aneurysms, which may be single or multiple, saccular or dissecting, and large or giant. They may be located extradurally on the cervical petrous ICA or cervical vertebral artery. Renal artery stenosis is the most common vascular lesion associated with NF1. The diagnosis is often made following rupture secondary to traumatic puncture or spontaneous dissections similar to Marfan syndrome, fibromuscular dysplasia, and Ehlers-Danlos syndrome type IV. In NF1 aneurysms, there is a female-to-male predominance of 5:1. The mutation involves the long arm of chromosome 17 and is transmitted as an autosomal dominant trait; in half the cases the disease is caused by a new mutation. The prevalence of NF1 is 1/3000 to 5000. The associated clinical diagnosis includes subcutaneous nodules, skin pigmentation, neurofibromatosis, schwannomas, gliomas, hamartomas, neurofibrosarcomas, skeletal abnormalities such as scoliosis, and cystic erosions. The vascular rupture often brings to attention patients with the diagnosis of cervical arteriovenous fistulas. Review of 100 consecutive patients with intracranial arterial aneurysms showed one case of NF1.

Fibromuscular Dysplasia

Fibromuscular dysplasia is characterized by multifocal dysplasia of vessel walls involving cervical branches of the aorta and can be associated with intracranial aneurysms. More than one third of patients have a family history of vascular disorders, including high blood pressure, migraine, impaired hearing, stroke, cerebral hemorrhages, or dissections. It has been suggested that fibromuscular dysplasia is inherited as a dominant trait with reduced penetrance in males. Therefore, a female-to-male predominance of 5.6:1 is encountered. Fibromuscular dysplasia causes irregular thickening of the vessel wall from proliferation of smooth muscle and fibrous tissue of the media. Angiographic changes of fibromuscular dysplasia are found in about 15% of patients with a spontaneous dissection of the carotid or vertebral artery. To a similar extent, arterial aneurysms, including dissecting arterial aneurysms, are known to be associated with this disease (Fig. 23-72). Multiplicity is more often encountered in females than in males. The prognosis of SAH in this female group is worse, with a higher degree of vasospasm. Frequent locations are the ICA, the anterior communicating artery, or the vertebral artery. Renal artery involvement tends to precede involvement of the carotids.

Marfan Syndrome and Other Rare Familial Syndromes

Marfan syndrome is an autosomal dominant disease resulting from a mutation on chromosome 15. The affected gene encodes for fibrillin-1, a microfibril component involved in the extracellular matrix. Disease prevalence is approximately 1/10,000 individuals. Approximately 30% of cases arise as sporadic mutations. Marfan syndrome causes ocular, skeletal, and cardiovascular abnormalities. The usual cause of death in children is aortic or mitral insufficiency, and in young adults it is aortic dissection. Patients with minor forms can survive to adulthood. Aneurysms are usually large or fusiform and can be both intradural and extradural.

Pseudoxanthoma elasticum and familial tumoral calcinosis may also manifest as a neurovascular pathologic process, with dysplastic changes in the large vessels and cavernous ICA, intracranial stenoses, and intradural aneurysms of the ICA. The disease prevalence is about 1/100,000. It is genetically heterogeneous, with autosomal dominant and autosomal recessive types.

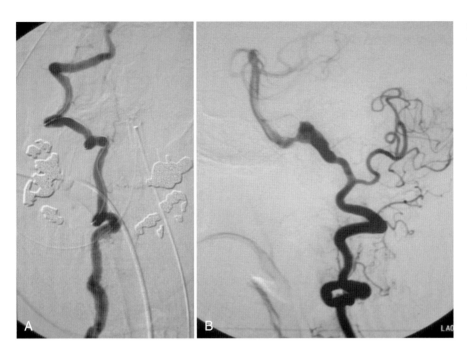

■ **FIGURE 23-72** **A** and **B,** Fibromuscular dysplasia with a dissecting vertebral artery aneurysm that was treated by parent vessel occlusion. Note the severe elongation and increased tortuosity of the vertebral artery harboring the aneurysm.

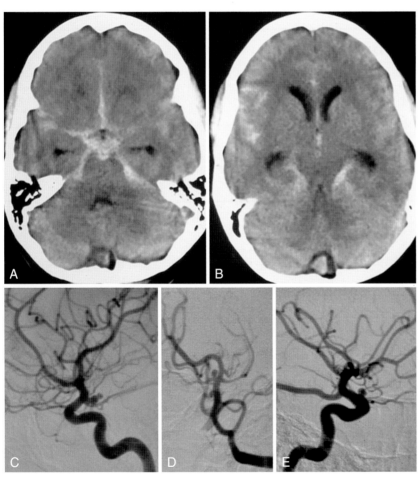

■ **FIGURE 23-73** See Box 23-1, Evaluation of a Ruptured Aneurysm, for an explanation of this figure.

ANALYSIS

In aneurysmal lesions of the brain, the first step in diagnosis is to identify the type of aneurysm, then the underlying disease, as far as possible. The analysis and report should include the features necessary to decide on surgical versus endovascular approaches and any risk factors associated with either approach.

Acute SAHs are emergencies that require prompt treatment. Incidental aneurysms, however, require a more scrutinized approach to determine the exact size, location, and underlying cause of the disease.

A sample report for Figure 23-73 is presented in Box 23-1.

BOX 23-1   Sample Report: Evaluation of a Ruptured Aneurysm

PATIENT HISTORY

A 48-year-old woman presented with an acute onset of severe headaches. On physical examination she was drowsy, not fully oriented to time, and had nuchal rigidity and photophobia. Given her symptoms of meningism, a subarachnoid hemorrhage was suspected and she was sent for emergency cranial CT.

TECHNIQUE

Unenhanced CT was performed with axial 4-mm-thick orbitomeatal sections from the occipital foramen to the sellar region, and 8-mm-thick sections from the sellar region to the vertex employing a conventional (non-helical) acquisition mode on a 4-detector row CT.

FINDINGS

Cranial computed tomography (CCT) demonstrates SAH with blood in the basal cisterns, the suprasellar cistern, the ambient cistern, and the right sylvian fissure (Fig. 23-73). There is more blood on the right compared with the left hemisphere. Ventricular dilatation is not present; there is no blood within the ventricles or in the parenchyma. The distribution of hemorrhage suggests an aneurysm of the right side. Further angiographic evaluation is necessary. On DSA, three aneurysms are found. There is a small, berry-type aneurysm at the origin of the right

SCA that is directed superiorly with a narrow communication with the SCA and a mean diameter of approximately 3 mm. There are no daughter aneurysms present on this aneurysm. No signs of localized vasospasm or active bleeding are found. After injection of the right internal cerebral artery, a posterior communicating aneurysm with an irregular shape and an upward directed daughter aneurysm can be seen. The aneurysm originates superior to the origin of the posterior communicating artery and the neck is narrow in comparison to the dome. Its size is 6×4 mm. There is no vasospasm. Injection in the left ICA demonstrates a round, berry-type aneurysm that originates from the ICA just superior to the ophthalmic artery. This aneurysm measures 3 mm, has a rather broad base toward the ICA, and shows no daughter aneurysm. There is a direct "fetal" origin of the PCA from the ICA on the left side. No vasospasm is present.

IMPRESSION

The blood distribution and the configuration clearly identify the right posterior communicating artery aneurysm as the acutely ruptured aneurysm that has to be treated first. The multiplicity of aneurysms should raise the suspicion of a familial or vessel wall disease that should be specifically sought after in subsequent studies.

KEY POINTS: DIFFERENTIAL DIAGNOSIS

■ Classical berry-type or saccular aneurysms have to be distinguished from dissecting, "partially thrombosed," and infectious aneurysms, because they exhibit a different natural history and require different treatment strategies.

■ Saccular aneurysms are the major cause for subarachnoid hemorrhage (SAH) and are typically present as focal outpouchings of the vessel wall close to branching sites of arteries. "Partially thrombosed" aneurysms present with mass effect, not SAH, owing to repetitive intramural hemorrhages that lead to onion-skin layers of hemorrhage of different ages within the vessel wall.

■ Intracranial dissecting vasculopathies are usually fusiform and may be associated with stenotic segments proximal to the dissected segment. They present with SAH or ischemic events and, once having bled, have a high propensity for rebleeding. Therapy should therefore be aimed at a complete occlusion of the dissected vessel segment.

■ Infectious and traumatic aneurysms are located distally on the vascular tree. Infectious aneurysms are often associated with cerebral edema in the clinical context of septicemia. Traumatic aneurysms typically present days to weeks after a significant trauma.

SUGGESTED READINGS

Berenstein A, Lasjaunias P, Ter Brugge KG. Surgical Neuroangiography, 2nd ed., Vol 2, Clinical and Endovascular Treatment Aspects in Adults. Springer, Berlin, Springer, 2004.

Bracard S, Anxionnat R, Picard L. Current diagnostic modalities for intracranial aneurysms. Neuroimaging Clin North Am 2006; 16:397-411.

Dammert S, Krings T, Moller-Hartmann W. Detection of intracranial aneurysms with multislice CT: comparison with conventional angiography. Neuroradiology 2004; 46:427-434.

Krings T, Mandell DM, Kiehl TR, et al. Intracranial aneurysms: from vessel wall pathology to therapeutic approach. Nature Rev Neurol 2011; 7:547-559.

Krings T, Piske R, Lasjaunias P. Intracranial arterial aneurysm vasculopathies: targeting the outer vessel wall. Neuroradiology 2005; 47:931-937.

Mizutani T, Kojima H, Asamoto S, Miki Y. Pathological mechanism and

three-dimensional structure of cerebral dissecting aneurysms. J Neurosurg 2001; 94:712-717.

Molyneux AJ, Kerr R, Stratton I, et al. International Subarachnoid Aneurysm Trial (ISAT) of neurosurgical clipping versus endovascular coiling in 2143 patients with ruptured intracranial aneurysms: a randomised trial. Lancet 2002; 360:1267-1274.

Rhoton AL Jr. Aneurysms. Neurosurgery 2002; 51:121-158.

Schievink WI. Intracranial aneurysms. N Engl J Med 1997; 336:28-40.

Stehbens WE. Etiology of intracranial berry aneurysms. J Neurosurg 1989; 70:823-831.

Wiebers DO, Whisnant JP, Huston J, et al. Unruptured intracranial aneurysms: natural history, clinical outcome, and risks of surgical and endovascular treatment. Lancet 2003; 362:103-110.

Zhao WY, Krings T, Alvarez H, et al. Management of spontaneous hemorrhagic intracranial vertebrobasilar dissection: review of 21 consecutive cases. Acta Neurochir (Wien) 2007; 149:585-596.

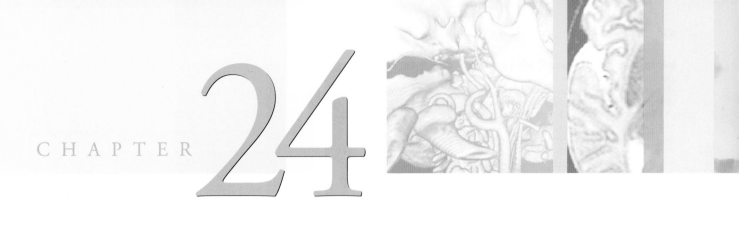

CHAPTER 24

Vascular Malformations

Timo Krings, Sasikhan Geibprasert, Vitor M. Pereira, Sirintara Pongpech,
Pakorn Jiarakongmun, and Pierre L. Lasjaunias

Four major types of primary malformations of the vascular systems can be identified: arterial, arteriovenous, capillary, and venous. Each of these malformations manifests intrinsic primary abnormalities and each causes derivative secondary change in the rest of the vascular system. Classically, these vascular malformations are grouped into four categories (1) the dural and pial arteriovenous malformations and shunts, (2) cavernous malformations (cavernomas), (3) capillary telangiectasias, and (4) developmental venous anomalies.

ARTERIOVENOUS MALFORMATIONS AND FISTULAS

Types

Pial Malformations

Arteriovenous shunts correspond to an abnormal capillary bed with a shortened arteriovenous transit time. The shunts are located in the subpial space, are fed by arteries that normally feed the brain parenchyma, and are drained by pial veins. Two categories of arteriovenous shunts—arteriovenous malformations (AVMs) and the arteriovenous fistulas (AVFs)—may be differentiated by their different angioarchitecture at the transition between feeding artery and draining vein.

AVMs are characterized by a network of abnormal channels (the nidus) interposed between the arterial feeder(s) and the draining vein(s). The shunts may be small (micro-AVMs) with a nidus less than 1 cm in diameter and normal size arteries and draining veins, or the shunts may be larger (macro-AVMs) with nidi larger than 1 cm in diameter and enlarged feeding arteries and draining veins. AVMs may be compartmentalized into portions fed and drained by separate vessels, as documented by angiography or at surgery. In many cases of pial AVMs the separate compartments exhibit differing internal angioarchitecture with more fistulous or more glomerular nidal appearances (see later) within the different compartments (Fig. 24-1).

AVFs consist of direct, fistulous transitions from an artery into a vein. They, too, can be classified as micro-AVF or macro-AVF depending on the size of the feeding artery. The AVFs are found almost exclusively on the *surface* of the brain or the spinal cord. Pial AVFs appear to be relatively frequent in children and rare in adults (Fig. 24-2).

Lesion Topography

Topographic location of an AVM is best assessed by combining the cross-sectional and the angiographic information. Lesions in

most locations recruit predictable arterial feeders and specific draining veins. One assumes that the primary defect is at the capillary level. Thus, both the arterial tree from which the feeders originate and the venous system that drains the lesion are, a priori, assumed to be normal. However, they may change their appearance secondarily in response to the alterations in flow and hemodynamics caused by the AVM. Analysis of arterial feeders and venous drainage accurately delineates the topography of the various compartments involved. Several general types of lesion can be differentiated on the basis of their distinct locations. Attention must also be paid to any alteration in the patterns of venous drainage caused by venous thrombosis.

Arteriovenous Malformations that Involve the Cortex

Cortical arteriovenous lesions involve the cortex, are fed exclusively by cortical arteries, and drain into superficial veins (unless secondary thrombosis of cortical veins shunts the venous flow into alternate pathways). These lesions are also designated sulcal AVMs (Fig. 23-3).

Cortical-subcortical arteriovenous lesions recruit cortical arteries and drain into superficial veins but may also drain into the deep venous system if the transcerebral venous system is patent. These lesions are also designated gyral AVMs (Fig. 23-4). In both cortical (sulcal) and cortical-subcortical (gyral) lesions, some regions of the cortex drain to deeply located veins that should not be considered as true parts of the deep venous system. Such vessels include the medial veins of the temporal lobe and the basal vein of Rosenthal, the veins of the cerebellar vermis, and the precentral cerebellar veins.

Corticoventricular arteriovenous lesions correspond to the classic pyramidal malformations that are based on the cortex and reach the ventricular wall at their apex. These malformations are fed by both cortical and perforating arteries and drain to both superficial and deep veins. Corticocallosal AVMs belong to the corticoventricular group (Fig. 23-5). They have the same venous characteristics but do not recruit perforating arteries. Corticocallosal AVMs drain into the subependymal veins and later into the deep venous system. The arterial supply to the corpus callosum is linked to the cortical arterial network, even though it may simulate perforating arterial channels in the supraoptic region and choroidal arteries at the splenium.

Deep-Seated Arteriovenous Lesions

Deep-seated lesions are located in the depth of the telencephalon, diencephalon, brain stem, or cerebellum (Fig. 23-6). The

■ **FIGURE 24-1** Glomerular versus fistulous arteriovenous malformation. Whereas on MRI glomerular AVMs can be perceived as a tangle of abnormal vessels within the brain parenchyma (**A, B**), fistulous AVMs are typically recognized by their large venous pouch that may demonstrate a mixed signal depending on the flow properties within the pouch (**C, D**). The superselective injection demonstrates the nidus aspect in the glomerular AVM whereas in the fistulous AVMs the direct transition from the artery into the massively enlarged venous pouch can be visualized.

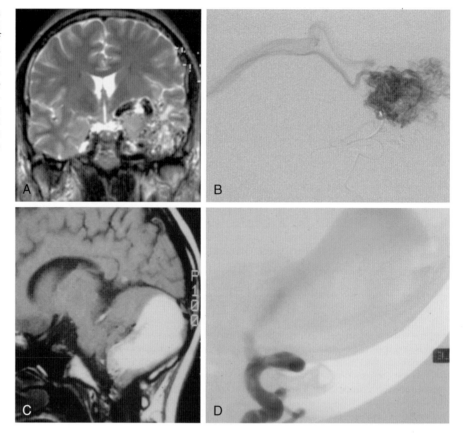

■ **FIGURE 24-2** Four different fistulous AVMs. These types of AVMs are, owing to their clinical symptomatology, most often encountered in the pediatric age group. When multiple fistulas occur, the possible diagnosis of Osler's disease (hereditary hemorrhagic telangiectasia) has to be discussed. Most often, these fistulas are single-hole fistulas (i.e., multiple feeding arteries converging at one single spot into the enlarged venous pouch). Clinical manifestations are due to venous congestion that may lead to hydrodynamic disorders in the pediatric population. Spontaneous thrombosis may also cause life-threatening mass effect.

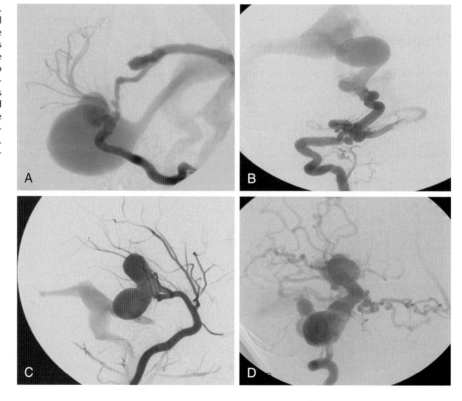

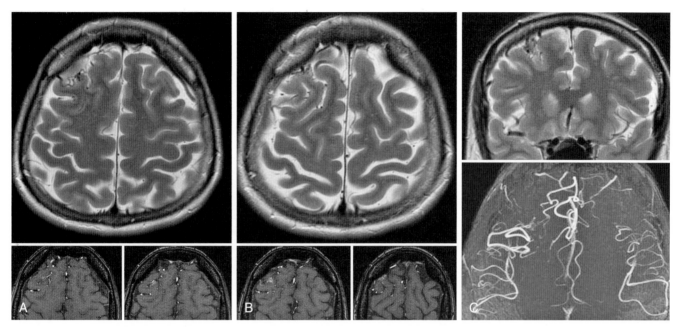

■ **FIGURE 24-3** A to C, Cortical micro-AVM. On T2W images the cortical location of this small AVM can be best appreciated on the coronal cuts; however, the axial slices also demonstrate the abnormal tangle of vessels. The axial raw data of the TOF sequence and their reconstruction demonstrate the asymmetric number of flow voids and the abnormal cortical vessels in the right frontal lobe, suggesting the diagnosis.

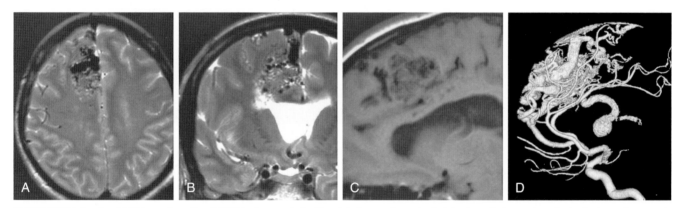

■ **FIGURE 24-4** A to D, This corticocallosal AVM had a massively dilated thalamostriate vein draining into the internal cerebral vein that subsequently led to unilateral hydrocephalus. On MRI, the flow voids can be well appreciated on T2W images (**A, B**) while on T1W nonenhanced studies (**C**) the AVM signal is typically hypointense.

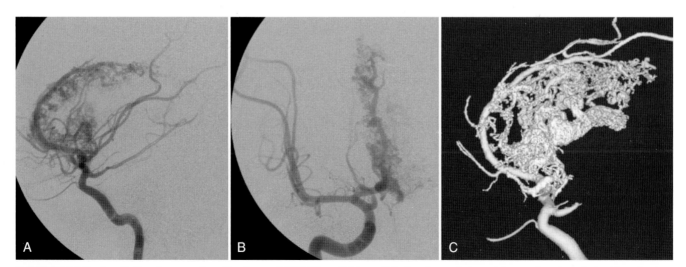

■ **FIGURE 24-5** A to C, Cingular or corticocallosal type of AVM. These AVMs are linked to the cortical arterial network and are drained into the deep venous system. In this case the type of feeding arteries are "en passage" rather than terminal-type feeders.

■ **FIGURE 24-6** A to D, Infratentorial micro-AVM of the pons. On FLAIR-weighted images a hyperintensity can be seen that corresponds to a small glomerular AVM that is fed by three separate pontine perforators. The 3D rotational angiography demonstrates well the glomerular aspect of this AVM.

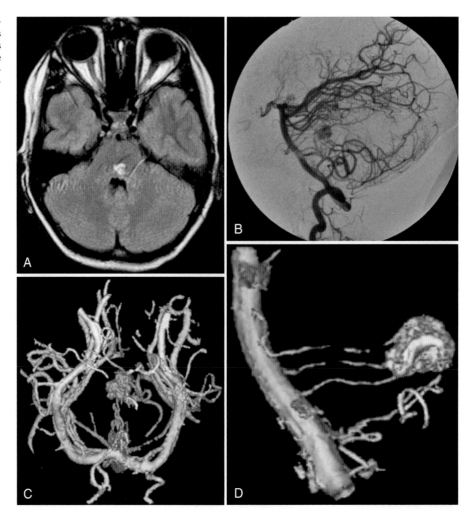

nidi involve the deep nuclei, and the arterial and venous connections are along the long fiber tracts. The deeply seated arteriovenous lesions recruit perforating arteries exclusively and drain into the deep venous system. They may use transcerebral veins, if patent, as direct venous outlets or as collateral pathways. Arteriovenous lesions of the lenticular and striate nuclei may recruit transcortical arteries from the insular branches of the middle cerebral artery. Arteriovenous lesions of the dentate nucleus may recruit hemispheric collaterals of the cerebellar arteries. MRI and angiography will be able to distinguish these deep-seated lesions from cortical-subcortical lesions, particularly because the dominant supply of the deep intracerebral lesions arises from the perforators.

Arteriovenous Lesions of the Choroid Plexus

Choroid plexus AVMs are important to recognize because they are anatomically extracerebral lesions accessible to surgical and endovascular therapy. Choroidal arteriovenous lesions are fed primarily by choroidal arteries and by subependymal arterial feeders arising from the circle of Willis, including the anterior thalamoperforate arteries arising from the posterior communicating arteries that course through the walls of the third ventricle to reach its roof and the adjacent choroid fissure (Fig. 23-7). By definition, choroid plexus arteriovenous lesions have no cortical arterial supply. They drain via ventricular veins, with occasional recruitment of transcerebral veins. These extra-axial lesions can be distinguished from intra-axial AVMs by angiographic criteria.

Epidemiology

The incidence of brain AVMs is difficult to estimate. Figures from small communities and autopsy series suggest that 0.14% to 0.8% of the population may present with a brain AVM in a given year. In adults, symptomatic brain AVMs appear to be about one tenth as frequent as intracranial arterial aneurysms. The risk of hemorrhage is estimated to be about 2% to 4% per year for "unruptured" brain AVMs but 8% to 17% per year for brain AVMs that have bled previously. Overall, the major morbidity or mortality of brain AVMs is about 1% per year.

Pathophysiology

The vascular malformation and the rest of the vasculature evolve with age. Assessment of a vascular malformation, therefore, requires consideration of (1) the presumably congenital defect that expresses itself as a malformation and (2) the response of the individual host harboring the malformation. AVMs are believed to be initially stable lesions, which become destabilized over time owing to hemodynamic increases in venous flow or mechanical compromise resulting in decreased venous outflow. Destabilization of the AVM leads to hemorrhage. Destabilization of the brain leads to seizures or progressive neurologic deficits.

The vessels surrounding the AVM are affected by the congenital malformation and by the hemodynamic alterations it produces. These secondary, acquired effects influence the clinical presentation and outcome. Pial AVMs may be found incidentally or because of headache, seizures, or hemorrhage. Children, especially those with high-flow fistulas, may manifest somatic

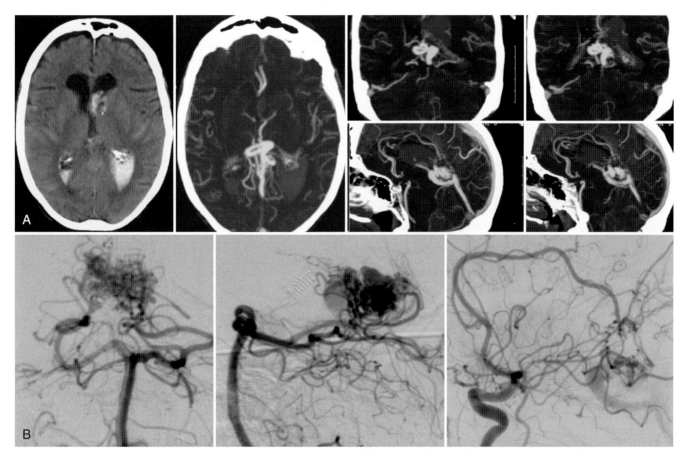

■ **FIGURE 24-7** Acute intraventricular hemorrhage in a 68-year-old woman without prior history of hypertension led to CTA that was able to demonstrate a choroidal type AVM with large venous outpouchings (**A**). CTA demonstrates a tangle of pathologic and enlarged vessels as a sign for the AVM that was verified on DSA (**B**). Typical for a choroidal AVM, feeders are recruited from the pericallosal artery via the limbic arch and from the lateral posterior choroidal arteries of the posterior cerebral artery.

symptoms and psychomotor retardation when venous congestion is a prominent feature of the malformation. Headaches are more commonly seen in children and are typically pseudomigrainous. AVMs in occipital locations and AVMs that have transdural supply, venous ectasia, and venous congestion show increased incidence of headaches. Most seizures associated with brain AVMs are focal and may reflect venous congestion or small hemorrhages that irritate healthy brain tissue near the brain AVM.

Pathology

The normal adult brain does not express growth factors such as vascular endothelial growth factor (VEGF) or transforming growth factor-β (TGF-β). These factors may be present in AVMs and may be induced by proliferation of new vessels, hemodynamic stress, ischemia, and/or hemorrhage. VEGF is predominantly expressed in the subendothelial layer and media of vessels in AVMs. Ultrastructurally, brain AVMs show preservation of mature vessel walls with phenotypic alterations due to high flow and hemodynamic stress, including arterial, nidal, and venous aneurysms. In contrast to the ultrastructure of cavernous malformations (CCM), AVMs maintain normal vessel wall and structural integrity with endothelial cell denudation. There may be intense laminin expression localized in and around the internal elastic lamina. Type IV collagen seems to be expressed intensely in the subendothelium at the level of the basal lamina. Type III collagen is observed in the media and perivascular tissue. Immunohistochemical analyses on activin, myosin, and smoothelin indicate

the disappearance of contractile properties in vascular smooth muscle cells of AVM vessels due to the hemodynamic stress of turbulent blood flow through these lesions. The levels of certain proteinases are increased in the endothelial/periendothelial cell layer of cerebral AVMs, consistent with vascular remodeling and instability within the AVM. Endothelial cells cultured from AVMs have reduced secretion of endothelin-1, a molecule involved in vascular cell phenotypes, and demonstrate increased proliferation.

On histopathology, "classic" cerebral AVMs consist of a tangle of abnormal arteries and veins with no intervening capillary bed. Gliotic and nonfunctional brain parenchyma may be present between the abnormal vascular channels. The walls of the feeding arteries show abnormal lamination with reduplication, interruption, and distortion of the internal elastic lamina, focal increase of arterial muscle fibers, and focal thinning of the muscularis to form arterial aneurysms. The walls of the veins are typically thickened by collagenous tissue. There may be secondary signs of vascular degeneration, including fibrosis, atheroma, and calcification. The surrounding cortex shows neuronal loss and increase in fibrillary glia. The neural tissue originally present between the abnormal blood vessels is restricted to thin gliotic bands, with no identifiable neurons. Signs of prior hemorrhage, such as hemosiderin-laden macrophages, may be present.

Classification

The Spetzler-Martin classification of pial brain AVMs is based on the size of the AVM, the pattern of venous drainage, and the

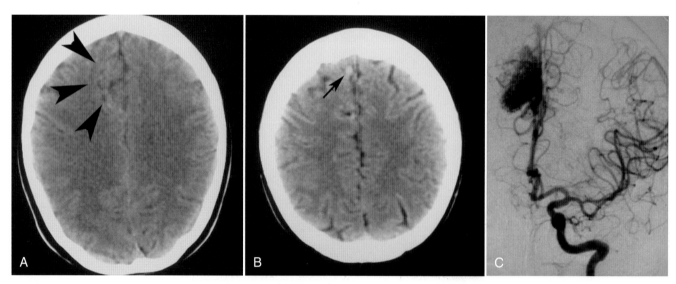

■ FIGURE 24-8 This patient presented to the emergency department with a first-ever seizure. **A** and **B,** Routine non–contrast-enhanced cranial CT revealed an ill-defined area of gray matter/white matter differentiation in the right frontal lobe (*arrowheads*) and a tubular extra-axial structure (*small arrow*) extending to the superior sagittal sinus, indicative of a vascular malformation with a large draining vein. This was verified on DSA (**C**).

eloquence of the portions of brain adjacent to the AVM. The classification was devised to anticipate the risk of treating brain AVMs surgically but has been extended to predict the (presumed) natural history of the entire group of AVMs. We believe this generalization to be improper because (1) the classification does not assess the special characteristics of an AVM in an individual patient (e.g., associated aneurysms), (2) the classification does not recognize that an AVM with high-grade risk for surgery is not necessarily dangerous to the patient, and (3) the classification does not allow assessment for alternate therapy by endovascular techniques and radiosurgery.

To determine whether endovascular therapies are suitable for a brain AVM, one must assess the angioarchitecture of the malformation, including the nature of the feeding artery, the number of separate compartments of the malformation, any arterial or venous ectasias near to or within the malformation, and the nature of the venous drainage. There are two basic types of feeding artery. *Direct arterial feeders* end in the AVM. *Indirect arterial feeders* supply the normal cortex and also supply the AVM "en passage" via small vessels that arise from the normal artery (see Fig. 24-5). Intranidal arterial aneurysms or venous varices indicate weak points in the system. Drainage into the deep venous system and stenoses that restrict venous outflow indicate increased risk of spontaneous hemorrhage. A long pial course of the draining vein may indicate that venous drainage is restricted over a large area, increasing the risk of venous congestion and subsequent epilepsy. Conversely, a short vein that drains almost directly into a dural sinus is unlikely to interfere with the normal pial drainage.

Imaging
CT
Small AVMs may be difficult to discern (Fig. 24-8). Larger AVMs usually display (1) tangled "serpiginous" parenchymal vessels that appear slightly dense due to blood pooling and (2) large draining veins in the subarachnoid space. Calcifications are present in about one third of brain AVMs. Focal hemorrhage, focal mass, or focal atrophy may also be present. Contrast enhancement opacifies the enlarged feeding arteries, the tangle of vessels in the parenchyma, and the dilated draining veins.

MRI
T2-weighted (T2W) imaging shows punctate to linear flow voids in the subarachnoid space over the brain, reflecting the dilated surface vessels. Within the brain, the punctate flow voids often lie within hyperintense, gliotic parenchyma. This gliosis may extend to the surrounding brain tissue. T1-weighted (T1W) imaging shows highly variable signal within the AVM, due to turbulent flow, blood degradation products, and the variable flow rate in the veins (Fig. 24-9). There is usually intense contrast enhancement of the vessels themselves. T2*-weighted images may detect smaller areas of hemorrhage.

MRA
"Static" magnetic resonance angiographic (MRA) sequences (such as time-of-flight [TOF] and phase contrast [PC] MRA) may detect the lesion but do not detail the angioarchitecture of the malformation (see Fig. 24-3). Static MRA provides little information about the presence of flow-related or intranidal aneurysms or the direct/indirect nature of the feeding arteries. Venous stenoses and ectasias are poorly displayed due to turbulent flow. Static MRA also fails to define the hemodynamics of the AVM, including the principal feeding arteries, the early venous drainage pattern, and the flow velocity.

High-resolution, 3D, dynamic contrast-enhanced MRA provides greater information about the velocity and direction of blood flow through each component of the AVM and can confirm the diagnosis of an AVM suggested by prior conventional MRI and MRA (Fig. 24-10). Complex subtraction techniques help to eliminate artifactual signal resulting from intraparenchymal hemorrhage. However, caution must be taken in very fast-flow AVMs, because the rapid flow results in poorer contrast of the feeding arteries compared with normal vessels and draining veins (Fig. 24-11).

Functional imaging methods such as blood oxygenation level–dependent contrast (BOLD) fMRI and perfusion imaging may give additional information about the pathophysiology of these AVMs (Fig. 24-12).

Conventional Digital Subtraction Angiography
Conventional catheter angiography remains the study of choice to evaluate all potential feeding arteries, including external

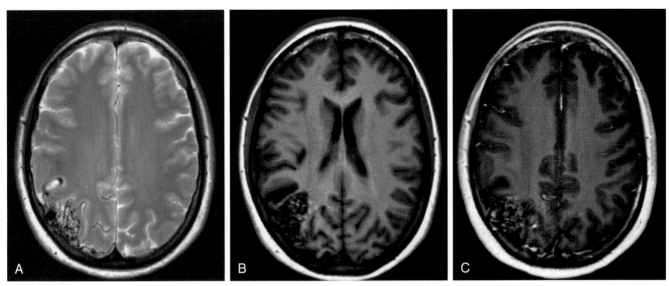

■ **FIGURE 24-9** **A** to **C,** MR aspect of a cortical AVM. A conglomeration of dilated vascular masses can be seen on both T2W (**A**) and T1W (**B, C**) images. The signal (especially on T1W sequences) depends on the velocity and direction of flow with both flow-void and/or enhanced areas. Remnants of recent or old bleeding have to be specifically sought using T2W GRE sequences (not shown) because AVMs that have bled once have a higher propensity to rebleed. FLAIR and T2W sequences should be evaluated for perifocal gliosis. Classically, the cortical AVMs extend wedge shaped into the subcortical areas within a sulcus.

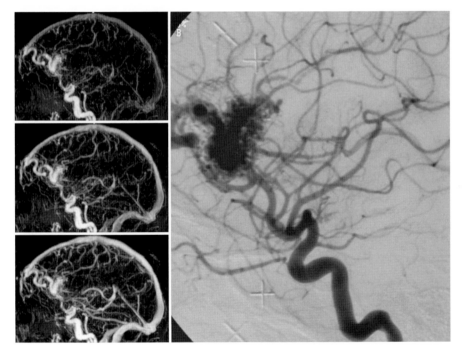

■ **FIGURE 24-10** Contrast-enhanced dynamic MRA can depict the large feeding vessels, the size of the nidus, its location, and the major draining veins. Pure morphologic classifications are therefore possible using this technique.

carotid branches that can supply the AVM via dural and leptomeningeal collaterals. Digital subtraction angiography (DSA) also provides a full assessment of the other vascular territories to rule out multiple shunts that may indicate an underlying systemic disease (e.g., hereditary hemorrhagic telangiectasia) or a syndromic disease such as cerebrofacial arteriovenous metameric syndrome. DSA should define the angioarchitecture of all feeding arteries, determine whether the shunt is a direct or indirect type, and display all significant arterial dilatations, stenoses, and associated flow-related aneurysms (Fig. 24-13). DSA should define the nidus, including its size, fistulous versus glomerular nature, intranidal aneurysms, false aneurysms (in case of hemorrhagic AVMs),

associated angioectasia, and neoangiogenesis. DSA should also display all of the draining veins to resolve deep versus superficial patterns of drainage, length of the pial segments, venous ectasias, and any stenoses that might cause flow restriction. DSA is paramount, therefore, for ascertaining the risk posed by an individual brain AVM and for selecting the therapy best suited for that specific AVM (Fig. 24-14).

Two conditions merit special imaging consideration:

1. *The acute hemorrhage that obscures an AVM.* A small AVM may be completely obscured by the mass effect of an acute hematoma. In the setting of acute hemorrhage, therefore, the

■ **FIGURE 24-11** The value of MR contrast-enhanced angiography is shown in this case. Whereas classic MR sequences such as T2W and T1W images (**A, B**) are able to show only a dilated basal vein of Rosenthal (*arrowhead,* **A**), the dynamic aspect of the contrast-enhanced MRA (**C, D**) is clearly able to depict the early arteriovenous shunt into the basal vein of Rosenthal and the venous filling of the straight and transverse sinuses in the early arterial phase, which is suggestive of a large shunting volume.

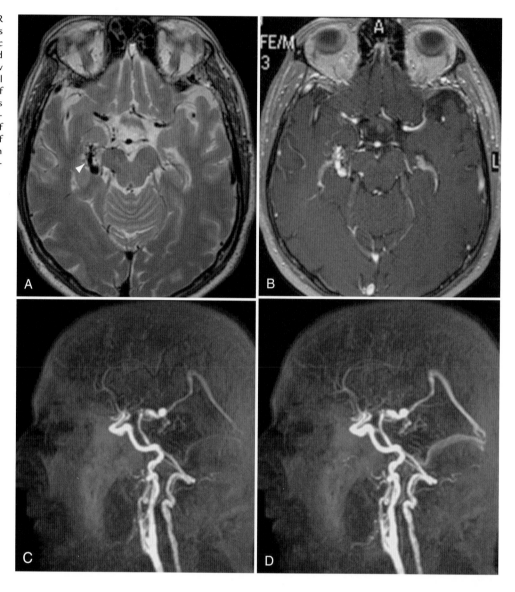

initial CT, MR, MRA, and DSA may be insufficient to rule out an AVM, even if contrast enhancement is used. For these reasons, a second DSA should be performed after the clot has cleared, especially if the patient is a child or the clot was atypical in appearance.

2. *Post-treatment evaluation.* Patients presenting with a treated AVM are evaluated for the completeness of occlusion and restoration of flow previously diverted toward the shunt (steal phenomenon). In these cases, dynamic contrast-enhanced MRA may be sufficient to separate the arterial and venous phases and document the presence of any persistent early filling of the draining veins. If the MRA shows an early vein, the AVM is not completely occluded. If dynamic contrast-enhanced MRA fails to demonstrate an early-filling vein, it may still be necessary to use the superior spatial resolution of DSA to ensure that the shunt is completely obliterated (Fig. 24-15).

Differential Diagnosis

Two significant entities must be considered in the differential diagnosis of cerebral AVMs: (1) cerebral proliferative angiopathy and (2) segmental vascular syndromes with brain AVMs.

Cerebral Proliferative Angiopathy

Cerebral proliferative angiopathy (CPA, diffuse nidus type AVM) is a clinical entity distinct from the "classic" brain AVMs in its clinical presentation, natural history, angioarchitecture, and treatment. CPA is present in 2% to 4% of all brain AVMs. It is more common in females by 2:1 and presents at a mean age of 20 years. Seizures, headaches, and transient ischemic attacks are far more frequent in CPA than in classic AVMs, whereas hemorrhages are exceedingly rare. On CT and MRI, CPA presents as a diffuse network of densely enhancing vascular spaces intermingled with normal brain parenchyma. T1W and T2W images show small, widely distributed flow voids that may involve multiple lobes or the entire hemisphere (Fig. 24-16). In most cases, the primary lesion extends from the surface into the basal ganglia and thalamus and involves more than one vascular territory. Compared with the size of the nidus, relatively few draining vessels are seen on CT or MRI, and these are only moderately enlarged. Perfusion-weighted MRI demonstrates perfusion abnormalities far beyond the boundaries of the morphologic malformation seen on conventional MR sequences, so the disease actually affects the entire hemisphere. The nidus shows increased cerebral blood volume, slightly decreased time to peak (TTP), and

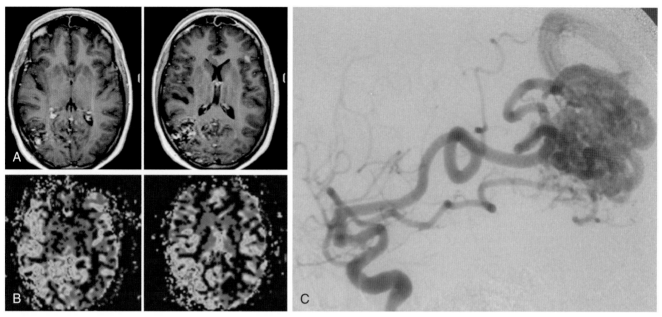

■ FIGURE 24-12 A to C, This 27-year-old woman underwent MRI due to recurrent and worsening headaches and repeated episodes of speech arrest followed by confusion. MRI demonstrated a right parietal AVM that, owing to its location, was unable to explain the clinical symptoms of recurrent speech arrests in this right-handed patient. Functional MRI was performed to localize the speech-related areas and demonstrated bilateral representation of areas responsible for naming located in the pars triangularis of the inferior frontal gyrus (Broca's area and its contralateral homologue). A perfusion MRI demonstrated an increased flow not only within the AVM but also in its vicinity, namely, those areas that were activated during the speech tasks. Owing to these results it was hypothesized that the high shunting volume of the AVM led to a reduced capillary transit time in the vicinity of the AVM and therefore to the recurrent speech arrests. After embolization achieved a significant reduction of the shunting volume the patient was free of symptoms. The remainder of the AVM was treated with gamma knife radiosurgery.

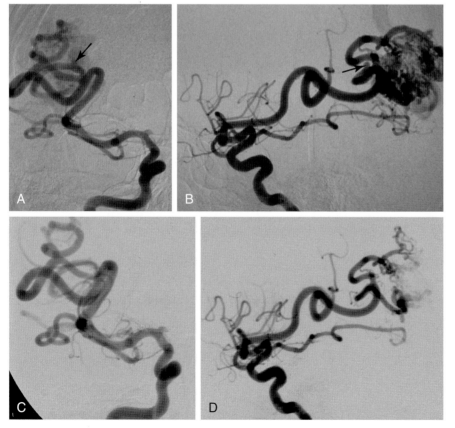

■ FIGURE 24-13 Effects of embolization on the remodeling of the feeding vessels. In this AVM an aneurysm can be seen in each division of the two major feeding arteries (*arrows* in **A** and **B**). Six weeks after initial embolization with significant flow reduction, the aneurysms are no longer seen, which is indicative of its flow-related nature (**C, D**).

■ **FIGURE 24-14** Right temporal AVM before (**A, B**) and after treatment (**C to E**) with super-selective glue injection demonstrating a markedly reduced size of the nidus and an enhanced flow in other cortical areas immediately after the intervention.

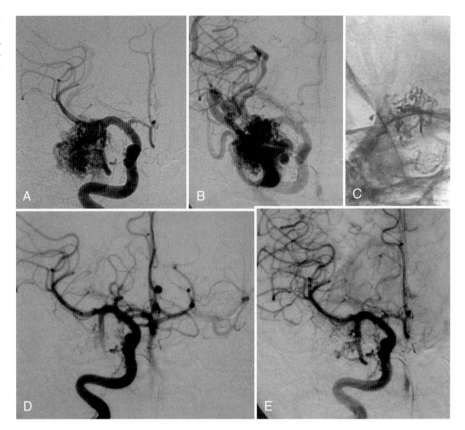

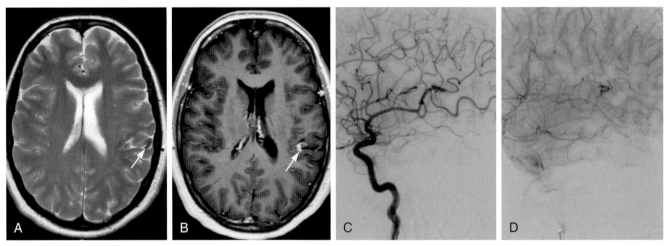

■ **FIGURE 24-15** Effects of gamma knife surgery. Three years before this MRI, stereotactic radiation of a left parietal AVM was performed. In the control image, a hemosiderin stain and persistent contrast enhancement in the area of the former AVM can be seen (*arrows* in **A** and **B**). DSA confirmed the complete occlusion of the AVM (**C, D**), but a slight area of hyperperfusion resembling the contrast enhancement on MRI was seen. Because no early-draining vein could be visualized, the treatment was, however, considered completed.

prolonged mean transit time (MTT). Remote from the nidus, in normal-appearing cortical and subcortical areas, the TTP is increased and the blood volume is decreased, indicating remote, widespread hypoperfusion (Fig. 24-17). Angiography shows no dominant feeders. Instead, CPA is fed by multiple arteries that are not enlarged or are only moderately enlarged. Unlike classic AVMs, all arteries of the affected region contribute equally to the malformation. Stenoses of the proximal arteries are present in 40% and affect the internal carotid artery (ICA) and the proximal

horizontal segments of the middle cerebral artery (M1) and anterior cerebral artery (A1). Most cases show transdural supply to both the malformation and the normal brain tissue. The nidus has a classic appearance with scattered areas of "puddling" of contrast medium within what looks like capillary ectasias. These persist into the late arterial and early venous phases. The nidus is usually fuzzy, poorly circumscribed, and larger than 6 cm in diameter. Intranidal vessels show a capillary angioectasia. Perinidal angiogenesis is often present and difficult to distinguish from

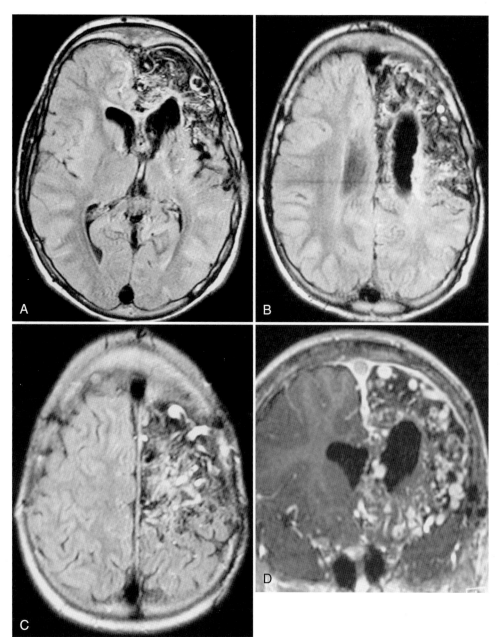

■ **FIGURE 24-16** FLAIR-weighted images (**A-C**) and T1W MR image post contrast (**D**) in a 15-year-old boy with recurrent seizures, disabling head-aches, and transitory ischemic attacks. A diffuse network of densely enhancing vascular spaces can be seen through-out the frontal lobe. Normal brain tissue seems to be dispersed along the vascular malformation. The size of the malformation is atypical for an AVM. These findings correspond with the diagnosis of cerebral proliferative angiopathy.

the nidus proper. There is no high-flow fistulous component to the arteriovenous shunt, so early opacification of draining veins is uncommon. The size of the draining veins, the "shunt volume," and the time until the veins are visualized never "correspond" to the size of the nidus. Histopathology demonstrates the pres-ence of normal-appearing neural tissue intermingled between these vascular channels. Perivascular gliosis is only mild. There is additional capillary angiogenesis within the subcortical region (Fig. 24-18). The implication is that the brain tissue within the "nidus" of the CPA is functional, similar to the brain tissue found between the abnormal vascular channels of capillary telangiec-tasia. This alters therapeutic strategies. Because these lesions appear to result from ischemia, therapy should be directed toward revascularization procedures, such as burr-hole therapy, not at the lesion proper.

The name "cerebral proliferative angiopathy" implies that new vessel formation is an important component of the disease. This is very different from classic AVMs. Meningeal vessels con-tribute to the lesion directly and contribute to the healthy brain tissue bilaterally via supratentorial and infratentorial transdural supply. Presumably the angiogenesis is induced by the (relative) cortical ischemia demonstrated with perfusion-weighted MRI, although the signaling mechanism remains unknown. It is not related to previous hemorrhage and does not suggest increased risk of hemorrhage in the future.

The combination of segmental stenoses of proximal arteries and distal angioectasia suggests that the pathogenesis of this lesion may be abnormal proliferation of the vessel wall. In their 1975 classification of vascular lesions in childhood and infancy, Mulliken and Glowacki differentiated between (1) vascular

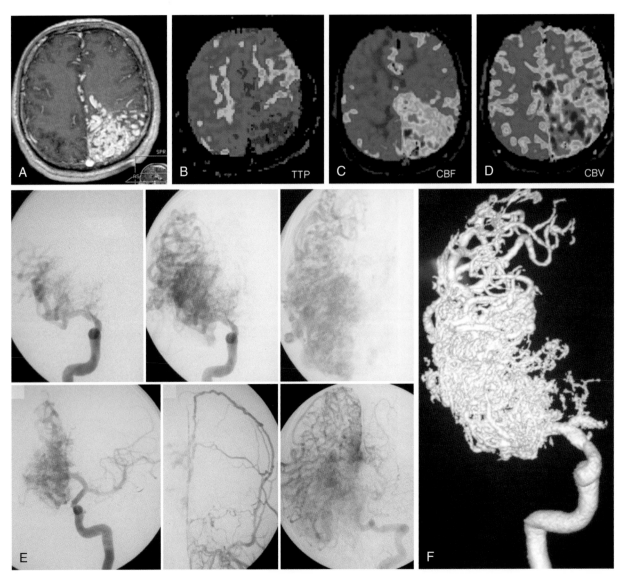

■ **FIGURE 24-17** Cerebral proliferative angiopathy. T1W (**A**) and perfusion MRI with time to peak (TTP), cerebral blood volume (CBV), and cerebral blood flow (CBF) maps in a 11-year-old girl with headaches demonstrating a large left frontoparietal nidus with brain parenchyma intermingled between the vascular spaces. Perfusion-weighted MRI demonstrates an increase in cerebral blood volume (**D**) and flow (**C**), with hypervascularization within the nidus and decreased times to peak (**B**) in the area surrounding the nidus, indicating the ischemic nature of the disease. **E, F,** Angiography in the early arterial phase demonstrates the absence of dominant feeders and the equal contribution of many different arteries. The contrast dynamics reveal persistence of contrast material in the malformation and no early venous drainage. Transdural supply testifies for the proliferative component of the disease while injection into the vertebral artery demonstrates diffuse neoangiogenesis in other cortical areas.

lesions that demonstrate cellular proliferation and endothelial hyperplasia ("hemangiomas" or true vascular *tumors* as in PHACES syndrome) and (2) vascular lesions that have normal endothelial turnover but structural abnormalities of the capillary, venous, lymphatic, or arterial channels (e.g., vascular *malformations* like brain AVMs). CPA can be regarded as an intermediate or transitional form between these two major types of vascular lesion. CPA exhibits both proliferative features (less prominent than in hemangiomas) and malformative features (less prominent than in true AVMs).

Segmental Vascular Syndromes with Brain AVMs

The significance of concurrent AVMs of the face, retina, and brain was first recognized in Lyon, France, by Bonnet, Dechaume, and Blanc, who reported two cases in 1937. Six years later,

Wyburn-Mason published a detailed analysis of all similar case reports and nine new cases. The association of retinal, facial, and cerebral vascular malformations became known as Bonnet-Dechaume-Blanc syndrome in France and continental Europe and as Wyburn-Mason syndrome in the English literature.

Recent genetic/biologic contributions suggest that disorders of neural crest and cephalic cell migration may be the link common to all components of this syndrome. The neural crest and neural plate share a common lineage from cells of the lateral border of the developing neural plate (i.e., the neural folds). Under inductive influence of the adjacent epithelium (and possibly mesoderm) these cells develop into neural crest cells, hence their common metameric origin with the cells of the hindbrain. The insult producing the underlying lesion has to be before the migration occurs and thus before the fourth week of development.

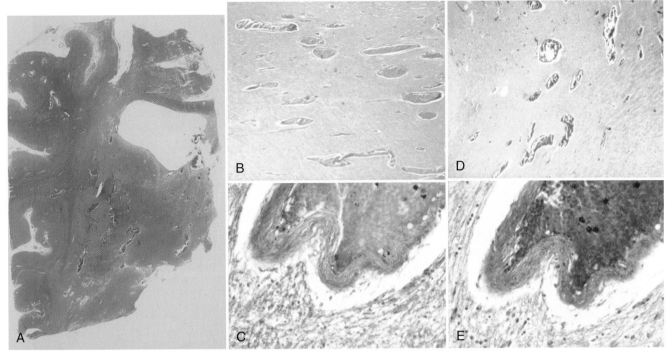

■ FIGURE 24-18   Histologic specimens of cerebral proliferative angiopathy. Paraffin-embedded tissues shown here were stained with hematoxylin and eosin (**A, B**), orcein van Gieson (**C**), and Masson trichrome (**D, E**). In **A**, a coronal cut through the right hemisphere at the level of the frontal horn and the striatum demonstrates intraparenchymal vascular proliferation with dilated and irregular arterioles that are otherwise histologically normal. These dilated vascular channels are located preferentially in regions with low cellular density (white matter tracts and between the basal ganglia). The venous vessel walls demonstrate collagenous thickening of the veins. Mild perifocal gliosis is seen directly surrounding the vessels, but normal-appearing neuronal tissue can be seen intermingled between the vascular channels.

In accord with the metameric concept of neural crest development, we have proposed a rational classification of regional AVMs that reflects the putative underlying disorder and coined the acronym CAMS (cerebrofacial arteriovenous metameric syndrome). Depending on the specific structures involved, distinct CAM syndromes can be identified. CAMS 1 indicates a midline prosencephalic (olfactory) group with involvement of hypothalamus, corpus callosum, hypophysis, and nose. CAMS 2 indicates a lateral prosencephalic (optic) group with involvement of the optic nerve, retina, parieto-temporal-occipital lobes, thalamus, and maxilla (Fig. 24-19). CAMS 3 indicates a rhombencephalic (otic) group, with involvement of the cerebellum, pons, petrous bone, and mandible (Fig. 24-20). CAMS 3 is located in a strategic position at the crossroads between the complex cephalic segmental arrangements and the relatively simplified spinal metamers, so it exhibits transitional characteristics. More extensive insult will lead to overlapping territories producing a complete prosencephalic phenotype (CAMS 1+2) or bilateral involvement.

Considered as a metameric lesion, intracranial AVMs are one of the most common findings in CAMS patients. The cerebral AVMs in CAMS may involve the corpus callosum, the olfactory region, and the hypothalamus in continuity (CAMS 1); the optic chiasm, thalamus, the cortex around the calcarine fissure (CAMS 2); or the cerebellum (CAMS 3). Infrequently they present as multiple scattered lesions in the same segmental distribution. Considering the angioarchitecture of cerebral AVMs in CAMS, certain findings differ from "classic" AVMs: the AVM nidus in CAMS is a cluster of small vessels with intervening normal brain tissue, some degree of angiogenesis, and a rather small shunting volume. Transdural arterial supply can be present. Progressive enlargement of these cerebral AVMs is one of the special observations in CAMS, suggesting that AVMs in CAMS are not static

processes within the segment that carry the embryonic defect. Multifocality is another typical aspect of CAMS AVMs.

DURAL ARTERIOVENOUS FISTULAS
Dural arteriovenous fistulas (DAVFs) are abnormal connections between arteries that would normally supply the meninges, the bone, and the muscle, but not the brain, and small venules situated within the walls of the dural sinuses.

The term *dural arteriovenous shunts* (DAVSs) is preferred by many authors, because the etiology of these lesions is unclear, especially in children. The term *dural arteriovenous malformations* (DAVMs) is no longer used.

Epidemiology
DAVFs account for 10% to 15% of all intracranial arteriovenous shunts. A male predominance is observed for aggressive DAVFs.

Pathophysiology
Adult-type DAVFs are acquired lesions, postulated to be sequelae of sinus thrombosis, subsequent recanalization, and development of secondary arteriovenous shunts from either neovascularization or enlargement of preexisting physiologic connections within the sinus walls. Many studies have shown that venous hypertension and local hypoxia will stimulate angiogenesis through hypoxia-inducible factor-1α (HIF-1α) and through multiple vascular growth factors, predominantly vascular endothelial growth factor (VEGF), basic fibroblast growth factor (bFGF), and transforming growth factor-α (TGF-α). No genetic, heritable form of adult DAVF is known. Initial reports of an association

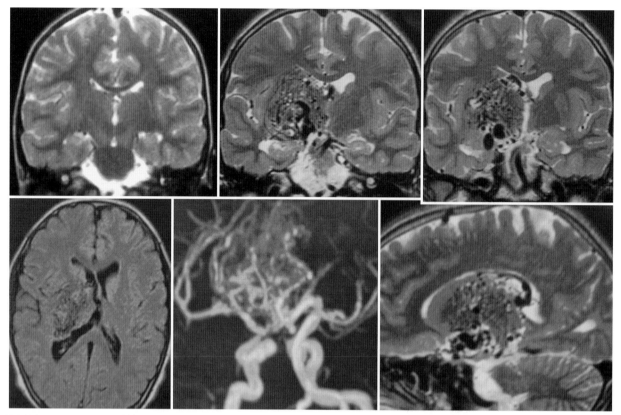

■ **FIGURE 24-19** A 15-year-old boy presented to the emergency department after a seizure; evaluation revealed a large hypothalamic AVM. Six years before this admission an MRI was performed because he harbored a retinal racemose angioma. At that time the thalamic area was normal, but in the present MRI a diffuse AVM of the thalamus can be seen. The de-novo appearance, the aspect of the normal brain tissue intermingled with the pathologic blood channels, and the concurrence with a retinal AVM strongly suggest lateral prosencephalic cerebrofacial arteriovenous metameric (CAMS 2) syndrome.

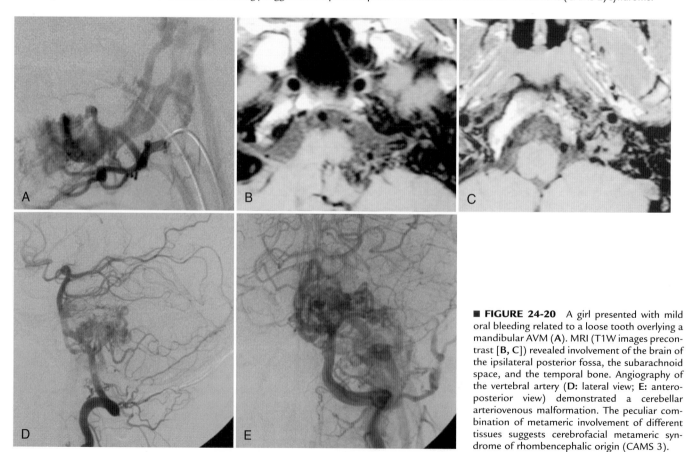

■ **FIGURE 24-20** A girl presented with mild oral bleeding related to a loose tooth overlying a mandibular AVM (**A**). MRI (T1W images precontrast [**B, C**]) revealed involvement of the brain of the ipsilateral posterior fossa, the subarachnoid space, and the temporal bone. Angiography of the vertebral artery (**D**: lateral view; **E**: antero-posterior view) demonstrated a cerebellar arteriovenous malformation. The peculiar combination of metameric involvement of different tissues suggests cerebrofacial metameric syndrome of rhombencephalic origin (CAMS 3).

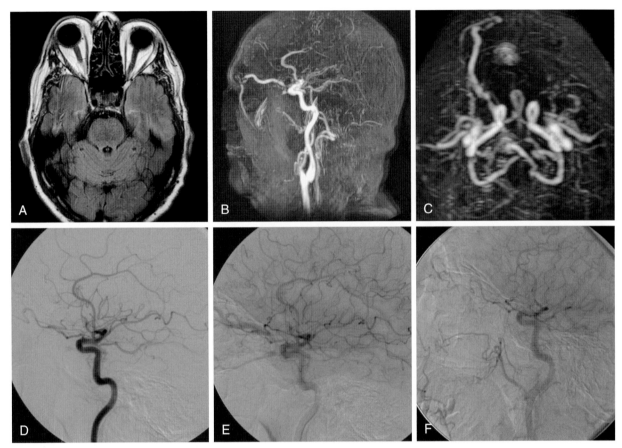

■ **FIGURE 24-21** A 53-year-old man experienced sudden, nontraumatic chemosis and bulging of his right eye that can be well appreciated on the FLAIR-weighted image (**A**). Because of the clinical symptoms a carotid-cavernous DAVF was suspected. Dynamic contrast-enhanced MR angiography was performed and demonstrated filling of the ophthalmic vein in the early arterial phase without filling into cortical veins (**B, C**), suggesting a benign, spontaneous carotid-cavernous DAVF that was verified on DSA (**D, E**). **F,** Right common carotid angiography during external compression of the right eye globe shows complete obliteration of the shunt flow in the ophthalmic vein without any rerouting of the venous drainage into the cortical veins. The patient was managed with external globe compression, which spontaneously thrombosed the DAVF.

between DAVFs and hereditary hemorrhagic telangiectasia (HHT)-2 appear to be coincidence, because DAVFs are found in less than 1% of HHT-2 patients, similar to their incidence in the general population.

Pathology

Histologic studies of DAVFs involving the transverse-sigmoid sinuses indicate that the essential abnormality is a connection between the arteries and dural veins within the walls of the venous sinus through small vessels averaging about 30 μm in diameter. These so-called crack-like vessels are part of the venous system. Sinus thrombosis with evidence of recanalization was also identified in many cases, and the intima of the dural arteries and the dural veins was thickened within the sinuses.

DAVFs are most commonly located in the transverse-sigmoid sinuses (30% to 50%), followed by the cavernous sinus (19% to 40%) (Fig. 24-21), tentorium (10% to 15%), superior sagittal sinus (6% to 8%), anterior cranial fossa (2% to 5%), foramen magnum (1% to 2%), and the deep venous system (<1%). Multiple lesions are present in 10% to 15%.

Classification and Grading

The most widely used classifications of DAVFs were proposed by Borden and by Cognard (Table 24-1). The major feature determining proper treatment is the presence of cortical or spinal venous reflux. DAVFs are called benign when there is no cortical or spinal venous reflux (Borden type I, Cognard types I and IIa)

(Fig. 24-22). DAVFs are called aggressive or malignant when they show cortical or spinal reflux (higher grade on both classification systems).

Clinical Presentation

The presenting symptoms may be benign or aggressive, depending on the lesion's location and the presence of cortical or spinal venous reflux. Benign clinical presentations include ocular symptoms of chemosis and proptosis, pulsatile tinnitus, headaches, and cranial nerve deficits from cavernous sinus syndrome (see Fig. 24-22). Aggressive clinical presentations are intracranial hemorrhage, seizures, dementia, alteration of consciousness, and focal nonhemorrhagic neurologic symptoms due to venous congestion. DAVFs in specific locations, such as the ethmoidal (anterior cranial fossa), tentorial, falcine, vein of Galen, and spinal DAVFs, always have cortical or spinal venous reflux with increased rates of aggressive clinical presentation: 79% to 97% for tentorial lesions and 68% to 88% for anterior cranial fossa lesions. Conversely, DAVFs at the cavernous sinus and sigmoid sinus rarely are aggressive. Cortical or spinal venous reflux is associated with a 10.4% annual mortality rate, an 8.1% annual hemorrhage rate, and a 6.9% annual event rate for nonhemorrhagic neurologic deficits. Discovery of venous reflux indicates need for urgent treatment to completely disconnect the reflux (Fig. 24-23). Patients harboring multiple lesions have twice the risk of developing cortical venous reflux.

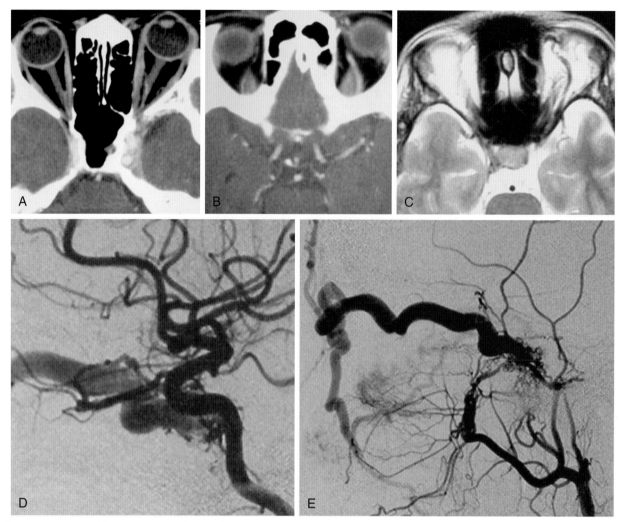

■ **FIGURE 24-22**   Carotid-cavernous DAVF (Cognard type I). On contrast-enhanced CT (**A, B**), the dilated cavernous sinus and the dilated superior ophthalmic vein can be seen; the latter is also well perceived on a T2W axial image (**C**) that demonstrates a flow void larger than on the contralateral side. Angiography reveals filling of the cavernous sinus via the recurrent meningeal branch from the ophthalmic artery and inferolateral trunk from the carotid artery (**D**). There is also filling of the fistula via branches of the internal maxillary artery and middle meningeal artery (**E**). There is no cortical venous reflux.

TABLE 24-1.   Classifications of Dural Arteriovenous Fistulas

Borden Classification

1	Venous drainage directly into dural venous sinus or meningeal vein
2	Venous drainage into dural venous sinus with CVR
3	Venous drainage into subarachnoid veins (CVR only)

Cognard Classification

I	Venous drainage into dural venous sinus with antegrade flow
IIa	Venous drainage into dural venous sinus with retrograde flow
IIb	Venous drainage into dural venous sinus with antegrade flow and CVR
IIa+b	Venous drainage into dural venous sinus with retrograde flow and CVR
III	Venous drainage directly into subarachnoid veins (CVR only)
IV	Type III with venous ectasias of the draining subarachnoid veins
V	Venous drainage into the spinal perimedullary veins

CVR, Cortical venous reflux.

Imaging

CT and MRI

CT and MRI features depend on the location of the lesion. DAVFs of the cavernous sinus typically cause outward bulging of the cavernous sinus with "too many" flow voids, enlargement of the superior ophthalmic vein, exophthalmos, and possible enlargement of the extraocular muscles from venous congestion (see Fig. 24-22). Lesions located solely at the sigmoid sinus are often falsely negative on CT and MRI, so MRA is crucial for evaluation of patients presenting with pulsatile tinnitus and suspected DAVF.

Aggressive or malignant type DAVFs usually show dilated cortical veins (the pseudophlebitic pattern) with abnormal enhancing tubular structures or flow voids within the cortical sulci (Fig. 24-24). No true nidus is present within the brain parenchyma (Fig. 24-25). Hypodensity of the white matter on CT or high T2 signal on MRI indicates venous congestion or infarction, which may lead to secondary intracerebral hemorrhage (Fig. 24-26). Focal enhancement of the hypodense or T2-hyperintense areas may also be observed (Fig. 24-27). These findings may be partially reversible after treatment.

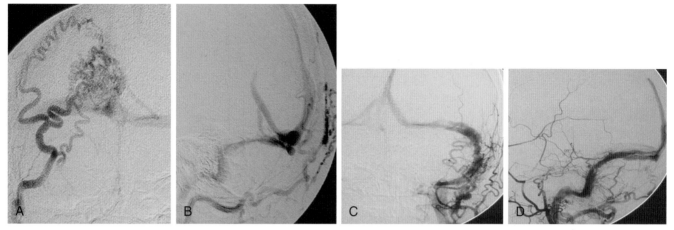

■ **FIGURE 24-23** DAVF type IIa. **A** to **D,** The venous drainage of this shunt is directed into the dural venous sinus, and there is retrograde flow; however, because of the missing cortical venous reflux these fistulas are still benign with a rather low risk of venous congestion and cortical hemorrhage. There are multiple dilated vessels entering the fistula at different points along the transverse sinus.

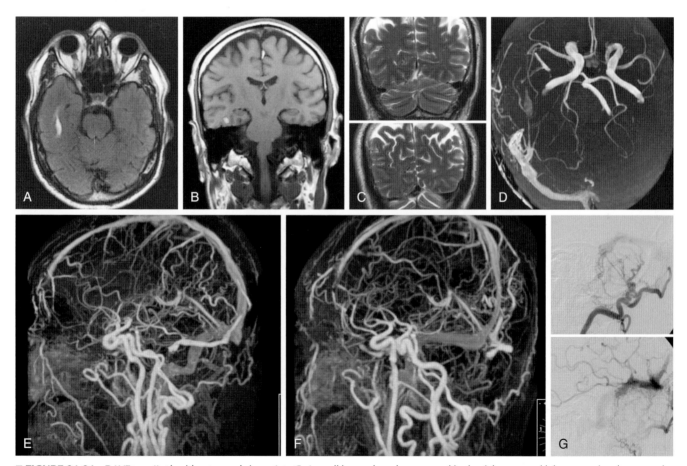

■ **FIGURE 24-24** DAVF type IIa+b with a trapped sinus. **A** to **C,** A small hemorrhage has occurred in the right temporal lobe suggesting the aggressive nature of these fistulas. On TOF angiographies the arterialized sinus can be well perceived (**D**). Dynamic contrast-enhanced MRA images in the late arterial phase demonstrate the "trapped" sinus that does not communicate with the torcular and therefore leads to corticovenous reflux (**E, F**). The fistula is well appreciated on superselective injection of the occipital artery, and is supplied mainly by the stylomastoid branches (**G**).

Hydrocephalus and tonsillar prolapse are present in rare cases, likely owing to venous hypertension in the superior sagittal sinus with impaired CSF absorption. On CT, subcortical curvilinear calcifications (Fig. 24-28) suggest chronic cortical venous reflux due to venous congestion or, perhaps, arterial hypoperfusion (Fig. 24-29). A few patients with DAVFs at the superior sagittal sinus or transverse sinus show sinus thrombosis with a hyperintense clot within the dural sinuses on T1W imaging.

Special Procedures
Angiography is the gold standard for characterizing the angioarchitecture and planning the treatment of patients with DAVF

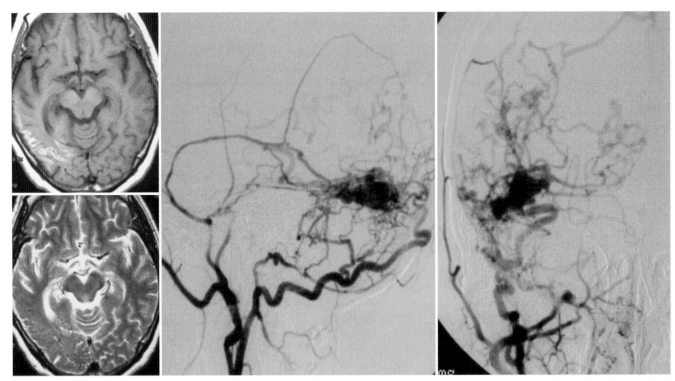

■ **FIGURE 24-25** DAVF type IIa+b. In this patient, a "trapped" sinus is present that hinders flow both antegradely and retrogradely. The arterialized blood, therefore, has to flow into those cortical veins that normally enter this part of the sinus. This has led in this case to a gyral T1 hyperintensity that may be related to slow-flowing blood or early calcifications.

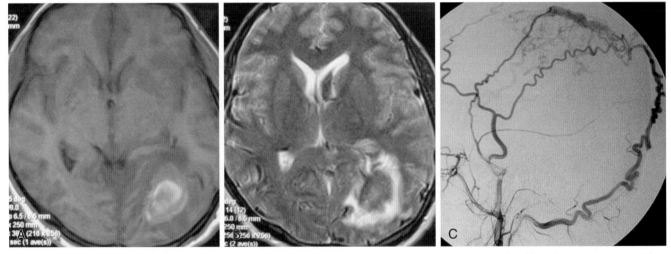

■ **FIGURE 24-26** A to C, Atypical hemorrhages should always lead to further diagnostic workup, which revealed in this patient a DAVF type IIa+b at the superior sagittal sinus that was fed at multiple different shunting zones by external carotid artery branches.

(Fig. 24-30). Diagnostic angiograms must include selective injections of both internal carotid arteries (ICAs), both external carotid arteries (ECAs), and at least the dominant vertebral artery. Common carotid angiograms should be avoided whenever possible. Whenever there is subarachnoid hemorrhage and no aneurysm or other cause can be identified, the ECAs should also be studied to rule out DAVF. Angiographic findings include early arteriovenous shunting from meningeal branches from the ICAs, ECAs, or vertebral arteries into either a sinus or cortical vein (Fig. 24-31). The venous drainage may then be normal antegrade flow or retrograde flow within the sinus or into the cortical veins. When there is cortical venous reflux, the venous

phase of the normal brain is often delayed and the cortical veins show a pseudophlebitic pattern. DAVFs located at the anterior cranial fossa, tentorium, superior petrosal sinus, and clival plexus may drain into dilated venous pouches (Fig. 24-32), ectatic veins (Fig. 24-33), or venous aneurysms (Fig. 24-34). These may rupture, causing subarachnoid or intraparenchymal hemorrhage, even in the absence of venous infarction. Stenosis or occlusion of the draining sinus is often seen with lesions involving the superior sagittal, transverse, and sigmoid sinuses and may reflect sinus thrombosis or intimal hyperplasia due to the high flow within the sinus from the arteriovenous shunting.

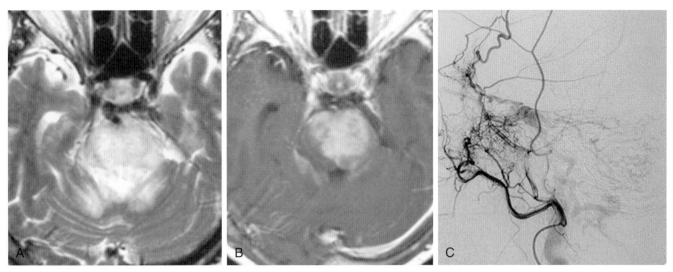

■ **FIGURE 24-27** A to C, Atypical findings in a patient with a DAVF type IIa+b. Venous congestion was relayed to the pons with subsequent massive contrast enhancement due to venous stagnation and/or venous ischemia.

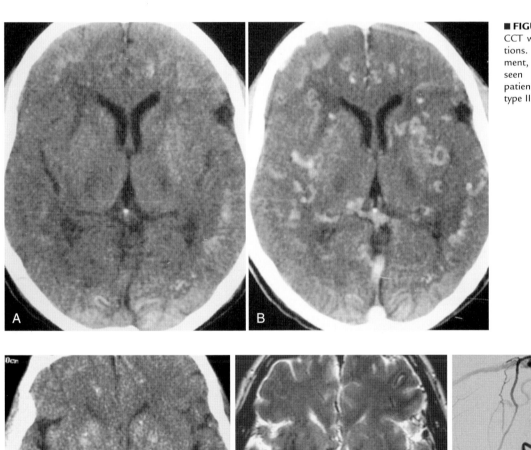

■ **FIGURE 24-28** A, Nonenhanced CCT with multiple cortical calcifications. B, After contrast enhancement, multiple dilated vessels can be seen in both hemispheres. The patient was found to have a DAVF type IIa+b on angiography.

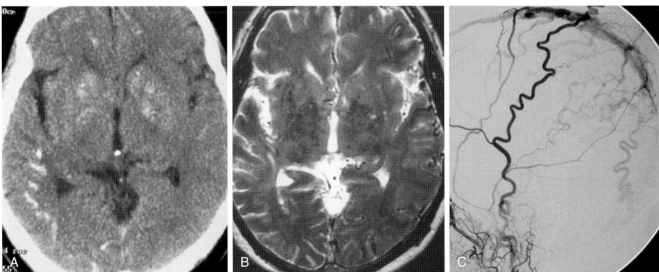

■ **FIGURE 24-29** DAVF type IIa+b. In this type the venous drainage is directed into a dural sinus and there is retrograde flow with corticovenous reflux. These fistulas may lead to venous congestion and subsequent hemorrhage. A to C, superior sagittal sinus DAVF. In the present case, the venous congestion of the contralateral hemisphere has led to multiple cortical calcifications that may be due to long-standing venous hypertension with venous wall calcifications. The calcifications do not represent the location of the shunt but rather the area that shows the most severe venous congestion.

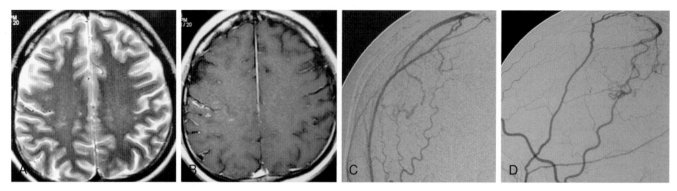

■ **FIGURE 24-30** DAVF type III. **A** to **D**, In this patient, venous drainage of the arteriovenous shunt is directed immediately into subarachnoid veins. Imaging findings on MRI are subtle with some dilated vessels seen on T2W images (**A**) and a hyperintensity on T1W images (**B**) that may be related to early calcifications or slow-flowing blood.

■ **FIGURE 24-31** DAVF type III. **A,** Contrast-enhanced CT demonstrates increased density of vessels on the left hemisphere, an early sign for an arteriovenous shunting. **B,** Three different shunting zones feed directly into pial veins in this patient.

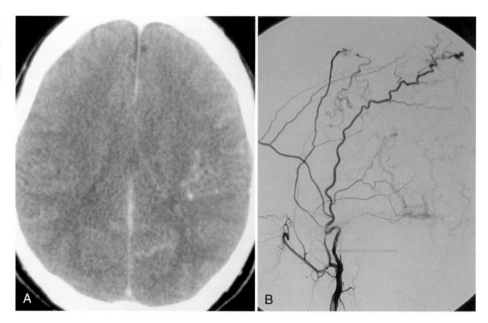

■ **FIGURE 24-32** DAVF type IV. **A** and **B,** Ethmoidal DAVF supplied mainly by branches of the ophthalmic artery. This type is present when a type III shunt has additional venous ectasias of the draining pial and subarachnoid veins. These are considered to be a sign for potential future hemorrhages and can be seen well on noninvasive imaging.

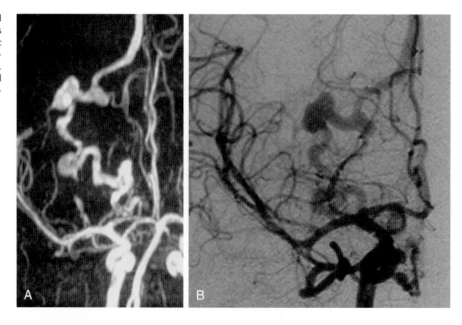

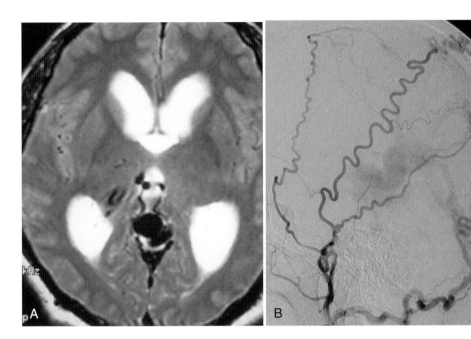

■ **FIGURE 24-33** A and B, DAVF type IV of the falx. On T2W images this may mimic a choroidal or vein of Galen AVM.

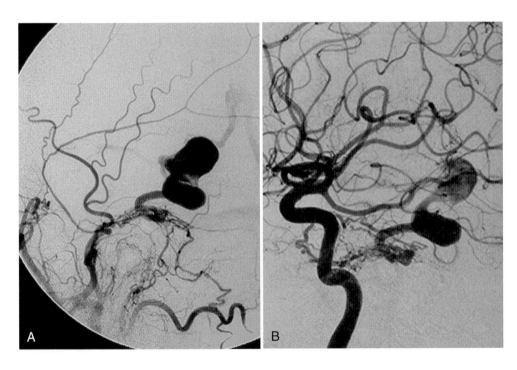

■ **FIGURE 24-34** A and **B,** DAVF type IV of the tentorium with dilated ectatic veins.

Treatment

DAVFs are usually treated first with endovascular therapies, with surgery reserved for refractory cases or residual portions of lesions. If the lesion drains into a vein or sinus that is used by the normal brain, cure may be achieved by obliterating the vein or sinus involved. Endovascular therapy may be accomplished by both transarterial and transvenous routes using diverse embolic materials chosen in accord with the size of the arterial feeders, the draining veins, and the drainage route of the shunt and brain. Surgery is often required for DAVFs located at the anterior cranial fossa, tentorium, and spinal canal and for aggressive DAVFs of the superior sagittal sinus or transverse sinus that have no other access routes. If the sinus is still patent and used by the normal brain, then it should always be preserved to avoid venous infarction or major hemorrhage.

Differential Diagnosis

In the diagnosis of cranial DAVFs, lesions of the cavernous sinus, ethmoids, tentorium, and foramen magnum require special comment.

Cavernous sinus DAVFs or indirect types of carotid-cavernous fistulas are shunts in the dura of the cavernous sinus. They are classified by their arterial supply as DAVFs of the meningeal branches of the ECA, ICA, or both. Cavernous sinus DAVFs show marked female predominance, likely related to hormonal factors. The presenting symptoms depend on the pattern of venous drainage. Drainage anteriorly into the superior and inferior ophthalmic veins most commonly causes ocular symptoms of chemosis, proptosis, and ophthalmoplegia. Drainage posteriorly through the inferior petrosal sinus may cause pulsatile tinnitus, although pulsatile tinnitus more commonly occurs with DAVFs of the transverse-sigmoid sinuses or jugular bulbs. Rarely, venous infarctions or hemorrhage may result from cortical venous reflux (1) from the sphenoparietal sinus into the superficial sylvian vein, medial temporal vein, or basal vein of Rosenthal and (2) from the superior petrosal sinus into the posterior fossa veins. Although the ocular symptoms are considered to be "benign," long-standing venous congestion and increased intraocular pressure may lead to secondary glaucoma and eventual blindness if left untreated. CT and MRI typically show bulging of the cavernous sinus with dilatation of the superior ophthalmic vein. Asymmetric dilatation of the sphenoparietal sinus, just inferior to the temporal pole, suggests mild cortical venous reflux. As in direct carotid-cavernous fistulas, CT and MRI do not identify the side of the lesion, because blood may shunt from side to side through intercavernous anastomoses. Dynamic gadolinium-enhanced MRA holds promise for noninvasive imaging, but the spatial resolution is not yet sufficient to replace DSA for evaluating DAVFs. DSA shows arterial supply to the DAVF from any meningeal branch of the ECA and ICA, including the middle meningeal artery, accessory meningeal artery, internal maxillary artery, ascending pharyngeal artery, inferolateral trunk, and meningohypophysial trunk. There are two large drainage compartments: (1) the anterior compartment connecting with the superior and inferior ophthalmic veins, the sphenoparietal sinus, and medial temporal vein and (2) the posterior compartment connecting to the superior and inferior petrosal sinuses. At least three intercavernous anastomoses interconnect the left and right cavernous sinuses. The main differential diagnosis for a cavernous sinus DAVF is a direct carotid cavernous fistula (CCF) (Figs. 25-35 and 25-36). Although the imaging characteristics and presentations may be similar, direct CCFs typically have a history of trauma and an audible bruit at the globe or temporal region. Cavernous sinus DAVFs are usually managed conservatively when they are clinically benign (see Fig. 24-21). Endovascular therapy is elected

for the initial treatment of aggressive lesions with cortical venous reflux. Because the cavernous sinus does not have any major role in drainage of the brain in a normal adult, DAVFs of the cavernous sinus can usually be cured by either transarterial or transvenous obliteration of the affected portion of the sinus. Surgical disconnection of the sphenoparietal sinus may also be contemplated if there is no endovascular route.

Ethmoidal DAVFs (anterior cranial fossa DAVF; cribriform plate DAVFs) are shunts located in the dura of the anterior cranial fossa. They are usually aggressive lesions and show male predominance. The presenting clinical feature is often a hemorrhage into the frontal lobe due to rupture of a dilated venous pouch or aneurysm. CT and MRI findings are often subtle with possible visualization of tubular enhancing structures or flow voids at the frontal cortical sulci, so cerebral angiography becomes necessary to show the DAVF. The arterial supply arises mainly from the ethmoidal branches of the ophthalmic artery. There is arteriovenous shunting into dilated frontal venous pouches that usually drain into the superior sagittal sinus.

Tentorial DAVFs are shunts located within the tentorium and are usually aggressive lesions with a male predominance. They have a wide range of clinical presentation, including benign pulsatile tinnitus, venous infarction, subarachnoid hemorrhage, and intraparenchymal hemorrhage, depending on their specific drainage pattern. The arterial supply of a tentorial DAVF always derives from the meningeal branches of the ICA, usually the meningohypophysial trunk or less commonly the lateral clival branch from the inferolateral trunk. Branches of the ascending pharyngeal artery occasionally contribute to the DAVF. The venous drainage can pass medially into the deep venous system and vein of Galen or laterally toward the superior petrosal sinus or the lateral veins of the brain stem and cerebellum. Rarely, a tentorial DAVF drains into the perimedullary veins of the cervical spine, causing symptoms of cervical myelopathy.

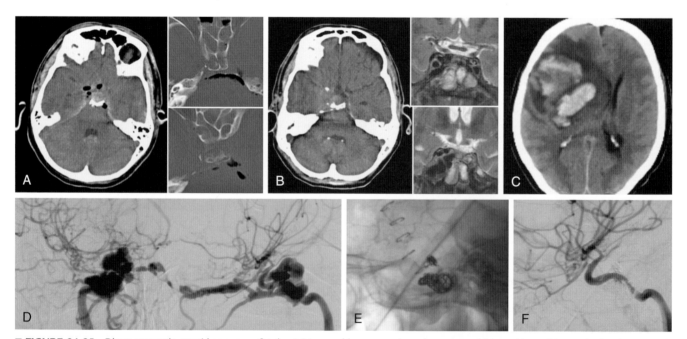

■ **FIGURE 24-35** Direct traumatic carotid-cavernous fistula. A 24-year-old man experienced a motor vehicle accident with massive head trauma. **A,** Initial CCT demonstrates pneumocephalus and a fracture of the sphenoidal sinus. A bone fragment pierces the cavernous sinus close to the presumed course of the internal carotid artery (ICA). **B,** Follow-up imaging 2 weeks after the trauma demonstrates bulging of the cavernous sinus that was verified on MRI: T2W coronal images show a massively dilated cavernous sinus on the right side with large flow voids (**C**). Angiography was scheduled for the next day; however, the patient bled in the night, which was thought to be due to venous congestion. **D,** Angiography demonstrated the carotid-cavernous fistula with pial reflux into the cortical veins. Two points of fistulation could be identified and were closed with tight packing of coils, resulting in reconstitution of flow in the ICA (**E, F**).

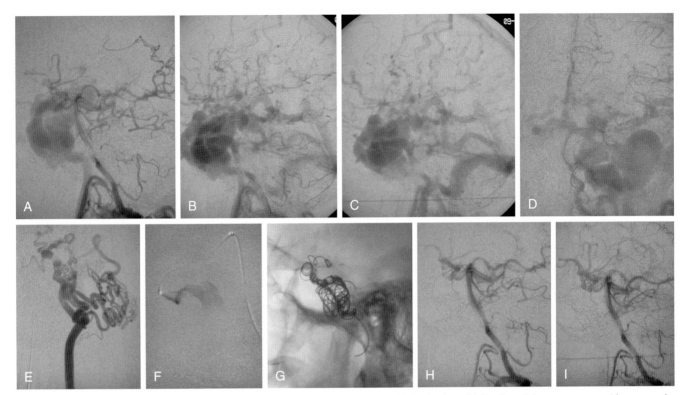

■ **FIGURE 24-36** A to I, This direct carotid-cavernous fistula was treated at an outside institution with ligation of the common carotid artery at the level of the neck that led to initially increased visual acuity. However, 2 months later symptoms recurred and the patient presented with chemosis, proptosis, and a loss of visual acuity. Angiography demonstrated complete occlusion of the carotid artery at the level of the neck and reconstitution of the internal and external carotid artery vascularization via dilated vessels of the neck (derived from the deep and ascending cervical arteries and the vertebral artery) as well as flow from the posterior circulation via the posterior communicating artery refilling the fistula. The point of fistulation was catheterized in a cross-over technique via the posterior communicating artery, and the fistula was completely occluded with coils while the flow in the distal internal carotid artery was preserved via the posterior communicating artery.

Foramen magnum DAVFs are shunts in the dura of the foramen magnum. A slight male predominance is observed within this group, and they present as either symptoms of cervical myelopathy when descending drainage into the perimedullary veins is observed (Fig. 24-37) or subarachnoid hemorrhage when there is ascending drainage into the posterior fossa veins with venous aneurysms. MRI reveals enlargement of the spinal cord with increased T2 signal intensity and enhancement on postgadolinium studies. The diagnosis is usually suggested when thin-slice T2W images show tubular structures surrounding the cord. There is usually dual arterial supply with feeders from (1) branches of the external carotid artery, usually the ascending pharyngeal artery, less commonly the occipital artery, and (2) radicular branches from C1-2 levels of the vertebral artery.

CAVERNOUS MALFORMATIONS

Cavernous malformations are vascular lesions composed of thin-walled, dilated capillary spaces with no intervening brain tissue. Cavernomas of the brain parenchyma appear to be different entities from cavernomas of the extra-axial compartment around the brain. Intra-axial cavernomas are typically angiographically silent, "grow" only through intralesional hemorrhage (Fig. 24-38), and are usually inherited through mutations of defined genes. Extra-axial cavernomas are usually hypervascular lesions with a potential for tumor growth and do not appear to be heritable genetic lesions. This section addresses the intra-axial cavernomas. The extra-axial cavernomas are discussed in greater detail in the section on differential diagnosis.

Other terms used for cavernous malformations include *cerebral cavernous malformation* (CCMs), *cavernous angioma*, *cavernous hemangioma*, and *angiographically occult vascular malformation*. The most common term is *cavernoma*.

Epidemiology

Cavernomas constitute about 9% of all central nervous system vascular malformations. The prevalence of intraparenchymal cavernomas is estimated to be about 0.5% based on MRI and autopsy studies of large cohorts of patients. Intra-axial lesions can be located at all locations within the central nervous system. Extra-axial locations are infrequent and may be located at the skull, the ventricles, and the cavernous sinus. Both sporadic and familial forms occur.

Clinical Presentation

Most cavernomas are incidental findings that tend to be stable over time. Only 20% to 30% become symptomatic, usually between the third and fifth decades of life. Symptoms include headaches, seizures, and focal neurologic deficits. Patients may present with acute "strokes" due to large intracerebral hemorrhages from cortical and subependymal lesions. The average risk of hemorrhage is quoted as 0.7% to 1.1% per lesion per year with increased rate of hemorrhage with increasing age, female gender, infratentorial lesion location, and prior hemorrhage. The risk for hemorrhage is slightly larger in the first trimester of pregnancy.

Pathophysiology

The etiology of these lesions is unclear. The sporadic cases are more commonly solitary lesions (>67%) than multiple (<33%). Sporadic lesions are reported to coexist with developmental venous anomalies (DVAs) in up to 33% and tend to develop within the territory drained by the DVA. Multiple case reports of de novo formation of cavernomas after radiation, in association with dural sinus thrombosis and in DAVSs with cortical venous reflux, suggest that hemodynamic changes resulting in increased venous pressure can trigger an underlying vascular or extraluminal defect, which may reveal itself as a cavernoma over time. Immunohistochemical studies show that cavernomas express proliferative indices and angiogenic growth factors, including VEGF in 37% to 97% of patients, TGF in 54% to 100% of patients, and platelet-derived growth factor (PDGF) in 95% of patients.

Familial cavernomas are more often multiple (50% to 73% of patients). They are inherited as autosomal dominant traits with incomplete penetrance and variable expression. Multiple-locus analysis of familial cavernomas has detected mutations at three different loci:

- *CCM1* on 7q21.2, accounting for 40% to 50% of cavernomas
- *CCM2* on 7p15-p13, accounting for 10% to 20% of cavernomas
- *CCM3* on 3q26.1-q27, accounting for 40% of cavernomas

Familial cavernomas are more prevalent in Hispanic-Americans than other ethnic groups.

In the familial form, new lesions appear at a rate of 0.2 to 0.4 lesion per patient-year. The prospective hemorrhage rate for familial cavernomas is 3.1%, and the new-onset seizure rate is 2.4% per patient-year.

The *CCM1* gene contains 16 coding exons that encode *KRIT1* (Krev Interaction Trapped1). More than 100 distinct *CCM1* mutations have been published, evenly distributed from exon 5 to exon 18. They are highly stereotyped because all lead to a premature termination codon. *CCM2* is a 10-exon gene, which encodes the MGC4607 protein (malcavernin) that contains a phosphotyrosine binding domain. The recently identified *CCM3* is a 7-exon gene that encodes PDCD10 (programmed cell death 10), a protein without any conserved functional domain known to be involved in apoptosis. Most *CCM2* and *CCM3* mutations involve early termination of the codon or are large deletions, also strongly suggesting that most of the defects are loss-of-function mutations.

Several studies have demonstrated the involvement of the *KRIT1* gene in angiogenesis and cell proliferation and its role in integrin signaling mechanisms that may be mediated by binding of the ICAP1α protein. *KRIT1* transcripts have also been detected in neural and epithelial cells during development and are associated with microtubules needed for arterial morphogenesis and identity. The interaction of *KRIT1* with various integrins suggests that *KRIT1* may help modulate the cytoskeleton and shape endothelial cell morphology and function in response to cell-matrix and cell-cell interactions. Loss of this targeting mechanism would lead to abnormal endothelial tube development and the subsequent appearance of cerebral cavernomas.

The *CCM2* gene (malcavernin) contains a phosphotyrosine binding (PTB) domain, similar to ICAP1α, suggesting an interaction between *KRIT1* and malcavernin and thus a common functional pathway. There have also been studies that showed malcavernin to be capable of sequestering *KRIT1* in the cytoplasm.

PDCD10/TFAR15 was initially identified as a gene upregulated in the TF-1 premyeloid cell line after growth factor deprivation and induction of apoptosis. Its role in the pathogenesis of cavernoma formation is unclear. As with *CCM1* and *CCM2*, in-situ hybridization shows *CCM3* mRNA expression in neuronal cells at embryonic and adult stages. Similarly, its expression coincides with the expression of *CCM2* in meningeal and parenchymal cerebral vessels. Apoptosis in smooth muscle cells has

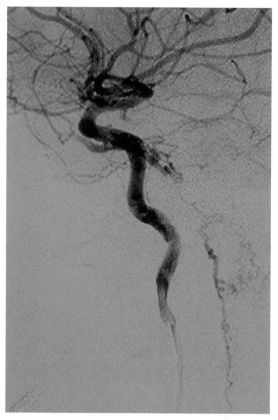

■ **FIGURE 24-37** DAVF type V of the cavernous sinus. In these patients, the arteriovenous shunt drains directly into the spinal perimedullary veins, leading to cervical and medullary venous congestion.

been shown to be mediated by a β_1-integrin signaling cascade, which may be the link with *CCM1* and *CCM2* in formation of cavernomas. Otherwise, little is still known about this gene product.

Because all three genes seem to be expressed in neurons rather than in blood vessels, the vascular phenotype should presumably result from a defect in signaling between these two juxtaposed structures. Several other proteins (i.e., neurophilin and VEGF) are closely linked with vascular and neuronal development. However, further studies are needed to determine whether the primary defects are vascular or neuronal.

Pathology

Cavernomas consist of a compact mass of sinusoidal vessels lying adjacent to each other with no intervening functional cerebral parenchyma. They vary from a few millimeters to several centimeters. On gross pathology, cavernomas appear as dark red, multilobular, nonencapsulated masses that are well circumscribed by the cerebral parenchyma. The lesion is often surrounded by reactive gliosis and hemosiderin deposits from minor, clinically silent hemorrhages (Fig. 24-39). Larger lesions may show areas of thrombosis with subsequent organization. Calcifications are found in a few cases. With recent hemorrhage, the cavernoma may be partially obliterated and lie at the periphery of the hematoma (Fig. 24-40).

Microscopically, cavernomas consist of endothelium-lined vascular sinusoids embedded in a dense collagenous matrix. Macrophages and hemosiderin pigment are present. There is no evidence of cellular proliferation and no capsule formation. Cavernomas are characterized by the absence of, or defects of, the blood-brain barrier. The tight junctions between the endothelial cells are poorly formed or absent, with gaps observed between

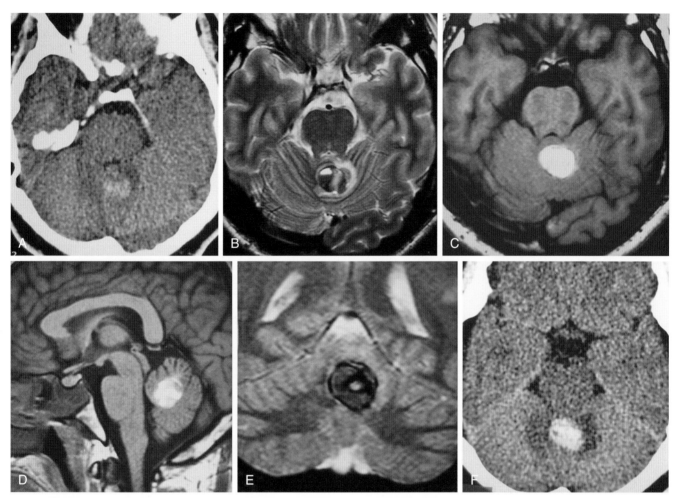

■ **FIGURE 24-38** Three days before first imaging the patient complained about sudden onset of dizziness. **A,** The CT demonstrated a slightly hyperdense lesion of the cerebellum that showed mixed intensities on MRI (**B-E**), suggesting a cavernoma with a recent hemorrhage. Seven days later the patient experienced a worsening of his symptoms with dizziness, vertigo, and vomiting. **F,** A second CT scan was done that showed enlargement of the hematoma and the surrounding edema.

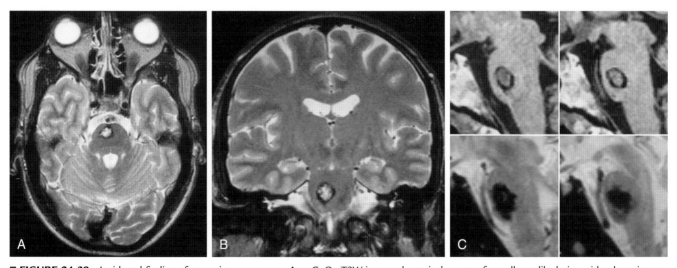

■ **FIGURE 24-39** Incidental finding of a pontine cavernoma. **A** to **C,** On T2W images the typical aspect of a mulberry-like lesion with a hyperintense core and a hypointense rim can be appreciated. T2W gradient-echo images demonstrate a prominent susceptibility effect (blooming). The mixed hyperintense and hypointense signals, surrounded by a rim of hypointense signal on T2W imaging, represent acute and chronic hemorrhage or calcifications and are the most commonly encountered appearances of cavernomas. The most important surgical information in brain stem cavernomas that have a unfavorable prognosis over time is whether the cavernoma reaches the surface. This information should never be obtained from gradient-echo sequences because they tend to overestimate the size of the cavernoma. In our experience, T1W images are best used to evaluate the exact extent of a cavernoma.

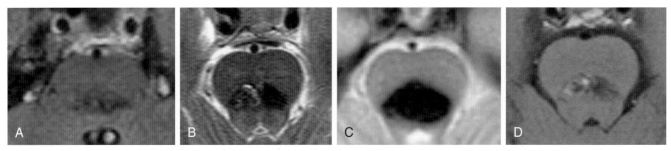

■ **FIGURE 24-40** A to D, Brain stem cavernoma on FLAIR-weighted images. A hypointensity can be seen that on T2W TSE sequences demonstrates an internal structure indicative of a true cavernoma. The size is overexaggerated on T2W gradient-echo sequences, whereas on T1W sequences the exact size of the cavernoma can be seen.

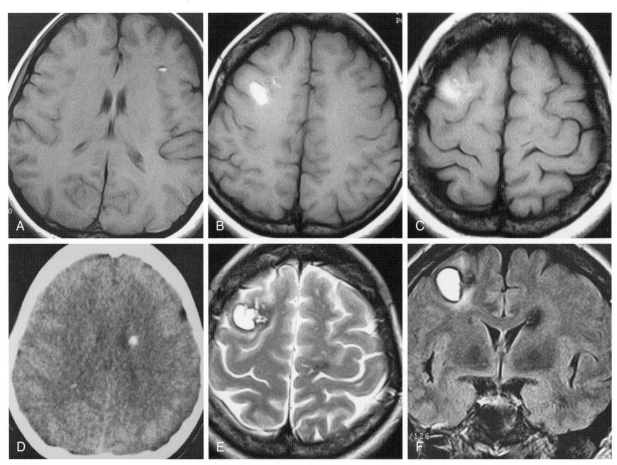

■ **FIGURE 24-41** A to F, A 37-year-old woman without a family history of cavernoma, cerebral hemorrhage, or sudden unexplained death presented with generalized tonic-clonic seizures. MRI demonstrated multiple cavernomas that were partly calcified.

the cells. No astrocytic foot processes and no normal nervous tissue are present within the lesion. Pericytes are rare.

Imaging
CT
Thirty to 50 percent of cavernomas are not detectable by CT. When visualized, they appear as rounded, hyperdense lesions (Fig. 24-41), with or without calcifications and acute hemorrhage (Fig. 24-42). They may show contrast enhancement and, perhaps, a concurrent DVA.

MRI
Cavernomas are best detected by MRI using T2W and T2*W gradient-echo sequences to demonstrate prominent susceptibility effect (blooming) (Fig. 24-43). Classically, cavernomas appear as a "popcorn" lesion consisting of a reticulated heterogeneous core surrounded by a hypointense hemosiderin rim (Fig. 24-44). Cavernomas have been classified into four types on the basis of their MR appearance. Type 1 lesions appear hyperintense on both T1W and T2W imaging, indicating acute hemorrhage. Type 2 (classic) lesions appear as mixed hyperintense and hypointense signals, surrounded by a rim of hypointense signal on T2W

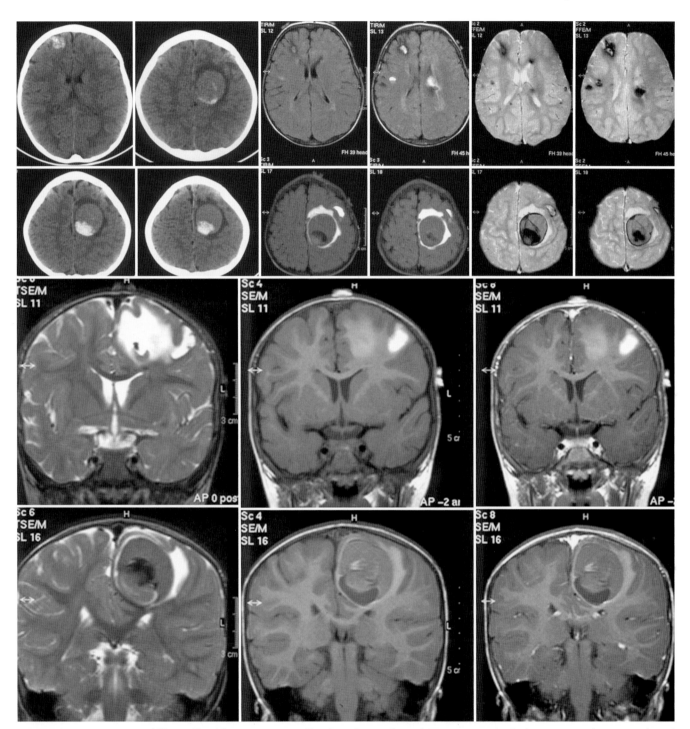

■ **FIGURE 24-42** A 6-year-old boy suffered from acute onset of hemiparesis. Unenhanced CT on presentation in the emergency department showed a partly hyperdense, partly hypodense lesion with perifocal edema and, some cuts deeper, a second lesion with calcifications. MRI revealed multiple cavernomas, one of which had acutely bled, leading to perifocal edema. The most sensitive sequence for detecting small cavernomas is the T2 gradient-echo sequence.

imaging, representing acute and chronic hemorrhage or calcifications. Type 3 lesions appear hypointense on both T1W and T2W images. Type 4 lesions have hypointense signal detected on only gradient-echo sequences and may correspond to precursors of mature cavernomas. Cavernomas of types 3 and 4 are usually asymptomatic. Fluid-attenuated inversion-recovery (FLAIR) and T2W MRI may show edema surrounding lesions with acute hemorrhage and contrast enhancement on post-gadolinium studies.

Susceptibility-weighted imaging is expected to show cavernomas better than present techniques. Use of susceptibility-weighted imaging may then show greater numbers of these lesions at smaller size in a greater proportion of the families of patients with heritable forms of cavernoma. MRI techniques, especially fiber tracking of the corticospinal tracts, have promising results in facilitating surgical removal of these lesions, particularly in paraventricular and brain stem lesions (Fig. 24-45).

■ **FIGURE 24-43** A to D, Solitary cavernoma of the temporal lobe in a patient presenting with medically intractable seizures.

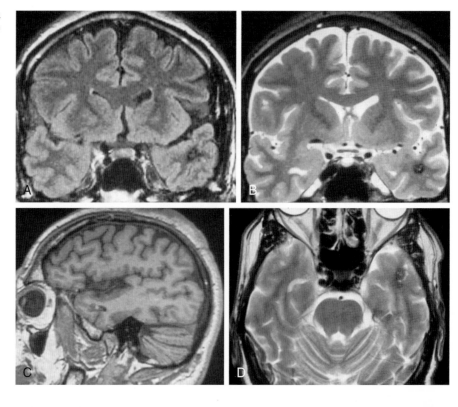

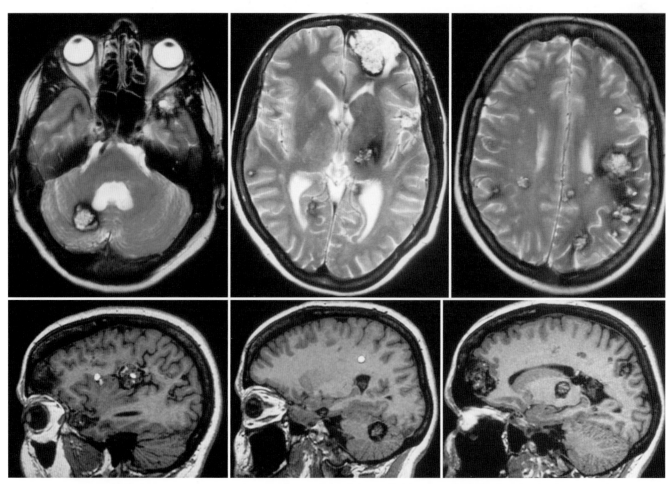

■ **FIGURE 24-44** Multiple cavernomas are present in approximately 60% of the familial forms and in 33% of nonfamilial lesions. In this patient, a familial form of cavernoma was present.

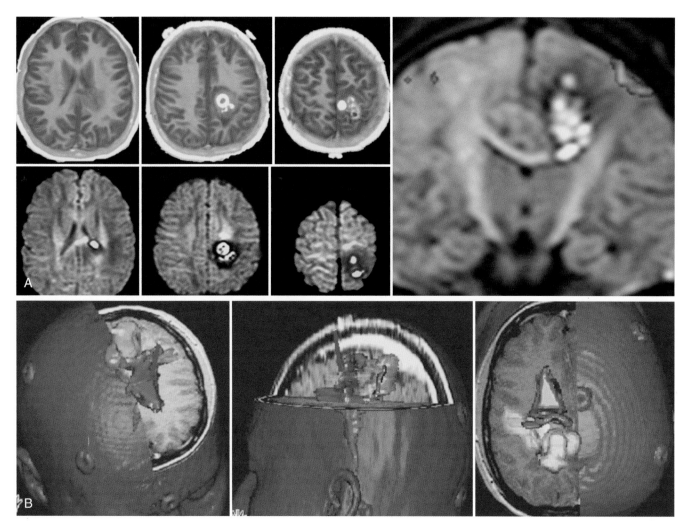

■ **FIGURE 24-45** **A** and **B,** New imaging techniques such as fiber tracking and functional MRI and their visualization in a navigation system have enabled safer resection, especially in those cavernomas that are located close to eloquent cortical areas such as the pyramidal tracts, the primary motor cortex, or the language areas.

DSA

Because cavernomas are angiographically occult, cerebral angiography is usually negative for the lesion but may reveal associated DVAs.

Treatment

Asymptomatic cavernomas are not treated. Surgical resection becomes indicated when lesions rebleed frequently or cause intractable seizures. Location of a cavernoma within the vicinity of a DVA may complicate the surgical access, since the venous anomaly must be left untouched. Convexity cavernomas are usually located in the glial tissue, facilitating the surgical approach. Cavernomas are usually resistant to radiotherapy, and radiosurgery is not generally accepted as standard treatment.

Differential Diagnosis

Extra-axial Cavernomas

Cavernous hemangiomas of the skull account for 7% to 10% of all benign skull tumors. They are far more common than capillary hemangiomas in this location. The vertebrae and the parietal and frontal bones are most often involved. The incidence is 2- to 4-fold higher in women than in men, with a peak incidence in the fourth decade. Patients usually present incidentally with a slowly growing mass. Headaches and painful swelling may be the leading symptoms and signs in some patients. If the frontal

or orbital bone is involved, cavernomas may cause proptosis or oculomotor deficits. Radiographic findings include a solitary lytic lesion with a sclerotic rim. A "honeycomb" trabecular or "sunburst" pattern with striations radiating from the center may also be seen. The lesions are usually sharply demarcated and involve both the inner and outer tables of the skull, best demonstrated with CT. On MRI the cavernoma is typically isointense on T1W images and hyperintense on T2W images. At angiography the tumors may show increased vascularity, typically with slightly prominent arterial feeders but no enlarged draining veins. Differential diagnoses include slowly growing tumors of the skull, such as meningiomas, fibrous dysplasia, osteoma, fibrohemangioma, and eosinophilic granuloma. The typical findings in the CT bone window, as described earlier, will usually lead to diagnosis.

Dural cavernous hemangiomas of the middle cranial fossa usually originate on the floor of the cavernous sinus and account for 2% to 3% of all cavernous sinus tumors. Other rare locations are the petrosal sinus and the torcular Herophili. There is a female predomination. The mean age at detection is 44 years. The presenting symptoms vary with cavernoma location but usually consist of cranial nerve deficits and headaches. Cavernous sinus lesions typically present with oculomotor deficits. Lesions in other locations may present as trigeminal neuralgia or facial nerve palsy. Acute symptoms are attributed to fresh bleeding within the cavernous hemangioma. On CT, these lesions are typically well circumscribed and hyperdense. They may erode or remodel the adjacent bone without the hyperostosis commonly seen in meningomas. They show intense, homogeneous contrast enhancement. On MRI, they may be hyperintense or hypointense on T1W images and show homogeneous contrast enhancement. On T2W imaging, cavernomas are mainly hyperintense but can be inhomogeneous. Angiography may show a mild contrast blush with multiple feeding arteries, but large draining veins are uncommon.

The major benign differential diagnoses are meningiomas and neurofibromas of the cranial nerves. On MRI, neurofibromas may have similar imaging characteristics but cavernous hemangiomas typically blush on angiography and show inhomogeneous structure on MRI. With the exception of the angioblastic subgroup, meningiomas can usually be distinguished by their signal characteristics. The major malignant differential diagnosis is metastases. These are distinguished by their bone destruction and the infiltration of the surrounding tissue, together with a history of a malignant primary tumor.

Dural cavernous hemangiomas outside the middle cranial fossa are extremely rare and are equally frequent in men and women. They usually occur at the tentorium and the dural convexity. A few lesions have been seen on the falx cerebri, close to the cerebellopontine angle and within the ventricular system. The presenting symptoms are usually headaches or dizziness. CT often shows well circumscribed, isodense to slightly hyperdense masses without adjacent edema or significant mass effect. Calcifications and homogeneous contrast enhancement are often seen. Areas of low density may be due to old thrombosis and/or cystic degeneration but are not typical findings for cavernous hemangiomas. The dural cavernomas usually do not have a peripheral low-signal hemosiderin rim nor a reticulated core on MRI. Instead, dural cavernomas enhance intensely and homogeneously after gadolinium administration.

TELANGIECTASIA

Capillary telangiectasia is a vascular malformation that consists of localized collections of abnormal thin-walled vascular channels interposed between normal brain parenchyma.

Epidemiology

Capillary telangiectasia is predominantly found in adults from the fourth to the eighth decades. They have not been described in children younger than 5 years old. There is no gender predilection. The true incidence is difficult to estimate owing to the asymptomatic nature of the lesion, but it is estimated to represent 16% to 20% of all intracranial vascular malformations in large autopsy series.

Pathophysiology

Most capillary telangiectases are incidental findings.

Pathology

Capillary telangiectasia is nearly always a single lesion but rarely can be multiple. It is significantly more frequent in the posterior fossa (60% to 70%), occurs mainly in the mid pons, and is often situated in the midline. It can also be found in the cerebral cortex and white matter. In the cerebellum, the middle cerebellar peduncles and the dentate nuclei are most often affected.

The affected brain parenchyma harbors a poorly defined group of pathologically dilated capillary blood vessels that vary in diameter. The vessels of telangiectases are interspersed within normal neural tissue, distinguishing them from cavernomas, which have no neural tissue between the dilated vessels. The arteries are normal. The walls of the pathologic capillaries are usually thin and devoid of muscle and elastic fibers, but there is no increase in the number of capillaries. Edema, gliosis, and signs of growth are typically absent on follow-up. Spontaneous hemorrhage is an extremely rare complication, reported in only a few cases. The rarity of spontaneous hemorrhage is confirmed by the almost universal absence of any signs of recent or old hemorrhage on MR images.

Imaging

CT and angiography are typically negative for telangiectasia. The lesions do not calcify and infrequently show an angiographic blush. Contrast-enhanced MRI is the only imaging modality that routinely displays capillary telangiectases (Fig. 24-46). Classic capillary telangiectasia appears as a T1-isointense, contrast-enhancing lesion (Fig. 24-47). The enhancement may be "fluffy" without apparent individual vessels or may demonstrate small radiating vessels that converge into a single larger collecting vein (Fig. 24-48). T2W and T2 FLAIR images may show the collector as a thin flow void but are otherwise normal. T2*W images may show hypointensity at the site of the lesion, presumably due to slowly flowing deoxygenated blood. The vascular malformation can be irregular in contour. The contrast enhancement is rapid, is of short duration, and typically disappears after 20 to 30 minutes (Fig. 24-49). Susceptibility-weighted imaging will likely display the telangiectasia well owing to the deoxygenated blood within the dilated capillaries.

Differential Diagnosis

In many cases the diagnosis of a capillary telangiectasia will remain speculative. Differential diagnoses include neoplasm, inflammation, infection, demyelination, and infarction. Key points that help to make the correct diagnosis are:

- Early contrast washout. A repeat MRI after 30 minutes should show persistent contrast enhancement in all lesions except capillary telangiectasia.
- Hypointensity on T2*W imaging, because vascular malformations are hypointense on these sequences
- Lack of mass effect and absence of change over time

DEVELOPMENTAL VENOUS ANOMALIES

DVAs are nonpathologic normal variations of the venous drainage. The anomalous veins drain the normal brain tissue along transmedullary venous anastomoses, where cortical differentiation has occurred. DVAs represent the extreme limit of variability in the transcerebral venous system, where convergence and concentration of the venous channels creates their classic angiographic features. Two types of DVAs are considered. Superficial DVAs consist of superficial medullary veins, which drain the deeper medullary regions into the cortical veins. Deep DVAs drain the subcortical territories into the deep venous collectors.

The previous terms *venous angioma* and *venous malformation* have been abandoned in the recent literature to distinguish these normal variations from true vascular malformations.

Epidemiology

DVAs are the most common cerebral vascular anomaly, with an incidence reported to be 0.5% to 2.6%. In large autopsy series, DVAs represent about 63% of all intracranial vascular lesions. There is no gender predominance.

Clinical Presentation

DVAs are rarely symptomatic. Most often they are discovered incidentally in patients who complain of headaches, seizures that do not correlate with electroencephalographic foci, focal neurologic deficits, and dizziness. Case reports of DVAs in patients with psychiatric symptoms of depression and eating disorders are most likely coincidental. Infratentorial DVAs may present with symptoms of gait disturbances and ataxia.

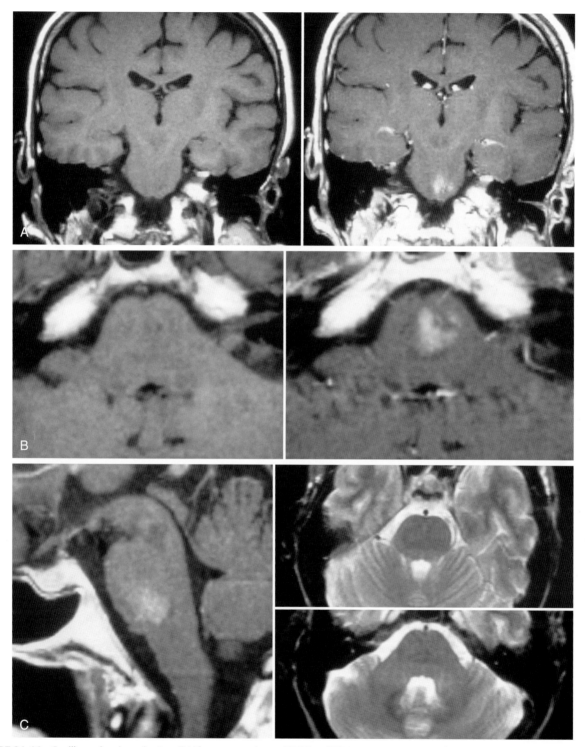

■ **FIGURE 24-46** Capillary telangiectasia. **A** to **C,** Whereas nonenhanced T1W and T2W sequences are normal, contrast-enhanced images demonstrate slight contrast enhancement in the pons without any appearance of mass effect. Individual vessels cannot be discerned. The contour is rather irregular.

The risk of hemorrhage from DVAs is about 0.22% per year but is higher during pregnancy and for DVAs of the posterior fossa. Cavernomas are reported to coexist with up to 33% of DVAs and tend to develop within the territory drained by the DVA. In cases with concurrent DVA and intracerebral hemorrhage there is usually an associated cavernoma. It has been argued that even in those cases where no cavernoma is found,

microcavernomas, and not the DVA, are the source of the bleeding.

Thrombosis of the venous collector of the DVA is a rare complication that may lead to venous infarction or even hemorrhage. In some cases, focal stenosis of the collecting vein may be observed at the point where the collector penetrates the dura to enter the dural sinus. The consequent stasis and pressure

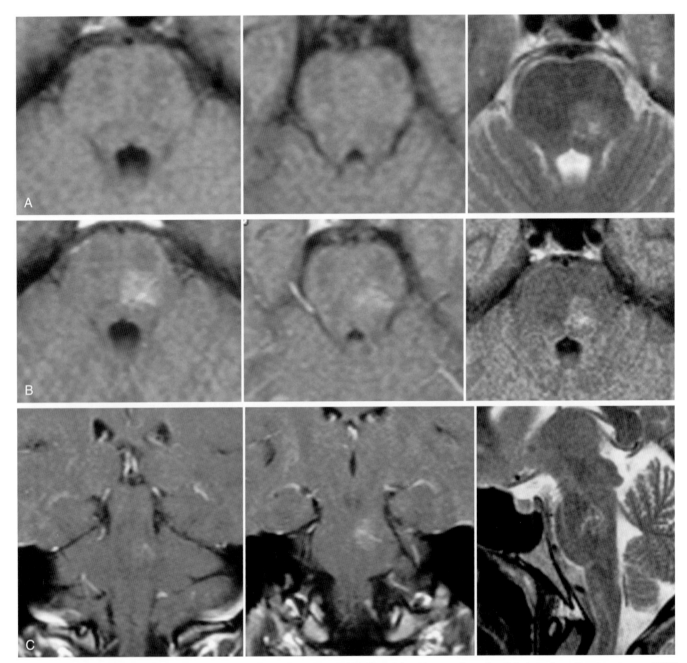

■ **FIGURE 24-47**   Capillary telangiectasia. **A** to **C,** In this patient, T2W and FLAIR-weighted images showed a slight hyperintensity; the aspect on T1W images after contrast administration is typical for capillary telangiectasia.

within the DVA precipitate thrombus formation. Treatment is usually conservative with anticoagulants.

DVAs may rarely be associated with AVMs and shunts. Because DVAs have reduced flexibility and capacity for altering venous pressure, the superimposed arteriovenous shunts may increase the risk of venous hemorrhage or infarction.

Pathophysiology

DVAs are believed to be adaptations to accidents occurring between Padget's fourth and seventh stages of embryogenesis (40- to 80-mm embryo), resulting in occlusion or maldevelopment of the superficial or deep veins. At these stages, the vascular system is plastic, so DVAs form as compensatory pathways recruiting and dilating preexisting transmedullary veins. Caver-

nomas coexist with up to 33% of DVAs and tend to develop within the territory drained by the DVA. However, there is currently no evidence that these malformations and the DVAs are genetically related. DVAs may also be associated with cortical dysplasias, pointing to a developmental defect of the vasculature in a confined region of the brain. Other lesions associated with DVAs include maxillofacial venous and lymphatic malformations, sinus pericranii, schizencephaly, and multiple mucocutaneous venous malformations.

Pathology

DVAs are characterized histologically by a composition of sometimes thickened and hyalinized veins with interspersed normal neural parenchyma. Approximately one third of these lesions are

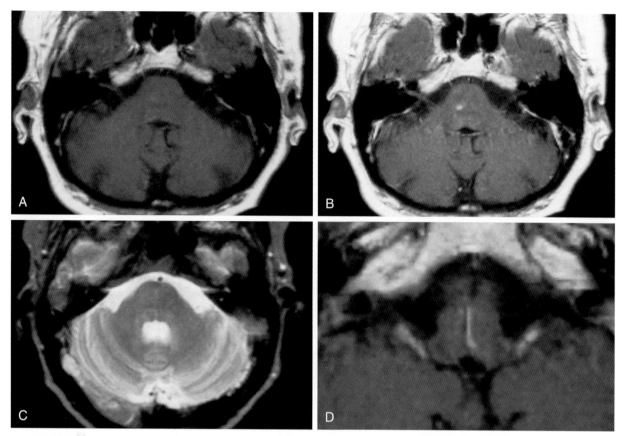

■ FIGURE 24-48 A to D, Capillary telangiectasia with a single large collecting vein in the pontomedullary junction.

located in the cerebellum and in the brain stem. The remaining two thirds are supratentorial.

Imaging

The venous collector of the DVA is usually detected as a thin transmedullary channel. Contrast-enhanced CT shows the collecting vein as a linear or curvilinear enhancement, typically coursing from the deep white matter to a cortical vein, a deep vein, or a dural sinus (Fig. 24-50). The tributary veins draining to the collector appear as a "*caput medusae*" (Fig. 24-51) converging to the linear enhancement. Concurrent cavernomas are variable in size and may show the typical "popcorn" center and hemosiderin rim.

On MRI, DVAs characteristically display a transhemispheric flow void on both T1W and T2W imaging (Fig. 24-52). Frequently, spatial misregistration artifact on proton density and T2W imaging creates contiguous, parallel channels of high and low signal. Spatial misregistration artifact will be absent, however, in cases where the draining vein courses parallel or perpendicular to the phase-encoding direction. In such cases, only a focal flow void within the brain parenchyma will be observed (Fig. 24-53). Contrast-enhanced MRI shows significant enhancement of the *caput medusae* of the medullary veins and of the venous collector, owing to the slow flow within them (Fig. 24-54). Susceptibility-weighted images are particular helpful in demonstrating the location and course of the DVA (Fig. 24-55).

In cases with complicated DVAs, MRI may show concurrent hemorrhage, cavernomas, or nonhemorrhagic venous infarction. MR angiography and venography may then be helpful to exclude a treatable arterial component of the lesion and to exclude focal stenosis of the terminal collecting vein at the point where it enters the dural sinus (Fig. 24-56).

Currently, DSA is reserved for patients with complications such as hemorrhage or infarction. Classic angiographic appearances include a *caput medusae* of transmedullary veins appearing during the early to mid-venous phase, draining into a single large venous collector (Fig. 24-57). The collector can extend to either the superficial or deep venous system, depending on the type of the DVA. In some cases, focal stenosis of the venous collector at the junction where it penetrates the dura to enter the dural sinus may be observed. This is better appreciated on rotational 3D angiography.

Treatment

Simple DVAs do not cause symptoms and do not require treatment. DVAs with concurrent hemorrhage should be studied to detect concurrent cavernomas, stenosis of the collector vein, or an associated shunting lesion. Whatever therapy is elected must preserve the DVA itself, because it constitutes the venous drainage for that portion of the brain.

Differential Diagnosis

Early opacification of DVAs, particularly DVAs located in the frontoparietal lobes, may appear as a capillary blush that represents rapid capillary transit time rather than true arteriovenous shunting. These early-opacifying DVAs must be differentiated from true AVMs. Whereas DVAs with rapid capillary transit time do well with conservative management, AVMs associated with DVAs have a 2% to 4% risk of hemorrhage per year along with higher chance for venous infarctions of the DVAs and therefore should always be treated.

Text continued on page 566

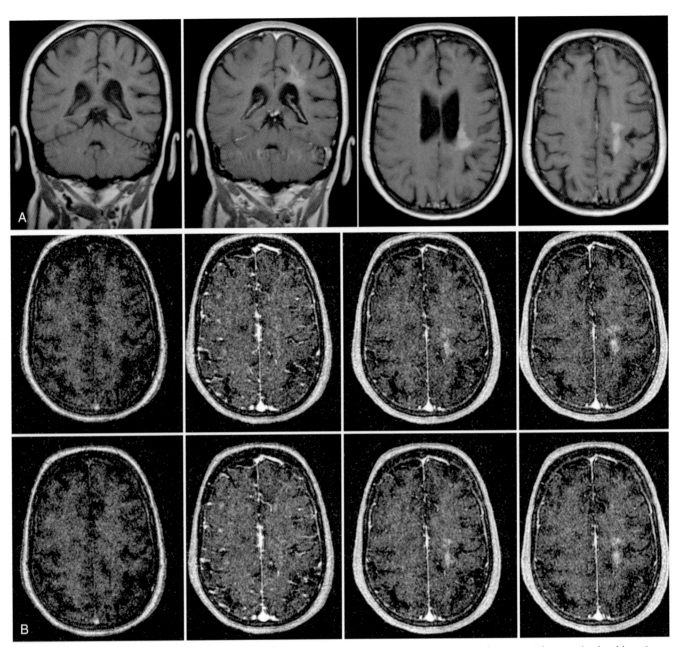

■ **FIGURE 24-49** A and B, Presumed supratentorial capillary telangiectasia with typical "fluffy" contrast enhancement that remained stable at 1 year follow-up. On dynamic contrast-enhanced imaging, there is a rapid filling of the vascular malformation; however, no large feeding vessels can be seen. The contrast agent stays in the lesion, and no large draining veins can be found. Contrast enhancement characteristics suggest a capillary telangiectasia.

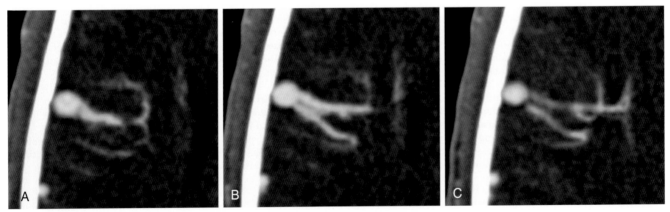

■ **FIGURE 24-50** A to C, CTA in a classic supratentorial DVA demonstrating the *caput medusae* as a fine network of radiating veins that converge into a single collecting vein that drains the white matter into a pial collecting vein.

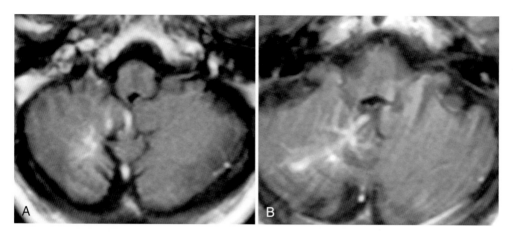

■ **FIGURE 24-51** A and B, MRI aspect of an infratentorial DVA with a large collector vein and a dispersed network of smaller contributing veins.

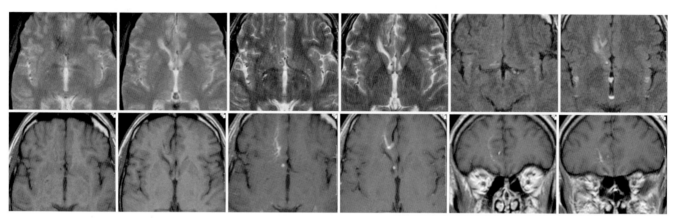

■ **FIGURE 24-52** MRI of a DVA. On T2W gradient-echo images a fine dispersed hypointensity can be seen, whereas on T2W TSE and FLAIR images some hyperintensity is demonstrated, suggesting some perifocal gliosis and slow-flowing blood. Whereas the nonenhanced T1W MRI is normal, contrast enhancement demonstrates the typical sign of fine, dispersed medullary vessels that drain the cortex into a transmedullary collector vein that drains into a subependymal vein of the right lateral ventricle.

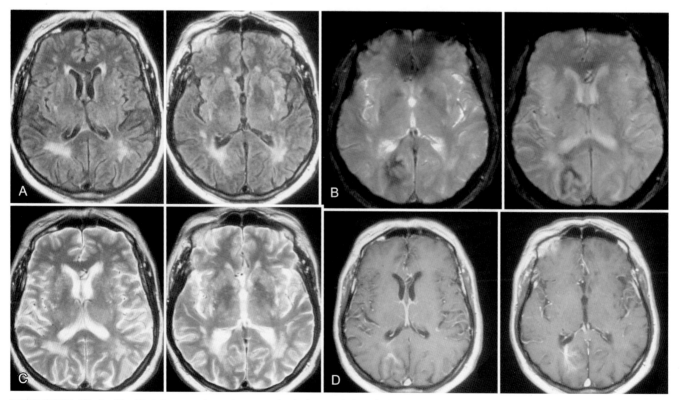

■ **FIGURE 24-53** In this elderly hypertensive patient, vascular leukoencephalopathy is present with a right occipital DVA that is hypointense on T2W gradient-echo images (**B**), presumably due to slow-flowing blood.

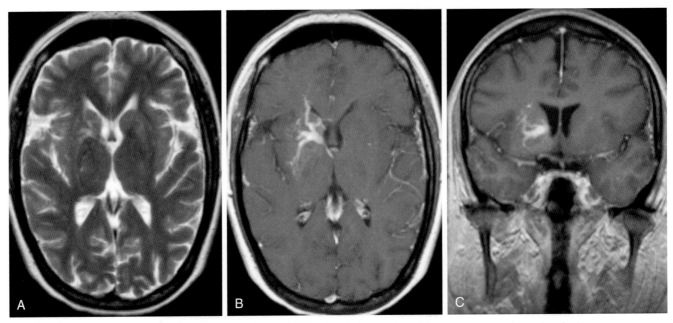

■ **FIGURE 24-54**   A to C, Typical MR aspect of a supratentorial DVA that drains the deep white matter into a subependymal vein.

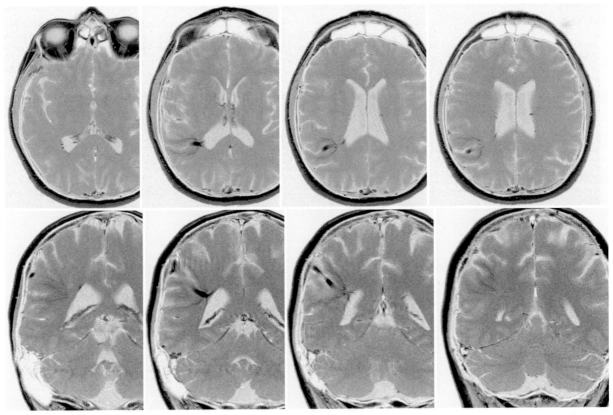

■ **FIGURE 24-55**   Superficial type of DVA. T2W gradient-echo MR sequences can depict nicely the venous anatomy of this transmedullary DVA with its white matter contributing veins.

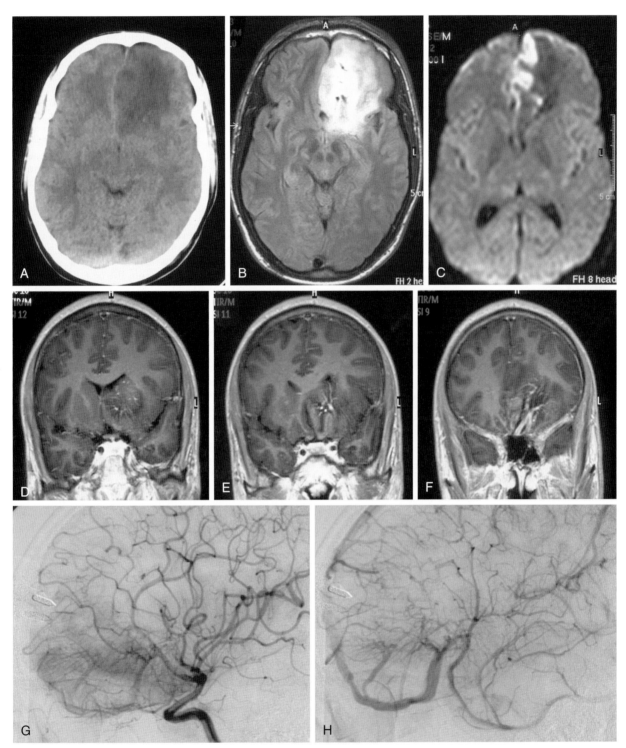

■ **FIGURE 24-56**   Although exceedingly rare, DVAs may cause symptoms due to venous congestion if their outflow is restricted. **A** to **H,** This patient came to the psychiatric department because of a sudden onset of personality change. CT (**A**) demonstrates a hypodensity of the left frontal lobe that did not suit a vascular territory (neither arterial nor venous). MRI demonstrates the edema that, as diffusion-weighted scans (**C**) verify, is of a congestive nature in its deep portion with some signs of cytotoxic edema on the outer rim, presumably owing to compressive effects of the small perforating arteries. T1W images after contrast administration (**D-F**) show a typical DVA that was confirmed on angiography (**G, H**), where, in addition, an outflow restriction of the DVA toward the superior sagittal sinus could be visualized, leading to congestive edema of the area that was drained by the DVA.

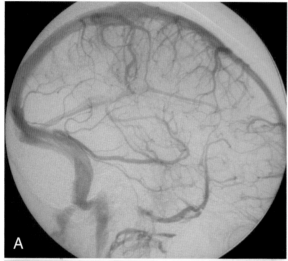

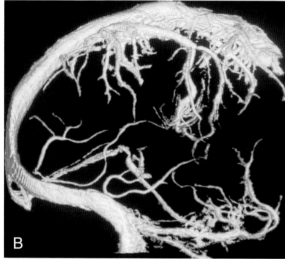

■ FIGURE 24-57 Angiography **(A)** and rotational angiography **(B)** demonstrate the classic inverse umbrella sign of the contributing veins that drain into the collecting veins that subsequently enter the superior sagittal sinus.

ANALYSIS OF VASCULAR MALFORMATIONS

In most cerebral vascular malformations, the first diagnostic clue and the most intriguing finding is the presence of pathologic vessels that may either be increased in number, dilated in their diameter, or encountered in atypical locations. Once these are identified, the type of vascular malformation has to be determined. This determines the risk of hemorrhage and is crucial for treatment planning. Capillary telangiectases do not bleed. DVAs become symptomatic only exceedingly rarely, so both may be considered nonaggressive lesions requiring no further therapy. However, capillary telangiectases and DVA may be associated with other vascular or nonvascular pathologic processes that do require further imaging. Pial and dural AVMs and cavernomas may require therapy, if risk factors such as pial reflux or previous hemorrhage are present. For these differential diagnoses, MRI is needed. The questions to be answered are the location of the vessels (intraparenchymal vs. subarachnoidal), the presence or absence of a shunt, and the presence or absence of old hemorrhages. High-resolution T2W sequences, T2*W sequences, and dynamic MR angiographies are thus the next diagnostic step. To plan subsequent treatment and to determine the exact nature of the vascular malformation in unclear cases, DSA is the third diagnostic step.

In acutely ruptured vascular malformations, the diagnostic approach is different. Once an atypical hemorrhage (atypical age, atypical location, atypical circumstances) is encountered, further diagnostic and therapeutic steps may become necessary while the most often encountered reasons for bleeding, such as hypertension, have to be ruled out. The primary role of the neuroradiologist is to determine whether a life-threatening situation is present that requires immediate surgical intervention (e.g., evacuation of an intraparenchymal hematoma, acute hydrocephalus after subarachnoid hemorrhage). In these cases, a fast imaging technique is needed, which in the majority of cases will be CT followed by CT angiography (CTA). With these modalities, large AVMs and most aneurysms can be found as the source of bleeding. If the hemorrhage is not life threatening, the most accurate diagnostic procedure is necessary and, depending on the distribution of the blood, MRI or DSA may be performed. In negative cases, however, imaging needs to be repeated because small cavernomas or micro-AVMs may be obscured in the acute setting by the intraparenchymal clot. A sample report for Figure 24-58 is presented in Box 24-1.

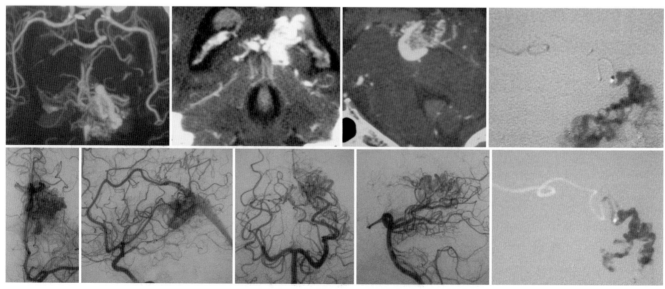

■ FIGURE 24-58   See Box 24-1 for an explanation of this figure.

BOX 24-1 Sample Report: Arteriovenous Malformation: Sample Report

PATIENT HISTORY

A 46-year-old man presented with acute headaches and loss of consciousness 1 hour before imaging.

TECHNIQUE

CT demonstrated an intraventricular hemorrhage, so CTA was immediately performed using 100 mL of nonionic contrast medium with an iodine concentration of 300 mg/mL (Fig. 24-58). The parameters for four-row multislice CT were 120 kV, 300 mA, 18 cm field of view, 512 × 512 matrix, collimation 4 × 1 mm, table speed 3.5 mm per rotation, and scanning time 0.75 second per rotation for a total scanning time of 28 seconds.

FINDINGS

An intraventricular hemorrhage seems to originate from the left lateral ventricle with blood in the fourth ventricle and mild ventricular dilatation. No intraparenchymal hemorrhage is noted. CTA demonstrates a

tangle of pathologically dilated vessels that pouch out into the lateral ventricle with a marked venous ectasia, which is the presumed origin of bleeding. Because of the pathologically dilated vessels, a shunting lesion can be expected; the location within the choroidal plexus suggests a choroidal AVM, which suggests involvement of the lateral posterior choroidal and anterior choroidal arteries as well as vessels of the limbic arch.

COMMENT

Angiography with injection into both the ICA and vertebral artery confirmed the diagnosis and demonstrated the false aneurysm as the point of rupture. Because a clear target could be identified, therapy was undertaken to prevent subsequent re-rupture. Superselective injection shows the glomerular aspect of the AVM. Subsequent glue cast documents the occlusion of this portion of the AVM, protecting the patient from further acute hemorrhage.

KEY POINTS: DIFFERENTIAL DIAGNOSIS

- Cerebral vascular malformations can be classified into the presumably inborn arteriovenous malformations (AVMs), capillary telangiectasia, cavernomas and developmental venous anomalies, and the presumably acquired dural arteriovenous shunts.
- AVMs are intraparenchymal arteriovenous shunts characterized by a network of abnormal channels (the nidus) interposed between the arterial feeder(s) and the draining veins. AVMs may be responsible for hemorrhage or seizures. They are fed by pial arteries and exhibit a tangle of abnormal blood vessels with varying degrees of contrast enhancement, depending on the flow.
- Dural arteriovenous fistulas are shunts between arteries and small venules situated within the dura mater. They are classified into benign fistulas with orthograde venous drainage and aggressive fistulas with retrograde venous flow into cortical veins.
- Capillary telangiectasia is an incidental vascular malformation composed of abnormally dilated capillaries interspersed within normal

neural tissue. It is typically located in the pons, silent on angiography, and detected only after contrast enhancement. It demonstrates early filling and early washout of contrast material.
- Cavernomas are vascular lesions composed of thin-walled, dilated capillary spaces with no intervening brain tissue. Cavernomas classically demonstrate mixed signal intensity cores and low signal hemosiderin rims on T1W and T2W images. They show variable contrast enhancement. A hallmark feature is their "blooming" on T2*W gradient-echo sequences owing to their hemosiderin content. They are silent on angiography and may present clinically as hemorrhage.
- Developmental venous anomalies are benign variations of the cortical venous drainage and are almost never symptomatic.

SUGGESTED READINGS

Berenstein A, Lasjaunias P, Ter Brugge KG. Surgical Neuroangiography, 2nd ed., Vol 2, Clinical and Endovascular Treatment Aspects in Adults. Berlin, Springer, 2004.

Bigner DD, McLendon RE, Bruner JM. Russell & Rubinstein's Pathology of Tumors of the Nervous System, 6th ed. London, Arnold, 1998.

Borden JA, Wu JK, Shucart WA. A proposed classification for spinal and cranial dural arteriovenous fistulous malformations and implications for treatment. J Neurosurg 1995; 82:166-179.

Cognard C, Gobin YP, Pierot L, et al. Cerebral dural arteriovenous fistulas: clinical and angiographic correlation with a revised classification of venous drainage. Radiology 1995; 194:671-680.

Gault J, Sarin H, Awadallah N, et al. Pathobiology of human cerebrovascular malformations: basic mechanisms and clinical relevance. Neurosurgery 2004; 55:1-16.

Geibprasert S, Pongpech S, Jiarakongmun P, et al. Radiologic assessment of brain arteriovenous malformations: what clinicians need to know. Radiographics 2010; 30:483-501.

Jellinger K. Vascular malformations of the central nervous system: a morphological overview. Neurosurg Rev 1986; 9:177-216.

Krings T, Geibprasert S, Luo B, et al. Segmental neurovascular syndromes in children. Neuroimaging Clin North Am 2007; 17:245-258.

Krings T, Hans FJ, Geibprasert S, Terbrugge K. Partial "targeted" embolisation of brain arteriovenous malformations. Eur Radiol 2010; 20:2723-2731.

Krings T, Ozanne A, Chng SM, et al. Neurovascular phenotypes in hereditary haemorrhagic telangiectasia patients according to age: review of 50 consecutive patients aged 1 day to 60 years. Neuroradiology 2005; 47:711-720.

Lasjaunias P, Landrieu P, Rodesch G, et al. Cerebral proliferative angiopathy: clinical and angiographic description of an entity different from cerebral AVMs. Stroke 2008; 39:878-885.

Stracke CP, Spüntrup E, Reinacher P, et al. Time resolved 3D MRA: applications for interventional neuroradiology. Intervent Neuroradiol 2006; 12:223-231.

Topper R, Jurgens E, Reul J, Thron A. Clinical significance of intracranial developmental venous anomalies. J Neurol Neurosurg Psychiatry 1999; 67:234-238.

Valavanis A, Wellauer J, Yasargil MG. The radiological diagnosis of cerebral venous angioma: cerebral angiography and computed tomography. Neuroradiology 1983; 24:193-199.

Craniocerebral Trauma

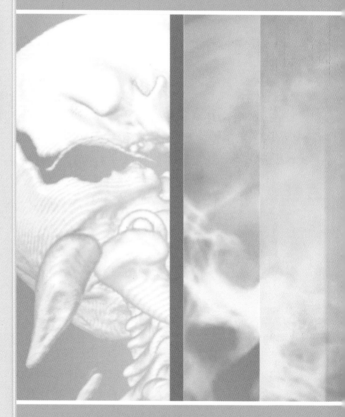

25

Fracture and Hemorrhage

Raymond Francis Carmody

Traumatic brain injury is common in all age groups and is a leading cause of death and disability, especially in young people. The National Center for Injury Prevention and Control estimates that 1.5 million individuals sustain traumatic brain injury in the United States each year. Of these, 50,000 die and 80,000 to 90,000 suffer long-term disability.[1] More than 5.3 million Americans currently are disabled by head injury.[2] The economic costs exceed $60 billion annually.[3] Caring for a victim of severe traumatic brain injury can cost more than a million dollars over a lifetime.

Traumatic brain injury is about twice as common in males as females; African-Americans are affected disproportionately.[4] Leading causes of traumatic brain injury are motor vehicle crashes, falls, and firearm use. Use of firearms causes 10% of all traumatic brain injuries but 44% of all deaths, because 90% of all gunshot wounds to the brain are fatal.

Neuroimaging is central to the initial diagnosis, management, and later follow-up of patients with head trauma. CT is the study of choice for initial imaging of acute head trauma. MRI is the preferred study for imaging subacute and chronic head injury. CT offers convenience, speed, and accuracy for diagnosing acute hemorrhage and mass effect and is usually sufficient for planning surgical intervention. Multislice CT using isotropic voxels provides superb coronal, sagittal, and oblique reformatted images without need to reposition the victim for additional imaging planes. MRI techniques such as diffusion tensor imaging and fiber tractography provide valuable prognostic information in the individual with chronic head injury.

The focus of this chapter is mainly on the imaging features of adult head trauma. The classification of head injury, mechanisms of injury, and pathophysiology are also discussed.

CLASSIFICATION OF HEAD INJURY

Traumatic brain injuries may be classified as primary or secondary and subclassified by the severity of injury. *Primary* brain injuries are those that occur at the time of impact and are a direct result of the traumatic force. Examples include contusions, diffuse axonal injury, intracerebral hematoma, and extra-axial hematomas. *Secondary* injuries are those that occur later as a consequence of the primary traumatic event and include vasospasm, infarction secondary to vascular compression and brain herniation, anoxic injury, fat embolism, and infection.[5] Severity is graded by either the clinical Glasgow Coma Scale (GCS) or the

CT-based Marshall score. When they are concordant, both are quite reliable. When they are discordant, additional imaging studies such as MRI should be considered. Clinical outcome is graded by the modified Rankin scale.

Glasgow Coma Scale

The severity of traumatic brain injury is usually classified according to the GCS (Table 25-1).[6] This standardized clinical test evaluates three parameters: (1) best eye-opening response, (2) best verbal response, and (3) best motor response. The scale ranges from 3 to 15, with 3 being an unresponsive, flaccid patient and 15 being a fully awake individual. Patients with GCS scores of 13 to 15 are considered to have minor head injuries; those with a score of 9 to 12 have moderate head injury; a score of 5 to 8 indicates severe head injury; and 3 to 4 indicates a very severe head injury.[7] The GCS score correlates well with morbidity and mortality.[8,9] For example, persistent vegetative state or death occurs in only 6% of patients with a GCS of 11 or higher but in 80% of those with a GCS of 5 or lower. The GCS score at 6 hours after injury predicts outcome more accurately than the immediate GCS score.[10] The GCS is less useful for assessing intoxicated trauma victims and infants. Metabolic conditions such as diabetic acidosis or hypoxia may skew the GCS score unfavorably.

The Marshall Score

The Marshall score utilizes the initial CT scan to assess the severity of diffuse head trauma (Table 25-2).[11] This score evaluates the perimesencephalic cisterns, the amount of midline shift, and the presence or absence of one or more surgical masses to assign patients to one of four groups of increasing severity. Individuals classified as having Diffuse Injury I (no visible pathology) have a mortality of 10%. Those with Diffuse Injury IV (midline shift >5 mm and no high- or mixed-density masses >25 mL) have a mortality rate greater than 50%. The Marshall classification allows certain subsets of patients to be directed toward specific types of therapy.[12]

The Modified Rankin Scale Score

The modified Rankin scale is used primarily to classify the level of disability in stroke patients[13] but can also be applied to head trauma victims (Table 25-3).[14] The scale ranges from 0 (no symptoms) to 6 (dead). This grading system assesses the functional outcome of the individual and looks at the whole patient in terms of limitations of activity and changes in lifestyle.[15]

TABLE 25-1. Glasgow Coma Scale

	Points
Eye Opening Response	
Spontaneous—open with blinking at baseline	4
To verbal stimuli, command, speech	3
To pain only (not applied to face)	2
No response	1
Verbal Response	
Oriented	5
Confused conversation but able to answer questions	4
Inappropriate words	3
Incomprehensible speech	2
No response	1
Motor Response	
Obeys commands for movement	6
Purposeful movement to painful stimulus	5
Withdraws in response to pain	4
Flexion in response to pain (decorticate posturing)	3
Extension response in response to pain (decerebrate posturing)	2
No response	1

TABLE 25-2. The Marshall Score: Diagnostic Categories of Abnormalities Visualized on CT

Category	Definition
Diffuse injury I (no visible pathologic process)	No visible intracranial pathologic process seen on CT
Diffuse injury II	Cisterns are present with midline shift 0-5 mm and/or: Lesion densities present No high- or mixed-density lesion >25 mL May include bone fragments and foreign bodies
Diffuse injury III (swelling)	Cisterns compressed or absent with midline shift 0-5 mm, no high- or mixed-density lesion >25 mL
Diffuse injury IV (shift)	Midline shift >5 mm, no high- or mixed-density lesion >25 mL
Evacuated mass lesion	Any lesion surgically evacuated
Nonevacuated mass lesion	High- or mixed-density lesion >25 mL, not surgically evacuated

From Marshall LF, Marshall SB, Klauber MR, et al. A new classification of head injury based on computerized tomography. J Neurosurg 1991; 75: S14-S20.

MECHANISMS OF HEAD INJURY

The two major types of head injury are blunt head trauma and penetrating injury. Blunt head injury is much more common. Penetrating head injuries, especially gunshot wounds, are more lethal. Severe traumatic brain injury from traffic accidents is becoming less common because of the use of modern protective devices such as seat belts and air bags.

Blunt Head Injury

Most forms of blunt traumatic brain injury are the result of *dynamic loading,* in which the forces acting on the head occur in less than 200 ms.[16] The most common type of dynamic loading is impact loading, in which a blunt object strikes the head or the head strikes an object. Examples would include objects that the head strikes in a motor vehicle accident (windshield, dashboard) or in a fall (ground, wall). With contact, a complex series of events occurs at the site of impact and remote from the point of contact. Directly at the point of impact the skull bends inward. Peripheral to the point of impact the skull bends outward. From the point of impact, shock waves propagate throughout the skull and brain at the speed of sound. The specific type and severity of brain injury depend on the mass and hardness of the object

TABLE 25-3. Modified Rankin Scale

Score	Description
0	No symptoms at all
1	No significant disability despite symptoms; able to carry out all usual duties and activities
2	Slight disability; unable to carry out all previous activities but able to look after own affairs without assistance
3	Moderate disability; requiring some help but able to walk without assistance
4	Moderately severe disability; unable to walk without assistance and unable to attend to own bodily needs without assistance
5	Severe disability; bedridden, incontinent, and requiring constant nursing care and attention
6	Dead

Data from Bonita R, Beaglehole R. Modification of Rankin Scale: recovery of motor function after stroke. Stroke 1988; 19:1497-1500.

struck and on the velocity at time of impact. As a result of inertial forces, the sudden deceleration of the head causes compressive forces at the site of impact and rarefaction in the tissues on the opposite side of the head.

Thus, the brain is exposed to three different types of strain: compressive, tensile, and shear. Bone, brain, and vascular tissue withstand compressive strain better than tensile strain, especially because brain tissue is essentially incompressible in vivo. Therefore, most injuries to the brain result from tensile and shear strains. Shear strains develop because different tissues like gray matter and white matter have different rates of acceleration/deceleration. Shear strains are especially frequent with rotational acceleration forces. The terms *coup* and *contrecoup* have been used for years to describe the type of lesion at the site of impact and opposite the site of impact, respectively. Some investigators eschew these terms as imprecise,[5] but they are convenient for descriptive purposes when categorizing the mechanism of a head injury. Compressive phenomena most often cause injury at the point of impact (*coup* injury), whereas rarefaction phenomena often cause more severe damage at sites distant from the site of impact (*contrecoup* injury). This concept holds not only for brain contusions but also for some extra-axial lesions, such as subdural hematoma.

Penetrating Head Injury

Penetrating traumatic brain injury may be the result of both intentional and unintentional events, including gunshot wounds, stabbings, and occupational events, such as nail gun injury. Stabbings and most occupational penetrating injuries result in low-velocity impacts over a relatively small area. The size of the offending object, the depth of penetration, and the trajectory are the key factors in determining the extent of injury. Bullets have far greater velocity and kinetic energy, so bullet wounds are much more devastating. Bullets damage brain tissue by laceration and crushing, shock waves, and cavitation. These phenomena are discussed more thoroughly in a subsequent section.

Pathophysiology

Blunt and penetrating trauma initially cause mechanical distortion of brain tissue. However, direct *primary* mechanical disruption of axons and instantaneous cell death is relatively uncommon in traumatic brain injury.[16] Instead, these injuries temporarily disrupt the integrity of the cell membrane, setting off a biochemical cascade that leads to *secondary* injury. Potassium leaks out of the cell. Sodium, calcium, and chloride diffuse in. High levels of intracellular calcium injure the cell and lead to delayed cell death. Additional cell damage is propagated by oxidative free radicals, glutamate,[17-19] and inflammatory events.[20] Excitatory amino acids, including glutamate and aspartate, are elevated after

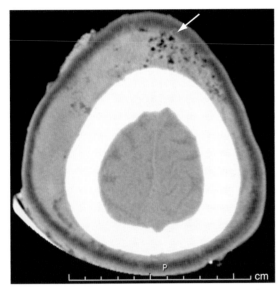

■ **FIGURE 25-1** Scalp hematoma in a 23-year-old man. CT shows large high-density mass in scalp on right. *Arrow* indicates air in the wound.

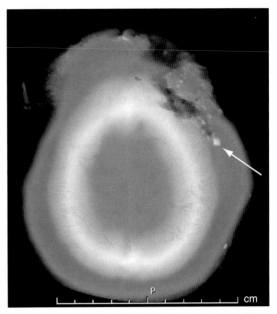

■ **FIGURE 25-2** Scalp and skull laceration in a 30-year-old man. CT demonstrates soft tissue and bone laceration, as well as foreign material (*arrow*) in the wound.

traumatic brain injury and can induce swelling, vacuolization, and death of neurons as well as astrocytic swelling.[21]

Scalp and Skull Injury
Scalp Injury

The scalp consists of five layers. From superficial to deep these are the skin, subcutaneous fibrofatty tissue, galea aponeurotica, loose areolar connective tissue, and periosteum.[22] Following head trauma, hemorrhage may accumulate in the subcutaneous, subgaleal, and subperiosteal compartments. Subcutaneous and subperiosteal hematomas are much more common in infants and may result from birth trauma. Subgaleal hematomas are the type most frequently seen in adults. Because the subgaleal space lies deep to the frontalis and occipitalis muscles but superficial to the temporalis muscles, subgaleal hemorrhages are often identified on noncontrast CT as crescentic or elliptical areas of high density superficial to the temporalis muscle (Fig. 25-1).

Lacerations of the scalp may accompany both penetrating and closed-head trauma. Any lacerations identified should be scrutinized for foreign material, which may be a source of infection (Fig. 25-2). Extensive scalp avulsion, or "degloving," is sometimes seen in unrestrained passengers ejected from moving vehicles (Fig. 25-3).

Skull Fractures

Skull fractures are present in only 25% of fatal head injuries at autopsy.[23] Patients with a skull fracture have a higher incidence of intracranial hematoma than those without fracture.[14] When a blunt object strikes the head, the local inbending causes a compressive strain on the outer table and a tensile strain on the inner table. Because bone is more susceptible to tensile strain, the fracture begins in the inner table.[16] It then propagates along the lines of least resistance. When the skull strikes a broad or flat object, as in a fall, a *linear* fracture commonly results (Fig. 25-4). *Depressed* fractures result from more intense forces delivered over a smaller area of impact. *Diastatic* fractures are linear fractures that intersect or occur along a suture line, causing diastasis of the suture. Reopening of a closed suture is a special form of fracture that may be called sutural diastasis. *Basal* skull fractures result from blows directly to the occiput or mastoid or from forces transmitted from blows to the face. They also frequently accompany gunshot injury.

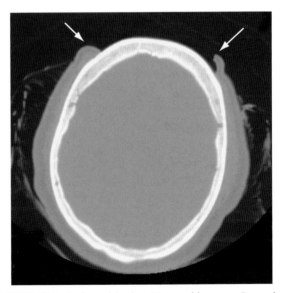

■ **FIGURE 25-3** Scalp avulsion in a 52-year-old woman. Bone window CT shows exposed calvaria. *Arrows* indicate scalp edges.

Noncontrast CT with bone algorithm is the study of choice for imaging all skull fractures (Figs. 25-5 and 25-6). It is important to study the scout image of the CT scan in addition to the individual slices, because linear skull fractures oriented precisely in the plane of CT section and concurrent trauma to the upper cervical spine may occasionally be imaged only on the scout view (Figs. 25-7 and 25-8). Linear fractures do not require specific treatment. However, they do indicate that substantial force was delivered to the skull, so detection of such fractures mandates careful search for accompanying intracranial contusion and hemorrhage. Linear fractures that cross the vascular grooves for the middle meningeal artery or dural venous sinuses are especially likely to cause epidural hematomas.

Depressed fractures are readily seen on CT and are likely to be associated with underlying brain injury. Depressed fractures

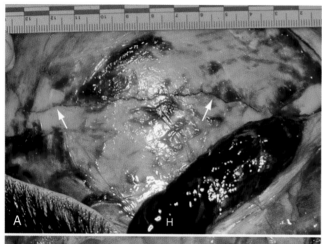

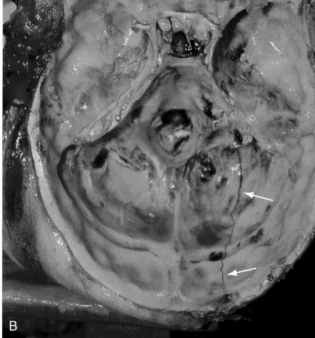

■ FIGURE 25-4 Linear skull fractures. Postmortem photographs. **A,** A large temporalis muscle hematoma (H) has been reflected away from the linear fracture line (*arrows*) that extends across the temporal squama. (See Fig. 25-17 for the internal view of this fracture line as it crosses the grooves for the ascending branches of the middle meningeal artery.) **B,** Left occipital fracture (*arrows*) and contrecoup fractures of both orbital roofs secondary to the occipital impact. (*Courtesy of John Deck, MD.*)

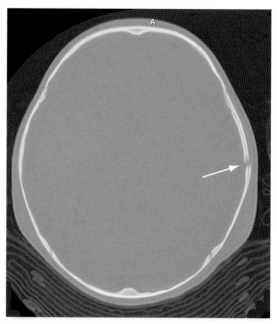

■ FIGURE 25-5 Linear skull fracture. A radiolucent line (*arrow*) is seen in the squamous temporal bone on bone window CT.

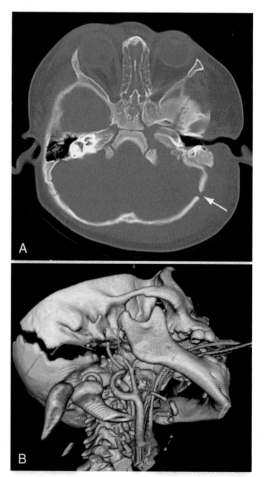

■ FIGURE 25-6 Diastatic lambdoid fracture in a 1-year-old boy. **A,** On bone window axial CT, the lambdoid suture is widened (*arrow*). **B,** 3D reformatted CT shows well-demonstrated fracture.

assume two forms: (1) the adjacent fragments may be angled inward at the fracture line without losing their relative position (Fig. 25-9) or (2) a section of bone may be displaced deep to the neighboring bone (subducted) leaving an open donor site and a double-thickness subduction zone (Fig. 25-10). Fractures depressed more than one full thickness of the skull need to be elevated,[24] so the degree of depression should be indicated in the report. Depressed fractures are most common in the frontal and parietal regions. Depressed fractures at the midline, crossing the superior sagittal sinus, carry risk for sinus thrombosis and subsequent venous infarction or hemorrhage. Infection, cerebrospinal fluid (CSF) leak, and post-traumatic epilepsy are other complications of depressed fractures.[25]

Basal skull fractures often require multiplanar thin-section CT for detection and display of their full extent. Axial slice thicknesses of 1 to 2 mm and coronal reformatted images are recom-

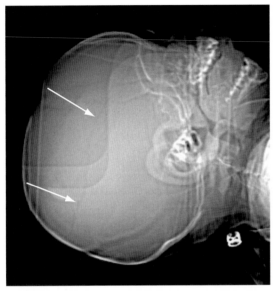

■ **FIGURE 25-7** Linear skull fracture seen on CT scout image only (*arrows*). Fracture was in the CT scan plane.

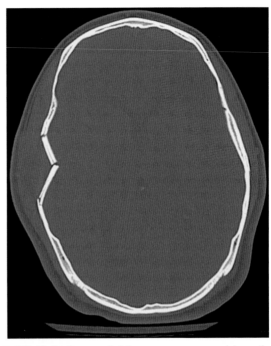

■ **FIGURE 25-9** Depressed right squamous temporal bone fracture. Fragments are bent inward but retain their relative position to the skull.

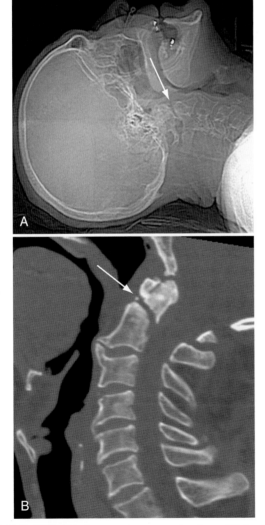

■ **FIGURE 25-8** C2 fracture that was missed on CT head scan. **A,** Scout radiograph shows fracture line (*arrow*). **B,** Follow-up CT of cervical spine demonstrates fracture (*arrow*).

mended. Cranial nerve injury and CSF rhinorrhea/otorrhea are common complications (Fig. 25-11). Pneumocephalus may follow fractures involving the frontal and sphenoidal sinuses (Fig. 25-12) or the mastoid portions of the temporal bones. Air-fluid levels in the paranasal sinuses suggest possible skull base fracture. Longitudinal fractures along the temporal bone may cause ossicular chain disruption (Fig. 25-13). Transverse fractures across the temporal bone may damage the seventh or eighth cranial nerves (Fig. 25-14).[26] Fractures of the cribriform plate may cause olfactory nerve injury and anosmia. The optic nerves, cavernous sinuses, and carotid arteries are susceptible to injury from sphenoid fracture. In cases of fracture through the carotid canal, CT angiography or MR angiography should be considered to rule out carotid dissection. Epidural abscess is a potential complication of fracture of the posterior wall of the frontal sinus or mastoid air cells. Meningitis, subdural empyema, and intracranial hypotension can result from meningeal tears.

Growing Skull Fracture
Also known as a leptomeningeal cyst, this lesion occurs exclusively in childhood; 90% are in children younger than age 3 years.[27-29] Growing fractures result when the dura deep to the fracture is torn and retracts, exposing the bony margins of the fracture to the pulsations of the arachnoid and subarachnoid CSF. Continued pulsations then erode the bone margins, enlarge the fracture, and permit the arachnoid and subarachnoid CSF to protrude into and through the enlarging fracture line. The presence of meninges in the fracture line interferes with osteoblastic activity and prevents fracture healing.[30] Growing skull fractures often originate from a diastatic parietal fracture but may develop at any site with fracture and torn dura. On plain radiographs, leptomeningeal cysts appear as elongate to ovoid radiolucent areas with smooth margins (Fig. 25-15). CT confirms the presence of a CSF-density cystic area at the fracture site (Fig. 25-16). Underlying brain injury is common, as are neurologic deficits, such as a contralateral hemiparesis.

Leptomeningeal cyst may be a sequela of a form of pediatric closed-head trauma known as the *cranial burst fracture.* This

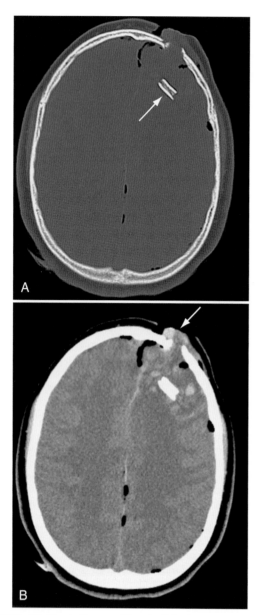

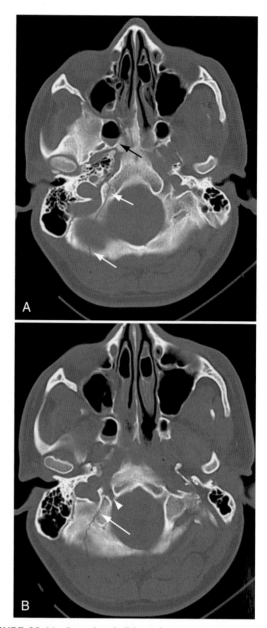

■ **FIGURE 25-10** A 13-year-old male following an ATV accident. **A,** Note subducted bone fragment (*arrow*) embedded deeply in frontal lobe. **B,** Soft tissue windows show brain tissue (*arrow*) herniating out of the bony defect. Pneumocephalus is present. ATV, All terrain vehicle.

■ **FIGURE 25-11** Posterior skull base fracture in a 21-year-old man. **A,** Fracture line extends through occipital bone on right (*white arrows*) and anteriorly into right sphenoidal sinus (*black arrow*), which has an air-fluid level. **B,** Fracture involves the right hypoglossal canal (*arrowhead*).

severe head injury consists of a widely diastatic fracture associated with dural laceration and extrusion of brain tissue outside the calvaria beneath an unbroken scalp.[31] The herniated cerebral tissue and dural tear may not be apparent on CT and require MRI for diagnosis.[28] Surgical repair of the defect is recommended to prevent further neurologic deterioration.[29] Because of its therapeutic implications, some investigators recommend MRI for all skull fractures with more than 4 mm of diastasis to exclude brain hernia. If the dura is intact, the fracture will heal and a leptomeningeal cyst will not develop.[27]

EXTRA-AXIAL HEMORRHAGE

The brain and the spinal cord are designated the *neuraxis. Intra-axial hemorrhage* is an umbrella term for hemorrhage within the brain and spinal cord. *Extra-axial hemorrhage* is an umbrella term for bleeding within the cranium but outside the brain or cord parenchyma. Therefore, extra-axial hemorrhages include any or all of epidural, subdural, subarachnoid, and intraventricular hemorrhages.

Closed-head trauma may cause extra-axial hemorrhage of any type or direct hemorrhage into the brain substance. As a rule, these are primary lesions, beginning at the time of injury. Although subarachnoid hemorrhage is a common finding with head trauma, epidural, subdural, and intracerebral hematomas are the usual expanding lesions that cause neurologic deterioration.

Epidural Hematoma

An epidural hematoma (EDH) is hemorrhage between the outer periosteal layer of the dura and the inner table of the skull, creating an epidural space.

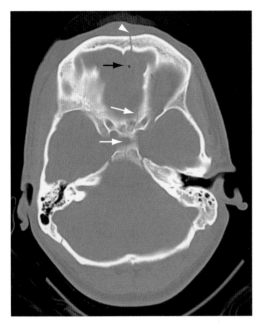

■ **FIGURE 25-12** Anterior skull base fracture. *White arrows* indicate fracture through the sella turcica and planum sphenoidale. A fracture through the frontal bone is also seen (*arrowhead*). There is a small amount of pneumocephalus (*black arrow*).

Epidemiology

Hemorrhage into the potential space between the periosteal dura and the inner table of the skull is seen in 2.7% to 4% of all traumatic brain injuries.[32] The leading causes of EDH are motor vehicle accidents, falls, and assaults, in that order. Associated skull fractures are present in 75% to 90% of cases. EDHs arise from tearing of a middle meningeal artery, middle meningeal vein, diploic vein, or dural venous sinus. Most EDHs occur in the squamous temporal region (Table 25-4), where the skull is thin and easily fractured, tearing the middle meningeal artery (Fig. 25-17). Frontal and parietal EDHs are less common. Because the dura is tightly adherent to the skull, epidural collections tend to be short and elliptical (Fig. 25-18). They seldom cross suture lines, where the dura is firmly attached to the inner table, unless the fracture also traverses the suture. Up to 50% of EDHs are accompanied by other intracranial injury, most commonly subdural hematoma, cortical contusions, and diffuse brain swelling. Less than 5% of adult EDHs occur in the posterior fossa.

Clinical Presentation

About half of all EDH patients suffer a period of loss of consciousness, followed by a lucid interval and then subsequent neurologic deterioration as the hematoma expands. If there are other intracranial injuries, the victim may remain unconscious from the time of the accident. In one series of 200 surgically treated EDHs, 23% had no loss of consciousness preoperatively.[33] Those individuals who remained conscious up to the time of surgery had a favorable outcome (only 4% unfavorable outcome) compared with those who were unconscious up to the time of surgery (10% mortality, 23% unfavorable functional recovery). Functional outcome was highly correlated with the GCS score at the time of admission (see Table 25-1). Other presenting symptoms include focal neurologic deficit, decerebrate posturing, and seizures.[32]

Imaging
CT

On noncontrast CT scans, acute EDHs typically appear as biconvex, hyperdense masses adjacent to the inner table of the skull

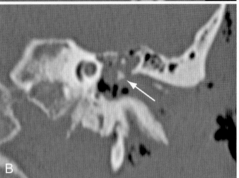

■ **FIGURE 25-13** Longitudinal left temporal bone fracture in a 56-year-old man. **A,** Axial CT shows fracture line (*arrows*) extending from mastoid into middle ear cavity. Incus (I) is dislocated from malleus (M). **B,** Coronal reformatted CT shows dislocated incus (*arrow*) in mesotympanum.

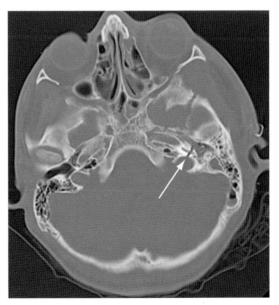

■ **FIGURE 25-14** Transverse left temporal bone fracture in a 15-year-old boy. Axial CT demonstrates fracture through basal turn of the cochlea (*arrow*), resulting in sensorineural hearing loss.

■ **FIGURE 25-15** Growing skull fracture. **A,** Diastatic fracture of left parietal bone. **B,** Skull radiograph 3¹/₂ months later shows widening of the fracture line. (Courtesy of Sandra Fernbach, MD.)

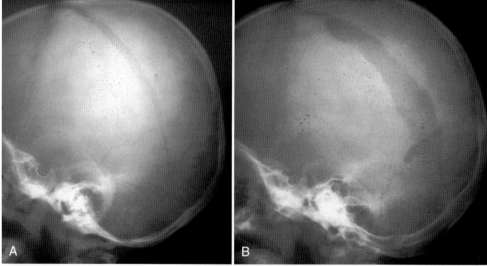

■ **FIGURE 25-16** Intradiploic leptomeningeal cyst in a 73-year-old woman. **A,** Axial bone window CT shows radiolucent defect in inner table of right parietal bone, with cavity indicated as CSF density in diploic space (*arrow*). **B,** Axial T2W MR image shows temporal lobe cortex (*arrow*) herniating into diploic CSF-filled space.

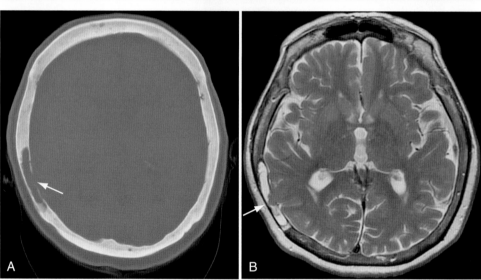

TABLE 25-4. Epidural Hematoma

Incidence	2.7%-4% of all traumatic brain injury patients and 9% of all patients in traumatic comas
Pathogenesis	Laceration of middle meningeal artery or vein, diploic veins, or dural venous sinus
Location	Temporoparietal region, 70%-80%; frontal and occipital area, 10%
Clinical Presentation	Coma, 25%-50%
	Lucid interval, 20%-47%
	Pupillary abnormalities
	Focal neurologic deficits
	Seizures
Associated Lesions	30%-50% of adult surgically evacuated epidural hematomas
	Skull fracture: 70%-95%
	Contusions
	Subdural hematomas
	Subarachnoid hemorrhage
	Diffuse brain swelling
Mortality	7%-12.5% of surgically evacuated epidural hematomas
Imaging Findings	High-density, biconvex mass on CT, usually in proximity of skull fracture
Indications on CT for Surgical Intervention	Hematoma 30 mL or greater
	Hematoma thicker than 15 mm
	Midline shift >5 mm

Data from Bullock MR, Chesnut R, Ghajar J, et al. Surgical management of acute epidural hematomas. Neurosurgery 2006; 58:S2-7-S2-15.

(Figs. 25-19 and 25-20). The CT attenuation of blood is related to the high electron density of the hemoglobin molecule and not the iron content. Clotted blood has a hematocrit of about 90%, whereas unclotted blood has a hematocrit of about 50%. On CT, areas of decreased attenuation within an EDH are thought to represent unclotted blood and indicate active bleeding (the swirl sign) (Fig. 25-21).[34] EDHs that result from a torn venous sinus may cross the falx or tentorium (Fig. 25-22) and thus be present in both the infratentorial and supratentorial compartments.[35]

MRI

On MRI, acute EDHs are usually isointense to brain on T1-weighted (T1W) images and isointense to hypointense on T2-weighted (T2W) images. Early subacute EDHs are hyperintense on T1W images and hypointense on T2W images (Fig. 25-23). Late subacute EDHs are typically hyperintense on both T1W and T2W imaging. The medially displaced dura is seen as a black line between the hematoma and compressed brain. MRI is rarely necessary to make the diagnosis of EDH, except occasionally for those that are located at the midline vertex, which are difficult to appreciate on CT.

Management

The management of EDHs has changed dramatically in recent decades.[36] Before CT almost all EDHs were surgically evacuated.

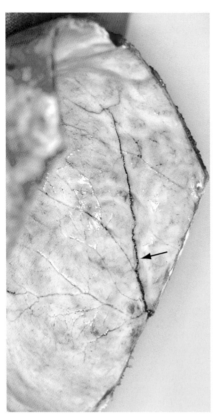

■ **FIGURE 25-17** Postmortem photograph shows a linear fracture line (arrow) crossing the grooves for the ascending branches of the middle meningeal artery (internal view of Figure 25-4A). *(Courtesy of John Deck, MD.)*

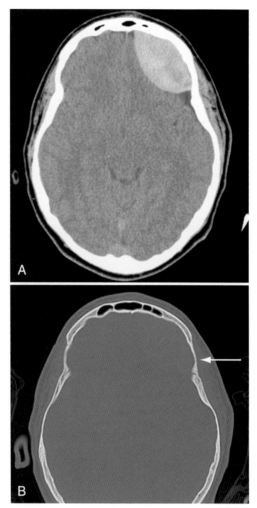

■ **FIGURE 25-19** Epidural hematoma in an 18-year-old boy. **A,** Axial CT shows high-density biconvex collection in left frontal region. **B,** Bone window CT shows subtle linear fracture (*arrow*).

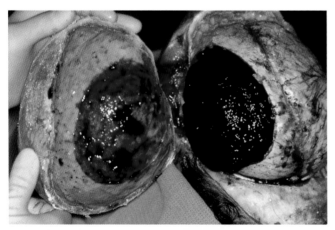

■ **FIGURE 25-18** Postmortem photograph of a large lentiform, sharply delimited "currant jelly" frontotemporal epidural hematoma. The dura is displaced inward, away from the inner table of the skull. *(Courtesy of John Deck, MD.)*

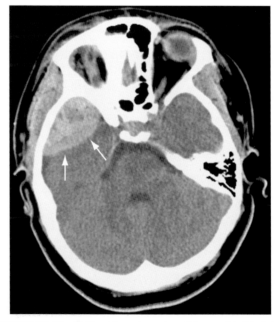

■ **FIGURE 25-20** Epidural hematoma in a 16-year-old girl. Axial CT demonstrates high-density collection in the right middle cranial fossa (*arrows*).

Now they can be followed with serial imaging studies, so more than 60% of EDHs can be managed nonsurgically.[37] Published neurosurgical guidelines specify which patients are suitable for nonoperative management[32]:

● An EDH greater than 30 mL should be surgically evacuated regardless of the patient's GCS score.
● An EDH less than 30 mL *and* with a thickness less than 1.5 cm *and* with a midline shift less than 5 mm in patients with a GCS score greater than 8 *without* focal deficit can be managed nonoperatively with serial CT and close neurologic observation in a neurosurgical center (Fig. 25-24).[32]
● The volume of an EDH can be approximated from the CT scan, using the formula $V = 0.5 \times L \times W \times H$.

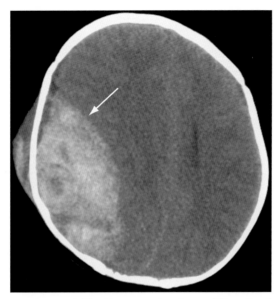

■ **FIGURE 25-21** Epidural hematoma in a 5-year-old boy. Unenhanced CT. *Arrow* indicates interface between brain and hematoma. Lower-density areas within the hematoma are the result of active bleeding (the swirl sign).

A lower threshold is used for operative management of middle cranial fossa EDHs, because these are more likely to cause uncal herniation and brain stem compression. Posterior fossa EDHs are usually evacuated, because mass effect in this compartment is poorly tolerated.[38]

In a study of 160 cases of EDHs treated conservatively, Sullivan and coworkers found that 23% enlarged, with a mean increase of 7 mm in width. The mean time to enlargement was 8 hours after injury. No EDH enlarged after 36 hours.[39] Of the EDHs that enlarged, 43% required surgical evacuation. Hence, close monitoring with CT is of paramount importance in the first 36 hours and especially in the first 8 hours. EDHs begin to decrease in size after the second week and in most patients will disappear completely after 4 to 6 weeks.

Subdural Hematoma

Subdural hematomas (SDHs) are misnamed because they actually represent hemorrhage into the innermost layer of the dura, designated the *dural border cell layer*. They are not hemorrhages into a potential subdural space, because there is no potential subdural space.[40,41]

Epidemiology
Subdural hemorrhages are seen in 12% to 29% of individuals with severe traumatic brain injury.[42] As with EDHs, the most common mechanisms of injury are motor vehicle accidents, falls, and assaults. In patients older than age 75 years, a fall is the most common cause of SDH.

Pathophysiology
SDHs arise from three sources: (1) rupture of a bridging cortical vein, (2) hemorrhagic contusion that breaks through the arachnoid, and (3) tear of a cortical artery or vein.[43] Most acute SDHs that are not associated with other intracranial injuries are thought to result from bridging vein rupture. Angular acceleration/deceleration of the head in the sagittal plane is the most common causative factor.[44] The bridging cortical veins course anteriorly and at an angle from the cortical surface of the frontal, parietal, and occipital lobes to the superior sagittal sinus (Fig. 25-25). This makes them particularly prone to rupture from a fall onto the occiput. The portion of the vein in the dural border

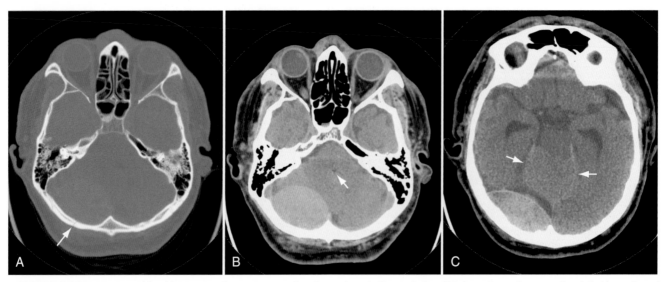

■ **FIGURE 25-22** Venous epidural hematoma from transverse sinus laceration. **A,** Bone window CT shows linear fracture of occipital bone (*arrow*). **B,** CT through posterior fossa demonstrates large infratentorial hematoma on right. Fourth ventricle (*arrow*) is compressed and displaced. **C,** Higher slice shows supratentorial component of hematoma. Upward herniation of cerebellar vermis (*arrows*) through the tentorial incisura is seen.

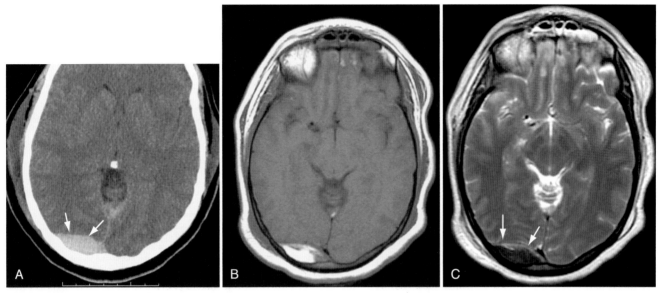

■ **FIGURE 25-23** Venous epidural hematoma, acute to early subacute phase. **A,** Unenhanced CT, day 2 post injury. High-density collection is seen in right occipital region (*arrows*). **B,** T1W MRI, day 4. Note bright signal in hematoma. **C,** T2W image shows low intensity in hematoma (*arrows*), consistent with intracellular methemoglobin.

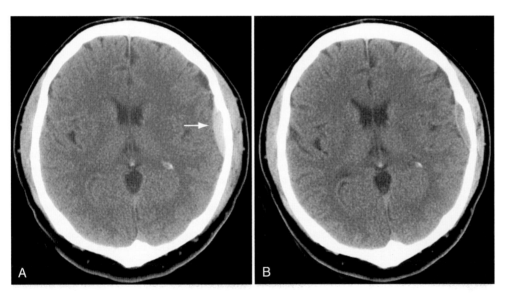

■ **FIGURE 25-24** Nonoperative management of a small epidural hematoma in a 29-year-old man. **A,** Initial CT demonstrates acute left frontal convexity hematoma (*arrow*). **B,** Follow-up CT shows resolving hematoma.

cell layer is thinner and more fragile than the subarachnoid segment, which accounts for the more frequent hemorrhage into the subdural compartment.[43] The dural border cell layer is composed of cells oriented like stacked plates with few cell-to-cell connections. For that reason it shears easily between cells along the plane of the layer. In the swine model, intracranial subdural hemorrhages may shear far caudally into the spinal canal in minutes.[45] It appears to be easier to shear along the dural border cell layer than to separate the periosteal dura from the inner table, so subdural hemorrhages typically appear to extend far more widely than do EDHs and typically spread over the surfaces of the hemispheres, along the falx, and under the occipital and temporal lobes (Fig. 25-26). Unlike EDHs, SDHs freely cross sutures and are inconsistently related to skull fracture. SDHs are likely to arise in relation to short loading times of 5 to 10 ms and are more likely to be contrecoup lesions.[16]

SDHs are classified as acute, subacute, or chronic, depending on the amount of time that has elapsed since the injury. However, there is no uniformity of terminology in the medical literature concerning the ages of SDHs. From the standpoint of neuroimaging, an SDH may be considered acute for up to 1 week, subacute for 1 to 3 weeks, and chronic when older than 3 weeks. The neurosurgical literature, however, tends to define acute SDH as an SDH in which the blood is still clotted and subacute SDH as an SDH in which the clot has lysed (which takes place over 48 hours to several days).[16] Using imaging studies to "date" an SDH is important for prognostic reasons and also may have significant forensic implications, especially in the case of suspected child abuse.

Clinical Presentation

Acute SDH

The typical patient with acute SDH presents with a GCS score of 8 or less (Table 25-5).[42] As with EDH, a lucid interval may be noted after the traumatic event, followed by neurologic deterioration. Mortality rates for acute SDH are typically in the range of

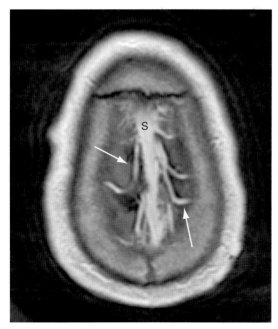

■ **FIGURE 25-25** Bridging cortical veins, as seen on a T1W gadolinium-enhanced MR image. *Arrows* indicate veins coursing anteromedially to enter the superior sagittal sinus (S).

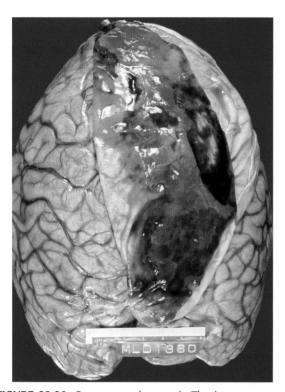

■ **FIGURE 25-26** Postmortem photograph. The dura mater covering the right cerebral convexity has been reflected to the left, revealing a sub-dural hematoma attached to the inner surface of the right convexity dura. This partially organized subdural hematoma is weeks old. *(Courtesy of John Deck, MD.)*

TABLE 25-5.	Subdural Hematoma
Incidence	11% of all head injury admissions and 21% of severe traumatic brain injury admissions
Pathogenesis	Tearing of bridging cortical vein, injured cortical artery, or bleeding from parenchymal injury
Location	Cerebral hemispheric convexities and interhemispheric fissure
	Rare in posterior fossa
Clinical Presentation	24% of all patients with traumatic brain injury who present with coma
	37%-80% of patients with acute subdural hematoma have a Glasgow Coma Scale score of 8 or less
	Lucid interval, 12%-38%
	Pupillary abnormality, 30%-50%
	Focal neurologic deficit
Associated Lesions	Contusions
	Parenchymal hematoma
	Subarachnoid hemorrhage, 14%-25%
	Epidural hematoma, 6%-14%
	Diffuse axonal injury
	Skull fracture is an inconsistent finding
Mortality	40%-60%, mainly due to associated lesions
Imaging Findings (CT)	Acute subdural hematoma: high-density, crescentic mass over cerebral convexity or sharply marginated, high-density mass in interhemispheric fissure
	Subacute subdural hematoma: often isodense to brain
	Chronic subdural hematoma: low density; may be biconvex
Imaging Findings (MRI)	Highly variable, depending on age of subdural hematoma
Indications on CT for Surgery	Hematoma >10 mm in thickness
	Midline shift >5 mm
	Falling Glasgow Coma Scale score
	Pupillary inequality
	Intracranial pressure >20 mm Hg

From Bullock MR, Chesnut R, Ghajar J, et al. Surgical management of acute subdural hematomas. Neurosurgery 2006; 58:S2-16-S2-24.

60% but vary widely.[46,47] Many of the survivors are permanently disabled. Acute SDHs are frequently accompanied by other intra-cranial injuries, such as diffuse axonal injury, intracerebral hematoma, and cortical contusions, and these additional lesions account for the poor outcome in most cases.[42] "Pure" SDHs have a much better prognosis. The mass effect exerted by an acute SDH may cause brain injury from herniation syndromes, increased intracranial pressure, and decreased cerebral blood flow, especially if the SDH expands rapidly. In addition to the size of the hematoma, bilaterality of the SDH, advanced patient age, and delayed surgical evacuation are associated with a poor outcome.[42]

Posterior fossa SDHs are rare in adults, probably because of restricted acceleration/deceleration of the cerebellum, as compared with the cerebral hemispheres.[48,49] In one series of 16 posterior fossa SDHs, the overall mortality rate was 56%: 100% for the nonoperated cases and 46% for those treated surgically.[50]

Imaging
CT

On noncontrast CT scans, acute SDHs typically have a high-density crescentic configuration (Fig. 25-27). Clotted blood in the subdural space may be indistinguishable from the adjacent skull if the images are viewed only on brain window settings. Hence, it is important to view CT scans of trauma victims at window widths intermediate between brain and bone settings to avoid missing thin SDHs (Fig. 25-28). Rarely, an acute SDH may be isodense to adjacent brain in individuals who are mark-edly anemic or when CSF leaks into the hematoma through a torn arachnoid. Occasionally, an acute SDH may have a more convex shape, if there are adhesions between the dura and arachnoid from prior trauma or infection (Fig. 25-29).

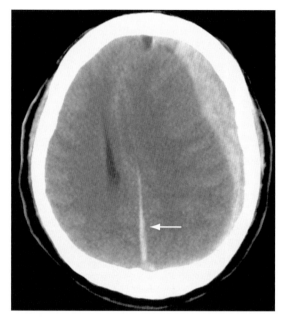

■ **FIGURE 25-27** Acute subdural hematoma. Unenhanced CT demonstrates high-density crescent-shaped collection over left frontoparietal region. A small interhemispheric hematoma is also present along the posterior falx (*arrow*).

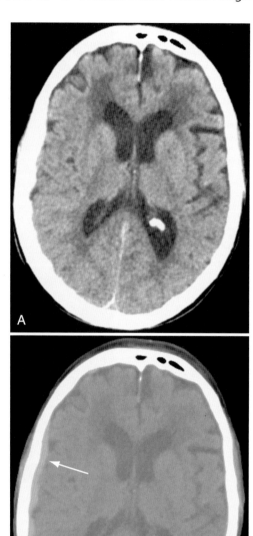

■ **FIGURE 25-28** Acute subdural hematoma in a 75-year-old woman. **A,** On unenhanced CT, at brain window width, hematoma is difficult to perceive. **B,** At intermediate window width, hematoma (*arrows*) becomes clearer.

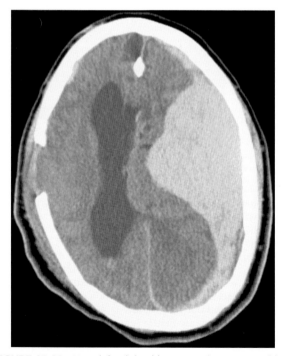

■ **FIGURE 25-29** Huge left subdural hematoma in a 55-year-old man. On unenhanced CT the hematoma has both a convex and a concave shape. An old craniotomy defect is seen on the right. Hypodensity of left occipital lobe indicates infarction as a result of posterior cerebral artery compression at the incisura due to temporal lobe herniation.

■ **FIGURE 25-30** Acute left suboccipital subdural hematoma in a 2-year-old boy. **A,** Unenhanced reformatted coronal CT demonstrates subdural collection (*arrow*) between occipital lobe and tentorium. **B,** Sagittal T1W MR image shows isointense hematoma (*arrow*), consistent with deoxyhemoglobin. On sagittal T2W FLAIR (**C**) and axial T2W (**D**) images the hematoma is markedly hypointense (*arrows*).

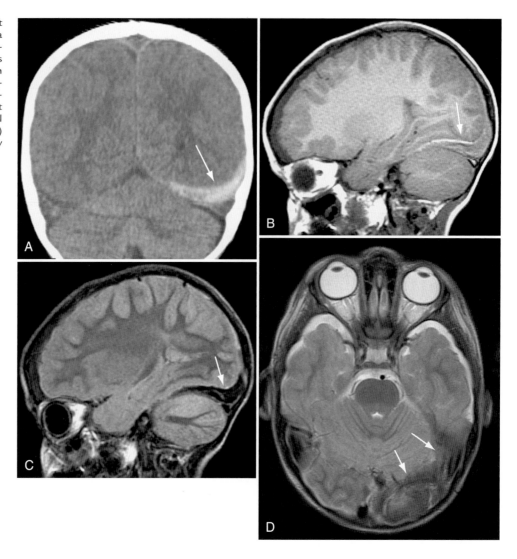

MRI

On MRI, the appearance of SDHs is highly dependent on the age of the collection. During the first few hours after the development of SDH, the hematoma has a high content of oxyhemoglobin, which is nonparamagnetic. At this stage the subdural collection will be nearly isointense or hypotense to adjacent brain tissue on T1W images and hyperintense on T2W and FLAIR images and T2W imaging. Hematomas at this stage are frequently termed *hyperacute.* By approximately 12 hours the oxygen has dissociated from the hemoglobin, and the resultant paramagnetic deoxyhemoglobin is isointense on T1W and markedly hypointense on T2W and T2*W imaging (Fig. 25-30). After 2 to 3 days, the deoxyhemoglobin starts to convert to intracellular methemoglobin, also a paramagnetic compound. Methemoglobin, with its five unpaired electrons, allows for proton-electron dipole-dipole interactions between the paramagnetic centers of the molecule and hydrogen atoms. This results in T1 shortening and, consequently, hyperintense signal with respect to brain on T1W imaging.[51] T2 shortening also occurs with intracellular methemoglobin, because the methemoglobin is unevenly distributed throughout the red cell. This heterogeneous local field strength causes protons diffusing into the cell to lose phase coherence on long repetition time, long echo time spin-echo sequences, which will, therefore, be markedly hypointense.[52]

Subacute SDH

As time passes, the unevacuated SDH undergoes predictable changes. After clot lysis, the red cells and debris may settle out in the dependent portion of the collection, producing a "hematocrit effect" (Fig. 25-31). At some point between 4 and 20 days the CT density of the SDH will approximate that of adjacent brain tissue.[5] These isodense SDHs are difficult to see on noncontrast CT, so secondary signs must be used to diagnose them correctly. These secondary signs include cortical gyri and sulci that do not extend out to the inner table, inward displacement of the gray matter/white matter junction (buckled white matter sign),[53] effacement of the ipsilateral lateral ventricle, and shift of the midline structures (Fig. 25-32). On contrast-enhanced CT an enhancing membrane on the inner surface of the hematoma becomes apparent, along with a small increase in attenuation value of the adjacent brain tissue (Fig. 25-33). Bilateral isodense SDHs are especially difficult to see, because midline shift is often absent (Fig. 25-34). In that case, the greatest clue may be (nearly) symmetric lateral ventricles that are simply too small for the patient's stated age.

Any question of possible isodense SDHs is readily resolved by MRI. During the early subacute stage (intracellular methemoglobin) the SDH is clearly evident, with increased T1 and decreased T2 signal intensity. In the late subacute stage, after

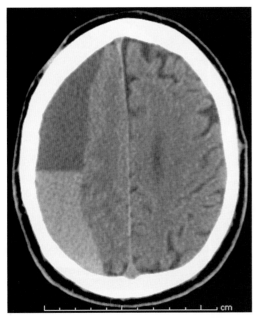

■ **FIGURE 25-31** Subacute subdural hematoma, hematocrit effect. Unenhanced CT demonstrates fluid-fluid level on right.

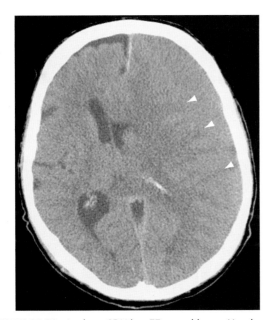

■ **FIGURE 25-32** Isodense SDH in a 77-year-old man. Unenhanced CT shows 18-mm left-to-right midline shift. *Arrowheads* indicate inward displacement of gray matter/white matter junction.

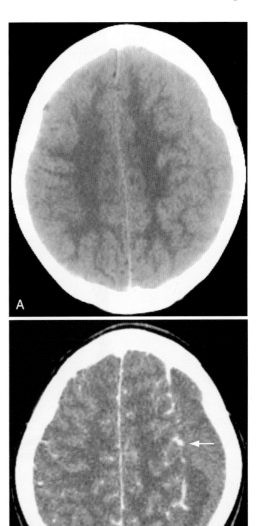

■ **FIGURE 25-33** Left convexity isodense subdural hematoma in a 10-year-old girl. **A,** Hematoma is poorly seen on unenhanced CT. **B,** On contrast-enhanced CT, brain/hematoma interface is clearly defined (*arrow*).

the red cells have lysed, the hematoma becomes hyperintense to brain on T2W images (Fig. 25-35).[51]

Chronic SDH
Subdural hematomas older than 2 to 3 weeks are considered to be chronic. Chronic SDHs are most common in older individuals. They may be the sequelae of untreated acute SDHs, but many appear to arise from repeated small hemorrhages that are clinically unapparent. In one fourth to one half of all cases there is no history of antecedent trauma.[54,55] Cerebral atrophy, as in elderly patients and alcoholics, causes the brain to separate from the inner table of the skull. This stretches the bridging veins and places them under greater tension, in position to tear after seem-

ingly insignificant trauma. Other predisposing factors include coagulopathy, epilepsy, and prior ventriculoperitoneal shunt placement. Slow bleeding from the low-pressure venous system allows for the formation of relatively large hematomas before they become symptomatic. Small hematomas often resorb spontaneously, but larger collections organize and become encapsulated within vascular membranes. Repeated bleeding from the friable vessels in these membranes may be the reason that some chronic SDHs continue to enlarge.[56]

The imaging appearance of chronic SDHs is variable. Typically, the subdural collection has CT attenuation between that of CSF and brain. Some are multiloculated, as a result of repeated episodes of bleeding and the formation of fibrous septations (Fig. 25-36). Blood products of varying ages are often found within the multiple compartments. The MR appearance of a chronic SDH reflects the age of the blood products contained therein. Most are hyperintense on both T1W and T2W owing to the

■ **FIGURE 25-34** Bilateral subacute subdural hematomas in a 47-year-old man who presented to the emergency department with papilledema. **A,** CT through the orbits shows elevation of both optic papillae (*arrows*). **B,** Slice through the lateral ventricles demonstrates 3.5-mm left-to-right shift. **C,** Higher slice shows small right convexity subacute hematoma (*arrows*) and larger left-sided subdural collection. Note inward displacement of the white matter on left. **D,** Microscopic view of the optic nerve head shows the edematous swelling of the papilla designated papilledema. *(Masson trichrome stain). (D, Courtesy of John Deck, MD.)*

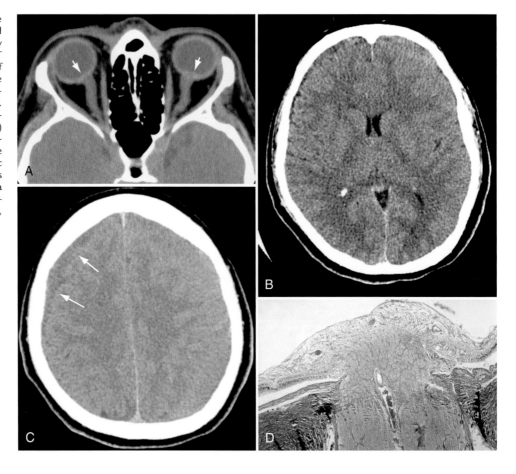

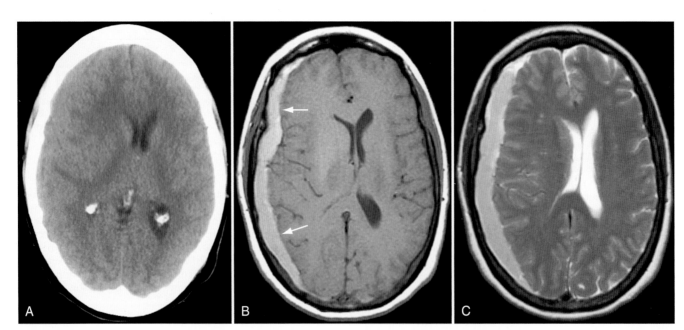

■ **FIGURE 25-35** Isodense subdural hematoma in a 68-year-old woman. **A,** Unenhanced CT. Hematoma is not visible. **B,** T1W MR image shows high signal intensity collection (*arrows*) over right cerebral hemisphere. **C,** T2W image shows increased signal in collection, consistent with extracellular methemoglobin.

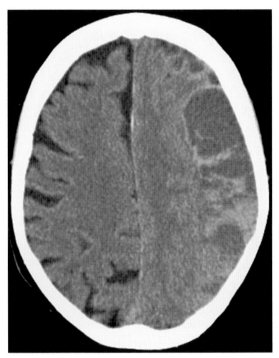

■ **FIGURE 25-36** Chronic subdural hematoma in an 89-year-old woman. Unenhanced CT demonstrates multiloculated fluid collections over left cerebral convexity, with blood products of different ages.

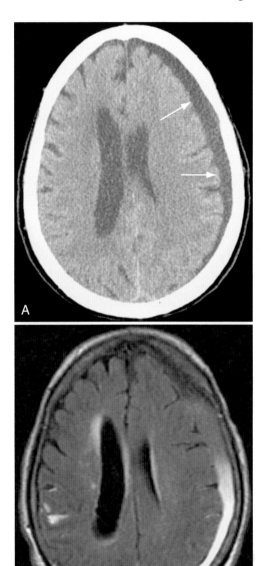

■ **FIGURE 25-37** Chronic subdural hematoma. **A,** Unenhanced CT demonstrates hypodense collection over left cerebral convexity (*arrows*). **B,** T2W FLAIR MR image shows mixed signal intensity collection, with layering of blood products.

extracellular methemoglobin in the collection. Fluid-fluid levels are common and are indicative of repeated hemorrhage (Fig. 25-37). Chronic SDHs may assume a biconvex shape (Fig. 25-38). Occasionally, a chronic SDH may calcify (Fig. 25-39).

Acute-on-Chronic SDH

Chronic SDHs displace the cortex from the dural membrane and cause the bridging veins to be under tension, making them more prone to tear. Moreover, the friable vascular membranes surrounding the SDH make them susceptible to re-hemorrhage. An acute SDH may form adjacent to the chronic collection (Fig. 25-40). This may occur after repeated trauma or after surgical evacuation of the original SDH.

Subdural Hygroma

Traumatic subdural hygromas arise from tears in the arachnoid membrane, with subsequent leakage of CSF into the subdural compartment. They typically appear 3 or more days after head trauma. On CT they have attenuation properties identical to CSF and may be indistinguishable from a chronic SDH. MRI can discriminate between these two entities, because hygromas have CSF signal intensity on all sequences (Fig. 25-41). The chronic SDH, in contrast, will have high signal on T1W images owing to the presence of methemoglobin. In most cases, hygromas are asymptomatic.

Traumatic Subarachnoid Hemorrhage

Bleeding into the CSF occurs as a result of head trauma.

Epidemiology

Head trauma is the most common cause of subarachnoid hemorrhage (SAH). Blood can enter the subarachnoid space from injury to the meninges (pia or arachnoid), contusion or laceration of the cerebral surface, or intraventricular hemorrhage (Fig. 25-42). In a patient with severe, nonpenetrating head injury, SAH is associated with a poorer outcome than the injury alone would

predict. Furthermore, larger amounts of SAH correlate with poorer prognosis.[57] Some investigators believe that traumatic SAH itself is not the cause of poor outcome but serves as a marker for more severe underlying brain injury.[58]

Imaging

On unenhanced CT, SAH manifests as areas of high attenuation within regions that normally contain CSF, including the basal cisterns, sylvian fissures, interhemispheric fissure, and cortical sulci. Small collections are often first demonstrated in the interpeduncular fossa or the posterior ends of the sylvian fissures (Fig. 25-43). SAH is more difficult to see on MRI but can be detected with fluid-attenuated inversion recovery (FLAIR) sequences (Fig. 25-44). Normally, CSF is hypointense on FLAIR sequences, whereas SAH has increased signal.[59] Care must be

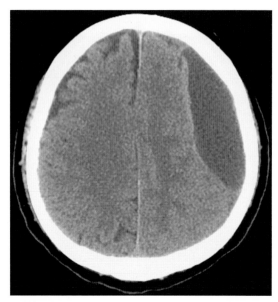

■ **FIGURE 25-38** Chronic subdural hematoma in a 64-year-old man. Unenhanced CT demonstrates biconvex low-density collection over left frontal lobe.

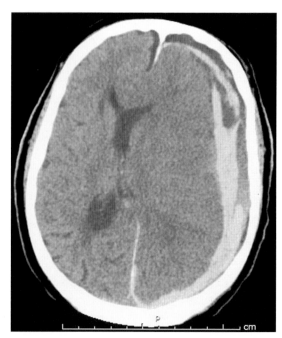

■ **FIGURE 25-40** Acute-on-chronic subdural hematoma. Unenhanced CT demonstrates bands of high and low density over left cerebral convexity.

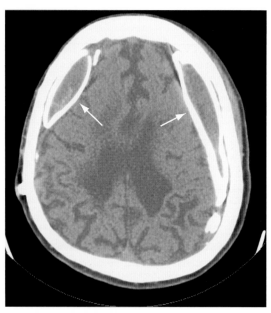

■ **FIGURE 25-39** Calcified subdural hematomas (*arrows*) in patient with extensive brain substance loss.

taken in interpreting the MRI in patients studied while receiving oxygen therapy, however. Oxygen, which has two unpaired electrons, is weakly paramagnetic and shortens T1 relaxation time. Oxygen diffuses rapidly out of the blood and into the CSF. Inhaled oxygen concentration of 100% increases the signal intensity of CSF by 4.0- to 5.3-fold, turning normal CSF "white" on FLAIR images.[60] Rescanning the FLAIR sequence after reducing the inhaled oxygen concentration to less than 30% for more than 5 minutes will return the FLAIR-white sulci to FLAIR-black sulci and prove that the increased signal intensity seen on the initial FLAIR images reflected increased oxygen tension in the CSF, not hemorrhage.[61] In one study, inhalation of 50% oxygen did not increase the CSF signal on FLAIR images.[62]

PARENCHYMAL INJURY AND HEMORRHAGE

This group of lesions includes contusion, intraparenchymal hematoma, and diffuse axonal injury.

Contusion

Contusions are primary neuronal and vascular injuries of the cortical surfaces, which may be thought of as bruises.

Pathophysiology

Contusions are the most common type of primary intra-axial lesion associated with trauma. On pathologic examination, contusions consist of punctate parenchymal microhemorrhages, edema, and necrosis. They are likely to occur at the crests of gyri, appear wedge shaped, and have their broad base against the pial surface (gliding contusions) (Fig. 25-45). Hemorrhage may extend up the Virchow-Robin spaces in a linear fashion and into the adjacent white matter.[23] Small, mild contusions may be nonhemorrhagic. *Coup contusions* occur at the point of impact, often from a small, hard object such as a pipe or hammer. *Contrecoup contusions* occur at a point distant, but not necessarily opposite, the point of contact.[16] The most common locations for cortical contusions include the inferior frontal lobes, the frontal poles, and the anterior temporal lobes (Table 25-6, Figs. 25-46 and 25-47). Cortical contusions are frequently bilateral, especially in the frontal lobes immediately above the cribriform plates and planum sphenoidale. Contusions are uncommon in the parietal lobes, occipital lobes, and cerebellum. Cerebral contusions are unlikely to cause severe impairment of consciousness. Instead, impaired consciousness is more likely to be caused by concomitant diffuse axonal injury or brain stem injury.

Imaging

CT

On a CT scan performed immediately after traumatic brain injury, cortical contusions may be subtle or invisible, unless quite large. Over the next hours to days, however, continued bleeding and edema formation increase their conspicuity, as well as the mass effect (Fig. 25-48). The contusions appear to "blossom

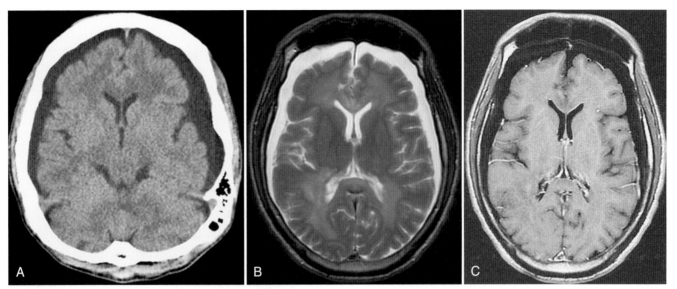

■ **FIGURE 25-41** Subdural hygroma. **A,** CT shows low-density fluid collections over both hemispheres. **B,** On T2W MRI, the fluid is isointense with CSF. **C,** Enhanced T1W image shows fluid collections that are isointense to CSF with no enhancing membranes surrounding fluid.

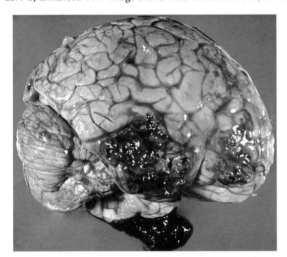

■ **FIGURE 25-42** Postmortem photograph. A thin film of subarachnoid hemorrhage extends over the cerebral convexity. Contrecoup contusions are seen along the anterior inferior temporal and frontal lobes. *(Courtesy of John Deck, MD.)*

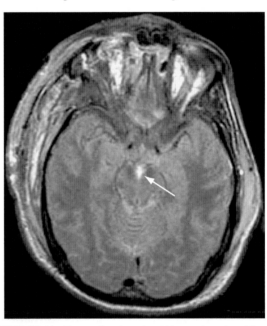

■ **FIGURE 25-44** Traumatic subarachnoid hemorrhage in a 46-year-old man. On T2W FLAIR image high signal intensity is seen in the interpeduncular fossa *(arrow)* and ambient cistern.

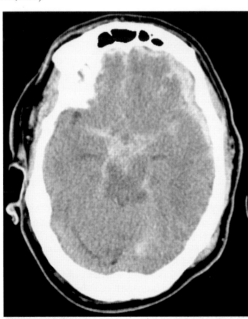

■ **FIGURE 25-43** Traumatic subarachnoid hemorrhage in a 57-year-old man. Unenhanced CT shows high-density material in basal cisterns. An acute left frontal subdural hematoma is also present.

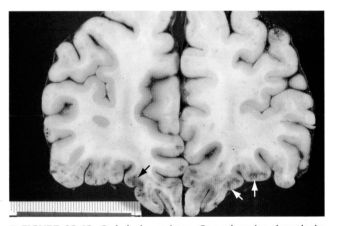

■ **FIGURE 25-45** Pathologic specimen. Coronal section through the frontal lobes. Multiple tiny hemorrhages along the orbital surfaces of both frontal lobes indicate bilateral contrecoup contusions *(arrows)*. Reddish discolorations along the sulci indicate mild subarachnoid hemorrhage. *(Courtesy of John Deck, MD.)*

TABLE 25-6. Contusions

Incidence	8% of all traumatic brain injuries, and 13%-35% of severe traumatic brain injuries
Pathogenesis	Punctate hemorrhaging at the crests of gyri resulting from blunt trauma
	Rupture of pial blood vessels
	Coup contusions: occur at the site of impact
	Contrecoup contusions: occur away from the site of impact
Most Common Locations	Frontal poles
	Orbital surfaces of the frontal lobes
	Temporal poles
	Lateral and inferior surfaces of the temporal lobes
Clinical Presentation	Unlikely to cause impairment of consciousness, unless large
	Tend to grow, especially over the first 48 hours, producing mass effect or increased intracranial pressure
Associated Lesions	Diffuse axonal injury
	Epidural hematoma
	Subdural hematoma
	Subarachnoid and intraventricular hemorrhage
	Skull fracture
Imaging Findings (CT)	Ovoid or irregular area of increased density, surrounded by edema
	Often enlarge with time, so must have serial scans
Imaging Findings (MRI)	Depend on age of lesion:
	Hyperacute: Iso- or low T1, high FLAIR, and high T2 signal (oxyhemoglobin)
	Acute: Iso- to low on T1, low on FLAIR and T2 (deoxyhemoglobin)
	Early subacute: High on T1, low on T2 (intracellular methemoglobin)
	Late subacute: High on T1, high on FLAIR and T2 (extracellular methemoglobin)
	Chronic: Low on T1 and T2 (hemosiderin)
Indications on CT for Surgery (somewhat controversial)	Parenchymal mass associated with neurologic deterioration
	Medically refractory intracranial hypertension
	Any lesion >50 mL
	Glasgow Coma Scale score of 6-8 and hematoma >20 mL, with midline shift >5 mm

From Bullock MR, Chesnut R, Ghajar J, et al. Surgical management of
   traumatic parenchymal lesions. Neurosurgery 2006; 58:S2-25-S2-46.

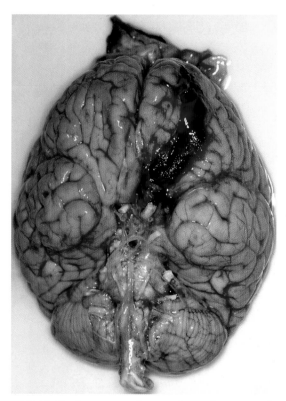

■ **FIGURE 25-46** Postmortem photograph. The linear contusion and hemorrhage along the inferior surface of the frontal lobe corresponded to a displaced fracture of the anterior cranial fossa. *(Courtesy of John Deck, MD.)*

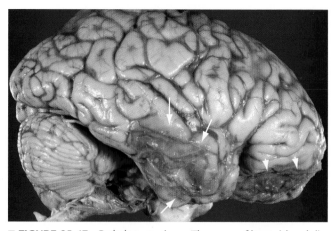

■ **FIGURE 25-47** Pathology specimen. The zones of brownish red discoloration indicate old contrecoup contusions of the anterior inferior temporal *(arrows)* and frontal lobes *(arrowheads)*. *(Courtesy of John Deck, MD.)*

or bloom." Accordingly, follow-up CT is extremely important, especially if the patient's neurologic status is deteriorating. The early CT appearance of a contusion may consist of only an area of decreased attenuation, representing edema. As oozing of blood into the lesion progresses, the involved area becomes hyperdense. A dark halo of edema often surrounds the hemorrhage. The edema may increase during the first week, so that serial CT scans may be warranted to look for increasing mass effect and early signs of herniation (Figs. 25-48 and 25-49).

MRI

MRI is more sensitive for cerebral edema and superior to CT for showing the true extent of contusions. The minimal number of sequences obtained in the TBI patient should include axial T1W, axial T2W, axial and sagittal FLAIR sequences, and a coronal T2*W gradient-recalled-echo sequence (because of its greater sensitivity to hemorrhage). As susceptibility-weighted imaging becomes available, the more sensitive susceptibility-weighted imaging will replace the T2*W gradient-recalled-echo sequence.[63] Initially, the contusion appears as an area of mild hypointensity on T1W images and hyperintensity on FLAIR and T2W images (Fig. 25-50). After about 12 hours the oxyhemoglobin in the hemorrhagic contusion is converted to deoxyhemoglobin, resulting in isointense to decreased signal on T1W images and markedly decreased signal on T2W images. Starting at about day 3, the intracellular deoxyhemoglobin is converted to methemoglobin, beginning at the periphery of the lesion and proceeding

toward the center. The intracellular methemoglobin has hyperintense signal on T1W images and hypointense signal on T2W images, as a result of T2 shortening. It is markedly hypointense on the T2*W gradient-recalled-echo sequences. As the hemorrhage liquefies and the red cells lyse, methemoglobin becomes extracellular, resulting in high signal on both T1W and T2W images (Fig. 25-51). This high signal from extracellular methemoglobin can persist for up to a year.[51]

When the contusion is about 2 weeks old, the edema begins to subside and there is an ingrowth of capillaries, astrocytes, and microglia.[16] Macrophages remove the necrotic tissue and blood products. With time, a shrunken, gliotic scar develops, sometimes containing residual hemosiderin-laden macrophages.

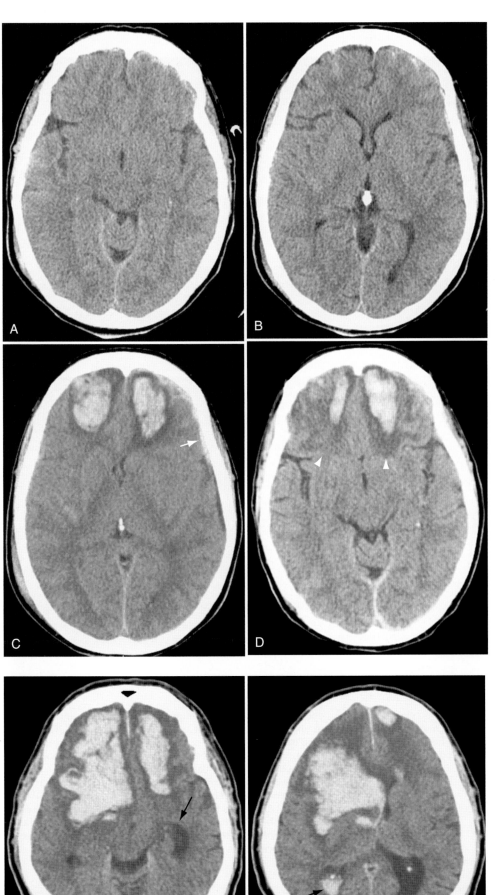

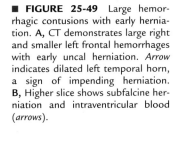

■ **FIGURE 25-48** Delayed hemorrhagic contrecoup contusions in a 61-year-old woman. **A** and **B,** Admission CT shows only trace of subarachnoid blood over frontal regions. **C,** Eight hours later, large bifrontal hemorrhages are seen. Small left frontal SDH (*arrow*) is present. **D,** After 18 hours, more edema (*arrowheads*) surrounds hemorrhages.

■ **FIGURE 25-49** Large hemorrhagic contusions with early herniation. **A,** CT demonstrates large right and smaller left frontal hemorrhages with early uncal herniation. *Arrow* indicates dilated left temporal horn, a sign of impending herniation. **B,** Higher slice shows subfalcine herniation and intraventricular blood (*arrows*).

■ **FIGURE 25-50** Small hemorrhagic contusion in 46-year-old man. **A,** Unenhanced CT demonstrates small area of hemorrhage surrounded by edema (*arrow*). **B,** On T1W MR image at 24 hours the lesion is hypointense (*arrows*). Contusion is mostly hyperintense on T2W imaging (not shown).

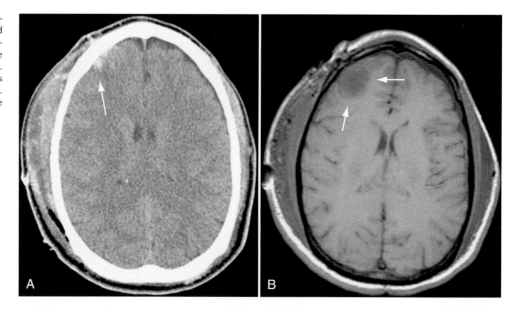

■ **FIGURE 25-51** Severe frontal hemorrhagic contusions in a 36-year-old man. T1W (**A**) and T2W (**B**) MR images were obtained 3 weeks after injury. Hyperintense signal is seen in both medial frontal lobes, representing extracellular methemoglobin.

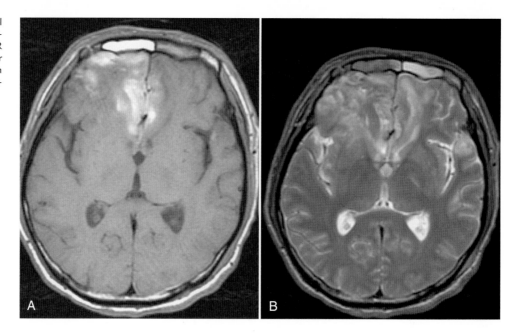

Imaging studies in this late phase show atrophic gyri, enlarged adjacent subarachnoid spaces, and enlargement of the ipsilateral lateral ventricle. There usually is residual hemosiderin in the tissues, so T1W images show slightly hypointense signal and T2W images show markedly hypointense signal.

Intraparenchymal Hematoma

Intraparenchymal hematoma (IPH) is bleeding into the brain tissue.

Pathophysiology

Not all IPHs arise from contusions. Some arise from penetrating injury, whereas others are the result of shear-strain injury to parenchymal vessels. A "pure" IPH is not in contact with the surface of the brain but may "point" toward the pial or ventricular surface and decompress into the subarachnoid or intraventricular space. Traumatic IPHs may be single but are often multiple. Most (80%-90%) occur in the frontal and temporal regions,[16] but they may also develop in the basal ganglia or cer-

ebellum. IPHs are less common than contusions and are found in about 15% of cases of traumatic brain injury.[16] Hematomas tend to dissect their way among neurons and along white matter tracts, whereas hemorrhagic contusions tend to expand in situ as a mixture of blood, damaged neurons, and edema.

Delayed intracerebral hematomas are hemorrhages that occur in an area of the brain that was normal on the initial CT scan. Delayed hematomas develop in 3.3% to 7.4% of cases of severe traumatic brain injury.[64] About 80% are present within 48 hours of injury, often in the same areas as the contusions.[16] Rarely, a delayed hematoma may first appear as long as a week after injury.

Imaging
CT and MRI

The CT appearance and evolution of IPHs are similar to those of hemorrhagic contusions (Fig. 25-52). Pure hematomas, however, tend to be more homogeneous than contusions. During the acute phase they are of uniform increased attenuation, with

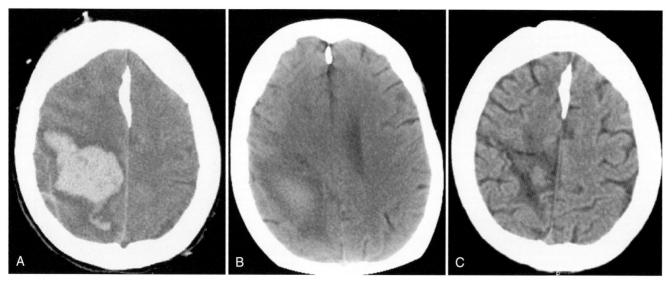

■ **FIGURE 25-52** Frontoparietal hematoma in a 52-year-old woman. **A,** CT demonstrates high-density lesion with mass effect. **B,** Appearance 2 months later. The hematoma is nearly isodense to cortex. **C,** Appearance 1 year later. Hematoma is replaced by gliotic area.

well-defined margins.[65] Subacute hematomas may exhibit a fluid-fluid level as blood components layer out, especially in patients who have been on anticoagulant therapy before trauma. On T2W imaging the dependent portion of the hematoma is hypointense (intracellular deoxyhemoglobin), whereas the supernatant is hyperintense.[51] Subacute hematomas have a surrounding rim of contrast enhancement on both enhanced CT and MRI. The enhancing rim is secondary to blood-brain barrier breakdown and to the appearance of vascular granulation tissue.[51] A key feature of the ring enhancement of simple IPH is that the ring forms *exactly* at the margin of the original hemorrhage, so it follows the contours of the original hemorrhage nearly exactly, although it becomes smaller as the hematoma resorbs.[66] After 6 to 12 months the blood products within the hematoma have been resorbed, leaving a slit-like cavity in the brain. The walls of this cavity are lined with hemosiderin-laden macrophages, causing decreased signal intensity on both T1W and T2W images. These linear remnants of old IPH are often designated *hemosiderin clefts.*

Diffuse Axonal Injury

Diffuse axonal injury (DAI) refers to disruption or shearing of axons as they course through the white matter of the brain. It can also be called shear injury, shearing injury, and traumatic axonal injury.

Epidemiology

DAI is present in 48% of cases of traumatic brain injury and frequently causes poor clinical outcome with permanent neurologic impairment.[67] Autopsy studies demonstrate DAI in 34% of fatal head injuries.[16] In individuals with mild traumatic brain injury (GCS score 13-15), MRI demonstrates subcortical white matter injury in 30%.[68]

Pathophysiology

Traumatic axonal injuries result from rotational acceleration of the head, which induces shear-strain deformation of the brain. Rotation in the coronal plane produces more frequent and severe injuries than sagittal rotation. Because different tissues in the brain accelerate at different rates, shear forces develop between them and disrupt the axons, which are particularly vulnerable to stretch injury (Fig. 25-53). DAI is produced by long impact loading (20-25 ms). Shorter loading times (5-10 ms) are more likely to cause SDHs.[16] Hence, DAI usually results from motor vehicle collisions, when the head strikes a resilient surface (e.g., padded dash, windshield). When the head strikes

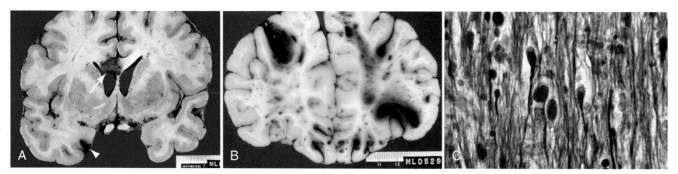

■ **FIGURE 25-53** Pathologic specimens. The sites of diffuse axonal injury are visible due to their associated hemorrhages. **A,** Coronal slice demonstrates injury of the corpus callosum (*arrow*) and a small cortical contusion (*arrowhead*). **B,** Coronal section through the frontal lobes. Multiple subcortical hemorrhages are frequently associated with diffuse axonal injuries. **C,** Histologic section. Silver stain demonstrates the disrupted axons as black retraction balls. *(Courtesy of John Deck, MD.)*

TABLE 25-7. Diffuse Axonal Injury

Incidence	48% of all traumatic brain injuries
Pathogenesis	Rotational acceleration of the head, which causes shear-strain deformation and disruption of axons
	20% are hemorrhagic
	80% are nonhemorrhagic
Most Common Locations	Subcortical white matter
	Corpus callosum, especially posterior body and splenium
	Dorsolateral brain stem
Clinical Presentation	*Milder cases:* brief period of unconsciousness, followed by cognitive impairment or psychiatric symptoms
	Severe cases: permanent vegetative state or severe disability
Associated Lesions	Subdural hematoma
	Hemorrhagic contusion
	Subarachnoid and intraventricular hemorrhage
	Epidural hematoma
Imaging Findings	*CT:* Detects only hemorrhagic lesions, which are typically 5-15 mm in diameter
	MRI: Increased signal intensity on FLAIR and diffusion-weighted sequences; decreased signal on gradient-recalled echo and susceptibility-weighted images

a hard surface, as in a fall, SDH and contusions are more likely to develop.

The gray matter/white matter junction is a common site of involvement. The corpus callosum is another. With lateral translation of the head, the motion of one cerebral hemisphere is restricted by the falx. The opposite hemisphere moves independently, causing stretch injury to the midline structures. The splenium is especially vulnerable, because it is in contact with the falx, which is broader posteriorly. The septum pellucidum and fornix may be injured where they join the corpus callosum.[67] Concurrent rupture of subependymal vessels may cause intraventricular hemorrhage. Whereas 80% of DAI lesions are nonhemorrhagic,[5] small hemorrhages are sometimes seen in the lobar white matter as well as in the splenium. With more severe trauma, lesions of the dorsolateral upper brain stem are seen. These may reflect tension by the large cerebellar hemispheres pulling on the narrow superior cerebellar peduncles.

Clinical Presentation
Patients with severe DAI are rendered unconscious at the time of impact. A lucid interval is not a feature, and these individuals either remain in a permanent vegetative state or are severely disabled. Milder cases may present after a brief period of unconsciousness, only later to experience difficulty concentrating, memory impairment, headache, depression, and abnormal neuropsychological testing (Table 25-7).[68]

Imaging
CT
CT is relatively insensitive for DAI and is positive in only 19% of nonhemorrhagic axonal shear injuries.[67] In those cases when it is abnormal, CT demonstrates discrete hypodense areas in the white matter, often at the gray matter/white matter junction. Other sites of involvement include the corpus callosum, corona radiata, internal capsule, and dorsolateral upper brain stem. Posterior fossa DAI lesions are very difficult to demonstrate on CT because of beam-hardening artifact. In one series, CT detected only 9% of brain stem lesions.[67] CT is much more sensitive for hemorrhagic DAI lesions, detecting 90% in one series (Fig. 25-54).[67]

MRI
MRI is superior to CT for detecting DAI and is used to search for DAI in the patient whose clinical condition is worse than what

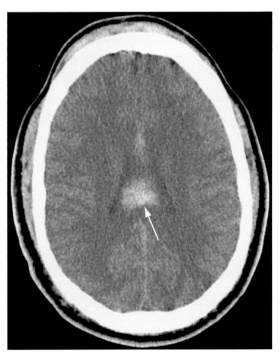

■ FIGURE 25-54 Diffuse axonal injury of corpus callosum. Unenhanced CT shows hemorrhage into body of corpus callosum (*arrow*).

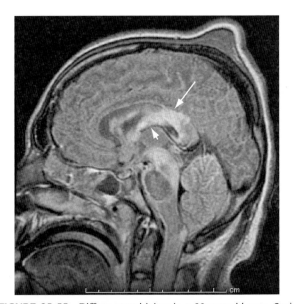

■ FIGURE 25-55 Diffuse axonal injury in a 20-year-old man. Sagittal FLAIR MR image shows increased signal intensity in corpus callosum (*arrow*), fornix (*arrowhead*), and dorsal brain stem. Subarachnoid hemorrhage is also evident.

would be expected by the CT scan. Whereas surgical management may not be changed, valuable prognostic information is gained. Sagittal FLAIR images are useful for examining the corpus callosum and fornix (Fig. 25-55) and have been shown to be superior to spin-echo T2W images for closed-head injury.[69] The superiority of FLAIR for DAI detection is related to its nulling of CSF signal, so the increased signal intensity of the lesion on FLAIR is not masked by the high signal from adjacent CSF. Gradient-recalled-echo sequences (T2*W GRE) are highly useful for detecting small hemorrhages (Fig. 25-56). These lesions may

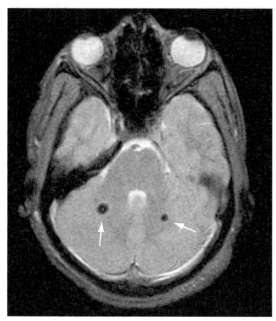

■ **FIGURE 25-56** Cerebellar diffuse axonal injury in a 13-year-old boy. Gradient-recalled-echo MR image shows focal low densities in cerebellum (*arrows*).

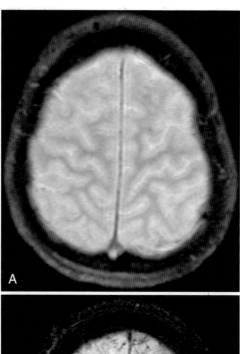

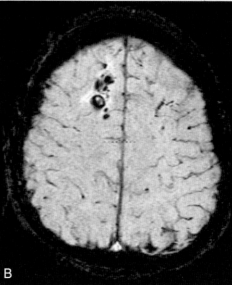

■ **FIGURE 25-57** Conventional gradient-recalled-echo (fast imaging with steady-state precession, 500/18, 15° flip angle, 78 Hz per pixel, 2 signals acquired, 4-mm thick sections) (**A**) and susceptibility-weighted (3D fast low-angle shot, 57/40, 20° flip angle, 78 Hz per pixel, 64 partitions, 1 signal acquired, 2-mm thick sections reconstructed over 4 mm) (**B**) MR images from the same brain region in a child with traumatic brain injury illustrating the increased ability of susceptibility-weighted imaging to detect hemorrhagic diffuse axonal injury. (*From Ashwal S, Babikian T, Gardner-Nichols J, et al. Susceptibility-weighted imaging and proton magnetic resonance spectroscopy in assessment of outcome after pediatric traumatic brain injury. Arch Phys Med Rehabil 2006; 87:12[Suppl 2].*)

remain visible as areas of decreased signal intensity (from hemosiderin) for years after injury.

Susceptibility-weighted imaging now detects many more areas of microhemorrhage than detected even by T2*W GRE imaging.[70,71] This will be the study of choice as it becomes more available (Fig. 25-57).

Diffusion-weighted MRI (DWI) adds valuable information when imaging DAI. In the acute and subacute stages, DAI lesions have decreased apparent diffusion coefficient, which appears to persist longer than it does in pure ischemic lesions.[72] Because of the restricted diffusion of water, foci of DAI have increased signal intensity on DWIs, reflecting cytotoxic edema (Fig. 25-58). Shaefer and associates found that DWI detected more DAI lesions than any other MR sequence tested and correlated well with initial GCS score as well as modified Rankin outcome scale score.[14] Huisman points out that measurements of fractional anisotropy values at sites where DAI is common may provide noninvasive surrogate markers for the severity of tissue injury and possible future outcome.[73] These data can be obtained even in the comatose or sedated patient, where clinical assessment is precluded. Arfanakis and colleagues used diffusion tensor imaging to evaluate 5 patients with mild traumatic brain injury.[74] They found that diffusion anisotropy was reduced in the internal capsule and corpus callosum early after injury. In a larger study, Inglese and coworkers examined 46 patients with mild traumatic brain injury with diffusion tensor imaging.[75] Their results were similar, in that fractional anisotropy was reduced in the corpus callosum, internal capsule, and centrum semiovale. These changes were seen in areas of normal-appearing white matter on MR images. In both of these studies whole-brain histogram analysis of mean diffusivity did not differ from control groups, indicating that the abnormalities of the diffusion tensor images caused by mild traumatic brain injury are restricted to specific areas. These studies support the limited histologic data available on mild cases of traumatic brain injury, which demonstrate microscopic evidence of DAI in 30%.[76]

MR spectroscopy can provide additional prognostic information in patients with DAI. Sinson and associates performed MR spectroscopy of the splenium in TBI patients and calculated the *N*-acetyl-aspartate (NAA)/creatine (Cr) ratio.[77] They found that a decreased NAA/Cr ratio correlated with the GCS outcome score: Twenty individuals with an NAA/Cr ratio of 1.53 ± 0.37 had a good neurologic outcome, whereas 10 patients with a ratio of 1.24 ± 0.28 had a poorer outcome. It is likely that the biochemical data provided by MR spectroscopy, as well as the information on structural white matter integrity provided by diffusion tensor imaging and susceptibility-weighted imaging, will be used increasingly to predict future outcome of patients with mild traumatic brain injury.

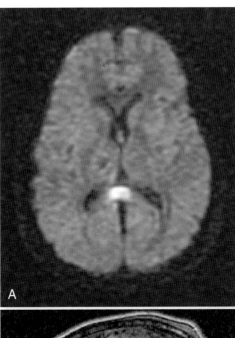

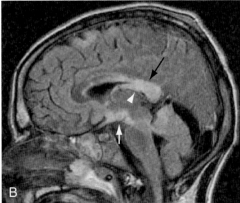

■ **FIGURE 25-58** A 16-year-old boy presented with diffuse axonal injury. **A,** Diffusion-weighted image shows high signal in splenium. **B,** Sagittal FLAIR image depicts lesions in corpus callosum (*black arrow*), fornix (*arrowhead*), and hypothalamus (*white arrow*).

PROJECTILE AND PENETRATING INJURY

Penetrating head trauma is conveniently divided into low-velocity and high-velocity injuries, because this variable has great prognostic significance. The science of wound ballistics uses the somewhat arbitrary figure of 1100 ft/s (335 m/s), the speed of sound in air, as the dividing line between low-velocity and high-velocity projectiles. Thus, all stab wounds (e.g., knives, ice picks, scissors, spikes) are low-velocity injuries. Handguns fall into both categories, depending on the caliber, and nearly all rifle bullets larger than .22 caliber are high-velocity rounds that cause high-velocity injuries.

Gunshot Injury
Epidemiology

Since 1990, gunshot wounds to the head have exceeded motor vehicle collisions as the leading cause of death from head trauma in the United States.[78] Engineering improvements in automobiles, such as air bags, seat belts, and anti-lock brakes, have made motor vehicles safer. Firearms are designed for maximum lethality and, sadly, age-adjusted death rates from firearm injury have increased nearly every year since 1985.[20]

Pathophysiology
Wound Ballistics

Wound ballistics is the study of the interaction of bullets with tissue. A basic understanding of this discipline is useful in evaluating gunshot injuries and in interpreting the imaging studies of these victims. The amount of damage caused by a bullet is a function of the mass of the slug and the square of its velocity (i.e., its kinetic energy). *Penetrating* injuries are those in which the bullet enters tissue, in this case the skull and its contents, and comes to a stop (Fig. 25-59). *Perforating* injuries occur when the bullet enters and exits the cranium. Perforating injuries carry a worse prognosis than penetrating wounds. Because the gelatinous brain tissue offers little resistance to a traversing bullet, it is not unusual for a slug to ricochet off the inner table of the skull and injure the brain at multiple sites before finally coming to rest. When a bullet enters the skull it causes two fractures—one of the outer table and a second of the inner table.[79] At the entrance wound the outer table fracture is smaller than the inner table fracture ("internal beveling"), a convenient way of identifying the entrance point. The same is true in reverse if the bullet leaves the skull, with the inner table fracture being smaller than the outer table defect ("external beveling") (Fig. 25-60). Also, bone and metal fragments are typically propelled into the brain tissue near the entrance wound.

As the projectile traverses tissue it is preceded by a shock wave, with pressures generated that can reach 60 atmospheres.[79] A hemorrhagic track is created along the path of the bullet, in which there is severe disruption of neural tissue and vessels. The size of this permanent track is typically three to four times larger than the diameter of the projectile (Fig. 25-61). A temporary cavity follows the bullet, and this cavity is up to 30 times larger than the diameter of the permanent track (Fig. 25-62). Expansion and contraction of the temporary cavity can propel brain tissue out of the skull and can also suck debris into the wound. The tremendous pressures generated within the cranial vault explain why fractures are often seen remote from the bullet track (Fig. 25-63).

In addition to hemorrhage along the permanent track, the temporary cavity causes stretch injury to neural tissue and axonal damage remote from the permanent cavity. The sudden and violent expansion of the temporary cavity may produce remote cortical contusions where the brain strikes bony surfaces or the tentorium. SDHs are a common occurrence after cranial gunshot injury (see Fig. 25-62). Vascular injury often leads to massive parenchymal, intraventricular, and subarachnoid hemorrhage. Laceration of dural venous sinuses leads to profuse hemorrhage that is difficult to control.[16] Traumatic aneurysms and arteriovenous fistulas are additional sequelae.

Imaging
CT

CT plays a crucial role in the evaluation of cranial gunshot injury. Careful analysis of the projectile path, the presence of foreign material in the brain (metallic fragments, bone), the size of the hematoma, and the amount of damaged brain tissue is paramount for surgical planning, if indicated. The initial CT also yields valuable prognostic information. Findings that predict a poor outcome include bihemispheric wounds, posterior fossa or brain stem involvement (Fig. 25-64), and a transventricular projectile path.[80] Obliteration of the basal cisterns is an ominous CT finding, because it indicates increased intracranial pressure and impending herniation. Diffuse hypodensity of brain tissue may be an indicator of hypoxic injury, because apnea is frequently an immediate sequela of cranial gunshot injury (Fig. 25-65).

MRI

MRI is rarely indicated in the initial evaluation of cranial missile wounds. Although most bullets in civilian use are

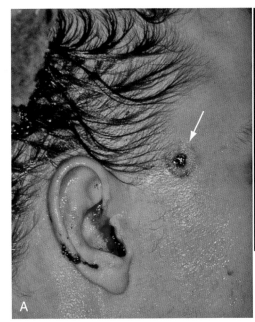

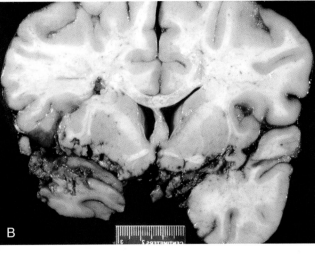

FIGURE 25-59 Postmortem photograph of a bullet wound. **A,** Contact bullet entrance wound anterior to the ear (*arrow*). **B,** Small caliber bullet track through the brain. (*Courtesy of John Deck, MD.*)

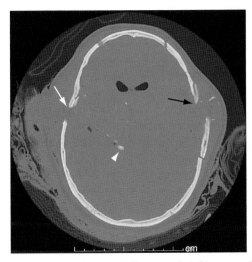

FIGURE 25-60 Perforating bullet wound. *White arrow* indicates entrance wound. *Black arrow* shows exit wound. Bone fragments are present in brain (*arrowhead*). Pneumocephalus is also present.

non-ferromagnetic, there is no practical way of knowing the composition of the projectile or its fragments in the acute trauma setting. Military ammunition is steel jacketed and is likely to tumble in a strong magnetic field. Logistical considerations also limit the use of MRI in the critically injured patient. In the subacute or chronic setting, where it is certain that no ferromagnetic material is lodged in the brain substance, MRI is useful in assessing the extent of tissue damage, especially DAI, for which it is more accurate than CT. If lead bullets remain in the head, MR images are less degraded than CT images, which suffer from severe streak artifacts.

Clinical predictors of a poor outcome include GCS score of 3 to 5, respiratory arrest and hypotension on admission,[80] and elevated intracranial pressure. The predictive value of GCS is limited on admission by alcohol or drug intoxication, medical sedation, hypotension, and intubation. Bullet trajectory is, of course, important; and in one study of patients with bihemispheric and transventricular wounds, 90% died and the other 10% had severe neurologic impairment.[81] Martins and coworkers reported 96% mortality with bihemispheric wounds and 97% for transventricular injuries.[82] The three victims who survived were in a persistent vegetative state.[82]

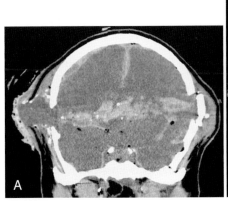

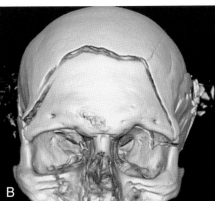

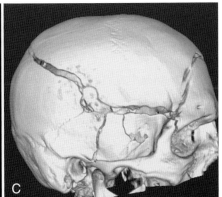

FIGURE 25-61 Hemorrhagic track from transverse gunshot injury to brain in a 31-year-old man. **A,** Coronal CT reformatted image. **B** and **C,** Reformatted 3D images demonstrate extensive skull fractures.

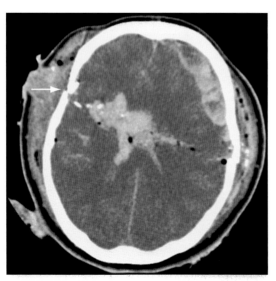

■ **FIGURE 25-62**   Hemorrhage into temporary cavity created by bullet. A left frontal subdural hematoma is also seen. *Arrow* indicates entrance site.

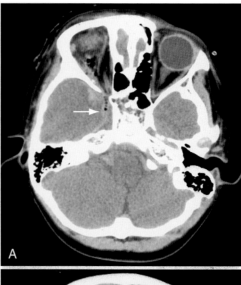

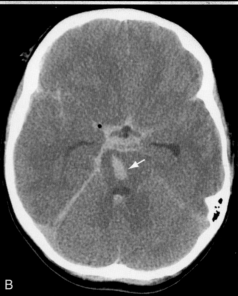

■ **FIGURE 25-64**   Fatal pellet gun injury in an 8-year-old boy. **A** and **B,** Pellet passed through right globe, superior orbital fissure, cavernous sinus (**A,** *arrow*), and brain stem (**B,** *arrow*).

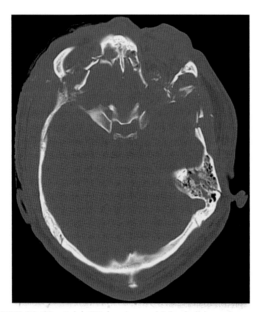

■ **FIGURE 25-63**   Axial CT showing multiple skull base fractures from gunshot wound to calvaria.

Delayed complications of cranial gunshot wounds include CSF leak, infection (meningitis, ventriculitis, brain abscess, osteomyelitis), and hydrocephalus. Moreover, 30% to 51% of patients have post-traumatic epilepsy.[83]

Stab Wounds
Pathophysiology
Stab wounds represent a smaller proportion of penetrating head trauma. Penetration typically occurs in the thinner bones of the skull, often the squamous temporal bones or orbital roofs.[20,84] In addition to the objects listed earlier, less common wounding objects include chopsticks, screwdrivers, hunting arrows, nails, and harpoons.[85-87] These injuries are characterized by lower levels of kinetic energy, so that shock waves and temporary cavities are not formed. Tissue destruction is limited to the immediate vicinity of the wound itself, unless a hematoma develops. Mortality rates are much lower than with gunshot wounds,

on the order of 17%.[88] Knife wounds that penetrate the skull produce a characteristic "slot fracture," in the shape of the blade. Skull penetration may not be evident on physical examination, so CT is indicated if cranial violation is a possibility.

Imaging
CT and MRI
The role of CT is to identify and document penetration of the skull, to assess hematoma formation and tissue damage, and to rule out retained foreign bodies (Fig. 25-66). Metallic foreign objects are usually easily seen, but wood is difficult to detect on CT.[89] Fresh wood is often aerated so it appears lucent, whereas wood left in situ for long periods becomes hydrated and less lucent.[90,91] Delayed complications of stab wounds are pseudoaneurysm and intracranial infection. If intracranial vascular injury is suspected, CT angiography is advisable. Once metallic foreign body has been ruled out with CT, MRI is more sensitive for evaluating tissue damage. Pseudoaneurysms may not be apparent on the immediate post-trauma study, so follow-up CT angiography or MRA at 7 to 14 days should be considered.

ANALYSIS

The examination of imaging studies on the head trauma victim should be an orderly and disciplined process. A "shotgun" approach is a sure-fire recipe for serious error. The exact order in which the various elements of a CT or MR image are reviewed is not important; what matters is consistency and thoroughness. The following are my preferences:

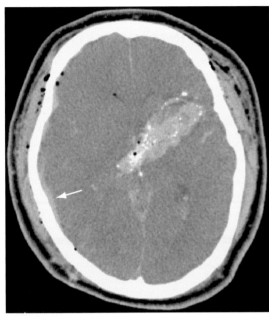

■ **FIGURE 25-65** Diffuse anoxic injury resulting from bihemispheric gunshot wound. CT demonstrates lack of gray matter/white matter differentiation. Hemorrhagic bullet track with multiple bone fragments is present. A small subdural hematoma is seen on right (*arrow*).

- Begin with the scout views, in case you forget to review them later. Especially evaluate the visualized portion of the cervical spine and nasopharynx for clues to concurrent spinal injuries that will simply not be included in the serial axial images obtained for the head itself. Search the scout views for fractures in the plane of the CT sections, because these may not be appreciable on axial imaging sections. Also look for orbital and paranasal sinus pathology that is associated with the trauma.
- Next evaluate the scalp at wide, soft tissue windows for lacerations and foreign bodies that may provide clues to the presence of trauma, sites of injury, and the trajectory or lines of force along which the trauma was applied.
- Then examine the bony structures. The skull is examined at a window width of 2000-4000 Hounsfield units (HU) on bone reconstruction algorithm images. A window width of 2000 HU is adequate for the calvaria, but 4000 HU is more appropriate for the petrous bones and otic capsules. If there is suspicion of fracture and one is not apparent on the axial slices, use reformatted coronal images from the axial data to see whether these demonstrate pathology less easily appreciated in the axial plane. The coronal reformatted images are of especially good quality when the axial slices are obtained with a multidetector CT at 0.5 mm. In the case of complex facial bone fractures, 3D reformatted images are obtained, because these may be helpful to the referring physician. I find 3D images to be interesting to look at but seldom do they add additional diagnostic information.

The intracranial contents are examined with the appropriate soft tissue windows and reconstruction algorithms. Intermediate windows are also viewed at the PACS workstation to rule out small extracerebral hematomas that would otherwise be obscured by the adjacent bone. It is critically important to visualize all parts of the head from the foramen magnum to the vertex. Any shift of the midline structures is measured and reported. If

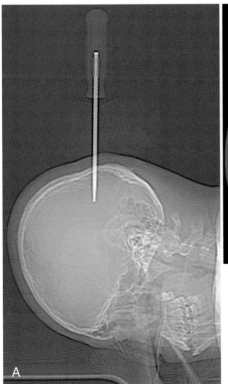

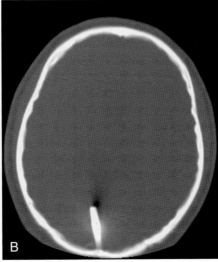

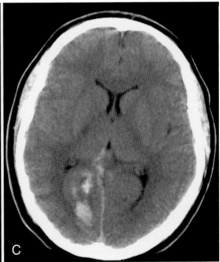

■ **FIGURE 25-66** Stabbing injury in a 16-year-old boy. **A,** CT scout image shows screwdriver imbedded in occiput. **B,** Bone window CT oriented face-up documents depth of penetration of blade. **C,** Soft tissue window CT oriented face-up discloses hematoma of occipital lobe.

an EDH or SDH is present, its thickness is measured. Places where subarachnoid hemorrhage is likely to accumulate, such as the interpeduncular fossa, tentorial notch, posterior ends of the sylvian fissures, and convexity sulci, are carefully scrutinized. It is also a good idea to vary the window settings when examining the bases of the frontal lobes and temporal tips, because hemorrhagic contusions are commonly seen in these regions and may be obscured by partial volume averaging. If a hemispheric mass is present, the suprasellar cisterns and uncus are inspected for evidence of herniation. If the uncus is medially displaced and encroaching on the adjacent brain stem, an immediate phone call is indicated.

Interpreting the MR images of the trauma patient differs only slightly from that of the routine brain MRI study. The sagittal FLAIR sequence is carefully scrutinized for evidence of shear injury. I pay particular attention to the corpus callosum, the brain stem, and the cortical/subcortical white matter on this sequence. The axial images are reviewed for signs of contusion, parenchymal hemorrhages, and extracerebral fluid collections. If an SDH is identified, I attempt to determine its age in addition to its size and location. This is best done by checking its signal intensity on both the T1W and T2W images, as described in prior sections of this chapter. With severe injuries the positions of the unci and cerebellar tonsils are observed for signs of herniation. A coronal T2*W gradient-echo sequence is routinely obtained, and this is checked for evidence of subtle parenchymal hemorrhages that might not be apparent on the spin-echo images. Susceptibility-weighted imaging sequences will likely substitute for these as they become more widely available. A sample report is shown in Box 25-1.

KEY POINTS: DIFFERENTIAL DIAGNOSIS

- Acute epidural hematomas are lens shaped and relatively restricted in extent, whereas acute subdural hematomas are crescent shaped and extend widely along the inner table on axial CT.
- Unless they are hemorrhagic, diffuse axonal injuries (shear injuries) are seldom seen on CT.
- Hemorrhagic contusions are dynamic lesions that "blossom" with time, so they require close CT or MRI follow-up.
- Bihemispheric or transventricular gunshot wounds have a very poor prognosis.

BOX 25-1 Sample Report: CT of Epidural Hematoma

PATIENT HISTORY

A male patient presented with a closed-head injury.

TECHNIQUE

CT head scan, without contrast, was done. Axial 3-mm slices were obtained from the skull base to the vertex.

FINDINGS

Examination of the skull shows a linear fracture of the left squamous temporal bone. This extends to the squamosal suture. A lens-shaped high-density extra-axial fluid collection is seen in the left middle cranial fossa, consistent with an epidural hematoma. This measures 9 mm in greatest thickness. The texture is homogeneously bright with no evidence of "swirling." The midline structures are shifted from left to right 4 mm, and there is no evidence of uncal herniation. No parenchymal hemorrhages are seen. A trace of subarachnoid blood is seen in the high convexity sulci on the left.

The posterior fossa structures are normal.

IMPRESSION

There is an acute left middle cranial fossa epidural hematoma with associated linear skull fracture and 4 mm midline shift.

SUGGESTED READINGS

Castillo M. Trauma. In: Neuroradiology Companion: Methods, Guidelines, and Imaging Fundamentals, 3rd ed. Philadelphia, Lippincott Williams & Wilkins, 2005, pp 44-58.

Gean AD. Imaging of Head Trauma. New York, Raven Press, 1994.

Grossman RI, Yousem DM. Head trauma. In: Neuroradiology: The Requisites, 2nd ed. St. Louis, Mosby, 2003, pp 243-272.

Provenzale J. CT and MR imaging of acute cranial trauma. Emerg Radiol 2007; 14:1-12.

Sehgal V, Delproposto Z, Haacke EM, et al. Clinical applications of neuroimaging with susceptibility-weighted imaging. J Magn Reson Imaging 2005; 22:439-450.

Thomas B, Somasundaram S, Thamburaj K, et al. Clinical applications of susceptibility weighted MR imaging of the brain—a pictorial review. Neuroradiology 2008; 50:105-116.

Zee CS, Go JL (eds). Imaging of head trauma. Neuroimag Clin North Am 2002; 12:165-343.

REFERENCES

1. National Center for Injury Prevention and Control. Traumatic Brain Injury. Available at www.cdc.gov/ncipc/factsheets/tbi. Accessed 6/15/2006.
2. Thurman D, Alverson C, Dunn K, et al. Traumatic brain injury in the United States: a public health perspective. J Head Trauma Rehabil 1999; 14:602-615.
3. Finkelstein E, Corso P, Miller T, et al. The Incidence and Economic Burden of Injuries in the United States. New York, Oxford University Press, 2006.
4. Langlois JA, Rutland-Brown W, Thomas KE. Traumatic Brain Injury in the United States: Emergency Department Visits, Hospitalizations, and Deaths. Atlanta, US Department of Health and Human Services, CDC, National Center for Injury Prevention and Control, 2004.
5. Gentry LR. Imaging of closed head injury. Radiology 1994; 191:1-17.
6. Teasdale G, Jennett B. Assessment of coma and impaired consciousness. Lancet 1974; 2:81-84.
7. Shepard S. Head trauma. eMedicine 2004; http://www.emedicine.com/MED/topic2820.htm. Accessed 5/28/2006.
8. Pal J, Brown R, Fleiszer D. The value of the Glasgow coma scale and injury severity score: predicting outcome in multiple trauma patients with head injury. J Trauma 1989; 29:746-748.

9. Asikainen I, Kaste M, Sarna S. Predicting late outcome for patients with traumatic brain injury referred to a rehabilitation programme: a study of 508 Finnish patients 5 years or more after injury. Brain Injury 1998; 12:95-107.

10. Waxman K, Sundine MJ, Young RF. Is early prediction of outcome in severe head injury possible? Arch Surg 1991; 126:1237-1241.

11. Marshall LF, Marshall SB, Klauber MR, et al. A new classification of head injury based on computerized tomography. J Neurosurg 1991; 75:S14-S20.

12. Foulkes MA, Eisenberg HM, Jane JA, et al. The Traumatic Coma Data Bank: design, methods, and baseline characteristics. J Neurosurg 1991; 75:S8-S13.

13. Van Swieten JC, Koudstaal PJ, Visser HJ, et al. Interobserver agreement for the assessment of handicap in stroke patients. Stroke 1988; 19:604-607.

14. Schaefer PW, Huisman TA, Sorensen AG. Diffusion-weighted MR imaging in closed head injury: high correlation with initial Glasgow coma scale score and score on modified Rankin scale at discharge. Radiology 2004; 233:58-66.

15. Wilson JT, Hareendran A, Grant M, et al. Improving the assessment of outcomes in stroke: Use of a structured interview to assign grades on the modified Rankin scale. Stroke 2002; 33:2243-2246.

16. Graham DI, Gennarelli TA, McIntosh TK. Trauma. In Graham DI, Lantos PL (eds). Greenfield's Neuropathology, 7th ed. London, Arnold, 2002, pp 822-898.

17. Arundine M, Tymianski M. Molecular mechanisms of glutamate-dependent neurodegeneration in ischemia and traumatic brain injury. Cell Mol Life Sci 2004; 61:657-668.

18. Baker AJ, Moulton RJ, MacMillan VH, Shedden PM. Excitatory amino acids in cerebrospinal fluid following traumatic brain injury in humans. J Neurosurg 1993; 79:369-372.

19. Obrenovitch TP, Urenjak J. Is high extracellular glutamate the key to excitotoxicity in traumatic brain injury? J Neurotrauma 1997; 14:677-698.

20. Vinas F, Pilitsis J. Penetrating head trauma. eMedicine, from WebMD: www.emedicine.com/med/topic2888.htm. Last updated June 20, 2006.

21. Dawodu ST. Traumatic brain injury: definition, epidemiology, pathophysiology. eMedicine 2007: http://www.emedicine.com/pmr/topic212.htm. Accessed 4/5/2007.

22. Kim PE, Go JL, Zee CS. Radiographic assessment of cranial gunshot wounds. Neuroimaging Clin North Am 2002; 12:229-248.

23. Hardman JM, Manoukian A. Pathology of head trauma. Neuroimaging Clin North Am 2002; 12:175-187.

24. Gruen A. Surgical management of head trauma. Neuroimaging Clin North Am 2002; 12:339-343.

25. Bullock MR, Chesnut R, Ghajar J, et al. Surgical management of depressed cranial fractures. Neurosurgery 2006; 58 (Suppl):S2-56-S2-60.

26. Swartz JD, Harnsberger HR. Imaging of the Temporal Bone. New York, Thieme, 1998, pp 318-344.

27. Johnson DL, Helman T. Enlarging skull fractures in children. Childs Nerv Syst 1995; 11:265-268.

28. Husson B, Pariente D, Tammam S, Zerah M. The value of MRI in the early diagnosis of growing skull fracture. Pediatr Radiol 1996; 26:744-747.

29. Kutlay M, Demircan N, Akin ON, Basekim C. Untreated growing cranial fractures detected in late stage. Neurosurgery 1998; 43:72-76.

30. Poussaint TY, Moeller KK. Imaging of pediatric head trauma. Neuroimag Clin North Am 2002; 12:271-294.

31. Ellis TS, Vezina G, Donahue DJ. Acute identification of cranial burst fracture: comparison between CT and MR imaging findings. AJNR Am J Neuroradiol 2000; 21:795-801.

32. Bullock MR, Chesnut R, Ghajar J, et al. Surgical management of acute epidural hematomas. Neurosurgery 2006; 58(Suppl):S2-7-S2-15.

33. Lee EJ, Hung YC, Wang LC, et al. Factors influencing the functional outcome of patients with acute epidural hematomas: analysis of 200 patients undergoing surgery. J Trauma 1998; 45:946-952.

34. Al-Nakshabandi NA. The swirl sign. Radiology 2001; 218:433.

35. Bor-Seng-Shu E, Aguiar PH, Almeida Leme RJ, et al. Epidural hematomas of the posterior fossa. Neurosurg Focus 2004; 16:1-4.

36. Hamilton M, Wallace C. Nonoperative management of acute epidural hematoma diagnosed by CT: the neuroradiologist's role. AJNR Am J Neuroradiol 1992; 13:853-859.

37. Shah MV. Conservative management of epidural hematomas: is it safe and is it cost effective? AJNR Am J Neuroradiol 1998; 20:115-116.

38. Bezicioglu H, Ersahin Y, Demircivi F, et al. Nonoperative treatment of acute extradural hematomas: analysis of 80 cases. J Trauma 1996; 41:696-698.

39. Sullivan TP, Jarvik JG, Cohen WA, et al. Follow-up of conservatively managed epidural hematomas: implications for timing of repeat CT. AJNR Am J Neuroradiol 1999; 20:107-113.

40. Haines DE. On the question of a subdural space. Anat Rec 1991; 230:3-21.

41. Haines DE, Harkey HL, Al-Mefty O. The "subdural" space: a new look at an outdated concept. Neurosurgery 1993; 32:111-120.

42. Bullock MR, Chesnut R, Ghajar J, et al. Surgical management of acute subdural hematomas. Neurosurgery 2006; 58(Suppl):S2-16-S2-24.

43. Depreitere B, Van Lierde C, Vander Sloten J, et al. Mechanics of acute subdural hematomas resulting from bridging vein rupture. J Neurosurg 2006; 104:950-956.

44. Generelli TA, Thibault LE. Biomechanics of acute subdural hematoma. J Trauma 1982; 22:680-686.

45. Orlin JR, Osen KK, Hovig T. Subdural compartment in pig: a morphologic study with blood and horseradish peroxidase infused subdurally. Anat Rec 1991; 230:22-37.

46. Jameson KG, Yelland JD, Surgically treated subdural hematomas. J Neurosurg 1972; 37:137-149.

47. Zumkeller M, Behrmann R, Heissler HE, et al. Computed tomographic criteria and survival rate for patients with acute subdural hematoma. Neurosurgery 1996; 39:708-712.

48. Raftopoulos C, Reuse C, Chaskis C, et al. Acute subdural hematoma of the posterior fossa. Clin Neurol Neurosurg 1990; 92:57-62.

49. Gean AD, Glastonbury C, Sonne C. Traumatic brain injury: Imaging update 2004. In: Mann FA (ed). RSNA 2004 Syllabus: Emergency Radiology. Oak Brook, IL, RSNA, 2004, pp 17-32.

50. Borzone M, Rivano C, Altomonte M, et al. Acute traumatic posterior fossa subdural hematomas. Acta Neurochir 1995; 135:32-37.

51. Gomori JM, Grossman RI, Goldberg HI, et al. Intracranial hematomas: imaging by high-field MR. Radiology 1985; 157:87-93.

52. Atlas SW, Mark AS, Grossman RI, Gomori JM. Intracranial hemorrhage: gradient-echo MR imaging at 1.5T. Radiology 1988; 168:803-807.

53. George AE, Russell EJ, Kricheff II. White matter buckling: CT sign of intracranial extra-axial mass. AJR Am J Roentgenol 1980; 135:1031-1036.

54. Hamilton MG, Frizzell JB, Tranmer BI. Chronic subdural hematoma: the role of craniotomy reevaluated. Neurosurgery 1993; 33:67-72.

55. Adhiyaman V, Asghar M, Ganeshram KN, Bhowmick BK. Chronic subdural hematoma in the elderly. Postgrad Med J 2002; 78:71-75.

56. Meagher RJ, Young WF. Subdural hematoma. eMedicine 2006. Available at http://www.emedicine.com/neuro/topic575.htm. Accessed 1/20/2007.

57. Greene KA, Marciano FF, Johnson BA, et al. Impact of traumatic subarachnoid hemorrhage on outcome in nonpenetrating head injury. J Neurosurg 1995; 83:445-452.

58. Mattioli C, Beretta L, Gerevini S, et al. Traumatic subarachnoid hemorrhage on the computerized tomography scan obtained at admission: a multicenter assessment of the accuracy of diagnosis and the potential impact of patient outcome. J Neurosurg 2003; 98:37-42.

59. Noguchi K, Ogawa T, Inugami A, et al. Acute subarachnoid hemorrhage: MR imaging with fluid-attenuated inversion recovery pulse sequences. Radiology 1995; 196:773-777.

60. Anzai Y, Ishikawa M, Shaw DW, et al. Paramagnetic effect of supplemental oxygen on CSF hyperintensity on fluid-attenuated inversion recovery MR images. AJNR Am J Neuroradiol 2004; 25:274-279.

61. Frigon C, Shaw DW, Heckbert SR, et al. Supplemental oxygen causes increased signal intensity in subarachnoid cerebrospinal fluid on brain FLAIR MR images obtained in children during general anesthesia. Radiology 2004; 233:51-55.

62. Braga FT, da Rocha AJ, Filho GH. Relationship between the concentration of supplemental oxygen and signal intensity of CSF depicted by fluid-attenuated inversion recovery imaging. AJNR Am J Neuroradiol 2003; 24:1863-1868.

63. Tong KA, Ashwal S, Holshouser BA, et al. Hemorrhagic shearing lesions in children and adolescents with post-traumatic diffuse

axonal injury: improved detection and initial results. Radiology 2003; 227:332-339.

64. Bullock MR, Chesnut R, Ghajar J, et al. Surgical management of traumatic parenchymal lesions. Neurosurgery 2006; 58(Suppl):S2-25-S2-46.

65. Young RJ, Destian S. Imaging of traumatic intracranial hemorrhage. Neuroimag Clin North Am 2002; 12:189-204.

66. Zimmerman RD, Leeds NE, Naidich TP. Ring blush associated with intracerebral hematoma. Radiology 1977; 122:707-711.

67. Gentry LR, Godersky JC, Thompson B. MR imaging of head trauma: review of the distribution and radiopathologic features of traumatic lesions. AJR Am J Roentgenol 1988; 150:663-672.

68. Mittl RL, Grossman RI, Hiehle JF, et al. Prevalence of MR evidence of diffuse axonal injury in patients with mild head injury and normal CT findings. AJNR Am J Neuroradiol 1994; 15:1583-1589.

69. Ashikaga R, Araki Y, Ishida O. MRI of head injury using FLAIR. Neuroradiology 1997; 39:239-242.

70. Haake EM, Xu Y, Cheng YN, Reichenbach JR. Susceptibility weighted imaging (SWI). Magn Reson Med 2004; 52:612-618.

71. Tong KA, Ashwal S, Obenaus A, et al. Susceptibility-weighted MR imaging: a review of clinical applications in children. AJNR Am J Neuroradiol 2008; 29:9-17.

72. Liu AY, Maldjian JA, Bagley LJ, et al. Traumatic brain injury: diffusion-weighted MR imaging findings. AJNR Am J Neuroradiol 1999; 20:1636-1641.

73. Huisman TA. Diffusion-weighted imaging: basic concepts and application in cerebral stroke and head trauma. Eur Radiol 2003; 13:2283-2297.

74. Arfanakis K, Haughton VM, Carew JD, et al. Diffusion tensor MR imaging in diffuse axonal injury. AJNR Am J Neuroradiol 2002; 23:794-802.

75. Inglese M, Makani S, Johnson G, et al. Diffuse axonal injury in mild traumatic brain injury: a diffusion tensor imaging study. J Neurosurg 2005; 103:298-303.

76. Adams JH, Graham DI, Jennett B. The structural basis of moderate disability after moderate traumatic brain damage. J Neurol Neurosurg Psychiatry 2001; 71:521-524.

77. Sinson G, Bagley LJ, Cecil KM, et al. Magnetization transfer imaging and proton MR spectroscopy in the evaluation of axonal injury: correlation with clinical outcome after traumatic brain injury. AJNR Am J Neuroradiol 2001; 22:143-151.

78. Sosin DM, Sniezek JE, Waxweiler RJ. Trends in death associated with traumatic brain injury, 1979 through 1992: success and failure. JAMA 1995; 273:1778-1780.

79. McDaniel T. Head and brain trauma. In Zimmerman RA, Gibby WA, Carmody RF (eds). Neuroimaging: Clinical and Physical Principles. New York, Springer-Verlag, 2000, pp 699-729.

80. Murano T, Mohr AM, Laver RF, et al. Civilian craniocerebral gunshot wounds: an update in predicting outcomes. Am Surgeon 2005; 71:1009-1014.

81. Grahm TW, Williams FC Jr, Harrington T, Spetzler RF. Civilian gunshot wounds to the head: a prospective study. Neurosurgery 1990; 27:696-700.

82. Martins RS, Siqueria MG, Santos MTS, et al. Prognostic factors and treatment of penetrating gunshot wounds to the head. Surg Neurol 2003; 60:98-104.

83. Weiss GH, Salazar AM, Vance SC, et al. Predicting posttraumatic epilepsy in penetrating head injury. Arch Neurol 1986; 43:771-773.

84. Deb S, Acosta J, Bridgeman A, et al. Stab wounds to the head with intracranial penetration. J Trauma 2000; 48:1159-1162.

85. Di Roio C, Jourdan C, Mottolese C, et al. Craniocerebral injury resulting from transorbital stick penetration in children. Childs Nerv Syst 2000; 16:503-507.

86. Lopez F, Martinez-Lage JF, Herrera A, et al. Penetrating craniocerebral injury from an underwater fishing harpoon. Childs Nerv Syst 2000; 16:117-119.

87. Litvak ZN, Hunt MA, Weinstein JS, et al. Self-inflicted nail-gun injury with 12 cranial penetrations and associated cerebral trauma. J Neurosurg 2006; 104:828-834.

88. De Villiers JC, Sevel D. Intracranial complications of transorbital stab wounds. Br J Ophthalmol 1975; 59:52-56.

89. Dalley RW. Intraorbital wood foreign bodies on CT: use of wide bone window settings to distinguish wood from air. AJR Am J Roentgenol 1995; 164:434-435.

90. Peterson JJ, Bancroft LW, Kransdorf MJ. Wooden foreign bodies: imaging appearance. AJR Am J Roentgenol 2002; 178:557-562.

91. Kantarci MK, Ogul H, Karasen RM. Detection of a giant wooden foreign body with multidetector computed tomography and multiplanar reconstruction imaging. Am J Emerg Med 2006; 25:211-213.

CHAPTER 26

Vascular Injury and Parenchymal Changes

Raymond Francis Carmody

The spectrum of cerebrovascular trauma includes arterial occlusion, dissection, pseudoaneurysm, arteriovenous fistula, vasospasm, and venous thrombosis. Vascular trauma is the most common cause of stroke in individuals younger than 45 years of age[1] and often has devastating consequences. Fortunately, newer diagnostic modalities such as CT angiography (CTA) have facilitated rapid diagnosis and treatment.

EXTRACRANIAL VASCULAR TRAUMA

Extracranial vascular trauma may be *blunt* or *penetrating*. Blunt vascular trauma is most likely to occur with motor vehicle accidents, whereas penetrating trauma is usually secondary to assault with a sharp object or firearm.

Blunt Trauma

Epidemiology

Blunt injury to the carotid and vertebral arteries is reported in fewer than 1% of motor vehicle collisions.[2] The injury may lead to disabling or lethal infarcts, especially in younger individuals. The true frequency of vascular injury is likely to be higher than reported, because 23% of patients with carotid or vertebral injury have no related symptoms at the time of presentation[3] and the diagnosis is often overlooked in the presence of concurrent severe head injuries.

Clinical Presentation

Vertebral artery dissections may present acutely or first become evident hours to weeks later.[4] Physical findings include neck hematoma, bruit, palpable thrill, and Horner's syndrome.[5] However, as many as 50% of patients with blunt carotid injury show no external evidence of neck trauma.[6] Damage to the intimal surface of the vessel can lead to platelet aggregation and subsequent embolization, so antiplatelet or anticoagulant drugs may be administered, provided there are no contraindications.[2] Frank dissections and occlusions may lead to embolism/infarction of the brain stem, cerebellum, and posterior cerebral artery territory.

Pathophysiology

The internal carotid artery is vulnerable to intimal tearing, dissection, and subsequent occlusion as a result of rapid acceleration/deceleration of the head (Fig. 26-1). Intimal tears tend to occur where the internal carotid artery becomes stretched over the transverse processes of the upper cervical vertebrae or where the artery enters the skull base. Traumatic intimal tears may heal spontaneously or progress to dissection/occlusion.

The long course of the vertebral artery through the foramen transversarium from C6 to C1 makes this vessel prone to traumatic dissection from motor vehicle accidents, sports injuries, and chiropractic neck manipulation. The C1-C2 articulation is the most mobile segment of the cervical spine, so C1-C2 is also the most common site of vertebral dissection. From C2 to C6, fracture-dislocation may injure the vertebral artery within the foramen transversarium, resulting in dissection or occlusion (Fig. 26-2).

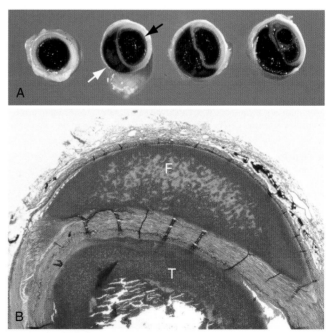

■ **FIGURE 26-1** Autopsy specimens. Dissecting hematoma of the internal carotid artery. **A,** Gross specimen cut in cross section. Black arrow indicates the true lumen. White arrow indicates the false lumen. **B,** Histologic section. The plane of dissection advances between the media and the adventitia. *(Masson trichrome stain). T,* true lumen; *F,* false lumen. *(Courtesy of John Deck, MD.)*

603

Imaging
CT Angiography

Multidetector CT angiography (MDCTA) is highly accurate for detecting blunt cerebrovascular injury, with sensitivities of 97.7% and specificities of 100%.[7,8] Therefore, MDCTA has replaced catheter angiography as a screening tool for blunt cerebrovascular injury at many level I trauma centers. Duplex ultrasonography, although accurate, cannot evaluate the carotid arteries at and above the skull base. Screening by MR angiography (MRA) presents logistical problems in the patient with multiple trauma, such as immediate MRI availability, lengthy examination time, patient motion, and incompatibility of many life support devices with MRI.

On contrast-enhanced CT, arterial injuries have varied appearances. With dissections, an intimal flap may be seen (Fig. 26-3), followed distally by tapering of the vessel. Maximum intensity pixel projection (MIPP) images confirm the abnormal morphology of the vessel lumen (Fig. 26-4). Pseudoaneurysms appear as collections of contrast material outside the wall of the injured artery (Fig. 26-5). Occlusions often present as a smoothly tapered artery that ends in a point. Thrombus may be seen as a filling defect within the artery (see Fig. 26-4C).

MR Angiography

Levy and associates showed that MRA has a sensitivity of 95% and a specificity of 99% for diagnosing *carotid* *artery* dissection.[9] However, the sensitivity was only 20% and specificity 100% for diagnosing *vertebral artery* dissection. The best MRA indicator of dissection was an apparent increase in the external diameter of the artery (Fig. 26-6). Additional helpful MRI signs were narrowing of the luminal flow void and detection of intramural hematoma (Fig. 26-7).

Penetrating Trauma
Epidemiology

Injury to the great vessels of the neck is much more common with penetrating wounds than with blunt trauma, with an incidence approaching 25%.[10] Gunshot and stab wounds are the most common mechanisms of penetrating injury. Blunt trauma and penetrating trauma cause similar lesions, including intimal flaps, dissection, occlusion, pseudoaneurysm, and arteriovenous fistula.

Clinical Presentation

For surgical purposes, penetrating neck wounds are divided into three zones, based on specific anatomic landmarks (Fig. 26-8). Zone I extends from the suprasternal notch to the cricoid cartilage. Zone II is the area from the cricoid cartilage to the angle of the mandible. Zone III extends from the angle of the mandible to the skull base.[11] Zone II injuries are the most amenable to surgical exploration, so surgery has been the preferred management of zone II injuries, until very recently, when

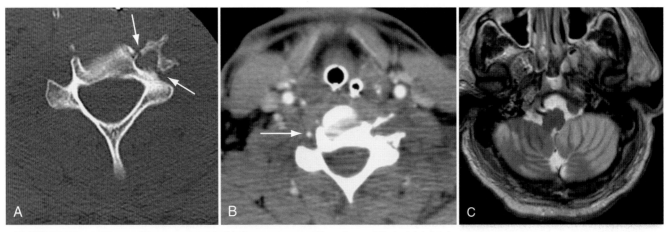

■ **FIGURE 26-2** A 39-year-old man presented with fracture-rotary subluxation at C6. **A,** Axial CT demonstrates fracture through the foramen transversarium of C6 (*arrows*). **B,** CTA shows occlusion of left vertebral artery at same level. Right vertebral artery is patent (*arrow*). **C,** T2W MR image demonstrates extensive cerebellar infarction, most likely due to anoxia, because it is bilateral.

■ **FIGURE 26-3** Traumatic internal carotid dissection in a 32-year-old woman. **A,** Axial CTA shows intimal flap (*arrow*). False lumen is on the medial side. **B,** Coronal MIP image. *Arrow* indicates flap.

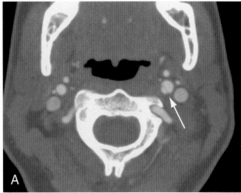

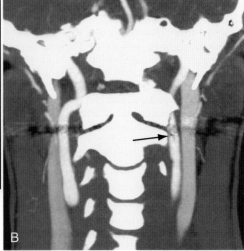

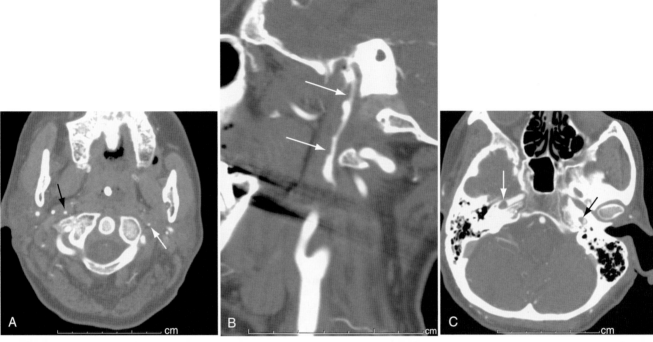

■ **FIGURE 26-4** Bilateral carotid dissection from a motor vehicle accident. **A,** Left internal carotid artery (*white arrow*) is markedly narrowed, as is right internal carotid artery (*black arrow*). **B,** Sagittal MIP image shows marked narrowing and irregularity of right carotid lumen (*arrows*). **C,** Higher slice shows thrombus (*white arrow*) in right petrous carotid and marked narrowing of left petrous carotid (*black arrow*).

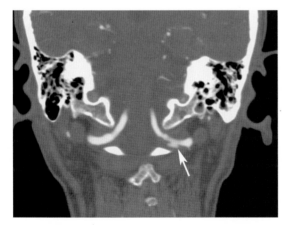

■ **FIGURE 26-5** Left vertebral artery pseudoaneurysm. Coronal MIP image demonstrates outpouching (*arrow*) from inferior surface of artery at the C1 level.

feasible, endovascular therapies are increasingly replacing surgical exploration.

Imaging
CT Angiography
MDCTA provides information on the status of the vascular structures, the trajectory of the missile, the integrity of the aerodigestive tract and other soft tissues, and the osseous structures (Figs. 26-9 and 26-10). Patients who are hemodynamically unstable require surgical exploration, regardless of the entry zone. MDCTA data, however, may reduce the number of negative neck explorations of penetrating injuries.

INTRACRANIAL VASCULAR TRAUMA
Intracranial vascular injury includes dissection, occlusion, hemorrhage, and fistula that involves the intracranial carotid and vertebral arteries, their branches, and any intracranial venous structures.

Epidemiology
Intracranial arterial injuries most commonly result from penetrating trauma or fractures of the skull base. The artery most commonly injured is the internal carotid artery. This may be affected at its entrance to the carotid canal or at its exit from the cavernous sinus beneath the anterior clinoid process.[12] Potential injuries include dissection, occlusion, pseudoaneurysm, and carotid-cavernous fistula.

Pathophysiology and Clinical Presentation
Dissection
Intracranial carotid dissection may extend up the supraclinoid segment to the carotid bifurcation and then into the proximal anterior and middle cerebral arteries. This subintimal lesion causes significant luminal narrowing. It may lead to infarction and/or subarachnoid hemorrhage (see Fig. 26-7).

Fistula
A tear in the cavernous portion of the internal carotid artery can cause a high-flow arteriovenous communication between the artery and the cavernous sinus: a carotid-cavernous fistula. Such tears usually result from fracture of the sphenoid bone in the region of the sella turcica or the anterior clinoid process. Nontraumatic carotid-cavernous fistulas can develop from rupture of a cavernous-carotid aneurysm. The consequent increase in venous pressure and retrograde venous outflow through the superior and inferior ophthalmic veins can cause severe ipsilateral proptosis and chemosis, with a bruit that can be heard over

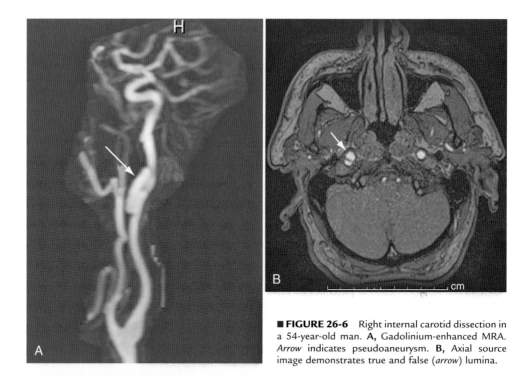

■ FIGURE 26-6   Right internal carotid dissection in a 54-year-old man. **A,** Gadolinium-enhanced MRA. *Arrow* indicates pseudoaneurysm. **B,** Axial source image demonstrates true and false (*arrow*) lumina.

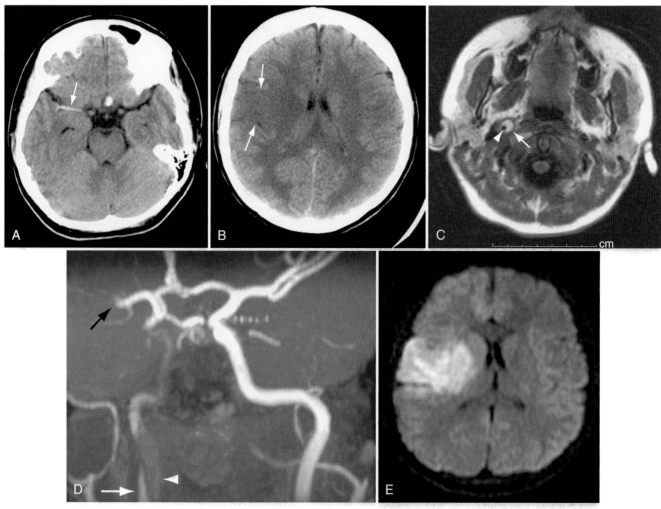

■ FIGURE 26-7   Right internal carotid dissection in a 12-year-old girl. **A,** Unenhanced CT shows dense right middle cerebral artery, consistent with thrombosis (*arrow*). **B,** CT a day later shows right frontal transcortical infarct (*arrows*). **C,** Axial FLAIR MR image on day 8 demonstrates intramural thrombus (*arrow*) surrounding lumen of internal carotid (*arrowhead*). **D,** Coronal oblique MRA shows clot in false lumen (*white arrow*), slow flow in true lumen (*arrowhead*), and occlusion of middle cerebral artery (*black arrow*). **E,** Diffusion-weighted MRI demonstrates extent of infarct.

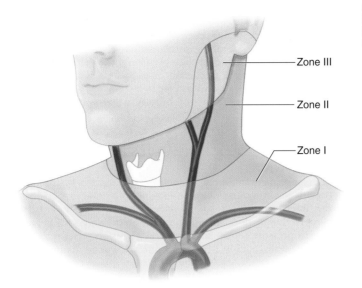

■ **FIGURE 26-8**   The three zones of the neck, for purposes of evaluating penetrating injury. *(From Nunez DB Jr, Torres-Leon M, Munera F. Vascular injuries of the neck and thoracic inlet: helical CT-angiographic correlation. Radio-Graphics 2004; 24:1087-1098.)*

Zone III

Zone II

Zone I

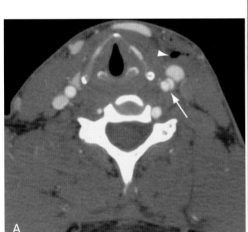

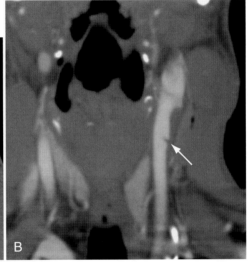

■ **FIGURE 26-9**   Stab wound to left anterior neck in a 29-year-old man. **A,** Axial CTA demonstrates dissection flap in left common carotid (*arrow*). *Arrowhead* indicates air in soft tissues. **B,** Coronal MIP CTA shows small intimal flap (*arrow*) in common carotid artery.

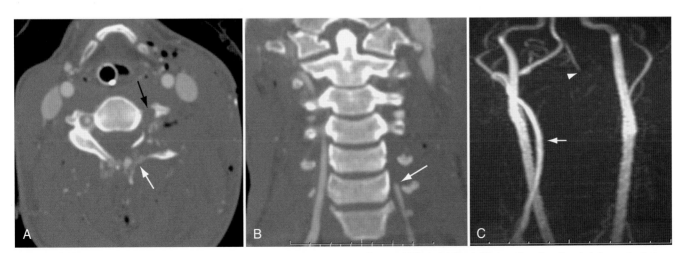

■ **FIGURE 26-10**   Gunshot wound with left vertebral occlusion. **A,** CTA shows shattered left C4 lamina (*white arrow*) and no flow in left vertebral artery (*black arrow*). **B,** Coronal CTA shows occlusion of left vertebral artery at C6 (*arrow*). **C,** Coronal MRA demonstrates no flow in cervical left vertebral artery. Note normal right vertebral artery (*arrow*). Left vertebral eventually reconstitutes at skull base (*arrowhead*).

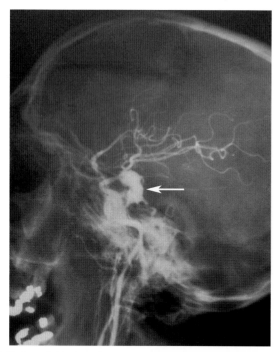

■ **FIGURE 26-11** Pseudoaneurysm from penetrating injury. Carotid arteriogram, lateral projection. Note large, irregular collection of contrast material originating from intracranial internal carotid (*arrow*).

the eye. Increased intraocular pressure and decreased retinal perfusion may cause vision loss.

Pseudoaneurysm

When injury disrupts all three layers of an arterial wall the resulting hemorrhage may become contained by the surrounding soft tissue. The blood within the hematoma remains in contact with turbulent flow in the parent artery.[5] With time, the wall of the hematoma organizes, becomes lined with fibrous tissue, and forms a pseudocapsule around the pseudoaneurysm. Pseudoaneurysms are unstable lesions that can rupture and present as sudden intracranial hemorrhage. They often rupture at 2 to 8 weeks after the traumatic event (Fig. 26-11) but may not rupture until years after the injury. Mortality after pseudoaneurysm rupture is 30% to 40%.[13] Treatment usually consists of occlusion of the lumen with detachable coils or trapping of the parent artery. Covered stents are a promising future alternative.

Imaging
Dissection

On conventional angiography or CTA the dissected segment is narrowed and irregular, sometimes tapering to occlusion. There may be intraluminal thrombus and/or pseudoaneurysm. MRI and MRA are also quite useful for demonstrating dissection. On T1-weighted (T1W) imaging, hemorrhage in the wall of the artery is frequently seen as increased signal intensity outside the narrowed lumen (subacute blood) (see Fig. 26-7C).

Fistula

In patients with carotid-cavernous fistula, contrast-enhanced CT may show dilatation of the ipsilateral superior ophthalmic vein (>4 mm), outward convexity of the cavernous sinus, engorgement of the extraocular muscles, proptosis, and preseptal soft tissue swelling. CTA may demonstrate irregularity of the cavernous carotid artery (Fig. 26-12). If the fistula has very high flow, CTA may also show involvement of both orbits. MRI and MRA more clearly depict the patterns of venous outflow, including the superior and inferior petrosal sinuses, emissary veins

to the pterygoid plexus, and sphenoparietal sinuses. Despite the recent advances in noninvasive imaging, catheter angiography with rapid filming rates is still required to demonstrate the location and size of the fistula definitively (see Fig. 26-12D) and to plan interventional therapy. Currently, the treatment of choice is transarterial occlusion of the fistula with detachable balloons. Advances in covered stent technology may allow for bridging the tear in the carotid artery while preserving vessel patency.[14,15]

ACUTE PHYSIOLOGIC CHANGES IN TRAUMATIC BRAIN INJURY

The assessment and management of traumatic brain injury require some understanding of cerebral physiology, specifically the interrelationships among cerebral blood volume (CBV), cerebral blood flow (CBF), intracranial pressure (ICP), mean arterial pressure (MAP), and cerebral perfusion pressure (CPP).

The normal adult ICP is 0 to 15 mm Hg. The adult intracranial volume is approximately 1500 mL. *Intracranial compliance* is defined as the change in intracranial volume divided by the change in ICP.[16] Treatment of head injury is based on how the treatment affects ICP and compliance.[16]

The skull is a rigid, nondistensible structure. In adults, the brain occupies 85% to 90% of intracranial volume, the CBV about 10%, and cerebrospinal fluid (CSF) the remaining 5%. As edema and hemorrhage expand the traumatized brain, the ICP rises. Initially, the increase in ICP is accommodated by displacement of CBV and CSF from inside to outside the skull. However, this compensatory mechanism is very limited. Further increases in intracranial mass effect cause a rapid increase in the ICP.

Cerebral perfusion pressure is the difference between the mean arterial pressure (MAP) and the intracranial pressure (ICP): CPP = MAP − ICP. Stated differently, CPP is the net pressure at which blood perfuses the brain. In a healthy individual with a normal MAP of 50 to 150 mm Hg, CBF is held constant through autoregulation by brain arterioles. When MAP falls below 50 mm Hg, compensatory mechanisms are no longer adequate. The CBF decreases, and ischemic injury is possible. Conversely, when MAP exceeds 160 mm Hg, excessive CBF may occur and lead to increased ICP. Autoregulation works well in the noninjured brain but is often impaired in the traumatized brain,[16] so ICP rises with intracranial injury. The brain has very limited tolerance for increases in ICP, especially rapid increases. Uncontrollable rise in ICP is the single most frequent cause of death in traumatic brain injury. The elevated ICP poses two dangers. First, increased ICP can lead to decreased CPP and ischemic infarction; indeed, 80% to 90% of patients who die of traumatic brain injury have evidence of ischemic injury at autopsy.[17] Second, very elevated ICP can lead to brain herniation.

Management of the acutely brain-injured patient requires control of ICP and maintenance of adequate CBF. In the adult, the ICP is ideally kept below 20 mm Hg. This is accomplished by elevating the head to 30 degrees, administering osmotic diuretics (mannitol), using hyperventilation to blow off CO_2, and draining CSF through a ventricular catheter. The CPP is kept at 60 mm Hg or higher to ensure adequate CBF. This is accomplished by keeping the patient euvolemic and supporting the patient's blood pressure.

CEREBRAL EDEMA

Cerebral edema is an increase in brain tissue volume resulting from an increase in tissue water content.[18] It may be focal or diffuse.

Pathophysiology

The pathogenesis of brain swelling after traumatic brain injury is unclear. Conventional wisdom held that vascular engorgement

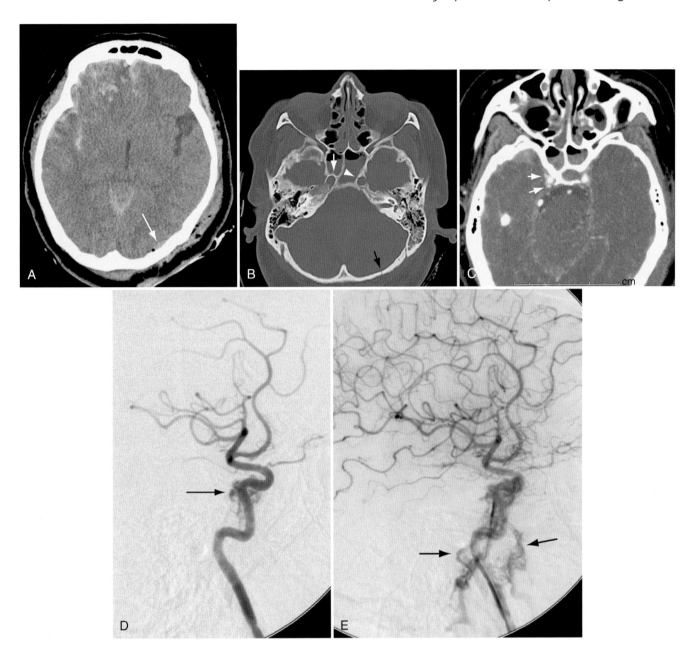

■ FIGURE 26-12 Traumatic carotid-cavernous sinus fistula in a 45-year-old woman. **A,** Unenhanced CT demonstrates extensive right frontal hemorrhagic contusion and a small left occipital epidural hematoma (*arrow*) with air. **B,** Bone window CT demonstrates right (*white arrow*) and left (*arrowhead*) carotid canal fractures and left occipital fracture (*black arrow*). **C,** CTA shows indistinctness of right cavernous carotid and early opacification of cavernous sinus (*arrows*). **D,** Lateral right carotid angiogram, early arterial phase, shows early opacification of cavernous sinus (*arrow*). **E,** Later image shows filling of inferior petrosal sinuses during arterial phase (*arrows*).

caused an increase in CBV that then elevated the ICP. However, the vascular engorgement "etiology" has not been substantiated in animal studies.[19] Until recently it had not been possible to measure brain water content or CBV in the living brain-injured patient. Brain tissue water content can now be calculated using phase-sensitive inversion recovery slices, from which a pure T1W image can be calculated.[20,21] The calculated T1W image is then converted into a brain water image. CBV is measured using a combination of stable xenon CT and contrast-enhanced CT.[22] The xenon CT scan is used to obtain CBF. Dynamic contrast-enhanced CT is used to determine mean transit time. CBV is then calculated from these two parameters using the equation: CBV = mean transit time × CBF.

Marmarou and colleagues studied 31 patients with severe traumatic brain injury who had determinations of both brain tissue water and CBV. They found that brain water was increased but CBV was actually decreased.[23] They concluded that the brain swelling associated with traumatic brain injury is caused by brain edema not increased CBV. An increase of only 1% in brain water content causes an increase in brain volume of 4.4%, which can elevate the ICP above 20 mm Hg.[24]

Imaging

The cerebral edema associated with severe traumatic brain injury is both intracellular (cytotoxic edema) and extracellular (vasogenic edema) (Fig. 26-13). MRI study of patients with diffuse brain injury showed restricted diffusion and decreased ADC values, indicating intracellular edema.[24] The CBF values of the study patients were all well above the ischemic threshold, eliminating ischemia as the cause of restricted diffusion.[24]

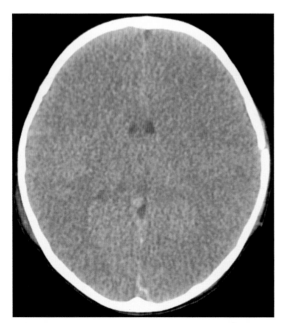

■ **FIGURE 26-13** Diffuse cerebral edema after closed-head injury in a 2-year-old boy. Unenhanced CT shows loss of gray matter/white matter discrimination, as well as small ventricles.

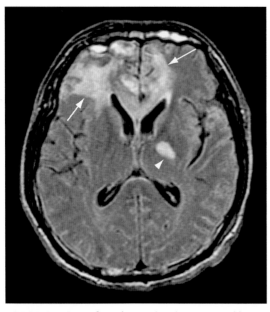

■ **FIGURE 26-14** Severe frontal contusions in a 36-year-old man. FLAIR MR image demonstrates vasogenic edema surrounding contusions (*arrows*). A diffuse axonal injury is seen in the left internal capsule (*arrowhead*).

Alternatively, in a case with focal brain injury, the core of a contusion and the area immediately surrounding it showed increased apparent diffusion coefficient, indicating vasogenic edema (Fig. 26-14). The brain more distant from the contusion showed decreased apparent diffusion coefficient, indicating cytotoxic edema. Thus, the cerebral edema seen in traumatic brain injury is both intracellular and extracellular, with cytotoxic edema predominating.

The mechanism by which the cytotoxic edema forms remains unknown but may be related to mitochondrial dysfunction.[24] The cellular edema develops slowly and becomes dominant at 1

or 2 weeks after injury.[25] The vasogenic edema is thought to result from breakdown in the blood-brain barrier immediately after traumatic brain injury. It predominates in the first hour or so after injury. Animal studies show that the blood-brain barrier is usually reestablished within 30 minutes after the trauma.[25] The type of edema present in traumatized brains therefore also varies with the time after injury.

ACQUIRED CEREBRAL HERNIATIONS

Herniation is displacement of brain tissue from one compartment into another. It is a dreaded complication of mass effect, regardless of the cause, because it may result in infarction, coma, or death. The major types of brain herniation include subfalcine, transtentorial, and tonsillar (Fig. 26-15). Transtentorial herniation is subdivided into lateral (uncal, hippocampal) and central types and then described as descending or ascending in accordance with the direction of brain shift. Most central transtentorial herniation is directed inferiorly, but significant ascending central herniation can result from masses situated inferior to the tentorium. Herniations are readily detected by both CT and MRI and must be recognized to prevent or limit serious neurologic sequelae (Table 26-1).

The sickle-shaped falx cerebri separates the two cerebral hemispheres. The falx is narrower anteriorly at its attachment to the crista galli and broader posteriorly at its attachment to the tentorium and internal occipital protuberance. The corpus callosum is located just below the inferior margin of the falx. The gap between the corpus callosum and falx is wider anteriorly and narrower posteriorly, so the genu lies farther from the free edge of the falx and the splenium closer to it. The cingulate gyrus, the pericallosal arteries, and the callosomarginal arteries lie to either side of the falx. Their relation to the free margin of the falx changes from anterior to posterior.

The tentorium cerebelli is a thick dural fold that divides the intracranial cavity into the supratentorial and infratentorial compartments. Posteriorly, the tentorium attaches to the skull along the course of the torcular and paired transverse venous sinuses. Laterally, the tentorium attaches to the superior crests of the petrous portions of the temporal bones and extends from there to the posterior clinoid processes bilaterally. Medially, the leaves of the tentorium form free margins that take the shape of a gothic arch. The apex of the arch lies posteriorly at the confluence of the falx and tentorium. From there, the tentorial leaves sweep anteriorly around the brain stem to insert onto the two anterior clinoid processes. The midbrain passes through the opening (incisura) of the tentorium. The superior vermis may enter into the incisura just behind the midbrain. The uncus and hippocampal gyrus of the medial temporal lobe slightly overhang the free margins of the tentorium laterally. The oculomotor nerves emerge from the interpeduncular fossa and run anteriorly in close proximity to the uncus. The trochlear nerves emerge from the posterior surface of the low midbrain and curve anteriorly just inferior to and immediately lateral to the free margins of the tentorium. The posterior cerebral arteries course posteriorly around the brain stem and over the free edge of the tentorium.

Pathophysiology
Subfalcine Herniation
Also known as midline shift, subfalcine herniation is the most common type of cerebral herniation. It is associated with unilateral frontal, parietal, or temporal lobe mass effect.[26] With subfalcine herniation, the anterior falx tilts to the contralateral side, away from the mass. The ipsilateral cingulate gyrus slides under the free margin of the falx (Fig. 26-16) and may bulge upward alongside the contralateral surface of the falx. The posterior portion of the falx is rigid and cannot shift significantly. Posterior subfalcine herniation of the cingulate gyrus displaces the corpus callosum downward. The ipsilateral lateral ventricle shows

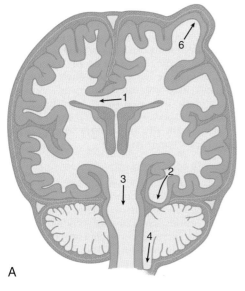

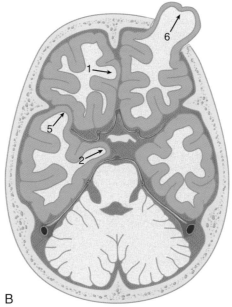

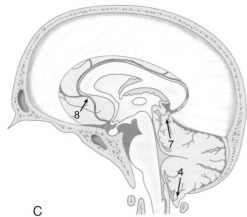

■ **FIGURE 26-15** Patterns of cerebral herniation. **A,** Coronal. **B,** Axial. **C,** Sagittal representations of the skull, dural portions, and brain. 1, Subfalcine; 2, uncal; 3, descending transtentorial; 4, tonsillar; 5, transalar; 6, external; 7, ascending transtentorial; 8, anterior cerebral artery branches (pericallosal and callosomarginal arteries. Vascular structures are shown in red. *(From Johnson PL, Eckard DA, Chason DP, et al. Imaging of acquired cerebral herniations. Neuroimag Clin North Am 2002; 12:217-228.)*

TABLE 26-1. Cerebral Herniation

Type of Herniation	Imaging Findings	Clinical Manifestations
Subfalcine herniation (midline shift; cingulate herniation)	Unilateral frontal, parietal, or temporal lobe mass effect or edema	Headache
	Anterior falx tilts away from the mass effect.	Contralateral weakness
	Ipsilateral cingulate gyrus is displaced beneath the free edge of the falx, pushing down the ipsilateral corpus callosum.	If severe, anterior cerebral artery infarction
		May progress to other forms of herniation
Uncal herniation (anterior lateral transtentorial herniation)	Unilateral supratentorial lesion, esp. middle fossa	Contralateral or ipsilateral hemiparesis (Kernohan's phenomenon)
	Displacement of the uncus; effacement of suprasellar cistern	CN III palsy (ipsilateral dilated pupil)
	Widening of ipsilateral ambient cistern; displacement and distortion of brain stem	Posterior cerebral artery infarction, if severe
Posterior (parahippocampal) herniation	Occipital or posterior temporal lobe mass	Parinaud syndrome (paralysis of upward gaze)
	Compression of posterior brain stem (tectum) by hippocampus	
Descending transtentorial herniation	Caudal descent of brain tissue through tentorial incisura due to large hemispheric or central mass effect	CN III paresis
	Duret hemorrhage	Decreasing level of consciousness
	Brain stem infarction	Coma
	Dilatation of contralateral temporal horn	Decerebrate posturing
	Hydrocephalus	Death
Ascending transtentorial herniation	Cerebellar mass or trapped fourth ventricle	Rapid onset of obtundation
	Effacement of superior cerebellar cistern	Death, if severe brain stem compression
	Upward displacement of superior vermis	
	Anterior displacement of pons	
Tonsillar herniation	Cerebellar tonsils >5 mm below foramen magnum	Increasing stupor
	Posterior fossa mass, or, descending transtentorial herniation	Coma
		Cerebellar infarction, if posteroinferior cerebellar artery compressed
		Death

From Johnson PL, Eckard DA, Chason DP, et al. Imaging of acquired cerebral herniations. Neuroimag Clin North Am 2002; 12:217-228.

evidence of compression. The mass effect causes hydrocephalus, leading to dilatation of the contralateral temporal horn. With severe midline shift, the cingulate gyri may develop pressure necrosis. Pinching of the pericallosal and callosomarginal arteries at the free edge of the falx may cause infarction of the parasagittal hemispheric structures (Fig. 26-17). Measuring the midline shift at the level of the septum pellucidum and reporting it in millimeters from the midline should be a standard feature of the CT or MRI report.

Lateral Transtentorial Herniation

Descending lateral transtentorial herniation signifies displacement of the uncus and/or hippocampal gyrus over the free edge of the tentorium into the suprasellar cistern, incisura, and perimesencephalic cistern. CT or MRI findings include obliteration of the ipsilateral suprasellar and perimesencephalic cisterns (Fig. 26-18), with compression, anteroposterior elongation, and caudal displacement of the brain stem. Uncal herniation typically results from a middle cranial fossa mass, such as an epidural hematoma. As the uncus herniates into the tentorial notch it

compresses the oculomotor nerve, causing an ipsilateral dilated pupil. The opposite cerebral peduncle is displaced laterally against the contralateral tentorial edge, producing pressure necrosis in the uncrossed corticospinal and corticobulbar tracts (Fig. 26-19). The free edge of the tentorium deeply indents the brain stem leaving a groove designated Kernohan's notch.[27] T2-weighted (T2W) and fluid-attenuated inversion recovery (FLAIR) MR sequences show increased signal intensity in the lateral aspect of the cerebral peduncle.[28] Clinical findings may include hemiplegia on the same side of the body as the middle fossa mass, a so-called false lateralizing sign.

Central Descending Transtentorial Herniation

Supratentorial mass effect far removed from the temporal lobes may lead to bilateral descending lateral transtentorial herniation. Generalized brain swelling, central masses, or large frontal, parietal, and occipital lobe lesions can cause descending central herniation. With hemispheric masses, subfalcine herniation usually precedes transtentorial herniation. The diencephalon, the mesencephalon, and both medial temporal lobes herniate downward into the tentorial hiatus. Cranial nerves and vessels become stretched, so third nerve palsy is common. Stretching and compression of the posterior cerebral arteries against the tentorial edge frequently results in occipital lobe infarction. Compression of the cerebral aqueduct causes hydrocephalus, which aggravates the herniation. The clinical picture progresses to stupor, decerebrate posturing, coma, and death.

Imaging
Descending Transtentorial Herniation

The CT and MRI findings of descending central transtentorial herniation include obliteration of the suprasellar and perimesencephalic cisterns, caudal displacement of the brain stem (best appreciated on sagittal MRI), and flattening of the pons and basilar artery against the clivus (Fig. 26-20). The mesencephalon is compressed laterally, elongated, and perhaps bowed into banana shape. In severe cases, imaging shows infarction of the occipital and temporal lobes, as well as portions of the brain stem (Fig. 26-21). With extensive infarction, loss of gray matter/white matter discrimination is seen in the cerebral hemispheres (Fig. 26-22). Caudal displacement of the brain stem causes stretch injury to the perforating arteries supplying

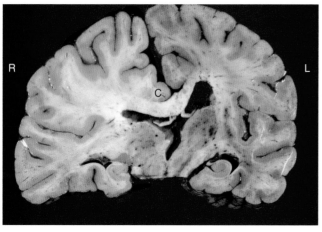

■ **FIGURE 26-16** Postmortem specimen of subfalcine herniation. Coronal section. Severe edema of the right cerebral hemisphere has caused midline shift with herniation of the cingulate gyrus (C) under the falx cerebri (falx not shown). *(Courtesy of John Deck, MD.)*

■ **FIGURE 26-17** Large left frontal hematoma in a 55-year-old woman. **A,** Unenhanced CT. Hematoma is causing massive shift of midline structures. **B,** Higher slice demonstrates bilateral anterior cerebral artery distribution infarcts (*arrows*).

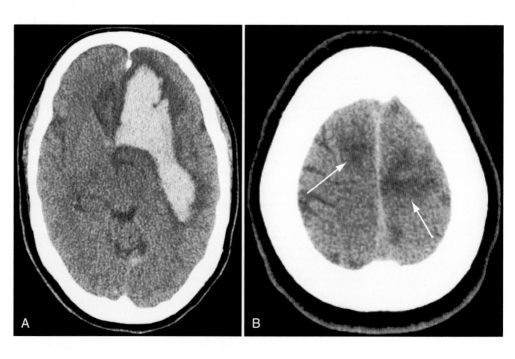

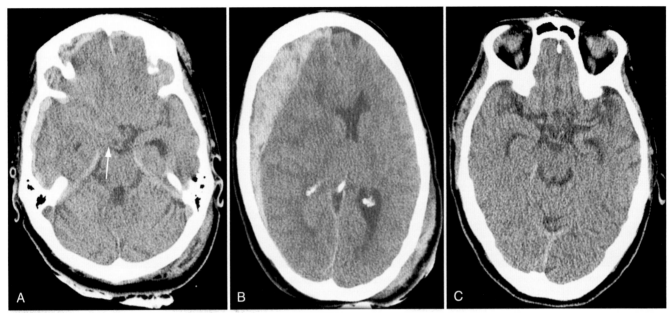

■ **FIGURE 26-18** A 59-year-old woman presented with a large subdural hematoma and uncal herniation. **A,** Medial border of right uncus is displaced nearly to the midline (*arrow*). **B,** Higher CT slice shows large right hemispheric hematoma. **C,** Three-month postoperative follow-up CT. Right temporal lobe is normal in appearance and location.

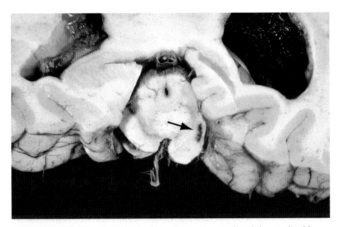

■ **FIGURE 26-19** Pathological specimen. A massive right cerebral hemorrhage has compressed the right lateral ventricle, ruptured into the ventricular system (as seen in the left lateral ventricle), caused the right medial temporal lobe to herniate into the incisura, and shifted the brainstem to the left. The shift has compressed the left cerebral peduncle against the free edge of the tentorium, causing injury and hemorrhage (*arrow*) to the midbrain (Kernohan's notch). *(Courtesy of John Deck, MD.)*

the pons and midbrain, resulting in Duret hemorrhages (Figs. 26-23 and 26-24). Duret hemorrhages portend a poor prognosis.

Ascending Transtentorial Herniation

Infratentorial masses such as cerebellar hematomas and edematous cerebellar infarcts may displace the superior vermis and hemispheres upward into the incisura. The tectal plate is compressed. The quadrigeminal plate cistern is obliterated, and the suprasellar cistern may be narrowed from behind. Severe ascending central herniation may cause deep notches in the upper surface of the cerebellum. Obstruction of the aqueduct and perimesencephalic cistern may cause hydrocephalus that partially balances the herniation (but increases the ICP). Shunting the dilated lateral ventricles may then increase

the pressure gradient across the incisura, aggravating the herniation.

CT or MRI typically shows obliteration of the superior cerebellar cistern by the herniated superior vermis. The quadrigeminal plate cistern is effaced, and the tectum is compressed (Fig. 26-25). The pons is displaced anteriorly against the clivus. In severe cases, midbrain compression may lead to periaqueductal necrosis.[29] Compression of the vein of Galen and the basal veins of Rosenthal causes further increase in ICP.

Tonsillar Herniation

In this condition, the cerebellar tonsils and medial cerebellar hemispheres are displaced caudally through the foramen magnum into the cervical spinal canal. Normally, the inferior tips of the cerebellar tonsils lie at or near the foramen magnum. In adults, they should not protrude more than 5 mm below the lower lip of the foramen magnum (Children: 6 mm).[30] Tonsillar herniation may be caused by a posterior fossa mass or by descending central transtentorial herniation.[31] Reich and coworkers found that two thirds of patients with upward transtentorial herniation and one half of those with descending transtentorial herniation also had tonsillar herniation.[31] Compression of the medulla oblongata against the foramen magnum by herniating cerebellar tonsils initially causes a decreased level of consciousness owing to pressure on the reticular activating system. Further compression leads to respiratory embarrassment from involvement of the respiratory centers. In turn, slower respirations raise the PCO_2 and increase ICP.

Tonsillar herniation is difficult to detect on axial CT scans. The medulla, surrounding CSF, and vertebral arteries should normally be resolved on good quality axial images through the foramen magnum. With herniation, the CSF spaces surrounding the brain stem are obliterated (Fig. 26-26A). MRI is far superior for diagnosing tonsillar herniation, especially midline and paramedian sagittal images (see Fig. 26-26B).

POST-TRAUMATIC CEREBRAL INFARCTION

Post-traumatic cerebral infarction is a well-recognized sequela of head trauma and is seen in 19% of patients with moderate or severe traumatic brain injury.[32]

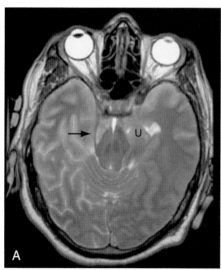

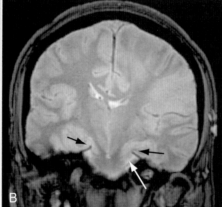

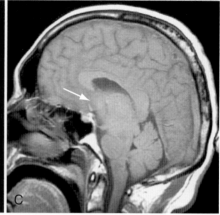

■ **FIGURE 26-20** Central herniation in a 42-year-old man. **A,** Axial T2W MR image demonstrates bilateral brain stem compression by uncal herniation. *Arrow* indicates tentorial edge. U, uncus. Brain stem is distorted. **B,** Coronal gradient-recalled-echo MR image shows downward herniation of both mesial temporal lobes (*white arrow*) through tentorium (*black arrows*). **C,** Sagittal T1W MR image shows brain stem compressed against clivus. *Arrow* indicates uncus interposed between clivus and mesencephalon.

■ **FIGURE 26-21** Severe closed-head injury in a 37-year-old man. **A,** Unenhanced CT shows brain stem compression and Duret hemorrhage (*arrow*). **B,** Axial FLAIR MRI demonstrates extensive posterior cerebral distribution infarction resulting from central herniation. **C,** Sagittal FLAIR shows extensive diffuse axonal injury in addition to infarcts. **D,** Diffusion-weighted imaging confirms the presence of acute infarction.

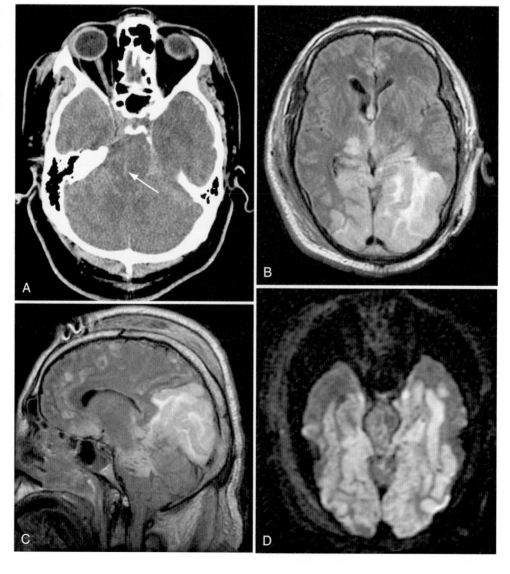

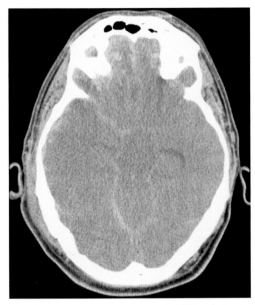

■ **FIGURE 26-22** Central herniation with diffuse infarction. Unenhanced CT shows lack of gray matter/white matter differentiation and frontal hemorrhagic contusion. Basal cisterns are obliterated.

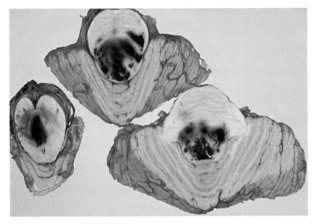

■ **FIGURE 26-23** Pathology specimen. Serial axial sections through the midbrain and upper pons show side-to-side compression of the midbrain and multiple Duret hemorrhages. *(Courtesy of John Deck, MD.)*

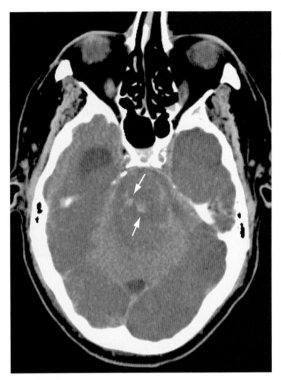

■ **FIGURE 26-24** Central herniation. Unenhanced CT shows central herniation, bilateral occipital lobe infarction, and Duret hemorrhages in brain stem (*arrows*).

Pathophysiology

Cerebral herniation may compress surface vessels against the free edges of the falx and tentorium, leading to secondary cerebral infarction, as discussed earlier. Infarction may also result from global hypoxia or hypoperfusion sustained at the time of injury, compressive ischemia from an overlying hematoma, arterial dissection, vasospasm, and/or fat embolism.[32] Decompressive craniectomy performed for control of ICP has been reported to cause middle cerebral artery infarction and lenticulostriate artery infarction.[32] Boundary zone (watershed) infarcts occur in the setting of hypotension, particularly when combined with elevated ICP.

In one series, mechanical shift or herniation of brain tissue accounted for 81% of post-traumatic cerebral infarctions.[33] Posterior cerebral artery territory infarction was the most commonly encountered, followed by middle cerebral artery infarction, then anterior cerebral artery infarction (Figs. 26-27 and 26-28).

Imaging

Whereas CT can detect most cases of post-traumatic cerebral infarction and identify its cause, MRI is usually more sensitive

and specific for detection and diagnosis. Diffusion-weighted MRI is able to detect an infarct within the first hour of its occurrence (Fig. 26-29).

LATE SEQUELAE OF HEAD TRAUMA

CT is the most practical and efficient procedure for evaluating acute traumatic brain injury, but MRI is superior for depicting the subacute and chronic changes of head injury. Even so, MRI underestimates the structural abnormalities that can persist even after mild TBI. Some of these lesions are microscopic or biochemical, so they are beyond the reach of current imaging techniques. Some inroads have been made with diffusion tensor imaging, functional MRI, and MR spectroscopy (see earlier), but correlation of these techniques with neurocognitive testing is still imperfect. Every year, 80,000 individuals sustain a traumatic brain injury severe enough to cause neurologic deficits, which are mainly cognitive. The disturbances in cognition that persist over time are a source of psychosocial, intellectual, and vocational impairment, often leading to depression and a sense of futility. To add to the problem, intellectual and memory impairment may be accompanied by the development of post-traumatic epilepsy. Having an imaging procedure that would predict outcome in these cases would greatly assist in planning and directing rehabilitation of these patients.[34] Accordingly, functional neuroimaging of traumatic brain injury has become an area of intense interest in recent years.

Encephalomalacia

Encephalomalacia refers to softening of brain tissue, whether it is secondary to hemorrhagic contusion, infarction, or diffuse axonal injury.

Pathophysiology

With time, areas of hemorrhagic contusion and necrosis become resorbed in an orderly succession, from the periphery inward. Within a day of injury, neutrophils begin infiltrating the lesion.

■ **FIGURE 26-25** Ascending transtentorial herniation in a 13-year-old boy. **A,** Sagittal FLAIR MRI demonstrates upward bulging of the vermis (*arrowheads*) and downward displacement of the cerebellar tonsils (*arrow*). Callosal diffuse axonal injury is also seen. **B,** Axial GRE shows multiple hemorrhagic contusions (*long arrows*) and cerebellar vermis protruding into tentorial notch (*short arrows*).

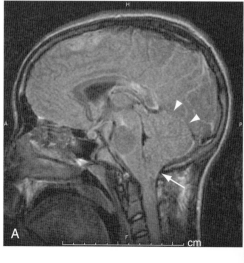

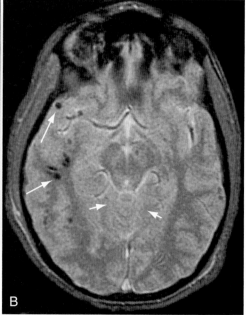

■ **FIGURE 26-26** Tonsillar herniation in a 24-year-old man. **A,** CT slice through foramen magnum shows tonsils (*arrows*) displacing cerebrospinal fluid and compressing brain stem. **B,** Finding is much more obvious on sagittal T1W MR image. Tonsils (*arrow*) are markedly herniated, medulla is compressed, and pons is flattened against clivus.

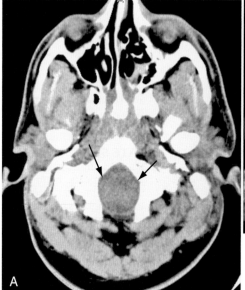

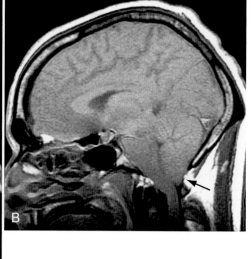

■ **FIGURE 26-27** Post-traumatic infarction in a 9-month-old girl. **A,** Admission CT shows acute right subdural hematoma and diffuse right hemisphere edema. **B,** Postoperative follow-up CT next day shows extensive infarction of right hemisphere.

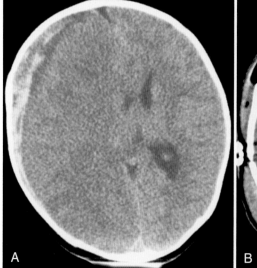

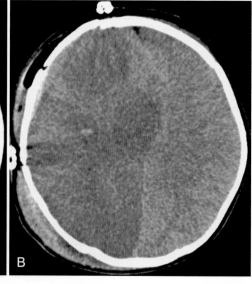

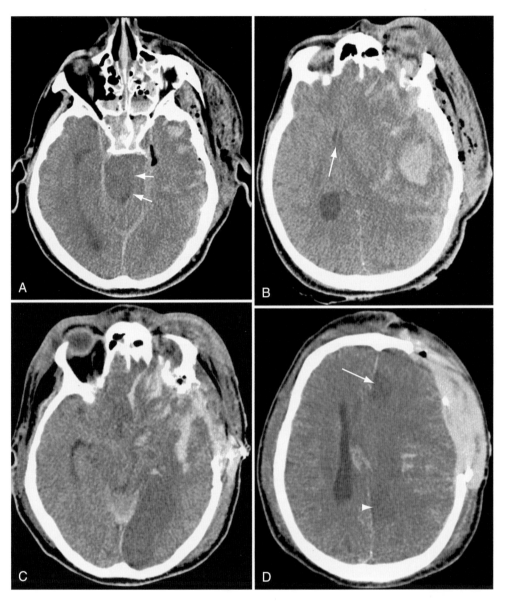

■ **FIGURE 26-28** Post-traumatic infarction in a 67-year-old man. **A,** Admission CT shows uncal herniation and brain stem compression (*arrows*). **B,** Higher slice demonstrates massive hemorrhagic contusion, subdural hematoma, and marked subfalcine herniation (*arrows*). **C** and **D,** Despite evacuation of the SDH, both anterior cerebral (**D,** *arrow*) and posterior cerebral (**D,** *arrowhead*) artery distribution infarcts are present.

By day 3, macrophages begin to remove necrotic debris. By about 1 week, reactive astrocytes surround the tissue, accompanied by an increased density of capillaries.[20] By 1 month after injury the damaged areas are intensely cellular, as a result of astrocytosis and microglial hyperplasia.[35] After 6 to 12 months a shrunken cystic cavity remains, lined with astrocytes and hemosiderin-laden macrophages. Cortical gyri in the area become atrophic. Adjacent CSF spaces enlarge, and there is often compensatory (atrophic) enlargement of the adjacent ventricle (Fig. 26-30). In cases of severe traumatic brain injury late findings may include widespread degeneration of subcortical white matter resulting from diffuse axonal injury.[35] Wallerian degeneration may cause secondary atrophy of the thalamus and brain stem by about 3 months after injury, if there has been widespread diffuse axonal injury.[35]

Imaging
MRI
On MRI, areas of encephalomalacia are hypointense on T1W imaging and hyperintense on T2W imaging (Fig. 26-31). On FLAIR series, areas of hyperintense gliosis are shown to surround the hypointense fluid-filled cavities. On sagittal MRI, thinning of

the corpus callosum indicates loss of crossing white matter tracts. The cerebellum can suffer diffuse injury, as demonstrated by quantitative MRI techniques. In a study of 16 children with moderate to severe traumatic brain injury, Spanos and associates found cerebellar atrophy in all subjects when compared with age-matched controls.[36] White matter volume loss exceeded gray matter loss.

MRI may show late sequelae of trauma even in cases of mild or moderate traumatic brain injury. MacKenzie and associates investigated 14 patients with mild or moderate traumatic brain injury and found that whole-brain atrophy was evident at an average of 11 months after trauma.[37] They also found that injuries that cause loss of consciousness lead to greater atrophy. Bigler and associates demonstrated progressive decline in hippocampal volume, as well as temporal horn enlargement in 94 patients with traumatic brain injury.[38]

Cranial Nerve Injury
Pathophysiology
Cranial nerves are especially vulnerable to traumatic injury because of their location at the skull base. Because the cranial nerves are tethered at their exit points through the neural

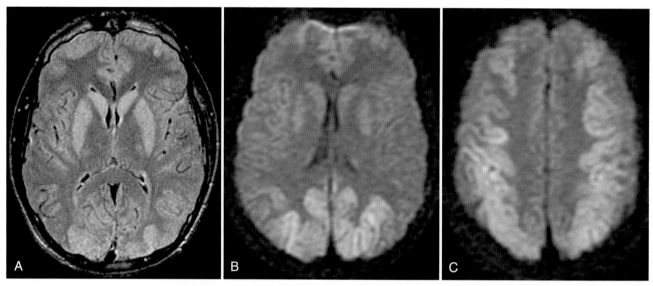

■ **FIGURE 26-29** Post-traumatic anoxia causing extensive infarction. **A,** Axial FLAIR MRI demonstrates increased signal in basal ganglia and occipital lobes. **B** and **C,** Diffusion-weighted images show extensive bilateral cortical infarction.

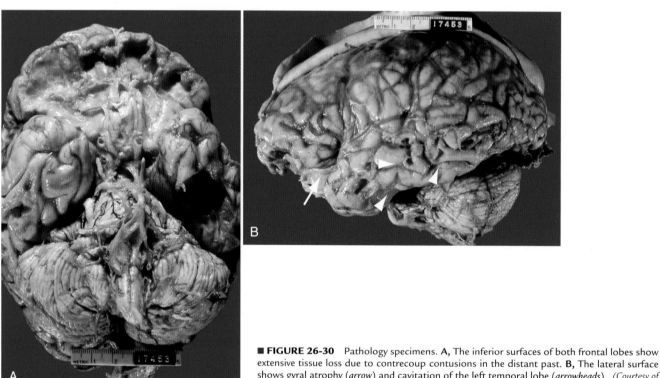

■ **FIGURE 26-30** Pathology specimens. **A,** The inferior surfaces of both frontal lobes show extensive tissue loss due to contrecoup contusions in the distant past. **B,** The lateral surface shows gyral atrophy (*arrow*) and cavitation of the left temporal lobe (*arrowheads*). *(Courtesy of John Deck, MD.)*

foramina, accelerations and decelerations that shift the brain may stretch them substantially. The most commonly injured cranial nerve (CN) is the olfactory nerve (CN I) (Table 26-2). Approximately 25% of victims of severe head injury will have post-traumatic anosmia, as a result of shearing of the olfactory nerves at the cribriform plate.[39] Post-traumatic anosmia is most likely to occur after occipital trauma (contrecoup injury) (Figs. 26-32 and 26-33) but is seen more commonly with frontal impacts, because frontal trauma is much more frequent (Fig. 26-34). Olfactory function returns in 14% to 39% of patients with head injury, as a result of the remarkable ability of olfactory neurons to regenerate.

The optic nerve most commonly suffers injury where it traverses the bony optic canal. A fracture of the lesser wing of the sphenoid bone that extends into the optic canal can transect the nerve (Fig. 26-35). Alternatively, the concussive force of trauma to this area may cause edema of the nerve and subsequent ischemic optic neuropathy.

Cranial nerves III and IV may sustain compressive injury as they course around the uncus in the event of uncal herniation. A traumatic carotid-cavernous sinus fistula may compromise CNs III, IV, V, and VI as they traverse the cavernous sinus.

An isolated CN VI palsy is common after severe head trauma and is usually a manifestation of increased ICP. The nerve becomes stretched as the brain stem is displaced caudally or becomes compressed by the basilar artery.[40] The clinical manifestation is an inability to abduct the ipsilateral eye.

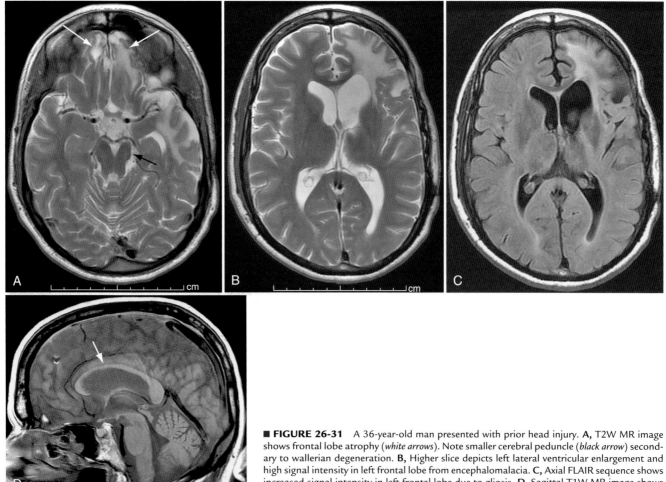

■ **FIGURE 26-31** A 36-year-old man presented with prior head injury. **A,** T2W MR image shows frontal lobe atrophy (*white arrows*). Note smaller cerebral peduncle (*black arrow*) secondary to wallerian degeneration. **B,** Higher slice depicts left lateral ventricular enlargement and high signal intensity in left frontal lobe from encephalomalacia. **C,** Axial FLAIR sequence shows increased signal intensity in left frontal lobe due to gliosis. **D,** Sagittal T1W MR image shows thinning of corpus callosum resulting from loss of brain substance (*arrow*).

TABLE 26-2. Cranial Nerve Injury

Cranial Nerve	Most Likely Type/Location	Clinical Manifestation
I. Olfactory	Cribriform plate fracture; contrecoup injury	Anosmia
II. Optic	Optic nerve canal fracture	Unilateral blindness
III. Oculomotor	Compression by uncus; cavernous sinus injury	Ptosis, dilated pupil; globe deviated downward
IV. Trochlear	Compression by uncus or parahippocampal gyrus	Vertical diplopia; outward deviation of eye
V. Trigeminal	Skull base fractures; facial fractures	Unilateral facial anesthesia; corneal anesthesia
VI. Abducens	Caudal displacement of brain stem causes stretching of nerve	Horizontal gaze diplopia; ipsilateral eye turns inward
VII. Facial	Temporal bone fracture involving facial nerve canal	Ipsilateral paralysis of facial muscles; loss of taste in anterior two thirds of tongue
VIII. Vestibulocochlear	Temporal bone fracture	Unilateral hearing loss Vertigo
IX. Glossopharyngeal	Penetrating injury to skull base; posterior skull base fracture	Loss of taste in posterior third of tongue Stylopharyngeus muscle
X. Vagus	Penetrating injury to skull base; posterior skull base fracture	Minor disturbance of palate, larynx, and pharynx
XI. Spinal accessory	Penetrating injury to skull base; posterior skull base fracture	Paralysis of sternocleidomastoid and trapezius muscles
XII. Hypoglossal	Occipital bone fracture; internal carotid dissection	Tongue deviates to side of injury

The facial nerve traverses the temporal bone through a long and convoluted bony canal, making it susceptible to injury with closed-head trauma. Facial nerve palsy is a common complication of temporal bone fracture, occurring in 7% to 10% of cases.[41] Seventy to 80 percent of temporal bone fractures are oriented along the long axis of the petrous bone (longitudinal fracture), 10% to 20% are oriented perpendicular to the long axis of the

petrous bone (transverse fractures), and 10% are mixed (oblique fractures). Facial nerve paralysis is most common with transverse fractures, especially ones that pass through the otic capsule.[42] Seventy-six percent of longitudinal fractures that result in CN VII palsy have bony impingement on the nerve or intraneural hematoma; 15% have nerve transection.[41] With transverse fractures, 92% have transected facial nerves and 8% have bony

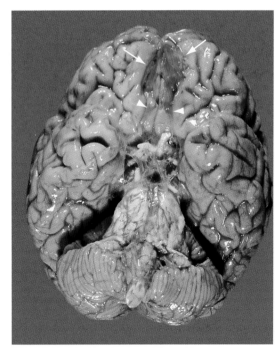

■ **FIGURE 26-32** Postmortem photograph shows chronic contrecoup contusions of the medial inferior surfaces of both frontal lobes (*arrows*) with severe tissue loss and destruction of the olfactory bulbs and tracts (*arrowheads*). (*Courtesy of John Deck, MD.*)

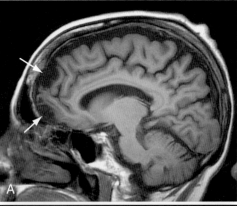

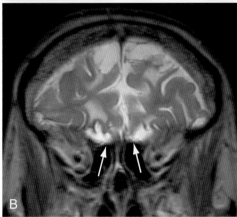

■ **FIGURE 26-33** Contrecoup injury to olfactory tracts in a 44-year-old woman. **A,** Sagittal T1W MR image shows frontal basal post-traumatic atrophy (*arrows*). **B,** Coronal T2W MR image shows loss of gyrus rectus and olfactory tracts (*arrows*).

impingement. Transverse fractures often begin at the foramen magnum and extend through the bony labyrinth, transecting the facial nerve in the fallopian canal.

Surgical management of traumatic facial nerve palsy is highly controversial, because most patients recover without surgery. Patients with delayed onset of facial palsy or incomplete paralysis have a good prognosis for full recovery.[43] Those individuals with immediate and complete paralysis have a poorer prognosis, usually reflecting nerve transection. These patients may benefit from nerve decompression, if it is performed during the first 14 days after injury.[41]

Injury to the vestibulocochlear nerve is also common with temporal bone fracture. In a series of 820 temporal bone fractures, Brodie and coworkers found hearing loss in 24%.[42] Of these, 21% had conductive hearing loss, 57% had sensorineural loss, and 22% had a mixed loss. Vertigo is a common sequela of temporal bone trauma and may be precipitated by injury to the vestibule, vestibular nerve, or vestibular aqueduct.[44]

Imaging
CT
Multidetector CT is the preferred modality for evaluating temporal bone trauma. Thin slices (1 mm or less) are acquired in the axial plane parallel to the hard palate. From these, coronal and sagittal images are reformatted. We prefer wide window settings (4000 HU) and bone algorithm reconstructions for viewing these images (Fig. 26-36). All portions of the intratemporal facial nerve canal are closely inspected in three planes, searching for fracture, areas of discontinuity, or bony impingement.

MRI
MRI is helpful in diagnosing intralabyrinthine hemorrhage, especially in the subacute and chronic stages.[44] The presence of methemoglobin results in a bright signal on T1W MR images. Fractures of the temporal bone, especially longitudinal fractures, may produce CSF otorrhea and subsequent meningitis.

Injury to cranial nerves IX to XII is uncommon after closed-head trauma. It is more likely to follow penetrating injury such as gunshot wounds.[18] Fractures of the posterior skull base or occipital condyle can injure the hypoglossal nerve where it traverses its canal. Ipsilateral palsy of cranial nerves IX to XII (Collet-Sicard syndrome) has been reported from posterior basal skull fracture[45] and Jefferson fracture.[46] Stretching trauma to the brain stem may also damage the root entry zones of the lower cranial nerves. This is shown by MRI.

Diabetes Insipidus
Diabetes insipidus (DI) is characterized by the excretion of large volumes of dilute urine, intake of excessive volumes of liquid, and hypernatremia. The criteria for the diagnosis of DI are urine output of 200 mL/hr or greater at a specific gravity of less than 1.005.[47]

Epidemiology
The incidence of DI immediately after moderate or severe traumatic brain injury is variously reported as 2.9% to 21.6%, depending on the criteria for diagnosis.[47,48] Most cases occur in patients with a Glasgow Coma Scale (GCS) score of 6 or lower, and the overall mortality in this group is 69%.[47] Most cases are transient, but permanent DI has been reported in 6.9% of victims of moderate or severe traumatic brain injury.[48]

Pathophysiology
Transient DI is thought to be the result of edema of the hypothalamic-posterior pituitary region, whereas permanent DI implies irreversible damage to the hypothalamic neurons or their projections to the posterior pituitary gland.[48]

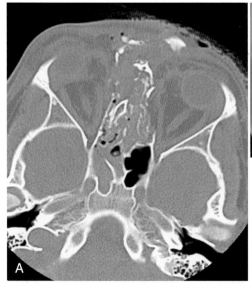

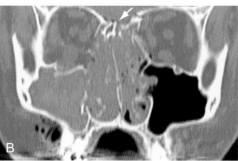

■ FIGURE 26-34 Severe naso-orbito-ethmoidal injury in a 16-year-old boy. **A,** Axial CT shows severely comminuted ethmoids, including the cribriform plate and both laminae papyraceae. **B,** Coronal reformatted CT depicts comminuted cribriform plate (*arrow*).

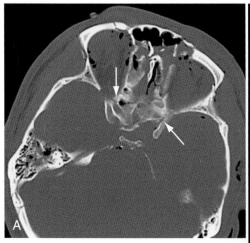

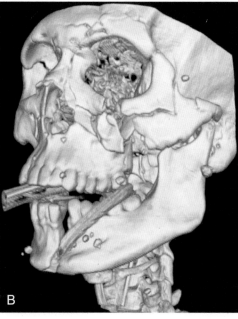

■ FIGURE 26-35 Facial smash injury in a 21-year-old man. **A,** Fractures of the lesser wing of the sphenoid extend into both optic nerve canals (*arrows*). **B,** 3D reformatted image depicts extent of fractures.

Imaging

Tien and coworkers described the MRI findings in two patients with post-traumatic DI.[49] In both cases, transection of the pituitary stalk was seen.

BRAIN DEATH PROTOCOLS

Under the Uniform Determination of Death Act adopted by all 50 states, a person is considered dead when there has been irreversible cessation of all functions of the entire brain, including the brain stem. The concept of "entire brain" distinguishes determination of death under this act from "neocortical death" or "persistent vegetative state."

For a person to be declared brain dead, a specific list of conditions must be met. The determination of brain death begins with the clinical neurologic examination. The cause of the coma must be ascertained, and all confounding factors must be removed. These include hypothermia (≤32°C), drug or alcohol intoxication, neuromuscular blocking agents, severe metabolic or electrolyte disturbances, and poisoning. The neurologic examination must document the presence of coma, the absence of brain stem reflexes, and apnea.[50] The apnea test must confirm the absence of respiratory movement over a period of 8 to 12 minutes after the victim is disconnected from the ventilator. If all these criteria are met, no further tests are required.

Imaging

If any part of the neurologic examination is equivocal and brain death is still suspected, confirmatory tests may be ordered. In patients who meet the clinical criteria (and restrictions) just mentioned, an electroencephalogram that shows no brain electrical activity over a period of 30 minutes is considered confirmatory evidence of brain death. Alternatively, a technetium blood flow study can be performed at the bedside. Absence of intracranial flow on the technetium brain scan confirms brain death (Fig. 26-37). Absence of blood flow to the brain as seen on MRI/MRA or CTA is also confirmatory (Fig. 26-38).

ANALYSIS

The diagnosis of brain herniation is one of the most critical a radiologist can make, because it has a profound effect on patient

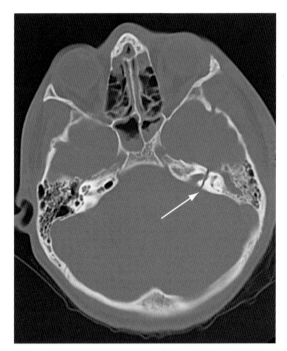

■ **FIGURE 26-36** Transverse temporal bone fracture in a 21-year-old man. CT demonstrates fracture line (*arrow*) perpendicular to long axis of petrous bone. Fracture crosses the facial nerve canal and the cochlea.

management. Although herniation is a relatively straightforward diagnosis on multiplanar MRI, it can be a bit more challenging on CT. Signs of herniation must be searched for on the CT scan of every victim of significant head trauma. This search begins with the lateral scout radiograph. If the patient is intubated, this implies a seriously ill or traumatized person. The scout film is scrutinized for skull and cervical spine fractures or dislocations, as well as foreign bodies. Occasionally, a malpositioned nasogastric tube is seen coiled in the hypopharynx, and the clinician is alerted to this finding.

After inspection of the scalp and skull at bone window/bone algorithm settings for fracture and foreign bodies, the posterior fossa is inspected. Is the fourth ventricle normal in size and position, or is it compressed and displaced caudally (Fig. 26-39)? Are the pontine and superior cerebellar cisterns normal or compressed? If the cerebellar tonsils can be visualized, are they in normal position? Is the pons displaced caudally? The mesencephalon should be surrounded by CSF and not effaced or distorted.

Turning next to the supratentorial compartment, one should look for mass effect. If present, is it sufficient to cause a shift of the midline structures? "Eyeballing" it is not adequate; the midline structures should be measured and any shift documented. Also, bihemispheric edema or masses can cause central herniation without a midline shift.

The key to the CT diagnosis of central or transtentorial herniation lies in the suprasellar cistern. On the normal scan, this area is filled with CSF and is symmetric. Is the medial border of the uncus normally located, or is it encroaching into the

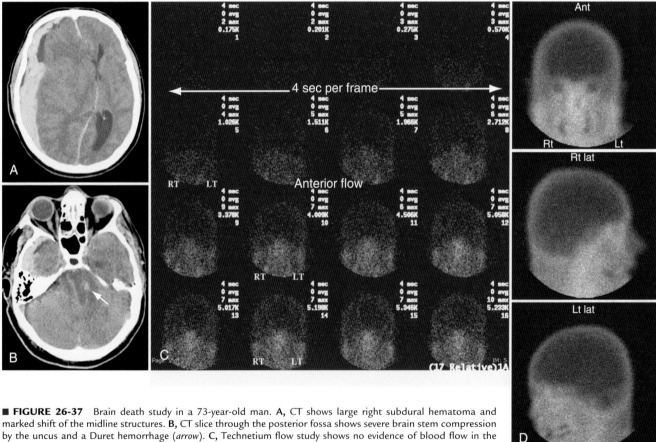

■ **FIGURE 26-37** Brain death study in a 73-year-old man. **A,** CT shows large right subdural hematoma and marked shift of the midline structures. **B,** CT slice through the posterior fossa shows severe brain stem compression by the uncus and a Duret hemorrhage (*arrow*). **C,** Technetium flow study shows no evidence of blood flow in the brain. **D,** Static images show no brain uptake.

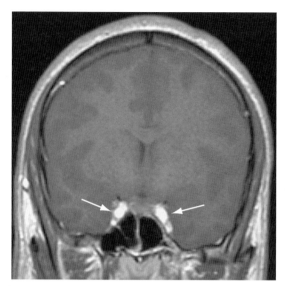

■ **FIGURE 26-38**   MRI confirmation of brain death in a 24-year-old man. Coronal T1W gadolinium-enhanced MR image shows blood flow to the skull base (*arrows*) but no intracranial flow.

cistern? If the hippocampus is medially displaced, is it compressing the brain stem? If there is unilateral uncal herniation, one should check the contralateral temporal horn, because dilatation of this structure is confirmatory evidence of herniation. If transtentorial herniation is present, then the mesencephalon and pons are inspected carefully for signs of Duret hemorrhage,

because this finding has ominous prognostic implications. If severe transtentorial herniation has been present for several hours or more, signs of posterior cerebral artery distribution infarction may be seen, manifested as low density or loss of gray matter/white matter discrimination in the occipital lobes.

The unfortunate patient whose CT scan is shown in Figure 26-39 sustained a severe closed head injury when he crashed his all-terrain vehicle. He was admitted with a GCS score of 3. Based on the results of this CT, as well as a careful, detailed neurologic examination, he was pronounced brain dead and was made an organ donor. No further imaging studies were required. A sample report of evaluation of brain death after a gunshot wound is given in Box 26-1.

SUMMARY

CT is the preferred tool for the initial evaluation of head trauma, because of its rapid scanning time, accuracy in detecting hemorrhage and fractures, and ability to depict mass effect. The decision for early surgical intervention can be made on the basis of CT alone. CTA is a rapid and accurate technique for diagnosing vascular injuries. MRI is useful in the subacute phase of care for detecting diffuse axonal injury. It is important to recognize the various types of brain herniation and to be able to identify them on CT as well as MRI. MRI is the procedure of choice for evaluating the late sequelae of head trauma. A working knowledge of the pathophysiologic alterations in cerebral blood volume, cerebral blood flow, tissue water (edema), intracranial pressure, and cerebral compliance that accompany traumatic brain injury permits more meaningful interpretation of the images, more relevant reporting of the results, and a more satisfying contribution to the clinical management of the patient.

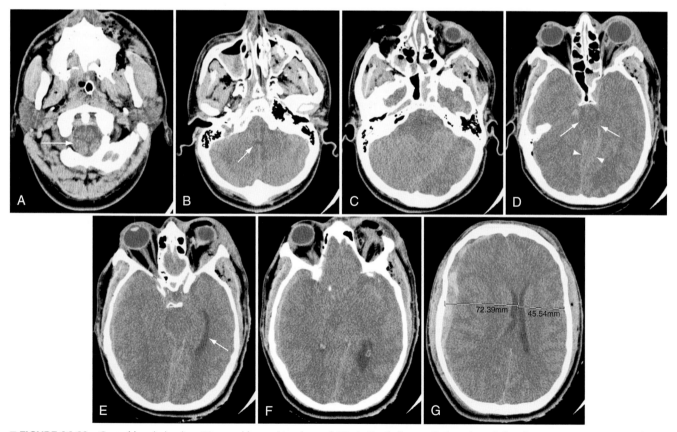

■ **FIGURE 26-39**   Central herniation in a 26-year-old man. Unenhanced CT. **A,** Cerebellar tonsils (*arrow*) are below foramen magnum. **B,** Fourth ventricle (*arrow*) is compressed and displaced caudally. **C,** Pontine cistern is obliterated, and pons is compressed against clivus. **D,** Mesencephalon (*arrows*) is compressed and distorted. Superior cerebellar cistern (*arrowheads*) is effaced. **E,** Left temporal horn (*arrow*) is dilated. **F,** Suprasellar cistern is completely obliterated. **G,** The septum pellucidum is shifted 13 mm to the left, and a hyperacute subdural hematoma is present on the right.

BOX 26-1　Sample Report: Nuclear Medicine Report of Brain Death

PATIENT HISTORY

A 26-year-old man had a gunshot wound to the neck and a GCS score of 3.

TECHNIQUE

Brain imaging was done using 25 mCi of ^{99m}Tc-labeled Neurolite IV.

FINDINGS

After the administration of the radiotracer, immediate flow images of the brain were obtained, followed by spot and anterior and lateral images of the brain.

There is no definite evidence for brain perfusion on the flow imaging. The delayed imaging shows no uptake in the brain tissue. The findings are consistent with brain death.

IMPRESSION

There was no evidence of brain perfusion, consistent with brain death. These findings were discussed with the trauma physician.

KEY POINTS: DIFFERENTIAL DIAGNOSIS

- Either MRA or MDCTA is appropriate for detecting arterial dissection, pseudoaneurysm, or occlusion.
- MRI is superior to CT for detection and characterization of brain herniations.
- Posterior cerebral artery distribution infarction is a common complication of transtentorial herniation.

SUGGESTED READINGS

Brown AW, Malec JF, McClelland RL, et al. Clinical elements that predict outcome after traumatic brain injury: a prospective multicenter recursive partitioning (decision-tree) analysis. J Neurotrauma 2005; 22:1040-1051.

Flanagan SR, Hibbard MR, Gordon WA. The impact of age on traumatic brain injury. Phys Med Rehabil Clin North Am 2005; 16:163-177.

Hagman P, Jonasson L, Maeder P, et al. Understanding diffusion MR imaging techniques: from scalar diffusion-weighted imaging to diffusion tensor imaging and beyond. RadioGraphics 2006; 26:S205-S223.

Hunter JV, Thornton RJ, Wang ZJ, et al. Late proton MR spectroscopy in children after traumatic brain injury: correlation with cognitive outcomes. AJNR Am J Neuroradiol 2005; 26:482-488.

Kelly WM. Cranial neuropathy. Neuroimag Clin North Am 1993; (1):1-206.

Kraus MF, Susmaras T, Caughlin BP, et al. White matter integrity and cognition in chronic traumatic brain injury: a diffusion tensor imaging study. Brain 2007; 130:2508-2519.

MacKenzie JD, Siddiqi F, Babb JS, et al. Brain atrophy in mild or moderate traumatic brain injury: a longitudinal quantitative analysis. AJNR Am J Neuroradiol 2002; 23:1509-1515.

Mirvis SE, Wolf Al, Numaguchi Y, et al. Post-traumatic cerebral infarction diagnosed by CT: prevalence, origin, and outcome. Am J Neuroradiol 1990; 11:355-360.

Newberg A, Alavi A, van Rhijn S, Reilly P. Radiologic diagnosis of brain death. JAMA 2002; 288:2121-2122.

Ropper AH, Gorson KC. Concussion. N Engl J Med 2007; 356:166-172.

Sinson G. He was never quite "himself" after that accident: exploring the long-term consequences of mild traumatic brain injury. AJNR Am J Neuroradiol 2001; 22:425-426.

REFERENCES

1. Hilton-Jones D, Warlow CP. The causes of stroke in the young. J Neurol 1985; 232:137-143.
2. Fabian TC, Patton JH Jr, Croce MA, et al. Blunt carotid injury: importance of early diagnosis and anticoagulant therapy. Ann Surg 1996; 223:513-525.
3. Rogers FB, Baker EF, Osler TM, et al. Computed tomographic angiography as a screening modality for blunt cervical arterial injuries: preliminary results. J Trauma 1999; 46:380-385.
4. Li MS, Smith BM, Espinosa J, et al. Nonpenetrating trauma to the carotid artery: seven cases and a literature review. J Trauma 1994; 36:265-272.
5. Larsen DW. Traumatic vascular injuries and their management. Neuroimag Clin North Am 2002; 12:249-269.
6. Yamada S, Kindt GW, Youmans JR. Carotid artery occlusion due to nonpenetrating injury. J Trauma 1967; 7:333-342.
7. Biffl WL, Egglin T, Benedetta B, et al. Sixteen-slice computed tomographic angiography is a reliable noninvasive screening test for clinically significant blunt cerebrovascular injuries. J Trauma 2006; 60:745-751.
8. Eastman AL, Chason DP, Perez CL, et al. Computed tomographic angiography for the diagnosis of blunt cervical vascular injury: is it ready for primetime? J Trauma 2006; 60:925-929.
9. Levy C, Laissy JP, Raveau V. Carotid and vertebral artery dissections: three-dimensional time-of-flight MR angiography and MR imaging versus conventional angiography. Radiology 1994; 190:97-103.
10. LeBlang SD, Nunez DB, Rivas LA, et al. Helical computed tomographic angiography in penetrating neck trauma. Emerg Radiol 1997; 4:200-206.
11. Nunez DB Jr, Torres-Leon M, Munera F. Vascular injuries of the neck and thoracic inlet: helical CT-angiographic correlation. RadioGraphics 2004; 24:1087-1098.
12. Le TH, Gean AD. Imaging of head trauma. Semin Roentgen 2006; 41:177-189.
13. Ivarez JA, Bambakidis N, Takaoka Y. Delayed rupture of traumatic intracranial pseudoaneurysm in a child following a gunshot wound to the head. J Craniomaxillofac Trauma 1999; 4:39-44.
14. Hachemi M, Jourdan C, Di Rio C, et al. Delayed rupture of traumatic aneurysm after civilian craniocerebral gunshot injury in children. Childs Nerv Syst 2007; 23:283-287.
15. Archondakis E, Pero G. Valvassori L, et al. Angiographic follow-up of traumatic carotid cavernous fistulas treated with endovascular stent graft placement. AJNR Am J Neuroradiol 2007; 28:342-347.
16. Shepard S. Head trauma. eMedicine 2004; http://www.emedicine.com/MED/topic2820.htm. Accessed 5/28/2006.

17. Isa R, Adnan WAW, Ghazali G, et al. Outcome of severe traumatic brain injury: comparison of three monitoring approaches. Neurosurg Focus 2003; 15:1-7.

18. Graham DI, Gennarelli TA, McIntosh TK. Trauma. In Graham DI, Lantos PL (eds). Greenfield's Neuropathology, 7th ed. London, Arnold, 2002, pp 822-898.

19. Marmarou A, Abd-Elfattah Foda M, van den Brink W, et al. A new model of diffuse brain injury in rats: I. pathophysiology and biomechanics. J Neurosurg 1994; 80:291-300.

20. Fatouros PP, Marmarou A. Use of magnetic resonance imaging for in vivo measurements of water content in human brain: method and normal values. J Neurosurg 1999; 90:109-115.

21. Fatouros PP, Marmarou A, Kraft KA, et al. In vivo brain water determination by T1 measurements: effect of total water content, hydration fraction, and field strength. Magn Reson Med 1991; 17:402-413.

22. Muizelaar JP, Fatouros PP, Schroder ML. A new method for quantitative regional cerebral blood volume measurements using computed tomography. Stroke 1997; 28:1998-2005.

23. Marmarou A, Fatouros P, Barazo P, et al. Contribution of edema and cerebral blood volume to traumatic brain swelling in head-injured patients. J. Neurosurg 2000; 93:183-193.

24. Marmarou A, Signoretti S, Fatouros P, et al. Predominance of cellular edema in traumatic brain swelling in patients with severe head injuries. J Neurosurg 2006; 104:720-730.

25. Barzo P, Marmarou A, Fatouros P, et al. Magnetic resonance imaging-monitored acute blood-brain barrier changes in experimental traumatic brain injury. J Neurosurg 1996; 85:1113-1121.

26. Johnson PL, Eckard DA, Chason DP, et al. Imaging of acquired cerebral herniations. Neuroimag Clin North Am 2002; 12:217-228.

27. Kernohan JW, Woltman HW. Incisura of the curs due to contralateral brain tumor. Arch Neurol Psychiatry 1929; 21:273-287.

28. Voyadzis JM, Panicker H, McGrail KM. Kernohan's phenomenon, resulting from a traumatic left acute subdural hematoma. Appl Radiol 2007; 35:34-35.

29. Coburn MW, Rodriguez FJ. Cerebral herniations. Appl Radiol 1998; 27:10-16.

30. Barkovich AJ, Wippold FJ, Sherman JL, Citrin CM. Significance of cerebellar tonsil position on MRI. AJNR Am J Neuroradiol 1986; 6:795-799.

31. Reich JB, Sierra J, Camp W, et al. Magnetic resonance imaging measurements and clinical changes accompanying transtentorial and foramen magnum brain herniation. Ann Neurol 1993; 33:159-170.

32. Marino R, Gasparotti R, Pinelli L, et al. Posttraumatic cerebral infarction in patients with moderate or severe head trauma. Neurology 2006; 67:1165-1171.

33. Server A, Dullerud R, Haakonsen M, et al. Post-traumatic cerebral infarction. Acta Radiol 2001; 42:254-260.

34. Strangman G, O'Neil-Pirozzi TM, Burke D, et al. Functional neuroimaging and cognitive rehabilitation for people with traumatic brain injury. Am J Phys Med Rehabil 2005; 84:62-75.

35. Adams JH, Jennett D, McLellan R, et al. The neuropathology of the vegetative state after head injury. J Clin Pathol 1999; 52:804-806.

36. Spanos GK, Wilde EA, Bigler ED, et al. Cerebellar atrophy after moderate-to-severe pediatric traumatic brain injury. AJNR Am J Neuroradiol 2007; 28:537-542.

37. MacKenzie JD, Siddiqi F, Babb JS, et al. Brain atrophy in mild or moderate traumatic brain injury: a longitudinal quantitative analysis. AJNR Am J Neuroradiol 2002; 23:1509-1515.

38. Bigler ED, Blatter DD, Anderson CV, et al. Hippocampal volume in normal aging and traumatic brain injury. AJNR Am J Neuroradiol 1997; 18:11-23.

39. Yousem DM, Oguz KK, Li C. Imaging of the olfactory system. Semin Ultrasound CT MRI 2001; 22:456-472.

40. Laine FJ, Smoker WRK. Cranial nerves III, IV, VI. Neuroimag Clin North Am 1993; 3:85-104.

41. Chang CY, Cass SP. Management of facial nerve injury due to temporal bone trauma. Am J Otol 1999; 20:96-114.

42. Brodie HA, Thompson TC. Management of complications from 820 temporal bone fractures. Am J Otol 1997; 18:188-197.

43. Massa N, Westerberg BD. Facial nerve, intratemporal bone trauma. eMedicine 2006; http://www.emedicine.com/Ent/topic160.htm. Accessed 3/26/2007.

44. Swartz JD, Harnsberger HR. Imaging of the Temporal Bone. New York, Thieme, 1998, pp 318-344.

45. Kato M, Tanaka Y, Toyoda I, et al. Delayed lower cranial nerve palsy (Collet-Sicard syndrome) after head injury. Injury Extra 2006; 37:104-108.

46. Connolly B, Turner C, DeVine J, Gerlinger T. Jefferson fracture resulting in Collet-Sicard syndrome. Spine 2000; 25:395-398.

47. Boughey JC, Yost MJ, Bynoe RP. Diabetes insipidus in the head-injured patient. Am Surg 2004; 70:500-503.

48. Agha A, Thornton E, O'Kelly P, et al. Posterior pituitary dysfunction after traumatic brain injury. J Clin Endocrinol Metab 2004; 89:5987-5992.

49. Tien R, Kucharczyk J, Kucharczyk W. MR imaging of the brain in patients with diabetes insipidus. AJNR Am J Neuroradiol 1991; 12:533-542.

50. Wijdicks EF. The diagnosis of brain death. N Engl J Med 2001; 344:121

Cysts and Tumors

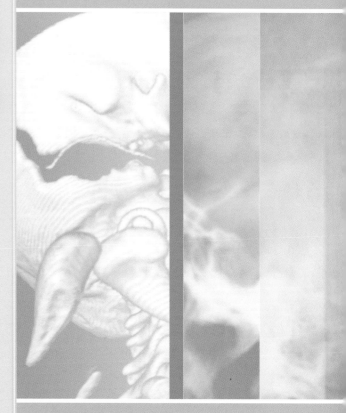

Intracranial Cysts and Cyst-Like Lesions

Cheng-Hong Toh and Mauricio Castillo

Non-neoplastic, noninfectious intracranial cysts are uncommon benign lesions of variable etiology and pathogenesis. The nomenclature for these lesions can be confusing. Single entities often have multiple names. Lesions with similar embryologic origins and histologic findings may be designated differently in different locations.

At present there is no established classification for intracranial cysts. Instead, they are often classified by their anatomic location and/or the nature of their lining membrane. In this chapter, we classify these cysts based on pathology as (1) cysts derived from endoderm, which include neurenteric cysts, Rathke's cleft cysts, and colloid cysts; (2) cysts derived from neuroectoderm, such as glioependymal cysts, ependymal cysts, and choroid plexus cysts; (3) congenital inclusion cysts, which include dermoid, epidermoid, and arachnoid cysts; and (4) pineal cysts.

Most of these cysts are asymptomatic. In symptomatic cases the clinical presentations are often related to the cyst's size and location. Most of these cysts have contents resembling cerebrospinal fluid (CSF), so their CT density and MR signal intensity will parallel that of CSF. The density and MR signal intensity of a cyst may be different from that of CSF when there is increased protein, other chemical compounds, or hemorrhage causing increase of CT attenuation or shortening of T1 and T2 relaxation times. Among these, the cysts with an *endodermal* lining have a tendency to retain secretory function. Their contents may cause marked increase in density and shortening of the T1 and T2 relaxation times, resulting in hyperdensity in precontrast CT and hyperintensity on T1-weighted (T1W) images.

Although some cysts have (nearly) specific features (e.g., a colloid cyst), the degree of confidence for preoperative diagnosis in the majority of these cysts is low. Diffusion-weighted imaging (DWI) is helpful to differentiate epidermoid cysts from other intracranial cysts and to increase detection of choroid plexus cysts.

Correct diagnosis of these cysts requires histologic examination, particularly immunohistochemistry, which can demonstrate the embryonic origin of the lesion. Ectodermal markers such as S-100 and glial fibrillary acidic protein (GFAP) are not present in an endodermal cyst. Endodermal-derived cysts typically stain positively for endodermal markers such as epithelial membrane antigen, cytokeratin, mucicarmine, periodic acid–Schiff, and carcinoembryonic antigen.

For a full discussion of the various intracranial cysts and cyst-like lesions, please visit www.expertconsult.com.

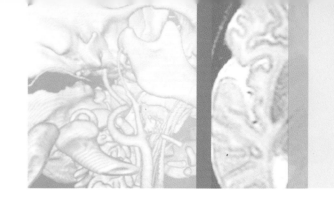

CHAPTER 28

Neuroepithelial Cysts, Porencephaly, and Perivascular Spaces

Lorne Rosenbloom and Thomas P. Naidich

Many pathologic processes present as cystic lesions of the brain. Noninfectious, non-neoplastic cysts of the brain parenchyma and ventricular system in children include porencephaly, neuroepithelial cysts, and enlarged perivascular spaces. These benign fluid spaces most commonly arise in utero from developmental defects or acquired insults.

Neuroepithelial cysts are histologically benign, smooth-walled cysts thought to arise from nests of neuroectodermal progenitor cells. Pathologically, they are characterized by a glial wall and an epithelial lining resembling ependyma or choroid plexus. Small cysts are usually asymptomatic. Large cysts do cause local mass effect. On imaging they appear as smooth, thin-walled, non-calcified, non-enhancing cavities containing a fluid that resembles CSF.

Porencephaly refers to a non-cystic cerebrospinal fluid–containing cavity that replaces normal brain parenchyma. Pathologically, there is no epithelial lining. Some authors classify porencephaly into two types: Porencephaly type I is thought to result from an encephaloclastic insult that occurs in utero, in premature newborns and in early infancy. The damaged area then evolves over time into a fluid-filled cavity. Porencephaly type II is thought to result from focal injury to the germinal matrix in early fetal life, disrupting the normal migration of subependymal neuroblasts to the surface of the developing hemisphere. This focal disruption creates a focal, often tubular cavity that extends across the full thickness of the brain from the ventricular system to the brain surface and is lined by dysplastic gray matter.

The clinical manifestations of porencephaly depend on the extent of the prenatal encephaloclastic event. The most common presenting signs are hemiparesis and epilepsy. When the insult is severe, spastic hemiplegia or tetraplegia may be present. There may be developmental delay, especially when the involvement is bilateral. When deeper midline structures are affected, there may be hypoplasia resulting in visual deficits.

Enlarged perivascular (Virchow-Robin) spaces are benign expansions of the fluid compartments that normally surround the blood vessels as they penetrate through the substance of the brain. They are generally asymptomatic, but may serve as a marker for underlying pathologic processes. Correlations have been reported between enlarged Virchow-Robin spaces and autism, childhood migraine, myotonic dystrophy, microangiopathic disease (in older adults), and traumatic brain injury. Enlarged perivascular spaces are also seen in patients with mucopolysaccharidoses and tuberous sclerosis.

For a full discussion of the pathophysiology and imaging of these spaces, please see the website www.expertconsult.com.

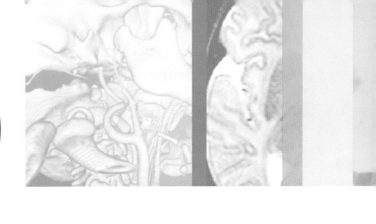

CHAPTER 29

Overview of Adult Primary Neoplasms and Metastatic Disease

James G. Smirniotopoulos, Alice B. Smith, John H. Rees, and Frances M. Murphy

The overwhelming majority of intracranial neoplasms are metastatic to the central nervous system (CNS). In a 2005 article, Nathoo, Chalavi, Barnett, and Toms wrote: "The incidence of metastases to the brain is estimated to be about 170,000/year in the USA, an incidence 10 times higher than that of primary malignant brain tumors."[1] However, the source that they quote in their review article, as the reference for this information, does not even mention the words "metastasis," "metastases," or "metastatic."[1-3]

Another article that is commonly quoted is a 2005 review by Gavrilovic and Posner, who wrote: "Thus, from epidemiologic studies, the incidence of brain metastases seems equal to or no more than twice that of gliomas. These data almost certainly underestimate the true incidence of brain metastases because some metastases are asymptomatic."[4]

However, a review by Arnold and Patchell indicated that the frequency of brain metastases had increased from 10% to 15% in the older literature to 20% to 40%—certainly much less than one half!

The point to be made is that the published literature has not yet established that metastatic disease—symptomatic or not—is the most common type of intracranial neoplasm, nor even the most common intra-axial tumor.

EPIDEMIOLOGY

Malignant disease outside the brain often comes to clinical attention because of CNS signs and symptoms. In addition, staging for extraneural primary tumors often, but not always, includes assessment of metastatic disease to significant "target organs": liver, lung, bone and marrow, and brain. Some experimental primary malignancy treatment protocols require initial staging to search for CNS lesions that would alter survival and therefore affect patient outcome. Neurologic findings typically occur in 25% to 50% of patients with extracranial malignancy at some time during their life. In addition, brain metastases are often symptomatic rather than incidental findings. The reasons for this

are that (1) most CNS metastases lodge in or near the cerebral cortex; (2) much of the cortex is clinically eloquent; (3) metastasis often creates a seizure focus; and (4) secondary effects of the tumor—increased intracranial pressure and vasogenic edema—produce symptoms and signs. These four situations may conspire to create the impression that metastatic neoplasms are more common than primary brain tumors. However, using population-based epidemiology, we should be able to actually assess the incidence and prevalence within a target population.

Gavrilovic and Posner reviewed metastatic disease and reported that metastases are up to 10 times more common than primary brain tumors.[4] Nathoo and associates estimated an incidence of 170,000 patients with metastatic disease per year.[5] However, the Central Brain Tumor Registry of the United States (CBTRUS) reported, in 2010, that the incidence of primary brain tumors is 18.71 cases/100,000/yr (7.19 malignant and 11.52 nonmalignant). This report predicts 62,930 new primary brain tumors occurring in the United States during 2010.[6] This would calculate to a primary to secondary tumor ratio of 3:5—certainly more metastasis, almost twice, but not overwhelmingly more, and obviously not a factor of 10.

The Swedish epidemiology study of hospital admissions showed a doubling of brain metastasis from 7 to 14/100,000 during the 2 decades from 1987 to 2006.[7] Again, compared with the CBTRUS data, this would be a primary to secondary ratio (at present) of 14/18.71, with primary tumors being more common. However, this is not a fair comparison, because the data come from two different populations: Sweden and the United States.

Materljan and colleagues reported a small population-based study (from Croatia) of 175 CNS tumors, showing primary neoplasms to be more common (11.8/100,000/yr) than metastases (9.9/100,000/yr).[8] Another population-based study from Croatia showed that 88% of intracranial tumors were primary, with an incidence rate of primary tumors of 11.8/100,000/yr.[9]

A study of asymptomatic human subject volunteers provides yet another potential surveillance mechanism. In several large

■ **FIGURE 29-1** **A,** Contrast-enhanced axial CT image shows a large irregular mass in the left kidney, which is the primary renal cell carcinoma (RCC). **B,** Frontal posteroanterior radiograph. There is an irregular left upper lobe mass, which is a pulmonary metastasis from the RCC. **C,** Sagittal T1W MR image. Many of the multiple small nodular lesions show T1 shortening from blood products. These are hemorrhagic metastases. **D,** Frontal posteroanterior radiograph. Follow-up study shows progression of the lung metastases with growth and newly visible lesions.

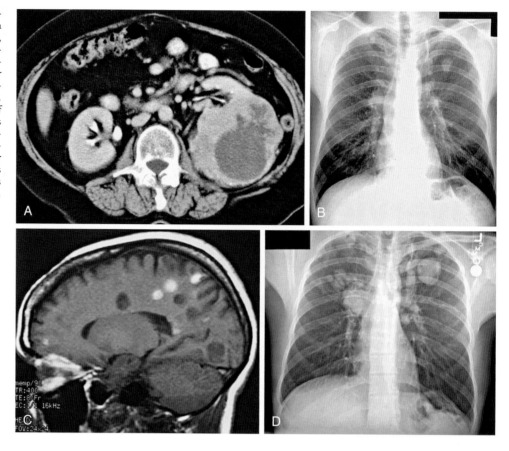

studies, including a meta-analysis of 16 projects with 19,559 subjects studied, the prevalence of unsuspected primary brain tumors was 0.7% (135 patients) but there were no cases of metastatic disease.[10] In a recent population-based study from Rotterdam, 2000 adults (aged 45 to 96 years, mean 63 years) were scanned with high-quality MRI at 1.5 Tesla.[11] There was one incidental metastasis, 1 incidental malignant primary brain tumor, and 31 (1.6%) incidental primary benign tumors (18 meningioma, 4 schwannoma, 6 pituitary adenoma). If we were to use this study, we could "prove" that primary tumors are 32 times more common than metastatic disease! So, if metastatic deposits are symptomatic, we find them when evaluating the symptoms. If a patient has certain cancers, we find the lesions with a staging examination. If the patient is asymptomatic, we will not find the metastasis, and the prevalence of these asymptomatic metastatic lesions is probably very low, unlike the prevalence of asymptomatic primary tumors.

CASCADE THEORY

How do extraneural malignancies reach the CNS? The "cascade theory" describes the sequence of events required for parenchymal CNS metastasis. Viable tumor cells must enter the systemic circulation to reach the brain. For example, a testicular tumor can spread into the venous system as well as the lymphatics. The sequence begins with passage of cells into the perinephric and para-aortic area—the normal venous and lymphatic drainage for the testis. From there, tumor cells travel through the inferior vena cava or the lymphatic drainage to the thoracic duct and then pass through the right side of the heart into the pulmonary circulation. The capillary bed in the lung will "trap" the tumor cells. However, some may become locally invasive in the lung

(a lung metastasis) and then travel through the pulmonary veins into the left side of the heart and then enter the systemic circulation. Alternately, tumor cells may bypass the "filtration bed" of the lung, through a right-to-left shunt or a patent foramen ovale. For gastrointestinal primary neoplasms, the sequence is one step more complicated. The portal venous blood drains into the liver, which is also a "filtration bed."[1] The case of renal cell carcinoma in Figure 29-1 shows a typical course of disease progression from primary tumor to lung to brain.

Theoretically, there should be lung metastasis before brain metastasis; and for a gastrointestinal malignancy, there should be liver metastasis before lung metastasis. However, on a practical level, these intermediate sites of metastatic disease may remain "occult" to conventional imaging. They would, or should, be visible with high-resolution imaging and are often seen at pathologic examination.

RATE, DELAY, SURVIVAL

Metastatic disease from non–small cell lung cancer and breast cancer occurs in 8% to 20% of patients. Metastases from lung cancer tend to occur earlier, with a median of 3 months, whereas breast cancer metastasis is found at a median of 42 months.[7] After the first hospitalization for brain metastasis, the median survival is only 3 months, and only 13% of patients will survive for a year.[7]

SCALP AND SKULL

Primary tumors of the skull vault are uncommon and include hemangioma, osteoma, Paget disease of bone, and fibrous dysplasia. Calvarial metastasis, as in other bones, may be lytic (e.g., Langerhans' histiocytosis, breast, lung) or blastic (e.g., breast,

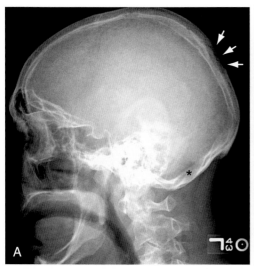

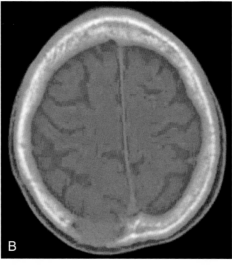

■ **FIGURE 29-2** **A,** Lateral skull radiograph. There are two lytic lesions: one is in the parietal region (*arrows*) and a second lesion is barely visible in the occipital bone (*asterisk*). **B,** Axial CT image. The parietal lytic lesion is just to the right of midline.

prostate, lymphoma, pancreas, carcinoid). Metastatic lesions to bone do not create or destroy bone directly. Instead, the metastasis may stimulate osteoclastic reabsorption, producing lytic lesions; or, there may be a desmoplastic tissue reaction in the bone, creating a dense "blastic" metastasis. Skull metastasis may be symptomatic or can produce painless swelling or deformity (Fig. 29-2).

In the skull base, primary tumors may arise from the nerves (schwannoma, neurofibroma) meninges (meningioma, hemangiopericytoma), pituitary gland (invasive adenoma), or the paranasal sinuses (inverting papilloma, squamous cell carcinoma, esthesioneuroblastoma). Clival neoplasms are only uncommonly metastatic, especially when that is the only bone involved, accounting for only 15% of cases.[12] Chordomas are the most common primary tumors of the clivus and probably the most common neoplasm overall in this bone. Primary chondrosarcomas arise most often from the synchondroses (e.g., the foramen lacerum region).

EXTRA-AXIAL METASTASIS

Dural metastases are found in almost 10% of patients dying with cancer.[13] In some cases, only dural metastases are present and they may mimic meningioma, hemangiopericytoma, or solitary fibrous tumor.[14] In men, dural metastases are mostly likely to be from prostate cancer; whereas in women, most dural metastasis arises from a breast tumor. Dural metastases may present years after the primary tumor; however, most often they are seen in the context of known extracranial cancers. Dural and/or calvarial bone metastasis are often compartmentalized by the tough dural membrane and may present as a biconvex or lenticular "epidural" lesion or a concavoconvex "subdural" lesion or involve only the skull and scalp (Figs. 29-3 and 29-4).[15]

Leptomeningeal metastasis, commonly called "carcinomatous meningitis," may be produced by both intracranial and systemic malignancies. The most common systemic primary cancer types, reported by Clarke and colleagues, included "breast (65 patients), lung (47), gastrointestinal (11), and melanoma (9)."[16] Some of these systemic cancers seed the cerebrospinal fluid (CSF) from an intracranial secondary metastatic deposit that contacts the ventricular or the pial surface of the brain. In many cases, the CSF spread appears without an obvious intraparenchymal lesion. CNS primary tumors that gain access to the ventricle or subarachnoid space will also seed the CSF. In children, these tumors include medulloblastoma (primitive neuroectodermal tumor or

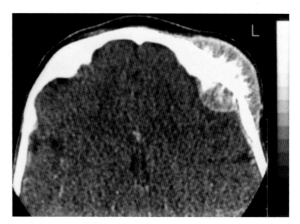

■ **FIGURE 29-3** Axial CT image shows a metastatic neuroblastoma to the calvaria. There is a spiculated "hair on end" periosteal new bone formation. The expansile metastasis is delimited and confined by the periosteum (dura) inside and by the periosteum outside, producing a biconvex mass.

PNET), ependymoma, intracranial germ cell tumors, and both benign choroid plexus papilloma and malignant choroid plexus carcinoma. In adult patients, CNS-to-CNS seeding occurs with primary CNS lymphoma, glioblastoma, and, occasionally, oligodendroglioma (Fig. 29-5).

INTRA-AXIAL METASTASIS

The vast majority of intra-axial metastasis are distributed by blood flow (hematogenous dissemination).[4] Arterial spread is more common than venous spread: the latter is associated with pelvic malignancies migrating through the valveless veins of the vertebral Batson plexus.[17] Most metastatic deposits will be peripheral, rather than deep, in or near the gray matter/ white matter junction and cerebral cortex. The deep gray matter (basal ganglia and thalamus) may also host metastases, usually associated with other lesions in a more typical peripheral gray-white junction location (Fig. 29-6). Multiple lesions that are clustered in the periventricular region or other primarily white matter locations should suggest multifocal glioma, primary CNS lymphoma or toxoplasmosis, or a leukoencephalopathy.

■ **FIGURE 29-4** Noncontrast (**A**) and postgadolinium (**B**) axial T1W MR images of metastatic neuroendocrine carcinoma, showing the biconvex shape created by the dural-limited tumor spread.

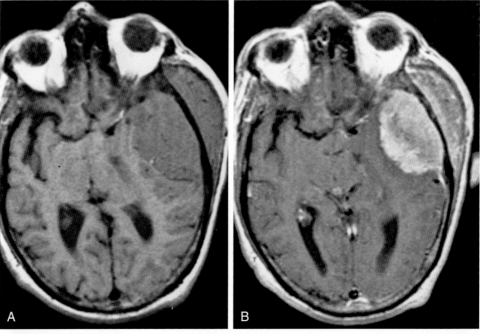

■ **FIGURE 29-5** Glioblastoma multiforme with leptomeningeal spread. Postgadolinium axial (**A**) and coronal (**B**) MR images show diffuse abnormal enhancement of the basal cisterns and sulci. **C,** Axial MR image shows an intra-axial heterogeneous (necrotic) lesion in the right posterior frontal lobe and a more superficial lesion on the left. **D,** Coronal MR image shows spread of the glioblastoma multiforme from the right to the left, with abnormal enhancement of the corpus callosum. The right-sided (probably primary) tumor infiltrates the cortex to spread into the subarachnoid space.

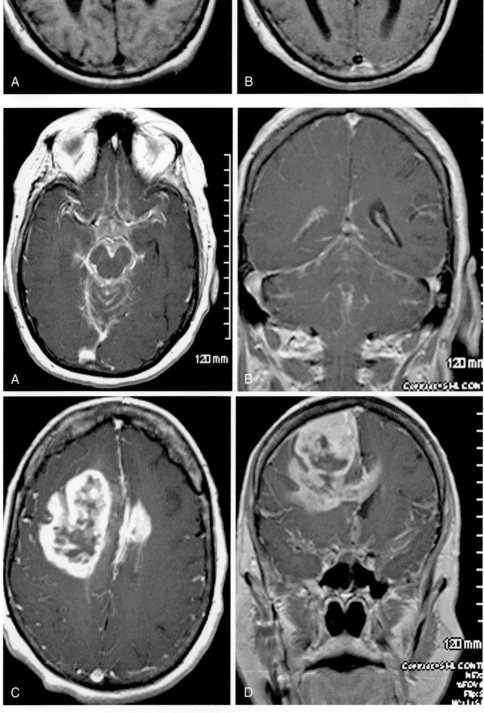

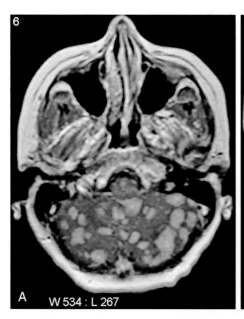
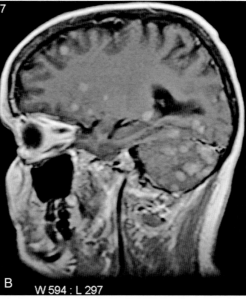

■ **FIGURE 29-6** Axial (**A**) and sagittal (**B**) T1W postgadolinium MR images show a multitude of small nodular enhancing lesions. Supratentorially, these are not only subcortical but also in the deep gray matter (basal ganglia).

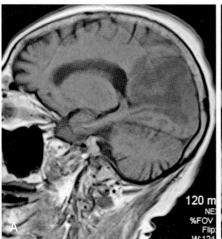
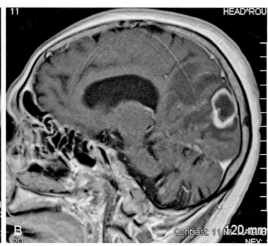

■ **FIGURE 29-7** Sagittal T1W MR images of metastatic breast cancer without (**A**) and with (**B**) contrast. There is only a single and relatively large lesion. The lesion has a smooth, rounded appearance, with very extensive intra-axial vasogenic edema. The differential diagnosis would include not only a primary astrocytoma (e.g., glioblastoma multiforme) but potentially an abscess or even cysticercosis.

In considering the routine surveillance of known cancer patients, there is also an increased incidence of developing a second primary tumor within the CNS. This creates the potential for misinterpretation of a new brain lesion as metastatic rather than as a second primary lesion. One review from Memorial Sloan-Kettering Cancer Center noted that 3% of all malignant gliomas presented as a second primary tumor in a patient with a previous cancer.[18] Some second primary tumors are related to prior radiation treatment of the original primary tumor. This has been shown for both meningioma and gliomas and should correlate with known treatment portals.[19] Long-term survivors of childhood leukemia who had received whole-brain irradiation are at particular risk, in addition to adults with pituitary, cavernous sinus, or other skull base lesions who may develop a meningioma as a second primary tumor.[20,21]

DIFFERENTIAL DIAGNOSIS OF GLIOMA VERSUS METASTASIS

Metastatic disease commonly presents as multiple small (<3 cm) round and well-demarcated nodular lesions with bright enhancement and perilesional edema. Most lesions will be supratentorial

and in or near the gray matter/white matter junction. However, 5% to 15% of primary cerebral gliomas will be multifocal; and primary CNS lymphoma (PCNSL) is commonly multifocal. These primary lesions, however, tend to have irregular and indistinct margins and are more often in the deeper white matter of the centrum semiovale or the periventricular white matter, including expansion of the corpus callosum.

The differential diagnosis becomes more difficult with a solitary lesion. Multiple series have shown that, on initial presentation, roughly half (40% to 60%) of patients will have only a solitary metastasis. These solitary lesions may suggest a primary glial tumor (glioblastoma multiforme) (Fig. 29-7), or they may mimic an abscess (Fig. 29-8). In addition to using diffusion imaging, MR spectroscopy may help distinguish abscess from necrotic neoplasm (see Fig. 29-9D). Conversely, 5% to 15% of gliomas will be multifocal (Fig. 29-9).[22] Although metastatic deposits are usually in or near the gray matter (see Fig. 29-6), the lesions from multifocal glioblastoma are in the deep white matter, which is a potentially useful feature for differential diagnosis. Another cause of multifocal neoplastic lesions is primary CNS lymphoma, which is multifocal in 20% to 30% of immunocompetent patients and up to two thirds

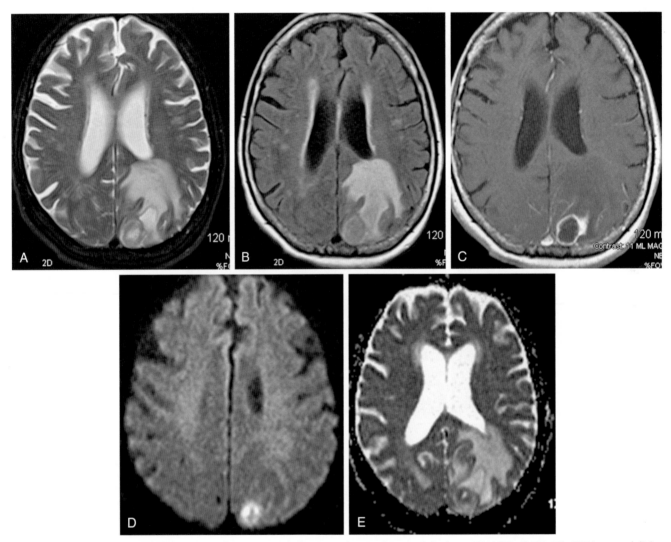

■ **FIGURE 29-8** Axial MR images showing solitary metastasis from an adenocarcinoma of the lung: T2W (**A**), FLAIR (**B**), T1W postgadolinium (**C**), diffusion-weighted (**D**), and apparent diffusion coefficient (ADC) map (**E**). This solitary metastasis mimics the appearance of an abscess—including ring enhancement and restricted diffusion (dark on ADC and bright on diffusion-weighted) images.

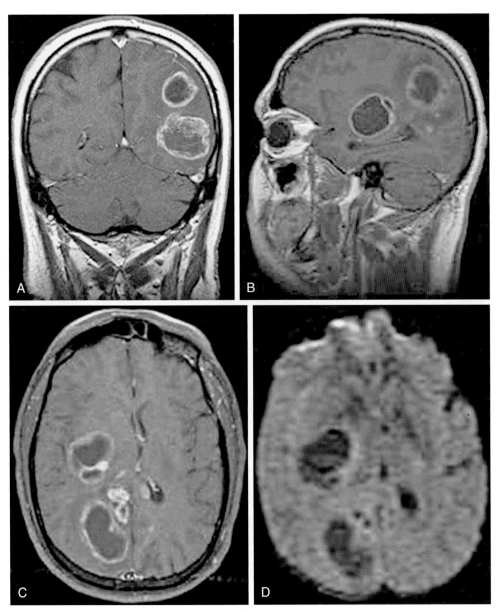

■ **FIGURE 29-9** Multifocal primary glioblastoma multiforme. Coronal (**A**), sagittal (**B**), and axial (**C**) T1W postgadolinium MR images show multiple ring-enhancing lesions that are mostly in the deep white matter. These are largely smooth and thin rings, with some thicker and/or solid regions of enhancement. **D**, Diffusion-weighted image shows very low signal from tumor necrosis, a potential for differential diagnosis from abscess.

of immune-suppressed patients with human immunodeficiency virus.[23,24] Primary and secondary lymphomas are "small, round, blue cell" tumors. In the setting of multiple lesions, we should suggest PNCSL when the lesions are periventricular or in the corpus callosum location, have low signal on T2-weighted imaging, and show a correlated restricted diffusion in the solid areas of the lesion (Fig. 29-10).

Metastases are usually well delimited, both pathologically and on imaging. Both PCNSL and gliomas, especially astrocytomas, are infiltrating neoplasms. Testing the "perilesional signal abnormality" may reveal this infiltration and would mitigate against a secondary tumor. Perilesional perfusion (regional cerebral blood volume) may be increased and apparent diffusion coefficient values may be decreased in both lymphoma and diffuse astrocytomas. Both of these tumors infiltrate into perilesional regions of "vasogenic edema," which actually includes a mixture of neoplastic tissue and interstitial water.[25] In addition, the fluid-attenuated inversion recovery (FLAIR) technique may be useful in detecting infiltrated cortical gray matter, a sign of primary glial tumors.[26] MR spectroscopy may also demonstrate infiltration when the peritumoral choline/*N*-acetyl-aspartate ratio is greater than 1.11.[27]

Spontaneous hemorrhage in cerebral metastasis occurs with deposits from several primary tumors: breast and lung (presumably due to their overall frequency), thyroid, choriocarcinoma, renal cell carcinoma, and metastatic melanoma (Figs. 29-11 and 29-12). Amyloid angiopathy may also produce synchronous or metachronous hemorrhages. Perilesional vasogenic edema, blood products of various chemistries and signal intensities, as well as heterogeneous rather than concentric patterns of signal, should suggest multifocal neoplastic hemorrhage and mitigate against amyloid vascular disease.

CHOROID PLEXUS AND VENTRICLE

Primary choroid plexus tumors are very uncommon—less than 2% of all primary brain tumors. Over 85% of choroid plexus

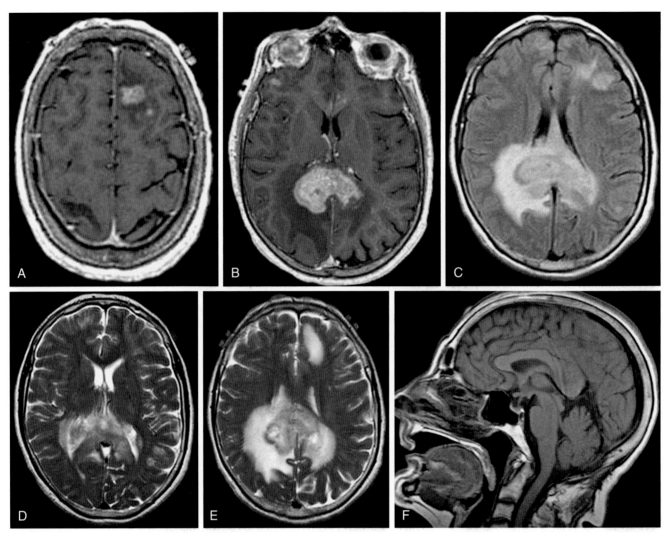

■ **FIGURE 29-10**   *Primary CNS lymphoma.* **A** and **B,** Axial T1W postgadolinium MR images. There are multiple lesions: one is left frontal and subcortical and another is in the splenium of the corpus callosum. Additional images show how the corpus callosum lesion has lower signal on FLAIR (**C**) and T2W (**D** and **E**) images. **F,** The sagittal T1W image helps localize the posterior lesion within the splenium of the corpus callosum.

primary tumors present in the first decade. Adult patients may have a meningioma of the choroid plexus, and that is usually in the lateral ventricle trigone. Because of its rich vascularity, the choroid plexus may receive hematogenous metastasis. Less than 5% of patients with cancer develop choroidal metastasis, which accounts for less than 10% of all intraventricular tumors. The lateral ventricle, having the most choroidal tissue, is the most common part affected. In adult patients choroidal metastases are much more common than primary choroid neoplasms. Primary choroidal plexus carcinoma may mimic an adenocarcinoma histologically, but these typically present in the first 5 years of life. Any adult with a diagnosis of "choroid plexus carcinoma" should be carefully evaluated for adenocarcinoma of extraneural origin. The occult primary tumor could be renal cell carcinoma or lung, gastric, or ovarian carcinoma. The most common source of choroidal metastasis is the kidney (usually renal cell carcinoma), representing one third to two thirds of primary sites disseminating to the choroid plexus.[28] This unusual relationship suggests either a "good soil" mechanism or an affinity or "tropism" for renal cell carcinoma to the choroid plexus.

A fourth ventricle choroid plexus mass, presenting in the adult patient, should also suggest a possible choroid plexus metastasis (Fig. 29-13).

SUMMARY

The most common intracranial neoplasms are probably primary tumors, especially when pooling pituitary and common extra-axial tumors such as meningioma and schwannoma. This is due to the prevalence of both symptomatic and asymptomatic meningiomas and schwannomas in the extra-axial space and gliomas, mostly astrocytomas, within the brain parenchyma. Metastatic disease may affect the skull and scalp, the dura and CSF spaces, the parenchyma, and the choroid plexus. Although we see metastatic disease often, any differential diagnosis of multiple lesions must also include primary neoplasms such as diffuse astrocytomas and primary CNS lymphoma. In a comparable manner, the differential diagnosis of any solitary brain or dural mass—once infection and demyelination have been considered—should include possible metastatic disease as well as primary neoplasms.

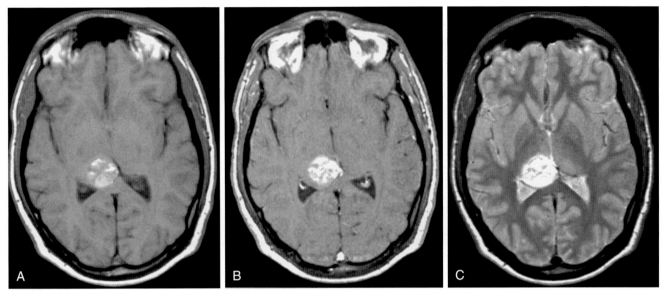

■ **FIGURE 29-11** Metastatic melanoma in the thalamus (pulvinar) with hemorrhage. Axial MR images. **A,** Noncontrast image shows heterogeneous hyperintensity (T1 shortening) from blood products within the lesion. **B,** Postcontrast image clearly shows enhancement that "fills in" the lesion, representing solid portions of the metastatic neoplasm. **C,** FLAIR image shows hyperintensity, unlike the low signal seen in Figure 29-10.

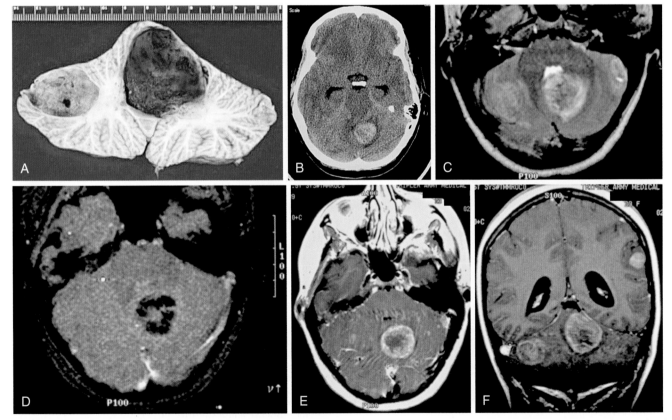

■ **FIGURE 29-12** Metastatic melanoma with multiple lesions, including the cerebellum. **A,** Gross photograph shows two lesions: a right peripheral and a larger, mostly hemorrhagic lesion on the left that involves the pons. **B,** Axial noncontrast CT scan shows a round hyperattenuating lesion. Corresponding contrast-enhanced axial (**C**), T2W (**D**), and gradient-recalled-echo (**E**) MR images show a rounded mass with heterogeneous enhancement. The central low signal on the gradient-recalled echo image is consistent with acute hemorrhage. **F,** Coronal T1W enhanced image shows both cerebellar lesions and a small cortical lesion in the left parietal lobe.

■ **FIGURE 29-13** Renal cell carcinoma, metastatic to the choroid plexus. Sagittal (**A**) and axial (**B**) T1W postgadolinium MR images show an intensely enhancing mass in the choroid plexus of the fourth ventricle.

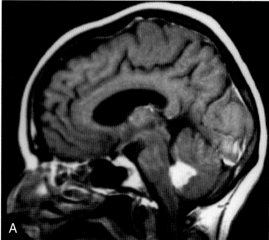 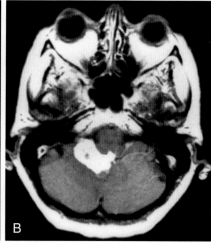

KEY POINTS

- Metastases are often solitary (40% to 50%).
- Primary glioblastoma multiforme (5% to 15%) and primary lymphoma (34% to 65%) are multiple.
- CSF dissemination arises from both brain primary and extra-CNS neoplasms.

- Primary intra-axial and metastatic tumors may be distinguished by examining the perilesional white matter, which is frequently infiltrated by primary tumors, showing increased perfusion and lower apparent diffusion coefficient values as compared with "pure" vasogenic edema surrounding metastasis.

SUGGESTED READINGS

Preusser M, Capper D, Ilhan-Mutlu A, et al. Brain metastases: pathobiology and emerging targeted therapies. Acta Neuropathol 2012; 123:205-222.

Fidler IJ. The role of the organ microenvironment in brain metastasis. Semin Cancer Biol 2011; 21:107-112.

Beasley KD, Toms SA. The molecular pathobiology of metastasis to the brain: a review. Neurosurg Clin N Am 2011; 22:7-14.

Waerzeggers Y, Rahbar K, Riemann B, et al. PET in the diagnosis and management of patients with brain metastasis: current role and future perspectives. Cancer Biomark 2010; 7:219-233.

Geiger TR, Peeper DS. Metastasis mechanisms. Biochim Biophys Acta 2009; 1796:293-308.

Kirsch M, Schackert G, Black PM. Metastasis and angiogenesis. Cancer Treat Res 2004; 117:285-304.

REFERENCES

1. Nathoo N, Chahlavi A, Barnett GH, et al. Pathobiology of brain metastases. J Clin Pathol 2005; 58:237-242.
2. Landis SH, Murray T, Bolden S, et al. Cancer statistics, 1999. CA Cancer J Clin 1999; 49:8-31.
3. Landis SH, Murray T, Bolden S, et al. Cancer statistics, 1998. CA Cancer J Clin 1998; 48:6-29.
4. Gavrilovic IT, Posner JB. Brain metastases: epidemiology and pathophysiology. J Neurooncol 2005; 75:5-14.
5. Nathoo N, Toms SA, Barnett GH. Metastases to the brain: current management perspectives. Expert Rev Neurother 2004; 4:633-640.
6. Central Brain Tumor Registry of the United States. Analyses of the NPCR and SEER data, 2004-2006. Available online at http://www.cbtrus.org/factsheet/factsheet.html.
7. Smedby KE, Brandt L, Bäcklund ML, et al. Brain metastases admissions in Sweden between 1987 and 2006. Br J Cancer 2009; 101:1919-1924.
8. Materljan E, Materljan B, Sepic J, et al. Epidemiology of central nervous system tumors in Labin area, Croatia, 1974-2001. Croat Med J 2004; 45:206-212.
9. Dobec-Meic B, Pikija S, Cvetko D, et al. Intracranial tumors in adult population of the Varazdin County (Croatia) 1996-2004: a population-based retrospective incidence study. J Neurooncol 2006; 78:303-310.
10. Morris Z, Whiteley WN, Longstreth WT Jr, et al. Incidental findings on brain magnetic resonance imaging: systematic review and meta-analysis. BMJ 2009; 339:b3016.
11. Vernooij MW, Ikram MA, Tanghe HL, et al. Incidental findings on brain MRI in the general population. N Engl J Med 2007; 357:1821.
12. Pallini R, Sabatino G, Doglietto F, et al. Clivus metastases: report of seven patients and literature review. Acta Neurochir (Wien) 2009; 151:291-296.
13. Laigle-Donadey F, Taillibert S, Mokhtari K, et al. Dural metastases. J Neurooncol 2005; 75:57-61.
14. Laidlaw JD, Kumar A, Chan A. Dural metastases mimicking meningioma: case report and review of the literature. J Clin Neurosci 2004; 11:780-783.
15. Maroldi R, Ambrosi C, Farina D. Metastatic disease of the brain: extra-axial metastases (skull, dura, leptomeningeal) and tumour spread. Eur Radiol 2005; 15:617-626.
16. Clarke JL, Perez HR, Jacks LM, et al. Leptomeningeal metastases in the MRI era. Neurology 2010; 74:1449-1454.
17. Vider M, Maruyama Y, Narvaez R. Significance of the vertebral venous (Batson's) plexus in metastatic spread in colorectal carcinoma. Cancer 1977; 40:67-71.
18. Maluf FC, DeAngelis LM, Raizer JJ, et al. High-grade gliomas in patients with prior systemic malignancies. Cancer 2002; 94:3219-3224.
19. Neglia JP, Robison LL, Stovall M, et al. New primary neoplasms of the central nervous system in survivors of childhood cancer: a report from the Childhood Cancer Survivor Study. J Natl Cancer Inst 2006; 98:1528-1537.

20. Rabin BM, Meyer JR, Berlin JW, et al. Radiation-induced changes in the central nervous system and head and neck. RadioGraphics 1996; 16:1055-1072.

21. Sadetzki S, Modan B, Chetrit A, et al. An iatrogenic epidemic of benign menigioma. Am J Epidemiol 2000; 151:266-272.

22. Showalter TN, Andrel J, Andrews DW, et al. Multifocal glioblastoma multiforme: prognostic factors and patterns of progression. Int J Radiat Oncol Biol Phys 2997; 69:820-824.

23. Zhang D, Hu LB, Henning TD, et al. MRI findings of primary CNS lymphoma in 26 immunocompetent patients. Korean J Radiol 2010; 11:269-277.

24. Küker W, Nägele T, Korfel A, et al. Primary central nervous system lymphomas (PCNSL): MRI features at presentation in 100 patients. J Neurooncol 2005; 72:169-177.

25. Rollin N, Guyotat J, Streichenberger N, et al. Clinical relevance of diffusion and perfusion magnetic resonance imaging in assessing intra-axial brain tumors. Neuroradiology 2006; 48: 150-159.

26. Tang YM, Ngai S, Stuckey S. The solitary enhancing cerebral lesion: can FLAIR aid the differentiation between glioma and metastasis? AJNR Am J Neuroradiol 2006; 27:609-611.

27. Server A, Josefsen R, Kulle B, et al. Proton magnetic resonance spectroscopy in the distinction of high-grade cerebral gliomas from single metastatic brain tumors. Acta Radiol 2010; 51: 316-325.

28. Hassaneen W, Suki D, Salaskar AL, et al. Surgical management of lateral-ventricle metastases: report of 29 cases in a single-institution experience. J Neurosurg 2010; 112:1046-1055.

30

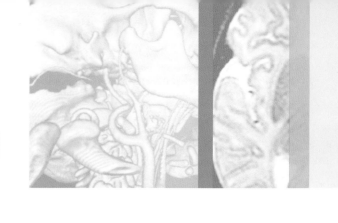

Meningeal Neoplasms

John H. Rees

The meningeal coverings of the human brain are composed of three distinct anatomic structures, each of which has two component layers.

The outermost and thickest layer is the dura mater (L. "tough mother"), which is composed of an outer layer, which functions as the periosteum of the inner table of the calvaria, and the deeper meningeal layer. This deeper layer infolds and forms the walls of the dural sinuses and the dural reflections of the brain compartments such as the falx cerebri, the tentorium cerebelli, and the diaphragma sella. This deeper meningeal layer also infolds to form a number of smaller canals and compartments including Meckel's cave, which houses the trigeminal or semilunar ganglion, and Dorello's canal, which allows passage of the sixth cranial nerve from the cisternal space to the lateral wall of the cavernous sinus. The cavernous sinus is a complex venous labyrinth in the lateral parasellar region formed from reflections of the inner layer of the dura. Similarly, the optic sheath is a cylindrical structure surrounding and protecting the optic nerves. The internal auditory canal is lined by this inner meningeal layer of dura as well.

The innermost layers, the pia mater and the arachnoid (Gr. "spider-like"), are relatively thin and are referred to collectively as the leptomeninges (Gr. *lepto,* "thin").

The arachnoid, which coats the inner surface of the dura, is also composed of two layers: the more superficial or arachnoid cap layer and the deeper arachnoid trabecular layer. These layers vary in thickness in different regions of the brain. The pia mater, which is innermost and immediately covers the brain, is composed of two layers: the epipia and the intima pia. Between the arachnoid and the pia is the subarachnoid space, which is filled with cerebrospinal fluid and is variable in size, enlarging to form the subarachnoid cisternal spaces at the base of the brain and narrowing over the cerebral convexities.[1]

The embryology of the meninges is a subject of ongoing study, with some believing that the dura mater is of mesodermal origin and that the leptomeninges are of ectodermal origin.[2] Comparative studies in birds show that the leptomeninges are at least partially of neural crest origin.[3,4] In any case, meningeal tissues and the neoplasms they give rise to are capable of exhibiting a wide range of mesodermal, ectodermal, and even neuroectodermal characteristics.

The term *meningeal neoplasms,* therefore, encompasses a broad group of extra-axial intracranial neoplasms that arise from any of the meningeal coverings of the brain:

- Meningothelial neoplasms or meningiomas
- Nonmeningothelial mesenchymal neoplasms, both benign and sarcomatous
- Melanocytic neoplasms
- Glial tumors of the leptomeninges
- Tumors of hematopoietic origin
- Miscellaneous neoplastic and non-neoplastic masses and cysts

MENINGIOMAS

In 1922, Harvey Cushing introduced the term *meningioma* to refer to a disparate group of intracranial, extra-axial neoplasms, which had been previously referred to by many different names, most commonly dural endotheliomata. Sixteen years later, Dr. Cushing and Dr. Louise Eisenhardt solidified the diagnostic nomenclature with their monograph entitled *Meningiomas.* They described their experience with 313 tumors, codifying 22 different histologic subtypes of this tumor, and providing convincing clinical and pathologic evidence that these different tumors were all variants of a single entity.[5]

Despite subsequent advances, particularly in the fields of molecular biology, much of their work has withstood the test of time. The generally accepted cell of origin of meningioma is the arachnoid cap cell, which is found in the most superficial layer of the arachnoid tissues. The arachnoid origin was first suggested by Bright in 1831,[5] then more conclusively demonstrated by Cleland in 1864.[5] In 1902, Schmidt[5] pursued a more detailed dissection, allowing the observation that these tumors arose from the most superficial layer of the arachnoid or, according to current terminology, the arachnoid cap cells. Arachnoid cap cells are most commonly found on the surface of the brain in association with dural sinuses and dural reflections but are also present in the tela choroidea, which extends throughout the ventricular system of the cerebrum. The arachnoid component of the tela choroidea gives rise to the less common intraventricular meningioma. Rarely, meningiomas are found elsewhere in the body, including intraosseous, intracerebral nondural,[6] and pulmonary locations.[7] The histogenesis of these tumors is uncertain; however, it is hypothesized that these distant or ectopic meningiomas may arise from arachnoid tissue associated with nerve sheaths or from ectopic meningothelial cells or possibly from pluripotential stem cells.

Epidemiology

Meningiomas are one of the most common intracranial neoplasms, representing approximately 25% of all new brain tumor diagnoses per year.[8] There is roughly a 1.5 to 2.0 female-to-male ratio, and the peak age at diagnosis is 60 to 70 for men and 70 to 80 for women. Interestingly, the female preponderance is not present in atypical and pediatric meningiomas but is increased to 8 to 10:1 in spinal meningiomas. Female preponderance is also lacking in Africans and African Americans, who, as a group, have a slightly higher incidence of meningiomas than persons of either European or Asian descent.[9,10] Incidence values vary in different studies, but a large meta-analysis gives the figure of 2.6 per 100,000 overall, and this is increased to 3.1 per 100,000 in those of African heritage.[11]

Meningiomas may be subdivided into many different categories according to histology, location, degree of biologic aggressivity, morphology, and demographic features. The classification scheme that has the most clinical relevance in terms of treatment, prognosis, and natural history is that adopted by the World Health Organization (WHO) in its 2007 revision of brain tumor taxonomy,[12] which divides meningiomas into three categories: benign, atypical, and malignant or anaplastic.

Benign—WHO grade I: 80% to 90%
- 1. Histologic atypia is lacking (e.g., increased mitotic index)
- 2. Certain specific histologic subtypes include meningothelial, fibroblastic, transitional, psammomatous, microcystic, lymphoplasmacytic, angiomatous, secretory, and metaplastic
- 3. Benign typical meningiomas may, and frequently do, exhibit invasion of adjacent soft tissues and bone, but brain invasion is indicative of at least grade II

Atypical—WHO grade II: 8% to 10%
- 1. Mitoses greater than 4 per 10 high-power fields
- 2. Certain histologic subtypes: clear cell and chordoid
- 3. Brain invasion. There has been an evolution of opinion regarding brain invasion. In the absence of frank anaplasia, meningiomas that exhibit brain invasion have been shown to be prognostically similar to atypical grade II, rather than malignant grade III, tumors. In the previous WHO classification, brain invasion alone connoted malignant or grade III, whereas in the latest edition it merits a grade II designation.
- 4. Three of five specific histologic findings, including spontaneous necrosis, hypercellularity, sheeting architecture, small cell formation with a high nuclear to cytoplasmic ratio, and/or macronucleoli

Malignant—WHO grade III: 1% to 2%
- 1. Frank anaplasia
- 2. Certain histologic subtypes: rhabdoid, and papillary
- 2. Mitotic index greater than 20 per 10 high-power fields, necrosis, and direct brain invasion

The 22 histologic subtypes initially proposed by Cushing and Eisenhardt have coalesced into 13 that have been incorporated into the WHO category, as just noted. In addition to the 4 atypical subtypes in WHO grade II (clear cell and chordoid) and grade III (papillary and rhabdoid), there are 9 other distinct histologic patterns recognized by WHO 2007; several of these also exhibit distinct imaging features. Varying degrees and admixtures are also seen, as well as other variations that are not judged to represent distinct subtypes at this point. In addition to histologic variations, meningiomas may also be differentiated by gross morphology. Most meningiomas assume a rounded morphology indicative of a radial growth pattern, but a small subset of meningiomas exhibits a flattened or en plaque morphology.

Neither WHO grade nor histologic subtype is the sole determinant of clinical outcome. Location and size at presentation are also important factors. Meningiomas occur most commonly in the parasagittal region (25%), followed by high convexities (19%); sphenoid ridge (17%); suprasellar, posterior fossa, and olfactory groove (each 8% to 9%); middle fossa/Meckel's cave; tentorial, and peritorcular regions (each 3% to 4%); and intraventricular, foramen magnum, and optic sheath (each 1%).

In addition to its effect on both neurologic symptoms and surgical therapy, there is evidence that meningiomas arising in different locations represent distinct subtypes, which may exhibit different demographics and different underlying genetic etiology. One example is the greater tendency to manifest perilesional edema associated with frontotemporal and occipital meningiomas. An example of demographic differences based on location is the high percentage of female patients with meningiomas overlying the greater sphenoid wing.

The age of the patient is also important. Some data suggest that meningiomas arising in younger individuals are more aggressive, although definitive statistical evidence has not been collected.[13-15]

Even grade I meningiomas frequently invade adjacent soft tissues and bone (but not brain and generally not arterial walls). Invasion makes complete resection more difficult and predisposes to local recurrence. Invasion of dural sinuses, such as the superior sagittal sinus, is a significant negative prognostic feature, even if the tumor is histologically grade I. En plaque morphology is usually associated with grade I histology and is typically seen in the skull base, sphenoid, and orbital regions. Surgically, curative local resection is more difficult to achieve with en plaque tumors; and therefore they have a greater tendency to recur.

Etiology

The etiology of meningiomas is multifactorial. There is clear evidence that local irradiation is associated with an increased incidence of meningiomas. Head trauma was believed by Cushing to be causative; however, this has not been confirmed and remains controversial.[16]

Viral particles of many types are found within the genetic material of meningiomas, which provides circumstantial evidence for an etiologic role in their growth. For example, papovaviruses such as BK and SV40, as well as adenovirus DNA, have been found in meningiomas. The exact role, if any, that viral genetic material plays in meningioma origin and/or growth remains uncertain.[17]

Pathophysiology

The genetic basis for meningiomas is currently under intensive ongoing study.[18] As in many other neoplasms, meningiomas are believed to arise by a multi-hit mechanism of genetic damage or abnormality, possibly involving damage or absence of a suppressor gene, as well as amplification or abnormality of an active pro-oncogene.[19] The most common genetic abnormality associated with meningioma is that found on chromosome 22q12, which is implicated in neurofibromatosis type 2 (NF2). Meningiomas are part of the NF2 syndrome, which is associated with multiple inherited schwannomas, meningiomas, and ependymomas, giving rise to the mnemonic MISME, pronounced "miss me." NF2 is associated with abnormal gene function at chromosome 22q12, which codes for a protein named merlin or schwannomin. Merlin's function is still under study, but it is believed to regulate cell-cell contact inhibition and also to play a role in cell morphology. Inactivation would therefore result in cells with altered morphology and impaired contact inhibition. *NF2* mutations are seen in patients with NF2 and also in more than half of patients with sporadic meningiomas. It has also been shown that other chromosome 22 mutations distinct from the *NF2* locus are common in meningiomas, suggesting that there may be another tumor suppressor locus on chromosome 22 distinct from that which encodes for merlin.[20,21] Some data suggest that different subpopulations of meningiomas based both on histology (transitional and fibrous) and location (anterior skull base) may be more likely to show merlin inactivation than others. Meningothelial tumors only rarely show reduced expression of merlin, and radiation-induced meningiomas also are associated with decreased likelihood of chromosome 22q12 abnormalities but are more likely to display structural abnormalities of chromosome 1p.

Chromosomal and genetic abnormalities that have been found in patients with meningiomas and particularly in patients with higher grade II and grade III meningiomas include dicentric or ring chromosomes, absence or alterations in 1p, 3p, 6q, 9p, 10q,[22] and 14q[23], and amplifications in 17q and 20q. These abnormalities may be associated both with origination of the meningothelial neoplasm and possibly also progression in grade.

Other specific genetic changes associated with atypical (grade II) and malignant or anaplastic (grade III) meningiomas include expression of the enzyme telomerase, which allows cells to maintain telomere length over multiple cell division cycles.[24] Proteins associated with increased angiogenesis, including tenascin and vascular endothelial growth factor, are also found in higher-grade meningiomas. In one group, 25% of malignant meningiomas showed deletions of the *CDKN2A* locus on chromosome 9p21. Other specific findings include the loss of the *NDRG2* gene on chromosome 14q11.2 and the gain of the *RPS6KB1* gene on chromosome 17q23 (Fig. 30-1).

It is fair to say that although many genetic findings associated with meningioma origination and progression to higher grade have been discovered, further work and study is expected to broaden our understanding of the developmental pathways of these tumors.

Meningiomas express a wide variety of cell surface proteins and receptors, including hormonal receptors.[25] Vimentin is virtually always present, and epithelial membrane antigen (EMA) reactivity is seen in the majority of cases. EMA is somewhat more specific than vimentin, which is generally diffusely positive but nonspecific. Claudin-1 may be useful in addition to EMA for ambiguous cases.

The role of hormonal receptors in meningioma growth is complex and not fully understood. Estrogen, progesterone, and androgen receptors may be found in meningiomas. Immunopositivity for progesterone is by far more common than other hormone receptors.[26] Progesterone receptors have been shown to stimulate meningeal cell growth in vitro culture, and progesterone receptor inhibitors have been shown to have the opposite effect. In addition, the extent of progesterone receptor expression appears to be inversely proportional to tumor grade and proliferation.[27] Accordingly, benign tumors are more likely to express immunoreactivity to progesterone receptor antigens (50% to 80%). Estrogen receptors are somewhat less commonly expressed than progesterone receptors. The relationship between gender and hormonal receptor status remains an area of ongoing study.[28]

Other immunohistochemical markers seen in meningiomas include somatostatin, prolactin, and growth hormone receptors. Overall, there is no specific marker or pattern of markers that is universally diagnostic of meningothelial neoplasms.

Pathology

Histologic features of meningiomas are variable and reflect the dual mesenchymal and epithelial nature of the arachnoid cap cells that are believed to be of neural crest origin. Secretory meningiomas, for instance, are highly epithelial with glandular elements. Other meningiomas may contain primarily mesenchymal derivatives such as fatty elements (lipomeningioma) or even cartilage and bone. The category metaplastic meningioma can be subdivided because it refers to the tendency of some meningiomas to express specific mesenchymal cell types such as osseous, lipoid, and chondroid, and these features may occasionally provide distinct imaging features. Other meningiomas contain numerous small cysts (microcystic or humid meningiomas).

Each different subtype has specific histologic criteria, several of which may be present in one tumor but which is then categorized on the basis of dominant or majority features.

Imaging
Radiography

Meningiomas exhibit several imaging features that may be seen on plain radiographs. Meningiomas may stimulate hyperostosis in underlying bone, which is believed secondary to secretion of factors that stimulate osteoblasts. This is also observed on nuclear medicine bone scintiscans as increased radiotracer deposition. As meningiomas grow through the calvaria, they may produce an exophytic hyperostosis in the scalp referred to as "hair-on-end" appearance (Fig. 30-2). Finally, meningiomas may contain psammomatous regions, and if dense enough these may be seen as hazy areas of calcification.

Angiography

Although less commonly used today, angiography was once the mainstay of diagnostic evaluation of intracranial tumors. Meningiomas are distinctive owing to their primary arterial supply from the middle meningeal branch of the external carotid artery or secondarily by posterior meningeal artery branches (Fig. 30-3). They also typically show early brisk arterial filling

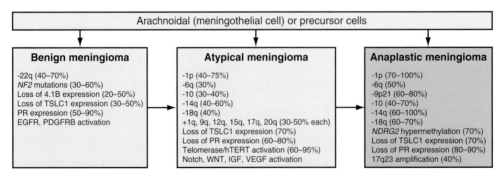

■ **FIGURE 30-1** Genetic model of meningioma tumorigenesis and malignant progression. EGFR, Epidermal growth factor receptor; hTERT, telomerase reverse transcriptase; IGF, insulin-like growth factor; *NDRG2*, N-Myc downstream regulated gene 2; PDGFRB, platelet-derived growth factor receptor, beta polypeptide; PR, progesterone receptor; TSLC1, tumor suppressor in lung cancer-1; VEGF, vascular endothelial growth factor. (*From Louis DN, Ohgaki H, Wiestler OD, Cavenee WK. WHO Classification of Tumors of the Central Nervous System. Albany, NY, World Health Organization Publications Center, 2007.*)

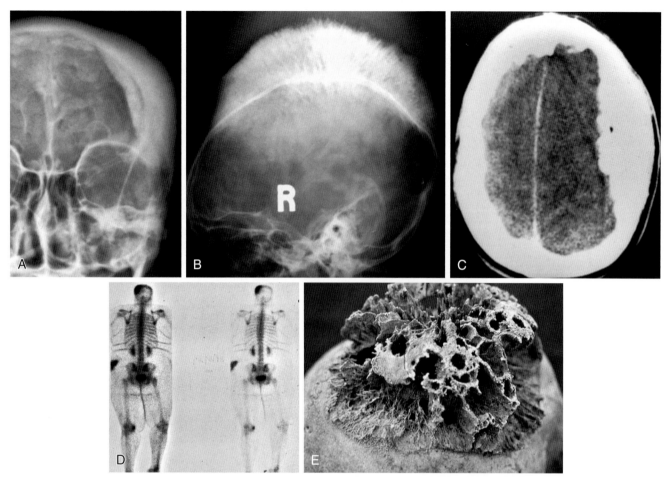

■ **FIGURE 30-2** Osseous manifestations of meningiomas in different patients. Frontal and lateral skull radiographs (**A, B**), and axial CT image (**C**) show prominent hyperostosis with typical hair-on-end appearance. Bone scintiscan (**D**) shows increased radiotracer uptake. Postmortem skull (**E**) shows marked, coarse, hyperostotic changes.

and delayed venous washout, sometimes referred to as the "the in-law sign" because of the pattern of arriving early and staying late. Angiographic visualization of meningiomas is currently performed primarily in order to perform preoperative embolization, which has been shown to decrease blood loss in difficult cases. Angiographic venous phase or MR venographic images may also be important to document impingement on dural sinuses (Fig. 30-4).

CT

On CT, meningiomas are generally hyperdense to brain parenchyma and enhance briskly and uniformly. If histologic variants are present, different imaging appearances may predominate. Microcystic meningioma may exhibit low density nearer to water. If lipomatous metaplasia has occurred, fatty density is seen (Fig. 30-5). Psammomatous calcifications may be present, giving a hazy sand-like appearance, whereas coarse calcifications may be observed with osseous metaplasia. Hyperostosis generally reflects thickening of bone adjacent to the tumor. Perilesional edema may be seen as low density following white matter tracts. Some meningiomas, presumably after many years, may become densely calcified throughout.

MRI

The great majority (80% to 90%) of meningiomas are grade I, and this figure may be higher if small asymptomatic tumors are included. The majority of these tumors display typical meningothelial histology without metaplastic or other atypical features. Typical imaging features consist of a rounded, smooth

and well-circumscribed extra-axial mass that is broad based against the dural surface. These lesions show dense and homogeneous enhancement, frequently with adjacent dural thickening and enhancement described as the "dural tail" (Fig. 30-6). This dural tail has been found to be reactive in most cases and may not represent extension of the neoplasm. It is suggestive but not specific for meningioma, and it is commonly seen in other dural-based tumors as well.[29,30] Most common locations include the frontal convexities and the falx as well as the sphenoid wing. Other typical but less common locations include the orbital sheath, the tentorium cerebelli, the petroclinoid ligaments, the cavernous sinuses, and the olfactory grooves (Fig. 30-7).

If any of several less common histologic variants are present, the MRI signal characteristics may vary, following water (Fig. 30-8), fat, or bone signal intensity. Central sand-like or psammomatous calcification is relatively common and will be hypointense on MRI (Fig. 30-9). Markedly prominent vascularity in an otherwise benign meningioma may be designated as an angiomatous meningioma (Fig. 30-10).

Morphologic variations range from rounded to flattened, or en plaque, configurations. Perilesional edema may be present to varying degrees, and some studies suggest that this is more common in frontal than occipital tumors. Although present in all three grades, perilesional edema may be somewhat more common and more exuberant in higher-grade tumors and may be associated with increased likelihood of local recurrence after surgical resection (Fig. 30-11).

Text continued on page 651

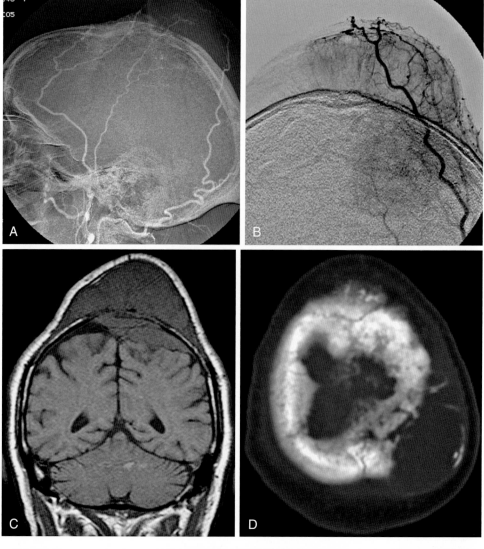

■ **FIGURE 30-3** Angiographic images (**A**, **B**) show typical middle and posterior meningeal artery supply to this large transcalvarial meningioma. Coronal T1W MR image (**C**) shows the substantial intracalvarial and extracalvarial soft tissue components of this mass and axial CT scan (**D**) shows the intact but altered bony structure at the tumor site.

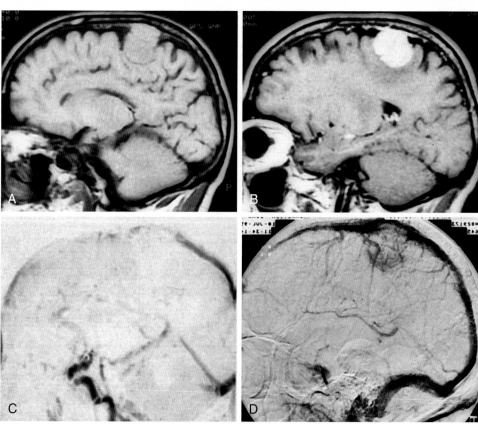

■ **FIGURE 30-4** Sagittal T1W images before (**A**) and after (**B**) administration of gadolinium and early and late venous phase angiograms (**C**, **D**) showing meningioma impinging on superior sagittal sinus.

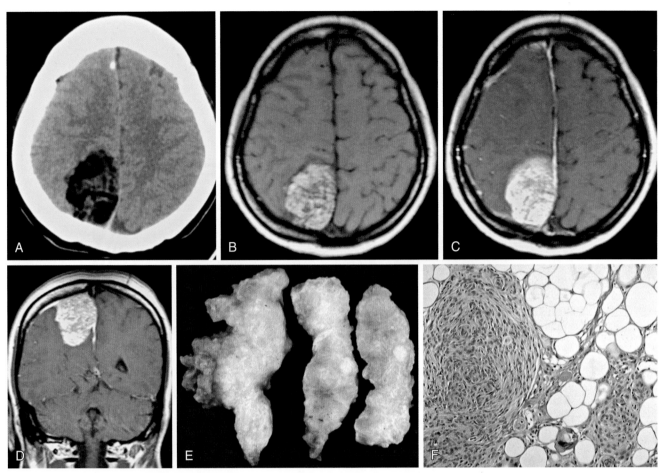

■ **FIGURE 30-5** Lipomeningioma. Low density is seen on noncontrast CT (**A**). Fatty high T1 signal intensity is seen on a nonenhanced T1W image (**B**), which is somewhat less obvious on postgadolinium axial and coronal T1W MR images (**C, D**). Gross pathologic specimen (**E**) shows typical yellow fatty tissue, and hematoxylin and eosin–stained (×100) microscopic specimen (**F**) shows lipid globules.

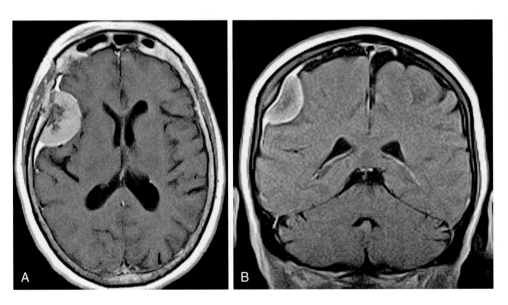

■ **FIGURE 30-6** Axial (**A**) and coronal (**B**) postgadolinium T1W MR images show dense homogeneous enhancement and a "dural tail." Some hyperostosis is also present. The dark signal intensity centrally is due to psammomatous or sand-like calcifications.

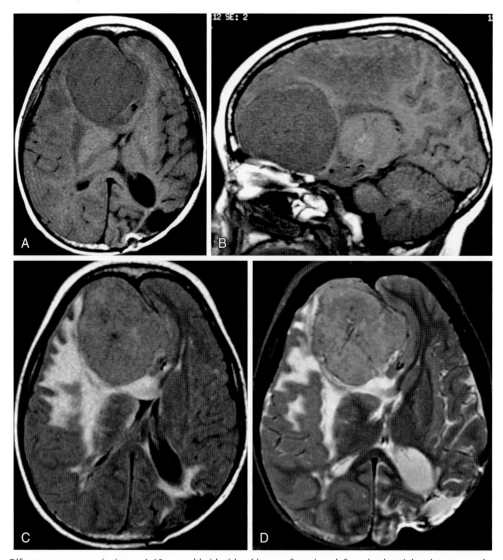

■ **FIGURE 30-7**   Olfactory groove meningioma. A 13-year-old girl with a history of previous left parietal peripheral neuroectodermal tumor and sub-sequent chemotherapy and radiation therapy presented with a headache that had been increasing in severity over the previous 2 weeks. Axial and sagittal T1W MR images (**A, B**) show a large extra-axial mass centered in the anteroinferior left frontal region with significant midline shift. Axial FLAIR (**C**) and T2W MR (**D**) images show prominent perilesional edema as well as postsurgical encephalomalacia in the left parietal lobe. Surgical excision followed by pathologic evaluation revealed olfactory groove meningioma with significant atypia classified as WHO grade II.

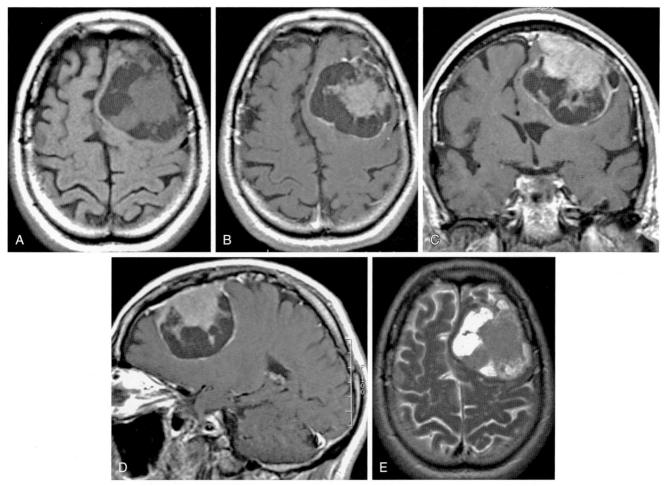

■ **FIGURE 30-8** Cystic meningioma. Axial T1W noncontrast (**A**) and axial (**B**), coronal (**C**), and sagittal (**D**) postgadolinium and axial T2W (**E**) MR images show left frontal meningioma with prominent cystic regions typically located deep to the dural surface.

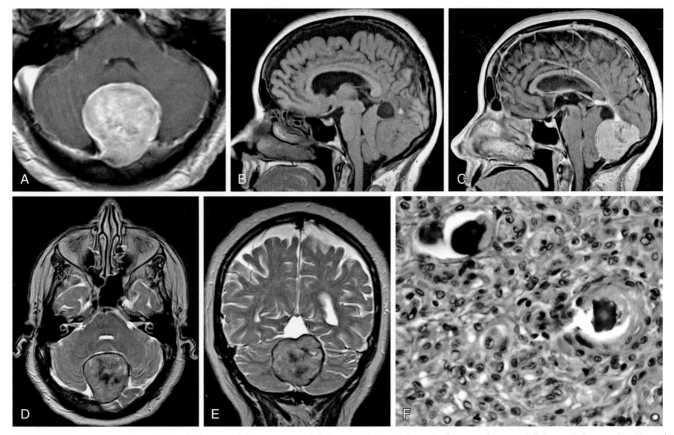

■ **FIGURE 30-9** Psammomatous meningioma. Axial T1W postgadolinium MR image (**A**), sagittal pre- and postgadolinium MR images (**B, C**), and axial and coronal T2W MR images (**D, E**) show hazy low signal intensity, as well as a dural tail in this posterior fossa meningioma. The histologic slide (**F**) shows the sand-like calcification or psammoma body.

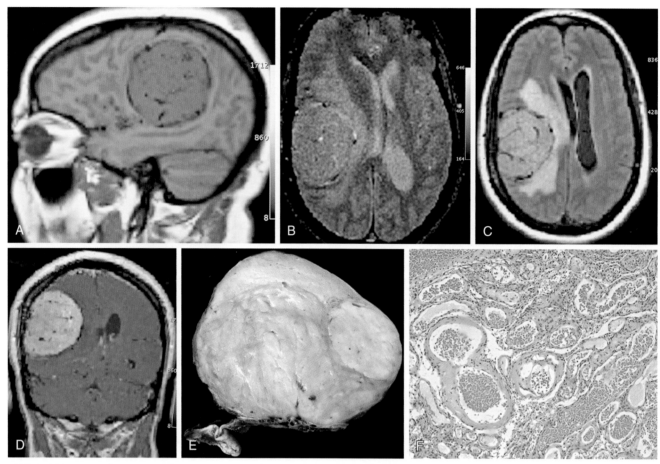

■ **FIGURE 30-10** Angiomatous meningioma. A 53-year-old woman presented with left upper extremity symptoms. Sagittal T1 (**A**), axial T2 (**B**), FLAIR (**C**), and coronal postgadolinium T1W (**D**) MR images display a highly vascular right frontoparietal mass with dense homogeneous enhancement with prominent vascular flow voids. Gross (**E**) and microscopic (**F**) pathologic sections also show an unusually prominent vascular pattern.

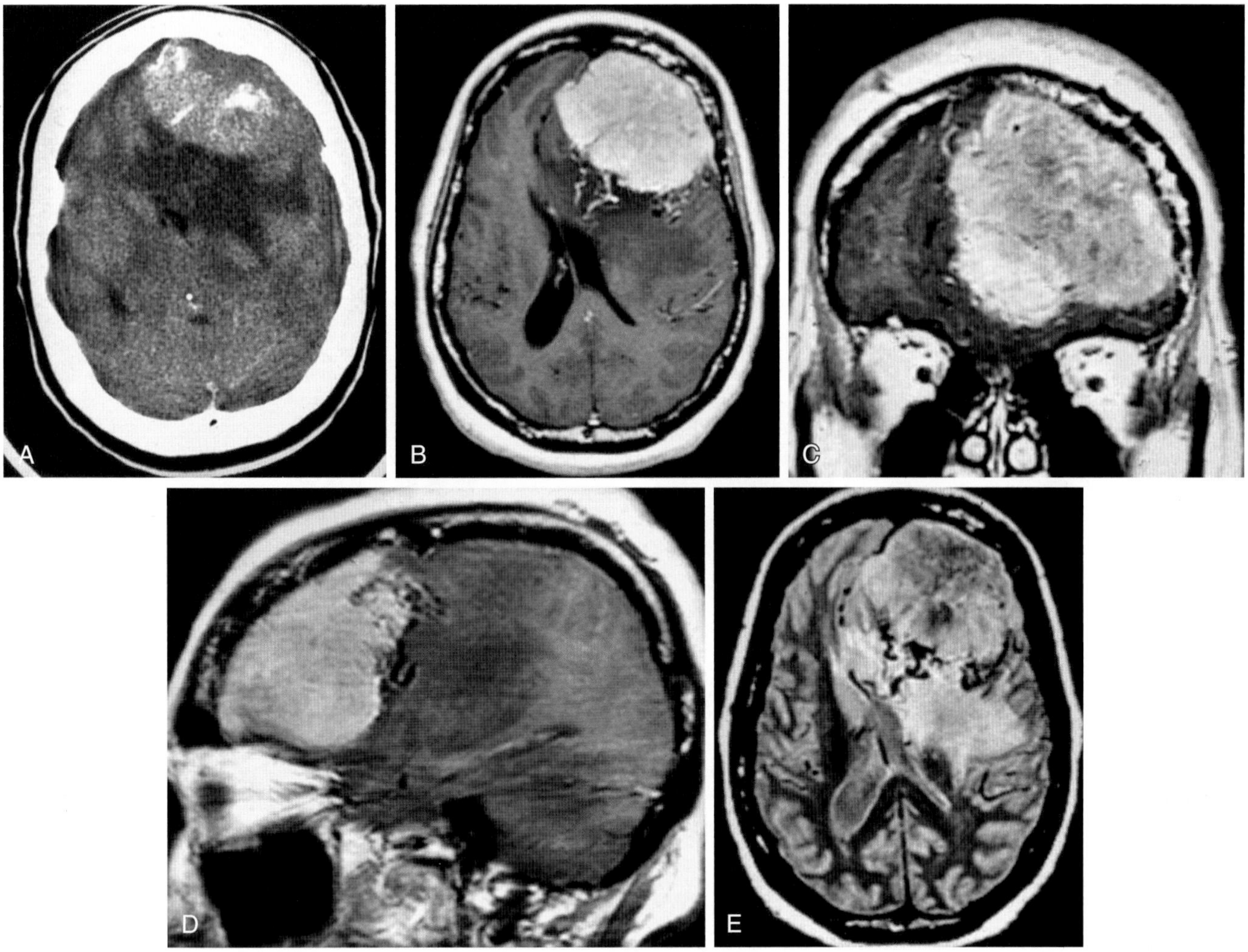

■ **FIGURE 30-11** Malignant meningioma, WHO grade III. This tumor shows increased density on a nonenhanced CT image (**A**) and diffuse relatively homogeneous enhancement on postgadolinium axial (**B**), coronal (**C**), and sagittal (**D**) T1W and axial proton density (**E**) MR images. Note the irregular margins, prominent vascularity, and exuberant perilesional edema, all of which are nonspecific but atypical for benign meningioma.

Meningioma location is usually dural based but may also be intraventricular, usually in the atrium of the lateral ventricles. Intraventricular meningiomas are most commonly typical grade I benign lesions (Fig. 30-12) but may occasionally be atypical grade II (Fig. 30-13) or even malignant grade III lesions.

Atypical (grade II) meningiomas, such as clear cell (Fig. 30-14) and chordoid (Fig. 30-15) subtypes, or malignant (grade III) meningiomas, including subtypes papillary (Fig. 30-16) and rhabdoid (Fig. 30-17), may be indistinguishable from "vanilla" or grade I tumors. Not uncommonly, however, they may display greater irregularity in margins and in overall morphology and may be seen to invade brain parenchyma. Florid perilesional edema is somewhat more common in higher-grade meningiomas as well. Atypical imaging features do sometimes but not invariably follow atypical histologic patterns.

Special Procedures
Meningiomas may show increased radiotracer deposition in bone scintigraphy due to hyperostosis in adjacent bone, or the tumor may itself accumulate radiotracer due to intrinsic ossification.

MENINGIOANGIOMATOSIS
Meningioangiomatosis is a rare meningovascular lesion or hamartoma that is usually located in the cortex and/or leptomeninges and may be associated with NF2.

Epidemiology
This lesion is often sporadic but is also found in patients with NF2 or central neurofibromatosis. If sporadic, it is most often a single lesion or mass, but when associated with NF2 it may be present in multiple locations. Meningioangiomatosis usually presents in children or young adults.

Clinical Presentation
Clinical presentation is either as an associated finding in patients with known or suspected NF2[31] or sporadic, as an unsuspected finding in a patient with seizure, headache, or other neurologic symptom.[32] Sporadic meningioangiomatosis appears to be genetically distinct from NF2, although both may be related to abnormality on different loci on chromosome 22.[33]

Pathophysiology
Meningioangiomatosis is a hamartomatous proliferation of meningothelial and vascular elements that may involve both the leptomeninges and the brain cortex but does not extend into white matter.

The histogenesis of this lesion is unknown. When it is sporadic it is caused by a genetic defect on chromosome 22 distinct from the NF2 lesion on chromosome 22q12. Meningiomas may be found adjacent to or within an area of meningioangiomatosis, and it is not known if the meningioma arises concurrently or secondarily within the lesion.[34] When present, the meningioma

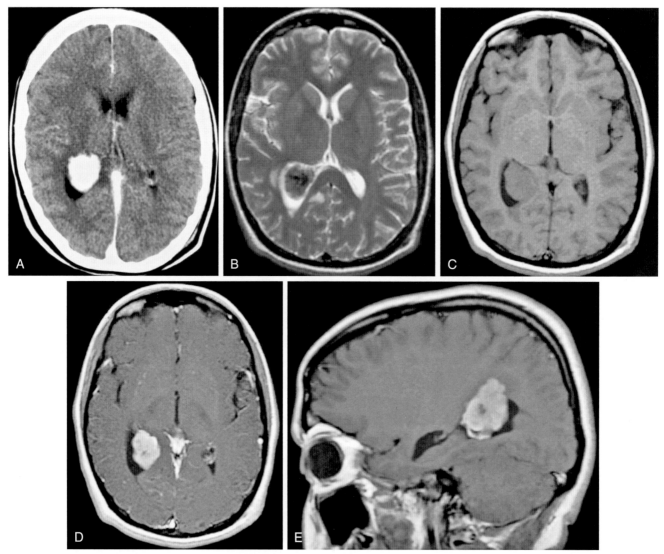

■ **FIGURE 30-12** Intraventricular meningioma, WHO grade I, in a 16-year-old girl with recurrent syncope. Contrast-enhanced CT image (**A**) shows an ovoid, well-circumscribed, densely enhancing mass in the atrium of the right lateral ventricle. Axial T1W (**B**), T2W (**C**), and axial and sagittal post-gadolinium (**D, E**) MR images show a densely enhancing mass with some low signal intensity on T2 weighting, suggesting calcification. Pathologic examination revealed typical meningothelial meningioma.

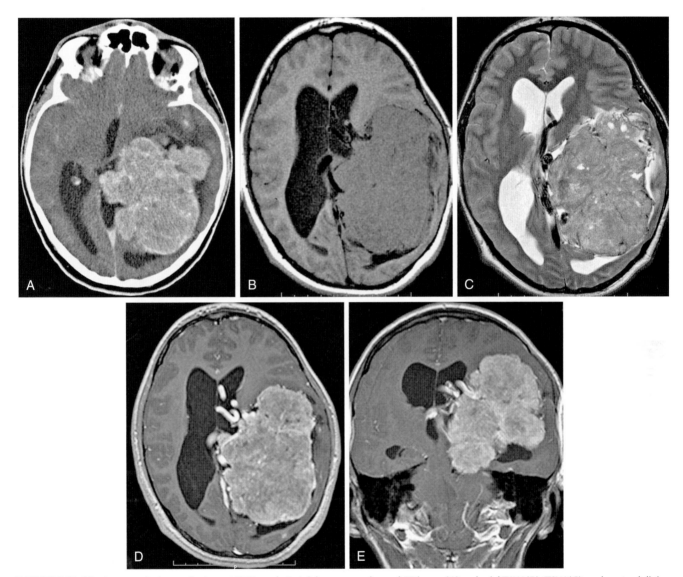

■ **FIGURE 30-13** Intraventricular meningioma, WHO grade II. Axial contrast-enhanced CT image (**A**) and axial T1W (**B**), T2W (**C**), and postgadolinium axial (**D**) and coronal (**E**) T1W MR images show a large mass centered at the atrium of the left lateral ventricle with somewhat irregular margins and diffuse but slightly heterogeneous enhancement. Atypical imaging features correspond, in this case, but not always, with atypical histology.

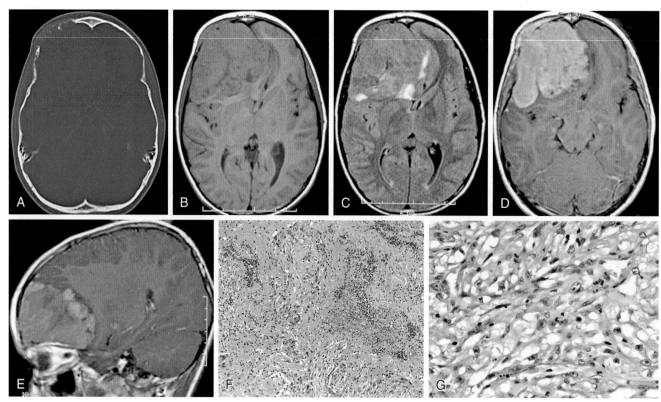

■ **FIGURE 30-14**   Meningioma, clear cell subtype, WHO grade II. An 11-year-old boy presented with a palpable abnormality of the right forehead. CT with bone windows (**A**) demonstrates bone invasion and destruction. Axial T1 (**B**) and FLAIR (**C**) MR images show a large, somewhat irregular mass that is slightly heterogeneous with perilesional edema. Axial (**D**) and sagittal (**E**) postgadolinium T1W MR images show moderate, diffuse, but somewhat heterogeneous enhancement. Photomicrographs taken after staining with hematoxylin and eosin at 100× (**F**) and 400× (**G**) show meningothelial cells with round to ovoid nuclei, multiple prominent nucleoli, and clear cytoplasm. Multiple mitotic figures are seen as well as foci of necrosis, thereby meeting criteria for WHO grade II.

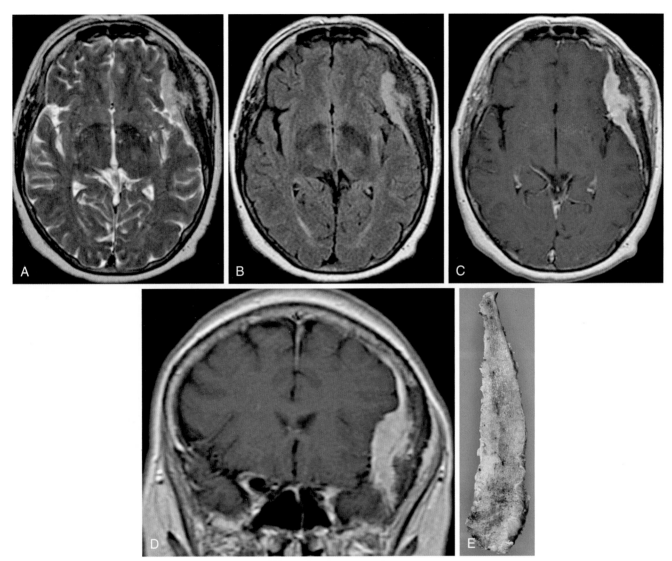

■ **FIGURE 30-15** Intraosseous meningioma, chordoid subtype, WHO grade II, in a 65-year-old woman with confusion, amnesia, and a palpable left temporal lesion. Axial T2W (**A**), FLAIR (**B**), and axial (**C**) and coronal postgadolinium T1W (**D**) MR images reveal expansion of the temporal bone (**E**) with an en plaque–enhancing dural lesion and extension into scalp and temporalis muscle. Pathologic examination reveals "nests and cords of cells embedded in a mucoid matrix" with a moderate mitotic index, as well as extensive invasion of scalp and dura.

may commonly show brain invasion, but the prognosis in these cases is better than expected for an invasive meningioma.

Pathology
On pathologic examination there are diffusely thickened and/or nodular cortical regions occasionally with evidence of hemosiderin staining and/or calcifications.

Different examples of meningioangiomatosis display a spectrum between more cellular and more vascular histology. The cellular examples consist of clustered spindle-shaped cells that are believed to be meningothelial, arising in a perivascular location with more nearly normal blood vessels. The more vascular lesions are less cellular and show blood vessels with thickened and calcified vessel walls.[35] Immunohistochemical staining shows an array of results, with virtually all cases positive for vimentin, many positive for EMA, and some positive for neuron-specific enolase (NSE) and some for glial fibrillary acidic protein (GFAP).[36] These results are not cohesive, and the histogenesis of this lesion remains uncertain.

Imaging
CT
Focal cortical thickening, possibly with gyriform calcifications can be seen on CT.

MRI
On MRI there may be focal regions of cortical thickening and signal changes, possibly with hypointense regions indicating previous hemorrhage and/or calcifications (Fig. 30-18).

HEMATOPOIETIC AND HISTIOCYTIC NEOPLASMS OF THE MENINGES
Neoplasms of hematopoietic tissue may arise primarily within the meninges and include lymphoma, histiocytic tumors, and plasma cell neoplasms. Dural lymphoma is discussed separately in the next section on primary meningeal lymphoma. Additional names for these disorders include primary leptomeningeal lymphoma, dural plasmacytoma, dural myeloma, myelomatous

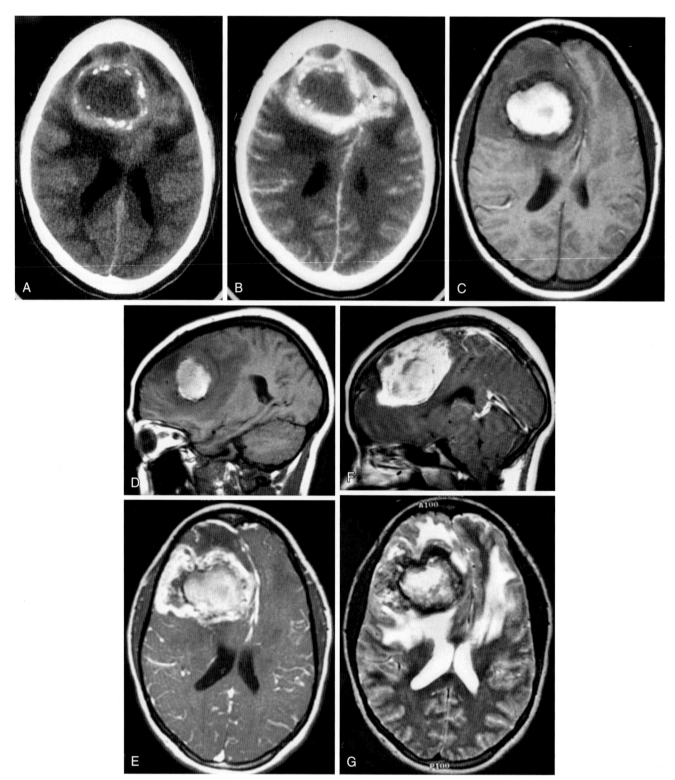

■ **FIGURE 30-16** Papillary meningioma, WHO grade III, in a 16-year-old girl with headache, confusion, and syncope. CT scan without contrast (**A**, **B**) shows a large right frontal mass with ring calcifications and central necrosis. Axial (**C**) and sagittal (**D**) unenhanced T1W MR images show bright T1 signal presumably owing to blood products in the necrotic center. Postgadolinium axial (**E**) and sagittal (**F**) T1W MR images demonstrate the ring enhancement and mass effect of the tumor. Axial T2W MR image (**G**) demonstrates extensive perilesional edema and necrotic center. Microscopic evaluation reveals sheets of polyhedral cells that form papillary-like structures with fibrovascular cores, as well as widespread necrosis and foci of calcification.

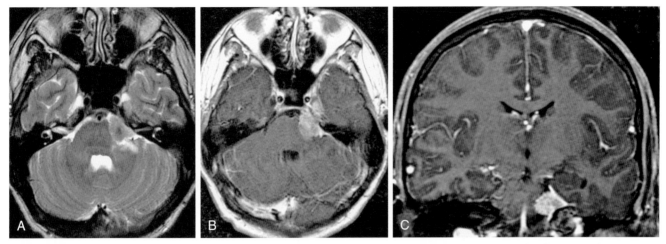

■ **FIGURE 30-17** Rhabdoid meningioma, WHO grade III, in a 19-year-old man with facial numbness in V1 and V2 distribution. Axial T2W (**A**) and axial (**B**) and coronal (**C**) T1W postgadolinium MR images reveal an enhancing, extra-axial, dural-based mass in the left cerebellopontine angle extending into the left Meckel cave, with slight perilesional edema. Pathologic evaluation revealed spindle and epithelioid cells with ovoid to elongated nuclei. Immunohistochemistry showed markedly increased MIB-1 positivity.

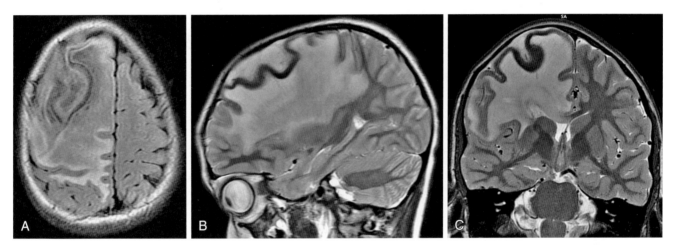

■ **FIGURE 30-18** Meningioangiomatosis. This patient is a 10-year-old boy with an 8-year history of worsening seizure disorder. Axial FLAIR (**A**), sagittal (**B**), and coronal T2W (**C**) MR images show cortical thickening and hypointensity with extensive underlying edema. After surgical resection, pathologic evaluation revealed meningothelial cells and vascular elements, with microscopic hemorrhage and dystrophic cortical calcifications.

meningitis, Langerhans cell histiocytosis, non–Langerhans cell histiocytoses, Rosai-Dorfman disease, Erdheim-Chester disease, and intracranial Castleman's disease.

Pathophysiology

The histogenesis of primary tumors of hematopoietic cells found in the leptomeninges without detectable primary site elsewhere is problematic because hematopoietic and histiocytic cells do not normally arise in the CNS or more particularly in the leptomeninges. Histiocytic masses such as Langerhans cell histiocytosis as well as the non–Langerhans cell histiocytoses, Rosai-Dorfman disease (Fig. 30-19),[37] Erdheim-Chester disease (Fig. 30-20),[38] and Castleman's disease (Fig. 30-21)[39] are of uncertain histogenesis but may arise within the hematopoietic system and deposit on the dura for reasons that are not presently understood. Dural plasmacytoma (Fig. 30-22) is a solitary mass of neoplastic monoclonal plasma cells that may be related to systemic monoclonal gammopathy or multiple myeloma. Dural chloroma (Fig. 30-23) is the name used for a focal solid deposit of leukemic cells, which may also be referred to as a granulocytic sarcoma.

Pathology

Each of these various lesions has distinctive clinical, gross pathologic, and histologic characteristics that are discussed more fully elsewhere[40] and are identical to those found in similar lesions elsewhere in the body.

Imaging

Imaging characteristics of these lesions are nonspecific and very similar to those for meningioma, being rounded or lobulated, well-circumscribed dural-based masses that are somewhat hyperdense on noncontrast CT, with dense uniform enhancement.

PRIMARY MENINGEAL LYMPHOMA

Primary meningeal lymphoma refers to lymphoma arising in meningeal tissues without a demonstrable primary site elsewhere. Additional names include primary leptomeningeal lymphoma, dural lymphoma, primary CNS lymphoma, and B-cell type non-Hodgkin's lymphoma.

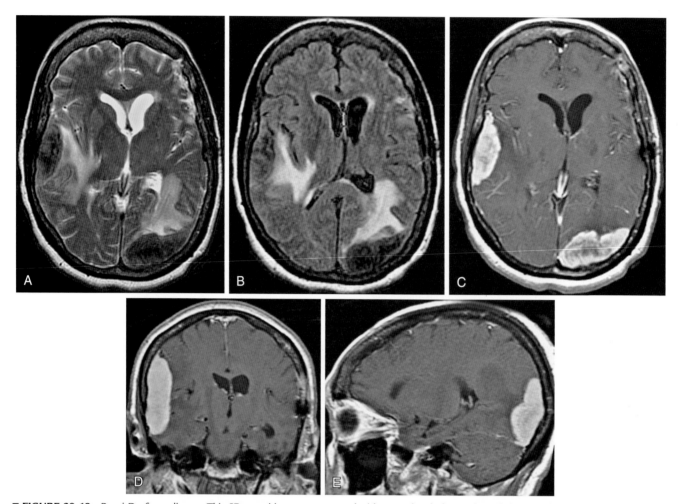

■ **FIGURE 30-19** Rosai-Dorfman disease. This 57-year-old woman presented with severe headaches and was believed to have multiple meningiomas based on imaging. Surgery and pathologic evaluation revealed histiocytes and plasma cells. Axial T2 (**A**), FLAIR (**B**), and axial (**C**), coronal (**D**), and sagittal (**E**) postgadolinium T1W MR images show densely enhancing, dural-based masses with moderate perilesional edema.

Epidemiology

Approximately 7% of primary intracranial lymphomas present as a primary site in the brain coverings. They are usually leptomeningeal, with dural primary lesions being much less common.[41]

Clinical Presentation

Clinical presentation varies widely from focal neurologic deficits to other more global CNS symptoms depending on site and extent of involvement.

Pathophysiology

The existence of primary meningeal lymphoma is problematic owing to the absence of lymphatic tissue in the CNS. Assuming that no primary site is found elsewhere and that no occult site is believed to exist elsewhere, it is presumed that malignant transformation occurs in cells that invade or migrate into dural or leptomeningeal tissues. It could also be argued that the malignant transformation occurs elsewhere, perhaps in a systemic location, with subsequent hematogenous dissemination. One theory is that the development of leptomeningeal specific adhesion molecules results in their presentation as primary leptomeningeal tumors, although this has not been proven. Extensive immunohistochemical and genetic analysis has been performed in the attempt to determine if there is a distinct intracranial

clonal population, and examples are described that support the concept of primary CNS origin of at least some of these neoplastic cell lines.

Pathology

Gross pathology of these lesions varies from a diffuse thickening and infiltration to a focal mass resembling a meningioma.

The majority of primary CNS lymphomas are Epstein Barr–negative diffuse large B-cell lymphomas, although T-cell lymphoma has been reported.[41] There is a wide range of possible histologies of intracranial and meningeal lymphoma just as there is elsewhere in the body. Various classification schemes exist and are evolving to accurately organize and stratify these lesions by their clinical and pathophysiologic behavior.

Common features are dense collections of lymphoid cells that are frequently perivascular and frequently embedded in a reticulin network. Follicular or pseudofollicular patterns are described particularly in dural or leptomeningeal lymphoma in distinction from other CNS sites. Cellular morphology and degree of pleomorphism may vary widely. Most CNS lymphomas are B-cell non-Hodgkin's lymphoma and display a variety of cellular patterns, including centroblastic, anaplastic, immunoblastic, and T-cell/histiocyte-rich variants.

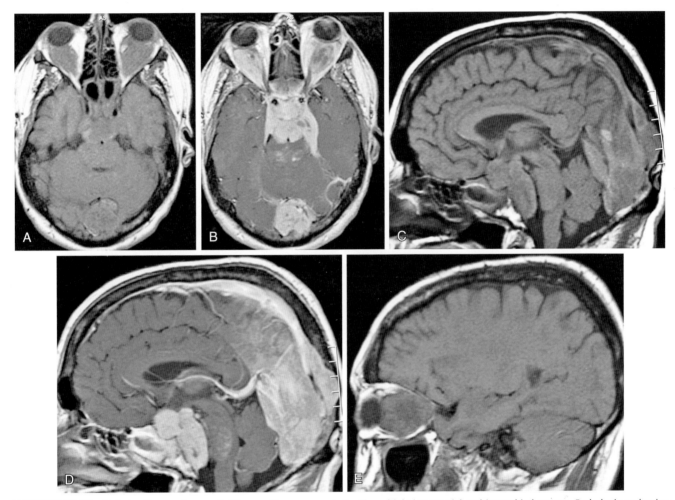

■ **FIGURE 30-20** Erdheim-Chester disease. A 37-year-old man presented with multiple intracranial and intraorbital masses. Pathologic evaluation revealed a histiocytic lesion with fibrosis. Axial nonenhanced (**A**) and postgadolinium (**B**), sagittal nonenhanced (**C**) and postgadolinium (**D**), and sagittal nonenhanced image targeting the orbit (**E**) reveal multiple, densely enhancing, well-circumscribed dural-based masses.

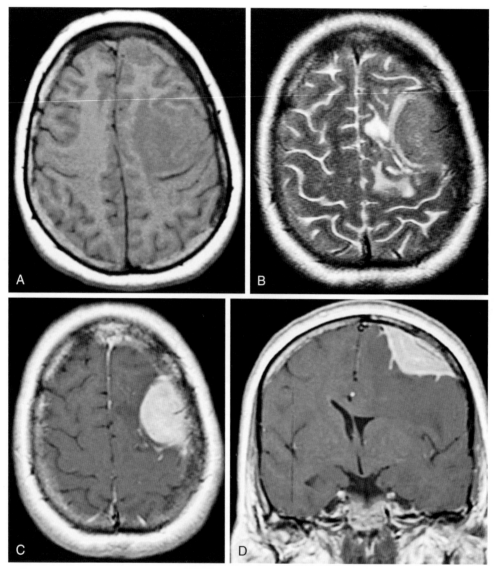

■ **FIGURE 30-21** Castleman's disease of dura in a 37-year-old woman with headache. Axial T1W (**A**), T2W (**B**), and postgadolinium axial (**C**) and coronal (**D**) T1W MR images show a moderate to large dural-based mass, relatively isointense to brain, with homogeneous enhancement. These imaging features would be perfectly typical for meningioma; however, pathologic examination revealed a monoclonal lymphocytic mass consistent with Castleman's disease.

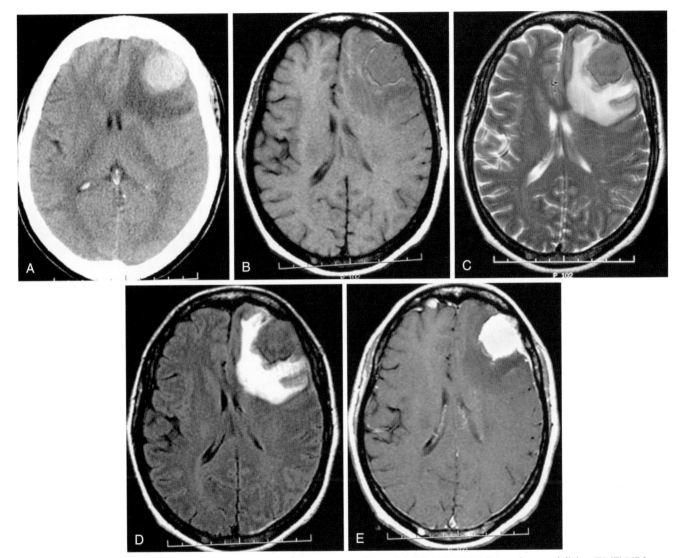

■ **FIGURE 30-22** Plasmacytoma of dura. Axial postcontrast CT image (**A**) and T1W (**B**), T2W (**C**), FLAIR (**D**), and postgadolinium T1 (**E**) MR images reveal a rounded, dural-based mass with perilesional edema and dense homogeneous enhancement.

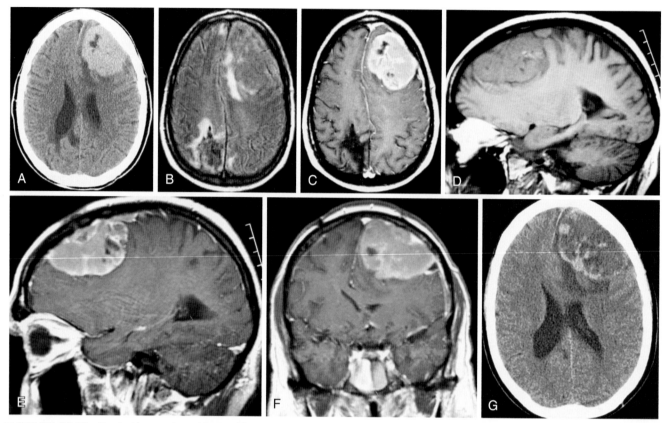

■ **FIGURE 30-23** Dural chloroma in a 45-year-old man with acute myelogenous leukemia. Axial contrast-enhanced CT image (**A**) and FLAIR (**B**), postgadolinium T1W (**C**), sagittal unenhanced (**D**) and postgadolinium (**E**), and coronal postgadolinium (**F**) MR images reveal a large, densely enhancing dural-based mass with small areas of nonenhancement. After chemotherapy, a contrast-enhanced CT scan (**G**) shows only minimal residual rim enhancement, indicating subtotal tumor necrosis.

Imaging

Imaging of meningeal lymphomas is relatively nonspecific (Fig. 30-24). Morphologic patterns range from diffuse or en plaque to focal and mass-like. They are generally denser than brain on noncontrast CT and enhance uniformly.

PRIMARY MESENCHYMAL NEOPLASMS OF THE MENINGES

Both benign and malignant mesenchymal neoplasms may arise in meningeal tissues. Names for these neoplasms include dural chondroma, dural chondrosarcoma, angiosarcoma, leiomyoma, leiomyosarcoma, fibrosarcoma, osteoma, osteosarcoma, leptomeningeal sarcoma or sarcomatosis, meningeal or leptomeningeal sarcoma or sarcomatosis, lipoma, and liposarcoma. Two specific entities, hemangiopericytoma and solitary fibrous tumor, are discussed separately in later sections.

Clinical Presentation

These tumors may present as a variety of symptoms, most commonly headache and/or seizure, depending on size and location.

Pathophysiology

The histogenesis of the wide variety of both benign and malignant mesenchymal neoplasms that may arise in the meningeal tissues is controversial. Theories include metaplasia and neoplastic transformation of fibroblasts versus neoplastic transformation of residual primitive mesenchymal cells. In either case, virtually the full range of mesenchymal tumors found elsewhere may arise primarily within the meninges, albeit rarely.

Malignant mesenchymal tumors of the meninges have been associated with viral infections such as human immunodeficiency virus and Epstein-Barr virus in several cases, suggesting a possible protumoral effect.[42]

Pathology

The histology of mesenchymal tumors varies with cell type and, in general, resembles the histologic features of the same type found elsewhere.

Imaging

Imaging features of mesenchymal neoplasms of the meninges may be nonspecific or may display features related to their histology. For instance, lipoma will show imaging features of fat, including marked low density on CT and high T1 signal intensity on MRI. Chondromas (Fig. 30-25)[43] and chondrosarcomas (Fig. 30-26) may show characteristic patterns such as flocculent or curvilinear calcifications. Angiosarcomas may show a permeative pattern of bone invasion and destruction with prominent vascular flow voids. Other tumors may be nonspecific such as Ewing's sarcoma[44] and undifferentiated sarcomas.[45,46]

HEMANGIOPERICYTOMA

Hemangiopericytoma (HPC) is a highly vascular neoplasm most commonly found extracranially, particularly in the pelvis, retroperitoneum, and lower extremities. The intracranial variety is almost always seen as a dural-based mass similar to meningioma. As the name suggests, the cell of origin was originally believed to be the pericyte, which is a cell type found adjacent to blood vessels throughout the body, although this is no longer

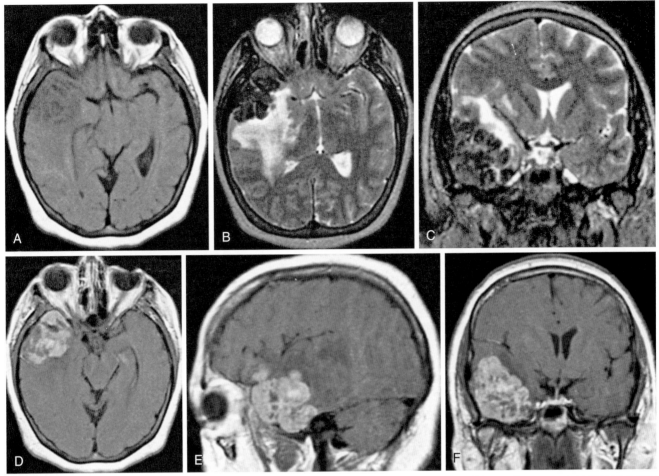

■ **FIGURE 30-24** Dural lymphoma in a 56-year-old woman with new-onset seizure and no previous history of a tumor. Axial T1W (A), T2W (B), coronal T2W (C), and postgadolinium axial (D), sagittal (E), and coronal T1W (F) MR images display a lobulated extra-axial mass in the right middle fossa with exuberant perilesional edema and slightly heterogeneous enhancement. Pathologic examination revealed follicular B-cell lymphoma.

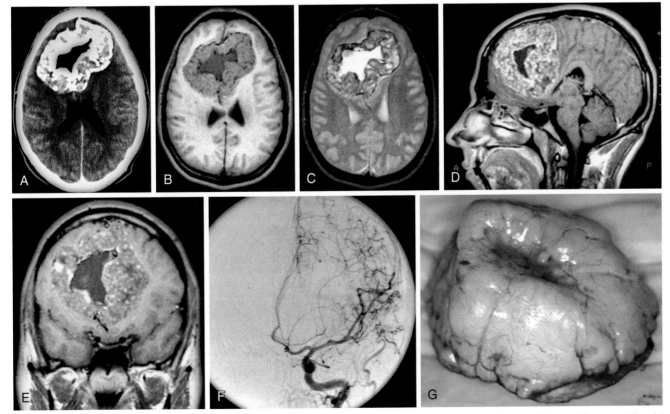

■ **FIGURE 30-25** Chondroma of the falx in a 26-year-old man with retro-orbital headache and memory loss. Imaging studies reveal large partially calcified mass centered on the anterior falx cerebri. Axial nonenhanced CT image (A), axial T1W (B), T2W (C), postgadolinium sagittal (D), and coronal T1W (E) MR images, and angiographic image (F) show displacement of the anterior cerebral artery. Gross pathologic specimen (G) shows glistening cartilaginous tumor.

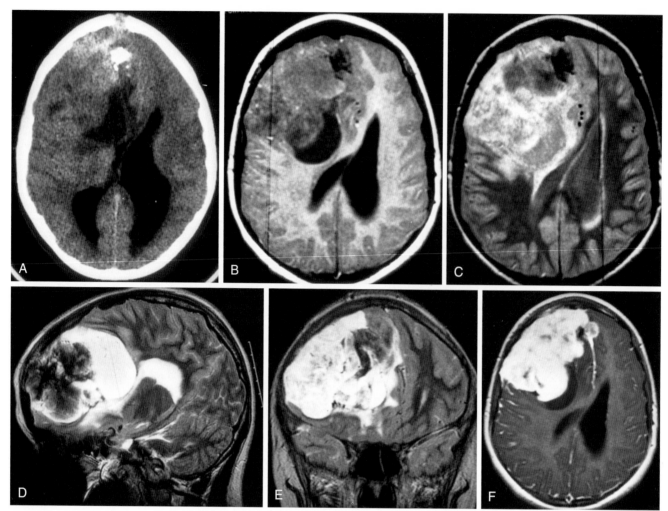

■ **FIGURE 30-26**   Chondrosarcoma of dura. A 13-year-old girl with a 1½-year history of headaches and 2-week history of proptosis was noted to have papilledema on ophthalmoscopic examination. Imaging studies displayed a large lobulated extra-axial mass in the left frontal region with some calcification and dense enhancement: axial nonenhanced CT image (**A**) and axial T1W (**B**), FLAIR (**C**), sagittal (**D**) and coronal T2W (**E**), and postgadolinium axial T1W (**F**) MR images. Pathologic diagnosis was mesenchymal meningeal chondrosarcoma.

considered certain, and the exact histogenesis of these tumors is unknown.

Percival Bailey initially described the intracranial HPC in 1928 as an angioblastic meningioma, and this nomenclature was repeated by Cushing and Eisenhardt in 1938. The extracranial variety was first described in 1942, but it was not until 1954 that the similarity between intracranial and extracranial varieties was clarified. Still, the tendency to classify intracranial HPCs as angioblastic meningiomas persisted until the late 1980s when immunohistochemical, ultrastructural, and other studies confirmed that it was not a meningothelial neoplasm but was, in fact, identical to HPCs found elsewhere in the body. The term *angioblastic meningioma* is no longer used, and this neoplasm is not to be confused with *angiomatous meningioma,* which is a histologic subtype of the grade I meningiomas.

Epidemiology

HPCs are rare and comprise less than 0.5% of new intracranial tumors per year. They have a peak incidence in the fifth decade and are slightly more common in males than females. Pediatric examples occur rarely. There is an infantile type, occurring in children younger than 1 year of age, that may have a more favorable prognosis than tumors occurring in older children and

adults.[47] This does not apply to all early childhood HPCs, unfortunately (Fig. 30-27).

Clinical Presentation

The clinical presentation is similar to that of meningiomas, primarily headache, possibly with a focal neurologic deficit. In addition, however, endocrine disturbances may be seen and are of two types. Hypoglycemia may be present in 30% to 40% of patients and is believed due to insulin-like growth factor secreted by the tumor.[48] In addition, osteomalacia has been reported, and although the exact etiology is unknown, it is believed to be related to phosphate loss in urine, similar to that seen in other phosphaturic mesenchymal tumors.[49]

Pathophysiology

In terms of biologic aggressivity, HPCs may either be grade II or grade III neoplasms according to WHO criteria, and therefore have significantly greater morbidity than the great majority of meningiomas. Five-year survival is reported as 90% or more; however, 15-year survival is less than roughly 40%, reflecting their tendency to recur locally and also to metastasize elsewhere in the body, both in a somewhat delayed manner.[50]

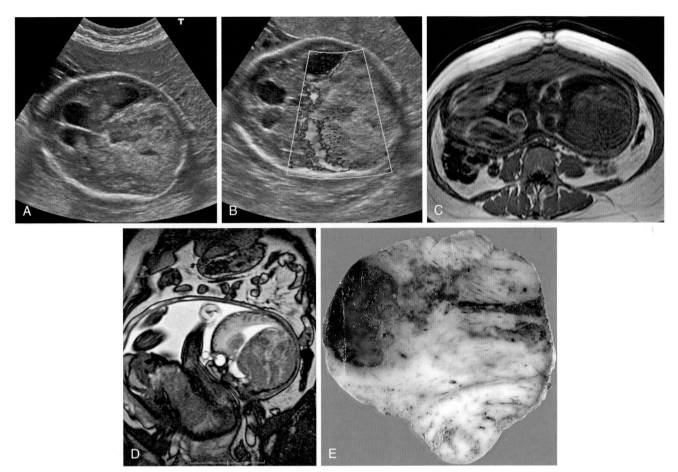

■ **FIGURE 30-27** Fetal hemangiopericytoma. Ultrasonography performed at 33 weeks' gestation shows a large, relatively hypovascular, posterior fossa mass (**A, B**), and subsequent T1W (**C**) and T2W (**D**) fetal MR images show a heterogeneous tumor with marked mass effect and obstructive hydrocephalus. Gross pathologic specimen (**E**) shows small focal areas of hemorrhage. Neuropathologic evaluation revealed marked pleomorphism, elevated mitotic index, and focal areas of hemorrhage and necrosis, suggesting a high-grade lesion.

Preliminary genetic study of these tumors has revealed rearrangements of 12q13 and, less consistently 19q13, 6p21, and 7p15,[51] as well as deletion of the *CDKN2A* tumor suppressor gene.[52] Some or various combinations of these defects are likely to give rise to this neoplasm; however, elucidation of a more definitive pathway will require further work.

Immunohistochemical analysis shows most HPCs to be positive for vimentin, CD99, factor XIIIa, Leu-7, and BCL-2, with partial positive staining for EMA and claudin and variable results for CD34. HPCs appear to be related to but distinct from the solitary fibrous tumor of the meninges (see later), which also mimics meningioma in imaging appearance.[53]

Pathology

HPCs are moderately cellular tumors with prominent branching vascular channels referred to as a staghorn vascular pattern. The predominant cell type is oval spindle cells, with occasional hypocellular areas and also areas of increased nuclear pleomorphism and atypia, multinucleated giant cells, and necrosis. Distinction between grade II and grade III is based on these features as well as on the presence of more than five mitoses per high-power field.

Imaging

HPCs are hyperdense on noncontrast CT but may be heterogeneous. They do not exhibit hyperostosis or intratumoral calcification and may have a narrow dural base. Bone erosion may be seen in roughly half.[54] They exhibit diffuse enhancement on both MRI and CT, which may be heterogeneous (Fig. 30-28). Some examples exhibit increased vascular flow voids on MRI; however, this is not always seen.[55] A reactive dural tail may be present.

SOLITARY FIBROUS TUMOR OF THE MENINGES

A solitary fibrous tumor (SFT) is an uncommon spindle cell neoplasm initially described originating in the visceral pleura of the lungs in 1931. Since then, it has been found in a variety of extrapleural sites, including the meninges, with a total number of more than 60 reported cases. The true incidence may be higher because of previous difficulty differentiating an SFT from both fibrous meningioma and HPC. This differentiation, particularly from HPC, is critical because the prognosis for SFT, with the exception of a few higher-grade examples, is very good, with a high likelihood of complete cure if the lesion is fully excised.

Epidemiology

Usually a tumor of adults, SFT has been reported in children.

Clinical Presentation

Clinical presentation is nonspecific and variable, depending on the size and location of the tumor, ranging from headache, to focal neurologic deficit, to exophthalmos.

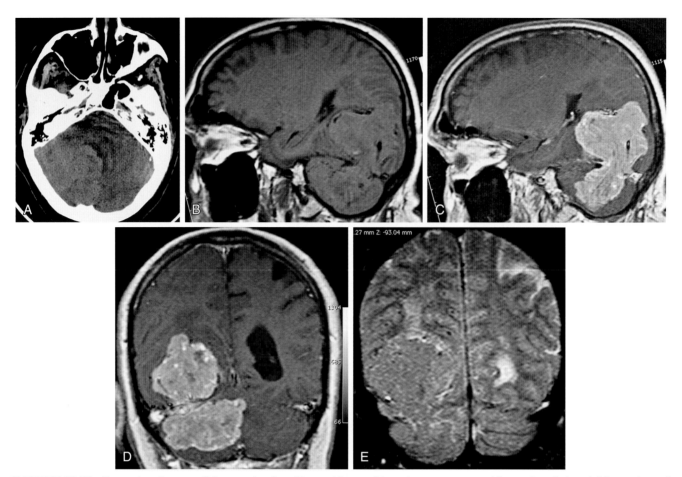

■ **FIGURE 30-28** Hemangiopericytoma of the tentorium in a 65-year-old man with weakness, nausea, vomiting, and confusion. Axial nonenhanced CT image (**A**) shows hyperdense mass above and below the right tentorium cerebelli. Sagittal T1W (**B**) and sagittal (**C**) and coronal (**D**) postgadolinium T1W and coronal T2W (**E**) MR images show a large, lobulated transtentorial mass with diffuse but slightly heterogeneous enhancement.

Pathophysiology

Meningeal SFT is a mesenchymal neoplasm that may be confused with fibrous meningioma and HPC. SFTs are strongly reactive for CD99, and this is also expressed by dural border cells, suggesting that this may be the cell of origin. SFTs are also nearly uniformly strongly reactive for CD34, and this is an important diagnostic criterion. Genetic analysis of SFT of the pleura has shown rearrangement of chromosome 12q13-15, and this is also seen in HPCs, providing further evidence that these tumors may be related.[56] Other study of SFTs elsewhere in the body has shown them to be karyotypically diverse,[57] with varied chromosomal and structural defects.

Clinically most SFTs are benign and do not recur unless incompletely resected.[58] There are reports of SFTs that display gross invasion of brain, dura, and bone.[59] Histologic features of necrosis and a high mitotic index have been described, and these tumors follow a more aggressive clinical course.[60]

Pathology

The SFT displays a range of histologic features that may resemble either fibrous meningiomas or HPCs. They consist of slender spindle cells embedded in a mesh of eosinophilic collagen bands in a characteristic lace-like pattern. More coalescent collagen bundles may also be present as well as areas of hyalinization. Prominent thin-walled vessels in a branching, or staghorn, pattern may be present that overlap in appearance with HPC.[53]

Immunohistochemically, SFTs express vimentin, as do meningiomas and HPC. They do not express either EMA or S-100, and this differentiates them from meningioma. SFTs overlap with HPC in that both express CD99 and BCL-2 but differ in that only SFTs are strongly positive reaction for CD34. Fibrous meningioma may resemble SFT histologically but will also lack strong CD34 positivity.[61]

Imaging

In general, SFTs are dense on noncontrast CT and densely enhancing on both CT and MRI and therefore may be indistinguishable from meningioma or HPC based solely on imaging findings. In one study, SFTs occasionally displayed heterogeneous enhancement and mixed T2 signal intensity, and these features may help provide some imaging differentiation. Calcification is not typically seen; however, bone invasion was present in one third of cases. Angiographic findings include abnormal tumor vessels and delayed tumor blush (Fig. 30-29).[62]

PRIMARY LEPTOMENINGEAL GLIAL AND NEURONAL NEOPLASMS

Neoplasms of glial origin may rarely arise from a primary site within the leptomeninges, presumably from heterotopic nests of glial tissue. The diagnosis is based on pathologic identification of a glial neoplasm either focally or diffusely involving the leptomeninges without clinical, imaging, or autopsy evidence of an intra-axial glial primary tumor. The dedicated and exhaustive search for a small or possibly occult intra-axial primary lesion is an essential component of the diagnosis. The origin

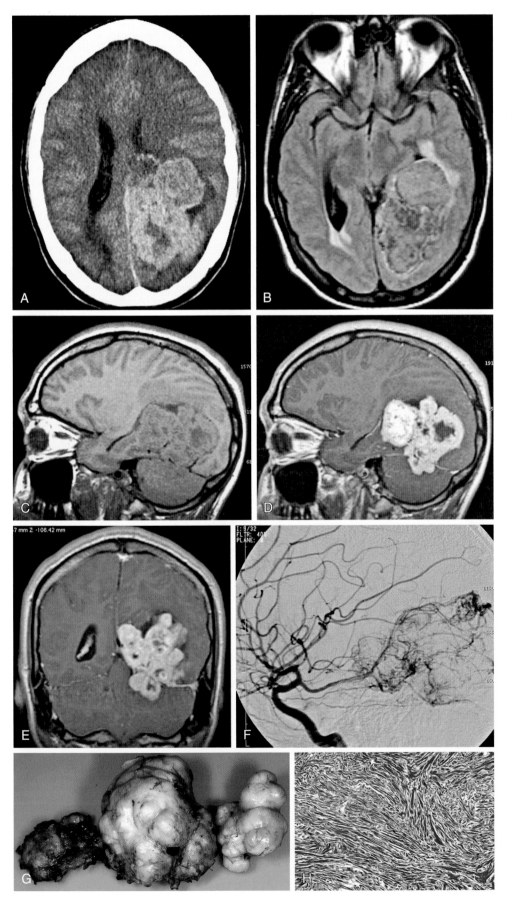

■ **FIGURE 30-29** Solitary fibrous tumor. Imaging reveals a large lobulated transtentorial mass with areas of central nonenhancement on contrast-enhanced (**A**), axial FLAIR (**B**), sagittal unenhanced (**C**), and sagittal (**D**) and coronal (**E**) postgadolinium T1W MR images. Angiography (**F**) reveals primary vascular supply from a hypertrophied anterior choroidal artery with abnormal neovascularity in more distal vessels. Gross pathologic specimen (**G**) displays complex nodular morphology, and trichrome stain (**H**) shows the marked prominence of fibrous connective tissue stained blue.

of leptomeningeal tumors that display neuronal or neuroectodermal differentiation is uncertain.

Alternate names include primary leptomemeningeal astrocytoma,[63] primary leptomeningeal glioblastoma, primary leptomeningeal oligodendroglioma (Fig. 30-30),[64] primary leptomeningeal gliosarcoma (Fig. 30-31), primary leptomeningeal gliomatosis,[65,66] primary leptomeningeal ependymoblastoma,[67] primary leptomeningeal ganglioglioma, meningeal glioma, primary leptomeningeal primitive neuroectodermal tumor,[68] (Fig. 30-32), and dural esthesioneuroblastoma (Fig. 30-33).

Epidemiology

This is an extremely rare category of neoplasms whose low incidence has not allowed for definitive demographic conclusions.

Clinical Presentation

Clinical presentation may be due to seizure, headache, or other more generalized neurologic symptoms due to increased intracranial pressure. Diagnosis is rare before death, and successful therapies are not currently available. The prognosis for most patients with these rare neoplasms is poor.

Pathophysiology

Heterotopic nests of non-neoplastic glial and neuronal tissues have been described within the leptomeninges on routine autopsy of up to 1% of normal patients and 25% of patients with other brain developmental abnormalities.[69] It is believed that, just as with intra-axial neoplasms, a cascade of genetic events can lead to the development of a neoplastic cell line within these cells.

Pathology

Gross pathologic examination may vary from a focal or nodular mass in the meningeal tissues to a diffuse thickening with focal mass.

The microscopic evaluation of these tumors reveals a spectrum similar to that found in intra-axial glial neoplasm, including elements of astrocytoma, oligodendroglioma, glioblastoma, gliosarcoma, and, in at least one case, ependymomatous elements. Neuroblastoma and neuroectodermal tumors, although rare, may also be seen as primary dural masses.

Imaging

The imaging findings of primary leptomeningeal glial neoplasms may vary from a focal enhancing meningeal mass to a diffuse thickening and enhancement that may be very subtle. Important differential diagnostic considerations include a wide variety of more common entities such as en plaque meningioma, leptomeningeal spread of a systemic primary neoplasm or of a CNS primary tumor, as well as a variety of non-neoplastic conditions, including meningitis, sarcoid, and other diseases of meningeal thickening.

■ **FIGURE 30-30** Oligodendrogliomatosis of leptomeninges. A 12-year-old boy presented with acute onset of inability to walk or talk. Initial diagnosis was meningoencephalitis, but subsequent imaging studies display diffuse leptomeningeal thickening and enhancement on axial (**A, B**) and sagittal (**C, D**) unenhanced and postgadolinium MR images. Findings at surgery and pathologic evaluation indicate grade III to IV oligodendrogliomatosis without intra-axial involvement.

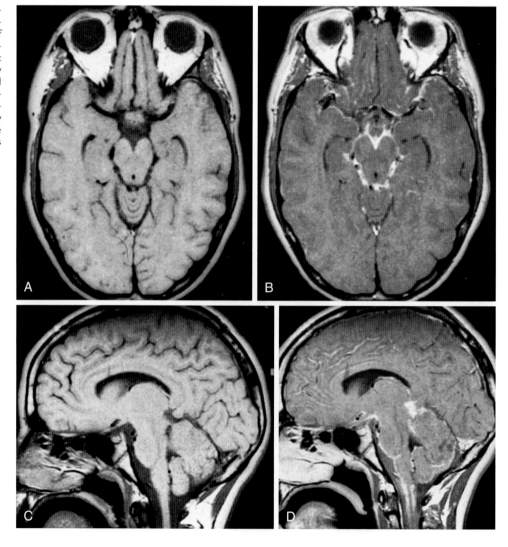

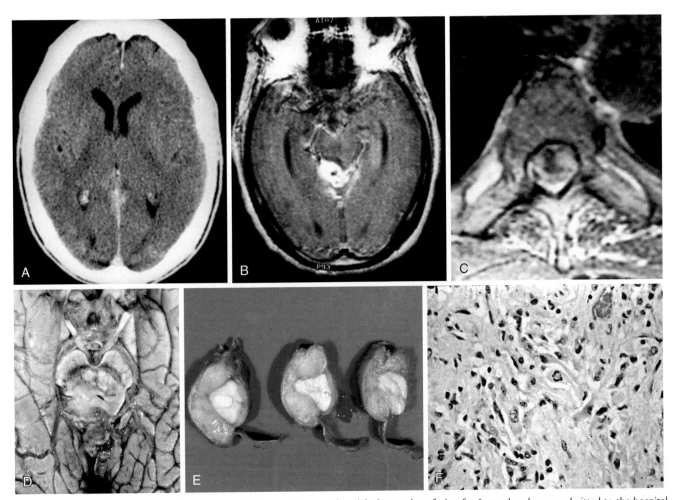

■ **FIGURE 30-31** Leptomeningeal gliosarcoma in a 53-year-old man with weight loss and confusion for 6 months who was admitted to the hospital for recurrent grand mal seizures. Imaging studies display irregular nodular areas of leptomeningeal thickening in the brain and spine without intra-axial abnormality. Initial contrast-enhanced CT shows barely visible surface enhancement on the posterior falx (**A**). Axial postgadolinium MR images at the midbrain (**B**) and in the spine (**C**) show leptomeningeal thickening and enhancement, and corresponding pathologic sections (**D, E**) show solid tumor thickening in the same regions. Histologic slide shows irregular spindle cells, nuclear pleomorphism, and central mitotic figure (**F**). Positive staining for glial fibrillary acidic protein helped confirm the diagnosis of leptomeningeal gliosarcomatosis.

■ **FIGURE 30-32** Primitive neuro-ectodermal tumor (PNET) of dura. This infant presented with a palpable mass behind the right ear (**A**). CT revealed a transcalvarial mass with bone destruction that is partially calcified (**B**) and enhances densely (**C**). Axial T1W (**D**), T2W (**E**), and post-gadolinium axial (**F**) and coronal (**G**) T1W MR images demonstrate a large well-circumscribed transcalvarial mass extending from the posterior fossa to the right retroauricular region. The tumor displays enhancement with a nonenhancing central region.

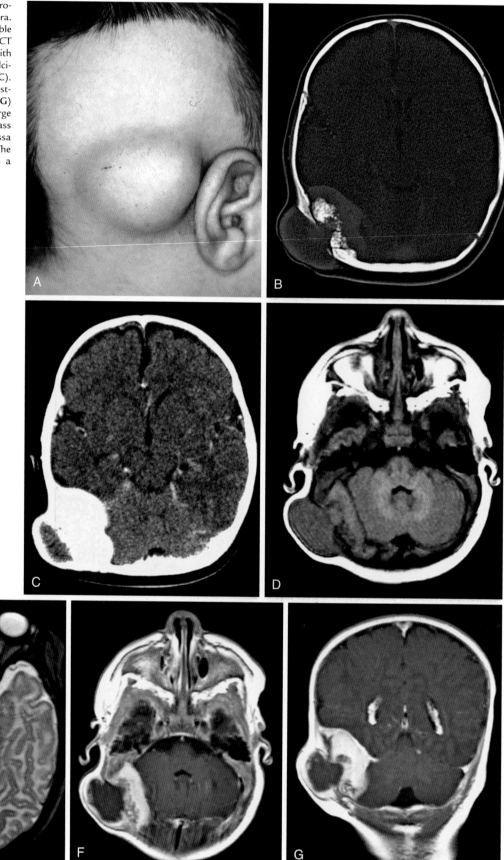

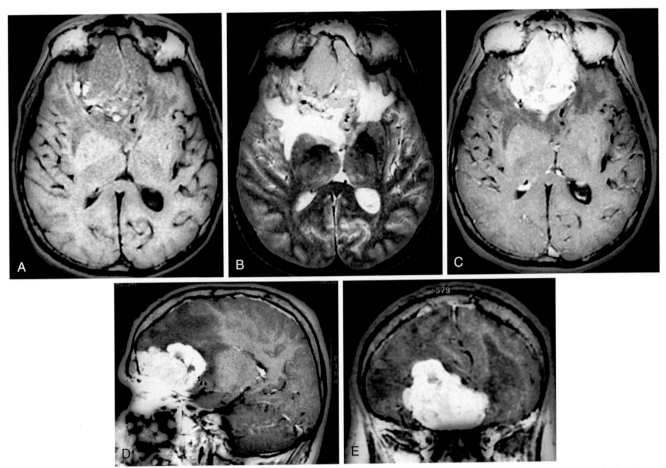

■ **FIGURE 30-33** Esthesioneuroblastoma in a 58-year-old man with a history of headache and acute psychotic episode. Imaging reveals dural-based tumor in the frontal midline on axial T1W (**A**), T2W (**B**), and postgadolinium axial (**C**), sagittal (**D**), and coronal (**E**) MR images with perilesional edema, possible brain invasion, and some extension into the sinuses. Extensive pathologic evaluation reveals malignant neoplasm with neuroblastoma and some glandular features. Immunohistochemical staining was positive for neuron-specific enolase and cytokeratin. This is most likely an unusual variation on esthesioneuroblastoma arising in components of the olfactory tracts as they passed through the dura in the region of the cribriform plate.

PRIMARY MELANOCYTIC NEOPLASMS OF THE MENINGES

Tumors of melanocytic origin may arise solely or primarily within the leptomeningeal or dural membranes. They may be referred to as meningeal melanocytoma (Fig. 30-34), primary meningeal malignant melanoma (Fig. 30-35), primary leptomeningeal melanomatosis or melanoblastosis (Fig. 30-36), neurocutaneous melanosis, diffuse melanocytosis, melanotic neuroectodermal tumor of infancy (Fig. 30-37), and melanotic progonoma.

Epidemiology

Melanocytic primary tumors of the meninges display significant variation in demography, arising both congenitally and sporadically in children, young adults, and the elderly. No clear epidemiologic patterns have been established.

Clinical Presentation

The clinical presentation may vary from acute seizures to headache to more focal neurologic deficits, depending on the location of the lesion. There may be an association between skin lesions and more diffuse melanocytic CNS processes in some patients. The nevus of Ota is a rare congenital hyperpigmentation in the distribution of the V1 and V2 segments of the trigeminal dermatome. In some rare cases, patients with nevus of Ota,

also referred to as oculodermal melanosis, have developed intracranial melanotic lesions, including melanocytoma, melanoma, and melanoblastosis.

Pathophysiology

Virchow first described diffuse leptomeningeal melanoma in 1859, and Rokitansky reported neurocutaneous melanosis in 1861. Superficial or cutaneous melanocytes arise from portions of neuroectoderm that give rise to the neural crest and are found normally in the leptomeninges. These cells are distinct from central melanocytes, which arise within the neural tube and produce neuromelanin. Neoplastic transformation may occur, giving rise to several different morphologic tumor types of varying degrees of malignancy and biologic aggressivity.

Cutaneous melanocytes may also be present in pigmented tumors, including pigmented meningioma and schwannoma.

Pathology

Gross appearances may vary, but it is characteristic to see a dark tarry mass or covering in the affected area or, in the case of a diffuse neoplasm, throughout the coverings of the neuraxis.

Microscopic features vary widely across the spectrum of primary meningeal melanocytic neoplasms; however, the presence of distinctive melanin is almost always diagnostic. Rarely,

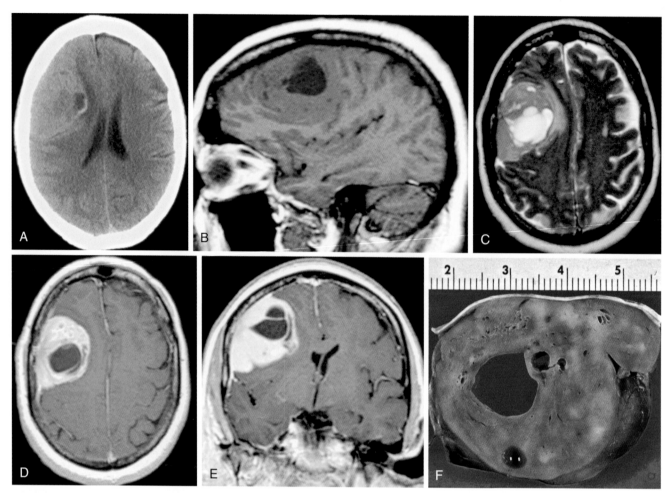

■ **FIGURE 30-34**   Melanocytoma of dura in a 64-year-old woman with right-sided headache and left facial droop. Initial nonenhanced CT (**A**) shows a hyperdense extra-axial mass with focal low density in the right frontal region. Sagittal T1W (**B**), axial T2W (**C**) and postgadolinium axial (**D**) and coronal (**E**) T1W MR images show densely enhancing dural-based mass with nonenhancing cavity and enhancing dural tail. Pathologic evaluation indicates low-grade melanocytic neoplasm, and gross specimen (**F**) correlates well with imaging findings.

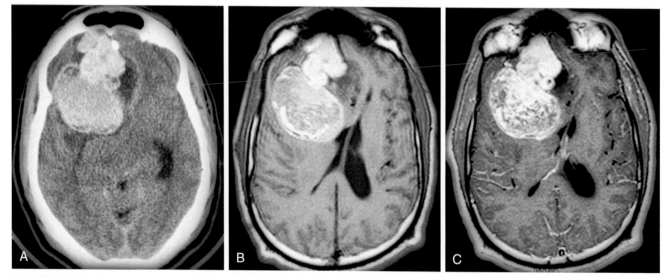

■ **FIGURE 30-35**   Malignant melanoma of dura. A 45-year-old man with a history of headaches for 2 months was found unconscious with dilation of the right pupil. Initial contrast-enhanced CT (**A**) shows large, lobulated, enhancing right frontal mass with significant mass effect. **B** and **C**, Axial MR images before and after administration of gadolinium show marked T1 hyperintensity on the unenhanced images with some additional hyperintensity on the postgadolinium images owing to paramagnetic T1 shortening.

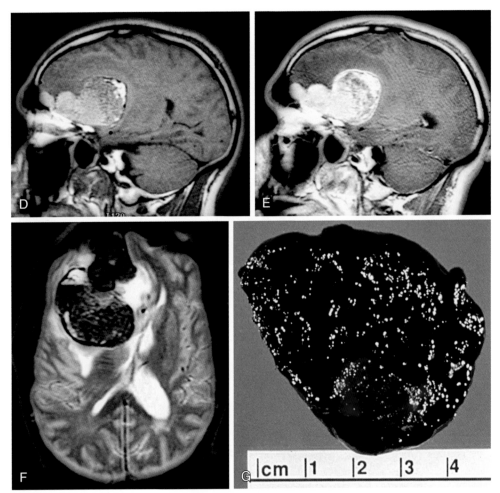

■ **FIGURE 30-35, cont'd**   D and E, Sagittal MR images before and after administration of gadolinium show marked T1 hyperintensity on the unenhanced images with some additional hyperintensity on the postgadolinium images owing to paramagnetic T1 shortening. Axial T2W MR image (**F**) shows marked hypointensity also due to paramagnetic effect. Pathologic specimen (**G**) shows typical dark tarry surface.

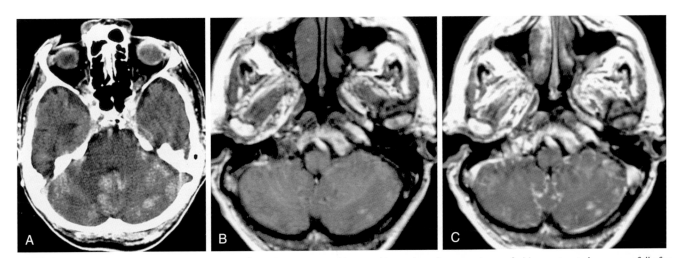

■ **FIGURE 30-36**   Primary leptomeningeal melanoblastosis. A 79-year-old man with ataxia and progressive confusion was treated unsuccessfully for fungal and mycobacterial meningitis and subsequently died. Initial contrast-enhanced CT image (**A**) shows patchy enhancement of cerebellar fissures. Axial pregadolinium T1W (**B**) and postgadolinium axial (**C**) T1W MR images show diffuse irregular surface enhancement throughout the posterior fossa.

Continued

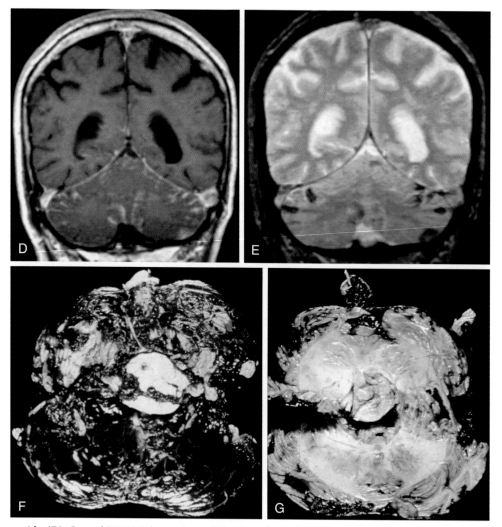

■ **FIGURE 30-36, cont'd** (D), Coronal T1W MR image shows diffuse irregular surface enhancement throughout the posterior fossa. Coronal T2W MR image (E) shows patchy areas of hypointensity due to paramagnetic effect. Gross pathologic specimens (F, G) show tarry coating on the surface of the cerebellar hemispheres without intra-axial involvement.

melanocytic lesions may be amelanotic, and the diagnosis in these cases relies on immunohistochemistry.[70]

Melanocytoma is a low-grade, well-differentiated, well-circumscribed lesion composed of clusters of slightly elongated melanocytes containing variable amounts of melanin. No invasion of adjacent tissues is seen, nor is there significant atypia or mitotic activity.[71] Both melanin-producing cells and pigment-filled melanophages may be present. Rarely, melanocytomas may be pigment free, and diagnosis in these cases rests on immunohistochemical characteristics. Although rare, melanocytomas seen in association with congenital nevus of Ota may be found in the region of Meckel's cave that harbors the trigeminal ganglion as well as along the convexity dura.[72]

Malignant primary melanoma may arise as a focal mass[73] or as diffuse melanomatosis and is composed of sheets or clusters of malignant cells with frank invasion of adjacent structures, including brain parenchyma.[74]

Neurocutaneous melanosis is an embryonal neuroectodermal dysplasia characterized by an excessive proliferation of melanin-producing cells in the skin and in the leptomeninges, either as focal masses or as a diffuse benign melanocytosis.[75]

Progression to malignant leptomeningeal melanomatosis is believed to occur in half of all patients. Diffuse malignant transformation may also be referred to as melanoblastosis or melanomatosis.[76]

Melanocytic neuroectodermal tumors are rare pigmented tumors of neuroectodermal origin that may arise in a variety of locations, usually in the head and neck region and occasionally from the leptomeninges.[77] In the past, these tumors have been referred to as melanotic progonomas.[78]

Imaging

All lesions may show hyperintense signal on noncontrast T1-weighted (T1W) MRI owing to slight paramagnetic effect of melanin. Melanocytoma and primary melanomas arise as a focal dural-based mass lesion with diffuse, usually homogeneous enhancement. The diffuse melanocytic neoplasms may display a spectrum of malignancy and yet overlap considerably in imaging appearance with diffuse enhancement and leptomeningeal thickening. Diffuse fluid-attenuated inversion recovery (FLAIR) hyperintensity may be seen in association with diffuse neurocutaneous melanosis.[79]

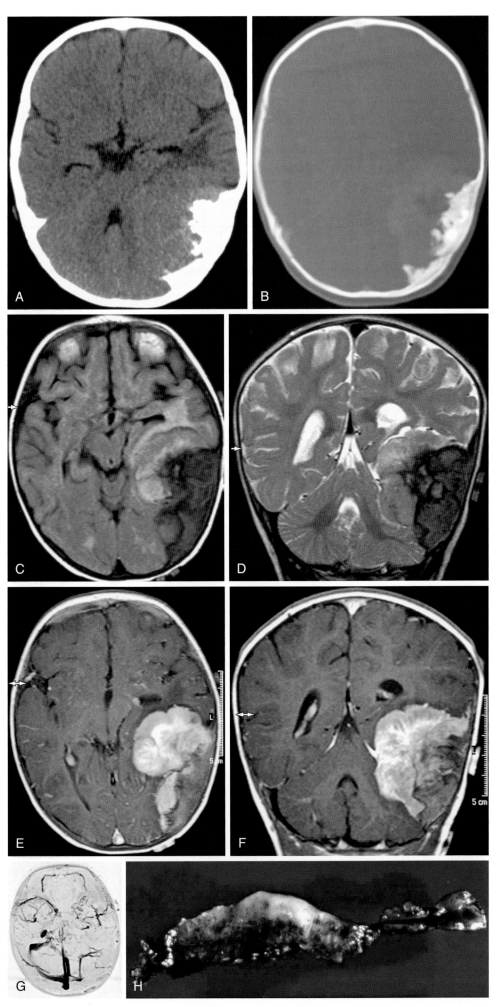

■ **FIGURE 30-37** Melanotic neuro-ectodermal tumor of infancy (melanotic progonoma). A 14-month-old boy presented with new-onset seizures and left facial weakness. On initial nonenhanced CT there is a large slightly hyperdense mass in the left posterior fossa (**A**) with an irregular calcified base (**B**) Axial FLAIR (**C**) and coronal T2W (**D**) MR images show hypointensity in a large irregular dural-based mass, suggesting a paramagnetic effect. Postgadolinium axial (**E**) and coronal (**F**) T1W MR images display diffuse enhancement of the solid portion of the tumor excepting the calcified base. MR venographic image (**G**) shows apparent obstruction on the left sigmoid sinus. Surgical specimen (**H**) shows some dark tarry material on the surface of the mass.

KEY POINTS

- The most common meningeal neoplasms are meningiomas, and of these, the great majority are typical in both imaging appearance and in their relatively benign clinical course.
- Typical benign meningiomas may have imaging features indistinguishable from the uncommon atypical and the rare malignant meningiomas.
- Other than meningiomas, there are a wide variety of primary and metastatic neoplasms which may present as meningeal masses, only a few of which may display distinctive imaging features.

- The etiology and pathogenesis of meningiomas, as well as most other less common meningeal neoplasms, remain the subject of active ongoing research and study. Like neoplasms in other areas of the body, currently available information suggests a multifactorial causative basis involving embryologic, genetic, and environmental factors in most cases.

Box 30-1   Sample Report: Olfactory Groove Meningioma (see Fig. 30-10)

PATIENT HISTORY

A 53-year-old woman presented with weakness of the left upper extremity.

COMPARISON STUDIES

No comparison studies are available at this institution.

TECHNIQUE

MRI was first performed as a multiplanar multisequence noncontrast study including sagittal T1W, axial T1W, T2W, T2W FLAIR, and gradient recalled echo T2*W, and axial diffusion-weighted images with apparent diffusion coefficient map, Following intravenous administration of Gd-chelate contrast agent, additional triplanar sagittal, axial, and coronal T1W series were obtained.

CONTRAST

0.1 mL per kg Gadavist I.V. for a total administered dose of 7.5 mL.

FINDINGS

MRI discloses a large (5 × 6 × 6 cm), sharply marginated right frontoparietal mass that has a broad base upon the convexity dura. The mass invaginates deeply into the underlying frontal and parietal opercula,

displaces the temporal operculum inferiorly, and is associated with marked vasogenic edema of the underlying brain. The combined mass of effect of the lesion and edema substantially compresses the right lateral ventricle and shifts the midline from right to left approximately 1.2 cm. There is no evidence of downward transincisural herniation. The mass shows prominent flow voids that appear to originate from the midpoint of its dural base. It shows prominent vessels along its deep surface (dome) and a well-defined cleavage plane from the underlying brain. There is marked, nearly homogeneous contrast enhancement that emphasizes the prominence and radial distribution of the tumor vascularity. No other lesion is identified. These features strongly suggest a diagnosis of right convexity meningioma. Differential diagnoses include other dural-based masses such as dural lymphoma and dural metastases.

IMPRESSION

Right hypervascular mid-convexity frontoparietal contrast-enhancing dural-based mass with substantial vasogenic edema of the underlying brain and midline shift of 1.2 cm from right to left. The imaging features are most strongly suggestive of meningioma. Differential diagnoses include other dural-based masses such as dural lymphoma and dural metastases.

SUGGESTED READINGS

Cushing H, Eisenhardt L. Meningioma. New York, Hafner, 1938 (reprinted 1962).

Kaye AH, Laws ER Jr (eds). Brain Tumors: An Encyclopedic Approach, 2nd ed. Edinburgh, Churchill Livingstone, 2001.

Louis DN, Ohgaki H, Wiestler OD, Cavenee WK. WHO Classification of Tumors of the Central Nervous System. Albany, NY, World Health Organization Publications Center, 2007.

McLendon RE, Rosemblum MK, Bigner DD (eds). Russell & Rubinstein's Pathology of Tumors of the Central Nervous System, 7th ed. London, Hodder Arnold, 2006.

Parent A. Carpenter's Human Neuroanatomy, 9th ed. Baltimore, Williams & Wilkins, 1996.

REFERENCES

1. Parent A. Carpenter's Human Neuroanatomy, 9th ed. Baltimore, Williams & Wilkins, 1996.
2. O'Rahilly R, Muller F. The meninges in human development. J Neuropathol Exp Neurol 1986; 45:588-608.
3. Le Douarin NM, Kalcheim C (eds). The neural crest, formation of the meninges. In The Neural Crest, 2nd ed. Cambridge, Cambridge University Press, 1999.
4. Catala M. Embryonic and fetal development of structures associated with the cerebrospinal fluid in man and other species: I. The ventricular system, meninges and choroid plexuses. Arch Anat Cytol Pathol 1998; 46:153-169.
5. Cushing H, Eisenhardt L. Meningiomas. New York, Hafner, 1938 (reprinted 1962).
6. Ishigaki D, Arai H, Sasoh M, et al. Meningioma in the posterior fossa without dural attachment. Neurol Med Chir 2007; 47:364-366.
7. Cesario A, Galetta D, Margaritora S, Granone P. Unsuspected primary pulmonary meningioma. Eur J Cardiothorac Surg 2002; 21:553-555.
8. Claus EB, Bondy ML, Schildkraut JM, et al. Epidemiology of intracranial meningioma. Neurosurgery 2005; 57:1088-1095; discussion 1088-1095.
9. Fan KJ, Pezeshkpour GH. Ethnic distribution of primary central nervous system tumors in Washington, DC, 1971 to 1985. J Natl Med Assoc 1992; 84:858-863.
10. Preston-Martin S, Paganini-Hill A, Henderson BE, et al. Case-control study of intracranial meningiomas in women in Los Angeles County, California. J Natl Cancer Inst 1980; 65:67-73.

11. Kaye A, Laws E. Brain Tumors, 2nd ed. Edinburgh, Churchill Livingstone, 2001, pp 719-720.

12. Louis DN, Ohgaki H, Wiestler OD, Cavenee WK. WHO Classification of Tumors of the Central Nervous System. Albany, NY, World Health Organization Publications Center, 2007.

13. Caroli E, Russillo M, Ferrante L. Intracranial meningiomas in children: report of 27 new cases and critical analysis of 440 cases reported in the literature. J Child Neurol 2006; 21:31-36.

14. Liu Y, Li F, Zhu S, et al. Clinical features and treatment of meningiomas in children: report of 12 cases and literature review. Pediatr Neurosurg 2008; 44:112-117.

15. Gupta R, Suri V, Jain A, et al. Anaplastic meningioma in an adolescent: a report of a rare case and brief review of literature. Childs Nerv Syst 2009; 25:241-245.

16. Phillips LE, Koepsell TD, van Belle G, et al. History of head trauma and risk of intracranial meningioma: population-based case-control study. Neurology 2002; 58:1849-1852.

17. Longstreth WT Jr, Dennis LK, McGuire VM, et al. Epidemiology of intracranial meningioma. Cancer 1993; 72:639-648.

18. Ragel BT, Jensen RL. Molecular genetics of meningiomas. Neurosurg Focus 2005; 19:E9.

19. Zang KD. Meningioma: a cytogenetic model of a complex benign human tumor, including data on 394 karyotyped cases. Cytogenet Cell Genet 2001; 93:207-220.

20. Dumanski JP, Rouleau GA, Nordenskjold M, Collins VP. Molecular genetic analysis of chromosome 22 in 81 cases of meningioma. Cancer Res 1990; 50:5863-5867.

21. Wozniak K, Piaskowski S, Gresner SM, et al. *BCR* expression is decreased in meningiomas showing loss of heterozygosity of 22q within a new minimal deletion region. Cancer Genet Cytogenet 2008; 183:14-20.

22. Rempel SA, Schwechheimer K, Davis RL, et al. Loss of heterozygosity for loci on chromosome 10 is associated with morphologically malignant meningioma progression. Cancer Res 1993; 53(10 Suppl):2386-2392.

23. Simon M, von Deimling A, Larson JJ, et al. Allelic losses on chromosomes 14, 10, and 1 in atypical and malignant meningiomas: a genetic model of meningioma progression. Cancer Res 1995; 55: 4696-4701.

24. Simon M, Bostrom JP, Hartmann C. Molecular genetics of meningiomas: from basic research to potential clinical applications. Neurosurgery 2007; 60:787-798; discussion 787-798.

25. Takei H, Bhattacharjee MB, Rivera A, et al. New immunohistochemical markers in the evaluation of central nervous system tumors: a review of 7 selected adult and pediatric brain tumors. Arch Pathol Lab Med 2007; 131:234-241.

26. Ding YS, Wang HD, Tang K, et al. Expression of vascular endothelial growth factor in human meningiomas and peritumoral brain areas. Ann Clin Lab Sci 2008; 38:344-351.

27. Blankenstein MA, Verheijen FM, Jacobs JM, et al. Occurrence, regulation, and significance of progesterone receptors in human meningioma. Steroids 2000; 65:795-800.

28. Korhonen K, Salminen T, Raitanen J, et al. Female predominance in meningiomas cannot be explained by differences in progesterone, estrogen, or androgen receptor expression. J Neuro-oncol 2006; 80:1-7.

29. Guermazi A, Lafitte F, Miaux Y, et al. The dural tail sign—beyond meningioma. Clin Radiol 2005; 60:171-188.

30. Rokni-Yazdi H, Sotoudeh H. Prevalence of "dural tail sign" in patients with different intracranial pathologies. Eur J Radiol 2006; 60:42-45.

31. Omeis I, Hillard VH, Braun A, et al. Meningioangiomatosis associated with neurofibromatosis: report of 2 cases in a single family and review of the literature. Surg Neurol 2006; 65:595-603.

32. Jallo GI, Kothbauer K, Mehta V, et al. Meningioangiomatosis without neurofibromatosis: a clinical analysis. J Neurosurg 2005; 103(4 Suppl):319-324.

33. Takeshima Y, Amatya VJ, Nakayori F, et al. Meningioangiomatosis occurring in a young male without neurofibromatosis: with special reference to its histogenesis and loss of heterozygosity in the *NF2* gene region. Am J Surg Pathol 2002; 26:125-129.

34. Kim NR, Choe G, Shin SH, et al. Childhood meningiomas associated with meningioangiomatosis: report of five cases and literature review. Neuropathol Appl Neurobiol 2002; 28:48-56.

35. Wiebe S, Munoz DG, Smith S, Lee DH. Meningioangiomatosis: a comprehensive analysis of clinical and laboratory features. Brain 1999; 122:709-726.

36. Wang Y, Gao X, Yao ZW, et al. Histopathological study of five cases with sporadic meningioangiomatosis. Neuropathology 2006; 26: 249-256.

37. Franco-Paredes C, Martin K. Extranodal Rosai-Dorfman disease involving the meninges. South Med J 2002; 95:1101-1102.

38. Lachenal F, Cotton F, Desmurs-Clavel H, et al. Neurological manifestations and neuroradiological presentation of Erdheim-Chester disease: report of 6 cases and systematic review of the literature. J Neurol 2006; 253:1267.

39. Coca S, Salas I, Martinez R, et al. Meningeal Castleman's disease with multifocal involvement: a case report and review of literature. J Neuro-Oncol 2008; 88:37-41.

40. Johnson MD, Powell SZ, Boyer PJ, et al. Dural lesions mimicking meningiomas. Hum Pathol 2002; 33:1211-1226.

41. Shenkier TN. Unusual variants of primary central nervous system lymphoma. Hematol Oncol Clin North Am 2005; 19:651-664.

42. Morgello S, Kotsianti A, Gumprecht JP, Moore F. Epstein-Barr virus–associated dural leiomyosarcoma in a man infected with human immunodeficiency virus. Case report. J Neurosurg 1997; 86: 883-887.

43. Colpan E, Attar A, Erekul S, Arasil E. Convexity dural chondroma: a case report and review of the literature. J Clin Neurosci 2003; 10:106-108.

44. Guzel A, Tatli M, Er U, et al. Multifocal Ewing's sarcoma of the brain, calvarium, leptomeninges, spine and other bones in a child. J Clin Neurosci 2008; 15:813-817.

45. Uluc K, Arsava EM, Ozkan B, et al. Primary leptomeningeal sarcomatosis; a pathology proven case with challenging MRI and clinical findings. J Neuro-Oncol 2004; 66:307-312.

46. Buttner A, Pfluger T, Weis S. Primary meningeal sarcomas in two children. J Neuro-Oncol 2001; 52:181-188.

47. Herzog CE, Leeds NE, Bruner JM, Baumgartner JE. Intracranial hemangiopericytomas in children. Pediatr Neurosurg 1995; 22: 274-279.

48. Sohda T, Yun K. Insulin-like growth factor II expression in primary meningeal hemangiopericytoma and its metastasis to the liver accompanied by hypoglycemia. Hum Pathol 1996; 27:858-861.

49. Beech TJ, Rokade A, Gittoes N, Johnson AP. A haemangiopericytoma of the ethmoid sinus causing oncogenic osteomalacia: a case report and review of the literature. Int J Oral Maxillofacial Surg 2007; 36:956-958.

50. Mena H, Ribas JL, Pezeshkpour GH, et al. Hemangiopericytoma of the central nervous system: a review of 94 cases. Hum Pathol 1991; 22:84-91.

51. Henn W, Wullich B, Thonnes M, et al. Recurrent t(12;19)(q13;q13.3) in intracranial and extracranial hemangiopericytoma. Cancer Genet Cytogenet 1993; 71:151-154.

52. Ono Y, Ueki K, Joseph JT, Louis DN. Homozygous deletions of the *CDKN2/p16* gene in dural hemangiopericytomas. Acta Neuropathol 1996; 91:221-225.

53. Perry A, Scheithauer BW, Nascimento AG. The immunophenotypic spectrum of meningeal hemangiopericytoma: a comparison with fibrous meningioma and solitary fibrous tumor of meninges. Am J Surg Pathol 1997; 21:1354-1360.

54. Chiechi MV, Smirniotopoulos JG, Mena H. Intracranial hemangiopericytomas: MR and CT features. AJNR Am J Neuroradiol 1996; 17:1365-1371.

55. Akiyama M, Sakai H, Onoue H, et al. Imaging intracranial haemangiopericytomas: study of seven cases. Neuroradiology 2004; 46:194-197.

56. Donner LR, Silva MT, Dobin SM. Solitary fibrous tumor of the pleura: a cytogenetic study. Cancer Genet Cytogenet 1999; 111:169-171.

57. Torabi A, Lele SM, DiMaio D, et al. Lack of a common or characteristic cytogenetic anomaly in solitary fibrous tumor. Cancer Genet Cytogenet 2008; 181:60-64.

58. Brunori A, Cerasoli S, Donati R, et al. Solitary fibrous tumor of the meninges: two new cases and review of the literature. Surg Neurol 1999; 51:636-640.

59. Cassarino DS, Auerbach A, Rushing EJ. Widely invasive solitary fibrous tumor of the sphenoid sinus, cavernous sinus, and pituitary fossa. Ann Diagn Pathol 2003; 7:169-173.

60. Ogawa K, Tada T, Takahashi S, et al. Malignant solitary fibrous tumor of the meninges. Virchows Arch 2004; 444:459-464.

61. Suzuki SO, Fukui M, Nishio S, Iwaki T. Clinicopathological features of solitary fibrous tumor of the meninges: an immunohistochemical

reappraisal of cases previously diagnosed to be fibrous meningioma or hemangiopericytoma. Pathol Int 2000; 50:808.

62. Weon YC, Kim EY, Kim HJ, et al. Intracranial solitary fibrous tumors: imaging findings in 6 consecutive patients. AJNR Am J Neuroradiol 2007; 28:1466-1469.

63. Ng HK, Poon WS. Primary leptomeningeal astrocytoma. J Neurosurg 1998; 88:586-589.

64. Rogers LR, Estes ML, Rosenbloom SA, Harrold L. Primary leptomeningeal oligodendroglioma: case report. Neurosurgery 1995; 36:166-168; discussion 169.

65. Debono B, Derrey S, Rabehenoina C, et al. Primary diffuse multinodular leptomeningeal gliomatosis: case report and review of the literature. Surg Neurol 2006; 65:273-282; discussion 282.

66. Riva M, Bacigaluppi S, Galli C, et al. Primary leptomeningeal gliomatosis: case report and review of the literature. Neurol Sci 2005; 26:129-134.

67. Wada C, Kurata A, Hirose R, et al. Primary leptomeningeal ependymoblastoma: case report. J Neurosurg 1986; 64:968-973.

68. Begemann M, Lyden D, Rosenblum MK, et al. Primary leptomeningeal primitive neuroectodermal tumor. J Neuro-oncol 2003; 63:299-303.

69. Cooper IS, Kernohan JW. Heterotopic glial nests in the subarachnoid space; histopathologic characteristics, mode of origin and relation to meningeal gliomas. J Neuropathol Exp Neurol 1951; 10:16-29.

70. Bussone G, La Mantia L, Vaghi MA, et al. Amelanotic leptomeningeal melanoblastosis. Ital J Neurol Sci 1990; 11:171-175.

71. Ahluwalia S, Ashkan K, Casey AT. Meningeal melanocytoma: clinical features and review of the literature. Br J Neurosurg 2003; 17:347-351.

72. Rahimi-Movaghar V, Karimi M. Meningeal melanocytoma of the brain and oculodermal melanocytosis (nevus of Ota): case report and literature review. Surg Neurol 2003; 59:200-210.

73. Kiecker F, Hofmann MA, Audring H, et al. Large primary meningeal melanoma in an adult patient with neurocutaneous melanosis. Clin Neurol Neurosurg 2007; 109:448-451.

74. Rosenthal G, Gomori JM, Tobias S, et al. Unusual cases involving the CNS and nasal sinuses: Case 1. Primary leptomeningeal melanoma. J Clin Oncol 2003; 21:3875-3877.

75. Plikaitis CM, David LR, Argenta LC. Neurocutaneous melanosis: clinical presentations. J Craniofac Surg 2005; 16:921-925.

76. Arunkumar MJ, Ranjan A, Jacob M, Rajshekhar V. Neurocutaneous melanosis: a case of primary intracranial melanoma with metastasis. Clin Oncol (Royal College of Radiologists) 2001; 13:52-54.

77. Latham K, Podda S, Wolfe SA. Melanocytic neuroectodermal tumor of infancy: excision and primary palatal repair at 7 months of age. J Craniofac Surg 2007; 18:450-454.

78. Anagnostopoulos DI, Everard GJH. Melanotic progonoma of the skull. J Neurol Neurosurg Psychiatry 1972; 35:88-91.

79. Hayashi M, Maeda M, Maji T, et al. Diffuse leptomeningeal hyperintensity on fluid-attenuated inversion recovery MR images in neurocutaneous melanosis. AJNR Am J Neuroradiol 2004; 25:138-141.

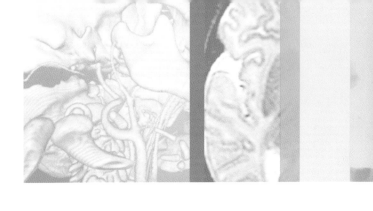

31

Vascular and Hematopoietic Neoplasms

Benjamin C. Lee

The focus of this chapter is on tumors that are vascular or of blood cell origin. These include hemangioblastoma, hemangiopericytoma, primary central nervous system (CNS) lymphoma, intravascular lymphoma, leukemia, and plasmacytoma. These neoplasms combined make up fewer than 10% of CNS tumors.

HEMANGIOBLASTOMA

Hemangioblastoma is a benign vascular tumor composed of endothelial and stromal cell components that can occur throughout the neural axis. The majority of these tumors are sporadic (75%), with the remaining associated with von Hippel-Lindau (VHL) disease.[1] It is also referred to as capillary hemangioblastoma and is the most common primary intraparenchymal tumor to occur in the posterior fossa in adults.

Epidemiology

Sporadic hemangioblastomas have their onset at an average age of 35 years and are more common in men. In patients with VHL they present an average of 10 years earlier. Sporadic cases are usually solitary lesions that can recur, whereas lesions associated with VHL are often multiple. There is no difference between sporadic and VHL-associated tumors with respect to recurrence or dissemination.[1]

Clinical Presentation

The clinical presentation often includes headache, ataxia, nausea, vomiting, and focal neurologic deficits. Symptoms depend on the size and location of the tumor. Hemangioblastomas can be found throughout the neural axis but are most common in the posterior fossa (44%-72% in the cerebellum, 13%-44% in the spine).[2-4] Patients may also present with subarachnoid hemorrhage.

The majority of mass effect is from the associated cyst rather than the tumor; the larger the tumor, the more likely it is to produce an associated cyst. Cysts grow at a rate several times that of the solid tumor and reach a volume almost always several times the volume of the causative tumor.[5]

In VHL, ocular hemorrhage secondary to a retinal lesion is often the first manifestation of disease.

Secondary polycythemia may be seen secondary to increased erythropoietin production.

Pathophysiology

Tumor growth is variable, and both the solid and the cystic component can cycle through periods of growth and stability.[5]

The VHL gene is a tumor suppressor gene on chromosome 3 (3p25-26) found in patients with VHL disease.[6]

Local growth factors such as vascular endothelial growth factor, placental growth factor, epidermal growth factor, and platelet-derived growth factor, as well as their respective receptors, have been shown to be elevated in patients with hemangioblastomas.[7-9]

The pathogenesis and cell of origin are not known.

Pathology

Hemangioblastomas have a dense vasculature and grossly appear reddish brown to yellowish. The cyst fluid is xanthochromatic and rarely hemorrhagic. The cyst wall is made of benign neuronal glial cells (usually compressed brain).

A small, highly vascular mural nodule is associated with a much larger fluid-filled cyst situated near the surface of the cerebellum. Approximately 20% of tumors are purely solid.

Foamy to clear stromal cells are interspersed with endothelium-lined vascular channels.

Imaging
CT

The most common finding (60%) is a cerebellar cyst with a mural nodule isodense to brain on nonenhanced CT. The mural nodule is often found adjacent to the pial surface. The lesion can be purely solid. On postcontrast imaging, the solid component enhances avidly. Faint marginal enhancement may be seen around the cyst that likely reflects compressed cerebellum.[10] Feeding arteries may be seen on CT angiography.

MRI

Early hemangioblastoma has prolonged T1 and T2 relaxation times and is indistinguishable from other masses. Later, it develops cystic components with adjacent flow voids. The cystic component has a high T2 signal equal to or higher than that of cerebrospinal fluid (CSF).[11] An enhancing mural nodule is often near the pial surface. Vasogenic edema may be seen around the tumor. Gradient-recalled-echo imaging may demonstrate areas of susceptibility if there has been hemorrhage (Fig. 31-1).

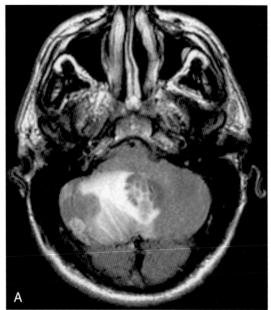

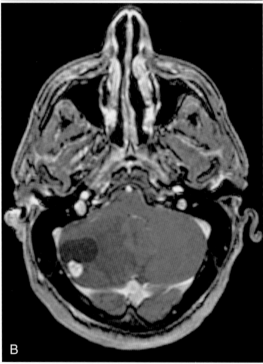

■ **FIGURE 31-1** Hemangioblastoma. **A,** Axial FLAIR imaging demonstrates a cyst with a mural nodule in the right cerebellar hemisphere. Surrounding vasogenic edema and mass effect are present. **B,** Axial T1W post-gadolinium MR image demonstrates an avidly enhancing nodule with an associated cyst (same patient as in **A**). The nodule abuts the pia. The cyst does not enhance.

MR perfusion demonstrates increased cerebral blood volume with poor return to baseline (Fig. 31-2).

Special Procedures

With angiography, the cyst is seen as an avascular mass. A mural nodule or solitary nodule is seen as a hypervascular mass with prolonged blush. Arteriovenous shunting may or may not be seen. Angiography may find hypervascular nodules not clearly seen on CT.[10]

Thallium-201 spectroscopy shows a high uptake of tracer during the early phase and almost no retention during the delayed phase. Washout of radiotracer is faster in comparison with gliomas.

KEY POINTS: HEMANGIOBLASTOMA

■ Hemangioblastoma is the most common primary intraparenchymal infratentorial tumor in adults and often presents as a solid and cystic mass, although purely solid and purely cystic lesions occur as well.
■ An important differential factor in patients with von Hippel-Lindau disease is hemangioblastoma versus metastatic renal cell carcinoma.
■ Differential diagnosis also includes juvenile pilocytic astrocytoma in younger patients (patients with hemangioblastoma are usually older unless they have von Hippel-Lindau disease).

HEMANGIOPERICYTOMA

Hemangiopericytoma is a malignant tumor originating from the pericytes of Zimmerman around capillaries and postcapillary venules. The intracranial tumor arises from meningeal capillary pericytes and is also called an angioblastic meningioma. This tumor is also found in the skin and the musculoskeletal system.[12]

Epidemiology

There is a male predominance of 50% to 70%. The average age range at presentation is 38 to 42 years.

Clinical Presentation

Intracranial hypertension and headache are the most common features, but presentation may be related to location of tumor with motor and sensory deficits or seizures. Intracranial hemorrhage may also occur.[13]

There is a strong tendency for local recurrence and metastases outside the central nervous system (CNS) in comparison with meningioma. Hematogenous metastasis occurs to bone, lungs, and liver, in descending order of frequency.[14] Metastasis also occurs to the kidney, pancreas, and adrenal glands.

The recurrence rate is higher than that for meningioma, with a mean recurrence-free period of 47 to 78 months. The median time to recurrence is 65 months.

Hemangiopericytoma may also cause oncogenic osteomalacia.[15]

Pathophysiology

The World Health Organization classifies hemangiopericytoma as a mesenchymal, nonmeningothelial tumor.

Pathology

The intracranial location is similar to that of meningioma with approximately 15% of hemangiopericytomas found in the posterior fossa.[16] Most tumors have dural attachments. There are also reports of tumors in sellar, suprasellar, and pineal regions.[17] Very rarely they can be purely intraparenchymal.[14]

Hemangiopericytomas consist of numerous vascular channels with plump endothelial nuclei. Branching vessels may show a typical "staghorn" appearance with surrounding oval and spindle-shaped pericytes.

Imaging

Hemangiopericytoma can be indistinguishable from meningioma on imaging.

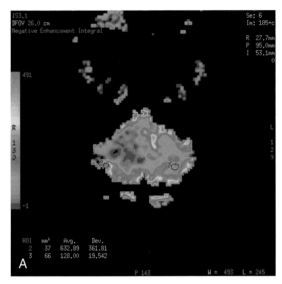

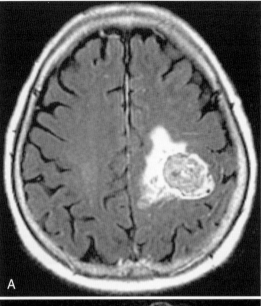

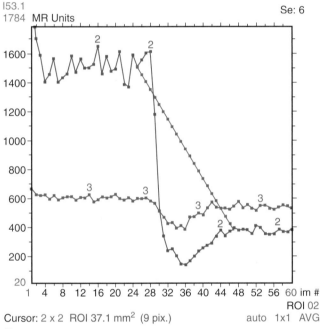

■ **FIGURE 31-2** Hemangioblastoma perfusion. **A,** MR perfusion color map demonstrates increased blood volume in a region of solid tumor. **B,** Hemangioblastoma perfusion. MR perfusion cerebral blood volume graph demonstrates increased blood volume with poor return to baseline corresponding to the solid lesion in **A**.

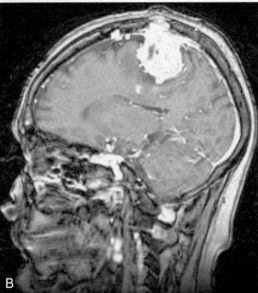

■ **FIGURE 31-3** Hemangiopericytoma. **A,** Axial FLAIR demonstrates an isointense lesion with surrounding vasogenic edema in the left perirolandic region. **B,** Hemangiopericytoma. Sagittal T1W postcontrast MR image demonstrates a heterogeneously enhancing dural based mass (same patient as in **A**) with "mushrooming" into the parenchyma and erosion through the skull. There is an associated dural tail.

CT

Intracranial lesions are often heterogeneous, hyperdense, dural-based multilobulated lesions that, unlike meningioma, are not associated with calcifications (although rare tumor calcification has been reported) or hyperostosis and typically show heterogeneous enhancement. Low-density cystic and necrotic areas may be identified. Adjacent bone erosion is seen in greater than 50% of cases. Over half of hemangiopericytomas may have an associated dural tail.[18]

The lesion usually shows broad-based dural attachment; however, a narrow-based attachment favors hemangiopericytoma rather than classic meningioma.[18]

The presence and degree of edema and mass effect are not necessarily related to the size and/or location of the lesion.

Aggressive-appearing features include apparent parenchymal invasion (mushrooming), irregular or polylobulated borders, bone erosion, and heterogeneous contrast enhancement.

MRI

MRI features are also similar to those of meningioma. The lesion is often multilobulated and predominantly isointense to cortical gray on T1- (T1W) and T2-weighted (T2W) sequences. Enhancement is more heterogeneous than meningioma. Surrounding vasogenic edema may be mild to moderate (Fig. 31-3). More than half of hemangiopericytomas are associated with a dural tail. Prominent internal vascular flow voids may be present.[18,19]

MR venography may demonstrate occlusion of dural sinuses by the mass. MR spectroscopy at short echo time may reveal a

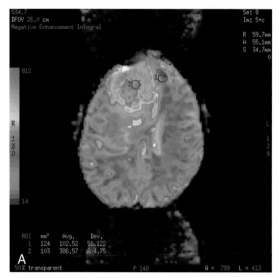

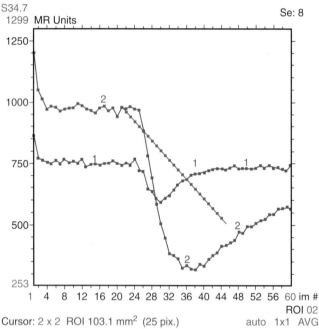

■ **FIGURE 31-4** Hemangiopericytoma. **A,** MR perfusion color map demonstrates increased cerebral blood volume in the tumor, particularly around the periphery. **B,** MR perfusion cerebral blood volume graph demonstrates an increase in blood volume with poor return to baseline consistent with an extra-axial mass.

larger peak at 3.56 ppm secondary to higher levels of myoinositol, in contradistinction to meningioma.[20] MR perfusion demonstrates increased cerebral blood volume with poor return to baseline, consistent with an extra-axial mass (Fig. 31-4).

Special Procedures
The usefulness of angiography has been debated in the literature. Marc and colleagues considered the following angiographic features to be characteristic: dural arterial supply with few arterial feeders from which a myriad of small corkscrew vessels arise; dense tumor stain, slow circulation, and slow venous drainage.[21] Alen and coworkers also found hemangiopericytoma to have a dense tumor stain with delayed venous drainage.[14] Guthrie, however, reported that angiography was not helpful in the diagnosis.[22]

Preoperative embolization of hemangiopericytoma can help reduce substantial intraoperative blood loss that can occur with these very vascular tumors.

KEY POINTS: HEMANGIOPERICYTOMA

- Hemangiopericytoma may mimic meningioma on imaging but occurs more often in males and usually without associated calcification or hyperostosis.
- Narrow-based dural attachment favors hemangiopericytoma over meningioma.

PRIMARY CNS LYMPHOMA
Primary CNS lymphoma is an extranodal non-Hodgkin's lymphoma (NHL), usually a diffuse large B-cell lymphoma that affects the CNS. The majority of CNS lymphomas are primary lesions (93%). The remaining are secondary lymphomas metastatic to the CNS.

Epidemiology
The incidence of primary CNS lymphoma is highest in the sixth to seventh decades in immunocompetent individuals and in the fourth to fifth decades in the immunocompromised individual. This tumor is also seen with frequency in the first decade because it is the most common intracranial mass lesion in pediatric patients with AIDS. There is a 2 : 1 to 1 : 1 male : female ratio.

The prevalence of primary CNS lymphoma substantially increased 2 decades ago but has only slightly increased in the past decade and currently represents up to 7% of intracranial tumors.[23,24] The past increase was partly secondary to the AIDS epidemic as well as immunosuppression in solid organ transplant recipients. There was also a threefold increase in primary CNS lymphoma in immunocompetent patients, an increase that was independent of improved imaging and detection. This finding was thought to be related to a fundamental biologic change in the disease, because the intermediate grade of primary CNS lymphoma was not seen after 1983. The tumor appears to have become more histologically aggressive.[24]

Secondary lymphoma involving the CNS occurs less often since the advent of effective chemotherapy and, when present, affects the dura mater and leptomeninges more often than brain parenchyma. Hodgkin's lymphoma rarely affects the CNS, and, if so, it does so late in the disease.[25]

Clinical Presentation
Primary CNS lymphoma presents as nonspecific neurologic findings, including focal symptoms, personality and cognitive changes, headaches, nausea, and vomiting. Symptoms are related to the size and location of the intracranial mass or masses. It may be preceded by a neurologic prodrome that may be misdiagnosed as multiple sclerosis.[23]

In HIV patients, the presence of primary CNS lymphoma is an AIDS-defining illness. Two percent of AIDS patients develop this tumor at some point in their disease.

Pathophysiology
Primary CSN lymphoma is a densely cellular tumor with a distinct affinity for perivascular extension and predilection for the periventricular region.[26] Diffuse microscopic disease is almost always present, which accounts for the ability of this tumor to produce distant disease and local recurrences.

Virtually all of these tumors are B-cell lymphomas (98%). The exact etiology is unknown because the brain has no endogenous lymphoid tissue.[27] It is generally agreed that CNS lymphoma and systemic extracerebral NHL share the same cell of origin. There are two theories as to the origin of this tumor: (1) lymphocytes are attracted to the CNS by infection or inflammation and there undergo a transformation event, and (2) B lymphocytes that are already carrying a CNS-specific binding marker are activated, proliferate, and undergo neoplastic transformation.

There appears to be an association with infectious agents. Epstein-Barr virus genetic material has been found in over 90% of cases in immunocompromised patients.[23] Cytomegalovirus has also been associated.

Pathology

Most lesions are supratentorial (75%) and have a predilection for the cerebral hemispheres, followed by basal ganglia, corpus callosum, and cerebellum. Leptomeningeal involvement occurs in about 12% of cases. Dural involvement is rare in primary CNS lymphoma. One percent of tumors occur in the spinal cord.[23,24,27]

Primary CNS lymphoma is frequently surrounded by edema, commonly spreads to leptomeninges and subpial regions, and is multifocal in almost 50% of cases. Focal necrosis and hemorrhage are common.[25]

Histology demonstrates monotonous, closely packed blue cells with a high degree of cellularity. Infiltrates are seen far beyond the borders of the grossly observed mass. Necrosis and hemorrhage are much more frequent in the lesions of immunocompromised patients.[26]

Neoplastic cells tend to cluster along vascular channels, a phenomenon that supports the theory that CNS lymphoma spreads diffusely through the brain by way of the perivascular spaces.[26] A vasculitis-like appearance on histopathology may be seen because of tumor infiltrating the blood vessel walls. This angiocentric growth pattern—tumor cells forming multiple, thick layers around the host vessels and widening of the perivascular space—is one of the histopathologic hallmarks of the disease.

Immunohistologic analysis is essential to the diagnosis. Antibodies are directed at common leukocyte antigens, pan-B antigens, and pan-T antigens. Tumors typically contain a population of atypical pleomorphic B cells mixed with reactive T cells. Even though primary CNS lymphoma is considered monoclonal, the lesion virtually always contains at least two cell populations, one of which is neoplastic and the other one reactive.

In general, lymphomas are divided into low-grade, high-grade, and possibly intermediate-grade NHL. No intermediate-grade cases have been reported since 1983. Today almost half of CNS lymphomas are of the high-grade, large-cell, immunoblastic subtype.[24]

The CSF may show elevated protein and decreased glucose levels. Cytology will often be negative.

Imaging

CT

Imaging features depend on the immune status of the patient. In an immunocompetent patient, primary CNS lymphoma appears hyperdense on noncontrast CT and demonstrates solid homogeneous enhancement. In immunocompromised patients it tends to be multicentric, hypoattenuated on unenhanced CT, and characterized by ring enhancement on contrast-enhanced CT.[26,28,29]

Deep gray nuclei are the classic location, but only 33% of CNS lymphomas occur in the region and most occur in cerebral white matter. Cerebral white matter of the frontal lobes is the most common location, followed by the temporal, parietal, and occipital lobes in decreasing order of frequency.

One of more characteristic features of primary CNS lymphoma is the tendency to abut the ependyma, the meninges, or both.[30] This feature supports the theory that the lesion originated in the periadventitial cells of penetrating arterioles in the perivascular spaces.

Primary CNS lymphoma is one of the neoplasms that classically can have a "butterfly" appearance when it involves the corpus callosum, along with glioblastoma multiforme and demyelinating disease. It does not show calcification except after treatment.

Negative findings from a CT examination do not exclude the diagnosis. Therefore, MRI is the imaging modality of choice.

MRI

Primary CNS lymphoma is a well-demarcated, round, oval, or rarely gyral-shaped mass that is T1 hypointense to isointense relative to gray matter and produces relatively little mass effect for size. Hypointensity to isointensity on T2W images likely reflects increased nuclear-to-cytoplasmic ratio in these densely packed and highly cellular tumors. This also results in reduced diffusion and low apparent diffusion coefficient values (Fig. 31-5). Less commonly the lesions show T2 hyperintensity relative to gray matter. T2 hypointensity, when seen, helps to differentiate CNS lymphoma from gliomas and demyelinating disease.[26,29,30]

A ring pattern is typical of immunocompromised patients with CNS lymphoma and is caused by a T2 hypointense, densely cellular rim surrounded by edema.[26] The central portion of this ring correlates with necrosis. On T1W imaging, this same rim appears slightly hyperintense relative to surrounding hypointense edema and exhibits intense ring-shaped contrast enhancement, which may be smooth or irregular and may have associated enhancing mural nodules.

Findings of irregular, sinuous, or even gyral-like contrast enhancement suggest primary CNS lymphoma rather than toxoplasmosis, which typically has smooth peripheral ring enhancement.[26]

With MR perfusion, cerebral blood volume is higher than in toxoplasmosis or tumefactive demyelinating lesions but lower than that of glioblastoma multiforme.[31]

Proton MR spectroscopy reveals a decreased N-acetyl-aspartate peak and an increased choline/creatine ratio. In addition, a high lipid resonance on MR spectroscopy may differentiate primary CNS lymphoma from glioma. A lactate peak may be identified.[32]

Special Procedures

Primary CNS lymphoma has various angiographic appearances: avascular mass, focal blush in the late arterial-to-capillary phase that persists well into the venous phase, arterial encasement, dilated deep medullary veins, and tumor neovascularity. Dural supply may be seen in lesions involving dura or leptomeninges.

PET

Increased metabolism of tumor causes rapid uptake of radiotracer carbon-11 methionine, which is seen on PET in areas that extend beyond the areas of enhancement seen on CT/MRI.[33]

SPECT

Thallium-201 SPECT can help distinguish lymphoma from toxoplasmosis. Lymphoma is hypermetabolic, whereas toxoplasmosis is isometabolic to hypometabolic.

With thallium-201 SPECT and PET, false-positive and false-negative findings occur, usually due to errors in interpretation. Sometimes the lesion does not demonstrate as much uptake, and other nonmalignant lesions such as bacterial abscess and progressive multifocal leukoencephalopathy may show hypermetabolism.

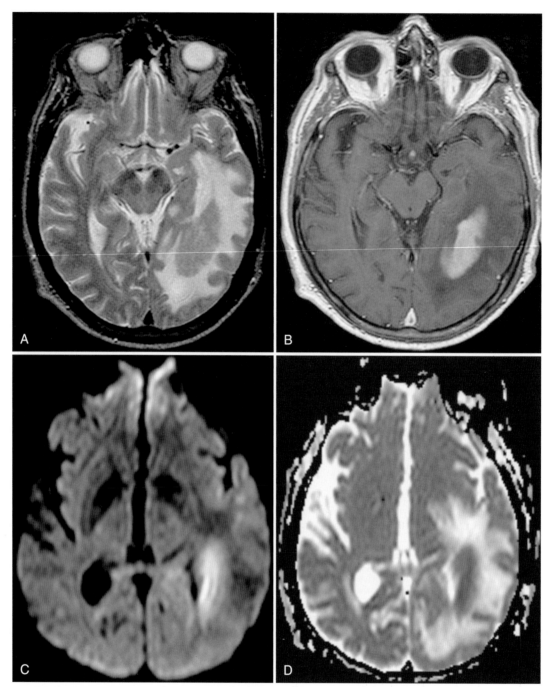

■ **FIGURE 31-5** Primary CNS lymphoma. **A,** Axial T2W MR image demonstrating a T2 hypointense lesion in the left temporal-occipital region. **B,** Axial T1W postcontrast MR image of same lesion in **A** demonstrates avid enhancement. **C,** Axial DW image of the same lesion demonstrates reduced diffusion consistent with high nuclear-to-cytoplasmic ratio and increased cellularity of the tumor. **D,** Axial apparent diffusion coefficient (ADC) map corresponding to DW image in **C** demonstrates decreased ADC values in the region of the tumor.

KEY POINTS: PRIMARY CNS LYMPHOMA

- Imaging features of primary CNS lymphoma depend on the immune status of the patient.
- The classic location is the deep gray nuclei, but this is seen less than a third of the time. Other locations include cerebral white matter and corpus callosum. Dural involvement is rare and is more often seen in secondary NHL to the CNS.
- Primary CNS lymphoma has an affinity for the perivascular spaces as well as subpial and subependymal regions.

- CT may reveal a hyperdense mass. T2W imaging often shows low signal in the mass, and it may demonstrate reduced diffusion. These findings are related to the high nuclear-to-cytoplasmic ratio and increased cellularity of the tumor.
- MR perfusion demonstrates increased cerebral blood volume in comparison to toxoplasmosis, but it is not as elevated as in glioblastoma multiforme.

INTRAVASCULAR LYMPHOMA

Intravascular lymphoma is a systemic NHL that involves the CNS with malignant lymphocytes adhering to the intima of arteries and arterioles, as well as affecting capillaries and venules. It is predominantly of B-cell origin, but T-cell intravascular lymphoma has been reported. In addition to the CNS, there is a predilection for skin. Alternate names include malignant angioendotheliomatosis, proliferating angioendotheliomatosis, intravascular malignant lymphomatosis, or angiotrophic large-cell lymphoma.

Epidemiology

This is a very rare entity, with fewer than 50 reported cases and fewer than 25 case reports.[34] There is a slight male predominance with age of onset at 63 years (range, 41-79). The average survival from onset of symptoms is 7 to 13 months. Poor prognosis may be related to delayed diagnosis.

Clinical Presentation

Progressive subacute dementia is the most common neurologic manifestation (75% of cases).[34] Focal deficits and seizures are less common. Progressive deterioration is the rule, but a spontaneous regression or even resolution without treatment is possible. CSF analysis may demonstrate an elevated protein level.

Skin changes include raised plaques and nodules on the extremities and trunk. Other sites of involvement include liver, spleen, and lymph nodes.

Pathology

Massive intravascular growth of lymphoid cells is present with predilection for CNS and skin. It may affect other organs as well.[34]

Macroscopically, small and sometimes hemorrhagic infarcts of varying ages are equally distributed throughout the brain and spinal cord, affecting cortex and subcortical white matter.[34]

Microscopically there is distention and occlusion of many small and intermediate size cerebral and meningeal arteries, arterioles, capillaries, and venules by proliferating noncohesive neoplastic mononuclear cells. Tumor cells are sometimes found outside vessels within brain parenchyma with adjacent localized destruction.[35,36]

Imaging
CT

Focal bilateral, asymmetric low densities are seen preferentially in supratentorial white matter at its junction with the cortex. A more periventricular distribution of low densities has also been described. The initial CT may be normal or show only cortical atrophy.[37]

MRI

There is involvement of the deep white matter in up to 45% of cases as well as less common involvement of the cortex and basal ganglia, demonstrated by high T2 signal lesions that correlate with edema and gliosis. Over a third have infarct-like lesions, with high T2 signal lesions in gray matter in a vascular territory with little or no edema. Lesions may also be seen infratentorially (Fig. 31-6). Partial hemorrhagic transformation can be detected.[38,39]

Meningeal or dural enhancement usually overlies enhancing parenchymal lesions. There are enhancing parenchymal masses in fewer than a third of cases. Contrast enhancement is variable either as an infarct-like gyriform enhancement or as a homogeneous moderately enhancing lesions.[40]

Changing appearances of the disease on MRI may be related to disturbed venous outflow, possibly secondary to free floating intravascular lymphoma cells. Infarct-like lesions may be related to complex lesions of the arteries, capillaries, and veins.[41]

Diffusion restriction has been reported. Hemorrhage may be seen on gradient-recalled-echo imaging.

Spinal cord involvement is also seen. A focal high signal on T2 imaging corresponds to ischemic necrosis seen on histology by occlusive intravascular aggregation. Moderate nodular meningeal enhancement along the cauda equina has been observed.

Special Procedures

Angiography is noncontributory and may mimic cerebral vasculitis.

KEY POINTS: INTRAVASCULAR LYMPHOMA

■ Intravascular lymphoma presents most often as progressive subacute dementia.
■ Vascular obstruction leads to multiple infarct-like lesions in multiple vascular territories. The lesions may or may not enhance.

LEUKEMIA

Leukemia is a heterogeneous group of hematologic malignancies. Neoplastic cells proliferate at an undifferentiated or partially differentiated stage of maturation. Alternate names include granulocytic sarcoma, chloroma, myeloblastoma, and extramedullary leukemic tumors. *Granulocytic sarcoma* is the preferred term over *chloroma* because not all lesions are green in color on gross pathologic examination.

Epidemiology

The majority of patients (60%) are younger than 15 years of age. There is a slight male predominance. Leukemia is almost twice as prevalent in whites as in nonwhites. A CNS complication will occur in 25% to 50% of patients.[42]

Clinical Presentation

CNS disease may be from direct leukemic involvement, underlying leukemic effects on immune or hematopoietic systems (anemia, alterations in hemostasis, infection), or anti-leukemia therapy itself.

CNS involvement is usually meningeal but can be parenchymal.[42] When it involves the meninges, it can affect the dura, leptomeninges, or both diffusely or focally. Leptomeningeal disease presents with signs and symptoms of increased intracranial pressure, including headache, nausea, vomiting, irritability, lethargy, and papilledema. Other symptoms include cranial nerve palsies, myelopathy, auditory symptoms, vertigo, ataxia, and hallucinations. Nonmeningeal disease is rarer and includes intracranial solid tumors composed of primitive precursors of the granulocytic series of white blood cells, which includes myeloblasts, myelocytes, and promyelocytes.

Granulocytic sarcoma occurs primarily in acute myelogenous leukemia but also may be seen in other myeloproliferative disorders. It is occurring with greater frequency because of improved anti-leukemia therapy and longer remission in acute myelogenous leukemia.[43] Skin, bone, and soft tissue are far more commonly affected with granulocytic sarcoma than is the CNS.

Intracranially, granulocytic sarcoma may be parenchymal or dural based. When dural based, it can be difficult to distinguish from meningioma. Rarely, granulocytic sarcoma can precede systemic leukemia.[44]

Orbital disease presents as focal intraconal and extraconal masses, which can be bilateral. Extraocular muscle infiltration, optic nerve infiltration, and intraocular involvement of the

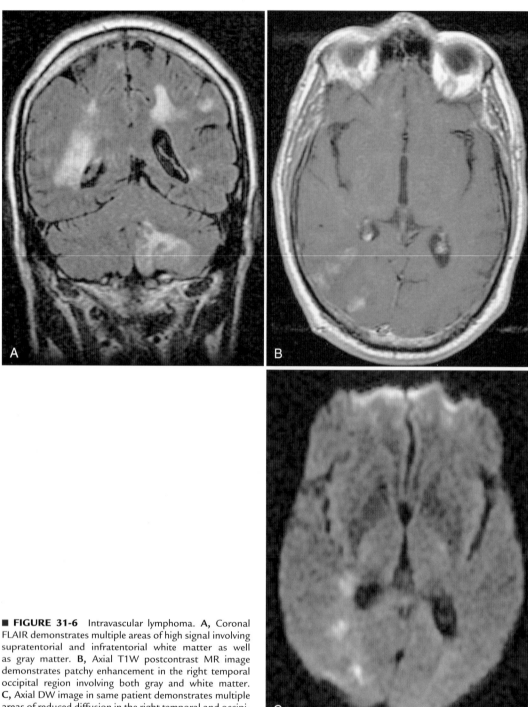

■ **FIGURE 31-6** Intravascular lymphoma. **A,** Coronal FLAIR demonstrates multiple areas of high signal involving supratentorial and infratentorial white matter as well as gray matter. **B,** Axial T1W postcontrast MR image demonstrates patchy enhancement in the right temporal occipital region involving both gray and white matter. **C,** Axial DW image in same patient demonstrates multiple areas of reduced diffusion in the right temporal and occipital lobes.

anterior chamber, ciliary body, choroid, or retina are also seen.[45] Granulocytic sarcoma also arises in the paranasal sinuses, nasopharynx, and skull base.

Complications

Hematologic events occur most commonly in acute leukemia resulting from a hypercoagulable state or bleeding diathesis or disseminated intravascular coagulation. Intracranial hemorrhage and cerebral infarction may be complications of the disease or secondary to treatment. Hemorrhage is more common than infarction in leukemia patients.[42] Venous thrombosis may be seen with chemotherapy (L-asparaginase) in addition to a

hypercoagulable state from leukemia itself. A vasculitis related to leukemia, leukemia treatment, or secondary infection may also occur.

Leukemia patients are more susceptible to infection because of abnormal or decreased granulocytes, mucosal damage from chemotherapy, corticosteroid treatment, and diminished mucociliary clearance. Viral, bacterial, and fungal infections are of concern, especially fungal sinus disease such as aspergillosis or mucormycosis, which can spread rapidly intracranially.[46] Abscesses can be difficult to distinguish from granulocytic sarcoma.

Anti-leukemia agents can be neurotoxic, and this can be difficult to distinguish from the other CNS complications of leukemia.[42] Methotrexate treatment can lead to disseminated necrotizing leukoencephalopathy, which results in multifocal demyelination, coagulative necrosis, glial loss, and axonal swelling, particularly in the white matter of the centrum semiovale. Radiation treatment is thought to potentiate chemotherapeutic toxicity. Radiation treatment may also lead to the development of cavernous angiomas.

Leukemia patients are also at increased risk for a second primary intracranial neoplasm.

Pathology

The typical granulocytic sarcoma is green because of high levels of myeloperoxidase. However, not all are green, and 30% are white, gray, or brown depending on the state of oxidation of myeloperoxidase or the different cellular enzyme concentrations.[42,47]

This rare tumor is composed of immature granulocytes. Granulocytic sarcoma can be confused with large cell lymphoma because of similar histopathology. Immunohistochemical tests are needed for accurate diagnosis.

Imaging

CT

On nonenhanced CT, granulocytic sarcoma is isodense to hyperdense and enhances avidly (Fig. 31-7A). Rim enhancement mimicking an abscess may also occur.[42,48]

Leukoencephalopathy on nonenhanced CT demonstrates periventricular white matter hypodensity. Calcifications may be seen in basal ganglia and subcortical white matter. Mineralizing microangiopathy describes the necrosis and calcification seen in the basal ganglia. Calcification occurs in the walls of cerebral blood vessels.

Intraspinal leukemic meningitis on myelograms or CT myelograms is seen as clumping and thickening of the cauda equina.[49] Abnormal nodular enhancement in the subarachnoid space, enhancement and thickening of nerve roots, or abnormal enhancement along the pial surface of the spinal cord may also be seen.

MRI

Imaging is not 100% sensitive, so a normal MRI does not exclude CNS involvement with certainty. MRI is more sensitive than CT in detecting treatment-related lesions, and screening with MRI has been proposed to detect early adverse treatment-related changes.

MRI is more sensitive than CT for assessing subarachnoid involvement. Leukemic involvement of the subarachnoid space is manifested by an abnormal appearance of the CSF or nerve roots or abnormal enhancement of the meninges. There may be nodular subarachnoid enhancement or abnormal cisternal or pial enhancement.[42]

Granulocytic sarcoma is isointense to hyperintense on T1 weighting, is isointense to slightly hyperintense on T2 weighting, and enhances avidly (see Fig. 31-7B). Cysts and necrosis are not typical but may occur. Multiple lesions as well as intraspinal and paraspinal involvement have been reported.[50]

The differential diagnosis of abnormal meningeal enhancement in leukemia is broad and includes infectious and inflammatory meningitides, irritation from intrathecal chemotherapy, or hemorrhage. Diffuse dural infiltration is a less common finding than leptomeningeal disease and is seen on MRI as dural thickening and abnormal dural enhancement.[42]

Bone marrow infiltration with replacement of normal hematopoietic elements and fat is seen. MRI reveals diffusely diminished signal intensity of vertebral body bone marrow. Marrow will revert if remission occurs. MRI of successful bone marrow transplant 40 to 90 days after transplant shows

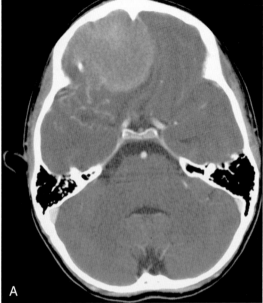

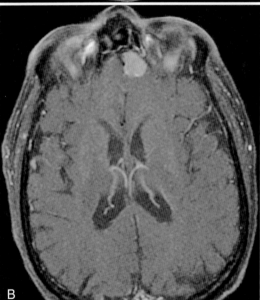

■ **FIGURE 31-7** Granulocytic sarcoma. **A,** Axial CT postcontrast image demonstrates a large enhancing mass in right frontal lobe with mass effect. **B,** Axial T1W postcontrast MR image of a different patient with an avidly enhancing left frontal lobe lesion.

alternating zones of high signal centrally (fat) with intermediate signal peripherally (reconstituted hematopoietic elements) on T1 weighting. If this band pattern does not develop or if marrow remains low signal, this is suggestive of failure of the graft or relapse.[51]

MRI of treatment-related leukoencephalopathy presents as multlifocal areas of high T2 signal intensity, typically in an anterior and posterior periventricular distribution. Enhancement can sometimes be seen early in the course. Mild changes may be seen even before onset of symptoms. Occasionally, severe cases of treatment-related leukoencephalopathy can appear large and mass-like, mimicking neoplasm.[52]

On MRI there may be abnormal enhancement and high T2 signal intensity in the ependyma and subependymal white matter surrounding the entrance site of the Ommaya reservoir in patients receiving intraventricular chemotherapy.

PLASMACYTOMA

Plasmacytoma is a neoplasm of plasma cell origin producing monoclonal immunoglobulins without evidence for systemic disease (i.e., multiple myeloma). It arises from bone (skull), dura, or, rarely, brain parenchyma. These tumors also have been reported to occur in the sella.

Alternate names include solitary craniocerebral plasmacytoma, solitary dural plasmacytoma, and plasmacytoma-revealing multiple myeloma.

Epidemiology

It is important to distinguish systemic disease from solitary craniocerebral plasmacytoma, which is extremely rare with only a few case reports in the medical literature. The treatment and prognosis are very different for multiple myeloma in comparison with solitary craniocerebral plasmacytoma, which demonstrates good response to surgery and radiation therapy.[53-55] Systemic development of solitary dural plasmacytoma into multiple myeloma has not been described.[56]

Clinical Presentation

Intracranial manifestations include diffuse leptomeningeal disease, solitary dural lesion without invasion of adjacent parenchyma, intra-axial tumor without attachment to dura or bone, or, rarely, an invasive tumor that grows from the subcutaneous tissue or dura into the brain parenchyma.[53]

Solitary intracranial plasmacytoma most often presents in the fifth decade of life as intracranial hypertension and focal neurologic signs.

Sellar lesions can present as symptoms and signs similar to a nonfunctioning pituitary adenoma and may also have cranial nerve involvement.[57]

Pathology

There is a relatively uniform, diffuse infiltration of plasmacytoid cells, of variable differentiation, within meningeal tissue. Immunohistologic staining may show restrictive reactivity with the immunoglobulin κ light chain and γ heavy chain.

Imaging

CT

Skull lesions are lytic and expansile, involving the diploic space as well as the inner and outer tables. They demonstrate diffuse homogeneous enhancement. Intratumoral calcifications (bone destruction) may or may not be present.[53]

Dural plasmacytomas are rounded or lobulated hyperdense lesions that homogenously enhance.[53-55]

MRI

Skull lesions are slightly heterogeneous expansile masses that erode bone. On MRI, a solitary intracranial plasmacytoma is hypointense to brain on T1W sequences and isointense to hyperintense on T2W sequences. They demonstrate homogeneous enhancement (Fig. 31-8).[53]

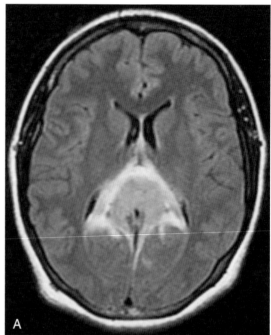
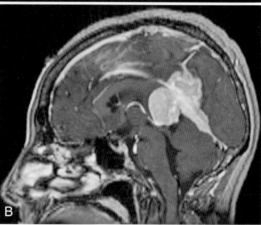

■ **FIGURE 31-8**　Solitary intracranial plasmacytoma. **A,** Axial FLAIR image demonstrates a T2 isointense to hyperintense extra-axial mass arising from the falx and tentorium and abutting the splenium. A mild amount of surrounding vasogenic edema is present. **B,** Sagittal T1W postcontrast MR image in the same patient demonstrates an avidly enhancing multilobulated extra-axial mass.

Plasmacytomas can closely mimic meningiomas because they occur more often in women, occur in middle to late life, and are found in similar locations.

Special Procedures

On angiography there is an avascular space-occupying lesion, although some report tumor staining.

ANALYSIS

In many instances, the key to diagnosing and differentiating the various entities will be suggested by the patient's medical history. A patient with VHL disease with a solid and cystic mass likely has a hemangioblastoma, although renal cell carcinoma metastasis is in the differential diagnosis. In patients who are immunosuppressed with an intracranial mass, primary CNS lymphoma is suggested, although the differential diagnosis includes infections such as toxoplasmosis. Leukemic patients with an intracranial mass may have a granulocytic sarcoma, but in this case one also needs to consider treatment-related toxicities and infections.

Important distinguishing characteristics include location of the mass—whether it is intra-axial or extra-axial. Signal characteristics on MRI may also provide important clues to the diagnosis (Table 31-1). Contrast enhancement may not be as helpful, because all these entities demonstrate enhancement. MR perfusion also is not helpful in making a distinction between these entities because they all may demonstrate increased cerebral blood volume and leaky capillaries due to blood-brain barrier breakdown. MR perfusion is helpful in distinguishing between these entities and other causes such as abscess. Morphology of the lesion may also provide clues to the diagnosis.

Sample reports are presented in Boxes 31-1 to 31-3.

TABLE 31-1. Differential Diagnosis of Vascular and Hematopoietic Tumors: Imaging Features

Primarily Extra-axial Location
Hemangiopericytoma
Solitary intracranial plasmacytoma
Leukemia

Primarily Intra-axial Location
Primary CNS lymphoma
Hemangioblastoma
Intravascular lymphoma

Hypointense on T2W Sequences
Primary CNS lymphoma

Reduced/Restricted Diffusion
Primary CNS lymphoma
Intravascular lymphoma (infarcts secondary to vascular occlusion)

Enhancing Nodule with Associated Cyst
Hemangioblastoma

BOX 31-1   Sample Report: Hemangioblastoma

PATIENT HISTORY

A 25-year-old man presented with a history of von Hippel-Lindau disease and headaches, nausea, and vomiting.

TECHNIQUE

Multiplanar T1, T2, FLAIR, and diffusion-weighted MR images of the brain were performed before and after the intravenous administration of gadolinium.

COMPARISON STUDIES

Unenhanced and enhanced head CT scans were obtained from earlier the same day.

FINDINGS

When compared with the previous CT scan there is re-demonstration of an approximately 1-cm enhancing nodule within the right cerebellum with an associated cyst measuring approximately 2.5 cm in diameter. The nodule abuts the pial surface, and the cyst does not demonstrate any enhancement. T2W and FLAIR images demonstrate surrounding edema. Mass effect is noted with compression of the fourth ventricle. There is no hydrocephalus at this time and no evidence for upward or downward herniation. There is no evidence of reduced diffusion.

IMPRESSION

A 1-cm enhancing nodule with a 2.5-cm associated cyst is present in the right cerebellum. The nodule abuts the pial surface. Given the patient's history of VHL, this likely represents a hemangioblastoma. Renal cell carcinoma metastasis is also a possibility, and correlation with renal imaging is recommended.

BOX 31-2   Sample Report: Primary CNS Lymphoma

PATIENT HISTORY

A 77-year-old woman with no significant past medical history presented with altered mental status, headaches, nausea, and vomiting.

COMPARISON STUDY

An unenhanced head CT was performed earlier the same day.

TECHNIQUE

Multiplanar T1W, T2W, FLAIR, and diffusion-weighted MR images of the brain were performed before and after the intravenous administration of gadolinium. MR perfusion and MR spectroscopy were performed and interrogated the lesion.

FINDINGS

There is an approximately 3-cm lesion centered in the region of the left basal ganglia. This lesion was identified on the prior noncontrast head CT as a hyperdense mass. On T1W images, the mass is isointense to gray matter. On T2W and FLAIR sequences, the mass demonstrates low signal intensity. Surrounding areas of T2 hyperintensity are seen consistent with vasogenic edema. The lesion has reduced diffusion on diffusion-weighted imaging. Postcontrast images reveal solid enhancement of the lesion with extension along the ependyma of the left lateral ventricle. MR perfusion demonstrates elevated blood volume, and MR spectroscopy at an echo time of 288 ms shows reduced *N*-acetyl-aspartate and elevated choline as well as a lipid peak.

IMPRESSION

An enhancing mass demonstrating T2 hypointensity and reduced diffusion is centered in the region of the left basal ganglia. Enhancement extends along the ependyma of the adjacent lateral ventricle. MR perfusion and MR spectroscopy are suggestive of neoplasm. Overall, the findings are consistent with primary CNS lymphoma.

BOX 31-3   Sample Report: Hemangiopericytoma

PATIENT HISTORY

A 45-year-old man presented with headache.

COMPARISON STUDY

An unenhanced head CT was done earlier the same day.

TECHNIQUE

Multiplanar T1W, T2W, FLAIR, and diffusion-weighted MR images of the brain were performed before and after the intravenous administration of gadolinium.

FINDINGS

A right parasagittal, extra-axial, heterogeneously enhancing multilobulated mass measuring approximately 3.5 cm in diameter is identified overlying the right parietal lobe. An enhancing dural tail is seen. The mass is isointense on T1W and T2W sequences. It was noted on the prior CT to not have any calcifications or adjacent bony hyperostosis. The inner table of the skull adjacent to the mass has been eroded. There is T2 hyperintensity in the adjacent parietal lobe white matter that likely represents vasogenic edema.

IMPRESSION

A heterogeneously enhancing extra-axial mass overlies the right parietal lobe with adjacent inner table bone erosion. In conjunction with the findings from the prior unenhanced head CT, this lesion is compatible with a hemangiopericytoma. The differential diagnosis includes dural metastasis.

SUGGESTED READINGS

Chiechi MV, Smirniotopoulos JG, Mena H. Intracranial hemangiopericytomas: MR and CT features. AJNR Am J Neuroradiol 1996; 17:1365-1371.

Choyke PL, et al. von Hippel-Lindau disease: genetic, clinical, and imaging features. Radiology 1995; 194:629-642.

Ginsberg LE, Leeds NE. Neuroradiology of leukemia. AJR Am J Roentgenol 1995; 165:525-534.

Hochberg FH, Baehring JM, Hochberg EP. Primary CNS lymphoma. Nat Clin Pract Neurol 2007; 3:24-35.

Johnson BA, et al. The variable MR appearance of primary lymphoma of the central nervous system: comparison with histopathologic features. AJNR Am J Neuroradiol 1997; 18:563-572.

Koeller KK, Smirniotopoulos JG, Jones RV. Primary central nervous system lymphoma: radiologic-pathologic correlation. RadioGraphics 1997; 17:1497-1526.

Provenzale JM, et al. Craniocerebral plasmacytoma: MR features. AJNR Am J Neuroradiol 1997; 18:389-392

Pui MH, Fletcher BD, Langston JW: Granulocytic sarcoma in childhood leukemia: imaging features. Radiology 1994; 190:698-702.

Wanebo JE, et al. The natural history of hemangioblastomas of the central nervous system in patients with von Hippel-Lindau disease. J Neurosurg 2003; 98:82-94.

Williams RL, et al. Cerebral MR imaging in intravascular lymphomatosis. AJNR Am J Neuroradiol 1998; 19:427-431.

REFERENCES

1. Choyke PL, et al. von Hippel-Lindau disease: genetic, clinical, and imaging features. Radiology 1995; 194:629-642.
2. Filling-Katz MR, et al. Central nervous system involvement in Von Hippel-Lindau disease. Neurology 1991; 41:41-46.
3. Lamiell JM, Salazar FG, Hsia YE. von Hippel-Lindau disease affecting 43 members of a single kindred. Medicine (Baltimore) 1989; 68:1-29.
4. Maher ER, et al. Clinical features and natural history of von Hippel-Lindau disease. Q J Med 1990; 77:1151-1163.
5. Wanebo JE, et al. The natural history of hemangioblastomas of the central nervous system in patients with von Hippel-Lindau disease. J Neurosurg 2003; 98:82-94.
6. Latif F, et al. Identification of the von Hippel-Lindau disease tumor suppressor gene. Science 1993; 260:1317-1320.
7. Bohling T, et al. Expression of growth factors and growth factor receptors in capillary hemangioblastoma. J Neuropathol Exp Neurol 1996; 55:522-527.
8. Stratmann R, et al. Putative control of angiogenesis in hemangioblastomas by the von Hippel-Lindau tumor suppressor gene. J Neuropathol Exp Neurol 1997; 56:1242-1252.
9. Wizigmann-Voos S, et al. Up-regulation of vascular endothelial growth factor and its receptors in von Hippel-Lindau disease-associated and sporadic hemangioblastomas. Cancer Res 1995; 55:1358-1364.
10. Seeger JF, et al. Computed tomographic and angiographic evaluation of hemangioblastomas. Radiology 1981; 138:65-73.
11. Sato Y, et al. Hippel-Lindau disease: MR imaging. Radiology 1988; 166:241-246.
12. Nunnery EW, et al. Hemangiopericytoma: a light microscopic and ultrastructural study. Cancer 1981; 47:906-914.
13. Feldman ZT, et al. Haemangiopericytoma presenting with intracerebral haemorrhage: case report and review of literature. Acta Neurochir (Wien) 1991; 112:151-153.
14. Alen JF, et al. Intracranial hemangiopericytoma: study of 12 cases. Acta Neurochir (Wien) 2001; 143:575-586.
15. Sandhu FA, Martuza RL. Craniofacial hemangiopericytoma associated with oncogenic osteomalacia: case report. J Neurooncol 2000; 46:241-247.
16. Younis GA, et al. Aggressive meningeal tumors: review of a series. J Neurosurg 1995; 82:17-27.
17. Morrison DA, Bibby K. Sellar and suprasellar hemangiopericytoma mimicking pituitary adenoma. Arch Ophthalmol 1997; 115:1201-1203.
18. Chiechi MV, Smirniotopoulos JG, Mena H. Intracranial hemangiopericytomas: MR and CT features. AJNR Am J Neuroradiol 1996; 17:1365-1371.
19. Cosentino CM, et al. Giant cranial hemangiopericytoma: MR and angiographic findings. AJNR Am J Neuroradiol 1993; 14:253-256.
20. Barba I, et al: Magnetic resonance spectroscopy of brain hemangiopericytomas: high myoinositol concentrations and discrimination from meningiomas. J Neurosurg 2001; 94:55-60.
21. Marc JA, et al. Intracranial hemangiopericytomas: Angiography, pathology and differential diagnosis. Am J Roentgenol Radium Ther Nucl Med 1975; 125:823-832.
22. Guthrie BL, et al. Meningeal hemangiopericytoma: histopathological features, treatment, and long-term follow-up of 44 cases. Neurosurgery 1989; 25:514-522.
23. Hochberg FH, Baehring JM, Hochberg EP. Primary CNS lymphoma. Nat Clin Pract Neurol 2007; 3:24-35.
24. Miller DC, et al. Pathology with clinical correlations of primary central nervous system non-Hodgkin's lymphoma. The Massachusetts General Hospital experience 1958-1989. Cancer 1994; 74: 1383-1397.
25. Zimmerman RA. Central nervous system lymphoma. Radiol Clin North Am 1990; 28:697-721.
26. Johnson BA, et al. The variable MR appearance of primary lymphoma of the central nervous system: comparison with histopathologic features. AJNR Am J Neuroradiol 1997; 18:563-572.
27. Hochberg FH, Miller DC. Primary central nervous system lymphoma. J Neurosurg 1988; 68:835-853.
28. Lee YY, et al. Primary central nervous system lymphoma: CT and pathologic correlation. AJR Am J Roentgenol 1986; 147:747-752.
29. Koeller KK, Smirniotopoulos JG, Jones RV. Primary central nervous system lymphoma: radiologic-pathologic correlation. RadioGraphics 1997; 17:1497-1526.
30. Roman-Goldstein SM, et al. MR of primary CNS lymphoma in immunologically normal patients. AJNR Am J Neuroradiol 1992; 13:1207-1213.
31. Cha S. Perfusion MR imaging of brain tumors. Top Magn Reson Imaging 2004; 15:279-289.
32. Harting I, et al. Differentiating primary central nervous system lymphoma from glioma in humans using localised proton magnetic resonance spectroscopy. Neurosci Lett 2003; 342:163-166
33. Ogawa T, et al. Methionine PET for follow-up of radiation therapy of primary lymphoma of the brain. RadioGraphics 1994; 14:101-110.
34. Martin-Duverneuil N, et al. Intravascular malignant lymphomatosis. Neuroradiology 2002; 44:749-754.
35. Wach M, et al. Intravascular B-cell lymphoma in a 38-year-old woman: a case report. Ann Hematol 2001; 80:224-227.
36. Kanda M, et al. Intravascular large cell lymphoma: clinicopathological, immuno-histochemical and molecular genetic studies. Leuk Lymphoma 1999; 34:569-580.
37. Knight RS, Anslow P, Theaker JM. Neoplastic angioendotheliosis: a case of subacute dementia with unusual cerebral CT appearances and a review of the literature. J Neurol Neurosurg Psychiatry 1987; 50:1022-1028.
38. Hashimoto H, et al. Presymptomatic brain lesions on MRI in a patient with intravascular malignant lymphomatosis. J Neuroimaging 1998; 8:110-113
39. Liow K, et al. Intravascular lymphomatosis: contribution of cerebral MRI findings to diagnosis. J Neuroimaging 2000; 10:116-118.
40. Williams RL, et al. Cerebral MR imaging in intravascular lymphomatosis. AJNR Am J Neuroradiol 1998; 19:427-431.
41. Amagasaki K, et al. Malignant intravascular lymphomatosis associated with venous stenosis: case report. J Neurosurg 1999; 90: 355-358.
42. Ginsberg LE, Leeds NE. Neuroradiology of leukemia. AJR Am J Roentgenol 1995; 165:525-534.

43. Stork JT, et al. Recurrent chloromas in acute myelogenous leukemia. AJR Am J Roentgenol 1984; 142:777-778.

44. Barnett MJ, Zussman WV. Granulocytic sarcoma of the brain: a case report and review of the literature. Radiology 1986; 160:223-225.

45. Banna M, Aur R, Akkad S. Orbital granulocytic sarcoma. AJNR Am J Neuroradiol 1991; 12:255-258.

46. Zinreich SJ, et al. Fungal sinusitis: diagnosis with CT and MR imaging. Radiology 1988; 169:439-444.

47. Pui MH, Fletcher BD, Langston JW. Granulocytic sarcoma in childhood leukemia: imaging features. Radiology 1994; 190:698-702.

48. Pomeranz SJ, et al. Granulocytic sarcoma (chloroma): CT manifestations. Radiology 1985; 155:167-170.

49. McAllister MD, O'Leary DH. CT myelography of subarachnoid leukemic infiltration of the lumbar thecal sac and lumbar nerve roots. AJNR Am J Neuroradiol 1987; 8:568-569.

50. Vinters HV, Gilbert JJ. Multifocal chloromas of the brain. Surg Neurol 1982; 17:47-51.

51. Stevens SK, Moore SG, Amylon MD. Repopulation of marrow after transplantation: MR imaging with pathologic correlation. Radiology 1990; 175:213-218.

52. Ball WS Jr, Prenger EC, Ballard ET. Neurotoxicity of radio/chemotherapy in children: pathologic and MR correlation. AJNR Am J Neuroradiol 1992; 13:761-776.

53. Provenzale JM, et al. Craniocerebral plasmacytoma: MR features. AJNR Am J Neuroradiol 1997; 18:389-392.

54. Mantyla R, Kinnunen J, Bohling T. Intracranial plasmacytoma: a case report. Neuroradiology 1996; 38:646-649.

55. Vaicys C, et al. Falcotentorial plasmacytoma: case report. J Neurosurg 1999; 91:132-135.

56. Haegelen C, et al. Dural plasmacytoma revealing multiple myeloma: case report. J Neurosurg 2006; 104:608-610.

57. McLaughlin DM, et al. Plasmacytoma: an unusual cause of a pituitary mass lesion: a case report and a review of the literature. Pituitary 2004; 7:179-181.

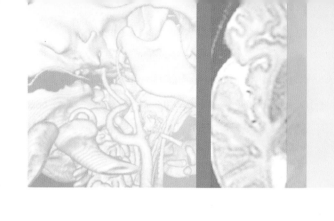

CHAPTER

32

Intra-Axial Neoplasms

Alice B. Smith and James G. Smirniotopoulos

Primary neoplasms of the central nervous system (CNS) are relatively infrequent, accounting for 16.5 to 18 cases per 100,000 person-years. However, they are a significant health concern.

Primary CNS neoplasms are histologically diverse and may arise from neuroepithelial tissue (e.g., astrocytic tumors, oligodendroglial tumors, ependymal tumors, embryonal tumors) or the hematopoietic system (primary CNS lymphoma). Neuroepithelial tissue consists of glial cells, neuronal cells, neuroblastic cells, pineal parenchymal cells, and residual embryonal cells. Most intra-axial neoplasms are of glial origin, accounting for 40% to 50% of primary CNS neoplasms.[1] The glial neoplasms arise from astrocytes, oligodendrocytes, ependymal cells, or their derivatives in the choroid plexus. The ganglion cell tumors (ganglioglioma, gangliocytoma) are composed of abnormal neoplastic neuronal cells or of a combination of neuronal and astrocytic elements.

Primary CNS neoplasms are graded according to the World Health Organization (WHO) classification system. The high-grade glial neoplasms are differentiated from the low grade on pathology by the presence of increased cellularity, increased mitotic activity, necrosis, and vascular proliferation. In a surgical series of stereotactic brain biopsies—consisting of 5000 specimens—the most common intra-axial brain masses were high-grade primary neoplasms (36%), low-grade primary neoplasms (33%), metastasis (8%), lymphoma (5%), demyelinating inflammatory lesions (3%), infarcts (2%), and abscesses (1%).[2,3]

Imaging plays an integral role in the detection, diagnosis, and management of these lesions, and advanced imaging, such as perfusion and MR spectroscopy, may help narrow the differential diagnosis and assist in post-treatment follow-up. However, the limitations of conventional MRI and advanced imaging must be kept in mind when interpreting the results. Conventional MRI is currently limited in its ability to demarcate the exact margins of infiltrative tumors, to accurately grade the neoplasm, and to monitor early changes after treatment. An example of the limitation of advanced imaging is in the evaluation of MR spectroscopy where there are no unequivocal cutoff metabolite peaks that clearly differentiate a neoplastic lesion from a non-neoplastic one, and low-grade neoplasms may have spectra that are similar to high-grade neoplasms, lymphoma, and metastases (i.e., elevation in choline [Cho], reduction in N-acetyl aspartate [NAA], and presence of a lipid/lactate peak). Tumefactive demyelinating lesions may show this pattern as well. However, in a review by

Al-Okaili and associates, it was found that a Cho/NAA cutoff ratio of 2.2 could reliably separate high-grade neoplasms from low-grade neoplasms and non-neoplastic lesions.[3]

Perfusion-weighted imaging may be of benefit in assessing angiogenesis induced by neoplasms. The vessels formed in a neoplastic process tend to be abnormal and leaky, thus resulting in increased permeability parameters on perfusion MRI. Several studies have demonstrated a correlation of tumor blood volume with the grade of neoplasm.[4-6] Law and colleagues observed that a relative cerebral blood volume (rCBV) threshold value of 1.75 provided a sensitivity of 95% and positive predictive values of 87% for distinguishing between high- and low-grade gliomas.[4] Because metastases tend to induce angiogenesis as well, the perfusion parameters of metastatic lesions tend to overlap with high-grade neoplasms.

Recent research has demonstrated that diffusion tensor imaging (DTI) has important potential benefits in surgical planning owing to the ability to detect white matter tracts in the region of the neoplasm.[7,8] The ability to assess whether the neoplasm has shifted the tracts versus infiltrating them is important information for the neurosurgeon and can assist in determining the method of approach and the extent of resection that is possible.

PILOCYTIC ASTROCYTOMA

Pilocytic astrocytoma is a slowly growing, well-circumscribed neoplasm classified by the WHO as a grade I glioma.

In the past, pilocytic astrocytomas were also referred to as "spongioblastoma polare" owing to their histologic resemblance to the spongioblastic cells of the fetus. This term is no longer in use. Pilocytic astrocytoma is also called "juvenile" pilocytic astrocytoma—a prefix no longer required. In addition, some refer to pilocytic astrocytomas by their location (i.e., optic nerve glioma, hypothalamic glioma).

Epidemiology

Pilocytic astrocytomas are the most common form of glioma in childhood and most frequently develop in the first two decades of life; 80% occur in patients younger than 20 years old.[9] Rarely, they arise in patients older than 50. They comprise 5% to 10% of all gliomas, and there is no strong gender predilection. However, some series have reported a slightly higher incidence in females (11:9). Pilocytic astrocytoma may arise anywhere

692

within the neuraxis, but within the pediatric population (<15 yr) they arise more frequently infratentorially and comprise 85% of all cerebellar neoplasms in the pediatric age group.[9] Other common sites are the optic nerve, optic chiasm and hypothalamus, basal ganglia, and thalamus.

Pilocytic astrocytomas are associated with neurofibromatosis type 1 (NF-1), occurring in 15% to 21% of patients with this disease.[9] In these patients the intraconal optic nerve and chiasm are most commonly involved (Fig. 32-1). The majority of optic

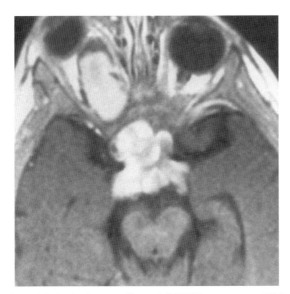

■ **FIGURE 32-1** Optic nerve glioma. Axial T1W postcontrast MR image from a patient with neurofibromatosis type 1 demonstrates an enhancing mass involving the optic nerve and chiasm.

pathway gliomas occur before 6 years of age, and there is a female predominance (2:1).

Pilocytic astrocytomas have benign biologic behavior with a survival rate of up to 94% at 10 years.[9] Disseminated disease and recurrence are very rare. Interestingly, when metastatic disease occurs, it can do so without increased mortality, unlike metastases from higher-grade neoplasms (Fig. 32-2).

Clinical Presentation

The clinical presentation depends, in part, on the location of the lesion. Pilocytic astrocytomas may present as focal neurologic signs or nonlocalizing signs such as headache, macrocephaly, endocrinopathy, or increased intracranial pressure due to mass effect or ventricular obstruction. Those involving the cerebellum can cause clumsiness, worsening headache, nausea, and vomiting. Seizures are uncommon because these lesions do not often involve the cerebral cortex. Those that involve the optic nerve/chiasm may result in visual loss, and those involving the hypothalamus may result in hypothalamic/pituitary dysfunction. Occasionally, the hypothalamic lesions result in the diencephalic syndrome—emaciation despite normal/slightly decreased appetite, alert appearance, hyperkinesis, irritability, and normal or accelerated growth.

Pathophysiology

Pilocytic astrocytomas are associated with NF-1, and approximately 15% of patients with NF-1 will develop a pilocytic astrocytoma, most commonly of the optic nerve. Pilocytic astrocytomas are a major source of morbidity in patients with NF-1. Cytogenetic studies of sporadic pilocytic astrocytomas have demonstrated a loss of genetic material of the long arm of chromosome 17(17q), which is near the same locus as the *NF1* tumor suppressor gene.[10] Other chromosomal mutations have been found on chromosomes 7, 8, 11, 19, and 21.[11]

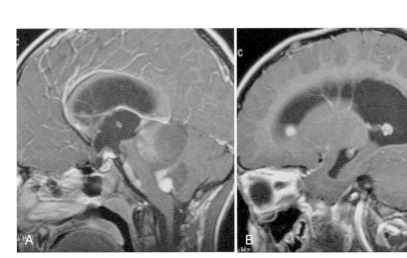
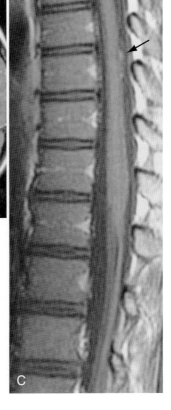

■ **FIGURE 32-2** Disseminated pilocytic astrocytoma. **A,** Sagittal postcontrast T1W MR image demonstrates a cystic lesion with an enhancing nodule in the posterior fossa. **B,** Sagittal postcontrast T1W MR image demonstrates an enhancing nodule in the anterior aspect of the lateral ventricle. **C,** Sagittal postcontrast T1W MR image of the spine reveals enhancing nodules (*arrow*) along the posterior aspect of the spinal cord.

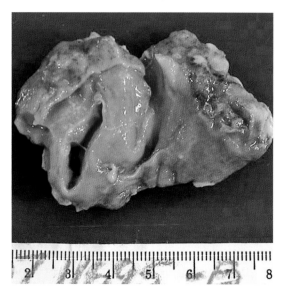

■ **FIGURE 32-3** Pilocytic astrocytoma. Bisected gross specimen reveals a soft, gelatinous, pink cystic mass.

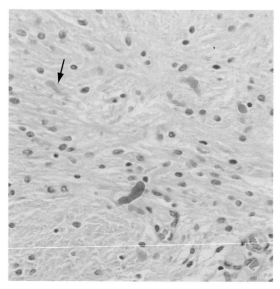

■ **FIGURE 32-4** Pilocytic astrocytoma. H&E stain demonstrates numerous Rosenthal fibers (*arrow*).

Pilocytic astrocytomas typically maintain their WHO grade I histology, tending toward degenerative changes over time rather than evolving into a more aggressive lesion. Rarely, progression to a malignant lesion has been reported; however, these tumors tend to have a better prognosis than glioblastoma multiforme and are referred to as anaplastic pilocytic astrocytoma. Most of the pilocytic astrocytomas that underwent malignant change had previously been irradiated, and it is possible that radiation may have been a factor in the malignant degeneration. Occasionally, pilocytic astrocytomas may seed the cerebrospinal fluid (CSF) and neuraxis, and in these cases the hypothalamus is usually the primary site rather than the cerebellum.

Pathology

On gross pathology, pilocytic astrocytomas are soft, well-circumscribed lesions. Fluid accumulation ("cyst formation") is commonly seen (Fig. 32-3). In older lesions, hemosiderin or calcium may be seen. Calcification tends to occur more often in tumors arising from the optic nerve or hypothalamic-thalamic regions. Lesions involving the optic nerve result in elongation and fusiform widening of the nerve.

Pilocytic astrocytomas have increased capillary vascularity and low to moderate cellularity. In long-standing neoplasms the vessels may become hyalinized and glomeruloid. A biphasic pattern of two astrocyte populations having varying proportions of compact bipolar cells with Rosenthal fibers (nonfilamentous electron-dense masses) and loose-textured multipolar cells with microcysts and eosinophilic granular bodies/hyaline droplets is seen (Figs. 32-4 and 32-5). The presence of eosinophilic granular bodies is thought to indicate slow growth and low histologic grade and is associated with an improved prognosis. Neoplastic changes involving the cyst wall have been reported.[12] Infiltration into the surrounding tissues may be seen but is usually shallow, especially in comparison with the adult or diffuse astrocytomas. This occurs more frequently in tumors involving the optic nerve and chiasm, and, commonly, there is poor demarcation between tumor and normal tissue. Pilocytic astrocytomas involving the cerebellum may infiltrate the leptomeninges, resulting in fixation of the cerebellar folia and filling of the sulci (Fig. 32-6).

On immunohistochemical evaluation, pilocytic astrocytomas are usually strongly and nearly diffusely positive for glial fibrillary acidic protein (GFAP), which is an intermediate filament found in the cytoplasm of astrocytes. S-100 protein, which is found in

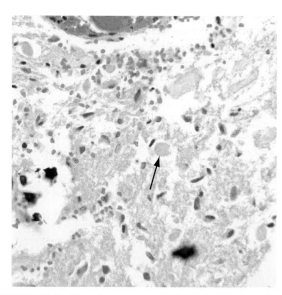

■ **FIGURE 32-5** Pilocytic astrocytoma. H&E stain reveals eosinophilic granular bodies (*arrow*).

all cells derived from the neural crest, is also positive. MIB-1 (a nuclear marker of proliferation) rates are usually low.

Imaging

Pilocytic astrocytomas are well-circumscribed lesions that enhance on postcontrast imaging. Fluid formation is common, and the classic description is that of a "cyst and nodule" (Fig. 32-7). Occasionally, calcification (up to 25%) may be seen and hemorrhage has been reported (Figs. 32-8 and 32-9). Pilocytic astrocytomas occasionally may enhance in a ring-like pattern, suggesting the morphology of a higher-grade neoplasm. In these cases, location (cerebellum) and age (<15 years) may suggest benign fluid, rather than necrosis, as the cause of the ring enhancement.

Four imaging patterns of pilocytic astrocytomas have been described: (1) enhancing mural nodule and nonenhancing cyst, (2) enhancing cyst wall and enhancing mural nodule, (3) "necrotic" mass with central nonenhancing region, and

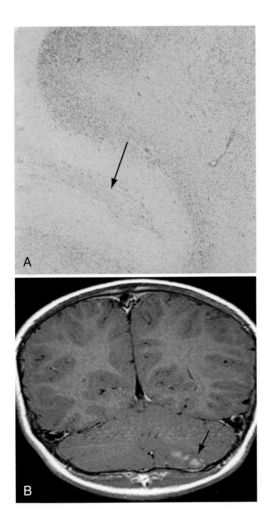

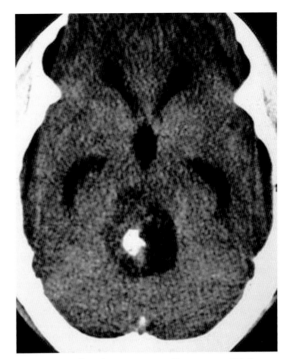

■ **FIGURE 32-8** Pilocytic astrocytoma. Noncontrast CT demonstrates a hypoattenuating lesion in the posterior fossa. A focus of high attenuation is present consistent with calcification.

■ **FIGURE 32-6** Pilocytic astrocytoma. **A,** H&E stain demonstrates the pilocytic astrocytoma "filling in" the subarachnoid space (*arrow*). **B,** Corresponding coronal postcontrast T1W MR image demonstrates an enhancing lesion in the inferior aspect of the left cerebellar hemisphere.

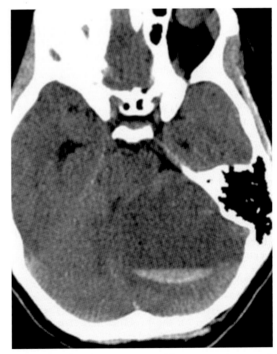

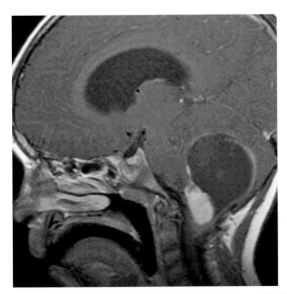

■ **FIGURE 32-7** Pilocytic astrocytoma. Sagittal postcontrast T1W MR image demonstrates the classic "cyst and nodule" appearance of a pilocytic astrocytoma in the posterior fossa. Thin rim enhancement is seen involving the cyst wall.

■ **FIGURE 32-9** Pilocytic astrocytoma. A low-attenuation mass lesion is present within the left cerebellar hemisphere consistent with a cyst, which has a fluid-fluid level consistent with hemorrhage.

(4) predominantly solid mass with minimal or no cyst.[12] Cyst wall enhancement does not necessarily imply there is tumor involvement, and removal of the cyst wall is not related to improved survival.[13,14] Some pilocytic astrocytomas may show thin rim enhancement from reactive gliosis surrounding the fluid.

CSF dissemination is rare (2%-12%) and increases in the setting of tumors located in the hypothalamus, in cases of partial resection, and in patients younger than 4 years old at the time of diagnosis. Dissemination tends to occur within the first 3 years after diagnosis.[15]

CT

On CT, pilocytic astrocytomas have the appearance of a solid nodule with associated fluid-filled "cyst." There may be little or no surrounding brain edema, which can provide a clue to the diagnosis. The majority will enhance after administration of a contrast agent, and the contrast agent may also accumulate within the cyst on very delayed imaging. Calcium may be seen in 20% to 25%, and hemorrhage rarely occurs.

MRI

On MRI, the solid portion of the neoplasm is typically isointense to hypointense on T1-weighted (T1W) imaging and hyperintense on T2-weighted (T2W) imaging to gray matter. The cystic portion is often hyperintense to CSF from protein (Fig. 32-10). The cyst contents do not suppress on FLAIR. The solid portion enhances on postcontrast imaging. Occasionally, the wall around the fluid may demonstrate rim enhancement. Rarely, leptomeningeal metastases may be seen.

In these low-grade tumors, MR spectroscopy demonstrates elevation in choline and a reduction in NAA, a pattern that is also seen in higher-grade neoplasms. There is minimal elevation in the lipid peak, and lactate peaks are elevated (Fig. 32-11). The elevation in lactate may represent alterations in mitochondrial metabolism or represent variability in glucose utilization rates among low-grade astrocytomas and not necrosis because necrosis is rare in pilocytic astrocytomas.[16]

Special Procedures

Evaluation of pilocytic astrocytomas by conventional angiography frequently demonstrates an avascular mass with peripheral displacement of normal vessels. Occasionally, neovascularity can be seen in the solid nodule.

PILOMYXOID ASTROCYTOMA

Pilomyxoid astrocytoma is a WHO grade II neoplasm that is closely related to pilocytic astrocytoma.

In the past, pilomyxoid astrocytomas were referred to as infantile pilocytic astrocytomas. The term pilomyxoid was introduced in 1999.

Epidemiology

The incidence of pilomyxoid astrocytomas is not known. It typically presents in infancy (median 10 months) but may be seen in older children and rarely in adults. There is no gender predilection.

Clinical Presentation

Pilomyxoid astrocytomas have nonspecific symptoms related to their location. They can occur anywhere along the neuraxis but have a predilection for the hypothalamus. The most common presenting symptoms are those related to increased intracranial pressure or parenchymal compression. Other reported symptoms include developmental delay, failure to thrive, altered level of consciousness, feeding difficulties, and generalized weakness. Pilomyxoid astrocytomas behave more aggressively than pilocytic astrocytomas, and they have a shorter progression-free and overall survival. They also have a higher rate of recurrence and CNS dissemination.[17]

There is currently no standard treatment for pilomyxoid astrocytomas. Treatment depends in part on location of the pilomyxoid astrocytoma. Those in the cerebellum are amenable to gross total surgical resection, whereas those in the hypothalamus are difficult to completely resect. Adjuvant chemotherapy may be

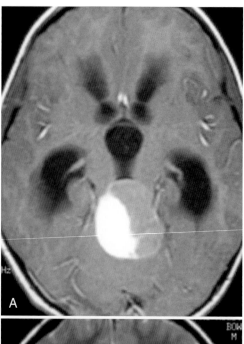

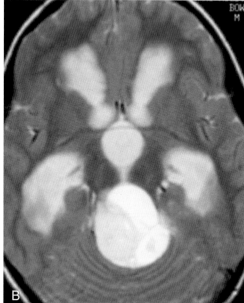

■ **FIGURE 32-10** Pilocytic astrocytoma. **A,** Axial postcontrast T1W MR image demonstrates a cyst with an enhancing mural nodule. **B,** T2W imaging demonstrates that the fluid within the cystic portion of the lesion is hyperintense to CSF. Hydrocephalus is present.

implemented in those cases of inoperable or partially resected gliomas.

Pathophysiology

Pilomyxoid astrocytomas are closely related to pilocytic astrocytomas. There have been occasional reports of pilomyxoid astrocytomas converting into pilocytic astrocytomas. The cell of origin is unclear. Reports describe it as having a close relationship to pilocytic astrocytoma, suggesting an astrocyte origin. However, it has been suggested that it may arise from the radial glia. No genetic abnormalities have been described.

These neoplasms behave more aggressively than pilocytic astrocytomas, with local recurrence (76% for pilomyxoid astrocytomas compared with 50% for pilocytic tumors) occurring

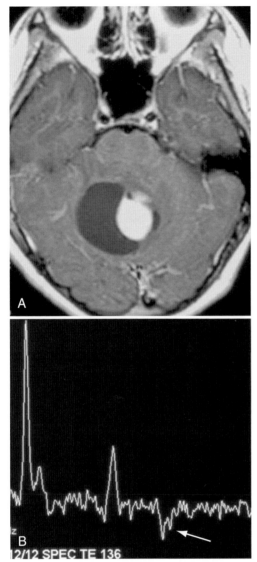

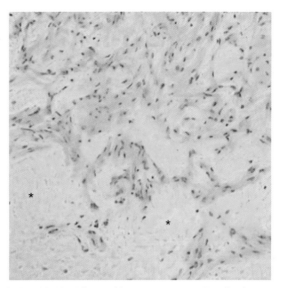

■ **FIGURE 32-12** Pilomyxoid astrocytoma. H&E stain demonstrates small piloid cells in a mucopolysaccharide matrix (*asterisks*).

■ **FIGURE 32-11** Pilocytic astrocytoma. **A,** Axial postcontrast T1W MR image demonstrates a cyst with an enhancing mural nodule. **B,** Single-voxel MR spectroscopy (TE = 136) placed in the region of the enhancing nodule demonstrates a more ominous-appearing MR spectroscopy pattern than would be expected for a grade I lesion. Choline level is elevated, NAA level is reduced, and lactate is present (*arrow*).

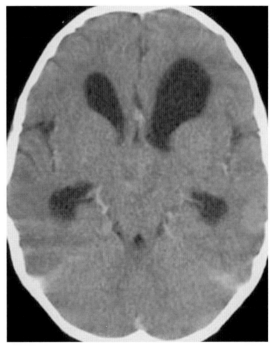

■ **FIGURE 32-13** Pilomyxoid astrocytoma. Contrast-enhanced CT demonstrates a minimally enhancing, solid, hypothalamic lesion. Hydrocephalus is present.

more frequently, despite having equal rates for gross total resection. CSF dissemination is relatively common, occurring in up to 14%.[18] In addition, 33% of patients with pilomyxoid astrocytoma died of their disease, compared with only 17% of patients with pilocytic astrocytoma.[18]

Pathology

Pilomyxoid astrocytomas are described as soft gelatinous masses. They have a prominent mucoid matrix and an angiocentric arrangement of bipolar tumor cells, resembling the perivascular rosettes seen in ependymomas (Fig. 32-12). Monomorphous piloid cells are present in a loose fibrillary and myxoid background. They do not demonstrate the Rosenthal fibers or eosinophilic granular bodies that are common in pilocytic astrocytomas. Rare mitotic figures may be seen. In some cases, infiltration of tumor cells into the surrounding neuropil occurs at the periphery of the neoplasm.[19]

Imaging

Pilomyxoid astrocytomas may occur anywhere along the neuraxis but are most common in the hypothalamic/chiasmatic region (76.9%).[20] On imaging, pilomyxoid astrocytomas are predominantly solid neoplasms, in contrast to the "cyst and nodule" frequently seen in pilocytic astrocytomas (Fig. 32-13). Pilomyxoid astrocytomas may occasionally demonstrate a minimal cystic component. On postcontrast imaging, pilomyxoid astrocytomas have been described as demonstrating homogeneous enhancement, although the number of cases in the literature is limited. Hydrocephalus is frequently present. Hemorrhage is rare, with only a few cases reported.[21,22]

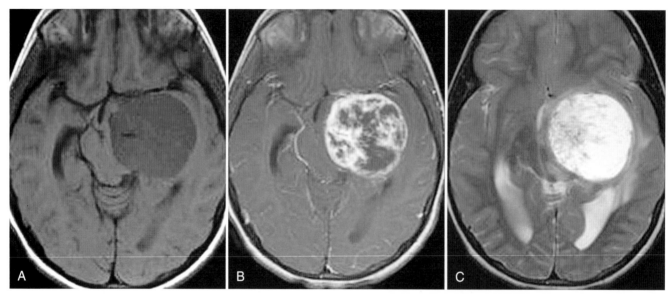

■ **FIGURE 32-14**   Pilomyxoid astrocytoma. **A,** Axial T1W MR image demonstrates a low-signal, well-circumscribed lesion in the left temporal lobe. **B,** On postcontrast imaging this particular lesion enhances heterogeneously. **C,** T2W MR image reveals high signal intensity.

MRI

Pilomyxoid astrocytomas are well circumscribed and "watery" and hypointense on T1W and hyperintense on T2W images (Fig. 32-14). They enhance after contrast agent administration, and they may demonstrate CSF dissemination. Necrosis is rare, and peritumoral edema is absent.

PLEOMORPHIC XANTHOASTROCYTOMA

Pleomorphic xanthoastrocytoma (PXA) is a WHO grade II neoplasm. Occasional examples have anaplastic features. Before immunostaining, PXAs were thought to be mesenchymal neoplasms of the meninges and brain.

Epidemiology

PXAs typically occur in children and young adults, with two thirds occurring before the age of 18 years; however, there have been rare reports of the lesions in older adults (age range: 5-82 years). These are uncommon neoplasms, accounting for less than 1% of astrocytic neoplasms.[1] There is no documented gender predilection. The majority occur in the supratentorial brain (98%), most commonly the temporal lobe (49%).[1]

Clinical Presentation

PXAs are superficially located and affect the cerebral cortex; thus, patients frequently present with a long history of seizures.

Pathophysiology

PXAs are occasionally associated with cortical dysplasia or with ganglionic lesions, suggesting that their formation may be promoted in malformative states. They have also been reported in patients with NF1, although no definite association with hereditary tumor syndromes has been demonstrated. Because of their typical superficial location, origin from subpial astrocytes is postulated. However, the histogenesis is unclear and there is the suggestion that this tumor may derive from bipotential precursor cells.[23]

Long-term survival in patients with PXAs is reported at 81% at 5 years and 70% at 10 years.[24] The degree of resection appears to be the best predictor of outcome, along with a low mitotic index. The tumor has a relatively high rate of recurrence; a malignant transformation occurs in up to 20%.[24]

Pathology

PXAs are peripherally located neoplasms and involve the leptomeninges (Fig. 32-15). Cyst formation is common, and a "cyst and nodule" appearance is common.

Pleomorphic xanthoastrocytomas have a variable histologic appearance, hence the name "pleomorphic." Mononucleated or multinucleated giant astrocytes with variable nuclear size and staining are seen. They have a dense reticulin network and lipid (xanthomatous) deposits within the tumor cells. The term *xanthoastrocytoma* refers to large cells with intracellular lipid accumulation (Fig. 32-16). Despite a circumscribed appearance, most PXAs demonstrate extension into the surrounding brain. Even though the tumor is frequently attached to the leptomeninges, dural invasion is uncommon. Necrosis within the tumor portends a poorer prognosis.[25] Mitoses are usually absent or rare; however, atypical PXAs demonstrate high mitotic activity and marked hypercellularity and necrosis. These may be considered grade III or anaplastic PXA.

Immunohistochemical analysis demonstrates the presence of glial fibrillary acidic protein (GFAP) and S-100 (present in cells derived from the neural crest); and neuronal markers such as synaptophysin (protein present in neurons in the brain and spinal cord that participate in synaptic transmission), class III β-tubulin (a neuronal marker), and NF proteins (play an important role in neuronal development) are also described. *TP53* is the tumor suppressor gene, and mutations occur in many human cancers. Analysis for the *TP53* mutation is negative or only focally positive. In one study of PXAs that demonstrated malignant progression, histochemical analysis revealed GFAP positivity in 100% and S-100 and TP53 were expressed in 67% but synaptophysin and NF protein were absent.[26] The MIB-1 index for PXAs is typically less than 1%.

Imaging

The classic imaging appearance of PXAs is that of a peripherally located "cystic" supratentorial mass. However, 52% do not have macroscopic fluid changes.[1] Lesions may be well circumscribed or poorly defined.

CT

On CT, the solid portion of the PXA is hyperattenuating and the cystic portion is hypoattenuating. The solid portion enhances on

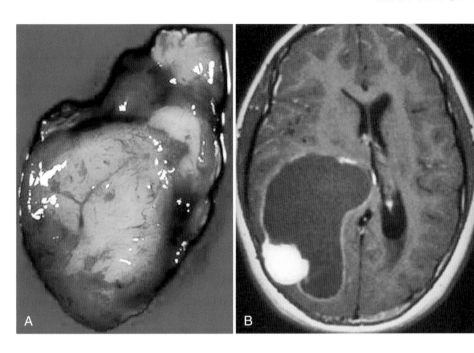

■ **FIGURE 32-15** Pleomorphic xantho-astrocytoma. **A,** Gross specimen of the solid nodular component demonstrates a seemingly well-demarcated lesion. **B,** Corresponding postcontrast T1W MR image reveals a cystic lesion with the enhancing mural nodule. The cystic lining enhances as well.

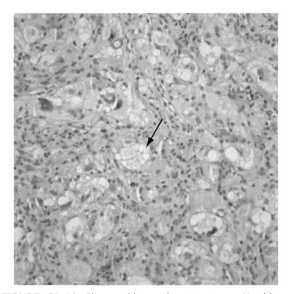

■ **FIGURE 32-16** Pleomorphic xanthoastrocytoma. Xanthic cells, expressed as vacuolization of the neoplastic cells, are shown (*arrow*).

postcontrast imaging. Calcification is rare (Fig. 32-17). Overlying skull remodeling, erosion, or lytic change is uncommon; when present it suggests slow progression of the tumor.

MRI
The solid portion of a PXA is isointense to gray matter on T1W and T2W images. Peritumoral edema may be seen, but it is uncommon. On postcontrast imaging the solid portion enhances (Fig. 32-18). Involvement of the leptomeninges is highly characteristic of PXA, and enhancement along the adjacent meningeal surface may be seen.

Special Procedures
PXAs are typically avascular on catheter angiography.

DIFFUSE ASTROCYTOMA
Diffuse astrocytomas are diffusely infiltrating primary brain neoplasms of astrocytic origin that are classified as WHO grade II. Diffuse astrocytomas are also referred to as low-grade diffuse astrocytomas and as grade II astrocytomas but most often simply as "astrocytoma."

Epidemiology
Diffuse astrocytomas are most common between the ages of 30 and 40 years. Ten percent occur earlier than the age of 20, and 30% occur after the age of 45 years. There is a slight male predominance (1.18:1). They represent 10% to 15% of astrocytic brain tumors and are more commonly supratentorial (2/3). The frontal and temporal lobes are the most frequently involved regions, and there is a relative sparing of the occipital lobes. This may merely reflect the relative size of these lobes.

Diffuse astrocytomas have a tendency toward malignant progression, with grade II becoming anaplastic astrocytoma, usually after a mean time interval of 4 to 5 years. The overall median survival is 6 to 10 years, and improved survival is seen in younger patients.

Clinical Presentation
The most common clinical presentation of diffuse astrocytoma is seizure. If the neoplasm occurs in the frontal lobe, then personality change may be the presenting symptom.

These lesions may grow slowly over several years, but over time almost all will progress to higher-grade gliomas (WHO grade III or IV). The management of these patients is debated. Some centers treat them aggressively; however, studies have not produced evidence of improved survival after radical surgery or early radiation therapy. Other centers have adopted a "watch and wait" policy with clinical and imaging surveillance.[27-29]

Pathophysiology
Diffuse astrocytomas probably arise from differentiated astrocytes or astrocytic precursor cells. Diffuse astrocytomas demonstrate slow growth and may nondestructively infiltrate the brain. The gemistocytic variant is prone to more frequent and more rapid progression to anaplastic astrocytoma (grade III) and glioblastoma (grade IV).

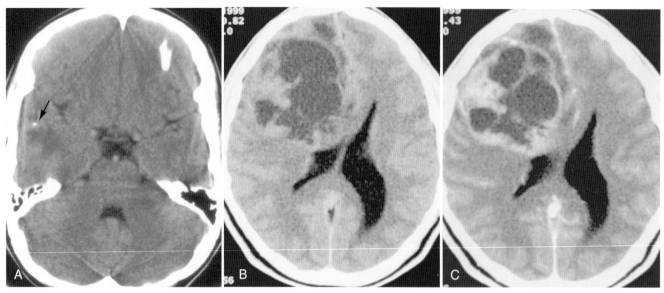

■ **FIGURE 32-17** Pleomorphic xanthoastrocytoma. **A,** Noncontrast CT demonstrates a mixed attenuation lesion in the right temporal lobe. A small focus of calcification is seen (*arrow*). **B,** Noncontrast CT from another patient demonstrates a large cystic and solid mass involving the right frontal lobe. **C,** Postcontrast CT demonstrates an enhancing nodule and enhancement of the cyst walls.

■ **FIGURE 32-18** Pleomorphic xanthoastrocytoma. **A,** T2W MR image demonstrates a cystic and solid lesion in the right temporal lobe. **B,** Note enhancement of the solid portion on a T1W postcontrast image.

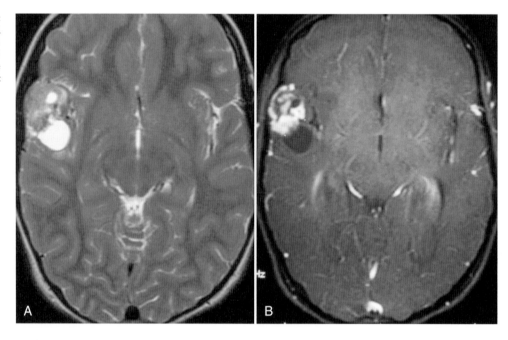

A genetic hallmark for these neoplasms is frequent *TP53* mutation, which is seen in greater than 60%. *TP53* is the gene that codes for the TP53 protein, an essential transcription factor. *TP53* mutations in grade II astrocytoma may be seen in patients with Li-Fraumeni syndrome, although these patients typically develop higher-grade neoplasms (III or IV). An association with inherited multiple enchondromatosis type 1 (Ollier disease) has also been noted. Overexpression of platelet-derived growth receptor-α is also reported. Chromosomal abnormalities are also reported (e.g., gain of 7q, 8q amplification, LOH 10p, 22q, chromosome 6 deletions).

Pathology
When visible grossly, diffuse astrocytomas may be yellow-white or gray masses. They are infiltrating lesions, so there is blurring of the anatomic boundaries (e.g., loss of gray matter/white matter demarcation). Involved and infiltrated structures are enlarged and distorted. There is no associated destruction of the tissue. Calcification and cysts may be present but are not common.

The fibrillary astrocytoma is the most common histologic subtype of diffuse astrocytoma. Gemistocytic (from the Greek *gemisto* meaning "stuffed") is the other common subtype, and it has a higher and more rapid rate of progression to glioblastoma (Fig. 32-19). Overall, the infiltrated white matter shows increased cellularity in comparison with the normal brain and occasional nuclear atypia is present. Mitotic activity is typically absent in grade II astrocytoma. No necrosis or neovascular proliferation is present. Infiltration of adjacent structures is seen. On immunohistochemistry, GFAP and S-100 protein are positive. The MIB-1 index is low, correlating with the low mitotic activity.

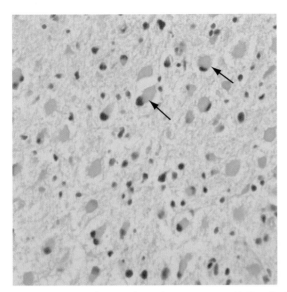

■ **FIGURE 32-19** Grade II gemistocytic astrocytoma. H&E stain demonstrates numerous gemistocytes (*arrows*).

Imaging

CT

Diffuse astrocytomas are typically isoattenuating to hypoattenuating masses. They do not enhance on postcontrast imaging and, when enhancement is present on follow-up examinations, suspicion should be raised for transformation to a higher-grade neoplasm. Calcification occurs in approximately 20%, and macroscopic cyst formation is rare.

MRI

Diffuse astrocytomas are low in signal on T1W imaging and may expand the white matter and adjacent cortex. They may cause loss of signal contrast between gray and white matter. On T2W imaging they are hypointense to hyperintense and may appear circumscribed. This is deceptive, because pathologically they are not discrete. Surrounding or spreading vasogenic edema is uncommon, and calcification, cysts, and hemorrhage are rare. They do not enhance on postcontrast imaging (Fig. 32-20).

MR spectroscopy should show an elevation of choline and a reduction in NAA. A high myoinositol (mI)/creatine (Cr) ratio is also present (0.82 ± 0.25).[30] On dynamic contrast-enhanced T2*W the rCBV is typically low and should be lower than values seen in the high-grade astrocytomas; rCBV is typically less than 1.75.[4] A study by Danchaivijitr and coworkers found that evaluation of the rCBV was able to distinguish between patients whose tumor did not transform to a higher grade and those whose tumor did over a 23-month observation period. In the nontransforming stable neoplasms the rCBV measurements remained low, whereas in those tumors that transformed, the mean rCBV value at the point of transformation was elevated to 5.36 ± 3.01. The elevated rCBV occurred before the development of contrast enhancement and may be an "early warning signal."[29]

An assessment of the utility of DTI in differentiating diffuse astrocytomas from anaplastic was performed by Goebell and associates, who found that the fiber tracts were better preserved along the periphery of low-grade (II) neoplasms, whereas the tracts tended to be disarranged (lower anisotropy) in high-grade gliomas. Within the center of both low- and high-grade gliomas the fractional anisotropy (FA) was low, which was consistent with a high degree of disorganization of myelinated fiber tracts.[31]

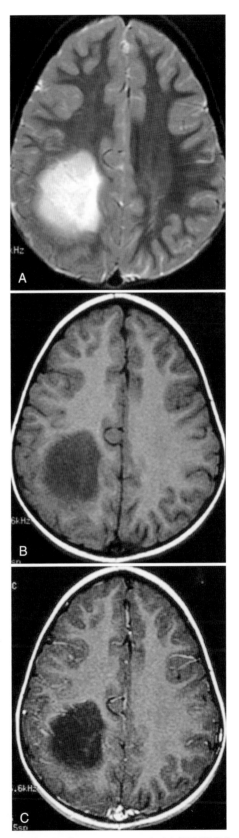

■ **FIGURE 32-20** Grade II astrocytoma. **A,** Axial T2W MR image demonstrates a relatively well-circumscribed hyperintense mass in the left parietal lobe. **B,** The lesion is hypointense on T1W imaging and does not demonstrate enhancement on the postcontrast image (**C**).

ANAPLASTIC ASTROCYTOMA

Anaplastic astrocytomas are WHO grade III, diffusely infiltrating neoplasms. They are also referred to as grade III astrocytomas. Confusing synonyms include "malignant astrocytoma," "malignant glioma," and high-grade astrocytoma. However, these terms have also been used for glioblastoma, which is a WHO grade IV lesion.

Epidemiology

Anaplastic astrocytomas primarily affect adults. The population-based registry data from the United States records a mean age at onset of 51 years, and there is a slight male predominance (1.31:1). The median survival after diagnosis is 2 to 3 years. These tumors can progress to glioblastomas, and the typical time to progression is 2 years.

Clinical Presentation

Patients with anaplastic astrocytomas typically present with neurologic deficits, seizures, and signs of increased intracranial pressure. Other symptoms include headaches and personality or behavioral changes. Treatment consists of resection and radiation therapy, either with or without chemotherapy.

Pathophysiology

Anaplastic astrocytomas may arise from a preexisting grade II astrocytic neoplasm or de novo. They infiltrate and spread along the white matter tracts but may also spread along the ependyma and leptomeningeal surfaces and within CSF.

There is a high incidence of *TP53* mutation (70%). Deletion of chromosome 6 is seen in 30% of cases. Loss of tumor suppressor genes on chromosomes 9, 13, or 19 may also lead to the formation of anaplastic astrocytomas.

Pathology

Anaplastic astrocytomas are infiltrating neoplasms that usually do not result in frank destruction of tissue. There is enlargement of the invaded structures. On gross inspection, they are difficult to distinguish from a grade II astrocytoma. Cysts and hemorrhage are uncommon and unlikely.

These tumors demonstrate increased cellularity, nuclear atypia, and significant proliferative activity (Fig. 32-21). The GFAP is positive, and the MIB-1 index is 5% to 10%. Microvascular proliferation and necrosis are absent (according to the current WHO revision of 2007).

Imaging

CT

On CT, anaplastic astrocytomas are low-attenuation masses whose borders are ill defined. Consistent with the absence of microscopic vascular changes, enhancement should not occur. The majority do not enhance on postcontrast imaging. In the older literature, up to 50% enhance. Hemorrhage and calcification are rare.

MRI

Anaplastic astrocytomas are hypointense or isointense mass lesions located within the white matter, but they may involve the overlying cortex, resulting in its expansion. On postcontrast imaging there is usually no enhancement. T2W images reveal a heterogeneously hyperintense mass (Fig. 32-22). MR spectroscopy demonstrates a decrease in NAA and an elevation in the

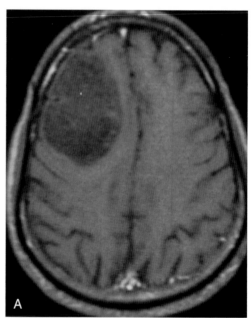

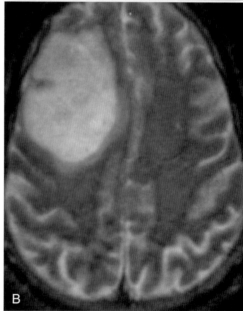

■ **FIGURE 32-22** Anaplastic astrocytoma. **A,** T1W postcontrast MR image demonstrates a nonenhancing, hypointense mass lesion within the right frontal lobe. **B,** On T2W imaging the lesion appears hyperintense and relatively circumscribed.

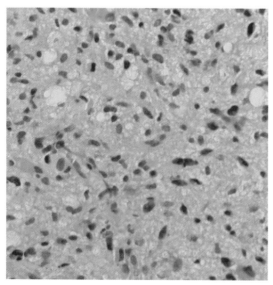

■ **FIGURE 32-21** Anaplastic astrocytoma. H&E stain demonstrates increased cellularity and nuclear pleomorphism.

Cho/Cr ratio. Lower mI/Cr ratios are seen than in low-grade gliomas (0.33 ± 0.16).[30] Some authors suggest that mI reflects well-differentiated astrocytic cells.

Sugahara and associates found mean maximum rCBV values of 5.84 in anaplastic astrocytomas.[32] Assessment with DTI reveals greater derangement of fiber tracts at the periphery of anaplastic astrocytomas, whereas in lower-grade astrocytomas they tend to be preserved.[31]

The imaging differential diagnosis includes diffuse astrocytomas grade II, and the imaging findings may be indistinguishable. Similar imaging findings may also be seen in oligodendrogliomas, and biopsy may be necessary to distinguish these possibilities.

GLIOBLASTOMA

Glioblastoma multiforme (GBM) is the most malignant of the neoplasms with a primary astrocytic differentiation. Because it was thought to arise from the most primitive precursor of the stromal cell population (the glioblasts) and its gross morphology is highly variable and complex, it was given the name "glioblastoma multiforme."[33] The name is somewhat of a misnomer because GBMs are currently thought to arise from progressive dedifferentiation of mature astrocytes and not from rests of immature glioblasts. Glioblastomas are also referred to as grade IV astrocytoma.

Epidemiology

Glioblastomas are the most frequent primary brain tumor, accounting for 12% to 30% of all intracranial neoplasms and 60% to 75% of the astrocytic tumors. Although they may present at any age, including newborns, the peak incidence is between 45 and 75 years of age. There is a slight male predominance (1.26 : 1).

Clinical Presentation

The clinical presentation of glioblastomas depends on the location of the tumor, but they typically present as signs of increased intracranial pressure (e.g., headache), and up to one third of patients experience seizures. Personality changes can also occur.

Surgical treatment of GBMs involves surgical debulking, which is typically followed by both radiation therapy and chemotherapy. Outcome, despite many treatment innovations, continues to be poor. The average survival from time of diagnosis varies significantly with patient age and tumor type (de novo vs. progression from previous low-grade astrocytomas) from 2 to 18 months. In patients younger than age 50, mean survival is less than 10 months and that drops to only 3 months in the eighth decade.[34]

Pathophysiology

GBMs are thought to arise from the progressive dedifferentiation of mature cells. They may arise from within a preexisting lower-grade astrocytoma or arise de novo. The genetics of GBMs that arise de novo are thought to differ from those that arise from a preexisting lower-grade glioma. Ironically, however, several authors continue to pursue bipotential precursor and neural stem cells or even the "brain tumor stem cell" as the culprits. A number of genetic abnormalities that predispose to the development of GBMs have been identified that may be acquired or inherited. Loss of tumor-suppressor genes on chromosomes 9, 10, 13, or 19 may lead to formation of a GBM. Allelic loss from chromosome 10 appears to be involved in up to 80% of GBMs.[35] Interestingly, chromosome 10 damage has not been found to be common in other neoplasms, which suggests that it may be unique to GBM.

The tumor suppressor gene *TP53*, located on the short arm of chromosome 17, is linked to the development of GBMs. At least 40% of GBMs have been shown to have this mutation, and it is thought to be involved in the progression of lower-grade to higher-grade astrocytomas.[36,37]

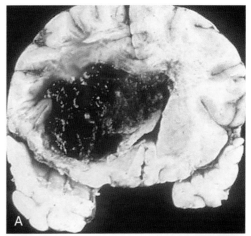

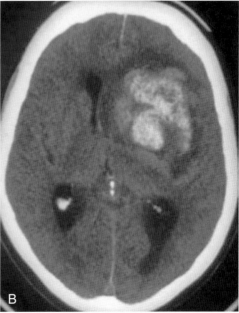

■ **FIGURE 32-23** Glioblastoma multiforme. **A,** Gross specimen shows a large hemorrhagic lesion involving the left frontal lobe. **B,** Corresponding noncontrast CT scan demonstrates the hemorrhagic lesion.

GBMs may disseminate via CSF spread; however, this is uncommon, occurring in less than 2% of patients.[38] Hematogenous spread is even less common, typically occurring almost exclusively in patients who have undergone surgery.

High-grade astrocytomas demonstrate rapid cell growth, leading to hypercellularity and requiring neovascularization. The tumor cells secrete several different paracrine substances, such as endothelial growth factor and rennin, resulting in rapid proliferation of new blood vessels. These vessels are structurally abnormal and do not form the blood-brain barrier. Owing to their "leaky" nature there is a brisk transudation of fluid into the extracellular space that translates into the spreading pattern of vasogenic edema seen on imaging.

Pathology

Glioblastomas are often large and typically solitary and unilateral, although they may infiltrate and cross the corpus callosum. They most commonly arise within the deep white matter but also may be seen in peripheral locations and may even appear to be dural based. The tumors are grayish, demonstrate necrosis, and typically have evidence of hemorrhage (Figs. 32-23 and 32-24). The tumor itself does not have distinct margins; however, areas of

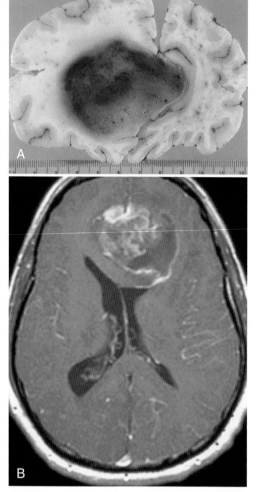

■ **FIGURE 32-24**   Glioblastoma multiforme. **A,** Gross specimen showing a large lesion involving the left frontal lobe with darker areas corresponding to hemorrhage. **B,** Corresponding postcontrast T1W image demonstrates a heterogeneously enhancing lesion in the left frontal lobe.

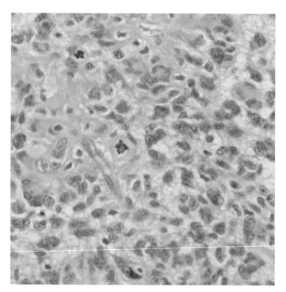

■ **FIGURE 32-25**   Glioblastoma multiforme. H&E stain demonstrates increased cellularity and nuclear pleomorphism.

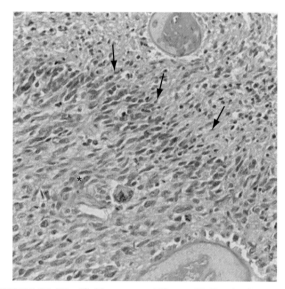

■ **FIGURE 32-26**   Glioblastoma multiforme. H&E stain demonstrates fusiform tumor cells arranged in a palisading fashion (*arrows*) around an area of necrosis (*asterisk*).

necrosis and intense vascular proliferation are often discrete, creating a deceptive appearance of demarcation.

Glioblastomas demonstrate nuclear atypia, cellular pleomorphism, mitotic activity, microvascular proliferation, and necrosis (Fig. 32-25). A distinctive histopathologic feature of GBM is pseudopalisading necrosis, where viable neoplastic cells align in an irregular border around regions of necrotic debris (Fig. 32-26). They are GFAP positive on immunohistochemical staining, and the MIB-1 index is increased (9%-31%).

Imaging

The imaging appearance of GBM is variable, as its name also reflects. The most commonly identified features include a mixture of hemorrhage and necrosis within the neoplasm. The typical imaging appearance is a supratentorial space-occupying lesion with proportionate mass effect and extensive surrounding vasogenic edema. Multifocality occurs in 4% to 6% of cases and may result from microscopic infiltration rather than multicentric origin.

CT

On noncontrast CT, uncomplicated glioblastoma is a low-attenuation lesion. Hemorrhage and necrosis can be seen, producing a grossly heterogeneous lesion. Cellular regions of tumor with

neovascularity show intense enhancement on postcontrast images (Fig. 32-27).

MRI

Glioblastomas are irregular and heterogeneous lesions that are isointense or hypointense on T1W images and are heterogeneous, often hyperintense masses on T2W images. The margins of the solid portions of the lesion are typically thick, and cavitation from necrosis is frequent. Hemorrhage may be present, and gradient imaging may reveal susceptibility secondary to hemorrhage (Fig. 32-28). Fluid secretion and "cyst" are distinctly uncommon in comparison to necrosis. On postcontrast imaging, irregular, thick enhancement is typically seen that may be ring, solid, nodular, or patchy (Fig. 32-29). However, one study found that up to one third of malignant gliomas did not enhance.[39] The pathologic grading is based on the most aggressive feature found regardless of their predominance. Nonenhancing GBMs may reflect tumors with only scattered microscopic

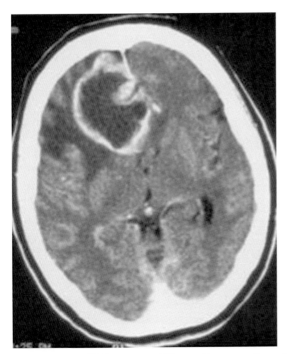

■ **FIGURE 32-27** Glioblastoma multiforme. Contrast-enhanced CT demonstrates a ring-enhancing lesion with surrounding low attenuation consistent with vasogenic edema and possible tumor infiltration.

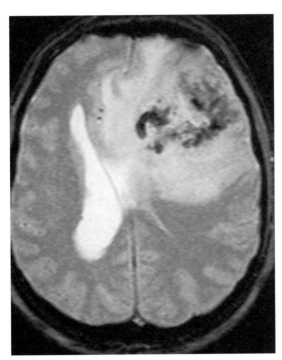

■ **FIGURE 32-28** Glioblastoma multiforme. An MPGR gradient image demonstrates a large mass lesion in the left frontal lobe with areas of low signal consistent with hemorrhage.

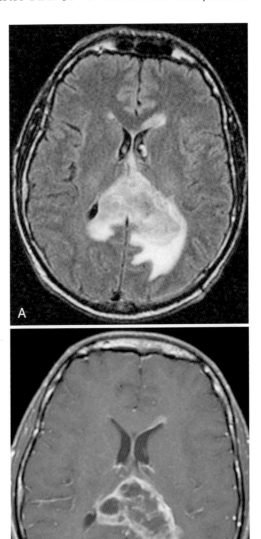

■ **FIGURE 32-29** Glioblastoma multiforme. **A,** Axial FLAIR image demonstrates an expansile lesion with heterogeneous signal involving the splenium of the corpus callosum. Increased T2 hyperintensity is seen adjacent to the lesion representing a combination of vasogenic edema and tumor infiltration. A second focus of hyperintensity is seen adjacent to the left frontal horn. **B,** Postcontrast T1W MR image demonstrates predominantly peripheral irregular enhancement. The smaller focus adjacent to the left frontal horn enhances as well, consistent with a multifocal glioblastoma multiforme.

changes, including those that arise from and within a lower-grade astrocytoma. MR spectroscopy demonstrates decreased NAA and occasional myoinositol. Choline level is increased, and a lipid/lactate peak may be present (Fig. 32-30).

On dynamic contrast-enhanced T2*-weighted (T2*W) imaging there is elevation of the maximum rCBV within portions of the tumor. Sugahara and coworkers found mean maximum rCBV values of 7.32 in glioblastomas (Fig. 32-31).[32]

The differential diagnosis on imaging includes tumefactive demyelinating lesions. An elevated rCBV would be compatible with GBM and not be seen in tumefactive demyelination, and perfusion-weighted imaging may show vessels coursing through a demyelinating lesion, which is not likely in a neoplasm, because these demyelinating lesions tend to occur along venous structures. Glioblastomas would, on the other hand, displace the vasculature. Abscesses are also in the differential diagnosis for heterogeneous ring lesions. These tend to demonstrate smoother borders, have thin and T2 hypointense rims, and typically demonstrate central regions of reduced diffusion from purulent

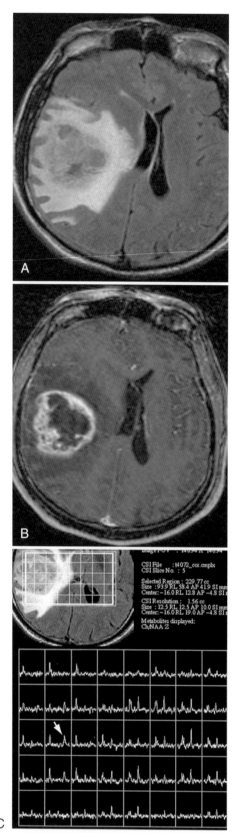

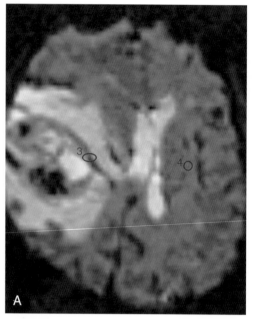

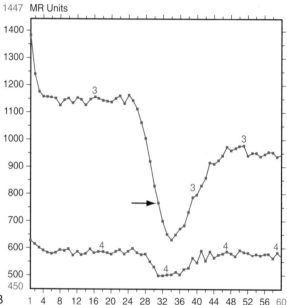

■ **FIGURE 32-31** Glioblastoma multiforme. **A,** T2*W MR image demonstrates areas of signal that decrease as contrast passes through. **B,** Perfusion imaging rCBV map demonstrates an elevated rCBV (*arrow*) in the region of interest placed along the periphery of the lesion.

■ **FIGURE 32-30** Glioblastoma multiforme. **A,** Axial FLAIR image demonstrates a heterogeneous mass lesion surrounded by T2 hyperintensity in the right hemisphere with associated midline shift. **B,** Postcontrast image demonstrates a ring-enhancing lesion. **C,** 3D MR spectroscopy demonstrates elevated choline and decreased NAA levels. Measurement voxels placed over the necrotic center demonstrate an elevated lipid/lactate peak (*arrow*).

material in contradistinction to glioblastomas, which show increased diffusion in necrosis (Fig. 32-32). However, there are reports of "cystic" glioblastomas demonstrating reduced diffusion, which may reflect hemorrhage, cytotoxic edema, thick sterile liquefaction, or secondary infection. In fact, one study reported that 12% of glioblastomas demonstrated reduced diffusion.[40]

Special Procedures

Glioblastomas appear as irregular hypervascular masses (consistent with the neovascularity seen on pathology) on conventional angiography, and there is a prominent tumor blush (Fig. 32-33). Tumor vessels have irregular caliber and branching patterns and may show puddling of contrast and pseudoaneurysms. Arteriovenous shunting and early draining veins are commonly seen.

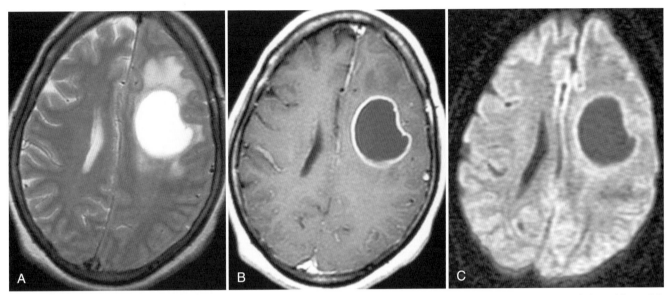

■ FIGURE 32-32 Glioblastoma multiforme. **A,** Axial T2W MR image of a biopsy-proven tumor demonstrates a hyperintense lesion with a mildly hypointense rim and surrounding vasogenic edema, which might suggest the possibility of an abscess. **B,** On T1W postcontrast imaging a thin enhancing rim is seen. However, the diffusion-weighted image (**C**) does not demonstrate reduced diffusion.

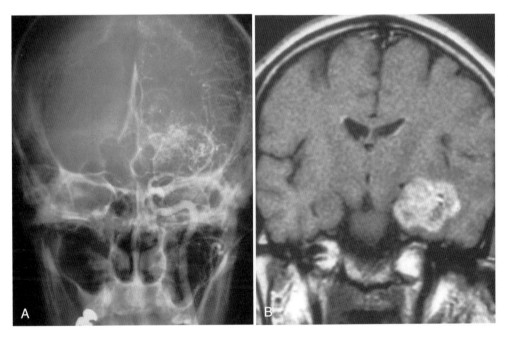

■ FIGURE 32-33 Glioblastoma multiforme. **A,** Left internal carotid injection demonstrates increased vascularity in the region of the left temporal lobe. **B,** Corresponding T1W postcontrast MR image demonstrates a heterogeneously enhancing mass.

An early draining vein on angiography is the radiographic correlate of a shortened mean transit time seen on MRI and CT perfusion.

GLIOMATOSIS CEREBRI

Gliomatosis cerebri is a diffuse, extensive neuroepithelial neoplasm of uncertain origin involving at least two cerebral lobes. Because of its typically aggressive behavior it is usually classified as a WHO grade III neoplasm. Many prominent neuropathologists believe that gliomatosis cerebri is fundamentally a diffuse astrocytoma. Gliomatosis cerebri has also been referred to as gliomatosis or diffuse cerebral gliomatosis.

Epidemiology

Gliomatosis cerebri is a rare neoplasm that affects a broad age range (neonate to elderly), but the peak incidence is between 40 and 50 years.[41,42] There is no gender predilection.

Clinical Presentation

The clinical presentation of gliomatosis cerebri is variable, depending on the region of brain involved. It can include dementia, seizures, gait disturbances, cranial nerve dysfunction, visual disturbances, sensory deficits, and symptoms of increased intracranial pressure. Gliomatosis is relentlessly progressive, and the prognosis is poor. One-year survival is 50% and decreases to 25% at 3 years (median survival, 38 months). Treatment is limited: gliomatosis responds poorly to chemotherapy and radiation therapy. Surgical decompression may be performed and corticosteroid therapy may provide some benefit.

Pathophysiology

The etiology of gliomatosis is controversial, and its histogenesis is unknown. Many postulate that it is a glioma (astrocytoma) with a tendency for widespread infiltration.[43,44] The karyotype is consistent with a clonal neoplasm arising from a single cell. *TP53*

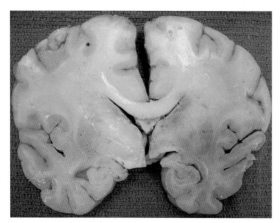

FIGURE 32-34   Gliomatosis cerebri. Gross specimen demonstrates expansion and infiltration of the white matter. The gray matter/white matter differentiation is not as defined as it is in the uninvolved left temporal lobe.

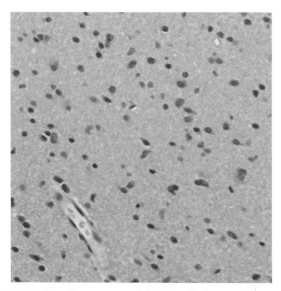

FIGURE 32-35   Gliomatosis cerebri. H&E stain demonstrates tumor cells that are diffusely infiltrative throughout the parenchyma.

mutation is found in gliomatosis, similar to that seen in diffuse astrocytoma.[45]

Pathology

On gross pathology, the involved areas are swollen and firm and the gray matter/white matter distinction is blurred (Fig. 32-34). However, the underlying brain architecture is largely preserved. It involves at least two lobes of the brain and is distinguished from multifocal glioma by the clear presence of continuity of cellular infiltration and a lack of demarcation from adjacent normal brain. Within the cerebral hemispheres, the white matter is always invaded and the cortex may be involved in up to 19% of cases.[46,47] No necrosis is present.

Some pathologists describe two types of gliomatosis. Type I is the classic form in which diffuse overgrowth of neoplastic cells is seen without a distinct mass lesion. In type II, both diffuse infiltration, and a focal mass, typically a high-grade glioma, are present.[47]

On histology, a proliferation of glial cells is seen with elongated, fusiform nuclei. The neuronal architecture is usually preserved unless the infiltration becomes particularly dense (Fig. 32-35). Microvascular proliferation and necrosis are absent.

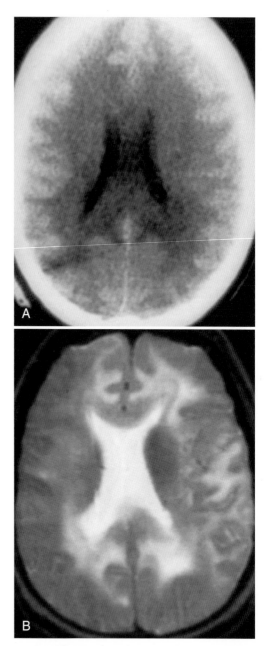

FIGURE 32-36   Gliomatosis cerebri. **A,** Axial noncontrast CT demonstrates low attenuation in the periventricular white matter that is most pronounced in the parietal lobes. **B,** Corresponding axial T2W MR image demonstrates patchy hyperintensity involving the periventricular and subcortical white matter. The abnormality is better appreciated with MRI.

Mitotic activity is low but variable. Immunohistochemistry demonstrates variable staining for GFAP and S-100, which are markers of astrocytes. The proliferation index (MIB-1) is 6% to 8%.

Imaging

CT

The CT findings of gliomatosis cerebri may be subtle with asymmetric low attenuation seen within the white matter (Fig. 32-36). No enhancement occurs on postcontrast imaging. If enhancement is seen, it may indicate malignant progression.

MRI

The MRI findings of gliomatosis are typically nonspecific, and the differential diagnosis includes encephalitis, demyelinating

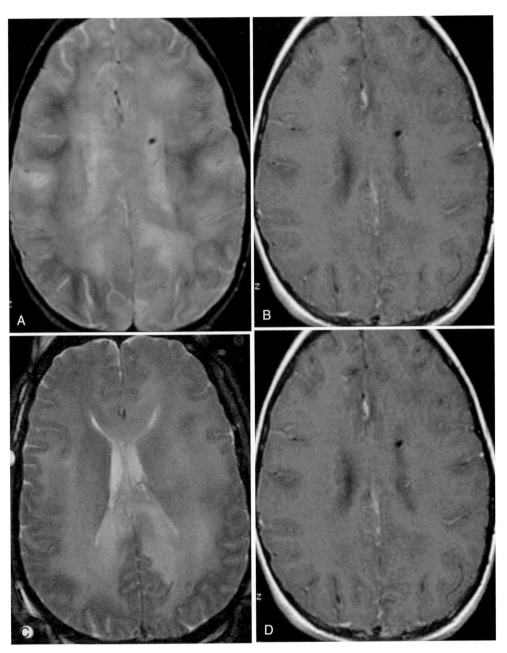

■ **FIGURE 32-37** Gliomatosis cerebri. **A,** Axial T2W MR image demonstrates patchy areas of T2 hyperintensity involving both the white and gray matter bilaterally. **B,** Postcontrast T1W MR image demonstrates no enhancement. **C,** Axial T2W image from another patient shows more confluent T2 hyperintensity. **D,** The postcontrast T1W image does not demonstrate enhancement.

processes, and ischemic changes. On T1W imaging isointensity or low signal intensity is present in the white matter, which corresponds to areas of hyperintensity (Fig. 32-37). Gray matter may also be involved. The lesion is infiltrative, and mass effect is mild. On postcontrast imaging there is typically minimal to no enhancement, and if enhancement is present it may indicate malignant progression.

The ability to direct the neurosurgeon to a biopsy site is important in gliomatosis. The region of greatest anaplasia determines patient outcome, and MR spectroscopy has been evaluated for its potential in directing biopsy. MR spectroscopy typically reveals an elevation of myoinositol and decreased NAA. A study by Saraf-Lavi and associates recommends that the mI/Cr and mI/NAA should be measured because they can be elevated even when the Cho/Cr is normal.[48] Choline is frequently normal or mildly elevated. Lipid and lactate peaks may or may not be seen. Their presence has been thought to be suggestive

of malignant progression, but large studies have demonstrated that the presence of lactate is not a reliable predictor of malignancy.[44,49] Low-grade (WHO II) lesions demonstrate a moderate Cho/NAA ratio increase (up to 1.3), whereas anaplastic lesions have a higher Cho/NAA increase ($\geq$2.5).[44] Targeting the area of maximum Cho/NAA may yield the most informative biopsy specimen.

Perfusion-weighted imaging reveals a low rCBV, reflecting the lack of vascular hyperplasia.[50]

OLIGODENDROGLIOMA AND ANAPLASTIC OLIGODENDROGLIOMA

Oligodendroglioma is a diffusely infiltrating and well-differentiated glioma classified as a WHO grade II neoplasm. Anaplastic oligodendroglioma is a highly cellular diffusely infiltrating glioma classified as a WHO grade III tumor.

Epidemiology

Oligodendrogliomas typically occur in adults and are rare in children; they make up less than 1% of pediatric CNS neoplasms.[51] The peak age at presentation is between 40 and 45 years, and there is a slight male predominance (1.1:1). It is the third most common glial subtype, accounting for 5% to 18% of all glial neoplasms.[52] It is most frequently located in the frontal lobe (50%-65%), and the temporal lobe is the second most common region affected (47%).[51,53] Multiple lobe involvement may occur.[53] In addition, these tumors may arise from the leptomeninges, where they are thought to arise from glial heterotopia.[54]

The WHO recognizes two forms of oligodendrogliomas: well-differentiated (grade II) and anaplastic (grade III). The prevalence of anaplastic oligodendrogliomas is variable among studies, ranging from 3.5% of malignant gliomas to 20% to 54% of oligodendroglial neoplasms.[51,55] Patients with the anaplastic variant tend to be slightly older (peak 6th and 7th decades) compared with those with the well-differentiated form. In addition, there may be a mixed population of neoplastic cells, including an astrocyte component. The exact mixture of neoplastic astrocytes and oligodendrocytes is variable; in some cases they are referred to as oligoastrocytomas or "mixed glioma."

Clinical Presentation

Oligodendrogliomas are thought to be more slowly growing neoplasms (even compared with grade II astrocytomas) and, therefore, they typically demonstrate a longer clinical history (in many cases 5 years or more).[51,52] Patients with oligodendrogliomas present with seizures (two thirds of cases), which reflects their tendency to involve the cortex, in contrast to astrocytomas, which are more likely to involve the deeper white matter, including the corpus callosum. Other symptoms include cognitive or mental changes, headache, or other signs of increased intracranial pressure. Treatment consists of surgical resection, and many patients experience a long progression-free period. Unfortunately, virtually all patients develop a recurrence. In some cases, malignant transformation to the anaplastic form or a glioblastoma multiforme may occur. Rarely, distant extraneural spread can occur, with the skeleton, lymph nodes, lung, pleura, and liver being the most common sites.

Pathophysiology

Genotyping of well-differentiated oligodendrogliomas has demonstrated a chromosomal loss of 1p (short arm) and 19q (long arm), suggesting inactivation of a tumor suppressor gene. Anaplastic oligodendrogliomas demonstrate more chromosomal deletions, involving chromosome 9p and 10.[51] Approximately 25% of anaplastic oligodendrogliomas demonstrate a deletion of a tumor suppressor gene (*CDKN2A*) found on the short arm of chromosome 9.[56]

Many oligoastrocytomas (30%-50%) have deletions of 1p and 19q alleles that are seen in oligodendrogliomas, but approximately 30% have genetic changes that are also seen in astrocytomas. This includes mutation of the *TP53* tumor suppressor gene and loss of heterozygosity of chromosome 10.[51,57] The anaplastic oligoastrocytoma is a WHO grade III neoplasm with the additional features of nuclear atypia, high mitotic activity, and increased cellularity. Chromosomal alterations, similar to those seen in the other oligodendroglial neoplasms, have been found.[51]

Pathology

Oligodendrogliomas are typically soft gray-pink neoplasms that, in many cases, extend superficially through the cerebral cortex to involve the pial surface (Fig. 32-38). Calcification is common and probably reflects long periods of slow growth.

Oligodendrogliomas are classified histologically as either well differentiated or anaplastic. A mixture of oligodendroglial and

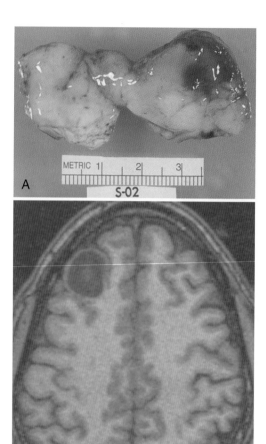

■ **FIGURE 32-38** Oligodendroglioma. **A,** Gross specimen. The red-tan soft tissue was described as "rubbery" on sectioning. This specimen is cut open revealing a focal area of hemorrhage. **B,** Axial T1 SPGR gradient image demonstrates the close approximation of the mass to the cortex.

astrocytic components may occur, and they may be diagnosed as oligoastrocytomas or "mixed glioma." Oligodendrogliomas are moderately cellular neoplasms that have uniformly round hyperchromatic nuclei surrounded by clear cytoplasm, giving the classic "fried egg" appearance on hematoxylin-eosin stain (Fig. 32-39). The perinuclear clearing may represent a fixation artifact. Microcalcifications (e.g., psammoma bodies) are seen in approximately 90% of oligodendrogliomas in adult patients. Endothelial proliferation and necrosis are not seen. However, these tumors may have a fine capillary network that resembles "chicken wire" and may cause spontaneous intratumoral hemorrhage. Anaplastic oligodendrogliomas have frequent mitoses and endothelial hyperplasia, as well as necrosis (Fig. 32-40). On immunohistochemical staining, oligodendrogliomas are S-100 positive. GFAP is usually negative; however, it may be present in some cell types (mini-gemistocytes and gliofibrillary oligodendrocytes). The MIB-1 index for oligodendrogliomas is less than 5%.

Involvement of the cortical gray matter is commonly seen: oligodendrogliomas are infiltrating neoplasms, and the normal neuronal cells within the cortex are "overrun" by the neoplastic oligodendroglial cells.[51]

Oligoastrocytomas are moderately cellular neoplasms composed of oligodendroglial and astrocytic components. Microcalcifications and cystic degeneration may be seen. No necrosis or endothelial proliferation is present, and there is little or no mitotic activity.

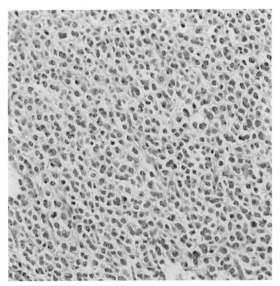

■ FIGURE 32-39 Oligodendroglioma. H&E stain demonstrates uniform cells with round nuclei with clear cytoplasm giving the "fried egg" appearance. Delicate capillaries are present, which are common in low-grade oligodendrogliomas.

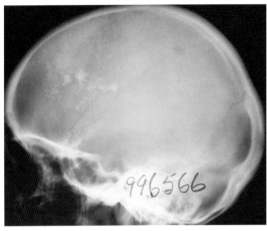

■ FIGURE 32-41 Oligodendroglioma. Plain radiograph demonstrates coarse calcifications in the frontal region.

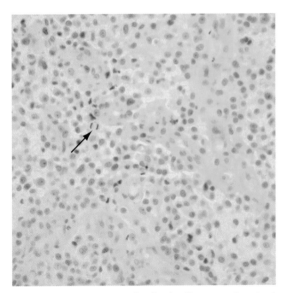

■ FIGURE 32-40 Anaplastic oligodendroglioma. H&E stain demonstrates increased cellularity, and mitoses are present (*arrow*).

Imaging

Oligodendrogliomas are typically sharply marginated lesions that extend to involve the cortex. Calcification is frequently present (Fig. 32-41). On postcontrast imaging, intense enhancement is uncommon and its presence suggests evolution to a higher histiologic grade or a different diagnosis. Oligodendrogliomas, as well as anaplastic oligodendrogliomas, may be multifocal.

CT

On CT, the majority of oligodendrogliomas are hypoattenuating to isoattenuating masses. Calcification is frequently present and is usually coarse and dense (Fig. 32-42). If the oligodendroglioma is exophytic, periosteal remodeling and erosion of the inner table of the calvaria may be noted (Fig. 32-43). Myxoid ("cystic") degeneration, and, rarely, hemorrhage may be seen (Fig. 32-44). After the administration of contrast, ill-defined enhancement

may be seen in up to 20% and suggests the possibility of a higher grade neoplasm.[53]

MRI

MRI provides better imaging of oligodendrogliomas than CT. These neoplasms are typically hypointense to gray matter on T1W images and hyperintense on T2W images. Heterogeneity of signal is common. Oligodendrogliomas tend to appear well circumscribed despite the fact that they are microscopically infiltrating neoplasms. Associated vasogenic edema is not common. Infrequently, a cyst-like pattern may be seen. On occasion, lesions within the frontal lobes may involve the corpus callosum, mimicking the appearance of a butterfly glioma. Oligodendrogliomas that have the 1p and 19q deletions are more likely to have ill-defined margins and calcifications, and they are more likely to be located within the frontal lobe and extend across the midline. T2* gradient imaging may demonstrate areas of "blooming" if calcification is present. However, CT is still more sensitive in finding this valuable differential feature of oligodendroglioma.

On postcontrast imaging, many oligodendrogliomas do not enhance (approximately 50%), or they may demonstrate a "lacy" enhancement pattern. The presence of enhancement suggests, but is not always indicative of, a more aggressive neoplasm; however, the absence of enhancement does not necessarily indicate a low-grade neoplasm. Perfusion imaging may reveal regions of elevated rCBV that may mimic a higher-grade neoplasm (Fig. 32-45). It must be emphasized that response to chemotherapy—and thus prognosis and survival—is more related to tumor genetics than any other factor. Biopsy and mutation analysis are essential to find the chromosome 1p and 19q mutations associated with response to therapy.

Anaplastic oligodendrogliomas have a more variable imaging appearance owing to the presence of necrosis and cystic degeneration (Fig. 32-46). Hemorrhage may also be seen. On postcontrast imaging they may demonstrate a ring-like enhancement mimicking a glioblastoma. On perfusion imaging, the higher-grade oligodendrogliomas demonstrate an increased rCBV.

MR spectroscopy of oligodendrogliomas demonstrates an elevation of choline and a reduction in NAA (Fig. 32-47). Anaplastic oligodendrogliomas also have increased Cho/Cr ratios and decreased NAA but may also have a lipid/lactate peak.

There are no imaging features to distinguish oligodendrogliomas and oligoastrocytomas. Calcification is not as common in the oligoastrocytomas (14%), and enhancement after administration of a contrast agent is more common (50%).[58]

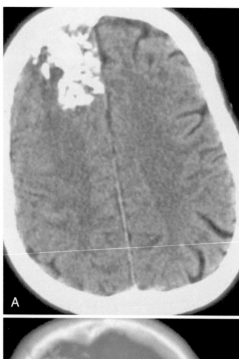

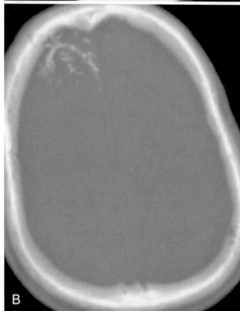

■ **FIGURE 32-42** Oligodendroglioma. Axial noncontrast CT in brain (**A**) and bone (**B**) windows demonstrates a coarsely calcified mass involving the right frontal lobe.

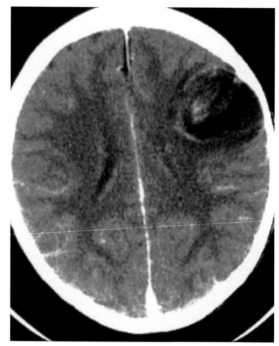

■ **FIGURE 32-43** Oligodendroglioma. Postcontrast axial CT demonstrates a low-attenuation, minimally enhancing lesion of the left frontal lobe that has resulted in remodeling of the adjacent calvaria.

GANGLIOGLIOMA AND GANGLIOCYTOMA

Gangliogliomas are WHO grade I or grade II neoplasms that contain both neoplastic neuronal and neoplastic glial components. The anaplastic form is uncommon and is a WHO grade III lesion. Gangliocytomas, on the other hand, do not have the glial component.

Gangliocytomas are also referred to as ganglioneuromas. The differentiation between gangliogliomas and gangliocytomas is histologic, and some group them together under the term *ganglion cell tumor.*

Epidemiology

Gangliogliomas have a peak incidence between the ages of 10 to 20 years of age, and 80% occur in persons younger than age 30 years.[1] They comprise 0.4% to 0.9% of intracranial neoplasms.[1,59] There is a slight male predominance. Gangliogliomas

are most commonly located in the temporal lobes, and the parietal and frontal lobes are the next most common locations. Many other locations have been described, including the pineal region, ventricles, cerebellum, brain stem, and the optic nerve and chiasm. Leptomeningeal spread has been reported but is rare.[60]

Gangliocytomas are also most common in children and young adults and account for 0.1% to 0.5% of brain neoplasms in this age group.[61] Gangliocytomas are located in both the cerebral hemispheres and the cerebellum and are most commonly found in the floor of the third ventricle.[1,61]

Clinical Presentation

Gangliogliomas and gangliocytomas occurring within the temporal lobes are the most common cause of chronic temporal lobe epilepsy, frequently causing partial complex seizures. These lesions are treated by gross total resection, typically resulting in cessation of seizure activity in the majority of patients. Other symptoms include headache and signs of increased intracranial pressure.

Patients have an excellent prognosis if the surgical resection is complete. If tumors are unresectable or aggressive, then chemotherapy and/or radiation therapy is used.

Pathophysiology

Gangliogliomas are slow-growing neoplasms and typically behave in a benign manner; however, on occasion, a malignant pattern is seen. In these cases, the astrocytic cells are less-differentiated anaplastic gangliogliomas (WHO grade III). The biologic behavior of these anaplastic gangliogliomas is variable, with some patients having extended survival after surgical resection and others dying as a result of diffuse dissemination. Malignant degeneration of gangliogliomas occurs in approximately 6% of cases.[1]

Pathology

Gangliogliomas and gangliocytomas are well circumscribed, often within the gray matter, and are either cystic masses with a mural nodule or solid. The solid portions are firm and gritty

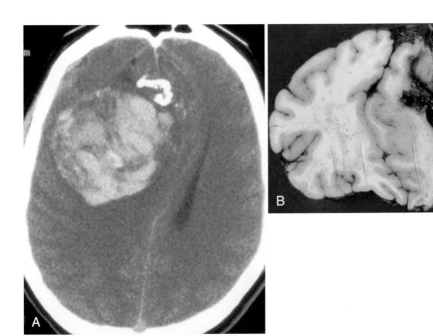

■ **FIGURE 32-44** Oligodendroglioma. **A,** Axial noncontrast CT
demonstrates a large area of hemorrhage in the right frontal lobe. An
area of increased density is seen anterior to the hemorrhage consistent
with calcification. **B,** Gross photograph demonstrates a hemorrhagic
lesion that abuts the cortex.

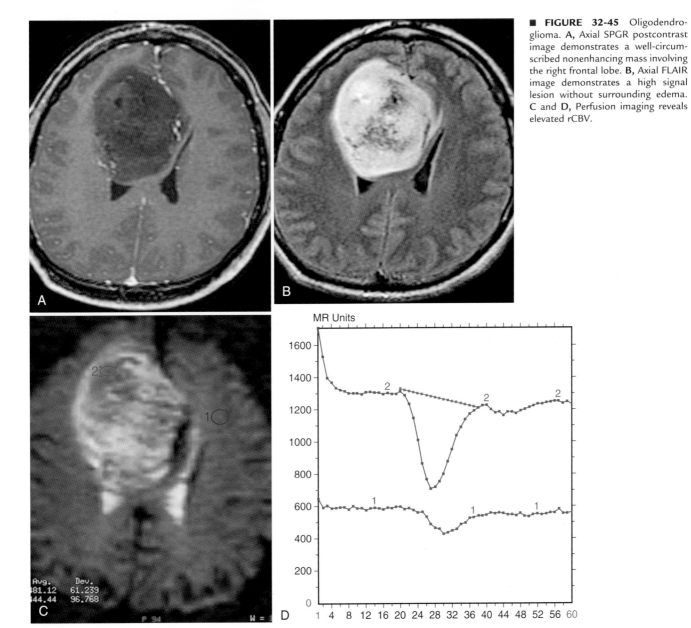

■ **FIGURE 32-45** Oligodendroglioma. **A,** Axial SPGR postcontrast
image demonstrates a well-circumscribed nonenhancing mass involving
the right frontal lobe. **B,** Axial FLAIR
image demonstrates a high signal
lesion without surrounding edema.
C and **D,** Perfusion imaging reveals
elevated rCBV.

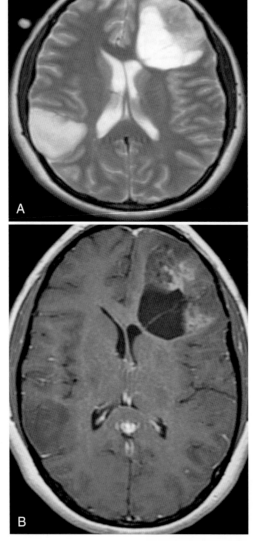

■ FIGURE 32-46 Multifocal anaplastic oligodendroglioma. **A,** Axial T2W image demonstrates a cystic and solid-appearing lesion involving the cortex of the left frontal lobe. A second high signal lesion involves the cortex of the right parietal lobe. **B,** Axial postcontrast T1W image demonstrates heterogeneous enhancement of the left frontal lesion. No enhancement is seen in the right parietal lesion.

owing to the presence of calcific deposits. Hemorrhage may occasionally be present.

Gangliogliomas are composed of mature ganglion cells and dysplastic neurons along with neoplastic glial cells. The glial component most often resembles a pilocytic or fibrillary astrocytoma, and, rarely, it may resemble a higher-grade astrocytoma. The glial component is absent in gangliocytomas. The abnormal ganglion cells may demonstrate characteristic binucleation and are often clumped together. The cells typically have large nuclei and prominent nucleoli, abundant cytoplasm, and frequently Nissl substance. Mitoses are rare. The neoplastic glial cells are GFAP positive. GFAP is a protein found in microfilaments of glial cells that helps distinguish them from nonglial tumors. Synaptophysin and neurofilament protein are also positive, representing the neuronal cell component of ganglioglioma. The MIB-1 index is low.

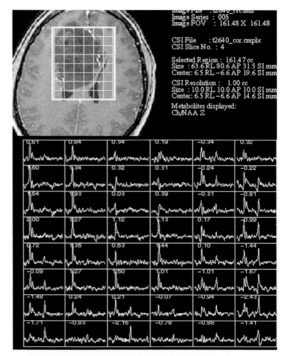

■ FIGURE 32-47 Oligodendroglioma. 3D-MR spectroscopy demonstrates elevation of choline and reduction in NAA. A small lactate peak is also present.

Imaging

Gangliogliomas and gangliocytomas are indistinguishable on imaging. They may be either solid or a combined cystic and solid mass. Only about 5% are cystic.[1,62]

CT

Gangliogliomas and gangliocytomas tend to be hypoattenuating or of mixed attenuation on CT imaging. In only about 15% of cases are they isoattenuating, and in another 15% they are hyperattenuating.[63] Calcification is a common finding (Fig. 32-48). On postcontrast imaging the enhancement pattern is variable. Remodeling of the skull may be seen in peripherally located lesions and reflects chronicity.

MRI

On MRI, gangliogliomas and gangliocytomas have a variable appearance but are commonly hypointense to isointense on T1W images and hyperintense on T2W images. Associated cortical dysplasia may be present. Postcontrast imaging demonstrates variable enhancement (Figs. 32-49 and 32-50). T2*W gradient imaging may demonstrate "blooming" if calcification is present. On MR spectroscopy an elevated Cho/Cr ratio has been described, suggesting increased membrane synthesis and degradation (Fig. 32-51).

DYSPLASTIC CEREBELLAR GANGLIOCYTOMA

Dysplastic cerebellar gangliocytoma is a cerebellar mass lesion that has features of both a malformation and a benign neoplasm. Recent investigations suggest that it is of hamartomatous origin, but debate continues as to the true nature of the lesion. It is classified as a WHO grade I tumor.[64] Dysplastic cerebellar gangliocytoma is also referred to by the eponym Lhermitte-Duclos disease or Lhermitte-Duclos-Cowden syndrome.

Epidemiology

Dysplastic cerebellar gangliocytoma is typically identified in young adults, with the average age at presentation being 34 years. No gender predilection has been described. It is often associated with Cowden disease, an autosomal dominant phakomatosis.

Clinical Presentation

Patients with dysplastic cerebellar gangliocytoma have symptoms related to increased intracranial pressure and hydrocephalus. Megalencephaly and mental retardation may also be present. Approximately 40% of patients present with a slowly progressive cerebellar syndrome; however, cerebellar signs may be mild or absent.[1,65] There are reports of asymptomatic patients, with the discovery of the lesion only on autopsy. Within the literature, there is variability in the duration of reported symptoms.[66] Treatment consists of surgical decompression of the ventricular system and partial or complete resection of the lesion. Patients frequently do well after surgery, but recurrences have been reported even after a long disease-free interval, requiring long-term follow-up.[67]

Pathophysiology

Dysplastic cerebellar gangliocytoma has a strong association with Cowden disease, which is an autosomal dominant hamartoma/phakomatosis syndrome. Patients with Cowden disease have an increased frequency of hamartomas and neoplasia of the CNS (glioma and meningioma), breast, colon, thyroid, and genitourinary organs. They also have a variety of mucocutaneous lesions (e.g., mucosal neuromas of the lips) and macrocephaly. The gene for Cowden disease has been localized to the long arm of chromosome 10 (10q23).[68]

The etiology of dysplastic cerebellar gangliocytoma is being debated. There is evidence that supports both a hamartomatous and a neoplastic origin. Support for a hamartomatous origin includes hypertrophy of the granular cell layer along with migrational arrest of the granular cells within the molecular layer.[69] Recurrence after surgical removal suggests a neoplastic etiology.

Pathology

Dysplastic cerebellar gangliocytoma consists of an area of sharply marginated enlarged cortex (Fig. 32-52). Usually only a portion of one cerebellar hemisphere is involved, but occasionally the involvement may extend to the vermis or rarely to the contralateral hemisphere.

Disruption of the normal cerebellar laminar structure, along with hypertrophic ganglion cells, is seen in dysplastic cerebellar gangliocytoma, resulting in expansion of the granular and molecular layers of the cerebellar cortex. Abnormally increased myelination is seen within the molecular layer, and a reduction in myelination of the central white matter of the cerebellar folia is frequently observed. There is no necrosis or mitosis, and malignant transformation has not been reported.

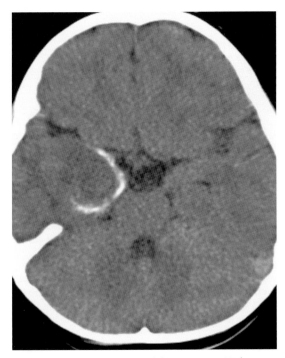

■ **FIGURE 32-48** Ganglioglioma. Axial noncontrast CT demonstrates a low-attenuation lesion in the right mesiotemporal lobe with a thin rim of calcification.

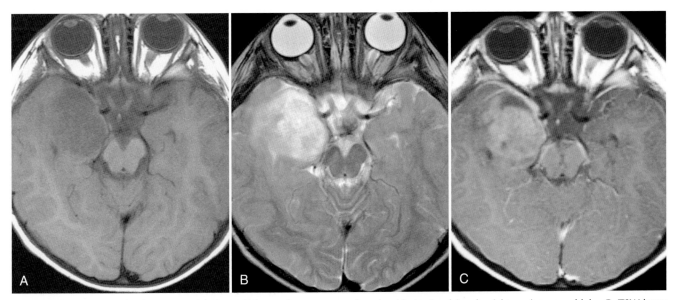

■ **FIGURE 32-49** Ganglioglioma. **A,** Axial T1W MR image demonstrates a low signal lesion involving the right mesiotemporal lobe. **B,** T2W image demonstrates lesion hyperintensity. **C,** On the postcontrast image the lesion heterogeneously enhances.

■ **FIGURE 32-50** Ganglioglioma. **A,** Axial T2W MR image demonstrates a heterogeneous-appearing lesion with cystic and solid components. **B,** The solid components enhance on postcontrast imaging.

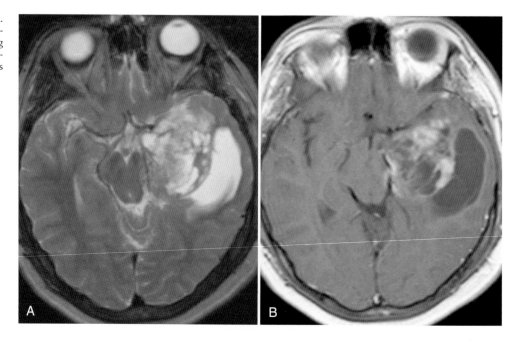

Imaging

CT

Dysplastic cerebellar gangliocytoma on CT is typically a hypoattenuating lesion found in the cerebellum, although it may occasionally be isointense. Calcification is uncommon and enhancement is not expected (Fig. 32-53).

MRI

On MRI, dysplastic cerebellar gangliocytoma results in expansion of the involved cerebellar hemisphere and has alternating bands of low and normal signal intensity on T1W imaging and bands of high or normal signal intensity on T2W imaging—the "tiger-striped" appearance (Fig. 32-54). T2*W gradient-recalled-echo images may demonstrate "blooming" if calcification is present. Rarely, lesions demonstrate enhancement on postcontrast imaging (Fig. 32-55). This is thought to occur as a result of vascular proliferation or the presence of anomalous veins.[70] On MR perfusion, elevated rCBV may be seen. Klisch and colleagues assumed that the hyperperfusion may be related to the histopathologic observation of numerous dilated thin-walled vessels within the lesion.[71] MR spectroscopy reveals slightly decreased NAA (10%), along with decreases in choline (30%-80%) and myoinositol (20%-50%).[71,72] In some cases, lactate has been reported but lipids are not increased. The elevation in lactate is speculated to be due to an abnormally high glucose metabolism.[71]

Special Procedures

Dysplastic cerebellar gangliocytomas are avascular masses on conventional angiography.

DYSEMBRYOPLASTIC NEUROEPITHELIAL TUMOR

Dysembryoplastic neuroepithelial tumors (DNETs) are WHO grade I supratentorial glial neuronal neoplasms involving the cerebral cortex or deep gray matter.

Epidemiology

DNETs occur predominantly in children and young adults, with the majority of patients being younger than 20 years old. They make up less than 1% of primary brain neoplasms. These are cortically located lesions and are most commonly found in the temporal lobe (usually the amygdala or hippocampus). Rarely, they may occur deep within the cerebral hemisphere, usually in the area of the caudate nucleus.[73]

Clinical Presentation

DNETs almost always present as partial complex seizure disorders in children and young adults, and they may be the cause of up to 20% of cases of medically refractory epilepsy in children and young adults.[74] Other neurologic signs or symptoms are uncommon.

Surgical removal is performed for seizure control, and the prognosis is excellent. Recurrences are rare, even if they are subtotally resected. However, one case of malignant transformation of a DNET has been reported that occurred 11 years after the initial resection.[75]

Pathophysiology

No consistent genetic alterations have been reported in DNETs.

Pathology

DNETs appear as an often wedge-shaped area of thickened cortex on gross pathologic evaluation and are mucin rich (Fig. 32-56).

The histologic hallmark of DNETs is the presence of the "specific glioneuronal element" (SGNE) with mature-appearing neurons "floating" among columns of oligodendroglial-like cells. Necrosis, mitoses, and endothelial hyperplasia are rare. Calcification and leptomeningeal involvement are common, as is adjacent cortical dysplasia.

The immunohistochemical features of DNETs include the presence of neuronal markers such as synaptophysin. GFAP is usually negative, and S-100 protein is positive in the oligodendroglial-like cells.

Three histologic forms of DNETs are described: complex, simple, and "nonspecific." The complex form is composed of the SGNE with glial nodules and a multinodular architecture. Focal areas of cortical dysplasia are commonly associated. The simple form consists of only the SGNE, and the "nonspecific" form does not have the SGNE but has the same clinical and neuroimaging features as complex DNET.[76,77]

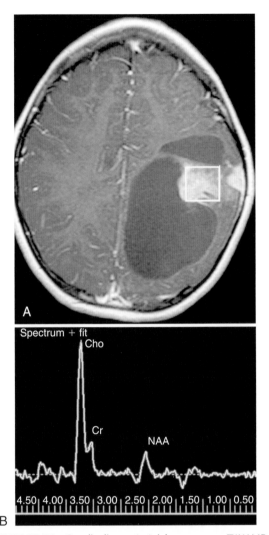

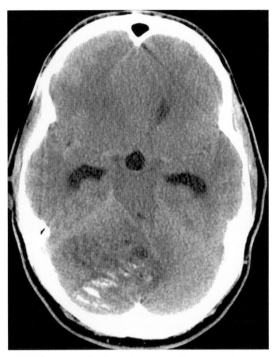

■ **FIGURE 32-53** Dysplastic cerebellar gangliocytoma. Noncontrast CT demonstrates expansion of the right cerebellar hemisphere by a low-attenuation lesion, resulting in compression of the midbrain and hydrocephalus. Linear calcifications are present.

■ **FIGURE 32-51** Ganglioglioma. **A,** Axial postcontrast T1W MR image demonstrates a predominantly cystic lesion with an enhancing nodule involving the left hemisphere. **B,** Single-voxel MR spectroscopy of the enhancing nodule demonstrates an elevated choline level and a markedly reduced NAA level.

Imaging
On imaging, DNETs tend to be well-circumscribed peripheral cortical wedge-shaped lesions, which are similar in imaging appearance to other low-grade glial tumors and ganglioglioma. The size is variable, ranging from involvement of a portion of a gyrus to up to 7 cm. Despite the potential for large size, there is minimal to no mass effect, and that may help in the differential diagnosis.

CT
DNETs are hypoattenuating, typically wedge-shaped lesions on CT. Occasionally, calcification may be present (Fig. 32-57). Like many other cortically based lesions, remodeling of the adjacent inner table of the skull may be evident.

MRI
On MRI, DNETs are hypointense on T1W images and hyperintense with a septated appearance on T2W images. They are well-demarcated, wedge-shaped lesions with a "bubbly" appearance. On fluid-attenuated inversion recovery (FLAIR) imaging they have a low or isointense signal with a surrounding bright rim. No surrounding T2 hyperintensity consistent with vasogenic edema is seen (Fig. 32-58). Approximately one third of DNETs enhance on postcontrast imaging.[1] MR spectroscopy demonstrates near-normal or diminished NAA, choline, and creatine.[78] Lactate may be present in some tumors.

PRIMARY CNS LYMPHOMA (PCNSL)
CNS lymphoma is an aggressive primary neoplasm of the CNS composed of B-cell lymphocytes.

Epidemiology
The prevalence of CNS lymphoma has increased in both immunocompetent and immunosuppressed patients over the past 3 decades and now represents 4% to 7% of primary CNS neoplasms; and in some centers it accounts for up to 15% of all brain

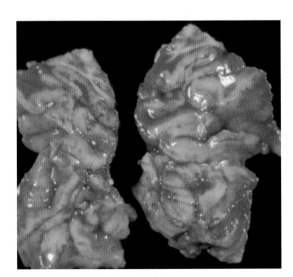

■ **FIGURE 32-52** Dysplastic cerebellar gangliocytoma. Gross specimen from the cerebellum demonstrates enlarged cerebellar folia.

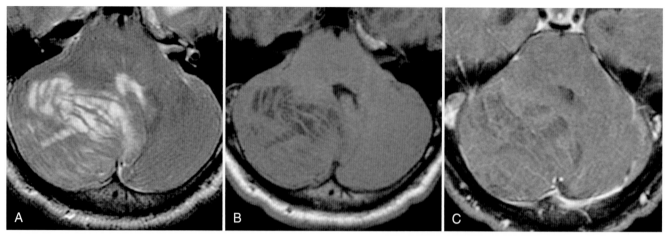

■ **FIGURE 32-54**   Dysplastic cerebellar gangliocytoma. **A,** Axial T2W image demonstrates expansion of the right cerebellar hemisphere and a striated "tiger stripe" hyperintense lesion. **B,** On T1W imaging the signal is low intensity. **C,** Postcontrast imaging reveals no enhancement.

■ **FIGURE 32-55**   Dysplastic cerebellar gangliocytoma. **A,** Axial T2W image demonstrates expansion of the left cerebellar hemisphere and increased signal that extends into the brachium pontis, vermis, and right cerebellar hemisphere. **B,** Postcontrast image reveals patchy enhancement.

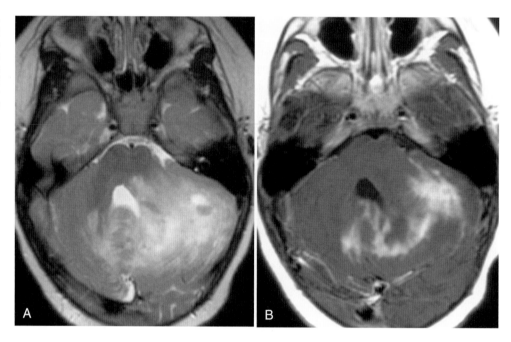

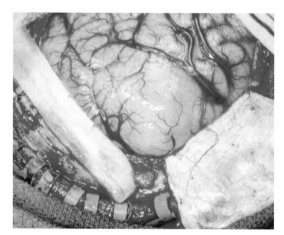

■ **FIGURE 32-56**   DNET. Intraoperative photograph demonstrates enlargement of a region of the cortex, with loss of the normal sulcal pattern.

tumors.[79,80] Primary CNS lymphoma in immunocompetent patients tends to occur at an older age (mean, 57 years), whereas those that occur in immunocompromised patients (HIV/AIDS and transplant) occur at a younger age (mean, 32 years).[81] In HIV-infected patients there is a male preponderance for primary CNS lymphoma, but in the immunocompetent group the male-to-female ratio is equal.[81]

Clinical Presentation

The most common clinical presentation is altered mental status and/or focal neurologic signs. Headache, neuropsychiatric symptoms, and seizure may be seen. The prognosis is typically poor but is better in immunocompetent patients, in patients with single lesions, in the absence of meningeal or periventricular tumor, and in patients younger than 60 years of age. Median survival for immunocompetent patients is 17 to 45 months but decreases to 2 to 6 months in patients with AIDS.

Treatment with corticosteroids and radiation usually results in a dramatic, but short-lived response, with the lesions appearing to "melt away," leading some to describe primary CNS lymphoma as the "ghost tumor." Current therapy consists of combined radiation therapy and chemotherapy.

Pathophysiology

The majority of CNS lymphomas are primary (93%) and occur within the brain as compared with the spinal cord. They are more common supratentorially than in the posterior fossa (3-9:1).[82,83] The origin of primary CNS lymphoma is controversial, because the CNS does not have lymphoid tissue. However, it is suggested that they arise from circulating lymphocytes that migrate into the brain. No genetic predisposition is recognized.

Patients with an acquired or inherited immunodeficiency have a predisposition for developing primary CNS lymphoma, and in these patients Epstein-Barr virus is associated with its development.

Pathology

Primary CNS lymphoma may appear as a single mass or as multiple masses on gross pathologic evaluation. Necrosis may be present if the patient is immune compromised. The lesions may be well defined or infiltrating (Fig. 32-59) and may involve the corpus callosum and extend along the ependymal surfaces. Secondary CNS lymphoma, in contrast, is most often extra-axial and occurs in the meninges.

Non-Hodgkin's B-cell lymphoma comprises nearly all CNS lymphomas (98%). T-cell lymphoma of the CNS occurs rarely.[84] Scant cytoplasm and prominent nuclei are present (Fig. 32-60). Cells are often arranged in an angiocentric pattern. Immunohistochemical staining for B-cell lymphoid markers (CD20 and CD79a) as well as T-cell markers (CD3) is useful. The MIB-1 is high.

Imaging

CT

Primary CNS lymphoma classically is a high-attenuation lesion on plain CT but may be isoattenuating (Fig. 32-61). Necrosis may be seen in immunocompromised patients, and hemorrhage is uncommon. On postcontrast imaging, homogeneous enhancement is usually seen in immunocompetent patients and ring enhancement is more common in immunocompromised patients.

MRI

Primary CNS lymphoma is isointense to hypointense to gray matter on T1W and T2W imaging. In immunocompetent patients

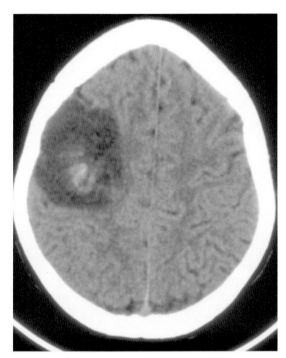

■ **FIGURE 32-57** DNET. Axial noncontrast CT demonstrates a well-demarcated region of low attenuation in the right frontal lobe. A gyral pattern of high attenuation is noted consistent with calcification.

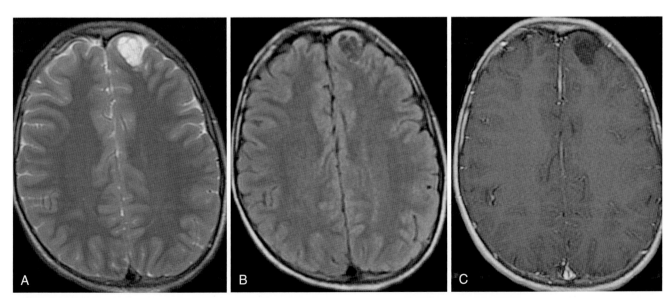

■ **FIGURE 32-58** DNET. **A,** Axial T2W MR image demonstrates a wedge-shaped, cortically based, high signal lesion in the left frontal lobe that has a "bubbly" appearance. **B,** FLAIR image demonstrates a hypointense lesion with a faint hyperintense rim. **C,** On postcontrast T1W imaging there is no enhancement.

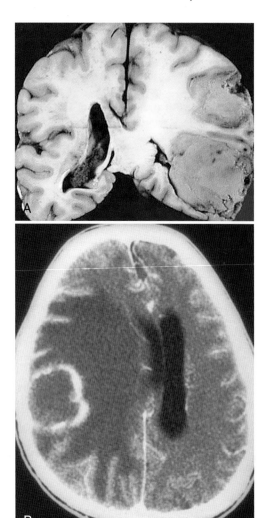

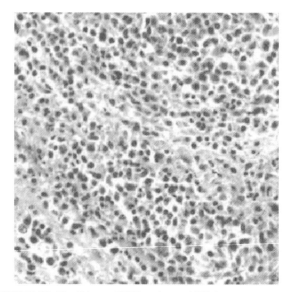

■ **FIGURE 32-60** Primary CNS lymphoma. H&E demonstrates numerous lymphocytes with prominent round-to-oval nuclei.

■ **FIGURE 32-59** Primary CNS lymphoma. **A,** Gross specimen demonstrates two discrete masses in the right cerebral hemisphere. **B,** Corresponding contrast-enhanced CT scan demonstrates a ring-enhancing lesion in the right cerebral hemisphere with a large degree of surrounding vasogenic edema for which the imaging differential diagnosis includes glioblastoma multiforme and abscess. This patient was HIV positive.

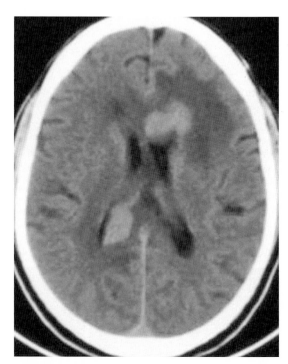

■ **FIGURE 32-61** Primary CNS lymphoma. Axial noncontrast CT from an immunocompetent patient demonstrates high-attenuation lesions in a characteristic periventricular location.

the signal is homogeneous, whereas in immunocompromised patients it is heterogeneous owing to necrosis and/or hemorrhage. On FLAIR imaging the lesions may be hyperintense, and mild surrounding edema is frequently present. Contrast enhancement is homogeneous and typically intense in immunocompetent patients (Figs. 32-62 and 32-63). In the immunocompromised patient, ring enhancement may be present owing to necrosis but homogeneous enhancement may also occur. Rarely, lesions may not enhance on postcontrast imaging. Perfusion imaging typically demonstrates an elevated rCBV (Fig. 32-64).

On diffusion-weighted imaging (DWI), lymphoma is hyperintense to gray matter and isointense to hypointense on apparent diffusion coefficient (ADC), consistent with reduced water diffusion and thus reflecting the highly cellular nature of these neoplasms, which results in decreased extracellular space in combination with scant cytoplasm and wide nuclei.

Distinguishing between primary CNS lymphoma and GBM may be difficult on conventional imaging. Even on DWI there are reports of GBMs demonstrating reduced diffusion.[85,86] Toh and coworkers investigated utilizing fractional anisotropy and the ADC and found that the fractional anisotropy and ADC values

of cerebral lymphoma were significantly lower than those of GBM.[87] However, deep, large, and homogeneously enhancing lesions are more likely to be primary CNS lymphoma than GBM. Here, again, CT can be valuable by showing fairly uniform hyperattenuation that can be diagnostic of primary CNS lymphoma.

In addition, distinguishing between CNS toxoplasmosis and lymphoma in patients with HIV infection can also be difficult. A study by Camacho and associates found that evaluating ADC values in these cases may be beneficial. They found that ADC values in toxoplasmosis are greater than those in lymphoma and that ADC values greater than 1.6 were seen only in toxoplasmosis.[88] MR spectroscopy has also been used to try to differentiate

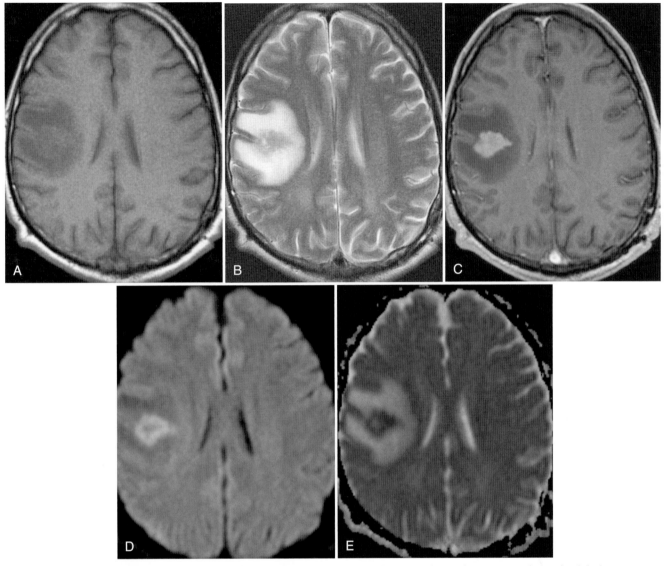

■ **FIGURE 32-62** Primary CNS lymphoma in an immunocompetent patient. **A,** Axial T1W MR image demonstrates a lesion that is isointense to gray matter and surrounded by low intensity vasogenic edema. **B,** T2W image reveals an isointense lesion. **C,** On postcontrast T1W imaging the lesion avidly enhances. **D,** DWI demonstrates a hyperintense lesion that is low in signal on the ADC map (**E**).

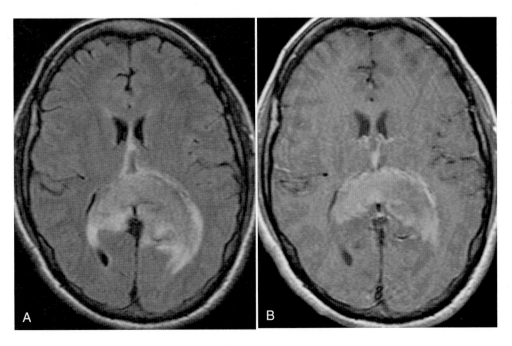

■ **FIGURE 32-63** Primary CNS lymphoma involving the corpus callosum. **A,** Axial FLAIR image demonstrates mildly hyperintense lesion expanding the splenium of the corpus callosum with a mild degree of surrounding edema. **B,** Postcontrast T1W image demonstrates relatively homogeneous enhancement.

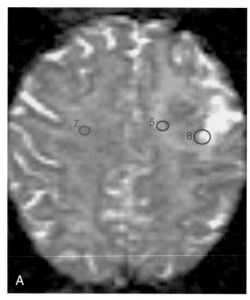

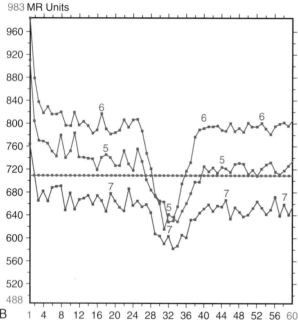

■ FIGURE 32-64 Primary CNS lymphoma. Perfusion imaging demonstrates elevated rCBV in the regions of interest placed around the lesion in the left frontal lobe.

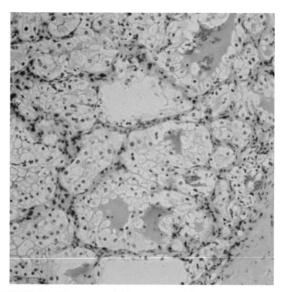

■ FIGURE 32-65 Hemangioblastoma nodule. H&E shows multiple small vascular channels similar to capillaries. Between the vascular spaces are pale pink polygonal "stromal cells." The densely pink areas are microcysts with proteinaceous fluid.

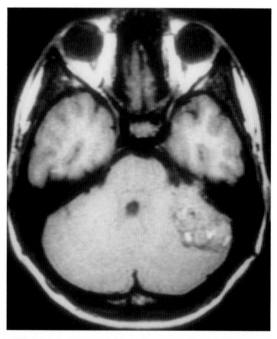

■ FIGURE 32-66 Hemangioblastoma. Axial T1W MR image shows a heterogeneous solid hemangioblastoma with focal hyperintensities and mostly peripheral curvilinear hypointensities.

lymphoma from toxoplasmosis. Lymphoma typically has elevated choline and decreased NAA, but if the voxel is placed in a necrotic region, lipid and lactate peaks may be seen, giving a similar spectroscopy as that of toxoplasmosis.

HEMANGIOBLASTOMA

Hemangioblastoma is a benign, WHO grade I lesion with a significant vascular component. Alternate names include Lindau tumor and capillary hemangioblastoma.

Epidemiology

Hemangioblastoma, although relatively common in the adult cerebellum, represents less than 3% of all intracranial tumors. Approximately one in four to five patients will have von Hippel-Lindau disease. For that reason, all patients with hemangioblastoma should be evaluated with abdominal imaging.

Clinical Presentation

Clinical presentation is typically due to mass effect. However, some patients present for evaluation of a known diagnosis or family history of von Hippel-Lindau disease. In some cases, the tumor may produce erythropoietic substances, causing relative or absolute polycythemia.

Pathophysiology

At least 50% of these tumors show genetic alterations with loss of heterozygosity. When associated with von Hippel-Lindau disease, there is a known mutation on chromosome 3p25-26.

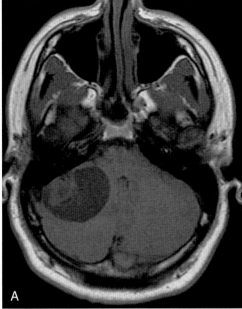

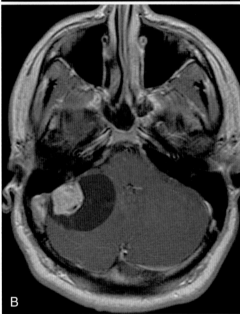

■ **FIGURE 32-67** Hemangioblastoma. Axial T1W (**A**) and axial post-contrast T1W (**B**) MR images demonstrate a cystic lesion with an enhancing mural nodule.

The derivation of these tumors is controversial: are they glial or vascular? Staining characteristics do not support a glial origin. Bleistein and coworkers suggest they arise from the embryonal vascular plexus.[89]

Pathology

These lesions are well demarcated and highly vascular. The solid components are often adjacent to a pial surface. The majority (more than 70%) will have a mixture of solid tissue and fluid. Fluid may be in a large, single or unicameral space or be interspersed between the solid elements. Intratumoral hemorrhage may be present, as well as fluid that may be straw colored or blood tinged. The tumor margin is well demarcated and usually without infiltration. The tumor may have intracellular lipid material, as well as blood and blood products (i.e., hemosiderin).

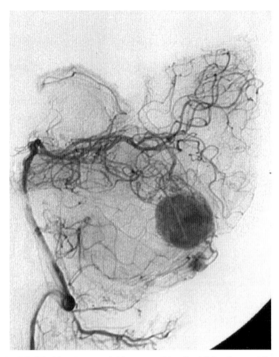

■ **FIGURE 32-68** Hemangioblastoma. Vertebral injection—mid to late arterial phase. There are two nodules, which demonstrate dense tumor blush, and an adjacent avascular region representing the fluid component.

Microscopically, this neoplasm consists of variable amounts of vascular tissue, varying in size between capillary and larger sinusoidal channels. Interspersed between the vascular spaces are "stromal cells" that are often large and pale staining (on H&E stain) with lipid-filled vacuoles (Fig. 32-65). These "clear cells" may mimic the appearance of metastatic renal cell carcinoma. Patients with von Hippel-Lindau disease are at considerable risk (>50% older than age 50) to develop a renal cell carcinoma. Despite this association, renal cell carcinoma metastasis to the cerebellum is uncommon, even in patients with von Hippel-Lindau disease. However, tumor-to-tumor metastasis from renal cell carcinoma into a hemangioblastoma has been frequently reported. Evaluation for a possible renal cell carcinoma metastasis should include a search for epithelial membrane antigen (EMA), which would be negative in hemangioblastoma. The origin and nature of the stromal cells is uncertain. They lack typical endothelial markers (von Willebrand factor, CD34, CD31). However, they may express vimentin, platelet-derived growth factor, and vascular endothelial growth factor. Hemangioblastoma does not express GFAP. Sclerosis, astrocytic gliosis, and Rosenthal fibers may be found about the tumor margin.

Imaging

CT

Hemangioblastomas usually have a clearly visible fluid component. However, they vary considerably in morphology, ranging from almost purely solid to large "cysts" with miniscule solid components.[90,91] The cyst fluid often has attenuation greater than CSF, either due to protein or infrequently from hemorrhage. The mural nodule has attenuation greater than brain, but calcification does not occur. CT angiography may show increased perfusion but often with a prolonged mean transit time. Solid areas typically enhance brightly after infusion of a contrast agent.

MRI

MRI demonstrates both the solid and fluid components of hemangioblastoma (Fig. 32-66). Slight T1 shortening from protein

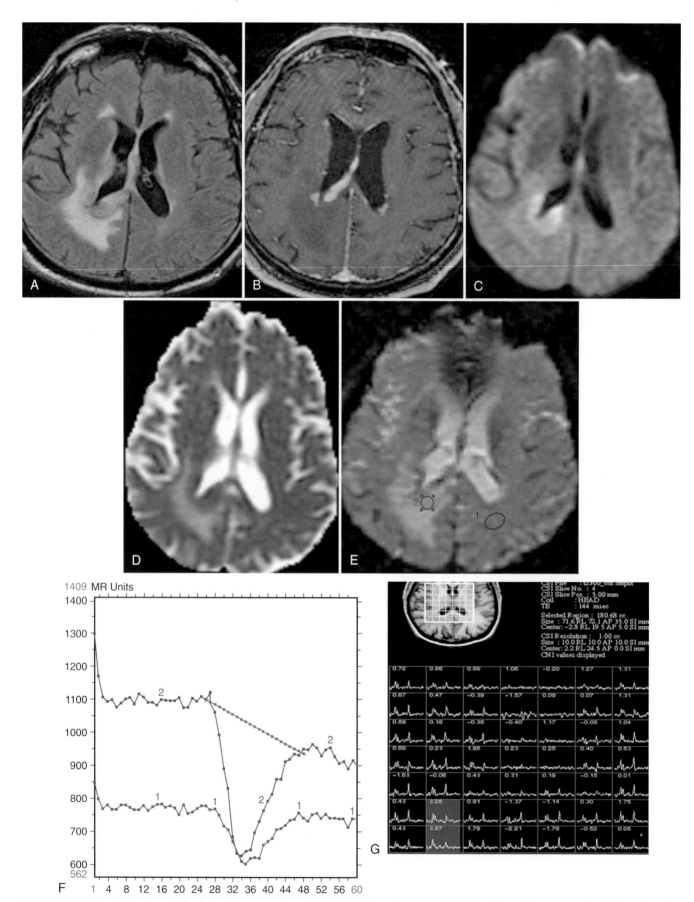

■ **FIGURE 32-69** **A,** A periventricular lesion demonstrated on MRI is slightly hyperintense on FLAIR imaging and has surrounding T2 hyperintensity with an imaging appearance consistent with vasogenic edema. **B,** On postcontrast imaging the lesion demonstrated enhancement. There was high signal on DWI (**C**) and low signal on the ADC map (**D**) consistent with reduced diffusion. **E, F,** Perfusion-weighted imaging revealed elevated rCBV values with greater than 50% return to baseline. **G,** MR spectroscopy demonstrated reduced NAA and a slight elevation of choline.

and/or blood products may increase the fluid signal above CSF. Lipid and/or methemoglobin in the solid portions may cause hyperintensities on T1W images. Hemangioblastoma may have increased ADC values and low signal on DWI. This may be due to the vascular spaces or microcysts within the solid tumor.[92] On T2W images, hemangioblastoma may demonstrate hypointensities from hemosiderin or flow voids in tumoral sinusoids as well as feeding/draining vessels.[91] As noted on CT, the solid portions of the tumor invariably show prominent enhancement after infusion of gadolinium (Fig. 32-67).

Special Procedures

Angiographically, these lesions may have one or two slightly dilated feeding arteries and a couple of medium-sized draining veins. The tumor blush in hemangioblastoma is often persistent into the venous phase and there may be delayed venous filling, both of which may mimic a meningioma (Fig. 32-68). Some clinicians have advocated therapeutic embolization of these lesions.

ANALYSIS

A sample report is presented in Box 32-1.

KEY POINTS: DIFFERENTIAL DIAGNOSIS

- CT is useful to assess the osseous response to the lesion and for evaluation of tumoral calcification.
- Those lesions that involve the cortex may have a similar imaging appearance, and many present with seizures.
- Imaging plays an integral role in the detection, diagnosis, and management of these lesions, and advanced imaging, such as perfusion-weighted MRI and MR spectroscopy, may help narrow the differential diagnosis and assist in post-treatment follow-up.

BOX 32-1 Sample Report: MRI for Evaluation of Altered Mental Status

PATIENT HISTORY

An 81-year-old man presented with altered mental status.

TECHNIQUE

Sagittal T1W, axial T2W, axial FLAIR, axial and coronal DWI, axial T1W precontrast and postcontrast, and coronal T1W postcontrast imaging was done along with 3D MR spectroscopy and perfusion-weighted imaging.

FINDINGS

FLAIR imaging demonstrates a slightly hyperintense to gray matter mass lesion predominantly involving the periventricular region of the body of the right lateral ventricle with surrounding T2 prolongation suggestive of vasogenic edema. On postcontrast imaging the lesion avidly and homogeneously enhances. A second smaller focus of enhancement and T2 hyperintensity is present adjacent to the frontal horn of the right lateral ventricle. On diffusion-weighted imaging the lesion along the body of the lateral ventricle demonstrates reduced diffusion.

Perfusion-weighted imaging reveals markedly elevated rCBV with a greater than 50% return to baseline. MR spectroscopy demonstrates a reduction in NAA, combined with a slight elevation in choline (Fig. 32-69).

IMPRESSION

This is an avidly enhancing periventricular lesion with reduced diffusion, elevated rCBV, and slight elevation in choline. These findings are most suggestive of primary CNS lymphoma.

COMMENT

Clues to the diagnosis in this case include the periventricular location, which narrows the differential diagnosis to lymphoma and GBM and, less likely, metastasis. The reduction in diffusion leads toward the diagnosis of lymphoma. Reduced diffusion is unlikely in GBM but may occur in some forms of metastasis. The elevated rCBV with greater than 50% return to baseline argues for a primary CNS neoplasm as opposed to a metastasis. The combination of these findings along with the homogeneous enhancement leads to the diagnosis of lymphoma.

SUGGESTED READINGS

Burger PC, et al. Surgical Pathology of the Nervous System and Its Coverings. Edinburgh, Churchill Livingstone, 2002, pp 160-378.

Ludeman L, et al. Comparison of dynamic contrast-enhanced MRI with WHO tumor grading for gliomas. Eur Radiol 2001; 11:1231-1241.

Perry JR. Oligodendrogliomas: clinical and genetic correlations. Curr Opin Neurol 2001; 14:705-710.

Tortosa A, et al. Prognostic implication of clinical, radiologic, and pathologic features in patients with anaplastic gliomas. Cancer 2003; 97:1063-1071.

Wessels PH, et al. Supratentorial grade II astrocytoma: biological features and clinical course. Lancet Neurol 2003; 2:395-403.

REFERENCES

1. Koeller KK, Henry JM. From the archives of the AFIP: superficial gliomas: radiologic-pathologic correlation. Armed Forces Institute of Pathology. RadioGraphics 2001; 21:1533-1556.
2. Tilgner J, Herr M, Ostertag C, Volk B. Validation of intraoperative diagnoses using smear preparations from stereotactic brain biopsies: intraoperative versus final diagnosis—influence of clinical factors. Neurosurgery 2005; 56:257-265; discussion 257-265.
3. Al-Okaili RN, Krejza J, Wang S, et al. Advanced MR imaging techniques in the diagnosis of intraaxial brain tumors in adults. RadioGraphics 2006; 26(Suppl 1):S173-S189.
4. Law M, Yang S, Wang H, et al. Glioma grading: sensitivity, specificity, and predictive values of perfusion MR imaging and proton MR spectroscopic imaging compared with conventional MR imaging. AJNR Am J Neuroradiol 2003; 24:1989-1998.
5. Aronen HJ, Pardo FS, Kennedy DN, et al. High microvascular blood volume is associated with high glucose uptake and tumor angiogenesis in human gliomas. Clin Cancer Res 2000; 6:2189-2200.
6. Aronen HJ, Gazit IE, Louis DN, et al. Cerebral blood volume maps of gliomas: comparison with tumor grade and histologic findings. Radiology 1994; 191:41-51.

7. Wieshmann UC, Symms MR, Parker GJ, et al. Diffusion tensor imaging demonstrates deviation of fibres in normal appearing white matter adjacent to a brain tumour. J Neurol Neurosurg Psychiatry 2000; 68:501-503.

8. Coenen VA, Krings T, Mayfrank L, et al. Three-dimensional visualization of the pyramidal tract in a neuronavigation system during brain tumor surgery: first experiences and technical note. Neurosurgery 2001; 49:86-92; discussion 92-93.

9. Koeller KK, Rushing EJ. From the archives of the AFIP: pilocytic astrocytoma: radiologic-pathologic correlation. RadioGraphics 2004; 24:1693-1708.

10. von Deimling A, Louis DN, Menon AG, et al. Deletions on the long arm of chromosome 17 in pilocytic astrocytoma. Acta Neuropathol 1993; 86:81-85.

11. Zattara-Cannoni H, Gambarelli D, Lena G, et al. Are juvenile pilocytic astrocytomas benign tumors? A cytogenetic study in 24 cases. Cancer Genet Cytogenet 1998; 104:157-160.

12. Pencalet P, Maixner W, Sainte-Rose C, et al. Benign cerebellar astrocytomas in children. J Neurosurg 1999; 90:265-273.

13. Beni-Adani L, Gomori M, Spektor S, Constantini S. Cyst wall enhancement in pilocytic astrocytoma: neoplastic or reactive phenomena. Pediatr Neurosurg 2000; 32:234-239.

14. Palma L, Guidetti B. Cystic pilocytic astrocytomas of the cerebral hemispheres: surgical experience with 51 cases and long-term results. J Neurosurg 1985; 62:811-815.

15. Mamelak AN, Prados MD, Obana WG, et al. Treatment options and prognosis for multicentric juvenile pilocytic astrocytoma. J Neurosurg 1994; 81:24-30.

16. Hwang JH, Egnaczyk GF, Ballard E, et al. Proton MR spectroscopic characteristics of pediatric pilocytic astrocytomas. AJNR Am J Neuroradiol 1998; 19:535-540.

17. Arslanoglu A, Cirak B, Horska A, et al. MR imaging characteristics of pilomyxoid astrocytomas. AJNR Am J Neuroradiol 2003; 24: 1906-1908.

18. Komotar RJ, Burger PC, Carson BS, et al. Pilocytic and pilomyxoid hypothalamic/chiasmatic astrocytomas. Neurosurgery 2004; 54:72-79; discussion 79-80.

19. Tihan T, Fisher PG, Kepner JL, et al. Pediatric astrocytomas with monomorphous pilomyxoid features and a less favorable outcome. J Neuropathol Exp Neurol 1999; 58:1061-1068.

20. Komotar RJ, Mocco J, Carson BS, et al. Pilomyxoid astrocytoma: a review. Med Gen Med 2004; 6:42.

21. Gottfried ON, Fults DW, Townsend JJ, Couldwell WT. Spontaneous hemorrhage associated with a pilomyxoid astrocytoma: case report. J Neurosurg 2003; 99:416-420.

22. Hamada H, Kurimoto M, Hayashi N, et al. Pilomyxoid astrocytoma in a patient presenting with fatal hemorrhage: case report. J Neurosurg Pediatr 2008; 1:244-246.

23. Powell SZ, Yachnis AT, Rorke LB, et al. Divergent differentiation in pleomorphic xanthoastrocytoma: evidence for a neuronal element and possible relationship to ganglion cell tumors. Am J Surg Pathol 1996; 20:80-85.

24. Giannini C, Scheithauer BW, Burger PC, et al. Pleomorphic xanthoastrocytoma: what do we really know about it? Cancer 1999; 85: 2033-2045.

25. Pahapill PA, Ramsay DA, Del Maestro RF. Pleomorphic xanthoastrocytoma: case report and analysis of the literature concerning the efficacy of resection and the significance of necrosis. Neurosurgery 1996; 38:822-828; discussion 828-829.

26. Marton E, Feletti A, Orvieto E, Longatti P. Malignant progression in pleomorphic xanthoastrocytoma: personal experience and review of the literature. J Neurol Sci 2007; 252:144-153.

27. Johannesen TB, Langmark F, Lote K. Progress in long-term survival in adult patients with supratentorial low-grade gliomas: a population-based study of 993 patients in whom tumors were diagnosed between 1970 and 1993. J Neurosurg 2003; 99:854-862.

28. van den Bent MJ, Afra D, de Witte O, et al. Long-term efficacy of early versus delayed radiotherapy for low-grade astrocytoma and oligodendroglioma in adults: the EORTC 22845 randomised trial. Lancet 2005; 366:985-990.

29. Danchaivijitr N, Waldman AD, Tozer DJ, et al. Low-grade gliomas: do changes in rCBV measurements at longitudinal perfusion-weighted MR imaging predict malignant transformation? Radiology 2008; 247:170-178.

30. Castillo M, Smith JK, Kwock L. Correlation of myo-inositol levels and grading of cerebral astrocytomas. AJNR Am J Neuroradiol 2000; 21:1645-1649.

31. Goebell E, Paustenbach S, Vaeterlein O, et al. Low-grade and anaplastic gliomas: differences in architecture evaluated with diffusion-tensor MR imaging. Radiology 2006; 239:217-222.

32. Sugahara T, Korogi Y, Kochi M, et al. Perfusion-sensitive MR imaging of gliomas: comparison between gradient-echo and spin-echo echo-planar imaging techniques. AJNR Am J Neuroradiol 2001; 22: 1306-1315.

33. Rees JH, Smirniotopoulos JG, Jones RV, Wong K. Glioblastoma multiforme: radiologic-pathologic correlation. RadioGraphics 1996; 16:1413-1438; quiz 1462-1463.

34. Salcman M. Survival in glioblastoma: historical perspective. Neurosurgery 1980; 7:435-439.

35. Westermark B, Nister M. Molecular genetics of human glioma. Curr Opin Oncol 1995; 7:220-225.

36. Wu JK, Ye Z, Darras BT. Frequency of p53 tumor suppressor gene mutations in human primary brain tumors. Neurosurgery 1993; 33:824-830; discussion 830-831.

37. Haapasalo H, Isola J, Sallinen P, et al. Aberrant p53 expression in astrocytic neoplasms of the brain: association with proliferation. Am J Pathol 1993; 142:1347-1351.

38. Vertosick FT Jr, Selker RG. Brain stem and spinal metastases of supratentorial glioblastoma multiforme: a clinical series. Neurosurgery 1990; 27:516-521; discussion 521-522.

39. Scott JN, Brasher PM, Sevick RJ, et al. How often are nonenhancing supratentorial gliomas malignant? A population study. Neurology 2002; 59:947-949.

40. Hakyemez B, Erdogan C, Yildirim N, Parlak M. Glioblastoma multiforme with atypical diffusion-weighted MR findings. Br J Radiol 2005; 78:989-992.

41. del Carpio-O'Donovan R, Korah I, Salazar A, Melancon D. Gliomatosis cerebri. Radiology 1996; 198:831-835.

42. Felsberg GJ, Silver SA, Brown MT, Tien RD. Radiologic-pathologic correlation. Gliomatosis cerebri. AJNR Am J Neuroradiol 1994; 15: 1745-1753.

43. Fallentin E, Skriver E, Herning M, Broholm H. Gliomatosis cerebri—an appropriate diagnosis? Case reports. Acta Radiol 1997; 38:381-390.

44. Bendszus M, Warmuth-Metz M, Klein R, et al. MR spectroscopy in gliomatosis cerebri. AJNR Am J Neuroradiol 2000; 21:375-380.

45. Mawrin C. Molecular genetic alterations in gliomatosis cerebri: what can we learn about the origin and course of the disease? Acta Neuropathol 2005; 110:527-536.

46. Jennings MT, Frenchman M, Shehab T, et al. Gliomatosis cerebri presenting as intractable epilepsy during early childhood. J Child Neurol 1995; 10:37-45.

47. Yip M, Fisch C, Lamarche JB. AFIP archives: gliomatosis cerebri affecting the entire neuraxis. RadioGraphics 2003; 23:247-253.

48. Bowen BC. Glial neoplasms without elevated choline-creatine ratios. AJNR Am J Neuroradiol 2003; 24:782-784.

49. Negendank WG, Sauter R, Brown TR, et al. Proton magnetic resonance spectroscopy in patients with glial tumors: a multicenter study. J Neurosurg 1996; 84:449-458.

50. Yang S, Wetzel S, Law M, et al. Dynamic contrast-enhanced T2*-weighted MR imaging of gliomatosis cerebri. AJNR Am J Neuroradiol 2002; 23:350-355.

51. Koeller KK, Rushing EJ. From the archives of the AFIP: oligodendroglioma and its variants: radiologic-pathologic correlation. RadioGraphics 2005; 25:1669-1688.

52. Mork SJ, Lindegaard KF, Halvorsen TB, et al. Oligodendroglioma: incidence and biological behavior in a defined population. J Neurosurg 1985; 63:881-889.

53. Olson JD, Riedel E, DeAngelis LM. Long-term outcome of low-grade oligodendroglioma and mixed glioma. Neurology 2000; 54:1442-1448.

54. Chen R, Macdonald DR, Ramsay DA. Primary diffuse leptomeningeal oligodendroglioma: case report. J Neurosurg 1995; 83:724-728.

55. Celli P, Nofrone I, Palma L, et al. Cerebral oligodendroglioma: prognostic factors and life history. Neurosurgery 1994; 35:1018-1034; discussion 1034-1035.

56. Cairncross JG, Ueki K, Zlatescu MC, et al. Specific genetic predictors of chemotherapeutic response and survival in patients with anaplastic oligodendrogliomas. J Natl Cancer Inst 1998; 90:1473-1479.

57. Reifenberger J, Reifenberger G, Liu L, et al. Molecular genetic analysis of oligodendroglial tumors shows preferential allelic deletions on 19q and 1p. Am J Pathol 1994; 145:1175-1190.
58. Shaw EG, Scheithauer BW, O'Fallon JR, Davis DH. Mixed oligoastrocytomas: a survival and prognostic factor analysis. Neurosurgery 1994; 34:577-582; discussion 582.
59. Castillo M, Davis PC, Takei Y, Hoffman JC Jr. Intracranial ganglioglioma: MR, CT, and clinical findings in 18 patients. AJNR Am J Neuroradiol 1990; 11:109-114.
60. Tien RD, Tuori SL, Pulkingham N, Burger PC. Ganglioglioma with leptomeningeal and subarachnoid spread: results of CT, MR, and PET imaging. AJR Am J Roentgenol 1992; 159:391-393.
61. Izukawa D, Lach B, Benoit B. Gangliocytoma of the cerebellum: ultrastructure and immunohistochemistry. Neurosurgery 1988; 22:576-581.
62. Zentner J, Wolf HK, Ostertun B, et al. Gangliogliomas: clinical, radiological, and histopathological findings in 51 patients. J Neurol Neurosurg Psychiatry 1994; 57:1497-1502.
63. Dorne HL, O'Gorman AM, Melanson D. Computed tomography of intracranial gangliogliomas. AJNR Am J Neuroradiol 1986; 7: 281-285.
64. Robinson S, Cohen AR. Cowden disease and Lhermitte-Duclos disease: characterization of a new phakomatosis. Neurosurgery 2000; 46:371-383.
65. Milbouw G, Born JD, Martin D, et al. Clinical and radiological aspects of dysplastic gangliocytoma (Lhermitte-Duclos disease): a report of two cases with review of the literature. Neurosurgery 1988; 22(1 pt 1):124-128.
66. Reeder RF, Saunders RL, Roberts DW, et al. Magnetic resonance imaging in the diagnosis and treatment of Lhermitte-Duclos disease (dysplastic gangliocytoma of the cerebellum). Neurosurgery 1988; 23:240-245.
67. Kulkantrakorn K, Awwad EE, Levy B, et al. MRI in Lhermitte-Duclos disease. Neurology 1997; 48:725-731.
68. Nelen MR, Padberg GW, Peeters EA, et al. Localization of the gene for Cowden disease to chromosome 10q22-23. Nat Genet 1996; 13:114-116.
69. Meltzer CC, Smirniotopoulos JG, Jones RV. The striated cerebellum: an MR imaging sign in Lhermitte-Duclos disease (dysplastic gangliocytoma). Radiology 1995; 194:699-703.
70. Awwad EE, Levy E, Martin DS, Merenda GO. Atypical MR appearance of Lhermitte-Duclos disease with contrast enhancement. AJNR Am J Neuroradiol 1995; 16:1719-1720.
71. Klisch J, Juengling F, Spreer J, et al. Lhermitte-Duclos disease: assessment with MR imaging, positron emission tomography, single-photon emission CT, and MR spectroscopy. AJNR Am J Neuroradiol 2001; 22:824-830.
72. Barkovich AJ. Pediatric Neuroimaging, 4th ed. Philadelphia, Lippincott Williams & Wilkins, 2005.
73. Cervera-Pierot P, Varlet P, Chodkiewicz JP, Daumas-Duport C. Dysembryoplastic neuroepithelial tumors located in the caudate nucleus area: report of four cases. Neurosurgery 1997; 40:1065-1069; discussion 1069-1070.
74. Pasquier B, Peoc HM, Fabre-Bocquentin B, et al. Surgical pathology of drug-resistant partial epilepsy: a 10-year-experience with a series of 327 consecutive resections. Epileptic Disord 2002; 4:99-119.
75. Hammond RR, Duggal N, Woulfe JM, Girvin JP. Malignant transformation of a dysembryoplastic neuroepithelial tumor: case report. J Neurosurg 2000; 92:722-725.
76. Daumas-Duport C. Dysembryoplastic neuroepithelial tumours. Brain Pathol 1993; 3:283-295.
77. Fernandez C, Girard N, Paz Paredes A, et al. The usefulness of MR imaging in the diagnosis of dysembryoplastic neuroepithelial tumor in children: a study of 14 cases. AJNR Am J Neuroradiol 2003; 24:829-834.
78. Vuori K, Kankaanranta L, Hakkinen AM, et al. Low-grade gliomas and focal cortical developmental malformations: differentiation with proton MR spectroscopy. Radiology 2004; 230:703-708.
79. Surawicz TS, McCarthy BJ, Kupelian V, et al. Descriptive epidemiology of primary brain and CNS tumors: results from the Central Brain Tumor Registry of the United States, 1990-1994. Neuro Oncol 1999; 1:14-25.
80. Koeller KK, Smirniotopoulos JG, Jones RV. Primary central nervous system lymphoma: radiologic-pathologic correlation. RadioGraphics 1997; 17:1497-1526.
81. Johnson BA, Fram EK, Johnson PC, Jacobowitz R. The variable MR appearance of primary lymphoma of the central nervous system: comparison with histopathologic features. AJNR Am J Neuroradiol 1997; 18:563-572.
82. Hochberg FH, Miller DC. Primary central nervous system lymphoma. J Neurosurg 1988; 68:835-853.
83. Remick SC, Diamond C, Migliozzi JA, et al. Primary central nervous system lymphoma in patients with and without the acquired immune deficiency syndrome: a retrospective analysis and review of the literature. Medicine (Baltimore) 1990; 69:345-360.
84. Bednar MM, Salerni A, Flanagan ME, Pendlebury WW. Primary central nervous system T-cell lymphoma: case report. J Neurosurg 1991; 74:668-672.
85. Batra A, Tripathi RP. Atypical diffusion-weighted magnetic resonance findings in glioblastoma multiforme. Australas Radiol 2004; 48:388-391.
86. Toh CH, Chen YL, Hsieh TC, et al. Glioblastoma multiforme with diffusion-weighted magnetic resonance imaging characteristics mimicking primary brain lymphoma: case report. J Neurosurg 2006; 105:132-135.
87. Toh CH, Castillo M, Wong AM, et al. Primary cerebral lymphoma and glioblastoma multiforme: differences in diffusion characteristics evaluated with diffusion tensor imaging. AJNR Am J Neuroradiol 2008; 29:471-475.
88. Camacho DL, Smith JK, Castillo M. Differentiation of toxoplasmosis and lymphoma in AIDS patients by using apparent diffusion coefficients. AJNR Am J Neuroradiol 2003; 24:633-637.
89. Bleistein M, Geiger K, Franz K, et al. Transthyretin and transferrin in hemangioblastoma stromal cells. Pathol Res Pract 2000; 196: 675-681.
90. Lee SR, Sanches J, Mark AS, et al. Posterior fossa hemangioblastomas: MR imaging. Radiology 1989; 171:463-468.
91. Ho VB, Smirniotopoulos JG, Murphy FM, Rushing EJ. Radiologic-pathologic correlation: hemangioblastoma. AJNR Am J Neuroradiol 1992; 13:1343-1352.
92. Quadery FA, Okamoto K. Diffusion-weighted MRI of haemangioblastomas and other cerebellar tumours. Neuroradiology 2003; 45: 212-219.

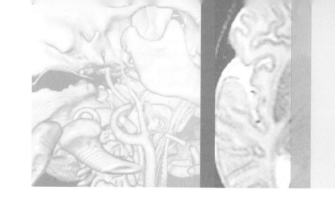

33

Sellar and Juxtasellar Tumors

Alice B. Smith and Soonmee Cha

The sellar region is defined by the sella turcica and its contents. The parasellar region has no precise boundaries but is considered to be the area surrounding the sella turcica, including the cavernous sinus. Many diverse lesions involve the sellar and juxtasellar regions, including primary benign and malignant neoplasms, metastases, perineurial spread of tumor, and direct invasion from adjacent tumors. The most common lesions are pituitary macroadenomas, craniopharyngiomas, meningiomas, metastasis, and hypothalamic-optic gliomas, which together account for about 75% of lesions in this area.[1] Aneurysms clearly must be considered in the differential diagnosis of this region but are discussed elsewhere.

The size and exact location of the lesion determine patient symptoms. Differentiating lesions in this region may be difficult, especially for larger lesions where the point of origin is no longer certain. Placing the origin as either sellar or parasellar at least assists in narrowing the differential diagnosis.

PITUITARY ADENOMA

The most common intrasellar lesion is an adenoma of the adenohypophysis (anterior lobe of the pituitary gland). Rarely, an adenoma may arise from the neurohypophysis (posterior lobe of the pituitary gland). Pituitary adenomas are defined by their size as microadenomas (<10 mm) or macroadenomas (>10 mm). Macroadenomas are further described as invasive when they break through the sellar floor or extend into the cavernous sinus.

Epidemiology

The incidence of pituitary adenomas ranges from 2% to 27% in the general population. They occur with greater frequency in females than males and most commonly arise in patients between 20 and 50 years of age.[1] Adenomas are the most common of the sellar lesions, accounting for up to 90% of neoplasms that involve this region.[2]

Clinical Presentation

Microadenomas frequently come to clinical attention because of hormonal secretion. Prolactin is the hormone most frequently elevated (25%) and can result in infertility, amenorrhea, and galactorrhea in women and decreased libido and impotence in men. Growth hormone–secreting adenomas result in acromegaly in adults and gigantism in children, whereas adrenocorticotropic hormone (ACTH)–secreting adenomas arising from the posterior pituitary or the neurohypophysial region cause Cushing's syndrome. Thyroid-stimulating hormone (TSH) and follicle-stimulating hormone/luteinizing hormone (FSH/LH)–secreting adenomas are rare. Twenty-five to 30 percent of pituitary microadenomas are nonfunctional.[1]

Macroadenomas frequently do not elaborate hormones. Instead, they present at larger size with mass effect on the chiasm causing visual impairment, compression of the pituitary gland and/or stalk causing pituitary insufficiency, compression of the third ventricle and foramina of Monro causing hydrocephalus, or invasion of the cavernous sinus causing cranial nerve palsies. In males, prolactinomas may reach large size, because the symptoms are less readily identifiable than in females. Occasionally, mass effect on the infundibulum causes elevated prolactin levels, but in these cases the prolactin levels typically do not exceed 150 ng/mL. Overall, about 40% of macroadenomas invade the cavernous sinus to some extent but rarely cause cranial nerve palsy.[2]

Intratumoral hemorrhage can occur in up to 15% of adenomas (Fig. 33-1). Both microadenomas and macroadenomas can undergo a rapid increase in size in the event of pituitary apoplexy, which is an acute hemorrhage or infarction of a pituitary adenoma. Apoplexy results in acute symptoms, such as headache, vomiting, ocular motility disturbance, and possibly a sudden decrease in vision.[3] Seizures or decreased consciousness may also occur.

Pathophysiology

Pituitary adenomas arise from the adenohypophysis, or anterior pituitary gland. Traditional embryology describes the anterior pituitary as arising by invagination of the rostral stomadeum.[4] The pars distalis makes up the majority of the anterior lobe. A portion of the pars distalis also extends superiorly and contributes to the anterior aspect of the infundibulum. Therefore, the infundibulum is composed of components from both the anterior and posterior pituitary lobes, explaining the occurrence of occasional adenomas along the stalk.[4]

Pathology

Grossly, pituitary adenomas tend to be circumscribed but unencapsulated lesions. Microadenomas appear as small tan-brown nodules within a pituitary gland of normal size. Macroadenomas enlarge the pituitary gland.

Histologically, pituitary adenomas are classified as basophilic, eosinophilic, or null cell. However, this classification system has little clinical value and has now been replaced with a functional classification system that involves electron microscopy and immunohistochemistry.

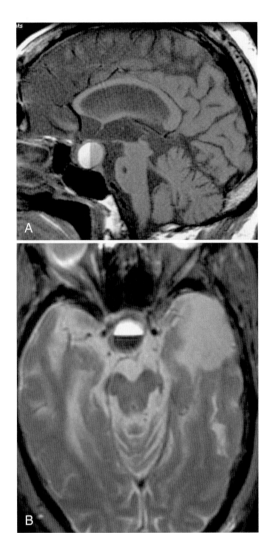

■ **FIGURE 33-1** Pituitary apoplexy. Sagittal T1W (**A**) and axial T2W (**B**) MR images demonstrate a fluid/fluid level within the sella. There is intrinsic T1 shortening as well as low signal on the T2W image consistent with blood products.

Microscopically, adenomas are composed of sheets of monomorphic cells. Prolactinomas may show psammomatous calcifications and amyloid deposits. Patients with pituitary apoplexy have hemorrhage and necrosis within the gland.

Pituitary adenomas also occur in up to two thirds of patients with multiple endocrine neoplasia (MEN) syndrome type I. In this familial syndrome, affected individuals develop tumors of the parathyroid glands, the pancreatic islet cells, and the anterior pituitary gland.

Imaging

The physiology central to all pituitary imaging is that the normal pituitary gland lies outside the blood-brain barrier. For that reason, administered contrast agents wash in and then wash out very rapidly. On contrast-enhanced CT and MRI, slowly enhancing lesions may first appear as negative (filling) defects within the normally enhancing residual gland and then as enhancing lesions within the now nonenhancing (washed out) normal gland. Detection of a pituitary lesion and localization of the lesion within the gland require careful synchronization of the imaging study to precise times after administration of a contrast agent.

CT

CT now plays a limited role in evaluating pituitary adenomas. On CT, microadenomas typically appear as hypodense regions within the gland. They may result in a focal thinning of the sellar floor, may increase the height of the gland to more than 9 mm, may bulge the diaphragma sellae superiorly, and may deviate the infundibulum away from the adenoma.

The appearance of macroadenomas varies with the size of the lesion. Nearly all (94%-100%) macroadenomas enlarge the sella turcica, but sellar enlargement is not specific for adenomas. Sellar enlargement has also been reported in more than 50% of nonadenomatous lesions involving the sella turcica, including meningiomas, craniopharyngiomas, and Rathke's cleft cysts.[5] On contrast-enhanced images, macroadenomas may appear isodense or hypodense as compared with the cavernous sinus. The imaging characteristics will also depend on the degree of necrosis and hemorrhage.

MRI

MRI can accurately demonstrate microadenomas as small as 3 mm and frequently succeeds in delineating even smaller lesions. Coronal and sagittal imaging are the most valuable for assessing microadenomas and macroadenomas. They are especially helpful for assessing cavernous sinus invasion and involvement of the optic nerves by macroadenomas. On T1-weighted (T1W) imaging, microadenomas are hypointense to isointense in comparison with the normal gland. They may deviate the infundibulum and bow the superior aspect of the gland superiorly. However, caution should be used when evaluating the tilt of the infundibulum, because some normal patients have infundibular deviation due to ectopic insertion of the infundibulum or eccentric gland position. Hemorrhage into the adenoma may cause T1 shortening. Suspected microadenomas may be evaluated by dynamic imaging, because they will enhance more slowly than the surrounding gland and therefore can be differentiated from the gland more easily (Fig. 33-2). On delayed contrast-enhanced MRI, the microadenomas will enhance like the gland itself and become difficult to distinguish. Still later, continued enhancement of the adenomas and washout of contrast from the gland may reverse the expected appearance, so the normal (now nonenhancing) gland is mistaken for the adenoma.

Macroadenomas are variable in their MRI appearance depending on the degree of necrosis and hemorrhage. They usually appear isointense to gray matter on T1W and T2-weighted (T2W) imaging, are hyperintense on fluid-attenuated inversion recovery (FLAIR) images, and show nearly constant heterogeneous contrast enhancement. They often show areas of cyst and hemorrhage, especially in the larger tumors. Coronal T2W images typically display the optic chiasm most clearly as a crescent of low signal crossing above the sella. The paired A1 segments of the anterior cerebral arteries pass immediately above the prechiasmal optic nerves or the chiasm itself. Compression of the chiasm by macroadenoma typically appears as elevation and thinning of the low signal "chiasmal crescent" with elevation of the flow voids of the A1 segments above it. Accurate detection of extension to the cavernous sinus is difficult. MRI is only 55% sensitive for invasion of the cavernous sinus. Invasion can be suspected when at least 50% of the cavernous segment of the internal carotid artery is surrounded by the macroadenoma. Unilateral carotid artery encasement is the most specific imaging sign of cavernous sinus involvement (Fig. 33-3A).[6] Characteristically, pituitary macroadenomas do not narrow the carotid artery, even when they encase it, whereas meningiomas of the cavernous sinus do narrow the carotid artery when they surround it. Therefore, preservation of normal caliber of an encased internal carotid artery suggests that the cavernous sinus has been invaded by a macroadenoma, rather than meningioma. This sign, however, is imperfect. Macroadenomas can also erode through

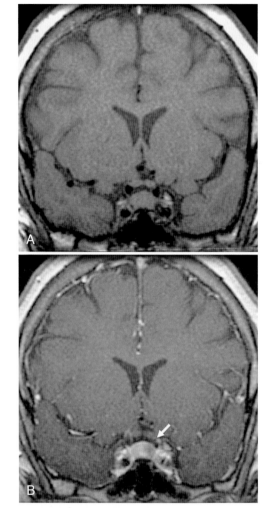

■ **FIGURE 33-2**   Pituitary microadenoma. Coronal T1W MR image without contrast (**A**) and early postcontrast T1W MR image (**B**) demonstrate a 7-mm focus of nonenhancement (*arrow*) consistent with a pituitary microadenoma.

the floor of the sella turcica. Large lesions may extend into the sphenoidal sinus and then through the sphenoidal sinus into the nasopharynx, mimicking carcinoma of the sphenoidal sinus or nasopharynx (see Fig. 33-3B). Because nasopharyngeal carcinomas also tend to narrow the internal carotid arteries, preservation of the caliber of these vessels again suggests pituitary macroadenoma. MR spectroscopy may show a choline peak or no metabolites at all.[7]

Other lesions that may mimic pituitary macroadenoma include lesions of the posterior pituitary gland, such as granular cell tumors and pituicytomas. In such cases, the best approach may be to demonstrate that the lesion arises from the anterior lobe of the pituitary, eliminating posterior pituitary lesions from consideration. Metastases to the pituitary gland are also included in the imaging differential for pituitary lesions, but, like posterior pituitary lesions, are much less common than macroadenomas.

Pituitary adenomas can be graded by their imaging appearance. Grade I adenomas are the microadenomas, which by definition are less than 1 cm. These do not enlarge the sella turcica, although they may cause focal erosions in the sellar floor. Grade II lesions are greater than 1 cm but remain within the sella or have suprasellar extension with no invasion of adjacent structures. Grade III lesions are locally invasive. Grade IV lesions are large tumors that invade extrasellar structures including bone, hypothalamus, and cavernous sinus.

Special Procedures

Conventional angiography is not part of the routine workup for pituitary adenoma. In cases of Cushing's disease when no adenoma is detected by imaging, transvenous catheter sampling of the inferior petrosal sinus for ACTH can assist in the diagnosis and determine the side of the adenoma for surgical resection.

PITUITARY CARCINOMA

Pituitary carcinomas are very rare lesions that arise from the adenohypophysis. They are distinguished from adenomas by the presence of systemic, subarachnoid, or brain metastasis.

Epidemiology

Pituitary carcinomas comprise 0.2% of adenohypophysial neoplasms. Approximately 140 cases have been reported thus far. Pituitary carcinomas are equally frequent in males and females.

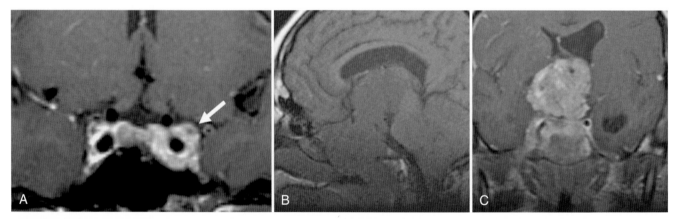

■ **FIGURE 33-3**   Invasive pituitary macroadenoma. Coronal T1W MR image (**A**) after gadolinium administration demonstrates extension of enhancing lesion around the left cavernous internal carotid artery (*arrow*). Sagittal T1W precontrast (**B**) and coronal T1W postcontrast (**C**) MR images of another patient demonstrate a large heterogeneously enhancing mass that expands the sella and extends inferiorly to involve the sphenoidal and ethmoidal air cells. No arterial narrowing is noted despite the large size of the lesion. However, the lesion results in hydrocephalus with enlargement of the left lateral ventricle.

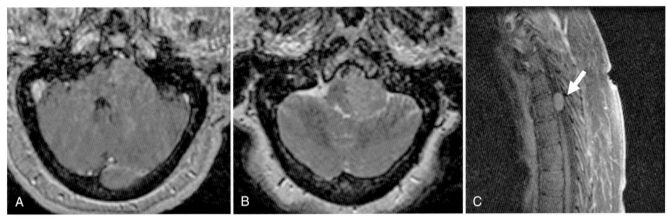

■ **FIGURE 33-4** A 63-year-old woman presented with a history of pituitary adenoma resection 10 years previously. Follow-up imaging initially was negative, but on recent follow-up a left cerebellopontine angle mass was noted (**A** and **B**). Biopsy was consistent with pituitary carcinoma. Imaging of the spine revealed multiple enhancing lesions, the largest of which was in the thoracic region (**C**, *arrow*).

The mean age at presentation is 44 years.[8] The diagnosis of pituitary carcinoma requires documentation of metastases. Patients typically survive about 4 years after lesion discovery.

Clinical Presentation
Pituitary carcinoma may first present as an invasive pituitary macroadenoma, only to demonstrate craniospinal or systemic metastases after a latent period of 5 to 10 years. The most common sites of hematogenous spread are liver and bone. Patients with craniospinal metastases tend to have a better prognosis than those with systemic spread. Pituitary carcinomas may secrete hormones, leading to endocrine imbalance. Their prognosis is then related to the endocrinologic subtype, with a worse prognosis for those secreting ACTH.[9]

Pathophysiology
Pituitary carcinomas may result from malignant transformation of benign adenomas. Chromosomal gains, especially additions to 14q, are likely involved with the malignant degeneration. In addition, pituitary carcinomas have *reduced expression* of the protein nm23, which normally prevents progression of the cell cycle and reduces the potential for metastasis.[8]

Like pituitary adenomas, pituitary carcinomas arise from adenohypophysial cells, so they can be difficult to differentiate from adenoma by histology. Features typical for malignancy, including nuclear pleomorphism, invasion, necrosis, and increased numbers of mitotic figures, are not reliable for distinguishing between the two.[8] This diagnosis cannot be made unless there is evidence of distant metastases.

Imaging
CT and MRI
Both CT and MRI reveal a lesion that mimics invasive macroadenoma. The only distinction on imaging is the presence of metastasis (Fig. 33-4).

GRANULAR CELL TUMORS
Granular cell tumors are benign tumors of the neurohypophysis that arise from the granular cell–type pituicytes. They are also known as choristomas, myoblastomas, and infundibulomas.

Epidemiology
Granular cell tumors are the most common primary tumor of the posterior pituitary gland. They most frequently present in the fifth decade and are twice as common in women as men.[10]

Clinical Presentation
Granular cell tumors are hormonally silent, so they usually present as masses. Most patients have visual complaints from compression of the optic chiasm.[10] Approximately 50% of patients show secondary signs of pituitary dysfunction, including hyperprolactinemia, which is presumed to result from compression of the pituitary stalk by the primary mass. Compression of the stalk impedes transport of pituitary-releasing hormones from the hypothalamus to the pituitary gland, leading to endocrine dysfunction (so-called stalk effect).

Pathophysiology
The cell of origin of granular cell tumors has not been identified definitively. Some evidence suggests that granular cell tumors originate from pituicytes. This is supported by the presence of glial fibrillary acidic protein (GFAP) within the tumor cells on electron microscopy. However, actual immunohistochemical staining for glial fibrillary acidic protein has been negative. There has been speculation that this may be explained by crowding of the cell cytoplasm by abundant lysosomes.[10]

Pathology
Granular cell tumors demonstrate abundant granular eosinophilic cytoplasm.

Imaging
CT
On CT, granular cell tumors are supra- and intrasellar masses, which are iso- to hyperdense to gray matter and show contrast enhancement. These imaging findings are nonspecific and can resemble pituitary macroadenomas, meningiomas, craniopharyngiomas, and hypothalamic-chiasmatic gliomas. Calcification within the lesion has been reported but is not a typical imaging feature.[10]

MRI
On MRI, granular cell tumors have a nonspecific appearance. They are hypointense to isointense to gray matter on both T1W and T2W imaging.[9] Granular cell tumors are vascular lesions, so MRI typically shows an enhancement within the sellar/suprasellar mass. Granular cell lesions do not cause significant edema in the surrounding brain. Their appearance is nonspecific, so imaging does not differentiate these tumors from other sellar/suprasellar lesions, including craniopharyngioma, pituitary adenoma, and meningioma. Absence of the posterior pituitary bright spot may provide a clue that the lesion originates from

the posterior pituitary gland, but absence of the posterior pituitary bright spot on incidental MRI is another nonspecific sign present in up to 20% of normal subjects.[9]

PITUICYTOMA

Pituicytomas are low-grade astrocytomas that involve the neurohypophysis, or posterior pituitary, and are histologically benign. They are also referred to as astrocytomas of the posterior pituitary.

Epidemiology

Pituicytomas are exceedingly rare. They occur from the third to the ninth decade and are more frequent in males.[11]

Clinical Presentation

Pituicytomas cause symptoms when they become large and exert mass effect on surrounding structures. This most frequently results in hypopituitarism and visual disturbance.

Pathophysiology

The posterior pituitary is an embryonic extension of the hypothalamus, so astrocytomas may develop in this region. They are low-grade astrocytomas but are histologically distinct from pilocytic astrocytomas.

Pathology

Pituicytomas are highly vascular tumors. Complete surgical resection is difficult, so local recurrence is common after resection. These tumors are composed of spindle-shaped cells with round-to-oval nuclei and fibrillary cytoplasm. The cells align around the vasculature in a pattern similar to the normal neurohypophysial architecture. Pituicytomas do not demonstrate immunoreactivity for neuroendocrine markers or pituitary hormones.[12] They do not exhibit Rosenthal fibers, microcysts, or granular bodies, so they are distinct from pilocytic astrocytomas.

Imaging
CT and MRI

On CT, pituicytomas are typically focal and well-circumscribed lesions located posteriorly within the sella turcica. They tend to demonstrate low signal on T1W images and high signal on T2W images. Cysts are uncommon. They enhance homogeneously after administration of a contrast agent.

Special Procedures

Because of the highly vascular nature of pituicytomas, angiography is beneficial for surgical planning. Prominent arterial feeders can be seen to arise from the hypophysial arteries. There is no supply from the external carotid artery, which is helpful in distinguishing these lesions from meningiomas.[12]

CRANIOPHARYNGIOMA

Craniopharyngiomas (Rathke's pouch tumor, craniopharyngeal duct tumor) are benign epithelial neoplasms of the suprasellar and sellar regions.

Epidemiology

Craniopharyngiomas represent 1% to 3% of intracranial tumors. They are equally frequent in males and females. Craniopharyngiomas may present at any age but demonstrate clear bimodal age peaks, with special frequency first in childhood and then in the fifth decade. More than half of craniopharyngiomas present in children and young adults. Craniopharyngiomas are the most common intracranial neoplasm of nonglial origin in the pediatric population.[13]

Clinical Presentation

Craniopharyngiomas usually present as headache, nausea, and visual symptoms due to compression of the optic pathway. Hypothalamic dysfunction and pituitary dysfunction are common. Up to 80% of children show endocrine dysfunction at the time of presentation, most frequently growth disturbance.[9] In adults, the most common presenting symptom is chronic headache.

Pathophysiology

Two complementary theories are offered for the development of craniopharyngiomas. Both help to understand the spectrum of craniopharyngiomas.

The embryologic theory postulates that craniopharyngiomas arise from squamous epithelial rests in the remnant of Rathke's pouch. Rathke's pouch is an upward invagination of the primitive oral cavity. The craniopharyngeal duct is the neck of Rathke's pouch (and the embryologic structure along which the adenohypophysis migrates). That origin would explain why craniopharyngiomas may be seen anywhere along the course of Rathke's pouch and the craniopharyngeal duct, including the third ventricle and nasopharynx. Very rarely, craniopharyngiomas may be purely intraventricular. This results when Rathe's pouch cells come in direct contact with the developing cerebral vesicle. The adamantinomatous variety of craniopharyngiomas most likely arises from this route. This variety is typically found in children.

The second theory is the *metaplastic theory*. The early depression that will lead to the mouth is called the stomodeum. The stomodeum contributes to the formation of the buccal mucosa. The metaplastic theory postulates that craniopharyngiomas arise from metaplasia of squamous epithelial cell rests, which are remnants of the area of the stomodeum that contributed to the buccal mucosa.[14] The squamous papillary craniopharyngiomas, which are most common in adults, are thought to arise by this route.

Pathology

Craniopharyngiomas consist of cystic and solid components and frequently show calcification. Multiple different cysts may be present, each appearing different because each contains a different proportion of cholesterol, methemoglobin, triglycerides, protein, and desquamated epithelium. The lesions are usually suprasellar, depress the diaphragma sellae, elevate the chiasm, and, when large, may obstruct the foramina of Monro to cause hydrocephalus. Large craniopharyngiomas typically extend far posteriorly into the depths of the interpeduncular fossa. They typically grow upward through the circle of Willis, displacing the vessels of the circle outward circumferentially. The adamantinomatous tumors have a tendency to encase adjacent arteries. Craniopharyngiomas have a variable relation to the pituitary stalk but usually displace it anteriorly.

Pathologically, craniopharyngiomas are divided into adamantinomatous and squamous papillary variants. The adamantinomatous type resemble the enamel-forming neoplasms of the oropharynx. They tend to be more cystic, calcify more frequently, and are most common in children. The squamous papillary form is often more solid, less frequently calcified, and more frequent in adults. However, most tumors have mixed features. Attempts to correlate pathology with imaging and recurrence rate have not proved fruitful.[15] Although craniopharyngiomas are histologically benign, slowly growing tumors, they are difficult to resect completely. They are often adherent to the pituitary stalk, the hypothalamus, the thalamoperforate vessels, and other small penetrating arteries and veins, so complete resection is difficult or impossible. For that reason they recur repeatedly, are locally aggressive, and may extend into the adjacent brain parenchyma. If the tumors are completely resected, recurrence is rare. With subtotal resection, however, only 47% of patients are disease free at 5 years.[9] Craniopharyngiomas can recur locally, along the surgical tract, and even distant from the original site, suggesting cerebrospinal fluid (CSF) seeding.[15]

Imaging

CT

On CT, craniopharyngiomas are round lobulated masses centered within the suprasellar cistern and occasionally involving the sella. Cystic areas are frequent (up to 85% of craniopharyngiomas) and are variable in attenuation, depending on their cholesterol content. Calcification is more frequent in childhood craniopharyngiomas (up to 90%) than adult tumors (50%-70%) and tends to be more prominent and chunkier in children than adults.[9] The calcification can be rim-like or conglomerate (Fig. 33-5). The solid portions of the tumor enhance markedly after contrast agent administration.

MRI

On MRI, the signal intensity of craniopharyngiomas is variable, depending on the cyst contents and degree of calcification. The

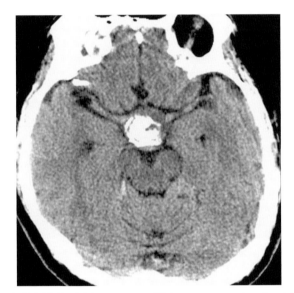

■ **FIGURE 33-5** Axial noncontrast CT demonstrates a densely calcified lesion in the suprasellar region consistent with a craniopharyngioma.

cystic components may show T1 shortening. After contrast agent administration, craniopharyngiomas usually show enhancement in the solid portions and rim enhancement about the cysts (Fig. 33-6). MR spectroscopy has been reported to be useful in distinguishing craniopharyngiomas from hypothalamic astrocytomas and pituitary adenomas. Craniopharyngiomas demonstrate peaks from 1 to 2 ppm, which correspond to the region for lipid and lactate. Astrocytomas will demonstrate elevated *N*-acetyl-aspartate (NAA) to creatine ratios, and adenomas demonstrate no brain metabolites.

Craniopharyngiomas commonly cause T2 prolongation along the optic tracts. This sign is nonspecific and has been reported in other pituitary region tumors, including meningiomas and metastases.[16] The high T2 signal may signify optic edema from compression by the tumor.

Special Procedures

Craniopharyngiomas are typically avascular on angiography and may be noted to encase or displace the vessels of the circle of Willis. Tumoral adhesion to vascular structures is one major reason for incomplete resection. After resection, sometimes long after resection, fusiform aneurysmal dilatation of adjacent arteries may be observed (Fig. 33-7). This has also been noted in other suprasellar tumors.[17]

METASTASIS, DIRECT TUMORAL SPREAD, AND PERINEURIAL SPREAD

Metastases can spread to the sellar-parasellar region by hematogenous spread, perineurial spread, or direct invasion. In hematogenous spread the tumor invades local blood vessels and rafts downstream to lodge in end-arteries of the sellar region. In perineurial spread the tumor invades the regional nerves and grows along their perineurium or endoneurium to reach a noncontiguous area.

Epidemiology

Hematogenous metastases to the pituitary and sellar region are uncommon, representing 0.14% to 28.1% of all brain metastases.[18] They most frequently originate from lung and breast carcinomas. Direct local invasion most commonly results from squamous cell carcinoma, nasopharyngeal carcinoma, and rhabdomyosarcoma. Perineurial spread is most frequent with squamous cell carcinoma and adenoid cystic carcinoma of the head and neck.

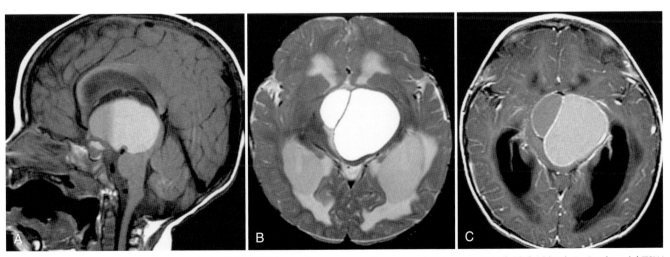

■ **FIGURE 33-6** Craniopharyngioma. **A,** Sagittal T1W MR image demonstrates a large suprasellar mass with a fluid/fluid level. **B,** On the axial T2W MR image enlargement of the ventricles consistent with hydrocephalus as a result of the mass effect is better appreciated. T2 prolongation surrounding the ventricles is consistent with transependymal flow. **C,** On the postcontrast image, enhancement of the cyst walls is noted.

■ FIGURE 33-7 Craniopharyngioma. Coronal T1W postcontrast (**A**) and axial T2W (**B**) MR images demonstrate a small lesion in the suprasellar region that has rim enhancement. This was resected and after pathologic study was confirmed to be a craniopharyngioma. Note the normal size of the carotid terminus on the right (*arrow,* **B**). Postoperative coronal T2W MR image (**C**) and 3D TOF MRA (**D**) demonstrate a fusiform aneurysm involving the carotid terminus on the right (*arrowhead,* **C**).

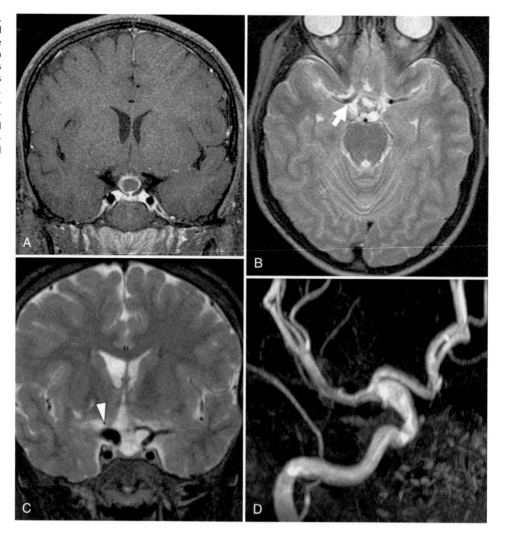

Clinical Presentation

About 40% of patients with hematogenous metastases develop diabetes insipidus. Visual deficits and hypopituitarism are also common.[18] Direct invasion by regional neoplasms usually causes symptoms from local mass effect. Perineurial spread may cause hypoesthesia and burning or stinging pain. Perineurial spread most frequently involves the fifth (trigeminal) and seventh (facial) cranial nerves, so it may be misdiagnosed as trigeminal neuralgia or Bell's palsy. It may be asymptomatic in up to 45% of patients. There may be a long latency period between development of perineurial spread and tumor treatment, with reports of perineurial spread manifesting as late as 45 years after resection of the original tumor.[20] Because perineurial spread changes the status of a lesion from resectable to nonresectable,[19] and because many patients retain normal nerve function on clinical examination, imaging studies must try to identify perineurial spread that escapes clinical detection.

Pathophysiology

Hematogenous metastases to this region most frequently go to the pituitary gland, infundibulum, and tuber cinereum, because these structures lie outside the blood-brain barrier. Metastases to the infundibulum cause visual disturbance by compression of the chiasm or endocrine disturbance by disruption of the hypothalamic-pituitary axis. Hematogenous metastases to the pituitary gland itself most commonly pass to the infundibulum and posterior lobe, rather than the anterior lobe of the pituitary,

because the posterior lobe is supplied directly through the inferior hypophysial branches of the internal carotid artery, whereas the anterior lobe is supplied indirectly via hypothalamic-portal vessels.[18] The cavernous sinus may be involved by direct extension from regional neoplasms such as nasopharyngeal carcinoma, by hematogenous metastases, or by perineurial spread. Tumors may spread along any nerve, but perineurial spread most commonly involves the fifth and seventh cranial nerves. Squamous cell carcinoma and adenoid cystic carcinoma are the two most common tumors to spread by perineurial extension, but melanoma, lymphoma, leukemia, basal cell carcinoma, and mucoepidermoid carcinoma also reach the sellar-parasellar region by this route. Perineurial spread usually indicates a poor prognosis and may change the lesion's status from resectable to nonresectable.

Pathology

The histology of the metastatic lesion is similar to that of the primary tumor. Microscopically, perineurial invasion demonstrates infiltration of the nerve involving either the perineurial or endoneurial tissue planes.

Imaging

CT

On CT, perineurial spread can be recognized by widening or destruction of the basal neural foramina, loss of the perineurial

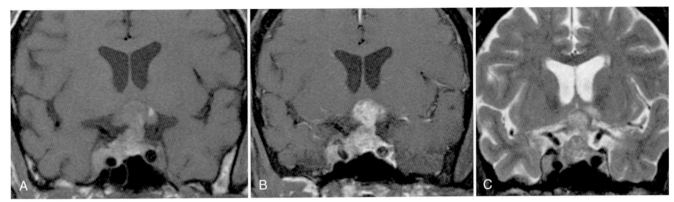

■ **FIGURE 33-8** Renal cell metastasis. T1W MR image (**A**) demonstrates a lesion with intrinsic T1 shortening involving the sella and suprasellar regions, as well as extension into the right cavernous sinus. The lesion enhances avidly after administration of a contrast agent (**B**) and has slightly hyperintense signal on the T2W MR image (**C**).

fat plane surrounding the nerves, and enhancement within the neural foramen after contrast agent administration. Growth of mass within the cavernous sinus bulges the lateral sinus wall outward. Normally, the lateral sinus wall is concave laterally. With a mass, it appears straightened or convex laterally. The internal carotid artery may be displaced, compressed, or occluded. There may be abnormal enhancement within the cavernous sinus.

MRI

Most pituitary metastases are difficult to distinguish from adenomas, especially if no other metastasis is identified. They typically appear as dumbbell-shaped intrasellar-suprasellar masses, indented at the level of the diaphragma sellae (Fig. 33-8). These lesions do not widen and remodel the sella because they grow too rapidly.[21] Instead, they may destroy the sphenoid bone and invade into the cavernous sinus, partially occluding it. The flow void from the cavernous segment of the internal carotid artery may be displaced. Flow through it may be reduced or obstructed.

Metastatic lesions are usually hypointense to isointense to gray matter on T1W imaging and hyperintense on T2W imaging. Metastases can enhance homogeneously or heterogeneously after contrast agent administration and occasionally show rim enhancement.

Perineurial spread is identified by isointense thickening of the nerve, loss of the normal intraforaminal fat plane, and concentric enlargement of the foramen on T1W images. Contrast-enhanced studies show increased nerve size, nerve enhancement, and widening of the cavernous sinus (Fig. 33-9). Fat suppression can help to identify the abnormal enhancement. Atrophy of the muscles supplied by the affected nerves is an important secondary sign of perineurial invasion. Because nasopharyngeal carcinoma is a common source of perineurial spread, imaging of the parasellar region should always include the nasopharynx.

LANGERHANS CELL HISTIOCYTOSIS

Langerhans cell histiocytosis is a reactive clonal disease of the macrophage-monocyte system. It can involve almost any organ.

Epidemiology

Langerhans cell histiocytosis is a rare disorder, seen in up to 2 per 100,000 people.[22] It most frequently affects children and adolescents but can occur in adults. There is no gender predilection.

Clinical Presentation

Involvement of the hypothalamic-pituitary axis by Langerhans cell histiocytosis most frequently results in diabetes insipidus. However, hypothalamic dysfunction, increased intracranial pres-

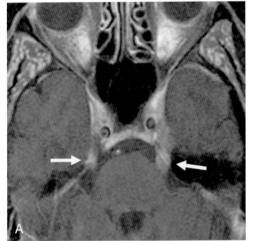

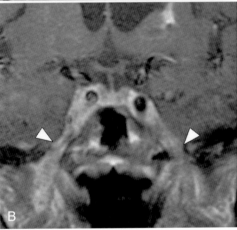

■ **FIGURE 33-9** Lymphoma with perineurial spread. **A,** Axial T1W post-contrast MR image demonstrates thickening and increased enhancement along the bilateral cisternal segment of the trigeminal nerve (*arrows*), and there is a prominence of the cavernous sinus. **B,** Abnormal enhancement and thickening of V3 extending through the foramen ovale is noted on this coronal image (*arrowheads*).

sure, visual disturbances, cranial nerve palsies, and seizures can also occur.

Pathophysiology

Langerhans cells are a dendritic cell line derived from bone marrow cells. The cells have antigen-presenting and

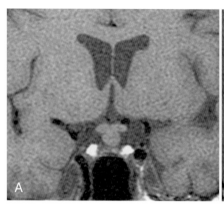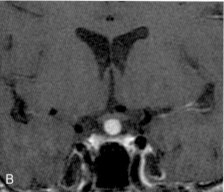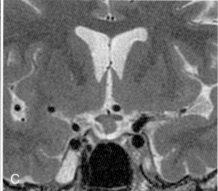

■ **FIGURE 33-10** Langerhans cell histiocytosis. Coronal imaging through the sellar region demonstrates enlargement of the infundibulum that is isointense to gray matter on T1W MRI (**A**) and enhances homogeneously on postcontrast imaging (**B**). The lesion is also noted to be isointense to gray matter on a T2W MR image (**C**).

antigen-processing properties[22] and are normally found in the pituitary and brain parenchyma. The pathophysiologic mechanism of Langerhans cell histiocytosis has not been elucidated.

Pathology
Grossly, Langerhans cell histiocytosis may appear as a discrete dural-based mass.

There is marked proliferation of Langerhans cell type histiocytes along with a mixed inflammatory response. Ultrastructurally, Langerhans cell histiocytes are characterized by Birbeck granules, which are tennis racquet–shaped intracytoplasmic structures.

Imaging
MRI

In Langerhans cell histiocytosis of the pituitary and hypothalamic region, MRI most frequently shows thickening of the infundibulum (>3 mm) and contrast enhancement (Fig. 33-10). The posterior pituitary bright spot may be absent. However, these findings are nonspecific and can also be seen in leukemia and lymphoma, granulomatous diseases such as sarcoid and tuberculosis, and neoplasms such as germinomas.

MENINGIOMA
Meningiomas are tumors that arise from rests of arachnoid cap cells within the meninges.[23]

Epidemiology
Meningiomas are the most common nonglial primary neoplasm of the central nervous system and the second most common neoplasm in the sellar region.[23] They are more frequent in females and typically occur between the ages of 20 and 60 years. They may be seen in children and in association with neurofibromatosis type 2.

Clinical Presentation
The clinical presentation of meningiomas depends on their location. They may arise in the cavernous sinus and present as a parasellar mass or along the planum sphenoidale, tuberculum sellae, anterior clinoid processes, or the diaphragma sellae, so they may also present as intrasellar or suprasellar masses. En plaque meningiomas along the sphenoid wing can present as a slowly progressive painless unilateral exophthalmos and occasionally numbness in the distribution of cranial nerves V1 and V2. Meningiomas that arise along the medial aspect of the sphenoid wing may encase the internal carotid and middle cerebral arteries and the optic nerves and chiasm. Planum sphenoidale meningiomas can grow posteriorly to involve the sella and infun-

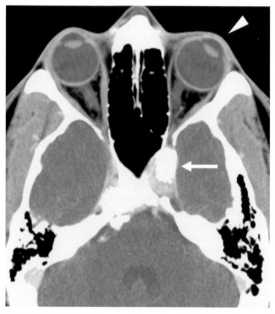

■ **FIGURE 33-11** Meningioma. A densely calcified mass is noted in the region of the left cavernous sinus (*arrow*). Note the abduction of the right eye, consistent with cranial nerve VI dysfunction (*arrowhead*).

dibulum, or they may exert mass effect on the cranial nerve causing deficits (Fig. 33-11).[24] Meningiomas arising from the tuberculum sellae comprise 5% to 10% of intracranial meningiomas. These present with visual and endocrinologic symptoms.

Pathophysiology
Meningiomas arise from a meningeal cell designated the arachnoid cap cell. They are graded as I to III by the World Health Organization (WHO). Grade I meningiomas are the most frequent and carry a 7% to 20% recurrence rate. Grade II meningiomas recur in 29% to 40% of patients. Grade III meningiomas are highly aggressive, rapidly growing tumors with a 50% to 78% recurrence rate. Twenty percent of meningiomas display aggressive histologic features. The pathologic criteria for higher-grade tumors include hypercellularity, loss of normal architecture, nuclear pleomorphism, increased mitotic index, tumor necrosis, and brain invasion. Approximately 0.1% of meningiomas demonstrate metastasis, usually to the lung and bone. The higher-grade meningiomas are more common in males and relatively more

common among meningiomas of children. Immunohistochemistry helps to confirm a diagnosis of meningiomas. Meningiomas are positive for epithelial membrane antigen (EMA) in approximately 80% of cases. Interestingly, progesterone receptors can be found in the cytoplasm of meningiomas.

The most common genetic abnormality associated with meningiomas is deletion along the long arm of chromosome 22 (22q deletion). There is an association of meningiomas with neurofibromatosis type 2 and a history of previous radiation therapy.

Pathology

Grossly, meningiomas are dural-based, sharply demarcated lesions. The appearance varies depending on the degree of cystic change, lipid content, calcification, and vascularity.

Meningiomas are composed of monomorphic cells. Rounded concretions of calcium called psammoma bodies are frequently seen. The three most common histologic subtypes of meningiomas are meningothelial, transitional, and fibroblastic meningiomas. The meningothelial form consists of densely packed cells arranged in sheets. Fibroblastic meningiomas consist of densely packed sheets of spindle cells, and transitional meningiomas have features common to both the fibroblastic and meningothelial forms.

Imaging

CT

Meningiomas tend to be homogeneously hyperdense on CT and typically show intense homogeneous enhancement after contrast agent administration (Fig. 33-12). Hyperostosis is common and appears to reflect local hypervascularity rather than bone invasion.[25] Fifteen to 20 percent of meningiomas demonstrate calcification. CT may be of benefit when evaluating for a small meningioma, because hyperostosis may be the only indication of the presence of the meningioma.[24] When meningiomas arise on the planum sphenoidale, the hypervascularity of the tumor softens the bony planum. The underlying air space of the sphenoidal sinus may balloon upward, elevating the base of the meningioma. The secondary expansion of the aerated sphenoidal sinus upward into the skull, beneath the meningioma, is designated pneumosinus dilatans (Fig. 33-13).

MRI

Meningiomas are hypointense to isointense on T1W images and isointense to hyperintense on T2W images. The signal characteristics of meningiomas may parallel those of normal brain so completely that even large tumors may be undetectable on noncontrast MRI. Meningiomas usually show homogeneous, moderate to intense contrast enhancement. There may be a central linear or fan-like zone of increased enhancement that corresponds to the vascular pedicle. The surface often shows a thin, more densely enhancing venous cap. In the cavernous sinus, fat saturation is beneficial on the postcontrast images (Fig. 33-14). A dural tail may be seen on the postcontrast images. However, a dural tail is not pathognomonic for meningioma, because the dural tail is only seen in up to 60% of meningiomas and because other dural-based lesions like schwannomas and hemangiopericytomas may also exhibit dural tails.

Approximately 15% of histologically benign meningiomas will have atypical imaging features such as heterogeneous enhancement, cyst formation, hemorrhage, and fatty degeneration.[25] There are no reliable imaging criteria to distinguish among the different grades of meningioma. If the meningioma is noted to mushroom into the brain, it may be said to have a degree of invasiveness suggesting a higher grade. The degree of associated vasogenic edema does not appear to correlate with tumor grade or size. The etiology of the vasogenic edema is controversial

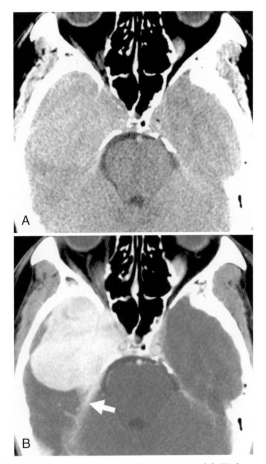

■ **FIGURE 33-12** Meningioma. **A,** Noncontrast axial CT demonstrates a slightly hyperdense mass within the right temporal fossa extending into the right cavernous sinus. **B,** Postcontrast image demonstrates a homogeneously enhancing lesion with a dural tail extending posteriorly along the tentorium (*arrow*).

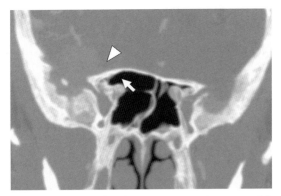

■ **FIGURE 33-13** Coronal CT demonstrates an enlargement of the right sphenoidal sinus (*arrow*) consistent with pneumosinus dilatans. An enhancing lesion is noted within the middle temporal fossa and along the right aspect of the planum sphenoidale (*arrowhead*).

and is probably the result of a combination of different mechanisms.[25]

In the rare case that a meningioma arises in the sella or close to it, the tumor may be difficult to differentiate from a pituitary adenoma. Demonstration of a plane separating the mass from the pituitary gland can help in this differentiation. Meningiomas also show a more rapid pattern of enhancement than do pituitary

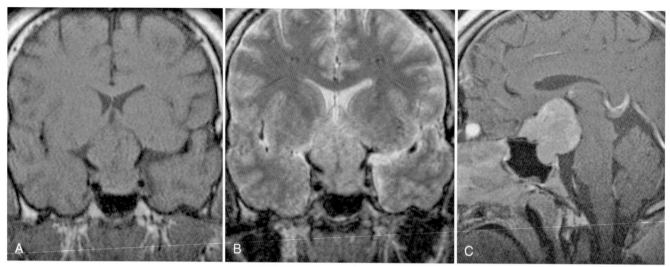

■ **FIGURE 33-14**   Meningioma. Coronal T1W (**A**) and T2W (**B**) MR images demonstrate a sellar and suprasellar lesion that is isointense to gray matter. On the sagittal T1 postcontrast MR image (**C**) the lesion shows relatively homogeneous enhancement.

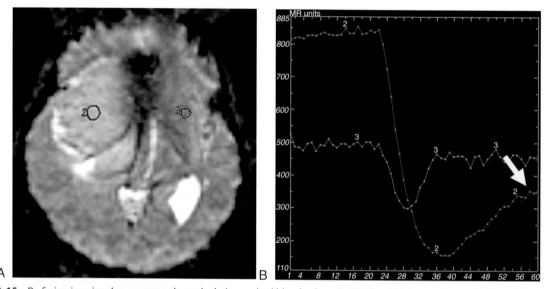

■ **FIGURE 33-15**   Perfusion imaging demonstrates elevated relative cerebral blood volume in ROI 2, which is over the meningioma (**A**). **B,** There is less than 50% return to baseline (*arrow*), which indicates a greater degree of intratumoral contrast agent leakage.

adenomas. Differentiation is important from a surgical standpoint, because meningiomas tend to bleed more at surgery. This may influence the choice of a transcranial versus a transsphenoidal approach to surgical resection.

On MR perfusion studies, meningiomas show an elevated relative cerebral blood volume (rCBV) in comparison with schwannomas (Fig. 33-15). On MR spectroscopy, 30% to 40% of meningiomas demonstrate an alanine doublet at 1.4 ppm, a marker of meningeal origin. MR spectroscopy does not demonstrate NAA within these tumors, because meningiomas are not tumors of neural origin. Choline may be elevated due to rapid membrane turnover.[26]

Meningiomas may extend out of the skull through the neural foramina, because arachnoid cells accompany the cranial nerves (Fig. 33-16). They may erode and enlarge the neural foramina and mimic a nerve sheath tumor. If the meningioma causes gross destruction of the foramina, it can mimic a malignancy.[24] Extraforaminal extension of meningioma may cause an infratemporal mass that presents as difficulty eating.

It is important to note the relationship of the parasellar meningiomas to the internal carotid artery. Meningioma can surround and *narrow* the artery. Occasional meningiomas even invade the outer wall of the artery (Fig. 33-17). They may follow the carotid artery inferiorly into the petrous canal. Neurologic deficits and cerebral ischemia due to reduced cerebral perfusion secondary to stenosis are very rare.

Special Procedures
On angiography, meningiomas have a tumor blush that appears early and persists late into the venous phase (Fig. 33-18). This is jokingly referred to as the "mother-in-law" effect. Preoperative embolization may be of benefit to reduce bleeding.

HEMANGIOPERICYTOMA
Hemangiopericytomas are very rare lesions of mesenchymal origin. They were previously called angioblastic meningiomas.

Epidemiology
Hemangiopericytomas are rare neoplasms, constituting less than 1% of all intracranial neoplasms. They occur at a mean age range of 37 to 44 years and have a slight male predominance.[27]

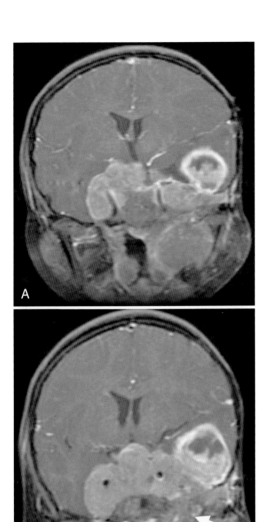

■ **FIGURE 33-16** **A** and **B,** Grade II meningioma in an 11-year-old boy showing extension into the infratentorial fossa via the foramen ovale (*arrow,* **B**).

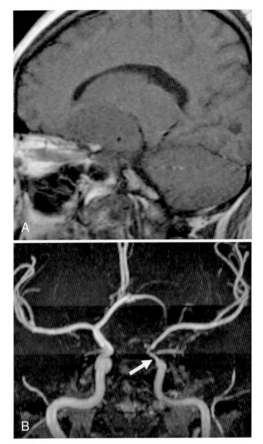

■ **FIGURE 33-17** Meningioma. Sagittal T1W MR image (**A**) demonstrates an isointense lesion along the planum sphenoidale. 3D TOF MRA (**B**) demonstrates narrowing of the left cavernous (*arrow*) and supraclinoid internal carotid arteries, as well as the left A1 segment.

Clinical Presentation

Hemangiopericytomas most commonly present as focal neurologic symptoms and hydrocephalus. The mean duration of symptoms is approximately 4 months. Intratumoral and intracerebral hemorrhage, cranial nerve deficits, hyperprolactinemia, and bitemporal hemianopsia have been reported.[27]

Pathophysiology

Hemangiopericytomas derive from the pericyte of Zimmerman, a leiomyoblastic cell situated around the capillaries. Because these are not the arachnoid cap cells, hemangiopericytomas are pathologically distinct from meningiomas. As a group they are more aggressive than meningiomas and may have late and distant metastases, typically to bone, lung, kidney, pancreas, liver, and adrenals. Hemangiopericytomas have a high rate of recurrence after resection. They are graded as WHO II or III based on the mitotic rate, degree of cellularity, nuclear pleomorphism, and hemorrhage and necrosis.

Pathology

Hemangiopericytomas tend to be large at presentation and frequently are greater than 4 cm. They commonly show a lobulated surface, whereas meningiomas tend to be more hemispheric. Hemangiopericytomas do not calcify and are not associated with hyperostosis but may have associated bone erosion.

Hemangiopericytomas consist of randomly oriented plump cells with scant cytoplasm. Irregularly shaped "staghorn" vessels are noted. Reticulin is abundant in most hemangiopericytomas, although in very highly cellular hemangiopericytomas it may be absent.

Imaging

CT

On CT, hemangiopericytomas are heterogeneous, hyperdense dural-based masses that show heterogeneous enhancement after contrast agent administration. They may be very difficult to distinguish from meningiomas on both CT and MRI.

MRI

Hemangiopericytomas are isointense on T1W images and isointense to slightly hyperintense on T2W images (Fig. 33-19). Prominent internal vessels may be seen as flow voids (Fig. 33-20). Postcontrast, they enhance and may show a dural tail. Hemangiopericytomas may demonstrate a broad or narrow dural base, whereas meningiomas typically have a broad dural attachment.[28]

On MR spectroscopy, hemangiopericytomas are reported to demonstrate an increased concentration of myoinositol.[27]

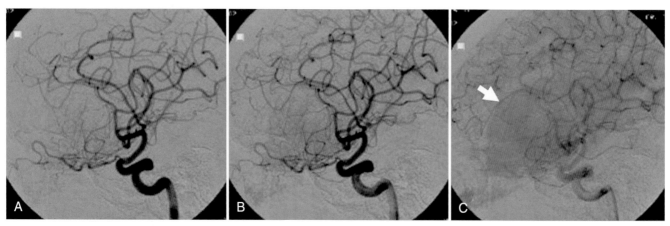

■ **FIGURE 33-18** Meningioma. Early (**A**) and midarterial (**B**) phase images demonstrate a vascular blush, which persists into the venous phase (**C**, *arrow*).

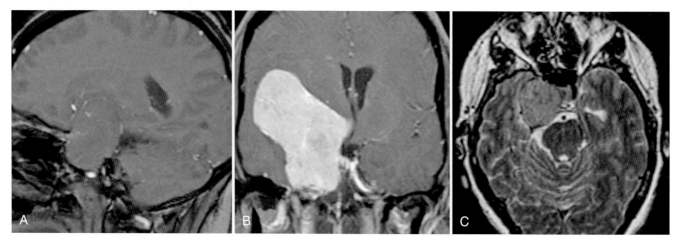

■ **FIGURE 33-19** Hemangiopericytoma. Sagittal T1W precontrast MR image (**A**) demonstrates a lesion that is isointense to gray matter and avidly enhances on the postcontrast MR image (**B**). On the axial T2W MR image (**C**) the lesion is noted to be isointense to gray matter.

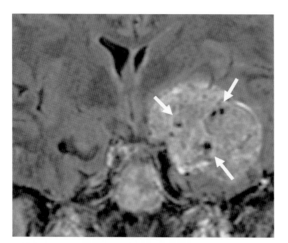

■ **FIGURE 33-20** Hemangiopericytoma. Coronal FLAIR imaging demonstrates a lesion involving the left temporal fossa as well as the suprasellar region. Prominent flow voids are noted (*arrows*).

Special Procedures

These lesions will have an early intense tumor blush on angiography owing to their highly vascular nature. Dual supply from the internal and external carotid arteries is reported with numerous corkscrew feeders being present. Due to the highly vascular nature of these lesions, preoperative embolization has been reported to be beneficial.

SCHWANNOMA

Schwannomas are encapsulated masses that arise from the perineurial Schwann cells that provide the myelin sheaths of peripheral nerves. They can arise along any nerve but occur more frequently on sensory nerves than on pure motor nerves. Schwannomas are also referred to as neurilemmomas. The malignant form has been referred to as malignant neurofibroma, neurosarcoma, malignant neurilemmoma, malignant nerve sheath tumor, and neurofibrosarcoma.

Epidemiology

Trigeminal schwannomas constitute less than 0.4% of intracranial tumors but are the most common schwannoma of the parasellar region. Schwannomas arising from cranial nerves III, IV, and VI are very rare.

Clinical Presentation

Trigeminal schwannomas can present as facial pain (sensory root of CN V) or trigeminal motor palsy and atrophy of the muscles of mastication (motor root of CN V). Patients with schwannomas of the other cranial nerves also present with loss of function of the affected cranial nerve or may be asymptomatic.

Pathophysiology

Schwannomas are WHO grade I tumors. They are usually isolated lesions except in the setting of neurofibromatosis type 2. On immunohistochemical testing, tumors originating from Schwann cells show positive reaction to the S-100 antigen. Mutations in the neurofibromatosis type 2 tumor suppressor gene are associated with the development of isolated schwannomas.

Pathology

Schwannomas are circumscribed encapsulated lesions and are most often tan. Larger and older tumors may undergo cystic degeneration. Trigeminal schwannomas may affect the portion of the nerve in the middle fossa (Meckel's cave) only, the portion in the high cerebellopontine angle only, or both together to form a dumbbell-shaped posterior fossa/middle fossa mass, with a "waist" where the mass is constricted by the petroclinoid ligament. Not uncommonly, the portion in Meckel's cave is solid whereas the portion in the posterior fossa is cystic. Trigeminal schwannomas may also extend through the foramen ovale into the infratemporal compartment, forming a mass below the skull base.

Schwannomas are spindle cell neoplasms composed of two tissue types: Antoni A and Antoni B. The Antoni A areas are hypercellular, compactly arranged regions of spindle cells. Antoni B regions are composed of looser myxomatous tissue that may give rise to cysts within the schwannomas. These cell types may align in palisades that are referred to as Verocay bodies. On average, smaller "younger" tumors have a higher proportion of Antoni A areas whereas larger "older" tumors show increasing proportions of Antoni B regions. Malignant schwannomas are rare. They are diagnosed on the basis of increased mitotic figures, necrosis, and perineurial extension along nerves. Epineural invasion and occasional invasion of adjacent structures help in making the diagnosis.[29]

Imaging

CT

On CT schwannomas tend to be smooth ovoid-lobulated isodense masses that partially mold themselves to the contours of the compartments in which they arise. They may bulge the lateral wall of Meckel's cave outward but remain confined within the cave. They typically displace the cavernous sinus and the internal carotid artery medially. They may enlarge the neural foramina, but the cortex of the foramen is usually maintained (Fig. 33-21). Schwannomas enhance homogeneously or heterogeneously, depending on the proportion of Antoni A and B areas. Trigeminal schwannomas may show enhancement of one portion of a dumbbell tumor, commonly the posterior fossa portion.

MRI

On MRI schwannomas have intermediate signal on T1W images. The T2W appearance depends on the proportion of Antoni A and Antoni B cells within the tumor. The hypercellular, compactly arranged Antoni A regions have low signal on T2W images, whereas the looser myxomatous Antoni B regions have tissue of high signal on T2W. These tumors may also exhibit cystic components, fatty degeneration, or hemorrhage (Fig. 33-22). It is difficult to differentiate the malignant schwannoma from the benign tumor by imaging alone. Rapid growth on serial images, extensive nerve involvement, and earlier erosion of basal neural foramina suggest malignancy.

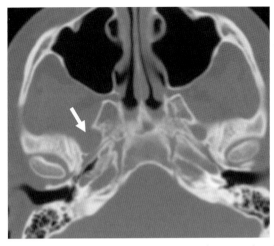

■ **FIGURE 33-21** Axial CT demonstrates a smooth concentric enlargement of the right foramen ovale (*arrow*). The patient had a schwannoma along the V3 segment of the trigeminal nerve.

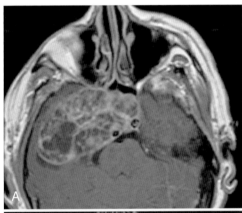

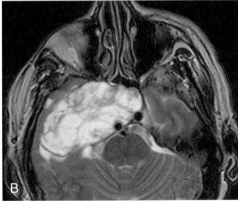

■ **FIGURE 33-22** Trigeminal schwannoma. **A,** Axial T1W postcontrast MR image demonstrates heterogeneous enhancement of a large lesion that is centered on the right cavernous sinus. **B,** On the T2W MR image the nonenhancing portion demonstrates high T2 signal consistent with cystic components of the lesion.

DERMOIDS AND EPIDERMOIDS

Epidermoid and dermoid tumors are slowly growing benign inclusion cysts that expand gradually over years. By definition, the epidermoid cyst contains a lining composed only of epidermal elements, whereas the dermoid cyst also contains elements of the dermis (including dermal adnexae).

Epidemiology

Epidermoids and dermoids constitute less than 5% of intracranial masses. There is a slight male predominance. Dermoids present slightly earlier in the second and third decades, whereas epidermoids tend to present later in the third to fourth decades.[30]

Clinical Presentation

Dermoids and epidermoids are slowly growing lesions that may produce only mild symptoms as a result of local mass effect. Most frequently, the complaint is of a chronic headache. Occasionally patients present with seizures. In the suprasellar region, these cysts can cause visual and endocrine disturbances by pressure on the optic apparatus and the pituitary stalk. Dermoid cysts may rupture, releasing irritant material that can cause a chemical meningitis.

Pathophysiology

Epidermoid and dermoid cysts are remnants of cutaneous tissue that have become misplaced during embryogenesis. They are thought to be an error of embryogenesis that occurs between the third and fifth weeks of gestation.[30] These inclusions may result from failure of the surface ectoderm to separate from underlying structures, from implantation of surface ectoderm, or from sequestration of surface ectoderm.

Pathology

Dermoid and epidermoid cysts tend to be unilocular lesions.

Epidermoid cysts characteristically lie off the midline rather than in the midline. They tend to be shiny, smooth, and waxy and are frequently described as "pearly." Dermoid cysts characteristically lie in the midline and form single encapsulated unilocular cysts. They typically have thicker linings than epidermoids and may contain dystrophic calcification. Dermoids are frequently described as "buttery" or "cheesy," with lipids floating within proteinaceous debris. Detection of a dermoid cyst suggests the potential of a related dermal sinus.

Epidermoids and dermoids are both composed of an internal layer of squamous epithelium covered by an external fibrous capsule and are both filled with keratinous material. Epidermoids are composed solely of epidermal elements (squamous epithelium), whereas dermoids also contain dermal elements (sebaceous and sweat glands and hair). Their lipid content arises from the sebaceous secretions of the dermal adnexae.

Imaging

CT

On CT epidermoids are hypodense, nonenhancing lesions that have attenuation similar to CSF. Dermoids have regions of lower attenuation (−60 HU to −90 HU) than epidermoids owing to their lipid content.[30] Calcification may be seen within the walls of both epidermoid and dermoid cysts, although it is less frequent in epidermoids. When dermoids rupture, areas of low attenuation can be seen throughout the ventricles and cisterns consistent with fat (Fig. 33-23). Epidermoids and dermoids are slowly growing and may exert pressure changes on surrounding structures.

MRI

The squamous cell lining of epidermoid cysts is usually too thin to be recognized by imaging, so the MRI appearance reflects the cyst content, not the wall. Epidermoids demonstrate T1 and T2 signal intensity that is similar to that of CSF. The cholesterol in epidermoids is not hydrolyzed, so there is T1 prolongation with low signal intensity. Otherwise-similar craniopharyngiomas have hydrolyzed cholesterol and therefore exhibit high signal intensity due to T1 shortening. The T2 signal intensity is variable. In epidermoids, T2W FLAIR usually show inhomogeneous signal intensities that are higher than CSF. Epidermoids characteristi-

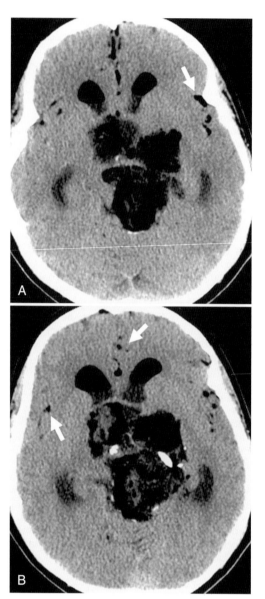

■ **FIGURE 33-23** **A,** Axial noncontrast CT demonstrates a low-attenuation suprasellar lesion (*arrow*) consistent with fat, along with small focal areas of calcification consistent with a dermoid. **B,** In addition, low attenuation is seen within the sulci consistent with fat droplets resulting from rupture of the dermoid (*arrows*).

cally show restricted diffusion with increased signal intensity on diffusion-weighted imaging (DWI) and low values of the apparent diffusion coefficient (ADC) (Fig. 33-24). Peritumoral parenchymal edema is typically not seen. On contrast-enhanced MRI, epidermoids may demonstrate faint rim enhancement, which may represent an inflammatory reaction. Epidermoids tend to engulf nerves and vessels rather than replace them.

Dermoids are also unilocular lesions but have a more complex cyst content and imaging appearance than epidermoids. They tend to occur along the midline. The thicker cyst wall may be visualized on imaging studies and enhance after contrast agent administration. The lipid content causes areas of T1 shortening, so dermoids may appear bright on T1W images. Occasional dermoids show no T1 shortening and may be difficult to differentiate from epidermoids. When a dermoid cyst is suspected, close radiologic examination for presence of a sinus tract or skeletal dysraphism is indicated. Dermoids can rupture, resulting in

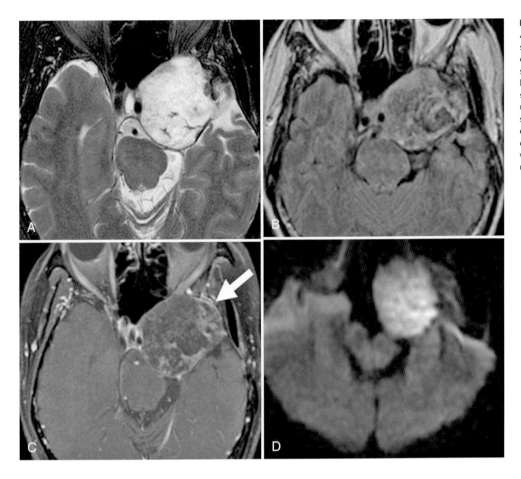

■ **FIGURE 33-24** Epidermoid. **A,** Axial T2W MR image demonstrates a lesion centered in the region of the left cavernous sinus that has signal intensity similar to that of CSF. **B,** However, on FLAIR imaging the signal within the lesion does not saturate, indicating that it is not the same as CSF. **C,** Minimal peripheral enhancement is noted on the postcontrast image (*arrow*). **D,** Diffusion-weighted imaging demonstrates reduced diffusion within the lesion.

chemical meningitis. Radiologic evidence for this is the presence of fat droplets within the subarachnoid spaces.

HEMANGIOMA

Hemangiomas are benign vascular tumors with numerous vessels composed of a single layer of endothelial cells devoid of smooth muscle or elastic membrane.

Epidemiology

Cavernous sinus hemangiomas are rare lesions. They are far more common in females than males (7 : 1) and tend to occur in middle age.

Clinical Presentation

Hemangiomas may cause symptoms by hemorrhage, encasement of neurovascular structures, and mass effect. Patients frequently present with headache and cranial nerve dysfunction, especially diplopia and ptosis. These tumors tend to increase in size during pregnancy.

Pathophysiology

Hemangiomas can arise within the compartments of the cavernous sinus (intracavernous) or from adjacent tissues (extracavernous). They are believed to grow by progressive ectasia of the blood vessels or by autonomous development at the edges of the lesion.[31]

Pathology

Grossly, hemangiomas appear as well-circumscribed vascular lesions.

Extra-axial hemangiomas have the same histologic features as intracranial lesions but different presentation and natural history.

The vascular channels are composed of a single layer of endothelial cells with no smooth muscle or elastic membranes. Calcification, hyaline degeneration, and cholesterol clefts can be seen within these lesions.

Imaging

CT

On CT, hemangiomas appear as well-demarcated lesions that have an enhancement pattern indistinguishable from meningiomas. They are isodense to hyperdense and enhance homogeneously after contrast agent administration. Intralesional calcifications are uncommon.

MRI

On MRI, hemangiomas are well-defined lesions that are isointense to hypointense on T1W images, are very hyperintense on T2W images, and show intense homogeneous enhancement after contrast agent administration (Fig. 33-25). Hemangiomas may be very difficult to distinguish from schwannomas and meningiomas by imaging criteria. On T2W imaging, however, hemangiomas tend to be far more hyperintense than meningiomas.

Special Procedures

Recognition that a parasellar lesion *could be* a hemangioma is very important, because hemangiomas may bleed severely during surgery and have a surgical mortality rate as high as 25%. Salaniti and associates reported use of labeled red cell blood pool scintigraphy to help differentiate hemangiomas from meningiomas. They found that hemangiomas show persistent increased activity on both early and delayed scintigraphy.[32]

At cerebral angiography, hemangiomas may show a vascular blush, typically in the late venous phase, or they may be

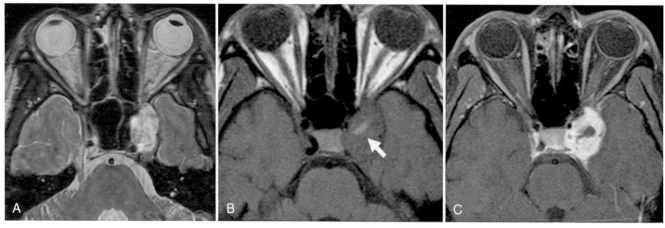

■ **FIGURE 33-25**   Hemangioma. **A,** Axial T2W MR image demonstrates a high signal intensity lesion within the left cavernous sinus. **B,** On the T1W MR image there is a focal area of T1 shortening within the lesion consistent with either hemorrhage or microcalcification. **C,** On postcontrast imaging the lesion avidly enhances except for the region of T1 shortening (*arrow,* **B**) seen on the noncontrast images.

avascular. They usually do not have well-formed feeding or draining vessels. However, feeder arteries may be seen arising from the cavernous portion of the internal carotid artery.

HYPOTHALAMIC AND OPTIC CHIASM GLIOMAS

Optic pathway gliomas and hypothalamic gliomas are both low-grade gliomas that arise in the same general area. They can be very difficult or impossible to differentiate by imaging and pathology, so they will be considered together.

Epidemiology

Optic gliomas account for about 5% of all brain tumors in children. Up to 70% of children with optic chiasm glioma have neurofibromatosis.[33] The malignant optic glioma tends to present in adults (most commonly in the sixth decade). They are very rare with fewer than 50 reported cases[34] and have no association with neurofibromatosis.

Optic and hypothalamic gliomas affect males and females equally.

Clinical Presentation

Optic gliomas can arise at any point along the optic apparatus from the intra-orbital portion of the optic nerve to the visual cortex. They may cause visual symptoms and endocrine dysfunction, most frequently disturbance of growth hormone leading to short stature.

Children with optic gliomas may have visual impairment and neurologic deficits (20%-30%). These lesions are associated with a high degree of morbidity and mortality. The prognosis tends to be better in children with neurofibromatosis.

Adult optic gliomas tend to be locally aggressive or malignant. Malignant optic gliomas present with symptoms similar to optic neuritis, but patients experience rapid progression to monocular blindness, possibly due to occlusion of the retinal artery or vein.[34] Malignant optic glioma is lethal. The expected survival is less than 1 year despite aggressive surgical treatment, radiation therapy, and/or chemotherapy.

Hypothalamic gliomas also present as visual disturbance, endocrine dysfunction, especially diabetes insipidus, and hydrocephalus. They are associated with a high degree of morbidity and mortality, although children with neurofibromatosis are reported to have a better prognosis.[33] Rarely, hypothalamic gliomas cause diencephalic syndrome, in which affected patients show failure to thrive with loss of appetite, vomiting, and emaciation.

Pathology

In childhood, the hypothalamic and optic gliomas are low grade, sometimes cystic neoplasms, either juvenile pilocytic astrocytomas (75%) or low-grade fibrillary astrocytomas (25%). In the adult, the optic gliomas are higher-grade tumors, often anaplastic astrocytomas or glioblastoma multiforme, with increased cellularity, increased mitotic rate, nuclear pleomorphism, and areas of necrosis.

Imaging
CT

On CT, optic and hypothalamic gliomas appear as suprasellar masses that are hypodense to gray matter. Cyst formation and calcification are rare.

MRI

On MRI, optic and hypothalamic gliomas tend to be hypointense to isointense relative to gray matter on T1W images and hyperintense on T2W images (Fig. 33-26). Contrast enhancement is variable but typically homogeneous. Extension to the optic radiations indicates that the lesion is an optic glioma, not a hypothalamic glioma. Patients with neurofibromatosis type 1 may show increased signal intensity in the optic tracts and radiations.

Malignant optic gliomas also tend to be hypointense to isointense on T1W imaging, to be hyperintense on T2W imaging, and to show intense contrast enhancement.

The nature of the optic glioma and its imaging appearance differ in children with and without neurofibromatosis type 1. In children with neurofibromatosis type 1, optic gliomas tend to be smaller, more frequently involve the orbital portion of the optic nerve, and less frequently cystic. In patients not affected by neurofibromatosis type 1, optic gliomas tend to be larger, more frequently involve the optic chiasm and hypothalamus, often extend beyond the optic pathways, and frequently have cystic components.

In malignant optic glioma, nonspecific enlargement of the optic nerve is typically seen, especially in the early stages.

CHORDOID GLIOMA

The chordoid glioma is a recently described low-grade neoplasm that occurs in the region of the anterior third ventricle and hypothalamus and is so named because it has a chordoma-like histology.

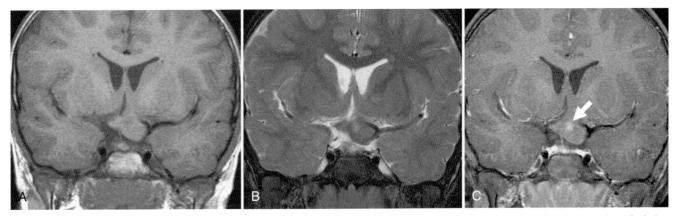

■ **FIGURE 33-26** Optic glioma. Coronal imaging demonstrates a lesion involving the left aspect of the optic chiasm, resulting in expansion. The lesion has signal characteristics similar to gray matter on both the T1W (**A**) and T2W (**B**) MR images and minimal enhancement on the postcontrast image (**C**, *arrow*).

Epidemiology

The incidence of chordoid glioma is not yet known owing to their recent description; however, they appear to be uncommon. Patients are usually adults, with a mean age of 46 years at the time of diagnosis. Chordoid gliomas are reported more frequently in females than males by 3:1.

Clinical Presentation

Patients with chordoid gliomas tend to present with symptoms related to local mass effect, such as headaches, hydrocephalus, hypothalamic dysfunction, and homonymous hemianopsia.

Pathophysiology

Chordoid gliomas are classified as WHO grade II. The cell of origin for these tumors is unknown, but it is suggested that they arise from subependymal tissue.[35,36] Although they are described as well-circumscribed lesions, they are frequently tightly adherent to the hypothalamus, leading to the idea that these tumors arise from the hypothalamus.

Pathology

Chordoid gliomas are soft mucoid tumors. These low-grade neoplasms are given the name chordoid glioma because their histologic appearance resembles a chordoma and they stain avidly with the glial cell marker glial fibrillary acidic protein (GFAP). The stroma is mucin rich. Vacuolization within the stroma can resemble physaliphorous cells. Even though this tumor is low grade, the prognosis tends to be poor, mainly owing to location and the difficulty of obtaining a complete surgical resection.[35]

Case reports have offered the possibility that the neoplasm arises from the subependymal tissue, whereas other possibilities include origin from the hypothalamus. This thought is supported by reports of the neoplasm being tightly adherent to the hypothalamus at the time of surgery.[35]

Imaging
CT

On CT, chordoid gliomas are well-circumscribed, oval masses in the region of the anterior third ventricle and hypothalamus. CT shows a hyperdense lesion.

MRI

Chordoid gliomas are hyperdense to gray matter on T1W images and enhance homogeneously after contrast agent administration. On T2W imaging they are slightly hyperintense.

GANGLIOGLIOMA

Gangliogliomas are benign lesions in which the neuronal and the glial elements each show evidence of neoplasia.

Epidemiology

Gangliogliomas most frequently occur in the temporal lobes and the region of the third ventricle. They are uncommon in the suprasellar region. Suprasellar gangliogliomas show a slight male predominance; the mean age at presentation is 20 years.[37]

Clinical Presentation

The most frequent symptom of suprasellar ganglioglioma is visual disturbance.

Pathophysiology

The majority of gangliogliomas are WHO grade I. No consistent genetic alterations are reported.

Pathology

Gangliogliomas are well-circumscribed lesions. Calcification and cyst formation are common.

Microscopically, dysmorphic, haphazardly arranged ganglion cells are noted in gangliogliomas. Occasionally, Rosenthal fibers may be seen.

Imaging
CT and MRI

The imaging findings of gangliogliomas in the suprasellar region are nonspecific. On T1W images they may be isointense to hypointense. On T2W imaging they tend to be hyperintense to gray matter. They typically show solid or ring enhancement. Approximately 60% of lesions will have some degree of cystic component.

GERMINOMA

Germinomas are the most common of the intracranial germ cell tumors. Most frequently they are located in the pineal and suprasellar regions.[38] Morphologically, they resemble germ cell neoplasms in the ovary or testis.

Epidemiology

Germinomas account for 0.5% to 2.1% of intracranial neoplasms and 60% of the intracranial germ cell tumors.[38] They present most frequently in the second and third decades of life. Germ cell tumors are most common in the pineal region and then the suprasellar region. In 5% to 10% of cases they are found in both

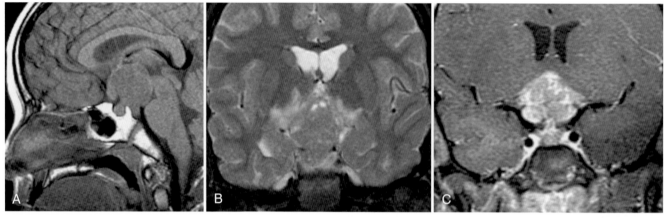

■ **FIGURE 33-27** Sagittal T1W (**A**) and coronal T2W (**B**) MR images demonstrate a predominantly suprasellar lesion that is similar in signal intensity to gray matter and demonstrates heterogeneous enhancement on the postcontrast image (**C**). This was pathologically proven to be a germinoma.

regions. Although pineal germ cell tumors are more common in males, suprasellar germ cell tumors are equally common in males and females.

Clinical Presentation

Germinomas are associated with symptoms of hypothalamic involvement such as emaciation and precocious puberty and often have associated visual or pituitary axis dysfunction, most commonly diabetes insipidus. They may be disseminated throughout the cerebrospinal axis at the time of diagnosis, but symptoms of spinal cord or cerebral cortical involvement are rare.

Pathophysiology

Germ cell tumors arise in midline locations as the result of neoplastic transformation of embryonic germ cells. These embryonic germ cells either migrated inappropriately or failed to migrate from these locations during embryonic development.

Up to 90% of germ cell tumors are associated with chromosomal anomalies. The i(12p) isochromosome on chromosome arm 12p is frequently seen in germ cell tumors in adults and adolescent males. Within the CNS, these lesions frequently have anomalies of the sex chromosomes, typically increased copies of chromosome X.[38]

Pathology

Germinomas tend to be solid lesions. The presence of hemorrhage is usually associated with the more aggressive forms of germ cell neoplasm, such as embryonal carcinoma, yolk sac tumor, and choriocarcinoma.

Germinomas are histologically similar to testicular seminomas and ovarian dysgerminomas. They are composed of large round tumor cells with well-defined borders and show surface staining for placental alkaline phosphatase.

Imaging
CT

On imaging studies, germinomas are infiltrating lesions that are usually isointense to brain parenchyma on T1W imaging and hyperintense on T2W imaging. They typically show homogeneous enhancement (Fig. 33-27). Because of the tendency of germ cell tumors to disseminate via the CSF, imaging of the entire craniospinal axis is necessary.

HYPOTHALAMIC HAMARTOMA

Hypothalamic hamartomas are rare congenital, nonneoplastic neuronal lesions that arise in the region of the tuber cinereum. There are two clinicoanatomic types of hypothalamic hamartomas, designated the parahypothalamic and the intrahypothalamic subtypes. The parahypothalamic form is a pedunculated lesion attached to the floor of the hypothalamus by a narrow base, whereas the intrahypothalamic is a sessile mass with a broad attachment to the hypothalamus.

Epidemiology

Hypothalamic hamartomas occur with equal frequency in males and females. Most patients present in the first or second decade of life.

Clinical Presentation

Hypothalamic hamartomas are commonly associated with isosexual precocious puberty and gelastic seizures.[39,40] Hamartomas less than 1 cm tend to present as precocious puberty, whereas those greater than 1 cm have a greater tendency to present with gelastic seizures.[40] In addition, the parahypothalamic hamartomas present as isosexual central precocious puberty more frequently than as gelastic seizures, whereas intrahypothalamic lesions present as gelastic seizures more frequently than with precocious puberty. The precocious puberty is thought to result from the direct neurosecretory process of the hamartoma; however, it may also arise from physical perturbation of the inhibitory pathways.[39] Gelastic seizures may result from connections with the limbic system and propagation of seizure activity or from the presence of an associated malformation.

Pathophysiology

Hypothalamic hamartomas are heterotopias. The neurons within the hamartoma are similar to normal hypothalamic neurons. Hypothalamic hamartomas may be associated with other congenital anomalies, suggesting that they arise as early as 4 weeks' gestation. They are the abnormality most frequently associated with duplication of the pituitary gland, which is an extremely rare malformation.[41]

Pathology

Hypothalamic hamartomas are pedunculated or sessile lesions that arise in the region between the mammillary bodies and the tuber cinereum.

These lesions are composed of neurons similar in morphology to hypothalamic neurons. Dysplastic neurons and glial cells may also be seen.

Imaging
CT

Hypothalamic hamartomas typically form solid, sometimes pedunculated hypothalamic-suprasellar masses that are isodense to gray matter and show no contrast enhancement.

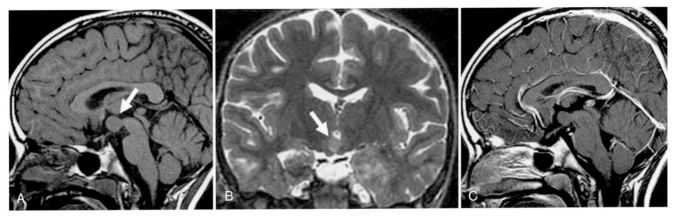

■ **FIGURE 33-28** Hypothalamic hamartoma. Sagittal T1W (**A**) MR image demonstrates enlargement of the hypothalamus that is isointense to gray matter and slightly hyperintense on a T2W image (**B**) (*arrows*). No enhancement is seen on a postcontrast image (**C**).

MRI

Hypothalamic hamartomas are typically solid lesions. On MRI, they show signal intensity similar to gray matter on all sequences and do not enhance (Fig. 33-28). Increased T2 signal and growth may signify malignant transformation, although recent studies have described increased T2 signal in lesions without malignant transformation.[42] Rarely, they may show cystic components. Other atypical features include giant hamartoma, prominent T2 prolongation, and lipomatous content. On MR spectroscopy the NAA and choline levels are relatively normal. Elevation of the myoinositol peak has been reported.[43]

LYMPHOMA

Primary CNS lymphoma is defined as extranodal lymphoma occurring in the CNS without evidence of involvement elsewhere. Lymphoma can also involve the parasellar regions via perineurial spread.

Epidemiology

The incidence of CNS lymphoma is increasing worldwide. In part, this may be due to its association with immunocompromised states, most predominantly human immunodeficiency virus (HIV) infection. Two to 12 percent of HIV patients will develop CNS lymphoma. Lymphoma of the pituitary gland is very rare, with only five cases reported.[44]

Primary CNS lymphoma can affect any age group; however, in immunocompetent patients, CNS lymphoma is most common in the sixth and seventh decades. The incidence is slightly higher in males than females (3 : 2).

Clinical Presentation

Patients with primary CNS lymphoma may demonstrate focal neurologic deficits, seizures, or evidence of increased intracranial pressure. Involvement of the sella may result in hypopituitarism.

Pathophysiology

CNS lymphoma is typically a B-cell lymphoma and has an association with the Epstein-Barr virus. No genetic predisposition to CNS lymphoma is known.

Pathology

Lymphoma may present as solitary or multiple masses. They may be firm, focally necrotic, hemorrhagic, or friable.

The majority of these tumors are B-cell lymphomas, although occasional tumors have T-cell origin (2%). Microscopically, there is a proliferation of diffusely infiltrating lymphoid cells.

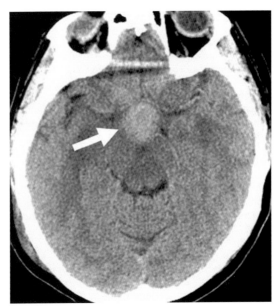

■ **FIGURE 33-29** Lymphoma. Noncontrast CT demonstrates a hyperdense suprasellar lesion (*arrow*), which was proven pathologically to be lymphoma.

Imaging

CT

On CT, primary CNS lymphoma tends to be hyperdense and show enhancement on postcontrast imaging (Fig. 33-29).

MRI

Primary CNS lymphoma typically is seen as isointense to hypointense on both T1W and T2W images and enhances on the postcontrast images. Lymphoma may involve the pituitary infundibulum, resulting in thickening and enhancement of the stalk (Fig. 33-30). Such cases may be difficult to distinguish radiographically from Langerhans cell histiocytosis, but patients with lymphoma are typically older. Leukemia and granulomatous disease such as tuberculosis and sarcoid are other differential diagnoses for lymphoma involving the infundibulum.

In the rare cases that lymphoma involves the pituitary gland, a dumbbell-shaped mass may be seen arising from the sella and extending superiorly through the diaphragma sellae into the suprasellar region. Such lesions may be mistaken for pituitary adenomas. The floor of the sella turcica may be eroded.

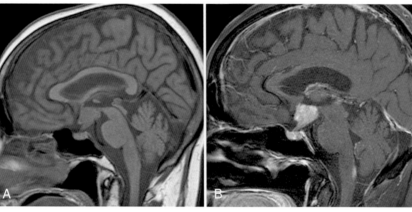
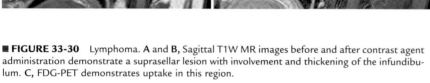
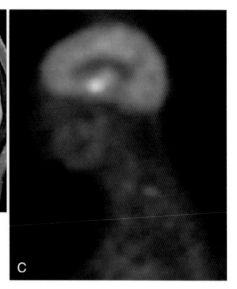

■ **FIGURE 33-30** Lymphoma. **A** and **B**, Sagittal T1W MR images before and after contrast agent administration demonstrate a suprasellar lesion with involvement and thickening of the infundibulum. **C**, FDG-PET demonstrates uptake in this region.

CHORDOMA

Chordomas are locally aggressive tumors of the skull base that arise from primitive notochordal remnants.

Epidemiology

Chordomas account for 1% of intracranial tumors. They are more frequent in males than females (2 : 1) and usually arise in the fourth decade.

Clinical Presentation

Chordomas are slow-growing neoplasms. The symptoms associated with these tumors depend on their location. However, more common symptoms are headaches and diplopia related to involvement of the cranial nerves, especially the abducens (CN VI).

Pathophysiology

Chordomas arise from primitive notochordal remnants and can appear anywhere along the course of the embryonic notochord. Intracranial chordomas account for 32% of chordomas. The remainder are spinal (32.8%) and sacral (29.2%).[45] Intracranial chordomas frequently arise along the upper clivus or along the caudal margin of the clivus. In 15% of cases they may arise unilaterally in the petrous apex, a finding that may make it difficult to distinguish them from chondrosarcomas. This may be the result of notochordal cells penetrating the skull base from different directions during early embryologic development. Chordomas are locally aggressive tumors that rarely metastasize.[45]

Pathology

Chordomas are multilobulated gelatinous tumors that are semitranslucent and have a gray coloration. Most lesions range from 2 to 5 cm.[45]

One of the histologic characteristics of chordomas is the physaliphorous cell, which has bubble-like vacuolated cytoplasm. Two histopathologic subtypes of chordoma are described: the typical chordoma and the chondroid chordoma. Typical chordomas have cells that are arranged in cords and are set in a pale mucopolysaccharide matrix. Regions of necrosis and hemorrhage can be seen as well as entrapped bone trabeculae. Mitoses are uncommon, even in those lesions that have metastasized.

The chondroid form refers to a histologic mimic that is not of true chondroid origin but is epithelially derived. The stroma resembles hyaline cartilage, and neoplastic cells are seen within lacunae. This form can resemble a low-grade sarcoma and is more likely to have intratumoral calcifications.

Chordomas can resemble chondrosarcomas histologically, with the greatest confusion occurring between the classic chordoma and the myxoid form of chondrosarcoma. Immunohistochemical staining can help to differentiate between the two. The cells of chondrosarcoma are chondrocytes and do not stain for cytokeratin or other epithelial markers.[46]

Imaging

CT

On CT, chordomas tend to form a well-circumscribed soft tissue mass in a central location. The lesion arises from the clivus and causes lytic bone destruction (Fig. 33-31). Lytic bone destruction can also be seen in metastatic lesions and in invasive adenomas, both of which are differential diagnoses for chordoma. Occasionally, intratumoral calcifications are seen. These are thought to represent sequestra from bone destruction, rather than dystrophic calcifications within the tumor.

MRI

On T1W imaging chordomas are isointense to hypointense lesions. They show very high signal intensity on T2W imaging, most likely due to the high fluid content within the vacuolated cellular components. Occasional foci of T1 shortening may be seen, which correspond to hemorrhagic foci or mucus. On contrast-enhanced MRI, chordomas demonstrate moderate to marked enhancement, which is frequently heterogeneous (Fig. 33-32). Less frequently, enhancement may be slight or absent. Fat-suppressed images help to display the tumor margins. Some investigators have tried to use imaging to differentiate chondroid chordomas from typical chordomas by imaging because the survival rate of patients with chondroid chordoma is better. In chondroid chordomas, cartilaginous foci have replaced the gelatinous matrix, shortening the T1 and T2 relaxation times versus typical chordomas. Chondrosarcomas typically arise from the cartilage at the junctions between bones, so they typically lie off midline along the petroclival suture. They can be a differential diagnosis when chordomas occur off the midline.

Evaluation of the relationship of chordomas to the surrounding vasculature is important for surgical planning. Up to 79% of intracranial chordomas displace or encase adjacent vasculature. However, they rarely narrow the involved vessel.[45] MR angiography is useful in evaluating this relationship.

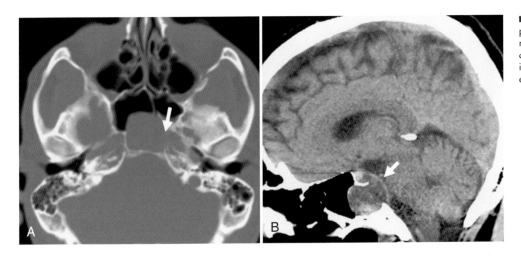

■ **FIGURE 33-31** Chordoma. Axial precontrast (**A**) and sagittal reformatted postcontrast (**B**) CT scans demonstrate an expansile lytic lesion involving the clivus (*arrows*) and extending into the sellar region.

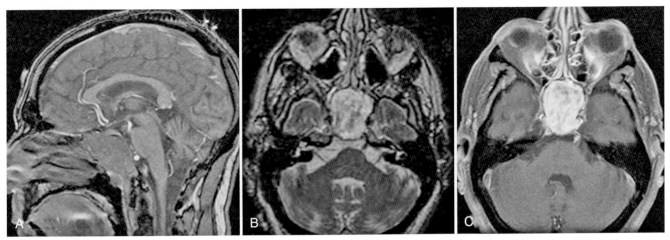

■ **FIGURE 33-32** Sagittal T1W FSPGR MR image (**A**) demonstrates an expansile mass involving the clivus and extending into the sella and suprasellar region. The lesion demonstrates T2 hyperintensity (**B**) with avid enhancement (**C**). Pathology was consistent with chordoma.

Special Procedures

The angiographic findings of chordoma are nonspecific. There is rarely any tumoral blush or abnormal tumor vascularity. Diagnostic angiography may be of benefit to better demonstrate any vascular narrowing or occlusion. Temporary balloon occlusion of the internal carotid artery may be of benefit in determining whether that artery can be sacrificed, if necessary, without significant neurologic impairment.[45]

CHONDROSARCOMA

Chondrosarcomas are malignant bone tumors that produce hyaline cartilage.

Epidemiology

Chondrosarcomas are most frequent in middle age but can occur at any age.

Clinical Presentation

Signs and symptoms of chondrosarcoma depend on the location of the lesion, but, typically, there is a history of headache and cranial nerve dysfunction, most frequently resulting in diplopia.

Pathophysiology

Chondrosarcomas most commonly arise in relation to synchondroses, so they are often seen along the petroclival synchondrosis. Occasionally, chondrosarcomas may be found along the midline in the region of the sphenoccipital synchondrosis and in the posterior nasal septum. These lesions grow slowly and rarely metastasize.

Pathology

Chondrosarcomas may be grossly well delineated. Necrosis and hemorrhage may be seen.

There are several histologic subtypes of chondrosarcomas. However, almost all skull base chondrosarcomas are of the conventional hyaline or myxoid subtypes or show a combination of both. The myxoid matrix can appear very similar to the matrix of classic chordoma. The chondrosarcoma cells may be found in strands that resemble the cord pattern of chordoma, and the vacuoles in some chondrocytes may resemble the physaliphorous cell. For those reasons, correct histologic diagnosis often depends on immunohistochemical stains. The cells of chondrosarcoma are chondrocytes and do not stain for cytokeratin or other epithelial markers.[46]

Imaging

CT

The CT appearance of chondrosarcomas varies with the degree of chondroid matrix. Usually there is a soft tissue component that appears dense. The tumor matrix commonly calcifies in the form of small ringlets or incomplete rings. The presence of calcifications with this morphology can help to distinguish chondrosarcoma from chordoma.

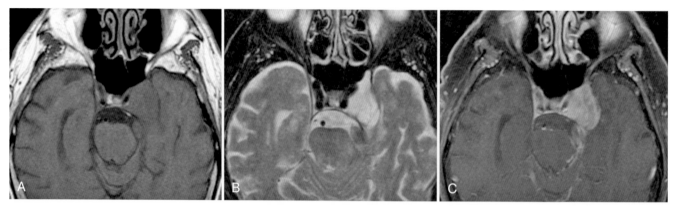

■ **FIGURE 33-33**   Axial images demonstrate a lesion involving the left cavernous sinus that was isointense on T1W (**A**) and hyperintense on T2W (**B**) MR images. Enhancement is seen on the postcontrast imaging (**C**). Pathologically this was proven to be chondrosarcoma.

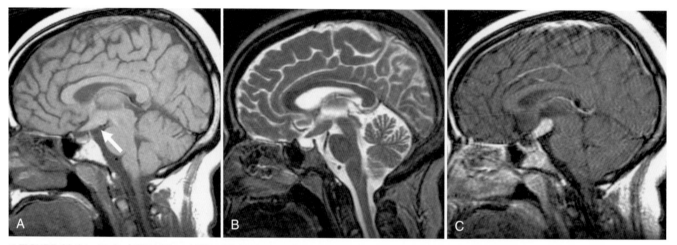

■ **FIGURE 33-34**   Sagittal T1W (**A**) and T2W (**B**) MR images demonstrate enlargement of the pituitary infundibulum (*arrow,* **A**). Postcontrast T1W image (**C**) demonstrates homogeneous enhancement of the abnormal enlargement.

MRI

Chondrosarcomas show intermediate signal intensity on T1W imaging, are fairly hyperintense on T2W imaging, and enhance after contrast agent administration (Fig. 33-33). They may be difficult to differentiate from a chordoma by MRI, although chordomas are typically thought to be midline lesions whereas chondrosarcomas more frequently are situated laterally along the synchondroses and the petroclival fissure. Unfortunately, occasional chondrosarcomas are midline and occasional chordomas are off midline.

ANALYSIS

A 31-year-old woman presented with a history of diabetes insipidus. An MRI was obtained for further evaluation (Fig. 33-34; Box 33-1). On imaging, enlargement and homogeneous enhancement of the pituitary infundibulum and the hypothalamic region were noted. The differential diagnosis for lesions in the sellar and parasellar region is very broad, but the ability to localize the lesion to the posterior aspect in the suprasellar region helps to narrow the diagnosis. One no longer has to consider sellar lesions or those occurring within the cavernous sinus. Also, avid enhancement and involvement of the pituitary infundibulum help exclude hypothalamic hamartoma.

In considering the lesions that involve the infundibulum and hypothalamic region, the differential diagnosis is still relatively broad. Neoplastic lesions in this region include lymphoma (Fig. 33-35), leukemia, germinoma (Fig. 33-36), metastasis, Langer-hans cell histiocytosis (Fig. 33-37), and hypothalamic glioma (Fig. 33-38). In addition, non-neoplastic processes such as sarcoid and tuberculosis also involve this region. However, germinoma and hypothalamic glioma are less likely, because these lesions tend to be more lobular on imaging. To further narrow the differential diagnosis, knowledge of patient history and physical examination findings, as well as results of other radiologic and laboratory studies, may help.

Patient age is of benefit. Hypothalamic glioma is a lesion that is most frequent in childhood and adolescence. Given that the patient is a young adult, the remainder of the lesions remain in the differential diagnosis. Other patient history and imaging/laboratory findings are beneficial. If there is a history of a primary neoplasm, then metastasis would be suggested. A history of sarcoid or tuberculosis especially if there are positive radiographic findings elsewhere can point toward these lesions as the possible cause. If either one of these entities is considered, a chest radiograph may be of benefit. Knowledge of laboratory findings, especially CSF studies, may help confirm the diagnosis.

In the case of this patient, she had an abnormal chest radiograph that showed findings consistent with sarcoidosis. In patients with sarcoid, the chest radiograph is positive in 90% of cases. In addition, the angiotensin-converting enzyme (ACE) level was elevated. This elevation is not as specific as chest radiograph findings, because ACE is elevated in only 60% of patients. Therefore, knowledge of the patient's laboratory and chest radiograph findings was able to help narrow the diagnosis to sarcoid and not a neoplasm.

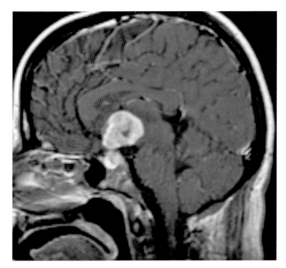

■ **FIGURE 33-35** Lymphoma.

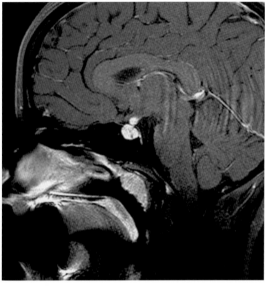

■ **FIGURE 33-37** Langerhans cell histiocytosis.

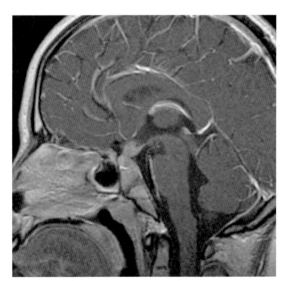

■ **FIGURE 33-36** Germinoma.

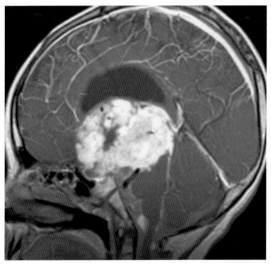

■ **FIGURE 33-38** Hypothalamic glioma.

BOX 33-1   Sample Report: MRI of Enlarged Infundibulum and Hypothalamus

PATIENT HISTORY

A 31-year-old woman presented with central diabetes insipidus.

COMPARISON STUDY

CT of the brain was done 15 days previously.

TECHNIQUE

The following were obtained through the sellar region: sagittal T1W precontrast and postcontrast, coronal T1W precontrast and postcontrast, and sagittal and coronal T2W images.

FINDINGS

Enlargement of the infundibulum and hypothalamic region is noted, which is isointense on both T1W and T2W imaging. The infundibulum is midline in location, and there is no involvement of the optic chiasm.

The posterior pituitary bright spot is not visualized on these images. The sella does not appear enlarged.

On postcontrast imaging there is avid and homogeneous enhancement of the infundibulum and hypothalamus. No other regions of abnormal enhancement are noted in the remainder of the visualized portions of the brain and sellar region. The visualized marrow signal is normal.

IMPRESSION

There is enlargement and homogeneous enhancement of the pituitary infundibulum and in the region of the hypothalamus. The differential diagnosis for this lesion is broad and includes neoplastic lesions such as lymphoma, leukemia, Langerhans cell histiocytosis, metastasis, and, to a lesser degree, germinoma; correlation with a systemic neoplastic process or CSF studies may be of benefit. Granulomatous diseases such as sarcoid or tuberculosis are also possibilities. A chest radiograph may be of assistance in further evaluation of these entities.

SUGGESTED READINGS

Alshail E, Rutka JT, Becker LE, Hoffman JH. Optic chiasmatic-hypothalamic glioma. Brain Pathol 1997; 7:799-806.

Choi SH, Kwon BJ, Na DG, et al. Pituitary adenoma, craniopharyngioma, and Rathke cleft cyst involving both intrasellar and suprasellar regions: differentiation using MRI. Clin Radiol 2007; 62:453-462.

Garnett MR, Puget S, Grill J, Sainte-Rose C. Craniopharyngioma. Orphanet J Rare Dis 2007; 2:18.

Huang BY, Castillo M. Nonadenomatous tumors of the pituitary and sella turcica. Top Magn Reson Imaging 2005; 16:289-299.

Johnsen DE, Woodruff WW, Allen IS, et al. MR Imaging of the sellar and juxtasellar regions. RadioGraphics 1991; 11:727-752.

Rennert J, Doerfler A. Imaging of sellar and parasellar lesions. Clin Neurol Neurosurg 2007; 109:111-124.

Sautner D, Saeger W, Ludecke DK. Tumors of the sellar region mimicking pituitary adenomas. Exp Clin Endocrinol 1993; 101:283-289.

Scheithauer BW, Gaffey TA, Lloyd RV, et al. Pathobiology of pituitary adenomas and carcinomas. Neurosurgery 2006; 59:341-353.

Simonetta AB. Imaging of suprasellar and parasellar tumors. Neuroimaging Clin North Am 1999; 9:717-732.

REFERENCES

1. Johnsen DE, Woodruff WW, Allen IS, et al. MR imaging of the sellar and juxtasellar regions. RadioGraphics 1991; 11:727-758.
2. Snyder PJ. Clinically nonfunctioning pituitary adenomas. Endocrinol Metab Clin North Am 1993; 22:163-175.
3. Rolih CA, Ober KP. Pituitary apoplexy. Endocrinol Metab Clin North Am 1993; 22:291-302.
4. Castillo M. Pituitary gland: development, normal appearances, and magnetic resonance imaging protocols. Top Magn Reson Imaging 2005; 16:259-268.
5. Donovan JL Nesbit GM. Distinction of masses involving the sella and suprasellar space: specificity of imaging features. AJR Am J Roentgenol 1996; 167:597-603.
6. Cottier JP, Destrieux C, Brunereau L, et al. Cavernous sinus invasion by pituitary adenoma: MR imaging. Radiology 2000; 215:463-469.
7. Sutton LN, Wang ZJ, Wehrli SL, et al. Proton spectroscopy of suprasellar tumors in pediatric patients. Neurosurgery 1997; 41:388-397.
8. Kaltsas GA, Nomikos P, Kontogeorgos G, et al. Clinical review: Diagnosis and management of pituitary carcinomas. J Clin Endocrinol Metab 2005; 90:3089-3099.
9. Huang BY, Castillo M. Nonadenomatous tumors of the pituitary and sella turcica. Top Magn Reson Imaging 2005; 16:289-299.
10. Schaller B, Kirsch E, Tolnay M, Mindermann T. Symptomatic granular cell tumor of the pituitary gland: case report and review of the literature. Neurosurgery 1998; 42:166-170; discussion 170-171.
11. Katsuta T, Inoue T, Nakagaki H, et al. Distinctions between pituicytoma and ordinary pilocytic astrocytoma: case report. J Neurosurg 2003; 98:404-406.
12. Brat DJ, Scheithauer BW, Staugaitis SM, et al. Pituicytoma: a distinctive low-grade glioma of the neurohypophysis. Am J Surg Pathol 2000; 24:362-368.
13. Shin JL, Asa SL, Woodhouse LJ, et al. Cystic lesions of the pituitary: clinicopathological features distinguishing craniopharyngioma, Rathke's cleft cyst, and arachnoid cyst. J Clin Endocrinol Metab 1999; 84:3972-3982.
14. Ruscalleda J. Imaging of parasellar lesions. Eur Radiol 2005; 15:549-559.
15. Eldevik OP, Blaivas M, Gabrielsen TO, et al. Craniopharyngioma: radiologic and histologic findings and recurrence. AJNR Am J Neuroradiol 1996; 17:1427-1439.
16. Saeki N, Uchino Y, Murai H, et al. MR imaging study of edema-like change along the optic tract in patients with pituitary region tumors. AJNR Am J Neuroradiol 2003; 24:336-342.

17. Sutton LN, Gusnard D, Bruce DA, et al. Fusiform dilatations of the carotid artery following radical surgery of childhood craniopharyngiomas. J Neurosurg 1991; 74:695-700.
18. Komninos J, Vlassopoulou V, Protopapa D, et al. Tumors metastatic to the pituitary gland: case report and literature review. J Clin Endocrinol Metab 2004; 89:574-580.
19. Nemzek WR, Hecht S, Gandour-Edwards R, et al. Perineural spread of head and neck tumors: how accurate is MR imaging? AJNR Am J Neuroradiol 1998; 19:701-706.
20. Caldemeyer KS, Mathews VP, Righi PD, Smith RR. Imaging features and clinical significance of perineural spread or extension of head and neck tumors. RadioGraphics 1998; 18:97-110; quiz 147.
21. Koshimoto Y, Maeda M, Naiki H, et al. MR of pituitary metastasis in a patient with diabetes insipidus. AJNR Am J Neuroradiol 1995; 16:971-974.
22. Prosch H, Grois N, Wnorowski M, et al. MR imaging presentation of intracranial Langerhans cell histiocytosis. AJNR Am J Neuroradiol 2004; 25:880-891.
23. Wood MW, White, RJ, Kernohan J. One hundred meningiomas found incidentally at necropsy. J Neuropathol Exp Neurol 1957; 16:337-340.
24. Laine FJ, Nadel L, Braun IF. CT and MR imaging of the central skull base: II. Pathologic spectrum. RadioGraphics 1990; 10:797-821.
25. Buetow MP, Buetow PC, Smirniotopoulos JG. Typical, atypical, and misleading features in meningioma. RadioGraphics 1991; 11:1087-1106.
26. Shino A, Nakasu S, Matsuda M, et al. Noninvasive evaluation of the malignant potential of intracranial meningiomas performed using proton magnetic resonance spectroscopy. J Neurosurg 1999; 91:928-934.
27. Fountas KN, Kapsalaki E, Kassam M, et al. Management of intracranial meningeal hemangiopericytomas: outcome and experience. Neurosurg Rev 2006; 29:145-153.
28. Chiechi MV, Smirniotopoulos JG, Mena H. Intracranial hemangiopericytomas: MR and CT features. AJNR Am J Neuroradiol 1996; 17:1365-1371.
29. Stone JA, Cooper H, Castillo M, Mukherji SK. Malignant schwannoma of the trigeminal nerve. AJNR Am J Neuroradiol 2001; 22:505-507.
30. Smirniotopoulos JG, Chiechi MV. Teratomas, dermoids, and epidermoids of the head and neck. RadioGraphics 1995; 15:1437-1455.
31. Sohn CH, Kim SP, Kim IM, et al. Characteristic MR imaging findings of cavernous hemangiomas in the cavernous sinus. AJNR Am J Neuroradiol 2003; 24:1148-1151.

32. Salanitri GC, Stuckey SL, Murphy M. Extracerebral cavernous hemangioma of the cavernous sinus: diagnosis with MR imaging and labeled red cell blood pool scintigraphy. AJNR Am J Neuroradiol 2004; 25:280-284.

33. Luh GY, Bird CR. Imaging of brain tumors in the pediatric population. Neuroimaging Clin 1999; 9:691-716.

34. Millar WS, Tartaglino LM, Sergott RC, et al. MR of malignant optic glioma of adulthood. AJNR 1995; 16:1673-1676.

35. Pomper MG, Passe TJ, Burger PC, et al. Chordoid glioma: a neoplasm unique to the hypothalamus and anterior third ventricle. AJNR Am J Neuroradiol 2001; 22:464-469.

36. Ricoy JR, Lobato RD, Báez B, et al. Suprasellar chordoid glioma. Acta Neuropathol (Berl) 2000; 99:699-703.

37. Shanop S, Kirsch E, Bannan P, Fabian VA. Ganglioglioma of the optic chiasm: case report and review of the literature. AJNR Am J Neuroradiol 2000; 21:1486-1489.

38. Tamaki N, Lin T, Shirataki K, et al. Germ cell tumors of the thalamus and the basal ganglia. Childs Nerv Syst 1990; 6:3-7.

39. Jung H, Ojeda SR. Pathogenesis of precocious puberty in hypothalamic hamartoma. Horm Res 2002; 57(Suppl 2):31-34.

40. Kollias SS, Ball WS, Prenger EC. Review of the embryologic development of the pituitary gland and report of a case of hypophyseal duplication detected by MRI. Neuroradiology 1995; 37:3-12.

41. Ng SM, Kumar Y, Cody D, et al. Cranial MRI scans are indicated in all girls with central precocious puberty. Arch Dis Child 2003; 88:414-418; discussion 414-418.

42. Amstutz DR, Coons SW, Kerrigan JF, et al. Hypothalamic hamartomas: correlation of MR imaging and spectroscopic findings with tumor glial content. AJNR Am J Neuroradiol 2006; 27:794-798.

43. Martin DD, Seeger U, Ranke MB, Grodd W. MR imaging and spectroscopy of a tuber cinereum hamartoma in a patient with growth hormone deficiency and hypogonadotropic hypogonadism. AJNR Am J Neuroradiol 2003; 24:1177-1180.

44. Kaufmann TJ, Lopes MBS, Laws E, Lipper MH. Primary sellar lymphoma: radiologic and pathologic findings in patients. AJNR Am J Neuroradiol 2002; 23:364-367.

45. Erdem E, Angtuaco EC, Van Hemert R, et al. Comprehensive review of intracranial chordoma. RadioGraphics 2003; 23:995-1009.

46. Rosenburg AE, Brown GA, Bhan AK, Lee JM. Chondroid chordoma: a variant of chordoma. Am J Clin Pathol 1994; 101:36-41.

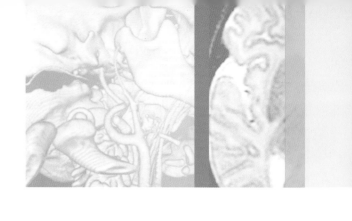

CHAPTER 34

Pineal Region Masses

John H. Rees and James G. Smirniotopoulos

The pineal gland is a unique neuroendocrine structure situated roughly in the center of the skull. It has been the subject of interest and speculation by anatomists and natural philosophers since ancient times, with references as far back as 800 BC.[1] Its modern name is based on its pine cone–like shape, and, for the same reason, the pineal was previously referred to as the conarium.[1] Historical theories detailing its function and purpose abound. As early as 300 BC, Herophilus and others believed that it was the seat of the mind and functioned as a sphincter to regulate the flow of thoughts.[1] Galen (circa AD 150) was convinced that it was a gland and proposed that the cerebellar vermis was actually the thought sphincter.[1] The noted philosopher and natural scientist René Descartes (c. 1750) was keenly interested in the pineal gland. Despite objections from his contemporaries such as the Dutch anatomist Caspar Bartholin, Descartes revived the concept that the pineal gland was the seat of the soul in his work *The Passions of the Soul* (1749).[1] François Magendie and other physicians of the same period resurrected the ancient notion that the pineal gland was a sphincter to control the flow of cerebrospinal fluid (CSF) rather than the flow of thought.[1] In 1763, Thomas Gibson in his *Epitome of Anatomy* described the pineal body as an endocrine gland, which leads us into present-day concepts.[1]

OVERVIEW

Embryogenesis and Maturation

The pineal gland, or epiphysis cerebri, evaginates from the posterior diencephalic roof during early embryonic life.[2] The mature gland hangs by the pineal stalk from the posterior roof of the third ventricle (Fig. 34-1). Within the pineal stalk is the pineal recess,[2] a passageway lined by ependymal cells and directly connected to the third ventricle. The gland is fully formed by around 1 year of age and gradually increases in size to age 2 years, after which it remains stable until age 20 years.[3] Throughout adult life there is a gradual decrease in melatonin synthesis and release, and gradual involution may occur, although this is variable.[4] Pineal parenchyma typically contains a variable quantity of calcific particles, called corpora arenacea ("brain sand"). Chemical analysis shows that these structures are composed of calcium phosphate, calcium carbonate, magnesium phosphate, and ammonium phosphate. As the gland ages and involutes, cysts occur within the pineal with increasing frequency. Most cysts measure less than 1 cm, with some larger cysts measuring up to 3 cm. Up to 40% of glands show various-sized cysts at autopsy, and a recent high-resolution MRI study showed pineal cysts in 23% of normal adults.[5] Some studies have shown slightly increased incidence of pineal cysts in females. Pineal cysts may remain stable, or they may increase or decrease in size over time.[6] Most pineal cysts are considered incidental and nonpathologic unless they exhibit untoward mass effect or other atypical features, such as hemorrhage. A recent study found a higher than predicted association between incidental-appearing pineal cysts and history of headache, although the existence of a causative etiology is lacking.[7]

Histology

Histologically, the pineal gland contains two main cell types. Primary pineal parenchymal cells are of a similar lineage as the photosensory cells of the retina, which display further evolution into neurosecretory cells. Combined immunohistochemical and ultrastructural data corroborate the dual neurosensory and neurosecretory nature of pineal parenchymal cells. Parenchymal cells stain positively for both synaptophysin and neurofilament protein. These specialized neurosecretory cells are contained within a multilobular and septated structure composed of leptomeningeal and glial elements. Glial cells within the pineal gland are primarily astrocytic, but ependymal elements and possibly choroidal cells may be present in fewer numbers. The cellular development of the human pineal gland recapitulates its development as a neurosecretory organ derived from photosensitive cells. In late intrauterine life, the gland is composed primarily of pigmented cells arranged in a rosette pattern similar to the developing retina. In subsequent postnatal development, pineal cells lose their pigmented components and develop positive reactivity for neuron-specific enolase.[8]

The external capsule of the pineal gland is leptomeningeal, of primarily arachnoidal tissue, and continuous and commingled with internal glial elements. There is extensive sympathetic innervation via the superior cervical ganglion with some parasympathetic innervation. True ganglion cells are present but are rare within the pineal gland. These cells rarely give rise to a true primary pineal ganglioglioma. Finally, the pineal gland is permeated by a dense capillary bed of vessels, without forming a blood-brain barrier.[1,9]

Pathophysiology

The most important function of the pineal gland is the elaboration and secretion of melatonin. Melatonin has at least two distinct functions. First, it regulates our diurnal cycle, whereby bodily functions are organized around a day-night schedule. The production of melatonin is stimulated by darkness and inhibited by light. How does this occur? In submammalian species, the pineal gland is a light-sensitive organ and has been referred to as the "third eye," which is thought to be related to the parietal eye of some ancient and primitive fish species. In some reptiles and amphibians, the gland is close to the skin surface in the back of the neck and receives direct stimulation from light that penetrates superficial tissues.[10] In the human, the pineal gland receives no direct photic input but retinohypothalamic tracts transmit light/dark information to the suprachiasmatic nucleus and then to the tuber cinereum of the hypothalamus. This information is subsequently conveyed in the medial forebrain bundle, leading into the inferomedial column of the spinal cord and thence to the superior cervical ganglion. Sympathetic fibers from the superior cervical ganglion follow the carotid vessels upward to the parasellar region and then track posteriorly to provide direct sympathetic input to the pineal gland (Fig. 34-2). Because of this circuitous pathway, the pineal gland is referred to as a neuroendocrine transducer, which transforms retinal light/dark signals into neuroendocrine secretions, in turn regulating other neural and somatic functions.[9] Abnormal melatonin production and release is implicated in a variety of conditions, including seasonal affective disorder, jet lag, narcolepsy, and other sleep disorders.[11]

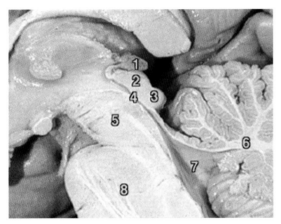

■ FIGURE 34-1 Pineal anatomy. 1, Pineal gland; 2, tectum of midbrain, superior colliculus; 3, tectum, inferior colliculus; 4, aqueduct of Sylvius; 5, tegmentum of midbrain; 6, cerebellum; 7, fourth ventricle; 8, pons.

Another major function of melatonin is to regulate sexual development, primarily by delaying the onset of puberty. Accordingly, pineal region tumors that suppress melatonin production occasionally present as precocious puberty.

Melatonin is secreted into the extracellular space with uptake by the dense capillary vascular bed. Although the pineal gland is not within the blood-brain barrier, the target organs for its endocrine products are solely within the brain. There is no direct tractal connection between the brain and the pineal gland, and the primary innervation of the pineal gland is sympathetic autonomic via the superior cervical ganglion, as discussed earlier. However, there is some parasympathetic innervation from the sphenopalatine and otic ganglia. In addition, some nerve fibers penetrate into the pineal gland via the pineal stalk (central innervation). Finally, neurons in the trigeminal ganglion innervate the gland with nerve fibers containing the neuropeptide pituitary adenylate cyclase–activating polypeptide (PACAP.)

Pineocytes produce melatonin in a four-step enzymatic pathway, using circulating tryptophan as raw material. This pathway functions primarily at night with diurnal regulation provided through sympathetic input that is informed by the retinohypothalamic connection just described.

In addition to melatonin, the normal pineal gland secretes serotonin, the immediate precursor of melatonin, as well as norepinephrine. Pineocytes also contain significant intracellular concentrations of other hypothalamic peptides such as thyroid-releasing hormone (TRH), luteinizing hormone releasing factor (LHRH), and somatostatin.

Epidemiology

Tumors in the pineal gland and adjacent region have historically been grouped together and at one time were collectively referred to as *pinealomas*. With better understanding, this term has been abandoned in favor of the more general term *pineal region masses*. These entities fall into four major categories: germ cell tumors, pineal parenchymal tumors, gliomas, and other neoplastic and non-neoplastic masses or cysts. Accurate epidemiologic information about pineal tumors is problematic owing to variations in classification and regional differences in biopsy protocols. Because germinomas, the most common tumor in this region, are exquisitely radiosensitive, many pineal region tumors have historically been treated with primary radiation therapy without histologic confirmation. Although this practice has

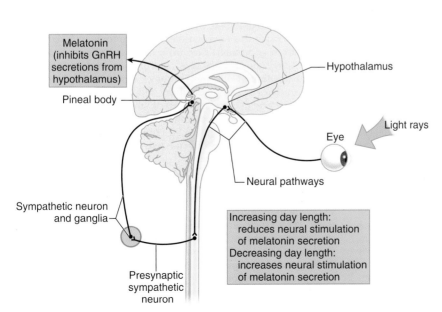

■ FIGURE 34-2 Schematic drawing of the pathway of light, which is converted to photic impulses that travel from the retina to the superior chiasmatic nucleus (SCN) down the brain stem into the cervical cord, out along sympathetic fibers to the superior cervical ganglion, and then back superiorly to the pineal gland. It is by this pathway that day-night cycles are "read" by the pineal gland, which then modulates the release of melatonin, creating our physiologic diurnal cycle.

produced good clinical results, it has made it more difficult to ascertain the true incidence of different tumor types. Large series historically suggest an overall incidence of pineal region tumors of 0.4 to 0.9 per 100,000/year,[12] which represents less than 1% of all new intracranial tumors per year in adults and between 3% and 8% of new pediatric brain tumors.[13] Of these, germ cell tumors are most common, accounting for 50% to 60% with an estimated incidence of approximately 0.4 per 100,000/year in the United States and Europe.[14] Next most common are tumors of pineocyte origin, which account for approximately 14% to 27% of pineal region masses,[15,16] with an estimated incidence of 0.1 to 0.2 per 100,000/year, representing 0.3% to 0.6% of new brain tumors in adults and 3% to 4% in children.[17]

Pineal region tumors have been found to exhibit significant geographic variation for reasons that are not known. There is a significantly increased incidence of germ cell tumors in Japan and to a lesser extent elsewhere in Far East Asia, with estimated three to four times as many germinomas as in the United States.[17] Although data are incomplete, true pineal parenchymal tumors do not appear to have major geographic variations in incidence.

Overall, pineal region tumors are more common in younger age groups. Germ cell tumors taken as a group have an average age at onset of 11 years. Pineal parenchymal tumors occur somewhat later and display a wider age range, with mean ages in different series from 22 to 36 and an age range between childhood and the eighth decade of life.[15]

Germ cell tumors of the pineal region are approximately three times more common in males,[18] although this figure is even higher in some series; however, in the suprasellar region this gender differential is not seen. Pineal parenchymal tumors do not display a convincing gender predilection overall, although a slight male bias has been reported in Japan.[17]

Of germ cell tumors, germinomas are most common, representing more than 50% in most series. Teratomas are next most common, representing 15% to 20% of intracranial germ cell tumors, followed by small numbers of endodermal sinus or yolk sac tumors, choriocarcinoma, and embryonal cell carcinoma, each of which contributes 3.5%, with the remaining 10% to 15% comprising germ cell tumors of mixed histology (Fig. 34-3).[15]

The histogenesis of intracranial germ cell tumors is unknown. It is hypothesized that primitive cells, which have already begun germ cell development along the urogenital ridge, are accidentally enfolded into the neural tube and subsequently become neoplastic.[18] Earlier and less differentiated embryonic germ cells may give rise to biologically more aggressive tumors. Why does this development of germ cell neoplasms occur specifically and most commonly in the pineal region and secondarily in the hypothalamic pituitary region? Although undoubtedly multifactorial, with some genetic factors playing a role, the production and storage of pineal melatonin and hypothalamic gonadotrophins in these regions is believed likely to play some role in their pathogenesis.[15]

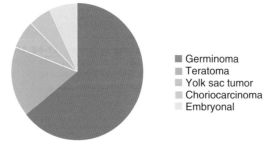

■ FIGURE 34-3 Relative proportions of different types of intracranial germ cell tumors from the Armed Forces Institute of Pathology.

Pineal parenchymal tumors comprise slightly less than a third of total pineal region masses and are divided between pineocytomas, 40%; pineoblastomas, 30%; and the rest with mixed pineoblastoma/pineocytoma histology. Pineal parenchymal tumors have an average age at onset somewhat later than germ cell tumors, with 22 years for pineoblastoma, 32 years for pineocytomas, and 36 years for mixed lesions.[17]

The majority of pineal parenchymal tumors are sporadic; however, some pineoblastomas occur in patients with a mutation in the *RB1* (retinoblastoma) gene. This association has given rise to the term *trilateral retinoblastoma,* referring to patients who have retinoblastomas in both eyes and also pineoblastoma. In general, in these patients the pineoblastoma develops approximately 24 months after diagnosis of the retinoblastoma.

Astrocytomas are uncommon tumors of the pineal region that typically arise from the tectum of the midbrain and secondarily involve the gland. Rare examples of true primary pineal astrocytomas and gangliogliomas arising from pineal glial and neuronal elements have been reported. Meningiomas may also arise in the pineal region and are referred to as falcotentorial meningiomas because they arise near the confluence of the falx cerebri and the tentorium cerebelli.

Non-neoplastic masses or cysts that affect the pineal gland include symptomatic pineal cysts, epidermoids, and the cavum velum interpositum, which, if large, may impinge on the pineal region. The medial diverticulum of the lateral ventricle is an uncommon cystic-appearing lesion that occurs in patients with severe hydrocephalus. Under great pressure, the lateral ventricle may rupture through the fornix, which forms its medial and weakest wall, creating a cystic mass in the pineal region. In childhood and infancy, the vein of Galen aneurysm may present in the pineal region. Dural-based processes such as lymphomas and other tumors of hematopoietic origin as well as uncommon lesions such as amyloidomas rarely present in the pineal region.

Clinical Presentation

Clinically, pineal region tumors or masses may present as a variety of signs and symptoms due to mass effect on adjacent structures. One common manifestation of pineal region masses is Parinaud's syndrome, first described by Henri Parinaud, an ophthalmologist working with Jean-Martin Charcot in Paris in the late 1800s. This syndrome is also referred to as pretectal syndrome, dorsal midbrain syndrome, and other less common eponyms. It is produced by downward mass effect of the pineal region on the tectum of the midbrain, which produces a variety of neuro-ophthalmologic symptoms due to oculomotor tracts passing through this region. Common symptoms include paralysis or paresis of upward gaze from impingement on the rostral medial longitudinal fasciculus and/or posterior commissure, eyelid retraction (Collier's syndrome) possibly resulting from excess superior rectus innervation, and levator palpebrae innervation, convergence retraction nystagmus, and impaired pupillary reaction to light sometimes with sparing of near light reactivity. Other less common findings include intermittent esotropia due to pseudoabducens palsy and convergence and accommodation insufficiency.[19]

In addition to neuro-ophthalmologic manifestations, generalized signs of increased intracranial pressure and hydrocephalus may be present due to obstruction of the aqueduct of Sylvius. These include headache, syncope, and other generalized symptoms. Mass effect on or invasion of the hypothalamic pituitary axis or impingement on the pineal gland itself may disrupt the normal regulation of melatonin production and secretion, producing precocious puberty, diabetes insipidus, and other endocrinopathies. Precocious puberty, in particular, is more commonly associated with germinomas and other germ cell tumors; this may be due to decreased circulating melatonin

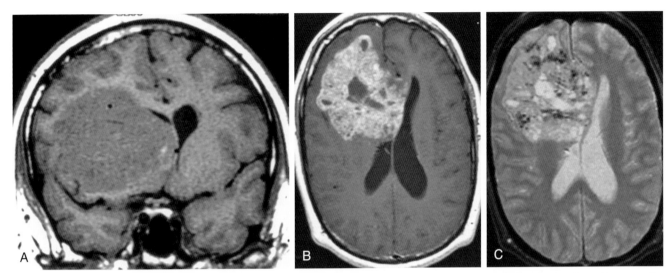

■ **FIGURE 34-4** Hemispheric germinoma in a 37-year-old man. The majority of intracranial germinomas occur in the pineal region, with a secondary locus in the pituitary hypothalamic region. A very small percentage, less than 5% of the total, occurs in other locations, including the skull base and within the cerebral hemispheres, as in this case. On coronal precontrast (**A**), axial postcontrast (**B**), and axial T2W (**C**) MR images there is a large, complex, solid and fluid mass with mass effect on the frontal horns and dense enhancement of the solid components. This imaging appearance is relatively nonspecific but on pathologic examination displayed typical histology for germinoma.

as well as increased gonadotropins such as human chorionic gonadotropin (hCG) secreted by the tumor.

GERMINOMA

Germinomas are intracranial tumors of germ cell origin. They are exquisitely radiosensitive neoplasms, with up to 80% to 90% curable by radiation therapy alone.[20] Therefore, noninvasive diagnosis, through a combination of imaging and serum and CSF analysis accompanied by clinical evaluation, is of vital importance. If noninvasive evaluation is not definitive, and tissue diagnosis is required, ventriculoscopy may provide a less invasive biopsy approach. This technique has been shown to provide adequate tissue sampling and allows for placement of a definitive ventriculostomy for treating hydrocephalus and even tumor debulking.

The term *pinealoma* is no longer used for this tumor because it was also applied to pineal parenchymal tumors in the older literature.

Epidemiology

Germinoma is the most common type of intracranial germ cell tumor, representing 50% to 60% in most series. These are usually midline tumors, with approximately 80% of germinomas arising in the pineal region and most of the remaining examples in the suprasellar or parasellar regions. Only rarely do they present elsewhere in the brain.[21] The average age at presentation is 11 years, and in the pineal region there is a marked male predominance. The male-to-female ratio of pineal region germinomas is approximately 2.5:1 overall, although much higher percentages of up to 4 to 5:1 or more have been reported in the Japanese population. In the United States, the incidence is estimated at 0.1 per 100,000/year,[22] whereas this may be twice as high in Japan. Significant differences in the incidence of pure germinomas have been reported in several large studies, with the greatest incidence reported in Japan, Korea, and the Republic of China.[23]

There is an increased incidence of germinomas and, to a lesser extent, other germ cell tumors in patients with Klinefelter's syndrome. This condition is characterized by an XXY karyotype and elevated gonadotrophic hormones, which may play a pathogenetic role in stimulating germ cell tumors.

Germinomas also have an increased frequency in patients with trisomy 21 (Down syndrome), although the causal mechanism is unknown. There is also a slight increase in germinomas in first-degree relatives of patients with a germ cell tumor, perhaps reflecting the presence of a shared pro-oncogene.

As noted, 10% to 20% of germinomas arise in the sellar region, and in this location there is no clear male predominance. Various studies have reported either an equal male-to-female ratio or a slight female predominance. In addition, a small number of germinomas are found scattered elsewhere throughout the neuraxis (Fig. 34-4).

Clinical Presentation

Germinomas may present with nonspecific signs such as headache, nausea, vomiting, and visual changes. In the case of sellar region tumors, visual changes may be due to invasion and mass effect on the optic chiasm. Parinaud's syndrome, characterized by paralysis of upward gaze, retraction nystagmus, and other visual signs results from mass effect on the midbrain tectum. An associated finding, hydrocephalus, may result from compression of the aqueduct of Sylvius.

Some patients may exhibit endocrinologic disturbance such as precocious puberty that may be due to suppression of melatonin but may also be secondary to direct release of hormones such as β-hCG by neoplastic cells. Precocious puberty occurs primarily in boys, with only a few rare cases in girls.

Diabetes insipidus may occur due to extension and impingement on the hypothalamic region and pituitary stalk, resulting in suppression of arginine vasopressin, also known as antidiuretic hormone. Increased serum and CSF levels of placental alkaline phosphatase (PLAP), β-hCG, and α-fetoprotein (AFP) are frequently present in blood and in CSF and serve as diagnostic markers and prognostic indicators.[24]

Less commonly with germinomas—compared with other germ cell tumors—hemorrhage may occur, resulting in pineal apoplexy.

Pathophysiology

The reader is referred to the general discussion of intracranial germ cell tumors at the beginning of this chapter.

Pathology

Pathologically, germinomas are typically firm, well-circumscribed solid masses that are whitish or tan (Fig. 34-5). Fluid ("cystic")

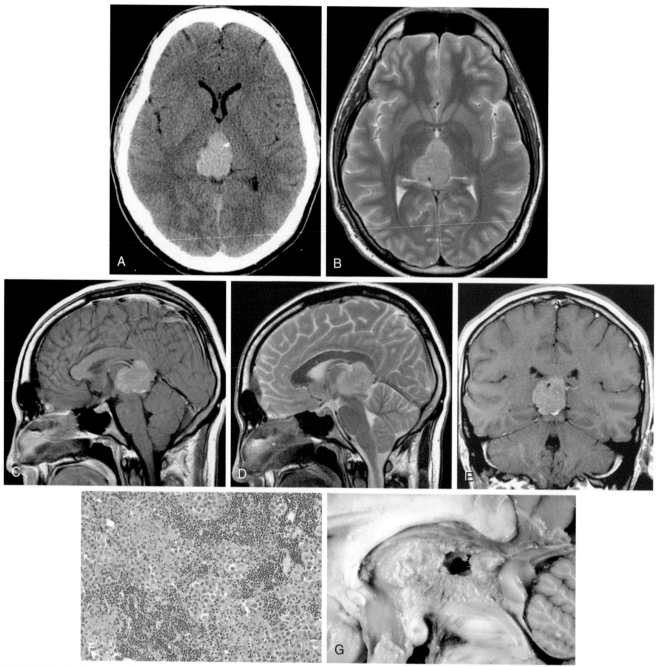

■ **FIGURE 34-5**   Pineal germinoma. A rounded but slightly lobular mass is shown that is hyperdense on noncontrast CT, with diffuse moderate homogeneous signal intensity and enhancement on MRI. **A,** CT image without contrast. **B,** Axial T2W MR image. **C,** Sagittal T1W MR image after gadolinium administration. **D,** Sagittal T2W MR image. **E,** Coronal T1W MR image after gadolinium administration. **F,** Histologic preparation shows typical biphasic histology of round mononuclear tumor cells engulfed in an inflammatory response consisting mainly of small lymphocytes, primarily both helper and killer T cells. **G,** Gross anatomic specimen shows relative location to brain stem and corpus callosum.

regions are seen in up to one third of cases, particularly in larger tumors. Germinomas, although usually round when small, preferentially grow in several directions, including inferiorly and posteriorly into the posterior fossa, superiorly and anteriorly into the third ventricle, and anteriorly and inferiorly into the hypothalamic, chiasmatic, and suprasellar regions.

CSF dissemination may affect the adjacent margins of the tentorium and/or the suprasellar cistern and hypothalamus.

Histologically, pure germinomas are composed of germ cells intermixed with reactive lymphocytes arranged in sheets or lobules and embedded in a fibrovascular stroma. Germ cells are recognized by their large size, abundant clear or pink cytoplasm,

and vesicular nuclei with prominent eosinophilic nucleoli. A small percentage, perhaps 5%, may contain admixed syncytiotrophoblastic giant cells. These tumors show an increased rate of recurrence and decreased long-term survival.

Germinomas may also coexist with other types of germ cell elements to a varying degree. In cases where en bloc resection is incomplete; the exact breakdown of mixed cell versus pure germinomas remains an approximation.

The lymphocytic component is primarily T cell, including both helper and suppressor subtypes (see Fig. 34-5).

Immunohistochemical analysis shows OCT4 reactivity as the most helpful marker, followed by CD117 and PLAP.[25]

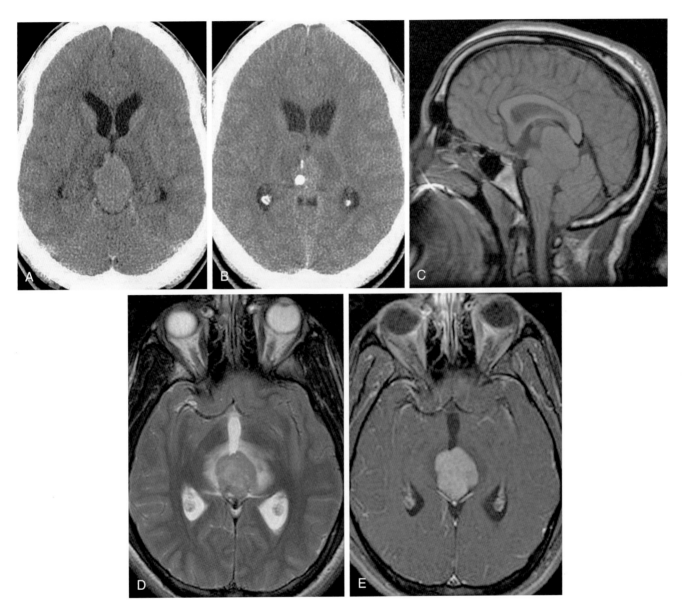

■ **FIGURE 34-6** Germinoma. On initial CT (**A, B**) there is a soft tissue mass surrounding and engulfing a coarse chunk of calcification. This pattern is considered typical for germinoma, which arises outside the densely calcified pineal parenchyma. **C,** Sagittal precontrast T1W MR image shows mass effect with inferior cerebellar tonsillar excursion through the foramen magnum. **D,** Axial T2W MR image shows the mass with surrounding edema. **E,** On postcontrast T1W MRI there is dense uniform enhancement. Note that the calcification clearly seen on CT is not detected by MRI.

Imaging

CT

On CT, the typical appearance of a germinoma is that of a hyper-attenuating mass in the pineal region that typically surrounds or "engulfs" the gland and any pineal calcification that is present (Fig. 34-6). Cysts are present in a third to a half of cases and are more clearly observed in larger tumors (Fig. 34-7). Dense uniform enhancement of the solid component is typical.[26]

MRI

On MRI, germinomas are typically homogeneous or partially "cystic" with signal intensity isointense to white matter on T1-weighted (T1W) images and slightly hyperintense on T2-weighted (T2W) images. After gadolinium administration, dense homogeneous enhancement is seen. Hemorrhage is uncommon in germinoma, as compared with other germ cell tumors.[27] Because any CSF dissemination must be detected, post-contrast imaging of the entire neuraxis is mandated once a primary tumor is discovered. Direct extension, either into the

posterior fossa, the third ventricle, or the hypothalamic pituitary region, may also be seen, particularly with larger tumors.

TERATOMA

A teratoma is a germ cell tumor composed of tissues representing two or three of the primary germ cell layers (i.e., endoderm, mesoderm, and ectoderm). Mature teratomas consist of cells that have reached an adult level of differentiation. Immature teratomas are composed, either completely or partially, of primitive incompletely differentiated cells. The term *malignant teratoma* refers to a neoplasm that develops from one of the mature germ cell components, such as a "signet cell" adenocarcinoma in an area of intestinal differentiation. This is also referred to as a somatic type malignant transformation.

Epidemiology

Teratoma is the second most common intracranial germ cell tumor, representing 15% to 20% of all intracranial germ cell tumors in most series. Teratomas are subcategorized as mature,

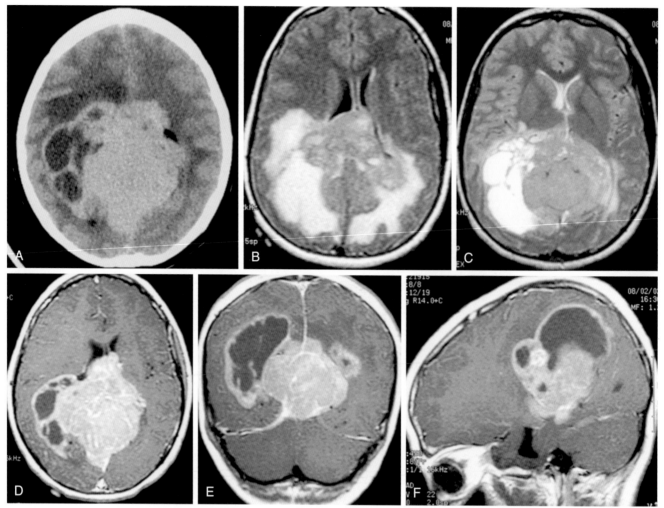

■ **FIGURE 34-7**   Large solid and cystic mass roughly centered on the pineal region in a 16-year-old boy. Selected images show irregular solid components that are hyperdense on noncontrast CT and relatively homogeneous in signal intensity and enhancement on MRI, with large cystic or fluid regions surrounded by enhancing capsule. **A,** Noncontrast CT image. **B,** Axial FLAIR MR image. **C,** Axial T2W MR image. **D to F,** Axial, coronal, and sagittal T1W MR images after administration of gadolinium.

immature, and malignant. Mature teratomas are most common, accounting for two thirds of all types, followed by immature teratomas. Malignant degeneration in a mature teratoma occurs much less commonly. Average age at diagnosis of a teratoma is 5 years, with a significant number presenting in the first year of life, or even on prenatal imaging studies such as ultrasonography or fetal MRI (Figs. 34-8 to 34-10). Teratomas are the most common intracranial tumor detected on prenatal imaging, either ultrasonography or fetal MRI. As with other germ cell tumors, there is a male predilection and the incidence is slightly higher in Japan, Korea, and the Republic of China.

Clinical Presentation
Clinical features are similar to those of germinomas and other pineal region masses as discussed earlier. One unique presentation is that of marked neonatal hydrocephalus.

Pathophysiology
The reader is referred to the general discussion of intracranial germ cell tumors at the beginning of this chapter.

Pathology
On gross examination a teratoma may exhibit heterogeneity both in morphology and also in tissue type. Solid cystic,

glandular, cartilaginous, and calcified elements may be present and visible, particularly in mature teratomas.

On pathologic examination, mature teratomas in the pineal region exhibit features similar to those found elsewhere in the body (Fig. 34-11). The tumors are frequently lobulated and complex or multiloculated and may be quite large. Representative areas of disorganized tissue from the three embryologic strata are sometimes seen with more completely developed visceral or skeletal structures. The presence of clumps of hair and sebaceous elements is not uncommon. Areas of less developed embryonal tissue may be evident.

Immature teratomas, the second most common intracranial variety, are characterized by poorly differentiated embryonal tissue, most commonly neuroepithelial, but they may also be related to other primitive germ layers. Immature teratomas have a higher incidence of CSF dissemination and local recurrence when excised, which contribute to their generally poorer prognosis. Their imaging and gross pathologic appearance is less characteristic than tumors with more differentiated embryonal tissue (Fig. 34-12).

Malignant teratoma is the least common variety of teratoma. This term refers to malignant degeneration of mature adult tissue types within the teratoma. An example would be adenocarcinoma arising from mature gastrointestinal or renal cells within a

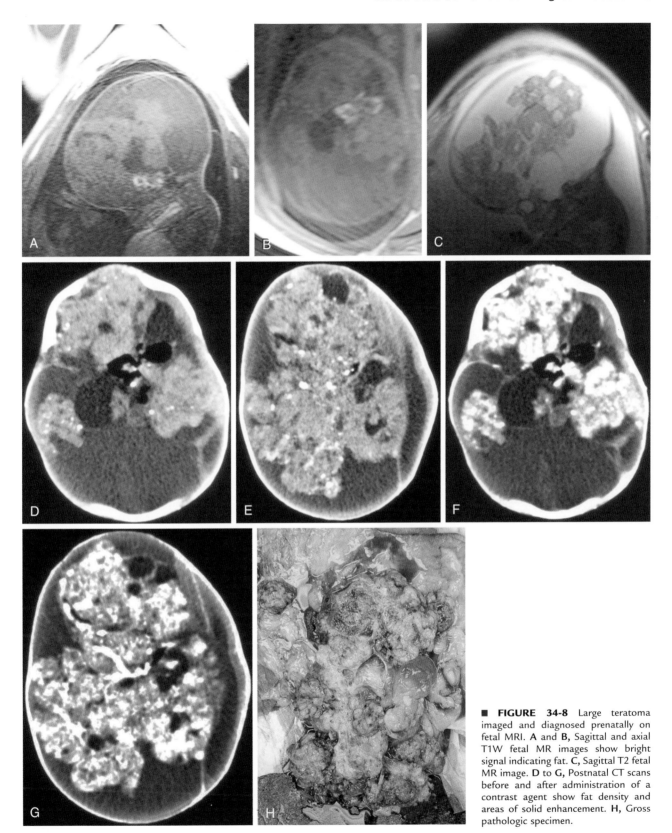

■ **FIGURE 34-8** Large teratoma imaged and diagnosed prenatally on fetal MRI. **A** and **B,** Sagittal and axial T1W fetal MR images show bright signal indicating fat. **C,** Sagittal T2 fetal MR image. **D** to **G,** Postnatal CT scans before and after administration of a contrast agent show fat density and areas of solid enhancement. **H,** Gross pathologic specimen.

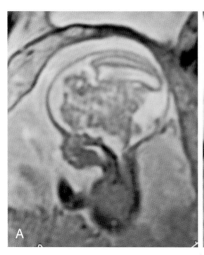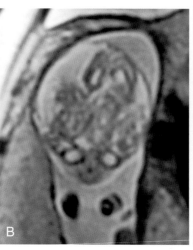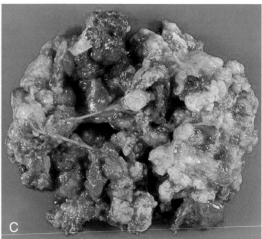

■ **FIGURE 34-9** Teratoma. Intrauterine fetal sagittal **(A)** and coronal **(B)** T2W MR image shows hydrocephalus and a large irregular central mass. Subsequent pathologic evaluation provides a diagnosis of teratoma. **C,** Gross pathologic specimen.

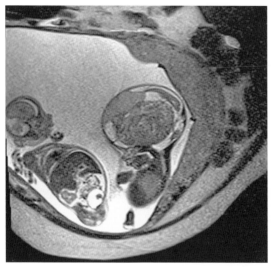

■ **FIGURE 34-10** Teratoma in twin gestation. Sagittal T2W fetal MR image shows hydrocephalus and large complex intracranial mass in twin A and no obvious abnormality on partially seen twin B. *(Case courtesy of Erin Simon Schwartz, MD.)*

teratoma. These secondary tumors may metastasize or recur locally and, although uncommon, are associated with a poorer prognosis.[15,28]

Imaging

Ultrasonography

On fetal ultrasonography, teratomas may display hydrocephalus and a large complex, centrally located mass consisting of solid cystic, fatty, and calcified elements.

Radiography

On plain radiographs, coarse irregular calcifications may be seen as well as a calcific structure such as a tooth or a bone (Fig. 34-13).

CT

CT examination may display a heterogeneous mass with attenuation characteristics typical for the wide variety of tissue types, including bone, fat, and soft tissue. Occasionally, partially formed

or completely formed organs or other somatic structures such as teeth are seen. The presence of small areas of lipid attenuation within a complex pineal region mass is virtually pathognomonic for a teratoma.

MRI

Similar to CT but in greater detail, MRI examination may reveal complex heterogeneous features such as fat, cartilage, bone, and incompletely formed tissues. Like on CT, the presence of small areas of lipid signal in a complex pineal region mass is virtually pathognomonic for a teratoma. If there is rupture of a compartment containing lipid a "fat-fluid level" may be seen in the ventricles (Fig. 34-14).

ENDODERMAL SINUS TUMOR

Intracranial endodermal sinus tumor is a rare highly malignant germ cell tumor, representing the malignant degeneration of cells related to the primitive yolk sac or endodermal sinus. Alternate names include yolk sac tumor, extragonadal yolk sac tumor, and nongerminomatous germ cell tumor.

Epidemiology

Endodermal sinus tumor represents 5% to 7% of intracranial germ cell tumors, with an average age at diagnosis of 14 years. Fifty percent of intracranial endodermal sinus tumors arise in the pineal region, with scattered cases occurring elsewhere. There is a male predominance of approximately 2:1. These tumors may present as hydrocephalus, hemorrhage, or mass effect. AFP is typically elevated in the CSF and serum.

Clinical Presentation

The clinical features are similar to those of other pineal region masses.

Pathophysiology

Like the other intracranial germ cell tumors, these tumors arise from primitive neoplastic germ cells that either migrate to the CNS, are abnormally enfolded into the neural tube during early embryonic life, or develop from pluripotential stem cells within the CNS.

Histologically, endodermal sinus tumor displays cuboidal to columnar epithelial cells arrayed in sheets, cords, tubules, and/or papillary projections fed by delicate fibrovascular stroma. Schiller-Duval bodies are perivascular epithelial-lined spaces

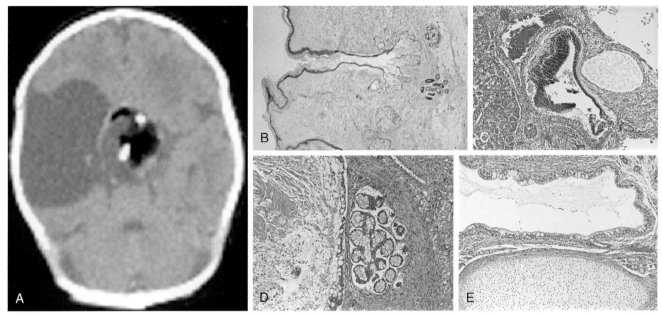

■ **FIGURE 34-11**   Mature teratoma. **A,** On CT scan the diagnosis of teratoma is virtually certain owing to the presence of fat, dense calcification, and solid tissues in a pineal region mass. Histologic preparations from this tumor reveal mature tissues of mature teratoma: sebaceous gland (**B**), primitive retina (**C**), primitive gut (**D**), and primitive lung (**E**).

with an outer layer of tumor cells. Another typical morphologic feature is the pseudoglandular structure composed of neoplastic cells with a prominent Golgi apparatus and endoplasmic reticulum. Laboratory studies reveal periodic acid–Schiff (PAS)-positive cytoplasmic bodies and AFP-reactive stromal globules. Positive immunoreactivity for AFP is characteristic for endodermal sinus tumors and also for the endodermal sinus tumor constituents of mixed germ cell neoplasms. This not surprising because AFP is directly synthesized by primitive yolk sac cells.[15,28]

Imaging
CT

CT displays a pineal region mass that is primarily somewhat hyperdense to brain. The mass may be heterogeneous and occasionally exhibits hemorrhage (Fig. 34-15).

MRI

Endodermal sinus tumors frequently demonstrate heterogeneous signal on MRI owing to hemorrhage and/or areas of necrosis. On postcontrast images, dense but occasionally heterogeneous enhancement is seen.

EMBRYONAL CARCINOMA

Embryonal carcinoma is a highly malignant tumor believed to be derived from primitive embryonic germ cells or pluripotential stem cells. It can be referred to as a nongerminomatous germ cell tumor or a malignant germ cell tumor.

Epidemiology

Embryonal carcinoma represents approximately 5% or less of all intracranial germ cell tumors. It has the oldest average age at onset (17 years) of all germ cell tumors. It is more common in males, and there is a slightly higher incidence reported in Far East Asian populations.

Clinical Presentation

Clinical presentation may be due to mass effect, hydrocephalus, or, less commonly, hemorrhage. Elevated serum and CSF levels of hCG are suggestive of this diagnosis.

Pathology

Embryonic carcinoma is a firm, fibrous highly vascular tumor that may be large at presentation and is reported to grow around vascular structures, complicating excision.

Cuboidal to polygonal cells with large vesicular nuclei arranged in sheets, cords, and semiglandular formations are seen on histologic examination. Diffuse cytokeratin reactivity is common, as well as PLAP reactivity with occasional AFP- and hCG-positive cells.[15,28]

Imaging
CT

A heterogeneous, large pineal region mass is seen that is hyperdense on precontrast images with dense but heterogeneous enhancement. The mass may contain cystic regions (Fig. 34-16).

MRI

A large heterogeneous, pineal region mass is evident with dense but heterogeneous enhancement. Cystic regions may be noted.

CHORIOCARCINOMA

Intracranial choriocarcinoma is a rare germ cell tumor composed of neoplastic cells related to gestational trophoblastic tissue. Alternate names include nongerminomatous germ cell tumor and extragonadal choriocarcinoma.

Epidemiology

These tumors represent 3% to 5% of intracranial germ cell tumors and have an average age at diagnosis of 8 years. Surprisingly, there is a male predominance of approximately 2 : 1. Seventy-five percent of intracranial choriocarcinomas arise in the pineal region with secondary sellar or parasellar locations and, rarely, other locations such as basal ganglia and frontoparietal lobes of the cerebral hemispheres.

Clinical Presentation

Clinical presentation may be due to mass effect and hydrocephalus as well as hemorrhage. Hormonal factors may result in

Text continued on page 769

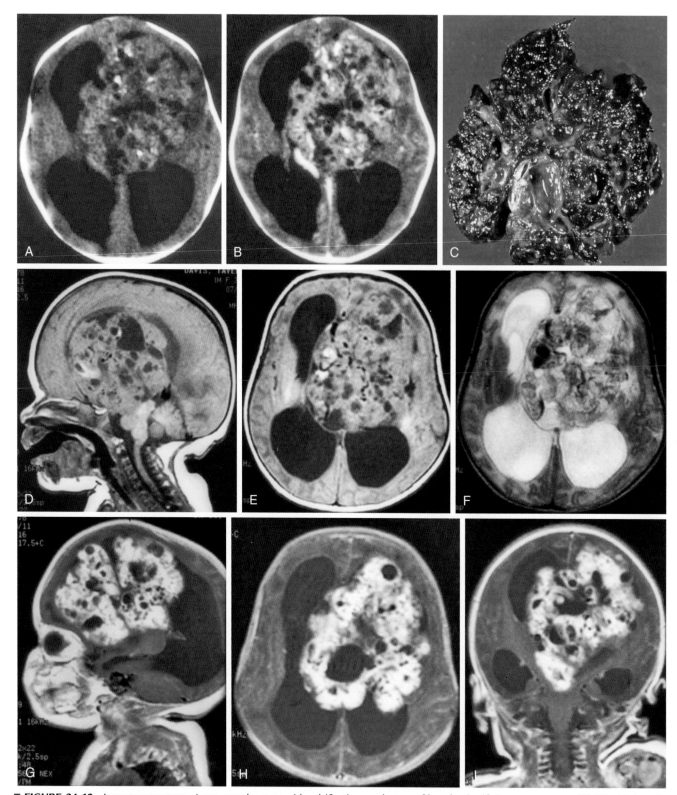

■ **FIGURE 34-12**   Immature teratoma. Large complex mass with calcifications and areas of low density (fat) on noncontrast CT (**A**) with irregular enhancement on postcontrast CT (**B**). Gross pathologic specimen (**C**) shows areas of fat and soft tissue as well as cystic-appearing regions. Sagittal (**D**) and axial (**E**) precontrast T1W MR images, axial T2W (**F**), and postcontrast sagittal (**G**), axial (**H**), and coronal (**I**) images further demonstrate the presence of fatty, soft tissue, and fluid components.

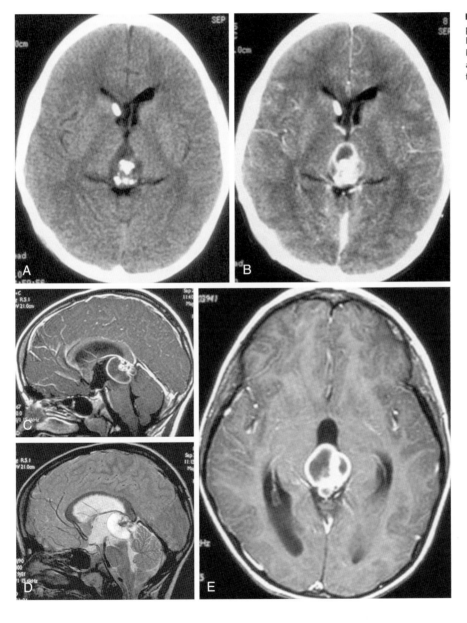

■ **FIGURE 34-13** Mature teratoma. Initial precontrast CT (**A**) shows coarse calcifications. Postcontrast CT (**B**) shows partial enhancement. Postcontrast sagittal T1W (**C**), sagittal T2W (**D**), and axial T1W (**E**) images show the solid and fluid components of this mature teratoma.

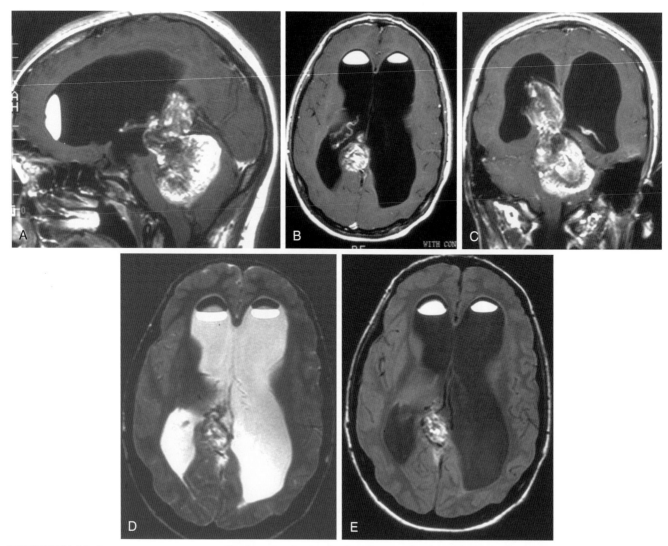

■ **FIGURE 34-14**   Large mature teratoma extending from the pineal region into the posterior fossa. There is rupture and fat-fluid level in the frontal horns with prominent chemical shift artifact. The images displayed include postcontrast sagittal (**A**), axial (**B**), and coronal (**C**) T1W MR images and axial T2W (**D**) and axial FLAIR (**E**) images.

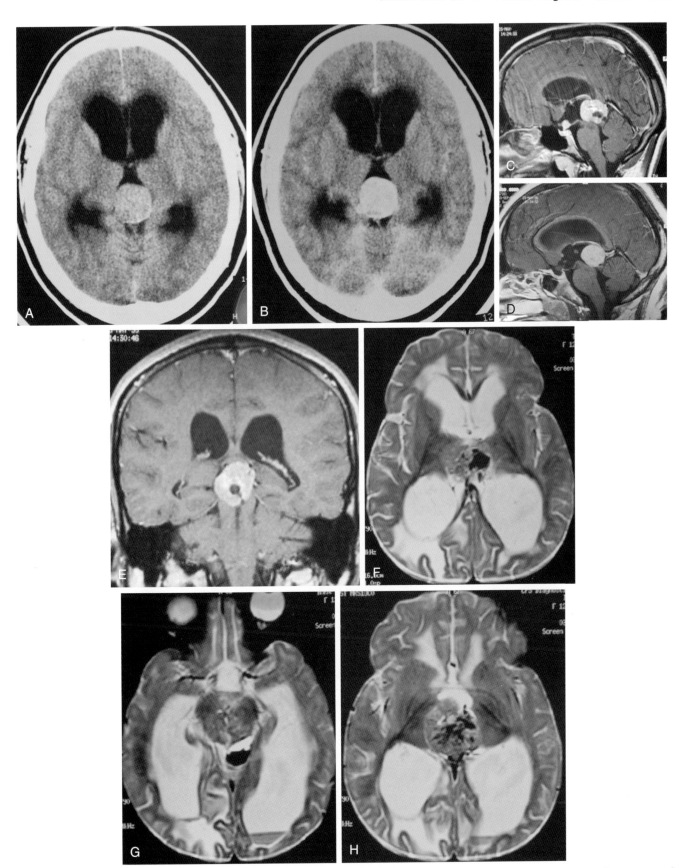

■ **FIGURE 34-15** **A** to **H,** Endodermal sinus or yolk sac tumor in two different patients. This rare neoplasm comprises only a small percentage of intracranial nongerminomatous germ cell tumors and is histologically identical to the tumor of the same name, also rare, that is more commonly found in the pelvis. **A-D,** In the first patient, precontrast (**A**) and postcontrast (**B**) CT scans and postcontrast sagittal MR image (**C**) show slight heterogeneity without definite overt hemorrhage, although intratumoral hemorrhage was documented pathologically. **E-H,** In the second patient, sagittal (**D**) and coronal (**E**) postcontrast T1W MR images and axial T2W (**F** to **H**) MR images demonstrate focal low signal intensity seen within the tumor that was confirmed to be hemorrhagic pathologically. There is a small fluid-fluid level in the occipital horns on the T2W images indicating some extratumoral hemorrhage has occurred and extended into the ventricles, possibly via the choroidal fissures.

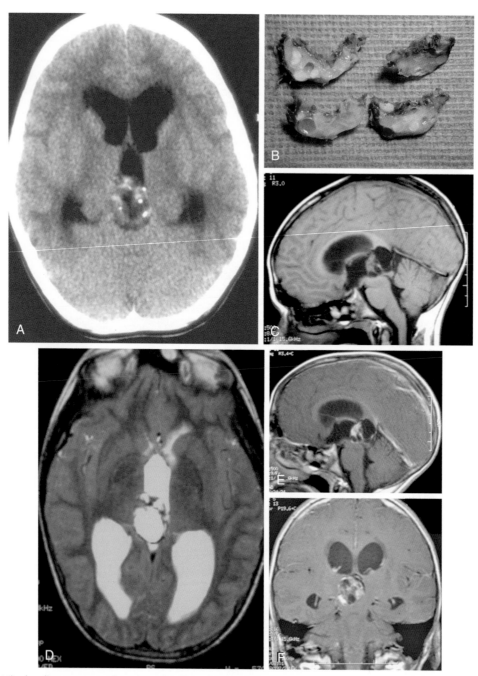

■ **FIGURE 34-16**   Mixed malignant germ cell tumor, primarily embryonal carcinoma. Selected images show solid and cystic or necrotic components with heterogeneity and possibly some hemorrhage and/or calcification. **A,** Axial CT scan. **B,** Gross specimen. **C,** Sagittal T1W MR image. **D,** Axial T2W MR image. **E,** Sagittal T1W MR image after administration of gadolinium. **F,** Coronal postcontrast T1W MR image.

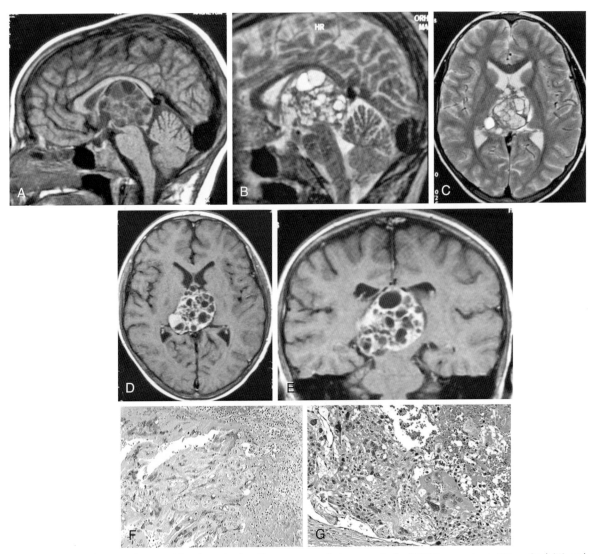

■ FIGURE 34-17 Pineal choriocarcinoma with other mixed malignant germ cell elements. Sagittal T1W noncontrast (**A**), sagittal (**B**) and axial (**C**) T2W, and postcontrast axial (**D**) and coronal (**E**) MR images show a solid and cystic mass in the pineal region that is lobulated but well circumscribed with mass effect but without obvious invasion of adjacent structures. **F** and **G,** Histologic slides stained with hematoxylin and eosin show typical features of choriocarcinoma with large multinucleated syncytiotrophoblasts adjacent to dense clusters of mononuclear cytotrophoblastic cells.

precocious puberty. Elevated serum and CSF levels of hCG, luteinizing hormone, and other hormones may provide diagnostic clues.

Pathophysiology

These tumors more commonly arise in the pelvis from trophoblastic tissue associated with gestation and at other extragonadal sites. Their rare intracranial occurrence is not fully understood, except that they represent a special lineage of germ cell differentiation. Primitive neoplastic germ cells either migrate to the central nervous system or are abnormally enfolded into the neural tube during early embryonic life or develop from pluripotential stem cells within the central nervous system.

Pathology

On gross inspection these tumors are well circumscribed, heterogeneous, and frequently hemorrhagic.

Syncytiotrophoblastic and cytotrophoblastic cells are arranged in bilayered structures interlaced with vascular sinusoids (Fig. 34-17). The syncytiotrophoblastic cells produce hCG. Other cells

are commonly immunoreactive with PLAP and cytokeratin antibody markers.[15,28]

Imaging

MRI

The most likely imaging appearance is a well-circumscribed, irregular or lobulated mass, usually in the pineal region. On CT, and to a greater extent on MRI, there may be heterogeneity, reflecting hemorrhage and possibly areas of necrosis. Calcification is less common (see Fig. 34-17).

PINEOCYTOMA

A pineocytoma is a tumor composed of well-differentiated pineal parenchymal cells, or pineocytes. The term *pinealoma* is no longer used.

Epidemiology

Thirty to 40 percent of all pineal parenchymal tumors are pineocytomas, which means that 10% to 15% of all pineal region tumors are pineocytomas.[16] The average age at presentation is 32 to 44 years, with a wide range in different studies.

■ **FIGURE 34-18** Pineocytoma with hemorrhage, pineal apoplexy. On initial CT scan (**A**) there is a solid mass in the pineal region with a layering fluid compartment extending posteriorly. This appearance is confirmed with precontrast (**B**) and postcontrast (**C**) axial T1W and sagittal postcontrast (**D**) images. The term *pineal apoplexy* can be used to refer to any significant acute hemorrhage in the pineal region and could apply to a tumoral hemorrhage or hemorrhage within a cyst.

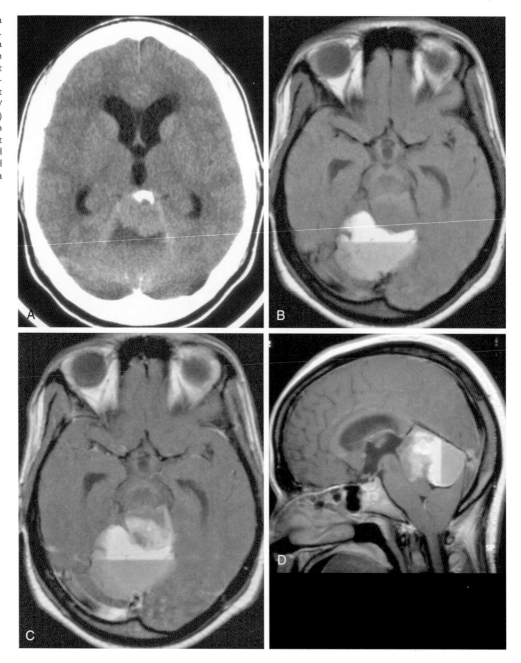

Clinical Presentation

Clinical features are similar to those of other pineal region masses (see earlier). Pineocytomas may present due to mass effect, with either hydrocephalus due to compression of the aqueduct of Sylvius or Parinaud's syndrome from compression of the tectum. Rarely, these tumors present as hemorrhage, resulting in pineal apoplexy (Fig. 34-18). Radiosurgery is increasingly used, with significant success.[29]

Pathophysiology

Genetic alterations include monosomy or loss of chromosome 22, deletions in distal 12q, and loss of chromosome 11. Pineocytomas are sporadic tumors without specific familial or syndromal associations.[15,28]

Pathology

Neoplastic cells surround irregular, acellular zones to form "pineocytomatous rosettes." In addition, these tumors are recog-

nized by the presence of expanded, irregular lobules, in contrast to the smaller, less cellular and more regular lobules of the gland. Neuronal and photoreceptor proteins are present, including synaptophysin and retinal S-antigen, likely reflecting the phylogenetic precursors of the normal pineocytes.

There is a variant known as pleomorphic pineocytoma, composed of typical areas admixed with large, hyperchromatic cells with pleomorphic nuclei.[15,28]

Imaging

CT

Pineocytomas are often hyperdense on noncontrast CT, are usually round, and may displace or disrupt the compact normal calcifications of the pineal gland (Fig. 34-19). Uniform or variable enhancement may be seen, and cysts may be present. Occasionally, the preexisting pineal calcification may be dispersed in a rim around the tumor—the "exploded pineal" sign.[30]

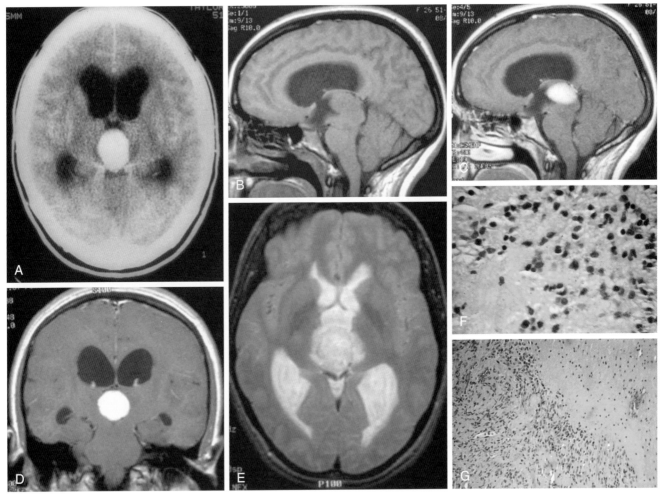

■ **FIGURE 34-19** Pineocytoma in a 26-year-old woman. Relatively nonspecific imaging features are displayed in this typical example of a rounded homogeneous and homogeneously enhancing pineal mass causing hydrocephalus. Axial postcontrast CT (**A**), sagittal precontrast (**B**) and postcontrast (**C**) T1W MR images, coronal postcontrast T1W (**D**) image, and axial T2W (**E**) image. Typical histologic features are seen on high- (**F**) and low- (**G**) power hematoxylin and eosin preparations.

MRI

On MRI, pineocytomas are usually hypointense on T1W images and hyperintense on T2W images with diffuse but heterogeneous enhancement (see Fig. 34-19). Hemorrhage may occur but is uncommon.[30]

PINEOBLASTOMA

Pineoblastoma is a primitive neuroectodermal tumor (PNET) related to medulloblastoma and other PNETs with unique features related to its cell of origin. It can be referred to as a primitive neuroectodermal tumor of the pineal region, trilateral retinoblastoma.

Epidemiology

As expected for an embryonic neoplasm, pineoblastomas occur in a younger age group than pineocytomas, with an average age at onset of 18.5 to 22 years in different series. The majority of cases are sporadic; however, some cases occur in patients with a mutation in the *RB* gene and either have a personal or family history of retinoblastoma. This association has given rise to the term *trilateral retinoblastoma*. These patients may have retinoblastomas in both eyes and an intracranial pineal region pineoblastoma. In the group with this *RB* mutation, pineoblastoma usually develops approximately 24 months after diagnosis of the retinoblastoma. The trilateral retinoblastoma syndrome is rare

but important and underscores the similarity between the retinal and pineal cell lines of differentiation (Fig. 34-20).

Clinical Presentation

Pineoblastomas may present as headache, nausea and vomiting, ataxia, and/or other generalized signs of increased intracranial pressure and hydrocephalus (see earlier). Bilateral papilledema has been reported in up to one third of cases.

Pathophysiology

A wide variety of genetic abnormalities have been identified in patients with pineoblastoma. As mentioned earlier, mutation in the *RB* gene accounts for a small number of cases. In addition, loss of chromosome 20 and rearrangements in chromosomes 1p and 1q have been reported. Similar to infratentorial PNET or medulloblastoma, unbalanced gain in 17q, deletions in 9q, 11q, and 16q, and monosomy 22 have been described, suggesting a common genetic pathway.

Pathology

Pineoblastomas may be somewhat more irregular than pineocytomas and may display evidence of brain invasion and/or CSF dissemination (Fig. 34-21). The CSF dissemination may be seen either as a gross infiltrating thickening of the leptomeninges or as fine nodular deposits (Fig. 34-22).[31]

■ **FIGURE 34-20** Pineoblastoma, trilateral retinoblastoma. This child had previously been diagnosed with bilateral retinoblastomas and was subsequently found to have this large pineal region tumor, which was subsequently shown to be a pineoblastoma. The pineoblastoma occurrence after bilateral retino-blastomas is referred to as trilateral retinoblastoma owing to the common cellular heritage of the two tumors and is associated with muta-tion of the retinoblastoma (*RB*) gene locus. **A,** Sagittal T1W MR image after administration of gado-linium shows a large, enhancing pineal region mass with some prob-able leptomeningeal spread to the posterior falx cerebri. Examples of bilateral retinoblastoma in different patients: CT scan (**B**) and gross specimens (**C**).

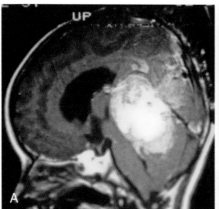
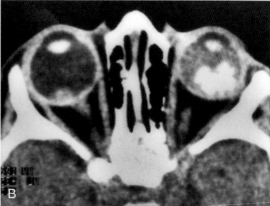
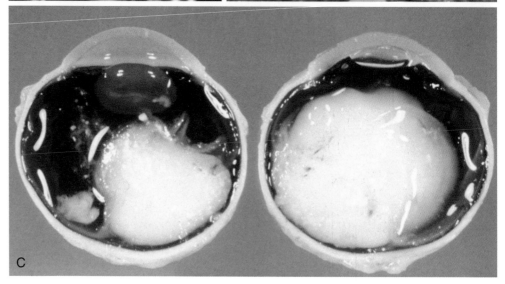

Pineoblastomas are densely cellular neoplasms composed pri-marily of small round cells with prominent nuclei and sparse cytoplasm. Mitoses and necrosis are usually present. Occasion-ally, either Homer-Wright or Flexner-Wintersteiner rosettes are observed.

On electron microscopy, pineoblastomas are composed of poorly differentiated neuroectodermal cells with few distinctive ultrastructural features.

Immunohistochemical reactivity for neuron-specific enolase and synaptophysin reflect neuroectodermal origins.[15,28]

Melanin pigment and occasionally mesenchymal elements are rarely present in pineoblastoma (Fig. 34-23).

Imaging

CT

On CT, pineoblastoma is typically a rounded and/or lobulated hyperdense mass centered in the pineal region. Calcification within the pineal gland may be forced outward by the growing mass, creating an "exploded" pattern of calcifications rather than a dense cluster noted in the normal gland or tumors that arise outside the gland. On postcontrast CT, dense homogeneous enhancement is typical. Cysts and, less commonly, areas of hem-orrhage are occasionally present.[30]

MRI

Pineoblastomas are isointense or slightly hyperintense to brain parenchyma on T2W images, and dense, homogeneous enhance-ment is seen. Heterogeneous signal and enhancement is present

in approximately one third of cases (Fig. 34-24). If the tumor is large, a more aggressive appearance may be seen, with invasion of adjacent structures.

Moderate to severe hydrocephalus is common, owing to com-pression of the aqueduct of Sylvius (Fig. 34-25).

Pineoblastomas may display CSF dissemination with spread to the third ventricle, the subarachnoid space, and the leptomen-inges of brain and spinal cord. Postcontrast imaging of the entire neuraxis is needed to exclude distant metastases.

PINEAL CYST

This benign fluid-filled cyst occurs within the pineal gland.

Epidemiology

Pineal cysts are a common incidental finding on MRI and at autopsy. They are typically diagnosed in young adults and are slightly more common in women than men. Recent high-resolu-tion MRI documents the prevalence of pineal cysts in healthy adults at 23%. Autopsy studies have suggested a prevalence of up to 40%.

Clinical Presentation

Usually incidental, these cysts may present as symptoms due to mass effect and hydrocephalus, such as headaches and visual changes (Fig. 34-26).

Rarely, spontaneous hemorrhage may occur into a pineal cyst, giving rise to acute symptoms of headache. This event has been termed *pineal apoplexy.*

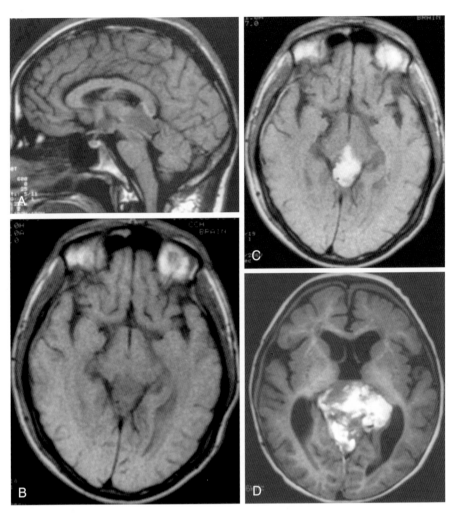

FIGURE 34-21 Two different examples of pineoblastoma with brain invasion. In the first case, shown on sagittal T1W (**A**), axial T1W precontrast (**B**), and axial T1W postcontrast (**C**) MR images, there is direct invasion of the brain stem by a relatively small primary tumor. In the second case (**D**) there is a larger heterogeneous mass that extends outward, causing hydrocephalus with invasion of at least the medial occipital lobe.

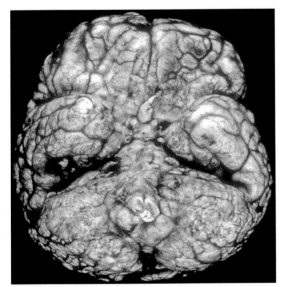

FIGURE 34-22 Pineoblastoma. Autopsy photograph shows extensive leptomeningeal spread on the undersurface of the brain centered in the pineal region.

Pathophysiology

The exact etiology of pineal cysts is unknown; however, they most likely represent cystic degeneration within the pineal gland beginning after sexual maturation. Death of pineal parenchymal cells leaves the glial structural elements that form the cyst walls (Fig. 34-27). Exact molecular triggers of pineal apoptosis that lead to cyst formation are not known.

The wall of a pineal cyst comprises three components: an inner gliotic layer, which may contain Rosenthal fibers and chronic blood products; a middle layer composed of pineal parenchymal cells; and an outer fibrous leptomeningeal layer.[28] This structure suggests that the cyst is formed when pineal cells become apoptotic within their lobular glial network.

The cyst fluid is proteinaceous and may contain varying amounts of chronic blood products.

Imaging
CT

On CT images, a pineal cyst usually measures between 0.5 and 3 cm and exhibits water attenuation; it has a thin regular wall. No enhancement will be seen other than in the wall of the cyst (< 2 mm) and the normal enhancement of the adjacent normal pineal parenchyma.

MRI

On MRI, a pineal cyst will follow fluid signal intensity on all sequences. On fluid-attenuated inversion recovery (FLAIR)

■ **FIGURE   34-23** Melanotic pineal PNET or pineoblastoma is a rare subtype of pineoblastoma. This example shows relatively nonspecific imaging features; however, there is some high T1 and low T2 signal suggesting the paramagnetic effects of melanin. **A,** Sagittal T1W MRI without gadolinium. Sagittal (**B**) and axial (**C**) T2W MR images. **D,** Gross autopsy specimen shows focal areas of purplish melanotic discoloration.

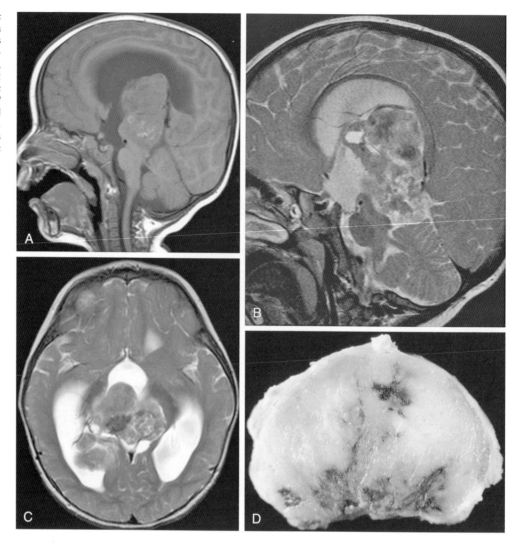

■ **FIGURE   34-24** Pineoblastoma. This pineoblastoma causes mass effect and hydrocephalus in the pineal region and also extends posteriorly into the fourth ventricle. On sagittal T1W MRI before (**A**) and after (**B**) administration of gadolinium there is slight signal heterogeneity centrally and slight nodular enhancement superiorly. This appearance is nonspecific and somewhat atypical for pineoblastoma, which usually enhances homogeneously.

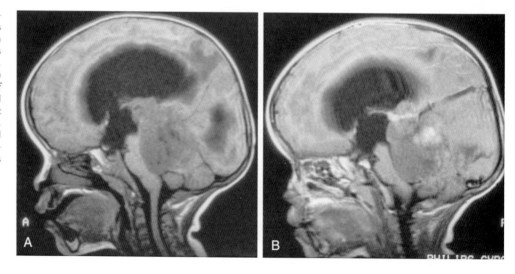

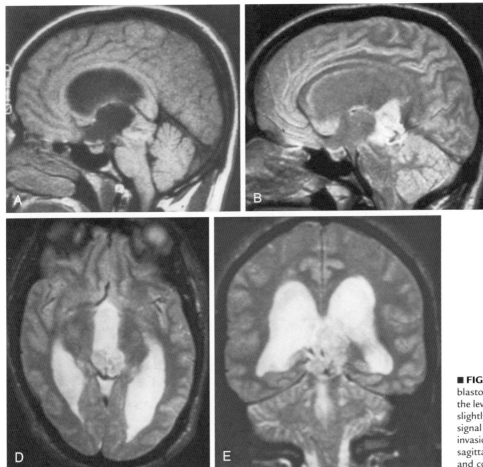

■ **FIGURE 34-25** This relatively small pineoblastoma causes obstructive hydrocephalus at the level of the aqueduct of Sylvius and displays slightly irregular morphology as well as some signal heterogeneity; however, no definite brain invasion is seen. Sagittal T1W precontrast (**A**), sagittal (**B**) and axial FLAIR (**C**), and axial (**D**) and coronal (**E**) T2W MR images are shown.

sequences, the cyst fluid may appear slightly hyperintense owing to proteinaceous material. After contrast administration, the cyst wall may show regular smooth enhancement measuring less than 2 mm in thickness (Fig. 34-28).

In cases of pineal apoplexy, the cyst will display signal intensity that will reflect the state of aging of the blood product, which is initially hyperintense, then hypointense, and then returns to simple fluid signal intensity (see Fig. 34-28).

GLIAL TUMOR OF THE PINEAL REGION
This neoplasm of glial cell origin arises either within the pineal gland itself or, more commonly, from adjacent structures such as the tectum of the midbrain. Other names include, among others, ganglioglioma, choroid plexus papilloma, astrocytoma, and juvenile pilocytic astrocytoma.

Epidemiology
These are uncommon tumors without specific syndromal or familial associations.

Clinical Presentation
Clinical presentation is similar to that seen in other pineal region masses.

Pathology
Glial tumors of the pineal region may display any glial phenotype. Pineal gland gliomas are exceedingly rare, but astrocytomas, gangliogliomas (Fig. 34-29), ependymomas, and choroid plexus neoplasms have been reported. Rather than representing a primary neoplasm, regional astrocytomas—arising in the tectum or elsewhere within the adjacent brain stem—are more likely to impinge on or secondarily invade pineal structures. These regional astrocytomas may be either the diffuse type or the juvenile pilocytic variety (Fig. 34-30). Oligodendrogliomas and at least one reported case of a fibrosarcoma have also been described in the pineal region (Fig. 34-31).

Imaging
The imaging features of different glial tumors of the pineal region will follow imaging features that these varied tumors display elsewhere.

PAPILLARY TUMOR OF THE PINEAL REGION
This is a newly described glial tumor of the pineal region.[32]

Pathophysiology
This glial tumor may be a specialized ependymoma arising from the subcommissural organ (Fig. 34-32).

Pathology
This tumor is characterized histologically by a papillary area consisting of columnar or cuboidal cells with clear cytoplasm and round or infolded nucleus.

Positive immunohistochemistry for cytokeratin and epithelial membrane antigen, vimentin, and neuron-specific enolase are

■ **FIGURE 34-26** A young adult presented with headache and altered mental status. She was found to have a 3-cm pineal cyst with some internal hemorrhage and mild hydrocephalus and was treated by ventriculoscopic drainage. **A,** CT scan. **B,** Sagittal nonenhanced T1W MR image showing intracystic hemorrhage and hydrocephalus. Sagittal T1W (**C**) and T2W (**D**) MR images after ventriculoscopic drainage show partial collapse and normal-sized third ventricle. *(Case courtesy of Alexander Mark, MD.)*

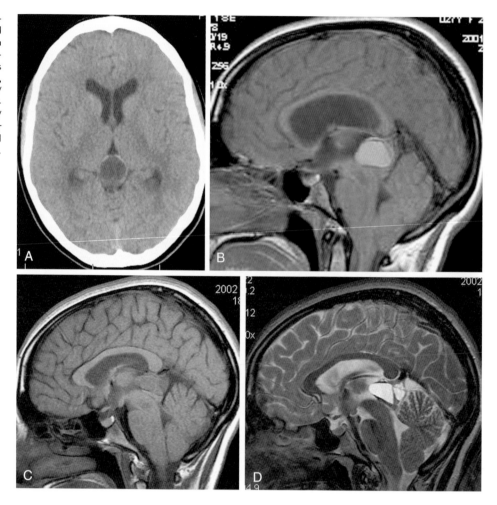

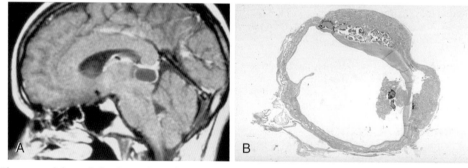

■ **FIGURE 34-27** The exact etiology of pineal cysts is not known, but they may represent the residua of involuting or apoptotic pineal parenchyma within its lobular glial architecture. The typical pineal cyst shows a thin, regular-enhancing rim measuring 1 to 2 mm at most without nodularity or visible solid component. The wall of a pineal cyst may be composed of three layers: an inner gliotic layer, a middle layer composed of flattened or degenerated pineal parenchymal cells, and an outer fibrous leptomeningeal layer. **A,** Typical incidental pineal cyst. **B,** Gross pathologic specimen of a benign pineal cyst.

characteristic and may aid in the differentiation from metastatic tumors.[15]

Imaging

CT

A papillary tumor of the pineal region may present on CT as a dense and densely enhancing mass in the pineal region.

MRI

On MRI, this tumor is isointense to slightly hyperintense on T2 weighting and densely enhancing after administration of gadolinium.

EPIDERMOID

An inclusion cyst composed of desquamating epithelium is called an epidermoid, a pearly tumor, or an epidermoid cyst.

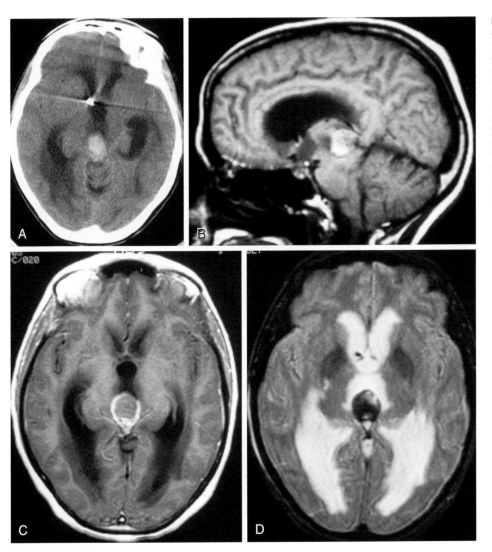

■ **FIGURE 34-28** Pineal cyst with chronic hemorrhage and granulation tissue removed surgically due to hydrocephalus and concern for possible solid neoplasm. **A,** Nonenhanced CT scan shows a hyperdense rounded mass in the pineal region and hydrocephalus. **B,** Sagittal nonenhanced T1W MR image shows some complex increased signal intensity. **C,** Axial T1W MR image after gadolinium administration shows an enhancing rim and solid or complex internal signal intensity. **D,** Axial T2W MR image shows some low signal intensity owing to the paramagnetic effect of chronic blood products such as hemosiderin.

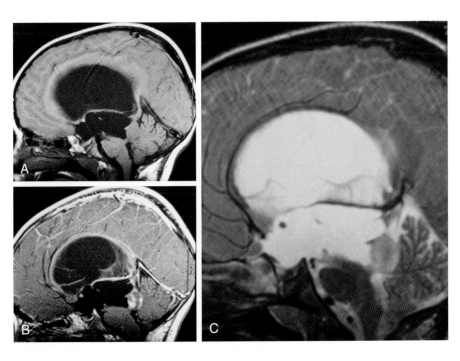

■ **FIGURE 34-29** Juvenile pilocytic astrocytoma arising in the tectum of a 7-year-old boy causes obstructive hydrocephalus at the level of the aqueduct of Sylvius and impinges on the pineal region. Sagittal T1W precontrast (**A**) and postcontrast (**B**) images and sagittal T2W (**C**) image.

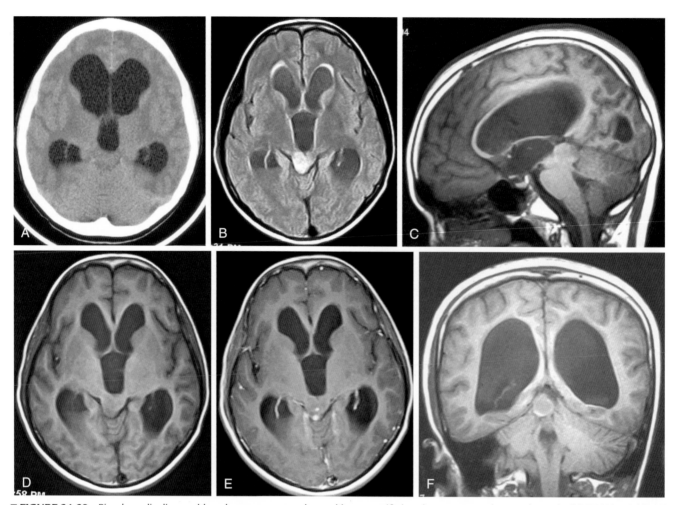

■ **FIGURE 34-30**   Pineal ganglioglioma, although rare, presents a thoroughly nonspecific imaging appearance in nonenhanced axial CT **(A)**, axial FLAIR **(B)**, noncontrast sagittal **(C)** and axial **(D)** T1 weighted images and postcontrast axial **(E)** and coronal **(F)** T1 weighted images.

Clinical Presentation

The clinical features of this lesion are similar to those of other pineal region masses.

Imaging

CT

Epidermoids are seen as hypodense and nonenhancing on CT.

MRI

On MRI these cysts generally follow fluid on T1W and T2W images but are bright on FLAIR and other inversion recovery sequences (Fig. 34-33).

CAVUM VELUM INTERPOSITUM

A cystic space formed by fluid trapped within the bilaminar velum interpositum above the third ventricle may impinge on the posterior third ventricle and pineal region. This lesion, by definition, is medial to the fornices, above the third ventricle, and below the lateral ventricles. It is a vertically thin triangle, with its base at the pineal and its point just posterior to the foramina of Monro.

Pathophysiology

In early fetal development, the neural tube develops lateral diverticula, which then extend posteriorly, then slightly inferiorly, and finally anteriorly, eventually leading to the mature adult ventricular configuration.

During this process the neural tube doubles back on itself, leading to a partially bilaminar roof of the third ventricle. This creates a potential space for the bilateral internal cerebral veins referred to as the velum interpositum. When fluid enters and becomes trapped in this potential space, this is referred to as "cavum velum interpositum."

Imaging

Ultrasonography

Cavum velum interpositum appears as a cyst in the pineal region on prenatal ultrasonography, usually with an inverted helmet shape.[33,34]

CT

CT images display a roughly triangular fluid structure overlying the posterior third ventricle without a solid component and without enhancement.

MRI

A cavum velum interpositum is a cystic space overlying the posterior third ventricle that follows a fluid signal on all sequences. It may be most clearly diagnosed on coronal T2W images when the internal cerebral veins can be seen within the dilated CSF space (Fig. 34-34).

ARACHNOID CYST

This intra-arachnoidal duplication cyst can be either congenital or developmental.[35]

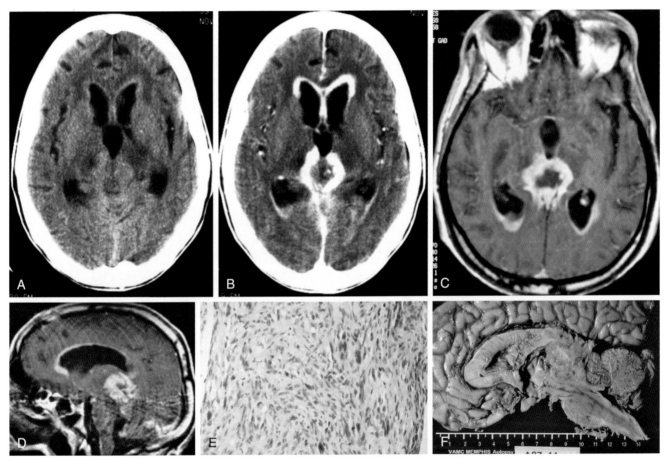

■ **FIGURE 34-31** Pineal region fibrosarcoma. Fibrosarcoma is a rare tumor that displays biphasic histology, including neuroepithelial and mesenchymal derivatives. Although controversial, it may be a variant of glioblastoma multiforme/gliosarcoma. This occurrence in the pineal region is vanishingly rare if not unique. This case was initially diagnosed as a probable germ cell tumor but was reclassified on further pathologic evaluation as a mixed glial mesenchymal tumor possibly of leptomeningeal origin. The imaging features are nonspecific, although the appearance of a ring-enhancing lesion with a thick wall would be considered suggestive of a high-grade glioma if it occurred within the cerebral hemispheres. Precontrast (**A**) and postcontrast (**B**) CT scans show a high-density ring lesion with subsequent ring enhancement. Axial (**C**) and sagittal (**D**) postcontrast images show a ring-enhancing mass with thick irregular walls and nonenhancing, likely necrotic center. **E,** Photomicrograph shows variable histology with pleomorphic nuclei and elongated spindle cells. **F,** Autopsy specimen confirms the poor prognosis associated with this lesion.

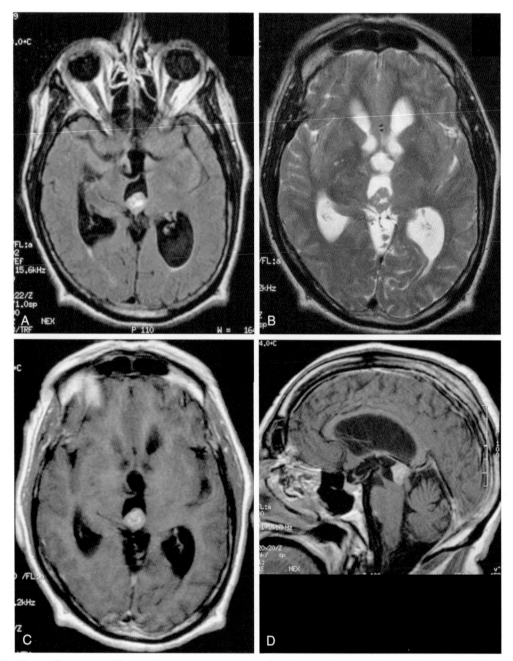

■ **FIGURE 34-32** The papillary tumor of the pineal region is a rare, recently described neoplasm that shows evidence of possible ependymal derivation and a papillary pattern on histologic examination. Imaging features are nonspecific in axial FLAIR (**A**), T2W (**B**), and T1W postcontrast axial (**C**) and sagittal (**D**) MR images.

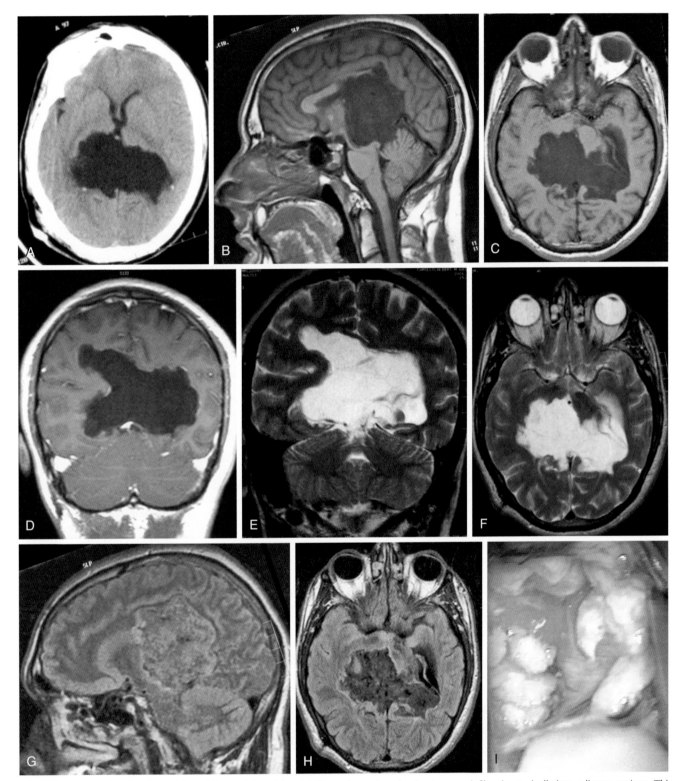

■ **FIGURE 34-33** Pineal region epidermoid cyst. Selected images show a large, low-density structure infiltrating typically into adjacent regions. This tumor follows fluid signal intensity on the T1W and T2W images but is slightly hyperintense on FLAIR sequences. The photograph of the gross specimen in **I** shows the typical opalescent appearance, hence the term *pearly tumor.* **A,** Axial CT. **B** and **C,** Sagittal and axial T1W MR images. **D,** Coronal T1W postcontrast MR image. **E** and **F,** Coronal and axial T2W MR images. **G** and **H,** Sagittal and axial FLAIR MR images. **I,** Surgical photograph.

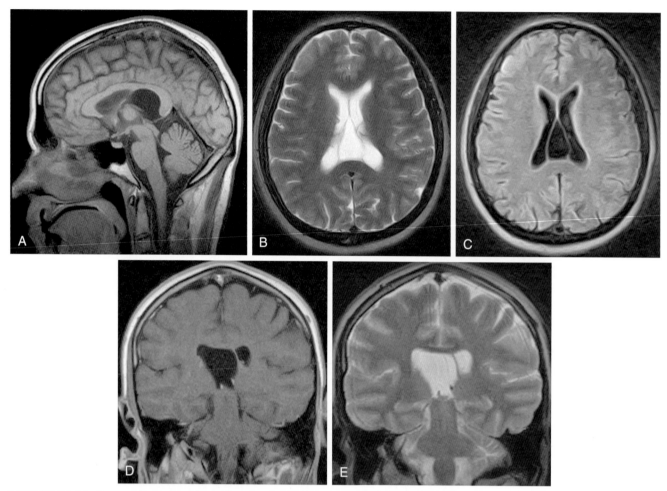

■ **FIGURE 34-34** Cavum velum interpositum. The velum interpositum is a potential space in the bilaminar roof of the third ventricle that occurs embryologically as the rostralmost neural tube folds posteriorly during normal brain development. When this space is fluid-filled, it is referred to as a cavum velum interpositum (CVP). **A,** On sagittal T1W MRI the CVP is seen as a cystic space overlying the posterior third ventricle, possibly bowing the forniceal arches forward slightly. **B** and **C,** On axial T2W and FLAIR images, the CVP forms an isosceles triangle with its base abutting the splenium of the corpus callosum. **D** and **E,** On coronal T1W and T2W images, CVP is definitively identified by the paired internal cerebral veins that normally traverse it. Note that in these coronal images from a different patient the CVP is asymmetric to the right.

Pathophysiology

Most commonly seen in the anterior middle fossa and posterior fossa, these benign CSF-containing collections are congenital and generally incidental, although there are reports of symptomatic mass effect and increase in size requiring resection and drainage.[36] They have been reported in the pineal region, but this is uncommon.

MEDIAL DIVERTICULUM OF THE LATERAL VENTRICLE

A pulsion diverticulum of the lateral ventricle extends through the crus of the fornix into the pineal region. It also can be called a ventricular diverticulum.

Pathophysiology

Patients with severe and long-standing obstructive hydrocephalus such as from aqueductal stenosis develop massive enlargement of the ventricular space. This leads to stretching of the fornix and dehiscence of fibers of the forniceal arches, which support the medial walls of the atria of the lateral ventricle. This may lead to unilateral or bilateral pulsion diverticula that extend into the pineal region and also into the superior cerebellar cistern but maintain direct communication with the intraventricular space. Originally described on CT, they may be more clearly displayed on MRI, which can be used to show the extension from

the medial wall of the atria, and often pulsatile flow can be demonstrated on flow-sensitive sequences (Fig. 34-35).[37]

Imaging
CT
CT displays a large cystic structure that extends through the medial wall of the atrium of the lateral ventricle into the pineal region and sometimes further inferiorly into the superior cerebellar cistern.[38]

MRI
On MRI this appears as a large CSF structure in the pineal region. Coronal images clearly display the communication with the atrium of the lateral ventricle, and pulsatile flow may be demonstrated on flow-sensitive sequences.[39]

AMYLOIDOMA

Focal accumulation of amyloid protein is referred to as an amyloidoma.

Pathophysiology

Amyloidoma is a focal deposit of extracellular protein that exhibits apple-green birefringence when stained with Congo red and viewed under a polarized light source. This condition has many variants but is commonly associated with overproduction of light-chain immunoglobulin in patients with multiple myeloma

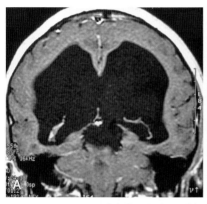 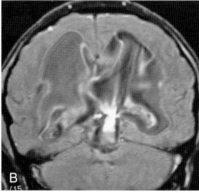 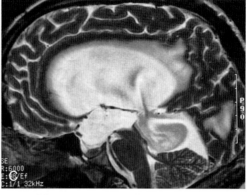

■ **FIGURE 34-35** Medial diverticulum of the lateral ventricle. Coronal postcontrast T1W (**A**), coronal flow sensitive (**B**), and sagittal T2W (**C**) images. There is marked hydrocephalus and there is a direct connection between the atrium of the left lateral ventricle and the superior cerebellar cistern, caused by rupture of the medial wall of the ventricle and the proximal forniceal arch.

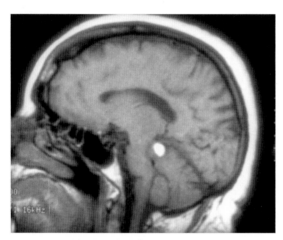

■ **FIGURE 34-36** Focal amyloid deposits or amyloidomas may occur in a wide variety of locations and present a nonspecific appearance. Sagittal T1W postcontrast MR image shows a homogeneous enhancing rounded tectal mass that was found to represent a focal amyloidoma.

or reactive protein in patients with chronic inflammatory conditions.[40]

Imaging
CT
On CT there is an isodense to hyperdense deposit with dense enhancement.

MRI
An amyloidoma may present as a mass or nodule isointense to cortex with dense enhancement (Fig. 34-36).

MENINGIOMA
This neoplasm is also called a meningothelial neoplasm or a falcotentorial meningioma.

Pathophysiology
Many histologic variants may be found.

Imaging
CT
A hyperdense mass that is dural based related either to the falx cerebri or to the tentorium cerebelli or both is evident.

MRI
There is an isointense mass with dense enhancement that is usually homogeneous, possibly associated with a dural tail (Fig. 34-37).[41]

ANALYSIS
Most of the neoplastic and cystic entities that occur in the pineal region contain nonspecific features; however, there are a number of more specific findings that must be looked for and analyzed (see Key Points).

Evidence of lipid material, low attenuation on CT, and high T1 signal intensity suggest a teratoma or sebaceous material in a dermoid tumor. Dermoid tumors should be unilocular with limited rim enhancement, whereas teratomas are more commonly multilocular with solid and cystic regions. Leakage from these tumors may result in a fat-fluid level in the ventricular system. Also, if tooth or bone is seen, even partially formed, the lesion should be a teratoma. If there is a large heterogeneous mass detected on prenatal ultrasonography or fetal MRI, then teratoma is considered most likely.

In contrast, if there is a homogeneous mass, especially if it is hyperdense on noncontrast CT, surrounding a central calcification, germinoma is most likely. If there are calcifications that appear eccentric, displaced, or exploded from a central location, a pineal parenchymal tumor, either pineocytoma or pineoblastoma, becomes a likely possibility.

Hemorrhage is nonspecific but, if seen, suggests a more aggressive "nongerminomatous germ cell tumor" such as choriocarcinoma and endodermal sinus tumor (yolk sac tumor). These lesions, although rare, are noted to have a somewhat higher incidence of hemorrhage.

The most common fluid-filled lesion is a simple pineal cyst, which may occur routinely in many normal people. Careful evaluation of size (<1-2 cm), wall thickness (<1-2 mm), enhancement pattern (no abnormal or nodular enhancement), and effect on adjacent structures (no hydrocephalus or displacement) will allow the interpretation of a probable incidental pineal cyst. If a cyst is larger or associated with any of the other findings listed, the differential becomes broader. If a cystic lesion shows slightly altered signal intensity, particularly on FLAIR images, it may be an epidermoid cyst. If there is evidence of flow artifact or possible connection to the atria of the lateral ventricles, then medial ventricular diverticulum should be considered. If the cystic lesion is triangular, related to the roof of the third ventricle, and particularly contains the internal cerebral veins, then a cavum velum interpositum is suggested.

Clinical information, when available, may also limit the differential diagnosis significantly. If there is a history of precocious puberty or other endocrinologic abnormalities, then germ cell tumors, particularly germinomas, become most likely. If there is a previous history or family history of retinoblastoma, then pineoblastoma or trilateral retinoblastoma should be suggested and genetic karyotyping should be performed.

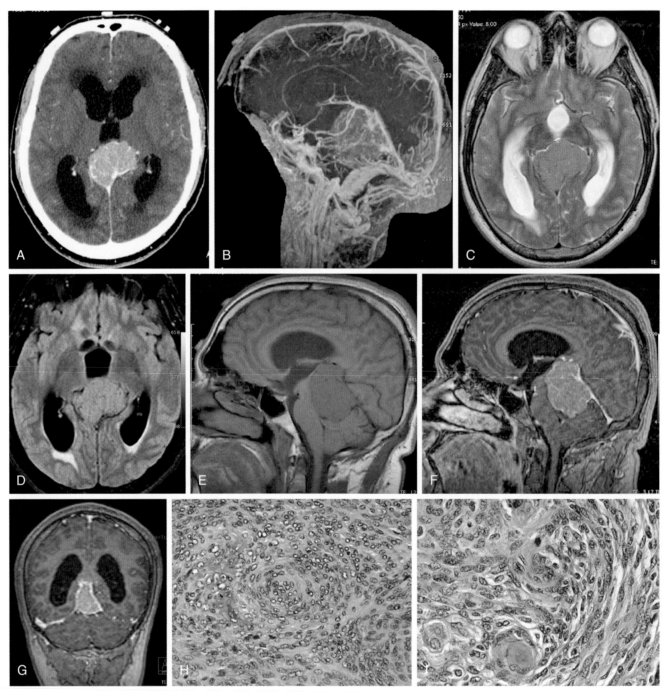

■ **FIGURE 34-37** Falcotentorial meningioma. Meningioma arising in the pineal region at the junction of the falx cerebri and the tentorium cerebelli shows typical although nonspecific imaging features of dense homogeneous enhancement on postcontrast axial CT (**A**) and on CTA sagittal reconstruction (**B**), as well as on postcontrast sagittal (**F**) and coronal (**G**) T1 weighted images. The tumor is relatively isointense on noncontrast axial T2 (**C**), axial FLAIR (**D**) and sagittal T1 (**E**) images. Photomicrographs (**H** and **I**) show a typical meningothelial pattern.

KEY POINTS: DIFFERENTIAL DIAGNOSIS

- Morphology—Is the mass rounded and well circumscribed, or is it irregular, lobular, and/or invasive to surrounding structures?
- Composition—Is the mass homogeneous in density (CT) and signal intensity (MRI) and enhancement (both)?
- If it is heterogeneous, what other components are visualized? Is there fat/lipid, calcification, or hemorrhage, or are other elements seen?

- If calcification is seen, is it typical pineal calcification (central and roughly rounded) or is it peripheral (exploded) or does it resemble tooth or bone?
- Are there other associated abnormalities such as hydrocephalus, ventricular fluid levels, or lesions elsewhere?

SUGGESTED READINGS

Graham DI, Lantos PL (eds). Greenfield's Neuropathology, 6th ed. London, Hodder Arnold, 1997.

Jinkins JR. Atlas of Neuroradiologic Embryology, Anatomy, and Variants. Philadelphia, Lippincott, Williams, & Wilkins, 2000.

Kaye AH, Laws ER Jr. Brain Tumors: An Encyclopedic Approach, 2nd ed. Philadelphia, Churchill Livingstone, 2001.

Kitay JI. Altschule MD. The Pineal Gland: A Review of the Physiologic Literature. Cambridge, Mass, Harvard University Press, 1954.

Louis, DN, Ohgaki K, Wiestler OD, Cavenee WK (eds). WHO Classification of Tumours of the Central Nervous System. Lyon, IARC, 2007, p 122.

Mclendon RE, Rosenblum MK, Bigner DD (eds). Russell and Rubinstein's Pathology of Tumors of the Nervous System, 7th ed. London, Hodder Arnold, 2006.

Parent A. Carpenter's Human Neuroanatomy, 9th ed. Baltimore, Williams & Wilkins, 1996.

Wolstenholme GEW, Knight J. The Pineal Gland. Edinburgh, Churchill Livingstone, 1971.

REFERENCES

1. Kitay JI. Altschule MD. The Pineal Gland: A Review of the Physiologic Literature. Cambridge, mass, Harvard University Press, 1954, preface and pp v-vi.
2. Jinkins JR. Atlas of Neuroradiologic Embryology, Anatomy, and Variants. Philadelphia, Lippincott, Williams & Wilkins, 2000, pp 237-238.
3. Sumida M, Barkovich J, Newton TH. Development of the pineal gland. AJNR Am J Neuroradiol 1996; 17:233-236.
4. Hasegawa A, Ohtsubo K, Mori W. Pineal gland in old age. Brain Res 1987; 409:343-349.
5. Pu Y, Mahankali S, Hou L, et al. High prevalence of pineal cysts in healthy adults demonstrated by high-resolution, noncontrast brain MR imaging. AJNR Am J Neuroradiol 2007; 28;1706-1709.
6. Barboriak DP, Lee L, Provenzale JM. Serial MR imaging of pineal cysts: implications for natural history and follow-up. AJR Am J Roentgenol 2001; 176:737-743.
7. Seifert CL, Woeller A, Valet M, et al. Headaches and pineal cyst: a case-control study. Headache 2008; 48:448-452.
8. Min KW, Seo IS, Song J. Postnatal evolution of the human pineal gland: an immunohistochemical study. Lab Invest 1987; 57:724-728.
9. Parent A. Carpenter's Human Neuroanatomy, 9th ed. Baltimore, Williams & Wilkins, 1995, p 638.
10. Kappers JA. The pineal organ: an introduction. In Wolstenholme GEW, Knight J (eds): The Pineal Gland, Edinburgh, Churchill Livingstone, 1971.
11. Saper CB, Scammell TE, Lu J. Hypothalamic regulation of sleep and circadian rhythms. Nature 2005; 437:1257-1263.
12. Zimmerman RA, Bilaniuk LT, Wood JH, et al. Computed tomography of pineal, parapineal, and histologically related tumors. Radiology 1980; 137:669-677.
13. Mena H, Nakazato Y, Jouvet A, Scheithauer BW. Pineal parenchymal tumors. In: WHO Classification of Tumours: Pathology, and Genetics of Tumours of the Central Nervous System. Lyon, IARC, 2000.
14. Jennings MT, Gelman R, Hochberg F. Intracranial germ-cell tumors: natural history and pathogenesis. Journal of Neurosurgery 1985; 63:155-167.
15. Louis DN, Ohgaki K, Wiestler OD, Cavenee WK (eds). In: WHO Classification of Tumours of the Central Nervous System. Lyon, IARC, 2007, p 122.
16. Schild SE, Scheithauer BW, Schomberg PJ, et al. Pineal parenchymal tumors, clinical, pathologic, and therapeutic aspects. Cancer 1993; 72:870-880.
17. Kaye AH, Laws ER Jr. Brain Tumors: An Encyclopedic Approach, 2nd ed. Churchill Livingstone, 2001, p 772.
18. Sano K. Pathogenesis of intracranial germ cell tumors reconsidered. J Neurosurg 1999; 90:258-264.
19. Liu GT, Volpe NJ, Galetta SL. Neuro-Ophthalmology. Philadelphia, WB Saunders, 2001 pp 604-605.
20. Endo H, Kumabe T, Jokura H, Tominaga T. Stereotactic radiosurgery followed by whole ventricular irradiation for primary intracranial germinoma of the pineal region. Minim Invasive Neurosurg 2005; 48:186-190.
21. Matsutani M, Sano K, Takakura K, et al. Primary intracranial germ cell tumors: a clinical analysis of 153 histologically verified cases. J Neurosurg 1997; 86:446-455.
22. Horowitz MB, Hall WA. Central nervous system germinomas: a review. Arch Neurol 1991; 48:652-657.
23. Suh YL, Koo H, Kim TS, et al. Neuropathology Study Group of the Korean Society of Pathologists. Tumors of the central nervous system in Korea: a multicenter study of 3221 cases. J Neuro Oncol 2002; 56:251-259.
24. Inamura T, Nishio S, Ikezaki K, Fukui M. Human chorionic gonadotrophin in CSF, not serum, predicts outcome in germinomas. J Neurol Neurosurg Psychiatry 1999; 66:654-657.
25. Hattab EM, Tu P-H, Wilson JD, Cheng L. OCT4 immunohistochemistry is superior to placental alkaline phosphatase (PLAP) in the diagnosis of central nervous system germinoma. Am J Surg Pathol 2005; 29:368-371.
26. Smirniotopoulos JG, Rushing EJ, Mena H. Pineal region masses: differential diagnosis. RadioGraphics 1992; 12:577-596.
27. Liang L, Korogi Y, Sugahara T, et al. MRI of intracranial germ-cell tumours. Neuroradiology 2002; 44:382-388.
28. Mclendon RE, Rosenblum MK, Bigner DD (eds). Russell and Rubinstein's Pathology of Tumors of the Nervous System, 7th ed. London, Hodder Arnold, 2006, pp 563-564.
29. Hasegawa T, Kondziolka D, Hadjipanayis CG, et al. The role of radiosurgery for the treatment of pineal parenchymal tumors. Neurosurgery 2002; 51:880-889.
30. Chiechi MV, Smirniotopoulos JG, Mena H. Pineal parenchymal tumors: CT and MR features. JCAT 1995; 19:509-517.
31. Lutterbach J, Fauchon F, Schild SE, et al. Malignant pineal parenchymal tumors in adult patients: patterns of care and prognostic factors. Neurosurgery 2002; 51:44-55; discussion 55-56.
32. Jouvet A, Fauchon F, Liberski P, et al. Papillary tumor of the pineal region. Am J Surg Pathol 2003; 27:505-512.
33. Chen CY, Chen FH, Lee CC, et al. Sonographic characteristics of the cavum velum interpositum. AJNR Am J Neuroradiol 1998; 19:1631-1635.
34. Eisenberg VH, Zalel Y, Hoffmann C, et al. Prenatal diagnosis of cavum velum interpositum cysts: significance and outcome. Prenatal Diagn 2003; 23:779-783.
35. Choi JU, Kim DS. Pathogenesis of arachnoid cyst: congenital or traumatic. Pediatr Neurosurg 1998; 29:260-266.
36. Thinakara-Rajan T, Janjua A, Srinivasan V. Posterior fossa arachnoid cyst presenting with isolated sensorineural hearing loss. J Laryngol Otol 2006; 120:979-982.
37. Mott M, Cummins B. Hydrocephalus related to pulsion diverticulum of lateral ventricle. Arch Dis Child 1974; 49:407-410.
38. Naidich TP, McLone DG, Hahn YS, Hanaway J. Atrial diverticula in severe hydrocephalus. AJNR Am J Neuroradiol 1982; 3:257-266.
39. Huh JS, Hwang YS, Yoon SH, et al. Lateral ventricular diverticulum extending into supracerebellar cistern from unilateral obstruction of the foramen of Monro in a neonate. Pediatr Neurosurg 2007; 43:115-120.
40. Lee J, Krol G, Rosenblum M. Primary amyloidoma of the brain: CT and MR presentation. AJNR Am J Neuroradiol 1995; 16:712-714.
41. Quinones-Hinojosa A, Chang EF, McDermott MW. Falcotentorial meningiomas: clinical, neuroimaging, and surgical features in six patients. Neurosurg Focus 2004; 14:e11.

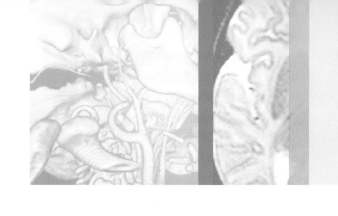

CHAPTER 35

Posterior Fossa Intra-Axial Tumors

Blaise V. Jones

Brain parenchyma of the posterior fossa includes the cerebellar hemispheres, vermis, pons, midbrain, and medulla oblongata. Neoplasms arising from these structures are a significant source of morbidity and mortality, especially in the pediatric patient. A clear understanding of the tumors that present in the posterior fossa is essential for the radiologist performing brain imaging in these patients.

Posterior fossa intra-axial neoplasms in children are dominated by the "Big Four" tumors: medulloblastoma, cerebellar pilocytic astrocytoma, brain stem glioma, and ependymoma. Of these, cerebellar pilocytic astrocytoma and medulloblastoma are by far the most common. Recognition of the relative incidence of the various posterior fossa intra-axial tumors that occur in children can significantly narrow differential considerations, as can an understanding of the typical age ranges in which these tumors present. In addition to the four major tumor types, several other less common posterior fossa intra-axial tumors are diagnosed in children. Some of these tumors have only recently been recognized as distinct entities. For example, a significant percentage of tumors previously diagnosed as medulloblastoma are now recognized to be atypical teratoid/rhabdoid tumors. Pilomyxoid astrocytomas were previously thought to represent a variant of pilocytic astrocytoma.

Clinical presentation of posterior fossa pediatric intra-axial tumors is fairly stereotypical. Signs and symptoms of increased intracranial pressure such as headache, vomiting, and papilledema are nearly ubiquitous. Cranial nerve palsies are frequently encountered, although sometimes only appreciated after the diagnosis has been made. In infants with patent cranial sutures, ventricular obstruction from posterior fossa tumors will result in macrocrania. Although many children with posterior fossa intra-axial tumors will be ataxic at presentation, recognition of cerebellar ataxia can be difficult in infants and toddlers. In addition, the signs and symptoms associated with posterior fossa tumors are more often encountered in children with non-neoplastic lesions. Indeed, the majority of children undergoing imaging for headache, vomiting, nystagmus, apnea, or facial nerve palsy have normal imaging studies.

Intra-axial posterior fossa tumors are frequently diagnosed in infants and toddlers, and the young age of the patients can restrict the treatment options available to the oncologist. As with most brain tumors, prognosis in this group is most closely related to the ability to achieve a gross total surgical resection. In those cases in which this is not possible the prognosis is often poor.

In this chapter six intra-axial neoplasms and one neoplastic/dysplastic lesion encountered in the posterior fossa in children are discussed and findings helpful in the distinction of these entities from one another on imaging are reviewed. However, extra-axial tumors and non-neoplastic lesions figure prominently in the differential diagnosis of posterior fossa intra-axial tumors in children. Neoplasms arising from extra-axial sources such as cranial nerves, choroid plexus, skull base, and meninges are often considered in the differential diagnosis of posterior fossa masses in children but are less commonly encountered than intra-axial tumors.

MEDULLOBLASTOMA

Medulloblastoma is a small cell neuroectodermal tumor of the cerebellum. It is the most common of the central nervous system (CNS) primitive neuroectodermal tumors (PNETs), a category of tumors composed of primitive small cells with multipotential differentiation. As such, some authors will refer to medulloblastoma as a posterior fossa PNET, emphasizing its similarity to primitive neuroectodermal tumors found in the supratentorial brain. The term *medulloblastoma* is based on the labeling of the primitive tumor cells as "medulloblasts."

Epidemiology

Medulloblastoma is primarily a tumor of young children, but it has been reported in all age ranges. It is the most common malignant brain tumor diagnosed in children and is the most commonly encountered of the pediatric posterior fossa tumors. It accounts for up to 25% of all pediatric brain tumors and close to 40% of posterior fossa pediatric brain tumors. Medulloblastoma is slightly more common in boys and is infrequently diagnosed in adults. When considering only pediatric patients, the mean age at diagnosis is just over 7 years. However, the distribution can be parsed further, with a typical presentation occurring in children 1 to 4 years of age and a variant group presenting at 6 to 9 years of age. Recent population studies have identified increased rates of diagnosis associated with birth in the autumn and winter and increased number of siblings.[1]

Clinical Presentation

The characteristic presentation of medulloblastoma is that of an infant or preschool-aged child with signs and symptoms of increased intracranial pressure caused by obstruction of the ventricular system at the level of the fourth ventricle. Such signs and symptoms include headache, irritability, nausea/vomiting, papilledema, and macrocephaly.[1] Symptoms caused by local effects of the tumor in the posterior fossa include cranial nerve palsies and ataxia. Vomiting may be the result of increased intracranial pressure or direct impingement of the tumor on the area postrema on the floor of the fourth ventricle. Less common presenting symptoms include neurologic deficits associated with spinal cord compression from metastatic disease, seizure, or precipitous neurologic decline due to intratumoral hemorrhage. Symptoms are generally short in duration before diagnosis, reflecting the rapid growth of the tumor.

Pathophysiology

The true cell of origin of medulloblastoma remains a point of some controversy and mystery. Some consider medulloblastoma to be a PNET, emphasizing common features found throughout this group of tumors thought to arise from primitive multipotential neuroepithelial cells. Others believe that these tumors originate from the external granular layer of the cerebellar vermis, either at their early location along the roof of the fourth ventricle or their later position more laterally. Still others have suggested more than one cell of origin, accounting for the various subtypes of medulloblastoma.

Over a third of medulloblastoma patients will have loss of genetic material from chromosome 17. Genetic defects have also been identified in chromosomes 1, 8, 9, 10, 11, and 16.[2] Nevoid basal cell carcinoma syndrome (NBCCS, Gorlin's syndrome), an autosomal dominant–inherited cancer syndrome caused by genetic mutations in the *PTCH* gene on chromosome 9, is associated with an increased risk for the development of medulloblastoma. Other clinical features of the syndrome that can be identified on imaging studies include odontogenic keratocysts of the jaw and calcifications of the falx cerebri. The latter may be present at a much earlier age than typical senescent meningeal calcifications. Medulloblastoma has also been reported in Li-Fraumeni syndrome, Rubenstein-Taybi syndrome, and Turcot's syndrome.[3]

Pathology

Medulloblastoma presenting in infants and preschool-aged children is almost invariably a midline tumor. It often appears to arise from the inferior medullary velum of the cerebellar vermis. The tumor exhibits a spherical pattern of growth, projecting into and enlarging the fourth ventricle. In contrast, medulloblastoma presenting in older children and adults is more characteristically found in the cerebellar hemispheres, sometimes mimicking a tumor of the cerebellopontine angle. These differences in tumor location are, to a certain extent, reflected in differences in histologic subtype.

Medulloblastoma is characterized as a grade IV tumor by the World Health Organization (WHO), with four major subtypes. The most commonly encountered subtype is *classic medulloblastoma*, characterized by monotonous sheets of round cells with abundant nuclei and scant cytoplasm (Fig. 35-1). The cells may form Homer-Wright rosettes, with tumor cells radially arranged around fibrillary processes. The *desmoplastic medulloblastoma* contains "pale islands" of cells with abundant neoplasm, surrounded by more primitive-appearing tumor cells. *Medulloblastoma with extensive nodularity and advanced neuronal differentiation* (nodular medulloblastoma) is almost exclusively diagnosed in children younger than 3 years of age, with tumor cells clustered in nodules surrounded by a fibrillary matrix. This histologic subtype is frequently identifiable by its

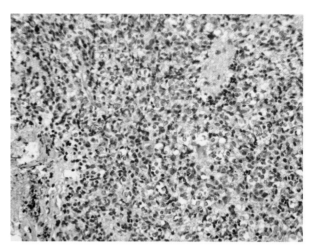

■ FIGURE 35-1 Medium-power photomicrograph of medulloblastoma demonstrates monotonous sheets of small cells with scant cytoplasm and multiple mitotic figures (H&E stain).

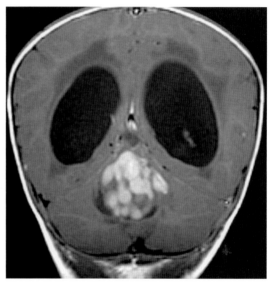

■ FIGURE 35-2 Coronal T1W MR image after contrast agent administration shows the grape-like clusters of solid enhancing tumor characteristic of nodular medulloblastoma.

clinical imaging appearance (Fig. 35-2). The least common of the four major subtypes is the *large cell medulloblastoma*, which contains large cells with abundant neoplasm and prominent nucleoli.[4,5]

Anaplastic features, encountered with some frequency in the large cell variant, portend a poor prognosis. The desmoplastic subtype has a better prognosis than the other subtypes, although it often is more difficult to surgically resect.

Imaging

CT

CT is often the first diagnostic imaging study performed on children subsequently diagnosed with medulloblastoma, and specific features on CT can increase confidence in the preoperative diagnosis. Unusual among posterior fossa tumors in children, solid portions of medulloblastoma are characteristically hyperattenuating at CT before contrast agent administration (Fig. 35-3); most other posterior fossa tumors of childhood are slightly hypoattenuating. This CT imaging feature is thought to reflect the high nuclear-to-cytoplasmic ratio and dense cellularity of the tumor. Up to 20% of medulloblastomas will demonstrate some

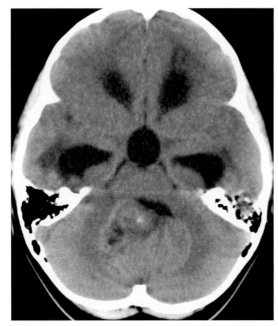

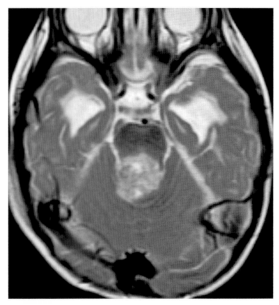

■ **FIGURE 35-4** Axial T2W MR image of medulloblastoma filling the superior aspect of the fourth ventricle. Although solid portions of the tumor are isointense relative to gray matter, the overall appearance is that of a hyperintense mass.

■ **FIGURE 35-3** Axial noncontrast CT of a 2-year-old with medulloblastoma. The tumor is isodense to gray matter in the cerebellar hemispheres, with a small focus of calcification anteriorly. It causes obstructive hydrocephalus, with periventricular interstitial edema evident at the margins of the frontal and temporal horns.

calcification at CT, but this is not a helpful differentiating finding. However, if calcifications are identified along the falx cerebri, a diagnosis of Gorlin's syndrome should be strongly considered. Although cyst formation is more typically associated with cerebellar astrocytoma, it is common to identify small cysts or regions of necrosis within a medulloblastoma; these may be more apparent on MRI. Also more apparent on MRI is the presence of vasogenic edema surrounding the tumor. Tumors that are primarily within the fourth ventricle will often elicit little or no surrounding vasogenic edema, but this is not a reliable distinguishing feature. Advanced CT techniques, including CT angiography and CT perfusion, have not been extensively applied in the evaluation of medulloblastoma.

MRI

MRI is the diagnostic study of choice in evaluation of medulloblastoma, allowing for multiplanar analysis and sensitive detection of characteristic features of the tumor itself and of metastatic lesions in the brain and spinal canal. The same features that cause high attenuation on CT can result in solid portions of the tumor appearing isointense relative to gray matter on T2-weighted (T2W) and fluid-attenuated inversion recovery (FLAIR) images. However, these sequences also emphasize small cystic foci within the tumor that are hyperintense relative to cerebrospinal fluid (CSF) within the ventricles. In addition, these tumors will appear relatively hyperintense juxtaposed to the middle cerebellar peduncles bordering the fourth ventricle (Fig. 35-4). Thus, the concept of the "dark on T2" medulloblastoma is misleading; it is more accurate to say that these tumors tend to be hypointense on T2W images *relative to other pediatric posterior fossa tumors.* Gradient-echo imaging will increase sensitivity for the detection of hemorrhage or calcifications, but hemorrhagic foci within these tumors are rare, and the detection of calcification is of little help in narrowing the differential diagnosis. On T1-weighted (T1W) images, medulloblastomas are typically isointense to hypointense, exhibiting variable degrees of enhancement after contrast agent administration.

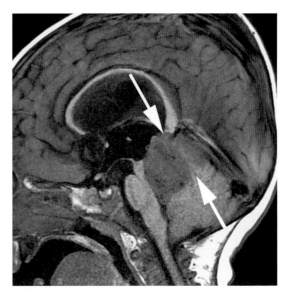

■ **FIGURE 35-5** Sagittal noncontrast T1W MR image showing the poor definition of the junction of tumor with the roof of the fourth ventricle (*arrows*), indicating the superior medullary velum as the site of origin of this medulloblastoma. The margin between the tumor and the floor of the fourth ventricle is much more clearly defined.

Upward of a third of children with medulloblastoma will have imaging evidence of subarachnoid spread of tumor at the time of diagnosis.[1,6] Although contrast enhancement is the primary means of identifying subarachnoid spread of tumor both in the cranial vault and in the spine, it should be recognized that some metastatic lesions will exhibit little or no enhancement. Contrast-enhanced sagittal images can often clearly demonstrate the base of the tumor arising from the "roof" of the fourth ventricle. This can be a key diagnostic clue to the correct diagnosis (Fig. 35-5); the less common ependymoma is much more likely to arise from the "floor" of the fourth ventricle, growing dorsally. Dynamic MR perfusion imaging can demonstrate increases in

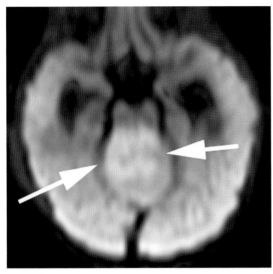

■ **FIGURE 35-6** DWI demonstrates restricted diffusion in the solid portions of this medulloblastoma (*arrows*).

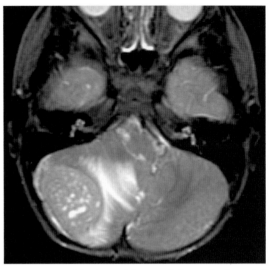

■ **FIGURE 35-8** Axial T2W MR image of desmoplastic medulloblastoma. The lateral location is unusual for classic medulloblastoma, but the desmoplastic subtype is often centered in the cerebellar hemispheres.

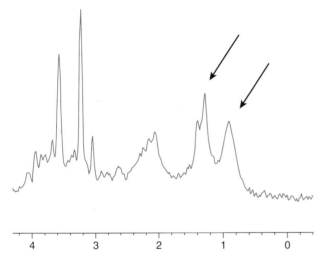

■ **FIGURE 35-7** MR spectroscopy of medulloblastoma. *Arrows* point to the resonance doublet of lipid and lactate, reflecting the anaerobic metabolism characteristic of this aggressive tumor.

blood flow associated with angiogenesis within high-grade tumors. Application of this imaging technique in the evaluation of medulloblastoma has been sporadic, and its impact on clinical decision-making in this diagnosis remains uncertain.

Diffusion-weighted imaging (DWI) characteristically demonstrates restricted diffusion within medulloblastomas (Fig. 35-6); and when compared with other intra-axial posterior fossa tumors in children, medulloblastoma shows a consistently greater degree of diffusion restriction.[7] In one study,[8] an apparent diffusion coefficient (ADC) value of less than 0.9×10^3 mm²/s was specific for medulloblastoma, relative to cerebellar astrocytoma and ependymoma.

MR spectroscopy is frequently employed in the preoperative evaluation of medulloblastoma. These tumors show a characteristically aggressive metabolite spectrum, with marked elevation of choline and suppression/absence of *N*-acetyl-aspartate (NAA) (Fig. 35-7). Lipid and lactate elevation can be seen as a manifestation of anaerobic metabolism in the tumor. Several authors have reported frequent elevation of taurine, at 3.3 ppm.[9] The anatomy

of the posterior fossa may lead to some degradation of spectroscopic quality, but multi-voxel spectroscopic imaging can help distinguish laterally based tumors (Fig. 35-8) from regions of adjacent edematous brain.

EPENDYMOMA

Ependymoma is a neoplasm of ependymal cells. These tumors can arise virtually anywhere along the neuraxis and have been reported in multiple regions outside the CNS. However, in the pediatric patient they are most frequently encountered within and around the fourth ventricle. Less commonly, childhood ependymomas are diagnosed in the cerebral hemispheres or spinal cord. It should be recognized that two other neoplasms with similar names, subependymoma and ependymoblastoma, do not represent subtypes of ependymoma. The subependymoma is a well-differentiated and slowly growing glioma that is most frequently encountered in the lateral ventricles of adults. The ependymoblastoma is a PNET that exhibits ependymoblastic rosettes and is typically found in the cerebral hemispheres in young children.

Epidemiology

Although reported in all age ranges, intracranial ependymomas are most frequently diagnosed in children, in whom they account for up to 15% of posterior fossa neoplasms. Slightly more common in boys, they are most frequently diagnosed between 1 and 5 years of age.

Clinical Presentation

Like other posterior fossa tumors, ependymomas most frequently present with headache, nausea, and vomiting. More specific indicators of posterior fossa disease, such as cranial neuropathies and ataxia, can also be encountered. Infants may present with lethargy and developmental delay.

Pathophysiology

In general, ependymomas are relatively well-differentiated tumors with multiple ultrastructural features. This accounts for their heterogeneous appearance on imaging and at gross inspection, as well as their relatively slow growth. The majority of posterior fossa ependymomas are classified as WHO grade II lesions. A small proportion of ependymomas will exhibit more aggressive features at histologic analysis, with dense cellularity

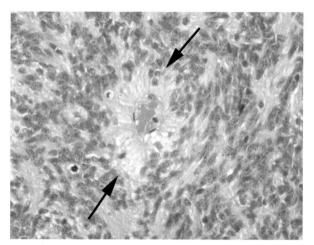

■ FIGURE 35-9 High-power photomicrograph of ependymoma with *arrows* pointing to a perivascular pseudorosette (H&E stain).

and prominent mitotic activity; these are termed *anaplastic ependymomas.*

Multiple chromosomal aberrations have been identified in association with ependymoma, including defects on chromosomes 1, 6, 9, 13, 16, 17, 19, 20, and 22.[10] There is a high incidence of spinal ependymomas in neurofibromatosis 2.

Pathology

Ependymomas are soft and well-delineated tumors on gross inspection, frequently with extension into fourth ventricular foramina. Grossly visible cystic foci and necrotic regions can be identified.

Four pathologic subtypes of ependymoma have been described. The *classic ependymoma* is characterized by a moderately cellular and lobular pattern of growth interrupted by perivascular pseudorosettes (Fig. 35-9). These structures demonstrate strong immunoreactivity for glial fibrillary acidic protein (GFAP). True ependymal rosettes can also be identified, characterized by columnar epithelium surrounding a distinct lumen. The rare tumors with a growth pattern resulting in extensive and complex epithelial surfaces have been termed *papillary ependymomas.* Another uncommon subtype is characterized by cells that have a prominent perinuclear halo and nuclear uniformity, called *clear cell ependymoma.* The fourth variant of ependymoma encountered in the posterior fossa in children is the *tanycytic ependymoma,* in which individual cells are markedly elongated with fibular processes resembling pilocytic astrocytoma. The familiar *myxopapillary ependymoma* is essentially restricted to an intraspinal location at the filum terminale.[4]

Imaging

CT

CT of posterior fossa ependymoma typically demonstrates a heterogeneous tumor filling and expanding the fourth ventricle, with extension laterally through the foramen of Luschka. Close to 50% of posterior fossa ependymomas will demonstrate calcification on CT (Fig. 35-10), and many will show regions of hemorrhage or necrosis. Enhancement is variable and irregular.

MRI

The MRI appearance of posterior fossa ependymoma reflects the heterogeneity of the tumor. T2W images demonstrate a tumor with solid components that are isointense or hyperintense to brain parenchyma, markedly hypointense regions reflecting hemorrhage and/or calcification, and cystic foci. A similar pattern is seen with FLAIR sequences (Fig. 35-11), with

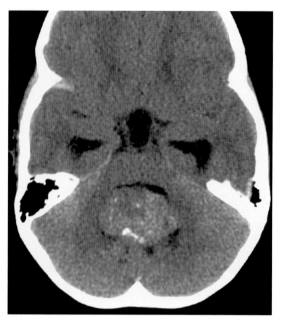

■ FIGURE 35-10 Fourth ventricular ependymoma on nonenhanced CT. Note punctate calcifications scattered throughout the lesion, which appears slightly hyperattenuating relative to cerebellar gray matter.

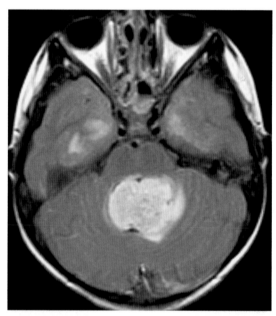

■ FIGURE 35-11 Axial FLAIR image of a fourth ventricular ependymoma in a 7-year-old. The tumor elicits little edema in the adjacent cerebellum.

pronounced hyperintense signal in cystic or necrotic regions. Hemorrhagic and calcified areas may demonstrate hyperintense signal on T1W images, and the heterogeneous and variable pattern of contrast enhancement exhibited on CT is duplicated with MRI. As with medulloblastoma, sagittal postcontrast imaging can be very helpful in demonstrating point of attachment of an intraventricular tumor (Fig. 35-12). When this point of attachment is from the dorsal brain stem with tumor growth into the ventricle itself, a diagnosis of ependymoma or exophytic brain stem glioma is likely.

DWI demonstrates restricted diffusion in infratentorial ependymoma but not as pronounced as in the more common

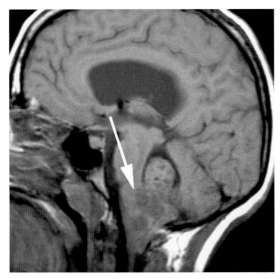

■ **FIGURE 35-12** Sagittal noncontrast T1W MR image of the fourth ventricular ependymoma with inferior extension through foramen magnum. *Arrow* points to site of attachment of tumor to the dorsal inferior aspect of the brain stem.

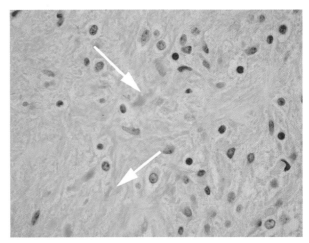

■ **FIGURE 35-13** High-power photomicrograph of a pilocytic astrocytoma with *arrows* pointing to characteristic Rosenthal fibers (H&E stain).

medulloblastoma. The degree of restriction is typically greater than in pilocytic astrocytoma,[8] and DWI will also show restricted diffusion in areas of necrosis.

MR spectroscopy in ependymoma usually demonstrates the recognizable pattern of diminished NAA and elevated choline. The degree of choline elevation is less than typically seen in medulloblastoma. Regions of necrosis may result in large resonance peaks at 1.1 to 1.3 ppm, reflecting the presence of lipids and lactate. Like the brain stem glioma, infratentorial ependymoma can demonstrate elevated levels of myoinositol, especially relative to pilocytic astrocytoma or medulloblastoma. The heterogeneity of ependymoma undermines the reliability of MR spectroscopy in differentiating this tumor from other commonly encountered infratentorial neoplasms.

PILOCYTIC ASTROCYTOMA

Pilocytic astrocytoma is a tumor composed of astrocytes that contain Rosenthal fibers and/or eosinophilic granular bodies. It is the single most common CNS neoplasm in children and is sometimes referred to as juvenile pilocytic astrocytoma. Other names are spongioblastoma polare and cerebellar astrocytoma.

Epidemiology
Pilocytic astrocytoma is a tumor of childhood, with over 80% of cases diagnosed before 20 years of age. Of these, most are diagnosed in children 5 to 15 years old. Over 60% of pilocytic astrocytomas are located in the posterior fossa, the majority in the cerebellar hemispheres.

Clinical Presentation
Like other tumors of the posterior fossa, pilocytic astrocytoma typically presents with headache, nausea, and vomiting. Ataxia and cranial neuropathies may also bring the child to medical attention. On careful evaluation, a more prolonged history of symptoms related to the posterior fossa can be elicited in many cases, reflecting the slow-growing nature of the tumor.

Pathophysiology
The treatment and therefore the understanding of the natural history of pilocytic astrocytoma are strongly dependent on its location in the CNS. Cerebellar tumors by and large are promptly resected after diagnosis; optic pathway lesions are rarely resected.

As a consequence, much of the knowledge of the natural history of these tumors is based on the behavior of supratentorial lesions, specifically those of the visual pathways.

With this understanding, it is generally accepted that the cerebellar pilocytic astrocytoma is a slow-growing neoplasm that has a strong tendency to develop cystic foci. Mass effect from these lesions is frequently a result of the large cystic foci, rather than solid portions of the tumor. Although supratentorial lesions are strongly associated with neurofibromatosis type 1 (NF1), cerebellar lesions are much more likely to be sporadic. Specific genetic markers and other syndromes have not been implicated.

Pilocytic astrocytomas are designated as grade I lesions by the WHO classification. If gross total resection can be achieved surgically, the long-term disease-free survival is well over 90%. Adjuvant therapy is rarely employed. Moreover, there are numerous reports of long-term survival in the face of subtotal resection, with some cases demonstrating regression of residual tumor.[11] However, there are also numerous reports of pilocytic astrocytoma presenting with widespread subarachnoid dissemination, as well as reports of progressive and essentially malignant behavior of these tumors. This variability in clinical behavior may be due to previously unrecognized tumor subtypes (see discussion of pilomyxoid astrocytoma) or unrecognized oncogenic stimulation in a small percentage of cases.

Pathology
Cerebellar pilocytic astrocytomas are soft and gray, with solid portions of the tumor often dwarfed by an associated thin-walled cyst. They appear well circumscribed and often cause significant mass effect on, and distortion of, the associated cerebellar hemisphere. Presence of vasogenic edema in surrounding parenchyma is inconsistent.

Although pilocytic astrocytomas appear well circumscribed on gross inspection, many lesions will demonstrate some degree of infiltration into the surrounding parenchyma. The tumor also has a tendency to break through the pia into the subarachnoid space and to infiltrate perivascular spaces. Despite these histologic characteristics, the degree and extent of infiltration into surrounding brain parenchyma is much less than that seen in other more aggressive astrocytoma subtypes.

The classic histologic feature of pilocytic astrocytoma is the Rosenthal fiber,[12,13] an eosinophilic worm-like or corkscrew-shaped structure representing intracellular bundles of astrocytic fibers (Fig. 35-13). They are GFAP positive. Although not exclusive to, or diagnostic of, pilocytic astrocytoma, these structures are a characteristic feature. Eosinophilic granular bodies are also

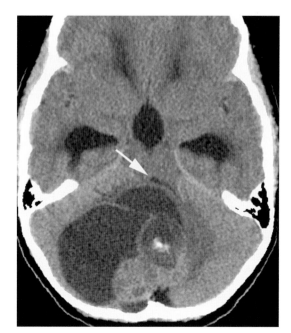

■ **FIGURE 35-14** Axial noncontrast CT image of a pilocytic astrocytoma of the right cerebellar hemisphere. The tumor is characterized by several large cysts with nodules of solid tissue, one of which has a focal calcification. *Arrow* points to the fourth ventricle, which is nearly completely effaced by the tumor.

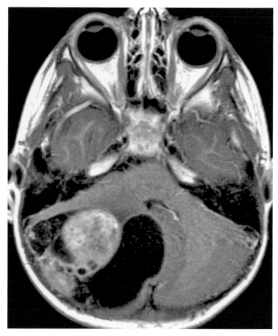

■ **FIGURE 35-15** Axial T1W MR image with gadolinium demonstrating the avid enhancement of the solid portions of this pilocytic astrocytoma.

identified within tumor cells. The tumors classically consist of two histologic regions; loosely organized microcystic regions with stellate astrocytes and compact tissue with fibrillary cells. The stellate cells typically contain the eosinophilic granular bodies, with Rosenthal fibers found in the compact tissue.[4]

Although pilocytic astrocytomas in the posterior fossa are most commonly found in the cerebellar hemispheres, these lesions may arise from the vermis, cerebellar peduncles, pons, and brain stem. Site of tumor origin is the primary factor affecting degree of resectability and associated morbidity and prognosis.

Imaging
CT

Pilocytic astrocytoma is recognized as one of several CNS tumors that exhibit the architecture of a nonenhancing cyst with an avidly enhancing mural nodule. This appearance can be recognized on both CT and MRI and is found in approximately one half of these tumors. Nearly as common is the appearance of a solid tumor with central necrosis, rather than thin-walled cyst formation. Less common in the posterior fossa is the homogeneously solid tumor, without any cystic or necrotic foci.

Typically large at the time of diagnosis (>3 cm), cerebellar pilocytic astrocytoma often elicit little or no surrounding vasogenic edema. Up to 20% of lesions may demonstrate some calcification, but this is not a helpful distinguishing feature. Evidence for intratumoral hemorrhage is rare. Solid portions of the tumor typically exhibit avid enhancement after intravenous contrast agent administration (Fig. 35-14).

These tumors characteristically cause some degree of obstructive hydrocephalus due to their mass effect on the fourth ventricle or the inferior aspect of the cerebral aqueduct. Evidence for the long-standing nature of the hydrocephalus and associated increased intracranial pressure can be recognized on CT by thinning of the calvaria. A relatively mild degree of periventricular edema may reflect a compensatory response to the presence of increased intraventricular pressure over an extended period of time.

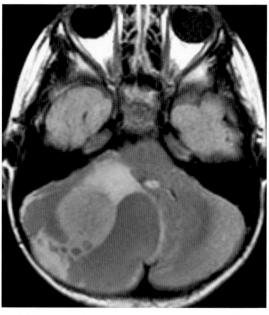

■ **FIGURE 35-16** The fluid in the cysts of this cerebellar pilocytic astrocytoma does not suppress to the same degree as the CSF in the ventricles and basal cisterns on this axial FLAIR image.

MRI

MRI features of pilocytic astrocytoma reflect histologic characteristics and parallel the appearance on CT. Solid portions of the tumor are isointense or hypointense relative to gray matter on T1W images and are slightly hyperintense to gray matter on T2W images.[13] The solid portions almost invariably enhance avidly after contrast agent administration (Fig. 35-15). The thin walls of the cysts will typically not demonstrate contrast enhancement, reflecting absence of tumor cells in the wall at histology. However, some cysts may be surrounded by enhancing tumor, likely representing regions of prior necrosis. Cystic foci typically follow CSF in signal on all pulse sequences (Fig. 35-16); necrotic

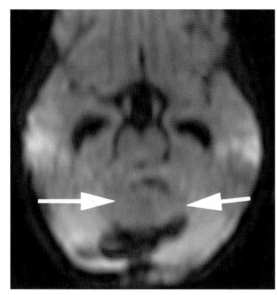

■ **FIGURE 35-17** DWI of pilocytic astrocytoma, showing no appreciable restricted diffusion (*arrows*). This is in stark contrast to the restricted diffusion demonstrated in medulloblastoma (compare with Fig. 35-6).

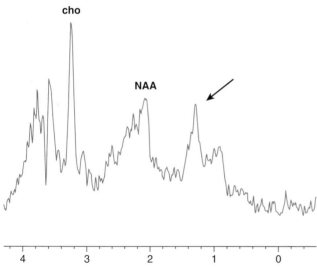

■ **FIGURE 35-18** Short-echo MR spectroscopy of pilocytic astrocytoma paradoxically shows an aggressive pattern of metabolite resonances in spite of the fully benign nature of the tumor: elevated choline (cho), depressed *N*-acetyl-aspartate (NAA), and a prominent lactate peak (*arrow*).

foci will usually be hyperintense to CSF on T2W images, FLAIR images, and DWI.

Evaluation of solid aspects of pilocytic astrocytoma with DWI demonstrates a lesser degree of diffusion restriction than is seen with medulloblastoma or ependymoma (Fig. 35-17).[8]

MR spectroscopy of pilocytic astrocytoma indicates a metabolically aggressive tumor (Fig. 35-18), despite the relatively benign prognosis of this lesion. NAA is dramatically suppressed, with elevation of choline and lactate. Myoinositol is usually not as elevated as in ependymoma.

PILOMYXOID ASTROCYTOMA

Pilomyxoid astrocytoma was first described as a tumor distinct from the more common pilocytic astrocytoma in 1999.[14] These astrocytic tumors were initially described as occurring nearly exclusively in the parasellar region in infants, with histologic features distinguishing them from the more common pilocytic astrocytoma. Other names for this tumor include pediatric astrocytoma with monomorphous pilomyxoid features, pilomyxoid glioma, and tanycytoma.

Epidemiology

Epidemiologic and demographic data regarding this newly described tumor are understandably fluctuant. Initially described as a tumor of infants, with a mean age at diagnosis of 16 to 18 months,[15] the age range appears to be shifting toward older children with the increased frequency of diagnosis.

Clinical Presentation

Pilomyxoid astrocytoma does not exhibit distinct features of clinical presentation relative to other posterior fossa tumors, presenting with nausea, vomiting, headache, or focal cerebellar signs such as ataxia and nystagmus. However, because these tumors are often diagnosed in infants, an additional presenting symptom can be failure to thrive.

Pathophysiology

There is some debate as to whether pilomyxoid astrocytoma represents an entity distinct from pilocytic astrocytoma or a variant subtype of that more common tumor. Distinct histologic features indicate that pilomyxoid astrocytoma should be considered a separate entity, with appropriate alterations in clinical management strategy. However, there has been report of recurrent pilomyxoid astrocytoma demonstrating histologic features of pilocytic astrocytoma at second biopsy, suggesting that the original tumor may have "matured" or "evolved" into the more common form.[16]

There is little debate regarding the more aggressive clinical course of pilomyxoid astrocytoma relative to pilocytic astrocytoma. Pilomyxoid astrocytoma demonstrates a higher rate of local recurrence and subarachnoid dissemination, with associated decrease in length of progression-free or disease-free survival. Accordingly, there has been greater use of adjuvant chemotherapy in the clinical management of children diagnosed with pilomyxoid astrocytoma, with radiation therapy held in abeyance owing to the young age of the affected patient population.

Unlike the characteristic biphasic histology of pilocytic astrocytoma, pilomyxoid astrocytoma demonstrates a monomorphous population of piloid astrocytes in an extensive myxoid background. The tumor cells typically lack the characteristic Rosenthal fibers and the eosinophilic granular bodies seen in pilocytic astrocytoma and often demonstrate an angiocentric growth pattern.[15]

Initially described as a tumor of the hypothalamic/chiasmatic region exclusively, pilomyxoid astrocytoma has been diagnosed in the posterior fossa and spinal cord as well.

Imaging
CT

Most reports of imaging in pilomyxoid astrocytoma have concentrated on findings at MRI. Unlike pilocytic astrocytoma, these tumors are rarely cystic and there are no reports of tumors containing calcifications.

MRI

Pilomyxoid astrocytomas are recognized as predominantly solid tumors on MRI, with hypointense signal on T1W sequences and hyperintense signal on T2W sequences. They exhibit homogeneous and avid enhancement after contrast agent administration (Fig. 35-19), and the majority will demonstrate adjacent or disseminated abnormal leptomeningeal enhancement. Although many will show regions of tumor necrosis, hemorrhage has not been reported in association with pilomyxoid astrocytoma.

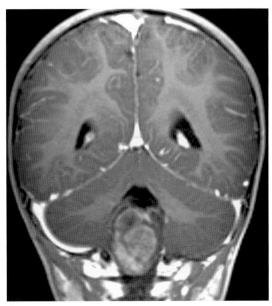

■ **FIGURE 35-19** Contrast-enhanced coronal T1W MR image of posterior fossa pilomyxoid astrocytoma.

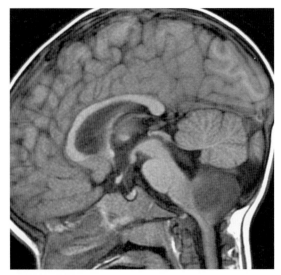

■ **FIGURE 35-20** Exophytic pontomedullary glioma. This low-grade tumor has a distinctly better prognosis than the more commonly encountered infiltrating pontine glioma.

Cystic foci can be recognized but are seen with much less frequency than in pilocytic astrocytoma.[17]

BRAIN STEM GLIOMA

Brain stem glioma is an infiltrating astrocytoma of the medulla, pons, or midbrain. Alternate names include pontine glioma, pontine astrocytoma, midbrain glioma, midbrain astrocytoma, and fibrillary astrocytoma.

Epidemiology

Brain stem gliomas account for up to 25% of posterior fossa neoplasms in children. They are almost all sporadic tumors, although there is an increased incidence in children with NF1.

Clinical Presentation

Infiltrating brain stem gliomas are most commonly diagnosed in children 3 to 10 years of age, equally distributed between males and females. Progressive cranial nerve palsies are characteristically diagnosed at presentation, as well as headache, nausea, vomiting, ataxia, and apneic episodes. However, the stratification of natural history associated with the craniocaudal distribution of these lesions (see later) is also seen in their initial clinical presentation. Superiorly located lesions, impinging on the cerebral aqueduct or tectum, typically present in the older half of this age range (6-10 years) as headache secondary to CSF obstruction; they may be dormant. Infiltrating pontine lesions classically cause pyramidal tract signs, ataxia, and nystagmus. Medullary lesions characteristically present as dysfunction of lower cranial nerves, which may cause apnea or swallowing difficulties.[18]

Pathophysiology

Brain stem glioma is an entity that is primarily defined by its location rather then unique structural, physiologic, or genetic features. The presumed cell of origin is the astrocyte, and the intrinsic characteristics of this tumor are not significantly different from those of infiltrating astrocytomas diagnosed in other regions of the brain. However, infiltrating fibrillary astrocytomas outside the brain stem are rarely diagnosed in children.

As indicated earlier, there is some stratification of clinical behavior and natural history dependent on location within the brain stem, such that most authors will distinguish midbrain and periaqueductal gliomas from those occurring within the pons,

which are, in turn, distinguished from those occurring at the cervicomedullary junction.[19]

Gliomas of the tectum and periaqueductal gray matter are typically indolent lesions with a clinical behavior more akin to dysplasia than neoplasia. Not truly posterior fossa tumors, these lesions will not be further considered here.

A significant proportion of gliomas arising in the medulla oblongata will be clearly defined lesions with a prominent dorsally exophytic pattern of growth, projecting into the cisterna magna and displacing the cerebellar vermis superiorly (Fig. 35-20). Tumors demonstrating this growth pattern are almost invariably pilocytic astrocytomas, with clinical and imaging features that parallel those of this lesion diagnosed elsewhere in the CNS.

Conversely, the diffuse and infiltrating brain stem glioma is a neoplasm of fibrillary astrocytes and comprises more than two thirds of all pediatric brain stem tumors. Because these tumors are poorly defined infiltrating lesions in the brain stem, complete surgical resection is rarely feasible. By and large they are resistant to treatment with radiation therapy or chemotherapy. Moreover, the young age at diagnosis and the compromise of vital functions caused by these tumors often limit the aggressiveness of chemotherapeutic or radiation treatment protocols. As a consequence, prognosis of these lesions is almost uniformly dismal.

Children diagnosed with NF1 frequently will exhibit regions of abnormal signal and altered morphology in the brain stem. These nonspecific signal abnormalities typically involute over time, without clinically significant sequelae. However, their presence can mask the development of an infiltrating glioma in the brain stem, a diagnosis that occurs with a slightly increased frequency in this phakomatosis. Fortunately, brain stem gliomas in children with NF1 exhibit a less aggressive natural history than sporadically occurring lesions.

Pathology

The infiltrating brain stem glioma considered here is most commonly centered within the pons but will often have extension superiorly into the midbrain, inferiorly into the medulla, and dorsally into the cerebellar peduncles. Although some tumors will have frankly exophytic foci, a diffuse and infiltrative pattern of growth predominates. Margins of the tumor are often difficult to distinguish by imaging or visual inspection, confounding attempts at accurate documentation of lesion size. However,

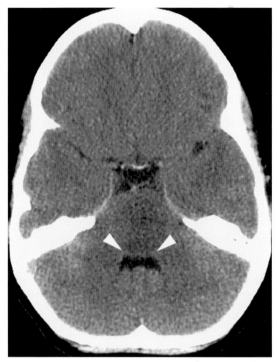

■ **FIGURE 35-21** Although there is subtle decreased density in the pons of this child with an infiltrating pontine glioma, the more helpful finding on this nonenhanced CT study is the flattening of the normal curved contour of the anterior fourth ventricle (*arrowheads*).

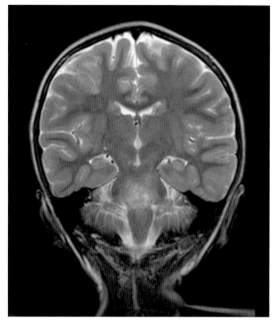

■ **FIGURE 35-22** Coronal T2W MR image of an infiltrating pontine glioma shows the characteristic irregular hyperintense signal and poorly defined margins.

most infiltrating pontine gliomas are 2 to 3 cm in diameter at presentation. They expand the pons and brain stem, often encasing vascular structures on the surface.

The microscopic features of an infiltrating brain stem glioma are dominated by hypercellularity and lack of normal structural organization. As they infiltrate into surrounding white matter, tumor cells encase axons, oligodendrocytes, and normal astrocytes. The tumor cells classically demonstrate some degree of nuclear atypia; low-grade lesions exhibit few if any mitotic figures and may be difficult to distinguish from reactive gliosis. However, infiltrating pontine gliomas are almost invariably anaplastic (grade III) at histology, with multiple mitotic figures, cellular pleomorphism, and necrosis.[4] Highly undifferentiated tumors with necrotic and hemorrhagic foci are considered grade IV lesions (glioblastoma multiforme).

Imaging
The diagnosis of infiltrating brain stem glioma is often made by imaging and clinical evaluation alone; small-volume needle biopsies of these lesions are rarely sufficient to make the diagnosis, and the eloquent location of these tumors makes more aggressive excisional biopsy or attempts at surgical resection imprudent. Inflammatory pathologic processes can mimic infiltrating pontine glioma,[20] and it is important for the imager to employ all techniques available to confidently make the correct diagnosis.

CT
Although hypercellular relative to normal white matter, the disorganization of infiltrating brain stem gliomas causes them to be subtly hypoattenuating on CT. The degree of attenuation difference may be very difficult to appreciate, especially in the presence of beam-hardening artifact in the posterior fossa. A more definitive finding on CT is the distortion of normal pontine morphology that can cause effacement of the prepontine cistern and distortion of the fourth ventricle (Fig. 35-21). Calcifications are

essentially unheard of in infiltrating brain stem glioma, and these lesions usually have minimal or delayed contrast enhancement. All of these factors hamper the ability to correctly diagnose these lesions on CT.

MRI
MRI is the modality of choice for the detection and diagnosis of infiltrating brain stem glioma. It is not only the most accurate means of identifying and characterizing these tumors, it is also the most sensitive modality for the detection of other posterior fossa neoplasms and non-neoplastic lesions that must be considered in the clinical differential diagnosis. Because histologic confirmation is frequently not obtained, it is essential that the MRI evaluation be as complete as possible, employing techniques that will allow for an accurate assessment and associated prognosis.

Infiltrating brain stem gliomas are hyperintense on T2W and FLAIR imaging (Fig. 35-22), reflecting the decreased organization and increasing intercellular space compared with the normally tightly compacted white matter of the pons and brain stem. The signal abnormality of the tumor typically fades into the surrounding white matter structures, without a clearly defined margin. This marginal indistinctness is frequently compounded by the presence of surrounding vasogenic edema. However, some lesions are more focally defined, appearing encapsulated (Fig. 35-23). Such a clearly defined appearance may indicate the less commonly encountered histology of pilocytic astrocytoma that may justify attempts at surgical resection or excisional biopsy. These are more often located in the medulla, dorsal pons, and midbrain (see Fig. 35-20).

Infiltrating brain stem gliomas demonstrate variable degrees of contrast enhancement. Some lesions will dramatically change in their pattern of enhancement over time, perhaps in response to treatment. Although there is a general trend toward more prominent enhancement in more aggressive lesions, the degree and extent of contrast enhancement cannot be relied on to determine lesion grade or predict response to therapy.

Most brain stem gliomas do not exhibit significantly restricted diffusion. However, the key differentiating factor between a

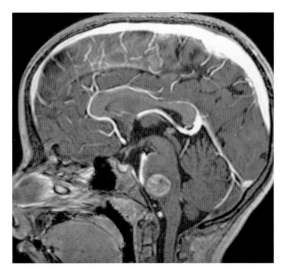

■ **FIGURE 35-23**   This sagittal T1W MR image with contrast indicates that this pontine glioma has well-defined margins and may be amenable to surgical resection.

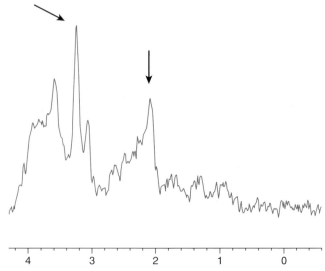

■ **FIGURE 35-25**   MR spectroscopy of an infiltrating brain stem glioma shows an aggressive metabolite pattern, with reduction of *N*-acetyl-aspartate (*vertical arrow*) and elevation of choline (*oblique arrow*).

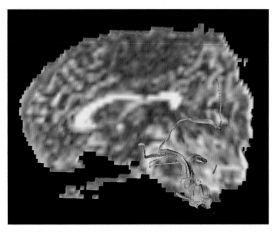

■ **FIGURE 35-24**   Diffusion tractography (DTI) was performed on white matter tracks in the medulla oblongata of this child with a pontine glioma, demonstrating dorsal displacement of the white matter tracts by the more ventrally situated tumor. DTI has been used to help guide surgical planning for these types of tumors.

potentially resectable lesion and the more common diffusely infiltrating glioma is the integrity of the ascending, descending, and crossing white matter tracts in the brain stem. Infiltrating tumors engulf these tracts, preventing any significant degree of resection without intolerable neurologic deficit. In contrast, exophytic or encapsulated lesions may primarily displace the normal white matter tracts. Limited experience suggests that multidirectional diffusion tractography techniques can distinguish between these patterns of white matter tract encasement versus displacement.[21,22] While it is reasonable to employ diffusion tensor imaging in the evaluation of all brain stem lesions, it is especially helpful in those that demonstrate features suggesting an encapsulated or exophytic nature (Fig. 35-24).

MR spectroscopy can provide valuable insight in the diagnosis of brain stem gliomas. Because these tumors will encase (rather than displace) normal brain tissue as they grow, MR spectroscopy may show some preservation of NAA in even high-grade lesions. However, choline levels will increase with increasing tumor grade and the presence of a lipid/lactate doublet suggests some degree of necrosis (Fig. 35-25). Encephalitis will

not exhibit the same degree of choline elevation and may be notable for increases in myoinositol.

Perfusion imaging techniques have been employed in the evaluation of infiltrating gliomas in the cerebrum in adults, with some success in predicting lesion grade.[23] These techniques are beginning to be employed in the pediatric population. Although it is rare to identify hemorrhage in a brain stem glioma at presentation, hemorrhage and/or necrosis in response to therapy is relatively common. Rarely, a brain stem tumor will present as massive life-threatening hemorrhage.

ATYPICAL TERATOID/RHABDOID TUMOR

This uncommon and aggressive tumor of young children is composed of rhabdoid cells, undifferentiated cells, and malignant mesenchymal or epithelial tissue. Other names include malignant rhabdoid tumor of brain, intracranial rhabdoid tumor, and CNS rhabdoid.

Epidemiology

Atypical teratoid/rhabdoid tumors are tumors of very young children, with the majority reported in children younger than 3 years of age. However, as this tumor has become diagnosed with more frequency, reports of older children with this tumor are increasing.

Clinical Presentation

Atypical teratoid/rhabdoid tumor is considered to be a mimic of medulloblastoma in its clinical, imaging, and histologic features. Like medulloblastoma, clinical onset tends to be rapid, with signs and symptoms of increased intracranial pressure (increased head circumference, irritability, vomiting, papilledema). Ataxia, seizures, cranial nerve palsies, and spinal cord symptoms due to metastatic disease have all been observed.

Pathophysiology

The cell of origin of atypical teratoid/rhabdoid tumors is not defined. One theory is that the tumor arises from meningothelial cells, which share characteristics with serosal cells, which may be related to renal rhabdoid tumors. Atypical teratoid/rhabdoid tumors is a complex tumor that contains a combination of epithelial, mesenchymal, and primitive neuroectodermal elements. The distinctive rhabdoid cells found in this tumor resemble those of malignant rhabdoid tumors of the kidney. Like a tera-

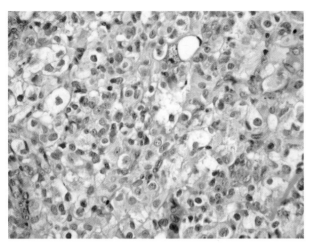

■ **FIGURE 35-26** High-power photomicrograph of atypical teratoid/rhabdoid tumor shows striking heterogeneity when compared with the more common medulloblastoma. Tumor cells are larger, with pale cytoplasm and prominent nucleoli (H&E stain).

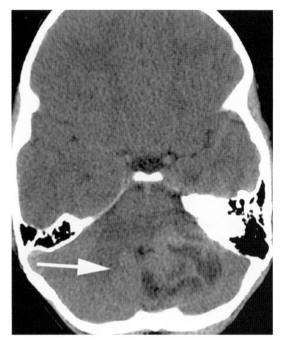

■ **FIGURE 35-27** An eccentrically located posterior fossa atypical teratoid/rhabdoid tumor appears notably heterogeneous (*arrow*) on this nonenhanced CT study.

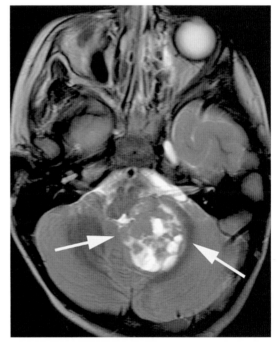

■ **FIGURE 35-28** Axial T2W MR image of atypical teratoid/rhabdoid tumor shows multiple solid and cystic foci within the tumor (*arrows*).

toma, multiple cell lines can be identified in these tumors by immunohistologic staining. However, none of the cell lines demonstrates significant differentiation/maturation. Like rhabdoid tumors of the kidney, atypical teratoid/rhabdoid tumor is associated with deletions and mutations of the rhabdoid tumor suppressor gene *INI1*, found on chromosome 22.[24] Some authors have identified differences in the types of mutations that occur in CNS tumors and renal tumors.

Atypical teratoid/rhabdoid tumors have been misdiagnosed as medulloblastoma in the past because of similar clinical features and dense cellularity at histology. However, these tumors are typically more heterogeneous, despite their lack of ultrastructural differentiation. Rhabdoid cells are considered a characteristic feature of this tumor. These cells are described as plump, with round or kidney-shaped nuclei and prominent nucleoli. Sheets of tumor cells are interspersed with fibrovascular septa (Fig. 35-26). Vacuolated cells can be interspersed, giving a "starry sky" appearance. These tumors invariably demonstrate immunoreactivity to vimentin and frequently stain positive for GFAP and cytokeratin.[4]

Because of their close association with medulloblastoma, atypical teratoid/rhabdoid tumors are classically thought of as posterior fossa tumors. However, a high percentage of tumors are supratentorial in origin or widely metastatic at presentation with an uncertain primary site.

Imaging
CT
Atypical teratoid/rhabdoid tumors can appear solid or heterogeneous on CT (Fig. 35-27). Like medulloblastoma, the dense cellularity of this tumor results in hyperattenuation relative to brain parenchyma on noncontrast studies. Calcifications may be present but are not a dominant feature. Close to 50% of tumors will demonstrate some hemorrhage. Solid portions enhance heterogeneously.

MRI
MRI features of atypical teratoid/rhabdoid tumors parallel those of medulloblastoma. Solid portions of the tumor often appear isointense to hypointense on T2W imaging, again reflecting dense cellularity (Fig. 35-28). However, the presence of calcification, hemorrhage, or regions of necrosis results in a heterogeneous signal pattern on most sequences. Surrounding vasogenic edema is a consistent feature. Solid portions of the tumor demonstrate moderate to marked enhancement and close to 50% of

lesions will demonstrate subarachnoid spread of disease (Fig. 35-29) at diagnosis.[25-27]

DYSPLASTIC CEREBELLAR GANGLIOCYTOMA
Dysplastic cerebellar gangliocytoma is a mass lesion of the cerebellum that has some features of a mixed glial-neuronal tumor but with a clinical pattern of behavior that is more characteristic of a hamartoma. Other names include Lhermitte-Duclos disease, purkinjeoma, cerebellar hamartoma, ganglioneuroma,

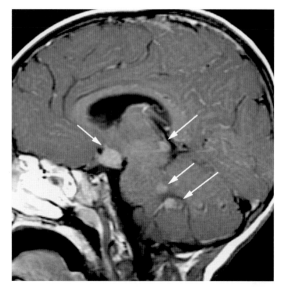

■ **FIGURE 35-29**   Enhancing tumor nodules (*arrows*) can be seen in the suprasellar cistern, abutting the tectum, and at the superior and inferior aspects of the fourth ventricle on contrast-enhanced T1W MRI in this infant with widespread atypical teratoid/rhabdoid tumor.

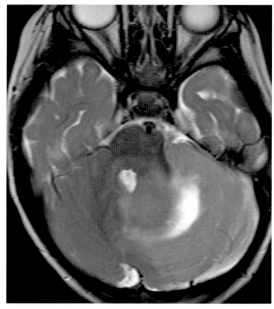

■ **FIGURE 35-30**   Axial T2W MR image of dysplastic cerebellar ganglio-cytoma (Lhermitte-Duclos disease). Like an infiltrating glioma of the brain stem, this lesion enlarges and distorts the cerebellar hemisphere, rather than displacing normal brain tissue.

benign hypertrophy of the cerebellum, ganglion cell tumor of the cerebellum, granular cell hypertrophy, neurocytoma myelini-cum, and gangliocytoma myelinicum diffusum.

Epidemiology
Dysplastic cerebellar gangliocytoma is an extremely rare entity, with approximately 100 cases reported in the literature. It is characteristically a lesion of young adults but has been reported in children.

Clinical Presentation
Although these lesions will occasionally present with cerebellar signs, they are more commonly diagnosed secondary to obstruc-tion of the fourth ventricle and associated increased intracranial pressure.

Pathophysiology
Dysplastic cerebellar gangliocytoma is associated with Cowden syndrome, an autosomal dominant inherited syndrome causing multiple hamartomas and associated with mutations of the *PTEN/MMAC* gene on chromosome 10. Other lesions of Cowden syndrome include gastrointestinal tract polyps, thyroid adeno-mas, cataracts, and oral papillomas.[28]

Strictly speaking, dysplastic cerebellar gangliocytoma lesions are not neoplasms but rather hamartomas. However, there has been report of a case in which anaplastic ganglioglioma devel-oped at the site of pathologically diagnosed dysplastic cerebellar gangliocytoma.[29]

Pathology
Dysplastic cerebellar gangliocytomas are typically pale relative to normal adjacent cerebellum, causing diffuse enlargement of the affected cerebellar hemisphere. Unlike focal tumors within the hemisphere, they do not flatten cerebellar sulci but result in enlarged and thickened cerebellar folia. Although they charac-teristically involve one hemisphere, they can be located in the vermis or cross the midline.

The major histologic features of dysplastic cerebellar ganglio-cytoma are replacement and enlargement of the internal granular layer of the cerebellum by large neurons with prominent nucle-oli. The cells lack the structural organization of normal Purkinje

cells and may be confused with glial cells, raising concern for an infiltrating glioma. Because they are neuronal cells, they are immunopositive for synaptophysin.

Imaging
CT
Dysplastic cerebellar gangliocytoma is nonenhancing and typi-cally hypodense relative to normal cerebellum on CT. Occasion-ally, the characteristic striations of this lesion can be appreciated on CT.

MRI
The thickened and enlarged cerebellar folia found in dysplastic cerebellar gangliocytoma results in a characteristic appear-ance on T2W MRI, with alternating lines of hyperintense and hypointense signal. The "striated" cerebellum is considered a

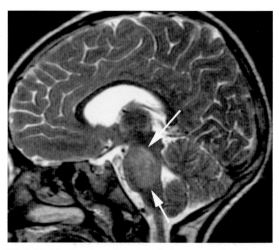

■ **FIGURE 35-31**   *Arrows* point to the lesion centered in the pons; the poorly defined margins and hyperintense signal on this T2W MR image are suggestive of infiltrating brain stem glioma.

pathognomonic appearance. Deeper portions of the lesion may appear considerably more bland (Fig. 35-30), lacking the corduroy appearance that is caused by the enlargement of cerebellar folia.

ANALYSIS

An analysis of the objective factors of patient age, lesion location, and lesion morphology can rapidly narrow the differential diagnosis of the posterior fossa mass in a child. Application of findings on DWI and MR spectroscopy can further specify the appropriate diagnostic considerations, as illustrated in the examples in Boxes 35-1 and 35-2.

KEY POINTS: DIFFERENTIAL DIAGNOSIS

- Medulloblastoma and pilocytic astrocytoma are two of the most common intracranial neoplasms diagnosed in children and comprise the majority of posterior fossa intra-axial tumors.
- Ependymoma and medulloblastoma are both primarily intraventricular neoplasms, with ependymoma growing dorsally from the floor of the fourth ventricle and the more common medulloblastoma growing ventrally from the roof.
- Although choroid plexus papilloma is in the differential diagnosis of a fourth ventricular neoplasm, in the pediatric population these lesions are more commonly found in the lateral ventricles.
- In older children (5-10 years old) medulloblastoma has a tendency to arise more laterally in the cerebellar hemispheres, often with variant histology (desmoplastic)
- Atypical teratoid/rhabdoid tumors often cannot be distinguished from medulloblastoma by imaging but classically occur in very young children (<18 months).
- MR spectroscopy can help distinguish infiltrating brain stem glioma from encephalitis by demonstrating a neoplastic, rather than reactive, metabolite pattern.
- Diffusion tractography may support the concept that a brain stem lesion is localized and therefore more amenable to surgical intervention.

BOX 35-1 Sample Report: MR Spectroscopy of Posterior Fossa Mass

PATIENT HISTORY

The patient is 11 years old, with a congenital immunologic deficiency. He presented acutely with nystagmus, and the lesion was inapparent on brain imaging 6 months previously.

FINDINGS

This is a lesion characterized by expansion of the pons with abnormal hyperintense signal on T2W images (Fig. 35-31). The lesion exhibits no enhancement (Fig. 35-32) and on MR spectroscopy shows only mildly diminished NAA and elevation of myoinositol (Fig. 35-33). Although the MR appearance is consistent with a diagnosis of infiltrating brain stem glioma, the patient is considerably older than most children diagnosed with this tumor. Moreover, the findings on MR spectroscopy suggest an inflammatory or reactive lesion rather than a neoplasm.

IMPRESSION

Coupled with the patient's susceptibility for atypical infectious disease, a presumptive diagnosis of brain stem encephalitis was made.

COMMENT

The patient was managed conservatively and had a complete recovery, with normalization of MRI.

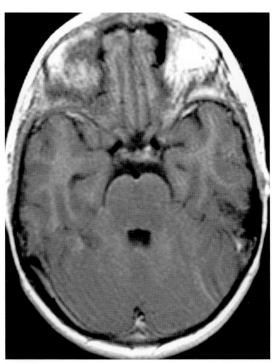

■ **FIGURE 35-32** Axial T1W MR image with contrast demonstrates no abnormal enhancement in the pontine lesion and surprisingly little architectural distortion.

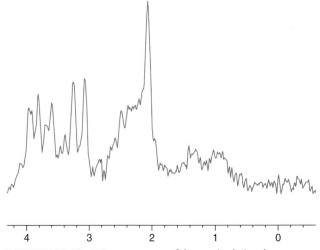

■ **FIGURE 35-33** MR spectroscopy of the pontine lesion demonstrates a benign pattern of metabolite resonances, inconsistent with an infiltrating glioma. Final diagnosis was encephalitis.

BOX 35-2 Sample Report: MRI of Posterior Fossa Mass

PATIENT HISTORY

A mass of the posterior fossa was identified on CT in a 2-year-old girl. CT study was obtained because of a history of a fall 2 weeks earlier. The child presented with vomiting.

TECHNIQUE

Contrast-enhanced MRI of brain was done with intravenous gadolinium (2.8 mL). Sagittal and axial precontrast T1W images and sagittal/axial/coronal T1W postcontrast images were obtained. Axial T2W, FLAIR, and diffusion-weighted images were done. Single voxel (8 mL) proton MR spectroscopy was performed over the lesion with short (35 ms) and long (288 ms) echo times. The study was performed under anesthesia.

FINDINGS

As noted on the prior CT, there is a large posterior fossa mass that is heterogeneous in signal intensity on all series, with a mild heterogeneous postcontrast enhancement. It exhibits a mild degree of diffusion restriction. It fills the mid and lower aspect of the fourth ventricle and extends through the foramen of Magendie into the upper cervical canal. There is also extension into the foramina of Luschka on both sides, left greater than right, without extension into the cerebellopontine angle. There is a well-defined plane between this mass and the dorsal aspect of the brain stem that is significantly flattened by the mass. Inferior extension extends to the mid body of C2. On postcontrast images the mass measures a maximum of 2.8 cm (anteroposterior) × 3.6 cm (transverse) × 5 cm (craniocaudad).

Short- and long-echo MR spectroscopy demonstrates elevated choline, absent NAA, and elevated lactate/lipid peak within the lesion.

There is obstructive hydrocephalus caused by the mass, with moderate to marked enlargement of the lateral and third ventricles and enlargement of the cerebral aqueduct; the degree of ventriculomegaly is similar to the prior CT. There is mild transependymal flow of CSF in a periventricular location. Since the prior CT there has been an intraventricular catheter placed via the right frontal approach with the tip in the region of the foramen of Monro.

Brain parenchymal signal intensity is otherwise normal. No CSF seeding is seen within the intracranial contents.

IMPRESSION

A midline intraventricular mass in the posterior fossa is causing obstructive hydrocephalus.

COMMENT

The imaging and MR spectroscopy characteristics are most consistent with an ependymoma. Less likely considerations would include atypical teratoid/rhabdoid tumor or medulloblastoma.

SUGGESTED READINGS

Biegel JA. Genetics of pediatric central nervous system tumors. J Pediatr Hematol Oncol 1997; 19:492-501.

Cha S. Update on brain tumor imaging: from anatomy to physiology. AJNR Am J Neuroradiol 2006; 27:475-487.

Chamberlain MC. Ependymomas. Curr Neurol Neurosci Rep 2003; 3:193-199.

Comstock B, Jarvik JG. A systematic literature review of magnetic resonance spectroscopy for the characterization of brain tumors. AJNR Am J Neuroradiol 2006; 27:1404-1411.

Hollingworth W, Medina LS, Lenkinski RE, et al. Brain tumors in children. Arch Neurol 1999; 56:421-425.

Schneider JF, Viola A, Confort-Gouny S, et al. Infratentorial pediatric brain tumors: the value of new imaging modalities. J Neuroradiol 2007; 34:49-58.

Tzika AA, Zarifi MK, Goumnerova L, et al. Neuroimaging in pediatric brain tumors: Gd-DTPA-enhanced, hemodynamic, and diffusion MR imaging compared with MR spectroscopic imaging. AJNR Am J Neuroradiol 2002; 23:322-333.

Wootton-Gorges SL, Foreman NK, Albano EA, et al. Pattern of recurrence in children with midline posterior fossa malignant neoplasms. Pediatr Radiol 2000; 30:90-93.

REFERENCES

1. Koeller KK, Rushing EJ. From the archives of the AFIP: medulloblastoma: a comprehensive review with radiologic-pathologic correlation. RadioGraphics 2003; 23:1613-1637.

2. Michiels EM, Weiss MM, Hoovers JM, et al. Genetic alterations in childhood medulloblastoma analyzed by comparative genomic hybridization. J Pediatr Hematol Oncol 2002; 24:205-210.

3. Amlashi SFA, Riffaud L, Brassier G, Morandi X. Nevoid basal cell carcinoma syndrome: relation with desmoplastic medulloblastoma in infancy: a population-based study and review of the literature. Cancer 2003; 98:618-624.

4. Burger PC, Scheithauer BW. Tumors of the Central Nervous System. Washington, DC, Armed Forces Institute of Pathology, 1994.

5. Provias JP, Becker LE. Cellular and molecular pathology of medulloblastoma. Neurooncol 1996; 29:35-43.

6. Chawla A, Emmanuel JV, Seow WT, et al. Paediatric PNET: presurgical MRI features. Clin Radiol 2007; 62:43-52.

7. Schubert MI, Wilke M, Muller-Weihrich S, Auer DP. Diffusion-weighted magnetic resonance imaging of treatment-associated changes in recurrent and residual medulloblastoma: preliminary observations in three children. Acta Radiol 2006; 47:1100-1104.

8. Rumboldt Z, Camacho DL, Lake D, et al. Apparent diffusion coefficients for differentiation of cerebellar tumors in children. AJNR Am J Neuroradiol 2006; 27:1362-1369.

9. Panigrahy A, Krieger MD, Gonzalez-Gomez I, et al. Quantitative short echo time 1H-MR spectroscopy of untreated pediatric brain tumors: preoperative diagnosis and characterization. AJNR Am J Neuroradiol 2006; 27:560-572.

10. Grill J, Avet-Loiseau H, Lellouch-Tubiana A, et al. Comparative genomic hybridization detects specific cytogenetic abnormalities in pediatric ependymomas and choroid plexus papillomas. Cancer Genet Cytogenet 2002; 136:121-125.

11. Steinbok P, Poskitt K, Hendson G. Spontaneous regression of cerebellar astrocytoma after subtotal resection. Childs Nerv Syst 2006; 22:572-576.

12. Wippold FJ 2nd, Perry A, Lennerz J. Neuropathology for the neuroradiologist: Rosenthal fibers. AJNR Am J Neuroradiol 2006; 27:958-961.

13. Koeller KK, Rushing EJ. From the Archives of the AFIP: Pilocytic astrocytoma: radiologic-pathologic correlation. RadioGraphics 2004; 24:1693-1708.

14. Tihan T, Fisher PG, Kepner JL, et al. Pediatric astrocytomas with monomorphous pilomyxoid features and a less favorable outcome. J Neuropathol Exp Neurol 1999; 58:1061-1068.

15. Komotar RJ, Mocco J, Carson BS, et al. Pilomyxoid astrocytoma: a review. Med Gen Med 2004; 6:42.

16. Ceppa EP, Bouffet E, Griebel R, et al. The pilomyxoid astrocytoma and its relationship to pilocytic astrocytoma: report of a case and a critical review of the entity. J Neurooncol 2007; 81:191-196.
17. Arslanoglu A, Cirak B, Horska A, et al. MR imaging characteristics of pilomyxoid astrocytomas. AJNR Am J Neuroradiol 2003; 24:1906-1908.
18. Jallo GI, Biser-Rohrbaugh A, Freed D. Brainstem gliomas. Childs Nerv Syst 2004; 20:143-53. Epub 2003 Dec 11.
19. Fisher PG, Breiter SN, Carson BS, et al. A clinicopathologic reappraisal of brain stem tumor classification: identification of pilocytic astrocytoma and fibrillary astrocytoma as distinct entities. Cancer 2000; 89:1569-1576.
20. Soo MS, Tien RD, Gray L, et al. Mesenrhombencephalitis: MR findings in nine patients. AJR Am J Roentgenol 1993; 160:1089-1093.
21. Chen X, Weigel D, Ganslandt O, et al. Diffusion tensor imaging and white matter tractography in patients with brainstem lesions. Acta Neurochir (Wien) 2007; Aug 23 [Epub ahead of print].
22. Tummala RP, Chu RM, Liu H, et al. Application of diffusion tensor imaging to magnetic-resonance-guided brain tumor resection. Pediatr Neurosurg 2003; 39:39-43.
23. Law M, Yang S, Wang H, et al. Glioma grading: sensitivity, specificity, and predictive values of perfusion MR imaging and proton MR spectroscopic imaging compared with conventional MR imaging. AJNR Am J Neuroradiol 2003; 24:1989-1998.
24. Takei H, Bhattacharjee MB, Rivera A, et al. New immunohistochemical markers in the evaluation of central nervous system tumors: a review of 7 selected adult and pediatric brain tumors. Arch Pathol Lab Med 2007; 131:234-241.
25. Arslanoglu A, Aygun N, Tekhtani D, et al. Imaging findings of CNS atypical teratoid/rhabdoid tumors. AJNR Am J Neuroradiol 2004; 25:476-480.
26. Meyers SP, Khademian ZP, Biegel JA, et al. Primary intracranial atypical teratoid/rhabdoid tumors of infancy and childhood: MRI features and patient outcomes. AJNR Am J Neuroradiol 2006; 27:962-971.
27. Parmar H, Hawkins C, Bouffet E, et al. Imaging findings in primary intracranial atypical teratoid/rhabdoid tumors. Pediatr Radiol 2006; 36:126-132.
28. Abel TW, Baker SJ, Fraser MM, et al. Lhermitte-Duclos disease: a report of 31 cases with immunohistochemical analysis of the PTEN/AKT/mTOR pathway. J Neuropathol Exp Neurol 2005; 64:341-349.
29. Takei H, Dauser R, Su J, et al. Anaplastic ganglioglioma arising from a Lhermitte-Duclos-like lesion. J Neurosurg (2 Suppl Pediatrics) 2007; 107:137-142.

CHAPTER 36

Cerebellopontine Angle and Internal Auditory Canal Neoplasms

Alice B. Smith and James G. Smirniotopoulos

The cerebellopontine angle (CPA) cistern is a cerebrospinal fluid (CSF)–filled space whose boundaries are made up by the pons and cerebellum medially, the petrous portion of the temporal bone laterally, and the tentorium superiorly. The Cranial nerves V through VIII pass through the upper portion of the cistern, whereas the cranial nerves IX through XI pass through the lower portion. The presenting symptoms of CPA lesions are usually not related to the histology of the lesion but to the nerves and other structures that the lesion affects.

Neoplasms occurring in this region make up 6% to 10% of all intracranial tumors in adults and only 1% of lesions in children.[1,2] The two most common lesions are the meningioma and the vestibular schwannoma. Indeed, meningiomas and schwannomas comprise approximately 90% of neoplasms in this region.[3] However, a variety of other lesions also make their home in the CPA region. These lesions arise within the cerebellopontine cistern or from related structures and include arachnoid cysts, nonacoustic schwannomas, and meningeal lesions. Embryologic remnants may also be found, including lipomas, epidermoid cysts, and neurenteric cysts. Lesions, such as chondromatous tumors, chordomas, paragangliomas, and endolymphatic sac tumors, involve the CPA by extension from surrounding structures such as the skull base and petrous apex. Exophytic brain stem neoplasms or ventricular tumors can also involve the CPA. Locating a point of origin along with knowledge of a lesion's morphology, CT density, MR intensity, and reaction of adjacent structures can help narrow the differential diagnosis.

SCHWANNOMA

Schwannomas are encapsulated lesions that arise from the Schwann cells of cranial, spinal, and peripheral nerves. Schwannomas are also referred to as neurilemmomas. Schwannomas arising from the vestibular nerves are currently referred to as vestibular or acoustic schwannomas but have also been known by the names acoustic neuroma, acoustic neurinoma, and neurilemmoma.

Epidemiology

Vestibular schwannomas are the most common lesions of the CPA, comprising up to 90% of lesions that occur within this region. For sporadic vestibular schwannomas, the age at presentation is typically between 30 and 40 years of age. In patients with neurofibromatosis type 2 the presentation is frequently earlier, usually in the second decade of life. Some reports describe no sex predilection; however, others report an increased prevalence in women of $2:1$.[1,4]

Clinical Presentation

Patients with schwannomas may present with loss of function of the affected cranial nerve or may be asymptomatic. Sensorineural hearing loss, especially high frequency, is the most common presentation in patients with vestibular schwannoma, whereas vertigo and balance problems are relatively uncommon. In patients with trigeminal schwannomas, the presenting symptoms may be facial pain or atrophy of the muscles of mastication.

Pathophysiology

In the majority of cases (>95%), schwannomas arise as sporadic lesions. However, schwannomas are also associated with neurofibromatosis type 2, which is an autosomal dominant syndrome with a mutation located on chromosome 22. These patients frequently have multiple schwannomas, and the presence of bilateral vestibular schwannomas is nearly pathognomonic for the disorder. In addition, these patients also have a propensity to develop meningiomas and ependymomas (Fig. 36-1).

Intracranial schwannomas most frequently arise from the sensory nerves, and of these the vestibular segment of the eighth cranial nerve is most common. The trigeminal nerve is the second most frequently involved cranial nerve, but these lesions are much less frequent.

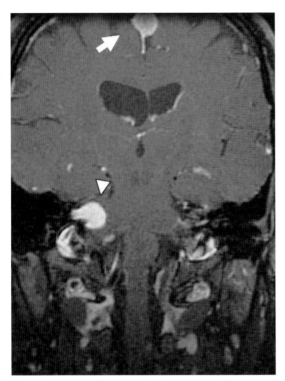

■ **FIGURE 36-1** Neurofibromatosis type 2. Coronal T1W MR image after gadolinium administration demonstrates an enhancing lesion within the right IAC (*arrowhead*) consistent with a vestibular schwannoma. In addition, a meningioma (*arrow*) is noted adjacent to the falx cerebri.

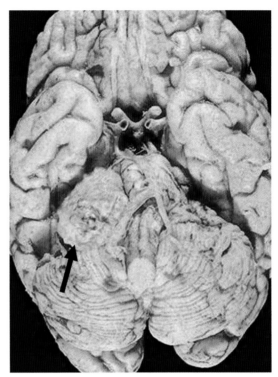

■ **FIGURE 36-2** Vestibular schwannoma. Gross specimen of the brain demonstrates a mass (*arrow*) with similar coloration to the adjacent brain that is displacing the brain stem.

Pathology

Schwannomas are well-circumscribed lesions that are most often tan (Fig. 36-2). The larger and older tumors may undergo benign cystic degeneration. They are spindle cell neoplasms that are composed of two tissue types, the Antoni A and Antoni B cells (Fig. 36-3). The Antoni A regions are hypercellular and compactly arranged. These areas account for a lower signal on T2-weighted (T2W) images. Antoni B regions are composed of looser myxomatous tissue, resulting in a brighter signal on T2W images. These areas are thought responsible for cystic changes within schwannomas. The imaging findings of schwannomas are dependent on the component of Antoni A or B cells. Antoni A and B tissues may align into palisades, which are referred to as the Verocay body.[5]

Immunohistochemical staining of schwannomas is positive for S-100, which is a protein found in cells derived from neural crest origin. They may be focally positive for glial fibrillary acidic protein (GFAP). GFAP is a member of the intermediate filament family that provides support and strength to astroglial cells.[5]

Imaging

CT

For the most part, MRI has replaced CT in the evaluation of CPA angle masses. When CT is utilized, thin-section (1.5 mm) imaging should be performed. The imaging characteristics of schwannomas on CT depend in part on the size of the lesion. Smaller schwannomas may not be readily visible on CT. In the case of vestibular schwannomas a small lesion arising along the intracanalicular portion of the nerve will be contained entirely within the internal auditory canal (IAC) and may not be readily visible by CT. As the lesion enlarges, it extends outward into the CPA and presents as a rounded mass that is either hypoattenuating or isodense to brain. This is referred to by some as the "ice cream

cone" pattern. Expansion of the IAC may be seen in up to 70% to 90%.[6] In addition, the intracanalicular lesions may "dumbbell" into the vestibule or cochlea, which is better appreciated on MRI.[7]

Larger lesions may have a heterogeneous appearance due to cystic degeneration. In fact, most, if not all, schwannomas larger than 2.5 cm become heterogeneous due to cystic and necrotic components.[8] On postcontrast imaging schwannomas demonstrate enhancement. Calcification is very rare within schwannomas and, if seen, should raise the suspicion of a meningioma. Thin-section (1.5 mm) imaging utilizing bone algorithm assists in visualizing the expansion of the IAC as well as any small calcifications within the lesion.

MRI

The utilization of thin-section (3 mm) MRI is beneficial in evaluation of most lesions of the CPA. Administration of a contrast agent is a necessary part of the examination because smaller lesions may be missed if contrast enhancement is not utilized.

The appearance of schwannomas on MRI, like CT, may vary with the tumor size. As the lesions become larger they may undergo cystic change, and this alters their signal characteristics. Typically, schwannomas are slightly hypointense to isointense on T1-weighted (T1W) imaging. However, T1 hyperintensity may be seen if there has been hemorrhage into the schwannoma or if regions of cystic degeneration contain proteinaceous material. These lesions enhance intensely after gadolinium infusion, and the degree of homogeneous enhancement depends on the amount of cystic change (Fig. 36-4). Schwannomas are typically hyperintense on T2W imaging, and if cystic degeneration is present more focal areas of increased signal will be seen. Expansion of the IAC may be seen in up to 70% to 90% of vestibular schwannomas (Fig. 36-5).[6] Approximately 5% of schwannomas may be associated with an arachnoid cyst that occurs between the neoplasm and the brain, suggesting that the mechanism of formation is peritumoral adhesions (Fig. 36-6).[9]

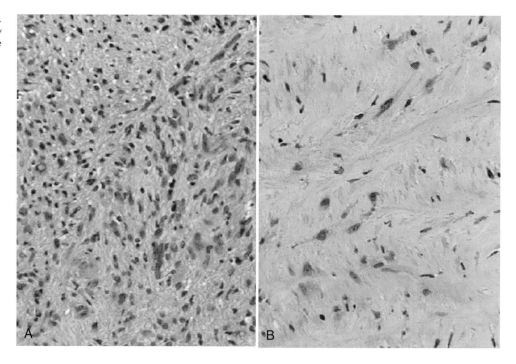

■ **FIGURE 36-3** Schwannoma. Antoni A cells **(A)** stain more darkly and are more compact than the more loosely arranged Antoni B cells **(B)**.

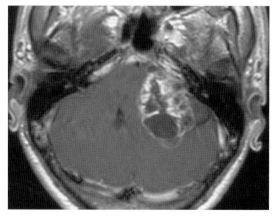

■ **FIGURE 36-4** Vestibular schwannoma. A large, heterogeneously enhancing mass is seen in the right CPA. Areas of nonenhancement correspond to regions of cystic degeneration.

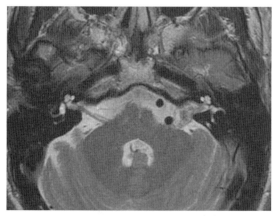

■ **FIGURE 36-5** Vestibular schwannoma. Axial T2W MR image demonstrates a heterogeneous-appearing lesion involving the left IAC that extends into the CPA. Widening of the left IAC is noted.

The major imaging differential diagnosis for schwannomas is the meningioma. Meningiomas may extend into the IAC and may be very difficult to distinguish from a schwannoma. However, the ability to center the lesion over the IAC greatly favors schwannoma. In general, schwannomas are usually more hyperintense on T2W images compared with meningiomas. They also tend to be more spherical as opposed to meningiomas, which are more often hemispheric. Meningiomas may occasionally result in expansion of the IAC, but this is much less common than with schwannomas.

If the lesion is large enough, MR spectroscopy has the potential to aid in differentiating the two lesions. Schwannomas have been noted to have elevated signal at 3.56 ppm representing myoinositol, as well as reduction in *N*-acetyl-aspartate (NAA) and elevation in choline. Meningiomas, on the other hand, demonstrate absence of NAA because they are not of neural origin, and an alanine peak may be noted at 1.55 ppm.[10] Evaluation of the brain stem with a 3D fast spin-echo heavily T2W sequence may

reveal a focus of increased signal intensity in the dorsal brain stem in the region of the vestibular nucleus unilateral to the lesion. This is thought to represent degeneration of the vestibular nucleus associated with a vestibular schwannoma and helps to suggest the diagnosis.[11] Relative cerebral blood volume (rCBV) has been evaluated as a means of differentiating meningiomas from schwannomas; however, there is some overlap between the two lesions. Studies have compared the rCBV ratios (rCBV of the lesion divided by the rCBV of normal white matter) and found the highest reported rCBV ratio in schwannomas to be 4.4, whereas in meningiomas the ratio typically ranges from 6 to 9.[12,13]

MENINGIOMA

Meningiomas arise from meningothelial cells, also known as arachnoid cap cells, and are the most common nonglial primary neoplasms of the central nervous system (CNS). They are the second most common lesion in the CPA after schwannomas.

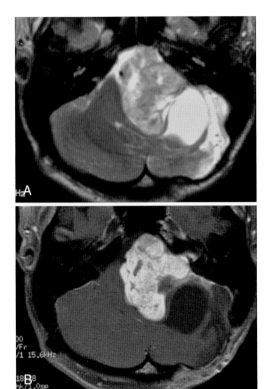

■ **FIGURE 36-6** Schwannoma and arachnoid cyst. Axial T2W **(A)** and T1W postcontrast **(B)** MR images through the CPA reveal a large vestibular schwannoma with a focal, well-circumscribed nonenhancing area of T2 hyperintensity posterior and lateral to the lesion consistent with an arachnoid cyst.

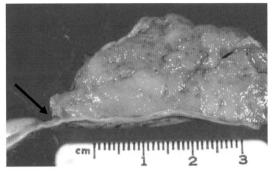

■ **FIGURE 36-7** Meningioma. Gross specimen demonstrates a well-circumscribed, hemispheric lesion with a broad base and dural attachment (*arrow*).

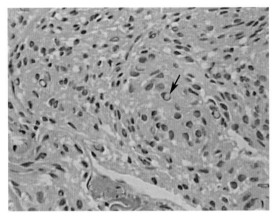

■ **FIGURE 36-8** Meningioma. Sheets of oval nuclei are noted with occasional intranuclear inclusions (*arrow*).

Epidemiology

Meningiomas comprise 10% to 15% of CPA masses. These lesions are more frequent in women, and the gender ratio ranges from 2:1 to 4:1 depending on the series. Meningiomas typically occur between the ages of 20 and 60 years, but these lesions have been found in children.[1,14,15] They are also found in association with neurofibromatosis type 2, in which case they are frequently multiple.

Clinical Presentation

The clinical presentation of meningiomas depends on their location and results from their mass effect on surrounding structures.

Pathophysiology

Meningiomas arise from meningothelial cells, which are also known as arachnoid cap cells. The World Health Organization (WHO) grades meningiomas from I to III. The most frequent form is grade I, which has a 7% to 20% recurrence rate. Grade II recurs in 29% to 40%. Grade III are highly aggressive, rapidly growing meningiomas that have a 50% to 78% recurrence rate. Twenty percent of meningiomas display aggressive histologic features, and the pathologic criteria for a higher grade include hypercellularity, loss of architecture, nuclear pleomorphism, mitotic index, tumor necrosis, and brain invasion. Metastasis can be seen in approximately 0.1% of meningiomas. Higher-grade meningiomas are more common in males and children.[16]

Immunohistochemistry is beneficial in making the diagnosis of meningiomas. In 80% of cases meningiomas are positive for epithelial membrane antigen. Interestingly, progesterone receptors can be found in the cytoplasm of meningiomas and may play a role in the proliferation of meningiomas in females. However, there is debate in the literature of whether these progesterone receptors are functional.[17]

A deletion on chromosome 22q is the most common genetic abnormality associated with meningiomas. There is an association of meningiomas with neurofibromatosis type 2 and also with a history of previous radiation therapy.

Pathology

Meningiomas are well-demarcated lesions with a broad dural base (Fig. 36-7). They are firm, rubbery lesions whose appearance varies depending on the degree of cystic change, lipid content, calcification, and vascularity. Meningiomas also frequently stimulate hyperostosis in adjacent bone.

Meningiomas are composed of monomorphic cells and have oval nuclei that may demonstrate intranuclear inclusions (Fig. 36-8). Psammoma bodies, which are rounded collections of calcium, may be seen interspersed between the cells. The three most common histologic subtypes of meningiomas are meningothelial, fibroblastic, and transitional. The meningothelial form consists of densely packed cells arranged in sheets. Fibroblastic meningiomas consist of densely packed sheets of spindle cells interwoven with collagen and reticulin. Transitional meningiomas have features common to both the fibroblastic and meningothelial forms.[1]

Imaging

CT

Meningiomas are usually homogeneously hyperattenuating, well-circumscribed, extra-axial lesions on CT. The center of the mass tends to be eccentric to the porus acusticus. Very rarely are they located entirely within the IAC. They are vascular lesions and, typically, homogeneously and intensely enhance after contrast agent administration. Fifteen to 20 percent will demonstrate calcification. Hyperostosis may be seen, which is not related to the presence of bone invasion, and is more likely related to local hypervascularity (Fig. 36-9).[18] In fact, CT may be of benefit when evaluating for a small meningioma because hyperostosis may be the only indication of its presence. However, detection of hyperostosis in the petrous bone may be more difficult than in other locations owing to the inherent density of this bone.

MRI

Meningiomas are hypointense to isointense on T1W imaging and avidly and homogeneously enhance on postcontrast imaging owing to their vascular nature. They are isointense to hyperintense on T2W imaging (Fig. 36-10), but there may be areas of hypointensity that correlate to regions of calcification. T2 hyperintensity may be seen within the adjacent brain parenchyma secondary to tumor-induced vasogenic edema. On postcontrast

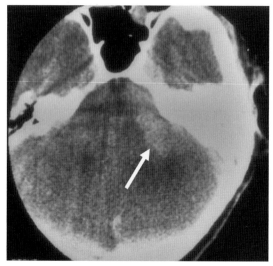

■ **FIGURE 36-9** Meningioma. Axial postcontrast CT demonstrates hyperostosis of the left petrous bone. An enhancing mass (*arrow*) adjacent to the petrous bone is consistent with a meningioma.

imaging a "dural tail" may be seen, but this is not pathognomonic for meningiomas and has been reported in other lesions adjacent to the dura, including both schwannomas and hemangiopericytomas. In addition, the dural tail is only seen in up to 60% of meningiomas.[19]

Atypical imaging features such as heterogeneous enhancement, cyst formation, hemorrhage, and fatty degeneration may be seen in approximately 15% of histologically benign meningiomas.[18] The degree of associated vasogenic edema does not appear to correlate with tumor grade or size. The etiology of the vasogenic edema is controversial and is probably the result of a combination of different mechanisms.[18]

MR perfusion demonstrates an elevated rCBV ratio, usually in the range of 6 to 9. Typically, there is less than 50% return to baseline because of the extra-axial nature of these lesions. This marked elevation in rCBV may be of some assistance in differentiating meningiomas from schwannomas, whose rCBV ratio values typically do not exceed 4, but there can be overlap.[12] Because of susceptibility artifact in the posterior fossa, obtaining perfusion studies in this region may be limited. MR spectroscopy may demonstrate an alanine doublet at 1.4 ppm, but, again, like perfusion, there may be limitations of spectroscopy in the posterior fossa owing to the surrounding osseous structures. Alanine is found in tumors of meningeal origin and may be seen in 30% to 40% of meningiomas. NAA is not visualized because these tumors are not of neural origin, and choline may be elevated due to rapid membrane turnover.[20]

The major imaging differential diagnosis for a CPA meningioma is the schwannoma. Meningiomas may extend into the IAC and may be very difficult to distinguish from a schwannoma. However, meningiomas are less likely to be centered over the IAC than a schwannoma and they do not tend to enlarge the IAC. Also, schwannomas are usually more hyperintense on T2W images than meningiomas. Meningiomas are more hemispheric as compared with schwannomas, which tend to be rounded. In addition, schwannomas demonstrate elevated myoinositol and present, but reduced, NAA.

Special Procedures

On angiography, meningiomas have a tumor blush that appears early and persists to the venous phase. This appearance is often jokingly referred to as the "mother-in-law" effect. One or more large meningeal vessels are typically noted feeding the meningioma. Preoperative angiography is beneficial to identify the vas-

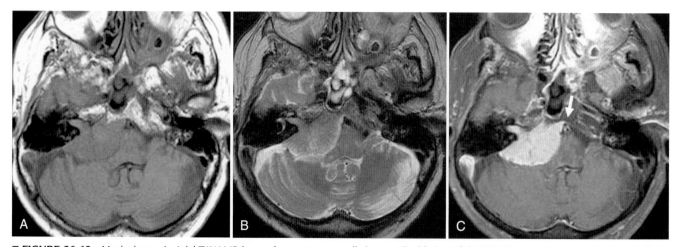

■ **FIGURE 36-10** Meningioma. **A,** Axial T1W MR image demonstrates a well-circumscribed lesion of the CPA that is isointense to brain and results in mass effect on the adjacent medulla and cerebellum. **B,** Axial T2W MR image demonstrates that the signal of the lesion is again relatively isointense to that of brain. **C,** On postcontrast imaging the lesion homogeneously enhances and a small dural tail is noted (*arrow*). The contrast agent helps to outline the extent to which the lesion involves the IAC.

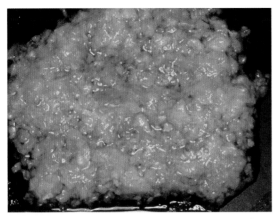

■ FIGURE 36-11 Gross image of an epidermoid cyst reveals the "pearly" appearance characteristically described in these lesions.

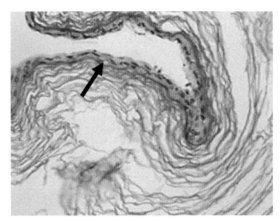

■ FIGURE 36-12 Epidermoid cyst. A thin lining of squamous epithelium is noted. Within the cyst, layer upon layer of keratin is noted, giving it an onionskin appearance.

cular supply and embolization may be of benefit to reduce bleeding during surgery.

EPIDERMOID CYST

Epidermoid cysts are benign, slow-growing ectoderm-lined inclusion cysts that gradually expand over the years. They have been referred to as cholesteatomas, owing to their high cholesterol content. However, this term is confusing because of the presence of other intracranial entities that are referred to by the same name; thus, use of this term should be avoided.

Epidemiology

Epidermoid cysts make up fewer than 5% of intracranial masses; however, they are the third most common mass lesion in the CPA. They typically present in the third to fourth decades.[21]

Clinical Presentation

These cysts grow slowly and may produce only mild symptoms as a result of local mass effect. Most frequently these symptoms consist of a chronic headache or facial pain. Although very rare, brain stem stroke resulting from stretching of the basilar artery has been reported.[22]

Pathophysiology

Epidermoid cysts are remnants of ectodermal tissue misplaced during embryogenesis that may result from failure of the surface ectoderm to separate from underlying structures, from implantation of surface ectoderm, or from sequestration of surface ectoderm. This probably occurs at 3 to 5 weeks of gestational age when the neural tube is closing.[21]

Pathology

Epidermoid cysts are unilocular lesions. They expand over decades as a result of accumulation of debris from the desquamation of the lining. They tend to be shiny, smooth, and waxy and are frequently described as "pearly" (Fig. 36-11). Scattered calcifications may be seen along the surface.

Epidermoid cysts are composed of an internal layer of squamous epithelium that is covered by an external fibrous capsule. They are filled with keratinous material that typically forms layers, giving an "onionskin" appearance (Fig. 36-12).

Imaging
CT

Epidermoid cysts are well-demarcated, unilocular lesions. The margins are typically scalloped and irregular due to molding around adjacent structures. On CT they are hypodense, nonenhancing mass lesions that have attenuation similar to CSF. The hypodensity is thought to be due to the high cholesterol and keratin content of the desquamated debris. Occasionally, they may have slightly lower attenuation numbers (−10 to −20), but these numbers are never low enough to be confused with fat. Even rarer, they may be hyperdense, which, like bronchogenic cysts, may be related to high protein content.[23] Hemorrhage within the cyst and elevated protein content are both suggested causes for this. On postcontrast imaging, epidermoid cysts typically do not enhance. On occasion, thin peripheral enhancement may be seen along the lining that may be due to an inflammatory response. The lobulated, irregular margins help distinguish them from arachnoid cysts, which usually have smooth margins. Epidermoid cysts tend to insinuate themselves around structures rather than displacing them; however, they may become adherent to these structures, making resection difficult.

MRI

MRI of epidermoid cysts usually demonstrates T1 and T2 intensity that is similar to CSF. However, high T1 signal intensity has been reported in some epidermoid cysts ("white epidermoids"). These lesions have a high lipid content composed of mixed triglycerides that contain unsaturated fatty acid residues.[24] Occasionally, low signal may be seen on T2W images that may be related to elevated protein content and increased viscosity, and these may also have increased signal on T1W images. Hemorrhage into arachnoid cysts has been reported, which alters the signal characteristics.[25] On fluid-attenuated inversion recovery (FLAIR) imaging, epidermoid cysts do not follow CSF, and they demonstrate reduced diffusion on diffusion-weighted imaging (Fig. 36-13). The finding of reduced diffusion is useful in postsurgical follow-up to assess for the presence of residual material. Both the FLAIR signal and reduced diffusion help to differentiate epidermoid cysts from arachnoid cysts, which follow CSF signal on all sequences. Unlike arachnoid cysts, epidermoid cysts tend to engulf nerves and vessels, rather than displace them, which can make surgical resection difficult. On MR spectroscopy, elevated lactate levels are seen within epidermoid cysts.[26]

Epidermoid cysts may have a lamellated appearance on MRI owing to layering of the accumulated desquamated material. The squamous cell lining of epidermoid cysts is usually too thin to be recognized by MRI. Peritumoral parenchymal edema is typically not seen. After the administration of gadolinium, these cysts may demonstrate thin rim enhancement, which may represent an inflammatory reaction.

■ **FIGURE 36-13** Epidermoid cyst. **A,** Sagittal T1W SPGR MR image demonstrates an irregularly marginated lesion in the region of the CPA. **B,** Axial T2W MR image again demonstrates the irregular margins. The signal is similar to CSF, but there is the subtle appearance of lamellation within the lesion. **C,** On the axial FLAIR image the signal does not completely saturate as would be expected with CSF. **D,** The diffusion-weighted image demonstrates high signal, which helps to confirm the diagnosis of an epidermoid.

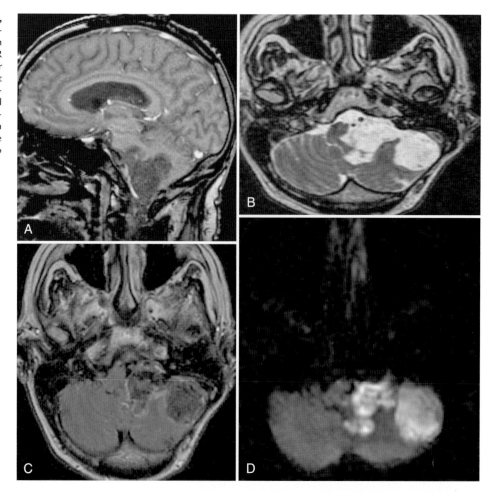

LIPOMA

Lipomas are non-neoplastic developmental lesions developing from the meninx primitiva, which is the precursor to the pia mater and arachnoid.

Epidemiology

Lipomas are rare in the CPA and make up approximately 0.14% of lesions in this area.[27]

Clinical Presentation

Lipomas are frequently asymptomatic, discovered only as incidental findings on imaging studies or at autopsy. When they are symptomatic, those within the CPA may cause slowly progressive cranial nerve symptoms. The most frequent symptoms are hearing loss, tinnitus, and dizziness. These lesions can entrap the cranial nerves, and this makes their resection difficult.

Pathophysiology

CPA lipomas are not associated with developmental CNS anomalies, unlike supratentorial lipomas, especially those involving the corpus callosum, which are frequently associated with anomalies.

On histologic examination lipomas have a variable quantity of fibrovascular tissue along with mature adipose cells. In addition, there are components of normal cranial nerves, including myelinated axons and glial cells.

Imaging

CT

On CT, lipomas are low-attenuation lesions with negative attenuation values (−50 to −100) consistent with fat (Fig. 36-14). They

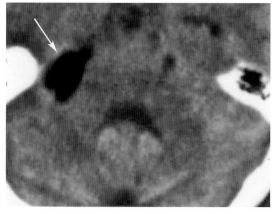

■ **FIGURE 36-14** Lipoma. Axial CT demonstrates a low-attenuation lesion in the right CPA (*arrow*) consistent with a lipoma.

do not demonstrate any internal contrast enhancement. CPA lipomas may be difficult to detect owing to beam hardening in this region.

MRI

On MRI, lipomas demonstrate T1 shortening consistent with fat (Fig. 36-15), and their signal will suppress on fat-saturation imaging. They do not enhance on postcontrast imaging. Vascular structures may occasionally be seen coursing through them.

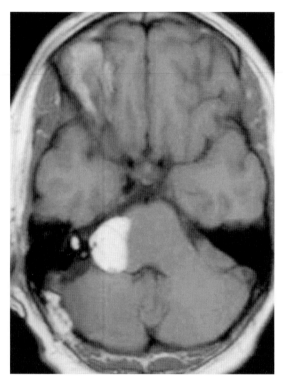

■ **FIGURE 36-15** Lipoma. Axial noncontrast T1W MR image demonstrates a hyperintense lesion in the right CPA consistent with a lipoma.

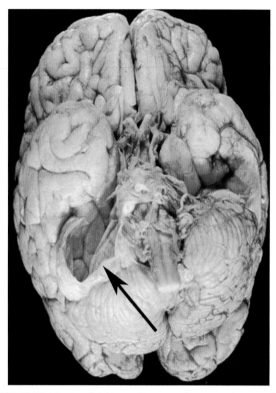

■ **FIGURE 36-16** Arachnoid cyst. Gross specimen reveals a membrane (*arrow*) that had surrounded an arachnoid cyst within the CPA. Distortion of the cerebellar hemisphere is noted from the mass effect that was exerted by the cyst.

ARACHNOID CYST

Arachnoid cysts are intra-arachnoid "pouches" that are filled with CSF.

Epidemiology

Arachnoid cysts comprise approximately 1% of intracranial lesions, but the exact incidence is unknown because many are asymptomatic throughout life and may go undetected. When they are symptomatic, they typically present in the first 2 decades of life. There is no known gender predilection.[28] Approximately 10% of arachnoid cysts are located in the posterior fossa. The remainder are located in the middle cranial fossa and suprasellar cistern.

Clinical Presentation

Arachnoid cysts may be asymptomatic or can produce symptoms related to mass effect. In the CPA the most frequent symptom is hemifacial spasm secondary to pressure on cranial nerve VII. Other symptoms include seizures, hydrocephalus, and increased intracranial pressure.

Pathophysiology

Arachnoid cysts are most frequently congenital in origin but may arise as the result of trauma, surgery, or subarachnoid hemorrhage. They may also develop adjacent to a mass. Congenital arachnoid cysts may result from duplication or splitting of the arachnoid membrane, creating a space between layers that fills with CSF. Arachnoid cysts are classified as either communicating or noncommunicating, depending on their relation with the subarachnoid space. Those that do not communicate or have inadequate communication with the subarachnoid space can result in mass effect. If surgical therapy is planned, distinguishing between a communicating and noncommunicating cyst is important. CT cisternography can assist in helping differentiate the two.

Rarely, hemorrhage can occur into the arachnoid cyst. This may be secondary to trauma. It is possible that even mild trauma may result in disruption of unsupported vessels surrounding the arachnoid cyst resulting in an increase in size and symptoms of mass effect due to bleeding.[29] Hemorrhage can result in enlargement of the cyst. Other causes of enlargement are thought to be due to the possibility of passive fluid diffusion into the cyst or a ball-valve mechanism. Active secretion from the cyst wall has also been speculated, but this is controversial.[30]

Pathology

Arachnoid cysts are well-marginated cysts with smooth walls that contain CSF (Fig. 36-16).

On microscopic evaluation the walls of the arachnoid cyst are composed of meningoendothelial cells as seen in normal arachnoid. The content of the cyst is CSF. On immunohistochemical studies they are positive for epithelial membrane antigen.

Imaging

CT

On CT, arachnoid cysts have attenuation values that match CSF. They are smooth lesions with rounded, convex margins that may exert mass effect on adjacent structures and may erode adjacent bone. Arachnoid cysts are avascular structures and, therefore, do not enhance on postcontrast imaging. In the rare case of intracystic hemorrhage, a blood/fluid level may be seen.

CT cisternography can be utilized to help distinguish between communicating and noncommunicating cysts. This involves the intrathecal administration of a contrast agent and evaluation of the presence of contrast agent within the cyst (Fig. 36-17). If no agent is initially seen, then delayed imaging is performed.

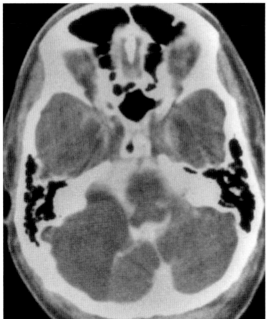

■ **FIGURE 36-17** Arachnoid cyst. CT cisternogram demonstrates an extra-axial lesion with attenuation similar to CSF occupying a majority of the inferior right cerebellar fossa. No contrast agent is noted entering the cyst.

MRI

Arachnoid cysts follow CSF signal on all imaging sequences. They are hypointense on T1W images, are hyperintense on T2W images, and do not demonstrate enhancement. Unlike epidermoid cysts, which have a similar appearance, they do not demonstrate reduced diffusion and they will suppress on FLAIR imaging (Fig. 36-18). In addition, arachnoid cysts displace adjacent structures, unlike epidermoid cysts, which engulf them. As noted in the section on CT imaging, in the rare case of hemorrhage into the cyst, a blood/fluid level can be seen.

Recent studies have investigated the utility of phase contrast (PC) cine MRI to evaluate whether an arachnoid cyst communicates with the subarachnoid space. Yildiz and associates found that PC cine MRI was a reasonable alternative to CT cisternography, by allowing visualization of flow jets between the cisterns and the cysts.[31] This provides an alternative to CT cisternography, which is an invasive procedure and exposes the patient to radiation.

NEURENTERIC CYST

Neurenteric cysts are rare, benign lesions of the CNS that are of endodermal origin. Neurenteric cysts are also referred to as enterogenous cysts, enteric cysts, endodermal cysts, gastroenterogenous cysts, gastrocytomas, intestinomas, and archenteric cysts.

■ **FIGURE 36-18** Arachnoid cyst. **A,** Axial T1W MR image demonstrates a smoothly marginated lesion within the right CPA that exerts mass effect on the adjacent structures. **B,** On T2W imaging the lesion follows CSF signal. **C,** Coronal FLAIR imaging demonstrates complete suppression of the signal from the cyst contents. **D,** On postcontrast imaging no enhancement is noted involving the cyst.

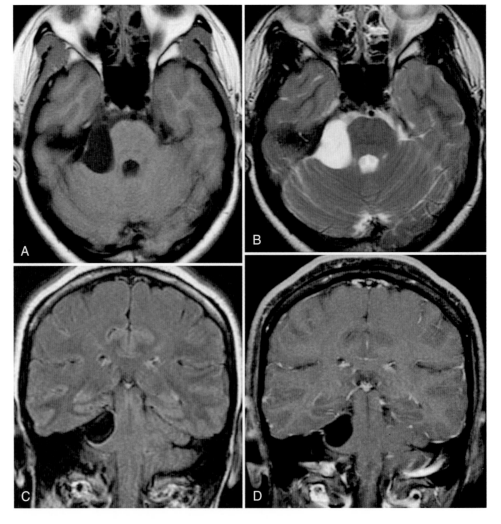

Epidemiology

Neurenteric cysts are very rare lesions with fewer than 60 reports documented in the literature.[32] They are more frequent in the spine but can occur intracranially. When they occur intracranially, they are more prevalent in the posterior fossa but may occur supratentorially as well. In the posterior fossa they are more common in the CPA and in the midline anterior to the brain stem. These lesions occur in all age groups, and there does not appear to be a gender predilection.

Clinical Presentation

Headache is the major presenting symptom for patients with neurenteric cysts. Less frequently, cranial nerve deficits have been reported.

Pathophysiology

The etiology of neurenteric cysts is uncertain. A theory that addresses the development of these lesions in the posterior fossa proposes that they arise during the time of notochordal development and that the notochord and foregut fail to separate. This results in primitive endodermal cells incorporating into the notochord.

Two histologic patterns have been described in neurenteric cysts. One pattern is composed of pseudostratified ciliated, columnar epithelium with few mucin-producing cells. This pattern corresponds to the respiratory features associated with these lesions (Fig. 36-19). The other pattern is simple, nonciliated epithelium with abundant mucin-producing cells corresponding to the gastrointestinal features attributed to these lesions.[32]

Immunohistochemical staining can demonstrate positivity for cytokeratin, epithelial membrane antigen, and carcinoembryonic antigen. Neurenteric cysts are negative for GFAP and S-100 protein, confirming their endodermal origin.[33]

Imaging

CT

On CT, neurenteric cysts within the CPA are typically hypodense, well-circumscribed, extra-axial lesions that can be mistaken for arachnoid cysts or cystic lesions of the posterior fossa. Occasionally, they may be isodense or hyperdense to brain. Among the limited case reports available, no contrast enhancement was identified on CT.[32]

MRI

The MRI appearance of neurenteric cysts varies depending on the protein content within the cyst. Most cysts are isointense to hyperintense to CSF on T1W imaging and hyperintense on T2W imaging (Fig. 36-20), unless the cyst contents are inspissated. They are typically hyperintense to CSF and brain on FLAIR. Neurenteric cysts may have mildly reduced diffusion, however, usually not to the degree seen in epidermoid cysts, which can help differentiate them from these lesions.[32] On postcontrast imaging, rim enhancement has been reported but is rare. Most of these lesions are less than 2 cm and are ovoid or lobulated.

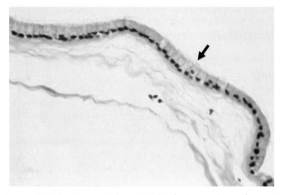

■ **FIGURE 36-19** Neurenteric cyst. Histologic specimen demonstrates pseudostratifed ciliated, columnar mucin-producing cell–poor epithelium, which corresponds to the respiratory features seen in these lesions.

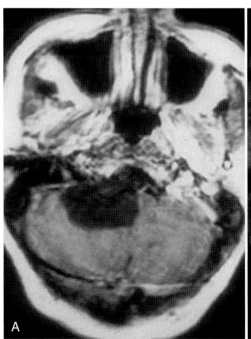
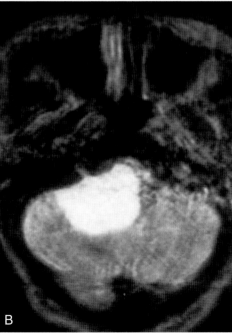

■ **FIGURE 36-20** Neurenteric cyst. Axial T1W MR image (**A**) reveals a hypointense nonenhancing lesion in the right CPA that on T2W imaging (**B**) is hyperintense. At pathology this was shown to be a neurenteric cyst.

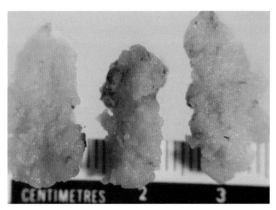

■ **FIGURE 36-21** Choroid plexus papilloma. Gross specimen reveals a tan lesion with an irregular "cauliflower" surface.

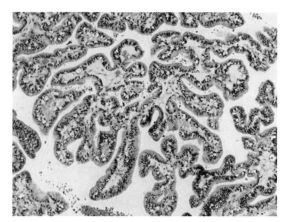

■ **FIGURE 36-22** Choroid plexus papilloma. Histologic specimen demonstrates the typical frond-like appearance of choroid plexus papillomas.

The imaging differential diagnosis for these lesions would include other cystic lesions of the posterior fossa, such as arachnoid and epidermoid cysts.

CHOROID PLEXUS PAPILLOMA
Choroid plexus papillomas are neoplasms derived from the neuroepithelial cells of the choroid plexus.

Epidemiology
Choroid plexus papillomas comprise 0.4% to 0.6% of intracranial tumors.[34] They are more common in children, where they mainly occur in the lateral ventricles. In adults they are more frequent within the fourth ventricle, from which they can extend laterally to the CPA through the foramen of Luschka. They can also arise primarily in the region of the CPA from embryonic rests located in this region. Fourth ventricular choroid plexus papillomas can be found evenly distributed within the age range from birth to 50 years and are more common in males (3:2), unlike the lateral ventricular tumors, which have no gender predilection.

Clinical Presentation
The presenting symptoms of choroid plexus papillomas are related to increased intracranial pressure and hydrocephalus. The hydrocephalus may result from a variety of causes, including CSF hypersecretion by the tumor, obstruction of CSF pathways by the tumor, or by impairment of CSF absorption at the arachnoid granulations due to proteinaceous or hemorrhagic material secondary to the choroid plexus papilloma.[35] In addition, neurologic deficits, seizures, cranial nerve deficits, and coma have been reported.

Pathophysiology
Choroid plexus papillomas are WHO grade I neoplasms. They have been reported to be associated with Aicardi's syndrome and Li-Fraumeni syndrome. Simian virus 40 (SV40) DNA sequences are present in about 50% of tumors. SV40 is a polyomavirus found in both monkeys and humans and is thought to have the potential to cause tumors. Hyperdiploidy with genes on chromosomes 7, 9, 12, 15, 17, and 18 have also been reported.[5]

Immunohistochemical evaluation reveals staining with antibodies to keratin and S-100 protein. S-100 protein is a protein that occurs within the CNS, in Schwann cells, and in satellite cells of ganglia.

Pathology
Choroid plexus papillomas are well-circumscribed, cauliflower-shaped lesions (Fig. 36-21). Cyst formation may be seen as well as areas of hemorrhage. These papillomas resemble the normal choroid plexus on histology. Fronds of fibrovascular tissue are noted that are surrounded by columnar cells (Fig. 36-22). There is minimal mitotic activity and cytologic atypia.

Imaging
CT

Choroid plexus papillomas are isodense to hyperdense lesions on CT, which may demonstrate areas of calcification or cysts. These are vascular lesions that enhance avidly after the administration of a contrast agent (Fig. 36-23). Hydrocephalus is frequent; and when choroid plexus papillomas involve the CPA, remodeling of the petrous bone may be seen.

MRI

On MRI, choroid plexus papillomas are typically isointense on T1W images and heterogeneously hyperintense on T2W images. On T2 weighting, regions of hypointensity may be identified that may represent calcifications or vascular structures. The lesions are irregular and lobulated, and multiple ventricle hydrocephalus is typically seen (Fig. 36-24). Flow voids may be seen within the lesion. Evaluation of the spine is recommended on postoperative imaging because CSF seeding may occur.

Special Procedures

Evaluation by angiography before surgical resection may be of benefit to identify the vascular supply. The fourth ventricular tumors are typically supplied by the choroidal branches of the posterior inferior cerebellar artery. Choroid plexus papillomas are very vascular, and preoperative embolization may be of benefit.

EPENDYMOMA
Ependymomas are glial neoplasms arising from differentiated ependymal cells lining the cerebral ventricles and the central canal of the spinal cord.

Epidemiology
Ependymomas comprise 3% to 9% of all neuroepithelial neoplasms and constitute approximately one third of all intracranial neoplasms in children younger than 3 years of age. Sixty percent of these lesions are infratentorial.[34] Even though they are more common in younger patients, they may present in any age group. Children typically have a worse prognosis than adults, owing in part to a greater propensity for these lesions to occur in the region of the fourth ventricle in children; and ependymomas in children have a greater likelihood of being of anaplastic

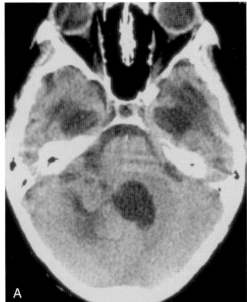

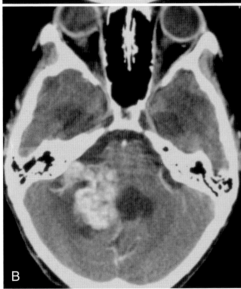

■ **FIGURE 36-23** Choroid plexus papilloma. **A,** Noncontrast CT reveals an irregularly shaped lesion within the right cerebellopontine cistern that is mainly isodense to brain. Dilation of the fourth ventricles and temporal horns is noted consistent with hydrocephalus. **B,** Postcontrast imaging demonstrates marked enhancement of the lesion.

histology. No definite gender predilection has been identified.[34]

Clinical Presentation

Ependymomas typically present with signs and symptoms related to increased intracranial pressure and hydrocephalus, such as nausea and vomiting. Lesions presenting in the fourth ventricle may also cause ataxia and paresis.

Pathophysiology

Ependymomas are graded as either WHO I, II, or III. Myxopapillary ependymomas and subependymomas are grade I. The grade II tumors consist of cellular, papillary, and clear cell variants, and the grade III ones are the anaplastic ependymomas. The myxopapillary ependymomas occur almost exclusively in the region of the conus medullaris and cauda equina of the spine in adults.

Limited data are available on the genetics of ependymomas. There is an increased incidence of spinal ependymomas in neurofibromatosis type 2 patients, but this is not the case for the intracranial ependymomas.

Pathology

Ependymomas are well-circumscribed lesions that fill the ventricular lumen. They tend to be grayish red. Hemorrhage and necrosis may be present.

Ependymomas are cellular tumors that demonstrate rare mitotic figures. Perivascular rosettes are the most characteristic feature (Fig. 36-25).[34] These lesions are considered WHO grade II; however, the anaplastic variety is a grade III. Hypercellularity, frequent mitoses, and endothelial hyperplasia are seen within the grade III ependymomas.

On immunohistochemical staining, GFAP and S-100 protein are usually positive. GFAP is a member of the intermediate filament family that provides support and strength to astroglial cells. S-100 protein is a protein that occurs within the CNS, in Schwann cells, and in satellite cells of ganglia.[5]

Imaging
CT

CT reveals a lesion that is isodense to brain parenchyma and has calcifications in about one half of cases. Occasionally, a blood/fluid level may be seen due to intratumoral hemorrhage. On postcontrast imaging, ependymomas avidly enhance, although this may be heterogeneous due to calcification, cyst formation, and hemorrhage (Fig. 36-26).

MRI

On MRI, ependymomas are typically isointense on T1W images and hyperintense on T2W images. They tend to be heterogeneous due to calcifications, cyst formation, and regions of hemorrhage. On postcontrast images they enhance, but this is typically heterogeneous (Fig. 36-27).

METASTASIS

The metastatic lesions that most commonly involve the leptomeninges of the CPA are from lung and breast cancer as well as melanoma.

Clinical Presentation

Metastatic lesions comprise approximately 1% of CPA lesions. Metastasis to the CPA typically presents as acute onset of cranial nerve symptoms that rapidly progress. Cranial nerves VII and VIII are the most frequently involved.

Pathology

The histology of the metastatic lesion is similar to that of the primary tumor.

Imaging
CT

On CT, metastatic lesions may mimic other CPA lesions, such as schwannomas and meningiomas. However, they will usually have a more aggressive appearance and typically other metastatic lesions will be present, which helps direct the diagnosis. They typically enhance after the administration of contrast media owing to their vascularity.

MRI

On MRI, metastatic lesions may mimic other CPA lesions, such as schwannomas and meningiomas. However, they will usually have a more aggressive appearance and typically other metastatic lesions will be present, which helps direct the diagnosis.

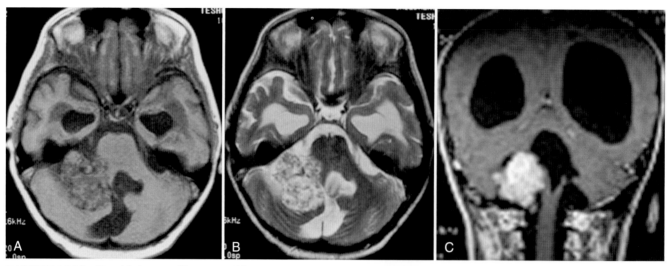

■ **FIGURE 36-24**   Choroid plexus papilloma. **A,** Axial T1W MR image demonstrates a slightly hypointense irregular lesion in the right CPA that exerts mass effect on the adjacent brain parenchyma. Hydrocephalus is evident, and hypointensity is noted adjacent to the temporal horns consistent with transependymal flow. **B,** On T2W imaging the lesion is heterogeneous. **C,** Coronal postcontrast imaging reveals an avidly enhancing mass.

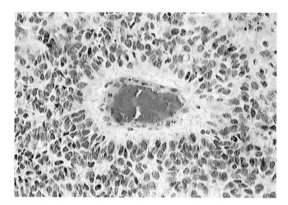

■ **FIGURE 36-25**   Ependymoma. Note the perivascular rosette, which is a characteristic feature of ependymomas.

They typically enhance after the administration of gadolinium. Edema may be noted in adjacent brain parenchyma. In the case of metastasis from melanoma, intrinsic T1 hyperintensity may be noted. Metastases from adenocarcinomas may demonstrate reduced diffusion on diffusion-weighted imaging and may mimic an abscess.

Evaluation of the rCBV ratio values in metastasis typically reveals a moderate elevation varying from 1.5 to 5. This may help in distinguishing metastasis from meningioma, whose rCBV ratio value is typically around 8.[12] MR spectroscopy demonstrates an elevation in choline along with a prominent lipid peak.[36]

PARAGANGLIOMA

Paragangliomas are locally invasive neoplasms of neural crest origin that arise from the chemoreceptor glomus bodies. They arise within the jugular foramen, either from the jugular bulb or Jacobson's or Arnold's nerve. Glomus tumor and chemodectoma are previously utilized names; however, *paraganglioma* is the term that is currently accepted.

Epidemiology

Paragangliomas are the second most common tumor arising from the region of the temporal bone, and from there they can extend into the CPA. The jugulotympanic paragangliomas are more fre-

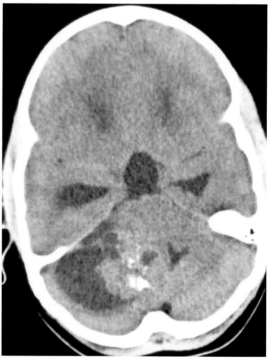

■ **FIGURE 36-26**   Ependymoma. Non–contrast-enhanced axial CT reveals a partially calcified lesion in the right CPA. Dilatation of the temporal horns and third ventricle are consistent with hydrocephalus.

quent in women (4:1) and typically occur in the fifth to sixth decades. In up to 10% of cases they can be multiple. The glomus jugulare and the carotid body tumors are the most common form of paragangliomas.[37]

Clinical Presentation

Patients with paragangliomas most frequently present with otologic symptoms, such as conductive hearing loss and pulsatile tinnitus. Cranial nerve palsies are present in only a minority of patients and tend to occur late in the course of the disease. Cranial nerve VII is the most commonly involved.

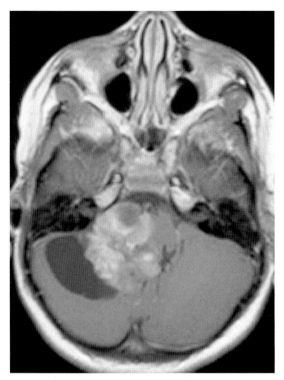

■ **FIGURE 36-27** Ependymoma. Axial T1W postcontrast MR image demonstrates a heterogeneously enhancing lesion that was proven pathologically to be an ependymoma. Posterior to the mass is a well-demarcated region of low signal most likely representing an arachnoid cyst.

The larger lesions can secrete norepinephrine or, less likely, adrenocorticotropic hormone, serotonin, calcitonin, or dopamine. Those that are hormonally active are referred to as functional paragangliomas and are estimated to occur in 1% to 3% of cases.[38] Symptoms such as hypertension, palpitations, and tachycardia from these functioning paragangliomas are less common than would be expected.

Pathophysiology
Paragangliomas grow slowly and rarely metastasize. Typically, they follow the path of least resistance and invade into the mastoid air cells, vascular channels, neural foramina, and eustachian tube.

Familial association of paragangliomas has been described, the majority of which (90%) arise from the carotid body. The mode of inheritance is autosomal dominant with incomplete penetrance and is secondary to the deactivation of a tumor suppressor gene on the long arm of chromosome 11. They may also be seen in association with von Hippel-Lindau disease and in multiple endocrine neoplasia types IIA and IIB.[37]

Pathology
Paragangliomas are well-defined lobulated lesions that are usually tan-gray to reddish purple (Fig. 36-28).

On histology, paragangliomas resemble pheochromocytomas and are composed of chief cells and sustentacular cells in a fibrovascular stroma. These cells are arranged in nests or lobules referred to as Zellballen (Fig. 36-29) that are surrounded by a single layer of sustentacular cells.

The most reliable marker for malignant degeneration is the presence of metastatic lesions. However, the presence of mitoses, vascular invasion, and central necrosis suggests a more aggressive lesion. A decreased number or absent sustentacular cells indicates a higher tumor grade.

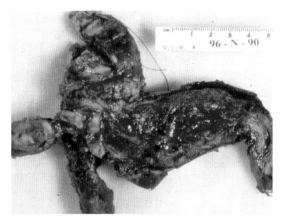

■ **FIGURE 36-28** Paraganglioma. Gross specimen reveals a reddish-brown neoplasm.

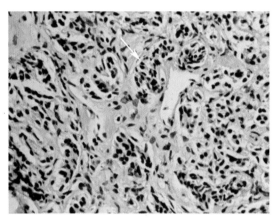

■ **FIGURE 36-29** Cells are arranged in nests or lobules referred to as Zellballen.

Immunohistochemical techniques are useful in the evaluation of paragangliomas. Chromogranins are structural proteins located within the neurosecretory granules of chief cells and are specific for neuroendocrine tumors. S-100 protein is a marker for the sustentacular cells.[5]

Imaging
CT

On CT, paragangliomas are well-defined soft tissue masses located at the jugular foramen. Because of their highly vascular nature, these lesions enhance avidly on postcontrast imaging. Evaluation of the temporal bone may demonstrate expansion and erosion of the jugular foramen (Fig. 28-30). Invasion into the mastoid air cells and middle ear may be identified, and ossicular chain destruction is a common finding. The tumor may spread laterally and destroy the facial nerve canal and infiltrate the facial nerve.[37]

MRI

On T1W images paragangliomas are hypointense, and they are hyperintense on T2W images. MRI of larger paragangliomas (>1 cm) typically reveals a "salt-and-pepper" pattern created by the numerous flow voids combined with foci of hemorrhage or slow flow. This finding, however, is not pathognomonic for paragangliomas because it may also be seen in other vascular tumors, such as metastasis. On postcontrast imaging these lesions avidly enhance, reflecting their vascular nature (Fig.

36-31). Their vascular nature also results in high rCBV on perfusion imaging. Paragangliomas may be multicentric and may occur either synchronously or metachronously, so it is important to evaluate the carotid body, glomus vagale, and glomus tympanicum.

Special Procedures

Angiography is useful in the evaluation of paragangliomas when the identity of the tumor is not obvious. These are highly vascular neoplasms that demonstrate an intense tumor blush and early draining veins. The most common arterial feeder is the ascending pharyngeal artery. Other frequent sources of vascular supply are the posterior auricular, stylomastoid, and occipital arteries. The intradural portion of the glomus jugulare may also be supplied by parenchymal branches of the posterior inferior cerebellar artery and the anterior inferior cerebellar artery. Preoperative embolization is useful owing to the highly vascular nature of these lesions.

CHORDOMA

Chordomas arise from primitive notochordal remnants and are locally aggressive tumors of the skull base.

Epidemiology

Chordomas account for 1% of intracranial tumors. They usually arise in the fourth decade and are more frequent in males than females (2 : 1).

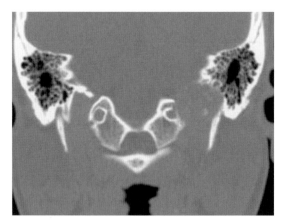

■ **FIGURE 36-30** Paraganglioma. Coronal CT reveals expansion and erosion of the left jugular foramen.

Clinical Presentation

Chordomas are slow-growing neoplasms. The symptoms associated with these lesions depend on their location.

Pathophysiology

Chordomas arise from primitive notochordal remnants and can appear anywhere along the course of the embryonic notochord. Intracranial chordomas account for 32% of chordomas, and the remainder occur in the spinal (32.8%) and sacral regions (29.2%). Intracranially, these lesions frequently arise in the midline along the upper clivus or along the caudal margin of the clivus. In 15% of cases they may arise unilaterally in the petrous apex, a finding that may make it difficult to distinguish them from chondrosarcomas. This may be the result of notochordal cells penetrating the skull base from different directions during early embryologic development. Chordomas are locally aggressive tumors that rarely metastasize.[39]

Pathology

Chordomas are multilobulated gelatinous tumors that are semitranslucent. Most lesions range from 2 to 5 cm.[39]

One of the histologic characteristics of chordomas is the physaliphorous cell, which has a bubble-like vacuolated cytoplasm. Two histopathologic subtypes of chordoma are described: the typical chordoma and the chondroid chordoma. Typical chordomas have cells that are arranged in cords that are set in a pale mucopolysaccharide matrix. Regions of necrosis and hemorrhage can be seen as well as entrapped bone trabeculae. Mitoses are uncommon, even in those lesions that have metastasized.

The chondroid form refers to a histologic mimic and is not of true chondroid origin but is epithelially derived. The stroma resembles hyaline cartilage, and neoplastic cells are seen within lacunae imitating chondrocytes. This form can resemble a low-grade sarcoma and is more likely to have intratumoral calcifications.

Chordomas can resemble chondrosarcomas histologically, with the greatest confusion occurring between the classic chordoma and the myxoid form of chondrosarcoma. Immunohistochemical staining can be of benefit to differentiate between the two.

Imaging
CT

On CT, chordomas tend to be well-circumscribed soft tissue masses in a central location. This lesion arises from the clivus

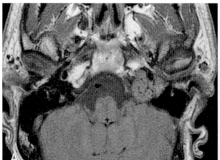
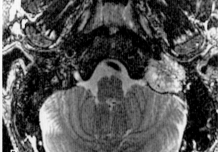
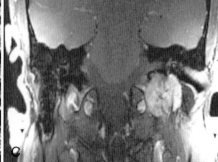

■ **FIGURE 36-31** Paraganglioma. **A,** Axial T1W MR image demonstrates an isointense lesion centered over the left jugular fossa. There are foci of hypointensity within the lesion consistent with flow voids. **B,** On T2W imaging the lesion is heterogeneously hyperintense, and again flow voids are noted. **C,** Coronal T1W postcontrast image reveals avid enhancement of the lesion.

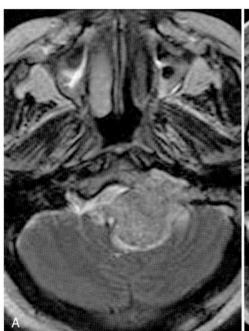
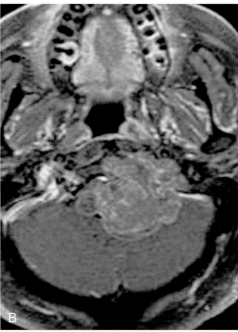

■ **FIGURE 36-32** Chordoma. **A,** Axial T2W MR image reveals a heterogeneously hyperintense lesion that involves the left aspect of the clivus. **B,** Axial T1W image with fat saturation at lower level through the clivus demonstrates heterogeneous enhancement along with greater involvement of the clivus in this location.

and usually has associated lytic bone destruction. Lytic bone destruction can also be seen in metastatic lesions and invasive adenomas, which are also in the differential diagnosis for this lesion. Occasionally, intratumoral calcifications are seen. These are thought to represent sequestra from bone destruction, rather than dystrophic calcifications within the tumor; however, both may occur.

MRI

On T1W images chordomas are isointense to hypointense lesions. They have very high signal intensity on T2W images, which is most likely due to the high fluid content within the vacuolated cellular components. Occasional foci of T1 shortening may be seen that correspond to hemorrhagic foci or mucus. On postcontrast imaging they demonstrate moderate to marked enhancement, which is frequently heterogeneous (Fig. 36-32). Less frequently, enhancement may be slight or absent. Utilization of fat suppression is beneficial in determination of the tumor margins. Some investigators have tried to differentiate chondroid chordomas from typical chordomas by imaging, because the survival rate of patients with chondroid chordoma is better. The chondroid chordoma has replacement of the gelatinous matrix by cartilaginous foci, which result in shortening of both T1 and T2 as compared with the typical chordomas. The differential diagnosis for chordomas on imaging includes chondrosarcoma, and these tumors can appear very similar especially when chordomas occur off the midline.

Evaluation of the relationship of chordomas to the surrounding vasculature is important for surgical planning. In up to 79% of intracranial chordomas the lesion was noted to displace or encase adjacent vasculature; however, they rarely narrow the involved vessel.[39] MR angiography is useful in evaluating this relationship.

Special Procedures

The angiographic findings of chordoma are nonspecific. There is rarely any tumoral blush or abnormal tumor vascularity. Diagnostic angiography may help to better determine the degree of vascular narrowing or occlusion, and temporary balloon occlusion of the internal carotid artery may be of benefit in determin-

ing whether that artery can be sacrificed, if necessary, without significant neurologic impairment.[39]

CHONDROSARCOMA

Chondrosarcomas are malignant bone tumors that produce hyaline cartilage.

Epidemiology

Less than 5% of chondrosarcomas occur in the head and neck region. These lesions are most frequent in middle age but can occur at any age. There is no reported sex predilection.

Clinical Presentation

Signs and symptoms of chondrosarcoma depend on the location of the lesion, but, typically, there is a history of headache and cranial nerve problems, most frequently diplopia.

Pathophysiology

Chondrosarcomas are most commonly found in the region of the skull base synchondroses, the most common of which is the petroclival synchondrosis. Occasionally, these lesions may be found along the midline in the region of the spheno-occipital synchondrosis and posterior nasal septum. They arise from remnants of embryonal cartilage or meningeal fibroblast metaplasia. These lesions grow slowly and rarely metastasize. Chondrosarcomas are associated with Ollier's disease and Maffucci's syndrome.

Cytogenetics are useful in distinguishing myxoid chondrosarcoma, which has a specific (t9;22) translocation, from chordoma, with which it can be confused on pathology.[40]

Pathology

Chondrosarcomas may be grossly well delineated, and the cut surface reveals a gray-white, glistening tumor parenchyma (Fig. 36-33). Necrosis and hemorrhage may be seen.

There are several histologic subtypes of chondrosarcomas; however, almost all skull base chondrosarcomas are of the conventional type, which consists of the hyaline or myxoid subtypes, or a combination of both. The myxoid matrix can appear similar to the matrix of classic chordoma, and the cells are found

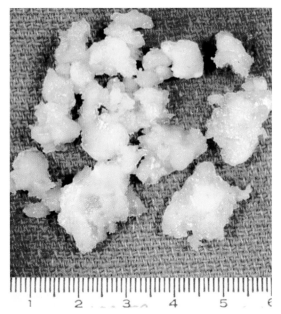

■ FIGURE 36-33 Chondrosarcoma. Gross specimen reveals white, glistening tumor parenchyma.

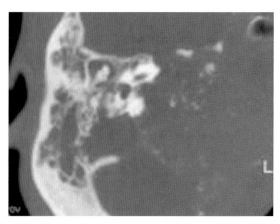

■ FIGURE 36-34 Chondrosarcoma. Axial noncontrast CT reveals erosion of the temporal bone and a large lesion demonstrating matrix calcification.

in strands that resemble the cord pattern of chordoma. The vacuoles in some chondrocytes may resemble the physaliphorous cell. Immunohistochemical stains are of benefit in differentiating between chondrosarcoma and chordoma. The cells of chondrosarcoma are chondrocytes and do not stain for cytokeratin or other epithelial markers.[41]

Imaging
CT
On CT, chondrosarcomas can have a varied appearance depending on the degree of chondroid matrix. Usually there is a soft tissue component that appears dense, and calcification of the tumor matrix is common and typically has the appearance of small ringlets or incomplete rings (Fig. 36-34).

The presence of calcifications with this morphology can be an imaging finding that can help distinguish chondrosarcoma from chordoma.

MRI
On T1W images chondrosarcomas are of intermediate signal and enhance after the administration of a contrast agent. These lesions are fairly hyperintense on T2W imaging (Fig. 36-35). On MRI, they may be difficult to differentiate from a chordoma, although typically chordomas are midline lesions and chondrosarcomas occur more frequently along fissures. In the skull base the petroclival fissure is frequently involved and this is located off the midline. Unfortunately, occasionally chondrosarcomas may be midline and chordomas off the midline so location is not always helpful.

ENDOLYMPHATIC SAC TUMOR
Endolymphatic sac tumors are papillary adenomatous tumors that are thought to originate from the middle third of the endolymphatic sac.

Epidemiology
Endolymphatic sac tumors are very rare neoplasms.

Clinical Presentation
Patients typically present with ipsilateral hearing loss. In addition, vestibular dysfunction and facial nerve palsy may be seen.

Pathophysiology
Endolymphatic sac tumors occur sporadically, but they are also associated with von Hippel-Lindau disease. They can occasionally be bilateral, and this is more frequent in those patients with von Hippel-Lindau disease. They are locally aggressive neoplasms, but metastasis is exceedingly rare, with only two cases reported of drop metastasis to the spine.[42] Endolymphatic sac tumors in patients who have von Hippel-Lindau disease are twice as likely to occur in females as compared with patients with sporadic endolymphatic sac tumors.

Two histopathologic categories of endolymphatic sac tumors are described. There is a follicular form that contains colloid-filled cysts and can mimic thyroid tissue. The papillary form consists of interdigitating papillary processes, which are embedded in dense fibrous tissue and may have evidence of hemorrhage. This form can resemble renal cell carcinoma.[5]

Immunohistochemical staining is useful in diagnosing endolymphatic sac tumors. These lesions stain positively for periodic acid–Schiff (PAS), S-100, cytokeratin, vimentin, and epithelial membrane antigen. S-100 protein is a protein that occurs within the CNS, in Schwann cells, and in satellite cells of ganglia. Vimentin is a member of the intermediate filament family of proteins and contributes to the cytoskeleton of cells. It is found in mesodermally derived cells.[5]

Imaging
CT
Endolymphatic sac tumors are locally aggressive, and, on CT, destruction of the retrolabyrinthine petrous bone is noted (Fig. 36-36). The margins of the bone appear motheaten, and intratumoral spiculated bone may be seen. On postcontrast imaging, avid enhancement is seen and central areas of cystic change or necrosis may be noted.

MRI
Endolymphatic sac tumors are heterogeneous in appearance on both T1W and T2W imaging. There may be focal regions of high signal intensity due to subacute hemorrhage, and low signal intensity may be seen due to calcification or hemosiderin. The presence of both blood- and protein-filled cysts, which are hyperintense on T1W and T2W images, offer a clue to the diagnosis. On postcontrast imaging, heterogeneous enhancement is noted (Fig. 36-37).

Owing to the rarity of drop metastasis from endolymphatic sac tumors, routine screening is unlikely to be cost effective. Evaluation of the spine should be performed if there are

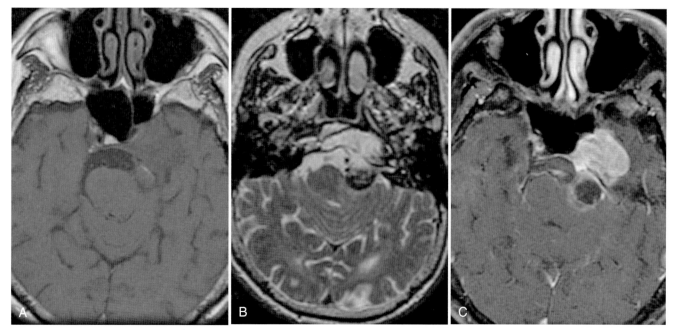

■ **FIGURE 36-35** Chondrosarcoma. **A,** Axial T1W MR image reveals a mass lesion centered at the petroclival synchondrosis that is isointense to muscle. The lesion results in mass effect on the pons and fourth ventricle. **B,** The lesion is hyperintense on T2W imaging. The focus of low signal intensity is consistent with hemorrhage. **C,** On postcontrast imaging the lesion heterogeneously enhances.

complaints of back pain, cauda equina syndrome, or radiculopathy.[42]

Special Procedures

Endolymphatic sac tumors are very vascular lesions. In a series of 12 patients examined by angiography by Mukherji and colleagues, all tumors received a substantial amount of their blood supply from the external carotid, with the ascending pharyngeal and stylomastoid arteries being the most common feeder arteries.[43] Two of the lesions were also supplied in part by the internal carotid artery.

CHOLESTEROL GRANULOMA

Cholesterol granulomas are expansile masses of the petrous apex. They have also been referred to as cholesterol cysts, giant cholesterol cyst, chocolate cysts, and xanthomas.

Epidemiology

Cholesterol granulomas are the most common primary petrous apex lesions. They typically take decades to grow and usually present in young to middle-aged adults.

Clinical Presentation

Cholesterol granulomas may present as sensorineural hearing loss. Other symptoms include tinnitus, hemifacial spasm, trigeminal neuralgia, facial numbness, and abducens palsy.

Pathophysiology

It has been previously proposed that cholesterol granulomas develop from obstructed air cells of the petrous apex. A vacuum can develop within the obstructed air cells, leading to rupture of blood vessels and resulting in hemorrhage into the air cell. The cholesterol crystals form from the degradation of the blood cells, and granulation tissue forms secondary to the repeated hemorrhage. However, a more recent hypothesis suggests that mucosal penetration occurs into the petrous apex, resulting in exposure of the bone marrow that results in hemorrhage.[44,45]

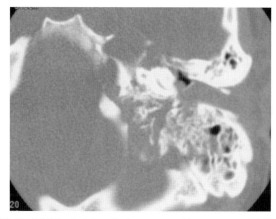

■ **FIGURE 36-36** Endolymphatic sac tumor. Noncontrast axial CT demonstrates a destructive lesion of the petrous bone with extension of the lesion into the mastoid air cells.

Pathology

Grossly, cholesterol granulomas are cystic masses that do not have an epithelial lining. They contain a brownish fluid containing old blood and cholesterol crystals, hence the name "chocolate cyst."

Cholesterol granulomas contain red blood cells in various stages of degradation. Hemosiderin-laden macrophages, cholesterol crystals, and chronic inflammatory cells are also found within these lesions.

Imaging

CT

CT of cholesterol granulomas reveals an expansile lesion of the petrous apex that is well defined and smoothly marginated.

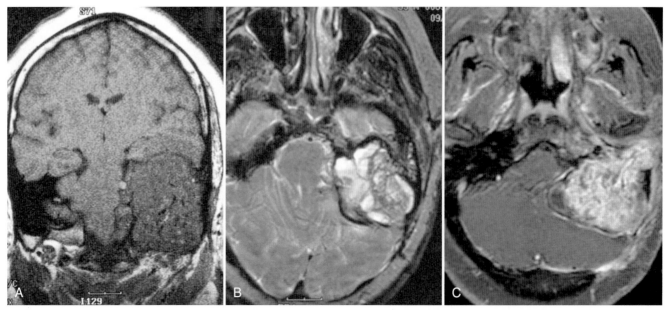

■ **FIGURE 36-37**   Endolymphatic sac tumor. **A,** Coronal T1W MR image reveals a lesion in the region of the left temporal bone. **B,** Axial T2W image reveals a heterogeneous lesion with areas of low signal suggestive of blood products. **C,** On axial postcontrast imaging the lesion demonstrates enhancement and is noted to involve the retrolabyrinthine temporal bone.

■ **FIGURE 36-38** Cholesterol granuloma. Axial T1W (**A**) and T2W (**B**) MR images demonstrate an expansile hyperintense lesion centered within the right petrous apex.

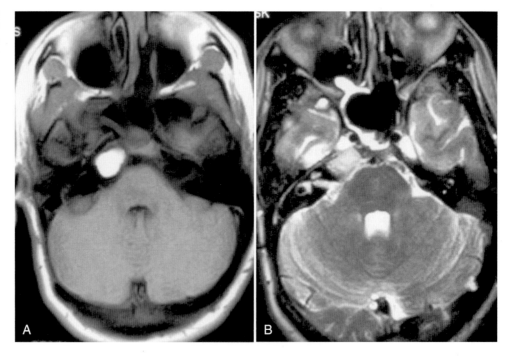

MRI

On MRI, cholesterol granulomas demonstrate hyperintensity on both T1W and T2W images. A low signal rim can be seen on the T2W images corresponding to hemosiderin deposition (Fig. 36-38). On postcontrast imaging, peripheral enhancement may be noted but there is no internal enhancement.

PEDUNCULATED (FOCAL) PONTINE GLIOMA

Focal pontine gliomas are gliomas that occupy less than 50% of the transverse area of the pons. When they are located in the periphery of the pons they may extend exophytically into the fourth ventricle or CPA.[3] Pontine gliomas fall under the category of brain stem glioma.

Epidemiology

Pontine gliomas are rare lesions that mainly affect children. They account for 10% to 15% of CNS lesions in childhood. The peak age at presentation for pontine gliomas is younger than 14 years, and there is an equal incidence between males and females. They only account for 2.4% of intracranial tumors in adults. In adults, pontine gliomas are more likely to remain focal and be of lower grade than in children.[3]

Clinical Presentation

Clinical presentation of brain stem gliomas includes cranial nerve deficits, disturbance of motor and sensory pathways, and ataxia. Hydrocephalus is uncommon.

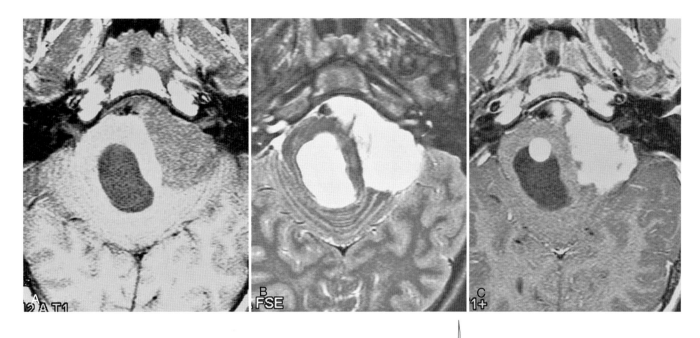

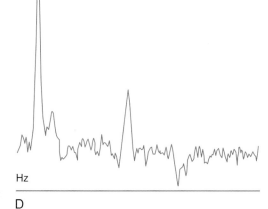

■ **FIGURE 36-39** Brain stem pilocytic astrocytoma. Axial T1W MR image (**A**) reveals a hypointense lesion involving the left CPA. On T2W imaging (**B**) the lesion is hyperintense and it demonstrates marked enhancement on the postcontrast image (**C**). **D,** MR spectroscopy demonstrates an elevation in choline and a reduction in *N*-acetyl-aspartate consistent with tumor metabolites.

Pathophysiology

Pontine gliomas may be either focal or diffuse. It is the focal form that is exophytic and may be found in the CPA. The focal variety has a better prognosis than the diffuse form, and 5-year survival reaches 75%.[3]

There is an association with neurofibromatosis. Currently, no genetic or molecular markers for brain stem gliomas have been identified.

The focal pontine gliomas usually have lower-grade histology than the diffuse forms and include the slow-growing fibrillary or the pilocytic astrocytoma.

Imaging

CT

On CT, brain stem gliomas are hypoattenuating masses, which have variable enhancement depending on grade.

MRI

Brain stem gliomas are hypointense on T1W imaging and hyperintense on T2W imaging. The solid portions of the tumor tend to enhance heterogeneously on postcontrast imaging. MR

spectroscopy reveals elevation of choline and reduction in NAA (Fig. 36-39).

LYMPHOMA

Primary CNS lymphoma is defined as extranodal lymphoma occurring in the CNS without evidence of involvement elsewhere.

Epidemiology

The worldwide incidence of CNS lymphoma has been increasing. This may be due in part to its association with immunocompromised states, most predominantly human immunodeficiency virus (HIV) infection. Two to 12 percent of HIV-infected patients will develop CNS lymphoma. However, CNS lymphoma confined to the CPA is very rare, with fewer than 20 cases reported.[3,46]

Any age group can be affected by primary CNS lymphoma. However, for those cases occurring in immunocompetent patients it is most common in the sixth and seventh decades. The incidence is slightly higher in males than females (3:2).

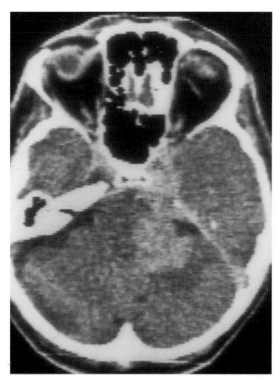

■ **FIGURE 36-40** Lymphoma. Noncontrast CT reveals a high density mass within the left CPA that extends anteriorly into the left cavernous sinus. At autopsy, the mass appeared to have started in the CPA and grown from there.

Clinical Presentation

Patients with primary CNS lymphoma may demonstrate focal neurologic deficits, seizures, or evidence of increased intracranial pressure.

Pathophysiology

There is no genetic predisposition to CNS lymphoma. CNS lymphoma is typically a B-cell lymphoma, and there is an association with the Epstein-Barr virus.

Pathology

Lymphoma may present as solitary or multiple masses. They may be firm, focally necrotic, hemorrhagic, or friable.

The majority of these tumors are B-cell lymphomas, although occasionally they can be of T-cell origin (2%). A proliferation of diffusely infiltrating lymphoid cells is seen at the microscopic level.[5] Immunohistochemical staining for CD20 and CD79a, which are B-cell lymphoid markers, is useful in evaluation. For the rare T-cell lymphoma, CD3 is a marker.[5]

Imaging

CT

On CT, primary CNS lymphoma tends to be hyperdense (Fig. 36-40) and enhance on postcontrast imaging.

MRI

Primary CNS lymphoma typically is seen as isointense to hypointense on both T1W and T2W images and has enhancement on the postcontrast images.

HEMANGIOBLASTOMA

Hemangioblastomas are benign meningeal tumors of uncertain origin. They have been referred to as Lindau tumors after the Swedish pathologist Arvid Vihelm Lindau, who first described them in 1926.

Epidemiology

Hemangioblastomas are relatively uncommon tumors, comprising 1% to 3% of all intracranial neoplasms. They occur within the cerebellum and less frequently the brain stem, spinal cord, and cerebral hemispheres. Rarely, they extend exophytically to involve the CPA. They most frequently occur between the fifth and sixth decade in sporadic cases, and there is a slight male predominance. Approximately one fourth of these patients have von Hippel-Lindau disease, and in these cases the tumors tend to present earlier, usually in the third to fourth decade.[3,47]

Clinical Presentation

The clinical presentation depends to a certain degree on the location of the lesion. Patients may present with symptoms secondary to CSF obstruction or cerebellar dysfunction. Approximately 10% of these patients will present with polycythemia secondary to production of an erythropoietin-like protein, but this is frequently asymptomatic.

Pathophysiology

Hemangioblastomas are WHO grade I neoplasms. These lesions usually grow within the parenchyma of the cerebellum, brain stem, or spinal cord. They receive their rich vascular supply from the pial vessels.

Most cases arise sporadically. Those associated with von Hippel-Lindau disease have been noted to demonstrate a defective tumor suppressor gene on chromosome 3p25-26.[5]

Pathology

Hemangioblastomas are typically well-circumscribed, cystic lesions with a mural nodule; however, they may be solid. The nodule tends to be reddish owing to its vascular nature, and the cyst contains a clear fluid. The nodule tends to be in a peripheral subpial location. Both pathologically and radiologically hemangioblastomas are described as four types. Type 1 is a simple cyst without a macroscopic nodule, type 2 is a cyst with a mural nodule, type 3 is a solid tumor, and type 4 is solid tumor with small internal cysts.[48]

Hemangioblastomas display a prominent capillary or sinusoidal vasculature with intermixed stromal cells. Mitotic activity and necrosis are not typically seen.

Imaging

CT

On CT, the cystic portion of the hemangioblastoma may appear as a region of low attenuation. If the hemangioblastoma results in CSF obstruction, hydrocephalus may be seen. After the administration of a contrast agent the solid portion avidly enhances.

MRI

On MRI, the solid portion of the hemangioblastoma is typically hypointense to isointense on T1W images and hyperintense on T2W images. The solid portion avidly enhances on the postcontrast imaging, but the cyst and its walls rarely enhance (Fig. 36-41). Complete imaging of the neural axis is recommended to rule out multiple lesions, especially in cases of von Hippel-Lindau disease. However, solitary lesions are associated with von Hippel-Lindau disease in 10% to 20% of cases.

Special Procedures

Hemangioblastomas are highly vascular lesions, and on angiography a highly vascular tumor blush is noted. Angiography can be useful for identifying the vascular supply of the lesion for surgical planning purposes. In addition, it may assist in finding smaller lesions.

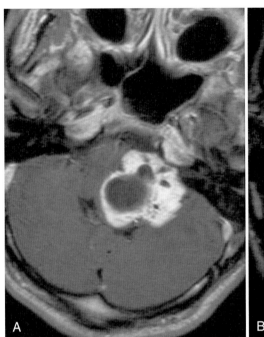
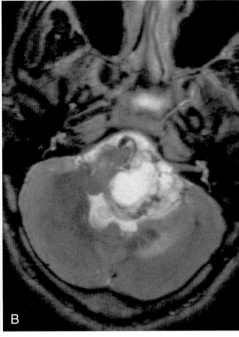

■ FIGURE 36-41 Hemangioblastoma. Axial postcontrast T1W **(A)** and axial T2W **(B)** MR images demonstrate a partially cystic lesion with avid enhancement that extends into the left CPA.

ANALYSIS

A 77-year-old man presented to the emergency department with a headache. A CT scan was obtained that revealed a hyperdense lesion in the left CPA. Inspection of the images in bone algorithm demonstrated erosion along the petroclival synchondrosis. MRI was obtained the next morning on which a mass lesion was noted extending into the left CPA. The lesion was heterogeneous on T2 weighting, involving the portion extending into the CPA, with low signal suggesting blood products. Abnormal signal was also identified within the clivus. On postcontrast imaging the portion centered over the petroclival synchondrosis avidly enhanced (see Fig. 36-35).

The key to making the diagnosis in this case is identifying where the lesion was centered. Once the petroclival synchon-drosis was recognized as being involved, the differential diagnosis was quickly narrowed to chondrosarcoma. Care should be taken in making this diagnosis because chordoma, which is typically thought of as being a midline lesion, can on occasion be eccentric and can have a similar imaging appearance to chondrosarcoma. The other major differential diagnosis for a hyperdense lesion in the CPA would be a meningioma, but one would not expect involvement of the petroclival synchondrosis by a meningioma. Metastases are uncommon in the CPA, but given the bone erosion this could be considered in the differential diagnosis if there is history of a primary cancer. A report of this case is presented in Box 36-1.

BOX 36-1　Sample Report: Cerebellopontine Angle Tumor

PATIENT HISTORY

A 77-year-old man presented with a history of headache and mass lesion noted in the CPA on CT.

COMPARISON STUDY

CT of the brain was done the previous day.

TECHNIQUE

Axial T1W images before and after gadolinium administration, 3D FSE T2W images, and coronal T1W post-gadolinium images were obtained through the region of the CPA. In addition, whole-brain post-gadolinium and FLAIR images were obtained.

FINDINGS

There is a mass lesion that demonstrates increased T2 signal and appears to be centered on the petroclival fissure on the left. Abnormal T2 prolongation is present in the clivus bilaterally, left greater than right. The mass extends posteriorly into the left CPA. At this point, the lesion becomes heterogeneous, with low signal on T2W imaging suggesting hemorrhage. The lesion results in distortion of the left aspect of the pons and the left brachium pontis. Increased T2 signal is noted within these structures, suggestive of secondary edema. On postcontrast imaging the majority of the lesion avidly enhances. The portion extending into the CPA only peripherally enhances. This may be secondary to the suspected hemorrhagic component.

The lesion is noted to extend anteriorly into the region of Meckel's cave and cavernous sinus. The left vertebral flow void courses adjacent and inferior to the left aspect of the lesion at its inferior margin, as does the basilar artery.

No regions of abnormal enhancement or T2 prolongation are noted within the supratentorial brain.

IMPRESSION

An enhancing lesion is centered over the left petroclival synchondrosis with extension into the left CPA. Given the location and imaging characteristics, this lesion most likely represents a chondrosarcoma. A chordoma arising in an eccentric location is a less likely diagnosis, as is a metastatic lesion.

KEY POINTS

- The ability to locate the point of origin of a lesion within the CPA can assist in narrowing the differential diagnosis.
- In most cases, MRI is the most beneficial imaging modality in the CPA owing in part to multiplanar acquisition and it is not limited by the beam-hardening artifact seen on CT.
- CT is useful to assess the osseous response to the lesion and for evaluation of tumoral calcification.
- Diagnostic angiography is of value for suspected vascular lesions that may require preoperative embolization.

SUGGESTED READINGS

Beskonakli E, Cayli S, Bostanci U, et al. Choroid plexus papillomas of the posterior fossa: extraventricular extension, intraventricular and primary extraventricular location: report of four cases. J Neurosurg Sci 1998; 42:37-40.

Liu P, Saida Y, Yoshioka H, Itai Y. MR imaging of epidermoids at the cerebellopontine angle. Magn Reson Med Sci 2003; 2:109-115.

Mulkens TH, Parizel PM, Martin JJ, et al. Acoustic schwannoma: MR findings in 84 tumors. AJR Am J Roentgenol 1993; 160:395-398.

Muzumdar DP, Goel A, Fatteprkar S, Goel N. Endolymphatic sac carcinoma of the right petrous bone in von Hippel-Lindau disease. J Clin Neurosci 2006; 13:471-474.

Zuccaro G, Sosa F. Cerebellopontine angle lesions in children. Child's Nerv Syst 2007; 23:177-183.

REFERENCES

1. Smirniotopoulos JG, Yue NC, Rushing EJ. Cerebellopontine angle masses: radiologic-pathologic correlation. RadioGraphics 1993; 13:1131-1147.
2. Zuccaro G, Sosa F. Cerebellopontine angle lesions in children. Childs Nerv Syst 2007; 23:177-183.
3. Bonneville F, Sarrazin JL, Marsot-Dupuch K, et al. Unusual lesions of the cerebellopontine angle: a segmental approach. RadioGraphics 2001; 21:419-438.
4. Kasantikul V, Netsky MG, Glasscock ME 3rd, Hays JW. Acoustic neurilemmoma: clinicoanatomical study of 103 patients. J Neurosurg 1980; 52:28-35.
5. Prayson R. Neuropathology. Philadelphia, Elsevier, 2005.
6. Wu EH, Tang YS, Zhang YT, Bai RJ. CT in diagnosis of acoustic neuromas. AJNR Am J Neuroradiol 1986; 7:645-650.
7. Salzman KL, Davidson HC, Harnsberger HR, et al. Dumbbell schwannomas of the internal auditory canal. AJNR Am J Neuroradiol 2001; 22:1368-1376.
8. Duvoisin B, Fernandes J, Doyon D, et al. Magnetic resonance findings in 92 acoustic neuromas. Eur J Radiol 1991; 13:96-102.
9. Tali ET, Yuh WT, Nguyen HD, et al. Cystic acoustic schwannomas: MR characteristics. AJNR Am J Neuroradiol 1993; 14:1241-1247.
10. Cho YD, Choi GH, Lee SP, Kim JK. (1)H-MRS metabolic patterns for distinguishing between meningiomas and other brain tumors. Magn Reson Imaging 2003; 21:663-672.
11. Okamoto K, Furusawa T, Ishikawa K, et al. Focal T2 hyperintensity in the dorsal brain stem in patients with vestibular schwannoma. AJNR Am J Neuroradiol 2006; 27:1307-1311.
12. Hakyemez B, Erdogan C, Bolca N, et al. Evaluation of different cerebral mass lesions by perfusion-weighted MR imaging. J Magn Reson Imaging 2006; 24:817-824.
13. Bonneville F, Savatovsky J, Chiras J. Imaging of cerebellopontine angle lesions: an update: II. Intra-axial lesions, skull base lesions that may invade the CPA region, and non-enhancing extra-axial lesions. Eur Radiol 2007; 17:2908-2920.
14. Buetow MP, Buetow PC, Smirniotopoulos JG. Typical, atypical, and misleading features in meningioma. RadioGraphics 1991; 11:1087-1106.
15. Russell EJ, George AE, Krieheff II, Budzilovich G. Atypical computed tomography features of intracranial meningioma: radiological-pathological correlation in a series of 131 consecutive cases. Radiology 1980; 135:673-682.
16. Mahmood A, Caccamo DV, Tomecek FJ, Malik GM. Atypical and malignant meningiomas: a clinicopathological review. Neurosurgery 1993; 33:955-963.
17. Carroll RS, Zhang J, Dashner K, Black PM. Progesterone and glucocorticoid receptor activation in meningiomas. Neurosurgery 1995; 37:92-97.
18. Buetow MP BP, Smirniotopoulos JG. Typical, atypical, and misleading features in meningioma. RadioGraphics 1991; 11:1087-1106.
19. Goldsher D, Litt AW, Pinto RS, et al. Dural "tail" associated with meningiomas on Gd-DTPA–enhanced MR images: characteristics, differential diagnostic value, and possible implications for treatment. Radiology 1990; 176:447-450.
20. Shino A NS, Matsuda M, Handa S, Inubushi T. Noninvasive evaluation of the malignant potential of intracranial meningiomas performed using proton magnetic resonance spectroscopy. J Neurosurg 1999; 91:928-934.
21. Smirniotopoulos JG, Chiechi MV. Teratomas, dermoids, and epidermoids of the head and neck. RadioGraphics 1995; 15:1437-1455.
22. Yilmazlar S, Kocaeli H, Cordan T. Brain stem stroke associated with epidermoid tumours: report of two cases. J Neurol Neurosurg Psychiatry 2004; 75:1340-1342.
23. Timmer FA, Sluzewski M, Treskes M, et al. Chemical analysis of an epidermoid cyst with unusual CT and MR characteristics. AJNR Am J Neuroradiol 1998; 19:1111-1112.
24. Horowitz BL, Chari MV, James R, Bryan RN. MR of intracranial epidermoid tumors: correlation of in vivo imaging with in vitro 13C spectroscopy. AJNR Am J Neuroradiol 1990; 11:299-302.
25. Chen CY, Wong JS, Hsieh SC, et al. Intracranial epidermoid cyst with hemorrhage: MR imaging findings. AJNR Am J Neuroradiol 2006; 27:427-429.
26. Nguyen JB, Ahktar N, Delgado PN, Lowe LH. Magnetic resonance imaging and proton magnetic resonance spectroscopy of intracranial epidermoid tumors. Crit Rev Comput Tomogr 2004; 45:389-427.
27. Tankere F, Vitte E, Martin-Duverneuil N, Soudant J. Cerebellopontine angle lipomas: report of four cases and review of the literature. Neurosurgery 2002; 50:626-631; discussion 631-622.
28. Passero S, Filosomi G, Cioni R, et al. Arachnoid cysts of the middle cranial fossa: a clinical, radiological and follow-up study. Acta Neurol Scand 1990; 82:94-100.
29. Ide C, De Coene B, Gilliard C, et al. Hemorrhagic arachnoid cyst with third nerve paresis: CT and MR findings. AJNR Am J Neuroradiol 1997; 18:1407-1410.
30. Samii M, Carvalho GA, Schuhmann MU, Matthies C. Arachnoid cysts of the posterior fossa. Surg Neurol 1999; 51:376-382.
31. Yildiz H, Erdogan C, Yalcin R, et al. Evaluation of communication between intracranial arachnoid cysts and cisterns with phase-contrast cine MR imaging. AJNR Am J Neuroradiol 2005; 26:145-151.

32. Preece MT, Osborn AG, Chin SS, Smirniotopoulos JG. Intracranial neurenteric cysts: imaging and pathology spectrum. AJNR Am J Neuroradiol 2006; 27:1211-1216.

33. Oyama H, Ikeda A, Inoue S, et al. Multiple neurenteric cysts in the posterior fossa and cervical spinal canal—case report. Neurol Med Chir (Tokyo) 2004; 44:146-149.

34. Koeller KK, Sandberg GD. From the archives of the AFIP. Cerebral intraventricular neoplasms: radiologic-pathologic correlation. Radio-Graphics 2002; 22:1473-1505.

35. Pencalet P, Sainte-Rose C, Lellouch-Tubiana A, et al. Papillomas and carcinomas of the choroid plexus in children. J Neurosurg 1998; 88:521-528.

36. Bulakbasi N, Kocaoglu M, Ors F, et al. Combination of single-voxel proton MR spectroscopy and apparent diffusion coefficient calculation in the evaluation of common brain tumors. AJNR Am J Neuroradiol 2003; 24:225-233.

37. Rao AB, Koeller KK, Adair CF. From the archives of the AFIP. Paragangliomas of the head and neck: radiologic-pathologic correlation. Armed Forces Institute of Pathology. RadioGraphics 1999; 19:1605-1632.

38. Borba LA, Al-Mefty O. Intravagal paragangliomas: report of four cases. Neurosurgery 1996; 38:569-575; discussion 575.

39. Erdem E, Angtuaco EC, Van Hemert R, et al. Comprehensive review of intracranial chordoma. RadioGraphics 2003; 23:995-1009.

40. Bjerkehagen B, Dietrich C, Reed W, et al. Extraskeletal myxoid chondrosarcoma: multimodal diagnosis and identification of a new cytogenetic subgroup characterized by t(9;17)(q22;q11). Virchows Arch 1999; 435:524-530.

41. Rosenberg AE, Brown GA, Bhan AK, Lee JM. Chondroid chordoma—a variant of chordoma: a morphologic and immunohistochemical study. Am J Clin Pathol 1994; 101:36-41.

42. Tay KY, Yu E, Kassel E. Spinal metastasis from endolymphatic sac tumor. AJNR Am J Neuroradiol 2007; 28:613-614.

43. Mukherji SK, Albernaz VS, Lo WW, et al. Papillary endolymphatic sac tumors: CT, MR imaging, and angiographic findings in 20 patients. Radiology 1997; 202:801-808.

44. Eisenberg MB, Haddad G, Al-Mefty O. Petrous apex cholesterol granulomas: evolution and management. J Neurosurg 1997; 86:822-829.

45. Jackler RK, Cho M. A new theory to explain the genesis of petrous apex cholesterol granuloma. Otol Neurotol 2003; 24:96-106; discussion 106.

46. Nishimura T, Uchida Y, Fukuoka M, et al. Cerebellopontine angle lymphoma: a case report and review of the literature. Surg Neurol 1998; 50:480-485; discussion 485-486.

47. Slater A, Moore NR, Huson SM. The natural history of cerebellar hemangioblastomas in von Hippel-Lindau disease. AJNR Am J Neuroradiol 2003; 24:1570-1574.

48. Lee SR, Sanches J, Mark AS, et al. Posterior fossa hemangioblastomas: MR imaging. Radiology 1989; 171:463-468.

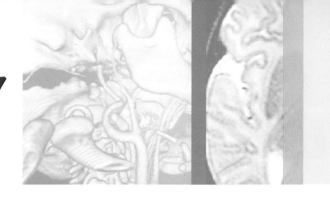

CHAPTER 37

Tumors of the Cranial/Spinal Nerves

Marc Taiwo Awobuluyi

Primary tumors of the cranial and spinal nerves derive from the cellular and extracellular support structures of the nervous system, rather than the functional neurons per se. The tumors are generally benign, slow growing, and often asymptomatic findings. Surgery is typically reserved for symptomatic cases and cases in which rare malignant transformation is suggested. Each of the tumors may arise sporadically or be part of the constellation of pathologic processes within specific genetic conditions.

Schwannomas account for 68% of intracranial neoplasms and 30% of primary spine tumors. Acoustic (vestibular) schwannomas are by far the most common among all intracranial nerve schwannomas. The incidences of nonvestibular schwannomas are as follows: cranial nerves (CNs) V >> IX > X > VII > XI > XII > III > IV > VI. CNs I and II do not exhibit schwannomas because they are not peripheral nerves but rather extensions of the central nervous system. *Neurofibromas* represent 5% of all benign soft tissue tumors.

In the United States, *optic nerve gliomas* represent 4% of orbital tumors, 4% of intracranial gliomas, and 2% of intracranial tumors. They also comprise two thirds of all primary optic nerve tumors.[1] Aggressive optic gliomas are a rare, unusual presentation of the more common adult astrocytoma.[2]

SCHWANNOMA

Schwannomas are benign, rare tumors of Schwann cells that invest the nerve sheaths of intracranial and extracranial peripheral nerves. They are also referred to as neuromas, neurilemmomas, and nerve sheath tumors.

Epidemiology

The mean age at presentation of isolated schwannomas is 35 to 45 years. In patients with neurofibromatosis type 2 (NF2), schwannomas may occur at a much younger age; acoustic schwannomas are the most common of these, occurring in more than 90% of patients with NF2. The rare ancient schwannoma variant occurs predominantly in elderly patients.[3] A male predominance has been reported only for isolated carotid space schwannomas (involving CNs IX, X, XI, or XII). No racial predilection has been reported.

Clinical Presentation

The clinical presentation of cranial schwannomas is variable and depends on the specific segment of the intracranial or extracranial nerve involved.

Schwannomas involving the oculomotor, trochlear, and abducens nerves are rare (Fig. 37-1). Presenting symptoms can include palsy of the affected muscle and ipsilateral cavernous sinus symptoms if the mass is in the cavernous sinus.[4,5]

Trigeminal Nerve Schwannoma

The tumor most commonly is an asymptomatic finding. Even large trigeminal nerve schwannomas of the deep face may be asymptomatic (Figs. 37-2 and 37-3). Atypical facial pain/paresthesias and masticator muscle weakness are less common presenting signs.

Facial Nerve Schwannoma

The most common presenting symptom of facial nerve schwannomas is hearing loss (present in ~70%). Slowly progressive facial nerve paralysis occurs in about 50%. Other less common presenting symptoms include ear and facial pain, hemifacial spasm, and, rarely, an acute onset of Bell's palsy–like facial paralysis. Cerebellopontine angle/internal auditory canal (CPA/IAC) facial nerve schwannomas most commonly present as sensorineural hearing loss, vertigo, and tinnitus. Tympanic and mastoid segment facial nerve schwannomas, if large, may present as an avascular retrotympanic mass in the setting of conductive hearing loss (Fig. 37-4).

Acoustic (Vestibular) Schwannoma

The most common symptom is sensorineural hearing loss. Small acoustic schwannomas may also present as tinnitus or disequilibrium. Larger acoustic schwannomas may cause facial and/or trigeminal neuropathy.

Jugular Foramen Schwannoma

The most common presentation of jugular foramen schwannomas (involving CNs IX > X > XI) is sensorineural hearing loss (90%). This presumably results from the superomedial vector spread of these tumors (Figs. 37-5 and 37-6). CN IX to XI

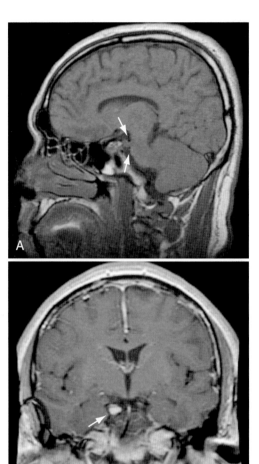

■ **FIGURE 37-1** **A,** Sagittal T1 MRI demonstrates enlargement of CN III at its root exit in the midbrain at the level of the tegmentum as it courses between the posterior cerebral and superior cerebellar arteries (*arrows*). **B,** Coronal T1W post-contrast (PC) image in the same patient demonstrates uniform enhancement of the CN III schwannoma within the suprasellar cistern (*arrow*) in this patient with NF2.

neuropathy occurs late in the disease progression. This may include glossopharyngeal dysfunction (e.g., hoarseness, difficulty swallowing, aspiration) and/or spinal accessory symptoms (e.g., trapezius atrophy). Hoarseness also may occur with involvement of the recurrent laryngeal branch of CN X. Other presenting signs and symptoms may include dizziness with cerebellar compression and jugular vein occlusion.

Hypoglossal Canal Schwannoma
These rare lesions most commonly present as ipsilateral hemitongue denervation (Fig. 37-7) and occasionally as tongue fasciculations in the subacute phase. Large lesions that extend along the prepontine cistern may produce multiple lower cranial neuropathies, involving any of CNs VII to XII.

Carotid Space Schwannoma
These tumors most commonly present as an asymptomatic posterolateral pharyngeal wall mass (nasopharyngeal and oropharyngeal [Figs. 37-8 and 37-9]) or an asymptomatic anterolateral

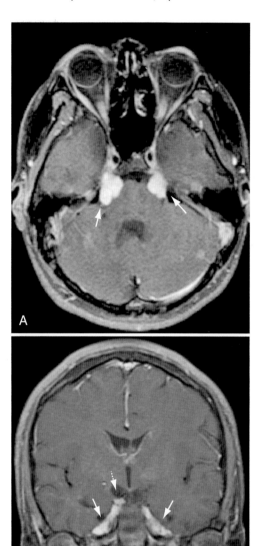

■ **FIGURE 37-2** **A,** Axial T1W PC fat-saturated MR image shows bilateral, avid, uniform enhancement and enlargement of the cisternal segments of CN V within the prepontine cistern. Lesions are consistent with CN V schwannomas in this patient with NF2. **B,** Coronal T1W PC fat-saturated MR image in the same patient demonstrates extension of the enhancing schwannomas to Meckel's cave bilaterally (*solid arrows*). Note additional right CN III schwannoma (*dashed arrow*).

neck mass (cervical). Other presenting signs and symptoms include Horner's syndrome, vocal cord paralysis, sleep apnea, and dysphagia.

Spinal Peripheral Schwannoma
The common presentation is radicular pain and, less commonly, paresthesias or progressive paraparesis (Fig. 37-10). Multiple schwannomas in patients with NF2 may be completely asymptomatic.

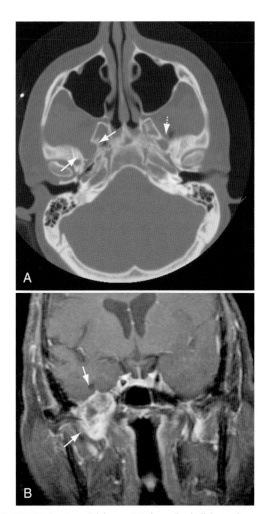

■ **FIGURE 37-3** **A,** Axial bone CT through skull base demonstrates enlargement of the right foramen ovale (*arrows*). Note the smooth remodeling typical of growth of a V3 schwannoma and normal appearance of the left foramen ovale (*dashed arrow*). **B,** Coronal T1W PC fat-saturated MR image in a different patient demonstrates a heterogeneously enhancing V3 schwannoma expanding the right foramen ovale, extending into the infratemporal fossa (*arrows*).

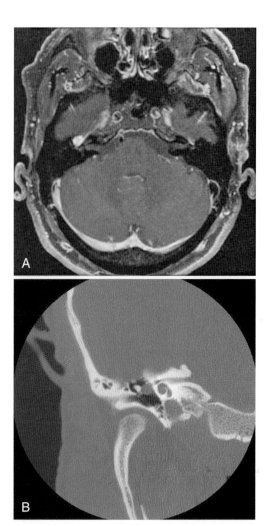

■ **FIGURE 37-4** **A,** Axial T1W PC fat-saturated MR image demonstrates uniformly enhancing CN7 schwannoma centered at the right geniculate ganglion. Enhancement also extended along the proximal anterior tympanic (horizontal) segment of CN VII. **B,** Coronal T-bone CT of same right ear demonstrates expansion of the CN VII canal, with extension of the mass into the middle ear and apposition with the ossicles.

Pathophysiology

The natural history of the majority of schwannomas is that of a slow-growing benign tumor. However, 10% of acoustic schwannomas demonstrate rapid growth (≥1 cm/yr). Malignant transformation is exceedingly rare.[6] Schwannomas commonly present as sporadic tumors but may present as part of the constellation of multiple inherited schwannomas, meningiomas, and ependymomas (MISME) in the setting of NF2. Multiple peripheral schwannomas may rarely occur in the absence of other NF2 features, and this is referred to as schwannomatosis.

The vast majority of schwannomas occur as a result of sporadic mutations. Sixty percent of sporadic vestibular schwannomas specifically demonstrate inactivation of the NF2 tumor suppressor gene through point mutations, loss of the NF2 locus on chromosome 22q, or loss of chromosome 22 entirely.[7,8] Carney complex is a rare autosomal dominant disease caused by mutation in the gene encoding the regulatory subunit of protein kinase A. The disease locus has been mapped to chromosome 17. Carney complex manifests as an array of pathologic processes, including melanotic schwannomas, cutaneous myxomas, potentially life-threatening cardiac myxomas, and pigmented adrenal tumors.[9]

Specific differential considerations should be made when evaluating schwannomas involving particular intracranial and extracranial peripheral nerves.

Differential Diagnostic Considerations
Trigeminal Nerve Schwannoma

Differential considerations include neurofibromas (typically the plexiform type in patients with NF1), masticator space sarcomas, and perineural spread of tumors such as squamous cell carcinoma.[10]

Facial Nerve Schwannoma

When involving the CPA/IAC these lesions may exactly mimic acoustic schwannomas. An important distinction is extension of tumor into the labyrinthine segment of CN VII, which makes the imaging diagnosis (Fig. 37-11). Additional differential considerations include normal enhancement along the geniculate ganglion and anterior tympanic segment of CN VII (from surrounding

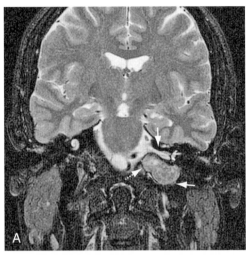
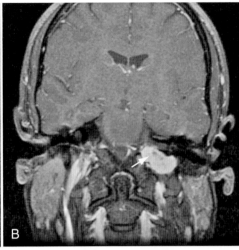

■ **FIGURE 37-5** **A,** Coronal T2W MR image demonstrates classic jugular foramen schwannoma as fusiform mass (*lower arrow*). Note relationship of superior component to the internal auditory canal (*arrow*). Inferiorly, the schwannoma extends into the nasopharyngeal carotid space (*dashed arrow*). **B,** Coronal T1W PC fat-saturated MR image in the same patient shows avid schwannoma enhancement with a central focus of cystic change (*arrow*). Note absence of high velocity flow voids.

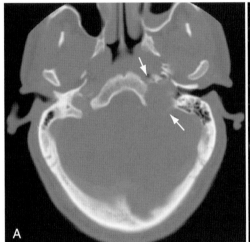
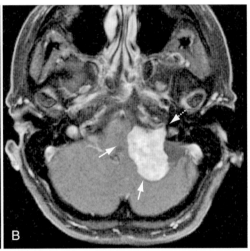

■ **FIGURE 37-6** **A,** Axial bone CT in same patient as Figure 37-5 demonstrates significant enlargement of the left jugular foramen (*arrows*). Note smooth and sharp margins, which are highly suggestive of a jugular foramen schwannoma. **B,** Axial T1W PC fat-saturated MR image in a different patient demonstrating a CN IX schwannoma within the left jugular foramen (*dashed arrow*) with significant medial extension, exerting mass effect on the brain stem and cerebellum (*arrows*).

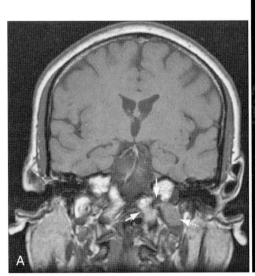
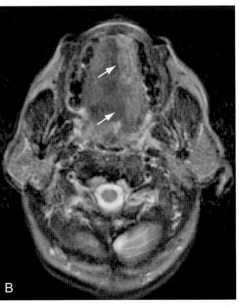

■ **FIGURE 37-7** **A,** Coronal T1W MR image shows schwannoma emerging from hypoglossal canal (*arrow*) and extending into the most cephalad portion of the nasopharyngeal carotid space (*dashed arrow*). Note normal marrow signal and cortex of the jugular tubercle and occipital condyle (*arrowhead*). **B,** Axial T2W MR image in the same patient demonstrates ipsilateral hemi-tongue atrophy.

■ **FIGURE 37-8 A,** Axial T2W MR image shows extensive central cystic change within right nasopharyngeal carotid space: CN X schwannoma. Sharp margins, absent high velocity flow voids, and the internal carotid artery draped over the anteromedial surface (*arrow*) are all consistent with the diagnosis of schwannoma. Note also anteromedial displacement of the parapharyngeal fat (*dashed arrow*). **B,** Coronal T1W PC fat-saturated MR image in the same patient shows ovoid enhancing mass with extensive cystic change (*arrows*), consistent with carotid space schwannoma.

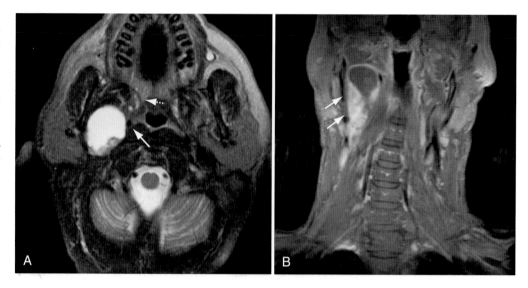

■ **FIGURE 37-9 A,** Axial T1W PC fat-saturated MR image shows enhancement of suprahyoid carotid space CN X schwannoma, with central intramural cystic change. Note anteromedial displacement of carotid vessels (*dashed arrow*) and posterolateral deflection/effacement of the jugular vein (*arrow*). **B,** Axial CT with contrast in same patient shows mild enhancement of the CN X schwannoma (*arrows*) with central areas of cystic change.

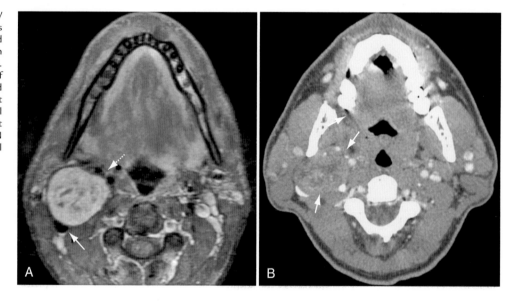

■ **FIGURE 37-10 A,** Coronal T1W PC fat-saturated MR image of lumbar spine demonstrating schwannoma of left L5 nerve root (*arrows*). **B,** Axial T2W MR image in a different patient shows schwannoma filling the left neural foramen (*arrow*) with a large eccentric cystic component (*dashed arrow*).

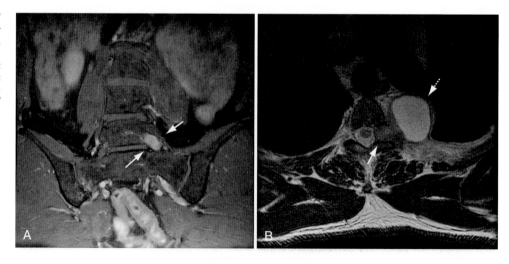

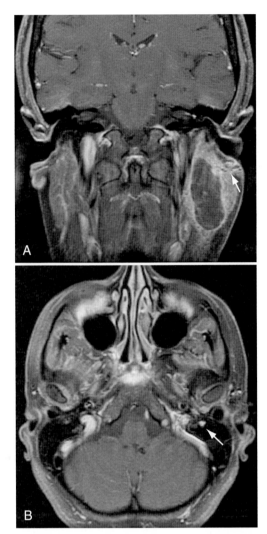

■ FIGURE 37-11 **A,** Coronal T1W PC fat-saturated MR image demonstrating a well-circumscribed cystic lesion within the left parotid gland representing cystic degeneration of a biopsy-proven CN VII schwannoma. *Arrow* denotes linear biopsy track. **B,** Axial T1W PC fat-saturated MR image in the same patient demonstrates smooth extension of the solid portion of the CN VII schwannoma within the distal facial canal.

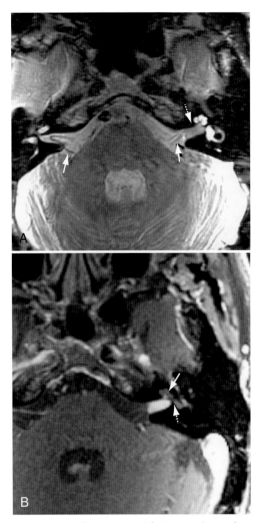

■ FIGURE 37-12 **A,** Thin-section axial T2W MR image demonstrates an intracanalicular-fundal acoustic schwannoma (*dashed arrow*) mildly enlarging the left internal auditory canal. Note the course of the proximal eighth nerves (*arrows*) and the increased T2 signal within the left cochlea. **B,** Axial T1W PC MR image in the same patient demonstrates uniform enhancement of the acoustic schwannoma with focal enhancement within the cochlear aperture (*arrow*). Note at the same time absent enhancement along the expected course of the labyrinthine segment of CN VII (*dashed arrow*), arguing against a CN VII origin.

arteriovenous plexus), perineural spread of parotid malignancy, facial nerve hemangioma, and Bell's palsy in the setting of herpetic infection.[11]

Acoustic (Vestibular) Schwannoma

The vast majority of these lesions arise from the inferior or superior division of the vestibular nerve, but they typically cause symptoms due to mass effect on the adjacent cochlear nerve.[12] Negative prognostic signs for recovery of hearing loss when imaging acoustic schwannomas include size 2 cm or larger and involvement of the IAC fundus or cochlear apparatus (Fig. 37-12). Principal differential considerations for intracanalicular acoustic schwannomas include the significantly less common facial nerve schwannoma, meningioma, and, specifically in the adult patient, metastasis and lymphoma.

Jugular Foramen Schwannoma

Slow venous flow in an asymmetrically enlarged jugular bulb may mimic a jugular foramen schwannoma. Other differential entities include glomus jugulare paraganglioma, jugular fora-

men meningioma, a large cerebellopontine angle acoustic schwannoma, and metastases/lymphoma involving the jugular foramen.[13]

Hypoglossal Canal Schwannoma

Differential considerations include glomus jugulare (when sufficiently large to invade the hypoglossal canal), metastases/lymphoma involving the hypoglossal canal (specifically in the context of surrounding marrow infiltration or lytic changes), and the uncommon persistent hypoglossal artery.[14]

Carotid Space Schwannoma

Differential considerations include neurofibroma (neurofibromatosis type 1 [NF1] association in 50%), carotid body paraganglioma (splays the internal carotid artery/external carotid artery; high-velocity flow voids when >2 cm), and glomus vagale paragangliomas of the nasopharyngeal carotid space (high-velocity flow voids when >2 cm).

Spinal Peripheral Schwannoma

Extruded disc fragments are commonly mistaken for schwannomas. However, with extruded discs the nerve root usually may be identified as a separate structure and enhancement is typically absent. Neurofibromas, meningiomas, and myxopapillary ependymomas are other tumors in the differential diagnosis.

Pathology

A resected schwannoma appears as an ovoid, tubular encapsulated mass eccentrically arising and expanding from the outer nerve sheath layer of the cranial nerve. Cysts may be present. Gross hemorrhage and frank necrosis are uncommon.

Histologically, schwannomas are benign encapsulated tumors composed of bundles of spindle-shaped Schwann cells with elongated nuclei. The cellular architecture consists of densely cellular regions of Antoni A cells—compact, elongated cells with occasional palisading ± loose, myxomatous regions of Antoni B cells. Large tumors may demonstrate intratumoral cystic change ± hemorrhage ± calcification. The rare ancient schwannoma variant is characterized by degenerative changes within the tumor typified by perivascular hyalinization, calcification, cystic necrosis, relative loss of Antoni type A tissue, and degenerative nuclei that may be misinterpreted as sarcomatous pleomorphisms. Schwannomas, in contrast to neurofibromas, demonstrate strong, diffuse immunostaining for S-100 protein (a neural crest marker antigen) and Leu-7 (CD57) but are endothelial membrane antigen (EMA) negative.

Schwannomas arise variably along the course of intracranial and extracranial peripheral nerves. The anatomic distribution of certain specific cranial nerves is of note:

- *Facial nerve schwannomas* located within the temporal bone (T-bone) are significantly more common than those within the CPA/IAC. Facial nerve schwannomas of the CPA/IAC, in turn, occur more commonly than intraparotid lesions.
- *Acoustic schwannomas* occur far more commonly along the vestibular division of CN VIII than the cochlear nerve, specifically arising from the glial–Schwann cell junction. Some authors report that these lesions more commonly arise from the inferior division of the nerve, but others report equal frequency for lesions from the superior and inferior divisions.
- Nasopharyngeal *carotid space schwannomas* may arise from CNs IX to XII. Schwannomas arising in the oropharyngeal carotid space to the aortic arch derive from the vagus nerve.[15]
- *Ancient schwannomas* are usually located deep in the head and neck, thorax, retroperitoneum, pelvis, and extremities of elderly patients.

Imaging

CT

Nonenhanced CT is the best imaging technique for delineating the classic bony changes of smooth foraminal/canal remodeling and scalloping associated with schwannomas. Atrophy of muscles innervated by the affected nerve may also be seen. Calcification and hemorrhage may be seen rarely.

Specific variations of facial nerve schwannomas deserve attention:

- *Tympanic (horizontal) segment facial nerve schwannoma* presents as a pedunculated mass deriving from the tympanic segment of CN VII, extending into the middle ear cavity (see Fig. 37-4). When large, a tympanic facial nerve schwannoma may laterally displace the ossicles.
- *Mastoid segment facial nerve schwannoma* may demonstrate a smooth, tubular morphology or a globular, irregular

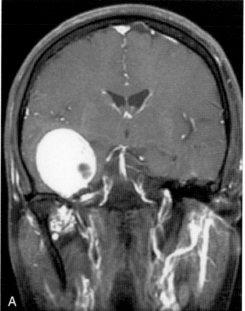

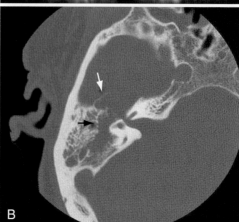

■ **FIGURE 37-13** **A,** Coronal T1W PC fat-saturated MR image demonstrates a large, avidly enhancing, greater superficial petrosal nerve schwannoma extending into the middle cranial fossa. Note absence of high-velocity flow voids despite large size. **B,** Axial temporal bone CT of the right ear demonstrates a large mass in the expected location of the geniculate ganglion. The mass thins the overlying temporal bone and expands into the middle cranial fossa (*arrow*). The mass also extends with lobulated, irregular margins along the expected course of the tympanic (horizontal) segment of CN VII (*black arrow*).

morphology (if it breaks into the mastoid air cells) (Fig. 37-13).

- *Greater superficial petrosal nerve* is just anteromedial to the geniculate fossa. Typically, whole-brain imaging is needed to fully characterize these lesions because facial nerve schwannomas involving this nerve often project into the middle cranial fossa (see Fig. 37-13).

Contrast-enhanced CT has a limited role (contrast-enhanced MRI should be obtained instead). Uniform enhancement of schwannomas is classic, except in areas of cystic change.

MRI

Typically, T1-weighted (T1W) lesions have low to intermediate signal intensity. Atrophy of muscles innervated by the affected nerve may also be seen. T2-weighted (T2W) images typically show lesions of high signal intensity relative to white matter (compared with meningiomas, which typically have low to intermediate T2 signal relative to white matter).

T1W post-contrast (PC) imaging typically demonstrates well-marginated, uniform contrast enhancement. Large lesions may demonstrate intratumoral cystic change. No high-velocity flow voids are seen even when lesions are large (compare with paragangliomas) (see Fig. 37-13).

Special Procedures
Angiography is usually unnecessary unless tumor histology is in doubt (typically the main differential considerations in this circumstance are paragangliomas and meningiomas). Schwannomas are typically avascular or demonstrate a fine vascular blush. Scattered contrast puddles are typically seen in the venous phase. No dominant feeding arteries or arteriovenous shunting is present.

NEUROFIBROMA
A neurofibroma is a localized, diffuse, or plexiform neoplasm of the nerve sheath. This can also be called a nerve sheath tumor.

Epidemiology
Whereas all three types of neurofibromas may be associated with NF1, the majority of localized and diffuse neurofibromas (90%) are sporadic. Plexiform neurofibromas, in contrast, are a characteristic and diagnostic feature of NF1, occurring in 25% of affected cases (Fig. 37-14). Peak presentation is at 20 to 30 years of age. There is no gender or racial predilection.

Clinical Presentation
The majority of neurofibromas in the head and neck are asymptomatic. Common symptoms of neurofibromas in the spine include pain, weakness, and sensory deficit.

Pathophysiology
Neurofibromas are slow-growing World Health Organization (WHO) grade 1 tumors. In the context of NF1 (von Recklinghausen's disease) they arise as a result of autosomal dominant inheritance or spontaneous mutation/loss of the *NF1* tumor suppressor gene on chromosome 17.[16] Malignant peripheral nerve sheath tumors (PNST) are WHO classification grade 3/4 and arise from malignant transformation of localized neurofibromas in 5% of NF1 patients but rarely arise de novo.[17] Sporadic neurofibromas are also believed to be due to *NF1* gene mutations but rarely undergo malignant transformation.

The major differential diagnoses for neurofibromas in the head, neck, and spine are schwannomas and meningiomas, the former of which may be indistinguishable from localized neurofibromas by imaging. Cystic degeneration, hemorrhage, and calcification, however, are more common with schwannomas. In the spine, additional differential considerations include meningoceles, neoplastic/inflammatory infiltration, and chronic interstitial demyelinating polyneuropathy.

Pathology
Localized neurofibromas are fusiform, firm, gray-white masses intermixed with the nerve of origin. *Plexiform neurofibromas are* tortuous, rope-like expansions of the affected nerve and resemble a "tangle of worms." *Malignant peripheral nerve sheath tumors* are fusiform, fleshy, tan-white masses with areas of necrosis and hemorrhage. Typically the affected nerve is thickened along its proximal and distal aspects owing to spread of tumor along the epineurium and perineurium.

Histologically, neurofibromas comprise all the components of the peripheral nerves, including fibroblasts, Schwann cells, and neurites. These cells are distributed in a loose stroma of collagen fibers and mucosubstance in which Schwann cells predominate. Localized neurofibromas typically have axons embedded within

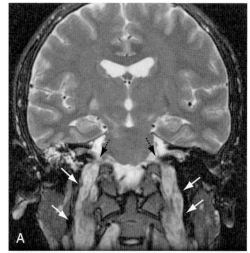

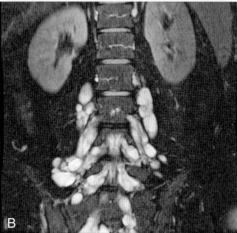

■ **FIGURE 37-14 A,** Coronal T2W fat-saturated MR image demonstrates large plexiform neurofibromas extending from the jugular foramina (*black arrows*) through the nasopharyngeal carotid spaces (*white arrows*). **B,** Coronal T2W fat-saturated MR image of the lumbar spine demonstrating extensive plexiform neurofibromas extending along the course of multiple nerve roots.

their substance. Plexiform neurofibromas grow within nerves, enlarging and elongating each fascicle. Malignant peripheral nerve sheath tumors are high-grade fibrosarcomas demonstrating fasciculated growth of spindle cells.

Neurofibromas may arise within or attach to nerve trunks anywhere in the skin, as well as any conceivable internal site, including intracranial peripheral nerves and intraspinal/paraspinal locations. Diffuse neurofibromas typically involve the subcutaneous tissues of the head and neck. Plexiform neurofibromas usually involve large nerve roots and within the head and neck most commonly involve the ophthalmic division of CN V in the context of NF1.

Imaging
CT
Nonenhanced CT shows smooth bony erosion (vertebral body scalloping or foramen/canal widening). Neurofibromas are isointense to nerve/spinal cord; and calcification, cystic change, and hemorrhage are rare. With the addition of a contrast agent, neurofibromas show variable mild-to-moderate, relatively homogeneous enhancement.

MRI

T1W images show similar intensity to nerves and spinal cord. T2W images have peripheral high signal with a central low/intermediate signal "target sign," which is suggestive but not pathognomonic for neurofibromas (seen less commonly with schwannomas). On T1W PC imaging there is variable mild-to-moderate relatively homogeneous enhancement.

Special Procedures

Malignant peripheral nerve sheath tumors and benign nerve sheath tumors may be metabolically active.[18]

OPTIC NERVE GLIOMA

An optic nerve glioma is a neoplasm of glial cell origin arising from the optic nerve. Alternate names include optic pathway tumor, juvenile pilocytic astrocytoma, and adult malignant optic glioma.

Epidemiology

The low-grade form of this neoplasm, benign (pilocytic) optic glioma, occurs most often in pediatric patients. The aggressive (fibrillary) glioma is most common in adults; it is frequently fatal, even with treatment. From 10% to 38% of pediatric patients with optic nerve glioma have NF1; conversely, 15% to 40% of children with NF1 have optic nerve glioma. Bilateral optic nerve gliomas are almost pathognomonic for NF1.[19] There is no distinct racial predilection to sporadic optic nerve glioma. Benign optic glioma has the same distribution as NF1. In pediatric patients there is a slight female predominance, whereas in adult patients the opposite is true.[1] In the pediatric population, the median patient age is 5 years, with 80% of patients presenting before age 15.[1] In adult patients, the age ranges from 22 to 79 years, with a mean age of 52 years.[2]

Clinical Presentation

In most young patients with optic glioma, the presenting symptom is painless proptosis. Optic atrophy is common, as is reduced visual acuity, although the latter may be a late symptom. A large lesion may compress the optic chiasm, causing nystagmus or other symptoms. In adult patients, bilateral vision loss is a common early finding because most lesions involve the optic chiasm.

Pathophysiology

The WHO classifies most pediatric optic nerve gliomas as grade I astrocytomas (pilocytic astrocytomas) because they are slow growing and tend not to metastasize. Twenty percent of optic gliomas that extend to the optic chiasm or beyond into the optic radiations, demonstrate a more aggressive course. When confined exclusively to the orbit, the lesion may mimic optic neuritis, pseudotumor, lymphoma, or optic nerve meningioma. When present, NF1 is associated with autosomal dominant inheritance and 100% penetrance but variable clinical expressivity.

Pathology

Gross pathology shows a tan-white tumor with smooth, fusiform, tubular enlargement of the optic nerve affected by the glioma. In patients with NF1, the tumor is often rounded with cystic changes that may be related to mucinous degeneration versus infarction.

Development of optic nerve gliomas occurs in stages, from generalized hyperplasia of glial cells in the nerve to complete disorganization with loss of neural landmarks in the nerve and nerve sheath. A reactive meningeal hyperplasia may be incited, making optic nerve glioma difficult to distinguish from a perioptic meningioma. In children without NF1, lesions tend to be expansile with intraneural infiltration. Childhood lesions with NF1 demonstrate central nerve sparing (allowing for preserved vision). Circumferential perineural infiltration occurs with arachnoid gliomatosis.

Histologically aggressive optic gliomas occurring in adults are either an anaplastic astrocytoma or a glioblastoma multiforme. Prominent features of these tumors include nuclear pleomorphism, numerous mitoses, and vascular endothelial proliferation.

In 66% of patients with NF1 with optic nerve glioma, the growth involves the intraorbital optic nerve. In 10% to 20%, the tumor is confined to the orbit, with the remainder of these patients showing involvement of the intracranial compartment. In the absence of NF1, the optic chiasm is most commonly involved, as is, less often, the intraorbital optic nerve.[20] Optic nerve gliomas may involve various portions of the retrobulbar visual pathway, including the optic nerve, chiasm, tracts, and radiations. Malignant lesions can invade the hypothalamus, basal ganglia, and internal capsule directly, or they may spread to the leptomeninges or subpial surfaces.

Imaging

CT

Contrast-enhanced CT can be used to characterize local involvement of optic nerve glioma within the orbit. However, MRI better demonstrates the extent of the lesion's intracranial growth.

In children, unenhanced CT typically reveals a marked, diffuse enlargement of the optic nerve, with characteristic kinking or bending. The enlargement may be tubular, fusiform, or excrescent. Areas of lucency may result from mucinous or cystic changes. Approximately 50% of the lesions demonstrate enhancement; this characteristic is more common with intracranial (especially retrochiasmatic) extension. Calcifications are rare (compare with optic nerve sheath meningiomas).

MRI

On T1W imaging optic nerve gliomas are usually isointense to the cortex and hypointense to white matter. Invariably, the lesions are hypointense to orbital fat. On T2W imaging lesions demonstrate a mixed appearance that is isointense to hyperintense relative to white matter and the cortex. On T1C+ imaging intense enhancement is common.

Classically, meningioma, the primary differential diagnostic consideration, is characterized by the "tram-track" sign, with enhancement of the periphery of the nerve/optic sheath unit. On the other hand, enhancement in optic nerve glioma is more uniform. Isolated enlargement of the optic nerve sheath also may present diagnostic difficulty; however, this enlargement can usually be distinguished by its signal characteristics, which follow fluid signal on all MRI pulse sequences.

The diagnosis may be made with a high degree of confidence when the enhancing lesion involves the optic chiasm and retrochiasmatic optic pathway.

ANALYSIS

Gliomas are specific to the central nervous system and as such only affect CN II (Fig. 37-15). Schwannomas and neurofibromas are limited to peripheral nerves, including CNs III to XII. Neurofibromas affecting the cranial nerves tend to be of the plexiform type and classically occur in the context of NF1, readily allowing their distinction from schwannomas of the cranial nerves (compare Fig. 37-5 with Fig. 37-14). The "target sign" seen on T2W is seen more commonly with neurofibromas but is not pathognomonic. Nerve sheath tumors in patients with NF1 are most likely neurofibromas. Nerve sheath tumors in patients with NF2 may be schwannomas or mixed tumors. In sporadic cases, cystic changes (see Fig. 37-10) calcifications or hemorrhage are all atypical for neurofibromas and favor schwannoma over the sometimes indistinguishable localized neurofibroma. A sample report is provided in Box 37-1.

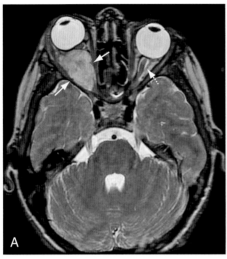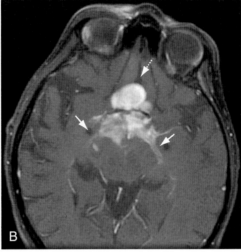

■ **FIGURE 37-15** **A,** Axial high resolution T2W MR image demonstrating large right optic nerve glioma filling the retrobulbar right orbit (*arrows*), causing right orbital proptosis. Note normal left optic nerve surrounded by cerebrospinal fluid (*dashed arrow*). **B,** Axial T1W PC MR image in a different patient demonstrates an optic glioma centered at the chiasm (*dashed arrow*) with extension along the optic tracts (*arrows*).

KEY POINTS: DIFFERENTIAL DIAGNOSIS

- Nerve sheath tumors in patients with NF1 are most likely neurofibromas.
- Nerve sheath tumors in patients with NF2 may be schwannomas or mixed tumors.

- Gliomas are specific to the central nervous system and thus involve only CN II.

BOX 37-1   Sample Report: Contrast-Enhanced MRI of the Head

PATIENT HISTORY

A 34-year-old man presented with a left-sided sensorineural hearing loss.

TECHNIQUE

Evaluation of the head was performed using noncontrast sagittal T1W, axial T1W, axial T2W, axial T2W FLAIR, axial diffusion-weighted (with ADC map) and axial gradient echo (susceptibility) sequences. The cisterns of the posterior fossa were evaluated with axial FIESTA series. Following intravenous administration of _____ mL of Gd-chelate contrast agent, additional high resolution axial and coronal T1W images were obtained through both internal auditory canals, followed by axial T1W images of the head.

FINDINGS

A heterogeneously enhancing mass fills and expands the left internal auditory canal and protrudes medially into the cerebellopontine angle cistern. The intracanalicular portion enhances nearly homogeneously. The cisternal portion shows nonenhancing zones that may represent cysts or necrosis. Small perilesional arachnoid cysts surround the mass and further expand the left CP angle cistern. The lesion extends superiorly to abut the origin and cisternal segment of CN V, but does not extend far enough inferiorly to affect the lower cranial nerves (CN IX-XII). The combined mass effect compresses the brachium pontis,

flattens the left side of the fourth ventricle, and deviates the fourth ventricle anteriorly and to the right. The compressed brachium pontis show mild edema. The lateral and third ventricles are moderately dilated consistent with hydrocephalus. No contralateral CP angle lesion or supratentorial lesion is identified. The left cochlea, vestibule, facial nerve canal, and petromastoid air cells are normal. The left transverse sinus, sigmoid sinus, and jugular bulb appear normal and smaller than those on the right. The vertebrobasilar arteries are of normal caliber and appear patent. There is no enlargement of the posterior inferior, anterior inferior, or superior cerebellar arteries to suggest aneurysm or high-flow vascular lesion.

IMPRESSION

The findings are most consistent with a left vestibular schwannoma with Antoni A histology in the intracanalicular component and Antoni B histology in the cisternal component. Perilesional arachnoid cysts surround the cisternal portion of the mass. The degree of hydrocephalus is greater than expected for the total mass effect on the fourth ventricle, likely signifying a component of hydrocephalus from high concentration of protein within the CSF. There is no imaging evidence of anatomic anomalies of the dural venous sinuses or structures of the petrous temporal and mastoid bones.

SUGGESTED READINGS

Addullah A, et al. The different faces of facial nerve schwannomas. Med J Malaysia 2003; 58:450-453.

Chateil JF, et al. MRI and clinical differences between optic pathway tumors in children with and without neurofibromatosis. Br J Radiol 2001; 74:24-31.

Colreavy MP, Lacy PD, Hughes J, et al. Head and neck schwannomas—a 10 year review. J Laryngol Otol 2000; 114:119-124.

Conti P, et al. Spinal neurinomas: retrospective analysis and long-term outcome of 179 consecutively operated cases and review of the literature. Surg Neurol 2004; 61:34-44.

Millar WS, et al. MR of malignant optic glioma of adulthood. Am J Neuroradiol 1995; 16:1673-1676.

Parnes LS, et al. Magnetic resonance imaging of facial nerve neuromas. Laryngoscope 1991; 101:31-35.

Rosenberg SI. Natural history of acoustic neuromas. Laryngoscope 2000; 110:497-508.

Sarma S, et al. Nonvestibular schwannomas of the brain: a 7-year experience. Neurosurgery 2002; 50:437-448.

REFERENCES

1. Hollander MD, FitzPatrick M, O'Connor SG, et al. Optic gliomas. Radiol Clin North Am 1999; 37:59-71.
2. Millar WS, Tartaglino LM, Sergott RC, et al. MR of malignant optic glioma of adulthood. AJNR Am J Neuroradiol 1995; 16:1673-1676.
3. Isobe K, Shimizu T, Akahane T, Kato H. Imaging of ancient schwannoma. AJR Am J Roentgenol 2004; 183:331-336.
4. Ginsberg F, Peyster RG, Rose WS, Drapkin AJ. Sixth nerve schwannoma: MR and CT demonstration. J Comput Assist Tomogr 1988; 12:482-484.
5. Katsumata Y, Maehara T, Noda M, Shirouzu I. Neurinoma of the oculomotor nerve: CT and MR features. J Comput Assist Tomogr 1990; 14:658-661.
6. Elias M, Balm A, Peterse J, et al. Malignant schwannoma of the parapharyngeal space in von Recklinghausen's disease: a case report and review of the literature. J Laryngol Otol 1993; 107:848-852.
7. Fontaine B, Sanson M, Delattre O, et al. Parental origin of chromosome 22 loss in sporadic and NF2 neuromas. Genomics 1991; 10:280-283.
8. Fontaine B, Hanson MP, VonSattel JP, et al. Loss of chromosome 22 alleles in human sporadic spinal schwannomas. Ann Neurol 1991; 29:183-186.
9. Casey M, Vaughan CJ, He J, et al. Mutations in the protein kinase A R1alpha regulatory subunit cause familial cardiac myxomas and Carney complex. J Clin Invest 2000; 106:R31-R38.
10. Yuh WT, Wright DC, Barloon TJ, et al. MR imaging of primary tumors of trigeminal nerve and Meckel's cave. AJR Am J Roentgenol 1988; 151:577-582.
11. Chung SY, Kim DI, Lee BH, et al. Facial nerve schwannomas: CT and MR findings. Yonsei Med J 1998; 39:148-153.
12. Schmalbrock P, Chakeres DW, Monroe JW, et al. Assessment of internal auditory canal tumors: a comparison of contrast-enhanced T1-weighted and steady-state T2-weighted gradient-echo MR imaging. AJNR Am J Neuroradiol 1999; 20:1207-1213.
13. Eldevik OP, Gabrielsen TO, Jacobsen EA. Imaging findings in schwannomas of the jugular foramen. AJNR Am J Neuroradiol 2000; 21:1139-1144.
14. Gomez Beldarrain M, Fernandez Canton G, Garcia-Monco JC. Hypoglossal schwannoma: an uncommon cause of twelfth-nerve palsy. Neurologia 2000; 15:182-183.
15. Gilmer-Hill HS, Kline DG. Neurogenic tumors of the cervical vagus nerve: report of four cases and review of the literature. Neurosurgery 2000; 46:1498-1503.
16. Aoki S, Barkovich AJ, Nishimura K, et al. Neurofibromatosis types 1 and 2: cranial MR findings. Radiology 1989; 172:527-533.
17. Gupta G, Maniker A. Malignant peripheral nerve sheath tumors. Neurosurg Focus 2007; 22:12.
18. Beaulieu S, Rubin B, Djang D, et al. Positron emission tomography of schwannomas: emphasizing its potential in preoperative planning. AJR Am J Roentgenol 2004; 182:971-974.
19. Listernick R, Charrow J, Greenwald MJ, et al. Optic gliomas in children with neurofibromatosis type 1. J Pediatr 1989; 114:788-792.
20. Kornreich L, Blaser S, Schwarz M, et al. Optic pathway glioma: correlation of imaging findings with the presence of neurofibromatosis. AJNR Am J Neuroradiol 2001; 22:1963-1969.

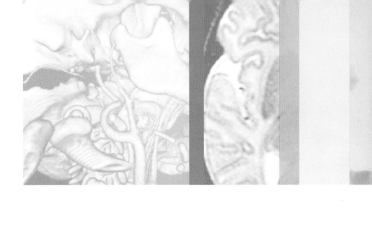

CHAPTER 38

Management of the Tumor Patient

Nicholas Butowski

Epidemiology

Primary brain cancer, those tumors that arise from the substance of brain itself, account for 1% of all cancers.[1,2] Approximately 14 per 100,000 people in the United States are diagnosed with primary brain tumors each year. Of these, roughly 7 per 100,000 are diagnosed with a primary malignant brain tumor and will account for approximately 2% of all cancer-related deaths. Brain tumors most commonly occur in the fifth and sixth decades of life but are the second most common form of cancer in childhood next to leukemia. Recently, there has been conjecture that the incidence of brain tumor is increasing. Analysis of this speculation is complicated by diagnostic discrepancies and ascertainment bias in registry data. However, after extensive review, this apparent increase is most likely due to factors such as better diagnostic procedures, improved access to medical care, and enhanced care for the elderly, all leading to greater detection rather than an actual increase in incidence. Nevertheless, more standardized and unbiased diagnosis and registration methods must become established and widely used before such speculation is truly resolved.

Metastases to the brain occur at some point in 10% to 15% of persons with cancer and are more common than primary brain tumors. Tumors arising in any other part of the body (most commonly from lung, breast, kidney, and skin) may metastasize to the brain; metastatic tumors to the brain are usually multiple, although a solitary metastasis can mimic a primary brain tumor.

Treatment

Treatment of most brain tumors is complex and will involve multiple medical personnel, including a neurosurgeon, neuro-oncologist, radiation oncologist, medical oncologist, and neurologist.

Before proceeding with a discussion of how specific brain tumors are treated it is useful to review several characteristics of brain tumors that distinguish them from other types of tumors.

- Most brain tumors range from a low- to high-grade type (the grade of each tumor is based on its microscopic features and determines the type of treatment and prognosis).
- Even the most aggressive or malignant brain tumors rarely metastasize outside the CNS.
- The location of a tumor often determines whether a neurologic deficit occurs.
- Even tumors regarded as slow growing or benign can produce symptoms as severe and life threatening as malignant tumors. This is because they may occur in a vital area of the brain or because when they reach a critical size there is no room for them to expand within the surrounding skull, which puts significant pressure on key structures.
- The brain has no lymphatic vessels to remove the treated or dead tumor, so the tumor may not appear to shrink on CT or MRI even if treatment is successful.
- Treatment of a tumor can result in a new neurologic deficit. For example, a temporary or permanent loss of function can occur after surgery and problems of brain swelling can occur during radiation treatments.
- Unless a dramatic, early and sustained improvement occurs after therapy, it may be difficult to determine the response to treatment. Treatments may produce temporary neurologic deterioration that might take weeks or months to improve.

For a full discussion of the treatment of specific brain tumors and some tumors of the spinal cord, please visit www.expertconsult.com.

The Phakomatoses

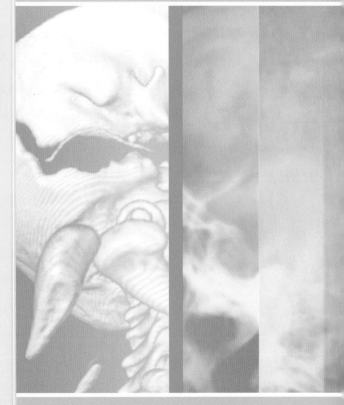

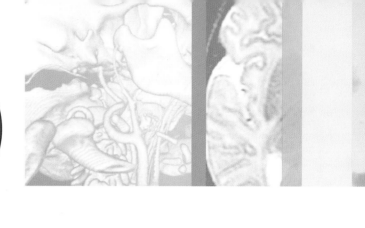

CHAPTER 39

Phakomatoses: Tumor Suppression Gene Defects

Noriko Aida, Tetsu Niwa, and Gen Nishimura

The phakomatoses, or neurocutaneous syndromes, include neurofibromatosis types 1 and 2 (NF1 and NF2), tuberous sclerosis complex (TSC), von Hippel-Lindau disease (VHL), ataxia-telangiectasia, and basal cell nevus syndrome (BCNS). All these disorders show a high frequency of tumor development. NF1, NF2, TSC, and VHL are attributed to a variety of tumor suppression genes. Ataxia-telangiectasia belongs to a group of chromosome breakage syndromes that result from deficient DNA repair. BCNS is caused by derangement of the hedgehog signaling pathway. Of surprise is the fact that the signaling pathway with a major role in early embryonic development is also responsible for tumor development.

NF1 is the most frequent of these syndromes, with estimated incidence of 1 in 2000 to 5000, and TSC is the second with an incidence of 1 in 5800. The others are relatively rare diseases. The clinical, genetic, molecular, pathogenic, and radiologic characteristics of these disorders are detailed. Key points in differential diagnosis for these disorders are emphasized. All disorders have a tendency to develop particular tumors with unique histologic characteristics in special anatomic regions. In addition, each disorder shows distinctive nontumoral associations. Radiologic examination readily enables us to delineate the highly characteristic combination of specific tumors with other associations and thus plays a pivotal role in the definitive diagnosis and management for affected individuals.

NEUROFIBROMATOSIS TYPE 1

NF1 is a common genetic disorder characterized by multiple tumors in the central and peripheral nervous systems, cutaneous pigmentation, and lesions of the vascular system and viscera. Additionally, there is a tendency for a variety of tissues to undergo malignant transformation.[1] It is also referred to as von Recklinghausen's disease, peripheral neurofibromatosis, and classic neurofibromatosis.

Epidemiology

NF1 is one of the most common genetic disorders, with an estimated prevalence of 1 in 2000 to 5000 individuals in most population studies, regardless of gender and ethnic background.[2]

Clinical Presentation

The National Institutes of Health (NIH) diagnostic criteria for NF1 are two or more of the following:

- Six or more café-au-lait spots whose greatest diameter is more than 5 mm in prepubertal patients and more than 15 mm in postpubertal patients
- Two or more neurofibromas of any type, or one or more plexiform neurofibromas
- Freckling of the axillary or inguinal region (Crowe's sign)
- An optic pathway tumor
- Two or more Lisch nodules (iris hamartoma)
- A distinctive osseous lesion such as sphenoid wing dysplasia or thinning of the cortex of the long bone (with or without pseudarthrosis)
- A first-degree relative (parent, siblings, or offspring) with NF1 according to the previously mentioned criteria

Only about half of children with NF1 meet the NIH criteria for diagnosis by 1 year of age, but almost all do so by age 8 because many features of NF1 increase in frequency with age.[3] Other clinical characteristics of NFI include learning disabilities, short stature, macrocephaly, and predisposition to developing neoplasia, such as gliomas, malignant peripheral nerve sheath tumors (MPNST), and myeloid malignancies.

Neurofibromas are classified as cutaneous (Fig. 39-E1A), subcutaneous, and plexiform, with the first two usually occurring in early adolescence and the latter being congenital (at least the diffuse type). Plexiform neurofibromas can become larger, progress to malignancy (usually MPNST), and may occur almost anywhere in the body. They commonly develop in the orbit and cause impaired ocular movement and exophthalmos. The neck is another common location.

Café-au-lait spots are benign pigmented lesions and are the first manifestation of NF1, usually becoming evident during the first year of life (Fig. 39-E1B). Freckling of the axilla will develop later in about two thirds of patients. Lisch nodules of the iris are best discernable by slit lamp examination. They begin to appear in childhood and are finally present in all NF1 patients.[4]

Skeletal manifestations include kyphoscoliosis, overgrowth or undergrowth of bones, bony rarefactions due to adjacent neurofibroma, and pseudarthrosis of the tibia.[1,5] Skull lesions include macrocephaly, lambdoid suture defect, and dysplasia of the greater sphenoidal wing.

Neurologic manifestations can be grouped into five major categories, including cognitive disabilities, intracranial tumors, tumors of the peripheral nerves, spinal nerve tumors, and cerebral infarction.[1] Thirty to 60 percent of children with NF1 have learning disabilities, and they tend to do better on verbal tasks than on performance tasks. Only 8% of patients with NF1 were reported to have an IQ less than 70.[1] Intracranial tumors include optic pathway gliomas, brain stem gliomas, and other hemispheric tumors. Tumors of the peripheral nerves are mainly neurofibromas, can arise at any age, and can involve any major nerve. Spinal nerve tumors generally develop slowly and are rare in children. Cerebral infarctions result from cerebrovascular occlusive disease, most commonly affecting the supraclinoid portion of the internal carotid artery or one of its major branches.[1]

Optic pathway glioma is the most common tumor of the central nervous system (CNS) in patients with NF1. It usually develops in the first 2 decades, with a peak incidence at around age 4 to 5 years. Although the reported incidence ranges from 15% to 23%, only approximately one half of the affected patients develop signs and symptoms.[1] The tumor may involve any portion of the optic pathway. Although optic pathway gliomas are an incidental finding in the majority of the children with NF1, they may result in progressive compromise of visual activity and may cause serious symptom. Precocious puberty may occur if the tumor extends to the hypothalamus. Spontaneous regression may occur and may be related to the NF1 gene activity as tumor suppressor. Therefore, aggressive therapy is not indicated without clinical or radiologic evidence of progression.[1,4,5] Astrocytomas may develop in the mesencephalic tectum, brain stem (especially medulla), cerebellum, and cerebral hemispheres.[5] NF-related brain stem gliomas show clinical courses different from those of isolated brain stem gliomas. They tend to have indolent courses and better long-term outcome. Although appropriate management for both optic pathway gliomas and other gliomas is still under discussion, conservative management with serial follow-up MRI is recommended.[4,5]

Another CNS manifestation in NF1 is bilateral, nearly symmetrical zones of myelin vacuolization (ZMVs) that appear as areas of hyperintensity on T2-weighted (T2W)/fluid-attenuated inversion recovery (FLAIR) images in 60% to 70% of patients. The details of MRI findings are discussed later in the section on imaging. These zones become apparent after infancy and tend to diminish or disappear with age. They have been given various names, such as histogenetic foci, neurofibromatosis bright objects, and hamartomatous lesions. Because these lesions are pathognomonic, several authors proposed to include them in the diagnostic criteria for pediatric patients. Their relationship with cognitive disabilities has been investigated by several authors and is still controversial. The anatomic location of ZMVs may be more important than their number. Particularly, myelin vacuolization in the thalamus might significantly correlate to neurophysiologic disability.[5,6]

The value of performing brain MRI for NF1 patients at the time of clinical diagnosis is controversial. It is useful in helping to establish the diagnosis in some and in identifying complications before they become clinically apparent in others, but clinical management is not affected by findings of intracranial lesions such as optic nerve thickening and ZMVs in asymptomatic patients.[5]

For the differential diagnosis of NF1, few disorders are ever confused with NF1 although more than 100 genetic diseases show café-au-lait spots or other features of NF1.

Pathophysiology

NF1 is transmitted in an autosomal dominant inheritance pattern with complete penetrance and variable expressivity. The disease is presumed to result from a loss-of-function mutation of the *NF1* gene. Approximately 50% of cases show de novo mutations. The reason for such a high mutational rate in the *NF1* gene remains unknown but might be due to its large size, genomic position, and unusual structure. Over 80% of new mutations have been found to be paternal in origin. Although more than 500 different

germline NF1 mutations have been reported, there have been few consistent relationships between the clinical phenotype and size, type, and location of the gene.[1,7] Currently, only two clear correlations have been observed: (1) a whole *NF1* gene deletion presents large numbers and early appearance of cutaneous neurofibromas, more frequent and more severe cognitive abnormalities, and sometimes somatic overgrowth with large hands and feet, and dysmorphic facial features; and (2) a 3-bp in-frame deletion of exon 17 does not present surface plexiform neurofibromas despite typical pigmentary features in NF1.

The *NF1* gene is mapped to chromosome 17q11.2 and is a tumor suppressor gene. It encodes neurofibromin, a cytoplasmic protein that is predominantly expressed in neurons, Schwann cells, oligodendrocytes, astrocytes, and leukocytes. The function of neurofibromin is not fully understood, but it appears to activate RAS guanosine triphosphatase (GTPase), thereby controlling cellular proliferation and acting as a tumor suppressor. Neurofibromin probably has other functional properties as well, including regulation of adenylylcyclase activity and intracellular cyclic adenosine monophosphate (AMP) generation. The pathogenic mechanisms of *NF1* gene mutations have been widely investigated, particularly focusing on tumor formation. Neurofibromas are considered to occur as a result of loss of the remaining wild-type NF1 allele. Loss of heterozygosity during fetal development may result in the formation of plexiform neurofibromas, whereas a second-hit mutation later in life could lead to development of cutaneous neurofibromas. Molecular studies for MPNSTs from NF1 patients have shown several tumor suppression gene mutations in addition to NF1 mutations, and these findings suggest that a second genetic event is required for the MPNST formation in NF1 patients.[7] In NF1 pilocytic astrocytomas (optic pathway tumors), no detectable neurofibromin expression or increased RAS activity is found. These reports suggest that astrocytoma formation in NF1 patients requires a second genetic hit (loss of NF1 expression).[7]

Pathology

Neurofibromas are grade I tumors of the WHO classification. They infiltrate the nerve and involve multiple Schwann cells. They may be ill defined at the margin and may assume a fusiform shape as a result of their intraneuronal growth. Cutaneous neurofibromas are the typical skin nodules. Plexiform neurofibromas may involve several locations, including the cranial and spinal nerves, peripheral nerves, and autonomic nervous system. The fronto-temporo-orbital region is one of the most common locations of these plexiform neurofibromas.

Optic pathway gliomas are usually fusiform, intradural masses that stretch rather than disrupt the overlying meninges. Macroscopically, the margin of the tumor may be difficult to separate from the normal nerve.

There are few pathologic reports on the histology of the bilateral symmetrical zones of hyperintensity. In these, myelin vacuolization and spongiform myelopathy have been reported.[8]

Most optic pathway gliomas are considered pilocytic astrocytomas, although those involving the optic nerves only are considered by some to be hamartomatous rather than neoplasm. Some optic pathway tumors can be highly malignant. Other gliomas also are most commonly pilocytic astrocytomas, but low-grade and high-grade tumors rarely may also develop.

Neurofibromas consist of multiple Schwann cells surrounding multiple axons with fibroblastic proliferation, some myelinated fibers, and a huge amount of connective tissue, especially collagen and elastin. They have a potential for anaplastic transformation (neurofibrosarcomas).

Imaging

Optic Pathway Gliomas and Other Gliomas

Astrocytomas are more common in NF1 patients than in the general population.[4] Although optic pathway gliomas (Figs. 39-1

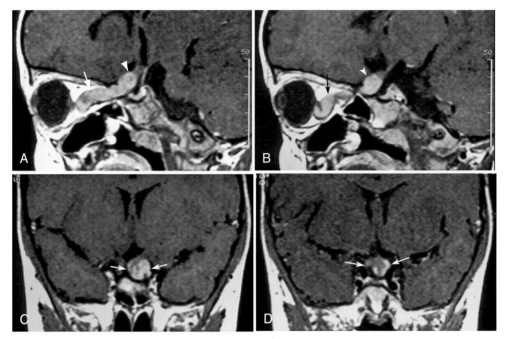

■ FIGURE 39-1 Neurofibromatosis type 1. Optic pathway glioma in a 3-year-old girl is evident on gadolinium-enhanced T1W sagittal (**A, B**) and coronal (**C, D**) MR images. Enlargement of the left optic nerve is seen in the intraorbital portion (*arrows*, **A, B**), prechiasmatic portion (*arrowheads*, **A, B**), and the optic chiasm (*arrows*, **C, D**). The tumor shows diffuse enhancement, and the optic nerve is markedly tortuous.

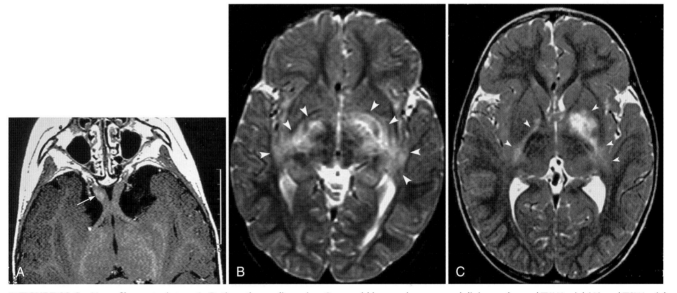

■ FIGURE 39-2 Neurofibromatosis type 1. Optic pathway glioma in a 2-year-old boy as shown on gadolinium-enhanced T1W axial (**A**) and T2W axial (**B, C**) MR images. Prechiasmatic portion of the right optic nerve shows mild enlargement and faint enhancement (*arrow*, **A**). T2W images reveal extended hyperintensity in the globi pallidi, internal capsule, and the optic tracts (*arrowheads*, **B, C**). It is impossible to determine whether this is a glioma or a zone of myelin vacuolization.

and 39-2) are the most common, astrocytomas may occur in the mesencephalic tectum, brain stem (Fig. 39-3), cerebellum, and cerebral hemispheres (see also Fig. 39-E2).[5] Imaging manifestations of these gliomas in NF1 patients are identical to those of patients without NF1.

CT

In optic pathway gliomas, enlargement of the optic nerve is readily identified, contrasting to the orbital fat on CT. Bone windows reveal enlargement of the optic canals. CT is less sensitive in evaluating the involvement of the optic tracts, the lateral geniculate bodies, and the optic radiations than MRI.

MRI

MRI is the best modality for assessing both intracranial and extracranial involvement of the optic pathway. T1-weighted (T1W) images particularly show distortion, enlargement, and sometimes elongation of the optic nerves, optic chiasm, and/or optic tracts (see Fig. 39-1). T2W/FLAIR sequences show abnormal hyperintensity extending posteriorly to the lateral geniculate bodies (see Fig. 39-2). The signal intensity of the lesions is variable on both T1W and T2W images. Enhancement of the lesions also is variable.[4,5]

Brain stem gliomas may be indistinguishable from UBOs. Both show high intensity on T2W images and may show mass effect without enhancement (see Fig. 39-3). Therefore, follow-up MRI

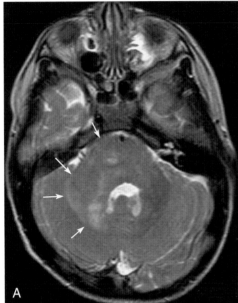

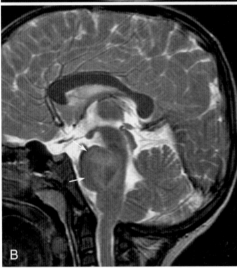

■ **FIGURE 39-3** Neurofibromatosis type 1. Brain stem glioma or unidentified bright objects in a 4-year-old boy as shown on axial (**A**) and sagittal (**B**) T2W MR images. Enlargement and ill-defined heterogeneous hyperintensity are seen in the pons, right middle cerebellar peduncle, and cerebellar white matter (*arrows,* **A, B**). It cannot be determined if this is a glioma or a zone of myelin vacuolation.

is mandatory. Apparent diffusion coefficient (ADC) could be reduced in the area of high-grade neoplasm.

Magnetic Resonance Spectroscopy

Proton MR spectroscopy (MRS) can help in differentiating between normal brain, ZMVs, and glioma.[5] On multivoxel proton MRS, ZMVs have shown elevated choline (Cho) levels, possibly reflecting increased myelin turnover; reduced creatinine (Cr); and normal *N*-acetyl-aspartate (NAA). Neoplasms show a Cho/Cr ratio greater than 2 and no NAA.[9] MRS may show metabolic abnormality even in normal-appearing areas of the brain,[5,9] and ADC is significantly higher in normal-appearing areas than in control subjects.[4,10]

Zones of Myelin Vacuolization

ZMVs are the most common intracranial lesions, occurring in about two thirds of NF1 patients and approximately 75% of children with NF1. The incidence rises to 90% in patients with

optic pathway glioma (see Fig. 39-2). Because a pathologic analysis has shown that they reflect myelin vacuolization, it is speculated that dysplasias of myelin are the cause of these lesions.[4] They are characteristic findings and appear to be pathognomonic, especially in pediatric patients.

ZMVs are typically multiple and commonly located in the white matter, splenium of the corpus callosum, hippocampi, basal ganglia (especially in the globus pallidus), internal capsules, thalami, brain stem, middle cerebellar peduncles, and cerebellar hemispheres (see Figs. 39-2 and 39-4).

CT

CT is not effective for detecting ZMVs, although a few of them can present as low-density lesions.

MRI

ZMVs are hyperintense on T2W, proton-density–weighted, and FLAIR images. They are usually isointense to slightly hypointense on T1W images (see Figs. 39-2 to 39-4) but sometimes may be hyperintense, particularly in the globus pallidus (see Fig. 39-4D and 39-E2B). Slight T1 shortening can also be observed in lesions of the brain stem and thalami. This has been suggested to relate to the presence of ectopic Schwann cells and melanocytes, to hypermyelination in hamartomatous or gliotic areas, to repair of vacuolized regions[11] and to microcalcifications.[8] But it tends to develop after the T2 prolongation appears and before the T2 prolongation disappears. This may mean that T1 shortening reflects delayed reactive formation of myelin.[11]

In general, ZMVs show neither contrast enhancement nor surrounding edema; yet mass effect may be present and transient enhancement has been reported in a few cases. Therefore, the differential diagnosis between myelin vacuolization and a low-grade neoplasm is difficult (see Figs. 39-2 and 39-3), so follow-up MRI is necessary. A neoplasm should be suspected when the lesion shows clear low signal with contrast enhancement on T1W images (see Fig. 39-E2).[5] Moreover, the biologic behavior of ZMVs cannot be predicted by imaging alone.[4] Benign-appearing lesions can evolve into neoplasms, whereas neoplastic-like lesions can decrease in size or disappear.

ZMVs are typically not found in infancy, increase in number and size until adolescence, and then attenuate, which might reflect myelin repair.[4,11]

Apparent diffusion coefficients (ADCs) are reported to be increased in ZMVs as compared with other areas of the brain in NF1 patients. Even the normal-appearing brain shows higher ADC values in patients with NF1 than in control individuals.[4,10]

MRS reveals spectra almost identical to those of normal brain but occasionally shows increased choline peak and decreased NAA levels, possibly due to increased myelin turnover.

Other Brain Lesions
MRI

Many NF1 patients have an increased volume of cerebral white matter with a large corpus callosum (Fig. 39-E3). These findings are postulated to result from increased size and number of axons.

Hydrocephalus is occasionally seen in NF1 patients. The causes of hydrocephalus include brain stem neoplasms adjacent to the aqueduct and benign aqueduct stenosis (Fig. 39-E4).[4]

Orbital and Calvarial Manifestations/ Plexiform Neurofibromas
CT

Bone dysplasias of the head and neck are common in NF1 patients and include defects of the sphenoid wing (Fig. 39-5A) and along the lambdoid suture (Fig. 39-E5). The latter has no clinical significance. Unilateral dysplasia of the sphenoid wings is characterized by hypoplasia or partial agenesis of the greater

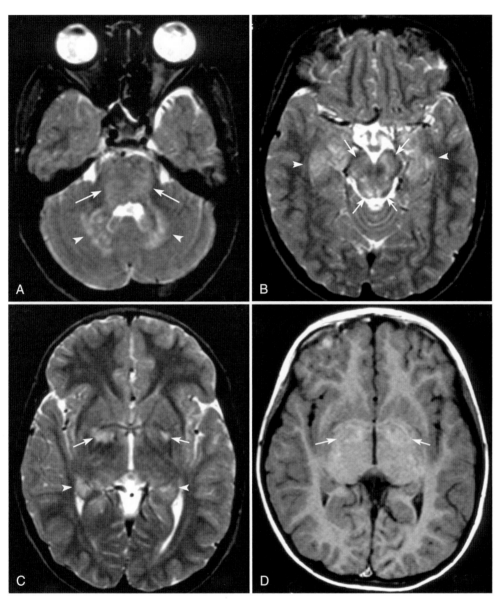

■ **FIGURE 39-4** Unidentified bright objects in a patient with neurofibromatosis type 1 evident on axial T2W (**A-C**) and T1W (**D**) MR images. T2W images show multiple hyperintense lesions in the pons (*arrows*, **A**), cerebellar dentate nuclei (*arrowheads*, **A**), and the midbrain (*arrows*, **B**). Bilateral hippocampi are slightly thickened and show T2 prolongation (*arrowheads*, **B, C**). Bilateral globi pallidi show as signal hyperintensity on a T2W image (*arrows*, **C**), and the peripheral areas of T2 prolongation are slightly hyperintense on a T1W image (*arrows*, **D**).

wing and partly of the lesser wing. As a result, the middle cranial fossa expands and the temporal lobe bulges through the bone defect. Pulsation of the temporal lobe may cause progressive pulsatile exophthalmos.[4,5] Rarely, there is enophthalmos instead.

Sphenoid wing dysplasia is almost always associated with plexiform neurofibromas of the orbit and periorbital region (see Fig. 39-5). Extension of plexiform neurofibromas to the cavernous sinus and the third to sixth cranial nerves is often observed. On CT, they are of low attenuation and do not show enhancement after administration of intravenous contrast material.

MRI

Plexiform neurofibromas present as heterogeneous masses, displaying mostly a low signal intensity compared with that of the brain parenchyma on T1W images and a high signal intensity on T2W images. However, the signal intensities are variable. T2W images typically show a peripheral high signal and a central low signal intensity compared with that of the muscle, called "target sign" (see Fig. 39-5B, C). The central hypointensity may reflect a dense central core of collagen.[4] After administration of intravenous contrast material, contrast enhancement of the tumor is variable but usually some parts of the tumor are enhanced (see Fig. 39-5D).

Vascular Dysplasia
CT

NF1 patients occasionally show dysplasia of the cerebral vasculature. The dysplasia is characterized by intimal proliferation resulting in arterial stenosis. The common and internal carotid arteries and the proximal middle and anterior cerebral arteries are usually involved (Fig. 39-E6).

Although vascular dysplasia is not easily detectable on standard CT or MRI, careful observation of flow voids may help to detect the narrowing of the cavernous or supraclinoid carotid arteries and proximal, middle, and anterior cerebral arteries. MR angiography is the modality of choice for screening the intracranial vascular dysplasia. Development of collateral vessels (moyamoya phenomenon) can be seen in these patients. Aneurysms and arteriovenous malformations are less common in NF1 patients.

Spinal Manifestations

Nontumoral spinal manifestations in NF1 patients include scoliosis, enlargement of the neural foramina (with or without lateral meningoceles), and posterior scalloping of the vertebral bodies. Both nerve sheath tumors and even spinal cord tumors may

■ **FIGURE 39-5** Neurofibromatosis type 1. Dysplasia of the left sphenoid wing with plexiform neurofibromatosis shown on a 3D CT image of the face and skull (**A**) and on T2W axial (**B**), coronal (**C**), gadolinium-enhanced T1W (**D**) MR images. Partial agenesis of the left greater sphenoid wing (*arrowheads,* **A**) and secondary expansion of the left orbit can be seen on CT. T2W images show multiple nodular and diffuse hyperintense lesions in the left orbit and extracranial region (*arrows,* **B, C**). Some nodular lesions show the target appearance (*arrowheads,* **B, C**). The lesions also show heterogeneous enhancement (**D**).

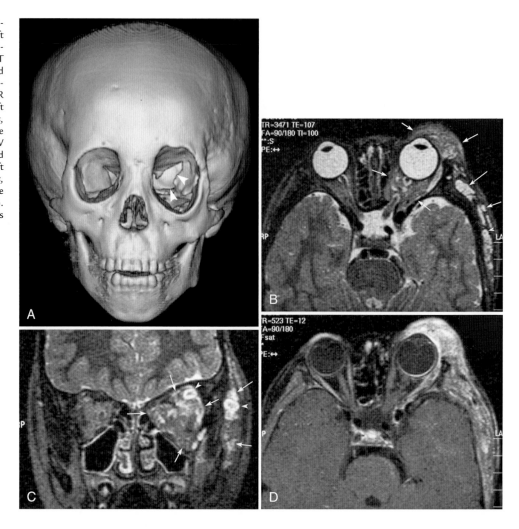

develop in NF1 patients but usually become symptomatic in older age.[5]

MRI

The role of the imaging study in NF1 patients with scoliosis is to clarify the underlying disorders: bone dysplasias, intradural lesions (tumors, cord tethering, syringohydromyelia), and paravertebral neurofibromas. Scoliosis in NF1 patients is most frequently the result of dysplasia of the vertebral bodies. Bone dysplasias are most clearly demonstrated on CT; yet, MRI also shows these changes and therefore is the modality of choice to identify both intrinsic spinal cord lesions and paravertebral tumors.

If an intramedullary tumor is found in a patient with NF1, it is likely to be an astrocytoma (commonly of low grade). The imaging findings of intramedullary astrocytoma in NF1 patients are identical to those in patients without NF1. If syringohydromyelia is found without an intraspinal mass in patients with NF1, a thin-slice contrast-enhancement MRI should be obtained to search for underlying intramedullary lesions.[4]

Nerve sheath tumors such as neurofibromas, plexiform neurofibromas, and MPNSTs may be found. Spinal/paravertebral neurofibromas are almost characteristic of NF1 patients. They may be single or multiple and unilateral or bilateral, and they may involve both intraspinal and extraspinal regions (dumbbell tumor) (Fig. 39-6). When small, the neurofibromas present as nodules along the nerve roots of the cauda equina on MRI. When large, they involve the neural foramina and extend into the paravertebral region.[4] As a result, the neural foramina are enlarged by bone erosion. On MRI, neurofibromas show a slight hyperintensity compared with the muscle on T1W images and

a peripheral hyperintensity with a relatively hypointense center on T2W images (see Fig. 39-6). This finding on T2W images is called a "target sign." Cord compression may occur if bilateral tumors grow at the same level.

MPNSTs occur in NF1 patients with a reported incidence of 10% to 15%.[4] Compared with benign neurofibromas, MPNSTs tend to be larger and relatively well circumscribed (see Fig. 39-6D, E). Increased internal heterogeneity has been reported to warrant a diagnosis of MPNST, although the finding is present in rare benign neurofibromas. The target sign is less common (see Fig. 39-6D, E). Local pain and rapid growth are most suggestive of malignant degeneration.[4]

NEUROFIBROMATOSIS TYPE 2

NF2 is a genetic disorder characterized by the development of a CNS tumor, especially bilateral vestibular schwannoma. It is also called central neurofibromatosis, bilateral acoustic neurofibromatosis, and neurofibromatosis type II. The term acoustic neuroma is considered incorrect, because the tumor most frequently arises from the vestibular division, not the cochlear division, of cranial nerve VIII.

Epidemiology

A recent update suggests that the incidence may be as high as 1 : 25,000, and at least higher than 1 : 100,000.[12]

Clinical Presentation

The most sensitive modified clinical diagnostic criteria for NF2 are as follows[13,14]:

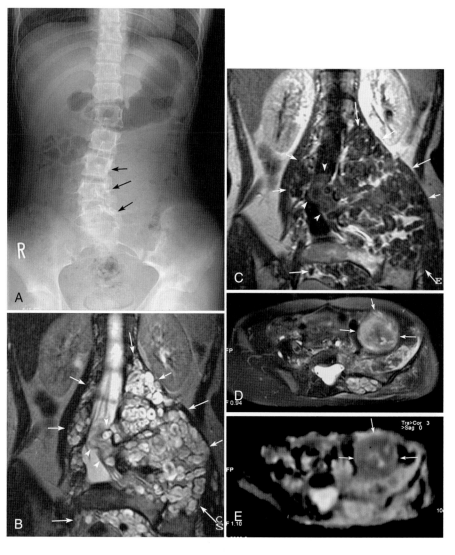

■ **FIGURE 39-6** Neurofibromatosis type 1. Lumbar scoliosis, multiple paravertebral neurofibromas, and development of a malignant peripheral nerve sheath tumor are shown on a radiograph of the lumbar spine (**A**), T2W (**B**) and gadolinium-enhanced T1W (**C**) coronal MR images, and follow-up axial T2W MR image (**D**) and apparent diffusion coefficient map (**E**) 3 years later. Numerous plexiform neurofibromas showing target signs are noted in the bilateral paravertebral regions and pelvis (*arrows,* **B, C**). Some tumors extend to the spinal canal (*arrowheads,* **B, C**). The lumbar spine shows secondary scoliosis with bone erosion (*arrows,* **A**). A follow-up MRI examination after 3 years shows an enlarged tumor with heterogeneous T2 prolongation and low apparent diffusion coefficient (*arrows,* **D, E**). The tumor was resected and proved to be a malignant peripheral nerve sheath tumor.

- Bilateral vestibular schwannomas
- A first-degree relative with NF2 *and*
  - Unilateral vestibular schwannoma *or*
  - Any two of: meningioma, schwannoma, glioma, neurofibroma, posterior subcapsular lenticular opacities*
- Unilateral vestibular schwannoma *and* any two of: meningioma, schwannoma, glioma, neurofibroma, posterior subcapsular lenticular opacities*
- Multiple meningiomas *and*
  - Unilateral vestibular schwannoma *or*
  - Any two of: schwannoma, glioma, neurofibroma, cataract

Beside bilateral vestibular schwannomas that affect almost all persons with NF2 by the age of 30 years, clinical features include schwannomas of other cranial, spinal, and peripheral nerves. Meningiomas are both cranial and spinal. Cord ependymomas and astrocytomas are observed occasionally. Generally, the mean age at onset of symptoms is the second decade of life and is reported to be 18 to 24 years. Although unilateral hearing loss is reported to be found in 35% to 44%, it is an uncommon symptom in NF2 children.[1,4,5] Intraspinal and paraspinal nerve sheath tumors are very common. Spinal nerve sheath tumor patients are more commonly symptomatic in NF2 (30%-40%) than in NF1 patients (only 1%-2%). Cataracts

*"Any two of" = two individual tumors or cataract.

(posterior subcapsular or cortical) are frequently seen and may be present in childhood.[1,5]

Age at diagnosis has been reported to be the strongest single predictor of the risk of mortality. Cataracts and cutaneous tumors are important clinical findings for early detection of affected children.[4,13] Other informative predictors of the risk for mortality include intracranial meningiomas, type of treatment centers, and type of constitutional NF2 mutations.[13]

Pathophysiology

NF2 is an autosomal dominant disorder with complete penetrance. The gene for NF2 is mapped on chromosome 22q11. Its gene product is called merlin (or schwannomin) and is a tumor suppressor. Merlin may regulate cell matrix attachment and cell adhesion. Therefore, a mutated merlin affects the cell adhesion, resulting in changes in the shape of the cell. Significant merlin expression is detected in Schwann cells, meningeal cells, lens, and nerves. This fact accounts for the high incidence of schwannomas, meningiomas, and cataracts in NF2 patients. Merlin expression is absent in almost all schwannomas, in many meningiomas, and in ependymomas in NF2 patients, indicative of a pivotal role of loss of heterozygosity in tumor development.

A large number of mutations have been documented. In general, patients with nonsense or frameshift (ultimately leading to premature stop codon) mutations show severe disease

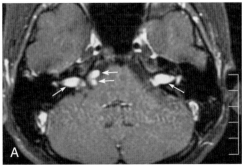
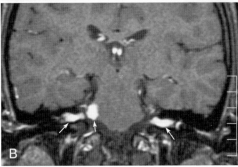

■ **FIGURE 39-7**   Bilateral vestibular schwannomas in neurofibromatosis type 2. Gadolinium-enhanced axial (**A**) and coronal (**B**) T1W MR images. Well-enhanced tumors (*arrows*) expand both internal auditory canals and extend into the cerebropontine angles.

phenotypes, those with missense mutations or in-frame deletions have mild disease, and those with slice-site mutations have variable disease severities. In contrast to NF1, large deletions of NF2 gene have been associated with a mild phenotype.

Pathology

Meningiomas are extra-axial nodular and calcified masses and are frequently multiple in NF2 patients.

Vestibular schwannomas initially manifest as round and solid masses that arise from the intracanalicular portion of the superior vestibular branch of the eighth cranial nerve. As they grow they expand the internal auditory canals and protrude medially into the cerebellopontine angle cisterns, forming the so-called ice cream cone appearance. About 40% of NF2-associated vestibular schwannomas show a lobular pattern that is uncommon in non-NF2 individuals.

In NF2, nerve sheath tumors commonly affect multiple locations (usually more than 10) and have intradural components. Spinal schwannomas may have cystic or hemorrhagic changes, develop from the posterior nerve roots, and may extend to the spinal cord.

The tumors of NF2 are derived from Schwann cells, meningeal cells, and glial cells, and all have benign histology. NF2-associated vestibular schwannomas tend to be more aggressive than non-NF2 tumors and show a higher degree of cell proliferation. NF2-associated meningiomas also have a higher degree of cell proliferation; they are usually of the fibroblastic variety. NF2-associated glial tumors are histologically not different from non-NF2 glial tumors.

Imaging
Intracranial Manifestations

As previously mentioned, the presence of bilateral vestibular schwannomas is the characteristic finding in NF2 patients (Figs. 39-7 and 39-8). Schwannomas occur on the other cranial nerves, spinal nerves, and peripheral nerves and tend to be multiple (see Fig. 39-8). Meningioma (often multiple) is the other hallmark (Fig. 39-9).

CT and MRI

In NF2 patients the CT and MRI findings of vestibular schwannomas are essentially similar to those in non-NF2 schwannomas. These tumors show a hypointensity to isointensity on T1W images and an isointensity to hyperintensity on T2W images. There is marked enhancement that may be homogeneous or heterogeneous, depending on the presence of cystic change within the tumor (see Figs. 39-7 and 39-8).

Meningiomas in NF2 patients are also similar in signal characteristics and location to those of non-NF2 meningiomas. Calcifications may occur (see Fig. 39-9).

If bilateral vestibular schwannomas are seen, or if NF2 is clinically suspected, contrast-enhanced whole-brain and spinal MRI examinations should be performed to search for other asymptomatic schwannomas or meningiomas. If a single schwannoma (particularly vestibular) or meningioma is found in a child, a contrast-enhanced brain MRI is recommended to search for other tumors, the presence of which gives an early diagnosis of NF2. When the diagnosis of NF2 has been made, repeat contrast-enhanced brain and whole spinal MRI examinations would show that new tumors may develop throughout life in NF2 patients.[4]

Spinal Manifestations

The characteristic spinal manifestations in NF2 patients include multiple paraspinal nerve sheath tumors (usually schwannomas, occasionally neurofibromas), intraspinal meningiomas, and intramedullary tumors (most commonly ependymomas and occasionally astrocytomas or schwannomas) (see Fig. 39-8).

MRI

Nerve tumors may be intramedullary or extramedullary. Schwannomas are usually multiple and often number more than 10. They are well defined and often show the "dumbbell" appearance due to intradural and extradural components. They are isointense on T1W images and hyperintense on T2W images with homogeneous contrast enhancement. They may cause enlargement of the neural foramina and vertebral scalloping by mechanical pressure, in contrast to bone changes in NF1 due to mesodermal dysplasia.[5]

Spinal meningiomas in NF2 patients show the same signal characteristics as those in non-NF2 meningiomas. They are extramedullary, are either intradural or extradural, and mainly occur in the thoracic region. They usually are isointense relative to the spinal cord both on T1W and T2W images with uniform contrast enhancement.[4,5] Postcontrast T1W images often show a "dural tail" sign. Dural tails are more prominent in NF2-associated meningiomas. A dural tail is useful for differentiating meningiomas from schwannomas in NF2 patients. Multiple tumors with local aggressiveness, fast and ubiquitous growth, and coexistence with schwannomas are characteristic features in NF2-associated meningiomas.[4,5]

Intramedullary ependymomas may be solitary, often involving the conus medullaris and filum terminale, or develop in multiple locations. They arise centrally in the cord and grow toward the surface of the cord. They show signal features similar to those in non-NF2 patients. Contrast-enhanced MRI is necessary to demonstrate the lesions. Spinal ependymoma may be indistinguishable from multifocal syringohydromyelia without contrast enhancement on MRI. Hematomyelia may be seen.[4,5]

TUBEROUS SCLEROSIS COMPLEX

TSC is classically defined by the clinical triad of mental retardation, epilepsy, and characteristic skin lesions. The clinical hallmarks are hamartomatous tumors in multiple organs such as the brain, kidney, heart, and skin. Alternate names include Bourneville's disease and Bourneville-Pringle syndrome.

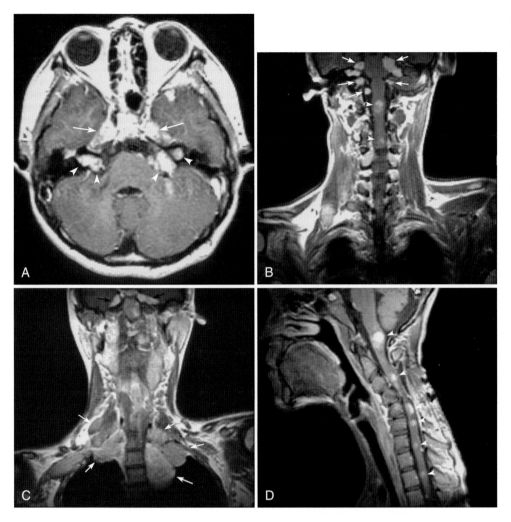

■ **FIGURE 39-8** Multiple cranial nerve schwannomas, paravertebral schwannomas, and multiple intramedullary tumors in a 14-year-old girl with neurofibromatosis type 2. Gadolinium-enhanced T1W axial brain (**A**), coronal (**B, C**), and sagittal (**D**) MR images of the cervicothoracic spine. Well-enhanced nodular tumors of multiple cranial nerves (*arrows,* **A, B**) as well as bilateral vestibular schwannomas (*arrowheads,* **A**) are noted. Large tumors in the bilateral paravertebral region are also seen (*arrows,* **C**). Sagittal and coronal images show multiple intramedullary tumors with gadolinium enhancement in the cervicomedullary junction and cervical cord (*arrowheads,* **B, D**).

Epidemiology

The incidence of TSC may be as high as 1 in 5800.[15] Neither racial nor gender predilection has been detected.

Clinical Presentation

The revised diagnostic criteria based on new genetic and clinical information are as follows:

● *Definite TSC:* Two major features or one major feature plus two minor features
● *Probable TSC:* One major feature plus one minor feature
● *Possible TSC:* One major feature or two or more minor features

Major features include:

● Facial angiofibromas or forehead plaque
● Nontraumatic ungual or periungual fibromas
● Hypomelanotic macules (three or more)
● Shagreen patch (connective tissue nevus)
● Multiple retinal nodular hamartomas
● Cortical tuber[1]
● Subependymal nodule
● Subependymal giant cell astrocytoma
● Cardiac rhabdomyoma, single or multiple
● Lymphangiomyomatosis[2]
● Renal angiomyolipoma[2]

Minor features are:

● Multiple randomly distributed pits in dental enamel
● Hamartomatous rectal polyps[4]
● Bone cysts[5]
● Cerebral white matter radial migration lines[1,3,5]
● Gingival fibromas
● Nonrenal hamartoma[4]
● Retinal achromic patch
● "Confetti" skin lesions
● Multiple renal cysts[4]

Additional criteria include:

1. Cerebral cortical dysplasia and cerebral white matter migration tracts occurring together are counted as one rather than two features of TSC.
2. When both lymphangiomyomatosis and renal angiomyolipomas are present, other features of tuberous sclerosis must be present before TSC is diagnosed.
3. White matter migration lines and focal cortical dysplasia are often seen in individuals with TSC; however, because these lesions can be seen independently and are relatively nonspecific, they are considered a minor diagnostic criterion for TSC.
4. Histologic confirmation is suggested.
5. Radiographic confirmation is sufficient.

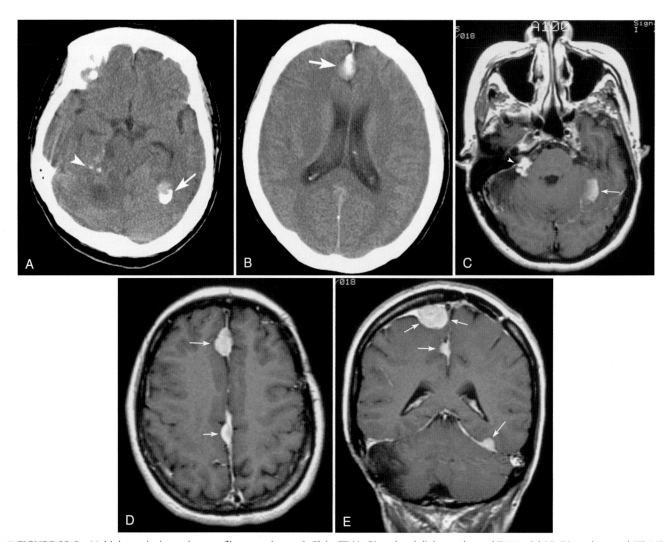

■ **FIGURE 39-9** Multiple meningiomas in neurofibromatosis type 2. Plain CT (**A, B**) and gadolinium-enhanced T1W axial (**C, D**), and coronal (**E**) MR images. Multiple enhanced meningiomas with dense calcification are noted along the left tentorium cerebelli and the falx cerebri (*arrows*, **A-E**). Partially resected vestibular schwannoma is seen in the right cerebellopontine angle (*arrowheads*, **A, C**).

The clinical manifestations of TSC show variable penetrance and vary considerably with respect to age at onset, severity, and rate of progression.[1] Four main clinical presentations are mental delay, seizures, cutaneous lesions, and tumors in various organs, including the brain.[1]

The diagnostic criteria for TSC consist of a set of major and minor diagnostic features.[16] No single feature in TSC is diagnostic; thus, an evaluation of all clinical features is necessary to make the diagnosis. Each manifestation in TSC appears at distinct developmental periods. For example, cortical tubers and cardiac rhabdomyomas develop during embryogenesis and thus are typical findings in infancy.

The neurologic manifestations include mental delay and seizures. The degree of mental delay varies greatly, and a significant proportion of affected youngsters develop autistic features. Fifty-five percent of affected individuals are reported to have an IQ greater than 70, whereas 30.5% have an estimated IQ less than 21. Approximately one third of patients diagnosed as having TSC on the basis of non-neurologic manifestations maintain a normal intelligence. Seizures occur at some time in all patients with mental delay. Almost all seizure types but absence seizure are seen in TSC. Infantile spasm is the most common seizure type during infancy. One fourth to one third of children presenting with infantile spasms are ultimately diagnosed as having TSC.[1]

Intracranial tumors are less frequent in TS than in neurofibromatosis. They are almost exclusively giant cell astrocytomas near the foramen of Monro. The incidence is reported to be 15% in a large series.[1] Giant cell astrocytomas are generally found in the first and second decades, with a peak incidence between 8 and 18 years of age and an equal incidence in both males and females.[17] There have been controversies in surgical treatment of giant cell tumors: some believe shunting for the obstructed lateral ventricle is sufficient, whereas others assert that the tumor should be resected to prevent possible degeneration to high-grade histology.[4]

Retinal hamartomas occur in about 50% of TSC patients.

Skin lesions include angiofibromas (adenoma sebaceum) (Fig. 39-E7A), hypopigmented macules (ash-leaf spots), so-called shagreen patch (connective tissue nevus) (Fig. 39-E7B), and ungual fibroma. Angiofibromas may be detected at any age but more often in late childhood and adolescence. Hypopigmented macules are generally detected in infancy or early childhood and are best demonstrated by Wood's light. Shagreen patch is identified with increasing frequency after 5 years of age.

In the kidney, angiomyolipomas develop in childhood, adolescence, or adulthood whereas renal cysts can be detected in infancy or early childhood. Cardiac rhabdomyomas occur in 50% of TSC patients, but they are of maximal size during intrauterine life or in early infancy and are clinically symptomatic only in this period; they usually regress spontaneously within 2 to 3 years.[1] Pulmonary lymphangiomyomatosis is found in adolescent girls or women with TSC.

No conclusive guidelines for surveillance have been established for TSC, but most specialized centers periodically perform brain and abdomen imaging to monitor development and progression of the lesions in the brain and kidneys.

Pathophysiology

TSC is an autosomal dominant disorder caused by a mutation in either of two disease-causing genes, *TSC1* or *TSC2*. A new mutation is responsible for up to 70% to 80% of affected individuals.

TSC1 and *TSC2* are tumor suppression genes. *TSC1* (encoding hamartin) is mapped on chromosome 9q34, and *TSC2* (encoding tuberin) is on chromosome 16p13.3. Hamartin and tuberin interact physically in vivo with each other, and inactivation of either is believed to prevent the formation of a functional protein complex that regulates cell proliferation and differentiation.[1] Molecular studies for *TSC1* and *TSC2* in patients with TSC have revealed a wide spectrum of mutations. *TSC2* mutations are more common than *TSC1* mutations in both familial and sporadic cases.[18] Although mutations of these two genes make up the vast majority of cases of TSC, 15% to 20% of patients who meet the clinical criteria for TSC have no identifiable mutations. Few differences in clinical phenotype have been noted between individuals with mutations of *TSC1* and those with *TSC2*, although the former seem to have less risk of intellectual impairment, a lower frequency of seizures, fewer subependymal nodules and cortical tubers, fewer retinal hamartomas, and fewer severe facial angiofibromas.[18] The latter may have a higher risk of renal cysts.

Tuberin and hamartin could be involved in cell regulation and differentiation. Intracranial abnormalities of TSC are postulated to result from an abnormal expression of genes within the cells of the germinal matrices. These stem cells cannot differentiate or migrate properly. The consequence is the presence of dysplastic lesions with dysplastic cells and disorganized tissue distributed from the subependymal region through the radial pathway in the white matter to the cerebral cortex.[17]

The tumor suppression gene mechanism in TSC is mostly consistent with classic Knudson's two-hit tumor suppressor model. Inactivation of both alleles of either *TSC1* or *TSC2* is responsible for the development of tumoral lesions in TSC. Loss of heterozygosity in *TSC1* or *TSC2* has been consistently observed in the majority of TSC-associated angiomyolipomas, cardiac rhabdomyomas, subependymal giant cell tumors, and lymphangiomyomatosis cells but has only rarely been found in cerebral cortical tubers. This fact may indicate either that inactivation of both alleles is not required for tuber pathogenesis or that only a subgroup of cells within a tuber is affected by the second hit.

Pathology

Brain lesions in TSC include cortical tubers and subependymal nodules, radial white matter abnormalities, and subependymal giant cell astrocytomas.

Cortical tubers may be large and flat or round and dimpled. They usually expand the affected gyri with a blurred gray matter/white matter junction. Adjacent subcortical white matter is consistently involved at the various degrees also. Cortical tubers may calcify, but calcification occurs less frequently in cortical tubers than in subependymal nodules. Cortical tubers develop most commonly in the supratentorial region, although 8% to 15% of TSC patients have cerebellar tubers.

Subependymal nodules are small, rounded or oval, and asymmetrically distributed lesions of the ventricular walls that protrude into the lateral ventricles, typically near the caudate nucleus along the striothalamic groove posterior to the foramen of Monro. Subependymal nodules located around the foramen of Monro differ biologically from the more posterior ones: they may enlarge and evolve into subependymal giant cell astrocytomas.

Typical white matter abnormalities in TSC are straight or curvilinear bands extending radially from the lateral ventricle to cortex across the cerebral mantle. These linear abnormalities may represent foci of hypomyelination and heterotopia along the pathway of neuronal migration and are pathologically identical to focal transmantle dysplasia.[5]

Every patient does not necessarily present with brain lesions, but all brain lesions are histologically characterized by so-called giant astrocytes or balloon cells, which are large abnormal cells that combine both neuronal and astrocytic features. Balloon cells are thought to have failed to differentiate at a very early embryonal stage and may represent markers of malformations due to abnormal stem cell differentiation.[17]

In cortical tubers there is disrupted cortical lamination with loss of demarcation between gray and white matter. This consists of bizarre giant cells, dense fibrillary gliosis, and diminished, disorganized myelin sheaths.[4] Adjacent subcortical white matter shows deficient myelination and gliosis.[5]

Subependymal nodules consist of swollen glial cells and giant or multinucleated cells with a covering layer of ependyma. They show calcification that begins after the first year of life and progresses with age.

Subependymal giant cell astrocytoma is a benign neoplasm, histologically characterized by typical cellular elements showing a combination of astrocytic and neuronal features.[5]

White matter abnormalities in patients with TSC are clusters of heterotopic cells containing bizarre cells, including giant neurons and balloon cells with areas of hypomyelination.[5]

Imaging

Subependymal Nodules

Ultrasonography

Transfontanelle ultrasonography may detect neonatal subependymal nodules as echogenic masses.[5]

CT and MRI

The appearance of subependymal nodules varies according to the patient's age (Figs. 39-10 and 39-11). They are rarely calcified in the first years of life but tend to be relatively dense compared with the low density of the surrounding white matter (see Fig. 39-10G). The number of calcified nodules increases with age, appearing on CT as hyperdense nodules that protrude into the ventricles (Fig. 39-12A); this is a very characteristic finding for TSC. On MRI, their appearance varies according to the amount of calcification and the stage of myelination of the surrounding white matter.[4] In neonates and very young infants, they are high signal on T1W and low signal on T2W images (see Fig. 39-10C-F).[19] As myelination progresses, they gradually become isointense to the surrounding white matter (Fig. 39-10H, I). In children, noncalcified subependymal nodules are easily detected on T1W images, contrasting to hypointensity of cerebrospinal fluid. On T2W images, they may be obscured by the hyperintense cerebrospinal fluid. Larger nodules show variably low signal intensity on T2W images depending on the extent of calcification.[17] Contrast enhancement is variable and has no clinical significance.[4]

Giant Cell Tumors (Subependymal Giant Cell Astrocytomas)

MRI

The diagnosis of a giant cell tumor is based on identification of a subependymal mass at the level of the foramen of Monro in a patient with known TSC (see Fig. 39-11). The mass is solid or

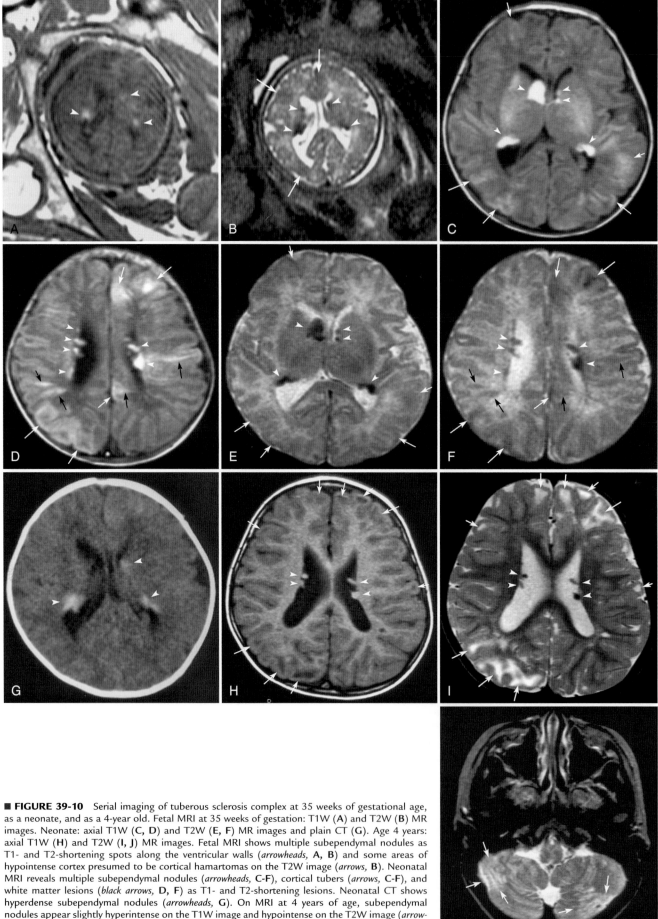

■ **FIGURE 39-10** Serial imaging of tuberous sclerosis complex at 35 weeks of gestational age, as a neonate, and as a 4-year old. Fetal MRI at 35 weeks of gestation: T1W (**A**) and T2W (**B**) MR images. Neonate: axial T1W (**C, D**) and T2W (**E, F**) MR images and plain CT (**G**). Age 4 years: axial T1W (**H**) and T2W (**I, J**) MR images. Fetal MRI shows multiple subependymal nodules as T1- and T2-shortening spots along the ventricular walls (*arrowheads, A, B*) and some areas of hypointense cortex presumed to be cortical hamartomas on the T2W image (*arrows, B*). Neonatal MRI reveals multiple subependymal nodules (*arrowheads, C-F*), cortical tubers (*arrows, C-F*), and white matter lesions (*black arrows, D, F*) as T1- and T2-shortening lesions. Neonatal CT shows hyperdense subependymal nodules (*arrowheads, G*). On MRI at 4 years of age, subependymal nodules appear slightly hyperintense on the T1W image and hypointense on the T2W image (*arrowheads, H, I*), whereas cortical hamartomas reveal subcortical T1 and T2 prolongation with broad gyri (*arrows, H, I*). Cerebellar cortical hamartomas are also noted (*arrows, J*).

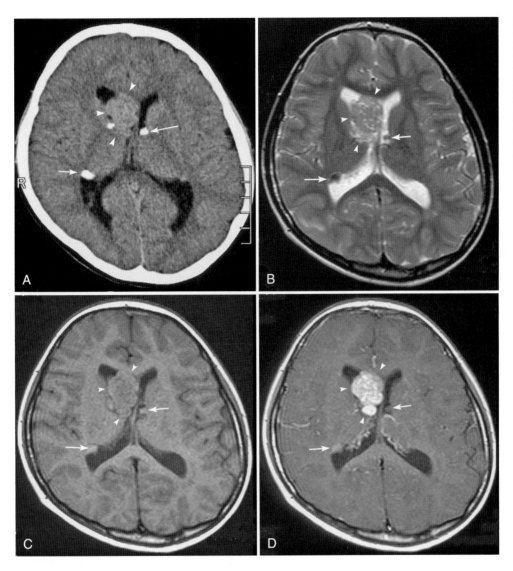

■ **FIGURE 39-11** Giant cell astrocytoma in tuberous sclerosis complex. Plain CT (**A**) and axial T2W (**B**), T1W (**C**), and gadolinium-enhanced T1W (**D**) MR images. A well-enhanced lobular tumor is noted near the right foramen of Monro (*arrowheads*, **A-D**). The tumor shows isodensity to slight hyperdensity to the gray matter on CT (**A**) and isointensity to the gray matter on MR images (**B, C**). Multiple subependymal nodules are seen (*arrows*, **A-D**).

occasionally cystic and shows a well-defined margin and a rich vascular supply. Calcifications are common; there is typically no surrounding edema. A size criterion has been proposed: subependymal lesions greater than 12 mm diameter should be classified as giant cell tumors[17]; yet increase in size of the tumor seems to be more reliable. On CT, a giant cell tumor appears as an isodense or slightly hyperdense nodule with calcification (see Fig. 39-11A). On MRI, it shows isointensity to hypointensity relative to those of the gray matter on T1W images and isointensity on T2W images (see Fig. 39-11B, C). Marked and homogeneous enhancement is usually seen on both CT and MRI (see Fig. 39-11D).

Cortical Tubers (Cortical Hamartomas)
Ultrasonography
In infants, transfrontanelle ultrasonography may demonstrate cortical hamartomas as hyperechoic lesions.[4]

CT
In neonates, on CT, cortical tubers are hypodense and are difficult to differentiate from surrounding unmyelinated brain. They may appear as lucencies within broadened cortical gyri. The lucencies diminish with age, so noncalcified tubers become difficult to identify in older children and adults. Calcification of the tubers is a common feature (Fig. 39-12A, E), and the number of calcified tubers increases with age.[4]

MRI
The MRI appearance of cortical tubers also depends on age (see Figs. 39-10 and 39-12). In neonates and very young infants they appear as hyperintense gyri compared with the surrounding parenchyma on T1W images and are hypointense on T2W images (see Fig. 39-10C-F). About 20% of affected gyri show enlargement.[17] The T1 and/or T2 shortening may extend through the cerebral mantle to the ventricles from the cortical tuber (white matter abnormalities) (see Fig. 39-10D, F).[4,19] There have been several hypotheses to explain the signal characteristics in affected neonates and younger infants, such as the contrast between a solid lesion and the relatively high water content in the immature brain. The signal characteristics change as myelination progresses. In older infants, tubers have a hypointense center on T1W images and a hyperintense center on T2W and FLAIR images (see Figs. 39-10H, I and 39-12F, G). The tubers show subcortical location, clearly contrasted to overlying cortex, and have poorly defined inner margins in all image sequences (see Fig. 39-10H, I and 39-12F, G). The tubers may show a similar intensity to that of the white matter on T1W images, but they usually remain hyperintense on T2W and FLAIR images in the mature brain (see Fig. 39-12F, G). FLAIR imaging is useful for clear demonstration of parenchymal (both cortical tuber and white matter abnormality) lesions in myelinated brain with TSC (see Fig. 39-12C, G).[4] Cortical tubers typically show no contrast enhancement unless degenerated and/or calcified.

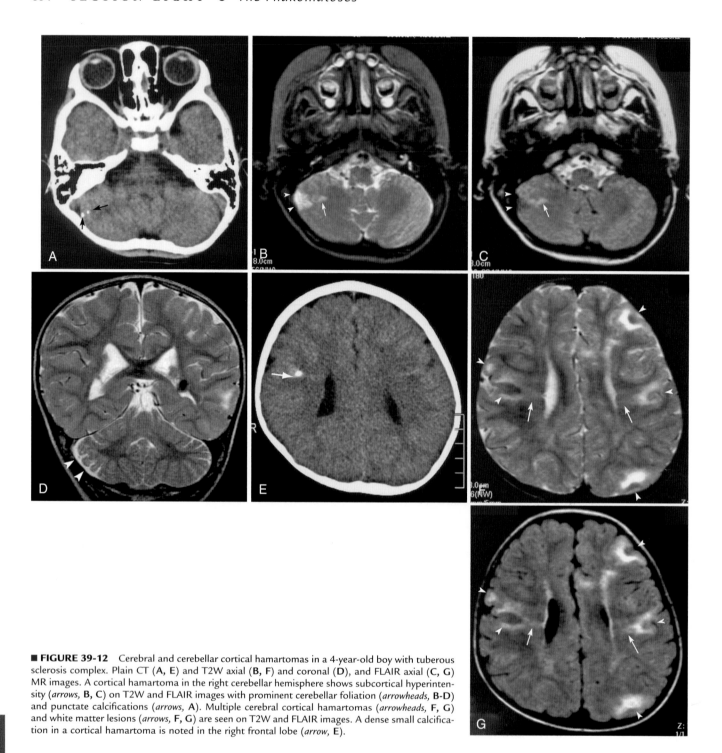

■ FIGURE 39-12 Cerebral and cerebellar cortical hamartomas in a 4-year-old boy with tuberous sclerosis complex. Plain CT (**A, E**) and T2W axial (**B, F**) and coronal (**D**), and FLAIR axial (**C, G**) MR images. A cortical hamartoma in the right cerebellar hemisphere shows subcortical hyperintensity (*arrows,* **B, C**) on T2W and FLAIR images with prominent cerebellar foliation (*arrowheads,* **B-D**) and punctate calcifications (*arrows,* **A**). Multiple cerebral cortical hamartomas (*arrowheads,* **F, G**) and white matter lesions (*arrows,* **F, G**) are seen on T2W and FLAIR images. A dense small calcification in a cortical hamartoma is noted in the right frontal lobe (*arrow,* **E**).

Cortical tubers are also found in the cerebellum, although less commonly than in the cerebrum. They may also calcify, and they are commonly associated with gliosis and focal cerebellar atrophy.[20]

TSC may also present as hemimegalencephaly that is either hemispheric or lobar/focal. Other findings such as contralateral tubers or subependymal nodules allow the diagnosis.[21] The histology of the cortical dysplastic lesion is still typical for TSC, with the characteristic giant astrocytes. Often, the lesion is diffusely calcified, so identification of an isolated diffusely calcified hemimegalencephaly requires, further investigation for possible TSC.

White Matter Abnormalities
CT and MRI
White matter abnormalities in TSC show the same signal characteristics as those of cortical tubers because both have similar histopathologic features. They appear hyperintense on T1W images and hypointense on T2W images in neonates and young infants (see Fig. 39-10D, F) and isointense to hypointense on T1W images and hyperintense on T2W, FLAIR, and proton density–weighted images in older children and adults (Fig. 39-10H, I and 39-12F, G). On CT, subtle hypodensity may rarely be recognizable unless the lesions calcify.

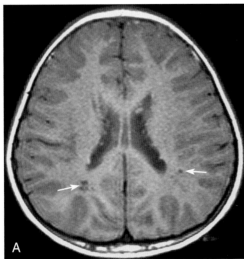

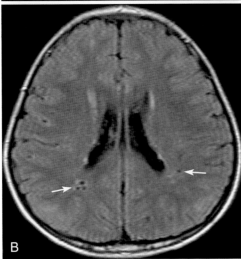

■ **FIGURE 39-13** Tuberous sclerosis complex: cystic white matter lesions. Axial T1W (**A**) and FLAIR (**B**) MR images. Small cystic lesions (*arrows*, **A, B**) are seen in the white matter. Multiple small subependymal nodules are also evident.

Other Lesions
MRI
On MRI, cystic lesions in the white matter are occasionally found (Fig. 39-13). Vascular abnormalities such as moyamoya-like vascular occlusion and cerebral aneurysm have been rarely reported.

Prenatal Imaging
Ultrasonography
High-resolution ultrasound examination of fetuses is used to search for cardiac tumors, particularly in affected families in which a disease-causing mutation has not been identified but the sensitivity is unknown. Cardiac tumors are generally not detected until the third trimester, but they may be seen as early as 20 weeks of gestation. Although 87% of fetuses with cardiac rhabdomyomas had TSC, only about half of the TSC patients have cardiac rhabdomyomas.

MRI
Fetal MRI may be of use in the evaluation for fetuses at 50% risk for TSC or when fetal ultrasonography shows a characteristic lesion such as a cardiac rhabdomyoma. It may demonstrate both cortical tubers and subependymal nodules with signal characteristics similar to those of neonates on postnatal MRI (T1, T2

shortening) (see Fig. 39-10A, B). The brain lesions are reported to be detected as early as 21 weeks of gestational age.

VON HIPPEL-LINDAU DISEASE
Von Hippel-Lindau (VHL) disease is characterized by retinal angiomas (hemangioblastomas); hemangioblastoma in the cerebellum, brain stem, and spinal cord; renal cysts and clear cell carcinoma of the kidney; pheochromocytoma; and endolymphatic sac tumor. Alternate names include CNS angiomatosis, familial cerebelloretinal angiomatosis, cerebelloretinal hemangioblastomatosis, Hippel disease, Hippel-Lindau disease, Lindau disease, and reticulocerebellar angiomatosis.

Epidemiology
The incidence of VHL disease is reported to be about 1 in 36,000 births per year with an estimated de novo mutation rate of 4.4 $\times 10^{-6}$ gametes per one generation.[22]

Clinical Presentation
Conventional clinical criteria for VHL disease are as follows[23]:

- A typical VHL tumor (hemangioblastoma, pheochromocytoma, or renal cell carcinoma and a positive family history.
- In isolated cases without a family history, two tumors (e.g., two hemangioblastomas or a hemangioblastoma and a visceral tumor)

The diagnostic criterion for isolated cases tends to delay diagnosis in many patients. Therefore, a diagnosis of VHL disease should be considered in all cases with retinal and CNS hemangioblastomas as well as in patients with familial, multicentric, or young-onset pheochromocytoma and renal cell carcinoma. A molecular genetic analysis allows early diagnosis of VHL disease in patients whose manifestations do not fulfill the conventional clinical diagnostic criteria.

Age at symptomatic presentation is usually between 18 and 30 years. Symptomatic disease in the pediatric age group is unusual. However, there is a considerable intrafamilial and interfamilial variability in disease presentation.[24]

CNS hemangioblastomas are the characteristic lesions of VHL disease. Their distribution was reported to be 63% in the cerebellum with a preference for the hemispheres, 5% in the brain stem, and 32% in the spinal canal. Cerebellar tumors may cause cerebellar signs such as ataxia and nystagmus and signs of high intracranial pressure due to occlusive hydrocephalus. Although spinal cord tumors can cause pain, sensory problems, and paresis, many affected patients remain asymptomatic.

Retinal angiomas (hemangioblastomas) are found in about 70% of patients with VHL disease. They may cause exudation and hemorrhage, leading to retinal detachment.

Another intracranial lesion is endolymphatic sac tumor. The tumor is seen in about 10% of affected individuals. They are usually asymptomatic but may cause deafness (often severe and of sudden onset).

Renal lesions include multiple renal cysts and renal cell carcinoma, especially clear cell carcinoma. Pheochromocytoma may present as hypertension or may be asymptomatic. Most pancreatic lesions are simple cysts. They are usually multiple and asymptomatic. Epididymal cysts or papillary cystadenomas are relatively common in males with VHL disease.

Pathophysiology
VHL disease is an autosomal dominant disorder with age-dependent penetrance and variable expression.[22] Almost all individuals with a VHL gene mutation express disease-related symptoms by age 65 years. VHL disease is caused by germline mutations in the *VHL* tumor suppressor gene mapped on chromosome 3p25-p26. It is widely believed that biallelic inactivation of the *VHL* tumor

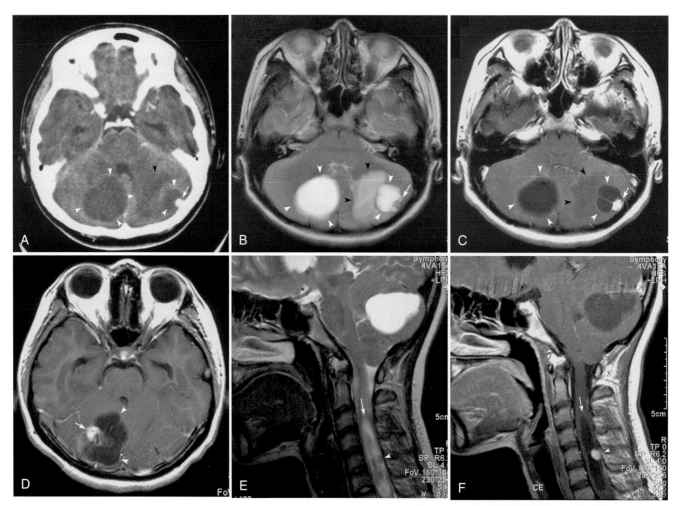

■ FIGURE 39-14 Von Hippel-Lindau disease. Multiple hemangioblastomas in the cerebellum and cervical spinal cord. Plain CT (**A**) and axial T2W (**B**) and gadolinium-enhanced T1W (**C, D**) images of the cerebellum and sagittal T2W (**E**) and gadolinium-enhanced T1W (**F**) MR images of the cervical spine. Multiple cystic lesions (*arrowheads, **A-D***) with well-defined enhanced nodules (*arrows, **A-D***) are noted in both cerebellar hemispheres. The lesion in the left hemisphere has surrounding edema (*black arrowheads, **A, B, C***). A longitudinal intramedullary cystic lesion (*arrows, **E, F***) with an enhanced mural nodule (*arrowheads, **E, F***) is also seen in the cervical spinal cord. The enhanced nodules are located on the surface of the cerebellum or spinal cord.

suppressor gene is an important step in the pathogenesis of tumors in VHL disease.

Complex genotype-phenotype associations are described, mainly based on the susceptibility of pheochromocytoma. Large deletions and truncating mutations typically predispose affected individuals to hemangioblastomas and renal cell carcinoma with low risk of pheochromocytoma (VHL type 1). Certain missense mutations develop VHL type 2, which is characterized by a high risk for pheochromocytoma and an ordinary risk for hemangioblastoma. VHL type 2 is further divided into three subgroups: type 2A is characterized by a low risk of renal cell carcinoma; type 2B has a high risk of renal cell carcinoma; and type 2C carries a risk for pheochromocytoma only.[23]

Pathology

Cerebellar hemangioblastoma is a hypervascular tumor of the pia mater. It may be solid or form a nodule on the superficial surface of a large cyst filled with secreted fluid. The nodule is not encapsulated and may infiltrate surrounding tissues, leading to hemorrhages.[5]

Spinal hemangioblastomas may occur anywhere in the spinal cord, with a preferential location in the conus medullaris and craniocervical junction. They are usually intramedullary but may be partially intramedullary and extramedullary, or rarely

extramedullary.[5] They are accompanied by syringomyelia in most cases.

Hemangioblastomas are benign (WHO grade I) and highly vasculized tumors. In hemangioblastomas, the stroma cells are neoplastic and the capillaries are assumed to grow secondarily into the tumors.

Imaging
MRI

Hemangioblastomas are best diagnosed with MRI. Postcontrast T1W imaging typically shows a brightly enhancing solid tumor or a nodular mass in the wall of a large cyst that is clearly demarcated from the surrounding tissue of the brain or spinal cord (Figs. 39-14 and 39-15). The cyst may show a variable intensity depending on protein or hemorrhagic content. The cyst wall does not enhance. If a nodule is large enough, CT may demonstrate the enhancing mass (Fig. 39-14A). The solid nodule usually shows T1 and T2 prolongation (see Fig. 39-14B, E). The nodules are located next to the cerebellar or spinal cord surface, and this finding is useful to differentiate hemangioblastoma from cerebellar pilocytic astrocytomas (see Figs. 39-14 and 39-15). Purely solid hemangioblastoma is not common. Large feeding and draining vessels in and near the tumor may be demonstrated by MRI and MR angiography.

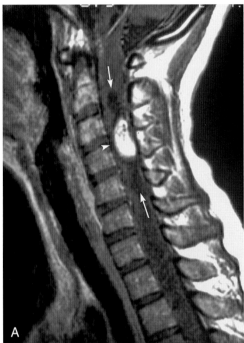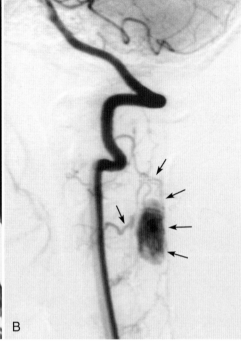

■ FIGURE 39-15 Hemangioblastoma in the cervical spinal cord in von Hippel-Lindau disease. Gadolinium-enhanced T1W sagittal MR (**A**) image and digital subtraction angiogram of vertebral artery (**B**). A well-defined enhanced nodule (*arrowhead,* **A**) is noted within the longitudinal cystic lesion (*arrows,* **A**) in the cervical cord. Angiography shows classic feature of a "cherry attached to its stalk" (*arrows,* **B**).

Spinal hemangioblastomas are often accompanied by syringomyelia. Without contrast enhancement, it is difficult to differentiate idiopathic syringomyelia from that caused by a hemangioblastoma. Although differentiation among syringomyelia, tumor cyst, and cord edema may be difficult, the degree of T2 prolongation may be helpful to differentiate cysts from edema; the cysts tend to show higher signal intensity with sharp margins (see Fig. 39-14E, F), whereas edema is less hyperintense with ill-defined margins.[4] Another typical MRI finding in hemangioblastomas is the presence of enlarged vessels, shown as serpiginous flow voids within and adjacent to the tumor.[4]

Endolymphatic sac tumors or papillary cystadenomas of the endolymphatic sac show bone destruction with scattered calcifications at the level of the vestibular aqueduct on CT. On MRI, they show heterogeneous intensity that is mainly isointense relative to the brain with areas of high intensity on T1W images and predominantly hyperintense with areas of low intensity on T2W images. Contrast enhancement is homogeneous or heterogeneous. A large tumor may show vascular flow voids.[4]

Special Procedures
The angiographic appearance of hemangioblastoma is characteristic, displaying tangles of tightly packed, wide vessels that are opacified in the early arterial phase. This finding may be called "cherry attached to its stalk" (see Fig. 39-17B). The angiographic finding is a very diagnostic feature of hemangioblastomas and is useful in differentiation from pilocytic astrocytomas.

ATAXIA-TELANGIECTASIA
Ataxia-telangiectasia is an autosomal recessive disorder characterized by progressive cerebellar ataxia, telangiectasia, immune defects, and a predisposition to malignancy. Other names include Louis-Bar syndrome, Border-Sedgwick syndrome, and cephalo-oculocutaneous telangiectasia.

Epidemiology
Ataxia-telangiectasia is a rare disorder, with an incidence of 1 in 40,000 to 100,000 individuals.[25] One to 3 percent of the general population may be carriers (heterozygotes).

Clinical Presentation
Cerebellar ataxia begins in early childhood. Truncal ataxia precedes appendicular ataxia. Other neurologic abnormalities include oculomotor apraxia, choreoathetosis, dystonia, hypotonia, dysarthria, and generalized muscle weakness.[25] Mental delay is usually absent. Unless telangiectasia manifests, a clinical diagnosis of ataxia-telangiectasia cannot be established with certainty; yet oculomotor apraxia points to an early diagnosis.

Oculocutaneous telangiectasia develops first, and the incidence is very high, close to 100%. Mucocutaneous telangiectasia typically develops between 3 and 5 years of age but may appear later.[26] Skin telangiectases (face, ears, neck, back of the hand, antecubital fossa, and popliteal fossa) subsequently develop. The combination of telangiectasia with cerebellar ataxia is pathognomonic for ataxia-telangiectasia.

Immune defects and thymic hypoplasia are noted. Recurrent episodes of sinopulmonary infection occur in most patients, leading to bronchiectasis and/or pulmonary arteriovenous fistulas.[26]

Malignancies develop with 100 to 1200 times higher incidence than in the general population of the same age. Lymphomas and leukemias are most common, particularly in younger patients.[26]

Death occurs frequently by the second or third decade of life as a consequence of airway infection and lymphoid tissue tumors.[25]

Pathophysiology
Ataxia-telangiectasia is an autosomal recessive disorder. The gene (*ATM,* ataxia-telangiectasia mutated) is mapped to chromosome 11q22.3. The *ATM* gene encodes a protein that plays a role in DNA repair and cell cycle checkpoint control after DNA damage; thus, ataxia-telangiectasia belongs to a group of chromosome breakage disorders and AT cells are abnormally sensitive to ionizing radiation.[26]

Pathology
Neuropathologic findings include atrophy of all cerebellar cortical layers with extensive Purkinje and granule cell loss, dentate

■ **FIGURE 39-16** Cerebellar atrophy in ataxia-telangiectasia. Sagittal T1W (**A**) and sagittal (**B, C**) and coronal (**D**) T2W MR images. Diffuse cerebellar cortical atrophy with prominent cerebellar folia is seen (*arrowheads*, **A-D**). Note the opacification of the maxillary sinus (*arrow*, **C**).

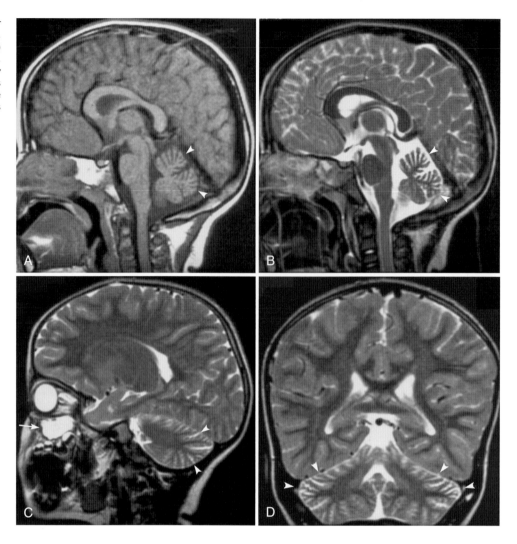

and olivary nuclei atrophy, neuronal loss of the substantia nigra and oculomotor nuclei, and spinal cord atrophy with degenerative changes in spinal motor neurons and dorsal root and sympathetic motor neurons. Telangiectatic vessels are seen in the leptomeninges.[25]

Imaging

Because of high sensitivity to irradiation in ataxia-telangiectasia, MRI is a modality of choice in the neuroimaging workup.[26]

The major neuroradiologic abnormality is cerebellar cortical atrophy, which presents with decreased size of the cerebellum, increased prominence of the cerebellar folia, and dilatation of the fourth ventricle (see Fig. 39-16).[25] Vermian atrophy is more prominent than hemisphere atrophy in the early stage. Patients with ataxia-telangiectasia show progressive panvermian cerebellar atrophy. In younger patients, the supratentorial system and brain stem tend to show no abnormality.[26,27] Older patients may show abnormal signals in the cerebral white matter, including T2 shortening suggesting multiple small hemorrhagic foci resulting from telangiectasia and high signals on T2 images possibly due to degenerative changes of the progeric type.[26,27]

Imaging findings of the paranasal sinuses vary from mucosal thickening to global sinus opacity with air-fluid levels to sclerotic bone changes. The combination of sinusitis and cerebellar atrophy in young patients raises a suspicion of ataxia-telangiectasia (see Fig. 39-16).[27]

BASAL CELL NEVUS SYNDROME

Basal cell nevus syndrome (BCNS) was first reported by Gorlin and Goltz in 1960 as a hamartomatous syndrome characterized by multiple basal cell carcinomas of the skin, odontogenic keratocysts of the mandible and maxilla, and bifid rib. It is marked by five major components: multiple nevoid cell carcinomas, jaw cysts, congenital skeletal abnormalities, ectopic calcifications, and plantar and palmar pits.[4] This syndrome is also referred to as nevoid basal cell carcinoma syndrome, Gorlin's syndrome, and Gorlin-Goltz syndrome.

Epidemiology

BCNS is very uncommon, and its prevalence is reported to be 1 in 57,000.[28] However, increased awareness of BCNS and better diagnosis have led to an increase in the prevalence up to 1 in 40,000 or even higher.

Clinical Presentation

Diagnostic criteria were proposed by Evans and associates.[29] The diagnosis rests on the presence of two major or one major plus two minor criteria:

Major criteria include:
- More than two basal cell carcinomas or one when younger than 30 years, or more than 10 basal cell nevi

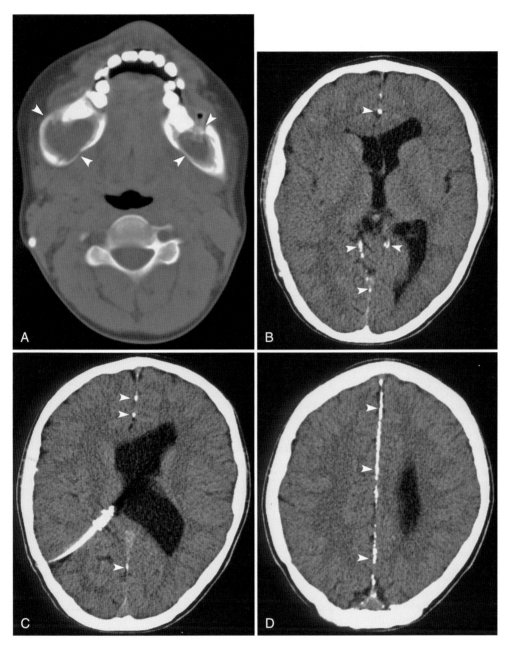

■ **FIGURE 39-17** Jaw cysts and calcifications in the dura mater of basal cell nevus syndrome. Plain CT images (**A-D**). Bone window CT of the mandible shows bilateral expanded cysts with thin cortex (*arrowheads,* **A**). Calcifications of the falx and tentorium cerebelli (*arrowheads,* **B-D**) are seen. A ventriculoperitoneal shunt tube for hydrocephalus is in place (**C**).

- Any odontogenic keratocyst (histology proven) or polyostotic bone cysts
- Three or more palmar or plantar pits
- Ectopic calcification: lamellar or early calcification of the falx (before 20 years of age)
- Family history of the syndrome

Minor criteria are:
- Rib anomalies (bifid, fused, missing) or vertebral anomalies (wedged, fused)
- Macrocrania (occipitofrontal circumference over 97th percentile) and frontal bossing
- Cardiac or ovarian fibroma
- Medulloblastoma
- Lymphomesenteric cysts
- Congenital malformations: cleft palate, polydactyly, ocular anomalies (cataract, coloboma, microphthalmia)

Also, childhood medulloblastoma with falx calcification suggests BCNS.[30]

Clinical findings in childhood are increased height, macrocephaly, macrosomia, and skeletal and dental abnormalities. Most patients (70%-90% in whites) develop basal cell carcinoma of the skin commonly during puberty. Other skin lesions include palmar and plantar pits and small keratin-filled cysts. Musculoskeletal anomalies, including malformations of the ribs and vertebral anomalies, are found in up to 75% of the patients. Other associations include renal anomalies, fibroma of the ovary and the myocardium, and mesenteric cysts.

Medulloblastoma is highly associated with BCNS, and the reported incidence ranges from 1% to 5% to 5% to 20% of patients. Conversely, 1% to 2% of all cases of medulloblastoma have BCNS. Medulloblastoma in BCNS occurs predominantly in boys and earlier than usual, during the first 2 years of life. Therefore, in patients who are diagnosed as having medulloblastoma before 5 years of age, BCNS should be carefully excluded.[4] Radiation therapy to patients with BCNS leads to subsequent appearance of neoplasms in the radiation field, most commonly basal cell nevus carcinomas.

Pathophysiology

BCNS is an autosomal dominant disorder, and its gene locus is mapped to chromosome 9q22.3. The gene is termed *patched* (*PTCH*) and is a tumor suppression gene. BCNS shows variable expressivity, complete penetrance, and no gender predilection. Thirty-five to 50 percent of patients represent new mutations.

Loss of normal copies of the gene in the tumors confirm that *PTCH* acts as a tumor suppressor gene in the cerebellum (medulloblastoma), skin (basal cell carcinoma), and tooth root (jaw cysts).

Imaging

The cardinal neuroimaging findings of BCNS include odontogenic keratocysts and calcifications of the intracranial dura (see Fig. 39-17).[27] Odontogenic keratocysts are usually multiple and present as expansile, sharply marginated cystic lesions in the maxilla and mandible (see Fig. 39-17A).[27] The intrinsic property of the cysts is a water density and water intensity on CT and MRI. The cysts seem to originate from the tooth roots. The overlying cortex is thinned. Ameloblastoma and squamous cell carcinoma may arise from the cysts.[31]

Lamellar calcification of the falx is a significant neuroimaging feature in early life and is ultimately found in 90% to 100% of adult patients (see Figs. 39-17B-D). Early dural calcification is also found in the diaphragma sellae, cerebellar tentorium, and petroclinoid ligament in 60% to 80%.[31] BCNS should be considered in any pediatric patients with such dural calcifications. Other calvarial and facial abnormalities include macrocephaly, frontal bossing, cleft palate (about 5%), and various ocular abnormalities (25%-33%).[31]

In BCNS patients, the incidence of medulloblastoma is high.[31] Imaging findings of medulloblastoma associated with BCNS are similar to those in nonsyndromic medulloblastoma. Other neoplasms of the CNS in BCNS patients include meningioma, astrocytoma, craniopharyngioma, and oligodendroglioma, all of which show radiologic appearances similar to those in individuals without BCNS.[4] Radiation-induced meningioma, schwannoma, sarcoma, and osteochondromas have been reported.

ANALYSIS

The very different clinical features and specific appearances of these diseases on imaging (CT and MRI) make any confusion very unlikely. NF1 and NF2 have been now clearly differentiated with well-defined criteria. Only exceptional instances of simultaneous occurrence in a single individual have been reported, when the patient has inherited both gene defects.[32]

A sample report is presented in Box 39-1.

BOX 39-1   Sample Report: MRI in a NF1 Patient

PATIENT HISTORY

An 8-year-old boy presented with a 5-day history of drowsiness and headaches. He had had MRI follow-up since age 22 months for clinical features of NF1 with right-sided papillary pallor on fundoscopy at age 4 years and slight right optic nerve enlargement on MRI that was stable over 4 years. No treatment was implemented. He also had severe scoliosis. Emergency CT disclosed right peri-insular cerebral hemorrhage that was evacuated. MRI was ordered to search for a cause.

TECHNIQUE

Sagittal and axial T1W, axial and coronal T2W, axial FLAIR, axial diffusion, axial T2*W, and triplanar T1W with gadolinium imaging was done.

FINDINGS

There was evidence of recent craniotomy with metallic artifacts. Postoperative/post-hemorrhagic changes were apparent in the region of the right insula and frontoparietal opercula, with high T2W/FLAIR signal and some restricted diffusion. Near-complete evacuation of the clot was demonstrated on T2*W images. T2W/FLAIR images also demonstrated characteristic features of NF1: bright signal of both hippocampi and zones of myelin vacuolization on medial inferior lentiform nuclei bilaterally, in the midbrain (left), in the dentate nuclei (bilaterally), and in the right cerebellar white matter, all unchanged from previous imaging.

Contrast T1W images demonstrate diffuse enhancement of brain tissue surrounding the insular-sylvian cistern, involving the frontoparietotemporal opercula. The enhancement is not so well demarcated and extends to the dura at the site of the previous surgery. There is a mild local mass effect. The topography is not consistent with an infarction but would rather suggest an infiltrative tumor/hematologic process. There is no abnormality to suggest a vascular malformation.

IMPRESSION

An infiltrative mass is surrounding the site of the hemorrhage. The hemorrhage and the location would be unusual for typical NF1 tumor such as a juvenile pilocytic astrocytoma. Malignant gliomas do occur in this context and should be considered, as well as a sarcoma.

COMMENT

Histology disclosed a sarcoma, treated with both radiation therapy and chemotherapy. Three years later, the tumor has recurred once. Non-neurogenic sarcomas, and other malignancies, do occur in NF1, even without the facilitating effect of previous radiation therapy.[33]

KEY POINTS: DIFFERENTIAL DIAGNOSIS

■ All diseases in this chapter have a tendency to develop particular tumors with unique histology in a specific anatomic region.

■ Radiologic examination readily enables us to delineate the highly characteristic combination of specific tumors with other associations, and thus plays a principal role in differential diagnosis.

■ Few disorders among the entities in this chapter would ever be confused, because each disease has characteristic radiologic findings in combination with unique clinical manifestations.

SUGGESTED READINGS

Baser ME, Evans DG, Gutmann DH. Neurofibromatosis 2. Curr Opin Neurol 2003; 16:27-33.

Braffman BH, Bilaniuk LT, Naidich TP, et al. MR imaging of tuberous sclerosis: Pathogenesis of this phakomatosis, use of gadopentetate dimeglumine and literature review. Radiology 1992; 183:227-238.

Choyke PL, Glenn GM, Walther MM, et al. von Hippel-Lindau disease: genetic, clinical, and imaging features. Radiology 1995; 194:629-642.

Crino PB, Nathanson KL, Henske EP. The tuberous sclerosis complex. N Engl J Med 2006; 355:1345-1356.

Glasker S. Central nervous system manifestations in VHL: genetics, pathology and clinical phenotypic features. Fam Cancer 2005; 4:37-42.

Gutmann DH, Aylsworth A, Carey JC, et al. The diagnostic evaluation and multidisciplinary management of neurofibromatosis 1 and neurofibromatosis 2. JAMA 1997; 278:51-57.

Herron J, Darrah R, Quaghebeur G: Intracranial manifestations of the neurocutaneous syndromes. Clin Radiol 2000; 55:82-98.

Inoue Y, Nemoto Y, Tashiro T, et al. Neurofibromatosis type 1 and type 2: review of the central nervous system and related structures. Brain Dev 1997; 19:1-12.

Trovo-Marqui AB, Tajara EH: Neurofibromin: a general outlook. Clin Genet 2006; 70:1-13.

REFERENCES

1. Maria BL, Menkes JH. Neurocutaneous syndromes. In Menkes JH, et al (eds). Child Neurology, 7th ed. Philadelphia, Lippincott Williams & Wilkins, 2006, pp 803-828.
2. Rasmussen SA, Friedman JM. NF1 gene and neurofibromatosis 1. Am J Epidemiol 2000; 151:33-40.
3. DeBella K, Poskitt K, Szudek J, Friedman JM. Use of "unidentified bright objects" on MRI for diagnosis of neurofibromatosis 1 in children. Neurology 2000; 54:1646-1651.
4. Barkovich AJ. The phakomatoses. In Pediatric Neuroimaging, 4th ed. Philadelphia, Lippincott Williams & Wilkins, 2005, pp 441-505.
5. Tortori-Donati P, Rossi A, Biancheri R. Phakomatosis. In Tortori-Donati P (ed). Pediatric Neuroradiology: Brain. Berlin, Springer-Verlag, 2005, pp 763-838.
6. Moore BD, Slopis JM, Schomer D, et al. Neuropsychological significance of areas of high signal intensity on brain MRIs of children with neurofibromatosis. Neurology 1996; 46:1660-1668.
7. Jancen LA, Gutman DH. NF1 and neurofibromatosis 1. In Epstein CJ, Erickson RP, Wynshaw-Boris A (eds). Inborn Errors of Development. New York, Oxford, 2004, pp 870-885.
8. DiPaolo DP, Zimmerman RA, Rorke LB, et al. Neurofibromatosis type 1: pathologic substrate of high-signal-intensity foci in the brain. Radiology 1995; 195:721-724.
9. Gonen O, Wang ZJ, Viswanathan AK, et al. Three-dimensional multivoxel proton MR spectroscopy of the brain in children with neurofibromatosis type 1. AJNR Am J Neuroradiol. 1999; 20:1333-1341.
10. Tognini G, Ferrozzi F, Garlaschi G, et al. Brain apparent diffusion coefficient evaluation in pediatric patients with neurofibromatosis type 1. J Comput Assist Tomogr 2005; 29:298-304.
11. Terada H, Barkovich AJ, Edwards MS, Ciricillo SM. Evolution of high-intensity basal ganglia lesions on T1-weighted MR in neurofibromatosis type 1. AJNR Am J Neuroradiol 1996; 17:755-760.
12. Evans DG, Moran A, King A, et al. Incidence of vestibular schwannoma and neurofibromatosis 2 in the North West of England over a 10-year period: higher incidence than previously thought. Otol Neurotol 2005; 26:93-97.
13. Baser ME, Friedman JM, Aeschliman D, et al. Predictors of the risk of mortality in neurofibromatosis 2. Am J Hum Genet 2002; 71:715-723.
14. Evans DG, Huson SM, Donnai D, et al. A clinical study of type 2 neurofibromatosis. Q J Med 1992; 84:603-618.
15. Osborne JP, Fryer A, Webb D: Epidemiology of tuberous sclerosis. Ann N Y Acad Sci 1991; 615:125-127.
16. Roach ES, Sparagana SP: Diagnosis of tuberous sclerosis complex. J Child Neurol 2004; 19:643-649.
17. Braffmann BH, Bilaniuk LT, Naidich TP, et al. MR imaging of tuberous sclerosis: pathogenesis of this phakomatosis, use of gadopentetate dimeglumine, and literature review. Radiology 1992; 183:227-238.
18. Dabora SL, Jozwiak S, Neal Franz D, et al. Mutational analysis in a cohort of 224 tuberous sclerosis patients indicates increased severity of TSC2, compared with TSC1, disease in multiple organs. Am J Hum Genet 2001; 68:64-80.
19. Baron Y, Barkovich AJ. MR imaging of tuberous sclerosis in neonates and young infants. Am J Neuroradiol 1999; 20:907-916.
20. Marti-Bonmati L, Menor F, Dosdá R. Tuberous sclerosis: differences between cerebral and cerebellar cortical tubers in the pediatric population. AJNR Am J Neuroradiol 2000; 21:557-560.
21. Griffiths PD, Gardner SA, Smith M, et al. Hemimegalencephaly and focal megalencephaly in tuberous sclerosis complex. AJNR Am J Neuroradiol 1998; 19:1935-1938.
22. Maher ER, Iselius L, Yates JR, et al. Von Hippel-Lindau disease: a genetic study. J Med Genet 1991; 28:443-447.
23. Maher ER. VHL and von Hippel-Lindau disease. In Epstein CJ, Erickson RP, Wynshaw-Boris A (eds). Inborn Errors of Development. New York, Oxford, 2004, pp 823-827.
24. Catapano D, Muscarella LA, Guarnieri V, et al. Hemangioblastomas of central nervous system: molecular genetic analysis and clinical management. Neurosurgery 2005; 56:1215-1221.
25. Kuljis RO, Xu Y, Aguila MC, Baltimore D. Degeneration of neurons, synapses, and neuropil and glial activation in a murine Atm knockout model of ataxia-telangiectasia. Proc Natl Acad Sci U S A 1997; 94:12687-12693.
26. Sardanelli F, Parodi RC, Ottenelo C, et al. Cranial MRI in ataxia-telangiectasia. Neuroradiology 1995; 37:77-82.
27. Edelstein S, Naidich TP, Newton TH. The rare phakomatosis. In Tortori-Donati P (ed). Pediatric Neuroradiology: Brain. Berlin, Springer-Verlag, 2005, pp 819-854.
28. Evans DG, Farndon PA, Burnell LD, et al. The incidence of Gorlin syndrome in 173 consecutive cases of medulloblastoma. Br J Cancer 1991; 64:959-961.
29. Evans DG,. Ladusans EJ, Rimmer S, et al. Complications of the naevoid basal cell carcinoma syndrome: results of a population based study. J Med Genet 1993; 30:460-464.
30. Stavrou T, Dubovsky EC, Reaman GH, et al. Intracranial calcifications in childhood medulloblastoma: relation to nevoid basal cell carcinoma syndrome. AJNR Am J Neuroradiol 2000; 21:790-794.
31. Gorlin RJ. Nevoid cell carcinoma syndrome. Dermatol Clin 1995; 13:113-125.
32. Wheeler PG, Sadeghi-Nejad A. Simultaneous occurrence of neurofibromatosis type 1 and tuberous sclerosis in a young girl. Am J Med Genet 2005; 133A:78-81.
33. Zöller MET, Rembeck B, Odén A, et al. Malignant and benign tumors in patients with neurofibromatosis type 1 in a defined Swedish population. Cancer 1997, 79:2125-2131.

Infection and Inflammation

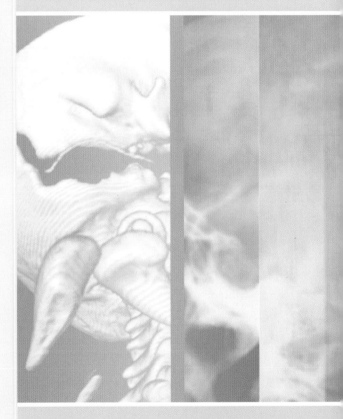

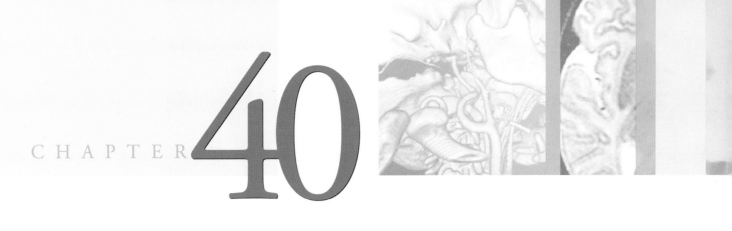

CHAPTER 40

Meningitis and Ventriculitis

Majda M. Thurnher

BACTERIAL MENINGITIS

Bacterial meningitis is an infectious inflammatory infiltration of the leptomeninges caused by bacteria. It can also be referred to as pyogenic meningitis and leptomeningitis.

Epidemiology

In the United States, bacterial meningitis is predominantly a disease of adults.[1-3] The most common (50%) cause of adult meningitis is *Streptococcus pneumoniae*. Other common causative organisms include *Neisseria meningitidis* and *Haemophilus influenzae*. Gram-negative bacillary meningitis shows an increased incidence in patients who have undergone neurosurgical procedures.[3] Successful vaccination against *H. influenzae* type B has markedly reduced the incidence of this infection in infants and children, leaving group B streptococci as the most common cause of bacterial meningitis and sepsis in the neonate. Group B streptococci are also an infrequent cause of meningitis in adults, especially in patients with diabetes mellitus, liver disease, prior stroke, breast cancer, and human immunodeficiency virus (HIV) infection.[2] *Citrobacter* is a distinct group of gram-negative bacilli that belong to the Enterobacteriaceae family. Citrobacter meningitis is frequent in neonates and young children but highly unusual in adults.

Clinical Presentation

The classic clinical features of meningitis include headache, neck stiffness, pyrexia, vomiting, and photophobia, followed by mental status changes. The definitive diagnosis is made by culture from blood or cerebrospinal fluid (CSF).

Pathophysiology

Bacteria may reach the meninges hematogenously, by direct spread from the sinuses or ears, or by direct inoculation after penetrating head trauma. Infection of the leptomeninges may then cause communicating or obstructive hydrocephalus, subdural effusions, arterial and venous infarctions, cerebritis, and ventriculitis. Arterial and/or venous infarctions result from the spread of the infection to small arteries and veins, with secondary spasm and thrombosis. Subdural effusions develop secondary to infection of the subarachnoid space.

Pathology

Pathologically, the meninges are congested. Purulent exudate is seen in the subarachnoid space and may fill the basal cisterns with pus. The brain becomes swollen. Meningitis starts when bacteria in the venous sinuses cause inflammation that impairs normal CSF drainage and may lead to hydrocephalus. In the early stages of infection, the pia and arachnoid mater become congested and hyperemic. Later, the leptomeninges become thickened and an inflammatory exudate can cover the brain, particularly in dependent regions such as the basal cisterns.

Congestion and hyperemia of the leptomeninges with exudates in the subarachnoid space are typical pathologic findings in meningitis.[4]

Imaging

CT

When meningitis is suspected clinically, CT is usually obtained before lumbar puncture to exclude a mass lesion or other signs of elevated intracranial pressure. Noncontrast CT is often normal in early cases of uncomplicated meningitis.[5] Later, the meninges may show contrast enhancement, suggesting inflammation. However, meningeal enhancement alone is not specific for meningitis (Fig. 40-1).

MRI

Fluid-attenuated inversion recovery (FLAIR) MR sequences appear to be the most sensitive technique for detecting meningeal diseases (Fig. 40-2). High signal in the subarachnoid space reflects high protein concentration in the CSF.[5-7] Contrast-enhanced T1-weighted (T1W) images typically show leptomeningeal enhancement (Fig. 40-3).

Neuroimaging detects the complications of meningitis, which include hydrocephalus, ventriculitis, empyema, venous sinus thrombosis, and infarctions.

Communicating hydrocephalus is a common complication, because the inflammatory debris may impede the flow and reabsorption of CSF.[8] The ventricles become distended. Transependymal "migration" of CSF appears as high signal intensity areas surrounding the portions of the ventricles that abut white matter. Pyogenic ventriculitis manifests as periventricular high signal on

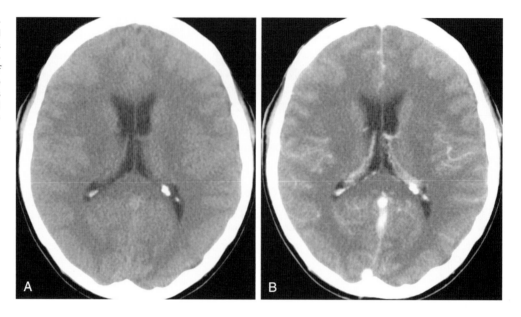

■ **FIGURE 40-1** Bacterial meningitis. A 35-year-old man presented with headache and neurologic signs of meningeal disease. **A,** Axial noncontrast scan shows obliteration of the sulci over the hemispheres. No enlargement of the ventricles was observed. **B,** Subtle meningeal enhancement was noted on contrast-enhanced CT scan.

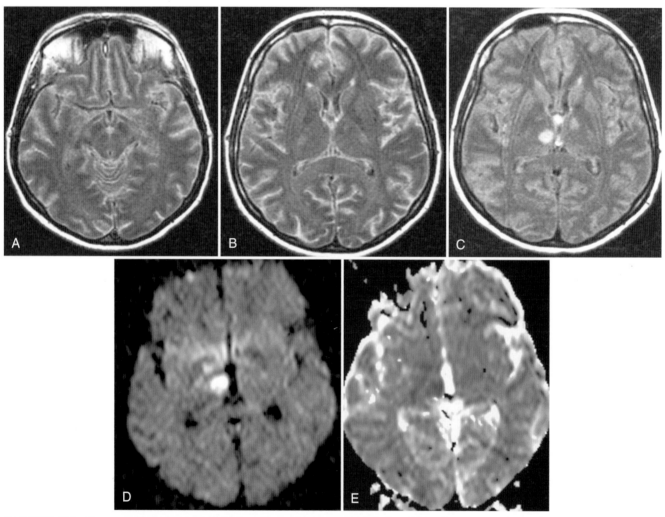

■ **FIGURE 40-2** *Streptococcus pneumoniae* meningitis in a 40-year-old woman. **A** to **C,** On axial FLAIR MR image (TR/TE/TI 10,000/130/2,100), high signal intensity is shown in the subarachnoid spaces, indicating a meningeal process. In addition, rounded hyperintensities were seen in both thalami (**C**). The trace DWI (**D**) and the ADC map (**E**) showed high signal with low ADC values, consistent with arterial infarctions and cytotoxic edema.

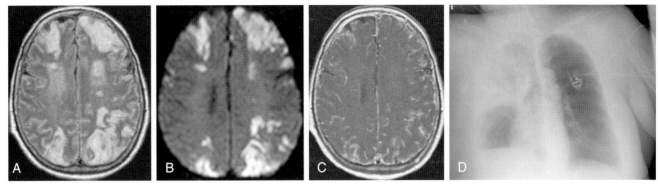

■ **FIGURE 40-3** Pneumococcal meningoencephalitis in a 50-year-old patient with pneumonia, fever, and seizures. **A,** Axial FLAIR-TSE MR image (TR/TE/TI 7385/130/2100) shows bilateral, symmetric, high signal intensity in the cortex and underlying white matter. **B,** Trace DWI shows high signal with low ADC values (not shown), indicating restricted diffusion. **C,** T1W contrast-enhanced MR image (TR/TE/flip° 20/2.1/35°) with magnetization transfer shows marked meningeal enhancement. **D,** Typical pattern of a lobar pneumonia was detected on chest radiography.

FLAIR MRI, ependymal enhancement, ventricular debris, and fluid-fluid levels within the ventricles.[9] Subdural effusions are typically sterile in meningitis; only 2% will form subdural empyemas. Venous thrombosis appears as high signal intensity within the venous sinuses on spin-echo sequences and absence of high signal within the sinuses on gradient-echo sequences. Such thromboses can lead to venous infarctions that do not conform to well-defined arterial territories and often manifest concurrent hemorrhage. Venous infarctions typically show high signal on T2-weighted (T2W) and FLAIR images as well as high signal on diffusion-weighted imaging (DWI) with low apparent diffusion coefficient (ADC). They are usually located cortically/subcortically close to the vertex and the thrombosed superior sagittal sinus. Occlusions or stenosis of the arteries may be detected on magnetic resonance angiography (MRA). Arterial infarctions have typical MR features and follow the expected arterial distributions (see Fig. 40-2).

EMPYEMA

Empyema is a collection of purulent material confined within the epidural or subdural space and can also be known as subdural empyema, epidural empyema, epidural abscess, or sinogenic intracranial empyema.

Epidemiology

Purulent subdural effusions occur most frequently in the second decade of life with a male-to-female ratio of 3:1.[10] The most common pathogens are *Streptococcus milleri,* other streptococci, enterococci, and gram-negative bacilli. Most subdural empyemas develop as complications of sinusitis, then otitis media. In one study, 6% of patients with otitis media had a subdural or epidural empyema.[11] Infratentorial empyema is an uncommon form of intracranial suppuration and is usually secondary to a neglected otogenic infection.[12] Only 41 cases of infratentorial empyema were described in the literature from 1966 through 2006.[12]

Clinical Presentation

Subdural empyema presents clinically as seizures, focal deficits, and progressive neurologic deterioration. Fever, vomiting, and meningismus may suggest meningitis. The clinical course is usually fulminant, with rapid development of coma. If the empyema is located in the frontal lobe, the only clinical signs may be subtle changes in personality or mood without focal neurologic symptoms. The clinical presentation of infratentorial empyema includes meningismus, altered level of consciousness, signs of raised intracranial pressure, draining ear, and pyrexia.[12]

Compared with subdural empyema, epidural empyema presents in a more subtle fashion, usually with several days of fever along with mental status changes and neck pain.[13]

Pathophysiology

Epidural empyemas tend to remain localized within the extradural space. Subdural empyemas commonly spread diffusely over the convexities and throughout the subdural space, because no anatomic constraints limit their spread.[10] Subdural empyema usually occurs in association with otorhinologic infection as a result of direct spread of infection or retrograde thrombophlebitis via bridging emissary veins. Because the bridging veins are valveless, thrombophlebitis can easily pass retrograde into the cavernous sinus and other dural venous sinuses. In the acute phase, a thin unencapsulated layer of pus covers the cerebral hemisphere. Retrograde thrombophlebitis produces early involvement of the cortex.

Pathology

Both epidural empyema and subdural empyema may be unilateral or bilateral. Epidural empyema has no barrier to bilateral spread and may cross the midline external to the dural venous sinuses. Subdural empyema may spread to both sides from a common source like the frontal sinuses or cross the midline under the falx.

Imaging

Ultrasonography

Ultrasonography can be used only in small infants when the fontanelles are still open.

CT

Subdural Empyema

In the acute phase of infection, subdural pus is not easy to identify on noncontrast CT. The detectability is increased with administration of a contrast agent. In this stage, the surface of the brain is bathed with a thin layer of anaerobic pus. Venous thrombosis can occur very quickly and lead to brain infarction and abscess.

Subdural empyema appears as a low-density subdural lesion on noncontrast CT and shows thick-walled marginal dural enhancement on contrast-enhanced CT.[14] CT shows displacement of the cortical surface, deflection of the gray matter/white matter interface (buckled white matter sign), deflection of the surface veins, and, perhaps, air bubbles within the collection. If sinusitis is present, the sinuses may appear opacified, with air-fluid levels and, perhaps, bony erosion. Venous stasis and thrombosis may produce hyperemia, which manifests as cortical swelling and minimal hyperdensity on noncontrast CT and as diffuse gyral enhancement on contrast-enhanced CT.

Postoperative empyema often demonstrates a thick-walled, well-defined lentiform collection with rim enhancement of the lesions indicating chronicity. In those cases, venous involvement will not be present, so cortical abnormalities will not be apparent.

Epidural Empyema

Epidural empyema can be recognized on noncontrast CT scans as a lens-shaped lesion of low density adjacent to the inner table of the skull. The skull may show evidence of prior trauma or surgery, focal osteomyelitis, or permeation by infection. Contrast-enhanced CT shows enhancement of the inner dural wall of the collection. Mass effect with effacement of sulci, ventricular compression, and ventricular displacement may be present.

MRI

Subdural empyema is usually crescentic, whereas epidural empyema is always lentiform. The pus within the subdural/epidural empyema is hypointense relative to the brain on T1W and hyperintense on T2W images. FLAIR MRI helps to distinguish infected effusions (high signal) from sterile hygromas (low signal) (Fig. 40-4A). The dura mater shows characteristically low signal on both T1W and T2W images, so identification of the low signal dura will help to distinguish a subdural empyema from an epidural empyema on both T1W and T2W imaging. On DWI, purulent subdural collections will show high signal due to restricted diffusion (Fig. 40-5D).[15] Epidural empyemas may show high, low, or inhomogeneous signal on DWI. The difference in pressure and other factors between the subdural and epidural spaces, as well as the content of empyemas, may be the causes of differences in the activity of pleomorphic leukocytes.

PYOGENIC PARENCHYMAL INFECTIONS

Cerebritis

Cerebritis is a purulent *nonencapsulated* parenchymal infection of the brain.

Epidemiology

The frequency of focal infections of the brain parenchyma varies among series, with a highest reported frequency of 19%.[16]

Clinical Presentation

Most patients present with late-stage cerebritis or abscess and clinical signs of an intracerebral mass lesion. The most common symptoms are fever, seizures, nausea, headache, and vomiting. Focal neurologic signs depend on the region of brain involved.

Pathophysiology

Cerebritis may arise by hematogenous spread of infection or by direct spread from an otogenic focus or meningitis. The infection goes through a stage of cerebral softening followed by liquefaction and central cavitation.

Pathology

Cerebritis is a localized, poorly demarcated area of parenchymal softening with foci of necrosis and petechial hemorrhage. Entry of the infective agent into the brain parenchyma causes an ill-defined area of coagulative necrosis with polymorphonuclear leukocyte infiltration of the center. An area of cerebritis consists of vascular congestion, prominent perivascular cuffing by inflammatory cells, petechial hemorrhage, and brain edema.

Swelling of endothelial cells, neutrophil infiltration, and small foci of necrosis are present in the early stage of cerebritis (1-2 days). Confluent necrotic foci, macrophages, and lymphocytes will be present in the late stage of cerebritis (2-7 days).

Imaging

The imaging features of cerebritis have not been reported widely due to the low number of patients who present clinically at that stage.

CT

In early cerebritis, noncontrast CT may show only a low-attenuation abnormality with sulcal effacement or ventricular compression. Contrast-enhanced CT may show mild patchy enhancement. In late cerebritis, hypodensity with increased mass effect and heterogeneous, peripheral enhancement will be apparent.

MRI

The early stage of cerebritis is characterized by a nonspecific, poorly demarcated area of high signal intensity on T2W imaging with heterogeneous patchy enhancement on contrast-enhanced MRI (Fig. 40-6).[17] There may be restricted diffusion and high signal on DWI (with low ADC values) (see Fig. 40-6D, E). Restricted diffusion may be due to hypercellularity, brain ischemia, or cytotoxic edema.[18]

Abscess

Brain (or cerebral) abscess is a focal, purulent *encapsulated* parenchymal infection of the brain. Abscess begins as a localized

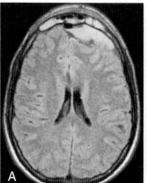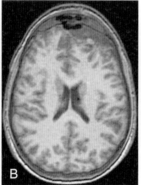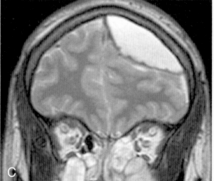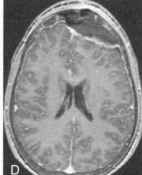

■ **FIGURE 40-4** Epidural empyema in a patient with left frontal sinusitis. **A,** Axial FLAIR-TSE MR image (TR/TE/TI 7385/130/2100) shows a hyperintense, lenticular lesion in the epidural space overlying the left frontal lobe. Medially displaced dura is recognized as a low signal intensity line between the lesion and the brain parenchyma. The left frontal sinus is opacified. The empyema is hypointense on an axial, precontrast T1W image (**B**) and hyperintense on a coronal T2W image (**C**). Gadolinium-enhanced T1W image (TR/TE/flip° 20/2.1/35°) shows marked enhancement of the dura with clear delineation of the epidural empyema (**D**).

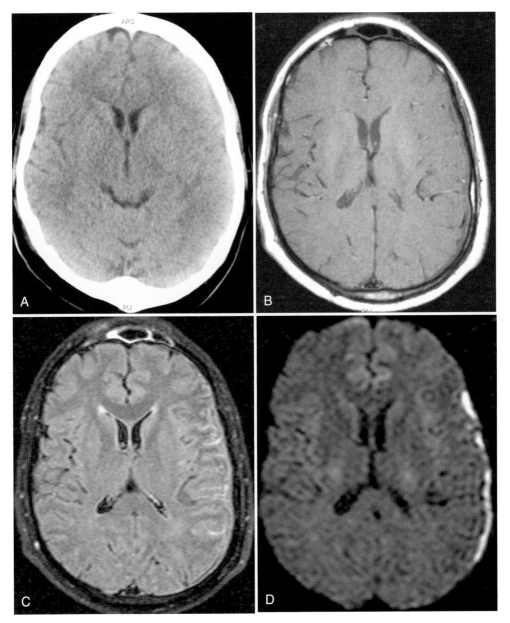

■ **FIGURE 40-5** Bacterial meningitis with subdural empyema. **A,** No abnormality was noted on the noncontrast CT of the brain. **B,** On a precontrast T1W image (TR/TE/flip° 20/2.1/35°), the dura is shown on the left side as a hypointense line. **C,** On axial FLAIR-TSE MR image (TR/TE/TI 7385/130/2100), high signal is demonstrated in the left subarachnoid spaces and in the subdural space overlying the left hemisphere. **D,** On trace DWI, the subdural collection has high signal, indicating restricted diffusion within purulent fluid: a subdural empyema.

region of cerebritis, which evolves into a collection of pus and immune cells surrounded by a collagenous capsule.

Epidemiology

Cerebral abscess accounts for up to 1% to 2% of all intracranial mass lesions in developed countries. In the past, abscess carried a high mortality. With modern imaging to detect, enumerate, localize, and characterize the lesions, the death rate is now very low. Each year 1500 to 2500 bacterial brain abscesses occur in the United States. The percentage is higher (8%) in developing countries. Although an abscess can occur at any age, most patients present in the third and fourth decades of life. Males are affected more often. Patients with immunodeficiency, intravenous drug abusers, alcohol abusers, and diabetics are at greater risk for developing brain abscesses.

The incidence of otogenic brain abscesses has significantly decreased over the years as otitis media has been managed more aggressively and as chronic otitis media becomes less common. Cerebellar abscess was seen in 6 of 70 (9%) cases of chronic suppurative otitis media.[19] Dental infections are a less common

cause of brain abscesses. When implicated, the dental infections have usually arisen in the molar teeth and lead to frontal lobe abscesses. Brain abscesses may also follow trauma, neurosurgery, or both. In 20% to 30% of brain abscesses, no obvious cause can be identified ("cryptic abscesses").[20]

Clinical Presentation

The clinical features of a cerebral abscess depend on lesion size, lesion location, virulence of the organism, and the patient's underlying condition. Usually there are signs of a rapidly expanding mass, including headache, drowsiness, confusion, seizures, hemiparesis, or speech difficulties. Fever is present in 50%. In a single series of patients with pneumococcal brain abscess, fever was found in only 29%, focal deficits in 86%, and headache in 81%.[21] Coma at presentation suggests an unfavorable outcome.[22]

Pathophysiology

Abscess arises by hematogenous dissemination, direct extension from the paranasal sinuses or mastoids, or concurrent

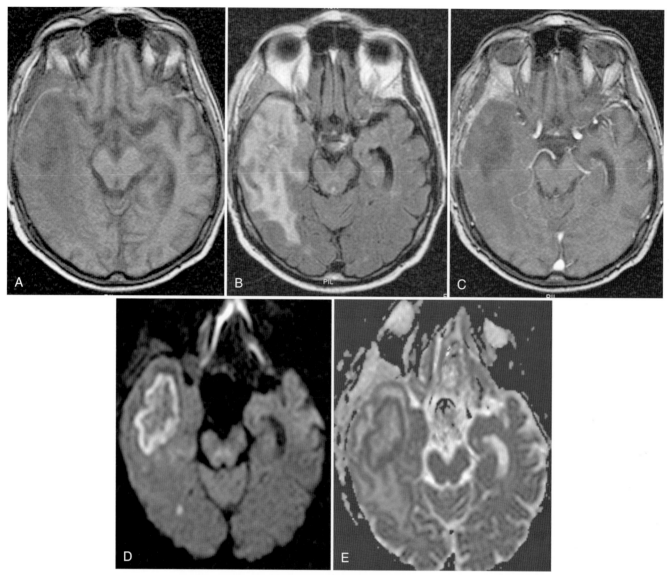

■ **FIGURE 40-6**   Early bacterial cerebritis (biopsy proven). This man presented with headache and fever. **A,** T1W MR image (TR/TE/flip° 20/2.1/35°) shows marked hypointensity in the right temporal lobe with mass effect and compression of the left temporal horn. **B,** On T2W MR image (TR/TE 2500/90) the lesion is hyperintense. **C,** Contrast-enhanced T1W image (TR/TE/flip° 20/2.1/35°) shows no enhancement. **D,** Trace DWI shows high signal on the periphery of the lesion, with low signal centrally. The ADC map (**E**) disclosed low ADC values at the margins and high ADC values in the center.

meningitis. Abscesses may be bacterial, fungal, or parasitic in origin. Numerous aerobic organisms (*Staphylococcus, Streptococcus, Proteus, Pseudomonas*) and anaerobic organisms (*Bacteroides* species, anaerobic streptococci) may cause brain abscess. De Louvois and associates have reported that *Streptococcus* species are the most common (74%) infective organisms isolated in central nervous system abscesses.[23] Fifty-four percent of the streptococci were *S. milleri.* The evolution of brain abscess from cerebritis to mature abscess can be divided into four stages: (1) early cerebritis (1 to 4 days); (2) late cerebritis (4 to 10 days); (3) early capsule formation (11 to 14 days); and (4) late capsule formation (>14 days).[24]

Pathology

In the early capsule stage, a necrotic liquefied core is surrounded by a thin capsule and peripheral gliosis. In the late capsule stage, the abscess capsule becomes thick and collagenous and the center begins to shrink.

Experimental study in dogs[25] demonstrated the evolution of an abscess. Early capsule formation was associated with the appearance of fibroblasts (by about day 5). Well-encapsulated lesions (14 days and older) showed five distinct histologic zones: (1) a well-formed necrotic center; (2) a peripheral zone of inflammatory cells, macrophages, and fibroblasts; (3) the dense collagenous capsule; (4) a layer of neovascularity associated with continuing cerebritis; and (5) reactive astrocytes, gliosis, and cerebral edema external to the capsule.[25]

Imaging

The imaging features depend on the abscess stage.

CT

Noncontrast CT shows a low-density mass with perifocal edema (Fig. 40-7A). On contrast-enhanced CT images, well-formed abscesses exhibit a smooth complete capsular ring (see Fig. 40-7B).[26] On CT, a ring blush may signify either late cerebritis or

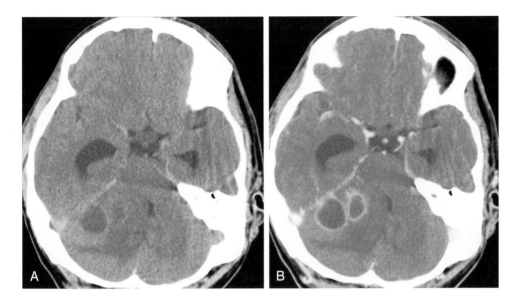

■ FIGURE 40-7 Cerebral abscesses in the posterior fossa after bacterial mastoiditis. **A,** Noncontrast CT shows a low density lesion and perifocal edema in the right cerebellum, with compression of the fourth ventricle. **B,** Contrast-enhanced CT shows two ring-enhancing abscesses.

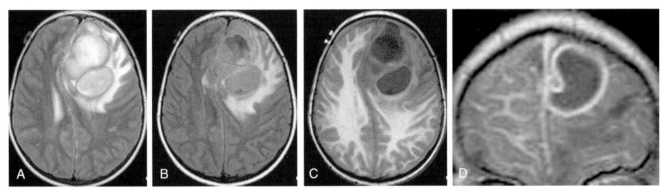

■ **FIGURE 40-8** Multiloculated brain abscess. **A,** Axial T2W MR image (TR/TE 2500/90) shows a multiloculated, right frontal mass with marked edema and midline shift from right to left. The high signal center and low signal rim indicate an abscess with a collagenous capsule. **B,** Axial FLAIR-TSE MR image (TR/TE/TI 7385/130/2100) and **(C)** axial T1W MR image (TR/TE/flip° 20/2.1/35°) show that the center of the mass is slightly hyperintense on FLAIR and hypointense on T1W imaging. **D,** Axial contrast-enhanced T1W MR image (TR/TE/flip° 20/2.1/35°) shows smooth ring enhancement of the multiloculated mass.

abscess. Demonstration of a complete ring on the noncontrast CT indicates the presence of a capsule and therefore defines the lesion as an abscess, not cerebritis.[25]

MRI

During the late stages of cerebritis, a collagenous capsule begins to form. This develops into a true capsule by the early abscess stage. On T2W imaging the capsule is visualized as a thin-walled, markedly hypointense ring with prominent surrounding edema (Fig. 40-8). On T1W imaging the wall is isointense or hyperintense, with a well-defined complete ring of enhancement indicative of a mature abscess (see Fig. 40-8A).[27] The proteinaceous, necrotic fluid within the abscess cavity is hyperintense to CSF on T1W and FLAIR images (see Fig. 40-8B). Because abscess capsules are better developed along the surfaces close to gray matter and thinner along the surfaces close to white matter, expanding abscesses tend to "point" toward the white matter and the underlying ventricles.[28]

Ring-enhancing brain lesions are nonspecific, so abscesses must be distinguished from other cystic lesions such as necrotic neoplasms. DWI helps in this differential diagnosis. In abscesses, the central collection of pus contains numerous white blood cells and highly viscous proteinaceous fluid. These cells and fluid restrict the diffusion of water molecules, so the lesion center appears markedly hyperintense on DWI and shows reduced ADC values. In cystic and necrotic tumors, the areas within the ring blush have low to intermediate DWI signal and elevated ADC values (Fig. 40-9).[29-31] This distinction is not pathognomonic, because cases of metastatic brain tumors with DWI hyperintensity and low ADC values have been described.[32] This is probably due to early tumor necrosis.

Perfusion MRI also helps to distinguish brain abscesses (which show a relative decrease in cerebral blood volume in enhancing capsule) from neoplasms, which demonstrate significantly elevated cerebral blood volume in enhancing peripheral parts.[33]

On MR spectroscopy, the main brain metabolites—*N*-acetylaspartate, creatine, and choline—are usually not detectable in abscesses. Instead, the spectra characteristically reveal peaks of acetate (at 1.92 ppm), succinate (at 2.4 ppm), and other amino acids (at 0.9 ppm), as well as lactate (at 1.3 ppm) (Fig. 40-10).[34] Aerobic organisms show spectra with the resonances of amino acids and lactate. Only anaerobic bacteria demonstrate the presence of additional acetate and succinate peaks.

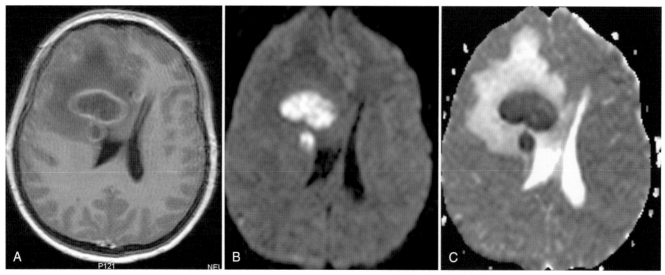

■ **FIGURE 40-9** Restricted diffusion in brain abscess. **A,** Axial gadolinium-enhanced T1W MR image (TR/TE/flip° 20/2.1/35°) shows two oval periph-erally enhancing lesions. The trace DWI (**B**) shows marked high signal within the abscess, and the ADC map (**C**) shows low ADC values due to restriction of diffusion by the proteinaceous material and pus.

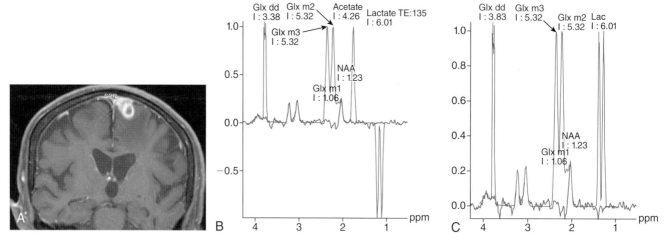

■ **FIGURE 40-10** Typical MR spectrum (MRS) of a brain abscess. **A,** Coronal T1W MR image (TR/TE/flip° 20/2.1/35°) shows a ring-enhancing lesion in the left frontal cortex. In-vivo proton MR spectra (PRESS) with long echo time (**B**) and short echo time (**C**) show signal resonances for acetate at 1.92 ppm, lactate (Lac), and the glutamate-glutamine complex (Glx), and a decrease in *N*-acetyl-aspartate (NAA).

With treatment, the necrotic center of the abscess typically shrinks progressively and the capsule shows decreasing hypoden-sity on T2W imaging. Decreasing signal intensity on DWI and increasing ADC values in the abscess cavity correlate with suc-cessful treatment (Fig. 40-11). The ring blush may persist for up to 8 months, so detection of the ring does not indicate treatment failure. Conversely, persistence or reappearance of DWI hyper-intensity and low ADC values correlate with reaccumulation of pus and do indicate treatment failure.[35] On MRS, the elimination of acetate and succinate peaks concordant with treatment seems to confirm a positive response to medical therapy.[36]

Pyocephalus

Pyocephalus is an inflammation of the ependyma of the ventricu-lar system with accumulation of suppurative fluid in the ventri-cles. Alternate names include pyencephalus, cerebral ventricular empyema, pyogenic ventriculitis, and ventricular empyema.

Epidemiology
Pyocephalus is an uncommon complication of acute pyogenic meningitis. The predisposing factors are head injury, brain surgery, CSF leak, ruptured abscess, and infected brain malformation.[37]

Clinical Presentation
Clinical signs and symptoms may be subtle, and the course can be indolent.

Pathophysiology
The pathogens that most frequently cause pyogenic ventriculitis are gram-negative bacteria and *Staphylococcus* species.[38] The frequency of gram-negative bacillary meningitis has increased steadily during the past 30 years. This is thought to reflect an increase in nosocomial meningitis after neurosurgical procedures.[39]

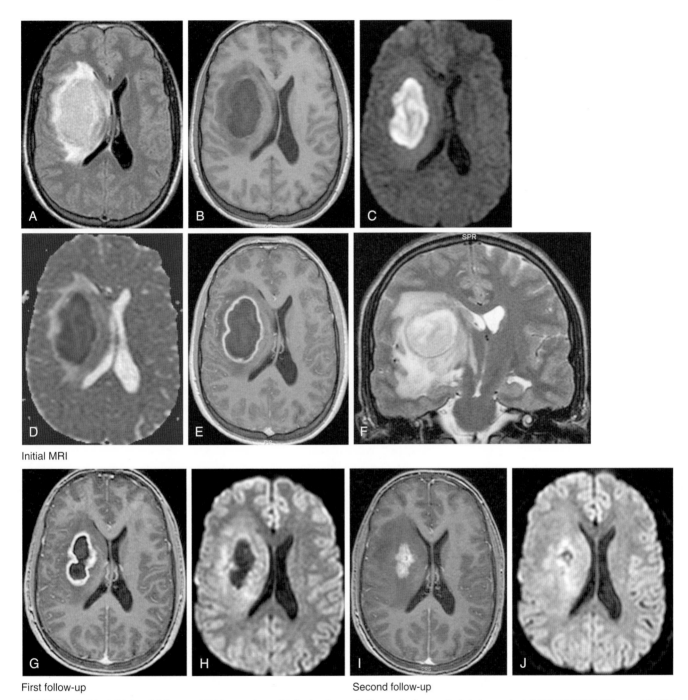

Initial MRI

First follow-up   Second follow-up

■ **FIGURE 40-11** Initial and follow-up MRI in a patient with brain abscess before and after surgical drainage. **A,** Axial FLAIR-TSE MR image (TR/TE/ TI 7385/130/2100). A mass of intermediate signal intensity with high signal perifocal edema compresses the right lateral ventricle and shifts the midline minimally. **B,** The mass has low signal intensity on an axial precontrast T1W MR image (TR/TE/flip° 20/2.1/35°). The cavity shows restricted diffusion on trace DWI (**C**) with low ADC values (**D**). **E,** The abscess capsule displays smooth peripheral enhancement on postcontrast T1W MR image (TR/TE/ flip° 20/2.1/35°). **F,** Coronal T2W MR image. The capsule show the low signal intensity typical for brain abscess. **G, H,** Three weeks after surgical drainage of the abscess cavity, follow-up MRI shows decreased abscess size (**G**). DWI now shows low signal within the abscess cavity, compatible with clear fluid (**H**). **I,** Six weeks later, the size of the abscess has decreased farther, indicating successful treatment. **J,** The remaining small abscess cavity shows only low signal on DWI. The enhancement seen on postcontrast T1W MR images at the second follow-up MR examination (**I**) represents a collagenous capsule collapsed around the smaller abscess cavity.

Pathology

Intraventricular sedimentation levels will be seen in the ventricles. Inflammation of ependymal and subependymal regions is also evident.

Imaging

CT

The increased protein and pus appear on CT as increased ventricular density, with fluid-debris levels in the dependent portions of the ventricles.[37,40] The walls of the ventricle are usually thickened from concurrent ependymitis. There may be loculation of the ventricles and hydrocephalus. Periventricular cerebral edema usually causes low density of the parenchyma. Contrast-enhanced CT typically shows enhancement of the ventricular walls and enhancement within any juxtaventricular cerebritis or abscess.

MRI

On MRI, characteristic features include altered signal of the intraventricular fluid, especially on FLAIR images; dependent debris; ependymal thickening and enhancement; hydrocephalus; periventricular hyperintensity from the hydrocephalus and/or periventricular inflammation; and leptomeningeal signal abnormality and enhancement reflecting concurrent meningitis (Fig. 40-12). In one series of 17 patients with pyogenic ventriculitis, the most frequent imaging sign of ventriculitis was intraventricular debris (94%).[38] In pyocephalus, T1W imaging often showed a nonlinear CSF-debris level, distinguishing dependent pus from the level straight line seen with acute hemorrhage or the "blood cast" of the ventricle seen with old clotted blood. Markedly restricted diffusion has been reported in dependent purulent intraventricular fluid (see Fig. 40-12C).[41] The ADC of frank pus will be significantly lower than white matter, whereas the ADC

■ **FIGURE 40-12** Pyocephalus in a child with proven bacterial meningitis. **A** and **B,** Axial FLAIR-TSE MR images (TR/TE/TI 7385/130/2100) shows high signal in the subarachnoid spaces, indicating meningeal disease. CSF analysis disclosed an increased cell count and other findings consistent with bacterial meningitis. Ventricular debris forms an irregular fluid-fluid interface in the dependent portions of both ventricles. **C,** High signal was demonstrated in the ventricles on trace DWI, indicating restricted diffusion in the purulent intraventricular fluid. **D,** Contrast-enhanced T1W MR image (TR/TE/flip° 20/2.1/35°) shows a fluid-fluid interface, with higher signal in the pus below the interface and lower signal in the CSF above it.

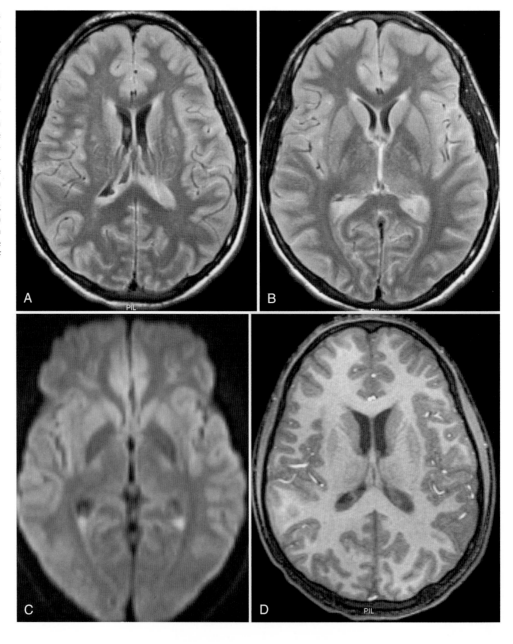

of dilute pus will be higher than that of white matter.[41] DWI can be useful for differentiating pyocephalus from intraventricular hemorrhage.

The DWI and FLAIR pulse sequences have proved to be the most effective for displaying pyocephalus. Of 20 MRI images in patients with ventriculitis, intraventricular abnormalities were shown by DWI in 19 (95%), by FLAIR sequences in 19 (95%), by T2W imaging in 13 (65%), and by contrast-enhanced T1W imaging in only 10 (50%).[42] Surprisingly, FLAIR imaging was superior to contrast-enhanced T1W imaging for detecting ventricular wall abnormalities.[42]

KEY POINTS: DIFFERENTIAL DIAGNOSIS

Pyogenic Meningitis
- MRI is the technique of choice for the detection of meningitis.
- FLAIR is the most sensitive MR technique for the detection of meningitis, showing characteristically high signal of the subarachnoid spaces.
- Complications such as hydrocephalus, venous sinus thrombosis with venous infarctions, arterial infarctions, and ventriculitis are common.
- Carcinomatous meningitis is a differential diagnosis but usually shows dural as well as leptomeningeal enhancement, permitting it to be differentiated from meningitis.

Empyema
- Subdural empyemas are usually associated with sinusitis.
- A crescentic shape indicates subdural empyema, whereas a lentiform shape indicates epidural empyema. These may both be present.
- High signal on T2W and T1W images in subdural or epidural collections suggests fluid with a high protein content (purulent fluid).
- Subdural empyemas have restricted diffusion and high signal on DWI (in contrast to clear collections).
- Epidural empyemas have variable signal on DWI.

Cerebritis
- Cerebritis is characterized by nonspecific features on CT (ill-defined low density area with peripheral enhancement) and cannot reliably be distinguished from neoplasms.
- High signal intensity on DWI is due to restriction of diffusion.

Abscess
- T2W images typically show a high signal intensity center and low signal intensity capsule.
- Fungal abscesses and tuberculomas usually show a low signal intensity center on T2W images.
- DWI can be used to help differentiate an abscess from a necrotic tumor. The center of an abscess shows high signal intensity on DWI, because the viscous content of the abscess cavity restricts diffusion of water. The necrotic centers of most neoplasms show low signal on DWI because the debris facilitates diffusion.
- Differential diagnoses for high signal on DWI include hemorrhagic metastases, metastases from adenocarcinoma of the lung, fungal abscesses, and tuberculoma.
- On perfusion MRI, an abscess has low cerebral blood volume, whereas necrotic neoplasms have high cerebral blood volume.

Pyocephalus
- The presence of ventricular debris is highly suggestive of ventriculitis.
- T1W imaging often shows a nonlinear fluid-fluid interface.
- Intraventricular hemorrhage often shows a straight level acutely or a blood cast of the ventricular system chronically.
- Pyogenic ventriculitis exhibits high signal on DWI, whereas intraventricular hemorrhage shows low signal on DWI.
- Periventricular enhancement may be seen in lymphomas and in cytomegaloviral ventriculitis (in human immunodeficiency virus–positive patients).

SUGGESTED READINGS

Adame N, Hedlund G, Byington CL. Sinogenic intracranial empyema in children. Pediatrics 2005; 116:461-467.

Anslow P. Cranial bacterial infection. Eur Radiol 2004; 14:E145-E154.

Barloon TJ, Yuh WT, Knepper LE, et al. Cerebral ventriculitis: MR findings. J Comput Assist Tomogr 1990; 14:272-275.

Castillo M. Magnetic resonance imaging of meningitis and its complications. Topics Magn Reson Imaging 1994; 6:53-58.

Castillo M. Imaging brain abscesses with diffusion-weighted and other sequences. AJNR Am J Neuroradiol 1999; 20:1193-1194.

Domingo P, Barquet N, Alvarez M, et al. Group B streptococcal meningitis in adults: report of twelve cases and review. Clin Infect Dis 1997; 25:1180-1187.

Falcone S, et al. Encephalitis, cerebritis, and brain abscess: pathophysiology and imaging findings. Neuroimaging Clin North Am 2000; 10:333-353.

Foerster BR, Thurnher MM, Malani PN, et al. Intracranial infections: clinical and imaging characteristics. Acta Radiol 2007; 48:875-893.

Garg M, Gupta RK, Husain M, et al. Brain abscesses: etiologic categorization with in vivo proton MR spectroscopy. Radiology 2004; 230:519-527.

Haykal H, Zamani A, Wang AM, Barsotti J. CT features of early *Listeria* monocytogenes cerebritis. AJNR Am J Neuroradiol 1987; 8:279-282.

Kanamalla US, Ibarra RA, Jinkins JR. Imaging of cranial meningitis and ventriculitis. Neuroimaging Clin North Am 2000; 10:309-331.

Moseley IF, Kendall BE. Radiology of intracranial empyemas, with special reference to computed tomography. Neuroradiology 1984; 26:333-345.

Nathoo N, Nadvi SS, van Dellen JR. Infratentorial empyema: analysis of 22 cases. Neurosurgery 1997; 41:1263-1268.

Osenbach RK, Loftus CM. Diagnosis and management of brain abscesses. Neurosurg Clin North Am 1992; 3:403-420.

Parmar H, Sitoh YY, Anand P, et al. Contrast-enhanced FLAIR imaging in the evaluation of infectious leptomeningeal diseases. Eur J Radiol 2006; 58:89-95.

Smith RR. Neuroradiology of intracranial infection. Pediatr Neurosurg 1992; 18:92-104.

Tung GA, Rogg JM. Diffusion-weighted imaging of cerebritis. AJNR Am J Neuroradiol 2003; 24:1110-1113.

Vachon L, Mikity V. Computed tomography and ultrasound in purulent ventriculitis. J Ultrasound Med 1987; 6:269-271.

Weingarten K, Zimmerman RD, Becker RD, et al. Subdural and epidural empyemas: MR imaging. AJR Am J Roentgenol 1989; 152:615-621.

REFERENCES

1. Schuchat A, Robinson K, Wenger JD, et al. Bacterial meningitis in the United States in 1995. N Engl J Med 1997; 337:970-976.

2. Dunne DW, Quagliarello V. Group B streptococcal meningitis in adults. Medicine (Baltimore) 1993; 72:1-10.

3. Lu CH, Chang WN, Chuang YC, Chang HW. Gram-negative bacillary meningitis in adult post-neurosurgical patients. Surg Neurol 1999; 52:438-443.

4. Parker JC Jr, Dyer MC. Neurologic infections due to bacteria, fungi and parasites. In Doris RL, Robertson DM (eds). Textbook of Neuropathology. Baltimore, Williams & Wilkins, 1985; pp 632-703.

5. Chang KH, Han MH, Roh JK, et al. Gd-DTPA-enhanced MR imaging of the brain in patients with meningitis: comparison with CT. AJNR Am J Neuroradiol 1990; 11:69-76.

6. Kastrup O, Wanke I, Maschke M. Neuroimaging of infections. NeuroRx 2005; 2:324-332.

7. Singer MB, Atlas SW, Drayer BP. Subarachnoid space disease: diagnosis with fluid-attenuated inversion recovery MR imaging and comparison with gadolinium-enhanced spin-echo MR imaging–blinded reader study. Neuroradiology 1998; 208:417-422.

8. Smith RR. Neuroradiology of intracranial infection. Pediatr Neurosurg 1992; 18:92-104.

9. Castillo M. Magnetic resonance imaging of meningitis and its complications. Topics Magn Reson Imaging 1994; 6:53-58.

10. Osborn MK, Steinberg JP. Subdural empyema and other suppurative complications of paranasal sinusitis. Lancet Infect Dis 2007; 7:62-67.

11. Penido Nde O, Borin A, Iha LC, et al. Intracranial complications of otitis media: 15 years of experience in 33 patients. Otolaryngol Head Neck Surg 2005; 132:37-42.

12. Van de Beck D, Campeau NG, Wijdicks EFM. The clinical challenge of recognizing infratentorial empyema. Neurology 2007; 69:477-481.

13. Tsai YD, Chang WN, Shen CC, et al. Intracranial suppuration: a clinical comparison of subdural empyemas and epidural abscesses. Surg Neurol 2003; 59:191-196.

14. Zimmerman RD, Leeds NE, Danziger A. Subdural empyema: CT findings. Radiology 1984; 150:417-422.

15. Tsuchiya K, Osawa A, Katase S, et al. Diffusion-weighted MRI of subdural and epidural empyemas. Neuroradiology 2003; 45:220-223.

16. Aladro Y, Ponce P, Santullano V, et al. Cerebritis due to *Listeria monocytogenes.* CT and MR findings. Eur Radiol 1996; 6:188-191.

17. Falcone S, et al. Encephalitis, cerebritis, and brain abscess: pathophysiology and imaging findings. Neuroimag Clin North Am 2000; 10:333-353.

18. Tung GA, Rogg JM. Diffusion-weighted imaging of cerebritis. AJNR Am J Neuroradiol 2003; 24:1110-1113.

19. Dubey SP, Larawin V. Complications of chronic suppurative otitis media and their management. Laryngoscope 2007; 117:264-267.

20. Mathisen GE, Johnson JP. Brain abscess. Clin Infect Dis 1997; 25:763-779.

21. Grigoriadis E, Gold W. Pyogenic brain abscess caused by *Streptococcus pneumoniae:* case report and review. Clin Infect Dis 1997; 25:1108-1112.

22. Tonon E, Scotton PG, Gallucci M, Vaglia A. Brain abscess: clinical aspects of 100 patients. Int J Infect Dis 2006; 10:103-109.

23. De Louvois J, Gortval P, Hurley R. Bacteriology of abscesses of the central nervous system: a multicentre prospective study. BMJ 1977; 2:981-984.

24. Haimes AB, Zimmerman RD, Morgello S, et al. MR imaging of brain abscesses. AJNR Am J Neuroradiol 1989; 10:279-291.

25. Britt RH, Enzmann DR, Yeager AS. Neuropathological and computerized tomographic findings in experimental brain abscess. J Neurosurg 1981; 55:590-603.

26. Miller ES, Dias PS, Uttley D. CT scanning in the management of intracranial abscess: a review of 100 cases. Br J Neurosurg 1988; 2:439-446.

27. Zimmerman RD, Weingarten K. Neuroimaging of cerebral abscesses. Neuroimaging Clin North Am 1991; 1:1-16.

28. Karampekios S, Hesselink J. Cerebral infections. Eur Radiol 2005; 15:485-493.

29. Guo AC, Provenzale JM, Cruz LCH, et al. Cerebral abscesses: investigation using apparent diffusion coefficient maps. Neuroradiology 2001; 43:370-374.

30. Kim YJ, Chang KH, Song IC, et al. Brain abscess and necrotic or cystic brain tumor: discrimination with signal intensity on diffusion weighted MR imaging. AJR Am J Roentgenol 1998; 171:1487-1490.

31. Stadnik TW, Chaskis C, Michotte A, et al: Diffusion-weighted MR-imaging of intracerebral masses: comparison with conventional MR-imaging and histologic findings. AJNR Am J Neuroradiol 2001; 22:969-976.

32. Holtas S, Geijer B, Stromblad LG, et al. A ring-enhancing metastasis with central high signal on diffusion-weighted imaging and low apparent diffusion coefficients. Neuroradiology 2000; 42:824-827.

33. Erdogan C, Hakyemez B, Yildirim N, et al. Brain abscess and cystic brain tumor: discrimination with dynamic susceptibility contrast perfusion-weighted MRI. J Comput Assist Tomogr 2005; 29:663-667.

34. Lai PH, Ho JT, Chen WL, et al. Brain abscess and necrotic brain tumor: discrimination with proton MR spectroscopy and diffusion-weighted imaging. AJNR Am J Neuroradiol 2002; 23:1369-1377.

35. Cartes-Zumelzu FW, Stavrou I, Castillo M, et al. Diffusion-weighted imaging in the assessment of brain abscesses therapy. AJNR Am J Neuroradiol 2004; 25:1310-1317.

36. Burtscher IM, Holtas S. In vivo proton MR spectroscopy of untreated and treated brain abscesses. AJNR Am J Neuroradiol 1999; 20:1049-1053.

37. Bakshi R, Kinkel PR, Mechtler LL, Bates VE. Cerebral ventricular empyema associated with severe adult pyogenic meningitis: computed tomography findings. Clin Neurol Neurosurg 1997; 99:252-255.

38. Fukui MB, Williams RL, Mudigonda S. CT and MR imaging features of pyogenic ventriculitis. AJNR Am J Neuroradiol 2001; 22:1510-1516.

39. Durand M, Calderwood S, Weber D, et al. Acute bacterial meningitis in adults: a review of 493 episodes. N Engl J Med 1993; 328:21-28.

40. Wormser G, Strashun A. Ventriculitis complicating gram-negative meningitis in an adult: diagnosis by radioisotope brain scanning and computerized tomography. Mt Sinai J Med 1980; 47:575-578.

41. Pezullo JA, Tung GA, Mudigonda S, Rogg JM. Diffusion-weighted MR imaging of pyogenic ventriculitis. AJR Am J Radiol 2003; 180:71-75.

42. Fujikawa A, Tsuchiya K, Honya K, Nitatori T. Comparison of MRI sequences to detect ventriculitis. AJR Am J Radiol 2006; 187:1048-1053.

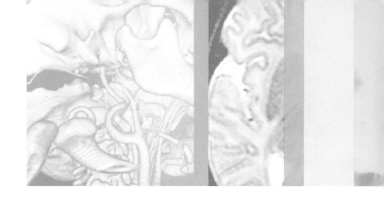

CHAPTER 41

Pyogens, Mycobacteria, and Fungus

Majda M. Thurnher

SYPHILIS AND NOCARDIA INFECTIONS

Neurosyphilis

Neurosyphilis is a chronic infection caused by the spirochete *Treponema pallidum*. When untreated, the disease progresses through three clinical stages designated primary, secondary, and tertiary syphilis. Alternate names include neurolues, syphilitic gumma, tabes dorsalis, and general paresis.

Epidemiology

After infection with *T. pallidum* about one third of patients with syphilis develop tertiary syphilis. One to 3 percent of AIDS patients present with neurosyphilis.[1]

Clinical Presentation

Neurosyphilis can occur weeks to decades after the initial infection. Most often it is asymptomatic. Symptomatic neurosyphilis may present in four forms: (1) meningovascular syphilis, (2) gummatous neurosyphilis, (3) paretic neurosyphilis, and (4) tabes dorsalis. Headache and focal neurologic deficits are characteristics of meningovascular neurosyphilis complicated by cerebral infarction. Personality changes, psychiatric symptoms, memory loss, and speech disturbances are typical for general paresis and diffuse parenchymal involvement. Neurosyphilis has an accelerated course in the AIDS population.[1]

Pathophysiology

In meningovascular syphilis the leptomeninges show thickening and perivascular lymphocytic infiltrates. The intracranial vessels show evidence of vasculitis that leads to stenoses and occlusions with ischemia and infarction. In one series, 23% of patients with syphilis showed evidence of cerebral infarctions.[2] In a second series, 43% of patients had cerebral infarction.[3] The infarctions primarily involved the basal ganglia, the middle cerebral artery territory, and branches of the basilar artery.[4] Large arteries show concentric or asymmetric stenoses. These may manifest as segmental constriction and occlusion of the supraclinoid carotid arteries.[5] Small arteries show focal stenosis and aneurysmal dilatations.

Syphilitic gummas represent a parenchymal form of neurosyphilis that results from cell-mediated immune response to *T. pallidum*.

Pathology

Meningovascular neurosyphilis is characterized by chronic meningitis with obliterative arteritis. Gummas are intraparenchymal lesions located close to the meninges.

Microscopic features of parenchymatous neurosyphilis include degenerative neuronal changes, gliosis, and scattered microglia.[6] Gummas are well-defined masses of granulation tissue surrounded by mononuclear epithelial and fibroblastic cells.

The arteries most commonly affected by meningovascular neurolues are the middle cerebral artery and branches of the basilar artery.[5]

Imaging
CT

One third of patients with neurosyphilis show normal CT scans. Others will show cerebral atrophy. In some patients, CT shows small infarcts as low-density areas that enhance in the subacute stage. Meningeal enhancement suggests meningovascular syphilis.

MRI

Meningovascular syphilis causes cerebral infarctions in 43% of patients.[3] Acute infarctions appear as zones of restricted diffusion with high signal intensity on diffusion-weighted imaging (DWI) and low apparent diffusion coefficient (ADC) values. Subacute and chronic infarctions appear as high signal lesions on T2-weighted (T2W) and fluid-attenuated inversion recovery (FLAIR) images. MR angiography shows the narrowing or occlusions of the vessels. Nonspecific focal or diffuse enhancement observed on enhanced MR images cannot distinguish meningovascular syphilis from meningitis of other origin.

In gummatous neurolues, gummas are usually hyperdense on CT and hyperintense on T2W MR images. On contrast-enhanced MRI, cortically located ring- or nodular-enhancing lesions with adjacent meningeal enhancement should raise suspicion of a possible syphilitic gumma.[7]

In general paresis, T2W and FLAIR images show cerebral atrophy and multiple high signal intensity lesions.

Nocardiosis

Nocardiosis is a bacterial infection caused by weakly gram-positive, filamentous *Nocardia* species.

Epidemiology

Most cases of nocardiosis occur as an opportunistic infection in immunocompromised patients. Nocardial infection is seen in less than 5% of renal transplant recipients. Fewer than 2% (0.3%-1.8%) of all infections in AIDS patients are due to *Nocardia*.[8] Fifty percent of patients with systemic nocardiosis have central nervous system (CNS) involvement.

Clinical Presentation

Clinical presentation mostly relates to the mass effect. Seizures are the first clinical sign in 30% of patients. The mortality rate of nocardial brain infection is approximately 80%.

Pathophysiology

Nocardia is a genus of gram-positive, rod-shaped bacteria. *N. asteroides* is responsible for approximately 80% of CNS nocardial infections.[9] Other pathogenic species include *N. farcinica*, *N. brasiliensis*, *N. transvalensis*, and *N. otitidis-caviarum*. *Nocardia* usually establishes a primary infection in the lung and spreads hematogenously to the CNS in 15% to 44% of cases. In one study of 30 *Nocardia* infections in HIV-positive patients, 73% of patients had pulmonary disease.[8] Solitary brain abscess is the most common form of CNS infection with *Nocardia*, but multiple lesions are found in about 38% of cases.

Pathology

Nocardial abscesses are more commonly supratentorial than infratentorial.[10]

Imaging
CT

Contrast-enhanced CT usually shows multiple or multiloculated ring-enhancing lesions with perifocal edema and mass effect (Fig. 41-1).[11]

MRI

The MR appearance of a nocardial abscess is similar to that of other pyogenic brain abscesses. The necrotic center is hyperintense on T2W imaging and hypointense on T1-weighted (T1W) imaging. The capsule has high T1 signal and low T2 signal and shows smooth peripheral enhancement on contrast-enhanced images. Nocardial CNS infection may also manifest as subependymal nodules and meningitis.[11] In one study, 92% of AIDS patients with nocardial CNS infection had imaging evidence of associated meningeal disease.[11] Of the nine patients, hydrocephalus was present in five, subependymal nodules were evident in five, and clinical evidence of meningitis occurred in three. Histologic examination of the small subependymal nodules revealed inflammatory cells consistent with ventriculitis/ependymitis and developing subependymal abscesses.[11] Nocardial abscesses may assume a characteristic "budding" appearance in which multiple, closely spaced, hematogenously disseminated abscesses conglomerate to create a budding appearance as they enlarge.[12] Diffusion-weighted images can show homogeneous hyperintensity within the lesion (Fig. 41-2). In limited case material of active nocardiosis, MR spectroscopy showed a rise in the mean choline/creatine ratio and a slight reduction in the mean *N*-acetyl-aspartate (NAA)/creatine ratio, with lactate and amino acid peaks consistent with bacterial abscess.[13]

CNS TUBERCULOSIS

Tuberculosis is a bacterial disease caused by organisms of the *Mycobacterium tuberculosis* complex. Most tuberculous infections of the CNS are caused by *M. tuberculosis*. Less frequently, other mycobacteria may be involved. Other terms associated with this disease include tuberculous meningitis, tuberculous granuloma, and tuberculoma.

Epidemiology

M. tuberculosis infects nearly 2 billion people—about one third of the world's population. Each year, nearly 9 million people develop active tuberculosis, the infectious form of the disease, and 2 million die. Tuberculosis has long been endemic in developing countries. Recently, tuberculosis has re-emerged as a public health problem in developed countries due to the rise of AIDS and the migration of infected populations from underdeveloped to developed countries. In 2006, a total of 13,767 cases of tuberculosis were reported in the United States (representing 4.6 per 100,000 population).

AIDS is considered the main risk factor for the development of tuberculosis.[14] In 2006 the percentage of tuberculosis cases known to be associated with human immunodeficiency virus (HIV) infection was 12.4% and the percentage of cases of tuberculosis with unknown HIV status was 31.7%. CNS involvement occurs in 2% to 5% of all tuberculosis patients and in up to 15% of AIDS patients.[15] It is known that tuberculosis may appear in

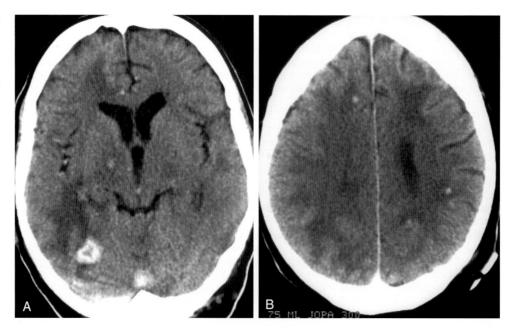

■ **FIGURE 41-1** *Nocardia* CNS infection in an HIV-positive individual. **A** and **B,** Contrast-enhanced CT shows multiple ring- and nodular-enhancing intraparenchymal lesions. The marked hypodensity of the white matter bilaterally is due to HIV encephalopathy.

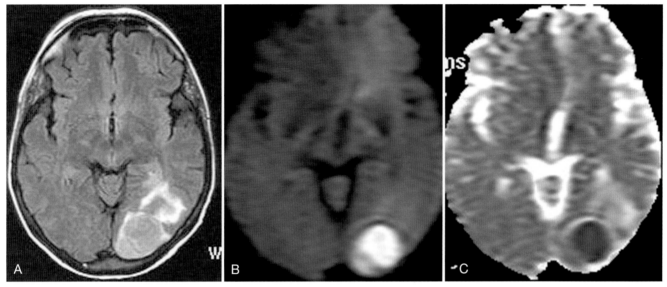

■ **FIGURE 41-2** *Nocardia* brain abscess in an immunocompetent woman. **A,** Axial FLAIR-TSE MRI (TR/TE/TI 7385/130/2100) shows a high signal intensity lesion in the left occipital cortex. **B** and **C,** High signal on DWI and low ADC value suggested a bacterial abscess. Biopsy, aspiration of the lesion cavity, and isolation of the organism confirmed the infection with *Nocardia*.

the early stages of immunodeficiency and that the clinical manifestations, management, and epidemiology are altered in AIDS patients.

Clinical Presentation

Tuberculous Meningitis

Tuberculous meningitis is usually characterized by a history of vague ill health with malaise, anorexia, fatigue, fever, myalgias, and headache for 2 to 8 weeks before presentation with meningeal irritation. With time, the headache worsens and becomes continuous. Neck stiffness is reported by about 25% of patients. Cranial nerve palsies occur in 20% to 30% of patients and may be the presenting manifestation of tuberculous meningitis. The sixth cranial nerve is most commonly affected. Optic nerve involvement may occasionally be dominant, with loss of vision. As the disease progresses, increasing evidence of cerebral dysfunction sets in, leading finally to lethargy, confusion, stupor, and coma. The terminal illness is characterized by deep coma, decerebrate or decorticate rigidity, and spasm.

Tuberculomas

Low-grade fever, headache, vomiting, seizures, focal neurologic deficits, and papilledema are characteristic clinical features of supratentorial tuberculomas.

Tuberculous Abscess

Clinical features of tuberculous abscess include partial seizures, focal neurologic deficits, and signs of increased intracranial pressure.

Calvarial Tuberculosis

Calvarial tuberculosis usually presents as a painless scalp swelling (Pott's puffy tumor). Involvement of the outer table and scalp may lead to a draining sinus. Neurologic deficits are uncommon. In one series of 42 cases of calvarial tuberculosis, the average duration of symptoms was 2.5 months.[16]

Pathophysiology

The infectious etiology of tuberculosis was definitively proven by Robert Koch, who discovered the tubercle bacillus in 1882.

CNS tuberculosis most commonly results from hematogenous spread of the infection from an outside focus. Tuberculous meningitis may also result from outward extension and rupture of a subpial or subependymal focus ("Rich focus") into the subarachnoid space. Rich and McCordock suggested that CNS tuberculosis develops in two stages:

1. Initially small tuberculous lesions (Rich's foci) develop in the meninges, the subpial or the subependymal surfaces of the brain or the spinal cord. These may remain dormant for years after initial infection.
2. Subsequent growth or rupture of one or more of these small tuberculous lesions causes the diverse forms of CNS tuberculosis. Rupture into the subarachnoid space or into the ventricular system results in meningitis.

Tuberculous meningitis is characterized by thick gelatinous exudates, which favor the meninges at the base of the brain. Tuberculous inflammation (vasculitis) of the vessels that traverse the subarachnoid space causes narrowing, occlusions of the vessels, and subsequent infarctions, usually affecting the middle cerebral artery territory and the small perforating arteries that supply the basal ganglia.[17] The meningeal involvement impairs cerebrospinal fluid flow and resorption, so communicating hydrocephalus is the most common complication of meningeal tuberculosis.[18] Villoria and colleagues report hydrocephalus in 51% of 35 patients with AIDS-related CNS tuberculosis.[19]

Parenchymal forms of the tuberculous infection include tuberculomas, tuberculous abscesses, and focal tuberculous cerebritis.

Tuberculous granulomas (tuberculomas) result from the hematogenous spread of infection or from the extension of meningitis into the parenchyma. Tuberculomas may be solitary or multiple, can occur anywhere in the brain, but are found predominantly in the supratentorial compartment.[19]

Tuberculous abscess is a true pyogenic lesion.

Focal tuberculous cerebritis is a rare form of tuberculosis.

Calvarial tuberculosis is another rare manifestation of extrapulmonary tuberculosis and usually occurs by hematogenous spread from the lungs. Because of the relatively low percentage of cancellous tissue in the bones of the cranium, calvarial tuberculosis is a rare condition. In some cases, extensive extradural granulations may cause thrombosis of the venous structures.

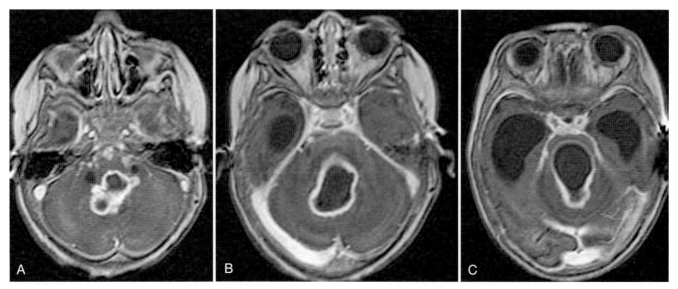

■ **FIGURE 41-3**   Severe tuberculous infection in a 5-year-old child. **A** to **C,** Contrast-enhanced T1W MRI (TR/TE/flip° 20/2.1/35°) shows meningeal enhancement, enhancement of the cranial nerves, ring-enhancing masses in the posterior fossa, and obstructive hydrocephalus.

Pathology

In tuberculosis, thick, gelatinous exudates will be present in the basal cisterns. Tuberculomas are firm, avascular, spherical granulomatous masses measuring 2 to 8 cm in diameter. They are well demarcated from the surrounding brain tissue, which is compressed around the lesion and shows edema and gliosis.

The thick, gelatinous basal exudate is composed of bacilli and small and large mononuclear cells, including epithelioid cells. It is histologically characteristic of tuberculosis. Tuberculomas are composed of caseous material with a thick collagen layer, in which tubercle bacilli can be demonstrated. The histopathologic diagnosis of tuberculous brain abscess is made with microscopic evidence of pus in the abscess cavity, microscopic changes in the abscess wall, and isolation of *M. tuberculosis.*

Imaging

Tuberculous Meningitis

Contrast-enhanced CT typically shows thick intensely enhancing basilar exudates. MRI shows such exudates at the base and over the convexity in 36% to 61% of cases (Fig. 41-3).[19-21] CT demonstrates infarcts in 20.5% to 38% of cases (Fig. 41-4), but MRI shows a significantly higher incidence. DWI helps to detect early infarcts. MR angiography helps to show tuberculous vascular pathology (see Fig. 41-4).[17] In the majority of patients, CT and MRI both show hydrocephalus as ventricular enlargement and ependymitis with abnormal enhancement of the ventricular ependyma (see Fig. 41-3). Enhancement of nerves indicates their involvement by tuberculosis.

Tuberculoma

The radiologic features of tuberculomas depend on the maturity of the lesion. On CT, mature granulomas are ring-enhancing lesions. They may show a "target sign" composed of a central calcification or punctate enhancement surrounded by a zone of hypodensity and a rim of enhancement, but other lesions such as toxoplasmosis, lymphoma, or brain abscess may show similar features.[22,23] On MRI, tuberculomas appear isointense with a hyperintense ring on T1W images and show variable signal on proton density and T2W images (Fig. 41-5). Some tuberculomas are hypointense on T2W images, possibly due to paramagnetic free radicals produced by macrophage activity.[24] Other tuberculomas have high signal on T2W imaging due to central

liquefactive necrosis. Kim and colleagues compared MR findings with pathologic features in tuberculomas and found that the outer enhancing portion consisted of a layer of collagenous fibers. Inflammatory infiltrates appeared on MRI as hypointense rings on T2W images. Central caseation necrosis appeared isointense or hypointense on all pulse sequences.[7] Healed tuberculomas do not enhance but may calcify. Recently, study of 52 intracranial tuberculomas with magnetization transfer (MT) imaging demonstrated that the nonenhancing cores of tuberculosis have a higher MT ratio (MTR) than do tumor necrosis or cysts.[25] The MTR of tuberculosis cores was also higher in tuberculomas than in abscesses, likely related to their higher cell content. However, MRI using MTR only slightly improves the diagnostic accuracy. In five patients, MTR improved the differentiation of solitary tuberculoma from low-grade glioma. In four patients, MTR successfully distinguished multiple tuberculomas from metastatic disease.

Tuberculous Abscess

Tuberculous abscesses demonstrate a typical imaging appearance of pyogenic abscesses: hyperintense on T2W MR images and hypointense on T1W MR images. Typically, tuberculous abscesses are multiloculated, are larger than tuberculomas, and show ring-like enhancement.[26]

Differentiation of tuberculous abscess from pyogenic abscess is important for patient management. A recent study has shown that, with MR spectroscopy combined with MT imaging, it might be possible to distinguish these two entities.[27] In that study, all pyogenic brain abscesses had lipid and lactate peaks and amino acid peaks. Patients with tuberculous abscesses had only lipid and lactate levels. The MT ratio from the wall of the pyogenic abscess was significantly higher than that from the tuberculous abscess wall. In another series of 28 tuberculomas, lipid peaks were seen in 86% of the tuberculomas.[28] Large resonances of fatty acids at 1.3 ppm and 0.9 ppm, assigned to a methylene group, and the terminal methyl groups of fatty acids described in tuberculomas, are due to the high lipid content of caseous material.[27]

Focal Tuberculous Cerebritis

Focal tuberculous cerebritis is characterized by intense gyral enhancement on CT (Fig. 41-6).[29]

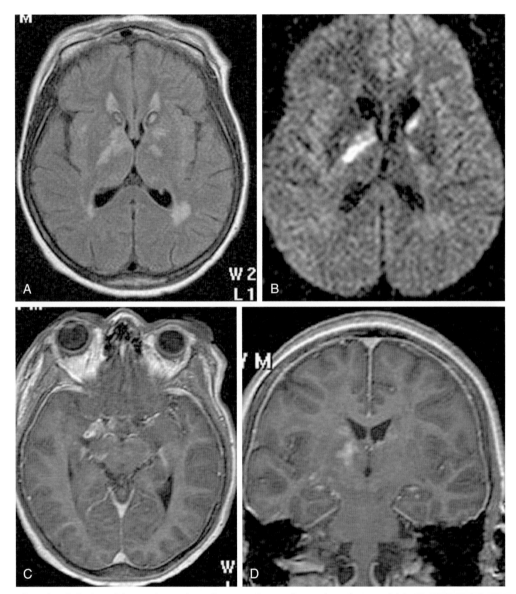

■ **FIGURE 41-4** Tuberculous infection of the CNS in a patient a few years after renal transplantation. **A,** Axial FLAIR-TSE MRI (TR/TE/TI 7385/130/2100) shows high signal intensity lesions in the basal ganglia. **B,** High signal on the trace DWI and corresponding low ADC values (not shown) suggest vascular lesions with cytotoxic edema. Contrast-enhanced T1W MRI (TR/TE/flip° 20/2.1/35°) in the axial (**C**) and coronal (**D**) planes shows ring-enhancing lesions in the basal cisterns (representing small tuberculomas in the subarachnoid space) and patchy enhancement in the right basal ganglia (subacute stage of small infarctions in the basal ganglia due to the spread of the tuberculous infection to the arteries).

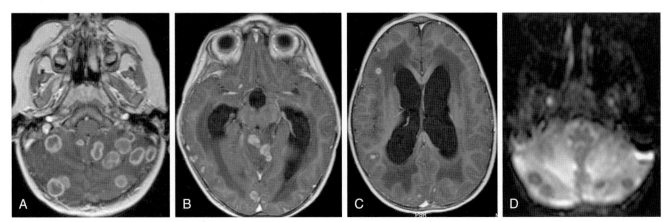

■ **FIGURE 41-5** Multiple CNS tuberculomas with obstructive hydrocephalus in a 3-year-old child. **A,** Axial FLAIR-FSE MRI (TR/TE/TI 7000/150/2100) shows edema surrounding multiple low signal intensity lesions in the cerebellum bilaterally. **B** and **C,** Contrast-enhanced T1W TSE MRI (TR/TE/flip° 20/4.6/25°) demonstrates ring enhancement of the posterior fossa lesions (**B**) but nodular enhancement of the supratentorial lesions (**C**). Dilatation of the ventricular system indicates obstructive hydrocephalus. **D,** Tuberculomas show low signal on axial trace DWI, indicating facilitated diffusion.

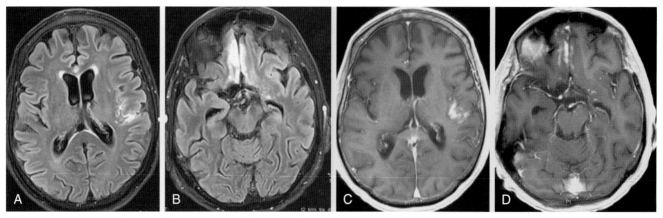

■ **FIGURE 41-6**   Tuberculous cerebritis in a 50-year-old man. Axial FLAIR-FSE MRI (TR/TE/TI 7000/150/2100) shows abnormal high signal intensity in the left parietal cortex (**A**) and bilateral frontal regions (**B**). **C** and **D**, Gyriform enhancement is observed on contrast-enhanced T1W TSE MRI (TR/TE/flip° 20/4.6/25°) MR images. CSF analysis confirmed the diagnosis of CNS tuberculosis.

Calvarial Tuberculosis

The presence of lytic lesions of the skull in a young individual in an endemic area suggests calvarial tuberculosis. Three types of tuberculous infection of the calvarial bones have been described on conventional radiography: perforating tuberculosis of the skull, diffuse tuberculosis of the cranium, and circumscribed sclerotic tuberculosis.[16] CT shows extracranial soft tissue swelling and bone destruction. Low density collection in the epidural space represents epidural granulation tissue. Rarely, MRI findings have been described in calvarial tuberculosis (Fig. 41-7). In one case report of calvarial tuberculosis, MRI showed evidence of extensive bilateral extradural granulations, bone destruction, and thrombosis of the anterior half of the superior sagittal sinus.[30]

CNS FUNGAL INFECTIONS
Cryptococcosis
Cryptococcosis is an infection caused by the saprophytic encapsulated yeast-like fungus *Cryptococcus neoformans*.

Epidemiology
According to the Centers for Disease Control and Prevention, 0.4 to 1.3 cases of cryptococcosis occur per 100,000 population per year in the United States. The infection rate is much higher in the AIDS population, with 2 to 7 cases per 1000 individuals per year. *Cryptococcus neoformans* is found in the droppings of wild birds, in eucalyptus trees, and in decaying wood that forms hollows in living trees. When dried bird droppings are stirred up, *Cryptococcus* disperses into the air and infects people who inhale the dust. CNS infection results from newly acquired infection that disseminates hematogenously from the primary site in the lung to the CNS. CNS cryptococcosis is the most common fungal infection in HIV-positive patients. Five to 10 percent of patients with AIDS develop CNS cryptococcosis. If left untreated, cryptococcal meningitis is fatal.

Clinical Presentation
The course of the infection is usually subacute or chronic. Most patients present with disseminated infection and signs of meningitis and meningoencephalitis, such as nausea, headache, dementia, irritability, confusion, and blurred vision.[31] Cases with no meningeal signs have been described.[32]

Pathophysiology
The CNS is a preferred site for cryptococcal infection, because soluble anti-cryptococcal factors present in serum are absent in cerebrospinal fluid.[33] The polysaccharide capsule of the cryptococcus hinders phagocytosis, impairs leukocyte migration, and does not release exotoxin. Therefore, the inflammatory response is minimal and little tissue necrosis will be present.

Cryptococcal meningitis is the most common manifestation of CNS cryptococcosis. The subarachnoid spaces become thickened and filled with multiple organisms and capsular material. Ependymal involvement causes occlusive hydrocephalus in approximately 50% of the cases. *Cryptococcus* extends along the Virchow-Robin perivascular spaces from the subarachnoid space into the basal ganglia, thalami, midbrain, and cerebellum.

The Virchow-Robin spaces become dilated, without involvement of the brain parenchyma. With disease progression, the dilated perivascular spaces become confluent and cystic lesions develop called "gelatinous pseudocysts," resembling soap bubbles. These lesions do not have a capsule and contain mucinous material and fungal organisms.

Cryptococcoma is the only parenchymal form of the cryptococcal CNS infection. The lesions result from the direct invasion of the brain by the fungus, with the development of a granulomatous reaction. One of the characteristic locations of cryptococcomas is the choroid plexus. Florid chorioid plexitis has been reported in an immunocompetent patient.

Pathology
In cryptococcal meningitis a grayish, mucinous exudate accumulates over the brain surface.

Cryptococcoma consists of a collection of fungi, inflammatory cells, and mucoid material.

Parenchymal lesions are most commonly found in the basal ganglia, the midbrain, the dentate nuclei of the cerebellum, and the choroid plexus.[34]

Imaging
Cryptococcal Meningitis
CT rarely shows meningeal enhancement. Contrast-enhanced T1W MR images demonstrate meningeal disease only in exceptional cases.[35]

Dilated Virchow-Robin Spaces
On MR images, widened perivascular spaces appear as multiple, bilateral, small round-to-oval lesions in the basal ganglia and midbrain. These show slightly higher signal than cerebrospinal fluid on T1W images and high signal on T2W images due to the mucoid material produced by the fungi (Fig. 41-8). Anatomically,

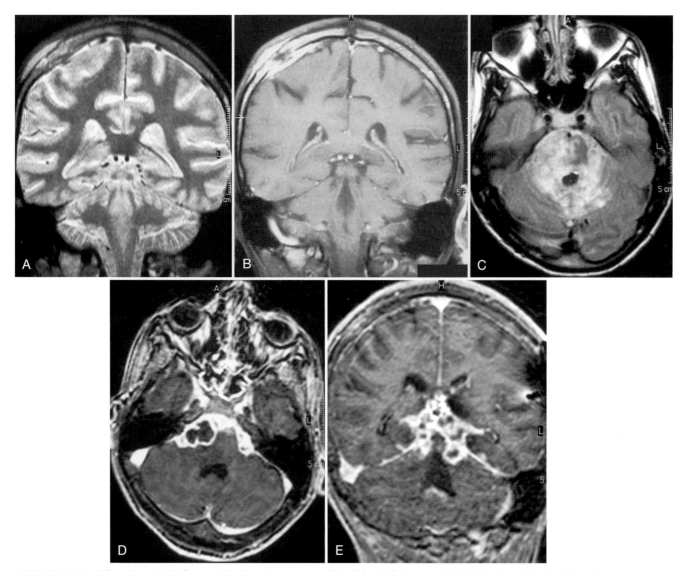

■ FIGURE 41-7 Tuberculous CNS infection with tuberculous osteomyelitis of the skull. **A,** Coronal STIR MRI shows high signal intensity in right parietal region. **B,** Contrast-enhanced T1W TSE MRI (TR/TE/flip° 20/4.6/25°) shows marked enhancement of the affected bone, scalp, and dura, with an epidural mass representing tuberculous osteomyelitis with extension of the infection to the soft tissue and the epidural space. Several months later, MRI showed abnormal signal (**C**) and marked meningeal enhancement (**D** and **E**), indicating tuberculous meningitis.

the perivascular spaces lie outside the brain, so there is no inflammatory response, no invasion of the brain parenchyma, and no contrast enhancement.

Gelatinous Pseudocysts
The MR appearance of gelatinous pseudocysts does not differ from dilated Virchow-Robin spaces. The mucinous material shortens the T1 relaxation time, so the lesions appear isointense to cortex. Enhancement and mass effect are absent (see Fig. 41-8).

Cryptococcoma
Cryptococcomas show low density on CT, low signal on T1W MR images, high signal on T2W MR images, higher signal than cerebrospinal fluid on FLAIR images, and a mosaic pattern on DWI (reflecting the inorganic structure of the lesion).[32] Contrast-enhanced studies usually demonstrate ring or nodular enhancement, which cannot be distinguished from granulomas of other origin (Fig. 41-9). One report describes calcification within a large ring-enhancing cryptococcoma.[36]

Aspergillosis
Aspergillosis is a group of diseases that includes invasive aspergillosis, allergic bronchopulmonary aspergillosis, and aspergilloma.

Epidemiology
Aspergillus species, especially *A. fumigatus*, are frequent pathogens in the CNS and account for 18% to 28% of all fungal brain abscesses. *Aspergillus* brain abscess is the most common CNS complication after bone marrow transplantation.[37] Aspergillosis has also been reported after cardiac, renal, and other organ transplantation, in acute leukemia, and in patients with glioblastoma multiforme who are on corticosteroid therapy.[38]

Clinical Presentation
Aspergillus infection of the CNS most commonly presents as headache, vomiting, convulsions, hemiparesis, cranial nerve deficits, paralysis, and sensory impairment of varying severity.[38] Patients are often afebrile or have only low-grade fever. Signs of meningeal disease and subarachnoid hemorrhage may signify a leaking mycotic aneurysm.

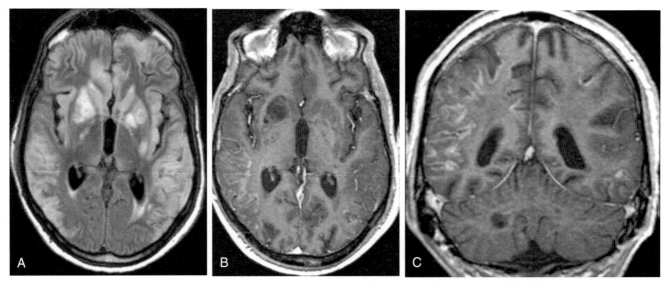

■ **FIGURE 41-8** *Cryptococcus neoformans* infection of the CNS in an HIV-positive individual. **A,** Axial FLAIR-FSE MRI (TR/TE/TI 7000/150/2100) shows high signal lesions in the basal ganglia bilaterally with swelling and hyperintensity of the cerebral cortex bilaterally. **B** and **C,** Axial and coronal contrast-enhanced T1W TSE MRI images (TR/TE/flip° 20/4.6/25°) shows nonenhancing, cystic lesions in the basal ganglia and right dentate nucleus, with linear enhancement of the affected cortex. The nonenhancing cystic lesions represent "gelatinous pseudocysts" filled with fungi and mucoid material. The cortical abnormalities represent cryptococcal meningoencephalitis.

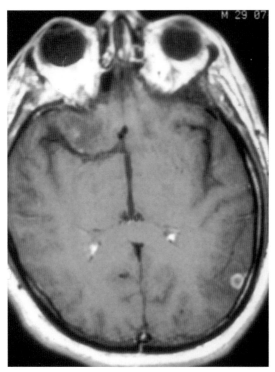

■ **FIGURE 41-9** Multiple cryptococcoma in an HIV-positive patient. Contrast-enhanced T1W SE MRI shows a ring-enhancing lesion in the left occipital cortex and a smaller nodular lesion in the right frontal region.

Pathophysiology

Cerebral aspergillosis is usually secondary to hematogenous spread from an extracerebral focus or contiguous spread from the paranasal sinuses. The infection may cause meningitis, abscess or granuloma, vascular invasion with thrombosis, infarction and hemorrhage, and aneurysm formation. The hyphal elements of *Aspergillus* are angioinvasive and penetrate the vessel walls to cause local thrombosis and infarction. Sterile infarctions become septic when the fungus erodes the wall of the vessel to extend into the brain parenchyma and cause inflammatory reaction and necrosis. Mycotic aneurysm is one of the most serious complications of fungal vasculitis.[39]

Pathology

Neuropathology discloses single or multiple abscesses, invasion of the blood vessels, and secondary thrombosis. Intracerebral aspergillomas show a central zone of hemorrhagic necrosis with sparse fungi.

Histologic sections of *Aspergillus* infection of the brain show hyphal forms of *Aspergillus* and parenchymal infiltration with vascular thrombosis due to fungal vascular invasion.

Aspergillus affects the lenticulostriate and thalamoperforate arteries, often leading to invasion of the basal ganglia, thalami and corpus callosum.

Imaging
CT

CT shows ring-enhancing lesions that are indistinguishable from other abscesses. Severely immunocompromised patients who are unable to mount an immune response may show ill-defined areas of low density with no enhancement.

MRI

MRI best displays the cerebral infarctions due to aspergillosis. T2W images usually show low signal centrally or peripherally due to blood breakdown products and accumulation of iron, magnesium, and manganese within the fungi (Figs. 41-10 and 41-11).[39,40] Low T2 signal is not specific for aspergillosis and may also be seen in tuberculomas, cysticercosis, and so on. In one series of 36 lesions, areas of low signal were seen centrally in 14 (39%) and peripherally in 8 (22%).[41] There is usually no contrast enhancement, owing to the patient's compromised immune state. Dietrich and colleagues observed faint enhancement in

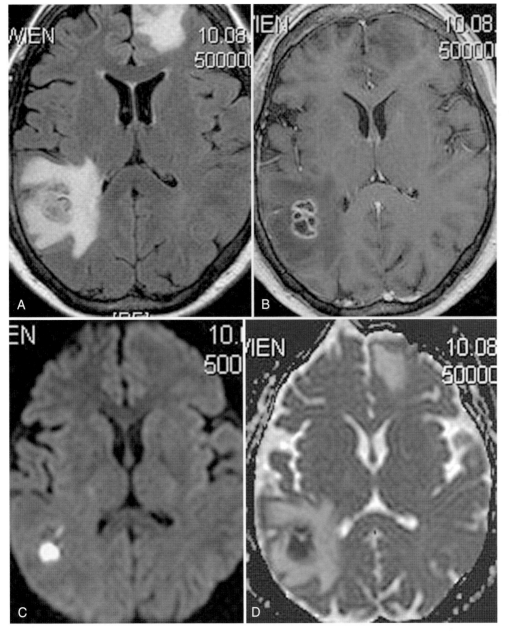

■ **FIGURE 41-10** *Aspergillus* infection of the CNS in a patient after bone marrow transplantation (BMT). **A,** Axial FLAIR-FSE MRI (TR/TE/TI 7000/150/2100) shows an inhomogeneously low signal intensity lesion with perifocal edema and a second lesion in the left frontal lobe. **B,** Contrast-enhanced T1W TSE MRI (TR/TE/flip° 20/4.6/25°) shows peripheral enhancement. **C** and **D,** The fungal abscess has restricted diffusion, with high signal on trace DWI MR image (**C**) and low signal on the ADC map (**D**).

■ **FIGURE 41-11** Cerebral aspergillosis in an immunocompromised patient. **A,** Axial T2W MRI shows multiple hyperintense lesions with central hypointensity in the left cerebral white matter, right parietal cortex, and occipital cortex. **B,** T1W MRI (TR/TE/flip° 20/4.6/25°) shows high signal intensities of subacute hemorrhage of the left lesion. The lesion in the right parietal cortex also shows a peripheral rim of hyperintensity. **C,** Contrast-enhanced T1W MRI (TR/TE/flip° 20/4.6/25°) shows ring- and nodular-enhancement of the fungal abscesses. **D,** Blood-sensitive MRI sequence clearly demonstrates multiple hemorrhagic lesions in cerebral aspergillosis. The imaging features of cortical and subcortical lesions, the hemorrhagic component, and the central, low signal on T2W imaging strongly suggest fungal cerebral infection.

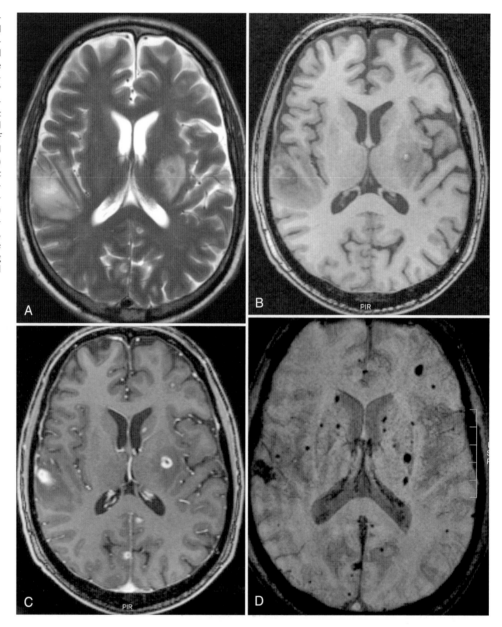

only 15 (42%) of 36 lesions in patients with bone marrow transplantation and cerebral aspergillosis.[41]

Gradient-echo T2*W imaging and diffusion-weighted images help to detect early hemorrhage and infarction from CNS aspergillosis (see Fig. 41-11).[42] DWI may also help to differentiate fungal from pyogenic brain abscesses (see Fig. 41-10).[43] On DWI, the signal from fungal abscess is usually inhomogeneous, whereas the signal from pyogenic abscesses is typically homogeneous. The ADC values of bacterial abscesses are usually lower (range: $0.11\text{-}0.76 \times 10^{-3}$ mm^2/s) than those measured in fungal lesions (range: $0.35\text{-}0.97 \times 10^{-3}$ mm^2/s),[43] perhaps owing to the lower cell density in fungal abscesses and, to a lesser extent, to the presence of hemorrhage. At present, no definitive ADC threshold is suggested for clinical use. In the appropriate clinical setting, imaging display of multiple lesions of the deep gray matter with heterogeneous appearance on T2W imaging and DWI should raise the suspicion of fungal infection of the CNS.

KEY POINTS: DIFFERENTIAL DIAGNOSIS

Syphilis
- Neurosyphilis must be ruled out in a young HIV-positive patient who presents with ischemic events, meningeal disease, and/or contrast-enhancing lesions of the cortex, even though symptomatic neurosyphilis is uncommon.
- In a young individual, foci of arterial narrowing and areas of infarction should be considered suggestive of lues.
- Ring-enhancing gummas are attached to the meningeal surface, whereas bacterial and fungal abscesses are usually located in the white matter or at the gray matter/white matter (corticomedullary) junction.

Nocardiosis
- Important clues to *Nocardia* infection are enhancing intraparenchymal lesions with additional subependymal nodules and evidence of meningitis.
- Renal transplant patients have increased risk for developing *Nocardia* infection.
- The coexistence of other infections, particularly parenchymal lesions of the lung, should indicate the possibility of a disseminated *Nocardia* infection.

CNS Tuberculosis
- Tuberculosis is common in HIV-positive patients.
- Tuberculous meningitis has a predilection for the basal regions of the brain.
- Tuberculomas commonly have low signal on T2W MR images (although low signal may also be present in fungal abscesses and lymphomas).
- Calvarial tuberculosis is characterized by soft tissue swelling and lytic bone lesions; the major differential diagnosis will be lymphoma of the scalp.
- Tuberculomas usually have low signal on DWI (see Fig. 41-5).

Cryptococcosis
- Bilateral nonenhancing cystic lesions isointense to CSF and located in the basal ganglia are highly suggestive of dilated Virchow-Robin spaces in cryptococcosis.
- Gelatinous pseudocysts are recognized as septated unencapsulated cystic lesions, which are commonly located in the basal ganglia, midbrain, and dentate nuclei of the cerebellum.
- Dilated Virchow-Robin spaces and gelatinous pseudocysts lie outside the brain parenchyma, so they do not show enhancement on CT or MRI.

Aspergillosis
- *Aspergillus* hyphae are angioinvasive and primarily cause sterile infarctions. These may subsequently become septic and necrotic.
- Ring-enhancing lesions show low signal centers on T2W images that are suggestive of fungal abscesses.
- In patients with bone marrow transplantation, aspergillosis will present as nonenhancing intracerebral lesions that are frequently hemorrhagic; the differential diagnosis should include toxoplasmosis.
- Fungal abscesses are usually smaller than bacterial abscesses and are commonly located in the gray matter (cortex and basal ganglia).
- Fungal abscesses show restricted diffusion (with high signal on DWI and low ADC values), but the signal is inhomogeneous compared with the typically homogeneous high signal seen in pyogenic abscesses.

SUGGESTED READINGS

Andreula CF, Burdi N, Carella A. CNS cryptococcosis in AIDS: spectrum of MR findings. J Comput Assist Tomogr 1993; 17:438-441.

Arbelaez A, Medina E, Restrepo F, Castillo M. Cerebral tuberculosis. Semin Roentgenol 2004; 39:474-481.

Centers for Disease Control and Prevention (CDC). Symptomatic early neurosyphilis among HIV-positive men who have sex with men—four cities, United States, January 2002-June 2004. MMWR Morb Mortal Wkly Rep 2007; 56:625-628.

Curry WA. Human nocardiosis: a clinical review with selected case reports. Arch Intern Med 1980; 140:818-826.

Dummer JS. Infections in solid organ transplant recipients. In Mandell GL, Bennett JE, Dolin R (eds). Principles and Practice of Infectious Diseases, 5th ed. Philadelphia, Churchill Livingstone, 2000, p 3155.

Gabelmann A, Klein S, Kern W, et al. Relevant imaging findings of cerebral aspergillosis on MRI: a retrospective case-based study in immunocompromised patients. Eur J Neurol 2007; 14:548-555.

Kiomehr F, Dadsetan MR, Rooholamini SA, et al. Central nervous system tuberculosis. Neuroradiology 1994; 36:93-96.

Popovich MJ, Arthur RH, Hemer E. CT of intracranial cryptococcosis. AJNR Am J Neuroradiol 1990; 11:139-142.

Thwaites GE, Tran TH. Tuberculous meningitis: many questions, too few answers. Lancet Neurol 2005; 4:160-170.

Tien RD, Chu PK, Hesslink JR, et al. Intracranial cryptococcosis in immunocompromised patients: CT and MR findings in 29 cases. AJNR Am J Neuroradiol 1991; 12:283-289.

Villoria FM, Fortea F, Moreno S, et al. MR imaging and CT of central nervous system tuberculosis in the patient with AIDS. Radiol Clin North Am 1995; 33:805-820.

Wehn SM, Heinz ER, Burger PC, Boyko OB. Dilated Virchow-Robin spaces in cryptococcal meningitis associated with AIDS: CT and MR findings. J Comput Assist Tomogr 1989; 13:756-762.

Yuh WTC, Nguyen HD, Gao F, et al. Brain parenchymal infection in bone marrow transplantation patients. CT and MR findings. AJR Am J Radiol 1994; 62:425-430.

Zetola NM, Klausner JD. Syphilis and HIV infection: an update. Clin Infect Dis 2007; 44:1222-1228.

REFERENCES

1. Katz DA, Berger JR, Duncan RC. Neurosyphilis, a comparative study of the effects of infection with human immunodeficiency virus. Arch Neurol 1993; 50:243-249.

2. Brightbill TC, Ihmeidan IH, Post MJ, et al. Neurosyphilis in HIV-positive and HIV-negative patients: neuroimaging findings. AJNR Am J Nuroradiol 1995; 16:703-711.

3. Peng F, Hua X, Zhongb X, et al. CT and MR findings in HIV-negative neurosyphilis. Eur J Radiol 2008; 66:1-6. Epub 2007; Jul 7.

4. Tien RD, Gean-Marton AD, Mark AS. Neurosyphilis in HIV carriers: MR findings in six patients. AJR Am J Radiol 1992; 158:1325-1328.

5. Holland BA, Perrett LV, Mills CM. Meningovascular syphilis: CT and MR findings. Radiology 1986; 158:439-442.

6. Parker JC Jr, Dyer MC. Neurological infection due to bacteria, fungi, parasites. In Davis RL, Robertson DM (eds). Textbook of Neuropathology. Baltimore, Williams Wilkins, 1985, pp 632-703.

7. Kim TK, Chang KH, Goo JM, et al. Intracranial tuberculoma: comparison of MR with pathologic findings. AJNR Am J Neuroradiol 1995; 16:1903-1908.

8. Uttamchandani RB, Daikos GL, Reyes RR, et al. Nocardiosis in 30 patients with advanced human immunodeficiency virus infection: clinical features and outcome. Clin Infect Dis 1994; 18:348-353.

9. Beaman BL, Beaman L: *Nocardia* species: host-parasite relationships. Clin Microbiol Rev 1994; 72:213.

10. Mamelak AN, Obana WG, Flaherty JF, Rosenblum ML. Nocardial brain abscess: treatment strategies and factors influencing outcome. Neurosurgery 1994; 35:622-631.

11. LeBlang SD, Whiteman ML, Post MJD, et al. CNS *Nocardia* in AIDS patients: CT and MRI with pathologic correlation. J Comput Assist Tomogr 1995; 19:15-22.

12. Shin JH, Lee HK. Nocardial brain abscess in a renal transplant recipient. Clin Imaging 2003; 27:321-324.

13. Soto-Hernandez JL, Moreno-Andrade T, Gongors-Rivera F, Ramirez-Crescencio MA. *Nocardia* abscess during treatment of brain toxoplasmosis in a patient with AIDS: utility of proton MR spectroscopy and diffusion-weighted imaging in diagnosis. Clin Neurol Neurosurg 2006; 108:493-498.

14. Moreno S, Baraia-Etxaburu J, Bouza E, et al. Risk for developing tuberculosis among anergic patients infected with HIV. Ann Intern Med 1993; 119:194-198.

15. Morgado C, Ruivo N. Imaging meningo-encephalitic tuberculosis. Eur J Radiol 2005;55:188-192.

16. Raut AA, Nagar AM, Muzumdar D, et al. Imaging features of calvarial tuberculosis: a study of 42 cases. AJNR Am J Neuroradiol 2004; 25:409-414.

17. Gupta RK, Gupta S, Singh D, et al. MR imaging and angiography in tuberculous meningitis. Neuroradiology 1994; 36:87-92.

18. Rovira M, Romero F, Torrent O, et al. Study of tuberculous meningitis by CT. Neuroradiology 1980; 19:137-141.

19. Villoria MF, de la Torre J, Fortea F, et al. Intracranial tuberculosis in AIDS: CT and MRI findings. Neuroradiology 1992; 34:11-14.

20. Tayfun C, Ücöz T, Tasar M, et al. Diagnostic value of MRI in tuberculous meningitis. Neuroradiology 1995; 6:380-386.

21. Whiteman M, Espinosa L, MJ, et al. Central nervous system tuberculosis in HIV-infected patients: clinical and radiographic findings. AJNR Am J Neuroradiol 1995; 16:1319-1327.

22. Welchman JM. Computerised tomography of intracranial tuberculomata. Clin Radiol 1979; 30:567-573.

23. Bargallo J, Berenguer J, Garcia-Barrionuevo J, et al. The "target-sign": is it a specific sign of CNS tuberculoma? Neuroradiology 1996; 38:547-550.

24. Sze G, Zimmerman RD. The magnetic resonance imaging of infection and inflammatory disease. Radiol Clin North Am 1988; 26:839-859.

25. Pui MH, Ahmad MN. Magnetization transfer imaging diagnosis of intracranial tuberculomas. Neuroradiology 2002; 44:210-215.

26. Yang PJ, Reger KM, Seeger JF, et al. Brain abscess: an atypical CT appearance of CNS tuberculosis. AJNR Am J Neuroradiol 1987; 8:919-920.

27. Gupta RK, Vatsal DK, Husain N, et al. Differentiation of tuberculous from pyogenic abscess with in vivo proton spectroscopy and magnetization transfer MR imaging. AJNR Am J Neuroradiol 2001; 22:1503-1509.

28. Jayasundar R, Singh VP, Raghunathan P, et al. Inflammatory granulomas: evaluation with proton MRS. NMR Biomed 1999; 12:139-144.

29. Jinkins JR. Focal tuberculous cerebritis. AJNR Am J Neuroradiol 1988; 9:121-124.

30. Sundaram PK, Sayed F. Superior sagittal sinus thrombosis caused by calvarial tuberculosis: case report. Neurosurgery 2007; 60:E776.

31. Berkefeld J, Enzensberger W, Lanferman H. *Cryptococcus* meningoencephalitis in AIDS: parenchymal and meningeal forms. Neuroradiology 1999; 41:129-133.

32. Awathi M, Patankar T, Shah P, Castillo M. Cerebral cryptococcosis: atypical appearances on CT. Br J Radiol 2001; 74:83-85.

33. Igel HJ, Bolande RP. Humoral defense mechanisms in cryptococcosis: substances in normal human serum, saliva and CSF affecting the growth of *Cryptococcus neoformans.* J Infect Dis 1966; 116:75.

34. Ruiz A, Post MJ, Bundschu CC. Dentate nuclei involvement in AIDS patients with CNS cryptococcosis: imaging findings with pathologic correlation. J Comput Assist Tomogr 1997; 21:175-182.

35. Arnder L, Castillo M, Heinz ER, et al. Unusual pattern of enhancement in cryptococcal meningitis: in vivo findings with postmortem correlation. J Comput Assist Tomogr 1996; 20:1023-1026.

36. Kamezawa T, Shimozuru T, Niiro M, et al. MRI demonstration of intracerebral cryptococcal granuloma. Neuroradiology 2000; 42:30-33.

37. Miaux Y, Ribaud P, Williams M, et al. MR of cerebral aspergillosis in patients who have had bone marrow transplantation. AJNR Am J Neuroradiol 1995; 16:555-562.

38. Nadkarni T, Goel A. Aspergilloma of the brain: an overview. J Postgrad Med 2005; 51:37-41.

39. Cox J, Murtagh FR, Wilfong A, et al. Cerebral aspergillosis: MR imaging and histopathologic correlation. AJNR Am J Neuroradiol 1992; 13:1489-1492.

40. Yamada K, Zoarski GH, Rothman MI, et al. An intracranial aspergilloma with low signal on T2-weighted images corresponding to iron accumulation. Neuroradiology 2000; 43:559-561.

41. Dietrich U, Hettmann M, Maschke M, et al. Cerebral aspergillosis: comparison of radiological and neuropathologic findings in patients with bone marrow transplantation. Eur Radiol 2001; 11:1242-1249.

42. Kami M, Shirouzu I, Mitani K, et al. Early diagnosis of central nervous system aspergillosis with combination use of cerebral diffusion-weighted echoplanar magnetic resonance image and polymerase chain reaction of cerebrospinal fluid. Intern Med 1999; 38:45-48.

43. Müller-Mang C, Castillo M, Mang TG, et al. Fungal versus bacterial brain abscesses: is diffusion-weighted MR imaging a useful tool in the differential diagnosis? Neuroradiology 2007; 49:651-657.

CHAPTER 42

Other Infections of the Brain

Majda M. Thurnher

ENCEPHALITIS

HIV Encephalitis

HIV encephalitis (HIVE) is direct infection of the brain with the human immunodeficiency virus (HIV). Alternate names include HIV-associated dementia (HAD) and HIV encephalopathy.

Epidemiology

Approximately 40 million people worldwide are infected with HIV. HIV-associated dementia (HAD) is now the most common cause of dementia worldwide among people aged 40 years or younger. Potent antiretroviral therapies have now reduced the incidence of HAD to as low as 10.5%.[1] Combinations of antiretroviral substances have been shown to increase the $CD4^+$ lymphocyte count and to decrease viral replication in plasma and lymph nodes to undetectable levels.

Clinical Presentation

HIV infection may lead to motor and cognitive deficits. The motor symptoms are usually mild and may manifest as a slowing of repetitive movements or difficulty with balance. Disabling HIV dementia presents as a slow decline in a patient's cognitive abilities with a characteristic triad of cognitive, behavioral, and motor dysfunctions.[2] Nearly 50% of HIV patients in the United States demonstrate neuropsychological testing performance that is below expectations compared to matched normative groups. HIV-associated neurocognitive disorders (HAND) can be subclassified into asymptomatic neurocognitive impairment (ANI), mild cognitive disorder (MND), and HIV-associated dementia (HAD).

Pathophysiology

HIV enters the central nervous system (CNS) early in the course of infection, possibly by using a cloak of human proteins to sneak into the cells (Trojan horse "stealth entry").[3] The brain then serves as an important reservoir for autonomous, self-sustaining, and persistent infection. Within the brain the virus resides primarily within microglia and macrophages.[4]

Pathology

Two neuropathologic consequences of cerebral HIV infection are multinucleated giant cell encephalitis (MGCE) and progressive diffuse leukoencephalopathy (PDL).[5] MGCE and PDL may be two ends of a broad spectrum of morphologic changes induced by HIV. MGCE is characterized by perivascular accumulation of inflammatory cells, predominantly microglia cells, monohistiocytes, and macrophages. In PDL, diffuse loss of myelin and axons with reactive astrocytosis and distinctive multinucleated giant cells are seen in the deep white matter.[5] New variants of HIVE have been reported recently, including severe leukoencephalopathy with intense perivascular macrophage and lymphocyte infiltration and chronic "burnt out" forms of HIVE.

The highest concentrations of HIV are found in the basal ganglia (especially the globus pallidus), subcortical regions, and frontal cortices.

Imaging

CT

The most common CT finding in HAD is *cerebral atrophy,* which may be central, peripheral, or mixed.[6,7] An early CT study of 200 patients reported that 37.5% of AIDS patients present with cerebral atrophy.[8] Other CT studies of HAD show progression of the atrophy over time. Cortical atrophy is found in 85% of symptomatic patients, suggesting that cortical atrophy may be relatively specific to patients with neuropsychological impairment. CT may also show hypodensities in the white matter bilaterally (Fig. 42-1).

MRI

MRI has documented reduction of gray matter volume in the basal ganglia and posterior cortex and generalized loss of volume in the white matter.[9]

White matter lesions are found in about 80% of HAD patients (range: 43%-100%) and usually assume any of four patterns: diffuse, patchy, focal, and punctiate.[10] These lesions are usually isointense or minimally hypointense on T1-weighted (T1W) imaging, have high signal on T2-weighted (T2W) imaging, and show no mass effect or enhancement (see Fig. 42-1). Two distinct patterns are observed on T2W imaging: (1) diffuse bilateral symmetrical high signal intensity in the white matter appears to represent HIV encephalopathy (see Fig. 42-1) and (2) patchy bilateral lesions with high T2 signal intensity in the gray and white matter appear to represent HIV encephalitis.[10] High signal intensity lesions may also be seen in the splenium of the corpus callosum and in the crura of the fornices.[11] Long-term studies show progressive increase in the white matter lesions with disease progression.[12-14] Fluid-attenuated inversion recovery (FLAIR) sequences are superior to T2W images for detection of

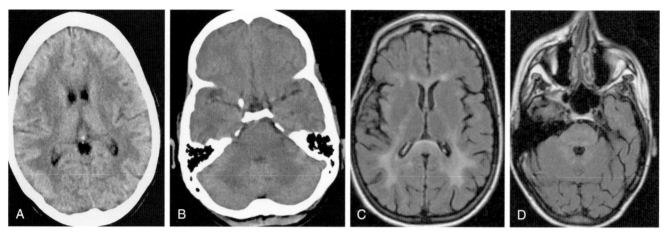

■ **FIGURE 42-1** HIV encephalopathy. This young HIV-positive patient had a high viral load level in the plasma and the CSF and a low CD4⁺ T lymphocyte count. **A** and **B,** Noncontrast CT scans show bilateral hypodensity in the white matter and in the posterior fossa. No enhancement was present on postcontrast scans (not shown). **C** and **D,** Axial FLAIR-TSE MRI (TR/TE/TI 7385/130/2100) scans show bilateral, symmetric high signal intensity abnormalities in the periventricular white matter (**C**) and brain stem (**D**). Enlarged ventricles and sulci are noted. Neuropsychological examinations were consistent with subcortical dementia.

white matter lesions, especially in periventricular and subcortical locations.[15] ¹H MR spectroscopy (MRS) is being used increasingly to detect early CNS involvement by HIV. Decreased N-acetyl-aspartate (NAA) and elevated choline (Cho) and myo-inositol (MI) levels (lower NAA/creatine [Cr] ratio, increased Cho/Cr ratio, increased MI/Cr ratio) in the basal ganglia or frontal white matter are seen in early HIV infection of the brain.[16] In HAD patients, perfusion MRI shows a statistically significant decrease in regional cerebral blood flow (rCBF) in the inferior lateral frontal cortices bilaterally with an increase in rCBF in the posteroinferior parietal white matter bilaterally.[17]

MRI and MRS have now been used in the clinical management of patients with HAD who are receiving potent antiretroviral therapy.[18-20] A combination of antiretroviral drugs in patients with HAD may result in stabilization or even regression of white matter signal intensity abnormalities observed on MR images.[19,20] The progression of white matter lesions on initial follow-up studies is likely the result of postinflammatory reactions due to immune reconstitutive effects after the initiation of highly active antiretroviral therapy (HAART).[20,21] Despite potent therapies, the neuronal damage appears to progress without clinical manifestations and the progression of cerebral atrophy is apparent on MR images.[20]

Progressive Multifocal Leukoencephalopathy
Progressive multifocal leukoencephalopathy (PML) is a subacute opportunistic infection caused by the JC polyomavirus (JCV, hence the name JCV infection).

Epidemiology
The JC virus was isolated in 1971 and named for the first patient in whom this virus was isolated.[22] Approximately 5% (0.7%-11%) of HIV patients will develop PML during the course of their illness.[23,24] PML may also occur in immunosuppressed patients with malignant diseases. Two cases of PML have been described recently in patients with multiple sclerosis who were treated with the α₄-integrin inhibitor natalizumab.[25]

Clinical Presentation
Common manifestations of PML include weakness, gait abnormalities, speech disturbance, cognitive disorders, headache, and visual impairment. Without treatment, the prognosis for PML is usually poor, with death occurring after 2.5 to 4 months. Only a small number of cases (7%-9%) have been reported to have a more benign clinical course with prolonged survival (>12

months) and associated improvement in clinical and radiographic abnormalities in the absence of specific therapy. About half the AIDS patients with PML will not experience benefit from HAART. However, PML can also develop in AIDS patients who are undergoing HAART.[26]

Pathophysiology
After initial infection, the JCV persists in the renal tubular epithelial cells. With reactivation of latent JCV in the kidneys and subsequent viremia, the JCV enters the brain and causes PML. JCV attacks the oligodendrocytes and causes their destruction and myelin loss.

Pathology
Demyelinated areas are recognized as discolorations of the white matter.

The histopathologic hallmark of PML is demyelination with enlarged oligodendroglial nuclei and bizarre astrocytes.[27] The central portion of the lesion is characterized by an almost total breakdown of the myelin sheath and by axonal damage, with an increase in the extracellular space; the most medial area of lesion development consists of oligodendrocytes with nuclear inclusions and partially destroyed myelin, with a relative sparing of axons.

PML is usually multifocal, and the lesions may occur in any location in the white matter, thalamus, brain stem, and cerebellum. In rare cases, PML may be limited to the posterior fossa.[28]

Imaging
CT
On CT, PML lesions are recognized as multifocal hypodense lesions without mass effect or enhancement (Fig. 42-2).

MRI
On T2W MR images, PML lesions are patchy, scalloped, high signal intensity white matter lesions with extension along the white fibers (Fig. 42-3).[24,28] Subcortical arcuate fibers are involved, mass effect is mild or absent, and peripheral, faint enhancement is a rare feature.[29-31] On T1W images, the PML lesions are markedly hypointense.[24,28] Magnetization transfer ratios (MTRs) can be used to differentiate between PML and lesions in HAD. The mean MTR value of PML lesions is significantly lower than that of HAD lesions (26.1% vs. 47.9%).[32] On DWI, different signal behavior between the lesion center and the extending margin has been observed (Fig. 42-4).[33] On apparent diffusion

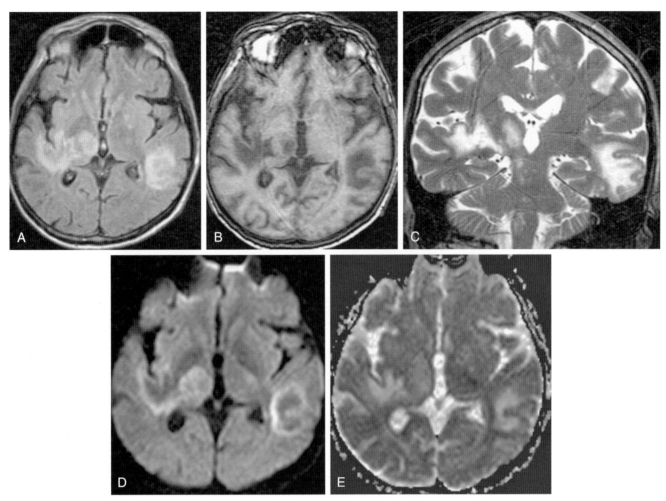

■ **FIGURE 42-2** Progressive multifocal leukoencephalopathy (PML). This AIDS patient presented to the emergency department with impaired consciousness. **A,** Axial FLAIR MRI (TR/TE/TI 6000/100/2000) shows multiple, scalloped, high signal intensity lesions in both cerebral hemispheres and in the right thalamus. **B,** On noncontrast T1W TFE MRI (TR/TE/flip° 20/2.1/35°), the lesions have markedly low signal. **C,** Coronal T2W MRI shows the scalloped pattern of the lesions caused by involvement of the arcuate subcortical "U fibers." **D** and **E,** Trace DWI images (**D**) and ADC map (**E**) show that the lesions have low signal centers with high signal margins (**D**), indicating elevated diffusivity in demyelinated PML lesions and cytotoxic edema along the active margins.

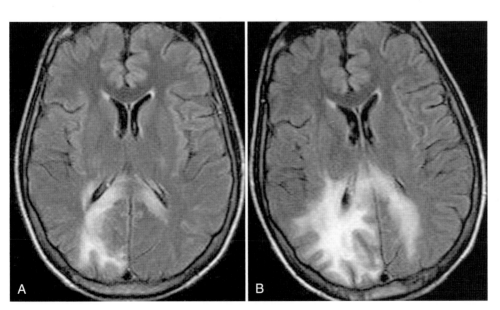

■ **FIGURE 42-3** Progressive multifocal leukoencephalopathy (PML). This HIV-positive patient did not respond well to highly active antiretroviral therapy (HAART). **A,** Axial FLAIR MRI (TR/TE/TI 6000/100/2000) shows scalloped high signal intensity lesions in the right occipital lobe with extension into the corpus callosum. PML was diagnosed with positive polymerase chain reaction for JC virus in the CSF, and HAART was initiated. **B,** Follow-up MR examination 6 weeks after HAART showed worsening of the abnormal signal intensity. The patient died 4 months after the initial diagnosis.

■ **FIGURE 42-4** Progressive multifocal leukoencephalopathy (PML) in an AIDS patient. The initial noncontrast (**A**) and contrast-enhanced CT scans (**B**) show multiple, scalloped, hypodense, nonenhancing lesions in the temporal lobes and left frontal lobe. **C,** FLAIR-TSE MRI (TR/TE/TI 7373/130/2100) shows abnormal high signal intensity in the left hemisphere, with no mass effect. (**D**) The T1W TFE MRI (TR/TE/flip° 10/3.5/10°) shows a low signal lesion with no enhancement. The CSF gave a positive polymerase chain reaction for JC virus.

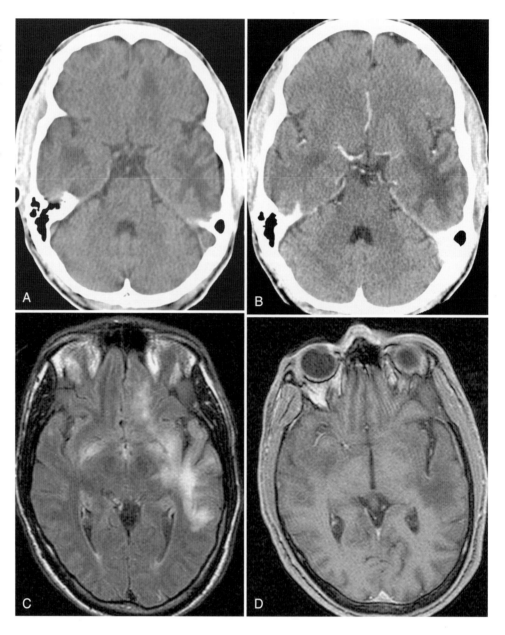

coefficient (ADC) maps, signal intensity was elevated in the central area, whereas at the lesion margins two areas were distinguished: (1) a newer portion, with reduced water diffusibility compatible with cytotoxic edema and (2) less recent portions with intermediate values.[33]

The ^{1}H spectra of PML lesions are characterized by significantly reduced NAA, lactate presence, and increased choline and lipids.[34,35] A decrease in NAA is the result of axonal loss, and the presence of lactate is related to cellular hypoxia. The increase in choline and lipid may reflect an accumulation of myelin breakdown products.

Although at present there is no specific therapy for PML, recent studies have shown clinical and radiologic improvement in patients with PML who underwent HAART.[36-38] In patients with prolonged survival regression or stabilization, MRI findings paralleled the suppression of virus replication and immune response recovery. Worsening of the MRI findings, with development of contrast enhancement, mass effect, and edema may be seen in some patients.[39] This phenomenon is known as immune reconstitution syndrome (IRIS) and is the result of a post-treatment inflammatory reaction due to the immune reconstitutive

effect. Atrophic changes and increased hypointensity on T1W images with concomitant low signal on FLAIR images in these patients represent leukomalacia and burnt-out PML lesions.

Cytomegalovirus Infection

This infection is caused by cytomegalovirus (CMV), a member of the herpesvirus family.

Epidemiology

According to published studies, 40% to 100% of the general population are infected with CMV. CMV infections have been described with increasing frequency in patients with AIDS, with up to 30% of patients showing neuropathologic evidence of CMV infection.[40] The incidence has decreased by more than 80% since the introduction of HAART.[41]

Clinical Presentation

Five distinct neurologic syndromes due to CMV infection have been described: retinitis, myelitis/polyradiculopathy, diffuse micronodular encephalitis, ventriculoencephalitis, and mononeuritis multiplex. In CMV infection, meningoencephalitis presents as fever, confusion, headache, and progressive dementia. Patients with ventriculoencephalitis have a more acute onset, with death usually occurring quickly. The infection of the CNS is difficult to diagnose while the patient is alive because CMV is difficult to culture from the cerebrospinal fluid (CSF). The recent development of the polymerase chain reaction technique has allowed isolation of CMV based on the presence of DNA within the CSF.[42]

Pathophysiology

CMV exists in latent form in about 90% of adults. CMV is a member of the herpesvirus family, and the infection in adults is a result of the reactivation of a latent infection, most commonly presenting as a mild infection that mimics mononucleosis. In immunocompromised patients CMV can produce a variety of clinical syndromes.

Pathology

Enlarged cells with distended nuclei that contain viral inclusions called "owl's eyes" are a pathologic hallmark of CMV encephalitis. Diffuse micronodular CMV encephalitis resembles HIV encephalitis histologically. Small microglial nodules and inclusion-bearing cytomegalic cells are widely distributed in the cortex, basal ganglia, brain stem, and cerebellum. In an autopsy series of 30 cases of CMV encephalitis, 76% of the patients had microglial nodules containing inclusion-bearing cells and 24% had CMV inclusions outside the nodules.[43] In ventriculoencephalitis, periventriculitis, and ependymal and subependymal necrosis, inclusion-bearing CMV cells are observed.[44]

Imaging
CT

Generalized atrophy is the most commonly reported CT abnormality, but it is a nonspecific finding often seen in AIDS patients.[45]

MRI

The most common imaging findings in patients with CMV encephalitis are cortical atrophy, periventricular enhancement, and diffuse white matter abnormalities.[45] Periventricular enhancement is not pathognomonic; it has been described in cases of lymphoma, toxoplasmosis, and other infections. White matter disease occurs as a result of inflammation of subependymal region and spread of the infection to the adjacent astrocytes of the white matter with infectious demyelination.[46,47] In six patients with pathologically confirmed CMV infection of the CNS, Hassine and associates found atrophy in three patients, subependymal nodular lesions without enhancement in two patients, and ventriculitis in one patient.[48]

Rarely, cerebral mass lesions due to CMV could be observed in AIDS patients. In one study, two cases of cerebral mass lesions due to CMV were described.[49] In both cases, a large contrast-enhancing mass was seen in the frontal lobe, with surrounding edema. CMV infection can also be present as *choroid plexitis*. In one reported case, a contrast-enhanced CT scan showed marked enhancement of the slightly enlarged right plexus. MRI confirmed the findings and the absence of enhancement of the ependyma.[50] The discrimination between HIV and CMV-associated CNS disease is often difficult using clinical and imaging findings. MRS could be potentially useful in such cases. In one study, MRS was used to distinguish HIV encephalitis from CMV encephalitis.[51] The findings suggest that a larger choline signal and a smaller NAA signal could be inferred within the white matter abnormalities due to HIV encephalitis/encephalopathy compared with CMV encephalitis.

Prion Diseases

Prion diseases are rare progressive neurodegenerative disorders that affect both humans and animals and are caused by prions.

They occur in humans as the various forms of Creutzfeldt-Jakob disease (sporadic [sCJD]; familial [fCJD], or variant [vCJD]), Gerstmann-Sträussler-Scheinker disease (GSS), fatal familial insomnia, and kuru. Another name for these diseases is transmissible spongiform encephalopathies (TSEs).

Epidemiology

Prion diseases are rare, with fewer than 2 per million individuals affected per year.[52] The elderly population is most commonly affected, with a peak incidence between 60 and 64 years of age. Prion diseases have also been demonstrated in young individuals.[53] The sporadic form of CJD seems to affect females more often than men (ratio: 2:1).[54,55] The majority of cases of CJD (about 85%) occur as sporadic disease, and a smaller proportion of patients (5%-15%) develop CJD because of inherited mutations of the prion protein gene. These inherited forms include Gerstmann-Sträussler-Scheinker syndrome and fatal familial insomnia.

Clinical Presentation

The sporadic form of CJD is characterized by rapidly progressive dementia. The patients suffer from myoclonic movements and both pyramidal (Babinski sign) and extrapyramidal symptoms (rigor, akinesia, choreatic movements).[56] Isolated cerebellar symptoms as early manifestations occur in only 5%.[55] The clinical features of vCJD include younger age at onset of disease and longer disease duration. Periodic sharp waves will be detected on electroencephalograms in cases of sCJD and will often be absent in vCJD cases. Common symptoms and signs in fatal familial insomnia include intractable insomnia, dysfunction of the autonomic system (hyperthermia, hypertension, tachycardia, tachypnea, hyperhidrosis), dementia, and motor paralysis.

Brain biopsy or autopsy is required to confirm the diagnosis. The detection of 14-3-3 protein in the CSF, an elevated concentration of neuron-specific enolase (NSE), and periodic sharp wave complexes on an electroencephalogram, along with clinical signs, usually allow for a probable diagnosis while the patient is still alive.[57-59]

Pathophysiology

A combination of various mechanisms leads to neuronal death in prion diseases, and the mechanism is still not completely understood. Fatal familial insomnia is a rare, autosomal dominant, inherited brain disease caused by a mutation in a protein called the prion protein (PrP).

Pathology
sCJD

The neuropathologic hallmark of sCJD is the highly disease-specific spongiform change in brain tissue accompanied by neuronal loss and astrogliosis and microgliosis. Spongiform changes are characterized by diffuse or focally clustered small round or oval vacuoles in the neuropil of the deep cortical layers, cerebellar cortex, or subcortical gray matter, which might become confluent.[60]

vCJD

The florid plaque is a neuropathologic hallmark of vCJD.[61] Widespread accumulation of PrP(res) will be detected on immunocytochemistry. Spongiform changes are most marked in the basal ganglia, whereas the thalamus exhibits severe neuronal loss and gliosis in the posterior nuclei.[61]

Fatal Familial Insomnia

In fatal familial insomnia, amyloid plaques are found in the thalamus and spongiotic changes are evident in the cortical areas. There is atrophy of the thalamus (with the mediodorsal and anterior ventral areas being more affected), and, with

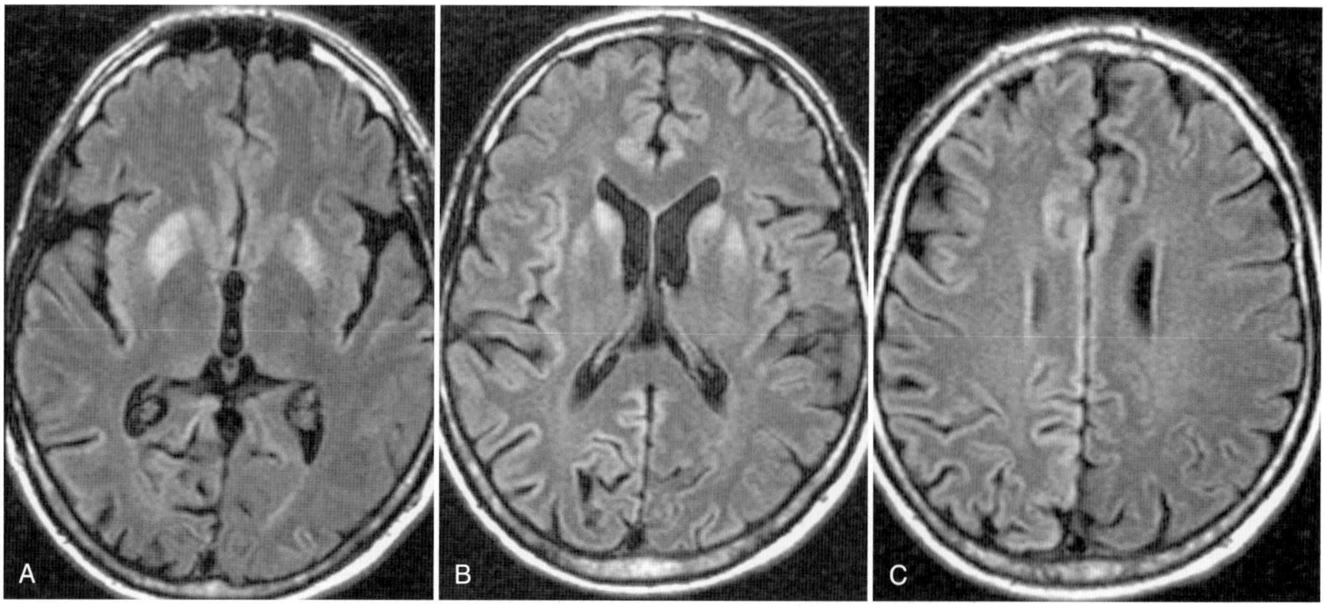

■ **FIGURE 42-5** Autopsy-proven Creutzfeldt-Jakob disease in a 50-year-old man. **A** to **C,** Axial FLAIR-TSE MRI (TR/TE/TI 7373/130/2100) shows abnormal high signal intensities in the region of the basal ganglia and in the left frontal and parietal cortex.

involvement of inferior olive, isolated cortical foci of spongiosis are present.

Imaging
MRI
sCJD
Typical MRI findings in sCJD are hyperintensity on T2W and FLAIR images in the cortex and basal ganglia (Fig. 42-5). Increased signal on diffusion-weighted imaging (DWI) and a low apparent diffusion coefficient (ADC) in the basal ganglia and cerebral cortex are also common.[62] These findings are more frequently seen in the head of the caudate nuclei, the putamen, the thalamus, the striatum, and the cortical gray matter. It has been speculated that the increased signal on DWI is related to decreased water diffusion by the spongiform changes. A decrease in NAA and elevation of MI have been demonstrated in the frontal white matter in a patient with fCJD and in the parietal and frontal white matter in a case of sCJD using a short echo time and a single-voxel technique.[63,64] Metabolic abnormalities have also been demonstrated in the pulvinar of the thalamus, with decreased NAA and significantly increased MI in vCJD.[65,66]

fCJD
MRI findings are quite variable but seem similar to those in sCJD, with signal abnormalities on T2W, FLAIR, and DWI in gray matter structures, such as the basal ganglia, the insula, and the cerebral cortex. Hyperintensity lesions on T1W imaging in the globus pallidus have also been reported both in fCJD and also in a case of sCJD.[67]

vCJD
The characteristic MRI abnormality in vCJD is hyperintensity on T2W sequences in the pulvinar nuclei, called the "pulvinar sign."[68] MRS findings in vCJD are characterized by marked metabolic changes in the thalamus, decreased NAA, and increased MI, reflecting the pattern of gray matter signal abnormalities seen on T2W and FLAIR images.[65,69]

Gerstmann-Sträussler-Scheinker Disease
In a patient with GSS, a reduced NAA/Cr ratio was found in the frontal cortex, the putamen, the cerebellar vermis, and in both hemispheres.[69]

Fatal Familial Insomnia
In fatal familial insomnia CT and MRI are normal or show nonspecific findings.

PET
In fatal familial insomnia, PET shows pronounced thalamic and limbic hypometabolism that becomes more widespread in the later stages of the disease.

Rasmussen's Encephalitis
Rasmussen's encephalitis is an inflammatory/autoimmunologic, unilateral, cortical inflammation with tissue destruction.

Epidemiology
Rasmussen's encephalitis is primarily a disease of childhood. In 80% of cases, patients are in the first decade of life. This disease has been also described in adults with minor variations.

Clinical Presentation
Patients frequently have episodes of epilepsia partialis continua and, much less frequently, generalized status epilepticus. The seizures are intractable despite aggressive medical management. Patients demonstrate a progressive motor deficit and mental deterioration that occur over several years. Most individuals with Rasmussen's encephalitis will experience frequent seizures and brain damage over the course of the first 8 to 12 months and then enter a phase of permanent, but stable, neurologic deficits. On electroencephalography, persistent temporal delta activity is observed early on, with multifocal spikes and background slowing later with disease progression. The outcome is much worse in adults than in children.[70]

Pathophysiology
The cause of Rasmussen's encephalitis is not yet clarified. A viral origin (CMV, slow virus, Epstein-Barr virus) has been discussed. There is convincing evidence that, in most patients, Rasmussen's encephalitis is an autoimmune disorder. In most patients it is not clear what triggers the abnormal immune response, although sometimes Rasmussen's encephalitis has occurred after an otherwise minor bacterial or viral infection or head injury.

Pathology

An atrophic hippocampus and an enlarged perisylvian cortical area will be seen on pathologic examination.

According to the latest pathologic reports, Rasmussen's encephalitis is the result of an autoimmune process with astrocytes as the primary target.[71] A specific feature is astrocytic apoptosis and subsequent loss of astrocytes. In addition, proliferation of microglia, neuronal degeneration, and marked perivascular lymphocytic infiltration are present.

Imaging

CT

A low attenuation area with local swelling is seen on precontrast CT scans in the temporal lobe. On follow-up CT, atrophic changes in the same area are observed.

MRI

On T2W sequences, high signal intensity abnormality and volume expansion will be seen in the cortex of the temporal or parietal lobe (Fig. 42-6). In the terminal stage, MRI shows destruction of the involved area with unilateral ventricular enlargement.

On MRS, decreased concentrations of NAA, indicative of neuronal loss, as well as increased MI, are detected in the atrophic cortex.

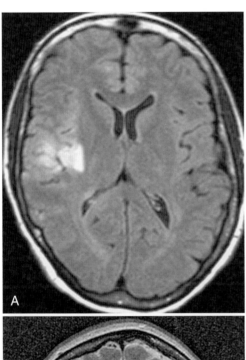

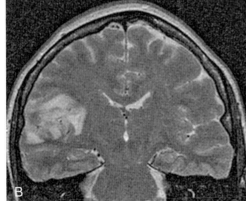

■ **FIGURE 42-6** Suspected Rasmussen's encephalitis. This 27-year-old woman presented with seizures. Axial FLAIR (**A**) and coronal T2W (**B**) MR images show abnormal high signal intensity affecting the cortex and underlying white matter of the right parietal region.

Herpes Simplex Encephalitis

Herpes simplex encephalitis (HSE) is a life-threatening disease caused by herpes simplex virus (HSV) infection of the CNS.

Epidemiology

HSE occurs as two distinct entities. In infants, children, and adults, HSE is caused by herpes simplex virus type 1 (HSV-1) and typically involves the temporal and frontal lobes. In neonates, brain involvement is more often diffuse and the usual cause is herpes simplex virus type 2 (HSV-2), which is acquired at the time of delivery.

HSE caused by HSV-1 is the most common cause of sporadic lethal encephalitis, which occurs in about 1 person per 250,000 to 500,000 population per year. In AIDS patients, the estimated frequency of HSV-1 infection is only 2% of autopsy cases.[72] In the absence of therapy, mortality exceeds 70% and prognosis is poor because only a minority of individuals return to normal function.

Clinical Presentation

The typical clinical presentation of HSE is acute onset of severe focal neurologic deficits, confusion, and seizures, with systemic signs of infection. Recurrent brain stem encephalitis associated with HSV has also been described.

Pathophysiology

Brain infection is a result of reactivation of latent infection by direct neuronal transmission of the virus from a peripheral site to the brain via the trigeminal or olfactory nerve.

Pathology

In immunocompetent patients, the infection usually results in necrosis of the temporal lobe and orbital surfaces of the frontal gyri, with sparing of the basal ganglia.

In sporadic HSE, the infection typically affects the temporal lobes, the orbital surfaces of the frontal lobes, the hippocampus, and the insular cortex. The cingulate gyrus and the posterior occipital cortex may be involved later with disease progression. The basal ganglia are usually not involved. In HIV-positive patients, the white matter may be predominantly involved, with sparing of the hippocampal region.

Imaging

CT

CT studies are frequently negative in the early stages of HSE. With disease progression (after 3-5 days), areas of low attenuation may be detected in the temporal lobes.[73]

MRI

The majority of patients with HSE will show signal abnormalities on scans, but normal MRI results have been reported in approximately 10% of polymerase chain reaction–positive patients who have HSE. On MRI, high signal intensity lesions will be observed on T2W images, with low signal on T1W images (Fig. 42-7). The FLAIR technique has been reported to be even more sensitive than T2W imaging in the detection of abnormalities due to HSV-1 infection, with the earliest imaging findings 48 hours after the onset of symptoms (see Fig. 42-7). Early on, enhancement is usually not apparent and gyriform enhancement on enhanced T1W images can be observed with disease progression (Fig. 42-8).[74] T2*W gradient-echo images may show a signal decrease caused by the magnetic susceptibility effect of hemoglobin degradation, suggesting a hemorrhagic component.

Magnetization transfer suppression techniques, after the administration of a contrast agent, have been shown to improve the detection of abnormalities associated with HSV-1 infection of the brain.[75] Enhanced T1W sequences with magnetization

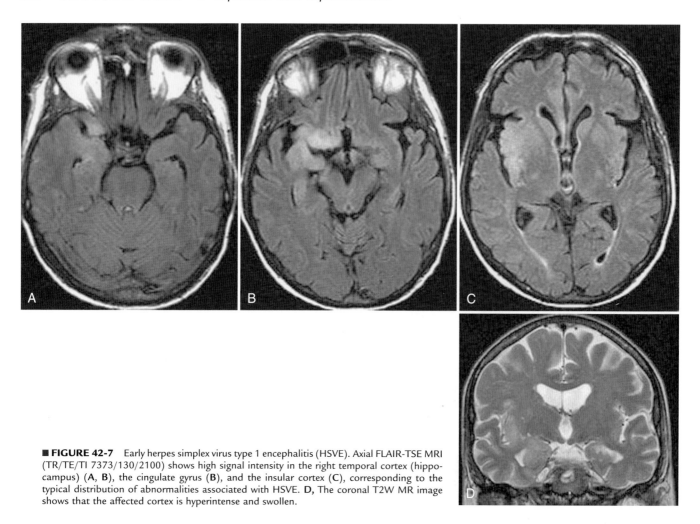

■ FIGURE 42-7 Early herpes simplex virus type 1 encephalitis (HSVE). Axial FLAIR-TSE MRI (TR/TE/TI 7373/130/2100) shows high signal intensity in the right temporal cortex (hippocampus) (**A, B**), the cingulate gyrus (**B**), and the insular cortex (**C**), corresponding to the typical distribution of abnormalities associated with HSVE. **D,** The coronal T2W MR image shows that the affected cortex is hyperintense and swollen.

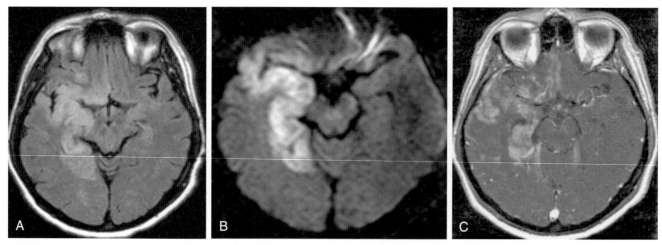

■ FIGURE 42-8 Subacute stage of extensive HSVE. **A,** Axial FLAIR-TSE MRI shows extensive high signal abnormalities in the right temporal lobe, right frontal lobe, and insula. **B,** Trace DWI also shows high signal, indicating restricted diffusion and cytotoxic edema. **C,** The postcontrast T1W MRI shows marked contrast enhancement.

transfer contrast revealed a greater degree of disease involvement than was apparent on the T2W image or on T1W imaging without magnetization transfer contrast (see Fig. 42-8).[75] This technique may be helpful in patients with a problematic diagnosis and atypical imaging findings. On DWI, two distinct types of findings are characteristic of HSV-1 encephalitis: lesions similar to cytotoxic edema and lesions similar to vasogenic edema (see Figs. 42-8 and 42-9).[76-79] The severity of the disease correlated well with the DWI findings in one study; the patients with lesions similar to cytotoxic edema had fulminating disease, whereas the others, with lesions similar to vasogenic edema, had a good outcome.

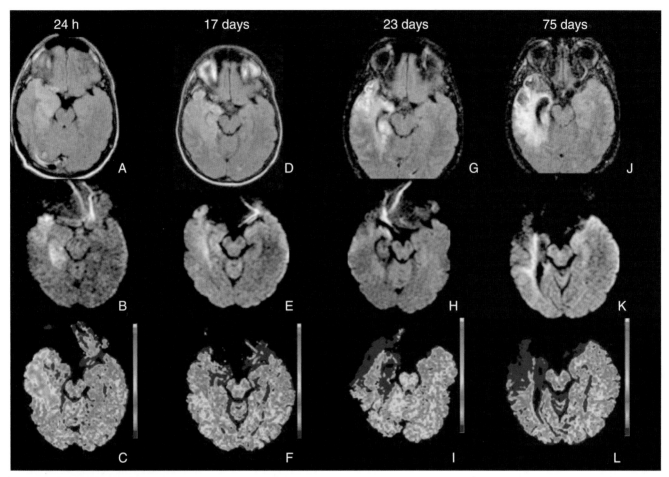

■ FIGURE 42-9 Initial and follow-up conventional MR sequences and DWI in a patient with HSVE. Initial MRI, performed 24 hours after the onset of symptoms, shows abnormal high signal in the right temporal lobe (**A**) with restricted diffusion and cytotoxic edema (**B**). The ADC map (**C**) shows red-orange areas of restricted diffusion. **D** to **F,** MRI examination performed 17 days later shows abnormal high signal intensity on the FLAIR image but a decrease in signal abnormality on DWI and the ADC map. **G** to **I,** MRI on the 23rd day after symptom onset shows high FLAIR signal and widening of the right temporal horn (beginning of atrophic changes). The ADC map now shows blue areas of atrophy in the previously affected regions. **J** to **L,** The last MR examination on the 75th day shows atrophic changes in the temporal lobe with elevated diffusion.

Varicella-Zoster Virus Encephalitis

Varicella-zoster virus encephalitis is a rare form of diffuse encephalitis caused by varicella-zoster virus (VZV). Other names include chickenpox, herpes zoster infection, and shingles.

Epidemiology

CNS infection with varicella is seen in only 1% of patients and can cause aseptic meningitis, cerebellar ataxia, transverse myelitis, encephalitis, Guillain-Barré syndrome, arterial ischemic strokes, and optic neuritis. Zoster infection of the CNS may cause chronic small vessel encephalitis, large vessel encephalitis, neuritis, myelitis, and herpes zoster ophthalmicus. Neuritis is common in immunocompetent individuals, whereas VZV encephalitis is common in immunosuppressed patients, especially in patients after organ or bone marrow transplantation. Every second patient, within 5 years after transplantation, will experience a VZV reactivation. Chronic VZV encephalitis is common in AIDS patients, occurring usually months after herpes zoster.

Clinical Presentation

Fever, vomiting, nausea, headache, seizures, and alterations in mental status are clinical symptoms in meningoencephalitis. Cranial nerve palsies will be seen in patients with herpes zoster.

Skin lesions may or may not be present (30% of patients with AIDS will not have skin lesions).

Pathophysiology

The VZV causes chickenpox (varicella) in childhood, remains latent in the dorsal root ganglia, and may be reactivated decades later to produce shingles (zoster) in adults. Reactivation occurs in immunocompromised situations. VZV encephalitis is predominantly a vasculopathy, involving small and large vessels.

Pathology

Multifocal necrotic changes will be seen at autopsy.

Histopathologically, small and large vessel alterations have been described, with necrosis and demyelination.

Imaging

CT

CT is usually negative.

MRI

MRI reveals large and small ischemic or hemorrhagic infarcts, often both, in the cortex and subcortical gray and white matter. MRI may show extensive necrosis of the basal ganglia and hydrocephalus. Subcortical, spherical, nonenhancing lesions that coalesce and develop enhancement with disease progression have been described and should raise suspicion for VZV infection.[80] A case of multifocal VZV leukoencephalitis has also been described in an AIDS patient. Multiple small, target-like lesions that coalesce into larger lesions have been described on MR images.

Lyme Encephalitis

Lyme disease is a multisystem and multistage infection caused by three species of tick-borne spirochetes in the *Borrelia burgdorferi* sensu lato genogroup. These include *B. burgdorferi* sensu stricto (North America and Western Europe), *B. afzelii* (Western Europe, Central Europe, and Russia), and *B. garinii* (Europe, Russia, and Northern Asia). Lyme neuroborreliosis is a frequent manifestation of disseminated Lyme disease and may develop either in the second or third stage of this multisystemic infection.

Epidemiology

Lyme borreliosis is the most prevalent tick-borne disease in Europe and North America, with more than 50,000 cases annually.

Clinical Presentation

In endemic areas, patients usually present in summer or fall with a characteristic triad of symptoms: (1) painful radiculoneuropathy, (2) cranial neuropathy (particularly facial neuropathy), and (3) meningitis. They usually report a rash or a flu-like illness 30 to 90 days before onset. The definitive diagnosis is made by the demonstration of intrathecal *Borrelia* infection in CSF culture, by an intrathecal concentration of *B. burgdorferi* antibody, or by polymerase chain reaction.[81,82]

Pathophysiology

As in another spirochetal disease, spirochetes in Lyme borreliosis penetrate the blood-brain barrier early in the infection after hematogenous dissemination. In the brain, focal vasculitis develops by activation of endothelial cells and the further release of inflammatory mediators. Neuroborreliosis has three clinical stages; second-stage neuroborreliosis is, in most patients, an acute self-limiting monophasic condition in contrast to the persisting chronic progressive nature of third-stage disease. In one study on 330 cases of neuroborreliosis, 10 clinical syndromes were described.[83] In stage II, the following forms of neuroborreliosis have been described: mononeuritis, polyneuritis (3%), meningoradiculitis cranialis et spinalis (29%), meningoradiculitis cranialis (9%), meningoradiculitis spinalis (37%), meningitis (4%), meningomyeloradiculitis (5%), and meningoencephaloradiculitis (4%).[83]

Cerebrovascular neuroborreliosis (1%), chronic progressive encephalomyelitis (6%), chronic mononeuritis, and polyneuritis (2%) are characteristic of stage III Lyme encephalitis.[83]

Pathology

CNS involvement in neuroborreliosis is associated with scattered perivascular mononuclear cell infiltrates in the cerebral cortex, sometimes accompanied by comparable focal changes in the leptomeninges.

Imaging

MRI

On MRI, high-signal lesions in the white matter on T2W images, simulating demyelinating or ischemic disease, are present (Fig. 42-10). On postcontrast T1W images, pial enhancement along the brain stem, tentorial enhancement, and interpeduncular leptomeningeal enhancement may be observed. The facial nerve is most frequently affected, but other cranial nerves can be affected also (Fig. 42-11).[84]

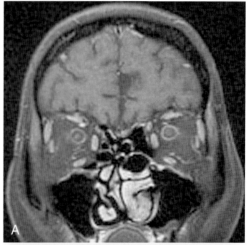

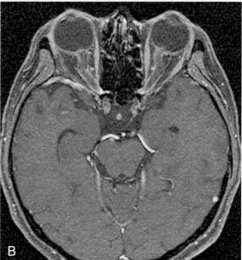

■ **FIGURE 42-10** Neuroborreliosis in a 31-year-old woman. Axial (**A**) and coronal (**B**) T1W MRI with fat suppression show bilateral enhancement of the optic nerves.

PARASITIC INFECTIONS
Toxoplasmosis

Cerebral toxoplasmosis results from infection by the intracellular protozoan *Toxoplasma gondii.*

Epidemiology

In the United States, 20% to 70% of adults are seropositive for toxoplasmosis.[8] Toxoplasmosis is a common opportunistic infection in HIV-positive patients and is found in 10% to 34% of all AIDS autopsies.[85] It is also a rare but severe complication in patients after bone marrow transplantation, usually appearing between the second and sixth post-transplant month.[86]

Clinical Presentation

Clinical signs and symptoms include headache, fever, seizures, focal neurologic deficits, altered mental status, and confusion.

Pathophysiology

After the acute infection, the latent form, called encysted bradyzoites, remains in the tissues until a decline in immunity. Rupture of the cysts releases the free tachyzoite, which causes acute illness. Encysted forms of *Toxoplasma* cannot be eradicated with therapy; thus, lifelong maintenance of therapy is necessary.

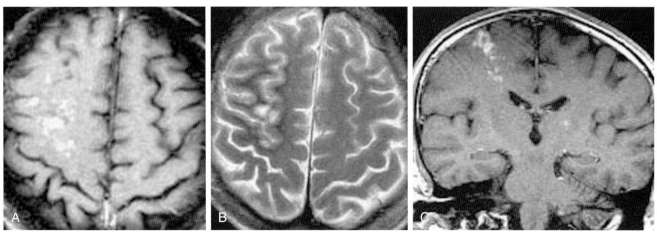

■ **FIGURE 42-11** Neuroborreliosis. **A** and **B**, Axial FLAIR and T2W MRI show abnormal high signal intensities in the right frontal white matter. **C**, Patchy enhancement was observed after gadolinium injection on coronal, postcontrast, T1W MR image. An additional contrast-enhancing area is observed in the left basal ganglia region.

Pathology

Toxoplasma abscesses will be recognized as intraparenchymal foci of coagulative necrosis.

In AIDS patients, *Toxoplasma* causes necrotizing encephalitis, and the lesions have three well-defined zones: a necrotic center, an intermediate zone, and a peripheral zone.[87] The central zone is an avascular zone with organisms and coagulative necrosis. The intermediate zone has blood vessels, extracellular and intracellular tachyzoites, and necrosis. The peripheral zone is characterized by the presence of numerous bradyzoites and only few tachyzoites. The lesions of toxoplasmosis do not have a capsule.

The most commonly affected areas are the basal ganglia and the corticomedullary junction.

Imaging
CT

On unenhanced CT, *Toxoplasma* lesions are hypodense with perifocal edema and mass effect. On postcontrast studies, solid, nodular, or ring-enhancing lesions are typically observed (Fig. 42-12). The use of a double-dose delayed technique significantly increases the number of detectable lesions.[88]

MRI

On T1W MR images, lesions of toxoplasmosis have isointense to low signal centrally. Signal intensity on T2W images depends on the stage of the lesion, which could be isointense, hypointense, or hyperintense (Fig. 42-13).[88,89] Lesions show ring or nodular enhancement after gadolinium application (see Figs. 42-12 and 42-13). They regress in size, mass effect, and enhancement under specific treatment. Full resolution may take 6 months, and calcifications or small areas of leukomalacia will be seen in healed lesions.[8]

In patients after bone marrow transplantation, MRI may reveal multiple, nonenhancing toxoplasmosis lesions with no or only mild edema.[90] Hemorrhagic transformation will often be seen.

Based on imaging findings on conventional MR sequences, cerebral toxoplasmosis cannot be distinguished from primary cerebral lymphoma. The number of lesions, signal intensities, location, and appearance on postcontrast images are not reliable factors in the differentiation between those two entities.

MRS has been introduced as a potentially useful technique in the differentiation between toxoplasmosis and lymphoma. However, the MRS pattern of the lesions of toxoplasmosis is nonspecific, consistent with anaerobic inflammation within the abscess (Fig. 42-14). An important variable for MR spectra is the maturity of the lesions, as well as the presence of necrosis. In lymphoma, an increase of lactate and lipids, as well as an elevated choline peak, has been described.[91] Because both lymphoma and toxoplasmosis contain necrosis, the compounds will be similar in MR spectra. The presence of lipids will be seen in both entities as a result of brain destruction.

Perfusion MRI is another potential, noninvasive method that may allow differentiation between toxoplasmosis and lymphoma in patients with AIDS. A prospective evaluation of 13 patients with focal brain lesions with perfusion MRI showed reduced rCBV in toxoplasmosis and increased rCBV in lymphoma.[92] Reduced rCBV in toxoplasmosis is probably due to a lack of vasculature within the abscess, whereas the hypervascularity of lymphoma is the reason for increased rCBV in lymphoma (Fig. 42-15).

A few studies have been performed using DWI to differentiate between toxoplasmosis and lymphoma.[93,94] Toxoplasmosis exhibited a wide spectrum of signal intensities on DWI, with ADC ratios ranging from 0.8 to 2.8, which had significant overlap with those of lymphoma.[94] Although ADC measurements cannot be reliably used for differentiation on a clinical basis, ADC ratios below 0.8 should favor lymphoma (see Fig. 42-15). The use of thallium-201 (^{201}Tl) brain SPECT in AIDS patients has been proven to be very helpful in distinguishing toxoplasmosis from lymphoma.[95,96] Thallium is a potassium analogue with uptake in active tissue.[95] After intravenous administration of thallium, increased activity is usually seen in the orbits, the base of the skull, the scalp, and the nasopharyngeal region. Normally, there is no uptake of ^{201}Tl in the brain. Positive ^{201}Tl brain SPECT is suggestive of CNS lymphoma, and negative uptake suggests infection (toxoplasmosis) in AIDS patients.[95] However, the reported accuracy and predictive values of this technique are variable. A combined approach with ^{201}Tl SPECT and the Epstein-Barr virus DNA polymerase chain reaction in CSF provides a high diagnostic accuracy for cerebral lymphoma.[97]

The potential use of fluorodeoxyglucose (FDG)-positron emission tomography (PET) to differentiate lymphoma from toxoplasmosis in AIDS patients has been also examined (Fig. 42-16).[98] The results of the studies have shown that FDG-PET can accurately differentiate lymphoma from infections.[99,100] The standardized uptake values over cerebral lesions were much higher in lymphomas than in the lesions of toxoplasmosis.[101]

■ **FIGURE 42-12** Cerebral toxoplasmosis in an HIV-positive patient. **A,** Noncontrast CT shows hypodensity in both frontal lobes. **B,** Contrast-enhanced CT shows a peripherally enhancing lesion with associated edema. **C,** Axial contrast-enhanced T1W TFE MRI (TR/TE/flip° 10/3.4/10°) demonstrates peripheral enhancement of the necrotic lesion and perifocal edema. **D,** The trace DWI shows central low signal and peripheral high signal within the toxoplasmic lesion.

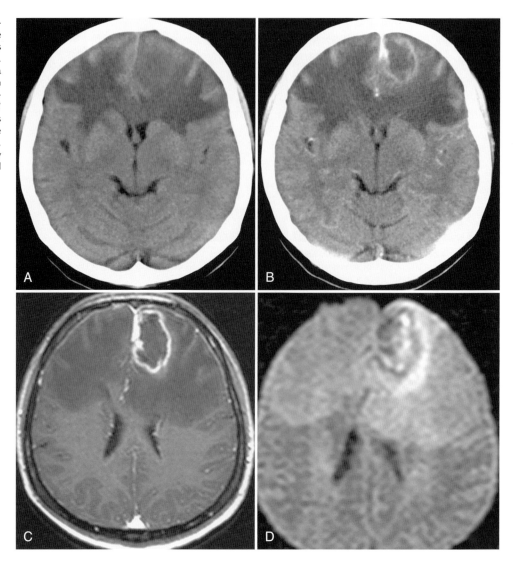

■ **FIGURE 42-13** Cerebral toxoplasmosis in an HIV-positive individual. Axial FLAIR-TSE (**A**) and T2W (**B**) MRI show a low signal intensity lesion with surrounding high signal edema located in the right basal ganglia.

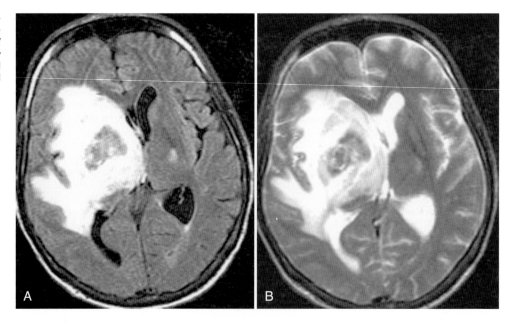

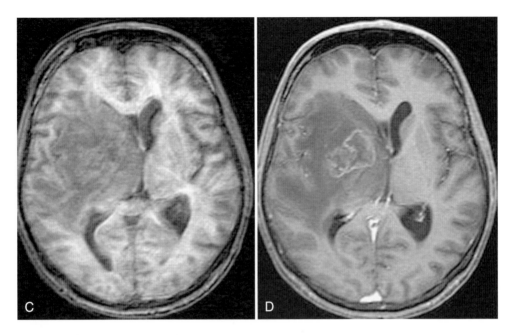

■ **FIGURE 42-13, cont'd** The non-contrast T1W MR image (**C**) and the contrast-enhanced T1W MR image (**D**) show inhomogeneously low signal and peripheral, irregular enhancement. These features and the findings of an FDG-PET scan (not shown) were consistent with toxoplasmosis. Ten days after the initiation of treatment, follow-up MR (not shown) showed decrease in lesion size and enhancement.

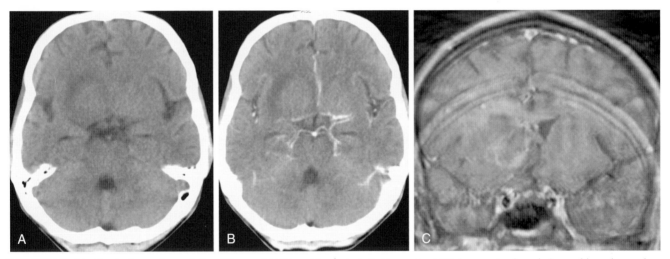

■ **FIGURE 42-14** Cerebral toxoplasmosis in a 37-year-old HIV-positive patient. **A,** Noncontrast CT shows an isodense lesion and hypodense edema in the right basal ganglia. **B,** Contrast-enhanced CT shows no contrast enhancement. **C,** Contrast-enhanced T1W MR image shows faint peripheral enhancement of the lesion.

Cysticercosis

Cysticercosis results from infection by the pork tapeworm *Taenia solium.* It is also known as *Cysticercus* infection, neurocysticercosis (NCC), taeniasis, or tapeworm infection.

Epidemiology

Cysticercosis is the most common parasitic infection of the CNS. *T. solium* is endemic in Mexico, South America, Asia, Africa, and Eastern Europe and is generally acquired by ingestion of undercooked pork. Cysticercosis may affect immunocompetent and immunocompromised individuals.

Clinical Presentation

Although most cases of neurocysticercosis are asymptomatic, seizures, other focal neurologic signs, and increased intracranial pressure can result.[102,103]

Seizures are the most common presentation of neurocysticercosis. Occasionally, a cyst grows larger than the usual 1 to 2 cm and produces symptoms of a mass lesion. Intracranial hypertension also occurs in patients with giant cysts and in those with a rare form of cysticercotic encephalitis.[104] Diagnosis of neurocysticercosis is typically made on the basis of neuroimaging studies and confirmatory serologic analysis.

Pathophysiology

Humans become a host for parasites after ingesting larvae from insufficiently cooked pork, and, subsequently, a tapeworm develops in the gastrointestinal tract. The worm attaches strongly to the mucosa of the upper small intestine by means of its suckers and hooks and produces only mild inflammation. The disease is then called taeniasis.

If a person ingests eggs in contaminated food or water, the person becomes the intermediate host. The invasive oncospheres in the eggs will be liberated by the action of gastric acid and intestinal fluids and will be released into the bloodstream. Once the larvae come into the blood, they spread to different

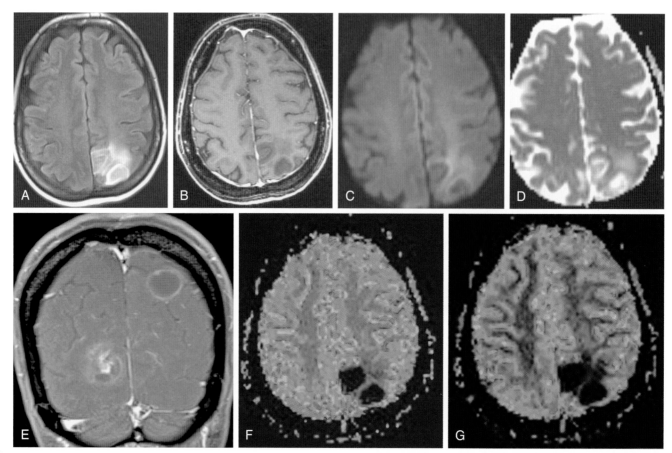

■ **FIGURE 42-15**   Cerebral toxoplasmosis in a 30-year-old woman with AIDS. **A,** Axial FLAIR-TSE MRI (TR/TE/TI 11,000/140/2,800) shows low signal intensity lesions with high signal intensity edema in the left parietal cortex. **B,** Contrast-enhanced T1W TFE MRI (TR/TE/flip° 10/3.4/10°) shows no contrast enhancement. **C** and **D,** The trace DWI (**C**) shows low signal intensity and the ADC map (**D**) shows high values, indicating facilitated diffusion. **E,** Coronal, contrast-enhanced T1W TFE MRI (TR/TE/flip° 10/3.4/10°) performed a few minutes later (delayed scan) shows peripheral enhancement of the necrotic toxoplasmic lesions. **F, G,** Perfusion MRI shows hypoperfusion of the necrotic toxoplasmic lesions.

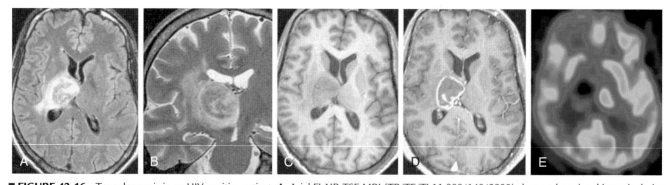

■ **FIGURE 42-16**   Toxoplasmosis in an HIV-positive patient. **A,** Axial FLAIR-TSE MRI (TR/TE/TI 11,000/140/2800) shows a low signal intensity lesion in the right basal ganglia. Coronal T2W MR image (**B**) and T1W MR image (**C**) show inhomogeneous low signal intensity. **D,** Contrast-enhanced T1W MR image shows peripheral enhancement of the lesion. **E,** No uptake was seen on FDG-PET, so toxoplasmosis was suspected.

organs. The incidence of CNS involvement is nearly 100%. This disease is called human cysticercosis.

There are four types of neurocysticercosis: parenchymal, subarachnoidal, intraventricular, and mixed. In the brain parenchyma, larvae develop over time into cysts that may measure 3 to 18 mm and contain a scolex.[105] The brain parenchyma reacts with minimal inflammation. With the appearance of cysts, death antigens and metabolites will be released and produce intense inflammation of the brain parenchyma. Over time, cysts collapse, degenerate, and calcify.[106]

The racemose form represents multiloculated subarachnoid cysts ("cluster of grapes") that may reach 9 cm.[106] These cysts do not have scolex and they usually do not calcify.

Pathology

Cysts are uniformly rounded or oval vesicles that vary from a few millimeters to 1 to 2 cm (rarely, several centimeters in diameter). Viable cysts will be recognized by their translucent membrane with a small 2- to 3-mm nodule, which represents the scolex.

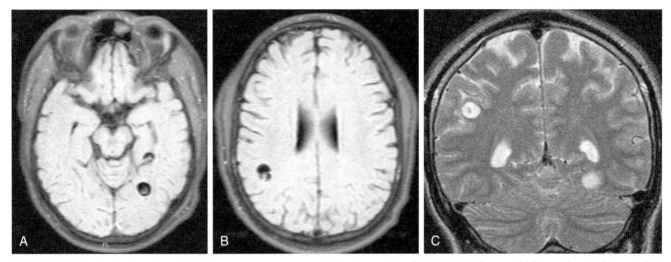

■ **FIGURE 42-17**   Cerebral cysticercosis. This young woman presented with seizures. **A** and **B,** T1W MRI shows multiple round, cystic lesions in both cerebral hemispheres. The cysts have CSF intensity, small intracystic nodules representing scolices, and no surrounding edema. **C,** On coronal T2W MRI, the cysts show high signal fluid with low signal scolices. Imaging findings are consistent with the parenchymal form of cysticercosis (early vesicular stage).

When the degeneration begins, the vesicular fluid becomes opaque and dense, and the edges of the cyst become irregular and shrink. Calcification begins in the cephalic portion; and, finally, a round, whitish, calcified nodule will be left.[104]

The cysticercosis lesions are commonly located at the junction of gray and white matter. In 10% to 15% of the affected individuals, the parasites are located in the subarachnoid spaces, most frequently around the sylvian fissure or in the basal cisterns.

Imaging
CT
Cysts appear on CT as hypodense lesions, with well-defined edges. Commonly there is a hyperdense nodule inside the cyst (parasite's scolex).[107] Contrast enhancement of the edges of the cyst and perilesional edema result from the inflammatory reaction due to the degeneration of the cysts. Over time, the cysts become isodense and show nodular or ring-like enhancement on postcontrast studies.[107] Characteristic calcifications are well demonstrated on CT and are slightly off center and spherical. Contrast enhancement and perilesional edema around old, calcified lesions suggest relapse.

MRI
MRI shows multiple cystic lesions, with signal intensities dependent on the different stages of the larval cycle. In the early vesicular stage, small nonenhancing cysts can be seen that are isointense to CSF on T1W and T2W imaging, with a mural nodule seen on T1W imaging (Fig. 42-17). As the larvae mature, a cyst wall becomes visible, with increasing T1W signal within the cyst relative to CSF. Edema and ring-like enhancement can then be visualized as the larvae die. Eventually, the cysts decrease in size and become calcified.

DWI was recently shown to be useful in the differentiation of degenerated cysticercosis lesions and intracranial tuberculomas.[108] ADC values for the vesicular and degenerating stages of cysticercus cysts were $1.66 \pm 0.29 \times 10^{-3}$ and $1.51 \pm 0.23 \times 10^{-3}$ mm^2/s, respectively, and were significantly higher than ADC values for all groups of tuberculomas and tuberculous abscesses.[108]

Echinococcosis
Echinococcosis is a human disease caused by the larval form of *Taenia echinococcus.* It can be called echinococcosis granulosus (EG), echinococcosis alveolaris (EA), or hydatid disease.

Epidemiology
Cystic echinococcosis is endemic in regions known for the raising of sheep and cattle (Middle East, Australia, New Zealand, South America, central and south Europe, and Turkey). Echinococcosis granulosus of the CNS may be primary or secondary and has been estimated to be approximately 2%.

CNS involvement in alveolar echinococcosis has been reported in about 5% of patients. The cycle of *E. multilocularis* involves carnivores (usually the red fox) as the final hosts. Rodents, dogs, cats, and humans can be accidental intermediate hosts.

Clinical Presentation
The clinical symptoms of cerebral echinococcosis include headache, seizure, increased intracranial pressure, and focal neurologic deficits. Papilledema is usually present in patients with intracranial hydatid cysts at the time of diagnosis.

Pathophysiology
The main species pathogenic for humans are *E. granulosus,* which causes cystic echinococcosis, and *E. multilocularis,* which causes alveolar echinococcosis.

In alveolar echinococcosis, when eaten by a human, the hexacanth embryo will be released into the duodenum and enter the intestinal wall. The embryos have hooklets and suckers with which they attach to the mucosa of the intestine with subsequent spread hematogenously into the liver. Echinococcosis multilocularis spreads from the primarily involved liver to other organs, such as the lungs, brain, and bone, which causes metastatic lesions.

Pathology
Lesions are usually distributed in the territory of the middle cerebral artery, especially in the parietal lobe. Most of the cysts

are located in the supratentorial regions and very rarely in the posterior fossa or in the ventricles.[109]

Alveolar Echinococcosis

Lesions of alveolar echinococcosis have alveolar structures composed of numerous irregular cysts (between 1 and 20 mm in diameter) that are not sharply demarcated from surrounding tissue. Necrosis and liquefaction of the inner area lead to the cystic central areas. The wall is irregularly thickened and partially calcified.

Cystic Echinococcosis

The hydatid cyst always starts as a fluid-filled cyst (type I), which may proceed to a type II lesion if daughter cysts and/or matrix develop. In some instances, the type II lesion becomes hypermature and, due to starvation, dies and becomes a mummified, inert calcified type III lesion.[110] The parasitic cyst consists of an inner germinal layer (endocyst) and an outer laminated layer (ectocyst). From the germinal layer, scolices, brood capsules, and daughter cysts are formed by endoproliferation (internal budding). The cysts in alveolar echinococcosis grow by external budding of the germinal membrane, with progressive infiltration of the surrounding tissue.[109]

Imaging

Cystic echinococcosis usually produces a single lesion, whereas multiple cerebral cystic echinococcosis is very rare. Cysts have CSF density on CT, CSF isointensity on MR images, a spherical form, and a thin wall. The two visible imaging components are the cyst and the pericyst. The pericyst is a peripheral capsule of the cyst, which is better delineated on MRI.[111]

On CT and MRI, alveolar echinococcosis appears as a solid or semisolid mass or as a multilocular cystic mass. Peripheral, ring-like, heterogeneous, nodular, and cauliflower-like enhancement patterns have been reported. Calcifications are a frequent finding (Fig. 42-18).[112-114]

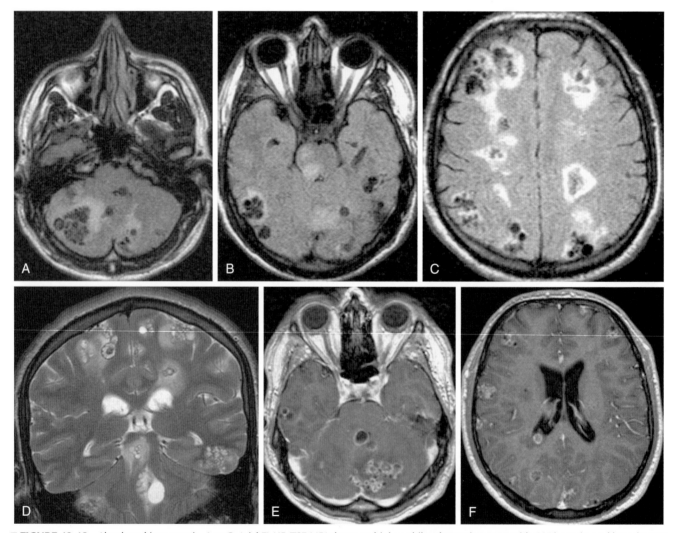

■ **FIGURE 42-18** Alveolar echinococcosis. **A** to **C**, Axial FLAIR-TSE MRI shows multiple multilocular cystic masses with CSF intensity and hyperintense perifocal edema in the posterior fossa (**A**) and in the supratentorial region bilaterally (**B**, **C**). **D**, The coronal T2W image confirms the presence of multiple small cysts. **E** and **F**, Contrast-enhanced T1W MR images show peripheral enhancement of the cauliflower-like lesions.

KEY POINTS: DIFFERENTIAL DIAGNOSIS

HIV Encephalitis

- Bilateral, symmetric, nonenhancing high signal intensity abnormalities of the white matter are typical of HIV encephalopathy; white matter lesions in progressive multifocal leukoencephalopathy (PML) will be asymmetric and multifocal.
- In HIV encephalitis nonenhancing high signal intensity lesions are present in the white matter.
- Because of extensive demyelination, PML lesions are markedly hypointense on T1W imaging whereas lesions in HIV encephalitis are isointense or slightly hypointense.
- Enhancement and progression of the white matter disease in a patient undergoing HAART represent an immune reconstitutive effect, not therapy failure.
- MR spectroscopy in the basal ganglia and white matter shows early changes in HIV encephalitis.

Progressive Multifocal Leukoencephalopathy

- PML is common in AIDS patients.
- PML lesions of the white matter are multifocal and scalloped.
- PML lesions normally do not show enhancement or mass effect.
- Under HAART, enhancement and a mass effect will be present in patients with PML who will have prolonged survival (immune response).

Cytomegalovirus Infection

- Imaging findings in CMV infection of the CNS are nonspecific. A definite diagnosis will usually be made by a positive polymerase chain reaction in CSF.
- Periventricular enhancement can be seen in CMV ventriculitis but can also be present in lymphoma and pyogenic ventriculitis.

Prion Diseases

- The clinical presentation of an adult patient with progressive dementia, cerebellar signs, myoclonus, or other abnormal movements, as well as a characteristic electroencephalogram, establishes the diagnosis of Creutzfeldt-Jakob disease (CJD) with good accuracy.
- In the appropriate clinical context, the MRI identification of a bilaterally increased pulvinar signal ("pulvinar sign") is a useful noninvasive test for the diagnosis of variant CJD.

Rasmussen's Encephalitis

- Young patients with Rasmussen's encephalitis have progressive untreatable seizures.
- Focal cortical swelling and T2W imaging signal abnormalities in the perisylvian region and temporal cortex are characteristic of the initial stage of the disease.
- Progressive atrophy will be characteristic of the second phase.

Herpes Simplex Encephalitis

- The temporal lobes, the hippocampi, the insular cortex, and the gyrus cinguli are typical locations for high signal intensity abnormalities on T2W and FLAIR imaging in herpes simplex encephalitis.
- Enhancement will not be present early on but will be apparent in the subacute stage.
- The most important differential diagnosis is low-grade tumor, which will not change signal intensities with time, as seen in herpes simplex encephalitis.
- On DWI, two patterns may be seen: restricted diffusion due to cytotoxic edema and elevated diffusion due to vasogenic edema.

Varicella-Zoster Encephalitis

- Patients with VZV involvement of the CNS often have characteristic skin lesions.
- Vascular lesions in the cortex and subcortical regions may suggest VZV vasculopathy.
- Differential diagnosis includes vasculitis and neurolues.

Toxoplasmosis

- CNS toxoplasmosis occurs commonly in HIV-positive patients and in patients after a bone marrow transplant (BMT).
- Lesions of toxoplasmosis may be hypointense, isointense, or hyperintense on T2W images.
- In BMT patients, toxoplasmosis lesions are often hemorrhagic.
- Conventional MRI sequences, DWI, and MR spectroscopy cannot reliably distinguish between toxoplasmosis and lymphoma.

Cysticercosis

- Cystic lesions with a mural, hyperdense nodule on CT that are CSF isointense on all MR sequences represent the vesicular form of neurocysticercosis.
- The degenerated form of cysticercosis (dead larva) will be recognized by enhancing lesions with perifocal edema on CT, which will be hyperintense to CSF on T1W imaging.

Echinococcosis

- A hydatid cyst should be suspected in a case of a single, large, thin-walled, spherical, nonenhancing CSF isointense cyst in the parietal region of the brain.

SUGGESTED READINGS

Antinori A, Larussa D, Cingolani A, et al. Prevalence, associated factors, and prognostic determinants of AIDS-related toxoplasmic encephalitis in the era of advanced highly active antiretroviral therapy. Clin Infect Dis 2004; 39:1681-1691.

Baskin HJ, Hedlund G. Neuroimaging of herpesvirus infections in children. Pediatr Radiol 2007; 37:949-963.

Berger JR. Progressive multifocal leukoencephalopathy. Curr Neurol Neurosci Rep 2007; 7:461-469.

Berger JR, Concha M. Progressive multifocal leukoencephalopathy: the evolution of a disease once considered rare. J Neurovirol 1995; 1:5-18.

Boivin G. Diagnosis of herpesvirus infections of the central nervous system. Herpes 2004; 11:48A-56A.

Budka H, Constanzi G, Cristina S, et al. Brain pathology induced by infection with the human immunodeficiency virus (HIV). Acta Neuropathol 1987; 75:185-198.

Castillo M, Thurnher M. Imaging viral and prion infections. Semin Roentgenol 2004; 39:482-494.

Davis LE, Hjelle BL, Miller VE, et al. Early viral brain invasion in iatrogenic human immunodeficiency virus infection. Neurology 1992; 42: 1736-1739.

DeBiasi RL, Kleinschmidt-DeMasters BK, Weinberg A, Tyler KL. Use of PCR for the diagnosis of herpesvirus infections of the central nervous system. J Clin Virol 2002; 25:S5-S11.

Garcia HH, Del Brutto OH, and the Cysticercosis Working Group in Peru. Neurocysticercosis: updated concepts about an old disease. Lancet Neurol 2005; 4:653-661.

Giudici B, Vaz B, Bossolasco S, et al. Highly active antiretroviral therapy and progressive multifocal leukoencephalopathy: effects on cerebrospinal fluid markers of JC virus replication and immune response. Clin Infect Dis 2000; 30:95-99.

Hainfellner JA, Budka H. Neuropathology of human immunodeficiency virus-related opportunistic infections and neoplasms. In Berger JR, Levy RM (eds). AIDS and the Nervous System, 2nd ed. Philadelphia, Lippincott-Raven, 1997, pp 461-515.

Halperin JJ. Central nervous system Lyme disease. Curr Neurol Neurosci Rep 2005; 5:446-452.

Halperin JJ, Luft BJ, Anand AK, et al. Lyme neuroborreliosis: central nervous system manifestations. Neurology 1989; 39:753-759.

Hill AF, Joiner S, Wadsworth JD, et al. Molecular classification of sporadic Creutzfeldt-Jacob disease. Brain 2003; 126:1333-1346.

Hinson VK, Tyor WR. Update on viral encephalitis. Curr Opin Neurol 2001; 14:369-374.

Hoffmann C, Ernst M, Meyer P, et al. Evolving characteristics of toxoplasmosis in patients infected with human immunodeficiency virus-1: clinical course and *Toxoplasma gondii*-specific immune responses. Clin Microbiol Infect 2007; 13:510-515.

Holland N, Power C, Mathews V, et al. Cytomegalovirus encephalitis in acquired immunodeficiency syndrome (AIDS). Neurology 1994; 44:1892-1900.

Kalayijan RC, Cohen ML, Bonomo RA, et al. Cytomegalovirus ventriculoencephalitis in AIDS: a syndrome with distinct clinical and pathologic features. Medicine (Baltimore) 1993; 72:67-77.

Langer-Gould A, Atlas SW, Green AJ, et al. Progressive multifocal leukoencephalopathy in a patient treated with natalizumab. N Engl J Med 2005; 353:375-381.

Lizerbram EK, Hesselink JR. Viral infections. Neuroimag Clin North Am 1997; 7:261-280.

Logigian EL, Kaplan RF, Steere AC. Chronic neurologic manifestations of Lyme disease. N Engl J Med 1990; 323:1438-1444.

Maschke M, Kastrup O, Diener HC. CNS manifestations of cytomegalovirus infections: diagnosis and treatment. CNS Drugs 2002; 16:303-315.

Meissner B, Köhler K, Körtner K, et al. Sporadic Creutzfeldt-Jacob disease: magnetic resonance imaging and clinical findings. Neurology 2004; 63:450-456.

Miravet E, Danchaivijitr N, Basu H, et al. Clinical and radiological features of childhood cerebral infarction following varicella zoster virus infection. Dev Med Child Neurol 2007; 49:417-422.

Offiah CE, Turnbull IW. The imaging appearances of intracranial CNS infections in adult HIV and AIDS patients. Clin Radiol 2006; 61: 393-401.

Parchi P, Giese A, Capellari S, et al. Classification of sporadic Creutzfeldt-Jacob disease based on molecular and phenotypic analysis of 300 subjects. Ann Neurol 1999; 46:224-233.

Prusiner SB. Prions. Proc Natl Acad Sci U S A 1998; 95:13363-13383.

Rasmussen T, Andermann F. Rasmussen's syndrome: symptomatology of the syndrome of chronic encephalitis and seizures: 35-year experience with 51 cases. In Luders H (ed). Epilepsy Surgery. New York, Raven Press, 1992.

Serpa JA, Yancey LS, White AC Jr. Advances in the diagnosis and management of neurocysticercosis. Expert Rev Anti Infect Ther 2006; 4:1051-1061.

Subsai K, Kanoksri S, Siwaporn C, et al. Neurological complications in AIDS patients receiving HAART: a 2-year retrospective study. Eur J Neurol 2006; 13:233-239.

Tien RD, Ashdown BC, Lewis DV Jr, et al. Rasmussen's encephalitis: neuroimaging findings in four patients. AJR Am J Roentgenol 1992; 158:1329-1332.

Tien RD, Feldberg GJ, Osumi AK. Herpesvirus infections of the CNS: MR findings. AJR Am J Roentgenol 1983; 158:1325-1328.

Türkdogan-Sözüer D, Özek MM, Sav A, et al. Serial MRI and MRS studies with unusual findings in Rasmussen's encephalitis. Eur Radiol 2000; 10:962-966.

Tüzün M, Altinörs N, Arda IS, Hekimoglu B. Cerebral hydatid disease: CT and MRI findings. Clin Imaging 2002; 26:353-357.

Tyler KL. Update on herpes simplex encephalitis. Rev Neurol Dis 2004; 1:169-178.

REFERENCES

1. Sacktor NC, Lyles RH, Skolasky MA, et al. HIV-associated neurologic disease incidence changes: multicenter AIDS cohort study, 1990-1998. Neurology 2001; 56:257-260.

2. Price RW, Sidtis JJ. Evaluation of the AIDS dementia complex in clinical trials. J Acquir Immune Defic Syndr 1990; 3:S51-S60.

3. Kramer-Hämmerle S, Rothenaigner I, Wolff H, et al. Cells of the central nervous system as targets and reservoirs of the human immunodeficiency virus. Virus Res 2005; 111:194-213.

4. Rausch DM, Davis MR. HIV in the CNS: pathogenic relationships to systemic HIV disease and other CNS disease. J Neuro Virol 2001; 7:85-96.

5. Kleihues P, Lang W, Burger PC, et al. Progressive diffuse leukoencephalopathy in patients with acquired immune deficiency syndrome (AIDS). Acta Neuropathol (Berl) 1985; 68:333-339.

6. Eloovara I, Poutiainen E, Raininko R, et al. Mild brain atrophy in early HIV-1 infection: the lack of association with cognitive deficits and HIV-specific intrathecal immune response. J Neurol Sci 1990; 99:121-136.

7. Poutiainen E, Eloovara I, Raininko R, et al. Cognitive performance in HIV-1 infection: relationship to severity of disease and brain atrophy. Acta Neurol Scand 1993; 87:88-94.

8. Levy RM, Rosenbloom S, Perrett LV. Neuroradiologic findings in AIDS: a review of 200 cases. AJR Am J Radiol 1986; 147: 977-983.

9. Aylward EH, Brettschneider PD, McArthur JC, et al. Magnetic resonance imaging measurement of gray matter volume reductions in HIV dementia. Am J Psychiatry 1995; 152:987-994.

10. Olsen WL, Longo FM, Mills CM, et al. White matter disease in AIDS: findings at MR imaging. Radiology 1988; 169:445-448.

11. Kieburtz KD, Ketonen L, Zettelmaier AE, et al. Magnetic resonance imaging findings in HIV cognitive impairment. Arch Neurol 1990; 47:643-645.

12. Cohen WA, Maravilla KR, Gerlach R, et al. Prospective cerebral MR study of HIV seropositive and seronegative men: correlation of MR findings with neurologic, neuropsychologic, and cerebrospinal fluid analysis. AJNR Am J Neuroradiol 1992; 13:1231-1240.

13. Post MJD, Levin BE, Berger JR, et al. Sequential cranial MR findings of asymptomatic and neurologically symptomatic HIV positive subjects. AJNR Am J Neuroradiol 1992; 13:359-370.

14. Post MJD, Berger JR, Duncan R, et al. Asymptomatic and neurologically symptomatic HIV-seropositive subjects: results of long-term MR imaging and clinical follow-up. Radiology 1993; 188:727-733.

15. Thurnher MM, Thurnher SA, Fleischmann D, et al. Comparison of T2-weighted and fluid-attenuated inversion-recovery fast spin-echo MR sequences in intracerebral AIDS-associated disease. AJNR Am J Neuroradiol 1997; 18:1601-1609.

16. Von Giesen HJ, Wittsack HJ, Wenserski F, et al. Basal ganglia metabolite abnormalities in minor motor disorders associated with human immunodeficiency virus type 1. Arch Neurol 2001; 58:1281-1286.

17. Chang L, Itti I, Itti L, et al. Changes in cerebral metabolism are detected prior to perfusion changes in early HIV-CMC: a coregistered (1)H MRS and SPECT study. J Magn Reson Imaging 2000; 12:859-865.

18. Chang L, Ernst T, Leonido-Yee M, et al. Highly active antiretroviral therapy reverses brain metabolite abnormalities in mild HIV dementia. Neurology 1999; 53:782-789.

19. Filippi CG, Sze G, Farber SJ, et al. Regression of HIV encephalopathy and basal ganglia signal intensity abnormality at MR imaging in patients with AIDS after initiation of protease inhibitor therapy. Radiology 1998; 206:491-498.

20. Thurnher MM, Schindler EG, Thurnher SA, et al. Highly active antiretroviral therapy for patients with AIDS dementia complex: effect on MR imaging findings and clinical course. AJNR Am J Neuroradiol 2000; 21:670-678.

21. DeSimone JA, Pomerantz RJ, Babinchak TJ. Inflammatory reactions in HIV-1-infected persons after initiation of highly active antiretroviral therapy. Ann Intern Med 2000; 133:447-454.

22. Padget BL, Walker DL, ZuRhein GM, et al. Cultivation of papova-like virus from human brain with progressive multifocal leukoencephalopathy. Lancet 1971; 1:1257-1260.

23. Von Einsiedel RW, Fife TD, Aksamit AJ, et al. Progressive multifocal leukoencephalopathy in AIDS: a clinicopathologic study and review of the literature. J Neurol 1993; 240:391-406.

24. Thurnher MM, Thurnher SA, Mühlbauer B, et al. Progressive multifocal leukoencephalopathy in AIDS: initial and follow-up CT and MRI. Neuroradiology 1997; 39:611-618.

25. Khalili K, White MK, Lublin F, et al. Reactivation of JC virus and development of PML in patients with multiple sclerosis. Neurology 2007; 68:985-990.

26. Tantisiriwat W, Tebas P, Clifford DB, et al. Progressive multifocal leukoencephalopathy in AIDS receiving highly active antiretroviral therapy. Clin Infect Dis 1999; 28:1152-1154.

27. Kastrup O, Machke M, Diener HC, et al. Progressive multifocal leukoencephalopathy limited to the brain stem. Neuroradiology 2002; 44:227-229.

28. Whiteman MLH, Post MJD, Berger JR, et al. Progressive multifocal leukoencephalopathy in 47 HIV-seropositive patients: neuroimaging with clinical and pathologic correlation. Radiology 1993; 187:233-240.

29. Kotecha N, George MJ, Smith TW, et al. Enhancing progressive multifocal leukoencephalopathy: an indicator of improved immune status. Am J Med 1998; 105:541-543.

30. Wheeler AL, Truwit CL, Kleinschmidt-DeMasters BK, et al. Progressive multifocal leukoencephalopathy: contrast enhancement on CT scans and MR imaging. AJR 1993; 161:1049-1051.

31. Woo HH, Rezai AR, Knopp EA, et al. Contrast-enhancing progressive multifocal leukoencephalopathy: radiological and pathological correlations: case report. Neurosurgery 1996; 39:1031-1035.

32. Ernst TE, Chang L, Witt MD, et al. Progressive multifocal leukoencephalopathy and human immunodeficiency virus–associated white matter lesions in AIDS: magnetization transfer MR imaging. Radiology 1999; 210:539-543.

33. Da Pozzo S, Manara R, Tonello S, Carollo C. Conventional and diffusion-weighted MRI in progressive multifocal leukoencephalopathy: new elements for identification and follow-up. Radiol Med (Torino) 2006; 111:971-977.

34. Chang L, Ernst T, Tornatore C, et al. Metabolite abnormalities in progressive multifocal leukoencephalopathy: a proton magnetic resonance spectroscopy study. Neurology 1997; 48:836-845.

35. Iranzo A, Moreno A, Pujol J, et al. Proton magnetic resonance spectroscopy pattern of progressive multifocal leukoencephalopathy in AIDS. J Neurol Neurosurg Psychiatry 1999; 66:520-523.

36. Tassie JM, Gasnault J, Bentata M, et al. Survival improvement of AIDS-related progressive multifocal leukoencephalopathy in the era of protease inhibitors. AIDS 1990; 13:1881-1887.

37. Teofilo E, Gouveia J, Brotas V, et al. Progressive multifocal leukoencephalopathy regression with highly active antiretroviral therapy. AIDS 1998; 12:449.

38. Shapiro RA, Mullane KM, Camras L, et al. Clinical and magnetic resonance imaging regression of progressive multifocal leukoencephalopathy in an AIDS patient after intensive antiretroviral therapy. J Neuroimaging 2001; 11:336-339.

39. Thurnher MM, Post MJD, Rieger A, et al. Initial and follow-up MR imaging findings in AIDS-related progressive multifocal leukoencephalopathy treated with highly active antiretroviral therapy. AJNR Am J Neuroradiol 2001; 22:977-984.

40. Setinek U, Wondrusch E, Jellinger K, et al. Cytomegalovirus infection of the brain in AIDS: a clinicopathological study. Acta Neuropathol (Berl) 1995; 90:511-515.

41. Salmon-Ceron D. Cytomegalovirus infection: the point in 2001. HIV Medicine 2001; 2:255-259.

42. Arribas JR, Clifford DB, Fichtenbaum CJ, et al. Level of cytomegalovirus (CMV) DNA in cerebrospinal fluid of subjects with AIDS and CMV infection of the central nervous system. J Infect Dis 1995; 172:527-531.

43. Morgello S, Cho E, Nielsen S, et al. Cytomegalovirus encephalitis in patients with acquired immunodeficiency syndrome: an autopsy study of 30 cases and a review of the literature. Hum Pathol 1987; 18:289-297.

44. Salazar A, Podzamczer D, Reñe R, et al. Cytomegalovirus ventriculoencephalitis in AIDS patients. Scand J Infect Dis 1995; 27:165-169.

45. Post MJD, Hensley GT, Moskowitz LB, et al. Cytomegalic inclusion virus encephalitis in patients with AIDS: CT, clinical, and pathologic correlation. AJNR Am J Neuroradiol 1986; 7:275-279.

46. Dorfman LJ. Cytomegalovirus encephalitis in adults. Neurology 1973; 23:136-143.

47. Hawley DA, Schaeffer JF, Schalz DM, et al. Cytomegalovirus encephalitis in acquired immunodeficiency syndrome. Am J Clin Pathol 1983; 80:874-877.

48. Hassine D, Gray F, Chekroun R, et al. Encéphalitides à CMV et VZV au cours du SIDA. J Neuroradiol 1995; 22:184-192.

49. Dyer JR, French MAH, Mallal SA. Cerebral mass lesions due to cytomegalovirus in patients with AIDS: report of two cases. J Infect 1995; 30:147-151.

50. Guermazi A, Miaux Y, Zagdanski AM, et al. Chorioid plexitis caused by cytomegalovirus in a patient with AIDS. AJNR Am J Neuroradiol 1996; 17:1398-1399.

51. Wilkinson ID, Miller RF, Paley MNJ, et al. Cerebral proton magnetic resonance spectroscopy in cytomegalovirus encephalitis and HIV leukoencephalopathy/encephalitis. AIDS 1996; 10:1443-1444.

52. Unterberger U, Voigtländer T, Budka H. Pathogenesis of prion diseases. Acta Neuropathol (Berl) 2005; 109:32-48.

53. Rosenburg C, Schulz-Schaeffer WJ, Meissner B, et al. Clinical course in young patients with sporadic Creutzfeldt-Jacob disease. Ann Neurol 2005; 58:533-543.

54. Meissner B, Köhler K, Körtner K, et al. Sporadic Creutzfeldt-Jacob disease: magnetic resonance imaging and clinical findings. Neurology 2004; 63:450-456.

55. Cooper SA, Murray KL, Hearth CA, et al. Sporadic Creutzfeldt-Jacob disease with cerebellar ataxia at onset in the UK. J Neurol Neurosurg Psychiatry 2006; 77:1273-1275.

56. Collins S, Boyd A, Fletcher A, et al. Recent advances in the premortem diagnosis of Creutzfeldt-Jacob disease. J Clin Neurosci 2000; 7:195-202.

57. Kretzschmar HA, Ironside JW, DeArmond SJ, et al. Diagnostic criteria for sporadic Creutzfeldt-Jacob disease. Arch Neurol 1996; 53:913-920.

58. Zerr I, Poochiari M, Collins S, et al. Analysis of EEG and CSF 14-3-3 proteins as aids to the diagnosis of Creutzfeldt-Jacob disease. Neurology 2000; 55:811-815.

59. Aksamit AJ Jr, Preissner CM, Hornburger HA. Quantification of 14-3-3 and neuron-specific enolase proteins in CSF in Creutzfeldt-Jacob disease. Neurology 2001; 57:728-730.

60. Budka H, Aguzzi A, Brown P, et al. Neuropathological diagnostic criteria for Creutzfeldt-Jacob disease (CJD) and other human spongiform encephalopathies (prion diseases). Brain Pathol 1995; 5:459-466.

61. Ironside JW, McCardle L, Horsburgh A, et al. Pathological diagnosis of variant Creutzfeldt-Jakob disease. APMIS 2002; 110:79-87.

62. Demaerel P, Sciot R, Robberecht W, et al. Accuracy of diffusion-weighted MR imaging in the diagnosis of sporadic Creutzfeldt-Jakob disease. J Neurol 2003; 250:222-225.

63. Bruhn H, Weber T, Thorwirth V, et al. In-vivo monitoring of neuronal loss in Creutzfeldt-Jacob disease by proton magnetic resonance spectroscopy. Lancet 1992; 337:1610-1611.

64. Waldman AD, Cordery RJ, McManus DG, et al. Regional brain metabolite abnormalities in inherited prion disease and asymptomatic gene carriers demonstrated in vivo by quantitative proton magnetic resonance spectroscopy. Neuroradiology 2006; 48:428-433.

65. Pandya HG, Coley SC, Wilkinson ID, et al. Magnetic resonance spectroscopy abnormalities in sporadic and variant Creutzfeldt-Jacob disease. Clin Radiol 2003; 58:148-153.

66. Galanaud D, Dormont D, Grabli D, et al. MR spectroscopic pulvinar sign in a case of variant Creutzfeldt-Jacob disease. J Neuroradiol 2002; 29:285-287.

67. de Priester JA, Jansen GH, de Kruijk JR, et al. New MRI findings in Creutzfeldt-Jacob disease; high signal in the globus pallidus on T1-weighted images. Neuroradiology 1999; 41:265-268.

68. Zeidler M, Sellar RJ, Collie DA, et al. The pulvinar sign on magnetic resonance imaging in variant Creutzfeldt-Jacob disease. Lancet 2000; 355:1412-1418.

69. Konaka K, Kaido M, Okuda Y, et al. Proton magnetic resonance spectroscopy of a patient with Gerstmann-Sträussler-Scheinker disease. Neuroradiology 2000; 42:662-665.

70. McLachlam RS, Girvin JP, Blume WT, Reichman H. Rasmussen's chronic encephalitis in adults. Arch Neurol 1993; 50:269-274.

71. Bauer J, Elger CE, Hans VH, et al. Astrocytes are a specific immunological target in Rasmussen's encephalitis. Ann Neurol 2007; 62:67-80.

72. Petito CK, Cho E-S, Lemann W, et al. Neuropathology of acquired immunodeficiency syndrome (AIDS): an autopsy review. J Neuropathol Exp Neurol 1986; 45:635-646.

73. Zimmerman RD, Russell EJ, Leeds NE, Kaufman D. CT in the early diagnosis of herpes simplex encephalitis. AJR Am J Radiol 1980; 134:61-66.

74. Enzmann DR, Ranson B, Norman D, Talberth E. Computed tomography of herpes simplex encephalitis. Radiology 1978; 129:419-425.

75. Burke JW, Mathews VP, Elster AD, et al. Contrast-enhanced magnetization transfer saturation imaging improves MR detection of herpes simplex encephalitis. AJNR Am J Neuroradiol 1996; 17:773-776.

76. Sener RN. Herpes simplex encephalitis: diffusion MR imaging findings. Comput Med Imaging Graph 2001; 25:391-397.

77. Küker W, Nägele T, Schmidt F, et al. Diffusion-weighted MRI in herpes simplex encephalitis: a report of three cases. Neuroradiology 2004; 46:122-125.

78. Heiner L, Demaerel P. Diffusion-weighted MR imaging findings in a patient with herpes simplex encephalitis. Eur J Radiol 2003; 45:195-198.

79. Sämann PG, Schlegel J, Müller G, et al. Serial proton MR spectroscopy and diffusion imaging findings in HIV-related herpes simplex encephalitis. AJNR Am J Neuroradiol 2003; 24:2015-2019.

80. Weaver S, Rosenblum MK, DeAngelis LM. Herpes varicella zoster encephalitis in immunocompromised patients. Neurology 1999; 52:193.

81. Stanek G, Strle F. Lyme borreliosis. Lancet Neurol 2003; 362:1639-1647.

82. Segal BM, Logigian EL. Sublime diagnosis of Lyme neuroborreliosis. Neurology 2005; 65:351-352.

83. Oschmann P, Dorndorf W, Hornig C, et al. Stages and syndromes of neuroborreliosis. J Neurol 1998; 245:262-272.

84. Nelson JA, Wolf MD, Yuh WT, Peeples ME. Cranial nerve involvement with Lyme borreliosis demonstrated by magnetic resonance imaging. Neurology 1992; 42:671-673.

85. Petito CK, Cho E-S, Lemann W, et al. Neuropathology of acquired immunodeficiency syndrome (AIDS): an autopsy review. J Neuropathol Exp Neurol 1986; 45:635-646.

86. Derouin F, Gluckman E, Beauvais B, et al. *Toxoplasma* infection after human allogenic bone marrow transplantation: clinical and serological study of 80 patients. Bone Marrow Transplant 1986; 1:67-73.

87. Post MJD, Chan JC, Hensley GT, et al. *Toxoplasma* encephalitis in Haitian adults with acquired immunodeficiency syndrome: a clinical-pathological-CT correlation. AJR Am J Roentgenol 1983; 140:861-868.

88. Post MJD, Sheldon JJ, Hensley GT, et al. Central nervous system disease in acquired immunodeficiency syndrome: prospective correlation using CT, MR imaging, and pathological studies. Radiology 1986; 158:141-148.

89. Post MJD, Tate LG, Quencer RM, et al. CT, MR, and pathology in HIV encephalitis and meningitis. AJR Am J Roentgenol 1988; 151:373-380.

90. Mueller-Mang C, Castillo M, Mang TG, et al. Fungal versus bacterial brain abscesses: is diffusion-weighted MR imaging a useful tool in the differential diagnosis? Neuroradiology 2007; 49:651-657.

91. Chinn RJS, Wilkinson ID, Hall-Craggs MA, et al. Toxoplasmosis and primary central nervous system lymphoma in HIV infection: diagnosis with MR spectroscopy. Radiology 1995; 197:649-654.

92. Ernst TE, Chang L, Witt MD, et al. Cerebral toxoplasmosis and lymphoma in AIDS: perfusion MR imaging experience in 13 patients. Radiology 1998; 208:663-669.

93. Camacho DL, Smith JK, Castillo M. Differentiation of toxoplasmosis and lymphoma in AIDS patients by using apparent diffusion coefficients. AJNR Am J Neuroradiol 2003; 24:633-637.

94. Schroeder PC, Post MJD, Oschatz E, et al. Analysis of the utility of diffusion-weighted MRI and apparent diffusion coefficient values in distinguishing central nervous system toxoplasmosis from lymphoma. Neuroradiology 2006; 48:715-720.

95. Ruiz A, Ganz WI, Post MJD, et al. Use of thallium-201 brain SPECT to differentiate cerebral lymphoma from *Toxoplasma* encephalitis in AIDS patients. AJNR Am J Neuroradiol 1994; 15:1885-1894.

96. Miller RF, Hall-Craggs MA, Costa DC, et al. Magnetic resonance imaging, thallium-210 SPECT scanning, and laboratory analyses for discrimination of cerebral lymphoma and toxoplasmosis in AIDS. Sex Transm Infect 1998; 74:258-264.

97. Antinori A, De Rossi G, Ammassari A, et al. Value of combined approach with thallium-201 single-photon emission computed tomography and Epstein-Barr virus DNA polymerase chain reaction in CSF for the diagnosis of AIDS-related primary CNS lymphoma. J Clin Oncol 1999; 17:554-560.

98. Villringer K, Jager H, Dichgans M, et al. Differential diagnosis of CNS lesions in AIDS patients by FDG-PET. J Comput Assist Tomogr 1995; 19:532-536.

99. Heald AE, Hoffman JM, Bartlett JA, et al. Differentiation of central nervous system lesions in AIDS patients using positron emission tomography (PET). Int J STD AIDS 1996; 7:337-346.

100. Hoffman JM, Waskin HA, Schifter T, et al. FDG-PET in differentiating lymphoma from nonmalignant central nervous system lesions in patients with AIDS. J Nucl Med 1993; 34:567-575.

101. O´Doherty MJ, Barrington SF, Campbell M, et al. PET scanning and the human immunodeficiency virus–positive patients. J Nucl Med 1997; 38:1575-1583.

102. Del Brutto OH, Sotelo J. Neurocysticercosis: an update. Rev Infect Dis 1998; 10:1075-1087.

103. Castillo M. Imaging of neurocysticercosis. Semin Roentgenol 2004; 39:465-473.

104. Garcia HH, Gonzales AE, Evans CAW, Gilman RH. *Taenia solium* cysticercosis. Lancet 2003; 362:547-556.

105. Escobar A. The pathology of neurocysticercosis. In Palacios E, Rodriguez-Carbajal J, Taveras JM, eds. Cysticercosis of the Central Nervous System. Springfield, IL, Charles C Thomas, 1983, pp 27-59.

106. Davis LE, Kornfeld M. Neurocysticercosis: neurologic, pathogenic, diagnostic and therapeutic aspects. Eur Neurol 1991; 31:229-240.

107. Nash TE, Neva FA. Recent advances in the diagnosis and treatment of cerebral cysticercosis. N Engl J Med 1984; 311:1492-1496.

108. Gupta RK, Prakash M, Mishra AM, et al. Role of diffusion weighted imaging in differentiation of intracranial tuberculoma and tuberculous abscess from cysticercus granulomas—a report of more than 100 lesions. Eur J Radiol 2005; 55:384-392.

109. Bükte Y, Kemanoglu S, Nazaroglu N, et al. Cerebral hydatid disease: CT and MR imaging findings. Swiss Med Wkly 2004; 134:459-467.

110. Lewall DB. Hydatid disease: biology, pathology, imaging and classification. Clin Radiol 1998; 53:863-874.

111. Tsitouridis J, Dimitriadis AS, Kazana E. MR in cisternal hydatid cysts. AJNR Am J Neuroradiol 1997; 18:1586-1587.

112. Senturk S, Oguz KK, Soylemezoglu F, Inci S. Cerebral alveolar echinococcosis mimicking primary brain tumor. AJNR Am J Neuroradiol 2006; 27:420-422.

113. Algros MP, Majo F, Bresson-Hadni S, et al. Intracerebral alveolar echinococcosis. Infection 2003; 31:63-65.

114. Al Zain TJ, Al-Witry SH, Khalili HM, et al. Multiple intracranial hydatidosis. Acta Neurochir (Wien) 2002; 144:1179-1185.

43

Multiple Sclerosis and Other Idiopathic Inflammatory-Demyelinating Diseases

Alex Rovira and Xavier Montalban

Idiopathic inflammatory-demyelinating diseases (IIDDs) represent a broad spectrum of central nervous system (CNS) disorders that can be differentiated on the basis of severity, clinical course, and lesion distribution, as well as imaging, laboratory, and pathologic findings. The spectrum includes monophasic, multiphasic, and progressive disorders ranging from highly localized forms to multifocal or diffuse variants.

Relapsing-remitting and secondary progressive multiple sclerosis (MS) are the two most common forms of IIDDs.[1] MS can also have a progressive course from onset (primary progressive and progressive relapsing MS). Some patients have a benign course with minimal or no disability years after onset (benign MS). Fulminant forms of IIDDs include a variety of disorders that have in common the severity of the clinical symptoms, an acute clinical course, and atypical findings on MRI. The classic fulminant IIDD is Marburg disease. Balo's concentric sclerosis, Schilder's disease, and acute disseminated encephalomyelitis (ADEM) can also present as acute and severe attacks.

Monosymptomatic IIDD, such as transverse myelitis, optic neuritis, and brain stem demyelinating syndromes are commonly the first manifestation of MS, although a percentage of patients never actually develop the disease. Patients with monofocal clinical syndromes and MRI evidence of brain lesions consistent with demyelination have an 88% chance of developing clinically definite MS over the subsequent 14 years, whereas clinically similar patients with normal brain MRIs have less than a 20% chance of such progression.[2] Hence, brain MRI is essential to target patients at high risk of early development of MS to select them for early immunomodulatory treatment.

Some IIDDs have a restricted topographic distribution, such as Devic's neuromyelitis optica (NMO), recurrent optic neuritis, and relapsing transverse myelitis, which can have a monophasic or, more frequently, a relapsing course. Other types of IIDDs occasionally present as a focal lesion that may be clinically and radiographically indistinguishable from a brain tumor. It is difficult to classify these tumefactive or pseudotumoral lesions within the spectrum of IIDDs. Some cases have a monophasic, self-limited course, whereas in others the tumefactive plaque is the first manifestation or appears during a typical relapsing form of MS. MRI of the brain and spine is the imaging technique of choice for diagnosing these disorders, and, together with the clinical and laboratory findings, can accurately classify them.

MULTIPLE SCLEROSIS

Multiple sclerosis is a chronic, persistent inflammatory-demyelinating disease characterized pathologically by areas of inflammation, demyelination, axonal loss, and gliosis scattered throughout the CNS. MS has a predilection for the optic nerves, brain stem, spinal cord, and cerebellar and periventricular white matter.

Relapses and progression are the two major clinical phenomena of prototypic MS. Relapses are considered the clinical expression of acute focal or multifocal inflammatory demyelination disseminated in the CNS. Remission of symptoms early in the disease is likely the result of remyelination, resolution of inflammation, and compensatory mechanisms such as redistribution of axolemmal sodium channels and cortical plasticity. These recovery mechanisms are less effective after recurrent attacks.

In parallel with the demyelinating episodes there may be damage to the exposed axons, leading to transection of the axons and retrograde neuronal degeneration. This process can be irreversible and is responsible for the accrual of disability that occurs as the disease progresses. Later in the disease, flares of inflammatory activity occur less frequently but the neurodegenerative process continues inexorably.

Epidemiology

MS is one of the most common neurologic disorders and the second cause of disability in Western countries in young white adults. It is relatively common in Europe, the United States, Canada, New Zealand, and parts of Australia but rare in Asia and in the tropics and subtropics of all continents. Within regions having a temperate climate, the incidence and prevalence of MS increase with latitude, both north and south of the equator. Multiple sclerosis is twice as common in women as in men; men have a tendency for later disease onset with a poorer prognosis. The incidence of MS is low in childhood, increases rapidly after the age of 18, reaches a peak between 25 and 35, and then slowly declines, becoming rare at 50 and older.[3] The disease affects approximately 1 million people between 17 and 65 years of age worldwide.

MS is usually not life shortening, but its socioeconomic importance is second only to trauma in young adults. The etiology of MS is still unknown, but it most likely results from an interplay between as yet unidentified environmental factors and susceptibility genes. Factors supporting a genetic influence include excess occurrence in Northern Europeans relative to indigenous populations from the same geographic location, familial aggregation, and lack of MS excess in adopted relatives of patients with MS.

The environmental epidemiology of MS is poorly understood. Although a direct causal link with diverse infectious agents has been suggested, such infectious agents may simply provide the appropriate milieu for the development of an autoreactive immune response directed against CNS myelin. Up to now, only Epstein-Barr virus (EBV) infection has been established as a strong, consistent risk factor. As compared with uninfected individuals, MS risk is about 10-fold higher among individuals who experienced an undiagnosed EBV infection in childhood and at least 20-fold higher among individuals who developed mononucleosis.[3]

Clinical Presentation

The clinical course of MS can follow different patterns over time but is usually characterized by acute episodes of worsening (relapses, bouts), gradual progressive deterioration of neurologic function, or a combination of both these features (relapsing MS). In a relatively small percentage of patients, the disease has a progressive course from onset without acute relapses (primary progressive MS).

Relapses or attacks typically present subacutely, with symptoms developing over hours to several days, persisting for several days or weeks, and then gradually abating. With time, the extent of recovery from these attacks often decreases, and baseline neurologic disability accumulates. The outcome in patients with relapsing forms of MS varies. About 50% of MS patients become dependent on a walking aid after 15 years of disease, whereas 10% remain free of any major disability after 25 years. The biologic basis of this variation in long-term clinical outcome is poorly understood. Neither symptom onset, nor gender, nor age at onset of symptoms predicts progression. However, increased attack frequency and poor recovery from attacks in the first year of clinical disease predict more rapid deterioration.[4] The number of T2-weighted (T2W) lesions on brain MRI also predicts attack frequency and long-term disability.[2]

Relapsing-Remitting and Secondary Progressive Multiple Sclerosis

Relapsing forms account for 85% of all MS. This clinical form typically presents as an acute, clinically isolated syndrome attributable to a monofocal or multifocal CNS demyelinating lesion. The presenting lesion usually affects the optic nerve (optic neuritis), spinal cord (acute transverse myelitis), brain stem (typically an internuclear ophthalmoparesis), and cerebellum (clumsiness and gait ataxia).

Some patients have brief, recurrent, stereotypical phenomena (paroxysmal pain or paresthesia, trigeminal neuralgia,

episodic clumsiness or dysarthria, and tonic limb posturing). Eventually, cognitive impairment, depression, vertigo, progressive quadriparesis and sensory loss, ataxic tremors, pain, sexual dysfunction, spasticity, bladder problems, and other manifestations of CNS dysfunction may become troublesome. Many MS patients describe fatigue that is worse in the afternoon. The onset of symptoms post partum, symptomatic worsening with increased body temperature (Uhthoff's symptom), and pseudo-exacerbation with fever are also frequent clinical features.

Over the following years, patients usually experience episodes of acute worsening of neurologic function, followed by variably complete recovery (relapsing-remitting course). Clinical and subclinical activity is frequent in this form. After several years of the relapsing-remitting course, more than 50% of untreated patients will develop progressive disability with or without occasional relapses, minor remissions, and plateaus (secondary progressive course).[1]

As long as the cause of MS remains unknown, causal therapy and effective prevention are not possible. Immunomodulatory drugs such as interferon-β, glatiramer acetate, mitoxantrone, and natalizumab can alter the course of the disease, particularly in the relapsing-remitting form, by reducing the number of relapses and the accumulation of lesions as seen on MRI, and by influencing the impact of the disease on disability. Patients with the secondary progressive form of MS, continuing relapses of activity, and pronounced progression of disability may also benefit from immunomodulatory or immunosuppressive therapy.

Primary Progressive and Progressive-Relapsing Multiple Sclerosis

Primary progressive forms comprise approximately 10% of MS cases. This form of MS begins as a progressive disease with occasional plateaus and relapses and temporary minor improvements. Progressive-relapsing MS follows a progressive course like primary progressive MS but shows clear acute relapses that may or may not be followed by full recovery.[1]

As compared with patients with the more common relapsing form of MS, patients with primary progressive MS tend to be older, show more rapid progression from onset, and are as likely to be male as female. The most common presentation by far is slowly progressing spastic paraparesis and, less frequently, progressive cerebellar, brain stem, visual, hemiplegic, and cognitive syndromes.[5]

According to the 2010 McDonald criteria (Table 43-1),[6] a diagnosis of primary progressive MS can be established if patients show insidious neurologic progression for at least 1 year associated with MS-like abnormalities on brain and/or spinal MRI, and/or oligoclonal bands on cerebrospinal fluid (CSF) study. In patients who present with progressive spastic paraparesis, it is mandatory to exclude structural or metabolic causes of myelopathy by appropriate laboratory studies and spinal MRI.

TABLE 43-1.   Diagnosis of MS with Disease Progression from Onset

---

1. One year of disease progression (retrospectively or prospectively determined)
2. *Plus* two of the three following criteria:
   a. Evidence for dissemination in space in the brain based on ≥1 T2 lesion in at least one area characteristic for MS (juxtacortical, periventricular, or infratentorial)
   b. Evidence for dissemination in space in the spinal cord based on ≥1 T2 lesion in the cord
   c. Positive CSF (isoelectric focusing evidence of oligoclonal IgG bands and/or increased IgG index).

CSF, cerebrospinal fluid.
From Polman CH, Reingold SC, Banwell B, et al. Diagnostic criteria for multiple sclerosis: 2010 revisions to the McDonald criteria. Ann Neurol 2010; 69:292-302.

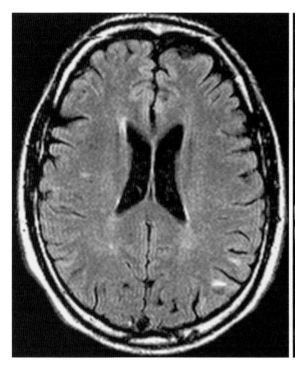
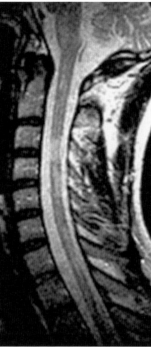

■ **FIGURE 43-1** Primary progressive MS. Transverse fast-FLAIR and FSE T2W sagittal MR images of the brain and cervical cord. The patient's severe disability (paraparesis) cannot be explained by the few demyelinating brain lesions but can result from the multiple demyelinating lesions within the cervical cord.

Compared with patients with the more frequent relapsing forms of MS, patients with primary progressive MS have smaller T2 lesion loads, smaller T2 lesions, slower rates of new lesion formation, and minimal gadolinium enhancement on brain MRI, despite their accumulating disability. The presence of extensive cortical damage, diffuse white matter tissue damage, and prevalent involvement of the spinal cord may partially explain this discrepancy between the MRI abnormalities and the severity of the clinical disease (Fig. 43-1).

Because patients with primary progressive MS may have less inflammation than those with relapsing MS, they may be less likely to respond to immunomodulatory therapies.

Benign Multiple Sclerosis

Benign MS accounts for about 20% of all cases of MS. These patients remain fully functional in all neurologic systems for at least 15 years after the onset of the disease. Factors that predict a benign course include onset with optic neuritis, female gender, onset before the age of 40, absence of pyramidal signs at presentation, duration of first remission more than 1 year, and only one exacerbation in the first 5 years after disease onset. Nevertheless, the form designated "benign" MS is often transient, because 50% to 70% of patients originally considered to have benign MS show significant clinical worsening or a shift to a secondary progressive disease course by 10 years after the baseline examination.

Patients with benign MS have few new or enlarging lesions on serial brain MRI studies, and such lesions that occur have a lower incidence of enhancement after use of a contrast agent (Fig. 43-2), as compared with the typical relapsing-remitting forms of MS associated with progressive disability (Fig. 43-3). Prediction of a benign MS course may have an impact on the decision to initiate immunomodulatory medication, because this treatment may be unnecessary or might at least be postponed for many years.

Multiple Sclerosis Variants

Marburg Disease

Marburg disease (also termed *malignant* MS) is a rare, acute MS variant that occurs predominantly in young adults. It is character-

ized by a confusional state, headache, vomiting, gait unsteadiness, and hemiparesis. This entity has a rapidly progressive course with frequent, severe relapses leading to death or severe disability within weeks to months, mainly from brain stem involvement or mass effect with herniation. Most of the patients who survive subsequently develop a relapsing form of MS. Because Marburg disease is often preceded by a febrile illness, this disease may also be considered a fulminant form of ADEM if it has a monophasic course. At the time of the clinical presentation, it can be difficult to find good predictors of whether the patient will follow a fulminant course, develop mild or severe MS, or even develop MS at all.

Pathologically, lesions of Marburg disease are more destructive than those of typical MS or ADEM and are characterized by massive macrophage infiltration, acute axonal injury, and tissue necrosis. Despite the destructive nature of these lesions, areas of remyelination are often observed. Neuropathologic studies suggest that this fulminant form of MS is often associated with deposition of immunoglobulins and pronounced complement activation at sites of active myelin destruction, which may support plasma exchange or mitoxantrone as treatment options when high-dose corticosteroids are not effective.

In Marburg disease, MRI typically shows multiple focal T2 lesions of varying size, which may coalesce to form large white matter plaques disseminated throughout the hemispheric white matter and brain stem (Fig. 43-4). Perilesional edema is often present. The lesions may show enhancement. A similar imaging pattern is also seen in ADEM.

A fulminant course can also be present in acute IIDDs showing a tumefactive or Balo-like lesion.

Schilder's Disease

Schilder's disease is a rare acute or subacute disorder that can be defined as a specific clinicoradiologic presentation of IIDD. It commonly affects children and young adults. The clinical spectrum of Schilder's disease includes psychiatric predominance, acute intracranial hypertension, intermittent exacerbations, and progressive deterioration. Imaging studies show

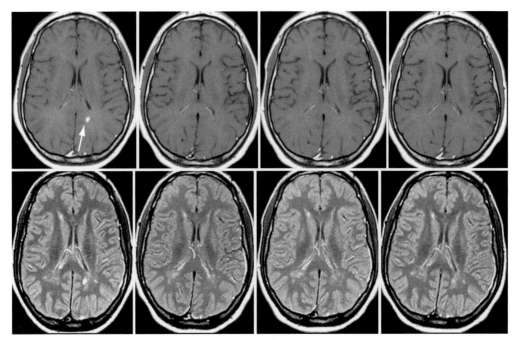

■ **FIGURE 43-2** Benign MS. Serial, contrast-enhanced T1W (*top row*) and T2W (*bottom row*) MR images of the brain obtained yearly in a patient with benign MS. Note the small number of new lesions that developed over the 3-year follow-up and the very low incidence of contrast enhancement (*arrow in the baseline scan*). (*From Cañellas AR, Gols AR, Izquierdo JR, et al. Idiopathic inflammatory-demyelinating diseases of the central nervous system. Neuroradiology 2007; 49:393-469.*)

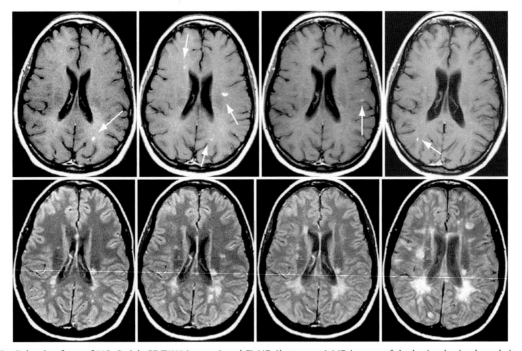

■ **FIGURE 43-3** Relapsing form of MS. Serial, CE T1W (*top row*) and FLAIR (*bottom row*) MR images of the brain obtained yearly in a patient with a typical relapsing form of MS and progressive disability. Note the new lesions that appeared during this 3-year follow-up, some of them showing gadolinium enhancement (*arrows*). (*From Cañellas AR, Gols AR, Izquierdo JR, et al. Idiopathic inflammatory-demyelinating diseases of the central nervous system. Neuroradiology 2007; 49:393-469.*)

large ring-enhancing lesions involving both hemispheres, sometimes symmetrically, and located preferentially in the parieto-occipital regions. These large, focal demyelinating lesions can resemble a brain tumor, an abscess, or even adrenoleukodystrophy. MR features that suggest possible Schilder's disease include large and relatively symmetric involvement of both

brain hemispheres, incomplete ring enhancement, minimal mass effect, restricted diffusivity, and sparing of the brain stem (Fig. 43-5).

Histopathologically, Schilder's disease consistently shows well-demarcated demyelination and reactive gliosis with relative sparing of the axons. Microcystic changes and even frank

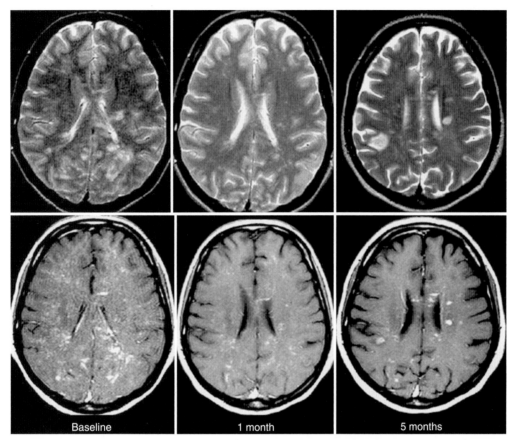

■ FIGURE 43-4 Marburg disease. Serial T2W (*top row*) and contrast-enhanced T1W (*bottom row*) MR images of the brain obtained in a patient with a final diagnosis of fulminant IIDD. Note multiple contrast-enhanced focal lesions diffusely involving the cerebral white matter. Some of the lesions are persistent, whereas others are new. The patient died 5 months after symptom onset. *(From Cañellas AR, Gols AR, Izquierdo JR, et al. Idiopathic inflammatory-demyelinating diseases of the central nervous system. Neuroradiology 2007; 49:393-469.)*

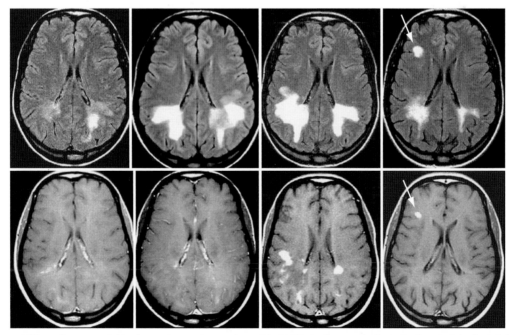

■ FIGURE 43-5 Schilder's disease. Serial brain MR images in a patient with Schilder's disease who later developed clinically definite MS. Transverse fast-FLAIR images (*top row*) and contrast-enhanced T1W (*bottom row*) images obtained serially over 6 months. Note the progressive appearance of large, bilateral, almost symmetric lesions in the posterior periventricular white matter. Despite considerable extension of the lesions there is no mass effect. The 6-month scan obtained during an episode of optic neuritis shows a new contrast-enhancing lesion in the right frontal white matter (*arrow*). A final diagnosis of relapsing-remitting MS was established. *(From Cañellas AR, Gols AR, Izquierdo JR, et al. Idiopathic inflammatory-demyelinating diseases of the central nervous system. Neuroradiology 2007; 49:393-469.)*

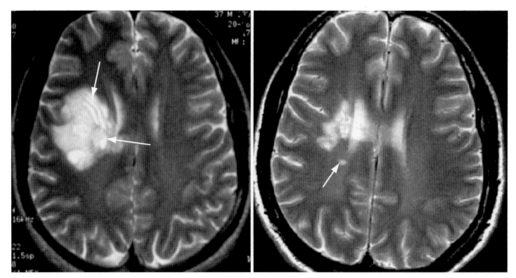

■ **FIGURE 43-6**   Balo-like lesion in a patient who converted to MS. Transverse T2W MR image of the brain shows a large focal lesion within the right frontal white matter. The striking lamellated pattern of alternating bands of demyelination and relatively normal white matter, reflecting either spared or remyelinated regions, is clear in this image (*arrows, left*). Note partial resolution of the large hemispheric lesion in a follow-up T2W MR image obtained 4 years after symptom onset and the presence of a new lesion (*arrow, right*).

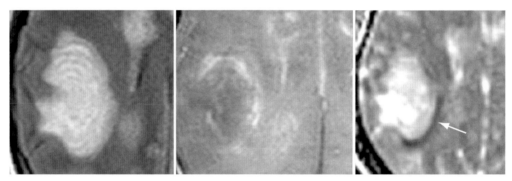

■ **FIGURE 43-7**   Balo-like lesion in patients with acute disseminated encephalomyelitis. Transverse T2W (*left*) and contrast-enhanced T1W (*middle*) MR images and apparent diffusion coefficient (ADC) map (*right*). Observe the alternating concentric bands, peripheral contrast uptake, and decreased peripheral diffusivity (*arrow*). *(From Cañellas AR, Gols AR, Izquierdo JR, et al. Idiopathic inflammatory-demyelinating diseases of the central nervous system. Neuroradiology 2007; 49:393-469.)*

cavitation can occur. The clinical and imaging findings usually show a dramatic response to corticosteroids.

Balo's Concentric Sclerosis

Balo's concentric sclerosis is thought to be a rare, aggressive variant of MS that can lead to death in weeks to months. The pathologic hallmarks of the disease are large demyelinated lesions showing a peculiar pattern of alternating layers of preserved and destroyed myelin. One possible explanation for the concentric alternating bands in this variant of MS may be that sublethal tissue injury is induced at the edge of the expanding lesion, which would then stimulate the expression of neuroprotective proteins to protect the rim of periplaque tissue from damage, thereby resulting in alternative layers of preserved and nonpreserved myelinated tissue.[7]

These alternating bands can be identified on T2W MRI, which typically shows concentric hyperintense bands corresponding to areas of demyelination and gliosis alternating with isointense bands corresponding to normal myelinated white matter (Figs. 43-6 and 43-7). This pattern can appear as multiple concentric layers (onionskin lesion), as a mosaic, or as a "floral" configuration. The center of the lesion usually shows no layering because of massive demyelination. Contrast enhancement and decreased diffusivity are frequent in the outer rings (inflammatory

edge) of the lesion (see Fig. 43-7). On MRI this Balo pattern can be isolated, multiple, or mixed with typical MS-like lesions.

Although Balo's concentric sclerosis was initially described as an acute, monophasic and rapidly fatal disease that resembled Marburg disease, large Balo-like lesions are frequently identified on MRI in patients with a classic acute or chronic MS disease course or in ADEM with a nonfatal course.

Tumefactive or Pseudotumoral IIDDs

Infrequently, IIDDs present as single or multiple focal lesions that can be clinically and radiographically indistinguishable from a brain tumor. This situation represents a diagnostic challenge and may require biopsy for definitive diagnosis, despite the clinical suspicion of demyelination. Given the hypercellular nature of these lesions, however, even the biopsy specimen may resemble a brain tumor. Large reactive astrocytes with fragmented chromatin (Creutzfeldt-Peters cells) are often present.

In some cases, pseudotumoral IIDDs are the first clinical and radiologic manifestation of MS. More commonly, tumefactive demyelinating plaques affect patients with a known diagnosis of MS (Fig. 43-8). In rare cases, pseudotumoral IIDDs have a relapsing course, with single or multiple pseudotumoral lesions appearing over time in different locations (Fig. 43-9).

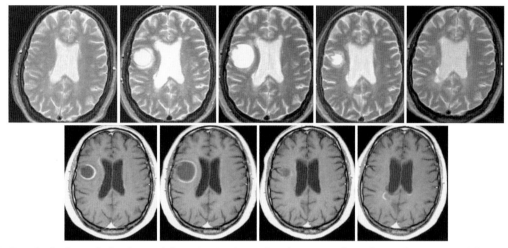

■ FIGURE 43-8 Tumefactive form of relapsing-remitting MS. T2W (*top row*) and contrast-enhanced T1W (*bottom row*) serial MR images of the brain acquired over 12 months in a patient with the relapsing-remitting form of MS. Note the initial increase and later decrease in size of the right frontal lobe pseudotumoral lesion, which is almost imperceptible on the 12-month scan. The lesion shows an open ring–enhancing pattern of contrast uptake, with the open margin facing the gray matter. The pseudotumoral lesion was asymptomatic.

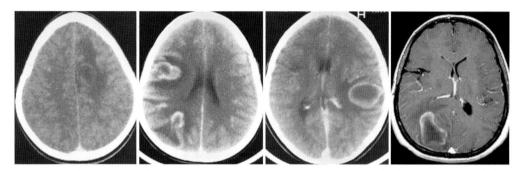

■ FIGURE 43-9 Tumefactive relapsing course. Serial contrast-enhanced CT and T1W MR images obtained in a 10-year-old girl who experienced several acute relapses over a period of several years related to pseudotumoral bihemispheric lesions. *(From Cañellas AR, Gols AR, Izquierdo JR, et al. Idiopathic inflammatory-demyelinating diseases of the central nervous system. Neuroradiology 2007; 49:393-469.)*

On CT or MRI the pseudotumoral plaques usually present as large, single or multiple focal lesions within the cerebral hemispheres. Clues that can help to differentiate these lesions from a brain tumor are the relatively minor mass effect and the presence of *incomplete* ring-enhancement on gadolinium-enhanced T1-weighted (T1W) images, with the open border facing the gray matter of the cortex or basal ganglia (Fig. 43-10),[8] sometimes associated with a rim of peripheral hypointensity on T2W sequences.

Diagnosis

All the diagnostic criteria for establishing the diagnosis of MS proposed in the past 50 years are based on three main principles: (1) demonstration of disease dissemination in space (DIS); (2) demonstration of disease dissemination in time (DIT); and (3) reasonable exclusion of alternative explanations for the clinical presentation.

These principles were codified in 1983 by the Poser committee,[9] which specified that the diagnosis of clinically definite MS could be based on either (1) occurrence of two attacks and clinical evidence of two lesions or (2) two attacks and clinical evidence of one lesion plus paraclinical evidence of a second lesion. MRI was not considered at that time because it was then a new, untested technique.

In 2001, new diagnostic criteria were published that incorporated a precisely defined role for MRI.[10] These 2001 McDonald criteria integrated MRI criteria into their scheme to demonstrate dissemination of demyelinating lesions in space (Table 43-2). To demonstrate this principle, brain MR images must meet the Barkhof-Tintoré criteria, in which a threshold of at least three of the following four features must be achieved: (1) one gadolinium-enhancing lesion or nine T2 hyperintense lesions if gadolinium-enhancing lesions are not present, (2) at least one infratentorial lesion, (3) at least one juxtacortical lesion, and (4) at least three periventricular lesions. When three of these four parameters are *not* fulfilled, the presence of two or more subclinical lesions consistent with MS on brain MRI plus CSF detection of oligoclonal bands or a raised IgG index are required to demonstrate DIS. DIT can be demonstrated with MRI when new lesions have developed at least 3 months after the clinical onset. This can be a gadolinium-enhancing lesion on a scan obtained more than 3 months after a clinically isolated syndrome if it is not associated with the initial clinical event. When the scan shows no new enhancing lesion, a subsequent scan is required to demonstrate new T2 and/or gadolinium-enhancing lesions. This criterion requires between one and three MR images to be performed, with a minimum delay between symptom onset and the first scan of at least 3 months.

In 2005, a consensus revision of the McDonald criteria based on new evidence was proposed (see Table 43-2).[13] Three major changes were introduced in the 2005 McDonald criteria. The first modification attempted to simplify the criteria for DIT. This was

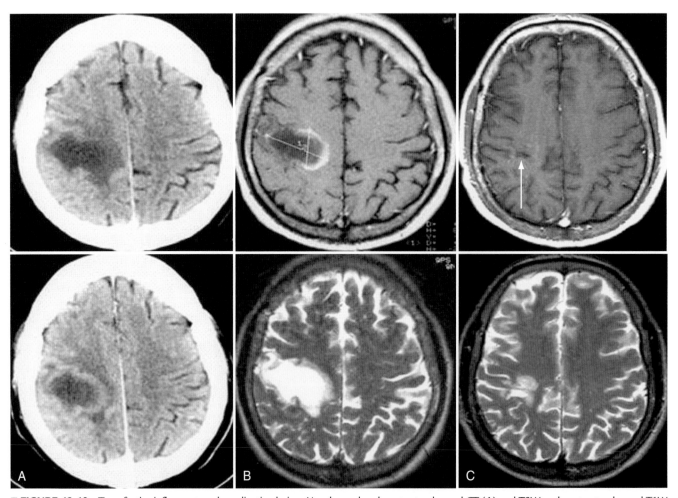

■ **FIGURE 43-10** Tumefactive inflammatory demyelinating lesion. Unenhanced and contrast-enhanced CT (**A**) and T2W and contrast-enhanced T1W MR images (**B**) of brain show a posterior frontal lesion with minimal surrounding vasogenic edema and no mass effect. Observe the ring-enhancing pattern of contrast agent uptake, with the open margin facing the cortical gray matter. A follow-up brain MR image performed 1 year later (**C**) shows almost complete resolution of the lesion. The necrotic focus (*arrow*) in the subcortical white matter corresponds to the site of a brain biopsy, which confirmed the diagnosis of inflammatory demyelinating lesion.

TABLE 43-2. MRI Criteria of Dissemination in Space (DIS) and Dissemination in Time (DIT) for Diagnosing MS

	McDonald 2001[10]	McDonald 2005[6]	McDonald 2010[13]
Dissemination in space (on either baseline or follow-up MRI)	Three or more of the following:	Three or more of the following:	≥1 lesion in each of ≥2 characteristic locations:
	9 T2 lesions or 1 Gd-enhancing lesion	9 T2 lesions or 1 Gd-enhancing lesion	
	3 or more PV lesions	3 or more PV lesions	PV
	1 or more JC lesions	1 or more JC lesions	JC
	1 or more PF lesions	1 or more PF lesions	PF
	A cord lesion can replace a brain lesion.	A cord lesion can replace an infratentorial lesion.	Cord
		Any number of cord lesions can be included in total lesion count.	All lesions in symptomatic regions excluded in BS and SC syndromes
Dissemination in time	A Gd-enhancing lesion at least 3 months after CIS onset	A Gd-enhancing lesion at least 3 months after CIS onset	A new T2 lesion on follow-up MRI regardless of timing of baseline scan
	A new T2 lesion relative to a prior scan, at least 3 months after CIS onset	A new T2 lesion relative to a baseline scan, obtained at least 30 days after CIS onset	Concomitant enhancing and nonenhancing lesions

Gd, gadolinium-enhancing lesion; PV, periventricular; JC, juxtacortical; PF, posterior fossa; BS, brain stem; SC, spinal cord; CIS, clinically isolated syndrome.
Modified from Swanton JK, Rovira A, Tintore M, et al. MRI criteria for multiple sclerosis in patients presenting with clinically isolated syndromes: a multicentre retrospective study. Lancet Neurol 2007; 6:677-686.

achieved by establishing the simple condition of demonstrating a new T2 lesion on a brain MR image at any time as compared with a reference scan done at least 30 days after the onset of the initial clinical event. The reason for selecting the 30-day time period was to exclude new T2 lesions occurring in the first few weeks after the onset of the first clinical episode, which would not be considered a new separate event. The second change proposed endeavored to better define the role of MRI of spinal cord lesions for demonstrating DIS.

A new version of the McDonald criteria (McDonald 2010)[6] proposed new MR imaging criteria, in which demonstration of DIS requires the presence of at least one asymptomatic T2 lesion in two of the four locations defined as characteristic for MS: juxtacortical, periventricular, infratentorial, and spinal cord, while demonstration of DIT requires demonstration of a new T2 lesion on a follow-up scan irrespective of the timing of the baseline scan, or concomitant enhancing and non enhancing lesions on a scan performed at any time after symptoms onset[11,12] (see Table 41-2). These criteria have shown similar (high) specificity for clinically definite MS and higher sensitivity when compared with the 2001 and 2005 McDonald criteria.

For optimal application of MRI criteria, scans must be technically adequate and well repositioned to permit fair comparisons between scans obtained at different times. Physicians involved in the diagnostic MRI evaluation must be provided with sufficient demographic and clinical information to properly interpret the imaging findings and be expert enough to recognize the full range of brain and spinal cord abnormalities that suggest the diagnosis of MS.

Pathophysiology

It is generally accepted that the sequence of events underlying the development of the inflammatory plaque in MS originates from a breach in the integrity of the blood-brain barrier via the interaction of integrins expressed on the surface of lymphocytes and adhesion molecules present on the endothelial surface of blood vessels. Genetic and environmental factors, such as a viral infection, may facilitate the entry of potentially pathogenic autoreactive T cells and antibodies into the CNS via blood-brain barrier disruption. Local CNS factors upregulate the expression of endothelial adhesion molecules, which further enhances the movement of pathogenic cells into the CNS. Proinflammatory cytokines within the CNS activate resident and hematogenous macrophages, which contribute to tissue injury and demyelination.

To propagate the inflammatory cascade, T cells that have entered the CNS need to be activated by specific antigens, which requires the presentation of antigenic peptides in the context of major histocompatibility complex (MHC) molecules. Therefore the presence of the so-called trimolecular complex consisting of the T-cell receptor, the processed antigen, and the MHC molecule is needed to activate the T cells, which will ultimately orchestrate multiple cellular and humoral responses that result in tissue injury and formation of an acute inflammatory-demyelinating lesion.

MS is remarkably heterogeneous, particularly when one considers the inflammatory mechanisms leading to tissue damage, patterns of demyelination, oligodendrocyte survival, extent of remyelination, and degree of axonal injury. Luchinetti and colleagues grouped focal active MS plaques into four types, I through IV, on the basis of the pathogeneses of the lesions. All four types are characterized by T cell– and macrophage-dominated inflammation:

Type I is distinguished by demyelination and macrophage-related products.
Type II is characterized by the presence of immunoglobulin and complement, which likely explains the good response to plasma exchange in patients with this pattern.

Type III lacks immunoglobulin and complement, yet it shows early loss of myelin-associated glycoprotein and no remyelination; in this type, demyelination has been attributed to oligodendrocyte dysfunction.
Type IV is distinguished by apoptosis of oligodendrocytes through DNA fragmentation.

The heterogeneous pathologic patterns have been related to specific MS variants. All patients with the Devic type of neuromyelitis optica have antibody-mediated tissue damage (type II), whereas all patients with the Balo type of concentric lesions have a distal oligodendrogliopathy (type III). Furthermore, primary oligodendrocyte degeneration (type IV) has only been found in patients with primary progressive MS disease.

In individual patients, this pathogenic heterogeneity disappears, because there is a striking homogeneity among lesions. For this reason it has been suggested that MS may represent a common name for different pathologic features.[13] This hypothesis has important therapeutic implications because specific therapies can be targeted to specific mechanisms.

Pathology

The pathologic hallmarks of MS lesions are (1) inflammation with T cells, B cells, and macrophages/microglia; (2) demyelination with oligodendrocyte loss during the chronic stage of the disease and varying degrees of remyelination; (3) axonal loss; and (4) gliosis with astrocyte proliferation and intense glial fiber production.

In general, MS plaques are centered on one or several medium-sized vessels and have a tendency to accumulate near the periventricular or outer surfaces of the brain and spinal cord. The lesions are usually round to oval but often show finger-like extensions in the periphery (Dawson's fingers) that follow the path of a small- or medium-sized vessel. On gross inspection, the plaques appear as gray discolored areas with a firm tissue texture. Neuropathologically, focal MS lesions can be divided into chronic and active plaques.

The Chronic MS Lesion

Chronic MS plaques vary in number and size (ranging from <1 mm to several centimeters). They are most conspicuous in the periventricular white matter around the angles of the lateral ventricles and at the floor of the fourth ventricle. The visual system, deep white matter, brain stem, and spinal cord are also commonly affected. These chronic inactive plaques are sharply circumscribed, are hypocellular, and show no evidence of active myelin breakdown. Fibrillary gliosis is prominent, and axonal density is manifestly reduced. Mature oligodendrocytes are markedly decreased or absent. Varying degrees of inflammation may still be present, particularly in the perivascular region.

In chronic MS plaques, remyelination is incomplete and restricted largely to their edge. These lesions are referred to as "shadow plaques" and consist of areas of reduced staining of myelin (myelin pallor) as a result of the decreased ratio between myelin sheath thickness and axonal diameter.

The Active MS Lesion

Active inflammatory demyelinating MS plaques are typically restricted to the white matter and are characterized by a mixture of lipid-laden macrophages and large reactive astrocytes, accompanied by varying perivascular inflammation. The affected areas show marked pallor of myelin staining with relative axonal preservation, although in areas where the damage is most severe the axons can be lost, be fragmented, or display irregular tortuous and clubbed profiles. Many macrophages become engorged with phagocytosed myelin remnants and debris. The so-called granular mitosis or Creutzfeldt-Peters cell is an unusual finding in reactive astrocytes in demyelination and other reactive processes. These structures have the appearance of large chromosomes arranged like mitotic figures but are actually small fragments of the nucleus. The Creutzfeldt-Peters cells may also suggest a diagnosis of glioma; however, the even distribution of the cells, the associated presence of large numbers of infiltrating macrophages in the setting of myelin loss, and relative axonal preservation should confirm that it is an inflammatory demyelinating disease and exclude the diagnosis of glioma.

Normal-Appearing Brain Tissue in MS

In addition to focal demyelinated plaques, diffuse global injury outside the focal MS lesions, referred to as normal-appearing brain tissue, is also found in the brains of MS patients. These abnormalities include diffuse astrocytic hyperplasia, patchy edema, and perivascular cellular infiltration, as well as axonal damage and microscopic focal lesions. In vivo demonstration of this widespread abnormality has been shown by several sophisticated MR techniques, such as MR spectroscopy (MRS), which reveals reduced *N*-acetyl-aspartate (NAA) and elevated creatine levels, magnetization transfer imaging, which demonstrates reduced magnetic transfer ratios, and diffusion-weighted imaging (DWI) sequences, which show increased diffusivity and decreased fractional anisotropy. These changes are more pronounced in the progressive forms of the disease, although they can also be detected in patients with clinically isolated syndromes suggestive of MS.

Gray Matter Pathology in MS

Although MS is considered a disease of the white matter, demyelination also can be found in the deep cerebral nuclei, cerebral cortex, and gray matter of the spinal cord and brain stem. Involvement of the cerebral cortex may contribute to neurologic and cognitive impairment, particularly in advanced disease stages, as a result of axon and dendrite transection, synapse loss, and neuron apoptosis. Cortical lesions differ from white matter plaques in several aspects. The lesions are hypocellular, contain fewer T lymphocytes, and show better preservation of overall tissue texture than do white matter lesions, suggesting less overall tissue injury.

Imaging
CT

The sensitivity of brain CT for detecting MS plaques is rather low but was the only method available for demonstrating these lesions before the advent of MRI. CT findings, such as areas of hypodensity or brain atrophy, appear late in the disease and are nonspecific. Active plaques may show varying contrast enhancement. Some active lesions become apparent only when high-dose, delayed contrast-enhanced CT scans are performed.

Contrast-enhanced CT may be the first imaging procedure used in patients with tumefactive pseudotumoral inflammatory-demyelinating brain lesions, because the clinical features may suggest a brain tumor. A finding of incomplete ring enhancement with the open margin abutting the gray matter should suggest the correct diagnosis,[8] because such findings are unusual for brain tumors and abscesses (see Fig. 43-10). Minimal or absent mass effect and a compatible clinical setting (young female, no history of cancer or brain infection) are additional clues.

CT can be useful for detecting brain or spinal cord lesions other than MS in patients with neurologic symptoms who cannot undergo MRI.

MRI
Conventional MRI Techniques
Brain

MRI is the most sensitive imaging technique for detecting MS plaques throughout the brain and spinal cord. Proton density

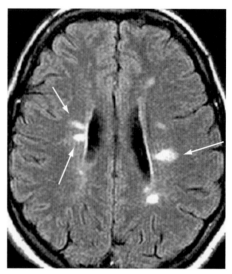

■ **FIGURE 43-11** Relapsing-remitting MS. Transverse fast-FLAIR MR image shows typical ovoid demyelinating plaques (*arrows*), whose major axis is perpendicular to the ventricular wall.

(PD)-weighted (PDW) or T2W MR images show areas of high signal intensity in the periventricular white matter in 98% of MS patients. MS plaques are generally round to ovoid and range from a few millimeters to more than 1 cm in diameter. They are typically discrete and focal at the early stages of the disease but become confluent as the disease progresses, particularly in the posterior hemispheric periventricular white matter (see Fig. 43-3). MS plaques tend to affect the deep white matter rather than the subcortical white matter, whereas small vessel ischemic lesions tend to involve the subcortical white matter more than the periventricular white matter. The total T2 lesion volume of the brain increases by 5% to 10% each year in the relapsing forms of MS.[14]

Both acute and chronic MS plaques appear bright on PDW and T2W sequences, reflecting their increased tissue water content. The signal increase indicates edema, inflammation, demyelination, reactive gliosis, and/or axonal loss in proportions that differ from lesion to lesion. The vast majority of MS patients have at least one ovoid periventricular lesion, whose major axis is oriented perpendicular to the outer surface of the lateral ventricles (Fig. 43-11). The ovoid shape and perpendicular orientation derive from the perivenular location of the demyelinating plaques (Dawson's fingers).

MS lesions tend to affect specific regions of the brain, including the periventricular white matter situated superolateral to the lateral angles of the ventricles, the callososeptal interface along the inferior surface of the corpus callosum, the corticojuxtacortical regions, and the infratentorial regions. Focal involvement of the periventricular white matter in the anterior temporal lobes is typical for MS and rarely seen in other white matter disorders (Fig. 43-12). The lesions commonly found at the callososeptal interface are best depicted by sagittal fast-FLAIR images; so this sequence is highly recommended for diagnostic MRI studies (Fig. 43-13).

Histopathologic studies have shown that a substantial portion of the total brain lesion load in MS is located within the cerebral cortex. Presently available MRI techniques are not optimal for detecting cortical lesions because of poor contrast resolution between normal-appearing gray matter and the plaques in question and because of the partial volume effects of the subarachnoid spaces and CSF surrounding the cortex. Cortical lesions are better visualized by 2D or 3D fast-FLAIR sequences and newer MR techniques such as double inversion recovery MR sequences,

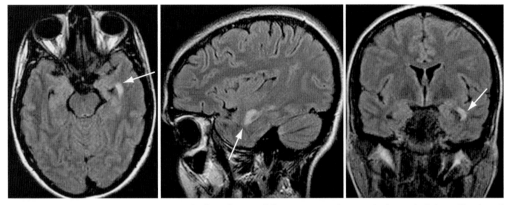

■ **FIGURE 43-12** Relapsing-remitting MS. Transverse, sagittal, and coronal fast-FLAIR MR images depict typical demyelinating plaques affecting the anterior temporal periventricular white matter on the left side (*arrows*).

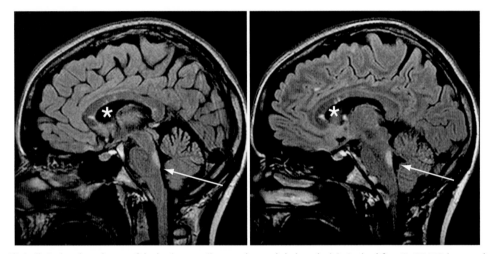

■ **FIGURE 43-13** Clinically isolated syndrome of the brain stem (internuclear ophthalmoplegia). Sagittal fast-FLAIR MR images show the symptomatic lesion located in the floor of the fourth ventricle (*arrows*) and subclinical lesions on the callososeptal interface (*asterisks*).

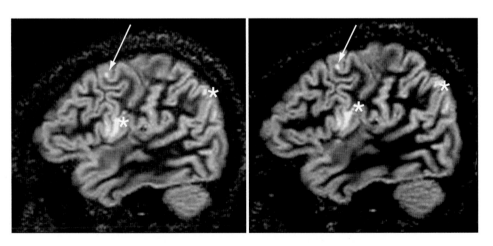

■ **FIGURE 43-14** Relapsing-remitting MS. Sagittal double inversion recovery MR images show small hyperintense lesions involving the posterior frontal cortex (*arrows*) and multiple juxtacortical lesions affecting the inferior frontal and parietal lobes (*asterisks*).

which selectively suppress the signal from white matter and CSF (Fig. 43-14); phase-sensitive inversion recovery sequences, which generates a high signal-to-noise ratio image; and very high resolution images obtained in high-field magnets.

Juxtacortical lesions that involve the U fibers are seen in two thirds of patients with MS. They are a rather characteristic finding in early stages of the disease and are best detected by

fast-FLAIR (Fig. 43-15) and contrast-enhanced T1W sequences (Fig. 43-16).

MS frequently affects the brain stem and cerebellum, leading to acute clinical syndromes, such as trigeminal neuralgia, internuclear ophthalmoplegia, vertigo, and ataxia. Later on, chronic damage to the posterior fossa causes chronic disabling symptoms such as ataxia and oculomotor disturbances. Acute

■ **FIGURE 43-15** Relapsing-remitting MS. Transverse FSE T2W (*left*) and fast-FLAIR (*right*) MR images. A juxtacortical lesion involving the inferior frontal lobe is better depicted on the fast-FLAIR image as compared with the FSE image (*arrow*).

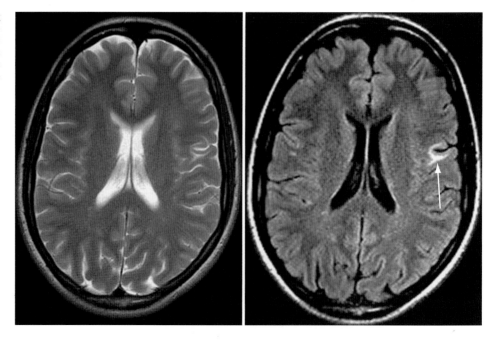

symptomatic lesions appear as well-defined, hyperintense focal lesions that enhance with contrast agent administration on T1W images (Fig. 43-17).

Posterior fossa lesions preferentially involve the floor of the fourth ventricle, the middle cerebellar peduncles, and the brain stem. Most brain stem lesions are contiguous with the cisternal or ventricular CSF spaces and range from large confluent patches to solitary, well-delineated paramedian lesions or discrete "linings" of the CSF border zones. Predilection for these areas is a key feature that helps to identify MS plaques and to differentiate them from focal areas of ischemic demyelination and infarction that preferentially involve the central pontine white matter (Fig. 43-18). Because of their short acquisition time and greater sensitivity, PDW and T2W fast spin-echo (FSE) sequences are preferred over conventional spin-echo or fast-FLAIR sequences for detecting posterior fossa lesions (Fig. 43-19).

Ten to 20 percent of T2 hyperintensities are also visible on T1W images as areas of low signal intensity compared with normal-appearing white matter. These so-called T1 black holes have a different pathologic substrate that depends, in part, on the lesion's age. The hypointensity is present in up to 80% of recently formed lesions and probably represents marked edema, with or without myelin destruction or axonal loss. In most cases the acute (or wet) "black holes" become isointense within a few months as inflammatory activity abates, edema resolves, and reparative mechanisms such as remyelination become active (Fig. 43-20). Less than 40% evolve into persisting or chronic black holes (Fig. 43-21).[15]

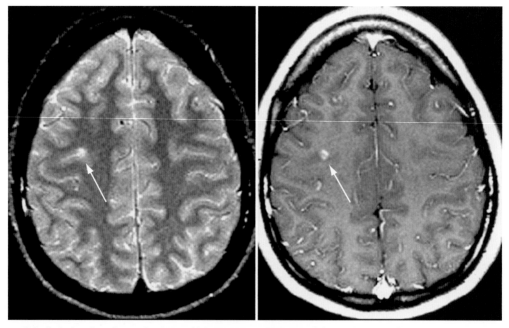

■ **FIGURE 43-16** Clinically isolated syndrome (optic neuritis). Transverse FSE T2W (*left*) MR image and contrast-enhanced T1W (*right*) image. A juxtacortical lesion in the frontal lobe is better visualized on the T1W image than on the T2W image (*arrows*).

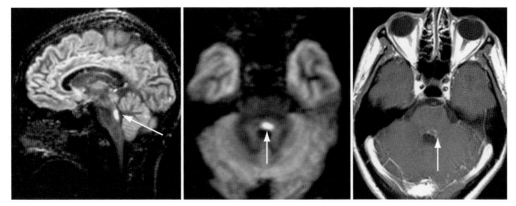

■ **FIGURE 43-17** Clinically isolated syndrome of the brain stem (internuclear ophthalmoplegia). Sagittal (*left*) and transverse (*middle*) double inversion recovery and contrast-enhanced T1W (*right*) MR images. The symptomatic lesion is clearly seen on the double inversion recovery sequence as a well-defined focal hyperintense area affecting the left medial longitudinal fasciculus and showing contrast uptake (*arrows*).

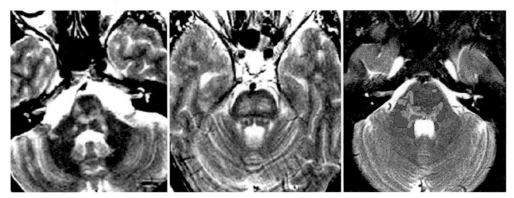

■ **FIGURE 43-18** Brain stem lesions. Transverse T2W MR images obtained in a patient with secondary progressive MS (*left*) and a patient with cerebral small vessel disease (*middle*). In MS, the lesions predominantly involve the periphery of the pons, whereas in the patient with small vessel disease the lesions mainly affect the central tegmentum. The image on the right is a probability map related to the most frequent locations within the pons of lesions responsible for acute inflammatory-demyelinating brain stem syndromes.

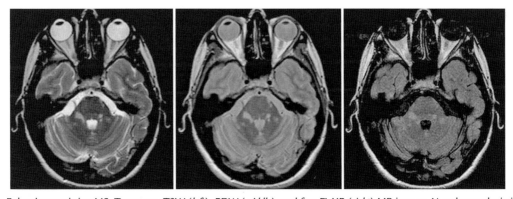

■ **FIGURE 43-19** Relapsing-remitting MS. Transverse T2W (*left*), PDW (*middle*), and fast-FLAIR (*right*) MR images. Note better depiction of the posterior fossa lesions in the T2W and PDW images as compared with the fast-FLAIR sequence.

Chronic "black holes" correlate pathologically with the most severe demyelination and axonal loss, indicating areas of irreversible tissue damage. Spin-echo T1-weighted sequences have a higher specificity than T2-weighted sequences for detecting lesions with irreversible tissue damage and may serve as surrogate markers of disability progression. Several clinical trials have shown significant reductions in the accumulation of new chronic black holes in patients treated with immunomodulatory drugs.

Chronic black holes are more frequent in patients with progressive disease than in those with relapsing-remitting disease (Fig. 43-22) and are more frequent in the supratentorial white matter as compared with the infratentorial white matter. They are rarely found in the spinal cord and optic nerves.

Spinal Cord

MS lesions of the spinal cord resemble those in the brain. The lesions can be focal (single or multiple) or diffuse and mainly affect the cervical cord segment. On sagittal scans, the lesions characteristically have a cigar shape and rarely exceed two vertebral segments in length. On cross section they typically occupy

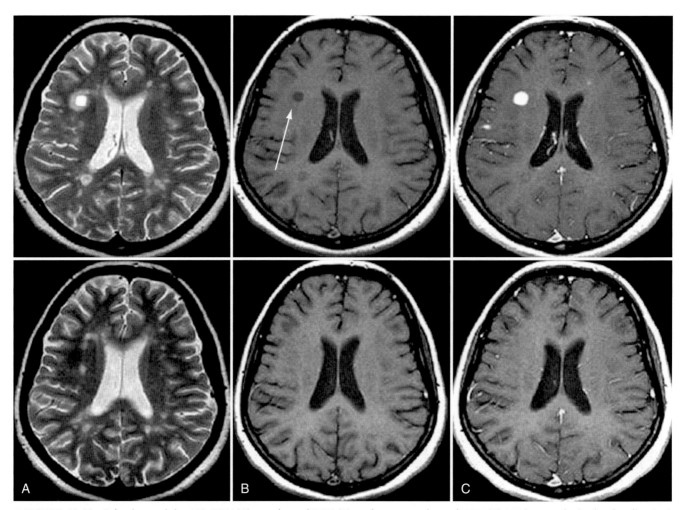

■ **FIGURE 43-20** Relapsing-remitting MS. T2W (**A**), unenhanced T1W (**B**), and contrast-enhanced T1W (**C**) MR images obtained at baseline (*top*) and 1 year later (*bottom*). Observe the active "black hole" (nodular enhancement) in the subcortical white matter of the right frontal lobe (*arrow*), which becomes isointense on T1W imaging with cessation of inflammatory activity (no enhancement).

the lateral and posterior white matter columns, extend to involve the central gray matter, and rarely occupy more than one half the cross-sectional area of the cord (Fig. 43-23).

Acute spinal cord lesions can produce a mild to moderate mass effect with cord swelling and may show contrast enhancement (Fig. 43-24). Active lesions are rarer in the spinal cord than the brain and are almost always associated with new clinical symptoms.

The prevalence of cord abnormalities is as high as 74% to 92% in established MS and depends on the clinical phenotype of MS. In clinically isolated syndromes, the prevalence of spinal cord lesions is lower, particularly if there are no spinal cord symptoms. Nevertheless, asymptomatic cord lesions are found in 30% to 40% of patients with a clinically isolated syndrome. The added value of performing spinal cord MRI in patients with a clinically isolated syndrome not involving the spinal cord has not been definitively established, but the presence of cord lesions may help to determine DIS, according to the 2010 McDonald criteria, at the time of the diagnosis.

In relapsing-remitting MS, the spinal cord lesions are typically multifocal. In secondary progressive MS the abnormalities are more extensive and diffuse and are commonly associated with spinal cord atrophy. In primary progressive MS, cord abnormalities are quite extensive as compared with brain abnormalities. This discrepancy may help to diagnose primary progressive MS in patients with few or no brain abnormalities.

MRI of the spinal cord can provide important diagnostic information in several clinical settings. Patients initially diagnosed with MS but showing signs or symptoms of myelopathy are typically evaluated by spinal cord MRI to exclude treatable lesions such as extrinsic compression, neoplasm, or vascular malformation. MRI demonstration of lesions of the spinal cord can strengthen the diagnosis of MS in patients fitting the clinical criteria for MS but with negative or equivocal brain MRI findings. Similarly, diagnostic certainty can be increased in patients with nonspecific brain findings, particularly those older than age 50 years, because asymptomatic cord lesions are relatively frequent in MS but rare with other white matter diseases. Proton-density and T2-weighted sequences combined with STIR sequences are more sensitive than single-echo T2-weighted spin-echo for detecting spinal cord lesions.

Gadolinium-Enhancing Lesions

Longitudinal and cross-sectional MRI studies have shown that the formation of new MS plaques is often associated with contrast enhancement, mainly in the acute and relapsing stages of the disease (Fig. 43-25).[16] The gadolinium (Gd) enhancement varies in size and shape but usually lasts from a few days to weeks. Incomplete ring enhancement on T1W Gd-enhanced images, with the open border facing the gray matter of the cortex or basal ganglia, is a common finding in active MS plaques and is a

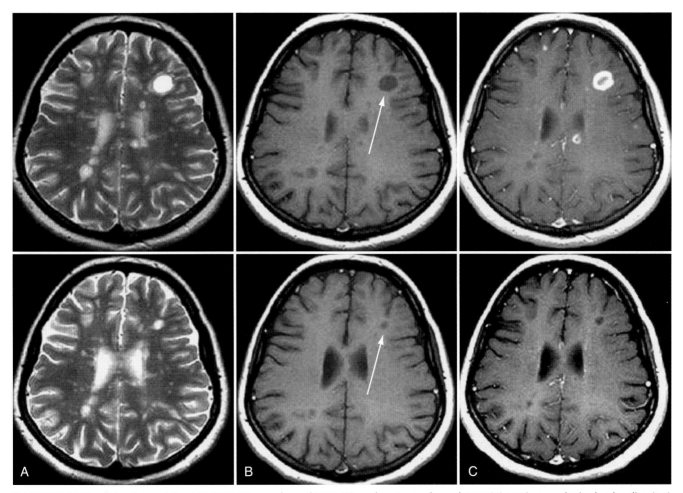

■ **FIGURE 43-21** Relapsing-remitting MS. T2W (**A**), unenhanced T1W (**B**), and contrast-enhanced T1W (**C**) MR images obtained at baseline (*top*) and 1 year later (*bottom*). Observe the active "black hole" in the subcortical white matter of the left frontal lobe (*arrow*), which shows a ring-enhancement pattern of contrast agent uptake. After 1 year, the lesion decreased in size (*arrow*) but remained hypointense on T1W images, indicating an irreversible "black hole."

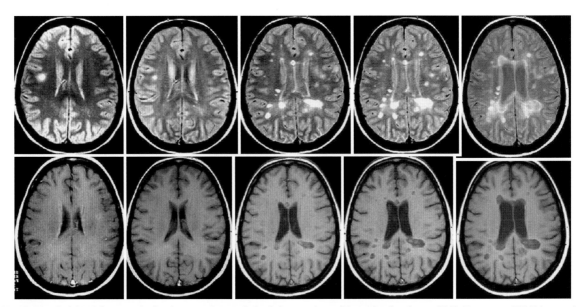

■ **FIGURE 43-22** Serial MR images obtained on a twice-yearly basis in a patient with a relapsing form of MS. Transverse PDW (*top row*) and T1W (*bottom row*) MR images. In addition to the increasing number of plaques within the hemispheric white matter, observe the increase in number and size of irreversible black holes and progressive brain volume loss.

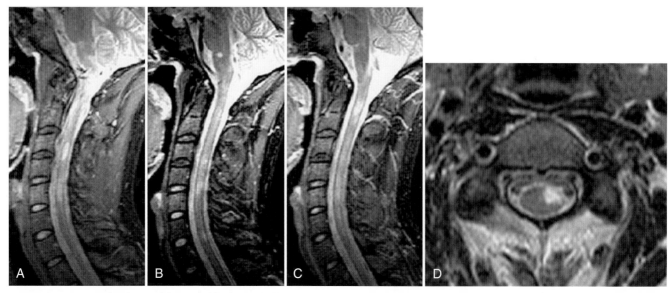

■ **FIGURE 43-23** Relapsing-remitting MS with plaques in the cervical spinal cord. Sagittal and transverse FSE T2W MR images. Observe the multiple small focal lesions that do not exceed two vertebral segments in length (**A, B, C**). One of the lesions occupies the left anterior white matter columns and does not affect more than half the cross-sectional area of the cord (**D**).

helpful feature for distinguishing between inflammatory-demyelinating lesions and other focal lesions, such as tumors or abscesses (Fig. 43-26).[8]

Focal enhancement can be detected before abnormalities appear on unenhanced T2W scans and can reappear in chronic lesions with or without a concomitant increase in size. Although enhancing lesions also occur in clinically stable MS patients, their number is much greater when there is concomitant clinical activity. Contrast enhancement is a relatively good predictor of further enhancement and of subsequent accumulation of T2 lesions but shows no (or weak) correlation with progression of disability and development of brain atrophy.

In relapsing-remitting and secondary progressive MS, enhancement is more frequent during relapses and correlates well with clinical activity. For patients with primary progressive MS, serial T2W studies show few new lesions and little or no enhancement with conventional doses of Gd, despite steady clinical deterioration.[5]

Contrast-enhanced T1W images are routinely used in the study of MS to provide a measure of inflammatory activity in vivo. The technique detects disease activity 5 to 10 times more frequently than clinical evaluation of relapses, suggesting that most of the enhancing lesions are clinically silent. Corticosteroid treatment shortens the period of enhancement. Subclinical disease activity with contrast-enhancing lesions is 4 to 10 times less frequent in the spinal cord than the brain, a fact that may be partially explained by the large volume of brain as compared with spinal cord. A double dose of gadolinium and a minimum of 10 to 15 minutes post-injection delay can increase the detection of active spinal cord lesions.

■ **FIGURE 43-24** Clinically isolated syndrome of the spinal cord (acute transverse myelitis). Unenhanced sagittal T1W FSE (*left*), T2W (*middle*), and contrast-enhanced T1W (*right*) MR images. A focal cervical spinal cord lesion is identified that produces a mild mass effect with swelling of the cord and peripheral uptake of contrast agent.

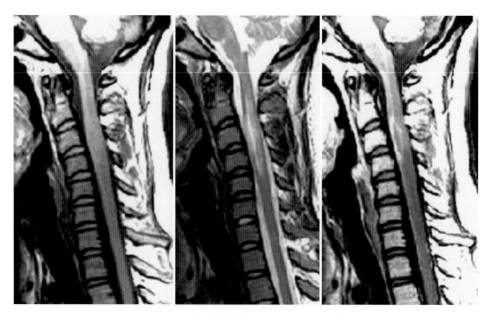

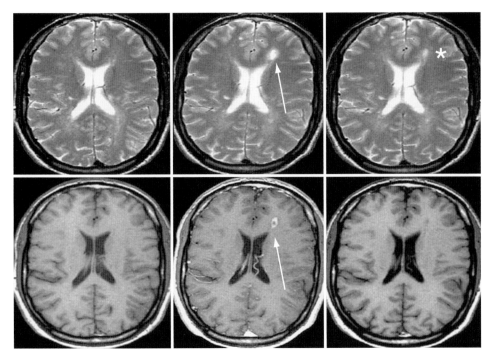

■ **FIGURE 43-25** Relapsing-remitting MS with new brain plaque formation. Transverse T2W (*top row*) and contrast-enhanced T1W (*bottom row*) brain MR images obtained serially at monthly intervals. Observe formation of a new plaque in the left frontal white matter showing transient contrast uptake (*arrow*). With cessation of inflammatory activity, the lesion on T2W imaging decreased in size but left a persistent hyperintense footprint (*asterisk*).

Optic Nerve Imaging

Optic neuritis can usually be diagnosed clinically. MRI is not necessary to confirm the diagnosis, unless there are atypical clinical features (e.g., no response to corticosteroids, long-standing symptoms). In these situations, brain and optic nerve MRI should be performed to rule out an alternative diagnosis, such as a compressive lesion.[17]

Coronal fat-saturated T2W images are the most sensitive MRI technique for depicting signal abnormalities. Focal thickening of the affected optic nerve reflects demyelination and inflammation (Fig. 43-27), which may persist for long periods despite improvements in vision and visual-evoked potential findings. Intense optic nerve enhancement seen on fat-suppressed contrast-enhanced T1W images is a consistent feature of acute optic neuritis (see Fig. 43-27). The length of the enhancing optic nerve segment on axial images correlates with the severity of visual impairment but does not predict the degree of visual recovery. In MS, signal abnormalities may also be seen in the absence of acute attacks of optic neuritis. In acute optic neuritis, noncontrast T1W images do not display *hypointense* lesions within the optic nerves.

Nonconventional MRI Techniques

Conventional MRI techniques (cMRI), such as T2W and Gd-enhanced T1W sequences, are highly sensitive for detecting MS plaques and can provide quantitative assessment of inflammatory activity and lesion load. cMRI-derived metrics have become established as the most important paraclinical tool for diagnosing MS, for understanding the natural history of the disease, and for monitoring the efficacy of experimental treatments. However, the correlation between the extent of lesions observed on cMRI and the clinical manifestations of the disease is weak and underlines the fact that cMRI techniques cannot demonstrate the entire spectrum of the disease. This clinicoradiologic mismatch or paradox may be partially explained by the limitations of cMRI, including (1) limited specificity for the various pathologic

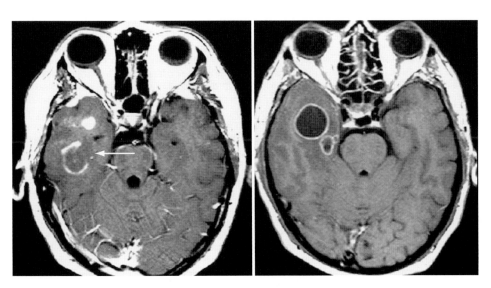

■ **FIGURE 43-26** Ring-enhancing pattern of contrast agent uptake. Contrast-enhanced T1W MR images obtained in a patient with relapsing-remitting MS (*left*) and a patient with glioblastoma multiforme (*right*). Both patients have focal lesions in the right temporal lobe. However, an incomplete ring-enhancing pattern of contrast agent uptake with the open margin facing the cortical gray matter of the hippocampus (*arrow*) is seen only in the patient with MS. In glioblastoma multiforme the lesions show a complete ring of enhancement despite contact with the cortical gray matter.

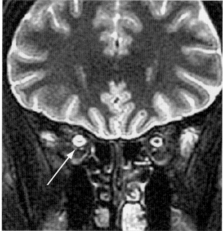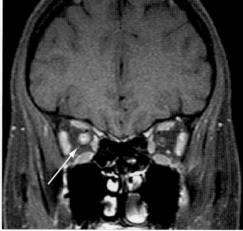

■ **FIGURE 43-27** Right optic neuritis. Coronal fat-suppressed T2W FSE (*left*) and fat-suppressed contrast-enhanced T1W (*right*) MR images. There is hyperintensity of the right optic nerve, with diffuse enhancement (*arrows*). (*From Cañellas AR, Gols AR, Izquierdo JR, et al. Idiopathic inflammatory-demyelinating diseases of the central nervous system. Neuroradiology 2007; 49:393-469.*)

substrates of MS; (2) inability to quantify the extent of damage in normal-appearing white matter; (3) inability to detect and quantify the extent of gray matter damage; (4) variability in the clinical expression of MS plaques in different anatomic locations (e.g., the spinal cord and optic nerve); and (5) inability to assess the effectiveness of reparative mechanisms in MS, such as cortical adaptive reorganization.

In the past few years, a huge effort has been made to overcome these limitations with nonconventional MR-derived metrics that can selectively measure the more destructive aspects of MS pathology and monitor the mechanisms of repair. These nonconventional MR-derived metrics include measures of CNS atrophy, magnetization transfer MRI, DWI, proton MR spectroscopy, and functional MRI (fMRI). These techniques are now being used to better understand the natural history of MS and to assess the effects of treatment.

CNS Atrophy

Atrophy of the brain and spinal cord is an important part of MS pathology and a clinically relevant component of disease progression.[18] Although this process is more severe in the progressive forms of the disease, it may also occur early in the disease process (see Fig. 43-22). In fact, early atrophy seems to predict subsequent development of physical disability better than do measures of lesion load. The etiology of CNS atrophy is multifactorial and likely reflects demyelination, wallerian degeneration, axonal loss, and glial contraction. CNS atrophy, which involves both gray and white matter, is a progressive phenomenon that worsens with increasing disease duration and progresses at a rate of 0.6% to 1.2% of brain loss per year. Quantitative measures of whole-brain atrophy, acquired by automated or semi-automated methods, display this progressive loss of brain tissue bulk in vivo in a sensitive and reproducible manner.

Subcortical brain atrophy is particularly well correlated to neuropsychological impairment, which can be explained by a disruption of frontal-subcortical circuits. Spinal cord atrophy is better correlated with motor disability.

Magnetization Transfer MRI

Magnetization transfer (MT) MRI affords a potential window into a macromolecular environment that is not directly visible with cMRI techniques. It provides one method for assessing the "invisible" disease within the so-called normal-appearing brain tissue. In MS, MT ratios (MTR) can be used to quantify the integrity of myelinated white matter in large areas of the brain.[19] In MS patients, decreased MTR most likely reflects demyelination and axonal loss, although this reduction may also be influenced by edema, gliosis, and inflammation. The cervical cord and optic nerve also show a decreased MTR in MS. The magnitude of MTR declines during the time of Gd enhancement predicts whether the lesion will evolve into a T1-hypointense lesion. This correlation indicates that the degree to which the MTR is altered is a marker of overall lesion severity. When initial MTR decreases are only modest, partial or complete MTR recovery is likely to occur in the next few months. This recovery of MTR values most likely reflects remyelination or simply resolution of edema and inflammation. Decreased MTR has also been detected in the normal-appearing brain tissue of patients with MS as compared with normal controls, supporting the concept of widespread brain tissue involvement. Decreases in MTR are more pronounced in patients with progressive disease but are also seen in relapsing-remitting MS and even at the time of the initial attack (clinically isolated syndrome). MTR decreases can predict the development of neurologic disability.

Diffusion-Weighted MRI

Disruption of white matter tracts and axonal membrane permeability lead to an increase in the apparent diffusion coefficient (ADC) and mean diffusivity (MD), measures of average molecular motion, as well as to a decrease in fractional anisotropy (FA), a measure of the directional preponderance of diffusion, which can be obtained with diffusion tensor imaging (DTI).

In MS, brain lesions may appear hyperintense on DWI owing to T2 shine-through effects; these can be separated from true restriction of diffusion using ADC mapping (Fig. 43-28). Typically, MS plaques show an increased MD or ADC and decreased FA when compared with the contralateral normal-appearing white matter. The ADC is especially high in contrast-enhancing lesions[20] and T1-hypointense lesions. The increased MD, increased ADC, and decreased FA are nonspecific findings, which reflect a variety of tissue changes such as demyelination, gliosis, inflammation, axonal contraction, and axonal loss. A transient decrease in ADC values may occur in acute MS plaques and likely reflects swelling of the myelin sheaths, reduced vascular supply leading to cytotoxic edema, or dense inflammatory cell infiltration (Fig. 43-29).

Areas of normal-appearing white matter that later develop overt lesions may exhibit a significant increase in MD values weeks before Gd enhancement, indicating that new inflammatory lesions are preceded by subtle, progressive diffusion alterations. An overall increase in MD and ADC and a decrease in FA have also been observed in normal-appearing brain tissue of MS patients, suggesting the presence of subtle microstructural changes (e.g., loss of barriers) in the normal-appearing brain

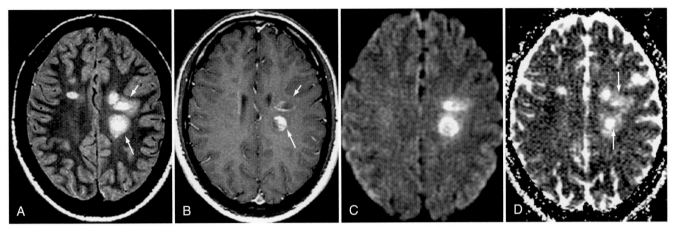

■ **FIGURE 43-28** MRI obtained in a patient with relapsing-remitting MS. Transverse PDW (**A**), contrast-enhanced T1W (**B**), and diffusion-weighted (**C**) MR images and ADC map (**D**). Acute enhancing lesions in the subcortical frontal white matter (*arrows*) are hyperintense on the PDW, T1W, and diffusion-weighted images. However, on the ADC map these lesions are hyperintense, indicating increased diffusivity. The hypersignal on the diffusion-weighted image corresponds to T2 shine-through effect. Only the periphery of the lesion has low diffusivity (low signal on the ADC map, *arrows*), which is likely related to dense inflammatory cell infiltration.

tissue that are not resolved by cMRI. Moderate correlations have been observed between overall DWI measures and neurologic disability and cognitive impairment.

Fiber tract disruption caused by the transection of lesions can be visualized on fiber tractography, supporting the concept of wallerian degeneration and axonal transection in MS disease (Fig. 43-30).

Proton MR Spectroscopy
In MS, proton MRS has provided evidence of active inflammatory demyelination and neuron/axon injury in both lesional and non-lesional brain tissues from the earliest stages of the disease.[21] In acute inflammatory-demyelinating lesions short- and long-echo proton MRS reveals increases in choline and lactate resonance intensities (Fig. 43-31). Changes in the resonance intensity of choline can be interpreted as a measure of increases in the steady state levels of membrane phospholipids released during active myelin breakdown. Increases in lactate may reflect primarily the metabolism of inflammatory cells. Short echo time spectra give evidence for transient increases in visible lipids (released during myelin breakdown) and more chronic increases in myo-inositol. These changes are consistently accompanied by substantial decreases in NAA since (1) NAA is a metabolite detected

almost exclusively in neurons and their processes in the normal mature brain and (2) decreases in NAA have been interpreted as a measure of axonal injury reflecting metabolic or structural changes. Glutamate levels may be elevated in acute lesions, suggesting a link between axonal injury in active lesions and glutamate excitotoxicity (see Fig. 43-31).

After the acute phase there is a progressive return of raised lactate resonance intensities to normal levels in focal lesions. In chronic lesions, persistent increases in the myoinositol resonance intensity may be related to microglial proliferation. Resonance intensities of choline and lipids typically return to normal over months. The signal intensity of NAA may remain decreased or show partial recovery, starting soon after the acute phase and lasting for several months (Fig. 43-32). The recovery of NAA may be related in various proportions to reversible metabolic changes in neuronal mitochondria, the resolution of edema, or changes in the relative partial volume of neuronal processes.

In MS patients, the metabolic abnormalities are not restricted to lesions but are found throughout the normal-appearing white matter. Notably, these include reduced NAA, which is thought to indicate axonal dysfunction or loss and is associated with functional impairment (Fig. 43-33).

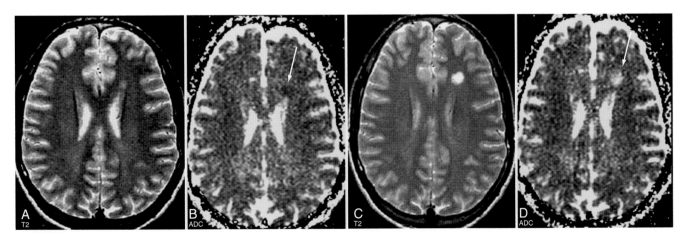

■ **FIGURE 43-29** New developing demyelinating plaque in a patient with relapsing-remitting MS. Initial MR image (**A**) shows a small T2 lesion in the left frontal periventricular white matter, which is hypointense on the ADC map (*arrow in B*). Lesion enlargement, which becomes hyperintense on the ADC map, is observed on the follow-up MR image obtained 7 days later (*arrow in D*).

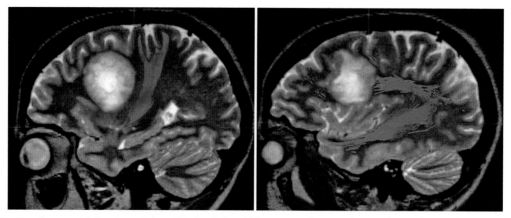

■ **FIGURE 43-30** Pseudotumoral inflammatory demyelinating lesion. MR tractography maps in a patient with a single tumefactive inflammatory-demyelinating lesion in the left frontal subcortical white matter who experienced conduction aphasia. Observe the gap between the lesion and the corticospinal tract (*blue, left*) and damage to the anterior segment of the arcuate fasciculus (*green, right*), which explain the symptoms.

Functional MRI

Patients with MS may exhibit symptomatic recovery even as they accumulate progressive tissue damage. This discrepancy may reflect the ability of the brain to compensate for tissue impairment or loss through a phenomenon known as "brain plasticity." In MS patients, fMRI shows increased magnitude of regional activation during task performance as compared with controls, suggesting that additional areas of the brain are recruited to help the brain adapt and/or compensate for damage (Fig. 43-34). These changes occur in the early phase of disease, are related to clinical symptoms and/or disability, and include increased activation of the ipsilateral and contralateral cortices on the basis of synaptic reorganization, recruitment of parallel existing pathways, and reorganization of more distant sites. The degree of fMRI abnormality correlates with the lesion burden detected by cMRI, supporting the notion that functional changes represent progressive consumption of the cerebral reserve capacity. In fact, as the disease progresses and brain reserve capacity is exceeded, patients show decreased activation relative to earlier in the disease process. This abnormal cortical activation pattern may change in response to both rehabilitation and pharmacologic agents. Therefore, in the future fMRI could be used as a tool for monitoring the efficacy of therapies that promote neuroplasticity.[22]

DEVIC'S NEUROMYELITIS OPTICA

Devic's neuromyelitis optica (NMO) is an uncommon and topographically restricted form of IIDD that is best considered to be a distinct disease rather than a variant of MS. NMO is characterized by severe unilateral or bilateral optic neuritis and complete transverse myelitis, which occur simultaneously or sequentially within a varying period of time (weeks or years), without clinical involvement of other CNS regions.

Epidemiology

The incidence and prevalence of NMO are unknown, but the condition likely accounts for fewer than 1% of IIDDs in whites. NMO affects females almost exclusively. The strong overrepresentation of females suggests that sex hormones play a more significant role than in other autoimmune diseases.[23] The median age at onset is late in the fourth decade, about 10 years later than typical MS. Up to 30% of Japanese IIDD patients have an opticospinal clinical form, which appears to be similar to relapsing NMO with respect to age of onset, MRI findings, CSF, and pathology. NMO appears to be a sporadic disease, although rare familial cases have been reported.

Clinical Presentation

The index events of new-onset NMO are severe unilateral or bilateral optic neuritis, acute myelitis, or a combination of these

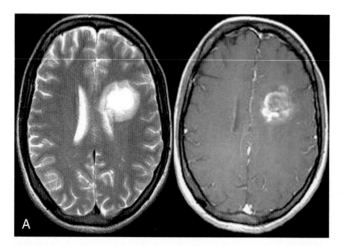
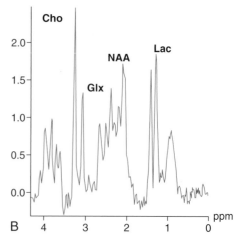

■ **FIGURE 43-31** Pseudotumoral inflammatory-demyelinating lesion. **A,** Transverse T2W (*left*) and contrast-enhanced T1W (*middle*) MR images in a patient with an acute pseudotumoral inflammatory-demyelinating lesion affecting the left frontal subcortical white matter (same patient as in Fig. 43-30). **B,** Proton spectrum obtained from the lesion (long echo time) (*right*) shows slight decrease in *N*-acetyl-aspartate (NAA) and increased choline (Cho), glutamate (Glx), and lactate (Lac).

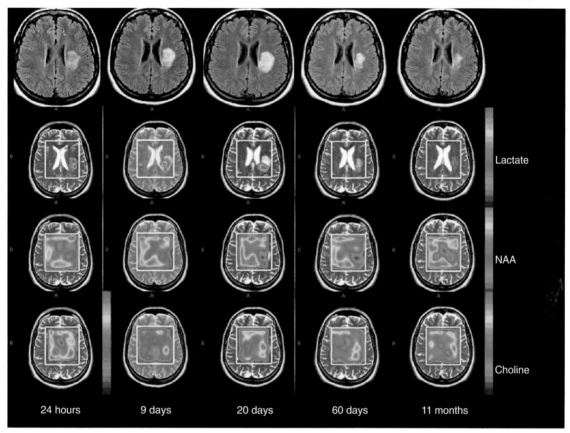

■ **FIGURE 43-32** Pseudotumoral inflammatory-demyelinating lesion. Serial proton MR spectroscopy of an acute large demyelinating lesion in the left centrum ovale obtained over a period of 11 months. Transverse fast-FLAIR images (*top row*) and lactate, *N*-acetyl-aspartate (NAA), and choline colored metabolic maps. Baseline examination shows slight decrease in NAA (*green-blue spots*), increased choline, and presence of lactate (*red spots*). NAA decrease and choline increase persisted over time, but lactate disappeared.

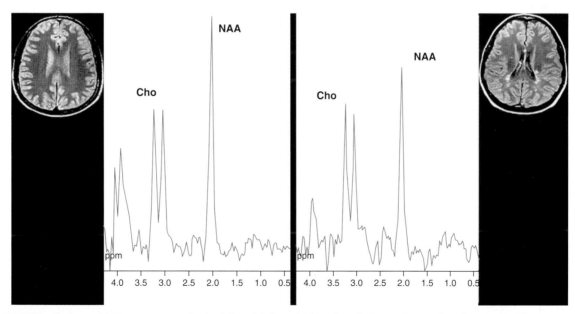

■ **FIGURE 43-33** Single-voxel MR spectroscopy obtained from left frontal lobe subcortical normal-appearing white matter. The spectra on the left were obtained in a normal volunteer and those on the right in a patient with relapsing-remitting MS. Observe decreased *N*-acetyl-aspartate (NAA) peak height in the MS patient.

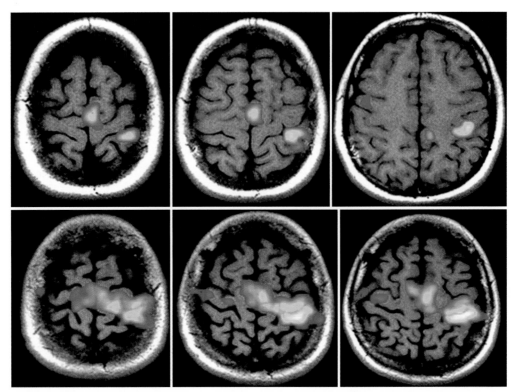

■ **FIGURE 43-34** Functional MRI in a normal volunteer (*top row*) and in a patient with secondary progressive MS (right hand movement stimulus) (*bottom row*). Observe the greater task-related activation in both the primary and supplementary motor areas in the patient as compared with the normal volunteer.

symptoms. The attacks of myelitis appear as complete transverse myelitis with severe bilateral motor deficits, sensory level, bowel and bladder dysfunction, pain, and significant residual neurologic injury. NMO attacks are generally more severe than those typical of MS. Approximately 85% of patients have a relapsing course with severe acute exacerbations and poor recovery, accumulating increasing neurologic impairment, and a high risk of respiratory failure and death due to cervical myelitis.[24]

Prediction of disease course at onset is desirable because those with relapsing disease require preventive immunosuppressive treatment (azathioprine, rituximab, corticosteroids). Patients who experience acute optic neuritis and myelitis simultaneously or within days of each other are much more likely to have a monophasic course. On the other hand, a relapsing course correlates with a longer interval between attacks, older age at onset, female sex, and less severe motor impairment after the myelitic onset. Although initial attacks are more severe in patients proven to have monophasic NMO, the long-term neurologic prognosis is somewhat better in this group because the patients do not accumulate disability from recurrent attacks. Within 5 years, 50% of patients lose functional vision in at least one eye or are unable to walk independently. Clinical features alone are insufficient to diagnose NMO; CSF analysis and MRI are usually required to confidently exclude other disorders. CSF pleocytosis (>50 leukocytes/mm³) is often present, whereas CSF oligoclonal bands are seen less frequently (20%-40%) than in MS patients (80%-90%).

A serum autoantibody marker for NMO (NMO-IgG) has been developed. The target antigen of NMO-IgG is aquaporin-4, a water channel located on the foot process of the astrocyte. It is associated with tight endothelial junctions and cerebral microvessels and plays a critical role in maintaining fluid homeostasis in the CNS. This autoantibody is reported to have a sensitivity of 73% and a specificity of 91% for NMO. It may be helpful

TABLE 43-3. Revised Diagnostic Criteria for Devic's Neuromyelitis Optica (NMO)

Optic neuritis
Acute myelitis
At least two of three supportive criteria:
   Contiguous MRI spinal cord lesion extending over ≥3 vertebral
     segments
   Brain MRI findings do not meet diagnostic criteria for multiple
     sclerosis
   NMO-IgG seropositive status

From Wingerchuk DM, Lennon VA, Pittock SJ, et al. Revised diagnostic criteria for neuromyelitis optica. Neurology 2006; 66:1485-1489.

for distinguishing this form of IIDD from MS and may predict relapse and conversion to NMO in patients presenting with a single attack of longitudinally extensive myelitis. NMO-IgG is also positive in 52% of patients with relapsing myelitis and in 25% of patients with recurrent idiopathic optic neuritis. These findings suggest that a sizeable proportion of these cases belong within the NMO spectrum, either as a variant or incompletely developed NMO.[25]

NMO-IgG has been detected with similar frequency in opticospinal MS and NMO cases, suggesting that they may be the same disorder.[25]

Wingerchuk and coworkers have proposed a revised set of criteria for diagnosing NMO (Table 43-3).[26] These new criteria remove the absolute restriction on CNS involvement beyond the optic nerves and spinal cord, allow any interval between the first events of optic neuritis and myelitis, and emphasize the specificity of longitudinally extensive spinal cord lesions on MRI and NMO-IgG seropositive status.

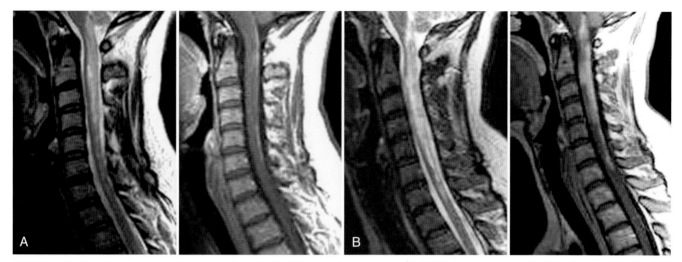

■ **FIGURE 43-35** Devic's neuromyelitis optica. Sagittal FSE T2W and contrast-enhanced T1W MR images of the cervical spinal cord obtained serially over a period of 4 months. Baseline examination (**A**) shows a large spinal cord lesion extending to the brain stem. Follow-up MR images acquired 4 months later (**B**) show lesion extension to the thoracic cord and persistent and more extensive contrast agent uptake.

Pathophysiology

Devic's neuromyelitis optica is a B-cell–mediated disorder that can coexist with diverse systemic autoimmune diseases such as systemic lupus erythematosus, Sjögren's syndrome, and autoimmune thyroiditis. The presence of prodromal factors such as fever, infections, and autoimmune abnormalities suggests that previous infectious-inflammatory events may be involved in the pathogenesis of the disease.[23]

The pathogenesis of NMO is incompletely understood, but immunopathologic and serologic observations implicate a circulating autoantibody as the principal effector of lesions. These primarily affect the perivascular spaces. In this scenario the classical complement pathway is activated and leads to recruitment of activated macrophages to the perivascular sites.[27] Increased vascular permeability and edema may contribute to parenchymal damage via secondary ischemia and may account for the typical central location of NMO plaques within the spinal cord.

Demyelinating lesions in NMO are, therefore, associated with deposition of perivascular immunoglobulin M, activation of the local complement cascade, and eosinophil infiltration. These findings suggest a role for humoral immunity in the pathogenesis of NMO that is strengthened by the common detection of NMO-IgG autoantibody.[27]

A possible explanation for the selective involvement of the spinal cord and optic nerve may be that these structures are particularly vulnerable to antibody-mediated injury due to the inherent weakness of the blood-brain barrier at these sites.[27] The increased blood-brain barrier permeability in the spinal cord may also be due to its vascular properties, with larger capillaries than those in the brain. Thus, on a background of an inflammatory process in the presence of extremely high antibody titers, lesions might preferentially, but not exclusively, affect the spinal cord and optic nerve.

Pathology

Acute spinal cord lesions demonstrate diffuse swelling and softening extending over several segments and occasionally the entire cord. These lesions reveal extensive demyelination across multiple spinal cord levels, necrosis of both gray and white matter, and extensive macrophage infiltration associated with large numbers of perivascular granulocytes, eosinophils, and T cells. There is a pronounced loss of oligodendrocytes within the lesions. Chronic lesions are characterized by gliosis, cystic degeneration, cavitation, and atrophy of the spinal cord and

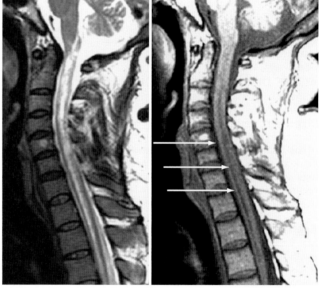

■ **FIGURE 43-36** Devic's neuromyelitis optica. Sagittal T2W and T1W MR images of the cervicodorsal spinal cord showing a long syrinx-like spinal cord lesion extending to the lower medulla (*arrows*).

optic nerves. A pronounced vasculocentric deposition of immunoglobulin and complement is present in active lesions, associated with prominent vascular fibrosis and hyalinization in active and inactive lesions.[27]

Imaging

MRI of the spinal cord shows extensive cervical or thoracic tumefactive myelitis, involving more than three vertebral segments on sagittal imaging and much of the cross section on axial T2W images, which sometimes enhance with Gd for several months (Fig. 43-35). In some cases, the spinal cord lesions are small at the onset of symptoms, mimicking those in MS, and then progress in extent over time. These lesions are usually located centrally, can progress to atrophy and necrosis, and may lead to syrinx-like cavities on T1W images (Fig. 43-36).

MRI of the brain can demonstrate unilateral or bilateral optic nerve enhancement during acute optic neuritis (Fig. 43-37). In

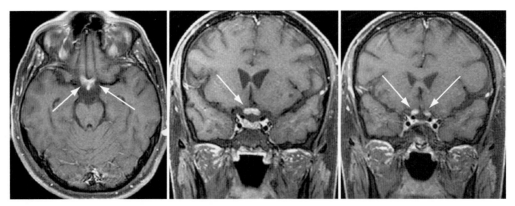

■ **FIGURE 43-37**   Devic's neuromyelitis optica. Transverse (*left*) and coronal contrast-enhanced T1W (*middle and right*) MR images in a patient with bilateral optic neuritis who had experienced an episode of myelitis a few months before. Observe contrast agent uptake at the intracranial segment of both optic nerves and optic chiasm (*arrows*). The patient met the diagnostic criteria of NMO.

contrast to MS, white matter lesions are absent or few in the early stages and are nonspecific. Over the next years serial studies may reveal an increasing number of cerebral white matter lesions but less than 10% ever meet MRI criteria for MS. Pediatric cases sometimes show diencephalic (hypothalamic), brain stem, or cerebral hemispheric lesions, which should be considered atypical for MS.[28] Hypothalamic lesions seem to be relatively specific for NMO and may be associated with clinical and laboratory evidence of hypothalamic endocrinopathy.

ACUTE DISSEMINATED ENCEPHALOMYELITIS

Acute disseminated encephalomyelitis (ADEM) is a severe, immune-mediated inflammatory disorder of the CNS that is usually triggered by an inflammatory response to viral or bacterial infections and vaccinations. It predominantly affects the white matter of the brain and spinal cord. In the absence of specific biologic markers, the diagnosis of ADEM is based on the clinical and radiologic features. Although ADEM usually has a monophasic course, recurrent or multiphasic forms have been reported, raising diagnostic difficulties in distinguishing these cases from MS.

Epidemiology
ADEM affects children more commonly than adults and, in contrast to MS, shows no sex predilection. The estimated incidence is 0.8 per 100,000 population per year. In 50% to 75% of cases, the clinical onset of disease is preceded by viral or bacterial infections, usually nonspecific upper respiratory tract infections. ADEM may also develop after a vaccination (postimmunization encephalomyelitis).[29] Although ADEM is relatively rare, it is becoming increasingly important, because vaccination schedules have expanded over the past years, particularly for children. Typically, there is a latency of 7 to 14 days between a febrile illness and the onset of neurologic symptoms. In the case of vaccination-associated ADEM, this latency period may be longer.

Clinical Presentation
Patients commonly present with nonspecific symptoms, including headaches, vomiting, drowsiness, fever, and lethargy, all of which are relatively uncommon in MS. The course of ADEM is usually monophasic, although recurrent and multiphasic forms also occur. In general, the disease is self-limiting and the prognostic outcome favorable.

Neurologic symptoms usually develop subacutely over a period of days and lead to hospitalization within a week. Although ataxia, altered level of consciousness, and brain stem symptoms are frequently present in both pediatric and adult cases, certain signs and symptoms appear to be age related. In childhood ADEM, long-lasting fever and headaches occur more frequently, whereas in adult cases motor and sensory deficits predominate.

According to the International Pediatric MS Study Group,[30] monophasic ADEM is defined as a multifocal clinical syndrome in patients with no history of a prior demyelinating event, including encephalopathic symptoms such as behavioral changes (e.g., irritability, lethargy) or altered consciousness (somnolence, coma). Recurrent ADEM requires a second ADEM attack more than 3 months after the initial event (one or more months after completion of corticosteroid therapy), involving the *same* anatomic area. Multiphasic ADEM requires a second ADEM attack with *new* areas of involvement. Symptoms evolving up to 3 months after the first ADEM attack should be considered a part of it and not recurrent or multiphasic ADEM.

Not infrequently, an ADEM attack is the first manifestation of the classic relapsing form of MS. In fact, 30% of patients who meet the ADEM criteria at initial presentation ultimately receive a diagnosis of MS. Hence, ADEM is likely to be overdiagnosed on the basis of the initial clinical presentation and MR findings. For this reason, a presumptive diagnosis of ADEM mandates close clinical and MRI follow-up (Fig. 43-38).

The first-line treatment for ADEM is intravenous high-dose corticosteroids, which, in nonresponsive cases, is followed by plasma exchange or immunoglobulins. Immunosuppressive agents, such as mitoxantrone or cyclophosphamide, should be considered as alternative therapies if anti-inflammatory treatment shows no clinical effect.

Pathophysiology
Two concepts have been proposed as pathogenic mechanisms in ADEM.[29] The inflammatory cascade concept implies a direct CNS infection with a neurotropic pathogen, resulting in CNS tissue damage and systemic leakage of CNS-confined autoantigens into the systemic circulation through a disintegrated blood-brain barrier. Once processed in systemic lymphatic organs, these autoantigens will lead to tolerance breakdown and to a self-reactive and encephalitogenic T-cell response. The activated T cells can invade the CNS and further perpetuate CNS inflammation.

The molecular mimicry concept proposes a structural homology between the inoculated pathogen and the host myelin proteins. This structural homology is not sufficient for a pathogen to be recognized as "self," which would result in immunotolerance. Antigen-presenting cells such as B cells or dendritic cells process the pathogen at the site of inoculation, leading to T-cell activation. Activated T cells may, in turn, cross-activate antigen-specific B cells. Activated T cells and B cells are both quite

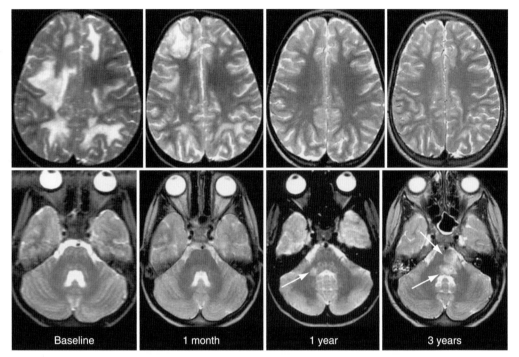

■ **FIGURE 43-38** Acute disseminated encephalomyelitis (ADEM) that will convert to MS. Serial brain MRI (T2W sequences) in a young patient in whom an initial diagnosis of ADEM was established. Note the development of new symptomatic T2 lesions within the middle cerebellar peduncle and brain stem (*arrows*) 1 and 3 years after symptom onset and complete disappearance of the subcortical supratentorial lesions identified in the first examination. A final diagnosis of clinically definite MS was established. *(From Cañellas AR, Gols AR, Izquierdo JR, et al. Idiopathic inflammatory-demyelinating diseases of the central nervous system. Neuroradiology 2007; 49:393-469.)*

capable of entering the CNS for routine immune surveillance. Thus, even after clearance of the pathogen, these antigen-specific cells may encounter the homologous myelin protein during their physiologic surveillance of the CNS, become reactivated by local antigen-presenting cells such as microglia, and cause an inflammatory immune reaction against the presumed foreign antigen.

Pathology

In patients who die acutely, the brain is swollen, is congested, and may show herniation. The freshly sliced brain shows little apart from swelling and, in some cases, several petechial hemorrhages; this contrasts to fatal cases of acute MS of comparable duration where lesions are visible macroscopically.

Microscopically, small, widely disseminated perivenous lesions are distributed throughout the cerebral hemispheres, brain stem, cerebellum, and spinal cord. The lesions are of similar histologic age, are most numerous in the white matter, but also affect the gray matter. Foci of myelin loss and infiltration by mononuclear cells (predominantly macrophages) are present. A distinctive feature is the long sleeves of perivenous demyelination surrounded by infiltrates of reactive microglia. Demyelination is restricted to the extended, sleeve-like hypercellular zones. Axons within demyelinated lesions, although preserved relative to myelin, may show tortuous and swollen profiles, sometimes with end bulbs indicating axonal interruption. Attempts to recover virus from the brain and demonstrate viral antigens or viral nucleic acid in affected neural tissue in ADEM have been negative, and the absence of typical viral infectious pathologic processes argues against direct invasion of the nervous system by virus as the cause of the disease.

Imaging

Unlike lesions in MS, the lesions of ADEM are often large, patchy, and poorly margined on MRI. There is usually asymmetric involvement of the subcortical and central white matter and cortical gray-white junction of both cerebral hemispheres, the cerebellum, brain stem, and spinal cord (Fig. 43-39). The gray matter of the thalami and basal ganglia is frequently affected, particularly in children, typically in a symmetric pattern.[30] Lesions confined to the periventricular white matter and corpus callosum are less common than in MS.

Four patterns of cerebral involvement have been proposed to describe the MRI findings in ADEM[30]: (1) ADEM with small lesions (<5 mm) (Fig. 43-40); (2) ADEM with large, confluent, or tumefactive lesions and frequent extensive perilesional edema and mass effect (Fig. 43-41); (3) ADEM with additional symmetric deep gray matter involvement (Fig. 43-42); and (4) acute hemorrhagic encephalomyelitis (Fig. 43-43). T1W images show Gd-enhancing lesions in 30% to 100% of patients.[30] The pattern of enhancement is variable: complete or incomplete ring-shaped, nodular, gyral, or spotty.

The spinal cord is involved in fewer than 30% of patients with ADEM,[30] predominantly in the thoracic region (see Fig. 43-39). The cord lesion is typically large, causes swelling of the cord, and shows variable enhancement. Most ADEM patients show partial or complete resolution of the MRI abnormalities within a few months after treatment. This evolution is positively associated with a final diagnosis of ADEM (see Fig. 43-39).

Because ADEM is usually a monophasic disease, the focal lesions would be expected to appear and mature simultaneously with the same appearance on contrast-enhanced MRI. They would be expected to resolve or remain unchanged, with no new lesions on follow-up MR images (Fig. 43-44). Not infrequently, however, new lesions are seen on follow-up MRI within the first month after the initial attack. This fact explains the mixed pattern of enhancing and nonenhancing lesions at the same time point.

Most MRI lesions appear early in the course of the disease, supporting the clinical diagnosis. In some cases there may be a

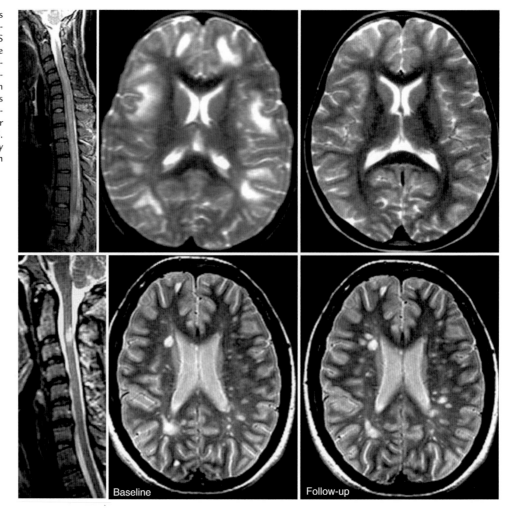

■ FIGURE 43-39 MRI differences between acute disseminated encephalomyelitis (ADEM) (*top row*) and MS (*bottom row*). Spinal cord lesions are extensive in ADEM and usually associated with large, poorly defined subcortical white matter lesions on brain MRI. In MS, symptomatic cord lesions are usually small and commonly associated with subclinical white matter brain lesions of the type seen in MS. In ADEM, longitudinal studies usually show resolution of lesions, whereas in MS new lesions appear.

delay of more than 1 month between the onset of symptoms and the appearance of lesions on MRI (see Fig. 43-40). Therefore, a normal brain MR image obtained within the first days after the onset of neurologic symptoms suggestive of ADEM does not exclude this diagnosis.

ACUTE DISSEMINATED ENCEPHALOMYELITIS VARIANTS
Bickerstaff's Encephalitis

Bickerstaff's encephalitis is a rare acute syndrome considered to be a subgroup of ADEM in which inflammation appears to be

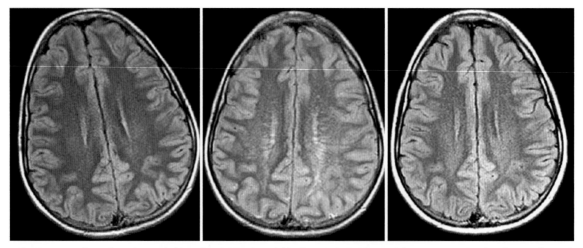

■ FIGURE 43-40 Acute disseminated encephalomyelitis (ADEM). Serial brain MRI (PDW images) in a young patient in whom a diagnosis of ADEM was established. Note absence of brain lesions in the first examination obtained 2 days after symptom onset (*left*) and appearance of multiple small periventricular lesions on a scan obtained 10 days later (*middle*). A follow-up scan taken 2 months later (*right*) demonstrates complete resolution of lesions.

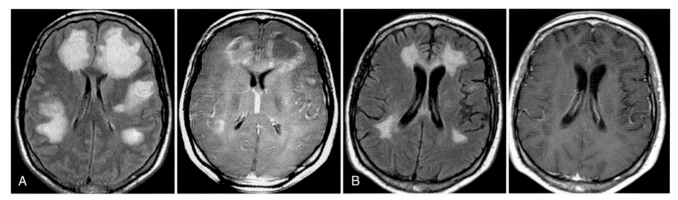

■ **FIGURE 43-41** Multiple tumefactive brain lesions in ADEM. Transverse fast-FLAIR and CE T1W sequences obtained 5 days after symptom onset (multifocal clinical syndrome associated with somnolence and behavioral changes) (**A**) show multiple large bihemispheric lesions with a Balo-like pattern and peripheral contrast agent uptake. Follow-up brain MR images obtained 1 year later (**B**) show size decrease, no contrast agent uptake, and no appearance of new lesions.

confined to the brain stem. The syndrome consists of localized encephalitis of the brain stem, commonly preceded by a febrile illness, and has a benign prognosis. T2W MRI usually shows an extensive high-signal intensity lesion involving the midbrain, the pons, and sometimes the thalamus. The clinical outcome is good and parallels resolution of the MRI lesions (Fig. 43-45). The pathogenesis of Bickerstaff's encephalitis is uncertain; however, the absence of CSF oligoclonal bands and resolution of the

clinical symptoms and MRI lesions suggest an inflammatory origin and make demyelination unlikely.

Acute Disseminated Necrohemorrhagic Leukoencephalitis

Acute disseminated necrohemorrhagic leukoencephalitis (acute hemorrhagic encephalomyelitis or Hurst's disease) is an uncommon condition that has been observed in patients of all ages. It

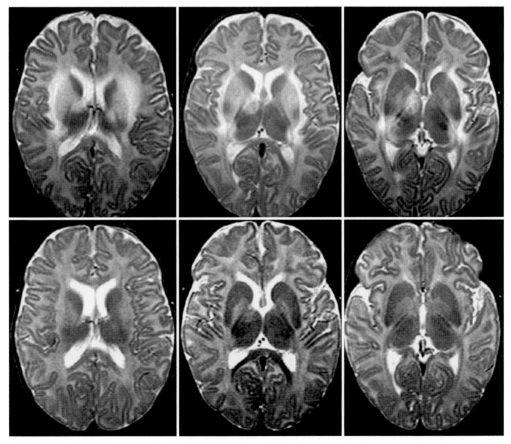

■ **FIGURE 43-42** Acute disseminated encephalomyelitis. Brain MRI in an 8-month-old boy shows diffuse, symmetric, hyperintense basal ganglia lesions on T2W images (*top row*) that completely disappeared 1 month later (*bottom row*). (*From Cañellas AR, Gols AR, Izquierdo JR, et al. Idiopathic inflammatory-demyelinating diseases of the central nervous system. Neuroradiology 2007; 49:393-469.*)

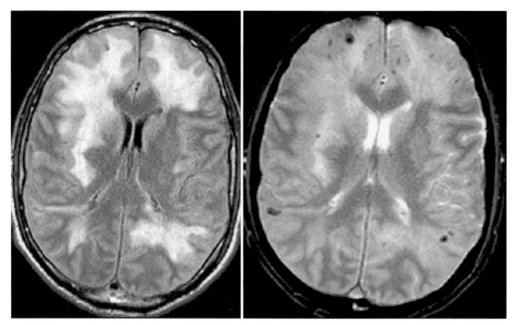

■ **FIGURE 43-43**   Acute hemorrhagic leukoencephalitis (Hurst's encephalitis). Axial FLAIR MR image shows an extensive abnormal signal affecting the periventricular and subcortical white matter (*left*), with acute hemorrhagic foci visualized as markedly hypointense areas within the white matter lesions on the T2*W GE MR image (*right*). *(From Cañellas AR, Gols AR, Izquierdo JR, et al. Idiopathic inflammatory-demyelinating diseases of the central nervous system. Neuroradiology 2007; 49:393-469.)*

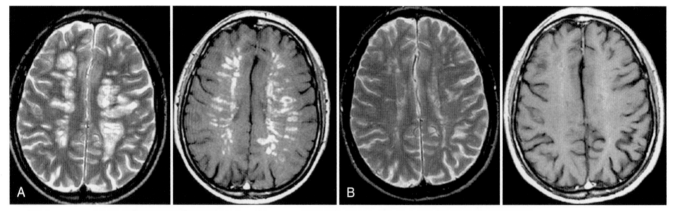

■ **FIGURE 43-44**   Acute disseminated encephalomyelitis. Transverse T2W and contrast-enhanced T1W MR images. Baseline scans show multiple enhancing periventricular and subcortical white matter lesions (**A**) that almost completely disappear on follow-up MR images obtained 12 months later (**B**).

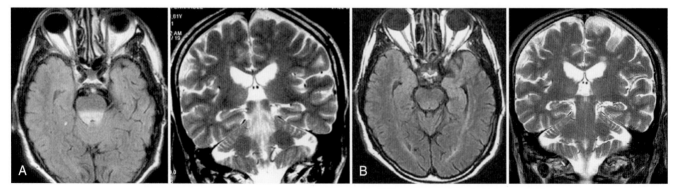

■ **FIGURE 43-45**   Bickerstaff encephalitis. Initial brain MRI (transverse fast-FLAIR and coronal FSE T2W sequences) shows an extensive brain stem lesion (**A**) that fully resolved in a follow-up study obtained 2 months later (**B**).

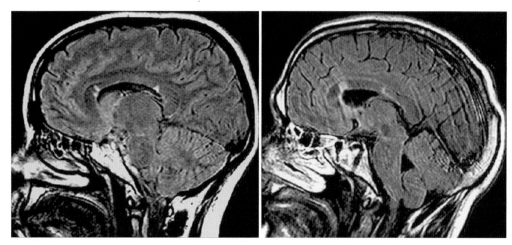

■ FIGURE 43-46 Corpus callosum lesions. Midsagittal fast-FLAIR MR images in a patient with relapsing-remitting MS (*left*) and a patient with cerebral autosomal dominant arteriopathy with subcortical infarcts and leukoencephalopathy (CADASIL). Observe the selective involvement of the callososeptal interface in the MS patient, whereas in CADASIL the lesions affect the entire corpus callosum width.

is thought to be a hyperacute form or the maximal variant of ADEM. This usually fatal disease manifests clinically as an abrupt onset of fever, neck stiffness, hemiplegia or other focal signs, seizures, and decreasing level of consciousness.[29] At autopsy, the brain is congested and swollen, sometimes asymmetrically, and herniation is frequent. Multiple petechial hemorrhages are distributed diffusely throughout the brain. The perivascular lesions chiefly consist of ball-like or ring hemorrhages surrounding necrotic venules, sometimes with fibrinous exudates within the vessel wall or extending into adjacent tissue. Perivenous demyelinating lesions, identical to those occurring in ADEM, may also be present. Perivascular cuffs of mononuclear cells, often with neutrophils, are seen. T2*W MR sequences show large regions of demyelination and petechial hemorrhages in the peripheral white matter of both cerebral hemispheres (see Fig. 43-43).

ANALYSIS
Differential Diagnosis between MS and Cerebral Small Vessel Disease

The changes identified by MRI in patients with MS are not disease specific. Other disorders can cause white matter lesions with imaging characteristics similar to those seen in MS. Nevertheless, the MRI pattern of brain MS is usually relatively specific when age, clinical information, and the full range of MRI abnormalities (including lesion number, distribution, size, shape, associated volume changes, and contrast enhancement) are taken into consideration. Even when only the number, location, and size of lesions are considered, the sensitivity and specificity for the diagnosis of MS is quite good, particularly after other diagnoses have been excluded by appropriate tests.

When lesions are found in the white matter, the most common differential diagnosis of MS is small vessel cerebrovascular disease. The prevalence of MS is only 1 per 1000 population, whereas small vessel disease is found in 5% to 10% of patients aged 20 to 40 years and nearly 100% of elderly people. In addition to the a priori chance of a white matter lesion being hypoxic-ischemic, several MRI features should suggest the diagnosis of MS, such as the following:

- *Involvement of the callososeptal interface of the corpus callosum.* The corpus callosum is frequently affected in MS owing to the large number of myelinated fibers within it. Callosal involvement is far less common with hypoxic-ischemic diseases, because the callosum has a unique double blood supply. However, the corpus callosum can be affected

in a significant proportion of patients with cerebral autosomal dominant arteriopathy with subcortical infarcts and leukoencephalopathy (CADASIL), Susac's syndrome, and severe subcortical arteriosclerotic encephalopathy. Small vessel diseases predominantly affect the central fibers of the corpus callosum, whereas MS typically affects the callososeptal interface (Fig. 43-46), at least in the early phases of the disease. Additional points of differential diagnosis include involvement of the deep gray matter of the basal ganglia and thalami in Susac's syndrome, preferential involvement of the external capsules and temporal lobes with multiple microhemorrhages in CADASIL, and the presence of lacunar infarctions in subcortical arteriosclerotic encephalopathy.
- *Involvement of U fibers.* The subcortical areas contiguous to the cortex contain the corticocortical association, or U, fibers. These tend to be spared in hypoxia, because they derive blood from both the cortical branches and the medullary arteries. In contrast, MS lesions are frequently seen at the corticomedullary junction (Fig. 43-47).
- *Involvement of the surface of the pons.* Pontine lesions are frequent in both MS and in small vessel diseases. The pontine lesions of MS are contiguous with the CSF spaces of the cisterns or ventricles (floor of the fourth ventricle), whereas small vessel disease lesions are usually located centrally. The central part of the pons may be particularly vulnerable to the effects of small vessel disease and hypoperfusion because this area corresponds to a vascular border zone, supplied by the anteromedial, lateral, and posterior groups of small penetrating arteries arising from the basilar and superior cerebellar arteries (see Fig. 43-18).
- *Presence of spinal cord lesions.* Spinal cord lesions are detected in more than 90% of MS patients, often without accompanying neurologic symptoms or signs. In contrast, patients with small vessel disease do not usually show cord abnormalities. Furthermore, incidental spinal cord lesions do not occur with aging and are rarely seen in other immune-mediated conditions (Fig. 43-48).

Differential Diagnosis between ADEM and MS
The lesions occurring in ADEM can resemble those of early MS. Discriminating features favoring the diagnosis of ADEM are poorly defined margins; relative absence of ovoid, corpus callosum, or periventricular lesions; relative symmetric involvement of the basal ganglia and thalamus, particularly in children; extensive spinal cord lesions; and no new lesion formation on

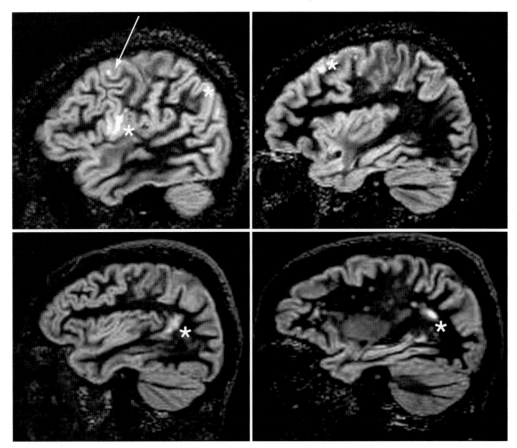

■ **FIGURE 43-47**   Corticojuxtacortical lesions. Sagittal double inversion recovery MR images in a patient with relapsing-remitting MS (*top row*) and a patient with cerebral small vessel disease (*bottom row*). In MS the lesions involve the posterior frontal cortex (*arrow*) and the inferior frontal and parietal juxtacortical white matter (*asterisks*). In the patient with small vessel disease, the lesions affect the subcortical white matter (*asterisks*) whereas no lesions are seen in the cortical gray matter or juxtacortical white matter.

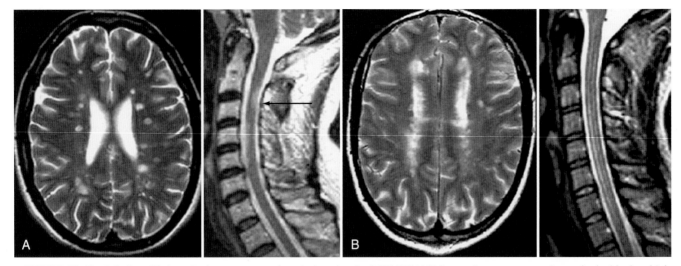

■ **FIGURE 43-48**   Spinal cord lesions. Brain transverse and cervical cord sagittal FSE T2W MR images in two young patients who had had multiple neurologic deficits disseminated in time and space. In both patients, multiple small periventricular white matter lesions are identified. The characteristics of the brain lesions are relatively similar in these two patients. In this situation, the presence of subclinical spinal cord lesions should suggest the diagnosis of MS (*arrow*). The final diagnosis was relapsing-remitting MS in the patient in **A**, and cerebral autosomal dominant arteriopathy with subcortical infarcts and leukoencephalopathy in the patient in **B**.

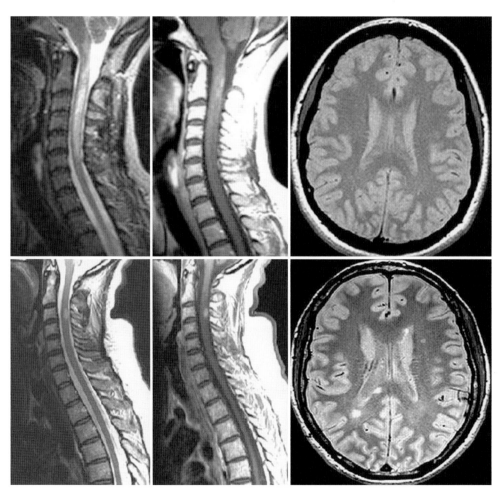

■ FIGURE 43-49 MRI differences between Devic's neuromyelitis optica (NMO) (*top row*) and MS (*bottom row*). Spinal cord lesions are extensive in NMO and usually associated with a normal brain MR image. In MS, symptomatic cord lesions are usually small and commonly associated with subclinical white matter brain lesions.

TABLE 43-4. Clinical, Biologic, and Radiologic Differences between Acute Disseminated Encephalomyelitis (ADEM) and Multiple Sclerosis (MS)

Criterion	ADEM	MS
Age	≤10 years	>10 years
Gender	Male = female	Male < female
Prior influenza	Very frequent	Variable
Encephalopathy	Required	Rare
Attacks	Fluctuate over 3 months	Separated by >1 month
Large MRI lesions	Frequent	Rare
Lesion margins	Poorly defined	Well defined
Deep gray matter	Frequently involved	Rarely involved
Spinal cord lesions	Extensive	Small
Longitudinal MRI	Resolution	New lesions
CSF white blood cell count >50/mm³	Frequent	Very rare
CSF oligoclonal bands	Variable	Frequent

TABLE 43-5. Clinical, Biologic, and Radiologic Differences between Devic's Neuromyelitis Optica (NMO) and Multiple Sclerosis (MS)

Criterion	NMO	MS
Female sex (%)	90	70
Age at onset (yr)	30-50	20-40
Topography	Optic nerve/spinal cord	Any
Symptomatic brain involvement	Uncommon and late	Common and early
Attack severity	Usually severe	Usually mild
Brain MRI	Normal/nonspecific	Abnormal
Spinal cord MRI	>3 segments, central	<1 segment, marginal
CSF cells	>50/mm³, PMNs	<50/mm³, lymphocytes
CSF oligoclonal bands	Usually negative	Usually positive
NMO-IgG	>70%	<10%
First-line treatment	Immunosuppressors	Immunomodulators

PMN, polymorphonuclear leukocytes.

follow-up MRI (see Fig. 43-39). The key clinical, biologic, and MRI features that can help to differentiate ADEM from MS are shown in Table 43-4.

Differential Diagnosis between NMO and MS

Key clinical characteristics that distinguish NMO from MS are the tendency for NMO to present as severe episodes of myelitis, which often, but not always, manifest as complete transverse myelitis, and severe episodes of optic neuritis, which often, but not always, result in incomplete recovery. The spinal cord lesions of NMO differ from those seen with MS. In NMO, MRI shows that the lesions usually extend vertically over three or more vertebral segments and commonly involve much of the cross section of the spinal cord. The brain is less frequently involved in NMO than MS. MRI of the brain is often normal with NMO, particularly early in the disease. When present, the brain lesions of NMO generally do not fulfill the Barkhof/Tintoré criteria for dissemination in space (Fig. 43-49). The key clinical, biologic, and MRI features that can help to differentiate NMO from MS are shown in Table 43-5.

Sample reports are presented in Boxes 43-1 and 43-2.

BOX 43-1   Sample Report: Risk for MS (Fig. 43-50)

PATIENT HISTORY

A 28-year-old woman presented with a 1-week history of blurred vision in the left eye, accompanied by pain on eye movement. The clinical diagnosis was unilateral optic neuritis. MRI was done to rule out subclinical demyelinating brain lesions suggestive of MS.

TECHNIQUE

Brain MRI was done that included transverse PDW and T2W FSE and fast-FLAIR sequences and unenhanced and contrast-enhanced T1W sequences (all transverse images were obtained with 5-mm slice thickness and no gap, covering the whole brain).

CONTRAST AGENT

A single dose of gadolinium (0.1 mmol/kg) was used with a scan delay of 7 minutes.

FINDINGS

Multiple (more than nine) small, focal, hyperintense lesions were evident on PDW/T2W sequences in the juxtacortical, subcortical, and periventricular brain white matter and in the left superior cerebellar peduncle.

Ring-enhancing contrast agent uptake is seen in several lesions identified on the PDW/T2W sequences.

IMPRESSION

Multiple, inflammatory, demyelinating, supratentorial and infratentorial white matter lesions of the type seen in MS, some of them with inflammatory activity. Lesions fulfill the McDonald 2010 multiple sclerosis criteria as this single-brain MRI scan demonstrates both dissemination in space (at least one asymptomatic lesion in three of the four characteristic locations, [juxtacortical, periventricular, posterior fossa]) and time (concomitant enhancing and nonenhancing lesions).

COMMENT

The present case corresponds to a typical patient who presents with a clinically isolated syndrome of the type seen in MS, involving the optic nerve. The diagnosis of optic neuritis is usually based on clinical features, and optic nerve MRI is not mandatory unless the clinical presentation is atypical. The main role of MRI is to assess the brain for asymptomatic lesions of the type seen in MS and to give an indication of the risk of subsequent development of MS.

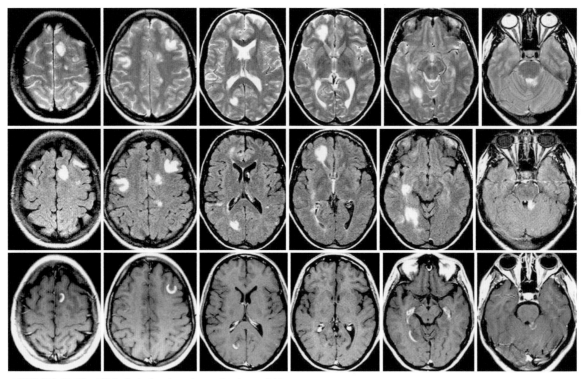

■ **FIGURE 43-50**   Clinically isolated syndrome (optic neuritis).

BOX 43-2   Sample Report: Role of MRI in Assessment of Treatment Efficacy in MS (Fig. 43-51)

PATIENT HISTORY

A 45-year-old woman presented with a previous diagnosis of relapsing-remitting MS. Interferon treatment was initiated 1 year earlier because of multiple relapses. Since the start of this treatment the patient experienced slight disability progression but clinical relapses could not be clearly demonstrated. The clinical diagnosis was secondary-progressive MS with inconclusive clinical activity. MRI was done to rule out inflammatory activity and assess disease progression and potential change in treatment.

COMPARISON STUDY

An MRI evaluation was done 14 months earlier.

TECHNIQUE

Brain MRI was done that included transverse PDW and T2W FSE sequences and transverse unenhanced and contrast-enhanced T1W sequences (all transverse images obtained with 3-mm slice thickness and no gap, covering the whole brain).

CONTRAST AGENT

A single dose gadolinium (0.1 mmol/kg) with scan delay of 7 minutes.

FINDINGS

The scan shows multiple, partially confluent hyperintense lesions on PDW/T2W sequences involving the subcortical and deep white matter

BOX 43-2   Sample Report: Role of MRI in Assessment of Treatment Efficacy in MS (Fig. 43-51)—cont'd

of both cerebral hemispheres. Many of the lesions (more than 10) show nodular/ring enhancement with gadolinium.

Ventricular and brain sulci enlargement is observed and is slightly more evident as compared with the previous scan. Compared with the previous scan, on PDW/T2W images several new lesions can be identified, most of them showing uptake of the contrast agent.

IMPRESSION

The study shows multiple, inflammatory, demyelinating, supratentorial and infratentorial white matter lesions of the type seen in MS, some of them new in comparison with the previous examination. Some of the new lesions show inflammatory activity. Associated with these focal MS plaques, evidence of a slight neurodegenerative component of the disease is demonstrated through the presence of brain volume loss, which has slightly progressed. The findings described indicate insufficient suppression of the inflammatory/demyelinating process (treatment failure).

COMMENT

The present case illustrates the role of MRI for assessing treatment efficacy in an MS patient. In MS, disease activity as evidenced by new and Gd-enhancing lesions is 5 to 10 times more frequent than clinical relapses. Based on this fact, it is obvious that the formation of new lesions with ongoing disease leads to an increase of the total T2 lesion burden, a measure that constitutes a more sensitive marker of disease progression than the clinical observation of a change in the severity of disability.

Combined assessment of new T2 lesions and Gd-enhancing lesions is now a frequently used composite measure (termed *combined unique lesion activity*) of focal disease activity in short- and long-term treatment trials for MS. This combined measure can also be used in daily management of MS patients to monitor treatment efficacy and to support treatment decisions in the individual patient. Accumulation of further lesions over time and/or the occurrence of Gd-enhancing lesions at a repeat examination certainly support insufficient suppression of the inflammatory/demyelinating process, while their absence argues for adequate treatment (concerning at least the antiinflammatory component). High standards regarding the reproducibility of image acquisition (identical technical parameters and repositioning) and interpretation are mandatory for reliable interpretation.

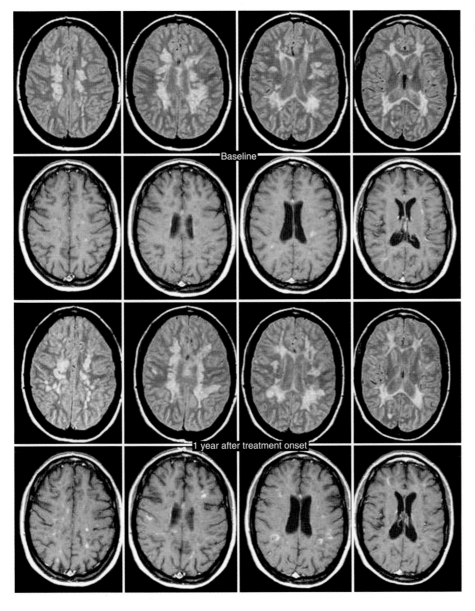

■ **FIGURE 43-51** Relapsing-remitting MS. Serial MRI obtained before and 1 year after initiating immunomodulating treatment (with interferon-β).

KEY POINTS: DIFFERENTIAL DIAGNOSIS

- *Between MS and Cerebral Small Vessel Disease. In MS:*
  - There is involvement of the callososeptal interface of the corpus callosum, U fibers, and the surface of the pons.
  - Spinal cord lesions are present.
- *Between ADEM and MS. In ADEM:*
  - Involvement of subcortical white matter and deep gray matter is predominant, with extensive lesions in the spinal cord and no new lesion formation.

- *Between NMO and MS. In NMO:*
  - Extensive spinal cord lesions are associated with no brain lesions or with brain lesions that are atypical for MS.

SUGGESTED READINGS

Bakshi R, Minagar A, Jaisani Z, Wolinsky JS. Imaging of multiple sclerosis: role in neurotherapeutics. NeuroRx 2005; 2:277-303.

Charil A, Yousry TA, Rovaris M, et al. MRI and the diagnosis of multiple sclerosis: expanding the concept of "no better explanation." Lancet Neurol 2006; 5:841-852.

Frohman EM, Racke MK, Raine CS. Multiple sclerosis—the plaque and its pathogenesis. N Engl J Med 2006; 354:942-955.

Ge Y. Multiple sclerosis: the role of MR imaging. AJNR Am J Neuroradiol 2006; 27:1165-1176.

Krupp LB, Banwell B, Tenembaum S. International Pediatric MS Study Group. Consensus definitions proposed for pediatric multiple sclerosis and related disorders. Neurology 2007; 68(16 Suppl 2): S7-S12.

Lassmann H, Bruck W, Lucchinetti C. Heterogeneity of multiple sclerosis pathogenesis: implications for diagnosis and therapy. Trends Mol Med 2001; 7:115-121.

Lucchinetti CF, Parisi J, Bruck W. The pathology of multiple sclerosis. Neurol Clin 2005; 23:77-105.

Lycklama G, Thompson A, Filippi M, et al. Spinal-cord MRI in multiple sclerosis. Lancet Neurol 2003; 2:555-562.

Miller D, Barkhof F, Montalban X, et al. Clinically isolated syndromes suggestive of multiple sclerosis: I. Natural history, pathogenesis, diagnosis, and prognosis. Lancet Neurol 2005; 4:281-288.

Noseworthy JH, Lucchinetti C, Rodriguez M, Weinshenker BG. Multiple sclerosis. N Engl J Med 2000; 343:938-952.

Tenembaum S, Chitnis T, Ness J, Hahn JS. International Pediatric MS Study Group. Acute disseminated encephalomyelitis. Neurology 2007; 68(16 Suppl 2):S23-S36.

REFERENCES

1. Lublin FD, Reingold SC. Defining the clinical course of multiple sclerosis: results of an international survey. National Multiple Sclerosis Society (USA) Advisory Committee on Clinical Trials of New Agents in Multiple Sclerosis. Neurology 1996; 46:907-911.

2. Brex PA, Ciccarelli O, O'Riordan JI, et al. A longitudinal study of abnormalities on MRI and disability from multiple sclerosis. N Engl J Med 2002; 346:158-164.

3. Ascherio A, Munger KL. Environmental risk factors for multiple sclerosis: I. The role of infection. Ann Neurol 2007; 61:288-299.

4. Weinshenker BG. Natural history of multiple sclerosis. Ann Neurol 1994; 36(Suppl):S6-S11.

5. Montalban X. Primary progressive multiple sclerosis. Curr Opin Neurol 2005; 18:261-266.

6. Polman CH, Reingold SC, Banwell B, et al. Diagnostic criteria for multiple sclerosis: 2010 revisions to the McDonald criteria. Ann Neurol 2011; 69:292-302.

7. Stadelmann C, Ludwin S, Tabira T, et al. Tissue preconditioning may explain concentric lesions in Balò's type of multiple sclerosis. Brain 2005; 128:979-987.

8. Masdeu JC, Quinto C, Olivera C, et al. Open-ring imaging sign: highly specific for atypical brain demyelination. Neurology 2000; 54:1427-1433.

9. Poser CM, Paty DW, Scheinberg L, et al. New diagnostic criteria for multiple sclerosis: guidelines for research protocols. Ann Neurol 1983; 13:227-231.

10. McDonald WI, Compston A, Edan G, et al. Recommended diagnostic criteria for multiple sclerosis: guidelines from the International Panel on the diagnosis of multiple sclerosis. Ann Neurol 2001; 50:121-127.

11. Montalban X, Tintoré M, Swanton J, et al. MRI criteria for MS in patients with clinically isolated syndromes. Neurology 2010; 74:427-434.

12. Rovira A, Swanton J, Tintoré M, et al. A single, early magnetic resonance imaging study in the diagnosis of multiple sclerosis. Arch Neurol 2009; 66:1-6.

13. Polman CH, Reingold SC, Edan G, et al Diagnostic criteria for multiple sclerosis: 2005 revisions to the "McDonald Criteria". Ann Neurol 2010; 58:840-846.

14. Lucchinetti C, Brück W, Parisi J, et al. Heterogeneity of multiple sclerosis lesions: implications for the pathogenesis of demyelination. Ann Neurol 2000; 47:707-717.

15. Bagnato F, Jeffries N, Richert ND, et al. Evolution of T1 black holes in patients with multiple sclerosis imaged monthly for 4 years. Brain 2003; 126(pt 8):1782-1789.

16. Cotton F, Weiner HL, Jolesz FA, Guttmann CR. MRI contrast uptake in new lesions in relapsing-remitting MS followed at weekly intervals. Neurology 2003; 60:640-646.

17. Rocca MA, Hickman SJ, Bö L, et al. Imaging the optic nerve in multiple sclerosis. Mult Scler 2005; 11:537-541.

18. Bermel RA, Bakshi R. The measurement and clinical relevance of brain atrophy in multiple sclerosis. Lancet Neurol 2006; 5:158-170.

19. Horsfield MA. Magnetization transfer imaging in multiple sclerosis. J Neuroimaging 2005; 15:58S-67S.

20. Rovaris M, Gass A, Bammer R, et al. Diffusion MRI in multiple sclerosis. Neurology 2005; 65:1526-1532.

21. De Stefano N, Bartolozzi ML, Guidi L, et al. Magnetic resonance spectroscopy as a measure of brain damage in multiple sclerosis. J Neurol Sci 2005; 233:203-208.

22. Pantano P, Mainero C, Caramia F. Functional brain reorganization in multiple sclerosis: evidence from fMRI studies. J Neuroimaging 2006; 16:104-114.

23. Ghezzi A, Bergamaschi R, Martinelli V, et al. Clinical characteristics, course and prognosis of relapsing Devic's neuromyelitis optica. J Neurol 2004; 251:47-52.

24. Wingerchuk DM, Weinshenker BG. Neuromyelitis optica: clinical predictors of a relapsing course and survival. Neurology 2003; 60:848-853.

25. Lennon VA, Wingerchuk DM, Kryzer TJ, et al. A serum autoantibody marker of neuromyelitis optica: distinction from multiple sclerosis. Lancet 2004; 364:2106-2112.

26. Wingerchuk DM, Lennon VA, Pittock SJ, et al. Revised diagnostic criteria for neuromyelitis optica. Neurology 2006; 66:1485-1489.
27. Lucchinetti CF, Mandler RN, McGavern D, et al. A role for humoral mechanisms in the pathogenesis of Devic's neuromyelitis optica. Brain 2002; 125(pt 7):1450-1461.
28. Pittock SJ, Lennon VA, Krecke K, et al. Brain abnormalities in neuromyelitis optica. Arch Neurol 2006; 63:390-396.
29. Menge T, Hemmer B, Nessler S, et al. Acute disseminated encephalomyelitis: an update. Arch Neurol 2005; 62:1673-1680.
30. Tenembaum S, Chamoles N, Fejerman N. Acute disseminated encephalomyelitis: a long-term follow-up study of 84 pediatric patients. Neurology 2002; 59:1224-1231.

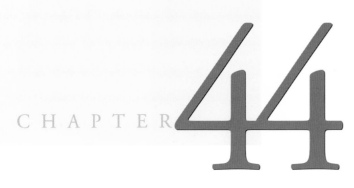
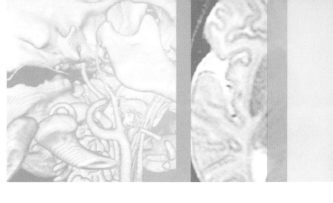

CHAPTER 44

Neurotoxicity Associated with Pediatric Malignancies

Nancy K. Rollins

Cancer is the most common cause of death in children up to 14 years of age; nearly 1 child in 600 will develop cancer. By 2010, 1 in 540 adults who are 20 to 34 years of age is predicted to be a survivor of childhood cancer with variable neurologic sequelae. The neurologic sequelae resulting from the therapy for childhood malignancy vary with the age at presentation, the site of origin of the malignancy, and the therapy. The most common pediatric malignancies associated with adverse neurologic affects are acute lymphoblastic leukemia (ALL), which accounts for approximately 25% of childhood malignancies, and brain tumors, accounting for about 20% of pediatric malignancies. The iatrogenic neurotoxicities may be due to chemotherapy—most often methotrexate (MTX), cranial irradiation, or bone marrow transplantation (BMT). The treatment for ALL involves multiple chemotherapeutic agents, the mainstay of which is MTX. Given intravenously, MTX crosses the blood-brain barrier, eradicating leukemic cells in the central nervous system (CNS), a common site of leukemic recurrence. MTX is also given sequentially via direct intrathecal injection to eliminate leukemic cells from the cerebrospinal fluid (CSF). Another chemotherapeutic agent used in ALL is the enzyme L-asparaginase, which is also associated with neurotoxicity but with a lower incidence and different pathophysiology and imaging abnormalities. Craniospinal irradiation is reserved for ALL patients with CNS relapse or for patients who cannot tolerate high-dose MTX; the doses given range from 1200 to 1800 cGy, which is considerably lower than that used for control of primary CNS malignancies.

Medulloblastoma is one of the most common CNS tumors of childhood. It is highly malignant with a propensity to disseminate along the neural axis. Control of medulloblastoma necessitates delivery of radiation to the craniospinal region. Unlike in other pediatric CNS tumors such as ependymoma and nonresectable pilocytic astrocytomas, which can often be controlled with conformational radiation therapy, whole-brain irradiation is needed in patients with medulloblastoma. The effects of cranial irradiation depend on the total dose to normal structures, radiation dose for each daily radiation treatment (daily fraction), combination of radiation therapy with other treatment modalities (chemotherapy and surgery), presence of hydrocephalus at presentation, and patient age when radiation is given. The neurologic impact on the brain from irradiation and chemotherapy is greatest in children younger than 3 years of age, and most therapeutic protocols withhold cranial irradiation until the patient reaches 3 years of age unless there is relapse or progression while the child is on chemotherapy. Allogenic BMT is used in the setting of very high-risk ALL or for those patients with a suboptimal response to chemotherapy. BMT is also used as treatment intensification for a variety of solid tumors of childhood. Complications of BMT include intracranial hemorrhage and strokes, reversible posterior leukoencephalopathy syndrome (PRES), graft-versus-host disease (GVHD), and infection. The focus of this chapter is on the most common pediatric iatrogenic neurotoxicities, which are those associated with treatment of leukemia (including BMT) and primary brain tumors of childhood.

For a full discussion of neurotoxicity in children, please visit www.expertconsult.com.

Aging and Degeneration

CHAPTER 45

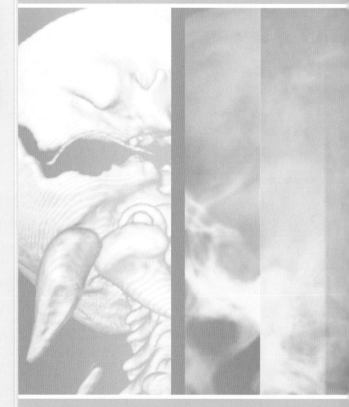

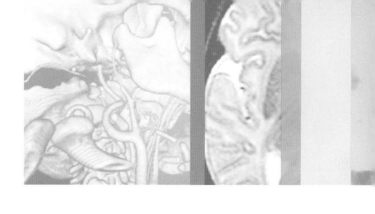

Neurodegeneration: Cerebrum

Basil H. Ridha and Tarek A. Yousry

Dementia is an acquired syndrome of progressive impairment of multiple cognitive domains (including memory), causing significant impairment of social and occupational functioning in the presence of normal consciousness.[1] Dementia should be differentiated from acute confusional state, or delirium, in which there is a transient reversible impairment of cognitive function, usually accompanied by fluctuating levels of consciousness. Both dementia and delirium are clinical syndromes and not diagnoses per se.

Most cases of dementia result from an underlying neurodegenerative disease. Most cases of delirium result, instead, from potentially reversible infective, inflammatory, or metabolic disturbances.

Mild cognitive impairment (MCI) is a transitional stage between normal aging and dementia.[2,3] Approximately 12% of MCI patients advance to frank dementia per year, with 50% doing so over the 5 years after diagnosis. Other MCI patients exhibit mild cognitive deficits that are not severe enough to warrant a diagnosis of dementia. Some of these may follow a benign course (the worried well) or prove to have reversible conditions, such as depression. Because MCI may be the early stage of a dementing illness, particularly Alzheimer's disease, MCI would be the ideal target for any therapy to modify or prevent disease progression.

An estimated 27.7 million people suffered from dementia in 2003 worldwide, of which 38% lived in the advanced economies.[4] The annual incidence of dementia is estimated to be 4.6 million cases, that is, a new case every 7 seconds, worldwide. With projected increases in life expectancy and the exponential increase of dementia with age, the prevalence of dementia is expected to double every 20 years to 81.1 million by 2040.[5] Because patients with dementia are heavy consumers of health care services and social care, this will have a significant impact on financial planning and policymaking for health care and social services. In addition, there is a high economic and psychosocial cost for the informal support required from family caregivers.[6]

The neurodegenerative diseases underlying dementia are defined by their underlying pathology. The common themes appear to be abnormal deposition of a normally soluble protein in the brain tissue (a proteinopathy) and/or a cerebrovascular abnormality. Alzheimer's disease is defined by (1) the extracellular deposition of insoluble Aβ, a peptide chain of 40 to 42 amino acids, resulting in extracellular amyloid plaques, and (2) the intracellular deposition of hyperphosphorylated tau protein, resulting in intraneuronal neurofibrillary tangles.[7] Other neurodegenerative diseases underlying dementia include vascular dementia, cortical Lewy body disease, frontotemporal lobar degeneration, and the prion diseases. Alzheimer's disease is the most common cause of dementia, followed by cortical Lewy body disease and vascular dementia. In individuals younger than age 60 years, frontotemporal lobar degeneration is the second most common cause of dementia after Alzheimer's disease. These pathologic processes may coexist with each other or even increase the likelihood of developing a second pathologic process. Mixed dementia (e.g. Alzheimer's disease and concurrent vascular dementia) is probably the most common form of all dementia overall.

For a full discussion of the neurodegenerative conditions underlying dementia and a review of their imaging features, please visit www.expertconsult.com.

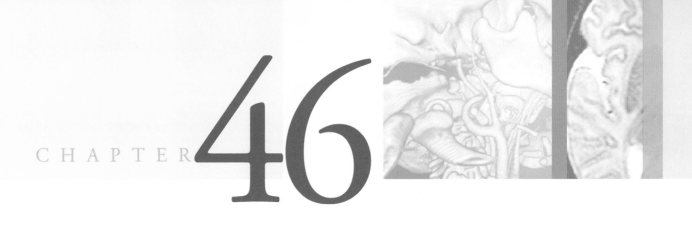

46

Neurodegeneration: Cerebellum and Brain Stem

Luke A. Massey and Tarek A. Yousry

In neurodegenerative diseases affecting primarily the brain stem and cerebellum, imaging is used to exclude other diseases that may mimic neurodegeneration, such as demyelination, vasculopathies, normal pressure hydrocephalus, and tumor, and to plan stereotactic surgery to control the symptoms of Parkinson's disease.[1] Advances in transcranial ultrasonography, MRI, functional imaging with positron emission tomography (PET), and single photon emission computed tomography (SPECT) offer hope that the diverse forms of neurodegeneration may soon be assessed directly. CT contributes little to the evaluation of neurodegenerative diseases, so it is not discussed further.

Neurodegenerative diseases become symptomatic in the later stages of adult life, so it is important to be able to distinguish these diseases from the effects of normal aging on brain volume and signal intensity. Age-related volume changes are usually diffuse with no regional predilection. Age-related changes in signal intensity largely reflect the deposition of metals, especially iron, within the brain. In the normal human brain, iron deposition is symmetric and geographic, affecting primarily the globus pallidus, the striatum, the substantia nigra (especially the pars reticulata), and the dentate nucleus of cerebellum. Quantitative techniques show that the highest concentrations of iron are found in the globus pallidus, red nucleus, substantia nigra, putamen, dentate, and caudate nuclei.[2] T2-weighted (T2W) MR images at 1.5 Tesla show normal, age-related hypointensities within the globus pallidus, substantia nigra pars reticulata, red nucleus, dentate, putamen, and the subcortical U fibers.[3] Postmortem studies with Perls' stain for ferric iron reveal that the areas of T2 hypointensity correlate with regions of intense Perls' staining. However, there is an imperfect match between the distribution of iron and the hypointensity on T2W images. Specifically, the putamen and caudate nucleus are less hypointense than would be expected from Perls' stain data, whereas the corpus callosum, other commissures, and internal capsule appear more hypointense than would be expected from Perls' stain data. However, MRI studies of the effect of age on T2 signal intensity within the deep gray nuclei are in agreement with the pathologic studies. There is no iron deposition at birth. Iron becomes deposited, in order, and causes low T2 signal intensity, in order, first within the globus pallidus, then the red nucleus and substantia nigra, and then the dentate nuclei of the cerebellum.[4] By age 25 years, these structures are all hypointense relative to cortical gray matter. During adult life the signal intensity within the red nucleus, dentate, and substantia nigra remain relatively stable. The pallidum becomes progressively more hypointense. The putamen becomes hypointense in the eighth and ninth decades. The thalamus and the caudate nucleus are not hypointense in healthy populations.[5]

For a full discussion of those neurodegenerative diseases that primarily affect the brain stem and cerebellum, please visit www.expertconsult.com.

Toxic and Metabolic Conditions

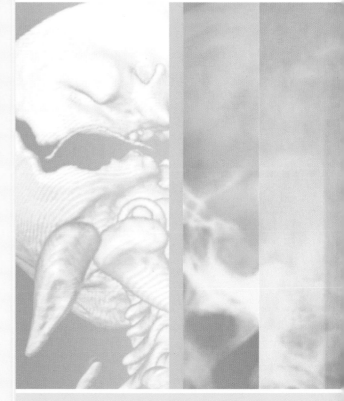

CHAPTER 47

Toxic and Metabolic Brain Disease

Benjamin Y. Huang

Toxic and metabolic brain disease encompasses a vast and heterogeneous group of disorders that can cause a great deal of confusion to both clinicians and radiologists. Diagnosis of these disorders can be challenging, because their clinical and imaging characteristics are often nonspecific. A number of systems have been proposed to classify these disorders and have been based on, among other things, clinical features, histologic features, and biochemical features. Each classification system has its own relative advantages and disadvantages, and no one system is perfect from an imaging standpoint.

Even the distinction between "toxic disorders" and "metabolic disorders" is often unclear. Most metabolic disorders cause brain injury through the actions of accumulated toxic substances within brain tissue and can therefore reasonably be considered to be forms of toxic disease. For instance, in phenylketonuria, deficiency of the enzyme phenylalanine hydroxylase, which is responsible for the metabolism of phenylalanine to tyrosine, results in accumulation of alternate phenylalanine breakdown products that are toxic to developing brain structures.

Conversely, external toxins cause brain injury by disturbing normal cellular metabolism. Therefore, one could just as reasonably consider toxic disorders to be acquired forms of metabolic disease. Regardless of what one ultimately calls these disorders, they all produce the same end result, namely, injury to brain tissue.

Perhaps the most straightforward method of categorizing this broad family of diseases is to divide them into those that are congenital and those that are acquired. Congenital metabolic diseases, also commonly referred to as inborn errors of metabolism, usually manifest in infancy or early childhood and include several families of disease, such as the mitochondrial disorders, lysosomal storage disorders, peroxysomal disorders, and Golgi complex disorders. These diseases are not discussed here.

Acquired metabolic disorders can occur in adults and children and can be related to nutritional deficiencies, abnormalities of glucose and electrolyte levels, impaired organ function (liver and renal failure), or the effects of exogenous toxins.

Exogenous toxins may exert their effects on tissue either directly or indirectly. With direct toxicity, a toxin is able to cause tissue injury on its own without requiring metabolism into another compound. Indirect toxicity results when substances that are not directly toxic to tissues are subsequently broken down into toxic metabolites.

Specific toxins tend to affect specific regions of the brain selectively. This so-called selective vulnerability seen in toxic and acquired metabolic disease reflects several important physiologic factors, including, but not limited to, (1) regional cerebral blood flow and oxygen demand, (2) neurotransmitter distribution, (3) specific chemical affinities and vulnerabilities, and (4) developmental maturation at the time of intoxication. Each of these factors plays a role in determining what structures in the brain are affected and, ultimately, the clinical syndrome that arises as a result of exposure to a particular toxin.

In this chapter we review several of the more common toxic and metabolic brain disorders seen in the adult population.

OSMOTIC MYELINOLYSIS

Osmotic myelinolysis is a neurologic disorder seen primarily in the setting of chronically malnourished alcoholics. It occurs when rapid changes in serum osmolality take place, and the most common scenario in which it is seen is aggressive iatrogenic correction of hyponatremia. The result is extensive demyelination classically within the pons but also affecting other sites in the brain. Alternate names include central pontine myelinolysis and osmotic demyelination syndrome.

Epidemiology

The exact incidence of osmotic myelinolysis is not known. The disorder occurs most commonly in middle-aged, chronically malnourished alcoholic patients, but it is also seen in patients made hyponatremic iatrogenically and in patients with severe liver disease.[1]

Clinical Presentation

Typically, patients initially present with encephalopathy as a result of hyponatremia. With intravenous sodium replacement, encephalopathy may show clinical improvement, but, subsequently, there is a neurologic decline over the next 48 to 72 hours. Symptoms may include quadriparesis or quadriplegia, pseudobulbar palsy, horizontal gaze palsies, seizures, and coma. Osmotic myelinolysis has an extremely poor prognosis, with only 5% to 10% of patients surviving beyond 6 months. Full recovery from the disorder has been reported, however.[2]

Pathophysiology

Rapid changes in serum osmolality are believed to cause disruption of the blood-brain barrier, resulting in accumulation of hypertonic fluid in the extracellular space. This ultimately results in extensive noninflammatory demyelination. It is unclear why the pons is preferentially involved, but it has been suggested that the close association of vascular gray matter with orthogonally arranged bundles of myelinated fibers in the pons causes increased susceptibility to compression from cellular edema.[2,3]

Pathology

Lesions caused by osmotic myelinolysis consist of circumscribed zones of demyelination appearing as regions of discoloration that are abnormally soft and granular, most commonly in the central portions of the upper pons, with involvement of the pontine nuclei and white matter of the base of the pons (Fig. 47-1). Extrapontine sites may also be involved, including the cerebellum, basal ganglia, thalamus, internal and external capsules, and subcortical white matter. The subpial and periventricular regions are spared. Exclusively extrapontine involvement is seen in up to 25% of cases.[4]

In the affected areas there is myelin loss with preservation of axons and neuronal cell bodies, which helps in distinguishing these lesions histologically from pontine infarcts. In later stages, infiltration by lipid-laden macrophages may be seen in the central portions of the lesions, with only scant lymphocytes. Oligodendrocytes are lost, but reactive astrocytes may be seen.[4]

Imaging

CT

CT demonstrates low density in affected areas, reflecting edema. The pons is the most commonly involved site, but lesions may also be seen in the basal ganglia, thalami, subcortical white matter, cerebellum, and middle cerebellar peduncles. The sensitivity of CT for pontine myelinolysis is low, because the pons is frequently obscured by streak artifact from the nearby petrous bone.[2]

MRI

In the acute phase, MRI demonstrates ovoid areas of T2-weighted (T2W) hyperintensity in the central portion of the pons with sparing of the ventrolateral aspect of the pons and the corticospinal tracts (Fig. 47-2). In some instances, the lesions may appear trident-shaped on axial images. No contrast enhancement is seen after gadolinium administration. In the subacute phase, usually 1 to 2 weeks after onset of symptoms, abnormalities may progress to involve the entire pons. Foci of restricted diffusion may also be evident. In 10% to 50% of cases, extrapontine involvement may be seen in the basal ganglia, thalami, cerebral peduncles, subcortical white matter, cerebellum, and cervicomedullary junction.[2,3] MR spectroscopy may demonstrate decreased *N*-acetyl-aspartate (NAA)/creatine (Cr) and increased choline (Cho)/Cr ratios within the pons. MR perfusion imaging can demonstrate increased perfusion on cerebral blood volume (CBV) maps.[5]

Patients who survive demonstrate residual signal abnormality or cavitation in the pons.[3]

HYPERGLYCEMIC HEMICHOREA-HEMIBALLISMUS

Hemichorea-hemiballismus (HCHB) is a syndrome associated with nonketotic hyperglycemia in patients with poorly controlled diabetes mellitus and is characterized by sudden onset of

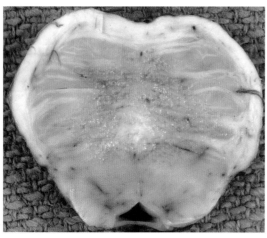

■ **FIGURE 47-1** Central pontine myelinolysis. Axial section through the base of the pons demonstrates discoloration and granularity in the central pons reflecting demyelination. The corticospinal tracts are spared. *(Courtesy of T. W. Bouldin, University of North Carolina, Chapel Hill, NC.)*

■ **FIGURE 47-2** Osmotic myelinolysis. **A,** Axial FLAIR image through the pons demonstrates diffuse pontine signal abnormality that spares the periphery of the pons and the corticospinal tracts. The cortex of the anterior temporal lobes are also involved. **B,** FLAIR image through the basal ganglia shows involvement of the basal ganglia, thalami, claustra, and insula.

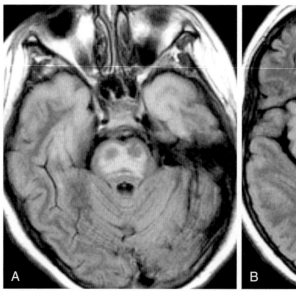
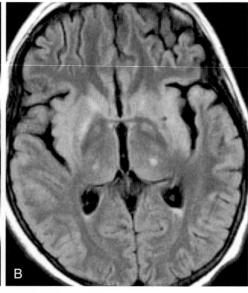

hemiballismus or hemichorea. This syndrome is also called hemi-ballismus-hemichorea, chorea-ballismus with nonketotic hyper-glycemia, and nonketotic hyperglycemia.

Epidemiology

HCHB is seen in poorly controlled diabetic patients with nonke-totic hyperglycemia and has been reported mostly in elderly women of Asian origin.[6] The entity is quite uncommon, and its exact incidence is not known.

Clinical Presentation

Affected individuals present with acute onset of random, jerking motions in the distal extremities (chorea), or sudden high-velocity flinging or kicking movements (ballismus). Involvement is usually unilateral but may occasionally be bilateral. Most patients will have an established diagnosis of diabetes mellitus, but in some cases HCHB may be the presenting feature of previ-ously undiagnosed diabetes. Blood sugar levels will be elevated and are typically greater than 200 mg/dL. Serum osmolarity may be normal or mildly elevated.[7] Symptoms are usually reversible with treatment of hyperglycemia, but the condition may rarely progress to coma and death. Chorea and ballismus are nonspe-cific symptoms and can also result from other conditions, includ-ing cerebrovascular disease, infections, drug toxicity, other metabolic disorders, neurodegenerative diseases, autoimmune disorders, and tumors.

Pathophysiology

Hyperglycemia results in global decreased regional cerebral blood flow, which is maximal in the basal ganglia. It is presumed that hyperglycemia and hyperviscosity of blood in diabetic patients causes ischemia in the striatum.[6] The decreased flow may contribute to decreased local amounts of the neurotransmit-ter γ-aminobutyric acid (GABA). Decreases in striatal GABA may allow increased pallidal activity, with resultant dyskinesia affect-ing the contralateral side of the body.[7]

The explanation for the specific imaging changes seen in HCHB remains controversial. Some believe that hyperglycemia causes partial ischemia in the basal ganglia with resultant micro-hemorrhage or reversible calcium influx. Alternative explana-tions include manganese accumulation in reactive astrocytes after ischemia, which would explain hyperintensity on T1-weighted (T1W) MR images but not high density on CT. Still others suggest protein desiccation during the course of wallerian degeneration is responsible for the imaging abnormalities.[8]

Histologically, the abnormal putamen contains multiple infarcts with reactive astrocytosis, fragmentation of axons, and myelin pallor. Punctate calcifications and scattered microhemor-rhages may be seen but are an inconstant finding.[6]

Imaging
CT
CT in patients with HCHB classically demonstrates increased density in the caudate, putamen, or both. Involvement is typi-cally unilateral but can be bilateral. When symptoms are unilat-eral, the lesions are located in the contralateral corpus striatum. Lesions typically resolve over time after treatment.[7]

MRI
MRI will typically demonstrate increased signal intensity in one of the basal ganglia on T1W images (Fig. 47-3).[7] Bilateral basal ganglia involvement can occasionally be seen. Hyperintensity on diffusion-weighted images with corresponding reduced appar-ent diffusion coefficients (ADC) may also be seen but may be reversible. Other entities that may produce hyperintensity in the basal ganglia on T1W imaging are manganese poisoning, pro-longed parenteral nutrition (presumedly due to deposition of manganese), and chronic liver failure.

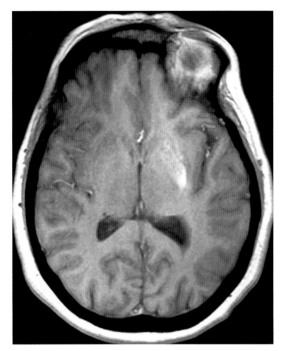

■ **FIGURE 47-3** Hyperglycemic hemichorea-hemiballismus. Axial unen-hanced T1W MR image shows asymmetric hyperintensity in the left basal ganglia (predominantly in the putamen).

Specific Procedures
Proton MR spectroscopy performed in the basal ganglia may demonstrate lactate elevation and decreased NAA, suggesting ischemia. Furthermore, several authors have reported decreased perfusion to the affected basal ganglia on SPECT imaging.[6]

DISORDERS OF IRON AND COPPER METABOLISM
Neurodegeneration with Brain Iron Accumulation
Neurodegeneration with brain iron accumulation (NBIA) is an autosomal recessive disorder characterized by dystonia, parkin-sonism, and brain iron accumulation. Classic and atypical forms of disease have been described. In the classic form, disease onset is early and symptoms are rapidly progressive. In the atypical form of the disease, onset is later in life and symptoms progress more slowly. Other names include Hallervorden-Spatz syndrome, Hallervorden-Spatz disease, and pantothenate kinase–associated neurodegeneration (PKAN).

Epidemiology
The exact prevalence of NBIA is not known. The disease occurs with equal frequency in males and females, and no race predilec-tion has been identified. Although NBIA is typically a disease of childhood, symptom onset during adulthood has been reported. The classic form of the disease usually presents by the age of 10. The atypical form presents in the second decade of life and occasionally in early adulthood.[9]

Clinical Presentation
The early-onset form of the disease presents in childhood with dystonia, dysarthria, rigidity, and choreoathetosis. Symptoms related to involvement of the corticospinal tract (spasticity, hyperreflexia) are also frequently observed. The most common presenting symptoms are gait or postural difficulties. In addition, most patients with the classic form of disease have clinical or electroretinographic evidence of retinopathy due to pigmentary

degeneration of the retina. Symptoms progress rapidly to severe disability by the age of 20, ultimately culminating in early death.

In the atypical form of the disease, symptoms are much more variable. Extrapyramidal symptoms occur less frequently than in the classic form, and the degree of dystonia and rigidity is generally less severe and progresses more slowly. Patients may remain ambulatory for up to 40 years after onset of symptoms. Spasticity, hyperreflexia, and clinical evidence of retinopathy are also less common. In a significant number of patients with the atypical form of disease, difficulty with speech may be the sole presenting feature, unlike patients with the classic form who almost never present initially with dysarthria (although they may develop it later in the disease course). Cognitive decline eventually resulting in dementia is prominent in atypical NBIA but is rare in the classic form.[9]

Pathophysiology

In the majority of patients with NBIA, the disease has been linked to a mutation in the *PANK2* gene located on chromosome 20p13. *PANK2* encodes a pantothenate kinase involved in the biosynthesis of coenzyme A from vitamin B_5. *PANK2* mutations are shown in all cases of classic NBIA and approximately one third of cases of the atypical form.[9] Although the genetic mutation causing most cases of the disorder has been identified, the exact mechanism of tissue injury is not known. It has been hypothesized that deficiency of *PANK2* leads to accumulation of cysteine-containing neurotoxic compounds in highly sensitive regions of the brain, resulting in tissue damage and edema. Accumulation of excess iron in normally iron-rich brain structures is suspected to be secondary to tissue damage in the disease.[10]

Pathology

Macroscopically, rusty-brown discoloration of the globus pallidus (particularly the internal segment) (Fig. 47-4) and reticular zone of the substantia nigra is seen.[4]

On microscopy, brownish yellow pigment is seen in the cytoplasm of nerve cells, microglia, and astrocytes from the globus pallidus (internal segment) and substantia nigra. Extracellular pigment is also present around blood vessels in the same areas. Pigment deposits give a strong reaction for iron and are periodic acid–Schiff (PAS) positive and Sudan black positive. Neuronal depletion is seen in the globus pallidus, in the reticular zone of the substantia nigra, and occasionally in the subthalamic nuclei and cerebellum. Reactive gliosis is also seen. A characteristic finding is the presence of rounded or oval structures known as spheroids, which represent axonal swellings.[4]

Imaging

CT

CT is generally not helpful in the diagnosis of NBIA. Although frequently normal, may demonstrate cerebral or cerebellar atrophy and mineralization of the basal ganglia, particularly the globus pallidus, probably reflecting deposition of iron-staining pigment.[11]

MRI

Findings on MRI in patients with NBIA correlate with the presence or absence of *PANK2* mutations. In patients with the *PANK2* mutation, the characteristic finding on MRI is the "eye of the tiger" sign, which consists of T2 signal hypointensity in the globus pallidus with a central region of T2 hyperintensity (Fig. 47-5). The low signal intensity of the globus pallidus reflects excess iron deposition, and the focus of hyperintensity centrally represents areas of loose tissue with vacuolization.[12] Enhancement in the globus pallidus after contrast agent administration is not seen. The earliest imaging finding is isolated T2 hyperintensity in the globus pallidus interna. Patients with this finding typically go on to develop the "eye of the tiger" sign within 3 years. Hypointensity in the reticular layer of substantia nigra on T2W images may also be seen in these patients.[10]

Patients without the *PANK2* mutation will not demonstrate the "eye of the tiger" sign. These patients may show T2 hypointensity alone in the globus pallidus. Cerebral and cerebellar atrophy and iron deposition in the red nucleus and dentate nucleus are common features in patients without the *PANK2* mutation.[9]

Specific Procedures

Proton MR spectroscopy in the globus pallidus demonstrates markedly decreased NAA.[13]

Wilson's Disease

Wilson's disease is a rare, autosomal recessive defect of copper metabolism that causes accumulation of abnormal amounts of copper in various tissues, with a predilection for involvement of

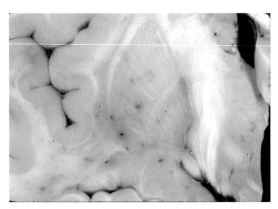

■ **FIGURE 47-4** Neurodegeneration with brain iron accumulation. Coronal section through the basal ganglia demonstrates rust-brown discoloration of the globus pallidus, most pronounced in its internal segment. *(Courtesy of T. W. Bouldin, University of North Carolina, Chapel Hill, NC.)*

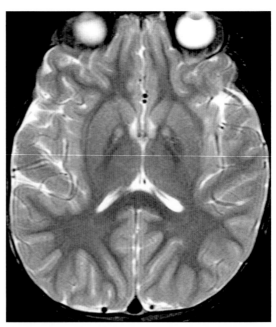

■ **FIGURE 47-5** Neurodegeneration with brain iron accumulation. Axial T2W MR image demonstrates symmetric foci of hyperintensity on a background of hypointensity of the globi pallidi. This is an example of the "eye of the tiger" sign.

the brain, kidney, and liver. Manifestations of Wilson's disease include liver disease and neurologic symptoms. Alternate names include hepatolenticular degeneration, progressive lenticular degeneration, and Westphal-Strümpell pseudosclerosis.

Epidemiology
Wilson's disease is inherited in an autosomal recessive fashion and affects between 1 in 30,000 and 1 in 100,000 individuals. Symptoms typically appear in the second or third decades of life, and there is a slight male predominance.

Clinical Presentation
Neurologic and neuropsychiatric abnormalities are the presenting signs in up to 50% of patients with Wilson's disease, and patients presenting with neurologic signs tend to be older than those with hepatic features alone. The neurologic abnormalities may include an akinetic-rigid syndrome similar to Parkinson's disease, tremor, ataxia, dystonia, choreiform movements, and pseudobulbar palsy. Changes in behavior, deterioration in school work, and worsening hand-eye coordination may appear before characteristic neurologic features arise. Other signs include drooling, dysarthria, and spasticity.

Wilson's disease may also present similarly to chronic hepatitis, as fulminant hepatic failure, or insidiously as cirrhosis and signs of portal hypertension. In patients presenting initially with liver disease, neurologic symptoms, if they do occur, usually occur 2 to 5 years later.

Characteristic Kayser-Fleischer rings, appearing as golden brown rings at the outer margin of the cornea caused by deposition of copper, and sunflower cataracts may be detected on slit lamp examination.

Diagnosis of Wilson's disease is usually confirmed on the basis of Kayser-Fleischer rings, decreased serum copper and ceruloplasmin levels, and increased 24-hour urinary copper excretion. Patients require lifelong treatment with de-coppering agents such as penicillamine, trientine, and zinc.[14,15]

Pathophysiology
The genetic defect responsible for Wilson's disease has been linked to chromosome 13q14.3. The gene *ATP7B* encodes a transmembrane protein, which plays a role in the transport of copper into cells, incorporation of copper into the plasma protein ceruloplasmin, and excretion of excess copper stores in the bile. Defects in *ATP7B* result in excess copper accumulation in tissues, most notably the liver and the brain.[15] Excess copper may combine with sulfhydryl, carboxyl, or amine groups and cause improper enzymatic activity, ultimately damaging cell structure. In addition, increased extracellular copper can cause oxidative stress, which leads to cell death.[16]

Pathology
On autopsy, the brain may appear normal externally, but on sectioning there will be shrinkage and brownish discoloration of the putamen (particularly the middle third) and caudate nuclei. Cysts may be present in the putamen, and the cerebral white matter may be softened and cystic. The globus pallidus, subthalamic nucleus, thalamus, and brain stem are often involved but less severely. Spongy degeneration in the cerebral cortex and white matter may also be seen.[4]

On histology, the brain will demonstrate an increase in the number of astrocytes (known as Alzheimer type 2 cells) within gray matter, swollen glia, liquefaction, and areas of spongiform degeneration, which is most pronounced in the putamina. Alzheimer type 2 cells are notable for enlarged, vesicular nuclei, and prominent nucleoli with inconspicuous cytoplasm. Macrophages may be seen within cystic regions and in nearby perivascular spaces. Perivascular and parenchymal granular copper deposits are evident on rhodanine or rubeanic acid stains.[17]

Neuronal loss and gliosis may be seen. Characteristic of Wilson's disease is the presence of Opalski cells—large cells containing fine granular cytoplasm and small, slightly abnormal nuclei—that are believed to represent degenerating astrocytes.[15,17]

Imaging
CT
On CT, patients with Wilson's disease demonstrate generalized atrophy. Hypodense lesions may be evident in the basal ganglia and frontal white matter. In general, CT is less sensitive than MRI for detecting gray and white matter abnormalities.[18]

MRI
Characteristic MRI findings in Wilson's disease are T1 hypointense and T2 hyperintense lesions, most commonly in the basal ganglia, with involvement most frequently in the putamina, followed by the caudate and globus pallidus. Lateral putaminal involvement is a characteristic feature. Thalamic involvement is also common and typically affects the lateral nuclei with relative sparing of the dorsomedial nuclei. Cerebellar involvement may also be seen, particularly in the superior and middle cerebellar peduncles. Involvement of the brain stem, in particular the midbrain, is also common and may be limited to the dorsal or periaqueductal regions (Fig. 47-6). Contrast enhancement with gadolinium is not typical.[18]

One sign considered characteristic of Wilson's disease is the "panda sign" in which T2W images demonstrate hyperintensity in the midbrain superimposed on low signal in the substantia nigra and red nucleus, giving the appearance of a panda face (see Fig. 47-6B). Pontine involvement with features similar to central pontine myelinolysis can also be seen.[14] Atrophy is common; and in addition to deep gray matter involvement, abnormalities in the cerebral white matter may be seen in approximately 25% of patients with Wilson's disease. White matter lesions are usually T2 hyperintense, are asymmetric, and have a frontal lobe predilection.[14] Signal changes have been shown to reverse with treatment, and improvement on follow-up MRI has been shown to correlate with clinical response to treatment.[16]

One report of MR spectroscopy in a patient with Wilson's disease describes the presence of lactate, a decreased NAA/Cr ratio, and a markedly increased ADC in a putaminal lesion.[14]

Patients presenting primarily with hepatic disease may demonstrate T1W hyperintensities in the striatal regions, as can be seen in other forms of chronic liver failure.[14]

DISORDERS RELATED TO ETHANOL ABUSE
Ethanol is the most widely used substance of abuse worldwide. In the United States, the prevalence of alcohol abuse is approximately 6% among males and 2% among females.[3] Long-term alcohol abuse is known to induce selective neuronal damage, but the exact mechanism of injury (direct toxicity vs. toxicity of breakdown products) is unknown. Among the most commonly recognized effects of chronic alcohol abuse seen on neuroimaging are cerebral atrophy and cerebellar atrophy. Cerebellar atrophy has a greater correlation with alcohol use and is typically more marked in the rostral vermis and adjacent superior cerebellar surfaces (Fig. 47-7). In addition, demyelinating lesions in the cerebral white matter, similar to those seen in multiple sclerosis, have been described. The pathogenesis of demyelination in these cases is unknown.[2]

A common finding in patients with alcoholic cirrhosis and other forms of liver failure is symmetric high-signal intensity in the basal ganglia (Fig. 47-8). This finding can be seen in the absence of signs of hepatic encephalopathy and is believed to be caused by the deposition of paramagnetic substances, including copper and manganese, which have bypassed the detoxification system of the liver. Manganese poisoning, which typically

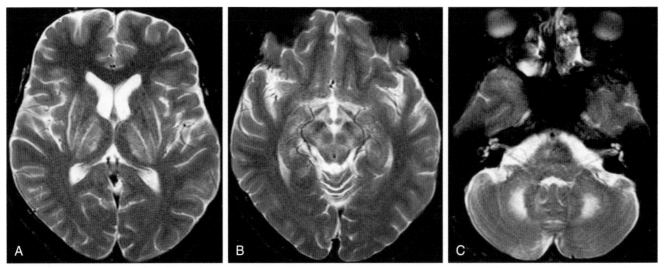

■ **FIGURE 47-6**   Wilson's disease. **A,** Axial T2W MR image through the basal ganglia demonstrates symmetric high signal intensity within the lentiform nuclei and thalamus. Hyperintensity is particularly marked along the lateral margins of the putamina. Note that the dorsomedial portions of the thalami are spared. **B,** Axial T2W MR image through the level of the midbrain demonstrates high signal intensity in the midbrain with superimposed low signal intensity within the red nuclei and substantia nigra, giving the characteristic "panda sign." **C,** Axial image through the level of the middle cerebellar peduncles demonstrates bilateral cerebellar and middle cerebellar peduncle hyperintensities.

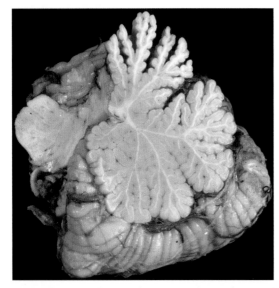

■ **FIGURE 47-7**   Cerebellar atrophy associated with chronic ethanol abuse. Sagittal section through the cerebellar vermis demonstrates atrophy predominantly involving the rostral vermis. *(Courtesy of T. W. Bouldin, University of North Carolina, Chapel Hill, NC.)*

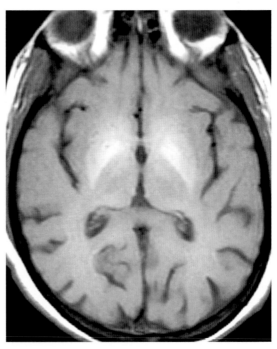

■ **FIGURE 47-8**   Liver failure. Axial unenhanced T1W image demonstrates symmetric hyperintensity in the lentiform nuclei, most pronounced in the globi pallidi.

presents as levodopa-resistant parkinsonism, and prolonged total parenteral nutrition (which is known to increase serum levels of manganese) also demonstrate similar basal ganglia hyperintensities on T1W MRI.[19]

In addition to having direct toxic effects on the brain, ethanol is associated with a number of clinical syndromes affecting the brain, including osmotic myelinolysis (discussed earlier), Wernicke encephalopathy, and Marchiafava-Bignami disease.

Wernicke Encephalopathy

Wernicke encephalopathy is a neurologic disorder that results from chronic thiamine deficiency. The disease is characterized by ocular abnormalities, ataxia, and confusion.[3] Korsakoff psychosis, also caused by chronic thiamine deficiency, is frequently

seen in conjunction with Wernicke encephalopathy and is characterized by more severe cognitive dysfunction and memory loss. The combination of these two entities is known as Wernicke-Korsakoff syndrome.

Epidemiology

The prevalence of Wernicke encephalopathy–specific changes at autopsy may be as high as 2.8% in the general population.[3,20] It is estimated that up to 80% of patients with the syndrome go undiagnosed.[20] Wernicke encephalopathy is predominantly a disease of alcoholics, but any condition that results in thiamine deficiency, including anorexia nervosa, gastrointestinal disorders, protracted parenteral therapy, hyperemesis gravidarum, AIDS, and hematologic malignancies, may cause it. Males are more likely to be affected, owing to the higher prevalence of alcoholism in the male population.

Clinical Presentation

Onset of symptoms may be abrupt or gradual. A classic triad of ocular abnormalities, ataxia, and confusion is seen in approximately 30% of cases.[3] Ocular disturbances may include nystagmus, abducens and conjugate gaze palsies, and ophthalmoplegia. Symptom improvement occurs with thiamine replacement.

If treatment with thiamine is not promptly initiated, the more severe symptoms of Korsakoff psychosis occur. The characteristic feature of Korsakoff psychosis is antegrade and retrograde amnesia, leading to confabulation. Some consider Korsakoff psychosis to be a chronic variant of Wernicke encephalopathy. If not treated, Wernicke encephalopathy has a mortality of up to 20%.[3]

Pathophysiology

Thiamine is involved in a number of cellular processes, including intermediate carbohydrate metabolism, maintenance of membrane integrity and osmotic gradients across cell membranes, redox equilibrium, and nucleic acid synthesis. Depletion of thiamine leads to cerebral lactic acidosis and edema with swelling of astrocytes, oligodendrocytes, myelin fibers, and dendrites. The periventricular regions utilize thiamine-dependent glucose and oxidative metabolism and are therefore susceptible to injury when thiamine deficiency occurs.[3]

Pathology

Lesions that are visible macroscopically as areas of congestion and petechial hemorrhage are seen in the subependymal regions around the third ventricle and aqueduct, the floor of the fourth ventricle, the pulvinar and dorsomedial thalamic nuclei, hypothalami, superior cerebellar vermis, and mammillary bodies (Fig. 47-9). In the later stages these areas will demonstrate brown discoloration and softening.[3,17]

In the acute stages, focal capillary dilatation, congestion, and endothelial swelling will be seen microscopically. Petechial hemorrhages and perivascular macrophages are also commonly seen. In the subacute and later stages, histologic findings include demyelination, fibrillary gliosis, capillary endothelial hyperplasia and proliferation, and petechial hemorrhages. Remyelination can occur if thiamine deficiency is corrected in the early stage. Neurons are relatively spared but may be shrunken. In the thalamus (most commonly the dorsomedial thalamic nuclei) there may be neuronal shrinkage without capillary changes.[3,17]

Imaging
CT

CT is generally not helpful in the diagnosis of acute Wernicke encephalopathy. Rarely, low density may be seen in the periventricular regions of the thalamus.[21]

MRI

MRI in acute Wernicke encephalopathy will demonstrate T2W hyperintensities located in the walls of the third ventricles, the pulvinars and dorsomedial nuclei of the thalami, the periaqueductal gray matter, the pineal regions, the floor of the fourth ventricle, and the mammillary bodies. Enhancement of these regions may be seen, and enhancement of the mammillary bodies is considered pathognomonic for Wernicke encephalopathy (Fig. 47-10). Microhemorrhages may be evident. Diffusion-weighted images may demonstrate hyperintensity with decreased ADCs in the involved regions, reflecting cytotoxic edema.[3]

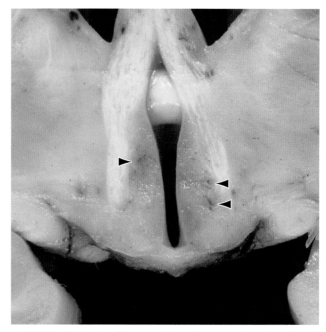

■ **FIGURE 47-9** Wernicke encephalopathy. Coronal section through the third ventricle demonstrates petechial hemorrhages along the walls of the third ventricle within the hypothalami (*arrowheads*). (*Courtesy of T. W. Bouldin, University of North Carolina, Chapel Hill, NC.*)

In patients with chronic Wernicke encephalopathy, signal abnormalities in the aforementioned regions may not be evident but there will be diffuse brain atrophy, particularly involving the fornices and mammillary bodies, with enlargement of the third ventricle.[3]

Specific Procedures

Proton MR spectroscopy performed during the acute stage of Wernicke encephalopathy may demonstrate lactate within the thalami.[20]

Marchiafava-Bignami Disease

Marchiafava-Bignami disease is a rare complication of chronic alcoholism characterized by necrosis of the corpus callosum. First described in 1903, the disease was initially linked to the consumption of massive amounts of an inexpensive red wine produced in the central regions of Italy. The disease is now linked to consumption of any type of alcoholic beverage. This disorder is also referred to as primary degeneration of the corpus callosum.

Epidemiology

Marchiafava-Bignami disease is a very rare condition and occurs primarily in middle-aged chronic alcoholics. The mean age at diagnosis is in the mid 40s. Males are more commonly diagnosed with the disease than females,[22] which is probably attributable to the higher rate of alcoholism among males. Rare cases have been reported in nonalcoholic patients.

Clinical Presentation

The disease may present in two forms. The acute form presents as marked neurologic changes, including seizures and coma, and is often fatal. In the chronic form of the disease, patients present with nonspecific neurologic signs, including cognitive impairment, gait disturbances, limb hypertonia, and dysarthria. The characteristic findings are signs of interhemispheric

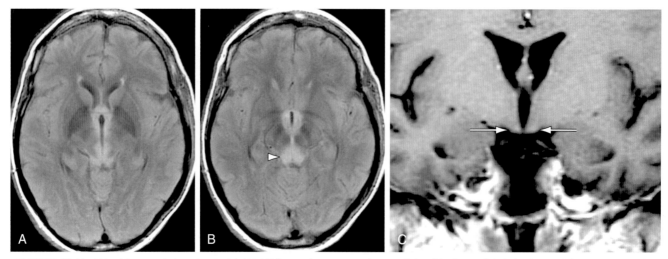

■ **FIGURE 47-10** Wernicke encephalopathy. **A,** Axial FLAIR image demonstrates increased signal in the medial thalami. **B,** Axial FLAIR image inferior to **A** demonstrates increased signal in the periaqueductal gray matter (*arrowhead*). **C,** Coronal gadolinium-enhanced T1W image demonstrates faint enhancement of the mammillary bodies (*arrows*).

disconnection.[2,3] In some cases, Marchiafava-Bignami disease may be difficult to distinguish from Wernicke encephalopathy and the two entities may coexist in the same patient.

Pathophysiology

The exact pathogenesis of tissue damage in Marchiafava-Bignami disease is not known. It is believed that a toxic agent contained in inexpensively produced red wines and malnutrition (particularly deficiencies of certain B vitamins) may play a role in the development of the disease.[3]

Pathology

Grossly, there may be edema, necrosis, and occasional hemorrhage in the corpus callosum. A pattern of necrosis is seen in which the middle layer of the corpus callosum degenerates (layered necrosis), which is a typical finding in the disease.[3] In the chronic phase, there is thinning of the corpus callosum, which may be focal.[2,3]

A well-demarcated band of demyelination is present in the lesions of the corpus callosum, and lesions may extend to involve the neighboring white matter of the centrum semiovale. Other white matter tracts including the anterior commissure and middle cerebellar peduncles may also be affected.[17]

Demyelination is seen, with relative, but incomplete, axonal sparing. There is reactive gliosis and vascular proliferation in the affected areas.[17]

Imaging
CT

The lesions of Marchiafava-Bignami disease may be difficult to see on CT. Larger lesions may be evident as areas of hypodensity in the corpus callosum.[2]

MRI

MRI is extremely useful in establishing the diagnosis of Marchiafava-Bignami disease. The typical findings are the presence of increased signal on T2W and FLAIR images without mass effect in the corpus callosum. Lesions may be seen in the genu, body, or splenium of the corpus callosum, and signal abnormalities may extend to involve the adjacent white matter (Fig. 47-11). In some instances, the entire corpus callosum may be involved, a finding that is associated with a poorer outcome.[22] The corpus callosum lesions are most easily appreciated in the sagittal or

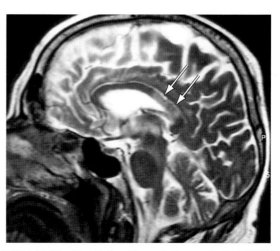

■ **FIGURE 47-11** Marchiafava-Bignami disease. Sagittal T2W image demonstrates increased signal intensity in the posterior body of the corpus callosum (*arrows*). (*From Arbalaez A, Pajon A, Castillo M. Acute Marchiafava-Bignami disease: MR findings in two patients. AJNR Am J Neuroradiol 2003; 24:1955-1957.*)

coronal planes. Similar lesions may be seen in the optic chiasm, anterior commissure, brachium pontis, and cerebral hemispheres. In the acute stages of disease, lesions may enhance peripherally. As time passes, the lesions begin to undergo cystic degeneration and the corpus callosum becomes atrophied.[3]

Specific Procedures

MR spectroscopy may show increased Cho/Cr ratios and lactate in the lesions.[3]

DISORDERS CAUSED BY OTHER EXOGENOUS TOXINS
Carbon Monoxide Poisoning

Carbon monoxide (CO) is a colorless, odorless, and tasteless gas that is the product of incomplete combustion of carbon-containing compounds. After carbon dioxide, CO is the most abundant atmospheric pollutant. Intoxication with carbon monoxide can result in toxicity to the central nervous system and heart similar to global anoxia. CO is also referred to as carbonic oxide, carbon oxide, flue gas, and exhaust gas, and the disorder has been called warehouse workers' headache.

Epidemiology

CO remains the leading cause of lethal inhalations in the United States and Europe. Poisonings may be accidental (often related to burning fuels in an enclosed and poorly ventilated area), but the majority of fatalities due to CO poisoning are suicidal. CO poisonings are more common in winter months.

Clinical Presentation

Symptoms of acute CO poisoning are nonspecific and include headache, nausea, vomiting, seizures, and syncope. Severe intoxications can lead to coma or death.[23] On physical examination, patients may demonstrate cherry-red lips and mucosa, cyanosis, or retinal hemorrhages, although these findings are uncommon.[23] Suspected CO poisoning can be confirmed by measuring blood carboxyhemoglobin levels. Hyperbaric oxygen is the treatment of choice in acute CO poisoning, but it needs to be initiated within 6 hours of exposure for maximum benefit.[24]

Among patients who recover from CO exposures, a delayed encephalopathy characterized by a temporary asymptomatic period of 2 to 3 weeks followed by recurrence of neurologic or neuropsychiatric symptoms may occur.[25]

Pathophysiology

CO binds hemoglobin 200 to 250 times more tightly than does oxygen, which results in formation of carboxyhemoglobin in favor of oxyhemoglobin in the blood. As a result, oxygen-carrying capacity is decreased. Furthermore, carboxyhemoglobin also acts by inhibiting the release of oxygen from remaining oxyhemoglobin molecules. This ultimately results in impaired oxygen delivery and tissue hypoxia.

In addition, CO binds directly to heme moieties of enzymes involved in mitochondrial oxidative phosphorylation and adenosine triphosphate synthesis (including the cytochrome oxidase system), resulting in impaired oxidative metabolism.[26]

The preferential effects on gray matter structures (in particular the globus pallidus) have been hypothesized to be due to the relatively high oxygen demands of gray matter relative to white matter. In addition, it has also been suggested that myocardial effects of CO result in hypotension, ultimately causing hypoperfusion injury to the brain, which preferentially affects the gray matter structures.[26]

Pathology

In acute CO poisoning, the brain is a deep pinkish red (Fig. 47-12). Petechial or larger hemorrhages may be seen, especially in the cerebral white matter. Well-circumscribed areas of softening are seen in the basal ganglia, most commonly in the inner segment of the globus pallidus.[17]

In long-term survivors of CO poisonings, diffuse atrophy and bilateral cystic lesions of the globus pallidus may be seen.[17]

Laminar necrosis and acute ischemic changes are also frequently seen in the cerebral cortex, hippocampi, and Purkinje cell layer of the cerebellum, and white matter lesions are common. White matter lesions consist of foci of demyelination, primarily in a perivascular distribution. Axons may be spared in some cases, and there is an associated glial reaction.[17]

Imaging
CT

The main CT finding in cases of acute CO poisoning is hypodensity in the globi pallidi (Fig. 47-13). Low-density lesions may also be evident in the cerebral and cerebellar white matter.

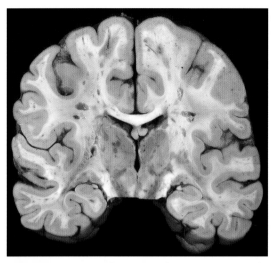

■ **FIGURE 47-12** Acute carbon monoxide poisoning. Coronal section demonstrates the brain to be deep pink and the overlying meninges to be "cherry red," secondary to the presence of carboxyhemoglobin. This patient also had multiple sclerosis (note the myriad lesions in the cerebral white matter and basal ganglia, reflecting multiple sclerosis plaques). *(Courtesy of T. W. Bouldin, University of North Carolina, Chapel Hill, NC.)*

MRI

MRI demonstrates symmetric hyperintensity in the globi pallidi on T2W images with associated hyperintensity on diffusion-weighted images (see Fig. 47-13). Evidence of hemorrhage in the globi pallidi may also be seen. In addition to the globus pallidus, the remainder of the basal ganglia can also be involved; and similar signal alterations can be seen in the cerebral cortex, hippocampi, cerebellum, and cerebral white matter.[24]

Delayed CO encephalopathy is characterized on MRI by confluent symmetric hyperintensity in the periventricular white matter and centrum semiovale on T2W images, which develops 2 to 3 weeks after recovery from acute CO poisoning.[27] Corresponding high signal intensity may also be seen on diffusion-weighted images.

Methanol Poisoning

Methanol (CH_3OH) is a clear, colorless fluid that smells and tastes similar to ethanol. Ingestion of methanol, as with ethanol, results in intoxication, but methanol itself is not highly toxic. Methanol's breakdown products, formaldehyde and formic acid, however, are extremely toxic and may cause a severe metabolic acidosis, blindness, encephalopathy, or even death. Methanol is also known as methyl alcohol, wood alcohol, and carbinol.

Epidemiology

Methanol is widely used in industry as a denaturant additive to ethanol and is also found in a number of commercially available products, including antifreeze, paint removers, windshield washer fluid, and various solvents. Poisonings are usually accidental and rarely the result of suicide attempts. Occasionally, methanol is consumed by alcoholics as an alternative to ethanol. Methanol poisoning has also been reported to occur with consumption of bootlegged alcohol and fraudulently adulterated alcoholic beverages.[28]

Clinical Presentation

After ingestion there is typically a latent period of 12 to 24 hours (sometimes lasting up to 72 hours). Initial CNS symptoms include headache, dizziness, weakness, and malaise. Patients may also complain of nausea, vomiting, and abdominal pain. Subsequently, blurred vision or complete blindness, often irreversible,

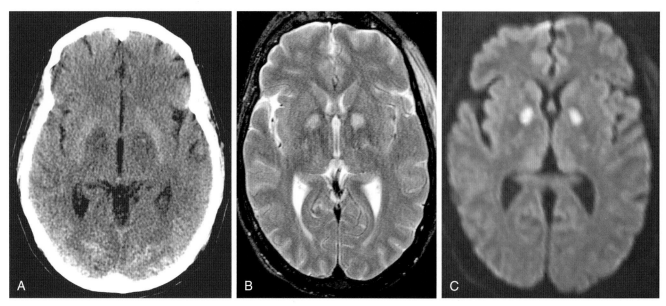

■ **FIGURE 47-13** Carbon monoxide poisoning. **A,** Axial NCCT image through the basal ganglia demonstrates symmetric hypodensity involving the bilateral globi pallidi. **B,** Axial T2W MR image in a different patient demonstrates symmetric hyperintensities in the bilateral globi pallidi. **C,** Corresponding diffusion-weighted image demonstrates hyperintensity in both globi pallidi consistent with restricted diffusion.

will develop, secondary to optic nerve necrosis and demyelination. With severe poisonings, seizure, obtundation, coma, and sometimes even death due to respiratory failure may occur. Diagnosis is based on history and the presence of metabolic acidosis with a high anion and osmolar gap and high serum methanol levels.[29]

Pathophysiology
Methanol is metabolized into formaldehyde in the liver by the enzyme alcohol dehydrogenase. This is subsequently metabolized into formic acid, the metabolite that is likely responsible for much of methanol's toxicity. Metabolism into formaldehyde is a relatively slow process, which likely explains the latent period observed in poisonings. Accumulation of formic acid results in a metabolic acidosis early on. In later stages, lactate may accumulate as a result of inhibition of the respiratory chain. The exact mechanism by which the metabolites of methanol damage tissues is not entirely clear. Tissue hypoxia caused by formate may explain its toxicity to the brain and optic nerves.[30] Optic nerve demyelination caused by formic acid may also explain the blindness associated with methanol intoxication.[29]

Pathology
Acute methanol poisoning causes brain swelling and congestion. Features similar to global hypoxic injury may be evident. Petechial hemorrhages may be seen. Necrosis of the cerebellar cortex and cystic or hemorrhagic necrosis of the putamina are seen.[4]

In survivors, residual foci of cavitation and yellow discoloration are seen. Degeneration of the retinal ganglion cells results in optic nerve atrophy and gliosis.[4]

There is putaminal necrosis and necrosis of all three layers of the cerebellar cortex. In the eyes, retinal ganglion cell destruction is seen; and in the optic nerves there is loss of axons and gliosis.[4,17]

Imaging
CT
CT demonstrates confluent low-attenuation lesions in the superficial white matter and in the putamina. Putaminal hemorrhages are typical.[29]

MRI
MRI of methanol intoxication characteristically demonstrates bilateral hemorrhagic putaminal necrosis, manifested as putaminal hyperintensity on T2W images with heterogeneous foci of low signal consistent with blood products. T1W images demonstrate variable signal. There may also be T2 signal hyperintensity in cerebral white matter (predominantly in the frontal lobes), likely reflecting edema. Subcortical white matter lesions, reflecting areas of necrosis, are also seen. Slight peripheral enhancement of putaminal lesions may be seen after gadolinium administration.[29] In the acute stage of intoxication, the optic nerves may appear normal but MRI performed in the subacute stage of methanol poisoning will demonstrate atrophy of the prechiasmatic optic nerves and optic chiasm.[31]

Ethylene Glycol Poisoning
Ethylene glycol is a clear, odorless, sweet-tasting liquid that is found in common consumer products including antifreeze, hydraulic brake fluids, household cleaners, and cosmetics. Ingestion of ethylene glycol and other glycol-containing compounds (diethylene glycol, propylene glycol) may result in a toxic encephalopathy, congestive heart failure, or renal failure.

Epidemiology
The incidence of ethylene glycol poisoning in the United States exceeds 5000 per year,[32,33] and it is estimated that ethylene glycol ingestion causes 40 to 60 deaths annually.[32,34] The majority of poisonings are accidental, but suicidal ingestions are not uncommon. Poisonings occur most commonly in adults, but nearly a fourth of poisonings occur in individuals younger than the age of 19 and more than 10% occur in children younger than age 6.[32]

Clinical Presentation
Acutely, patients present with symptoms similar to those of ethanol intoxication but without the odor of ethanol. Onset of symptoms is delayed, suggesting some lag between ingestion and conversion of ethylene glycol into its toxic metabolites. Laboratory evaluation may reveal serum electrolyte abnormalities with an osmol gap, and a metabolic acidosis will develop within 12 hours after ingestion. Three clinical stages develop

after ingestion: (1) At 30 minutes to 12 hours, neurologic symptoms including inebriation, nausea and vomiting, cranial nerve abnormalities, coma, and seizures develop; (2) at 12 to 24 hours a cardiorespiratory stage, characterized by blood pressure and heart rate elevations and signs of congestive heart failure, occurs; and (3) at 24 to 72 hours, renal failure may develop. Death may occur if prompt therapy with ethanol and hemodialysis is not initiated.[34]

Pathophysiology

Ethylene glycol is metabolized in the liver by alcohol dehydrogenase into glycoaldehyde, which is subsequently metabolized into a number of toxic metabolites, including glycolic acid, glyoxylic acid, formic acid, and oxalic acid, resulting in a profound metabolic acidosis.[34] The exact mechanism by which these metabolites cause damage to brain tissue remains unclear. Direct metabolite neurotoxicity or deposition of calcium oxalate crystals into tissues may play a role in brain injury.

Pathology

Acute intoxication produces meningeal congestion and cerebral edema, with occasional petechial hemorrhages.[4]

Birefringent calcium oxalate crystals are present in the cerebral vasculature, particularly in the mediobasilar regions of the brain, but crystals are not found in the brain parenchyma. Perivascular infiltrates with polymorphonuclear leukocytes, axonal swelling, and vacuolization with evidence of neuronal loss may be evident.[4,33]

Imaging

CT

CT may demonstrate diffuse cerebral edema early on. Hypodensities involving the basal ganglia, thalamus, midbrain, and pons may develop over the course of the next few days (Fig. 47-14). Hypodensity in the deep white matter may also be seen. Hypodensities may normalize by as early as 5 days after ingestion.[33] Hemorrhage in the globi pallidi has also been reported.[35]

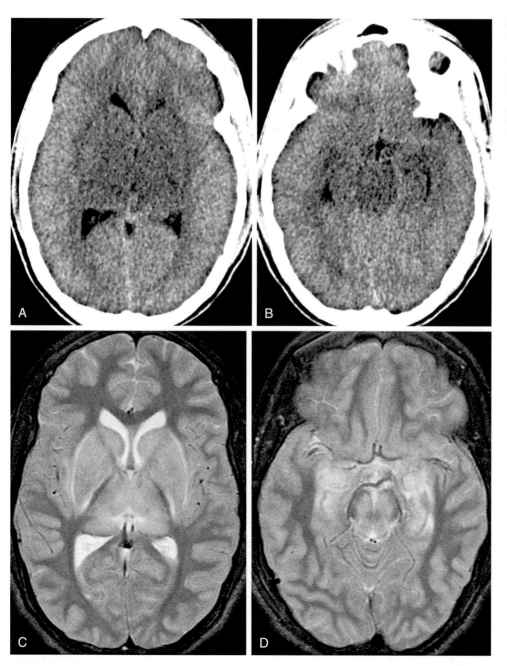

■ **FIGURE 47-14** Ethylene glycol poisoning. **A** and **B**, Axial NCCT images through the basal ganglia (**A**) and pons (**B**) demonstrate swelling and hypodensity throughout the basal ganglia, thalami, mesial temporal lobes, and pons. **C** and **D**, Corresponding T2W MR images demonstrate high signal intensity in these regions.

MRI

MRI may demonstrate T2 hyperintensity in the basal ganglia, thalamus, and brain stem (see Fig. 47-14). Necrosis may be seen in the putamen, and globus pallidus hemorrhage has also been reported.[35]

Cocaine Poisoning

Cocaine is an alkaloid compound derived from the coca plant with stimulant, local anesthetic, and vasoconstricting properties. Its pronounced psychotropic effects make it a popular drug of abuse. The effects of cocaine are due to a competitive blockade of dopamine and norepinephrine reuptake. Repeated use of cocaine produces persistent adaptation within the mesocortico-limbic system, leading to behavioral sensitization and addiction. Toxic effects of cocaine include stroke, intracranial hemorrhage, and seizures.[36]

Epidemiology

It is estimated that 25 to 30 million Americans have used cocaine, with 5 to 6 million using it regularly. Cocaine abuse is more prevalent among the urban poor, and young adults are the most common users.[37] In stroke patients younger than the age of 35, drug abuse is the most commonly identified predisposing condition. In a study of 422 cases of ischemic stroke in patients aged 15 to 44, 4.7% had drug abuse listed as the probable cause of stroke.[36] Neurologic complications can be seen with any of the usual forms of cocaine use, including snorting, smoking (crack cocaine), and intravenous use.

Clinical Presentation

Systemic effects of cocaine include dose-dependent increases in heart rate and blood pressure, which contribute, at least in part, to the neurologic effects of cocaine use. Among the most commonly reported neurologic complications of cocaine abuse are intracranial hemorrhages and ischemic strokes. Hemorrhages occur more frequently than ischemic strokes in cocaine users and may present as either subarachnoid hemorrhages or intraparenchymal hemorrhages.[36]

Cocaine can also provoke seizures and is known to exacerbate preexisting seizure disorders by reducing seizure thresholds. Cocaine may induce seizures by direct means, because seizures occur at high blood concentrations of cocaine, suggesting direct toxicity. Cocaine-induced seizures are resistant to most of the clinically used antiepileptic medications and can be life threatening.[36]

In addition to its neurologic effects, cocaine has been shown to be arrhythmogenic and may cause cardiomyopathy, which can contribute to sudden cardiac arrest and death.

Pathophysiology

Cerebral hemorrhages in abusers of cocaine may be due either to primary intracerebral hemorrhage or to bleeding from ruptured aneurysms and arteriovenous malformations. Increases in heart rate and blood pressure as a result of the sympathomimetic effects of cocaine are believed to increase the risk of hemorrhage from preexisting vascular anomalies, and some have suggested that cocaine users are at increased risk of aneurysm formation.[36]

Primary intracerebral hemorrhages in cocaine users are believed to be a result of cocaine's ability to shift the upper limit of cerebrovascular autoregulation toward lower blood pressure levels in hypertensive patients.[36]

Ischemic strokes are believed to be due to either cocaine-induced vasculitis or cerebral vasoconstriction. True vasculitis associated with cocaine abuse is rare, and the causal relationship between cocaine abuse and cerebral vasculitis is controversial. Cocaine also has been shown to promote platelet aggregation in vitro and may therefore promote thrombus formation, a property of the drug that may also contribute to increased stroke risk in cocaine abusers.[36]

Pathology

Histology in cases of cocaine-associated vasculitis demonstrates a non-necrotizing leukocytoclastic angiitis, with inflammatory infiltrates consisting of neutrophils and mononuclear cells.[38]

Imaging

Ultrasonography

Transcranial Doppler ultrasonography can demonstrate increased cerebrovascular resistance in cocaine abusers, which seems to persist over a month after use.[36]

CT

CT in patients with a history of cocaine abuse may demonstrate evidence of cortical infarcts and lacunar infarcts in the cerebral white matter, thalamus, midbrain, basal ganglia, and brain stem. Brain atrophy is common. In acute cases, patients may present with intraparenchymal cerebral hemorrhages or subarachnoid hemorrhage.[36,37]

MRI

Similar to the findings on CT, MRI may demonstrate evidence of cortical and lacunar infarcts. Acute infarcts will show restricted diffusion on diffusion-weighted imaging. White matter signal changes similar to those seen in patients with long-standing hypertension are typically seen.

Special Procedures

Conventional cerebral angiography may demonstrate beading of the intracranial arteries with multifocal areas of vasoconstriction, representing either vasculitis or multifocal spasm.[39] In cases of acute hemorrhage an underlying aneurysm or arteriovenous malformation should be sought.

MR angiography may demonstrate beading with multifocal stenoses of the intracranial vessels, compatible with vasculitis or vasoconstriction. Longstanding lifetime cocaine use appears to be associated with a greater likelihood of vasoconstriction.[39]

Perfusion-weighted imaging may demonstrate diminished regional cerebral blood volume (rCBV), reflecting vasoconstriction, after cocaine use.[40]

Poisoning with Toluene and Other Organic Solvents

Toluene is a highly volatile aromatic hydrocarbon used as a solvent in a number of products, including paint, lacquer, glue, ink, and cleaning fluid. It is a major component of spray paint, whose fumes may be inhaled to induce a euphoric state, and is therefore a popular substance of abuse. In addition to toluene there are a number of chemical compounds, including gasoline, propane, butane, alkyl halides, benzene, and nitrites, that may be inhaled as fumes or aerosols. Toluene is among the most commonly abused inhalants and is perhaps the most damaging to the CNS. Chronic abuse of toluene leads to an irreversible leukoencephalopathy, the most important feature of which is dementia.[41] Other names for toluene include methylbenzene and phenylmethane.

Epidemiology

The prevalence of inhalant abuse is quite high among younger children, and initiation of inhalant abuse tends to occur at a slightly earlier age than is seen with other substances of abuse. Up to 10% to 15% of young people in the United States report having used inhalants in some surveys, and the lifetime prevalence of inhalant abuse has been estimated to be 18%.[41] Inhalants are popular among adolescents for a number of reasons: they are legal, inexpensive, and easy to obtain because they are readily found in homes, offices, and stores. Boys are slightly more likely than girls to abuse inhalants. Use of organic solvents tends to decrease with increasing age.[42] Although adults may use inhalants less frequently than adolescents, inhalant abuse is not rare in the adult population. Adult intoxications may also be seen through occupational exposures.

Clinical Presentation

In the acute setting, low-level toluene exposure may manifest as fatigue, headache, paresthesias, and diminished reflexes. At higher levels of exposure, patients may become confused, euphoric, or hallucinatory. Obtundation or seizures can also occur. Chronic inhalant abuse will present as a leukoencephalopathy manifesting as cognitive deficits (which may progress to dementia), insomnia, anosmia, tremors, and tinnitus. Neurologic examination may reveal ataxia, tremors, hyperreflexia, and rigidity.[41,43]

Pathophysiology

Toluene appears to damage brain myelin, but the mechanism of injury remains unknown. Like other lipophilic substances, toluene is preferentially distributed in lipid-rich areas in the brain, which may explain why myelin is particularly susceptible to damage. It has been suggested that free radical–induced lipid peroxidation may be caused by toluene or one of its metabolites.

Pathology

Autopsy of chronic organic solvent abusers demonstrates cerebral atrophy. The brain may display patchy white matter discoloration, especially in the cerebellar, periventricular, and deep cerebral white matter, although this may be a subtle finding.[41,44] Thinning of the corpus callosum may also be noted.[41]

Microscopically, diffuse myelin pallor is seen in the cerebral and cerebellar white matter. Cerebellar involvement tends to predominate, particularly in the vermis. Axons are generally spared. In the cerebral hemispheres, the periventricular white matter is most affected and there is relative preservation of the subcortical U fibers. Reactive gliosis may also be evident. One of the earliest findings may be the presence of astrocytosis with perivascular PAS-positive macrophages.

Imaging
CT

CT findings in chronic toluene users include atrophy of the cerebrum, cerebellum, and brain stem. White matter changes, which are readily apparent on MRI, may not be evident on CT.[41]

MRI

The acute encephalopathy associated with toluene intoxication is usually reversible and is not associated with imaging changes.[41] Brain MRI in cases of chronic toluene inhalation demonstrates cerebral and cerebellar atrophy, white matter lesions, loss of gray matter/white matter differentiation in the cortex, thinning of the corpus callosum, and T1 and T2 hypointensity of the basal ganglia and thalami. White matter lesions may be multifocal or diffuse and may be seen in the cerebral (predominantly periventricular) and cerebellar white matter, internal capsule, brain stem, and upper cervical cord. The lesions are hyperintense on T2W images, probably reflecting gliosis, and are associated with a duration of abuse longer than 4 years.[43] In addition to the hypointensities in the basal ganglia and thalami, the red nuclei and substantia nigra may also demonstrate decreased signal. The basal ganglia hypointensity seen in chronic toluene abusers may be related to iron deposition or the partitioning of toluene into the lipids of cell membranes in the brain.

Lead Poisoning

Lead is a heavy metal that is toxic to multiple organ systems, including the CNS and peripheral nervous system, bones, blood, gastrointestinal tract, and kidneys. Symptoms typically occur with serum levels greater than 40 µg/dL (normal < 10 µg/dL), but adverse health effects have been documented at lower serum lead levels. Lead may produce an encephalopathy, which is almost invariably associated with levels greater than 100 µg/dL.[45] Alternate names for lead poisoning are lead encephalopathy, plumbism, saturnism, and painter's colic.

Epidemiology

Exposures to lead in the developed world have decreased dramatically with the elimination of lead-based paints, but poisonings continue to be seen in areas with older housing and in underdeveloped countries.[46] Children are much more commonly affected by lead poisoning for a number of reasons. Young children are prone to hand-to-mouth behaviors, which increase intake in environments with high lead exposures. Fractional gastrointestinal absorption of lead is also greater in infants and young children compared with adults, and absorption is also increased in the presence of certain nutritional deficiencies.[47]

Adult exposures tend to be occupational and are most frequently related to remodeling of old homes. Inhalation of lead-containing dusts is the main route of exposure in these cases.

Exposure through drinking water is also occasionally seen and is related to the use of lead-containing pipes in older homes. Lead may also be found in glazes, traditional medicines, and cosmetics.

Clinical Presentation

Encephalopathy due to lead poisoning can present as acute or chronic forms. The acute encephalopathy presents as headache, vomiting, ataxia, convulsions, and stupor. Severe poisonings can cause seizures, paralysis, coma, or even death.[46] Chronic lead poisoning can present as difficulties with memory and concentration, lethargy, irritability, headache, depression, dizziness, syncope, tremor, peripheral neuropathy, ataxia, and behavioral changes.[45,47] In adults, peripheral neuropathies (predominantly motor) tend to predominate over CNS effects, which is the opposite of what is observed in children. Furthermore, the peripheral nervous effects tend to reverse after cessation of exposure, whereas CNS effects do not.[47]

Lead poisoning also affects the gastrointestinal system, particularly in children, and may cause decreased appetite, nausea, vomiting, constipation, and abdominal pain. Low-level lead exposure has also been associated with hypertension in adults. Renal effects of acute lead poisoning include reversible deficits in proximal tubular reabsorption, prerenal azotemia, and interstitial fibrosis.[48] A microcytic anemia with accompanying basophilic stippling may also occur.[49]

In pregnant women, lead exposure has been associated with adverse outcomes of pregnancy, including an increased risk for spontaneous abortion, low birth weight, and postnatal developmental delay.[48]

Pathophysiology

Many of the neurotoxic effects of lead are a result of its ability to substitute for calcium in cellular processes. Cytotoxic effects include the induction of apoptosis, excitotoxicity, inhibition of mitochondrial respiration, inhibition of neurotransmission, and damage to endothelial and glial cells.[46] The adult brain is more resistant to the toxic effects of lead, potentially because of the ability of the mature brain to sequester lead away from its mitochondrial site of action within neurons.[45]

Pathology

In acute encephalopathy, the brain is typically swollen and congested. Petechial hemorrhages may occasionally be seen.[17] In chronic lead poisoning, extensive tissue destruction with cavitation is seen.[45]

Microscopically, edema, gliosis, hemorrhage, neuronal loss, and perivascular proteinaceous exudate can be seen.[45] Calcifications are observed in the walls of small and medium-sized vessels and perivascular spaces and may be seen in tissue from the cerebellum, cerebral cortex, gray matter/white matter junction, white matter, basal ganglia, and thalami. It has been postulated that the vascular calcifications observed represent the result of dystrophic calcification of incompletely cleared proteinaceous exudates. Calcifications are most pronounced in cerebellum, where they are concentrated in the granular layer, corpus medullare, and dentate nuclei.[50]

Imaging
CT

On CT, there are bilateral, symmetric hypodensities in the thalami, putamina, claustrum, and insula.[51] In chronic lead poisoning, intracranial calcifications, sometimes described as "curvilinear and speck-like,"[50] may be observed, involving the cerebellum, subcortical regions, thalami, and basal ganglia.[45]

MRI

On MRI, abnormalities may be observed in the thalami, putamina, claustrum, and insula.[51] Other authors have described lesions involving the gray matter and subcortical white matter of the cerebral hemispheres, particularly in the bilateral parasagittal occipital lobes. Callosal and brain stem lesions have also been described. The lesions are of low signal intensity on T1W images and high signal intensity on T2W images and do not enhance. Diffusion-weighted images are normal. Cerebellar edema and swelling may be observed that can occasionally mimic the appearance of a cerebellar mass. After chelation therapy, lesions may resolve on follow-up imaging.[45]

Mercury Poisoning

Mercury (Hg) is a heavy metal that exists in elemental, mercurous (divalent), and organic (methylated) forms and is toxic to humans. The elemental form of mercury, still used in industry and as a component of dental amalgam, is a volatile liquid at room temperature and is absorbed primarily through inhalation of its vapor. Organic mercury is found in two main forms: methyl mercury (CH_3Hg^+), used in the past as fungicide, and ethyl mercury ($CH_3CH_2Hg^+$), which is the active ingredient of thimerosal and was widely used until recently as a preservative in vaccines.

Epidemiology

Overt cases of mercury poisoning, both elemental and organic, are now rare. Exposure to elemental mercury is primarily occupational. Cases of chronic mercury vapor exposure were common in the hat-making industry in the 18th and 19th centuries, and mercury is still used in the medical field in thermometers and blood pressure cuffs and commercially in batteries, switches, and fluorescent lights. The greatest exposure of the general population to mercury vapor is from dental amalgams.[52]

Most modern exposures to organic mercury are through the ingestion of contaminated fish. The entity was first reported in 1956 when there was an epidemic traced back to the ingestion of fish from Minamata Bay in Japan, which had been contaminated with methyl mercury produced by a nearby factory. Organic mercury poisoning is therefore also referred to as Minamata disease.

Clinical Presentation

Elemental mercury poisoning is characterized by the triad of intentional tremor, gingivitis, and erethism (bizarre behavior characterized by excessive irritability). The kidney (nephrotic syndrome) and peripheral nervous system (neuropathy) are also target organs for the toxic effects of mercury vapor.[52]

Classic symptoms of organic mercury poisoning include perioral and extremity paresthesias, circumferential visual field constriction, and ataxia. Patients may also develop impairment of hearing and speech, muscle weakness, tremor, and abnormal eye movements. There is typically a latent period lasting weeks to months between mercury exposure and symptom onset.[52,53]

Pathophysiology

Mercury vapor is highly diffusible and lipid soluble, diffuses into all tissues in the body, and easily crosses the blood-brain barrier. The mercuric ion, Hg^{2+}, produced by oxidation of the mercury vapor within cells, is believed to be the chief toxic species in mercury vapor inhalation. Little is known about the distribution of inorganic mercury in the human brain.

Methylmercury is transported across the blood-brain barrier as a cysteine-bound complex. In the brain, methylmercury is partially broken down into inorganic mercury, but it is believed that it is the intact methylmercury species that is primarily responsible for brain damage in Minamata disease, as suggested by the differences in clinical presentation between inorganic and organic mercury poisoning. The exact mechanism of damage caused by methylmercury on the cellular level has not been well established but may be related to methylmercury's inhibitory effects on GABA receptors located on the outer cell surface of neurons. Effects on GABA may also explain the differential sensitivity of granule versus Purkinje cells in the cerebellum, because it has been observed that GABA receptors are more sensitive to blockade by methylmercury in granule cells than they are in Purkinje cells.[52] Apoptosis probably also plays a role in neuronal death induced by methylmercury, since ex vivo studies have shown that microtubule disruption occurs in cultured cells treated with methylmercury.[53]

The selective vulnerability of certain areas of the brain in methylmercury poisoning has also been attributed to differences in the repair capacities of neuronal cells. Observations in rat models have demonstrated impaired protein synthesis in cell populations that are damaged with methylmercury poisoning, with normal or even increased protein synthesis in spared cell populations.[52]

Pathology

Autopsy studies performed in patients with acute organic mercury poisoning demonstrate swelling of the brain and leptomeninges.

In acute methylmercury poisoning there is edema in the perivascular regions of the cerebral hemispheres with associated perivascular demyelination. Neurons may show swelling, acute shrinkage with cytoplasmic eosinophilia, and occasional ischemic changes. Areas predominantly affected include the calcarine region, the precentral and postcentral gyri, and the temporal transverse gyrus. Late findings in individuals who survive acute poisonings include secondary degeneration of the pyramidal tracts, internal sagittal stratum, and central cerebral white matter. Cerebellar changes are seen in deeper portions of the cerebellar hemispheres and include loss of granule cells with preservation of Purkinje cells.[53]

Imaging
CT

CT findings in patients with Minamata disease include atrophy of the calcarine cortex and of the cerebellar vermis and/or hemispheres.[54]

MRI

MRI in patients with chronic organic mercury poisoning demonstrates atrophy primarily involving the cerebellar vermis and hemispheres, calcarine cortex, and postcentral cortex. There will be significant dilatation of the calcarine fissure. These involved areas may demonstrate low signal intensity on T1W images and high signal intensity on T2W images.[55]

MEDICATION-INDUCED TOXIC DISORDERS

In addition to the just-discussed exogenous toxins there are a number of commonly used medications that are known to be toxic to the brain. These include, but are not limited to, immunosuppressant agents (cyclosporine and tacrolimus); chemotherapeutic agents (methotrexate, L-asparaginase, cisplatin, vincristine); antimicrobial agents (amphotericin B); and anticonvulsant agents (phenytoin and vigabatrin). In addition, there are several medications that are known to cause peripheral neuropathies with axonal degeneration. These include amiodarone, chloroquine, disulfiram, isoniazid, and nitrofurantoin.[17] Several central neurotoxic medications with well-described neuroimaging manifestations are discussed here.

Cyclosporine Toxicity

Cyclosporine is an immunosuppressive agent used in transplant patients to prevent and to control transplant rejection and graft-versus-host disease. The drug inhibits interleukin production by T cells by blocking the activity of calcineurin, which is a phosphatase that is essential in transcriptional activation of genes encoding interleukin-2, interleukin-4, and CD40L.[56] Cyclosporine is known to cause a syndrome similar to the posterior reversible encephalopathy syndrome.

Epidemiology

Cyclosporine neurotoxicity occurs in up to 60% of cyclosporine-treated patients[56] and may affect adult or pediatric patients.

Clinical Presentation

Symptoms of cyclosporine neurotoxicity typically manifest during the first month of treatment but may occur within hours or several months after the initiation of the drug.[57] Acute encephalopathy is associated with increased serum concentrations outside the normal therapeutic range but may also be seen with normal therapeutic serum concentrations. Patients may present with tremor, aphasia, ataxia, stroke-like episodes, paresthesias, mental status changes, seizures, or cortical blindness. Neurotoxic symptoms are usually reversible with withdrawal of the drug or a reduction in dose. In addition to acute toxicity, chronic neurotoxicity has been reported in patients on long-term treatment with blood cyclosporine concentrations in therapeutic target ranges. Chronic neurotoxicity tends to be longer lasting and persists beyond discontinuation of the agent.[56]

A virtually identical neurotoxic syndrome is also seen in patients taking the immunosuppressive agent tacrolimus (FK-506), which also acts by inhibiting the activity of calcineurin. Cisplatin has also been reported to produce abnormalities similar to those of the posterior reversible encephalopathy syndrome.[58] Early diagnosis of cyclosporine toxicity is essential because symptoms are reversible early on with prompt drug withdrawal; if diagnosed too late, however, neurotoxicity can become irreversible and fatal.[56]

Pathophysiology

The mechanisms of cyclosporine-induced neurotoxicity are poorly understood. Posited theories include physiologic effects of cyclosporine, including hypertension, vasoconstriction, or inhibition of mitochondrial function; toxicity caused by cyclosporine breakdown products; metabolic alterations associated with cyclosporine therapy (including hypomagnesemia and hypocholesterolemia); and direct vascular injury. Whether any one or a combination of these factors plays a role in the clinical and imaging features observed remains unclear. It has been suggested that the characteristic posterior location of lesions seen on imaging may result from regional differences in the distribution of adrenergic receptors, which are relatively sparse in the vertebrobasilar circulation. The lack of sympathetic innervation results in inability of these regions to initiate protective vasoconstriction in response to elevations in blood pressure. Ultimately, there may be loss of normal capillary integrity resulting in breakdown of the blood-brain barrier and leakage of fluid into the extracellular compartment appearing as vasogenic edema.[57] Occasional ischemic changes seen both pathologically and on imaging may be related to cyclosporine-induced vasospasm or inhibition of mitochondrial oxidative phosphorylation.[56]

The primary pathologic finding is vasogenic edema in the deep and subcortical white matter, most prominent in the occipital poles.[17,59] Areas of cortical ischemia, neuronal necrosis, and petechial hemorrhage may also be seen and are most pronounced in the arterial border zones and at the depths of the sulci.[59]

Imaging
CT

CT is generally less sensitive than MRI in demonstrating the lesions of cyclosporine neurotoxicity. The typical findings on CT are gray and white matter hypodensities, which are predominantly located in the posterior aspects of the cerebral hemispheres.[56]

MRI

On MRI, the typical changes observed in both cyclosporine and tacrolimus toxicity are similar to those seen in the posterior reversible encephalopathy syndrome associated with hypertensive encephalopathy and eclampsia. T2W images demonstrate areas of increased signal intensity involving the cortex and subcortical white matter (reflecting vasogenic edema), with lesions located predominantly in four major regions in the cerebral hemispheres: the occipital poles, the parietal region, the fronto-parietal junction, and the inferior temporo-occipital junction (Fig. 47-15).[59] Contrast enhancement is rarely seen and will appear as cortical enhancement with a stippled appearance in the regions of T2W signal abnormality.[59] Lesions typically resolve after cessation of cyclosporine therapy.

Occasionally, lesions will demonstrate restricted diffusion on diffusion-weighted imaging with ADC maps, suggesting the presence of cytotoxic edema and irreversible injury. In general, the presence of cytotoxic edema suggests tissue ischemia and portends a worse prognosis.[57]

Methotrexate Toxicity

Methotrexate is a cycle-specific chemotherapeutic agent that is used in the treatment of a number of neoplasms, including acute lymphocytic leukemia, primary CNS lymphoma, breast cancer, gastric cancer, and head and neck cancers. It is also used in the treatment of several autoimmune diseases, including rheumatoid arthritis, Crohn's disease, ankylosing spondylitis, and psoriasis, and in obstetrical treatment of ectopic pregnancies and gestational trophoblastic tumors. The drug inhibits cell replication by preventing folate conversion to tetrahydrofolic acid by the enzyme dihydrofolate reductase (DHFR), a necessary step in DNA synthesis. Methotrexate can be administered orally, intravenously, and intrathecally and readily crosses the blood-brain barrier and the CSF-brain barrier, making it useful in the treatment and prevention of CNS disease.[60]

Methotrexate has been implicated as a cause of neurotoxicity in patients undergoing chemotherapy, characterized by damage to the cerebral white matter. Another name for this disorder is amethopterin toxicity.

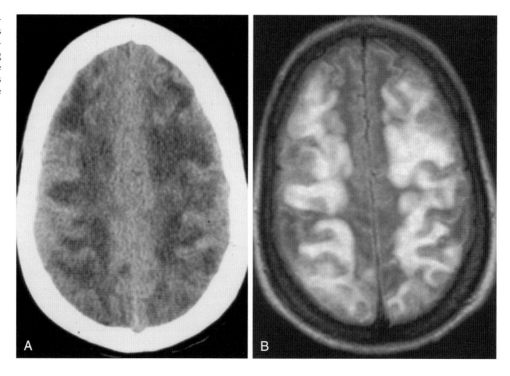

■ **FIGURE 47-15** Cyclosporine toxicity. **A,** NCCT image demonstrates hypodensity throughout the subcortical white matter. **B,** Corresponding T2W MR image demonstrates diffuse white matter hyperintensity as well as swelling and hyperintensity of the overlying cortical gray matter.

Epidemiology

The incidence of methotrexate neurotoxicity in children treated for acute lymphocytic leukemia ranges from 3% to 18% and varies with the dose and route of administration (intravenous vs. intrathecal), patient age (young age increases risk), and associated cranial irradiation.[60,61] In one study of patients being treated for primary CNS lymphoma, the incidence of neurotoxicity among those receiving methotrexate-based chemotherapies was 30%. Of note, the incidence of neurotoxicity was much higher in patients also receiving whole-brain irradiation compared with those receiving chemotherapy alone (46% vs. 4.5%, respectively) and was higher among patients older than 60.[62]

Clinical Presentation

Methotrexate can cause immediate, acute/subacute, or delayed neurotoxicity. Immediate methotrexate neurotoxicity presents within the first hours of high-dose intravenous or intrathecal administration as aseptic meningitis, transverse myelopathy, or stroke-like symptoms.[63]

Acute/subacute neurotoxicity occurs anywhere from several days to several weeks after methotrexate administration and usually results in seizures or stroke-like symptoms (including aphasia, weakness, sensory deficits, and ataxia). Symptoms are typically transient and resolve by 1 week.[60,61]

The delayed form appears several months to years after therapy. It is characterized by decline in cognitive functioning and is primarily described in association with combined treatment protocols of whole-brain irradiation and methotrexate-based chemotherapy. Median time from initiation of methotrexate therapy to symptom onset is approximately 15 months.[62] No effective therapy exists for the delayed form of the disease.[64]

Pathophysiology

Methotrexate may affect the brain via several metabolic pathways. Inhibition of DHFR inhibits DNA synthesis, which may impair the synthesis of numerous types of macromolecules, including myelin proteins and lipids. In addition, inhibition of DHFR leads to deficiency of S-adenosylmethionine, which is important in the maintenance of the myelin sheath. DHFR inhibition also leads to accumulation of homocysteine, which is believed to be directly toxic to vascular endothelium. Finally, methotrexate can cause elevated adenosine levels in the cerebrospinal fluid that may interfere with neurotransmitter synthesis.[63] The end result of one or more of these processes appears to be demyelination or microinfarction.

In the delayed form of the disease, damage is believed to be related to a necrotizing angiitis that may lead to ischemia, infarction, and necrosis, with eventual development of calcification. These changes are seen most frequently with combined modality therapy but can be seen in patients treated exclusively with methotrexate.[65]

Histologically, lesions demonstrate extensive necrosis or demyelination with surrounding edema and astrocytosis. Axons in affected areas are swollen but not destroyed. Inflammatory changes are not usually seen, and vascular changes are inconstant.[17]

Imaging
CT

CT of the brain in cases of methotrexate neurotoxicity may appear normal but commonly demonstrates areas of white matter hypodensity (Fig. 47-16). In cases of delayed neurotoxicity, CT may demonstrate areas of white matter hypodensity with associated subcortical calcifications.[65]

MRI

MRI abnormalities are not uncommon in otherwise asymptomatic patients receiving methotrexate therapy. Findings in asymptomatic patients consist of high-intensity areas in the periventricular white matter, which are seen in approximately 10% of patients on methotrexate. These changes may resolve several months after completion of therapy.[63]

In addition to the periventricular white matter changes commonly seen in asymptomatic patients, MRI performed in patients with acute neurotoxicity may demonstrate areas of T2 hyperintensity in the cerebral cortex, subcortical white matter,

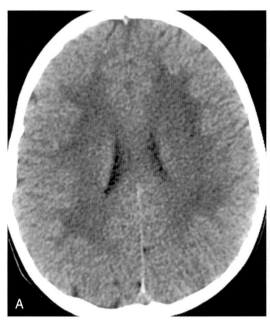 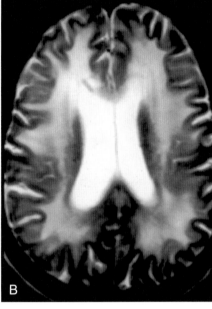

■ FIGURE 47-16 Chronic methotrexate toxicity. **A,** Axial NCCT image demonstrates diffuse confluent hypodensity involving the periventricular and central white matter. **B,** Axial T2W MR image in a different patient demonstrates confluent white matter hyperintensity and cerebral atrophy.

cerebellum, and thalamus (see Fig. 47-16). Restricted diffusion may be seen within these lesions.[60,61] Enhancement after gadolinium administration has been reported but is not generally present. Resolution of these abnormalities is typically seen after approximately 3 months.[63]

In the delayed form of methotrexate-associated neurotoxicity, MRI demonstrates diffuse white matter hyperintensities involving both the periventricular and subcortical white matter. Calcifications, when present, will demonstrate low signal intensity on the T2W images and high signal intensity on T1W images. Enhancement after gadolinium administration may be seen in the areas of calcification.[65]

Phenytoin Toxicity

Phenytoin is one of the most commonly used antiepileptic drugs.[66] Long-term phenytoin use is associated with cerebellar damage manifesting as cerebellar atrophy. Phenytoin is also known as fosphenytoin and is sold under the trade name of Dilantin.

Epidemiology

An estimated 873,000 prescriptions for phenytoin were issued during office visits in 2001, and it is estimated that as many as 25,000 cases of phenytoin intoxication present annually to emergency departments or result in hospitalizations in the United States annually.[67]

Clinical Presentation

Most adverse effects of phenytoin are associated with long-term ingestion, but acute intoxications do occur. Long-term side effects seen with chronic phenytoin use include gingival hyperplasia, skull thickening, and other dermatologic and hematologic complications. Chronic neurotoxicity can manifest as ataxia, nystagmus, slurred speech, and a sensory peripheral neuropathy.[68]

Pathophysiology

Phenytoin is believed to induce axonal atrophy and loss of Purkinje cells in the cerebellar cortex.[68] It is not entirely clear whether the drug alone is responsible for cerebellar damage or whether chronic seizures also play a role; however, reports of

cerebellar atrophy developing in patients on phenytoin for indications other than epilepsy suggest that the drug can cause cerebellar injury by itself.[66] In addition, it has been suggested that folate deficiency induced by inhibition of intestinal uptake by phenytoin may play a role in cerebellar atrophy.[69]

Loss of Purkinje cells and gliosis in the Bergmann cell layer of the cerebellum are the typical features of chronic phenytoin use.[17]

Imaging
CT

CT will demonstrate atrophy of the vermis, cerebellar hemispheres, and pons. Occasionally, cerebellar calcifications may be seen.

MRI

Atrophy involving the vermis, cerebellar hemispheres, and pons is the hallmark of chronic phenytoin toxicity (Fig. 47-17). Lesions within the splenium of the corpus callosum have also been reported in patients taking phenytoin for seizures. These lesions are hyperintense on T2W images and do not enhance.[69] Occasionally, the lesions in the corpus callosum may demonstrate reversible restricted diffusion on diffusion-weighted images.

ANALYSIS

In most cases of toxic brain disease, the offending toxin will be known or suggested by the patient's history or clinical setting. Rarely, the cause of encephalopathy will not be apparent clinically and neuroimaging may be helpful in pointing to a specific diagnosis. In certain instances, neuroimaging findings may be virtually pathognomonic (e.g., the "eye of the tiger" sign in NBIA) or at least allow one to narrow the list of differential considerations significantly.

Perhaps the most practical approach to image interpretation may be to classify diseases based on whether they primarily involve gray matter, white matter, or both (Table 47-1). Processes involving primarily gray matter often affect the deep gray matter structures over the cortex, and these include carbon monoxide poisoning, NBIA, and hyperglycemic HCHB. Further distinction can occasionally be made based on the specific gray

■ **FIGURE 47-17** Chronic phenytoin toxicity. Sagittal T1W (**A**) and coronal T2W (**B**) MR images demonstrate diffuse cerebellar atrophy.

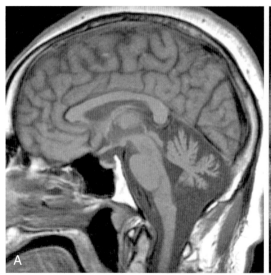
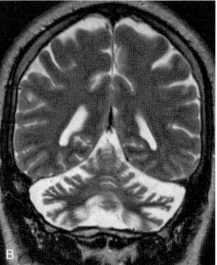

TABLE 47-1. Imaging Features Helpful in the Differential Diagnosis of Adult Toxic and Metabolic Brain Disease

Primarily Deep Gray Matter Involvement
Primarily globus pallidus involvement
  Carbon monoxide
  Cyanide
  Liver failure
  Neurodegeneration with brain iron accumulation
  Manganese
Ethylene glycol
Hyperglycemic hemichorea-hemiballismus

Primarily White Matter Involvement
Diffuse involvement
  Carbon monoxide (postanoxic leukoencephalopathy)
  Methotrexate (chronic)
Focal involvement
  Marchiafava-Bignami disease (primarily corpus callosum)
  Methotrexate (acute)

Gray and White Matter Involvement
Cocaine
Lead
Methanol (putaminal necrosis)
Osmotic myelinolysis
Toluene
Wilson's disease (primarily striatum)
Posterior reversible encephalopathy syndrome–like lesions
  Cisplatin
  Cyclosporine
  Tacrolimus (FK-506)

Cerebellar Calcifications
Fahr's syndrome
Hypoparathyroidism
Hyperparathyroidism
Hypothyroidism
Lead

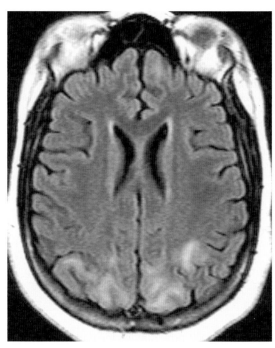

■ **FIGURE 47-18** Tacrolimus toxicity. Axial FLAIR image demonstrates high signal intensity in the cortex and subcortical white matter of the bilateral occipital lobes.

matter structures affected. For example, CO, cyanide, and NBIA primarily affect the globi pallidi, whereas ethylene glycol (diffuse basal ganglia and thalamic involvement) and hyperglycemic HCHB (neostriatal involvement) do not demonstrate a specific predilection for the globi pallidi.

Diseases affecting primarily white matter can be subdivided based on whether involvement is diffuse or whether lesions tend to be more multifocal (see Table 47-1). In many cases, both gray and white matter involvement are seen in a specific disease or toxic exposure. Often, the distribution of lesions is nonspecific, but in certain instances, such as in cases of cyclosporine and tacrolimus toxicity (Fig. 47-18), the pattern of brain involvement is helpful in suggesting a toxic etiology. Furthermore, when deep gray matter involvement predominates over cortical involvement, differential diagnosis can be narrowed based on the specific nuclei involved. For instance, Wilson's disease usually demonstrates primarily striatal involvement whereas methanol preferentially affects the putamina. Sample reports are presented in Boxes 47-1 to 47-3.

BOX 47-1 Sample Report: MRI of Wernicke Encephalopathy

PATIENT HISTORY

The patient is a 55-year-old man with a history of chronic alcohol abuse who presents with acute onset of mental status changes, ataxia, and ocular gaze palsies.

COMPARISON STUDY

An unenhanced head CT was done earlier the same day.

TECHNIQUE

Multiplanar T1W, T2W, TW2 FLAIR, and diffusion-weighted MR images of the brain were performed before and after the intravenous administration of 0.1 mmol/kg of gadobenate dimeglumine (Multihance).

FINDINGS

There is diffuse cerebral and cerebellar atrophy, most marked in the rostral vermis. T2W and FLAIR images demonstrate symmetric increased signal intensity along the walls of the third ventricles and the floor of the fourth ventricle, in the periaqueductal gray matter, in the pulvinars, and in the mammillary bodies (see Fig. 47-10). Gadolinium-enhanced T1W images show the enhancement of mammillary bodies. No signal abnormalities are seen on diffusion-weighted imaging.

IMPRESSION

The constellation of findings is compatible with Wernicke encephalopathy.

BOX 47-2 Sample Report: MRI of Carbon Monoxide Poisoning

PATIENT HISTORY

The patient is a 65-year-old man admitted for apparent suicide attempt by exhaust inhalation. By report the patient was found unresponsive and cyanotic within his garage with his car engine running.

COMPARISON STUDY

An unenhanced head CT was done earlier the same day.

TECHNIQUE

Multiplanar T1W, T2W, TW2 FLAIR, and diffusion-weighted MR images of the brain were performed before and after the intravenous administration of 0.1 mmol/kg of gadobenate dimeglumine (MultiHance).

FINDINGS

The globi pallidi, cerebellar hemispheres, and hippocampi demonstrate symmetric increased signal intensity on T2W and TW2 FLAIR images and decreased signal intensity on T1W images. Diffusion-weighted images demonstrate high signal intensity in these areas with decreased apparent diffusion coefficient (ADC) (see Fig. 47-13). No abnormal enhancement is seen after gadolinium administration.

IMPRESSION

Findings are compatible with anoxic brain injury due to carbon monoxide poisoning.

BOX 47-3 Sample Report: MRI of Cyclosporine Toxicity

PATIENT HISTORY

The patient is a 35-year-old man now 1 month status post renal transplant and currently on cyclosporine. He presented acutely to the emergency department with seizures and mental status changes.

COMPARISON STUDY

An unenhanced head CT was done earlier the same day.

TECHNIQUE

Multiplanar T1W, T2W, TW2 FLAIR, and diffusion-weighted MR images of the brain were performed before and after the intravenous administration of 0.1 mmol/kg of gadobenate dimeglumine (MultiHance).

FINDINGS

T2W and TW2 FLAIR images demonstrate increased signal intensity within the cortical gray matter and subcortical white matter of the bilateral occipital and parietal lobes and in the frontoparietal junctions (see Fig. 47-15). Several of these areas demonstrate slightly increased signal intensity on the diffusion-weighted images with reduced ADC, suggesting cytotoxic edema. After gadolinium administration, there is faint stippled cortical enhancement in the regions of signal abnormality.

IMPRESSION

Given the patient's history of cyclosporine use, the distribution of signal abnormalities within the posterior cerebral hemispheres is most suggestive of acute cyclosporine toxicity.

KEY POINTS: DIFFERENTIAL DIAGNOSIS

- Entities causing predominantly deep gray matter involvement include carbon monoxide, cyanide, ethylene glycol, NBIA, and hyperglycemic HCHB.
- Entities causing predominantly white matter involvement include methotrexate and Marchiafava-Bignami disease.
- Entities presenting with gray and white matter involvement include osmotic myelinolysis, Wilson's disease, and cocaine, lead, methanol, toluene, cyclosporine, and tacrolimus toxicity.
- Osmotic myelinolysis often involves the pons.

SUGGESTED READINGS

Arbalaez A, Pajon A, Castillo M. Acute Marchiafava-Bignami disease: MR findings in two patients. AJNR Am J Neuroradiol 2003; 24:1955-1957.

Clarkson TW, Magos L, Myers GJ. The toxicology of mercury—current exposures and clinical manifestations. N Engl J Med 2003; 349:1731-1737.

Gijtenbeek JMM, van den Bent MJ, Vecht CJ. Cyclosporine neurotoxicity: a review. J Neurol 1999; 246:339-346.

Hantson P, Duprez T. The value of morphologic neuroimaging after acute exposure to toxic substances. Toxicol Rev 2005; 25:87-98.

Lang CJ. The use of neuroimaging techniques for clinical detection of neurotoxicity: a review. Neurotoxicology 2000; 21:847-855.

Valk J, van der Knapp MS. Toxic encephalopathy. AJNR Am J Neuroradiol 1992; 13:747-760.

REFERENCES

1. Fraser CL, Arieff AI. Epidemiology, pathophysiology, and management of hyponatremic encephalopathy. Am J Med 1997; 102:67-77.

2. Scroop R, Sage MR, Voyvodic F, et al. Radiographic imaging procedures in the diagnosis of the major central neuropathological consequences of alcohol abuse. Australas Radiol 2002; 46:146-153.

3. Spampinato MV, Castillo M, Rojas R, et al. Magnetic resonance findings in substance abuse: alcohol and alcoholism and syndromes associated with alcohol abuse. Top Magn Reson Imaging 2005; 16:223-230.

4. Ellison D, Love S, Chimelli L, et al. Neuropathology: A Reference Text of CNS Pathology. London, Mosby, 2000.

5. Guo Y, Hu JH, Lin W, et al. Central pontine myelinolysis after liver transplantation: MR diffusion, spectroscopy and perfusion findings. Magn Reson Imaging 2006; 24:1395-1398.

6. Nath J, Jambhekar K, Rao C, et al. Radiological and pathological changes in hemiballism-hemichorea with striatal hyperintensity. J Magn Reson Imaging 2006; 23:564-568.

7. Lai PH, Tien RD, Chang MH, et al. Chorea-ballismus with nonketotic hyperglycemia in primary diabetes mellitus. AJNR Am J Neuroradiol 1996; 17:1057-1064.

8. Shan De, Ho DMT, Chang C, et al. Hemichorea-hemiballism: an explanation for MR signal changes. AJNR Am J Neuroradiol 1998; 19:863-870.

9. Hayflick SJ, Westaway SK, Levinson B, et al. Genetic, clinical, and radiographic delineation of Hallervorden-Spatz syndrome. N Engl J Med 2003; 348:33-40.

10. Hayflick SJ, Hartman M, Coryell J, et al. Brain MRI in neurodegeneration with brain iron accumulation with and without *PANK2* mutations. AJNR Am J Neuroradiol 2006; 27:1230-1233.

11. Boltshauser E, Lang W, Janzer R, et al. Computed tomography in Hallervorden-Spatz disease. Neuropediatrics 1987; 18:81-83.

12. Savoiardo M, Halliday WC, Nardocci N, et al. Hallervorden-Spatz disease: MR and pathologic findings. AJNR Am J Neuroradiol 1993; 14:155-162.

13. Sener RN. Pantothenate kinase-associated neurodegeneration: MR imaging, proton MR spectroscopy, and diffusion MR imaging findings. AJNR Am J Neuroradiol 2003; 24:1690-1693.

14. Sinha S, Taly AB, Ravishankar S, et al. Wilson's disease: cranial MRI observations and clinical correlation. Neuroradiology 2006; 48:613-621.

15. Ala A, Walker AP, Ashkan K, et al. Wilson's disease. Lancet 2007; 369:397-408.

16. Kim TJ, Kim IO, Kim WS, et al. MR imaging of the brain in Wilson disease of childhood: findings before and after treatment with clinical correlation. AJNR Am J Neuroradiol 2006; 27:1373-1378.

17. Esiri M, Perl D. Oppenheimer's Diagnostic Neuropathology: A Practical Manual. London, Hodder Arnold, 2006.

18. van Wassenaer-van Hall HN, van den Heuvel AG, Algra A, et al. Wilson disease: findings at MR imaging and CT of the brain with clinical correlation. Radiology 1996; 198:531-536.

19. de Bie RMA, Gladstone RM, Strafella AP, et al. Manganese-induced parkinsonism associated with methcathinone (Ephedrone) abuse. Arch Neurol 2007; 64:886-889.

20. Rugilo CA, Uribe Roca MC, Zurru MC, et al. Proton MR spectroscopy in Wernicke encephalopathy. AJNR Am J Neuroradiol 2003; 24: 952-955.

21. Antunez E, Estruch R, Cardenal C, et al. Usefulness of CT and MR imaging in the diagnosis of acute Wernicke's encephalopathy. AJR Am J Roentgenol 1998; 171:1131-1137.

22. Heinrich A, Runge U, Khaw AV. Clinicoradiologic subtypes of Marchiafava-Bignami disease. J Neurol 2004; 251:1050-1059.

23. Ely EW, Moorehead B, Haponik EF. Warehouse workers' headache: emergency evaluation and management of 30 patients with carbon monoxide poisoning. Am J Med 1995; 98:145-155.

24. O'Donnell P, Buxton PJ, Pitkin A, et al. The magnetic resonance imaging appearance of the brain in acute carbon monoxide poisoning. Clin Radiol 2000; 55:273-280.

25. Choi IS. Delayed neurologic sequelae in carbon monoxide intoxication. Arch Neurol 1983; 40:422-435.

26. Jaffe FA. Pathogenicity of carbon monoxide. Am J Forensic Med Pathol 1997; 18:406-410.

27. Chang KH, Han MH, Kim HS, et al. Delayed encephalopathy after acute carbon monoxide intoxication: MR imaging features and distribution of cerebral white matter lesions. Radiology 1992; 184:117-122.

28. Kuteifan K, Oesterle H, Tajahmady T, et al. Necrosis and haemorrhage of the putamen in methanol poisoning shown on MRI. Neuroradiology 1998; 40:158-160.

29. Blanco M, Casado R, Vazquez F, et al. CT and MR imaging findings in methanol intoxication. AJNR Am J Neuroradiol 2006; 27:452-454.

30. Jacobsen D, McMartin KE. Methanol and ethylene glycol poisonings: mechanism of toxicity, clinical course, diagnosis and treatment. Med Toxicol 1986; 1:309-334.

31. Hsu HH, Chen CY, Chen FH, et al. Optic atrophy and cerebral infarcts caused by methanol intoxication: MRI. Neuroradiology 1997; 39:192-194.

32. Watson WA, Litovitz TL, Rodgers GC, et al. 2004 annual report of the American Association of Poison Control Centers Toxic Exposure Surveillance System. Am J Emerg Med 2005; 23:589-666.

33. Morgan BW, Ford MD, Follmer R. Ethylene glycol ingestion resulting in brainstem and midbrain dysfunction. J Toxicol Clin Toxicol 2000; 38:445-451.

34. Armstrong EJ, Engelhart DA, Jenkins AJ, et al. Homicidal ethylene glycol intoxication—a report of a case. Am J Forensic Med Pathol 2006; 27:151-155.

35. Caparros-Lefebvre D, Policard J, Sengler C, et al. Bipallidal haemorrhage after ethylene glycol intoxication. Neuroradiology 2005; 47:105-107.

36. Neiman J, Haapaniemi HM, Hillbom M. Neurological complications of drug abuse: pathophysiological mechanisms. Eur J Neurol 2000; 7:595-606.

37. McEvoy AW, Kitchen ND, Thomas DGT. Intracerebral hemorrhage and drug abuse in young adults. Br J Neurosurg 2000; 14:449-454.

38. Merkel PA, Koroshetz WJ, Irizarry MC, et al. Cocaine-associated cerebral vasculitis. Semin Arthritis Rheum 1995; 25:172-183.

39. Kaufman MJ, Levin JM, Ross MH, et al. Cocaine-induced cerebral vasoconstriction detected in humans with magnetic resonance angiography. JAMA 1998; 279:376-380.

40. Kaufman MJ, Levin JM, Maas LC, et al. Cocaine decreases relative cerebral blood volume in humans: a dynamic susceptibility contrast magnetic resonance imaging study. Psychopharmacology 1998; 138:76-81.

41. Filley CM, Halliday W, Kleinschmidt-DeMasters BK. The effects of toluene on the central nervous system. J Neuropathol Exp Neurol 2004; 63:1-12.

42. Kurtzman TL, Otsuka KN, Wahl RA. Inhalant abuse by adolescents. J Adolesc Health 2001; 28:170-180.

43. Aydin K, Sencer S, Demir T, et al. Cranial MR findings in chronic toluene abuse by inhalation. AJNR Am J Neuroradiol 2002; 23:1173-1179.

44. Rosenberg NL, Kleinschmidt-DeMasters BK, Davis KA, et al. Toluene abuse causes diffuse central nervous system white matter changes. Ann Neurol 1988; 23:611-614.

45. Atre AL, Shide PR, Shinde SN, et al. Pre- and post-treatment MR imaging findings in lead encephalopathy. AJNR Am J Neuroradiol 2006; 27:902-903.

46. Lidsky TI, Schneider JS. Lead neurotoxicity in children: basic mechanisms and clinical correlates. Brain 2003; 126:5-19.

47. Bellinger DC. Lead. Pediatrics 2004; 113:1016-1022.

48. Kosnett MJ, Wedeen RP, Rothenberg SJ, et al. Recommendations for medical management of adult lead exposure. Environ Health Perspect 2007; 115:463-471.

49. Brodkin E, Copes R, Mattman A, et al. Lead and mercury exposures: interpretation and action. Can Med Assoc J 2007; 176:59-63.

50. Teo JG, Goh KY, Ahuja A, et al. Intracranial vascular calcifications, glioblastoma multiforme, and lead poisoning. AJNR Am J Neuroradiol 1997; 18:576-579.

51. Tüzün M, Tüzün D, Salan A, et al. Lead encephalopathy: CT and MR findings. J Comput Assist Tomogr 2002; 26:479-481.

52. Clarkson TW, Magos L. The toxicology of mercury and its chemical compounds. Crit Rev Toxicol 2006; 36:609-662.

53. Eto K. Minamata disease. Neuropathology 2000; 20(Suppl):S14-S19.

54. Matsumoto SC, Okajima T, Inayoshi S, et al. Minamata disease demonstrated by computed tomography. Neuroradiology 1988; 30:42-46.

55. Korogi Y, Takahashi M, Shinzato J, et al. MR findings in seven patients with organic mercury poisoning (Minamata disease). AJNR Am J Neuroradiol 1994; 15:1575-1578.

56. Serkova NJ, Christians U, Benet LZ. Biochemical mechanisms of cyclosporine neurotoxicity. Mol Interv 2004; 4:97-107.

57. Coley SC, Porter DA, Calamante F, et al. Quantitative MR diffusion mapping and cyclosporine-induced neurotoxicity. AJNR Am J Neuroradiol 1999; 20:1507-1510.

58. Ito Y, Arahata Y, Goto Y, et al. Cisplatin neurotoxicity presenting as reversible posterior leukoencephalopathy syndrome. AJNR Am J Neuroradiol 1998; 19:415-417.

59. Bartynski WS, Zeigler Z, Spearman MP, et al. Etiology of cortical and white matter lesions in cyclosporin-A and FK-506 neurotoxicity. AJNR Am J Neuroradiol 2001; 22:1901-1914.

60. Rollins N, Winick N, Bash R, et al. Acute methotrexate neurotoxicity: findings on diffusion-weighted imaging and correlation with clinical outcome. AJNR Am J Neuroradiol 2004; 25: 1688-1695.

61. Fisher MJ, Khademian ZP, Simon EM, et al. Diffusion-weighted MR imaging of early methotrexate-related neurotoxicity in children. AJNR Am J Neuroradiol 2005; 26:1686-1689.

62. Gavrilovic IT, Hormigo A, Yahalom J, et al. Long-term follow-up of high-dose methotrexate-based therapy with and without whole brain irradiation for newly diagnosed primary CNS lymphoma. J Clin Oncol 2006; 24:4570-4574.

63. Ziereisen F, Dan B, Azzi N, et al. Reversible acute methotrexate leukoencephalopathy: atypical brain MR imaging features. Pediatr Radiol 2006; 36:205-212.

64. Batchelor T, Loeffler JS. Primary CNS lymphoma. J Clin Oncol 2006; 24:1281-1288.

65. Lovblad KO, Kelkar P, Ozdoba C, et al. Pure methotrexate encephalopathy presenting with seizures: CT and MR features. Pediatr Radiol 1998; 28:86-91.

66. Tan EK, Chan LL, Auchus AP. Phenytoin cerebellopathy without epilepsy. Acta Neurol Scand 2001; 104:61-62.

67. Glick TH, Workman TP, Gaufberg SV. Preventing phenytoin intoxication: safer use of a familiar anticonvulsant. J Fam Pract 2004; 53:197-202.

68. Verity MA. Toxic disorders. In Graham DI, Lantos PL (eds). Greenfield's Neuropathology, 6th ed. London, Arnold, 1997, p 788.

69. Kim SS, Chang KH, Kim ST, et al. Focal lesion in the splenium of the corpus callosum in epileptic patients: antiepileptic drug toxicity? AJNR Am J Neuroradiol 1999; 20:125-129.

Hydrocephalus

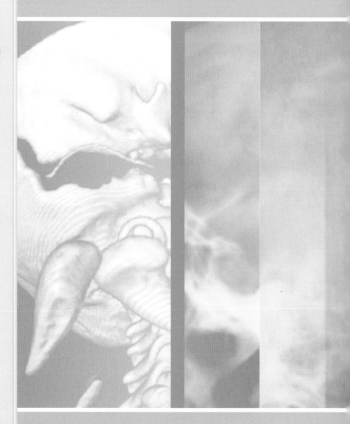

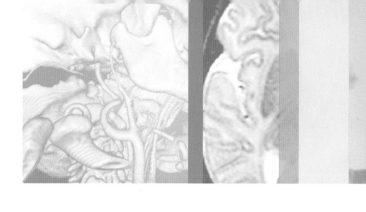

48

Classical Concepts of Hydrocephalus

Ramón E. Figueroa

Hydrocephalus ("water on the brain") is a condition in which there is excessive accumulation of cerebrospinal fluid (CSF) in the spaces of the intracranial compartment (cerebral ventricles, cisterns, and subarachnoid spaces). This accumulation of CSF results in distention of the cerebral ventricles and secondary increased intracranial pressure (ICP), which, if unresolved, leads to cerebral injury. Hydrocephalus results from an imbalance between the production of CSF, its circulation through the ventricles and subarachnoid spaces, and its reabsorption at distant sites, such as the arachnoid granulations of the dural venous sinuses.

The causes and effects of hydrocephalus in adults differ significantly from those seen with hydrocephalus in the pediatric age group. Pediatric hydrocephalus may be congenital (causes present at birth) or acquired (caused by internal or external factors after birth). Adult-onset hydrocephalus is typically an acquired condition caused by mechanisms that impair CSF flow through the ventricles or subarachnoid spaces, or that decrease CSF absorption. Adult-onset hydrocephalus may result from traumatic, vascular, inflammatory or neoplastic disease, with secondary increase in the ventricular volume and pressure. Adult-onset hydrocephalus is classified by the level at which the drainage of CSF is impaired: from the level of CSF production by the choroid plexus through its reabsorption into the dural sinuses, or, even the return of the venous blood to the right cardiac atrium.

There are two major subdivisions of adult hydrocephalus, which are generally designated "obstructive" and "communicating" hydrocephalus. *Obstructive hydrocephalus* is defined by obstruction of CSF flow at or proximal to the fourth ventricular foramina of Luschka and of Magendie. *Communicating hydrocephalus* is defined by obstruction of CSF flow outside the ventricular system, typically at the basal cisterns, convexity subarachnoid spaces, and/or the arachnoid granulations. Thrombosis of dural sinuses or other conditions producing dural sinus hypertension (arteriovenous fistulae, superior vena cava syndrome) can also cause communicating hydrocephalus.

According to the National Institute of Neurological Disorders and Stroke (NINDS), there is no current national registry or database for adult-onset hydrocephalus, resulting in a paucity of incidence and prevalence data in the medical literature.[1]

For a full discussion of the various forms of hydrocephalus in adults, please visit www.expertconsult.com.

CHAPTER 49

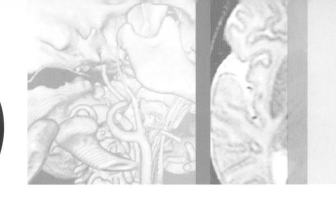

Emerging Concepts of Cerebrospinal Fluid Physiology and Communicating Hydrocephalus

Thomas P. Naidich

New data are modifying our classic concepts of cerebrospinal fluid (CSF) production, flow, and reabsorption.[1,2] Consequently, they are calling into question our present understanding of the cause and nature of hydrocephalus.[3-5] Classically, hydrocephalus has been considered to result from an imbalance in the formation, flow, or absorption of CSF with abnormally increased CSF volume and/or pressure. Increasingly, hydrocephalus is now believed to result from disordered pressure/volume relationships (compliance) within the intracranial-intraspinal compartments.[3-5] The information presented here builds on that in Chapter 48 to present some emerging concepts of CSF physiology and hydrocephalus. In some cases, the data appear conflicting. Nonetheless, it is hoped that a broader understanding of normal and deranged CSF physiology may lead to improved diagnosis and treatment of hydrocephalus in the future.

The following definitions are provided for a better understanding of the concepts discussed:

Cerebrospinal fluid is the fluid within the ventricles and cisterns of the intracranial and intraspinal spaces.

Interstitial fluid (ISF) is the extracellular fluid of the brain derived from the blood, the metabolic activity of the brain, and recycled CSF.

Compliance (C) is the ratio of the volume change (ΔV) to the pressure change (ΔP), given as $C = \Delta V / \Delta P$. In a highly compliant system, a large increase in volume will cause only a small change in pressure. In a rigid, less compliant system, a small increase in volume may lead to a large increase in pressure.

Hydrocephalus is a condition in which there is an increase in the total volume of CSF and in which that increased volume of CSF is associated with elevated intracranial pressure, presently, intermittently, or in the past (Fig. 49-1).

For a full discussion of current concepts of hydrocephalus and CSF physiology, please visit www.expertconsult.com.

Epilepsy

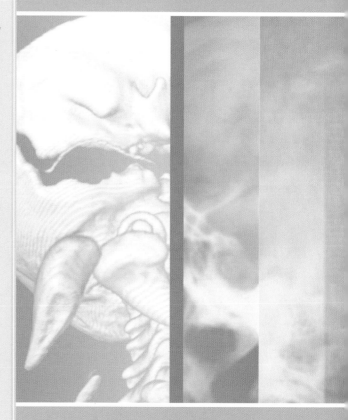

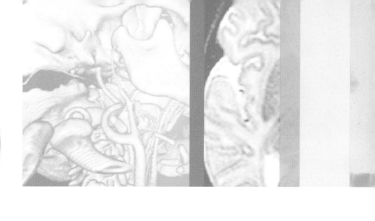

CHAPTER

50

Epilepsy

Puneet S. Pawha, John L. Ritter, and Richard A. Bronen

Seizures develop when cortical neurons undergo abnormal, excessive, hypersynchronous electrical discharges due to impaired regulation of neuronal excitation and inhibition. Epilepsy is a condition characterized by recurrent spontaneous seizures. It is a common disorder, present in 0.4% to 1% of the population.[1]

Seizures can be categorized as either partial or generalized. Partial seizures originate from a localized region of the brain. Generalized seizures involve both cerebral hemispheres simultaneously. Partial seizures are subdivided into complex partial seizures, with loss of consciousness, and simple partial seizures, without loss of consciousness. Partial seizures may generalize secondarily by spread from one area to another.

Seizure classification has therapeutic and prognostic implications for the care of the epilepsy patient. Some seizure classifications are clinical, like that used by the International League against Epilepsy (ILAE). These include findings on electroencephalography (EEG), patient age, and clinical seizure type to help categorize seizures. Other classifications are anatomic. The focus in this chapter is to address the anatomic substrates of seizures and epilepsy that are identifiable by neuroimaging. Clinical features and classifications are not discussed in detail.

Generalized epilepsy is usually well controlled by medication. Epilepsy associated with partial complex seizures is often medically intractable and may require surgery to achieve seizure control. Overall, 15% to 30% of adult patients with partial seizures are not well controlled with antiepileptic medication.[1] A major goal of epilepsy imaging is to identify an epileptogenic substrate or lesion that is amenable to surgery or other directed treatment. A second goal is to identify any syndromic cause of epilepsy.

MRI is the main modality of choice for evaluating patients with epilepsy, owing to its high soft tissue contrast, multiplanar imaging capability, lack of ionizing radiation, and higher sensitivity compared with CT. CT is useful in the initial evaluation of seizures, especially in the setting of trauma, acute focal neurologic signs, or fever. Published guidelines recommend that nonemergent MRI should be performed in most patients with epilepsy. Patients with febrile seizures and those with primary idiopathic generalized epilepsy do not need imaging unless there are complicating factors.

The sensitivity of MRI for detecting seizure foci is dependent on the population investigated. The sensitivity is relatively low for those with new onset of seizures but high for patients with medically refractory partial epilepsy. In one series of 300 consecutive patients with new-onset seizure, an anatomic substrate was identified by MRI in 14% (38/263).[2] In that study, all of the patients with an imaging abnormality had partial seizures. Patients with primary generalized seizures did not have imaging abnormalities. In another series of children with a new diagnosis of epilepsy, 13% (62/388) had a structural abnormality demonstrated by MRI.[3] Conversely, in patients with medically intractable epilepsy, the sensitivity of MRI has been reported as 82% to 86%.[4] In a series of 117 patients with refractory partial seizures who had surgery, the sensitivity for detecting anatomic substrates of seizure was 32% (35/109) for CT and 95% (104/109) for MRI.[4]

In surgical candidates, MRI is essential for identifying a structural lesion, localizing it, and demonstrating its relationship to eloquent regions of the brain. The MRI findings must be correlated with electrophysiologic and clinical data to avoid false-positive localization of the epileptogenic substrate.[5] When MRI findings and noninvasive electrophysiologic data are concordant, surgery may be undertaken without resorting to invasive electroencephalography. MRI also helps to prognosticate the potential for successful surgical control of seizures by identifying and characterizing the seizure substrate.[6] Postoperative MRI helps to localize electrode placement, identify surgical complications, and elucidate causes for treatment failure, such as recurrent or residual structural lesion.

EVALUATING THE PATIENT WITH SEIZURES
Current Concepts and Definitions

Complex partial seizures may arise from any portion of the cerebral cortex. The specific clinical manifestations depend on the region involved. By definition, the *epileptogenic region* or *zone* is the portion of tissue that, when removed, will result in a seizure-free state. Imaging workup is directed toward identifying the epileptogenic region. No single test perfectly defines the epileptogenic region, so clinical assessment, neuroimaging, EEG, and neuropsychological tests are used in conjunction to infer the localization and extent of the epileptogenic region. When all tests are concordant, there is a high likelihood that the epileptogenic region or a portion of it has been identified. CT, MRI, and pathologic evaluation can also identify the *epileptogenic lesion*, the anatomic substrate thought to be responsible for the epilepsy. The epileptogenic zone encompasses at least part of the epileptogenic lesion.

A few clinical terms are commonly used in epilepsy. Seizure *semiology* is the study and description of seizure signs and symptoms. An *aura* is a subjective or sensory simple partial seizure that may precede or herald a more severe complex partial or generalized seizure. An *automatism* is an intraictal repetitive motor activity often occurring during cognitive impairment, such as lip smacking. After a seizure, patients may experience transitory functional neurologic abnormalities referred to as *postictal phenomena*. A postictal unilateral neurologic deficit is referred to as a *lateralizing phenomenon*. A postictal phenomenon that is nonfocal and involves impaired cognition, psychosis, or amnesia is referred to as a *nonlateralizing* postictal phenomenon. *Postictal hemiparesis* is a common lateralizing sign called Todd's paralysis.

Clinical Correlates of Seizure Foci

Temporal lobe seizures can begin in the temporal lobe or generalize to the temporal lobe after originating elsewhere. The temporal lobe is the most common origin for complex partial seizures, both motor and sensory. A common temporal lobe motor seizure is dystonia of the contralateral upper extremity. Commonly reported temporal auras include visceral sensations, déjà vu, gustatory sensations, olfactory sensations, and staring. Automatisms may be present, often related to oroalimentary function, speech, facial expressions, or laughing. Postictal aphasia or amnesia can be seen.

Occipital seizures are characterized by visual and ocular symptoms, often with visual auras. Parietal seizures may include visual hallucinations, body movement sensations, and vertigo, but most do not have an identifiable aura. Frontal lobe seizures are poorly understood and have a wide variety of clinical presentations. They include unusual behavioral, sensory, autonomic, and hallucinatory patterns. Frontal motor seizures often result from involvement of the primary motor cortex. As opposed to temporal lobe seizures, which often have a long duration, frontal seizures may last only a few seconds. This brief period may be too short to permit adequate ictal SPECT injections (see later).

Study Protocols

Many factors determine which imaging protocols are "appropriate" or "optimal" for evaluating seizure disorders. These include patient age, the specific features of the population being imaged, and the imaging characteristics of the epileptogenic substrates expected at that age in that population. The imaging characteristics of normal brain change with age, so the optimal imaging protocol must also change with age. This particularly applies to the incompletely myelinated infant brain. The likely causes of epilepsy also vary with age, so imaging protocols must be optimized for the lesions most likely at each age (Table 50-1).

AGE DIFFERENCES

Infants

In infants younger than 18 months of age, myelination is still incomplete. The water content of the brain is higher, so fluid-attenuated inversion recovery (FLAIR) sequences are less useful for detecting areas of abnormal T2-weighted (T2W) signal. The interface between gray and white matter is usually indistinct on spoiled gradient-recalled-echo (SPGR) sequences, especially when the patient is younger than 6 months of age, so inversion recovery and fast spin-echo (FSE)/T2W sequences may be needed to optimize gray matter/white matter differentiation in these patients (Fig. 50-1). In neonates, infection, stroke and malformations of cortical development (MCD) are primary considerations, so attention is directed toward display of the cortex. Mesial temporal sclerosis is not a diagnostic consideration in this age group, so coronal oblique imaging through the hippocampus is not employed routinely. Diffusion-weighted imaging (DWI) and

TABLE 50-1. Causes of Epilepsy by Age at Seizure Onset

Cause	Age at Seizure Onset (yr)				
	0-2	3-20	21-40	41-60	>60
Metabolic abnormalities or inborn error of metabolism	X				
Cerebral anoxia	X				
Infection	X	X			
Congenital or developmental malformations	X	X			
Phacomatoses	X	X			
Hippocampal sclerosis		X			
Primary generalized seizures		X			
Vascular malformation		X	X		
Post-traumatic epilepsy		X	X	X	X
Tumor			X	X	X
Stroke				X	X

administration of gadolinium (Gd) may be useful in these patients, particularly in patients with new-onset seizures.

Mature Patients

In patients older than age 50 years, stroke and neoplasm are more common causes of new-onset seizure. Therefore, DWI is required to detect areas of ischemia; a contrast agent should be administered routinely to help detect neoplasms (Fig. 50-2). The frequency of hippocampal sclerosis is low in this population, so sequences tailored for evaluation of the hippocampus are not used routinely.

Patients 18 Months to 50 Years of Age

The patients most likely to be evaluated for medically refractory partial epilepsy are those between the ages of 18 months and 50 years. This population will have the highest yield for detection of structural pathology by MRI, including hippocampal sclerosis. These patients have completed myelination and can undergo detailed evaluation for subtle epileptogenic abnormalities. In this age group, special protocols are needed to increase the likelihood of identifying hippocampal sclerosis and cortical malformations.[7] Administration of a contrast agent is not needed routinely unless there is specific concern for tumor, vascular malformation, or infection. One notable exception to this is in the patient with hemiatrophy, where use of contrast enhancement may reveal the Sturge-Weber malformation.

TECHNIQUES

Evaluation of the Hippocampus

Slice Inclination

The coronal plane oriented perpendicular to the long axis of the hippocampus is ideal for assessing signal change within the hippocampus, abnormal hippocampal architecture, and hippocampal atrophy (Fig. 50-3).

Signal Intensity

FLAIR pulse sequences are most sensitive for detecting signal abnormalities of the hippocampus. However, it is best to use a combination of coronal FSE/T2W sequences and coronal FLAIR for assessing the hippocampus, because the normal hippocampus may appear slightly hyperintense as compared with neocortical gray matter on FLAIR sequences.[8]

Hippocampal Morphology

T1-weighted (T1W) gradient volume acquisitions (SPGR or MP-RAGE) are excellent for evaluating the morphology of the hippocampus. The raw data from these images can be reformatted

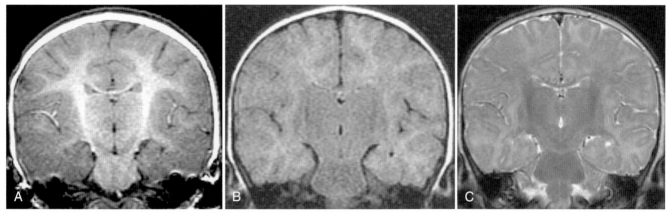

■ **FIGURE 50-1**   Immature myelination. **A,** Coronal spoiled gradient (SPGR) MR image obtained from a 4-month-old infant appears to demonstrate diffuse cortical thickening. There is poor differentiation between gray and white matter. This appearance, however, is due to the immature myelination, demonstrating the limited value of SPGR sequences before 12 months of age. **B,** Coronal FLAIR MR image from the same patient shows diffuse hyperintensity of the incompletely myelinated white matter. The utility of this sequence is also limited before 12 to 18 months of age. **C,** Coronal T2W FSE MR image from the same patient shows better gray matter/white matter differentiation.

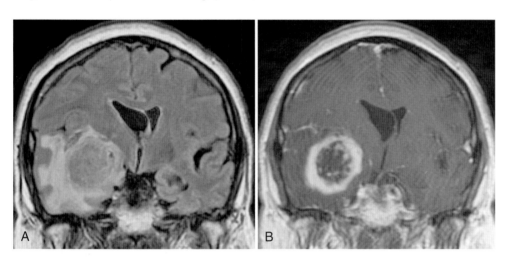

■ **FIGURE 50-2**   Right temporal lobe glioblastoma. **A,** Coronal FLAIR MR image of a 65-year-old patient who presented to the emergency department with new-onset seizures demonstrates a large medial right temporal lobe mass with surrounding vasogenic edema. **B,** Coronal T1W MR image post contrast agent administration shows thick irregular ring enhancement of the temporal lobe lesion. Pathology after resection confirmed this was a glioblastoma multiforme.

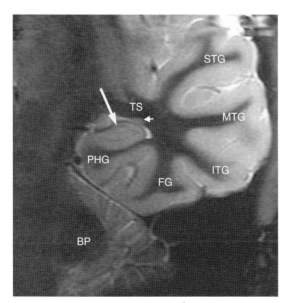

■ **FIGURE 50-3**   Normal coronal temporal lobe anatomy. Coronal inversion recovery MR image of normal temporal lobe anatomy. *Large arrow,* hippocampus; BP, brachium pontis (middle cerebellar peduncle); PHG, parahippocampal gyrus; TS, temporal stem; FG, fusiform gyrus; ITG, inferior temporal gyrus; MTG, middle temporal gyrus; STG, superior temporal gyrus; *small arrow,* tail of the caudate nucleus.

into any plane that is helpful for qualitative and volumetric analysis of the hippocampus.

Spectroscopy and Relaxometry

Spectroscopy and T2 relaxometry may be used for additional evaluation of the hippocampus and medial temporal lobes. T2 relaxometry obtained from multi-echo T2W sequences is especially useful in cases in which the findings on visual analysis are equivocal or for lateralizing the seizure focus when abnormalities are evident in both hippocampi.

Evaluation of Neocortical Structures and Malformations

Standard Evaluation

Cortical malformations may be difficult to detect without high-resolution techniques and pulse sequences that optimize gray matter/white matter differentiation. T1W gradient 3D volume sequences (SPGR or MP-RAGE) with thin slices can provide high spatial resolution with superb distinction between gray and white matter. Inversion recovery sequences can provide excellent corticomedullary contrast for detecting subtle thickening of the gray matter and indistinctness of the gray matter/white matter junction. FLAIR and T2W sequences are recommended to reveal any hyperintensity in the subcortical and deep white matter indicative of congenital malformation, as well as for detecting hyperintense cortical neoplastic, inflammatory, or gliotic abnormalities.

Further Assessment

High field magnets (3 T or greater) and high-resolution phased-array coils help to detect cortical malformations. Photographic image reversal of inversion recovery or T2W sequences may be helpful. Multiplanar or 3D reconstructions of volume-acquired data can demonstrate sulcal morphologic abnormalities, cortical dysplasia, indistinctness of the gray matter/white matter interface, and the relationship of developmental abnormalities to eloquent areas of the brain. However, the location and extent of cortical dysplasia identified by MRI may not correlate directly with the seizure semiology or the electrophysiologic data.[5]

MRI postprocessing techniques have advanced the quantitative and qualitative evaluation of epileptogenic abnormalities. Computerized segmentation of gray and white matter can detect developmental anomalies in epilepsy patients. Other image processing advancements such as curvilinear reformatting, texture analysis, and automated quantitative methods may be helpful in individual cases.

MESIAL TEMPORAL SCLEROSIS

The term *mesial temporal sclerosis* signifies scarring and volume loss of medial temporal structures: the hippocampus, the amygdala, and the parahippocampal gyrus (including the entorhinal cortex). Alternate names include hippocampal sclerosis and Ammon's horn sclerosis.

Epidemiology

Epilepsy affects 0.5% to 1% of the population. Up to 30% of cases are medically intractable or medically refractory, that is, seizures persist despite optimal medical therapy.[1] Temporal lobe epilepsy accounts for about 70% of intractable epilepsy. In patients undergoing surgery for intractable epilepsy, hippocampal sclerosis is found pathologically in 60% to 70%. MRI has also shown hippocampal sclerosis in patients with medically controlled, complex partial epilepsy and in relatives of epileptics without clinical seizures.

Clinical Presentation

Patients with hippocampal sclerosis often have a history of a childhood insult, usually complicated febrile seizure or encephalitis before the age of 5. After a quiescent period, recurrent temporal lobe seizures begin during the second decade. A subset of patients with medial temporal lobe epilepsy have *paradoxical medial temporal lobe epilepsy,* in which the MRI is normal. In this group, hippocampal gliosis occurs without neuronal loss. The postoperative outcome is somewhat poorer in this group than in classic hippocampal sclerosis.[9]

Dual pathology is the term to describe the coexistence of hippocampal sclerosis with another epileptogenic substrate. This occurs in 8% to 22% of surgical epilepsy patients.[10] The most frequent coexisting epileptogenic substrate is cortical dysgenesis. Dual pathology is associated with less favorable surgical outcome, unless both the hippocampus and the other substrate are resected. In this situation, a residual sclerotic hippocampus or a residual extrahippocampal substrate will become the epileptogenic source after the initial surgery.

Pathophysiology

The complex pathophysiology leading to hippocampal sclerosis is incompletely understood. Multiple factors may cause this condition. The "two-hit" hypothesis proposes that an initial precipitating injury (e.g., complicated febrile seizures or encephalitis) must occur in the presence of a predisposing factor (e.g., genetic disposition or developmental anomaly) that increases vulnerability. The presence of dual pathologic processes within the temporal lobe supports this proposal. Hippocampal sclerosis is associated with a second abnormality on MRI in 15% to 30% of

cases.[10] "Kindling," induction of a secondary seizure focus by repeated exposure from a primary seizure focus, may also contribute to the development of, or bilateral extension of, hippocampal sclerosis.

The hippocampus is a curved structure situated along the medial aspect of the temporal lobe. It can be divided into three regions by its morphology and relationship to the midbrain. The anterior, expanded region is called the *hippocampal head* or *pes hippocampus.* Three or four longitudinal striations groove the superior surface of the head, giving it the shape of fingers (the digitations of the pes hippocampi). The midregion is the cylindrically shaped *hippocampal body,* which lies adjacent to the midbrain. The posterior *hippocampal tail* rapidly narrows behind the brain stem.

In coronal sections, the hippocampus appears as two interlocking U-shaped layers of gray matter, the *dentate gyrus* and *cornu ammonis.* The cornu ammonis is divided into four segments: CA1, CA2, CA3, and CA4. CA1 is called the Sommer sector and is especially vulnerable to hypoxia. CA4 lies within the curve of the dentate gyrus and is also called the *end folium.* The cornu ammonis extends laterally to merge with the *subiculum,* which extends laterally, in turn, to merge into the neocortex of the *parahippocampal gyrus.* The convex ventricular surface of the hippocampus and dentate gyrus is covered with ependyma. A thin lamina of white matter between the ependyma and the superior surface of the hippocampus is designated the *alveus.* This is a major tangential communication pathway. The alveus passes medially over the dentate gyrus to form a free margin designated the *fimbria.* Together the alveus and the fimbria constitute the *fornix.* The *amygdala* is a gray matter structure located superomedial to the tip of the temporal horn of the lateral ventricle. The uncal recess of the temporal horn separates the amygdala from the hippocampal head. When the uncal recess is not visible, the alveus (i.e., the thin layer of white matter on the superior surface of the hippocampus) may help to separate the amygdala from the hippocampus.

Pathology

Mesial temporal sclerosis affects variable portions of the temporal lobe and may be unilateral, bilaterally asymmetric, or bilaterally symmetric. Ten to 20 percent of cases of hippocampal sclerosis are bilateral. Bilaterality is often associated with concurrent developmental anomalies. The sclerosis may affect the anterior hippocampus (head) most severely or extend the entire anteroposterior length of the hippocampus. Rarely, the amygdala is affected predominantly. The entire temporal lobe may be affected.

In hippocampal sclerosis there is usually loss of more than 50% of the neurons, notably loss of pyramidal cells in regions CA1, CA2, and CA4 and loss of granule cells within the dentate gyrus (Fig. 50-4). Hippocampal reorganization and changes in energy metabolism are also seen in hippocampal sclerosis. Findings of reorganization include abnormal axonal sprouting and loss of interneurons, which is thought to change the balance of neuronal excitation and inhibition.

Imaging

CT

CT does not display hippocampal sclerosis directly. In severe cases, it may demonstrate gross hippocampal atrophy, with enlargement of the adjacent temporal horn, small size of the hippocampal formation, and reduced size of the ipsilateral fornix.

MRI

MRI is the principal imaging modality used for evaluation of hippocampal sclerosis.

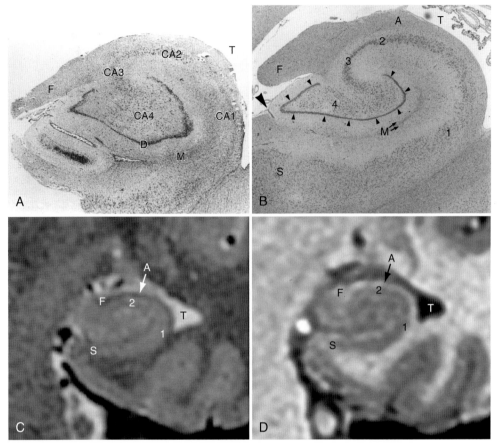

■ **FIGURE 50-4** Hippocampal sclerosis histology. **A,** Coronal histologic section of an adult hippocampus with hippocampal sclerosis. There is significant loss of pyramidal cells within the CA1 and CA4 fields. T, temporal lobe; F, fimbria; D, dentate gyrus; M, molecular strata of the dentate gyrus. **B,** Coronal histologic section of a normal adult hippocampus. S, subiculum; 1 to 4, CA1, CA2, CA3, and CA4 fields of the cornu ammonis, respectively; *small arrowheads,* dentate gyrus; M, molecular strata of the dentate gyrus; F, fimbria; A, alveus; *large arrowhead,* minimal residual hippocampal sulcus; T, temporal horn of the lateral ventricle. **C,** High-resolution thin-section coronal T2W MR image of a normal adult hippocampus. The general aspects of the hippocampal internal architecture are visible. S, subiculum; 1 and 2, CA1 and CA2 fields of the cornu ammonis; A, alveus; F, fimbria; T, temporal horn of the lateral ventricle. **D,** High-resolution thin-section coronal SPGR MR image of the same patient. S, subiculum; 1 and 2, CA1 and CA2 fields of the cornu ammonis; A, alveus; F, fimbria; T, temporal horn of the lateral ventricle. (*A, modified from Bronen RA, Cheung G, Charles JT, et al. Imaging findings in hippocampal sclerosis: correlation with pathology. AJNR Am J Neuroradiol 12:933-940, 1991, © by American Society of Neuroradiology; B from Kier EL, Kim JH, Fulbright RK, et al. Embryology of the human fetal hippocampus: MR imaging, anatomy, and histology. AJNR Am J Neuroradiol 18:530, 1997, © by American Society of Neuroradiology.*)

Visual Analysis

More than 75% of patients with surgically proven hippocampal sclerosis show prolonged T2 relaxation time (hyperintense signal on T2W images), hippocampal atrophy, and loss of the internal architecture of the hippocampus (Fig. 50-5). Other MRI findings associated with hippocampal sclerosis include loss of the digitations along the hippocampal head, dilatation of the adjacent temporal horn, atrophy of the white matter in the adjacent parahippocampal gyrus, increased T2 signal in the anterior temporal white matter, and secondary atrophy of the fornix and mammillary bodies due to degeneration of hippocampal tracts (Fig. 50-6). Overall, qualitative (i.e., visual) assessment of MRI detects hippocampal sclerosis with a sensitivity in the range of 75% to 90%.

Quantitative Methods

Quantitative MR methods, such as hippocampal volumetry and T2 relaxometry, increase the sensitivity for detecting hippocampal sclerosis to 90% to 95%. These quantitative methods are especially useful when hippocampal sclerosis occurs bilaterally without obvious T2 signal changes (Fig. 50-7). Proton MR spectroscopy may also be used quantitatively.

Hippocampal Volumetry

The criteria set forth by Watson and coworkers[11] are best for defining the anatomic boundaries needed to measure the volumes of the hippocampus and amygdala. Each center needs to establish its own normative data for hippocampal volume because the precise paradigm used in the quantitative imaging program varies from center to center. One needs to normalize for such variables as head size, patient age, patient gender, and the hemisphere imaged (right or left).

T2 Relaxometry

Quantitative measurements of T2 signal (T2 relaxometry) are obtained on a single-slice multi-echo sequence through the hippocampal body. The T2 signal is measurably elevated in approximately 70% of cases with hippocampal sclerosis.[12] Measurements of T2 relaxometry are particularly useful in detecting abnormalities of the amygdala (amygdala sclerosis), which may be difficult to identify on routine anatomic imaging.[13] Concurrent involvement of the amygdala in mesial temporal sclerosis reduces the likelihood that resective surgery will achieve a seizure-free outcome from 80% to 50%.[14]

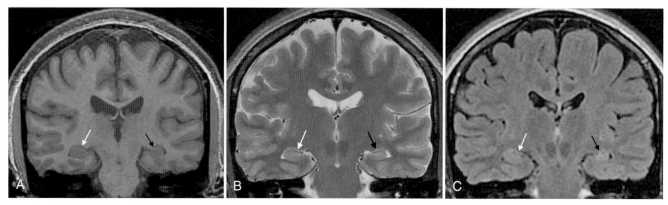

■ **FIGURE 50-5** Normal versus abnormal hippocampus. **A,** Coronal SPGR MR image from a patient with long-standing seizures shows a normal-sized right hippocampus (*white arrow*) in comparison with the smaller, atrophic left hippocampus (*black arrow*). **B,** Coronal T2W MR image of the same patient again shows the atrophy of the left hippocampus (*black arrow*), but without a significant signal difference from that of the right hippocampus (*white arrow*). **C,** Coronal FLAIR MR image demonstrates normal signal within the right hippocampus (*white arrow*) and also definitely depicts slight T2 prolongation within the atrophic left hippocampus (*black arrow*), suggesting mesial temporal sclerosis.

■ **FIGURE 50-6** Associated findings with hippocampal sclerosis. **A,** Coronal T2W MR image in a patient with left hippocampal sclerosis shows asymmetric thinning and atrophy of the left fornix (*black arrow*) compared with the normal right fornix (*white arrow*). **B,** A more anterior coronal T2W MR image of the same patient also shows atrophy of the left mammillary body (*black arrow*) as compared with the normal right mammillary body (*white arrow*).

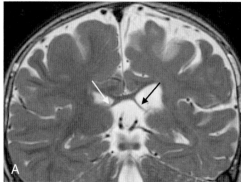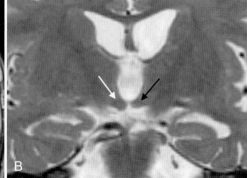

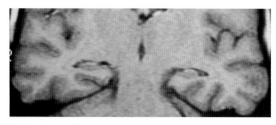

■ **FIGURE 50-7** Bilateral hippocampal sclerosis. Coronal SPGR MR image demonstrates bilateral atrophic hippocampi in a patient with bilateral mesial temporal sclerosis. Lack of asymmetry may hinder visual recognition.

MR Spectroscopy

Proton magnetic resonance spectroscopy (MRS) can be useful in evaluating the hippocampus and lateralizing a seizure focus. MRS of the hippocampus is typically performed using single voxel spectroscopy, which often includes some of the adjacent mesial temporal structures. The contralateral hippocampus is interrogated for comparison. The most important spectroscopic finding in mesial temporal sclerosis is decreased *N*-acetyl-aspartate (NAA). Reduced ratios of NAA to creatine or NAA to (choline + creatine) reflect metabolic dysfunction and/or neuronal loss. NAA may be a dynamic marker of neuronal dysfunction, rather than a simple sign of decreased numbers of neurons. Abnormally low NAA concentrations have been reported to recover in the unoperated temporal lobe after successful contralateral temporal lobectomy.[15] In patients with bilateral temporal lobe MRI abnormalities, reduced NAA ratios successfully lateralize the site of epileptogenesis in 65% to 96% of cases.[16] In temporal epilepsy

patients without MRI abnormalities, reduced NAA ratios have correctly lateralized the seizure focus in at least 20% of cases. Bilaterally reduced NAA to creatine ratios have been associated with failed resective surgery.

Quantitative methods have great value for research, allowing the investigator to test hypotheses correlating MRI data with clinical and pathologic data. Hippocampal volume has been correlated with cell loss, frequency of childhood febrile seizures, memory functions, duration of epilepsy, and successful surgical outcome.[17,18] One study correlated recurrent temporal lobe seizures with hippocampal volume loss, whereas generalized seizures were linked to progressive neuronal damage.[15] This study supports early intervention for seizure control to prevent progressive brain damage. Although quantitative MRI has many advantages for research, routine clinical use of quantitative measures faces some obstacles: operator time, the need for dedicated personnel, workstation, and software, and the requirement of a truly representative data sample of normal controls.

Neurotransmitters

Several neurotransmitters have been evaluated using proton spectroscopy, including glutamate, glutamine, and γ-aminobutyric acid (GABA). Future investigations may prove these techniques useful for elucidating neurochemical derangements in epilepsy syndromes and pharmacokinetic monitoring of medical therapy.

Diffusion MRI Techniques

DWI with its corresponding apparent diffusion coefficient (ADC) maps, diffusion tensor images (DTI), and fiber tract tra-

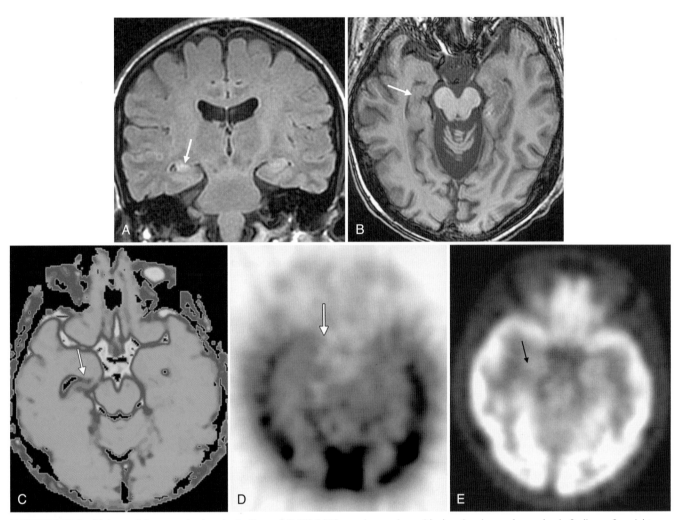

■ **FIGURE 50-8** Right mesial temporal sclerosis. **A,** Coronal FLAIR MR image in a patient with chronic seizures shows classic findings of mesial temporal sclerosis with an atrophic, hyperintense right hippocampus (*arrow*) compared with the left hippocampus with normal size and signal. **B,** Axial SPGR MR image of the same patient also demonstrates the atrophy of the right hippocampus (*arrow*) when compared with the normal left hippocampus. **C,** Diffusion tensor imaging (average diffusivity map) demonstrates increased average diffusivity within the abnormal right hippocampus (*arrow*). **D,** Axial interictal ^{99m}Tc HMPAO SPECT image demonstrates hypoperfusion of the right hippocampus/medial temporal lobe (*arrow*). **E,** Axial PET image shows subtly decreased glucose metabolism within the right medial temporal lobe (*arrow*).

jectography (FTT) also contribute to assessing mesial temporal sclerosis.

Diffusion-Weighted Imaging

Sclerotic hippocampi may show abnormally elevated ADCs,[19] even when conventional MRI is normal, likely reflecting early change. The ADCs of the abnormal hippocampi are higher than the ADCs of the corresponding contralateral hippocampi and higher than the ADCs from hippocampi of healthy volunteers. Interestingly, in patients with one sclerotic hippocampus, the ADCs of the contralateral normal-appearing hippocampi are higher than the ADCs of healthy volunteers. The ADC abnormalities in the contralateral normal-appearing hippocampi may resolve after resection of the ipsilateral abnormal hippocampus, suggesting that the biochemical change may be related to ongoing epileptic activity. In one study, ADC maps correctly lateralized the abnormality in 100% of patients. When the conventional MRI is nonlateralizing, however, the ADC values are also less helpful in lateralization.

Diffusion Tensor Imaging

DTI has shown reduced fractional anisotropy and increased mean diffusivity in the hippocampi on the side of seizure later-alization (Fig. 50-8) versus the contralateral normal-appearing hippocampus in control subjects.[20] Compared with normal controls, patients with hippocampal sclerosis and negative conventional MRI have higher mean diffusivity and low fractional anisotropy in the hippocampi bilaterally. Decreased fractional anisotropy values have also been demonstrated in the uncinate fasciculus on the side of seizure lateralization, suggesting that this tract has a role in the spread of temporal lobe seizures.

Fiber Tract Trajectography

Diffusion tensor fiber-tracking of major white matter tracts can be particularly helpful in surgical planning. In conjunction with functional MRI, tractography can demonstrate connectivity between noncontiguous functionally eloquent cortical regions. Connectivity mapping may improve understanding of seizure origin and spread and lead to innovative minimally invasive surgical strategies.

Functional MRI

In the planning of lesional resective surgery, many epilepsy centers use functional MRI (fMRI) to localize eloquent regions of the brain that should be preserved. Less frequently, functional mapping can be used to localize the activated cortex during an ictal seizure. fMRI uses blood oxygen level–dependent (BOLD) changes in T2* signal to demonstrate areas of increased neuronal activity and resultant increased perfusion. EEG and fMRI can be used in combination to obtain whole-brain maps of interictal epileptic spikes and their co-registered associated BOLD changes.

PET and SPECT

Radiotracer techniques are useful for detecting and evaluating areas where local metabolism is altered by present, recent prior, or remote seizure activity.

[18]F-fluorodeoxyglucose (FDG) positron emission tomography (PET) is used to map cerebral glucose metabolism. This study is usually performed in an interictal period. Routine FDG-PET has a sensitivity of more than 70% for lateralization of mesial temporal epilepsy. The epileptogenic temporal lobe demonstrates interictal hypometabolism, that is, decreased uptake of the glucose analogue. Hypometabolism may also occur in the contralateral temporal lobe and in ipsilateral extratemporal locations such as the frontoparietal cortex, basal ganglia, and thalamus. These additional areas, however, all demonstrate a lesser degree of hypometabolism compared with the epileptogenic temporal lobe. Bilateral asymmetric temporal lobe hypometabolism is commonly seen in mesial temporal epilepsy. One should keep in mind that antiepileptic medications, particularly barbiturates, can result in a global decrease in glucose metabolism.

The area of PET abnormality may be significantly larger than that requiring surgical resection. PET and SPECT do not give information about the nature of the underlying substrate but can help to focus the MRI interpretation, especially in cases of subtle MR findings.

PET with ^{11}C-flumazenil (FMZ) is a newer technique that has shown much promise. GABA is the most important inhibitory neurotransmitter. Flumazenil specifically binds to GABA receptors, which are decreased in mesial temporal sclerosis. Early studies have shown ^{11}C-FMZ abnormalities to be better localized than ^{18}F-FDG abnormalities,[21] so this technique may prove particularly useful in cases in which MRI is negative.

Single-photon emission CT (SPECT) and subtraction ictal-interictal SPECT co-registered to MRI (SISCOM) have been used. In epileptic patients, SPECT may be used to evaluate brain perfusion and to map regional cerebral blood flow (rCBF). SPECT can be performed using a number of different radiopharmaceuticals. The study acquires data in three dimensions, after which cross-sectional images can be generated in any plane by using filtered back-projection. Interictal SPECT characteristically demonstrates hypoperfusion in the epileptogenic region but has low sensitivity and specificity. Ictal SPECT demonstrates hyperperfusion in the epileptogenic region and has a very high sensitivity. The injection can be performed ictally, during the actual seizure, because the tracer is localized very quickly after injection. The actual imaging (data acquisition) can then be delayed up to 4 hours postictally, because the tracer remains localized at the original uptake site for long periods. This makes ictal SPECT far more feasible than ictal PET. Achieving an ictal injection, however, can be logistically challenging and requires a dedicated setup. SISCOM provides better localization than either ictal SPECT alone or qualitative comparison of ictal to interictal SPECT. This technique may be especially useful for patients in whom MRI is either negative or demonstrates diffuse or multifocal abnormalities.

Treatment Algorithm

Seizure therapy requires a multidisciplinary approach that integrates the imaging studies with clinical and paraclinical data to achieve correct seizure localization and plan correct therapy. At our institution, anterior temporal lobectomy is performed if EEG and MRI are concordant and there is no discordance of other lateralization testing (PET, SPECT, fMRI, neuropsychological testing, or intracarotid Amytal [WADA] procedure). If there is discordance, the patient proceeds to intracranial EEG for decisive localization. The exception to this algorithm is the rare case of concordance of EEG with PET but negative MRI study.

NEOCORTICAL TEMPORAL LOBE EPILEPSY

Neocortical temporal epilepsy can arise from any neocortical structures within the temporal lobe, including both the lateral and the basal temporal neocortical structures. The epileptogenic substrate may be neoplasm, vascular malformation, gliotic abnormalities, or malformations of cortical development but not mesial temporal sclerosis. Neoplasms that more frequently cause temporal lobe epilepsy include ganglioglioma, pleomorphic xanthoastrocytoma, dysembryoplastic neuroepithelial tumor (DNET), and oligodendroglioma, as well as the common low-grade glioma.

Malformations of Cortical Development

The term *malformations of cortical development* (MCD) is used to designate a group of anomalies characterized by disordered embryogenesis of the cerebral and cerebellar cortices, leading to alterations in the completeness of neuronal migration, the histochemical profiles of the migrating cells, the sharpness of definition of the interface between gray matter and white matter, the lamination of the cerebral and cerebellar cortices, and the size, number, and definition of the cortical gyri and sulci (folia and fissures for cerebellum). Because these malformations are dealt with in detail in other chapters, here the focus is on the MRI characteristics of MCDs in adults, how to differentiate among them, and how they relate to epilepsy. An alternate name is neuronal migration disorders.

Epidemiology

MCDs account for 10% to 50% of epilepsy cases in children and 4% to 25% of epilepsy cases in adults. MRI has led to increased recognition of developmental malformations as causes of epilepsy in children and young adults. Malformations of cortical development are often intrinsically epileptogenic. The extent of the epileptogenic zone can be more extensive than the area of MRI abnormality. Furthermore, the epileptogenic zone may not map directly to the malformation but may, in fact, be at a distance from the malformation.[5] Invasive electrophysiologic studies are often used to ensure concordance in the presurgical evaluation of these malformations (Fig. 50-9).

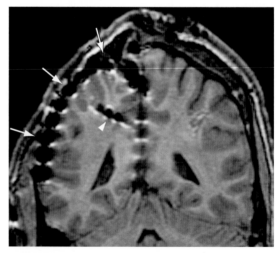

■ **FIGURE 50-9** Invasive monitoring. Coronal SPGR MR image of a patient with surface subdural electrodes (*arrows*), interhemispheric subdural electrodes, and a frontal lobe depth electrode (*arrowhead*) in place for accurate localization of the patient's seizure focus.

TABLE 50-2. MRI Findings in Malformations of Cortical Development

Blurring of gray matter/white matter junction
Irregularity of gray matter/white matter junction
Increased gray matter signal on T1W images
Cortical thickening
Macrogyria
Minigyria (polymicrogyria)
Paucity of gyri
Sulcal cleft and cortical dimple
Sulcal morphologic changes
Radial bands of hyperintensity
Gray matter heterotopia
Band heterotopia
Transmantle gray matter

The MRI features of developmental malformations may vary widely. Findings associated with cortical dysgenesis (Table 50-2) include cortical thickening, morphologic surface alterations, blurring of the normal gray matter/white matter interface, heterotopic gray matter, radial bands, and cerebrospinal fluid (CSF) clefts. Because many of these malformations are subtle, it is necessary to employ high-resolution imaging, which allows for optimal visualization of the corticomedullary junction (see earlier section on study protocols). The abnormalities may be focal, diffuse, unilateral, or bilateral and may be more widespread than the MRI visible anomaly. This scenario adds complexity to surgical decisions and planning, even when a distinct anatomic abnormality is identified on MRI. For these reasons, the preoperative evaluation of these malformations often includes invasive EEG.

Clinical Presentation
The most widely used classification of MCD was proposed by Barkovich and colleagues and consists of four categories.[22] The following outline is a brief modification of this scheme, directed toward imaging of MCD in the *adult* population:

I. Abnormal Neuronal and Glial Proliferation or Apoptosis
   A. Glial cell developmental neoplasms such as ganglioglioma, gangliocytoma, and dysembryoplastic neuroepithelial tumor
   B. Balloon cell cortical dysplasia
   C. Tuberous sclerosis
II. Abnormal Neuronal Migration
   A. Gray matter heterotopia
   B. Lissencephaly (agyria-pachygyria spectrum)
III. Abnormal Cortical Organization
   A. Polymicrogyria
   B. Schizencephaly
   C. Non–balloon cell cortical dysplasia
IV. Malformations of Cortical Development, Not Otherwise Classified

Because each classification group is based on the *earliest* stage of cortical development affected, abnormalities of later stages of development may be found in association with abnormalities of an earlier stage (the stage of disrupted development). For example, cortical organizational and neuronal migrational abnormalities may be associated with malformations of abnormal proliferation and those classified as abnormalities of neuronal migration may also exhibit associated malformations of cortical organization.

Tuberous Sclerosis and Focal Cortical Dysplasias
Abnormalities of neuronal proliferation are characterized by persistence and proliferation of large progenitor cells with both neural and glial characteristics, known as "balloon cells." Disorders resulting from the proliferation of these progenitor cells include balloon cell focal cortical dysplasia of Taylor, tuberous sclerosis, and hemimegalencephaly.

Tuberous sclerosis and balloon cell focal cortical dysplasia (type II focal cortical dysplasia) have similar imaging features.[23] Both disorders have hyperintense cortical lesions on T2W images, often with cortical thickening and radial bands extending toward the ventricle. Balloon cell focal cortical dysplasia consists of a single lesion, whereas tuberous sclerosis typically produces multiple cortical lesions. Tuberous sclerosis can also be distinguished by its characteristic subependymal nodules and clinical systemic manifestations (cardiac, renal, and dermatologic). Because balloon cell cortical dysplasia is a single T2 hyperintense lesion, the most important differential diagnostic consideration is often neoplasm. Cortical thickening, subcortical T2 prolongation, and radial bands may suggest a diagnosis of focal cortical dysplasia rather than neoplasm (Fig. 50-10). This differentiation may be crucial for surgical management.[23]

Focal cortical dysplasia of Taylor without balloon cells often has subtle imaging findings such as focal cortical thickening, abnormal sulcal morphology, and blurring of the gray matter/white matter interface.[24] Detection and characterization of these may require high-resolution imaging techniques. Non–balloon cell type focal cortical dysplasia typically does not demonstrate the T2 hyperintensity and radial bands seen with the balloon cell variety described earlier. However, there is overlap in their imaging findings, so each entity may mimic the other.

Gray matter heterotopias are ectopically located collections of neurons, which result from a failure of normal radial neuronal migration. These malformations are often genetic and may be sex linked. Some are caused by dysfunction of the microtubules essential for the migration of the neurons from the germinal matrix to the cortex along the radial glial unit. Heterotopic gray matter may be found in the periventricular, or subependymal, region, where it is typically nodular in morphology (Fig. 50-11). One X-linked form of bilateral periventricular nodular heterotopia is due to a mutation involving the filamin-1 gene, which encodes a protein important for cell locomotion. Another form of heterotopia, closely linked to lissencephaly, creates subcortical bands of heterotopic gray matter vaguely resembling a duplicated cerebral cortex. This form of subcortical laminar heterotopia results from defects in the gene doublecortin and may be called band heterotopia or double cortex syndrome.

Polymicrogyria can occur anywhere but is most common in the perisylvian region. Congenital bilateral perisylvian polymicrogyria typically presents as seizures, developmental delay, and pseudobulbar palsy. MRI demonstrates abnormally thickened cortex in the opercular regions and lining the sylvian fissures.[25] High-resolution imaging reveals multiple small (micro) gyri in the affected regions. Sulcal anomalies such as continuity of the sylvian and the rolandic fissures are often present and are best appreciated on parasagittal images. Polymicrogyria is associated with anomalous patterns of venous drainage, which may be visualized on contrast-enhanced MRIs.

Schizencephaly is a congenital malformation characterized by a full-thickness transcerebral column of gray matter oriented along a pial-ependymal seam. The outer surface of the column represents adjacent polymicrogyric cortex, the subarachnoid space, and its associated vasculature, which have been deeply folded inward to resemble a cerebral cleft. The deep surface of the column is often a diverticulum of the ventricle directed outward toward the surface. When the diverticulum is small, and the side walls of the cleft are closely apposed, the condition is designated closed-lip schizencephaly. Closed-lip schizencephaly has been associated with abnormalities of the gene *EMX2*. When there is associated hydrocephalus, the ventricular diverticulum is ballooned outward, separating the walls of the cleft widely. This condition is designated open-lip schizencephaly. The cortex

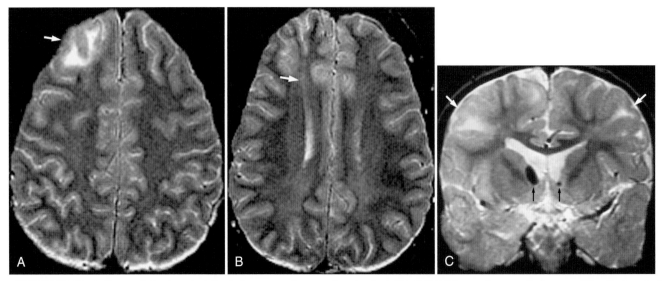

■ **FIGURE 50-10**   Balloon cell focal cortical dysplasia versus tuberous sclerosis. **A,** Axial T2W MR image shows a single area of focal subcortical hyperintensity within the anterior right frontal lobe. The adjacent cortex (*arrow*) is thickened. This patient had balloon cell focal cortical dysplasia. **B,** Axial T2W MR image of the same patient demonstrates a hyperintense band radiating from the ventricle (*arrow*). Radial bands can be seen with both balloon cell cortical dysplasia and tuberous sclerosis. **C,** Multiple areas of subcortical T2 hyperintensity are seen (a few of these are labeled with *white arrows*). There are also larger right and smaller left subependymal hypointensities consistent with calcified subependymal tubers (*small black arrows*).

■ **FIGURE 50-11**   Nodular gray matter heterotopia versus tuberous sclerosis. **A,** Axial T2W MR image of a young patient shows multiple small, focal periventricular lesions that are isointense to cortex (*arrows*). These nodules followed the signal of gray matter on all pulse sequences, consistent with foci of nodular heterotopic gray matter. **B,** Coronal SPGR MR image again shows the small bilateral subependymal lesions following the signal of gray matter (*arrows*). **C,** Coronal T2W MR image in a different patient demonstrates areas of T2 hypointensity within the subcortical white matter (*arrowhead*) and in a subependymal location within the lateral ventricle (*arrow*). Note the myelination is normal for the patient's age of 4 months. **D,** Coronal T1W MR image of the same 4-month-old shows multiple areas of hyperintensity within the subcortical and deep white matter (*arrowheads*) as well as subependymally within the lateral ventricles (*arrows*). Note that these areas of hyperintensity do not match the signal of gray matter.

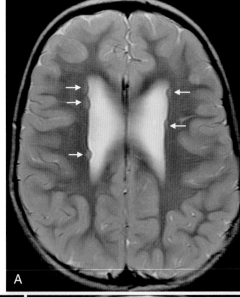

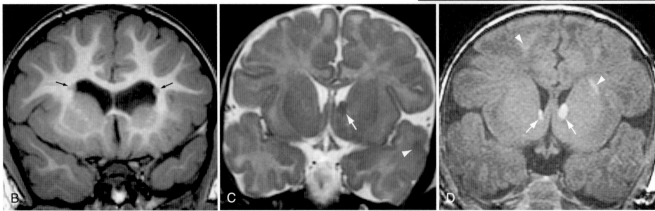

within and adjacent to the cleft is usually polymicrogyric (Fig. 50-12).

Neoplasms

The tumors responsible for chronic recurrent seizures tend to be small and well localized, with little or no perilesional edema. One third show no significant mass effect. They are typically peripheral, involve the cortical structures, and may remodel the inner table of the overlying calvaria. MRI has nearly 100% sensitivity for detecting epileptogenic neoplastic lesions[26] but is less accurate in predicting the tumor histology.

The majority of epileptogenic tumors occur in the temporal lobe. Indolent tumors such as *ganglioglioma, dysembryoplastic neuroepithelial tumor* (DNET), and low-grade glioma are often associated with chronic intractable seizures.

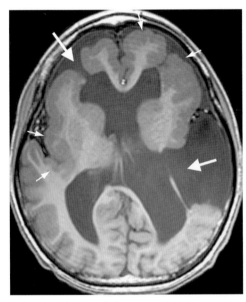

■ **FIGURE 50-12** Schizencephaly versus polymicrogyria. An axial SPGR MR image of this patient shows two large open-lipped schizencephalic clefts within the right frontal and left temporal lobes lined with thickened cortex (*large arrows*). Also note that the corresponding contralateral areas of the brain demonstrate areas of cortical thickening and multiple small gyri (*small arrows*).

Pleomorphic xanthoastrocytomas and *oligodendrogliomas* are also commonly associated with seizures. In the elderly, cerebral metastases are the most frequent neoplastic lesions associated with seizures.

Gangliogliomas and pleomorphic xanthoastrocytomas can present as solid and/or cystic masses and may demonstrate significant enhancement. They are peripherally located lesions and characteristically involve the leptomeninges. Gangliogliomas and mixed glial neoplasms have a predilection for the mesial temporal lobe and are an important cause of temporal epilepsy. Gangliogliomas and gangliocytomas usually occur in childhood through early adulthood (peak age, 10 to 20 years). They may be developmental in origin. They are characteristically mixed cystic-solid lesions, perhaps with an enhancing mural nodule, but can also be multicystic or predominantly solid. Calcifications are common. In the appropriate age group, imaging detection of a temporal lobe mass with cysts and calcification should raise consideration of these lesions (Fig. 50-13).

Oligodendrogliomas are typically peripherally located tumors that involve both the gray matter and the white matter of the frontal or frontotemporal lobes. Typical oligodendrogliomas are well-circumscribed nonenhancing tumors with relatively little vasogenic edema. Intratumoral calcification is common and best identified on CT or gradient-recalled-echo (GRE) MRI sequences (Fig. 50-14). Atypical oligodendrogliomas can enhance, can have cystic and hemorrhagic components, and may appear heterogeneous.

Dysembryoplastic neuroepithelial tumors (DNETs) are benign and slowly growing lesions, which some consider tumors and others classify as developmental abnormalities. They usually present in the temporal lobes of young patients. DNETs are typically well-defined multicystic lesions that appear hypointense on T1W and hyperintense on T2W. They typically do not enhance (although this is variable) and typically do not cause significant vasogenic edema (Fig. 50-15). Because of their peripheral location and slow rate of growth, they commonly remodel the calvaria.

VASCULAR MALFORMATIONS

Seizures are the primary clinical manifestation of vascular malformations. Seizures occur in 34% to 51% of cavernous malformations and 24% to 69% of arteriovenous malformations. The majority of capillary telangiectases and developmental venous anomalies (also known as venous angiomas) are clinically silent and not epileptogenic. MRI is quite sensitive in the detection of epileptogenic vascular malformations.

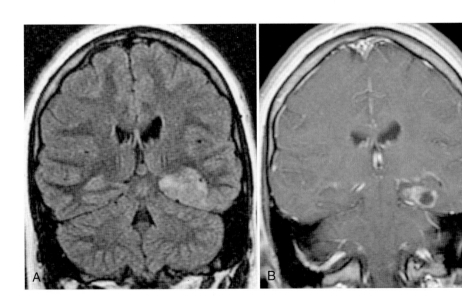

■ **FIGURE 50-13** Left temporal ganglioglioma. **A,** Coronal FLAIR MR image demonstrates a focal heterogeneous area of hyperintensity involving both cortex and white matter within the medial left temporal lobe with mass effect on adjacent structures. **B,** In the same patient, a coronal T1W MR image after administration of a contrast agent shows a heterogeneously enhancing, medial left temporal lobe mass with a cystic component.

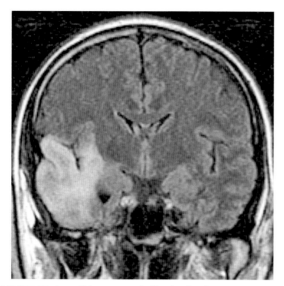

■ **FIGURE 50-14** Right temporal oligodendroglioma. Coronal FLAIR MR image shows enlargement of the lateral right temporal lobe with T2 prolongation and sulcal effacement. The abnormality involves both gray and white matter, resulting in loss of corticomedullary differentiation. There was no contrast enhancement of this area. This was a pathologically proven oligodendroglioma.

Cavernous malformations (cavernous hemangiomas, cavernous angiomas, cavernomas) are focal collections of sinusoidal vascular spaces filled with very slowly flowing blood. MRI characteristically demonstrates central hyperintensity (due to hemoglobin degradation products) and a peripheral hypointense hemosiderin rim (due to chronic leakage of blood products and, in some cases, remote hemorrhage) (Fig. 50-16). Cavernomas that have bled recently may show acute edema and be difficult to distinguish from hemorrhagic neoplasms or other hemorrhage. Cavernous malformations are particularly prone to produce seizures when a portion of the lesion or the surrounding hemosiderin ring touches the cortex. Hemosiderin itself may be epileptogenic. For that reason, some have advocated surgical resection of the surrounding hemosiderin-stained brain tissue, either primarily or in surgically refractory cases. The benefit of that is not yet clear. Developmental venous anomalies are often found in relation to cavernous malformations but do not themselves appear to induce seizures.[27]

Arteriovenous malformations are high-flow vascular malformations that manifest on MRI as curvilinear areas of signal void or enhancement. Enlarged feeding arteries and draining veins can usually be identified on routine imaging but are best evaluated with dedicated vascular imaging (Fig. 50-17). MR angiography can be performed using 3D time-of-flight technique, phase imaging, or time-resolved postcontrast imaging to display the arterial and venous phases separately. Angiography is often needed to fully evaluate and potentially treat these lesions.

GLIOSIS AND MISCELLANEOUS ABNORMALITIES

This category consists of a heterogeneous group of cerebral insults, most of which lead to neocortical gliosis. The disorders in this category can be divided by inflammatory/infectious, post-traumatic, and cerebrovascular causes. Resective surgery is usually less successful for neocortical gliosis than for hippocampal sclerosis. Rarely, a temporal lobe encephalocele may result in seizures and can also be included within this category. Regardless of its specific cause, the imaging appearance of gliosis is typically a region of T2 prolongation, often associated with

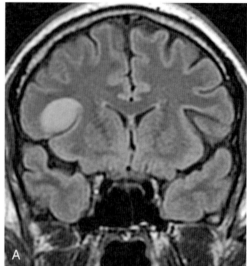

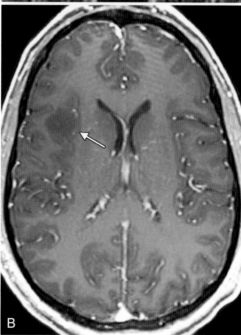

■ **FIGURE 50-15** Right frontal dysembryoplastic neuroepithelial tumor. **A,** Coronal FLAIR MR image obtained in a patient presenting with new-onset seizures demonstrates a well-circumscribed focal hyperintense lesion within the right frontal operculum. **B,** Axial SPGR MR image from the same patient shows no significant contrast enhancement within the mass (*arrow*). Histologic examination of the mass confirmed a dysembryoplastic neuroepithelial tumor.

volume loss. It can be focal or diffuse. Widespread cerebral gliosis and atrophy can be seen in such entities such as infantile hemiplegia, Sturge-Weber syndrome, and end-stage Rasmussen's encephalitis. Hypothalamic hamartoma can be regarded as a miscellaneous cause of seizures or as a malformation of cortical development.

Post-traumatic Seizures

The risk of developing seizures after an injury has been reported as 1.8% to 5% for civilians and up to 53% for war injuries. Post-traumatic seizures can be divided into *early-onset* and *late-onset* seizures. By definition, late-onset post-traumatic seizures begin at least 1 week after the initial traumatic event. Early-onset

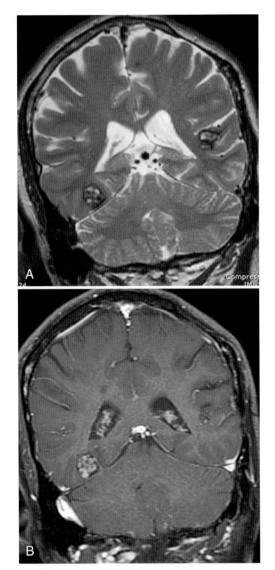

■ **FIGURE 50-16** Multiple cavernomas. **A,** Coronal T2W MR image from a patient with a history of seizures shows two separate lesions within both temporal lobes with central high signal and peripheral low signal. **B,** Coronal T1W MR image after administration of a contrast agent demonstrates mild central enhancement of the lesions. The findings are consistent with multiple cavernous angiomas.

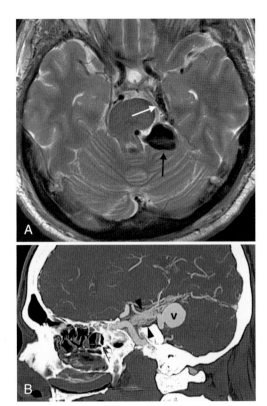

■ **FIGURE 50-17** Dural arteriovenous fistula. **A,** Axial T2W MR image obtained in a patient with new seizures demonstrates multiple small flow voids along the left tentorium, petrous apex, and petroclinoid ligament (*white arrow*). There is also a large, dilated vascular flow void within the left cerebellopontine angle with mass effect on adjacent structures (*black arrow*). **B,** Parasagittal CT angiogram image of the same patient again demonstrates the tiny vessels (*arrowheads*) extending along the left tentorium and petroclinoid ligament. Conventional angiography confirmed a dural arteriovenous fistula. The dilated vascular structure within the left cerebellopontine angle was a large venous varix (v) with venous drainage extending to an enlarged vein of Galen.

seizures have a favorable prognosis, but up to 25% of patients with late-onset seizures develop medically refractory epilepsy.

Contusion or shearing injury, often hemorrhagic, can cause cortical gliosis and/or hemosiderin deposition, which are the mechanisms for post-traumatic seizure generation and propagation. T2W GRE sequences are sensitive for detection of hemosiderin deposition and play an important role in the evaluation of post-traumatic epilepsy. Common sites of traumatic injury to the brain include the anteroinferior aspects of the frontal and temporal lobes. Circumstances that increase the risk of developing post-traumatic epilepsy are listed in Table 50-3.

Cerebrovascular Conditions

In patients older than age 50 years, *stroke* is the most common cause of seizures. The seizure may appear immediately as a result of cortical irritation, especially with hemorrhagic stroke, or it may appear later as a consequence of gliosis and hemosiderin deposition. The risk of developing chronic epilepsy is significantly greater when the onset of seizures is delayed after the

TABLE 50-3. Risk Factors for Post-traumatic Epilepsy

Age older than 65 years
Early post-traumatic seizures
Severe brain injury with loss of consciousness or post-traumatic amnesia
  lasting >24 hours
Intracranial hemorrhage (parenchymal or subdural)
Depressed skull fractures
Penetrating brain trauma
Residual intracerebral foreign bodies

cerebrovascular accident (just as is true for post-traumatic epilepsy).

Sturge-Weber syndrome (encephalotrigeminal angiomatosis) is a congenital neurocutaneous disorder characterized by a facial port-wine nevus in the trigeminal nerve distribution, leptomeningeal angiomatosis, recurrent seizures, mental retardation, and other neurologic deficits. Refractory epilepsy is the earliest, most common and most important clinical manifestation of the syndrome. Many patients appear relatively normal until the first major seizure and significantly impaired thereafter. Early on, therefore, antiepileptic therapy is directed toward *preventing* the first episode of prolonged seizures. Later, therapy is directed toward control of chronic seizures. Intractable cases may require surgical treatment by corpus callosotomy or hemispherectomy. Brain involvement may be unilateral or bilateral (but asymmetric),

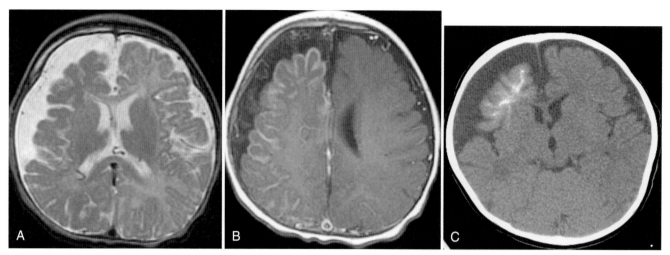

■ **FIGURE 50-18** Sturge-Weber syndrome. **A,** Axial T2W MR image of a pediatric patient with Sturge-Weber syndrome shows atrophy of the right frontal lobe but no MR evidence of calcification. **B,** Axial T1W MR image after administration of a contrast agent demonstrates classic pial enhancement of the right frontal lobe. **C,** Axial CT image of the same patient with calcification in the atrophic right frontal lobe.

with hemispheric atrophy, thickening of the overlying calvaria, and dilatation of the ipsilateral paranasal sinuses. CT and plain films may demonstrate tram-track gyriform calcification, which appears as linear low signal on MRI. These calcifications are thought to result from venous stasis that leads to chronic ischemia. Contrast-enhanced MRI reveals unilateral enlargement of the choroid plexus (reflecting redirection of venous flow to the deep venous system) and characteristic thick pial enhancement, reflecting the venous stasis and leptomeningeal angiomatosis (Fig. 50-18).

Inflammatory/Infectious

Infections of the central nervous system, including viral, bacterial, mycobacterial, fungal, and helminthic infections, can result in new-onset seizures in the acute phase as a result of the host's inflammatory reaction. Postinfectious or postinflammatory gliosis, however, can cause chronic epilepsy. In some developing nations, *cysticercosis* is one of the most common causes of new-onset partial seizures. In the active phase of infection, these lesions demonstrate ring enhancement and may have a characteristic central dot of low signal or enhancement (the scolex). In the inflammatory stage brought about by the dying parasite there is a variable degree of inflammatory edema in the surrounding parenchyma, which can induce seizures (Fig. 50-19). The lesions typically resolve on antiepileptic medication alone. Healing lesions may calcify, which is best shown on CT.

Rasmussen's encephalitis is characterized by intractable partial seizures, progressive neuropsychiatric deterioration, and mental retardation.[28] It is believed to result from chronic, immune-mediated cortical inflammation of one cerebral hemisphere. Progressive hemispheric atrophy and gliosis ensue. Rasmussen's encephalitis usually presents in children with *epilepsia partialis continua.* However, an adult form of the syndrome has been described. Early MRI findings include cortical and subcortical foci of T2 prolongation, which may be transient and migratory in this stage. In the late stages there is lobar or hemispheric atrophy with widespread gliosis (Fig. 50-20).[29] Crossed cerebellar diaschisis may result from degeneration of the corticopontocerebellar tracts.

Miscellaneous Lesions

Hypothalamic hamartomas can be divided into intrahypothalamic and parahypothalamic varieties.[30] Intrahypothalamic hamartomas are located within the hypothalamus and distort the

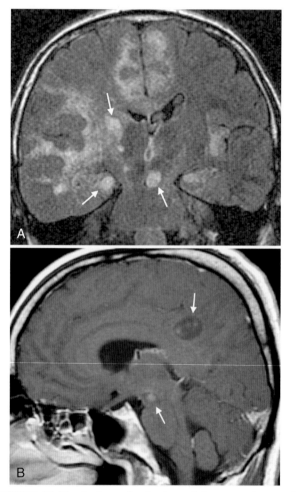

■ **FIGURE 50-19** Cysticercosis. **A,** Coronal FLAIR MR image of a patient with sudden onset of seizures shows multiple patchy regions of vasogenic edema throughout the cerebral hemispheres with more focal rounded hyperintense lesions (*arrows*) exerting mass effect on adjacent structures. **B,** Sagittal T1W postcontrast MR image demonstrates well-circumscribed cystic lesions (*arrows*) with a thin rim of peripheral enhancement and small areas of internal hyperintensity. Serologic testing for cysticercosis was positive.

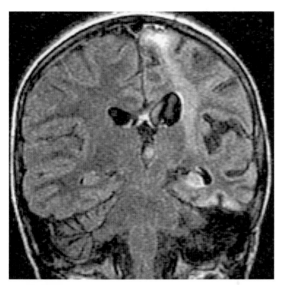

■ **FIGURE 50-20.** Rasmussen's encephalitis. Coronal FLAIR MR image of a young patient who had an initial episode of status epilepticus and then went on to develop chronic right hemiconvulsion syndrome. This image was obtained during a study 18 months after the initial event. There is diffuse atrophy of the left cerebral hemisphere with T2 hyperintensity within the white matter. The imaging findings and clinical course are consistent with Rasmussen's encephalitis.

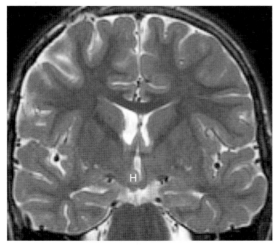

■ **FIGURE 50-21** Hypothalamic hamartoma. A coronal T2W MR image demonstrates a small well-circumscribed rounded focus (H) that is almost isointense to cortex and that is positioned just superior to the right mammillary body within the right hypothalamus and bulging into the third ventricle. Histologically this was a hypothalamic hamartoma and caused gelastic seizures.

third ventricle. These lesions are intrinsically epileptogenic and cause intractable seizures, typically, gelastic seizures (laughing seizures). Intrahypothalamic hamartomas may be located in the tuber cinereum or the floor of the third ventricle.[30] These patients present with precocious puberty (Fig. 50-21) more commonly than with seizures.

STATUS EPILEPTICUS AND BRAIN ISCHEMIA

Status epilepticus is a state in which a seizure continues for a prolonged period without clinical evidence of cessation or in which the seizure recurs after very brief intervals without return to baseline central nervous system function interictally.

Epidemiology

One-half to 1 percent of the population suffers from recurrent seizures. Status epilepticus occurs in approximately 0.1% of the population and is estimated to cause 180,000 episodes of status epilepticus per year in the United States. There is no gender preference. The age distribution is bimodal, with status epilepticus seen more frequently at both extremes of age.

Clinical Presentation

Status epilepticus is a clinical emergency with a high risk of morbidity and mortality. Patients can present with generalized convulsive status epilepticus (GCSE) or nonconvulsive status epilecticus (NCSE). NCSE is further subdivided into generalized (absence) or focal (complex partial) status epilepticus. Any form of status epilepticus can cause rapid widespread neuronal necrosis within the more vulnerable areas of the brain and consequent profound neurologic deficits.[31] The continued intense and prolonged muscle contractions of status epilepticus also lead to rhabdomyolysis, followed by acute renal tubular necrosis and renal failure. The muscle contractions release significant amounts of lactic acid, which, combined with hypoxia, cause a severe metabolic acidosis. The sustained muscle contractions can also lead to hyperkalemia with resulting cardiac arrhythmias and hyperpyrexia and endothelial damage and disseminated intravascular coagulation. Autonomic stimulation can also lead to hypoglycemia as well as early hypertension followed by hypotension.[31]

Pathophysiology

In humans and animal models, the areas of the brain most vulnerable to injury include the CA1 field, CA3 field, the hilus of the hippocampus, the amygdala, and the piriform cortex. The cerebral and cerebellar cortices and the thalamus are affected less severely.[32] The prolonged seizures are characterized by neuronal release of massive amounts of excitatory neurotransmitters, such as glutamate, aspartate, and acetylcholine. These excitatory neurotransmitters induce changes in permeability and ion homeostasis of cell membranes. The changes in cellular membrane permeability permit an influx of sodium and calcium and elevation of the extracellular potassium. This overloads the cell's ability to sequester calcium or transport the calcium back out of the cell, resulting in elevated intracellular concentrations of calcium. With the change in the osmotic gradient, free water rapidly flows into the cells, leading to neuronal and glial cell swelling, which may become irreversible, resulting in neuronal necrosis.[32]

Imaging

The MRI features reflect the underlying pathophysiologic processes. During the ictal phase, with the release of massive quantities of excitatory neurotransmitters, MRI demonstrates regional cerebral hyperperfusion. This hyperperfusion may be a result of increased glucose requirement owing to sustained overwhelming excitation. The changes in membrane permeability and osmotic gradients and the resulting movement of free water between intracellular and extracellular compartments restrict the diffusion of water protons. The ADC decreases and the signal intensity on DWI increases. There is also T2 prolongation in the affected areas (Fig. 50-22). Over time, the ADC values begin to normalize and the hyperintensity diminishes on the DW images. The T2 prolongation and edematous changes also slowly resolve and may be replaced by gliosis and loss of cortical volume. During the interictal period, regional hypoperfusion may be seen.[33]

The decreased ADC values and hyperintensity on DWI may not always portend subsequent neuronal death. With single seizures, the MRI changes are most often transient. In cases in which transient abnormal ADC values and DWI changes are seen

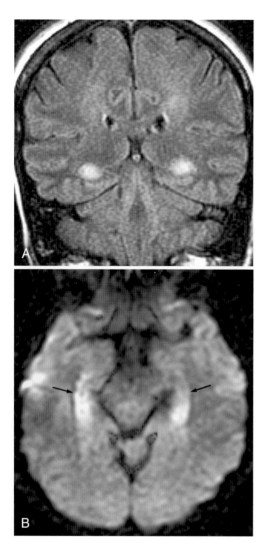

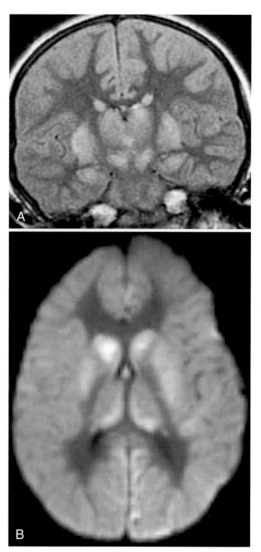

■ **FIGURE 50-22** Status epilepticus with diffusion abnormality. **A,** Coronal FLAIR MR image of a patient after status epilepticus demonstrates dramatic hyperintensity and mild enlargement of the bilateral hippocampi. The remainder of the cerebral hemispheres were spared. **B,** Axial diffusion-weighted image of the same patient shows restricted diffusion within the bilateral hippocampi (*arrows*). The areas of T2 hyperintensity and restricted diffusion were transient changes, which resolved on follow-up imaging of the patient.

■ **FIGURE 50-23** Status epilepticus with anoxic injury. **A,** Coronal FLAIR MR image of another patient after status epilepticus shows hyperintensity within the bilateral basal ganglia, thalami, subthalamic nuclei, and hippocampi. **B,** Axial diffusion image from the same patient demonstrates restricted diffusion corresponding to the areas of hyperintensity seen on the FLAIR image. The patient suffered an anoxic injury during status.

without T2 prolongation, the findings may indicate areas of reversible cellular change.[34] In the acute phase, the restricted diffusion and T2 prolongation can be mistaken for an infarct. However, use of perfusion imaging could help to differentiate these entities, because hyperperfusion (both increased regional cerebral blood flow and increased mean transit time) is seen acutely with seizures, whereas hypoperfusion is seen with infarctions.[33] With chronic seizures or status epilepticus, atrophy and gliotic changes can appear as early as 2 months to 1 year after the episode.[34]

Rarely, the contralateral cerebellar hemisphere demonstrates acute transient changes or chronic sequelae of status epilepticus. This phenomenon is designated crossed cerebellar diaschisis and is more frequently seen in cases of wallerian degeneration related to infarction. The cerebellum generally provides an inhibitory function through release of GABA from the Purkinje cells. In seizures, the massive release of excitatory neurotransmitters from the seizure focus demands corresponding release of inhibiting GABA from the Purkinje cells. This demand causes GABA

depletion and subsequent influx of calcium into the neurons. It also causes the same cascade of events described earlier: the changing cell membrane permeability, changing osmotic gradient, and rapid movement of free water. The inhibitory influence of the cerebellum is carried predominantly via the superior cerebellar peduncle.[32]

During status epilepticus, cerebral hypoxia can also occur. With prolonged seizure activity, glucose utilization is increased. The increased glucose requirement leads to regional hyperperfusion. However, the requirement for glucose may not be satisfied by the increased blood flow, leading to anaerobic glycolysis with decreased production of adenosine triphosphate and hypoxia. Hypoxia can also occur during the tonic phase of a seizure and its resulting apnea. This can result in MRI findings of acute anoxic injury (Fig. 50-23).[33]

ANALYSIS

Many epileptogenic abnormalities have subtle imaging findings. In addition to appropriate imaging protocols tailored to detect

TABLE 50-4. Systematic Approach to MRI Evaluation in Seizure Patients

Hippocampal size and signal abnormality; Hypothalamic hamartoma
Internal auditory canal and atrial asymmetry*
Periventricular heterotopia
Peripherial abnormalities
Obvious lesion†
Sulcal morphologic abnormalities
Atrophy
Gray matter thickening
Encephalocele of anterior temporal lobe

*Assess for the presence of head rotation when evaluating for hippocampal atrophy.
†Evaluate the obvious lesion last to avoid missing hippocampal sclerosis in cases of dual pathology.

these abnormalities, one needs to be familiar with common diagnostic pitfalls, including normal variations that may be mistaken for an epileptogenic abnormality. Given the wide variety of abnormalities that can result in seizures, a systematic approach is useful when interpreting MR images from a patient with epilepsy. One approach that can be followed utilizes the mnemonic HIPPO SAGE (Table 50-4).[35]

Normal Variations
Hippocampal Signal, Asymmetry, and Anatomic Variation
When interpreting FLAIR images, one must keep in mind that hippocampi may demonstrate mildly increased signal intensity compared with neocortical gray matter. This could potentially be misinterpreted as bilateral hippocampal sclerosis. Normal hippocampi should not be hyperintense to cortical gray matter on coronal T2W FSE images, which can serve a useful complementary role in this setting.

The size of the normal hippocampus is largest at its head and tapers as it extends posteriorly to the body and tail. Because the cross-sectional size of the hippocampus varies along its length, even a small degree of head rotation can create the false appearance of asymmetric hippocampal size. It is imperative to be aware of this variable, because atrophy is one of the key findings of hippocampal sclerosis. Correct interpretation depends on accurate alignment of the patient's head in the scanner and accounting for head rotation when determining whether there is hippocampal asymmetry (Fig. 50-24).

Variations in the configuration of the hippocampus can also potentially lead to difficulties in interpretation. The hippocampal body normally has a round or oval cross-sectional shape when imaged in the coronal plane. Occasionally, it may be more vertically oriented, which can be misdiagnosed as cortical dysgenesis. In cases of holoprosencephaly or dysgenesis of the corpus callosum there may be incomplete infolding of the dentate gyrus and cornu ammonis. On coronal imaging this manifests in a vertical configuration of the hippocampus with a shallow cleft on its medial side (Fig. 50-25).

Normal Variations Related to Gyral and Sulcal Configurations
Normal gyral and sulcal variations may occasionally be mistaken for an epileptogenic abnormality, typically, cortical dysgenesis. One should be familiar with the following normal variations to avoid misdiagnosis:

● Cortex surrounding the superior temporal sulcus on the right side is usually slightly thicker than that of the left side.
● Normal undulations of the cortex may give the appearance of cortical thickening on cross-sectional images, if the gyrus is parallel to the cross-sectional plane. As opposed to this

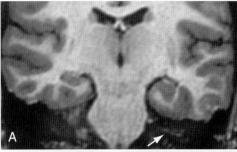
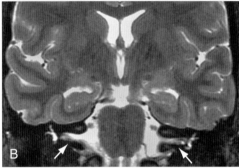

■ **FIGURE 50-24** Head rotation. **A,** Coronal SPGR MR image shows an asymmetric appearance of the hippocampi with the right appearing much smaller than the left. However, in this position, only the left internal auditory canal (*arrow*) can be seen, suggesting that the patient's head is rotated. **B,** Coronal T2W MR image of the same patient after repositioning shows symmetric hippocampi that are normal in size. Note that both right and left internal auditory canals can be identified on this single image (*arrows*).

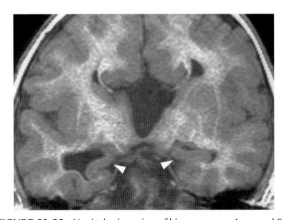

■ **FIGURE 50-25** Vertical orientation of hippocampus. A coronal SPGR MR image of a patient with agenesis of the corpus callosum demonstrates a vertical configuration of the hippocampi with shallow CSF clefts (*arrowheads*) as a result of incomplete infolding of the dentate gyrus and cornu ammonis.

potentially worrisome appearance of normal gyri, true cortical thickening should be visible on multiple images (usually at least three contiguous thin-section images) and can also be visualized in another plane (Fig. 50-26).
● The gyri surrounding the calcarine sulcus usually indents the occipital horn (in an area known as the calcar avis), giving rise to the appearance of thickened gyri, which can be asymmetric.
● The signal characteristics of gray and white matter in the infant with an incompletely myelinated brain can be confusing and are a possible source of misinterpretation. For example, the myelinated optic radiations surrounded by

■ **FIGURE 50-26** Pseudolesion versus perisylvian polymicrogyria. **A,** Coronal SPGR MR image shows a prominent area of gray matter on the right (*arrows*) that is suggestive of polymicrogyria. **B,** Sagittal SPGR MR image of the patient demonstrates that the coronal slice (*dashed line*) was taken along the edge of the vertical portion of the superior temporal gyrus resulting in the pseudolesion appearance. Note that the sylvian fissure (*arrows*) has a normal orientation and appearance. **C,** Coronal SPGR MR image demonstrates cortical thickening along the right sylvian fissure. In the inset, notice the appearance of tiny projections of gray matter extending into the adjacent white matter (*arrow*). These findings are typical of polymicrogyria, which is commonly located in the perisylvian region. **D,** Sagittal SPGR MR image of the same patient shows cortical thickening and multiple tiny gyri (*arrows*) along the left sylvian fissure. The sylvian fissure also appears contiguous with the central sulcus.

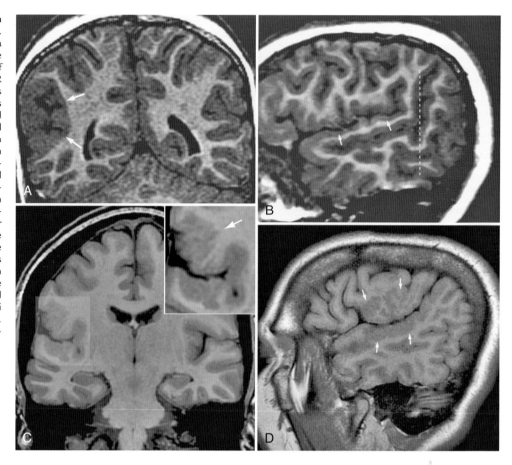

unmyelinated white matter could be mistaken for heterotopic gray matter (Fig. 50-27).

- The peri-rolandic gray matter is another region where normal anatomy may be misinterpreted for cortical dysgenesis. On coronal imaging there is poor distinction of gray and white matter and poor visualization of the peri-rolandic cortex compared with the rest of the frontal lobes. These variations appear to be due to a couple of factors. First, the gray matter surrounding the rolandic fissure is normally thinner than the rest of the neocortex. Second, the rolandic fissure and adjacent gyri are oriented parallel to the coronal plane. This may result in a peri-rolandic coronal slice either only imaging gray matter (resulting in the appearance of cortical thickening or a pseudomass) or volume averaging with white matter. Because of the difficulty interpreting this region on coronal images, reference to axial images should be performed.

CSF Collections

Cystic or CSF-containing structures are frequently encountered both in normal subjects and in the epilepsy population. These structures are isointense to CSF on all imaging sequences and do not demonstrate any contrast enhancement. Table 50-5 lists CSF structures that may be encountered during MRI evaluation for epilepsy and have no epileptogenic potential.

Perivascular spaces are frequently visualized in patients undergoing evaluation for epilepsy owing to the use of high-resolution imaging. Common locations of perivascular spaces include the subinsular zone (deep to the insular cortex), the anterior perforated substance and subcapsular zone (inferior to the basal ganglia), and the subcortical zone of the anterior temporal lobe. These can be asymmetric and may give pause to those unfamiliar with their appearance and typical locations. Although they are isointense to CSF, volume averaging effects may cause them to

appear slightly less hypointense than CSF on T1W images when they are small. Virchow-Robin spaces often have a feather-like, linear or oval configuration. Linear or punctate enhancement within these perivascular spaces represents the vessel and confirms the diagnosis. There should, however, be no other enhancement.

Choroidal fissure cysts and *arachnoid cysts* are commonly encountered in the temporal lobe and do not result in epilepsy. The *uncal recess* is the most anterior portion of the temporal horn and can be asymmetric in 60% of all subjects. The *hippocampal sulcal remnant* is a cystic normal variant seen in 10% to 15% of the normal population. This cyst is located in the hippocampus itself, between the cornu ammonis and the dentate gyrus and is the result of failure of a portion of the hippocampal sulcus to involute (Fig. 50-28).

Developmental Venous Malformations

Isolated developmental venous anomalies are not epileptogenic; however, developmental venous anomalies can be found in association with potentially epileptogenic abnormalities, such as malformations of cortical development (e.g., perisylvian polymicrogyria) and cavernous malformations.

Differential Diagnosis: Beware the Pitfalls!
Focal Lesions

Not uncommonly, we are faced with the challenge of differentiating cortical dysplasia from a neoplastic process. Both focal cortical dysplasia and neoplasms can demonstrate T2 prolongation in the subcortical white matter. Surgical strategies may differ for these entities, particularly if an epileptogenic lesion is located in an eloquent cortical region. MRI findings that favor cortical dysplasia over a neoplastic process include cortical thickening, homogeneous appearance of subcortical white

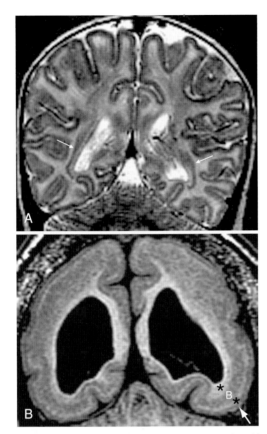

■ **FIGURE 50-27** Pseudo-band heterotopia versus true band heterotopia. **A,** Coronal T2W MR image of an infant demonstrates bilateral linear areas of signal (*arrows*) that are isointense to cortex within the occipital periventricular white matter. Although this appears similar to band heterotopia, these are actually the myelinated optic radiations surrounded by unmyelinated white matter. **B,** Coronal SPGR image demonstrates globally decreased sulcation and ventriculomegaly. The cortex (*arrow*) is thinned. There is a thick subcortical band (B) that is isointense to cortex and bounded on either side by white matter (*asterisk*). This is band heterotopia.

matter T2 hyperintensity, and the presence of a radial band extending from lesion to the ventricle. Neoplasms are more likely to occur in the temporal lobe, while a frontal location is more commonly seen in cortical dysplasias. The presence of subependymal nodules in addition to subcortical T2 hyperintense lesions should raise suspicion for tuberous sclerosis.

When encountering abnormal T2 hyperintensity in the hippocampus, we immediately think of hippocampal sclerosis; however, it is important to consider the possibility of neoplasm when certain imaging characteristics are present. It is not difficult to differentiate the two when the abnormal hippocampus is small, which is the cardinal finding of hippocampal sclerosis. However, the hippocampus is not small in all cases of hippocampal sclerosis. In these cases, the distinction is more challenging. Findings that raise suspicion for a neoplasm include heterogeneous signal changes and extension of signal changes beyond the hippocampus into the parahippocampal white matter (Fig. 50-29).

Dual Pathology

Dual pathology refers to the presence of both hippocampal sclerosis and an extrahippocampal epileptogenic abnormality and is discussed earlier in this chapter. Coexisting hippocampal sclerosis is not infrequent, particularly with developmental anomalies. Once an obvious epileptogenic abnormality is found, one can easily neglect to scrutinize the hippocampus, especially

TABLE 50-5. Nonepileptogenic CSF-Containing Structures

Perivascular Virchow-Robin spaces
Arachnoid cyst
Choroidal fissure cyst
Uncal recess of the temporal horn
Embryonic remnant of hippocampal sulcus

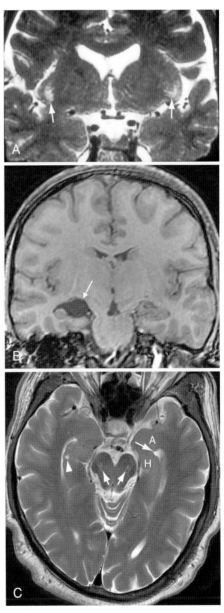

■ **FIGURE 50-28** Nonepileptogenic CSF-containing structures. **A,** Areas of hyperintensity (*arrows*) are noted on a coronal T2W MR image involving the bilateral insular subcortical white matter in this patient without seizures. These areas of hyperintensity are consistent with prominent Virchow-Robin spaces. **B,** Coronal SPGR MR image shows a prominent right choroidal fissure cyst (*arrow*) with mass effect and displacement of the right hippocampus and parahippocampal gyrus. **C,** Axial T2W MR image of a patient without a history of seizures demonstrates a tiny hippocampal sulcal remnant (*arrowhead*). The uncal recess (*long arrow*) of the temporal horn of the left lateral ventricle is well visualized between the amygdala (A) and the hippocampus (H). Prominent Virchow-Robin spaces (*short arrows*) are noted within the cerebral peduncles.

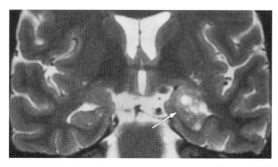

■ **FIGURE 50-29** Left hippocampal cystic mass. Coronal T2W MR image of a patient demonstrates an area of heterogeneous T2 hyperintensity involving the left hippocampus (*arrow*) but also extending beyond the margins of the hippocampus. No hippocampal atrophy is seen. These signs are consistent with neoplastic involvement and should not be confused with hippocampal sclerosis.

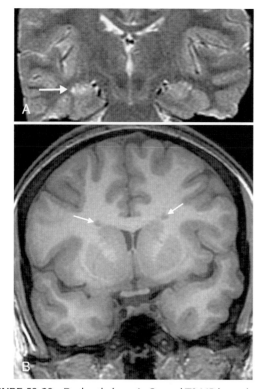

■ **FIGURE 50-30** Dual pathology. **A,** Coronal T2 MR image in a young patient with chronic seizures shows an atrophic right hippocampus with T2 hyperintensity (*arrow*), reflecting hippocampal sclerosis. **B,** Coronal SPGR MR image in the same patient also shows bilateral frontal periventricular white matter heterotopias (*arrows*).

if there are concordant clinical and paraclinical data. By the same token, if hippocampal sclerosis is found, one should also search the brain for other possibly subtle cortical abnormalities that may have been overlooked (Fig. 50-30). It is often necessary to surgically remove both lesions to attain a seizure-free outcome.

Developmental Malformations

Malformations of cortical development are often subtle and can be difficult to detect, even using high-resolution imaging. Furthermore, various malformations may sometimes be difficult to distinguish from one another.

Polymicrogyria can be quite difficult to distinguish from the spectrum of pachygyria/agyria (lissencephaly). Cortical thickening is seen on MRI in both of these entities. This appearance may

be bilateral and may appear as smooth cortices. Location and distribution pattern may help in differentiating the two. Polymicrogyria tends to occur in the gray matter surrounding the sylvian fissure or in the gray matter lining an abnormal CSF cleft in the brain (e.g., a schizencephalic cleft). Sagittal images may be particularly useful in identifying perisylvian polymicrogyria, which often results in a sylvian fissure that is continuous with the central sulcus. Although polymicrogyria may be bilateral, it is not typically as diffuse as pachygyria. Pachygyria, however, may affect the brain regionally (e.g., in the frontal lobes). Additionally, multiple tiny gyri can sometimes be visualized in cases of polymicrogyria, with the use of high-resolution imaging (Fig. 50-31).

The differential diagnosis for periventricular findings that are isointense to gray matter on T1W images include periventricular heterotopia, normal caudate nucleus, and subependymal hamartomas of tuberous sclerosis. True gray matter (both normal and heterotopic) follows the signal intensity of the cortex on all pulse sequences, not only T1W sequences. Regarding the caudate nucleus, the head is easily identified, allowing the identification of body and tail on subsequent slices and differentiation from heterotopia.

Hemispheric Changes

Asymmetry that involves an entire hemisphere can also pose a diagnostic challenge. Which is the abnormal side? Hemimegalencephaly may sometimes be mistaken for the hemiatrophic syndromes. In both processes, one cerebral hemisphere is larger than the other, one lateral ventricle is larger than the other, and there may be diffuse white matter hyperintensity. The two can be differentiated in the following manner: the enlarged ventricle is in the larger hemisphere in hemimegalencephaly, whereas ventricular enlargement in hemiatrophy occurs in the smaller hemisphere. Unlike hemiatrophy, hemimegalencephaly is associated with cortical thickening, sulcal abnormalities, heterotopias, and radial bands.

Transient Lesions

Interpretive pitfalls are particularly troubling when one is dealing with a focal transient signal abnormality. The potential exists for performing focal resective surgery for a transient abnormality or inadequate focal resection for a widespread epileptogenic region, as in Rasmussen's syndrome.

Transient "lesions" in patients with seizures can result from infections, from frequent or prolonged seizures, or as a result of rapid changes in antiepileptic medication dosage. Postictal signal changes can manifest as focal or multifocal signal abnormalities (T2 prolongation) and morphologic changes in the hippocampus or neocortical structures; these can be seen in the setting of recurrent or prolonged focal or febrile seizures. These areas may also have reduced diffusion. Whereas reduced diffusion may reflect ischemia, perfusion studies demonstrate increased cerebral blood flow as opposed to the decreased flow expected in an infarct. In Rasmussen's encephalitis, focal signal abnormalities not only may be temporary but can also change in location. Therefore, one should use caution in interpreting focal signal abnormalities in patients with active seizures, particularly when there is consideration for invasive studies or potential surgery.[36]

Transient focal signal abnormalities may also be seen in the splenium of the corpus callosum.[37] This rare lesion is seen in 0.5% of patients with seizure disorders. This transient abnormality demonstrates T2 hyperintensity and reduced diffusion and does not enhance after contrast agent administration. This abnormality is thought to result from an abrupt change in antiepileptic drug concentrations that, in turn, elevates the arginine vasopressin level, which is theorized to cause cytotoxic edema in the splenium (Fig. 50-32).

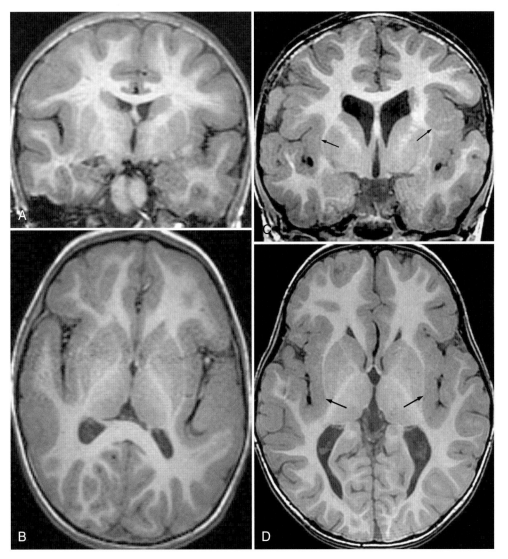

■ **FIGURE 50-31** Pachygyria versus bilateral perisylvian syndrome. **A,** Coronal SPGR MR image of a patient with pachygyria demonstrates diffusely thickened cortex throughout the frontal and temporal lobes. **B,** Axial SPGR MR image of the same patient confirms the diffuse cortical thickening with a paucity of sulci involving the frontal and temporal lobes (with sparing of the occipital lobes). **C,** In comparison, this patient with polymicrogyria demonstrates thickened cortex in the insula (*arrows*) and superior temporal lobe on a coronal SPGR MR image. Nodularity of the cortex predominantly localized to the opercula and the sylvian fissure is characteristic for this entity. **D,** Axial SPGR MR image of the same patient. Note that the area of cortical thickening is centered on the sylvian fissures while the remainder of the cerebral cortex is normal in thickness and demonstrates a normal sulcal pattern.

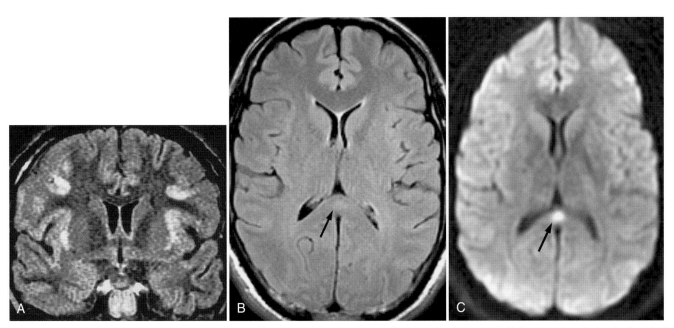

■ **FIGURE 50-32** Transient lesions. **A,** Coronal FLAIR MR image obtained in a postictal patient demonstrates multiple areas of cortical and subcortical T2 hyperintensity. **B,** An axial FLAIR MR image of a different patient shows a subtle area of T2 hyperintensity within the splenium of the corpus callosum (*arrow*). **C,** The axial diffusion image of the same patient confirms restricted diffusion within the splenium (*arrow*). This abnormality may be related to rapid changes in antiepileptic medication concentrations, resulting in cytotoxic edema.

Encephalocele

An uncommon cause of epilepsy is the anterior temporal lobe encephalocele. This may be overlooked if it is not considered, owing to its extra-axial location and its rarity. The basal temporal region should be scrutinized carefully. An encephalocele must be distinguished from the normal protrusions of brain parenchyma that can occur along the basal temporal lobes.

The MRI Report

Just as an MRI examination should be tailored for optimal detection and evaluation of potential epileptogenic abnormalities, the diagnostic report should likewise be focused on presence or absence of pertinent positive and negative findings relevant to this population. Below are a few guidelines in composing a relevant MRI report for a seizure evaluation.

Hippocampal Assessment

1. Are the hippocampi symmetric in size?
2. Is there signal change within the hippocampus?

3. In cases of hippocampal sclerosis:
   a. Is the process unilateral or bilateral?
   b. Is there another potentially epileptogenic lesion (i.e., dual pathology)?
   c. Note the presence of secondary changes of the temporal lobe white matter, fornix, mammillary bodies, etc., to support the diagnosis, especially in equivocal cases.

Nonhippocampal Abnormalities

1. Are there any focal lesions? Address the presence or absence of common epileptogenic substrates, such as focal or diffuse cortical abnormalities, gray matter heterotopia, or neoplasms.
2. Is there hemorrhage or evidence of prior hemorrhage (hemosiderin)?
3. Are there any foci of restricted diffusion?

Examples of normal and abnormal reports of MRI examinations done for the evaluation of seizures are presented in Boxes 50-1 and 50-2.

BOX 50-1   Sample Report: Normal MRI Report for Seizure Evaluation

PATIENT HISTORY

A 31-year-old woman presented with epilepsy.

COMPARISON STUDIES

There were no prior examinations for comparison.

TECHNIQUE

Multiplanar, multi-sequence unenhanced MR images of the brain were obtained on a 3-T scanner using a dedicated seizure evaluation protocol.

CONTRAST AGENT

No intravenous contrast agent was used.

FINDINGS

The hippocampi are symmetric in size and signal intensity. There are no areas of gray matter heterotopia, cortical thickening, or sulcal morphologic anomalies. Gray matter/white matter differentiation is well maintained.

There is no hydrocephalus, hemorrhage, mass, volume loss, or area of restricted diffusion.

IMPRESSION

This is a normal brain MRI examination using dedicated seizure protocol.

BOX 50-2   Sample Report: Abnormal MRI Report for Seizure Evaluation

PATIENT HISTORY

A patient presented with focal left-sided seizures.

COMPARISON STUDIES

There are no prior examinations for comparison.

TECHNIQUE

Multiplanar, multi-sequence unenhanced MR images of the brain were obtained on a 3-T scanner using a dedicated seizure evaluation protocol.

CONTRAST AGENT

No contrast agent was administered.

FINDINGS

The right hippocampal head, body, and tail are asymmetrically small, with loss of internal architecture and hyperintensity on long repetition

time imaging. There are secondary signs of hippocampal sclerosis, with ipsilateral temporal horn dilatation, and atrophy of the ipsilateral fornix and mammillary body.

The left hippocampus demonstrates normal size and signal characteristics.

There are no areas of gray matter heterotopia, cortical thickening, or sulcal morphologic anomalies. Gray matter/white matter differentiation is well maintained.

There is no hydrocephalus, hemorrhage, mass, volume loss, or area of restricted diffusion.

IMPRESSION

Findings are consistent with right-sided hippocampal sclerosis, with associated secondary findings.

KEY POINTS

- The sensitivity of MRI for detecting epileptogenic lesions decreases substantially when routine MRI techniques are used rather than a dedicated seizure protocol.
- In seizure patients, the sensitivity of MRI for detecting epileptogenic lesions is highest for medically refractory partial seizures and then decreases progressively for better controlled partial seizures, followed by new-onset seizures and then generalized epilepsy.
- A systematic approach for image interpretation should be used to avoid missing subtle epileptogenic lesions.

- Classic findings for hippocampal sclerosis consist of T2 prolongation and atrophy of the hippocampus on MRI, asymmetrically decreased temporal lobe metabolism on PET, decreased temporal lobe perfusion on interictal SPECT, and increased temporal lobe perfusion on ictal SPECT.
- Be careful to rule out a second associated pathologic process—dual lesions.
- In infants and adults younger than age 50 years, seizure evaluation and analysis of the MR images should focus on the hippocampus and the brain periphery (cortex).

SUGGESTED READINGS

Barkovich AJ, Raybaud CA. Malformations of cortical development. Neuroimaging Clin North Am 2004; 14:401-423.

Cascino GD, Jack CR (eds). Neuroimaging in Epilepsy: Principles and Practice. Boston, Butterworth-Heinemann, 1996.

Cascino GD, So EL, Buchhalter JR, Mullan BP. The current place of single photon emission computed tomography in epilepsy evaluations. Neuroimaging Clin North Am 2004; 14:553-561.

Henry TR, Votaw JR. The role of positron emission tomography with [18F] fluorodeoxyglucose in the evaluation of the epilepsies. Neuroimaging Clin North Am 2004; 14:517-535.

Kuzniecky R. Clinical applications of MR spectroscopy in epilepsy. Neuroimaging Clin North Am 2004; 14:507-516.

Kuzniecky R, Jackson GD (eds). Magnetic Resonance in Epilepsy: Neuroimaging Techniques, 2nd ed. Boston: Elsevier/Academic Press, 2005.

Spencer SS. When should temporal-lobe epilepsy be treated surgically? Lancet Neurol 2002; 1:375-382.

Spencer SS, Berg AT, Vickrey BG, et al. Predicting long-term seizure outcome after resective epilepsy surgery: the multicenter study. Neurology 2005; 65:912-918.

VanPaesschen W. Qualitative and quantitative imaging of the hippocampus in mesial temporal lobe epilepsy with hippocampal sclerosis. Neuroimaging Clin North Am 2004; 14:373-400.

Vattipally VR, Bronen RA. MR imaging of epilepsy: strategies for successful interpretation. Radiol Clin North Am 2006; 44:111-133.

REFERENCES

1. Sander JW. The epidemiology of epilepsy revisited. Curr Opin Neurol 2003; 16:165-170.

2. King MA, Newton MR, Jackson GD, et al. Epileptology of the first-seizure presentation: a clinical, electroencephalographic, and magnetic resonance imaging study of 300 consecutive patients. Lancet 1998; 352:1007-1011.

3. Berg AT, Testa FM, Levy SR, Shinnar S. Neuroimaging in children with newly diagnosed epilepsy: a community-based study. Pediatrics 2000; 106:527-532.

4. Bronen RA, Fulbright RK, Spencer DD, et al. Refractory epilepsy: comparison of MR imaging, CT, and histopathologic findings in 117 patients. Radiology 1996; 201:97-105.

5. Raymond AA, Fish DR, Sisodiya SM, et al. Abnormalities of gyration, heterotopias, tuberous sclerosis, focal cortical dysplasia, microdysgenesis, dysembryoplastic neuroepithelial tumour and dysgenesis of the archicortex in epilepsy: clinical, EEG and neuroimaging features in 100 adult patients. Brain 1995; 118:629-660.

6. Berkovic SF, McIntosh AM, Kalnins RM, et al. Preoperative MRI predicts outcome of temporal lobectomy: an actuarial analysis. Neurology 1995; 45:1358-1363.

7. McBride MC, Bronstein KS, Bennett B, et al. Failure of standard magnetic resonance imaging in patients with refractory temporal lobe epilepsy. Arch Neurol 1998; 55:346-348.

8. Hirai T, Korogi Y, Yoshizumi K, et al. Limbic lobe of the human brain: evaluation with turbo fluid-attenuated inversion-recovery MR imaging. Radiology 2000; 215:470-475.

9. Bronen RA, Fulbright RK, King D, et al. Qualitative MR imaging of refractory temporal lobe epilepsy requiring surgery: correlation with pathology and seizure outcome after surgery. AJR Am J Roentgenol 1997; 169:875-882.

10. Cendes F, Cook MJ, Watson C, et al. Frequency and characteristics of dual pathology in patients with lesional epilepsy. Neurology 1995; 45:2058-2064.

11. Watson C, Andermann F, Gloor P, et al. Anatomic basis of amygdaloid and hippocampal volume measurement by magnetic resonance imaging. Neurology 1992; 42:1743-1750.

12. Jackson GD, Connelly A, Duncan JS, et al. Detection of hippocampal pathology in intractable partial epilepsy: increased sensitivity with quantitative magnetic resonance T2 relaxometry. Neurology 1993; 43:1793-1799.

13. VanPaesschen W, Connelly A, Johnson CL, Duncan JS. The amygdala and intractable temporal lobe epilepsy: a quantitative magnetic resonance imaging study. Neurology 1996; 47:1021-1031.

14. Ho SS, Consalvo D, Gilliam F, et al. Amygdala atrophy and seizure outcome after temporal lobe epilepsy surgery. Neurology 1998; 51:1502-1504.

15. Tasch E, Cendes F, Li LM, et al. Neuroimaging evidence of progressive neuronal loss and dysfunction in temporal lobe epilepsy. Ann Neurol 1999; 45:568-576.

16. Kuzniecky R, Hugg JW, Hetherington H, et al. Relative utility of H-1 spectroscopic imaging and hippocampal volumetry in the lateralization of mesial temporal lobe epilepsy. Neurology 1998; 51:66-71.

17. Lencz T, McCarthy G, Bronen RA, et al. Quantitative magnetic resonance imaging in temporal lobe epilepsy: relationship to neuropathology and neuropsychological function. Ann Neurol 1992; 31:629-637.

18. Jack CR Jr, Sharbrough FW, Cascino GD, et al. Magnetic resonance image-based hippocampal volumetry: correlation with outcome after temporal lobectomy. Ann Neurol 1992; 31:138-146.

19. Wieshmann UC, Clark CA, Symms MR, et al. Water diffusion in the human hippocampus in epilepsy. Magn Reson Imaging 1999; 17:29-36.

20. Assaf BA, Mohamed FB, Abou-Khaled KJ, et al. Diffusion tensor imaging of the hippocampal formation in temporal lobe epilepsy. Am J Neuroradiol 2003; 24:1857-1862.

21. Hammers A. Flumazenil positron emission tomography and other ligands for functional imaging. Neuroimaging Clin North Am 2004; 14:537-551.

22. Barkovich AJ, Kuzniecky RI, Jackson GD, et al. A developmental and genetic classification for malformations of cortical development. Neurology 2005; 65:1873-1887.

23. Bronen RA, Vives K, Kim JH, et al. MR of focal cortical dysplasia of Taylor, balloon cell subtype: differentiation from low grade tumors. AJNR Am J Neuroradiol 1997; 18:1141-1151.

24. Chan S, Chin SS, Nordli DR, et al. Prospective magnetic resonance imaging identification of focal cortical dysplasia, including the non-balloon cell subtype. Ann Neurol 1998; 44:749-757.

25. Kuzniecky R, Andermann F, Guerrini R. Congenital bilateral perisylvian syndrome: study of 31 patients. Lancet 1993; 341:608-612.

26. Bronen RA, Fulbright RK, Spencer DD, et al. MR characteristics of neoplasms and vascular malformations associated with epilepsy. Magn Reson Imaging 1995; 13:1153-1162.

27. Töpper R, Jürgens E, Reul J, Thron A. Clinical significance of intracranial developmental venous anomalies. J Neurol Neurosurg Psychiatry 1999; 67:234-238.

28. Rasmussen T. Further observations on the syndrome of chronic encephalitis and epilepsy. Appl Neurophysiol 1978; 41:1-12.

29. Geller E, Faerber E, Legido A, et al. Rasmussen encephalitis: complementary role of multitechnique neuroimaging. AJNR Am J Neuroradiol 1998; 9:445-449.

30. Arita K, Ikawa F, Kurisu K, et al. The relationship between magnetic resonance imaging findings and clinical manifestations of hypothalamic hamartoma. J Neurosurg 1999; 91:212-220.

31. Wasterlain CG, Fujikawa DG, Penix L, Sankar R. Pathophysiological mechanisms of brain damage from status epilepticus. Epilepsia 1993; 34:S37-S53.

32. Men S, Lee DH, Barron JR, Munoz DG. Selective neuronal necrosis associated with status epilepticus: MR findings. AJNR Am J Neuroradiol 2000; 21:1837-1840.

33. Szabo K, Poepel A, Pohlmann-Eden B, et al. Diffusion-weighted and perfusion MRI demonstrates parenchymal changes in complex partial status epilepticus. Brain 2005; 128:1369-1376.

34. Bauer G, Gotwald T, Dobesberger J, et al. Transient and permanent magnetic resonance imaging abnormalities after complex partial status epilepticus. Epilepsy Behav 2006; 8:666-671.

35. Bronen RA, Fulbright RK, Kim JH, et al. A systematic approach for interpreting MR images of the seizure patient. AJR Am J Roentgenol 1997; 169:241-247.

36. Chan S, Chin SS, Kartha K, et al. Reversible signal abnormalities in the hippocampus and neocortex after prolonged seizures. AJNR Am J Neuroradiol 1996; 17:1725-1731.

37. Mirsattari SM, Lee DH, Jones MW, Blume WT. Transient lesion in the splenium of the corpus callosum in an epileptic patient. Neurology 2003; 60:1838-1841.

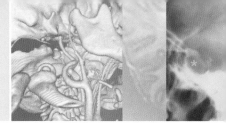

Index

A

Abducens nerve (CN VI), 351
  cisternal course, axial reconstructions, 358f
  cisternal segments, 357
  emergence, 298f
  intra-axial segments, 356-357
  medial border, 262
  MRI, 356-359
Aβ peptide, deposition (excess), *see website*
Abscesses, 87-88, 87f, 868-872
  clinical presentation, 869
  cryptic abscesses, 869
  CT, 870-871
  epidemiology, 869
  imaging, 870-872
  MRI, 871-872
  multiloculated brain abscess, 871f
  otogenic brain abscesses, incidence (decrease), 869
  pathology, 870
  pathophysiology, 869-870
Accessory cuneate nucleus (AC), 316f
Accessory nerve, cranial nerve roots, 353f
Acellular serum, correspondence, 390f
Acetate (elevation), single-voxel proton spectroscopy (usage), 39f
Acoustic neuroma, term (usage), 847
Acoustic schwannoma (vestibular schwannoma), 826
  anatomic distribution, 832
  differential diagnostic considerations, 831
  enhancement, 831f
AC-PC baseline of Talairach and Tournoux, 194f
Acquired cerebral herniations, 610-613
  ascending transtentorial herniation, 613
  central descending transtentorial herniation, 612
  descending transtentorial herniation, 612-613
  imaging, 612-613

Acquired cerebral herniations *(Continued)*
  lateral transtentorial herniation, 612
  pathophysiology, 610-612
  subfalcine herniation, 610, 612
  tonsillar herniation, 613
Active cerebritis, 88
Active MS lesion, 917-918
Acute anterior cerebral artery infarct, 33f
Acute cephalohematoma, *see website*
Acute cerebellar PICA infarction, 85f
Acute cerebral infarction, pathologic process, 18
Acute CTV, 477
Acute dissecting MCA aneurysm, subarachnoid hemorrhage (presence), 510f, 511f
Acute disseminated encephalomyelitis (ADEM), 932-934
  acute disseminated necrohemorrhagic leukoencephalitis, 935-937
  Balo-like lesion, 914f
  Bickerstaff's encephalitis, 934-935
  brain MRI, 935f
  clinical presentation, 932
  differential diagnosis, 937, 939
  enhancing periventricular/subcortical white matter lesions, 936f
  epidemiology, 932
  imaging, 933-934
  inflammatory demyelinating diseases, 50-51
  MRI differences, 934f
  multiple sclerosis
    clinical/biologic/radiologic differences, 939t
    conversion, 933f
  multiple tumefactive brain lesions, 935f
  pathology, 933
  pathophysiology, 932-933
  presentation, 91
  serial brain MRI, 934f
  spinal cord involvement, 933
  variants, 934-937
Acute disseminated necrohemorrhagic leukoencephalitis, 935-937
Acute epidural hematoma, 55f, 70f
  MRI appearance, 578

Acute global hypoxic injury, causes, 49-50
Acute hemorrhage, 390f, 394f
  contrast-enhanced CT (CECT), 389-390
  measure, 389
  vertebral artery dissection, 512f
    aneurysm indicators, 513f
Acute hemorrhagic leukoencephalitis (Hurst's encephalitis), 936f
Acute infarct detection, 424-426
  noncontrast CT, 417-418
Acute intraventricular hemorrhage, 533f
Acute ischemic changes, presence, 959
Acute ischemic lesion, 364f
Acute left hemibody numbness, presentation, *see website*
Acute left suboccipital subdural hematoma, 584f
Acute lymphoblastic leukemia (ALL), 944
  MRI, report sample, *see website*
  treatment, hemorrhagic complication, *see website*
Acute methotrexate toxicity
  occurrence, *see website*
  signal abnormalities, *see website*
Acute myelogenous leukemia, dural chloroma, 662f
Acute-on-chronic SDH, 587
  unenhanced CT, 588f
Acute-onset headache, presentation, 428f
Acute-onset right hemiplegia, 423f
Acute periventricular leukomalacia, 63f
  diagnosis, ultrasound evaluation (usage), 63
Acute psychotic episode, esthesioneuroblastoma, 671f
Acute right middle cerebral artery infarction, presentation, 86f
Acute right-sided hemiplegia, 425f
Acute stroke, 48f
  perfusion abnormality, patterns, 432t
Acute subarachnoid hemorrhage
  communicating hydrocephalus, *see website*
  detection, 6
  headache, acute onset, 69f
  presence, 458f
Acute subdural hematoma, 55f, 583f
  clinical presentation, 581-582